Success in the Classroom, in Clinicals, and on the NCLEX-RN®

Classroom

- Detailed lecture notes organized by learning outcome
- Suggestions for classroom activities
- Guide to relevant additional resources
- Comprehensive PowerPoint™ presentations integrating lecture, images, animations, and videos
- Classroom Response questions
- Image Gallery
- Video and Animation Gallery
- Online course management systems complete with instructor tools and student activities available in a variety of formats

PEARSON mynursinglab

- Saves instructors time by providing quality feedback, ongoing formative assessments and customized remediation for students
- Provides easy, one-stop access to a wealth of teaching resources, such as test item files, PowerPoint™ slides, and video suggestions
- A built-in electronic gradebook tracks students' progress on assessment and remediation activities

Clinical

- Suggestions for Clinical Activities and other clinical resources organized by learning outcome

Real Nursing Simulations Facilitator's Guide: Institutional Edition

- 25 simulation scenarios that span the nursing curriculum
- Consistent format includes learning objectives, case flow, instructions for set up, student debriefing questions and more
- Companion online course cartridge with student exercises, activities, videos, skill checklists, and reflective questions also available for adoption

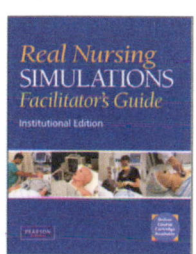

NCLEX-RN®

- Test Item Files with NCLEX®-style questions and complete rationales for correct and incorrect answers mapped to learning outcomes– available in TestGen, Par Test, and MS Word

D0023432

Instructor Resources

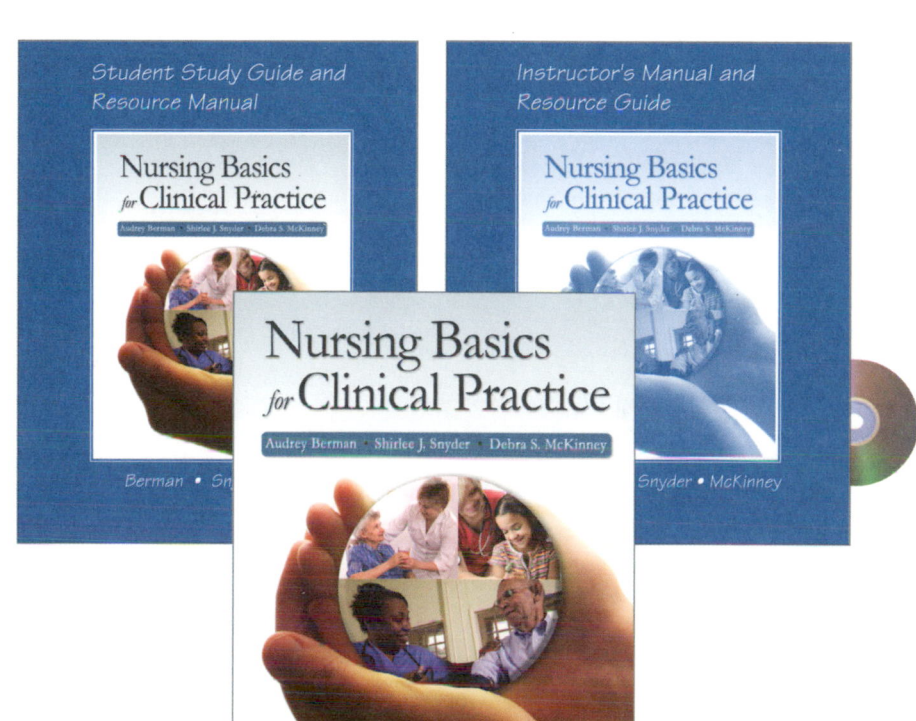

Student Study Guide and Resource Manual

Nursing Basics for Clinical Practice
Audrey Berman · Shirlee J. Snyder · Debra S. McKinney
Berman · Sn...

Instructor's Manual and Resource Guide

Nursing Basics for Clinical Practice
Audrey Berman · Shirlee J. Snyder · Debra S. McKinney
Snyder · McKinney

Nursing Basics for Clinical Practice
Audrey Berman · Shirlee J. Snyder · Debra S. McKinney
mynursingkit
www.mynursingkit.com

More information and instructor resources **visit** www.mynursingkit.com

Brief Table of Contents

EXPLORE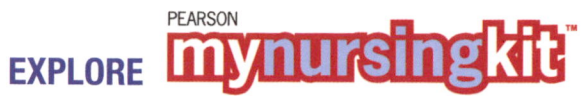

STEP 1: Register

All you need to get started is a valid email address and the access code below. To register, simply:

1. Go to **www.mynursingkit.com**. Click on the appropriate book cover.
2. In the "First-Time User" column, click "**Register**."
3. Read the **License Agreement** and **Privacy Policy**. If you accept, click "**I Accept**."
4. Under "**Do you have a Pearson account**?" select:
   • "**Yes**" if you have a Pearson account and know your Login Name and Password.
   • "**Not Sure**" if you do not know if you already have an account or do not recall your Login Name and Password.
   • "**No**" if you are sure you do not have a Pearson account.
5. Using a coin, scratch off the silver coating below to reveal your access code. Do not use a knife or other sharp object, which can damage the code.
6. Enter your access code in lowercase or uppercase, without the dashes, then click "**Next**."
7. Follow the on-screen instructions to complete registration.

After completing registration, you will be sent a confirmation email that contains your Login Name and Password. Be sure to save this email for future reference.

Your Access Code is:

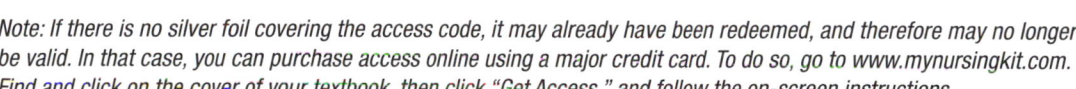

Note: If there is no silver foil covering the access code, it may already have been redeemed, and therefore may no longer be valid. In that case, you can purchase access online using a major credit card. To do so, go to www.mynursingkit.com. Find and click on the cover of your textbook, then click "Get Access," and follow the on-screen instructions.

STEP 2: Log in

1. Go to **www.mynursingkit.com**.
2. Find and click on the appropriate book cover. Cover must match the textbook edition used for your class.
3. Enter the Login Name and Password that you created during registration. If unsure of this information, refer to your registration confirmation email.
4. Click "**Login**."

Got technical questions?

Customer Technical Support: To obtain support, please visit us online anytime at http://247pearsoned.custhelp.com where you can search our knowledgebase for common solutions, view product alerts, and review all options for additional assistance.

SITE REQUIREMENTS
For the latest updates on Site Requirements, go to www.mynursingkit.com. Find and click on the cover of the book you are using. Click on "**Needs help?**" link at bottom of page. Under "**Technical Problems**" select the link "**What do I need on my computer to use this site?**"

Important: Please read the Subscription and End-User License agreement, accessible from the book website's login page, before using the *mynursingkit* website. By using the website, you indicate that you have read, understood, and accepted the terms of this agreement.

0136035485

Nursing Basics
for Clinical Practice

Nursing Basics
for Clinical Practice

AUDREY BERMAN PhD, RN, AOCN

SHIRLEE J. SNYDER EdD, RN

DEBRA S. MCKINNEY MSN, MBA/HCM, RN

Pearson

Boston   Columbus   Indianapolis   New York   San Francisco   Upper Saddle River
Amsterdam   Cape Town   Dubai   London   Madrid   Milan   Munich   Paris   Montreal   Toronto
Delhi   Mexico City   São Paulo   Sydney   Hong Kong   Seoul   Singapore   Taipei   Tokyo

Library of Congress Cataloging-in-Publication Data

Berman, Audrey.

   Nursing basics for clinical practice / Audrey Berman, Shirlee J. Snyder, Debra S. McKinney.

      p. ; cm.

   Includes bibliographical references and index.

   ISBN 978-0-13-603548-0

   1. Nursing. I. Snyder, Shirlee. II. McKinney, Debra S. III. Title.

   [DNLM: 1. Nursing Process. 2. Nursing—methods. 3. Nursing Care—methods.

WY 100 B4985n 2011]

   RT41.B3912 2011

   610.73—dc22

2009038339

Publisher: Julie Levin Alexander

Publisher's Assistant: Regina Bruno

Editor-in-Chief: Maura Connor

Senior Acquisitions Editor: Kelly Trakalo

Editorial Assistant: Lauren Sweeney

Development Editor: Tom Lochhaas

Managing Production Editor: Patrick Walsh

Production Liaison: Yagnesh Jani

Production Editor: Amy Gehl, S4Carlisle Publishing Services

Manufacturing Manager: Ilene Sanford

Design Director: Christy Mahon

Senior Art Director: Maria Guglielmo-Walsh

Interior and Cover Designer: Wanda España/Wee Design Group

Director of Marketing: David Gesell

Marketing Specialist: Michael Sirinides

Marketing Assistant: Crystal Gonzalez

Media Editor: Travis Moses-Westphal

Media Project Manager: Rachel Collett

Manager, Image Rights and Permissions: Zina Arabia

Manager, Visual Research: Beth Brenzel

Manager, Cover Visual Research and Permissions: Karen Sanatar

Image Permission Coordinator: Jan Marc Quisumbing

Composition: S4Carlisle Publishing Services

Printer/Binder: Courier Kendallville

Cover Printer: Lehigh Phoenix Color/Hagerstown

Cover Image: Courtesy of istockphoto.

Chapter Opener Images: Courtesy of istockphoto and shutterstock.

Notice: Care has been taken to confirm the accuracy of information presented in this book. The authors, editors, and the publisher, however, cannot accept any responsibility for errors or omissions or for consequences from application of the information in this book and make no warranty, express or implied, with respect to its contents.

    The authors and publisher have exerted every effort to ensure that drug selections and dosages set forth in this text are in accord with current recommendations and practice at time of publication. However, in view of ongoing research, changes in government regulations, and the constant flow of information relating to drug therapy and drug reactions, the reader is urged to check the package inserts of all drugs for any change in indications of dosage and for added warnings and precautions. This is particularly important when the recommended agent is a new and/or infrequently employed drug.

Pearson® is a registered trademark of Pearson plc.

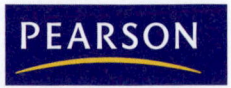

www.pearsonhighered.com

610.73
B516

10 9 8 7 6 5 4 3 2

ISBN 10:   0-13-603548-5

ISBN 13: 978-0-13-603548-0

About the Authors

AUDREY BERMAN

Audrey Berman received her BSN from the University of California–San Francisco and later returned to that campus to obtain her MS in physiologic nursing and her PhD in nursing. Her dissertation was entitled *Sailing a Course through Chemotherapy: The Experience of Women with Breast Cancer*. She worked in oncology at Samuel Merritt Hospital prior to beginning her teaching career in the diploma program at Samuel Merritt Hospital School of Nursing in 1976. As a faculty member, she participated in the transition of that program into a baccalaureate degree and in the development of the master of science in nursing program. Over the years, she has taught a variety of medical–surgical nursing courses in the prelicensure programs. She currently serves as the dean of nursing at Samuel Merritt College (an affiliate of Sutter Health).

Dr. Berman has traveled extensively, visiting nursing and health care institutions in Germany, Israel, Spain, Korea, Botswana, Australia, Japan, and Brazil. She serves on the board of directors for the Bay Area Tumor Institute. She is a member of the American Nurses Association and Sigma Theta Tau and is a site visitor for the Commission on Collegiate Nursing Education. She has twice participated as an NCLEX-RN® item writer for the National Council of State Boards of Nursing. She is certified as an advanced oncology nurse and as an AIDS educator and has presented locally, nationally, and internationally on topics related to nursing education, breast cancer, and technology in health care.

Dr. Berman authored the scripts for more than 35 nursing skills videotapes in the 1990s. She is the co-author of *Kozier & Erb's Fundamentals of Nursing* and *Skills in Clinical Nursing*.

Audrey Berman dedicates this edition to the real heroes in nursing education: the faculty. These men and women elect to spend their professional energies transmitting their knowledge, skills, and caring not just to clients, but to the extensions of their arms and minds—the generations of nurses to come. They are my colleagues, my friends, and my family.

SHIRLEE SNYDER

Shirlee J. Snyder graduated from Columbia Hospital School of Nursing in Milwaukee, Wisconsin, and subsequently received a bachelor of science in nursing from University of Wisconsin–Milwaukee. Because of an interest in cardiac nursing and teaching, she earned a master of science in nursing with a minor in cardiovascular clinical specialist and teaching from the University of Alabama in Birmingham. A move to California resulted in becoming a faculty member at Samuel Merritt Hospital School of Nursing in Oakland, California. Dr. Snyder was fortunate to be involved in the phasing out of the diploma and ADN programs and development of a baccalaureate intercollegiate nursing program. She held numerous positions during her 15-year tenure at Samuel Merritt College, including curriculum coordinator, assistant director–instruction, dean of instruction, and associate dean of the Intercollegiate Nursing Program. She is an associate professor alumnus at Samuel Merritt College. Her interest and experiences in nursing education resulted in Dr. Snyder obtaining a doctorate of education focused in curriculum and instruction from the University of San Francisco.

Dr. Snyder moved to Portland, Oregon, in 1990 and taught in the ADN program at Portland Community College for eight years. During this teaching experience she became interested in computer-assisted instruction (CAI) and initiated web-based assessment testing for student learning. She presented locally and nationally on topics related to using multimedia in the classroom and promoting ethnic and minority student success.

Another career opportunity in 1998 led her to the Community College of Southern Nevada in Las Vegas, Nevada, where Dr. Snyder was the nursing program director with responsibilities for the associate degree and practical nursing programs for five years. In 2003, Dr. Snyder returned to baccalaureate nursing education. She embraced the opportunity to be one of the nursing faculty teaching the first nursing class in the baccalaureate nursing program at the first state college in Nevada, which opened in 2002. She is currently the associate dean of the School of Nursing at Nevada State College in Henderson, Nevada.

Dr. Snyder is an advisory board member for the Nevada Geriatric Education Center and a member of the American Nurses Association, Sigma Theta Tau, and a variety of task groups addressing the Southern Nevada nursing shortage. She has been a site visitor for the National League for Nursing Accrediting Commission and the Northwest Association of Schools and Colleges. Dr. Synder is the co-author of *Kozier & Erb's Fundamentals of Nursing* and *Skills in Clinical Nursing*.

Dr. Snyder's experiences in nursing education and teaching keep her current in nursing and nursing education. She appreciates all she learns from the students she has taught and her past and present faculty colleagues.

Shirlee Snyder dedicates this edition to her husband, Terry J. Schnitter, for his unconditional love and support, and to her stepdaughter, Kelly, an awesome young woman, and caring mother, wife, and daughter who is diligently working on achieving her goal of becoming a nurse.

DEBRA MCKINNEY

Debra McKinney graduated from Saint Luke's Hospital School of Nursing in Bethlehem, Pennsylvania, with a diploma in professional nursing in 1977. She worked in pediatric and neonatal intensive care, emergency care, and adult critical care for 30 years. She obtained certification as a pediatric critical care nurse and contributed to research related to the use of extracorporeal membrane oxygenation in neonates as well as early work on use of liquid oxygen in pediatric clients.

After experiencing a back injury that limited her ability to walk, Mrs. McKinney subsequently obtained her bachelor of science in nursing from University of Phoenix in 2003, master of science in nursing and a master of business administration in health care management from University of Phoenix in 2007. She entered the field of nursing education in 2003 when she was asked to develop a practical nursing program in Northern Virginia.

Mrs. McKinney has developed curriculum for numerous schools of nursing at the practical and associate degree level. She consults with schools of nursing to assist in obtaining accreditation, revising curriculum, and correlating textbooks to syllabi. She teaches NCLEX® review courses for both the practical/vocational and professional nurse nationwide. She is currently an adjunct instructor for University of Illinois Global Campus and Axia College of University of Phoenix. However, the focus of her work today is writing a textbook to be used by schools of nursing using the concept-based pedagogy that is also the subject of her dissertation as she pursues a doctorate in education with a focus on curriculum design and instruction. Mrs. McKinney has developed many supplements for Pearson Prentice Hall, coauthored *Comprehensive Review of the NCLEX-PN®* with Mary Ann Hogan, and is currently writing several other nursing textbooks.

Mrs. McKinney is married and lives in the beautiful Myrtle Beach, South Carolina, area. She belongs to Sigma Theta Tau, National League for Nurses, National Association of Practical Nurse Education and Service, Committee of Practical Nurse Educators, and NANDA International.

Debra McKinney dedicates this edition to the men and women who are entering the profession of nursing, including her husband. The future of health care depends on each of these students who have chosen a difficult but highly rewarding career that places care of others over all else with the knowledge that real satisfaction comes from knowing they made a positive difference in the lives they touch. You are to be respected and admired for your decision.

Acknowledgments

We wish to extend a sincere thank you to the talented team involved in the development of this book: the contributors and reviewers who provided content and very helpful feedback; the nursing students, for their questioning minds and motivation; and the nursing instructors, who provided many valuable suggestions for this edition.

We would like to thank the editorial team at Pearson, including Kelly Trakalo, senior acquisitions editor, for never letting us forget our fundamental goals in writing this textbook; Tom Lochhaas, development editor, for his dedication to detail and knowledge as well as his willingness to teach and guide to help this book reach its full potential, and Lauren Sweeney, editorial assistant, who attended to the many details of making this book and its supplements happen. Many thanks to the production team of Patrick Walsh, production manager; Yagnesh Jani, production liaison; and Amy Gehl, S4Carlisle production editor, for producing this book with precision, and to the design team led by Maria Guglielmo-Walsh, creative director, for providing a truly beautiful design for this textbook.

As a nursing student begins on the path of a career in nursing, he or she also finds new opportunities unfolding as a light from within that brightens the path ahead. As students learn more about the field of nursing, they will explore and pursue areas of the field that they may have never imagined at the beginning of their journey. Now is your beginning—open your eyes and your mind to all of the wonderful opportunities in the field of nursing that are waiting to be pursued. You are the next generation of nursing.

Audrey Berman
Shirlee Snyder
Debra McKinney

Thank You

The authors wish to convey their special thanks to the many nurse contributors and reviewers who provided their unique knowledge and expertise to this project. Their insights, suggestions, eye for detail, and dedication to quality nursing education were evident and enabled us to prepare an accurate, relevant, and useful fundamentals textbook.

CONTRIBUTORS

Jan Joost
Front Range Community College
Chapter 1

REVIEWERS

Roberta P. Bartee, MS, RN, BC
Charity Delgado School of Nursing
New Orleans, LA

Holli Benge, MSN, RN
Tyler Junior College
Tyler, TX

Donna Bumpus, RN, MSN
Lamar University
Beaumont, TX

Karen A. Cassidy, RN, BSN, MHA
Dulles, VA

Charlene M. Chapman, RN, BSN
Pennsylvania Institute of Technology
Media, PA

Cynthia Lee Dols, RN, MN, PHN
College of St. Catherine
Minneapolis, MN

Cheryl Gardner, RN, BA
Bedford Hills, NY

Terry Girouard, MS, MSN, RN, BC
St. Joseph College
Standish, ME

Mary M. Goetteman, RN, Ed.D
Daytona State College
Daytona Beach, FL

Claudia Halie, RN, MSN
Corning Community College
Corning, NY

Judy R. Hembd, RN, MSN
Collin College
McKinney, TX

Eula Jackson, RN, BS, MSNEd, CNE, PhD
Reid State College
Evergreen, AL

Mary Ann Lubiejewski, MSN, RN
Mercyhurst North East
North East, PA

Kathi May, RN, BSN, M.Ed
Marshalltown Community College
Marshalltown, IA

Joseph Molinatti, Ed.D, RN
College of Mt. Saint Vincent
Bronx, NY

Mary-Rose Murray, RN, BSN, MSN
Midlands Technical College
Columbia, SC

Tricia O'Hara, RN, MSN
Gwynedd Mercy College
Gwynedd Valley, PA

VaLinda Pearson, PhD, RN, CRRN, CNE
College of St. Catherine
Minneapolis, MN

Patricia Poirier, PhD, RN, AOCN
University of Maine
School of Nursing
Orono, ME

Peggy Radke, RN, MSN
Central Community College
Grand Island, NE

Elizabeth Rohan, AAS, Nursing/RN
Wharton County Junior College
Wharton, TX

Connie Schroeder, MS, RN
Danville Area Community College
Danville, IL

Valerie Taylor, MSN, M.Ed
Lorain County Community College
Elyria, OH

Robyn Whitehair, MSN, ARNP-BC
Madisonville Community College
Madisonville, KY

SUPPLEMENT CONTRIBUTORS

Tracy Blanc, RN, BSN
Ivy Tech Community College
of Indiana
Terre Haute, IN
Instructor's Resource Manual

VaLinda Pearson, PhD, RN, CRRN, CNE
St. Catherine University
Minneapolis, MN
PowerPoint Slide Lecture

Gloria Jean Shover, RN, BSN, AHI
Erie Business College
Erie, PA
Student Workbook

Elizabeth Schneider, RN, MSN
MedVance Institute
Palm Springs, FL
TestBank

Preface

The practice of nursing is always evolving, especially in the face of what has been called the information age. As research adds more and more knowledge to our understanding of health, wellness and illness, nurses are challenged to remain current and keep up with evidenced based practice to always provide optimal client care.

As we look forward to national calls to reduce the cost of health care while maintaining quality nurses must be able to grow and evolve to meet the demands of a dramatically changing health care system. The nurse requires skills in information technology, maintaining cost-effectiveness of care, cultural competence in the face of increasing diversity in both clients and collaborative health care teams, and clinical decision making. They need to think critically and be creative in implementing nursing strategies in increasingly varied settings. They need skills in teaching, leading, managing, and implementing change. They need to be prepared to provide care in many different settings to clients across the life span—especially to the increasing numbers of older adults. They need to understand holistic healing modalities and complementary therapies. And, they need to continue their unique role that demands a blend of nurturance, sensitivity, caring, empathy, commitment, and skill founded on a broad base of knowledge.

Nursing Basics for Clinical Practice, addresses the concepts essential to the practice of nursing. These concepts include but are not limited to caring, wellness, health promotion, disease prevention, holistic care, multiculturalism, ethics, and advocacy. The content reflects the latest nursing research and the increasing emphasis on aging, wellness, and the need for every nurse to have an evidenced based practice while maintaining client safety as the first priority. We developed this text so that it can be used with a variety of nursing theories and conceptual frameworks.

STRUCTURE OF THE TEXT

The detailed table of contents at the beginning of the book makes its clear organization easy to follow. Continuing with a strong focus on nursing care, the book is divided into 8 units.

UNIT 1, The Nature of Nursing, clusters five chapters that provide comprehensive coverage of introductory concepts of nursing.

In **UNIT 2, The Nursing Process**, provides three chapters on the framework for problem solving used by nurses. Chapter 6 provides information to promote Critical Thinking. Chapter 7 describes each phase of the nursing process with emphasis on the interrelationship of each of the components. Chapter 8 assists students to improve the accuracy of documenting the nursing process in both the paper and electronic medical record. Starting in this unit and incorporated throughout the book, we refer to the NANDA 2009-2011 diagnoses.

UNIT 3 is **Development and Family Health** with emphasis on promoting health in each stage of the life span with special emphasis on both the geriatric client and the family.

In **UNIT 4, Integral Aspects of Nursing**, introduces students to those aspects of nursing that lay the foundation for all nurse client interactions including caring, communicating, teaching, and leading, managing, and delegating.

UNIT 5, Assessing Health, covers vital signs, health assessment, pain assessment and management, and diagnostic tests in four separate chapters so beginning students can understand normal assessment techniques and findings. Chapter 16, Vital Signs, begins to introduce students to the clinical procedures that they need to learn.

In **UNIT 6, Integral Components of Client Care**, the focus shifts to those components of client care that are universal to all clients, including asepsis, safety, hygiene, diagnostic testing, medications, wound care, and preoperative care.

UNIT 7, Promoting Psychosocial Health, includes 5 chapters that cover a wide range of areas that affect one's health. Sensory perception, self-concept, sexuality, spirituality, stress, and loss are all things that a nurse needs to consider to properly care for a client.

UNIT 8, Promoting Physiologic Health, discusses a variety of physiologic concepts that provide the foundations for nursing care. These include activity, exercise and sleep; nutrition; elimination; oxygenation and circulation; and fluid, electrolyte, and acid–base balance.

NURSING BASICS FOR CLINICAL PRACTICE
SETS THE FOUNDATION FOR SUCCESS IN NURSING!

A **Case Scenario** gives chapter content a clinically relevant perspective. Critical thinking questions around the case are provided at the end of the chapter.

CHAPTER

1

Principles of Nursing and Evidence-Based Practice

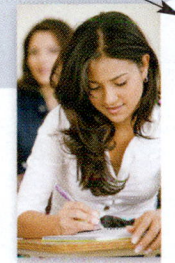

Rayna is beginning her career in nursing today. As she enters the nursing classroom for the first time, she is excited about the challenges to be met. She has wanted to be a nurse for a long time. Rayna was treated for a serious illness when she was young and watched all the things the nurses did for her to make her feel better, and decided she wanted to do the same thing for others. She has come to class ready to begin learning all the procedures a nurse needs to practice proficiently, and she is a little surprised that the first class revolves around nursing history and trends.

LEARNING OUTCOMES

After completing this chapter, you will be able to:

1. List four historical factors that influenced the history of nursing and explain how each factor impacted nursing practice.

2. List eight nursing leaders and briefly explain what they contributed to the practice of nursing.

3. Define nursing, including the eight essential aspects of nursing.

4. Identify four major areas within the scope of nursing practice.

5. Identify the purposes of the nursing practice acts and standards for nursing practice.

6. List 10 roles of the nurse, briefly explaining how the nurse would behave in each of these roles.

7. List six criteria of a profession and explain the professionalization of nursing.

8. List and describe Benner's stages of nursing expertise.

9. List at least three nursing organizations and describe the function of each.

10. List several types of nursing education programs and explain the purpose of each as it relates to entry into nursing practice.

11. State the importance of continuing education and list strategies for maintaining currency in nursing practice.

12. List the steps taken to protect the rights of human subjects when they participate in research.

13. Read a research article and critique it for relevance and scientific merit.

14. List seven nursing theorists and describe each theory.

2

Learning outcomes help identify critical concepts.

KEY TERMS

Assessing p151	Etiology p160	Nursing diagnosis p160	Quality improvement p183
Cephalocaudal p157	Evaluating p179	Nursing Interventions Classifications p175	Rapport p155
Collaborative care plan p169	Evaluation statement p181	Nursing Outcomes Classification p172	Rationale p169
Concept map p169	Goals p171	Planning p167	Risk factors p161
Critical pathway p169	Implementing p178	Policies p169	Sentinel event p183
Cues p139	Indicator p172	Priority setting p171	Sign p153
Data p151	Individualized care plan p168	Procedures p169	Standing order p169
Defining characteristics p161	Inference p159	Protocol p169	Symptom p152
Desired outcomes p171	Interview p155	Qualifiers p161	Taxonomy p160
Diagnosis p160	Multidisciplinary care plan p169	Quality assurance p183	Validation p159
Discharge planning p168			

Key Terms provide a study tool for learning new vocabulary. Page numbers are included for easy reference.

CLIENT-FOCUSED NURSING CARE, CRITICAL THINKING AND EVIDENCE-BASED PRACTICE

Nursing Care Plans help organize care around the nursing process.

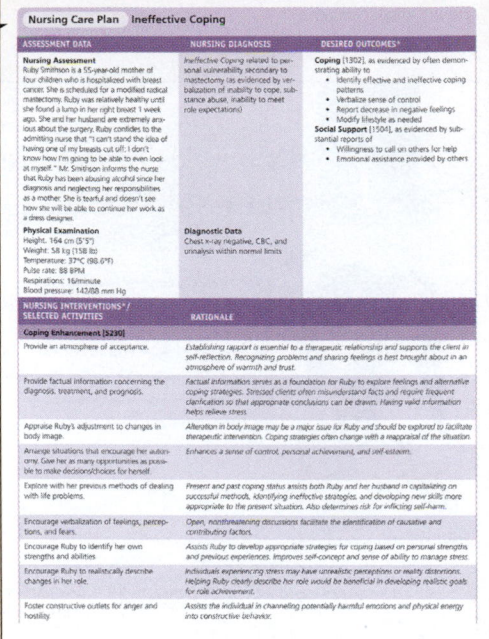

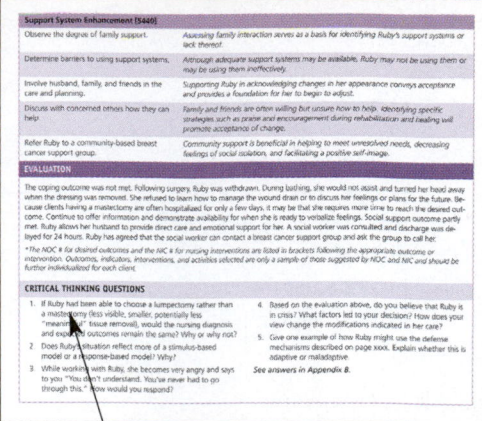

Critical Thinking Questions come at the end of each sample Nursing Care Plan to encourage further reflection and analysis.

Concept Maps! Sample concept maps throughout the textbook provide a visual representation of the nursing process, nursing care plans, and the relationships in different concepts.

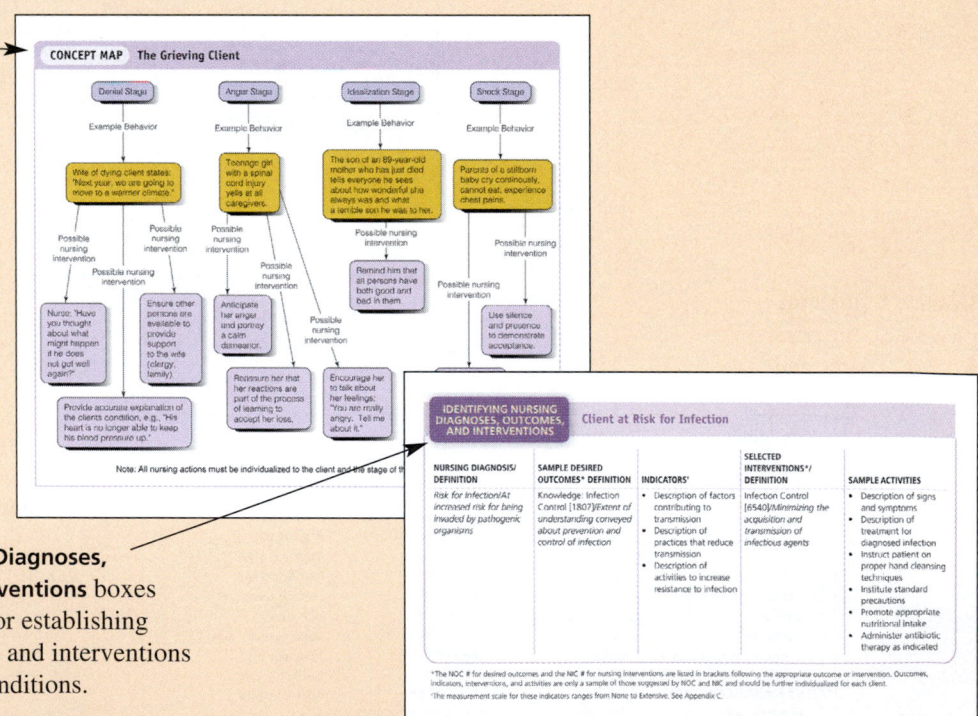

Identifying Nursing Diagnoses, Outcomes, and Interventions boxes provide guidelines for establishing diagnoses, outcomes and interventions for situations and conditions.

RESEARCH NOTES Evidence-Based Practice

Treatments once considered to be folk treatments, including acupuncture, therapeutic touch, and massage, are now being investigated for their therapeutic effect. The National Center for Complementary and Alternative Medicine at the National Institutes of Health provides up-to-date information on this line of research: http://nccam.nih.gov.

Research Notes focus on evidence-based practice. These boxes highlight relevant nursing research and implications for nursing care.

SUCCESS IN CLINICAL PRACTICE!

Step-by-step skills.
An easy-to-follow
format helps
students understand
techniques and
practice sequences.

Clearly labeled
Delegation boxes
assist you in
assigning tasks
appropriately.

Includes a complete
Equipment list for
easy preparation.

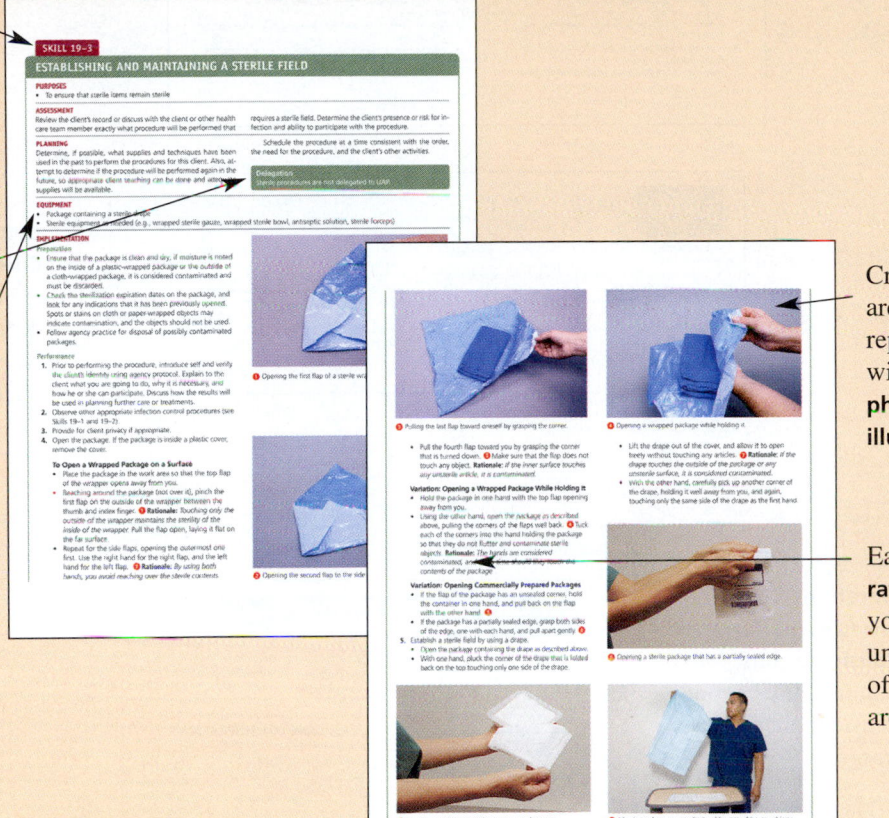

Critical steps
are visually
represented
with full-color
photographs and
illustrations!

Easy-to-find
rationales give
you a better
understanding
of why things
are done.

Practice Guidelines
provide summaries
of clinical do's and
don'ts.

Unique! **Drug Capsules** provide a brief
overview of drug information, nursing
responsibilities, and client teaching.

Assessment Interview boxes help students learn the type and range of what to ask in particular client situations.

ASSESSMENT INTERVIEW   Determining the Risk for Medication Nonadherence

- Are you having side effects from any of your medications?
- Do you think your medications are helping?
- Do you have "tools" to remind you to take your medication? Examples could be an alarm or environmental cues (e.g., 6:00 news).
- Is there someone at home who helps you with your medications?
- How many times per day are your medications prescribed?
- How many pills do you take every day?
- Are there any special storage requirements for your medications?
- How much do your medication requirements interfere with your lifestyle?
- How well are you able to follow special dosing requirements?
- How many doses of your medications have you missed over the last 3 days?

CULTURALLY COMPETENT CARE   Families

- Include cultural assessment of the client and family as part of overall assessment.
- Learn the rituals, customs, and practices of the major cultural groups with whom you come into contact. Learn to appreciate the richness of diversity and consider it an asset rather than a hindrance in your practice.
- Don't make assumptions about beliefs or practices.
- Ask about the client's use of cultural or alternative approaches to healing.
- Identify your personal biases, attitudes, prejudices, and stereotypes.
- Recognize that it is the client's (or family's) right to make their own health care choices. Explain in detail the client's condition and the treatment plan if the client is willing for you to do this.
- Convey respect and cooperate with traditional helpers and caregivers.

Culturally Competent Care boxes focus on how situations may have different approaches when considering the client's cultural heritage.

Home Care Considerations, Long Term Care Considerations (Unique!), and **Physician Office Considerations (Unique!)** help students think beyond the hospital and consider client issues in other client settings.

HOME CARE CONSIDERATIONS

In a home setting, the client's support people and caregivers are the ones who implement the plan of care; thus, its effectiveness depends largely on them.

LONG-TERM CARE CONSIDERATIONS

Clients in long-term care often reside in the facility for long periods of time and are, as such, inviting the health care provider into their home. Accommodating cultural differences in how they furnish their space is essential to the sense of home the client needs to feel comfortable in their space. Adding cultu... erations to the client's plan of care will improve client c...

BOX 4–1   Physician's Office Considerations

The physician's office or ambulatory care setting provides a unique opportunity to assess family interactions and function. The client is usually not as acutely ill as those requiring hospitalization, resulting in a family functioning under less stress and more normally. Who accompanies the client to the health care site? Do family members participate in health care discussions and decision making? Does the client bring family members into the examination room, or do family members stay in the waiting room? All of these assessment findings can help to demonstrate cultural beliefs of the family.

Lifespan Considerations highlight how nursing care is adapted for infants, children, adolescents, and elders.

LIFESPAN CONSIDERATIONS   Diagnosing

Children

Many developmental issues in pediatrics are not considered problems or illnesses, yet can benefit from nursing intervention. When applied to children and families, nursing diagnoses may reflect a condition or state of health. Assessment of the family system might lead the nurse to conclude that the family is ready and able, even eager, to take on the new roles and responsibilities of being parents. An appropriate diagnosis for such a family could be *Readiness for Enhanced Family Processes*, and nursing care could be directed to educating and providing encouragement and support to the parents.

Older Adults

Older adults tend to have multiple problems with com... physical and psychosocial needs when they are ill. If the n... has done a thorough, accurate assessment, nursing diagno... can be selected to cover all problems and, at the same time, ... oritize the special needs. As these conditions improve, ... other nursing diagnoses might require more attention. E... nursing diagnosis has specific expected outcomes and nurs... interventions. The client's strengths should be an essential ... sideration in all phases of the nursing process.

Client Teaching boxes give tips and tools to help clients facilitate self-care, monitor potential problems, perform prescribed therapies, and assist in other client teaching experiences.

CLIENT TEACHING   Preparing for Diagnostic Testing

- Instruct the client and family about requirements or restrictions (e.g., when and what to eat or drink, how long to fast).
- Provide information about what the client may feel (e.g., a temporary flushing and feeling of warmth when the dye is injected).
- Ask the client if a description or pictures of the involved equipment would help prepare him or her for the test.
- Encourage questions and dialogue about fears and apprehensions. Find out what the client may have heard about the test from others.
- Inform the client of the time period before the results will be available.
- Document teaching. Include the client's response. Record names of audiovisual and reading materials, if used.

Note: From A Manual of Laboratory & Diagnostic Tests, 7th ed., by F. Fischbach, 2004, Philadelphia: Lippincott Williams & Wilkins. Reprinted with permission.

UNDERSTANDING THE CHAPTER

The end of each chapter summarizes and applies chapter information.

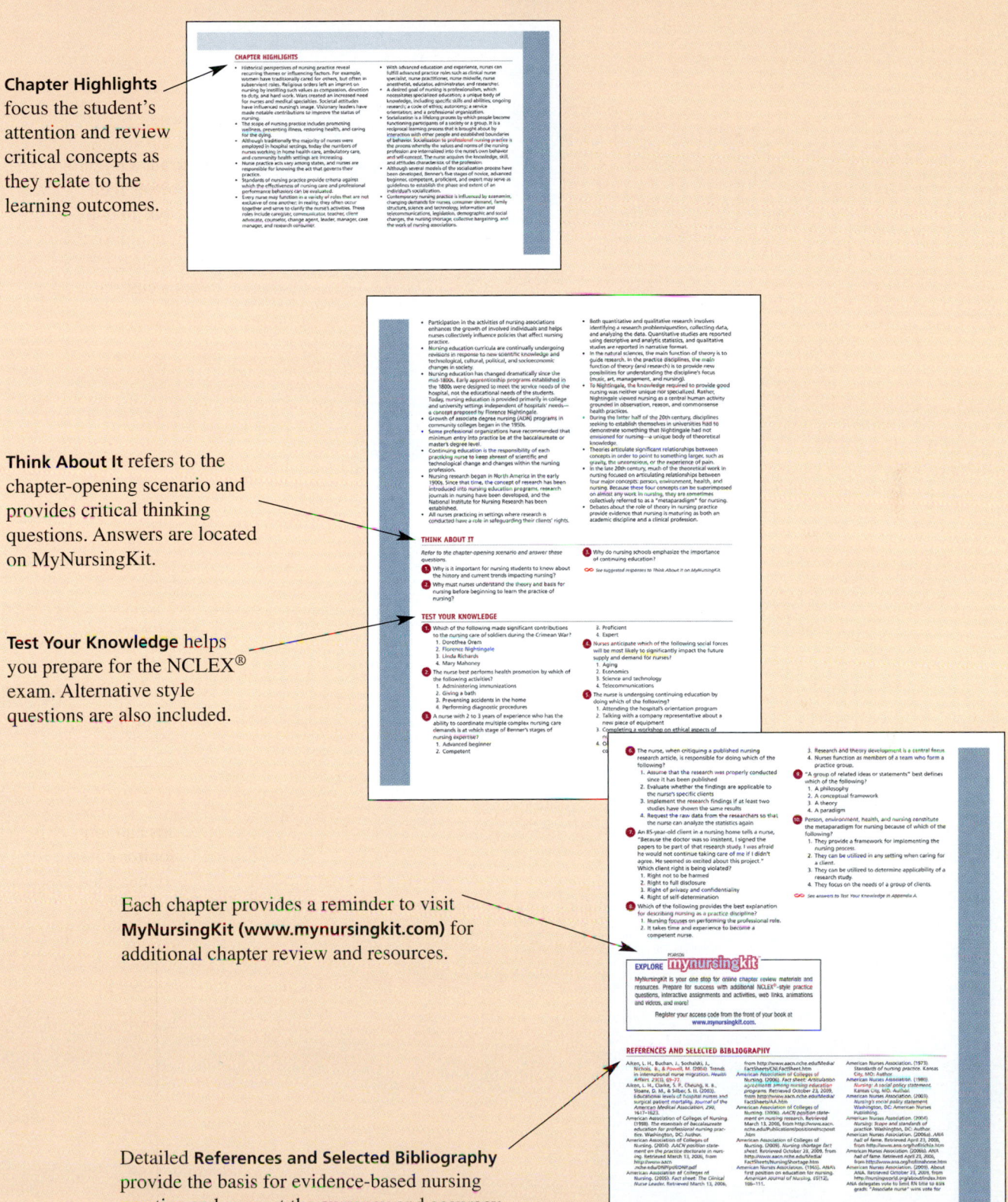

Chapter Highlights focus the student's attention and review critical concepts as they relate to the learning outcomes.

Think About It refers to the chapter-opening scenario and provides critical thinking questions. Answers are located on MyNursingKit.

Test Your Knowledge helps you prepare for the NCLEX® exam. Alternative style questions are also included.

Each chapter provides a reminder to visit **MyNursingKit** (www.mynursingkit.com) for additional chapter review and resources.

Detailed **References and Selected Bibliography** provide the basis for evidence-based nursing practice and support the currency and accuracy of textbook content.

Contents

The Nature of Nursing

Principles of Nursing and Evidence-Based Practice

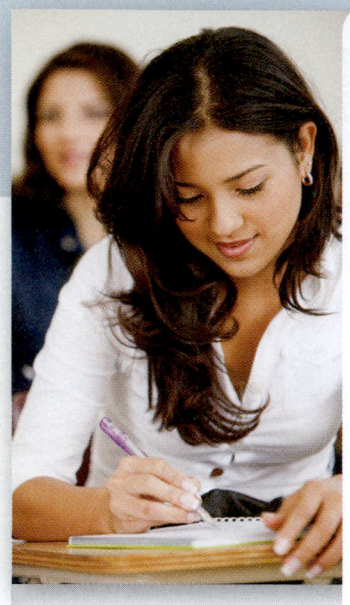

Rayna is beginning her career in nursing today. As she enters the nursing classroom for the first time, she is excited about the challenges to be met. She has wanted to be a nurse for a long time. Rayna was treated for a serious illness when she was young and watched all the things the nurses did for her to make her feel better, and decided she wanted to do the same thing for others. She has come to class ready to begin learning all the procedures a nurse needs to practice proficiently, and she is a little surprised that the first class revolves around nursing history and trends.

LEARNING OUTCOMES

After completing this chapter, you will be able to:

1. List four historical factors that influenced the history of nursing and explain how each factor impacted nursing practice.

2. List eight nursing leaders and briefly explain what they contributed to the practice of nursing.

3. Define nursing, including the eight essential aspects of nursing.

4. Identify four major areas within the scope of nursing practice.

5. Identify the purposes of the nursing practice acts and standards for nursing practice.

6. List 10 roles of the nurse, briefly explaining how the nurse would behave in each of these roles.

7. List six criteria of a profession and explain the professionalization of nursing.

8. List and describe Benner's stages of nursing expertise.

9. List at least three nursing organizations and describe the function of each.

10. List several types of nursing education programs and explain the purpose of each as it relates to entry into nursing practice.

11. State the importance of continuing education and list strategies for maintaining currency in nursing practice.

12. List the steps taken to protect the rights of human subjects when they participate in research.

13. Read a research article and critique it for relevance and scientific merit.

14. List seven nursing theorists and describe each theory.

HISTORICAL PERSPECTIVE OF NURSING

Factors Influencing the Evolution of Nursing

Nursing has undergone dramatic changes in response to societal needs and influences and will continue to change throughout the coming years. A look at nursing's beginnings reveals its continuing struggle for autonomy and professionalization. In recent decades, a renewed interest in nursing history has produced a growing amount of related literature. Recurring themes of women's roles and status, religious values, wars, societal attitudes, and visionary nursing leadership have influenced nursing practice in the past and will continue to have an effect on the future of the profession.

Traditional female roles of wife, mother, daughter, and sister have included caring and nurturing family members. Thus, nursing could be said to have its roots in the home. Additionally, women, who in general occupied a subservient and dependent role, were called on to care for others in the community who were ill. Generally, the care provided was related to physical maintenance and comfort. The traditional nursing role has always included humanistic caring, nurturing, comforting, and supporting.

Most early cultures developed special roles for those who practiced the healing arts. Often these roles were incorporated into other societal positions such as that of priest, priestess, witch, or shaman. These traditional healers provided care for centuries before the development of Western medicine. Many complementary and alternative health principles maintain these traditional healing roles and practices. In Western medicine, the role of the traditional healer suffered as a result of the influence of the church and early medical education. Traditional healers, particularly midwives, were favored targets of the medieval witch hunts that lasted from 1450 to about 1700 BC. Walpurga Hausmannin represents a typical victim of the witch hunts. A midwife for 19 years, Walpurga was burned at the stake after being accused of using witchcraft to kill a mother and newborn. At the same time, Western medicine was being developed in early European universities that likely excluded women. The result was a loss of traditional healing practices in Western medicine.

Religion has also played a significant role in the development of nursing. Although many of the world's religions encourage benevolence, it was the Christian value of "love thy neighbor as thyself" and Christ's parable of the Good Samaritan that had a significant impact on the development of Western nursing. During the third and fourth centuries, several wealthy matrons of the Roman Empire, such as Fabiola, converted to Christianity and used their wealth to provide houses of care and healing (the forerunner of hospitals) for the poor, the sick, and the homeless. The deaconess groups, which had their origins in the Roman Empire of the third and fourth centuries, were suppressed during the Middle Ages by the Western churches. However, these groups of nursing providers resurfaced occasionally throughout the centuries, most notably in 1836 when Theodore Fliedner reinstituted the Order of Deaconesses and opened a small hospital and training school in Kaiserswerth, Germany, where the most famous nurse in history, Florence Nightingale, received her "training" in nursing.

Wars have accentuated the need for nurses throughout history. Early armies were likely accompanied by individuals whose job was caring for the injured and dying. Modern nursing was born during the Crimean War (1854–1856) due to the inadequacy of care given to British soldiers, when Florence Nightingale was asked by Sir Sidney Herbert of the British War Department to recruit a contingent of female nurses to provide care to the sick and injured. Nightingale and her nurses transformed the military hospitals by setting up sanitation practices, such as hand washing and washing clothing regularly. Nightingale is credited with performing miracles; the mortality rate in the Barrack Hospital in Turkey, for example, was reduced from 42% to 2% (Donahue, 1996, p. 197). Since that time, war has continued to influence the development of nursing and changed the way clients suffering from traumatic injury are treated.

Society's attitudes about nurses and nursing have significantly influenced professional nursing. Before the mid-1800s, nursing was without organization, education, or social status; the prevailing attitude was that a woman's place was in the home and that no respectable woman should have a career. Nurses in hospitals during this period were poorly educated; some were incarcerated criminals. The *guardian angel* or *angel of mercy* image arose in the latter part of the 19th century, largely because of the work of Florence Nightingale during the Crimean War. After Nightingale brought respectability to the nursing profession, nurses were viewed as noble, compassionate, moral, religious, dedicated, and self-sacrificing. The image of the nurse as the physician's handmaiden arose in the early 19th century because women had yet to obtain the right to vote, family structures were largely paternalistic, and the medical profession portrayed increasing use of scientific knowledge that was viewed as a male domain. During the past few decades, the nursing profession has taken steps to improve the image of the nurse. In the early 1990s, the Tri-Council for Nursing (the American Association of Colleges of Nursing, the American Nurses Association, the American Organization of Nurse Executives, and the National League for Nursing) initiated a national effort titled "Nurses of America" to improve the image of nursing. More recently, the Johnson & Johnson Corporation contributed $20 million in 2002 to launch a "Campaign for Nursing's Future" to promote nursing as a positive career choice (Anonymous, 2003; Fitzpatrick, 2002).

Nursing Leaders

Nursing leaders have changed nursing practice throughout history and continue to guide the profession. Only a few of the notable nurses throughout history are described in this chapter, but there are many more who have influenced the practice of nursing. A timeline of these nursing leaders can be seen in Figure 1–1.

NIGHTINGALE (1820–1910)   Florence Nightingale improved the standards for the care of war casualties in the Crimea, earning her the title "Lady with the Lamp." Her efforts in reforming hospitals, stressing the need for cleanliness, encouraging holistic client care, and guiding public health policies made her the first nurse to successfully exert political pressure on government to improve health care. Through her contributions to nursing education—perhaps her greatest achievement—she is also recognized as nursing's first scientist-theorist for her work *Notes on Nursing: What It Is, and What It Is Not* (1860/1969). She was determined to become a nurse in spite of opposition from her family and the restrictive societal code for affluent young English women. She visited Kaiserswerth in 1847, where she received 3 months' training in nursing. In 1853 she studied in Paris with the Sisters of Charity, after which she returned to England to assume the position of superintendent of a charity hospital for ill governesses. She developed the Nightingale Training School for Nurses, which opened in 1860 and served as a model for other nurse training schools.

BARTON (1821–1912)   Clara Barton was a schoolteacher who volunteered as a nurse during the American Civil War,

organizing the nursing services. Barton is noted for her role in establishing the American Red Cross, which linked with the International Red Cross when the U.S. Congress ratified the Treaty of Geneva. Barton persuaded Congress in 1882 to ratify this treaty so that the Red Cross could perform humanitarian efforts in time of peace as well as times of war.

RICHARDS (1841–1930)   Linda Richards was America's first trained nurse. She graduated from the New England Hospital for Women and Children in 1873. Richards is known for introducing nurse's notes and doctor's orders. She also initiated the practice of nurses wearing uniforms (American Nurses Association, 2006a). She is credited for her pioneer work in psychiatric and industrial nursing.

MAHONEY (1845–1926)   Mary Mahoney was the first African American professional nurse. She graduated from the New England Hospital for Women and Children in 1879. She constantly worked for the acceptance of African Americans in nursing and for the promotion of equal opportunities (Donahue, 1996, p. 271). The American Nurses Association (2006b) gives a Mary Mahoney Award biennially in recognition of significant contributions in interracial relationships.

WALD (1867–1940)   Lillian Wald is considered the founder of public health nursing. Wald and Mary Brewster were the first to offer trained nursing services to the poor in the New York slums. Their home among the poor on the upper floor of a tenement, called the Henry Street Settlement and Visiting Nurse Service, provided nursing services, social services, and organized educational and cultural activities. Soon after the founding of the Henry Street Settlement, school nursing was established as an adjunct to visiting nursing.

DOCK (1858–1956)   Lavinia L. Dock was a feminist, prolific writer, political activist, suffragette, and friend of Wald. She participated in protest movements for women's rights that resulted in the 1920 passage of the 19th Amendment to the U.S. Constitution, which granted women the right to vote. In addition, Dock campaigned for legislation to allow nurses, rather than physicians, to control their own profession. In 1893, Dock, with the assistance of Mary Adelaide Nutting and Isabel Hampton Robb, founded the American Society of Superintendents of Training Schools for Nurses of the United States and Canada, a precursor to the current National League for Nursing.

SANGER (1879–1966)   Margaret Higgins Sanger, a public health nurse in New York, has had a lasting impact on women's health care. Imprisoned for opening the first birth control information clinic in America, she is considered the founder of Planned Parenthood. Her experience with the large number of unwanted pregnancies among the working poor was instrumental in addressing this problem.

BRECKINRIDGE (1881–1965)   After World War I, Mary Breckinridge, a notable pioneer nurse, established the Frontier Nursing Service (FNS). In 1918, she worked with the

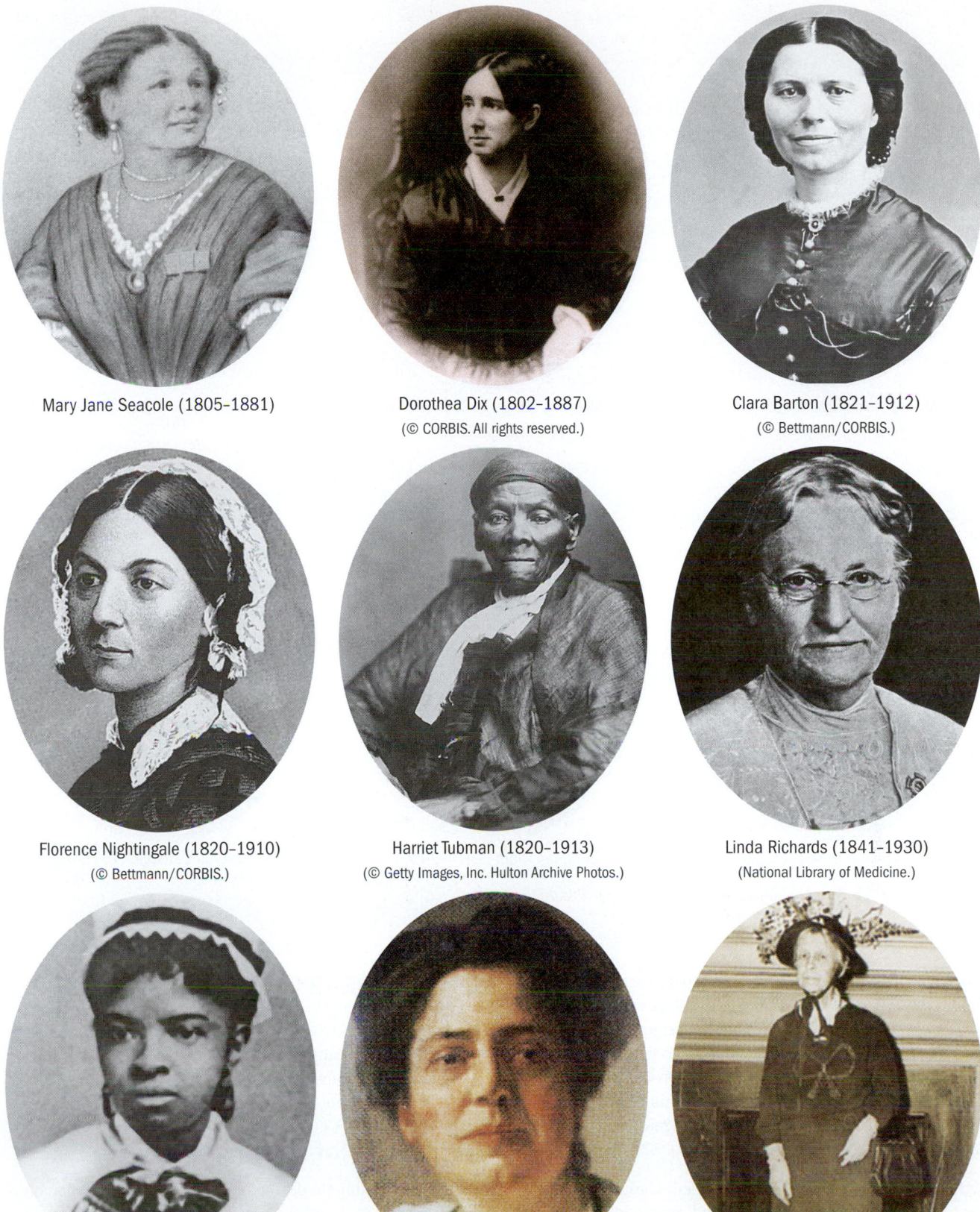

Mary Jane Seacole (1805–1881)

Dorothea Dix (1802–1887)
(© CORBIS. All rights reserved.)

Clara Barton (1821–1912)
(© Bettmann/CORBIS.)

Florence Nightingale (1820–1910)
(© Bettmann/CORBIS.)

Harriet Tubman (1820–1913)
(© Getty Images, Inc. Hulton Archive Photos.)

Linda Richards (1841–1930)
(National Library of Medicine.)

Mary Mahoney (1845–1926)
(© The New York Public Library.)

Lillian Wald (1867–1940)

Lavinia L. Dock (1858–1956)
(Courtesy of Teachers College, Columbia University.)

Figure 1–1 ⬭ Notable nurses throughout history.

(continued)

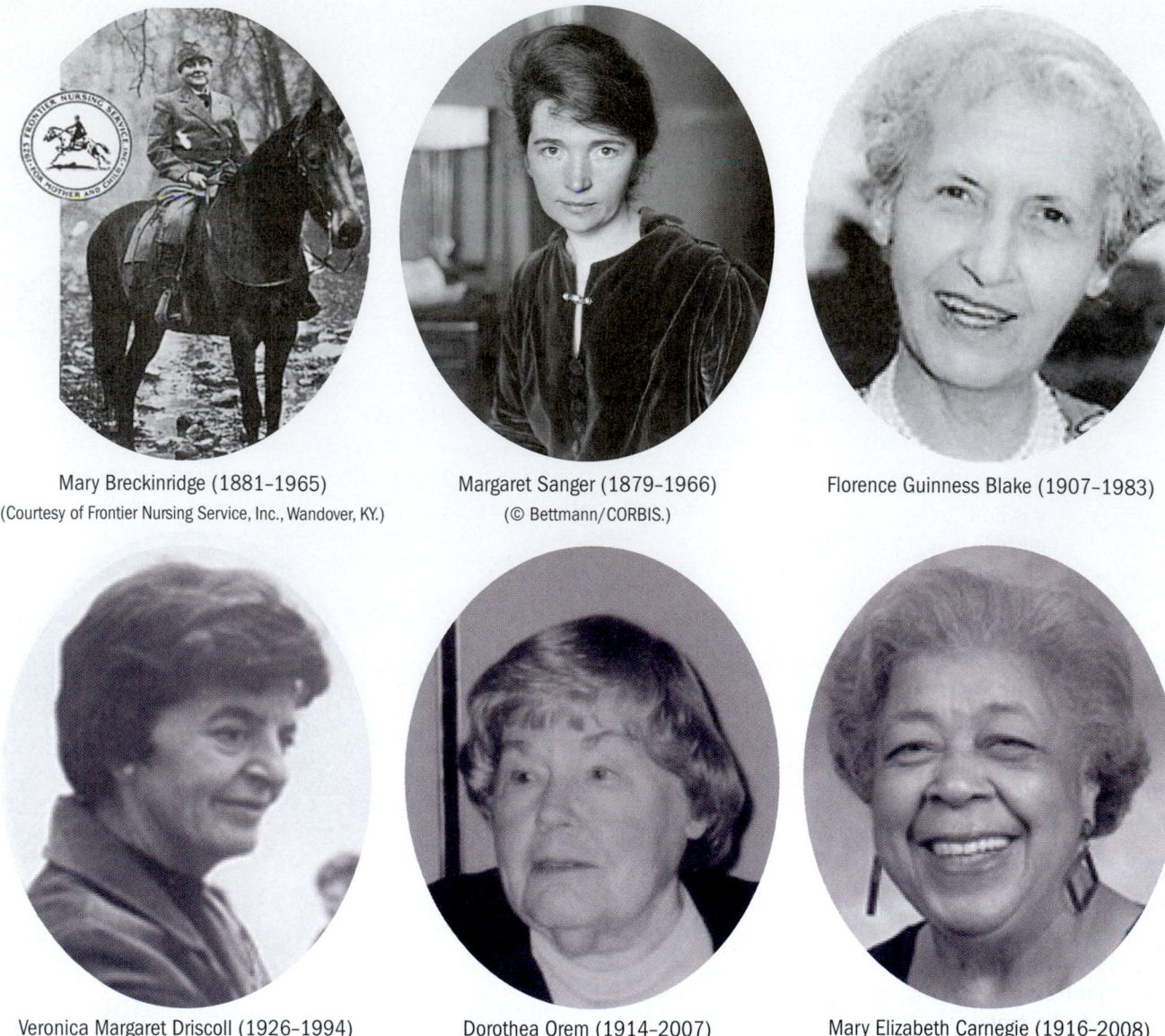

Mary Breckinridge (1881–1965)
(Courtesy of Frontier Nursing Service, Inc., Wandover, KY.)

Margaret Sanger (1879–1966)
(© Bettmann/CORBIS.)

Florence Guinness Blake (1907–1983)

Veronica Margaret Driscoll (1926–1994)

Dorothea Orem (1914–2007)

Mary Elizabeth Carnegie (1916–2008)

Figure 1–1 ○ Notable nurses throughout history. *(continued)*

American Committee for Devastated France, distributing food, clothing, and supplies to rural villages and taking care of sick children. In 1921, Breckinridge returned to the United States with plans to provide health care to the people of rural America. In 1925, Breckinridge and two other nurses began the FNS in Leslie County, Kentucky. Within this organization, Breckinridge started one of the first midwifery training schools in the United States.

CARNEGIE (1916–2008)   Mary Elizabeth Carnegie is known for breaking down racial barriers and preserving the history of African American Nurses. After noting the difference in treatment of white and black nurses, she pioneered for black nurses to be given full rights and responsibilities within the Florida State Nurses Association. She was a noted author, educator and researcher who was inducted into the American Nurses Association Hall of Fame.

CONTEMPORARY NURSING PRACTICE

Nursing continues to evolve and change. An understanding of contemporary nursing practice includes a look at definitions of nursing, recipients of nursing, scope of nursing, nurse practice acts, and current standards of clinical nursing practice.

Definitions of Nursing

Florence Nightingale defined nursing nearly 150 years ago as "the act of utilizing the environment of the patient to assist him in his recovery" (Nightingale, 1860/1969). Virginia Henderson wrote, "The unique function of the nurse is to assist the individual, sick or well, in the performance of those activities contributing to health or its recovery (or to peaceful death) that he would perform unaided if he had the necessary strength, will, or knowledge, and to do this in such a way as to help him gain independence as rapidly as possible" (Henderson, 1966, p. 3). Like Nightingale, Henderson described nursing in relation to the client and the client's environment. Unlike Nightingale, Henderson saw the nurse as concerned with both healthy and ill individuals, acknowledging that nurses interact with clients even when recovery may not be feasible, and mentioned the teaching and advocacy roles of the nurse. In the latter half of the 20th century, a number of nurse theorists developed their own theoretical definitions of nursing to describe what nursing is and the interrelationship among nurses, nursing, the client, the environment, and the intended client outcome. Certain themes are common to many of these definitions:

- Nursing is caring.
- Nursing is an art.
- Nursing is a science.
- Nursing is client centered.
- Nursing is holistic.
- Nursing is adaptive.
- Nursing is concerned with health promotion, health maintenance, and health restoration.
- Nursing is a helping profession.

Professional nursing associations have also examined nursing and developed their own definitions. In 1973, the American Nurses Association (ANA) described nursing practice as "direct, goal oriented, and adaptable to the needs of the individual, the family, and community during health and illness" (ANA, 1973, p. 2). In 1980, the ANA changed this definition of nursing to: "Nursing is the diagnosis and treatment of human responses to actual or potential health problems" (ANA, 1980, p. 9). In 1995, the ANA recognized the influence and contribution of the science of caring to nursing philosophy and practice. Their most recent definition of professional nursing is much broader and states: "Nursing is the protection, promotion, and optimization of health and abilities, preventions of illness and injury, alleviation of suffering through the diagnosis and treatment of human response, and advocacy in the care of individuals, families, communities, and populations" (ANA, 2003, p. 6).

Recipients of Nursing

The recipients of nursing are sometimes called consumers, patients, or clients. A **consumer** is an individual, a group of people, or a community that uses a service or commodity. People who use health care products or services are consumers of health care. A **patient** undergoes treatment and care, coming from a Latin phrase meaning "to suffer" or "to bear." Some nurses believe "patient" implies passive acceptance of the decisions and care of health professionals. Additionally, not all recipients of nursing care are ill, and nurses interact significantly with family members and significant others who provide support, information, and comfort in caring for the patient. For these reasons, nurses increasingly refer to recipients of health care as clients. A **client** is a person who engages the advice or services of another qualified person to deliver a service. The term "client" perceives the recipient of health care as an active participant who collaborates in his or her own care and takes responsibility for his or her own health needs.

Scope of Nursing

Nursing is a separate profession that functions in partnership with the medical model of health care. Nursing practice involves four areas: promoting health and wellness, preventing illness, restoring health, and caring for the dying.

PROMOTING HEALTH AND WELLNESS Wellness is a process that engages in activities and behaviors that enhance quality of life and maximize personal potential (Anspaugh, Hamrick, & Rosata, 2006). Nurses promote wellness in clients who are both healthy and ill. This may involve individual and community activities to enhance healthy lifestyles, such as improving nutrition and physical fitness, preventing drug and alcohol misuse, restricting smoking, and preventing accidents and injury in the home and workplace.

PREVENTING ILLNESS The goal of illness prevention is to maintain optimal health by preventing disease. Nursing activities that prevent illness include immunizations, prenatal and infant care, and prevention of sexually transmitted disease, to name just a few.

RESTORING HEALTH Restoring health focuses on the ill client, and extends from early detection of disease to helping the client during the recovery period. Nursing activities include the following:

- Providing direct care to the ill person, such as administering medications, baths, and specific procedures and treatments
- Performing diagnostic and assessment procedures, such as measuring blood pressure and examining feces for occult blood
- Consulting with other health care professionals about client problems
- Teaching clients about recovery activities, such as exercises that will accelerate recovery after a stroke
- Rehabilitating clients to their optimal functional level following physical or mental illness, injury, or chemical addiction

CARING FOR THE DYING This area of nursing practice involves comforting and caring for people of all ages who are dying. Nurses help clients live as comfortably as possible until their death, and support loved ones coping with the client's death. These nurses work in homes, hospitals, and extended care facilities. Some agencies, called *hospices*, are specifically designed for this purpose.

Settings for Nursing

In the past, the acute care hospital was the main practice setting open to most nurses. Today many nurses work in hospitals,

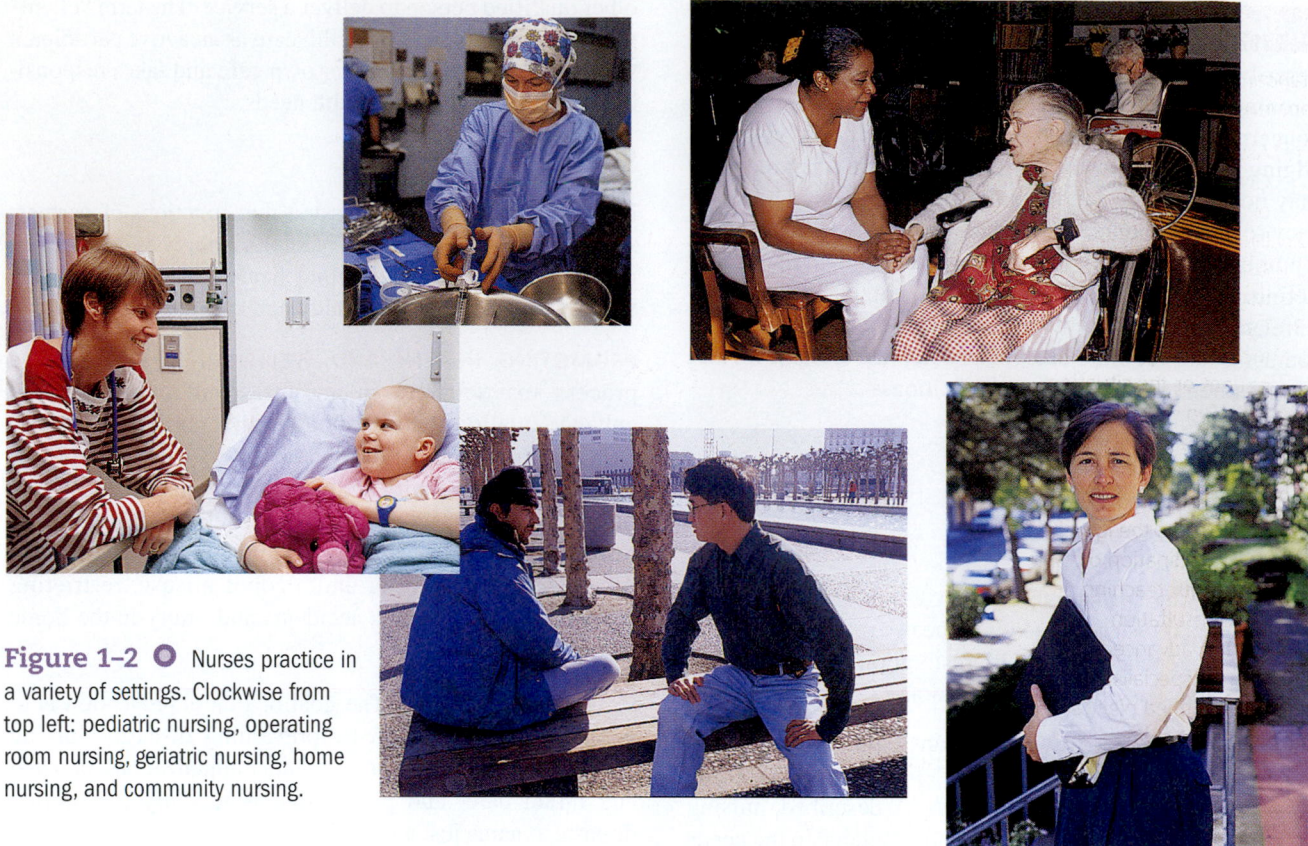

Figure 1–2 ○ Nurses practice in a variety of settings. Clockwise from top left: pediatric nursing, operating room nursing, geriatric nursing, home nursing, and community nursing.

but increasingly they work in clients' homes, community agencies, ambulatory clinics, long-term care facilities, health maintenance organizations (HMOs), and nursing practice centers (Figure 1–2).

Nurse Practice Acts

Nurse practice acts are legal acts that regulate the practice of nursing in the United States and Canada. Each state in the United States and each province in Canada has its own act. Although nurse practice acts differ in various jurisdictions, they all have a common purpose: to protect the public. Nurses are responsible for knowing and complying with their state's nurse practice act as it governs their practice.

Standards of Nursing Practice

Establishing and implementing standards of practice are major functions of a professional organization. The purpose of the ANA Standards of Practice is to describe the responsibilities for which nurses are accountable. The American Nurses Association developed **standards of nursing practice** that are generic in nature, by using the nursing process as a foundation, and provide for the practice of nursing regardless of area of specialization. Various specialty nursing organizations have developed specific standards of nursing practice for their area. For nurses in Canada, each province or territory establishes its own standards of practice. The ANA Standards of Nursing Practice describe behaviors expected in the professional nursing role (Box 1–1).

Roles of the Nurse

Nurses assume a number of roles when they provide care to clients. Nurses often carry out these roles concurrently, not exclusively of one another. For example, the nurse may act as a counselor and teacher while providing physical care. The roles required at a specific time depend on the needs of the client and aspects of the client's environment.

The caregiver role has traditionally included those activities that assist the client physically and psychologically while preserving the client's dignity. The required nursing actions may involve full care for the completely dependent client, partial care for the partially dependent client, and supportive-educative care to assist clients in attaining their highest possible level of health and wellness. Caregiving encompasses the physical, psychosocial, developmental, cultural, and spiritual levels. The nursing process provides nurses with a framework for providing care. A nurse may provide care directly or delegate it to other caregivers.

Communication is integral to all nursing roles. Nurses communicate with the client, support persons, other health professionals, and people in the community. In the role of communicator, nurses identify client problems and then communicate these verbally or in writing to other members of the health team. The quality of a nurse's communication is an important factor in nursing care. The nurse must be able to communicate clearly and accurately in order for a client's health care needs to be met.

| **BOX 1–1** | **ANA Standards of Nursing Practice** |

Standards of Practice for the Registered Nurse —describe a competent level of nursing care as demonstrated by the nursing process.

1. Assessment
   Collects comprehensive data pertinent to the patient's health or the situation.
2. Diagnosis
   Analyzes the assessment data to determine the diagnoses or issues.
3. Outcomes Identification
   Identifies expected outcomes for a plan individualized to the patient or the situation.
4. Planning
   Develops a plan that prescribes strategies and alternatives to attain expected outcomes.
5. Implementation
   Implements the identified plan.
   a. Coordination of care
   b. Health teaching and health promotion
   c. Consultation
      The advanced practice registered nurse and the nursing role specialist provide consultation to influence the identified plan, enhance the abilities of others, and effect change.
   d. Prescriptive authority and treatment
      The advanced practice registered nurse uses prescriptive authority, procedures, referrals, treatments, and therapies in accordance with state and federal laws and regulations.
   e. Treatment and evaluation
6. Evaluation
   Evaluates progress toward attainment of outcomes.

Standards of Professional Performance—describe a competent level of behavior in the professional role.

7. Quality of Practice
   Systematically enhances the quality and effectiveness of nursing practice.
8. Education
   Attains knowledge and competency that reflects current nursing practice.
9. Professional Practice Evaluation
   Evaluates one's own nursing practice in relation to professional practice standards and guidelines, relevant statutes, rules, and regulations.
10. Collegiality
    Interacts with and contributes to the professional development of peers and colleagues.
11. Collaboration
    Collaborates with patient, family, and others in the conduct of nursing practice.
12. Ethics
    Integrates ethical provisions in all areas of practice.
13. Research
    Integrates research findings into practice.
14. Resource Utilization
    Considers factors related to safety, effectiveness, cost, and impact on practice in the planning and delivery of nursing services.
15. Leadership
    Provides leadership in the professional practice setting and the profession.

Note: Reprinted with permission from American Nurses Association, *Nursing: Scope and Standards of Practice,* © 2004 Nursebooks.org, Silver Spring, MD.

As a teacher, the nurse helps clients learn about their health and the health care procedures they need to perform in order to restore or maintain their health. The nurse assesses the client's learning needs and readiness to learn, sets specific learning goals in conjunction with the client, enacts teaching strategies, and measures learning. Nurses also teach unlicensed assistive personnel (UAP) to whom they delegate care, and they share their expertise with nurses and other health professionals.

A **client advocate** acts to protect the client. In this role the nurse may represent the client's needs and wishes to other health professionals, such as relaying the client's wishes for information to the physician. They also assist clients in exercising their rights and help them speak up for themselves.

Counseling is the process of helping a client to recognize and cope with stressful psychologic or social problems, to develop improved interpersonal relationships, and to promote personal growth. It involves providing emotional, intellectual, and psychologic support. The nurse counsels individuals with normal adjustment difficulties and focuses on helping the person develop new attitudes, feelings, and behaviors by encouraging the client to look at alternative behaviors, recognize the choices, and develop a sense of control.

The nurse acts as a **change agent** when assisting clients to make modifications in their behavior. Nurses also act to make changes in a system, such as clinical care, if it is not helping a client return to health. Nurses also help to change the profession of nursing and the health care system by becoming involved in nursing organizations that work for political changes.

A **leader** influences others to work together to accomplish a specific goal. The leader role can be employed at different levels: individual client, family, groups of clients, colleagues, or the community. Effective leadership is a learned process requiring an understanding of the needs and goals that motivate people, the knowledge to apply the leadership skills, and the interpersonal skills to influence others.

The nurse manages the nursing care of individuals, families, and communities. The nurse **manager** also delegates nursing activities to ancillary workers and other nurses, and supervises and evaluates their performance. Managing requires knowledge about organizational structure and dynamics, authority and accountability, leadership, change theory, advocacy, delegation, and supervision and evaluation.

Nurse case managers work with the multidisciplinary health care team to measure the effectiveness of the case management plan and to monitor outcomes. Each agency or unit specifies the role of the nurse case manager. The role of case manager varies between different institutions. The case manager may work with primary or staff nurses to oversee the care of a specific caseload or function as the primary nurse providing some level of direct care to the client and family. Insurance companies have also developed a number of roles for nurse case managers. Regardless of the setting, case managers help ensure that care is oriented to the client, while controlling costs.

Nurses often use research to improve client care. In a clinical area, nurses need to (a) have some awareness of the process and language of research, (b) be sensitive to issues related to protecting the rights of human subjects, (c) participate in the identification of significant researchable problems, and (d) be a discriminating consumer of research findings.

With further nursing education there are many roles for fulfilling expanded career roles, such as those of nurse practitioner, clinical nurse specialist, nurse midwife, nurse educator, nurse researcher, and nurse anesthetist. These roles allow greater independence and autonomy as well as contributing to the future of nursing (Box 1–2).

NURSING AS A PROFESSION

Nursing has gained recognition as a profession. **Profession** has been defined as an occupation that requires extensive

---

BOX 1–2   Selected Expanded Career Roles for Nurses

Nurse Practitioner

A nurse who has an advanced education and is a graduate of a nurse practitioner program. These nurses are certified by the American Nurses Credentialing Center in areas such as adult nurse practitioner, family nurse practitioner, school nurse practitioner, pediatric nurse practitioner, or gerontology nurse practitioner. They are employed in health care agencies or community-based settings. They usually deal with nonemergency acute or chronic illness and provide primary ambulatory care.

Clinical Nurse Specialist

A nurse who has an advanced degree or expertise and is considered to be an expert in a specialized area of practice (e.g., gerontology, oncology). The nurse provides direct client care, educates others, consults, conducts research, and manages care. The American Nurses Credentialing Center provides national certification of clinical specialists.

Nurse Anesthetist

A nurse who has completed advanced education in an accredited program in anesthesiology. The nurse anesthetist carries out preoperative visits and assessments, and administers general anesthetics for surgery under the supervision of a physician prepared in anesthesiology. The nurse anesthetist also assesses the postoperative status of clients.

Nurse Midwife

An RN who has completed a program in midwifery and is certified by the American College of Nurse Midwives. The nurse gives prenatal and postnatal care and manages deliveries in normal pregnancies. The midwife practices in association with a health care agency and can obtain medical services if complications occur. The nurse midwife may also conduct routine Papanicolaou smears, family planning, and routine breast examinations.

Nurse Researcher

Nurse researchers investigate nursing problems to improve nursing care and to refine and expand nursing knowledge. They are employed in academic institutions, teaching hospitals, and research centers such as the National Institute for Nursing Research in Bethesda, Maryland. Nurse researchers usually have advanced education at the doctoral level.

Nurse Administrator

The nurse administrator manages client care, including the delivery of nursing services. The administrator may have a middle management position, such as head nurse or supervisor, or a more senior management position, such as director of nursing services. The functions of nurse administrators include budgeting, staffing, and planning programs. The educational preparation for nurse administrator positions is at least a baccalaureate degree in nursing and frequently a master's or doctoral degree.

Nurse Educator

Nurse educators are employed in nursing programs, at educational institutions, and in hospital staff education. The nurse educator usually has a baccalaureate degree or more advanced preparation and frequently has expertise in a particular area of practice. The nurse educator is responsible for classroom and often clinical teaching.

Nurse Entrepreneur

A nurse who usually has an advanced degree and manages a health-related business. The nurse may be involved in education, consultation, or research, for example.

Doctor of Nursing Practice

A doctorate in nursing provides the nurse with a clinical practice focus more than the more traditional research focus found in other doctorate programs. The nurse who holds a doctorate in nursing practice functions as a clinical nurse specialist in the area of expertise and helps to improve the quality of care provided to clients through direct client care, improvement of policies and procedures, development of programs aimed at prevention and minimizing complications, and teaching others providing care for clients at the bedside. Areas of specialization include pediatrics, obstetrics, diabetes mellitus, ostomy, heart disease, and cancer, to name only a few.

education or a calling requiring special knowledge, skills, and preparation. A profession is generally distinguished from other kinds of occupations by (a) its requirement of prolonged, specialized training to acquire a body of knowledge pertinent to the role to be performed; (b) an orientation of the individual toward service, either to a community or to an organization; (c) ongoing research; (d) a code of ethics; (e) autonomy; and (f) a professional organization. Specialized education is an important aspect of professional status. In modern times, the trend in education for the professions has shifted toward programs in colleges and universities. In the United States today, there are five means of entry into registered nursing: hospital diploma, associate degree, baccalaureate degree, master's degree, and doctoral degree. The ANA recommends the baccalaureate degree as the entry level for professional practice. Conversely, the National Organization for Associate Degree Nursing (N-OADN) supports ADN preparation as the entry level into registered nursing (N-OADN, 2009). As a profession, nursing is establishing a well-defined body of knowledge and expertise.

A service orientation differentiates nursing from an occupation pursued primarily for profit. Many consider altruism (selfless concern for others) the hallmark of a profession. Nursing has a tradition of service to others. This service, however, must be guided by certain rules, policies, or codes of ethics. Today, nursing is an important component of the health care delivery system.

Increasing research in nursing is contributing to nursing practice. In the 1940s, nursing research was at a very early stage of development. In the 1950s, increased federal funding and professional support helped establish centers for nursing research. Most early research was directed to the study of nursing education. In the 1960s, studies were often related to the nature of the knowledge base underlying nursing practice. Since the 1970s, nursing research has focused on practice-related issues.

Nurses have traditionally placed a high value on the worth and dignity of others. The nursing profession requires integrity of its members; that is, a member is expected to do what is considered right regardless of the personal cost. Ethical codes change as the needs and values of society change. Nursing has developed its own codes of ethics and in most instances has set up means to monitor the professional behavior of its members. See Chapter 2 ∞ for additional information on nursing ethics.

A profession is autonomous if it regulates itself and sets standards for its members. Providing autonomy is one of the purposes of a professional association. If nursing is to have professional status, it must function autonomously in the formation of policy and in the control of its activity. To be autonomous, a professional group must be granted legal authority to define the scope of its practice, describe its particular functions and roles, and determine its goals and responsibilities in delivery of its services. To practitioners of nursing, autonomy means independence at work, responsibility, and accountability for one's actions.

Operation under the umbrella of a professional organization differentiates a profession from an occupation. **Governance** is the establishment and maintenance of social, political, and economic arrangements by which practitioners control their practice, their self-discipline, their working conditions, and their professional affairs. Nurses, therefore, need to work within their professional organizations. The American Nurses Association is a professional organization that "advances the nursing profession by fostering high standards of nursing practice, promoting the economic and general welfare of nurses in the workplace, projecting a positive and realistic view of nursing, and by lobbying the Congress and regulatory agencies on health care issues affecting nurses and the public" (ANA, 2009). There are a large number of nursing organizations, some devoted to nursing specialties such as obstetrics, pediatrics, or operating room nursing, while others represent specific roles of nursing such as leadership, research, and clinical practice.

SOCIALIZATION TO NURSING

The standards of education and practice for the profession are determined by the members of the profession. The education of the professional involves a complete socialization process, more far reaching in its social and attitudinal aspects and its technical features than is usually required in other kinds of occupations. **Socialization** can be defined simply as the process by which people (a) learn to become members of groups and society and (b) learn the social rules defining relationships into which they will enter. Socialization involves learning to behave, feel, and see the world in a manner similar to other persons occupying the same role as oneself (Hardy & Conway, 1988, p. 261). The goal of professional socialization is to instill in individuals the norms, values, attitudes, and behaviors deemed essential for survival of the profession.

Benner's model (2001) describes five levels of proficiency in nursing based on the Dreyfus general model of skill acquisition. The five stages, which have implications for teaching and learning, are novice, advanced beginner, competent, proficient, and expert. Benner writes that experience is essential for the development of professional expertise (Box 1–3).

One of the most powerful mechanisms of professional socialization is interaction with fellow students. Within this student culture, students collectively set the level and direction of their scholastic efforts. They develop perspectives about the situation in which they are involved, the goals they are trying to achieve, and the kinds of activities that are expedient and proper, and they establish a set of practices congruent with all of these. Students become bound together by feelings of mutual cooperation, support, and solidarity. Box 1–4 includes the National Student Nurses' Association, Inc. Code of Academic and Clinical Conduct.

BOX 1–3   Benner's Stages of Nursing Expertise

Stage I, Novice

- No experience (e.g., nursing student).
- Performance is limited, inflexible, and governed by context-free rules and regulations rather than experience.

Stage II, Advanced Beginner

- Demonstrates marginally acceptable performance.
- Recognizes the meaningful "aspects" of a real situation.
- Has experienced enough real situations to make judgments about them.

Stage III, Competent

- Has 2 or 3 years of experience.
- Demonstrates organizational and planning abilities.
- Differentiates important factors from less important aspects of care.
- Coordinates multiple complex care demands.

Stage IV, Proficient

- Has 3 to 5 years of experience.
- Perceives situations as wholes rather than in terms of parts, as in Stage II.
- Uses maxims as guides for what to consider in a situation.
- Has holistic understanding of the client, which improves decision making.
- Focuses on long-term goals.

Stage V, Expert

- Performance is fluid, flexible, and highly proficient.
- No longer requires rules, guidelines, or maxims to connect an understanding of the situation to appropriate action.
- Demonstrates highly skilled intuitive and analytic ability in new situations.
- Is inclined to take a certain action because "it felt right."

Note: Benner, Patricia, from *Novice to Expert: Excellence and Power in Clinical Nursing Practice, Commemorative Edition*, 1st ed. © 2001. Electronically reproduced by permission of Pearson Education, Inc., Upper Saddle River, New Jersey.

BOX 1–4   National Student Nurses' Association, Inc. Code of Academic and Clinical Conduct

Preamble

Students of nursing have a responsibility to society in learning the academic theory and clinical skills needed to provide nursing care. The clinical setting presents unique challenges and responsibilities while caring for human beings in a variety of health care environments.

The Code of Academic and Clinical Conduct is based on an understanding that to practice nursing as a student is an agreement to uphold the trust with which society has placed in us. The statements of the Code provide guidance for the nursing student in the personal development of an ethical foundation and need not be limited strictly to the academic or clinical environment but can assist in the holistic development of the person.

A Code for Nursing Students

As students are involved in the clinical and academic environments we believe that ethical principles are a necessary guide to professional development. Therefore within these environments we:

1. Advocate for the rights of all clients.
2. Maintain client confidentiality.
3. Take appropriate action to ensure the safety of clients, self, and others.
4. Provide care for the client in a timely, compassionate and professional manner.
5. Communicate client care in a truthful, timely and accurate manner.
6. Actively promote the highest level of moral and ethical principles and accept responsibility for our actions.
7. Promote excellence in nursing by encouraging lifelong learning and professional development.
8. Treat others with respect and promote an environment that respects human rights, values and choice of cultural and spiritual beliefs.
9. Collaborate in every reasonable manner with the academic faculty and clinical staff to ensure the highest quality of client care.
10. Use every opportunity to improve faculty and clinical staff understanding of the learning needs of nursing students.
11. Encourage faculty, clinical staff, and peers to mentor nursing students.
12. Refrain from performing any technique or procedure for which the student has not been adequately trained.
13. Refrain from any deliberate action or omission of care in the academic or clinical setting that creates unnecessary risk of injury to the client, self, or others.
14. Assist the staff nurse or preceptor in ensuring that there is full disclosure and that proper authorizations are obtained from clients regarding any form of treatment or research.
15. Abstain from the use of alcoholic beverages or any substances in the academic and clinical setting that impair judgment.
16. Strive to achieve and maintain an optimal level of personal health.
17. Support access to treatment and rehabilitation for students who are experiencing impairments related to substance abuse and mental or physical health issues.
18. Uphold school policies and regulations related to academic and clinical performance, reserving the right to challenge and critique rules and regulations as per school grievance policy.

Note: Adopted by the NSNA House of Delegates, Nashville, TN, on April 6, 2001. Reprinted with permission.

FACTORS INFLUENCING CONTEMPORARY NURSING PRACTICE

To understand nursing as it is practiced today, and as it will be practiced tomorrow, requires an understanding of some of the social forces currently influencing the profession. These forces include economic, consumer demands, family structure, science and technology, information and communications, legislations, demography, the current nursing shortage, collective bargaining, and nursing associations. Each of these forces usually affect the entire health care system, and nursing, as a major component of that system, cannot avoid the effects. Greater financial support provided through public and private health insurance programs has increased the demand for nursing care as people who could not afford health care in the past are increasingly using such health services as emergency department care, mental health counseling, and preventive physical examinations. An increasing number of clients rely on government support such as **Medicare** (health insurance for those over 65 or disabled individuals) and **Medicaid** (health insurance for those not covered by Medicare who are medically indigent) to cover the cost of health care. In 1982, the Medicare payment system to hospitals and physicians was revised to establish reimbursement fees according to the client's medical diagnosis. This classification system is known as diagnostic-related groups (DRGs). The system has categories that establish pretreatment diagnosis billing categories. With the implementation of this legislation, clients in hospitals are more acutely ill than before and clients once considered sufficiently ill to be hospitalized are now treated at home. Reimbursement for services no longer covers 100% of the cost, resulting in higher costs for medical care. These changes present challenges to nurses. Currently, the health care industry is shifting its emphasis from inpatient to outpatient care with preadmission testing, increased outpatient same-day surgery, post-hospitalization rehabilitation, home health care, health maintenance, physical fitness programs, and community health education programs. As a result, more nurses are being employed in community-based health settings, such as home health agencies, hospices, and community clinics.

Consumers of nursing services have become an increasingly effective force in changing nursing practice. On the whole, people are better educated and have more knowledge about health and illness than in the past. Consumers are more aware of the ethical and moral issues raised by poverty and neglect, making them more vocal about the needs of minority groups and the poor. The public's concepts of health and nursing have also changed. Most now believe that health is a right of all people, not just a privilege of the rich. Increasingly, the consumer is an active participant in making decisions about health and nursing care.

New family structures are influencing the need for, and provision of, nursing services. More people are living away from the extended family and the nuclear family, and the family breadwinner is no longer necessarily the husband.

Today, many single men and women rear children, and in many two-parent families both parents work. It is also common for young parents to live at great distances from their own parents. These young families need support services, such as day-care centers.

Advances in science and technology affect nursing practice. Nurses must be knowledgeable about new medications and treatments, biotechnology, and other new technologies as well as the needs of clients receiving them. Nurses will need to expand their knowledge base and technical skills as they adapt to meet the new needs of clients. As technologies change, nursing education changes, and nurses require increasing education to provide effective, safe nursing practice.

The information superhighway, or Internet, has already affected health care, with more and more clients becoming well informed about their health concerns. People with chronic health conditions or battling life-threatening disease are the hungriest information seekers (DeLenardo, 2004). As a result, nurses may need to interpret Internet sources of information for clients and their families. Because not all of the Internet-based information is accurate, nurses need to become information brokers so they can help people access high-quality, valid websites; interpret information; and help clients evaluate the information and determine if it is useful to them.

Telecommunications is the transmission of information from one site to another, using equipment to transmit information in the form of signs, signals, words, or pictures by cable, radio, or other systems (Chaffee, 1999, p. 27). Greenberg (2000) explains that terms with the prefix *tele*, meaning distance, are used to describe the many health care services provided via telecommunications. The common denominators of teleservices are distance and technology. Telehealth uses telecommunication technology to provide long-distance health care. It can include using videoconferencing, computers, or telephones. Telenursing occurs when the nurse delivers care through a telecommunication system. Examples of telenursing include the nurse who telephones clients at home to assess their progress or to answer questions, the nurse who participates in a video teleconference where consultants or experts at various sites discuss a client's health care plan, and the nurse who uses videophone technology to assess a client living in a rural area.

Legislation about nursing practice and health matters affects both the public and nursing. Changes in legislation relating to health also affect nursing. For example, the Patient Self-Determination Act (PSDA) requires that every competent adult be informed in writing on admission to a health care institution about his or her rights to accept or refuse medical care and to use advance directives.

Demography is the study of population, including statistics about distribution by age and place of residence, mortality (death), and morbidity (incidence of disease). From demographic data, the needs of the population for nursing services can be assessed. Demographics indicate an increased population in North America with a higher proportion of older adults. The population is shifting from rural to urban settings. Mortality and morbidity studies help to better identify risk factors. As demographic factors change, nursing must change to meet the shifting needs of consumers.

The multiple factors influencing the current nursing shortage (Box 1–5) are different from previous nursing shortages. Registered nurses make up the largest group of health care providers. Fewer nurses, however, are entering the workforce, and certain geographic areas are experiencing acute nursing shortages. The supply is inadequate to meet the demand, especially for specialized nurses (e.g., critical care), and it is anticipated to worsen during the next 20 years (National League for Nursing, 2007). Addressing the nursing shortage requires collaborative activities among health care systems, policy makers, nursing educators, and professional organizations. Recommendations include but are not limited to:

- Develop mechanisms for nursing students to progress into and through educational programs more efficiently and quickly.
- Recruit young people to nursing early (e.g., grade school).

BOX 1–5   **Factors Affecting the Nursing Shortage**

Aging Nurse Workforce

- Number of nurses under age 30 decreasing
- Number of nurses age 40–49 increasing with 40% older than 50 by 2010
- New graduates entering workforce at an older age and will have fewer years to work

Aging of Nursing Faculty

- As nursing faculty retire, nursing programs may have fewer faculty to educate future nurses

Reduced Entry of Younger People into Nursing

- Reduction in nursing program enrollments

Aging Population

- Individuals 65 and older to double between 2000 and 2030
- Increasing health care needs of aging population

Increased Demand for Nurses

- Increased acuity of hospital clients requiring skilled and specialized nurses
- Shorter hospital stays resulting in transfer of clients to long-term care and community settings, creating increased demand for nurses in the community

Workplace Issues

- Inadequate staffing
- Heavy workloads
- Increased use of overtime
- Lack of sufficient support staff
- Inadequate wages
- Difficulty recruiting and retaining nurses

- Improve the nurse's work environment: Provide greater flexibility in work hours, reward experienced nurses who serve as mentors, ensure adequate staffing, and increase salaries.
- Increase nursing education funding.

NURSING ORGANIZATIONS

Professional nursing organizations have provided leadership that affects many areas of nursing. As nursing has developed, an increasing number of nursing organizations have formed. These organizations are at the local, state, national, and international levels. The organizations that involve most nurses in the United States are the American Nurses Association, the National League for Nursing, the International Council of Nurses, and the National Student Nurses' Association. The American Nurses Association represents the interests of all nurses in the United States and is politically active in furthering the cause of nursing at the local, state, and federal level. The National League for Nursing is the voice for nursing education. The International Council of Nurses is a federation of more than 120 national nurses associations with a goal of advancing the socioeconomic status of nurses and providing a unified international voice for nursing. The number of nursing specialty organizations is also increasing, for example, the Academy of Medical Surgical Nursing, the American Association of Nurse Anesthetists, the National Black Nurses Association, and the National Association of Pediatric Nurse Practitioners. Participation in the activities of nursing associations enhances the growth of involved individuals and helps nurses collectively influence policies affecting nursing practice. It also helps members to meet **continuing education** requirements in order for nursing practice to remain current.

NURSING EDUCATION

Nursing education is controlled from within the profession through state boards of nursing and national accrediting bodies. The traditional focus of nursing education was to teach the knowledge and skills that would enable a nurse to practice in the hospital setting. However, as nursing responds to new scientific knowledge and technological, cultural, political, and socioeconomic changes in society, nursing education curricula are revised to meet the needs of nurses working in a changing environment. Programs of nursing study are increasingly based on a broad knowledge of biological, social, and physical sciences as well as the liberal arts and humanities. Nursing curricula now have a greater focus on critical thinking and the application of nursing and supporting knowledge to health promotion, health maintenance, and health restoration as provided in both community and hospital settings.

At the present time, there are two types of entry-level generalist nurses: the registered nurse (RN), and the licensed practical or vocational nurse (LPN, LVN). Responsibilities and licensure differ for these two levels. The majority of new RNs graduate from diploma, associate degree, or baccalaureate nursing programs. There are also generic master's and doctoral programs that lead to eligibility for RN licensure. LPN/LVNs generally graduate from diploma programs.

Although these programs vary considerably, all RNs in the United States take the same licensing examination. The National Council Licensure Examination (NCLEX®-RN and NCLEX®-PN) is administered in each state. The successful candidate becomes licensed in that particular state even though the examinations are of national origin. Multistate licensure is now available through the Nurse Licensure Compact (NLC) for those states participating in the compact. Nurses from other countries may be granted registration by endorsement after successfully completing the NCLEX®. Both licensure and registration must be renewed regularly to remain valid. The legal right to practice nursing requires not only passing the licensing examination but also verifying that the graduate has completed a prescribed course of study in nursing. Individual states may have additional requirements. All U.S. nursing programs require approval by their state board of nursing.

Types of Nursing Educational Programs

There are many different educational programs available for nurses. Some of the educational offerings include practical or vocational nursing programs, registered nursing programs, advanced degree programs such as graduate nursing programs, and those programs aimed at continuing education for practicing nurses.

Practical or vocational nursing programs are provided by community colleges, vocational schools, hospitals, or other independent health agencies. These programs usually last 9 to 12 months and provide both classroom and clinical experiences. At the end of the program, the graduate takes the NCLEX®-PN to obtain a license as a practical or vocational nurse. Licensed practical/vocational nurses practice under the supervision of a registered nurse in a hospital, nursing home, rehabilitation center, or home health agency. LPNs (LVNs) usually provide basic direct technical care to clients. There is no difference between an LPN and an LVN. Most of the country uses the term LPN, while some areas use the term LVN.

Registered nurse programs include three routes that lead to RN licensure: diploma, associate degree, and baccalaureate programs. Each has both positive and negative features associated with them.

The three-year diploma programs were the dominant nursing programs from the late 1800s until the mid-1960s. In the United States, diploma programs are hospital-based educational programs that provide a rich clinical experience for nursing students and are often associated with colleges or universities.

Community college/associate degree nursing programs, which arose in the early 1950s, were the first educational programs for nursing that were systematically developed from planned research and controlled experi-

mentation. The low tuition and open-door policy of these colleges made higher education more accessible to all by offering the first two years of a four-year college program. Associate degree programs are offered in the United States primarily in community colleges although some 4-year colleges also have ADN programs. The graduating student receives an ADN or an associate of arts (AA), associate of science (AS), or associate in applied science (AAS) degree with a major in nursing.

Baccalaureate nursing programs are located in senior colleges and universities and are generally four years in length. The curricula offer courses in the liberal arts, sciences, humanities, and nursing. Graduates must fulfill both the degree requirements of the college or university and the nursing program before being awarded a baccalaureate degree. The usual degree awarded is a bachelor of science in nursing (BSN). Partially in response to the significant shortage of RNs, U.S. schools have also established accelerated BSN programs. The programs may include summer semesters in order to shorten the length of time required to complete the curriculum or may be a modified curriculum especially designed for students who already have a baccalaureate degree in another field. These "second-degree" or "fast-track" BSN programs can be completed in 12 to 18 months of continuous study.

Many baccalaureate programs also admit registered nurses who have diplomas or associate degrees. Online programs for the RN pursing advanced education are becoming increasingly popular. Many accept transfer credits from other accredited colleges and universities and offer students the opportunity to take challenge examinations when the students believe they have the knowledge or skills taught in a course. These programs are referred to as BSN completion, BSN transition, 2 + 2, or RN-BSN programs.

The growth of university nursing programs encouraged the development of graduate study in nursing. In 1953, the newly established National League for Nursing encouraged educators to develop programs for master's degrees in nursing. The major emphasis of the programs was research and specialization for teaching and administration. The first "clinical" master's degree (in psychiatric nursing) was offered at Rutgers University in New Jersey in 1954. Today, master's programs generally take from 1.5 to 2 years to complete. Degrees granted are the master of arts (MA), master in nursing (MN), master of science in nursing (MSN), and master of science (MS).

Doctoral programs in nursing, which award the degrees of doctor of philosophy (PhD), doctor of nursing science (DNS or DNSc), or nursing doctorate (ND), began in the 1960s in the United States. These programs further prepare the nurse for advanced clinical practice, administration, education, and research. Content and approach vary among doctoral programs. Some focus on the usual clinical areas, such as medical–surgical nursing, and others emphasize such nontraditional areas as transcultural nursing. Some programs emphasize theory development, and all emphasize research.

BOX 1–6	Twenty-One Competencies for the 21st Century

- Embrace a personal ethic of social responsibility and service.
- Exhibit ethical behavior in all professional activities.
- Provide evidence-based, clinically competent care.
- Incorporate the multiple determinants of health in clinical care.
- Apply knowledge of the new sciences.
- Demonstrate critical thinking, reflection, and problem-solving skills.
- Understand the role of primary care.
- Rigorously practice preventive health care.
- Integrate population-based care and services into practice.
- Improve access to health care for those with unmet health needs.
- Practice relationship-centered care with individuals and families.
- Provide culturally sensitive care to a diverse society.
- Partner with communities in health care decisions.
- Use communication and information technology effectively and appropriately.

- Work in interdisciplinary teams.
- Ensure care that balances individual, professional, system, and societal needs.
- Practice leadership.
- Take responsibility for quality of care and health outcomes at all levels.
- Contribute to continuous improvement of the health care system.
- Advocate for public policy that promotes and protects the health of the public.
- Continue to learn and help others learn.

Note: From *Recreating Health Professional Practice for a New Century*, by E. H. O'Neil and the Pew Health Professions Commission, 1998, San Francisco: Pew Health Professionals. Reprinted with permission.

Entry to Practice

In 1965, the ANA endorsed the BSN as the entry level for professional practice. According to the ANA's proposal, only the baccalaureate graduate would be licensed under the legal title registered nurse. The graduate with an associate degree in nursing would be considered a technical nurse and be licensed under the legal title associate nurse (AN). The ANA proposal sparked sharp debates among graduates, students, and educators, some of whom perceive that it undervalues associate degree (AD) graduates. As a result, the National League for Nursing (NLN) has suggested that the title of associate nurse be replaced by registered associate nurse. However, this suggestion has not eliminated the controversy; many argue that AD graduates have held the title registered nurse since the inception of these ADN programs and should retain that title.

Perspectives about entry into practice are changing. For example, the American Association of College of Nursing (AACN) (2006) provides a fact sheet that informs of AACN's support for articulation. The organization supports articulation from associate degree programs to baccalaureate and higher degree programs and desires to strengthen collaboration between ADN and BSN programs.

Continuing Education

The term "continuing education" (CE) refers to formalized experiences designed to enlarge the knowledge or skills of practitioners. Compared with advanced education programs, which result in an academic degree, CE courses tend to be more specific and shorter. Participants may receive certificates of completion or specialization.

Continuing education is the responsibility of each practicing nurse. Constant updating and growth are essential to keep abreast of scientific and technological change and changes within the nursing profession. Some state laws require nurses to obtain a certain number of CE credits to renew their licenses, but even nurses practicing in states that do not require CEs

have an ethical responsibility to maintain their competence through continuing education (Box 1–6). Continuing education can be obtained by attending a seminar, reading a nursing magazine article, or attending a webinar (a seminar held online).

In-Service Education

An in-service education program is administered by an employer and is designed to upgrade the knowledge or skills of employees. For example, an employer might offer an in-service program to inform nurses about a new piece of equipment, specific isolation practices, or methods of implementing a nurse theorist's conceptual framework for nursing. Some in-service programs are mandatory, such as cardiopulmonary resuscitation and fire safety programs.

NURSING RESEARCH AND EVIDENCE-BASED PRACTICE

Today, nurses are actively generating, publishing, and applying research in practice to improve client care and enhance nursing's scientific knowledge base. Recently, there has been increased emphasis on the importance of **evidence-based practice (EBP)**, that is, the use of some form of substantiation for making clinical decisions. This substantiation, or evidence, can arise from tradition, authority, experience, trial and error, logic or reason, or research. In evidence-based practice (EBP), the nurse integrates research findings with clinical experience, the client's preferences, and available resources in planning and implementing care. Such practice can help control cost by focusing on substantiated yet individualized approaches to care.

Although the focus for all nurses is use of research findings in practice, the degree of participation in research depends on the nurse's educational level, position, experience, and practical environment. In 1985, the U.S. Congress passed

BOX 1–7	**Quantitative Research Process**

- *State a Research Question or Problem.* The researcher narrows a broad area of interest to a circumscribed problem that specifies exactly the intent of the study.
- *Define the Study's Purpose or Rationale.* This is what the researcher intends to do with the research problem identified. The study purpose includes what the researcher will do, who the participants will be, and where the data will be collected.
- *Review the Related Literature.* The investigator determines what is known and what is not known about the problem by conducting a thorough review of the literature.
- *Formulate Hypotheses and Define Variables.* A hypothesis is a prediction of the relationship among two or more variables. Hypothesis formulation requires not only sufficient knowledge about a topic to predict the outcome of the study but also operational definitions, definitions that specify the instruments or procedures by which concepts will be measured.
- *Select a Research Design to Test the Hypothesis.* A research design is the overall plan for conducting the study to answer the research questions or test the research hypotheses.
- *Select the Population, Sample, and Setting.* The researcher chooses the study population, selects a sample, and decides on the setting where the sample can be found.

- *Conduct a Pilot Study.* A trial run of the research procedure is conducted on a few participants to assess the adequacy and feasibility of the data collection plan. By identifying any problems or flaws during the pilot study, the investigators can refine the proposed plan and strengthen the research methodology.
- *Collect the Data.* The research process relies on empirical data, or information collected from the observable world.
- *Analyze the Data.* In this step, the collected data are organized, coded, and analyzed for the purpose of answering the research question or testing the hypotheses.
- *Communicate Conclusions and Implications.* Implicit in conducting research is the requirement to share the knowledge generated with others, either through publication in professional journals or by reporting the results at professional conferences. Interpreting the results, communicating the findings, and suggesting directions for further study conclude the research process. The summary reports of research also include a discussion of any limitations in applying the particular findings to the broader population.

a bill creating a National Center for Nursing Research in the National Institutes of Health (NIH) to house the research activities conducted by the Division of Nursing at the Department of Health and Human Services (DHHS). In 1993, the Center for Nursing Research was promoted to the National Institute for Nursing Research (NINR), gaining equal status with other institutes within the NIH.

Quantitative Research

Quantitative research progresses through systematic, logical steps according to a specific plan to collect information, often under conditions of considerable control, that is analyzed using statistical procedures. Quantitative research is often viewed as "hard" science and uses deductive reasoning and the measurable attributes of human experience. The steps involved in conducting a quantitative research study are outlined in Box 1–7.

The Qualitative Approach

The qualitative approach is often associated with naturalistic inquiry, which explores the subjective and complex experiences of human beings. "Naturalistic investigation emphasizes understanding the human experience as it is lived, usually through careful collection and analysis of qualitative materials that are narrative and subjective" (Polit & Beck, 2005, p. 16). Data collection and its analysis occur concurrently (Box 1–8). Using the inductive method, data are analyzed by identifying themes and patterns to develop a theory or framework that helps explain the processes under observation.

BOX 1–8	**The Qualitative Research Process**

- The intent of qualitative research is to thoroughly describe and explain a phenomenon.
- The researchers collect narrative data through interviews or observation.
- These data are transcribed and often result in hundreds of pages that need to be organized and interpreted.
- These narrative data may be organized around some type of categorization scheme such as concepts, actions, or themes.
- Finally, the themes of the data are integrated to present a description or theory.

Protecting the Rights of Human Subjects

Because nursing research usually focuses on humans, a major nursing responsibility is to be aware of, and to advocate on behalf of, clients' rights in all types of research studies, whether qualitative or quantitative. All clients must be informed and understand the consequences of consenting to serve as research participants. The client needs to be able to assess whether an appropriate balance exists between the risks of participating in a study and the potential benefits, either to the client or to the development of knowledge. All nurses who practice in settings where research is being conducted with human subjects or who participate in such research play an important role in safeguarding the rights of human subjects (Box 1–9).

- Right not to be harmed
- Right to full disclosure
- Right of self-determination
- Right of privacy and **confidentiality**

Critiquing Research Reports

If nurses are to use research, they must conduct a critical appraisal of research reports published in the literature. A research critique enables the nurse, as a research consumer, to evaluate the scientific merit of the study and decide how the results may be useful in practice. A critique involves intensive scrutiny of a study, including its strengths and weaknesses, statistical and clinical significance, and the generalizability of the results.

Polit and Beck (2005) propose that the following elements be considered in a critique of quantitative research:

- *Substantive and theoretical dimensions.* The nurse evaluates the significance of the research problem, the appropriateness of the conceptualizations and the theoretical framework of the study, and the congruence between the research question and the methods used to address it.
- *Methodologic dimensions.* This pertains to the appropriateness of the research design, the size and representativeness of the study sample as well as the sampling design, **validity** and **reliability** of the instruments, adequacy of the research procedures, and the appropriateness of data analytic techniques used in the study.
- *Ethical dimensions.* The nurse must determine whether the rights of human subjects were protected during the course of the study and whether any ethical problems compromised the scientific merit of the study or the well-being of the subjects.
- *Interpretive dimensions.* For these dimensions, the nurse needs to ascertain the accuracy of the discussion, conclusions, and implications of the study results. The findings must be related back to the original hypotheses and the conceptual framework of the study. The implications and limitations of the study should be reviewed, together with the potential for replication or generalizability of the findings to similar populations.
- *Presentation and stylistic dimensions.* The manner in which the research plan and results are communicated refers to the presentation and stylistic dimensions. The research report must be detailed, logically organized, concise, and well written.

Reports of qualitative research are critiqued for their relevance to other persons or situations with the same characteristics as those studied and for usefulness in extending theory and nursing knowledge. A well-done qualitative study will have results that "ring true" to the reader.

NURSING THEORIES AND CONCEPTUAL FRAMEWORKS

As a profession, nursing is involved in identifying its own unique body of knowledge essential to nursing practice—nursing science. To identify this knowledge base, nurses must develop and recognize concepts and theories that are specific to nursing.

Introduction to Theories

Theory has been defined as a supposition or system of ideas that is proposed to explain a given phenomenon. Theories are also used to describe, predict, and control phenomena. Concepts are often called the building blocks of theories. A conceptual framework is a group of related ideas, statements, or concepts. The term *conceptual model* is often used interchangeably with "conceptual framework" and sometimes with "grand theories," those that articulate a broad range of the significant relationships among the concepts of a discipline (Fitzpatrick & Whall, 2005).

In the late 20th century, much of the theoretical work in nursing focused on articulating relationships among four major concepts: person, environment, health, and nursing. Because these four concepts can be superimposed on almost any work in nursing, they are sometimes collectively referred to as a *metaparadigm* for nursing. The term originates from two Greek words: *meta*, meaning "with," and *paradigm*, meaning "pattern." These four concepts include:

- **Client** – recipient of nursing care (individuals, families, groups, and communities).
- **Environment** – the internal and external surroundings that affect the client.
- **Health** – the degree of wellness or well-being that the client experiences.
- **Nursing** – the attributes, characteristics, and actions of the nurse providing care on behalf of, or in conjunction with, the client.

The work of American nurse theorists reflects a wide range of ideas about people, health, values, and the world. Each nurse theorist's definitions of these four major concepts vary in accordance with scientific and philosophical orientation, experience in nursing, and the effects of that experience on the theorist's view of nursing.

Purposes of Nursing Theory

Direct links exist among theory, education, research, and clinical practice. In many cases, nursing theory guides knowledge development and directs education, research, and practice although each influences the others (Fitzpatrick & Whall, 2005). The interface between nursing experts in each area helps to ensure that work in the other areas remains relevant, current, useful, and ultimately influences health.

Because nursing theory was used primarily to establish the profession's place in the university, it is not surprising that nursing theory became more firmly established in academia than in clinical practice. In the 1970s and 1980s, many nursing programs identified the major concepts in one or two nursing models, organized these concepts into a conceptual framework, and built the entire curriculum around that framework. The unique language in these models was typically introduced into program objectives, course objectives, course descriptions, and clinical performance criteria. The purpose was to elucidate the central meanings of the profession and to improve the status of the profession. Although all nursing programs are organized around concepts, many nursing programs have abandoned theory-driven conceptual frameworks.

Nurse scholars have repeatedly insisted that nursing research identify the philosophical assumptions or conceptual frameworks from which it proceeds. New theoretical perspectives provide an essential service by identifying gaps in the way we approach specific fields of study such as symptom management or quality of life. Different conceptual perspectives can also help generate new ideas, research questions, and interpretations.

Where nursing theory has been employed in clinical settings, its primary contribution has been the facilitation of reflecting, questioning, and thinking about what nurses do. Because nurses and nursing practice are often subordinate to powerful institutional forces and traditions, the introduction of any framework that encourages nurses to reflect on, question, and think about what they do provides an invaluable service.

Overview of Selected Nursing Theories

The nursing theories discussed in this chapter vary considerably (a) in their level of abstraction; (b) in their conceptualization of the client, health/illness, environment, and nursing; and (c) in their ability to describe, explain, or predict phenomena. The theories were chosen to help demonstrate how nursing has advanced from Florence Nightingale's time to the current practice of nursing. Research into other nursing theories is strongly encouraged to increase one's understanding of the theoretical implications for nursing practice.

NIGHTINGALE'S ENVIRONMENTAL THEORY Florence Nightingale, often considered the first nurse theorist, defined nursing almost 150 years ago as "the act of utilizing the environment of the patient to assist him in his recovery" (Nightingale, 1860/1969). She linked health with five environmental factors: (1) pure or fresh air, (2) pure water, (3) efficient drainage, (4) cleanliness, and (5) light, especially direct sunlight. Deficiencies in these five factors produced lack of health or illness. Nightingale also stressed the importance of keeping the client warm, maintaining a noise-free environment, and attending to the client's diet in terms of assessing intake, timeliness of food, and its effect on the person.

PEPLAU'S INTERPERSONAL RELATIONS MODEL Hildegard Peplau, a psychiatric nurse, introduced her interpersonal concepts in 1952. Central to Peplau's theory is the use of a therapeutic relationship between the nurse and the client. The nurse–client relationship evolves in four phases. During the *orientation* phase the client seeks help and the nurse assists the client to understand the problem and extent of help needed. The client assumes a posture of dependence, interdependence, or independence in relation to the nurse during the *identification* phase while the nurse's focus is to assure the client that the nurse understands the interpersonal meaning of the client's situation. The *exploitation* phase is when the client derives full value from what the nurse offers, using available services based on self-interest and needs. Power shifts from the nurse to the client. Finally during the *resolution* phase, old needs and goals are put aside and new ones are adopted. To help clients fulfill their needs, nurses assume many roles: stranger, teacher, resource person, surrogate, leader, and counselor. Peplau's model continues to be used by clinicians when working with individuals who have psychologic problems.

OREM'S GENERAL THEORY OF NURSING Dorothea Orem's Self Care theory includes four related concepts: self-care, self-care agency, self-care requisites, and therapeutic self-care demand. Self-care refers to those activities an individual performs independently throughout life to promote and maintain personal well-being. Self-care agency is the individual's *ability* to perform self-care activities. It consists of two agents: a self-care agent (an individual who performs self-care independently) and a dependent care agent (a person other than the individual who provides the care). Most adults care for themselves, whereas infants and people weakened by illness or disability require assistance with self-care activities.

Self-care requisites, also called self-care needs, are measures or actions taken to provide self-care. There are three categories of self-care requisites:

- Universal requisites are common to all people. They include maintaining intake and elimination of air, water, and food; balancing rest, solitude, and social interaction; preventing hazards to life and well-being; and promoting normal human functioning.
- Developmental requisites result from maturation or are associated with conditions or events, such as adjusting to a change in body image or to the loss of a spouse.
- Health deviation requisites result from illness, injury, or disease or its treatment. They include actions such as seeking health care assistance, carrying out prescribed therapies, and learning to live with the effects of illness or treatment.

Therapeutic self-care demand refers to all self-care activities required to meet existing self-care requisites, or in other words, actions to maintain health and well-being (Figure 1–3).

Self-care deficit results when self-care agency is not adequate to meet the known self-care demand. Orem's self-care deficit theory explains not only when nursing is needed

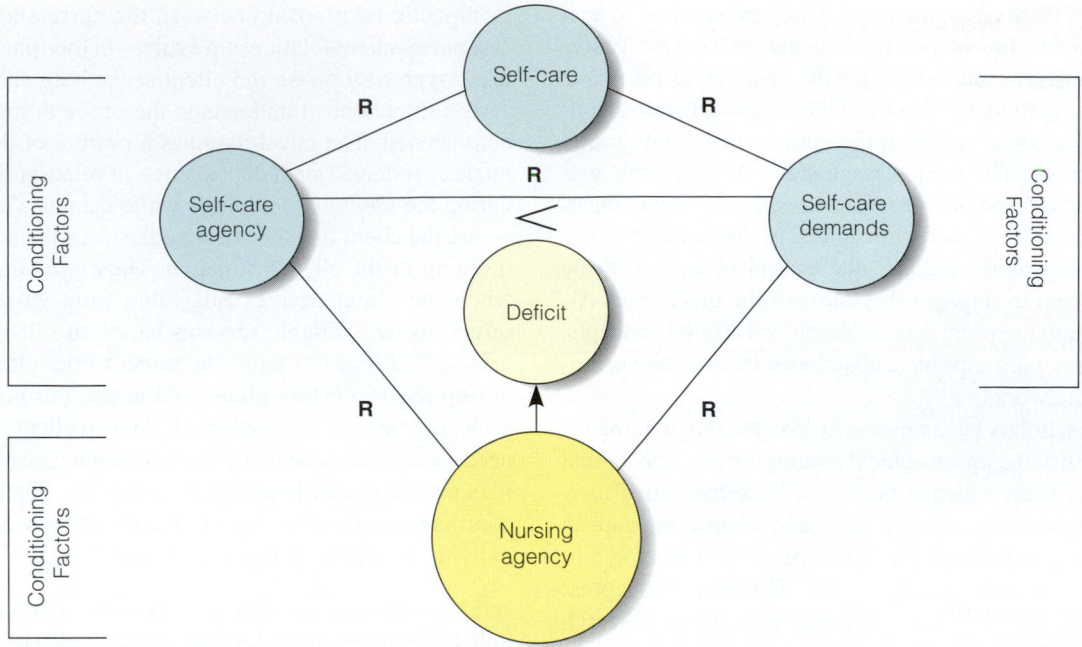

Figure 1–3 ● The major components of Orem's self-care deficit theory. R indicates a relationship between components; < indicates a current or potential deficit where nursing would be required.

but also how people can be assisted through five methods of helping: acting or doing for, guiding, teaching, supporting, and providing an environment that promotes the individual's abilities to meet current and future demands. The five methods of helping discussed for self-care deficit can be used in each nursing system.

Orem identifies three types of nursing systems:

- **Wholly compensatory** systems are required for individuals who are unable to control and monitor their environment and process information.
- **Partly compensatory** systems are designed for individuals who are unable to perform some, but not all, self-care activities.
- **Supportive-educative** (developmental) systems are designed for persons who need to learn to perform self-care measures and need assistance to do so.

NEUMAN'S SYSTEMS MODEL   Betty Neuman (Neuman & Fawcett, 2002), a community health nurse and clinical psychologist, developed a model based on the individual's relationship to stress, the reaction to it, and reconstitution factors that are dynamic in nature. Reconstitution is the state of adaptation to stressors. Neuman views the client as an open system consisting of a basic structure or central core of energy resources (physiologic, psychologic, sociocultural, developmental, and spiritual) surrounded by two concentric boundaries or rings that help the client defend against a stressor. There are two lines of defense; the normal line of defense, which represents the person's state of equilibrium or the state of adaptation developed and maintained over time and considered normal for that person, and the flexible line

of defense, which is dynamic and can be rapidly altered over a short period of time. Neuman categorizes stressors as intrapersonal stressors, those that occur within the individual (e.g., an infection); interpersonal stressors, those that occur between individuals (e.g., unrealistic role expectations); and extrapersonal stressors, those that occur outside the person (e.g., financial concerns). The individual's reaction to stressors depends on the strength of the lines of defense. Betty Neuman's model of nursing is applicable to a variety of nursing practice settings involving individuals, families, groups, and communities. The model is used in many countries and to direct nursing administration and research programs.

LEININGER'S CULTURAL CARE DIVERSITY AND UNIVERSALITY THEORY   Madeleine Leininger, a nurse anthropologist, put her views on transcultural nursing in print in the 1970s and then in 1991 published her book *Culture Care Diversity and Universality: A Theory of Nursing*. Leininger states that care is the essence of nursing and the dominant, distinctive, and unifying feature of nursing. She emphasizes that human caring, although a universal phenomenon, varies among cultures in its expressions, processes, and patterns; it is largely culturally derived.

WATSON'S HUMAN CARING THEORY   Jean Watson (2005) believes the practice of caring is central to nursing; it is the unifying focus for practice. Her major assumptions about caring are shown in Box 1–10. Watson's theory of human caring has received worldwide recognition and is a major force in redefining nursing as a caring-healing health model.

BOX 1–10	Watson's Assumptions of Caring

- Human caring in nursing is not just an emotion, concern, attitude, or benevolent desire. Caring connotes a personal response.
- Caring is an intersubjective human process and is the moral ideal of nursing.
- Caring can be effectively demonstrated only interpersonally.
- Effective caring promotes health and individual or family growth.
- Caring promotes health more than does curing.
- Caring responses accept a person not only as they are now, but also for what the person may become.
- A caring environment offers the development of potential while allowing the person to choose the best action for the self at a given point in time.

- Caring occasions involve action and choice by nurse and client. If the caring occasion is transpersonal, the limits of openness expand, as do human capacities.
- The most abstract characteristic of a caring person is that the person is somehow responsive to another person as a unique individual, perceives the other's feelings, and sets one person apart from another.
- Human caring involves values, a will and a commitment to care, knowledge, caring actions, and consequences.
- The ideal and value of caring is a starting point, a stance, and an attitude that has to become a will, an intention, a commitment, and a conscious judgment that manifests itself in concrete acts.

Note: From J. Watson, personal communication, September 22, 2002. Also see the website: http://currentnursing.com/nursing_theory/Watson.htm

Critique of Nursing Theory

Nursing scholars continue to debate whether grounding our research in the best theories from other disciplines is good or bad. Some think this detracts from the development of nursing as a separate discipline; others argue that nursing research becomes more relevant when informed by scholarship that addresses larger social concerns.

Most things in the world have both positive and negative implications. Technology can be used for good or for evil. Theory can be used to broaden our perspectives in nursing and facilitate the altruistic and humanistic values of the profession. At the same time, rational and predictive theory can produce language and social practices that are superimposed onto the lives of vulnerable patients and do violence to the fragility of human dignity. As a lens, theory can either illuminate or obscure. As a tool, theory can either liberate or enslave.

CHAPTER HIGHLIGHTS

- Historical perspectives of nursing practice reveal recurring themes or influencing factors. For example, women have traditionally cared for others, but often in subservient roles. Religious orders left an imprint on nursing by instilling such values as compassion, devotion to duty, and hard work. Wars created an increased need for nurses and medical specialties. Societal attitudes have influenced nursing's image. Visionary leaders have made notable contributions to improve the status of nursing.
- The scope of nursing practice includes promoting wellness, preventing illness, restoring health, and caring for the dying.
- Although traditionally the majority of nurses were employed in hospital settings, today the numbers of nurses working in home health care, ambulatory care, and community health settings are increasing.
- Nurse practice acts vary among states, and nurses are responsible for knowing the act that governs their practice.
- Standards of nursing practice provide criteria against which the effectiveness of nursing care and professional performance behaviors can be evaluated.
- Every nurse may function in a variety of roles that are not exclusive of one another; in reality, they often occur together and serve to clarify the nurse's activities. These roles include caregiver, communicator, teacher, client advocate, counselor, change agent, leader, manager, case manager, and research consumer.

- With advanced education and experience, nurses can fulfill advanced practice roles such as clinical nurse specialist, nurse practitioner, nurse midwife, nurse anesthetist, educator, administrator, and researcher.
- A desired goal of nursing is professionalism, which necessitates specialized education; a unique body of knowledge, including specific skills and abilities; ongoing research; a code of ethics; autonomy; a service orientation; and a professional organization.
- Socialization is a lifelong process by which people become functioning participants of a society or a group. It is a reciprocal learning process that is brought about by interaction with other people and established boundaries of behavior. Socialization to professional nursing practice is the process whereby the values and norms of the nursing profession are internalized into the nurse's own behavior and self-concept. The nurse acquires the knowledge, skill, and attitudes characteristic of the profession.
- Although several models of the socialization process have been developed, Benner's five stages of novice, advanced beginner, competent, proficient, and expert may serve as guidelines to establish the phase and extent of an individual's socialization.
- Contemporary nursing practice is influenced by economics, changing demands for nurses, consumer demand, family structure, science and technology, information and telecommunications, legislation, demographic and social changes, the nursing shortage, collective bargaining, and the work of nursing associations.

- Participation in the activities of nursing associations enhances the growth of involved individuals and helps nurses collectively influence policies that affect nursing practice.
- Nursing education curricula are continually undergoing revisions in response to new scientific knowledge and technological, cultural, political, and socioeconomic changes in society.
- Nursing education has changed dramatically since the mid-1800s. Early apprenticeship programs established in the 1800s were designed to meet the service needs of the hospital, not the educational needs of the students. Today, nursing education is provided primarily in college and university settings independent of hospitals' needs—a concept proposed by Florence Nightingale.
- Growth of associate degree nursing (ADN) programs in community colleges began in the 1950s.
- Some professional organizations have recommended that minimum entry into practice be at the baccalaureate or master's degree level.
- Continuing education is the responsibility of each practicing nurse to keep abreast of scientific and technological change and changes within the nursing profession.
- Nursing research began in North America in the early 1900s. Since that time, the concept of research has been introduced into nursing education programs, research journals in nursing have been developed, and the National Institute for Nursing Research has been established.
- All nurses practicing in settings where research is conducted have a role in safeguarding their clients' rights.

- Both quantitative and qualitative research involves identifying a research problem/question, collecting data, and analyzing the data. Quantitative studies are reported using descriptive and analytic statistics, and qualitative studies are reported in narrative format.
- In the natural sciences, the main function of theory is to guide research. In the practice disciplines, the main function of theory (and research) is to provide new possibilities for understanding the discipline's focus (music, art, management, and nursing).
- To Nightingale, the knowledge required to provide good nursing was neither unique nor specialized. Rather, Nightingale viewed nursing as a central human activity grounded in observation, reason, and commonsense health practices.
- During the latter half of the 20th century, disciplines seeking to establish themselves in universities had to demonstrate something that Nightingale had not envisioned for nursing—a unique body of theoretical knowledge.
- Theories articulate significant relationships between concepts in order to point to something larger, such as gravity, the unconscious, or the experience of pain.
- In the late 20th century, much of the theoretical work in nursing focused on articulating relationships between four major concepts: person, environment, health, and nursing. Because these four concepts can be superimposed on almost any work in nursing, they are sometimes collectively referred to as a "metaparadigm" for nursing.
- Debates about the role of theory in nursing practice provide evidence that nursing is maturing as both an academic discipline and a clinical profession.

THINK ABOUT IT

Refer to the chapter-opening scenario and answer these questions.

1. Why is it important for nursing students to know about the history and current trends impacting nursing?

2. Why must nurses understand the theory and basis for nursing before beginning to learn the practice of nursing?

3. Why do nursing schools emphasize the importance of continuing education?

∞ *See suggested responses to Think About It on MyNursingKit.*

TEST YOUR KNOWLEDGE

1. Which of the following made significant contributions to the nursing care of soldiers during the Crimean War?
   1. Dorothea Orem
   2. Florence Nightingale
   3. Linda Richards
   4. Mary Mahoney

2. The nurse best performs health promotion by which of the following activities?
   1. Administering immunizations
   2. Giving a bath
   3. Preventing accidents in the home
   4. Performing diagnostic procedures

3. A nurse with 2 to 3 years of experience who has the ability to coordinate multiple complex nursing care demands is at which stage of Benner's stages of nursing expertise?
   1. Advanced beginner
   2. Competent

   3. Proficient
   4. Expert

4. Nurses anticipate which of the following social forces will be most likely to significantly impact the future supply and demand for nurses?
   1. Aging
   2. Economics
   3. Science and technology
   4. Telecommunications

5. The nurse is undergoing continuing education by doing which of the following?
   1. Attending the hospital's orientation program
   2. Talking with a company representative about a new piece of equipment
   3. Completing a workshop on ethical aspects of nursing
   4. Obtaining information about the facility's new computer charting system

6. The nurse, when critiquing a published nursing research article, is responsible for doing which of the following?
1. Assume that the research was properly conducted since it has been published
2. Evaluate whether the findings are applicable to the nurse's specific clients
3. Implement the research findings if at least two studies have shown the same results
4. Request the raw data from the researchers so that the nurse can analyze the statistics again

7. An 85-year-old client in a nursing home tells a nurse, "Because the doctor was so insistent, I signed the papers to be part of that research study. I was afraid he would not continue taking care of me if I didn't agree. He seemed so excited about this project." Which client right is being violated?
1. Right not to be harmed
2. Right to full disclosure
3. Right of privacy and confidentiality
4. Right of self-determination

8. Which of the following provides the best explanation for describing nursing as a practice discipline?
1. Nursing focuses on performing the professional role.
2. It takes time and experience to become a competent nurse.

3. Research and theory development is a central focus.
4. Nurses function as members of a team who form a practice group.

9. "A group of related ideas or statements" best defines which of the following?
1. A philosophy
2. A conceptual framework
3. A theory
4. A paradigm

10. Person, environment, health, and nursing constitute the metaparadigm for nursing because of which of the following?
1. They provide a framework for implementing the nursing process.
2. They can be utilized in any setting when caring for a client.
3. They can be utilized to determine applicability of a research study.
4. They focus on the needs of a group of clients.

∞ *See answers to Test Your Knowledge in Appendix A.*

EXPLORE 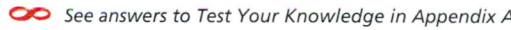 PEARSON mynursingkit™

MyNursingKit is your one stop for online chapter review materials and resources. Prepare for success with additional NCLEX®-style practice questions, interactive assignments and activities, web links, animations and videos, and more!

Register your access code from the front of your book at **www.mynursingkit.com.**

REFERENCES AND SELECTED BIBLIOGRAPHY

Aiken, L. H., Buchan, J., Sochalski, J., Nichols, B., & Powell, M. (2004). Trends in international nurse migration. *Health Affairs, 23*(3), 69–77.

Aiken, L. H., Clarke, S. P., Cheung, R. B., Sloane, D. M., & Silber, S. H. (2003). Educational levels of hospital nurses and surgical patient mortality. *Journal of the American Medical Association, 290,* 1617–1623.

American Association of Colleges of Nursing. (1998). *The essentials of baccalaureate education for professional nursing practice.* Washington, DC: Author.

American Association of Colleges of Nursing. (2004). *AACN position statement on the practice doctorate in nursing.* Retrieved March 13, 2006, from http://www.aacn.nche.edu/DNP/pdf/DNP.pdf

American Association of Colleges of Nursing. (2005). *Fact sheet: The Clinical Nurse Leader.* Retrieved March 13, 2006, from http://www.aacn.nche.edu/Media/FactSheets/CNLFactSheet.htm

American Association of Colleges of Nursing. (2006a). *Fact sheet: Articulation agreements among nursing education programs.* Retrieved October 23, 2009, from http://www.aacn.nche.edu/Media/FactSheets/AA.htm

American Association of Colleges of Nursing. (2006b). *AACN position statement on nursing research.* Retrieved March 13, 2006, from http://www.aacn.nche.edu/Publications/positions/rscposst.htm

American Association of Colleges of Nursing. (2009). *Nursing shortage fact sheet.* Retrieved October 23, 2009, from http://www.aacn.nche.edu/Media/FactSheets/NursingShortage.htm

American Nurses Association. (1965). ANA's first position on education for nursing. *American Journal of Nursing, 65*(12), 106–111.

American Nurses Association. (1973). *Standards of nursing practice.* Kansas City, MO: Author.

American Nurses Association. (1980). *Nursing: A social policy statement.* Kansas City, MO: Author.

American Nurses Association. (2003). *Nursing's social policy statement.* Washington, DC: American Nurses Publishing.

American Nurses Association. (2004). *Nursing: Scope and standards of practice.* Washington, DC: Author.

American Nurses Association. (2006a). *ANA hall of fame.* Retrieved April 23, 2006, from http://www.ana.org/hof/richla.htm

American Nurses Association. (2006b). *ANA hall of fame.* Retrieved April 23, 2006, from http://www.ana.org/hof/mahome.htm

American Nurses Association. (2009). About ANA. Retrieved October 23, 2009, from http://nursingworld.org/about/index.htm

ANA delegates vote to limit RN title to BSN grads: "Associate nurse" wins vote for technical level. (1985). *American Journal of Nursing, 85*(9), 1016, 1017, 1020, 1022, 1024, 1025.

Anonymous. (2003). Image change boosts US nurse recruitment. *Australian Nursing Journal, 11*(3), 16.

Anspaugh, D. J., Hamrick, M. H., & Rosata, F. D. (2006). *Wellness: Concepts and applications.* New York: McGraw-Hill.

Battey, L. (2004). The struggle for lives in Iraq. *RN, 67*(12), 32.

Baumann, S. L. (2004). Similarities and differences in experiences of hope. *Nursing Science Quarterly, 17*, 339–344.

Benner, P. (2001). *From novice to expert: Excellence and power in clinical nursing practice* (commemorative ed.). Upper Saddle River, NJ: Prentice Hall Health.

Brady, M., Leuner, J. D., Bellack, J. P., Loquist, R. S., Cipriano, P. F., & O'Neil, E. H. (2001). A proposed framework for differentiating the 21 Pew competencies by level of nursing education. *Nursing and Health Care Perspectives, 22*(1), 30–35.

Brown, E. L. (1948). *Nursing for the future: A report prepared for the National Nursing Council.* New York: Russell Sage Foundation.

Burge, P., Price, C., Cronin, S. N., Dolan, L., Kramer, J., & Ober, J. (2004). "Grow your own": A responsible approach to addressing the nursing shortage. *Nursing Economics, 22*(3), 155–156.

Campbell, E. T. (2005). Child abuse recognition, reporting and prevention: A culturally congruent approach. *Journal of Multicultural Nursing & Health, 11*(2), 35–40.

Cashion, A. K., Driscoll, C. J., & Sabek, O. (2004). Emerging genetic technologies in clinical and research settings. *Biological Research for Nursing, 5*(3), 159–167.

Chaffee, M. (1999). A telehealth odyssey. *American Journal of Nursing, 99*(7), 27–32.

Coffman, M. J. (2004). Cultural caring in nursing practice: A meta-synthesis of qualitative research. *Journal of Cultural Diversity, 11*(3), 100–109.

Committee on the Grading of Nursing Schools. (1934). *Nursing schools today and tomorrow.* New York: National League of Nursing Education.

DeLenardo, C. (2004). Web-based tools steer patient-focused care. *Nursing Management, 35*(12), 60–64.

Dobratz, M. C. (2004). Life-closing spirituality and the philosophic assumptions of the Roy adaptation model. *Nursing Science Quarterly, 17*, 335–338.

Donahue, M. P. (1996). *Nursing: The finest art. An illustrated history* (2nd ed.). St. Louis, MO: Mosby.

Donahue, M. P. (1996). *Nursing: The finest art.* St. Louis, MO: Mosby.

Dowling, M. (2004). Exploring the relationship between caring, love and intimacy in nursing. *British Journal of Nursing, 13*(21), 1289–1292.

Doyle, R. (2005). Nurses in short supply. *Scientific American, 292*(1), 32.

Erci, B., Sayan, A., Tortumluoglu, G., Kilic, D., Sahin, O., & Güngörmüs, Z. (2003). The effectiveness of Watson's caring model on the quality of life and blood pressure of patients with hypertension. *Journal of Advanced Nursing, 41*, 130–139.

Evans, G. D. (2003). Clara Barton: Teacher, nurse, Civil War heroine, founder of the American Red Cross. *International History of Nursing Journal, 7*, 75–82.

Fawcett, J. (2005). *Contemporary nursing knowledge: Analysis and evaluation of nursing models and theories* (2nd ed.). Philadelphia: F. A. Davis.

Fest, G. (2003a, October 13). Shining light. *Mountain West Nurse Week,* pp. 14–16.

Fest, G. (2003b, October 27). A beacon of change. *Mountain West Nurse Week,* pp. 10–13.

Fitzpatrick, J. J., & Whall, A. L. (2005). *Conceptual models of nursing: Analysis and application* (4th ed.). Upper Saddle River, NJ: Pearson Prentice Hall.

Fitzpatrick, M. A. (2002). "I" is for image. *Nursing Management, 33*(6), 6.

Fondiller, S. H. (2001). From the archives: Nursing's pioneers in the associate degree movement. *Nursing and Health Care Perspectives, 22*(4), 172–174.

Freud, S. (1949). *An outline of psycho-analysis* (J. Strachey, Trans.). New York: W. W. Norton. (Original work published 1940)

Girard, N. J. (2003). Men and nursing. *AORN Journal, 77*(4), 728–730.

Godkin, J., & Godkin, L. (2004). Caring behaviors among nurses: Fostering a conversation of gestures. *Health Care Management Review, 29*(3), 258–267.

Goldmark, J. (1923). *Nursing and nursing education in the United States.* New York: Macmillan.

Gordon, S., & Nelson, S. (2005). An end to angels. Moving away from the virtue script toward a knowledge-based identity for nurses. *American Journal of Nursing, 105*(5), 62–69.

Graber, D. R., & Mitcham, M. D. (2004). Compassionate clinicians: Take patient care beyond the ordinary. *Holistic Nursing Practice, 18*(2), 87–94.

Granger, B. B. (2003). How to make nursing research work for you. *Nursing, 33*(11), 47–49.

Greenberg, M. E. (2000). The domain of telenursing: Issues and prospects. *Nursing Economics, 18*(4), 220–223.

Hardy, M. E., & Conway, M. E. (1988). *Role theory: Perspectives for healthy professionals* (2nd ed.). Norwalk, CT: Appleton & Lange.

Henderson, V. (1966). *The nature of nursing: A definition and its implications for practice, research, and education.* New York: Macmillan.

Henderson, V. A. (1991). *The nature of nursing: Reflections after 25 years.* New York: National League for Nursing Press.

Hicks, L. L., Rantz, M. J., Petroski, G. F., & Mukamel, D. B. (2004). Nursing home costs and quality of care outcomes. *Nursing Economics, 22*, 178–192.

Holder, V. L. (2003). From hand maiden to right hand: The Civil War. *AORN Journal, 78*(3), 448–464.

Holder, V. L. (2004). From handmaiden to right hand—World War I and advancements in medicine. *AORN Journal, 80*(5), 911–923.

Honor Society of Nursing, Sigma Theta Tau International. (2001). *Nurses for a healthier tomorrow. Facts about the nursing shortage.* Retrieved June 19, 2006, from http://www.nursesource.org/facts_shortage.html

Hood, L. J., & Leddy, S. (2003). *Leddy & Pepper's conceptual bases of professional nursing* (5th ed.). Philadelphia: Lippincott.

Howard, V. B., & Tasota, R. J. (2004). How to spell relief for the nursing shortage: S-t-u-d-e-n-t-s. *Nursing, 34*(9), 32hn14–32hn16.

International Council of Nurses. (2009). *About the International Council of Nurses.* Retrieved October 23, 2009, from http://www.icn.ch/abouticn.htm

King, I. M. (1981). *A theory for nursing: Systems, concepts, process.* Albany, NY: Delmar.

King, I. M. (2006). Imogene M. King's theory of goal attainment. In M. E. Parker, *Nursing theories and nursing practice* (2nd ed., pp. 235–244). Philadelphia: F. A. Davis.

Lasiuk, G. C., & Ferguson, L. (2005). From practice to midrange theory and back again: Beck's theory of postpartum depression. *Advances in Nursing Science, 28*, 127–136.

Leininger, M. M. (2006). Madeline M. Leininger's theory of culture care diversity and universality. In M. E. Parker, *Nursing theories and nursing practice* (2nd ed., pp. 309–320). Philadelphia: F. A. Davis.

Leininger, M. M. (Ed.). (1991). *Culture care diversity and universality: A theory of nursing.* New York: National League for Nursing Press.

Leininger, M., & McFarland, M. R. (2002). *Culture care diversity and universality: A theory of nursing* (3rd ed.). New York: McGraw-Hill.

Liu, K. (2003). Breakthroughs in cancer gene therapy. *Seminars in Oncology Nursing, 19*(3), 217–226.

Malloch, K., & Porter-O'Grady, T. (2005). *Introduction to evidence-based practice in nursing and health care.* Sudbury, MA: Jones & Bartlett.

Mee, C. L. (2004). Postcards from the past: A salute to nursing specialties. *Nursing, 34*(1), 43–44.

Melnyk, B. M., & Fineout-Overholt, E. (2004). *Evidence-based practice in nursing and healthcare.* Philadelphia: Lippincott Williams & Wilkins.

Meyers, S. (2003). Real men choose nursing. *Hospitals & Health Networks, 77*(6), 72–77.

Military District of Washington. (n.d.). *The Nurses Memorial at Arlington Cemetery section 21.* Retrieved January 23, 2005, from http://www.mdw.army.mil/content/anmviewer.aspa-39

Montag, M. L. (1951). *The education of nursing technicians.* New York: Putnam.

Munhall, P. L. (Ed.). (2006). *Nursing research: A qualitative perspective* (4th ed.). Boston: Jones & Bartlett.

National Commission on Nursing Implementation Project (NCNIP). (1987). *Timeline for transition into the future: Nursing education system for two categories of nurse.* Milwaukee, WI: Author.

National Institute of Nursing Research. (2009). *About NINR. Mission of the National Institute of Nursing Research. Scientific goals and objectives* (Objective 1.1). Retrieved October 23, 2009, from http://ninr.nih.gov/

National League for Nursing Accrediting Commission. (2005). *Directory of accredited nursing programs.* New York: Author.

National League for Nursing. (2000). *Educational competencies for graduates of associate degree nursing programs.* Sudbury, MA: Jones & Bartlett.

National League for Nursing. (2007). Tri-Council for Nursing policy statement: Strategies to reverse the new nursing shortage. Retrieved October 23, 2009, from http://www.nln.org/

National Organization for Associate Degree Nursing. (2009a). *Position statement in support of associate degree as preparation for the entry-level registered nurse.* Retrieved October 23, 2009, from https://www.noadn.org/about/mission-and-goals.html

National Organization for Associate Degree Nursing. (2009b). *Associate degree nursing (ADN) facts.* Retrieved October 23, 2009, from http://www.noadn.org/pdfs/AssociateDegreeNursing.pdf

National Student Nurses' Association House of Delegates. (2001). *The code of academic and clinical conduct.* Nashville, TN: Author.

Nelson, R. (2004). The nurse poachers. *Lancet, 364,* 1743.

Neuman, B., & Fawcett, J. (2002). *The Neuman systems model* (4th ed.). Upper Saddle River, NJ: Prentice Hall.

Nightingale, F. (1969). *Notes on nursing: What it is, and what it is not.* New York: Dover. (Original work published 1860)

O'Neil, E. H., & the Pew Health Professions Commission. (1998). *Recreating health professional practice for a new century.* San Francisco: Pew Health Professions Commission.

Orem, D. E. (1971). *Nursing: Concepts of practice.* Hightstown, NJ: McGraw-Hill.

Orem, D. E., Taylor, S. G., & Renpenning, K. M. (2001). *Nursing: Concepts of practice* (6th ed.). St. Louis, MO: Mosby.

Overbay, J. D., & Aaltonen, P. M. (2001). A comparison of NLNAC and CCNE accreditation. *Nurse Educator, 26*(1), 17–22.

Parse, R. R. (1994). Quality of life: Sciencing and living the art of human becoming. *Nursing Science Quarterly, 7*(1), 16–21.

Parse, R. R. (2004). Person-centered care. *Nursing Science Quarterly, 17,* 193.

Parse, R. R. (2006). Rosemarie Rizzo Parse's human becoming school of thought. In M. E. Parker, *Nursing theories and nursing practice* (2nd ed., pp.187–194). Philadelphia: F. A. Davis.

Parse, R. R. (Ed.). (1999). *Illumination: The human becoming theory in practice and research.* Boston: Jones & Bartlett.

Peplau, H. E. (1952). *Interpersonal relations in nursing.* New York: Putnam.

Polit, D. F., & Beck, C. T. (2005). *Essentials of nursing research: Methods, appraisal, and utilization* (6th ed.). Philadelphia: Lippincott, Williams & Wilkins.

Powers, B. A., & Knapp, T. R. (2005). *Dictionary of nursing theory and research* (3rd ed.). New York: Springer.

Rogers, M. E. (1970). *An introduction to the theoretical basis of nursing.* Philadelphia: F. A. Davis.

Rogers, M. E. (1994). The science of unitary human beings: Current perspectives. *Nursing Science Quarterly, 7*(1), 33–35.

Rosenberg, S. (2006). Utilizing the language of Jean Watson's caring theory within a computerized clinical documentation system. *Computers, Informatics, Nursing, 24,* 53–56.

Roy, C. (1997). Future of the Roy model: Challenge to redefine adaptation. *Nursing Science Quarterly, 10*(1), 42–48.

Roy, C. (1999). *The Roy adaptation model* (2nd ed.). Upper Saddle River, NJ: Prentice Hall.

Sand-Jecklin, K. E., & Schaffer, A. J. (2006). Nursing students' perceptions of their chosen profession. *Nursing Education Perspectives, 27,* 130–136.

Schuyler, C. B. (1992). Florence Nightingale. In F. Nightingale, *Notes on nursing: What it is, and what it is not* (commemorative ed., pp. 3–17). Philadelphia: Lippincott.

Stein, M., & Deese, D. (2004). Addressing the next decade of nursing challenges. *Nursing Economics, 22*(5), 272–279.

Sutters, K. A., Miaskowski, C., Holdridge-Zeuner, D., Waite, S., Paul, S. M., Savedra, M. C., et al. (2005). Time-contingent dosing of an opioid analgesic after tonsillectomy does not increase moderate-to- severe side effects in children. *Pain Management Nursing, 6,* 49–57.

Tomey, A. M., & Alligood, M. R. (2006). *Nursing theorists and their work* (6th ed.). St. Louis, MO: Mosby.

Tourville, C., Ingalls, K. (2003). The living tree of nursing theories. *Nursing Forum, 38,* 21–30, 36.

Vetter, M. J., Bristow, L., & Ahrens, J. (2004). A model for home care clinician and home health aide collaboration: Diabetes care by nurse case managers and community health workers. *Home Healthcare Nurse, 22,* 645–648.

Vietnam Women's Memorial Foundation. (2009). *During the Vietnam era....* Retrieved October 23, 2009, from http://www.vietnamwomensmemorial.org/pages/frames/vwmp.html

Watson, J. (2005). *Caring science as sacred science.* Philadelphia: F. A. Davis.

Watson, J. (2006–07 in process). *Nursing: The philosophy and science of caring. Revised & updated edition.* Boulder: University Press of Colorado.

Watson, J. (2008). *From carative factors to clinical caritas processes.* Retrieved October 23, 2009, from http://www2.uchsc.edu/son/caring/content/evolution.asp

Watson, J., & Smith, M. C. (2002). Caring science and the science of unitary human beings: A trans-theoretical discourse for nursing knowledge development. *Journal of Advanced Nursing, 37,* 452–461.

Whitten, P., Doolittle, G., Mackert, M., & Rush, T. (2003). Telehospice: End-of-life care over the lines. *Nursing Management, 34*(11), 36–39.

Woodham-Smith, C. (1950). *Florence Nightingale.* London: Constable & Co.

Wooten, J. M., & Ross, V. M. (2005). How to make sense of clinical research. *RN, 68*(1), 22–27.

Legal and Ethical Aspects of Nursing

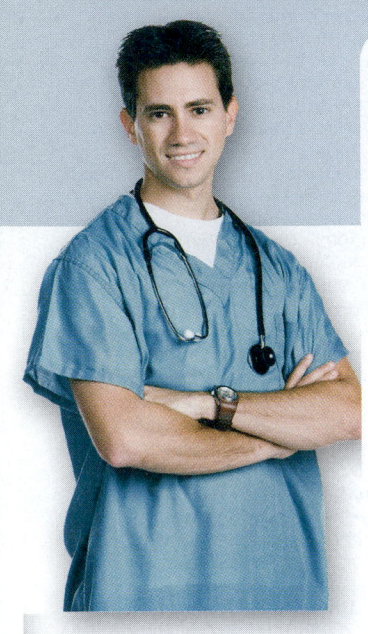

Bakaar is a student nurse spending his first day in a clinical facility. During the morning he observes a cardiac resuscitation and the placement of a chest tube and helps to transfer a client to the intensive care unit. Going to lunch, while in the elevator with several of his classmates, he excitedly begins to tell them what he did this morning, but his instructor signals for him to be quiet. When they get off the elevator, the instructor takes him aside and reminds him of the importance of maintaining client confidentiality. As he is driving home at the end of the day, he can't wait to tell his fiancé everything he experienced but wonders if he can legally discuss his day.

LEARNING OUTCOMES

After completing this chapter, you will be able to:

1. List the sources of laws in nursing and describe how nursing practice is licensed and regulated.

2. Give examples of areas of potential liability in nursing, including crimes, intentional torts, unintentional torts, malpractice, and negligence.

3. Describe the impact of the Health Insurance Portability and Accountability Act compliance on nursing practice.

4. List six strategies by which nurses can protect themselves from legal actions.

5. List the essential elements of informed consent and describe its purpose.

6. List four actions required of student nurses to reduce their legal liability.

7. Identify strategies nurses may employ to help clients clarify their values.

8. List six purposes of the nursing code of ethics.

9. Identify strategies nurses can employ to make ethical decisions.

10. Give examples of nurses acting as client advocates.

KEY TERMS

Fidelity p43	Injury p29	Morality p42	Standards of care p28
Foreseeability p29	Invasion of privacy p30	Negligence p28	Tort p28
Gross negligence p28	Justice p43	Nonmaleficence p43	Unprofessional conduct p32
Harm p29	Law p27	Responsibility p33	Values p40
Health care proxy p38	Liability p33	Right p33	Veracity p43
Implied consent p36	Libel p30	Slander p30	
Informed consent p36	Malpractice p28		

LEGAL ISSUES

Nurses must know the basics of legal concepts because nurses are accountable for their professional judgments and actions. Understanding the laws that regulate and affect nursing practice is essential to ensuring that the nurse's decisions and actions are consistent with current legal principles and to protect the nurse from liability. Accountability is a primary concept in the practice of nursing.

General Legal Concepts

Guido (2009) defines **law** as "the sum total of rules and regulations by which a society is governed. As such, law is created by people, and exists to regulate all persons." The primary sources of laws in the United States include the Constitution, statutes, administrative agencies, and decisions of the courts known as common law. Laws enacted by any legislative body are called statutory laws. If federal and state laws conflict, federal law supersedes. State laws supersede local laws.

There are several types of law. The two main types are public law and private or civil law. Public law refers to the body of law that deals with relationships between individuals and the government. Criminal law is a major segment of public law, dealing with actions against the safety and welfare of the public such as homicide, theft, and manslaughter. Private law, or civil law, deals with relationships among private individuals and includes contract law and tort law. Contract law enforces agreements among individuals while tort law defines and enforces duties and rights among private individuals not based on contractual agreements. Examples of tort law that affect nursing include negligence, malpractice, invasion of privacy, and assault or battery.

There are two kinds of legal actions: civil or private actions and criminal actions. Civil actions deal with relationships among individuals in society such as when a client sues a physician for malpractice. Criminal actions deal with disputes between an individual and society as a whole such as a person convicted of killing another. The major difference is the potential outcome for the defendant. If the defendant is found guilty in a civil action, they will be charged a sum of money. If the defendant is found to be guilty in a criminal action the client may lose money, be jailed, or could potentially be executed if the charges are serious

enough. A nurse found guilty in a criminal action could potentially lose licensure to practice nursing.

There are generally five steps involved in a lawsuit. A document, called a complaint, is filed by the plaintiff who claims their legal rights have been infringed upon by the defendant. A written response, called an answer, is made by the defendant. Both parties participate in discovery, in an effort to obtain all the facts of the situation. The trial is then held allowing both sides to present all relevant facts to a judge or jury. The judge renders a decision or the jury reaches a verdict. If the outcome is unsatisfactory to either party, they may appeal for another trial. It is the plaintiff's responsibility to demonstrate the wrongdoing of the defendant, called the burden of proof.

A nurse may be called to testify in a legal action and should seek the advice of an attorney before providing testimony. A nurse may also be asked to provide testimony as an expert witness if the nurse has special training, experience, or skill in a relevant area. In this case, the nurse offers an opinion on some issue within the area of expertise in order to help a judge or jury understand the appropriate standard of care.

Regulation of Nursing Practice

The regulation of nursing is a function of state law. State legislatures pass statutes that define and regulate nursing, called nurse practice acts. These acts must be consistent with constitutional and federal laws. After the statutes are passed, an administrative agency is given authority to create rules and regulations to enforce the statutory law. The administrative agency that is formed in most states to regulate nursing is the state board of nursing, which frequently functions under the state department of health. The state board of nursing writes rules and regulations to implement and enforce the nurse practice act (Guido, 2009).

Protection of the public is the legal purpose for defining the scope of practice, licensing requirements, and standards of care. Nurses who know and follow their nurse practice act and standards of care provide safe, competent nursing care.

NURSE PRACTICE ACTS Each state has a nurse practice act that legally defines and describes the scope of nursing practice and legally controls nursing practice through licensure requirements. Advanced practice nurses require additional licensure. While nurse practice acts are similar, they do differ somewhat from state to state. They may differ in the scope of practice or in licensing requirements. It is the nurse's responsibility to know and comply with the nurse practice act in the state in which they practice. Each nurse should receive a copy of the state's nurse practice act when the nurse's license is issued; it can be easily accessed on the state board of nursing's website.

CREDENTIALING **Credentialing** is the process of determining and maintaining competence in the nursing practice in order to maintain standards of practice and accountability for the educational preparation of its members. Credentialing includes licensure, certification, and accreditation.

A license is a legal permit that a government agency grants to individuals to engage in the practice of a profession and to use a particular title. Nursing licensure is mandatory in all states. For a profession or occupation to obtain the right to license its members, it must demonstrate a need to protect the public's safety or welfare, the profession is clearly delineated as a separate, distinct area of work, and there is proper authority to assume the obligations of the licensing process such as the state board of nursing. Each state has a mechanism by which a license can be granted as well as issues for which a license can be revoked for just cause.

In the last decade technological changes have brought about the need for a change in the way nurses are licensed. Telehealth is the delivery of health services over distances and includes nurses who care for clients over the Internet or over the phone. The old model of licensure required nurses to hold a license in every state where their clients lived. In response to this expanded role of nurses, the National Council of State Boards of Nursing (NCSBN) developed a new regulatory model named the mutual recognition model, which allows for multistate licensure. This allows nurses to practice across state lines while holding one license in their state of residence. A nurse may license in the state of residence and work in any state that has an interstate compact without having to relicense. However, nurses practicing in other states through the interstate compact has an obligation to understand the regulations that exist in the states where they practice nursing and must be licensed in their state of residence. As of 2009, 23 states have implemented the Nurse Licensure Compact for RNs and LVN/LPNs. The NCSBN website provides current information about the states that have passed NLC legislation and those states that are pending adoption of the legislation.

Certification is a voluntary practice for validating that an individual nurse has met the minimum standards of nursing competence in specialty areas such as maternal–child health, pediatrics, mental health, gerontology, or critical care nursing. National certification may be required to become licensed as an advanced practice nurse.

Another function of state boards of nursing is to ensure that schools preparing nurses maintain minimum standards of education. Depending on the state, the state board of nursing must either approve or accredit the program. This is a legal requirement in order for graduates of the program to be eligible for licensure. Schools may also choose to voluntarily accredit from a private organization such as the National League for Nursing Accrediting Commission (NLNAC) and the Com-

mission on Collegiate Nursing Education (CCNE). Maintaining voluntary accreditation is a means of informing the public and prospective students that the nursing program has met certain criteria. Some states require that nursing programs be both state approved/accredited and accredited by a national accrediting agency.

STANDARDS OF CARE **Standards of care** are the skills and learning commonly possessed by members of a profession to protect the consumer (Guido, 2009). These standards are used to evaluate the quality of care nurses provide and, therefore, become legal guidelines for nursing practice. There are internal and external standards. Internal standards of care include "the nurse's job description, education, and expertise as well as individual institutional policies and procedures" (Guido, 2009). External standards include nurse practice acts, professional organizations, nursing specialty-practice organizations, and federal organizations and federal guidelines. It is vital for nurses to know their institution's policies and procedures and nurse practice act. They also need to remain competent through reading professional journals and attending continuing education and in-service programs. Again, the purpose of knowing and practicing nursing's standards of care is to protect the client/consumer. Nurses who do not continue to learn quickly find that their practice endangers the people they care for.

Areas of Potential Liability in Nursing

CRIMES AND TORTS A crime is an act, intentional or unintentional, committed in violation of public criminal law and punishable by a fine or imprisonment. Crimes are classified as either a felony (a crime of a serious nature) or a misdemeanor (an offense of a less serious nature). A nurse who accidentally administers a lethal dose of a medication can be accused of manslaughter, a term used in some areas to describe second-degree murder.

A **tort** is a civil wrong committed against a person or a person's property and usually litigated in court by civil action between individuals. In other words, the person claimed to be responsible for the tort is sued for damages.

Unintentional Torts Negligence and malpractice are examples of unintentional torts that may occur in the health care setting. **Negligence** is misconduct or practice that is below the standard expected of an ordinary, reasonable, and prudent person. Such conduct places another person at risk for harm. **Gross negligence** involves extreme lack of knowledge, skill, or decision making that the person clearly should have known would put others at risk for harm. **Malpractice** is "professional negligence" or negligence that occurred while the person was performing as a professional. Five elements must be present for a case of nursing malpractice to be proven:

- **Duty** – The nurse must have a relationship with the client that involves providing care and following an acceptable standard of care.
- **Breach of duty** – There must be a standard of care that is expected in the specific situation that the nurse

failed to observe. This is the failure to act as a reasonable, prudent nurse under the same circumstances.

- **Foreseeability** – A link must exist between the nurse's act and the injury suffered.
- **Causation** – It must be proved that the harm occurred as a direct result of the nurse's failure to follow the standard of care and that the nurse could have or should have known that failure to follow the standard of care could result in such harm.
- **Harm** or **injury** – The client must demonstrate some type of harm or injury as a result of the breach of duty.

If all five of these factors are present, the judge or jury will then assign damages, an amount of money assigned to be paid to the client by the nurse with the goal of assisting the injured party to regain his or her original position as far as financially possible.

To defend against a malpractice lawsuit the nurse must prove that one or more of the five required elements are not met. There is a limit to the amount of time that can pass between occurrence and recognition of harm, known as the statute of limitations. The time period varies by state and the type of suit but is generally one to two years, although pediatric clients have six months after turning 21 years old (18 in some states) to determine that they suffered harm from a medical event.

Several legal doctrines or principles relate to negligence. *Respondeat superior* is one doctrine in which the lawsuit will also name the employer who can be held liable if they failed to provide adequate human and material resources for nursing care, failed to properly educate nurses on the use of new equipment or procedures, or failed to orient nurses to the facility. *Res ipsa loquitur* (the thing speaks for itself) is used in cases where the harm cannot be traced to a specific health care provider or standard but does not normally apply, such as when an instrument is left in the client during surgery. A potential defense might be contributory or comparative negligence if the client was at least partially responsible for the injury, such as when clients choose not to follow health care advice.

CLINICAL ALERT

The best defense against a malpractice claim is to know your nursing responsibilities, the scope of practice of members of your health team, and deliver care according to standards of care.

To avoid malpractice, nurses must recognize those nursing situations in which negligent actions are most likely to occur and take measures to prevent them (Box 2–1). The most common situation is medication errors. Other common situations include falls, ignoring a client's complaint, failure to answer a call bell, and incorrectly identifying clients.

CLINICAL ALERT

- To be a client advocate, you must know about the medications being administered. Know why the client is receiving the medication, the dosage range, possible adverse effects, toxicity levels, and contraindications.
- Never give a medication that you did not prepare.
- Assess clients for fall potential. Document nursing measures taken to protect the client.
- Monitor both physical and psychosocial status of the client. Document observations and interventions.

BOX 2–1   Categories of Negligence that Result in Malpractice

Failure to follow standards of care, including failure to

- Perform a complete admission assessment or design a plan of care.
- Adhere to standardized protocols or institutional policies and procedures (e.g., using an improper injection site).
- Follow a physician's verbal or written orders.

Failure to use equipment in a responsible manner, including failure to

- Follow the manufacturer's recommendations for operating the equipment.
- Check equipment for safety prior to use.
- Place equipment properly during treatment.
- Learn how equipment functions.

Failure to communicate, including failure to

- Notify a physician in a timely manner when conditions warrant it.
- Listen to a client's complaints and act on them.
- Communicate effectively with a client (e.g., inadequate or ineffective communication of discharge instructions).
- Seek higher medical authorization for a treatment.

Failure to document, including failure to note in the patient's medical record

- A client's progress and response to treatment.
- A client's injuries.
- Pertinent nursing assessment information (e.g., drug allergies).
- A physician's medical orders.
- Information on telephone conversations with physicians, including time, content of communication between nurse and physician, and actions taken.

Failure to assess and monitor, including failure to

- Complete a shift assessment.
- Implement a plan of care.
- Observe a client's ongoing progress.
- Interpret a client's signs and symptoms.

Failure to act as a patient advocate, including failure to

- Question discharge orders when a client's condition warrants it.
- Question incomplete or illegible medical orders.
- Provide a safe environment.

Note: Adapted from "Nurses, Negligence, and Malpractice," by E. M. Croke, 2003, *American Journal of Nursing, 103*(9), pp. 54–63.

Intentional Torts Intentional torts differ from unintentional torts because intentional torts do not require the element of harm that unintentional torts require. No harm need be caused by intentional torts for liability to exist, and no witnesses are needed because there is no standard involved. Four intentional torts related to nursing are assault and battery, false imprisonment, invasion of privacy, and defamation (libel and slander).

Assault is an attempt or threat to touch another person unjustifiably. Assault is an act that causes the person to believe a battery is about to occur. For example, a nurse who threatens a client with an injection after the client refuses to take the medication orally would be committing assault.

Battery is the willful touching of a person, the person's clothes, or even something the person is carrying that may or may not cause harm. In order for it to be considered battery, the touching must be wrong in some way, such as touching that is done without permission, that is embarrassing, or that causes injury. An example is a nurse who changes a client's saturated dressing if the client declined to have the dressing changed at this time. All nursing care requires the consent of the client unless the client is incompetent to make decisions autonomously, in which case the guardian must give consent. If the nurse is uncertain whether the client is competent to refuse care, the nursing supervisor or physician should be consulted. Battery exists when there is no consent, even if the plaintiff was not asked for consent. Unless there is implied consent, such as a life-threatening emergency, a procedure performed on an unconscious client without informed consent is battery.

False imprisonment is the "unjustifiable detention of a person without legal warrant to confine the person" (Guido, 2009). False imprisonment accompanied by forceful restraint or threat of restraint is battery. The client must not be detained against the client's will. The client has the right to leave even if it may be detrimental to the client's health. In this instance, the client can leave by signing an AWA (absence without authority) or AMA (against medical advice) form. Restraining a client can be construed as false imprisonment if the client is competent to decline restraints. To guide nurses in such dilemmas, agencies usually have clear policies regarding the application of restraints (see Chapter 20 ∞).

Invasion of privacy is a direct wrong of a personal nature. It injures the feelings of a person and does not take into account the effect of revealed information on the reputation of the person in the community. The right to privacy is the right of individuals to withhold themselves and their lives from public scrutiny. It can also be described as the right to be left alone. Liability can result if the nurse breaches confidentiality by passing along confidential client information to others or intrudes into the client's private domain. There is a delicate balance between the need of a number of people to contribute to the diagnosis and treatment of a client and the client's right to confidentiality. In most situations, necessary discussion about a client's medical condition is considered appropriate, but unnecessary discussions and gossip are considered a breach of confidentiality. Necessary discussion in-volves only those engaged in a client's care. This topic is discussed further in the next section of this chapter.

CLINICAL ALERT

Never discuss client situations in the elevator, cafeteria, or other public areas inside or outside of the facility.

Most jurisdictions have a variety of statutes that impose a duty to report certain confidential client information. Four major categories are vital statistics, infections and communicable diseases, child or elder abuse, and violent incidents.

The client must be protected from use of the client's name or likeness for profit (such as photographs), unreasonable intrusion (such as students observing procedures), public disclosure of private facts (giving private information to reporters who may call if the client was involved in a public event), and putting a person in a false light (such as publishing information that is offensive and untrue). Individual facilities have release forms clients may sign to allow photography using their image, should this be necessary, and verbal consent should always be obtained before allowing students to observe a procedure.

Defamation is a communication that is false or made with a careless disregard for the truth and results in injury to the reputation of a person. Both libel and slander are wrongful actions that come under the heading of defamation. **Libel** is defamation by means of print, writing, or pictures. Writing in the nurse's notes that a physician is incompetent because he didn't immediately respond to a call is an example of libel.

Slander is defamation by spoken word, stating unprivileged or false words by which a reputation is damaged, such as one nurse telling a client that their physician is incompetent or advising clients to find another physician. Only the person being defamed may bring a lawsuit, and a third party must be involved. If a nurse privately tells another nurse that their actions are incompetent, this would not be considered slander.

PRIVACY OF CLIENT HEALTH INFORMATION AND HIPAA The Health Insurance Portability and Accountability Act (HIPAA) is a federal law passed in 1996. Some of the goals of HIPAA include allowing people with preexisting medical conditions to transfer their health insurance from one provider to another when they change jobs, reduce fraud and abuse in health insurance and health delivery, promote the use of medical savings accounts, improve access to long-term care, and simplify the administration of health insurance. The goals of HIPAA important for this chapter are the goals of establishing national standards to protect personal health information, to

LONG-TERM CARE CONSIDERATION
Entering a Client's Room

When working in long-term care facilities, entering the client's room is similar to entering the client's home. Knock before entering the room and wait for the client to provide permission for entry if the client is competent to make choices.

place obligations on health care providers and health plans to protect health information, to provide clients greater access to their medical records, and to give clients more control over how their personally identifiable health information is used. HIPAA also provides rules about how health information can be electronically transmitted.

Protected Information   The privacy rule, a component of HIPAA, protects all individually identifiable health information held or transmitted by a physician or health care provider. Individually identified health information is information that could reasonably identify the person it belongs to, such as demographic date, in electronic or paper form. The common term for this individually identified health information is personal health information (PHI).

PHI is information that relates to the individual's past, present, or future physical and mental health status, health care provided to the client, payments made for health care, and information that identifies the client or is reasonable to believe it might identify the client. PHI may include name, address, birth date, admission or discharge date, telephone numbers, e-mail address, social security number, insurance group or plan numbers, vehicle identification, driver's license number, device identifiers, biometrics, photographs, or any unique identification number. While there are some exclusions, the rule covers most of the information nurses have access to in the client's medical records.

Who Must Comply with the Privacy Rule?   All health care providers, including student nurses, must comply with HIPAA. This includes health insurance providers, clearinghouses (those who act as middlemen between providers and health insurance companies), and anyone who is given access to the client's medical records. Furthermore, the American Recovery and Reinvestment Act (ARRA) of 2009 extended the need for compliance of those companies who do business with health care providers. Examples may include health information exchange organizations, legal associates, or contracted vendors who maintain information technology.

Nurses may communicate freely with other health care providers about treatment, payment, and other medical information on a "need to know" basis. In other words, if a nurse requires a consultation with another nurse, it is acceptable to discuss medical information because there is a "need to know." In the course of consulting with another nurse, only the minimum necessary (the smallest amount of information required) should be disclosed. For example, if a nurse working on the pediatric unit becomes aware that a celebrity, relative, or neighbor was treated and released in the emergency room and decides to look up the person's medical record on the hospital computer, this nurse has broken the HIPAA privacy rule and could face sanctions because there was no need for this nurse to access this medical record.

In order for a physician's office to bill insurance for payment, the client must sign a release authorizing the office to share PHI with the medical insurance company. If the client declines to give this permission, information cannot be sent to the medical insurance company. Most medical offices would then require the client to be responsible for her or his bill.

Clients' Rights under HIPAA   The privacy rule provides for several client rights and the need for health care providers to respect those rights. See Table 2–1 for a list of clients' rights and examples of how these rights are met in health care.

TABLE 2–1	Clients' Rights Under HIPAA Privacy Act
CLIENTS' RIGHTS	**EXAMPLES OF COMPLIANCE**
Clients have the right to receive notice of the privacy practice of the health care agency.	Clients are given a notice of the hospital's privacy practices when they are admitted to the hospital and are required to sign a form that they read and understood this notice.
Clients have the right to request an accounting of health information disclosures.	All health care facilities have "Request for Accounting of PHI" forms that clients may request and complete in order to be provided a list of agencies that were given any of their PHI.
Clients have the right to make amendments to their medical records.	If clients disagree with something a provider wrote in the medical record, clients have the right to add a note of their own clarifying the situation to their satisfaction.
Clients have the right to inspect and copy their health information.	Clients sign a form if they want to see, or receive a copy of, their medical record. Access to medical records cannot be denied to clients.
Clients have the right to receive confidential communications about their health information.	If a facility provides the option for a client to calls or e-mails requesting health care information or advice, the facility must set up the communication equipment to be secure from accidental disclosure whether to a hacker or someone eavesdropping.
Clients have the right to request restrictions on use or disclosure of PHI.	A client may request that specific information, such as HIV status or pregnancy, not be disclosed to agencies such as life or health insurance companies.
Clients have the right to complain to both the health care facility and the Department of Health and Human Services.	If the client has reason to believe that his or her PHI is being treated carelessly, the client may complain to both the facility and the Department of Health and Human Services (HHS), which will trigger an investigation into the practices of the facility.

Penalties for Noncompliance Regulation and monitoring for compliance has been transferred from the Department of Health and Human Services (HHS) to the Federal Communication Commission (FCC). The FCC was given increased funding and staff to strengthen enforcement monitoring by the American Recovery and Reinvestment Act (ARRA), and it has the authority to impose fines if a facility fails to comply with the privacy rule. Fines have been increased by ARRA. Fines increase with repeated offenses and are considerably higher if the breach of confidentiality is determined to be knowingly disclosed. The highest fine and imprisonment are reserved for intent to sell, transfer, or use identifiable health information for commercial advantage, personal gain, or malicious harm (U.S. Department of Health and Human Services, 2003).

Strategies for Maintaining Confidentiality Protecting clients' confidentiality has been an important responsibility for nursing long before creation of HIPAA, but it is important to be aware of identifying information that is protected under the law but may not be initially perceived as health information, such as social security number, fingerprints, and so on. Customary practices, such as writing the client's name and room number on a white board hung at the nurse's desk, are an invasion of client privacy and can no longer be done. Nurses must constantly consider whether their actions are invading clients' right to privacy.

A nurse is not authorized to give information about clients over the phone unless the client has signed a form giving permission for PHI to be shared with that person. Because there is no way of ensuring that the person on the phone is the person they claim to be, many hospitals provide a unique identifier number to family members. When family members call to receive updates on client's condition, they provide the unique identifier so the nurse knows that the person calling is in fact a member of that client's family. Calls from the media seeking updates on a client's condition, no matter how innocent the request may seem, need to be referred to the facility supervisor or the media relations department. During end of shift reports, or client rounds, nurses must verify that no one is within hearing distance, and speak softly. Some facilities limit visitors when rounds or report are in progress. Any paperwork with client PHI printed on it must be shredded, not just casually placed in the trash can where it can fall into others' hands.

When using a computer, passwords that contain numbers, characters, and letters are preferable to passwords that are easy to break such as 1234, your family or dog's name, or your birth date. A password should never be shared with anyone or posted where it can be accessed. The importance of logging off the computer before leaving it unattended—even if the user plans to be gone for only a second—should be emphasized. Nurses have access to a great deal of private information, and it is easy for a visitor to slip behind the desk when all the nurses are busy and view protected information. Computer monitors should be positioned so that visitors cannot see the information the nurse is viewing. Computer access is tracked within facilities, so nurses should never view client information that they have no right to view.

Overall, nurses must always recognize the unfettered access to personal information that they are privy to. This information must be protected with care, and nurses must recognize that they are legally liable for maintaining confidentiality of PHI.

LOSS OF CLIENT PROPERTY Loss of client property, such as jewelry, money, eyeglasses, and dentures, is a constant concern to hospital personnel. Agencies prefer to take less responsibility for property and request clients sign a waiver on admission relieving the hospital and its employees of any responsibility for property and request they send anything of value home. Situations arise in which the client cannot sign a waiver and the nursing staff must follow prescribed policies for safeguarding the client's property. Nurses are expected to take reasonable precautions to safeguard a client's property, and they can be held liable for its loss or damage if they do not exercise reasonable care.

UNPROFESSIONAL CONDUCT **Unprofessional conduct** includes incompetence or gross negligence, conviction for practicing without a license, falsification of client records, and illegally obtaining, using, or possessing controlled substances. Most nurse practice acts name unprofessional conduct as one of the grounds for actions against the nurse's license. Having a personal relationship with a client, especially a vulnerable client, may be considered unprofessional conduct because nurses are responsible for retaining their professional boundaries (ANA, 2001, P.11). Certain acts may constitute a tort or crime in addition to being unprofessional conduct.

Unethical conduct may also be addressed in nurse practice acts. Unethical conduct includes violations of professional ethical codes, breach of confidentiality, fraud, or refusing to care for clients of specific socioeconomic or cultural origins.

REPORTING CRIMES, TORTS, AND UNSAFE PRACTICES The Healthcare Integrity and Protection Data Bank (HIPDB) was created for reporting of civil judgments or criminal convictions related to health care and licensure or certification actions. Another data bank, the National Practitioner Data Bank (NPDB) was established to identify incompetent and unprofessional health care practitioners. The information in these two data banks is not accessible by the public but can be accessed by state licensing boards, health maintenance organizations, hospitals, and professional organizations. The data banks are examples of a nationwide effort to protect the public and to identify and track professionals found liable of malpractice or actions taken against their license. Nurses at all levels of nursing practice can be reported to national data banks.

Nurses may need to report nursing colleagues or other health professionals for practices that endanger the health and safety of clients. For instance, alcohol and drug use, theft from a client or agency, and unsafe nursing practice should be reported. Reporting a colleague is not easy. The person reporting may feel disloyal, incur the disapproval of others, or perceive that chances for promotion are endangered. When reporting an incident or series of incidents, the nurse must be careful to describe observed behavior only and not make inferences as to what might be happening. The accompanying Practice Guidelines can be used for reporting a crime, tort, or unsafe practice.

Reporting these events is referred to as "whistle-blowing." Many states have laws that prevent wrongful termination of whistle-blowers by employers. In some states, it is mandatory for a nurse with knowledge of someone's unprofessional conduct to report that behavior to the state board of nursing. In addition, reporting illegal, unethical, or incompetent performance is an ethical expectation.

Contractual Arrangements in Nursing

A **contract** is an agreement, written or oral, between two or more competent persons on sufficient consideration to do or not to do some lawful act, such as the agreement made between the nurse and the employer. The contract is considered to be *expressed* when the two parties discuss and agree, orally or in writing, to terms and conditions during the creation of the contract such as during the employment interview. An *implied* contract is one that has not been explicitly agreed to by the parties but that the law nevertheless considers existing. For example, the nurse is expected to be competent and to follow hospital policies and procedures, even if these expectations were not written or discussed. Likewise, the hospital is expected to provide the necessary supplies and equipment needed to provide competent nursing care.

LEGAL ROLES OF NURSES   The nurse's legal role includes provider of services, employee or contractor for service, and citizen. As providers of services, nurses are expected to deliver safe and competent care. Implicit in this role are several legal concepts including standards of care, liability, and contractual obligations.

Liability means nurses are legally responsible for their obligations and actions and will make financial restitution

for wrongful acts. A nurse is expected to practice, and direct the practice of others, in a way that will cause no harm to the client and maintain standards of care. If the nurse carries out the order of a physician, the responsibility and liability for the action belongs to the nurse. The nurse should never do anything that the nurse believes may be injurious to the client. The standards of care the nurse acts on, or fails to act on, are legally defined by nurse practice acts in every state. Nursing actions are judged by the rule of reasonable and prudent action. This is defined as what a reasonable and prudent professional with similar preparation and experience would do in similar circumstances. The nurse is also bound to provide care within the limitations and terms specified by the nurse practice act. For example, the nurse cannot write orders independently on a client's chart because this would be outside the bounds specified in the nurse practice act.

Contractual obligations refer to the nurse's duty to provide care. The nurse holds a contractual obligation to the client to deliver safe care and to the employer, such as the hospital or nursing home, in which the nurse represents and acts for the facility and therefore must function within the policies of the employing agency. The contractual obligation is established by the presence of an expressed or implied contract, or in some circumstances such as private duty nursing, may be established by a written fee for service contract. This legal relationship with the employer creates the doctrine known as *respondeat superior*, or "let the master answer." In other words, the employer assumes responsibility for the conduct of the employee and can be held responsible for the employee's actions. However, the nurse remains liable and will not prevail if the employee's actions are extraordinarily inappropriate or beyond those expected or foreseen by the employer such as criminal actions committed by the nurse. Nurses can be held liable for failure to act as well. The nurse is also required to respect the rights and responsibilities of other health care participants and should not adversely affect their practice, such as denouncing another care provider to the client.

The nurse also carries the rights and responsibilities of any other citizen in this country. Rights of citizenship protect clients from harm and ensure consideration for their personal property rights, rights to privacy, confidentiality, and other rights discussed later in this chapter. These same rights apply to nurses. An understanding of the roles of the nurse, and the rights and responsibilities that accompany these roles, promotes legally responsible conduct and practice. A **right** is a privilege or fundamental power to which an individual is entitled unless revoked by law or given up voluntarily; a **responsibility** is the obligation associated with a right.

COLLECTIVE BARGAINING   The collective bargaining process involves a certified bargaining agent, such as a union, trade association, or a professional organization that represents employees and participates in the formalized decision making process with employers to negotiate conditions of employment including wages, benefits, working environment, and work hours. When collective bargaining breaks down because an agreement cannot be reached, the employees may call a strike. A strike is an organized work stoppage by a group of employees to express a grievance, enforce a demand for changes in conditions of employment, or solve a dispute with management. Strikes provide moral dilemmas for many nurses because the actions taken by the nurses can affect the safety of people. Each nurse, facing a strike, must make an individual decision to cross or not cross a picket line. Nursing students may face this same decision if a clinical agency used for the learning experience is involved in a strike.

Legal Protections in Nursing Practice

Laws and strategies are in place to protect the nurse against litigation. Good Samaritan acts protect nurses when assisting at the scene of an emergency. Other safeguards include providing safe, competent practice by following the nurse practice act and standards of practice. Accurate and complete documentation is also a critical component of legal protection for nurses.

GOOD SAMARITAN ACTS   Good Samaritan acts are laws designed to protect health care providers who provide assistance at the scene of an emergency against claims of malpractice, unless it can be shown that there was a gross departure from the normal standard of care or willful wrongdoing on their part. Gross negligence usually involves further injury or harm to the person. For example, an automobile may strike an injured child left on the side of the road when the nurse leaves to obtain help.

Most state statutes do not require citizens to render aid to people in distress. Such assistance is considered more of an ethical than a legal duty. To encourage citizens to be "Good Samaritans," most states have now enacted legislation releasing individuals from legal liability for injuries caused under such circumstances, even if the injuries resulted from negligence of the person offering emergency aid. It is important, however, to check your state's statute since some states (e.g., Vermont) require people to stop and aid persons in danger.

It is generally believed that a person who renders help in an emergency, at a level that would be provided by any reasonably prudent person under similar circumstances, cannot be held liable. The same reasoning applies to nurses, who are among the people best prepared to help at the scene of an accident. If the level of care a nurse provides is of the caliber that would have been provided by any other nurse, then the nurse will not be held liable. However, nurses are held to a higher level than the layperson because nurses are expected to know more.

Guidelines for nurses who choose to render emergency care include: limiting their actions to what is normally considered first aid, if possible; not performing actions that the nurse does not know how to do; offering assistance but not insisting; sending someone to call or go for additional help; not leaving the scene until the injured person leaves or another qualified person takes over; and never accepting any form of compensation.

PROFESSIONAL LIABILITY INSURANCE   Nurses are increasingly being advised to carry their own liability insurance because of the increase in the number of malpractice lawsuits against health professionals. Most hospitals have liability insurance that covers all employees, including nurses. However, some smaller facilities, such as walk-in clinics, may not. Thus, nurses should always check with the employer at the time of hiring to see what coverage the facility provides. A physician or hospital can be sued because of the negligent conduct of a nurse, and the nurse can also be sued and held liable for negligence or malpractice. Because hospitals have been known to countersue nurses when they have been found negligent and the hospital was required to pay, nurses are advised to provide their own insurance coverage and not rely on hospital-provided insurance. Furthermore, if nurses provides care in their personal lives, such as providing first aid to friends of their children, they are not covered by hospital-provided insurance. Nurses, including student nurses, should use extreme caution when asked for medical advice from friends or neighbors, as they will be held to the same standards as when they are practicing in the hospital. Further, diagnosing a neighbor's illness is outside the scope of a nurse's practice and can result in a lawsuit.

Liability insurance coverage usually defrays all costs of defending a nurse, including the costs of retaining an attorney. The insurance also covers all costs incurred by the nurse up to the face value of the policy, including a settlement made out of court. In return, the insurance company may have the right to make the decisions about the claim and the settlement.

Nursing faculty and nursing students are also vulnerable to lawsuits. Students and teachers of nursing employed by community colleges and universities are not likely to be covered by the insurance carried by hospitals and health agencies. It is advisable for nursing students to check with their school about the coverage that applies to them. Faculty members are increasingly choosing to carry their own malpractice insurance. Liability insurance can be obtained through the American Nursing Association or private insurance companies. Nursing students can also obtain insurance through the National Student Nurses' Association. In some states, hospitals do not allow nursing students to provide nursing care without liability insurance or a signed disclaimer placing the responsibility of the student's actions while in the clinical setting on the student.

CARRYING OUT A PHYSICIAN'S ORDERS   Nurses are expected to analyze procedures and medications ordered by the physician. It is the nurse's responsibility to seek clarification of ambiguous or seemingly erroneous orders from the prescribing physician. Clarification from any other source is unacceptable and regarded as a departure from competent nursing practice.

If the order is neither ambiguous nor apparently erroneous, the nurse is responsible for carrying it out. For example, if the physician orders oxygen to be administered at 4 liters per minute, the nurse must administer oxygen at that rate, and not at 2 or 6 liters per minute. If the orders state that the client is not to have solid food after a bowel resection, the nurse must ensure that no solid food is given to the client.

Nurses are expected to question specific types of orders, including any order the client question, such as a medication the client believes is incorrect. The nurse is responsible for clarifying orders after a client's condition has changed. The nurse is expected to update the physician of significant changes in the client's condition, and this may require a change in standing orders. The nurse needs to use extreme caution in recording verbal orders to avoid miscommunication. Simple but important safeguard measures include recording the time, date, physician's name, the order, and the circumstances that occasioned the call to the physician, and reading the order back to the physician, documenting that the physician confirmed the order as the nurse read it back. The nurse should question any order that is illegible, unclear, incomplete, or incorrect.

PROVIDING COMPETENT NURSING CARE   Competent practice is one of the most important legal safeguard for nurses. Nurses need to provide care that is within the legal boundaries of their practice and within the boundaries of agency policies and procedures. Nurses therefore must be familiar with their job description, which may differ from agency to agency. Every nurse is responsible for ensuring that their education and experience are adequate to meet the responsibilities delineated in the job description.

Competency also involves care that protects clients from harm. Nurses need to anticipate sources of client injury, educate clients about hazards, and implement measures to prevent injury.

Application of the nursing process is another essential aspect of providing safe and effective client care. Clients need to be assessed and monitored appropriately and involved in care decisions. All assessments and care must be documented accurately. Effective communication can also protect the nurse from negligence claims. Nurses need to approach every client with sincere concern and include the client in conversations. In addition, nurses should always acknowledge when they do not know the answer to a client's questions, telling the client they will find out the answer and then follow through.

Methods of legal protection are summarized in the accompanying Practice Guidelines.

DOCUMENTATION   The client's medical record is a legal document and can be produced in court as evidence. The chart may serve as a reminder to witnesses, because the event may have occurred months or years prior to the court case. Poor documentation, rather than incompetent care, is frequently the cause of damages being awarded. Nurses must provide accurate and complete documentation of the nursing care provided because if it isn't documented, in the eyes of the court, it didn't happen. Insufficient or inaccurate assessments and documentation can hinder proper diagnosis and treatment and result in injury to the client. Chapter 8 ∞ discusses documentation in further detail.

> **PRACTICE GUIDELINES**   **Legal Protection for Nurses**
>
> - Function within the scope of your education, job description, and nurse practice act.
> - Follow the procedures and policies of the employing agency.
> - Build and maintain good rapport with clients.
> - Always check the identity of a client to make sure it is the right client.
> - Observe and monitor the client accurately. Communicate and record significant changes in the client's condition to the physician.
> - Promptly and accurately document all assessments and care given.
> - Be alert when implementing nursing interventions, and give each task your full attention and skill.
> - Perform procedures correctly and appropriately.
> - Make sure the correct medications are given in the correct dose, by the right route, at the scheduled time, and to the right client.
> - When delegating nursing responsibilities, make sure that the person who is delegated a task understands what to do and that the person has the required knowledge and skill.
> - Protect clients from injury.
> - Report all incidents involving clients.
> - Always check any order that a client questions.
> - Know your own strengths and weaknesses. Ask for assistance and supervision in situations for which you feel inadequately prepared.
> - Maintain your clinical competence. For students, this demands study and practice before caring for clients. For graduate nurses, it means continued study to maintain and update clinical knowledge and skills.

THE INCIDENT REPORT   An incident report (also called an unusual occurrence report or event report) is an agency record of an accident or unusual occurrence. Incident reports are used to make all the facts available to agency personnel, to contribute to statistical data about accidents or incidents, and to help health personnel prevent future incidents or accidents. All accidents are usually reported on incident forms. Some agencies also report other incidents, such as the occurrence of client infection or the loss of personal effects.

The nurse should document the client's name (some facilities use initials or identification number in lieu of name); date, time, and place of incident; the facts of the incident written objectively without conclusions or blame; the client's account of the incident using quotes; identification of all witnesses; and any equipment involved by number or medication by name and dosage. The report should be completed as soon as possible and filed according to agency policy. Because incident reports are not part of the client's medical record, the facts of the incident should also be noted in the medical record. Do not record that an incident report has been completed in the client record because the facts are already documented in the chart. The purpose of the report form is to alert the risk manager to the event.

The person who identifies that the incident occurred should complete the incident report. This may not be the same person actually involved with the incident. For example, the nurse who discovers that an incorrect medication has been administered completes the form even if it was another nurse who administered the medication.

Incident reports are often reviewed by an agency risk management committee, which decides whether to investigate the incident further. Nurses may be required to answer such questions as what they believe precipitated the accident, how it could have been prevented, and whether any equipment should be adjusted.

When an accident occurs, the nurse should first assess the client and intervene to prevent injury. If a client is injured, nurses must take steps to protect the client, themselves, and their employer. Most agencies have policies regarding accidents. It is important to follow these policies.

Selected Legal Aspects of Nursing Practice

Within nurses' legal roles there are a number of situations where the nurse, as client advocate, must act to assure that the client is informed and protected. Some of these situations include informed consent, delegation of duty to others, and reporting client abuse. The nurse also has the legal duty to report other nurses who are functioning in an unsafe manner, such as an impaired nurse.

INFORMED CONSENT   **Informed consent** is a legal agreement by a client to accept a course of treatment or a procedure after being provided complete information. There are two types of consent: express and implied. **Express consent** may be oral or written. The more invasive the procedure and/or the greater the potential risk to the client, the greater the need for written permission. **Implied consent** exists when the individual's nonverbal behavior indicates agreement such as when a spouse is allowed into the treatment room, indicating to the health care provider that private health information may be discussed in front of the spouse. Consent is also implied in a medical emergency when an individual cannot provide express consent because of physical condition.

The person performing the procedure is responsible for obtaining informed consent. The client must be informed of the diagnosis or condition requiring treatment, the purpose of the treatment, what the client can expect to experience, benefits and risks of treatment, advantages and disadvantages of alternatives to this particular treatment, and prognosis if not treated. The law says that a "reasonable amount" of information required for the client to make an informed decision is what any other reasonable physician or practitioner would disclose under similar circumstances (Quallich, 2005).

In order for the consent to be obtained legally, three major elements must be included.

- The client must give consent voluntarily and must not feel coerced. Sometimes fear of disapproval

> **CULTURALLY COMPETENT CARE** **Obtaining Informed Consent**
>
> Southeast Asians and American Indians may have a group perspective regarding decision making and may believe that another member of their family or tribe should make the decision for them regarding a procedure. In order to provide culturally competent care, ask the clients if there is someone they would like to be present when information or discussion of health care treatment occurs.

from a health professional can be the motivation for giving consent, and this is not voluntary consent. Coercion invalidates the consent. Therefore, the person obtaining consent must invite and answer questions from the client.

- The client must be capable and competent to understand what he or she is told. Illiteracy continues to present a challenge as it pertains to recognizing and understanding words commonly used in consent forms. If the client cannot read, the consent form must be read to the client and the client must state understanding before signing the form. Use of technical terms and medical terminology can result in the client's failure to adequately understand what he or she is being told. Another consideration for informed consent is language barriers for those who do not speak English. It is important to always provide an independent interpreter who can provide information in the client's primary language.

- The client must be competent to make health care decisions. If given sufficient information, a competent adult can make decisions regarding health care. A competent adult is a person over 18 years of age who is alert and oriented. A client who is confused, disoriented, or sedated is not considered functionally competent, and a legal guardian or representative must make decisions for the client.

Three groups of people cannot provide consent: minors, clients who are unconscious, and mentally ill persons. Parents or guardians must sign consent for minors and adults who have the mental capacity of a child. In some states, minors are allowed to give consent for such procedures as blood donations, treatment for substance abuse, treatment for mental health problems, and treatment for reproductive health concerns such as sexually transmitted infections or pregnancy (Brent, 2001). In addition, emancipated minors may give consent for themselves. An emancipated minor is someone under 18 years of age who is married, pregnant, a member of the military, or living independently. These statutes may vary by state. An unconscious person, or someone who has been injured in a way that would preclude the person from being considered competent, cannot sign a consent form. Usually the closest adult relative, depending on local statutes, will sign the consent for the client. In a life-

CULTURALLY COMPETENT CARE	Overcoming a Language Barrier

Health institutions have a legal responsibility and an ethical obligation to ensure that residents who do not speak English are informed regarding procedures or treatments. Using a translator is not foolproof and can result in errors. The best translator is one trained in the use of medical terminology. A telephone translator service, often available 24 hours every day, is available if there is no one physically present in the hospital. Brief the translator on the subject to be covered, the scope of services needed, and the importance of translating all parties' words as accurately as possible. Ask if the interpreter knows of any cultural beliefs that could affect the encounter, and verify that the translator has signed a form requiring confidentiality of information. Introduce the interpreter to the client and, depending on agency policy, you may need to obtain a signed consent from the client to use a translator. Speak to the client, not the translator. Take your time, speak slowly, and observe body language of the client. Ask questions as appropriate and ask the client to repeat any instructions provided to confirm understanding. Document that the client gave consent to the use of an interpreter and the full name and title of the interpreter. Document if the interpreter is a professional or a family member.

Modified from *RN* vol. 60, no. 10, pp. 67–69. *RN* is a copyrighted publication of Advanstar Communications Inc. All rights reserved.

threatening emergency the law generally agrees that consent is implied to provide necessary care if a relative is unknown or unreachable. Those judged mentally ill by professionals require a legal guardian or close relative to sign consent forms.

When all three elements of informed consent are present, the client may sign the form. Usually the client signs a form provided by the agency or facility that is a record of the informed consent, not the informed consent itself. The nurse may be asked to obtain the client's signature and witness the form. The nurse's signature confirms three things: the client gave consent voluntarily, the signature is authentic, and the client appeared competent to give consent. The nurse advocates for the client by verifying that the client received enough information to give consent. If the client has questions or if the nurse has doubts that that client understands, the nurse must notify the health provider performing the procedure. The nurse is not responsible for explaining the medical or surgical procedure and could be liable for giving incorrect or incomplete information or interfering with the client–provider relationship.

Informed consent also applies to nurses providing bedside care. The nurse relies on orally expressed consent or implied consent for most nursing interventions. It is imperative to remember the importance of explaining all nursing procedures, ensuring that the client understands, and obtaining permission.

The right of consent also involves the right of refusal (Guido, 2009). Remind clients that they can change their minds and cancel the procedure at any time because the right to refuse continues even after signing the consent. It is important to verify that the client is aware of the pros and cons of refusal and is making an informed decision. The nurse needs to notify the health provider of the client's refusal and document the refusal in the chart.

Documentation is an important aspect of informed consent. Document the client's concerns or questions, along with notification of the health care provider. Document when the client states understanding and record any teaching as a result of nursing-related questions. Any special circumstances, such as use of an interpreter, should also be documented.

DELEGATION   The American Nurses Association (2007) defines **delegation** as "the transfer of responsibility for the performance of an activity from one person to another while retaining accountability for the outcome." Competent unlicensed assistive personnel (UAP) can assist the nurse, thereby allowing the nurse to perform functions appropriate to only the nurse's scope of practice, but the task assigned must be appropriate to the UAP's knowledge and ability. From a legal perspective, the nurse's authority to delegate is based on laws and regulations. Nurses must be familiar with their nurse practice act to determine if delegation is permitted, what can be delegated, and any guidelines explaining the nurse's responsibility when delegating (Sheehan, 2001).

In addition to knowing their own scope of practice, nurses must also understand the scope of practice of the UAP, which may vary depending on the facility's policies and procedures. Thus, the nurse must know the employer's policies and procedures for delegation, the UAP's job description, and the UAP's skill level. The NCSBN has provided "five rights of delegation" to help nurses make delegation decisions (see Chapter 15 ∞). Remember, while the nurse delegates the performance of the task, the accountability for the outcome remains with the nurse (Zimmerman & Jackson, 2004).

OTHER LEGAL ASPECTS OF NURSING PRACTICE

Violence, Abuse, and Neglect   Violent behavior can include domestic violence, child abuse, elder abuse, or any number of other situations in which one person behaves violently toward another. Nurses can often identify and assess cases of violence against others and are often included as mandated reporters, meaning the nurse is required by law to report the situation to the proper authorities. See Chapter 9 ∞ for additional information about child abuse and Chapter 10 ∞ for elder abuse.

The Americans with Disabilities Act   Passed by the U.S. Congress in 1990 and fully implemented in 1994, this law prohibits discrimination on the basis of disability in employment, public services, and public accommodations. The nurse is instrumental in helping clients understand the opportunities provided by this law (Watson, 2000, p. 199). The purposes of the act are to provide a clear and comprehensive national mandate for eliminating discrimination against individuals with disabilities, to provide clear, strong, consistent, enforceable standards addressing discrimination against individuals with disabilities, and to ensure that the federal government plays a central role in enforcing standards established under the act.

Controlled Substances U.S. laws regulate the distribution and use of controlled substances such as narcotics, depressants, stimulants, and hallucinogens. Misuse of controlled substances leads to criminal penalties (see Chapter 22 ∞).

The Impaired Nurse The term impaired nurse refers to a nurse whose ability to perform the functions of a nurse is diminished by chemical dependency on drugs or alcohol or by mental illness (Blair, 2002). Approximately 3% to 6% of nurses may practice while impaired because of chemical dependency or psychiatric illness, and alcohol is the number one substance abused (Trossman, 2003, p. 27). More than half of nurses who abuse substances began abusing them before they finished their nursing education (Danis, 2004). As a result, resolutions have been passed by nursing organizations to ensure that nurses and student nurses with chemical dependencies receive treatment and support, not discipline and derision (Trossman, 2003). Employers must have sound policies and procedures for identifying and intervening in situations involving an impaired nurse, with the primary concern of protecting the client as well as identifying the problem quickly so appropriate treatment can be instituted.

Sexual Harassment Sexual harassment is a violation of the individual's rights and a form of discrimination, defined as "unwelcome sexual advances, requests for sexual favors, and other verbal or physical conduct of a sexual nature" (EEOC, 2009, section 1604.11). The victim or the harasser may be male or female, and the victim does not have to be of the opposite sex.

Abortion Abortion laws provide specific guidelines for nurses about what is legally permissible. The Supreme Court of the United States held that the constitutional rights of privacy give a woman the right to control her own body to the extent that she can abort her fetus in the early stage of pregnancy. In 1989 a Supreme Court decision banned the use of public funds or facilities for performing or assisting with abortions. Many statutes also include conscience clauses, upheld by the Supreme Court, designed to protect nurses and hospitals from participating, in an action they find morally wrong, without retaliation or discrimination.

DEATH AND RELATED ISSUES The nurse's role in legal issues related to death is prescribed in the laws of the region and the policies of the health care institution. These laws determine such things as the legality of removing feeding tubes from a person in a chronic vegetative state or do-not-resuscitate orders that specify the extent of life-sustaining measures. Clients who wish to donate organs create complex issues as well in terms of what medications, treatments, or equipment must be continued until harvesting of the organs. Many of these issues spark strong ethical concerns.

Advance Health Care Directives Advance health care directives include a variety of legal and lay documents that allow persons to specify aspects of care they wish to receive should they become unable to make or communicate their preferences. The Patient Self-Determination Act implemented in 1991 requires all health care facilities receiving Medicare and Medicaid reimbursement to recognize advance directives, ask clients whether they have advance directives, and provide educational materials advising clients of their rights to declare their personal wishes regarding treatment decisions, including the right to refuse medical treatment. It is important for clients and families to recognize that they always have the right to change their advance directives. Nurses need to assure that clients and families have an accurate understanding of life-sustaining measures.

There are two types of advance health care directives: the living will and the health care proxy or surrogate. The living will provides specific instructions about what medical treatment the client chooses to omit or refuse in the event that the client is unable to make those decisions. The **health care proxy**, also called a durable power of attorney for health care, is a notarized or witnessed statement appointing someone else to manage health care treatment decisions when the client is unable to do so.

Autopsy Autopsy or postmortem examination is an examination of the body after death. The law describes under what circumstances an autopsy must be performed, such as when death is sudden or occurs within 48 hours of admission to a hospital. The organs and tissues of the body are examined to establish the exact cause of death, to learn more about the disease, and to assist in the accumulation of statistical data. It is the responsibility of the physician to obtain consent for an autopsy from the decedent before death or the next of kin. In some instances, such as a suspicious death, no consent is required.

Certification of Death Certification of death is a formal determination of death and must be performed by a physician, coroner, or nurse, depending on local regulations. The granting of authority to nurses to pronounce death is regulated by state laws and may be limited to nurses in long-term care, home health, and hospice agencies. By law, a death certificate must be completed when a person dies; it is usually signed by the physician and filed with a local health or government office. The family is given a copy to use for legal matters, such as insurance claims.

Do-Not-Resuscitate Orders (DNR) Do-not-resuscitate (DNR) orders or "no code" orders may be written by the physician for clients who have a terminal condition, irreversible illness, or expected death. A DNR order is generally written when the client or proxy has expressed the wish for no resuscitation in the event of a respiratory or cardiac arrest. Many physicians are reluctant to write such an order if there is conflict within the family. A DNR order is written to indicate the goals of treatment has changed from restorative to palliative measures that will keep the client comfortable and allow for a dignified death without use of further life-sustaining measures. The American Nurses Association (ANA) (2003) recommends that: the competent client's values and choices be given priority over family or health care provider's values; when the client is incompetent, an advance directive or proxy decision maker acts for the client; a DNR order may be written only after a discussion between the client, the client's family, and designated decision maker and the health care team; the DNR orders must be clearly documented, reviewed, and updated periodically in order to meet standards of the Joint Commission on Accreditation of Healthcare Organizations; and that the DNR order is separate from other aspects of a client's care and does not imply that other types of care should be withdrawn. The ANA also recommends a process to help resolve conflicts between clients, their families, and health care professionals, usually in the form of ethics committees. Many states permit clients living at home to arrange special orders so that emergency technicians called to the home in the event of a cardiopulmonary arrest will respect the DNR order. Some states allow the physician to specify types of care to be provided under the DNR order, such as comfort care only, medications only, defibrillation only, or CPR without intubation. Other states allow for only full resuscitation or no resuscitation.

Euthanasia   Euthanasia is the act of painlessly putting to death persons suffering from incurable or distressing disease. It is sometimes referred to as "mercy killing." Regardless of compassion and good intentions or moral convictions, euthanasia is legally wrong in many parts of the United States and can lead to criminal charges of homicide or to a civil lawsuit for withholding treatment or providing an unacceptable standard of care. Euthanasia is not to be confused with withdrawing life-support measures. Euthanasia is putting a person to death, not allowing them to die. Voluntary euthanasia refers to situations in which the dying individual desires some control over the time and manner of death and is illegal in most states. Oregon passed the Death with Dignity Act in 1994 allowing physician-assisted suicide (voluntary euthanasia) if two physicians agree with the terminal diagnosis and conclude the client is of sound mind to make the decision to be helped to die. The law took effect in November 1997. North Carolina, Utah, and Wyoming do not have statutes criminalizing voluntary euthanasia. Ohio's supreme court has ruled that assisted suicide is not a crime, and Virginia has no real case law on the matter. The remaining 44 states criminalize voluntary euthanasia.

Inquest   An inquest is a legal inquiry into the cause or manner of a death. The inquest is conducted under the jurisdiction of a coroner or medical examiner. A **coroner** is a public official, not necessarily a physician, appointed or elected to inquire into the causes of death. A medical examiner is a physician and usually has advanced education in pathology or forensic medicine. Agency policy dictates who is responsible for reporting deaths to the coroner or medical examiner.

Organ Donation   Under the Uniform Anatomical Gift Act and the National Organ Transplant Act in the United States, people 18 years or older and of sound mind may make a gift of all or any part of their own bodies for the following purposes: for medical or dental education, research, advancement of medical or dental science, therapy, or transplantation. The donation can be made by a provision in a will or by signing a card-like form. This card is usually carried at all times by the person who signed it. The person can revoke the gift either by destroying the card or by revoking the gift orally in the presence of two witnesses. Nurses may serve as witnesses for people consenting to donate organs. In many states, if there is no valid donor document, health care workers are required to discuss with survivors of a potential organ donor the option to make an anatomical gift. Survivors are obliged to grant or withhold donations in accordance with their knowledge of the donor's views on anatomical gifts.

Legal Responsibilities of Student Nurses

Nursing students are responsible for their own actions and liable for their own acts of negligence committed during the course of clinical experiences. When they perform duties that are within the scope of professional nursing, such as administering an injection, they are legally held to the same standard of skill and competence as a registered professional nurse. Lower standards are not applied to the actions of nursing students.

CLINICAL ALERT

Students do not practice on their instructor's or another nurse's license. Each nurse and nursing student is responsible and accountable for providing safe client care. As a result, students should never do anything they are not competent to do.

Nursing students are not considered employees of the agencies in which they receive clinical experience because these nursing programs contract with agencies to provide clinical experiences for students. In cases of negligence involving such students, the hospital or agency (e.g., public health agency) and the educational institution may be held liable for negligent actions by students.

Nursing students need to be aware that most state boards of nursing require a reporting of prior criminal history when applying for licensure. A person with past felony or certain misdemeanor offenses may be denied licensure even though that individual graduated from an approved nursing program. Nursing students who are unsure of their personal situation are advised to contact their state board of nursing for more information.

Students in clinical situations must be assigned learning experiences within their capabilities and be given reasonable guidance and supervision. Nursing instructors are responsible for assigning students to the care of clients and for providing reasonable supervision. Failure to provide reasonable supervision, or the assignment of a client to a student who is not prepared and competent, can be a basis for liability.

To fulfill responsibilities to clients and to minimize chances for liability, nursing students need to make sure

---

LIFESPAN CONSIDERATIONS
The Omnibus Budget Reconciliation Act

Children

The Omnibus Budget Reconciliation Act of 1993 (OBRA 93) created the Pediatric Vaccine Distribution Program (known as Vaccines for Children [VFC] Program). States are required to establish a program for purchase and distribution of pediatric vaccines to program-registered providers who immunize certain specified groups of children without charge for the vaccine.

Older Adults

The Omnibus Budget Reconciliation Act (OBRA) was passed in 1990 and lists requirements for ensuring quality of care in skilled nursing facilities. These requirements mainly affect older adults, but also pertain to any resident in a long-term or skilled nursing facility. These standards were developed to enhance the quality of life of each resident and to focus on achieving the highest practical physical, mental, and psychosocial well-being for residents of these facilities. Requirements from OBRA include a quality assessment and assurance committee that meets quarterly to discuss resident's condition and make appropriate revisions; a physician visit at least every 30 days for 3 months then every 90 days, a registered nurse in the facility who works at least 40 hours per week, rehabilitation services for each resident, nurse's aides with special training on abuse and neglect, availability of social workers, careful monitoring and reevaluation of psychotropic drugs, and residents' rights must be recognized and honored.

---

they are prepared to carry out the necessary care for assigned clients, ask for help or supervision in situations in which they feel inadequately prepared or incompetent, and comply with agency policies at their clinical site and those supplied by the school of nursing.

Students who work as part-time or temporary nursing assistants or aides must also remember that legally they can perform only those tasks that appear in the job description of a nurse's aide or assistant. Even though a student may have received instruction and acquired competence in administering injections or suctioning a tracheostomy tube, the student cannot legally perform these tasks while employed as an aide or assistant. While acting as a paid employee, the student is covered for negligent acts by the employer, not by the school of nursing.

VALUES, ETHICS, MORALITY, AND ADVOCACY

Nurses deal with intimate and fundamental human events such as birth, death, and suffering. They must decide the morality of their own actions when they face the many ethical issues that surround such sensitive areas. The nurse–client relationship requires nurses to provide support and advocate for clients and families who are facing difficult choices and

who are living the results of choices others made for them. Issues such as cost containment and the nursing shortage are creating new moral problems and intensifying old ones, making it more critical than ever for nurses to make sound moral decisions. Nurses must develop sensitivity to ethical dimensions of nursing practice and examine their own values in addition to understanding how values influence their decisions. Nurses need to think ahead about the moral problems they are likely to face. This section explores the influences of values and moral frameworks on the ethical dimensions of nursing practice and the nurse's role as client advocate.

Values

Values are enduring beliefs or attitudes about the worth of a person, object, idea, or action. Values are important because they influence decisions and actions, including nurses' ethical decision making. Even though they may be unspoken and perhaps even unconsciously held, questions of value underlie all moral dilemmas. Of course, not all values are moral values. For example, people hold values about work, family, religion, politics, money, and relationships, to name just a few. Values are often taken for granted. In the same way that people are not aware of their breathing, they usually do not think about their values; they simply accept them and act on them. Values may be grouped into value sets held by an individual. People organize their set of values internally along a continuum from most important to least important, forming a value system. Value systems are basic to a way of life, give direction to life, and form the basis of behavior—especially behavior that is based on decisions or choices.

Values consist of beliefs and attitudes, which are related, but not identical, to values. People have many beliefs and attitudes, but only a small number of values. **Beliefs** (or opinions) are interpretations or conclusions that people accept as true. They are often based more on faith than fact and may or may not be true. Beliefs do not necessarily involve values. For example, the statement "If I study hard I will get a good grade" expresses a belief that does not involve a value. By contrast, the statement "Good grades are really important to me so I must study hard to obtain good grades" involves both a value and a belief. **Attitudes** are mental positions or feelings toward a person, object, or idea. An attitude lasts over time, whereas a belief may last only briefly. Attitudes have thinking and behavioral aspects.

Values are learned through observation and experience. As a result, they are heavily influenced by a person's sociocultural environment—that is, by societal traditions; by cultural, ethnic, and religious groups; and by family and peer groups. Nurses should keep in mind the influence of values on health (see Chapter 5 ∞). Although people derive values from society and their individual subgroups, they internalize some or all of these values and perceive them as personal values. People need societal values to feel accepted, and they need personal values to have a sense of individuality.

PROFESSIONAL VALUES   Nurses' professional values are acquired during socialization into nursing from codes of ethics, nursing experiences, teachers, and peers. The American Association of Colleges of Nursing (AACN), (1998) identified five values essential for the professional nurse. Altruism is a concern for the welfare and well-being of others, reflected by the nurse's concern for the welfare of clients and other health care providers. Autonomy is the right to self-determination, reflected by the nurse's respect of the client's rights to make decisions. Human dignity is respecting the uniqueness of individuals, displayed when the nurse respects the cultures, beliefs, and perspectives of others. Integrity is acting in accordance with an appropriate code of ethics and accepted standards of practice, shown when the nurse is honest and provides care based on an ethical framework acceptable within the profession. Social justice is upholding moral, legal, and humanistic principles, reflected when the nurse treats all clients equally.

Other behaviors that reflect professional behaviors include advocating for clients, taking risks on behalf of clients and colleagues, mentoring other professionals, and planning care in collaboration with clients and families. Nurses have professional behavior when they protect the client's privacy, honor the rights of clients and families to make decisions, and provide information to clients so they are able to make informed decisions. Nursing professionals must be honest and seek to remedy errors made by themselves or others, demonstrate accountability for their actions, and document care honestly and accurately.

VALUES CLARIFICATION   Values clarification is a process by which people identify, examine, and develop their own individual values. A principle of values clarification is that no one set of values is right for everyone. When people can identify their values, they can retain or change them and thus act based on freely chosen, rather than unconscious, values. Values clarification promotes personal growth by fostering awareness, empathy, and insight (Box 2–2). Therefore, it is an important step for nurses to take in dealing with ethical problems.

Nurses and nursing students need to examine the values they hold about life, death, health, and illness. One strategy for gaining awareness of personal values is to consider one's attitudes about specific issues such as abortion or euthanasia, asking: "Can I accept this, or live with this?" "Why does this bother me?" "What would I do or want done in this situation?" Nurses use critical thinking (see Chapter 6 ∞) to reflect on various viewpoints and previous experiences that may have influenced their own current values.

Clarifying Client Values   To plan effective care, nurses need to identify clients' values as they influence and relate to a particular health problem. For example, a client with failing eyesight will probably place a high value on the ability to see, and a client with chronic pain will value comfort. Normally, people take such things for granted. For information about health beliefs and values, see Chapter 5 ∞. When clients hold unclear or conflicting values that are detrimental to their health, the nurse should use values clarification as an intervention. Behaviors that may indicate the need for values clarification include ignoring a health professional's advice, inconsistent communication or behavior, numerous admissions for the same problem, or confusion or uncertainty about what course of action to take.

Processes that may help clients clarify their values include listing alternatives and examining possible consequences of choices. To determine if the client chose freely, ask "Did you have any say in that decision?" or "Do you have a choice?" Determine how clients feel about the choice they made and affirm the choice by asking how they will share the choice with others. Once the client has made a choice, the nurse needs to determine if the client is prepared to act on the decision. To determine whether the client acts with a pattern, ask how many times the client has done this before or if she or he would act that way again in the future. When implementing these steps, the nurse assists the client to think each question through, but does not impose personal values. The nurse rarely, if ever, offers an opinion

---

BOX 2–2	**Values Clarification**

Choosing (cognitive)

Beliefs are chosen

- Freely, without outside pressure
- From among alternatives
- After reflecting and considering consequences

Example: A person learns about energy resources, production, and consumption; the greenhouse effect; and other environmental issues, including ways to minimize use of and to recycle limited resources.

Prizing (affective)

Chosen beliefs are prized and cherished

Example: The person is proud of the belief that he or she has an obligation to participate in some way in reducing environmental waste.

Acting (behavioral)

Chosen beliefs are

- Affirmed to others
- Incorporated into one's behavior
- Repeated consistently in one's life

Example: The person participates in the city recycling program for household waste, uses public transportation rather than driving a personal car when possible, helps organize recycling in the workplace, and is active in legislative and political activities related to environmental issues.

Note: From Values and Teaching, 2nd ed. (p. 47), by L. Raths, M. Harmin, and S. Simon, copyright 1978. Adapted and reprinted with permission of the authors.

when the client asks for it—and then only with great care or when the nurse is an expert in the area. Since each situation is different, what the nurse would choose in his or her own life may not be relevant to the client's circumstances.

Morality and Ethics

The term **ethics** has several meanings in common use. It refers to (a) the study of morality, (b) the practices or beliefs of a certain person, and (c) the expected standards of moral behavior of a particular group as described in the group's formal code of professional ethics. Nurses have been viewed as the most ethical professionals in many recent Gallup polls (Gallup, 2007). Bioethics is ethics as applied to human life or health (e.g., to decisions about abortion or euthanasia). Nursing ethics refers to ethical issues that occur in nursing practice. The American Nurses Association (ANA) revised *Scope and Standards of Practice* (2003) holds nurses accountable for their ethical conduct. Professional Performance Standard 12 relates to ethics (Box 2–3).

Morality (or morals) is similar to ethics, and many use the terms interchangeably. **Morality** usually refers to private, personal standards of what is right and wrong in conduct, character, and attitude. Sometimes the first clue to the moral nature of a situation is the tendency to respond to the situation with words such as *ought, should, right, wrong, good,* and *bad.* Moral issues are concerned with important social values and norms; they are not about trivial things.

Nurses should distinguish between morality and law. Laws reflect the moral values of a society, and they offer guidance in determining what is moral. However, an action

---

<table>
<tr><td>**BOX 2–3**</td><td>**ANA Standards of Professional Performance**</td></tr>
</table>

Standard 12: Ethics

Measurement Criteria

- Uses the Code for Nurses with Interpretive Statements (ANA, 2001) to guide practice.
- Delivers care in a manner that preserves patient autonomy, dignity, and rights.
- Maintains patient confidentiality within legal and regulatory parameters.
- Serves as a patient advocate assisting patients in developing skills for self-advocacy.
- Maintains a therapeutic and professional patient–nurse relationship with appropriate professional role boundaries.
- Demonstrates a commitment to practicing self-care, managing stress, and connecting with self and others.
- Contributes to resolving ethical issues of patients, colleagues, or systems as evidenced in such activities as participating on ethics committees.
- Reports illegal, incompetent, or impaired practices.

Note: Reprinted with permission from American Nurses Association, *Nursing: Scope and Standards of Practice* © 2004 Nursebooks.org, Silver Spring, MD 20910.

---

can be legal but not moral, or can be moral but illegal. Nurses should also distinguish between morality and religion as they relate to health practices, although the two concepts are related. Common instances of differences in moral perspectives on health involving religious beliefs include blood transfusions, abortion, sterilization, and contraceptive and safer sex counseling.

MORAL DEVELOPMENT, FRAMEWORK, AND PRINCIPLES

Moral development is the process of learning to tell the difference between right and wrong and of learning what ought and ought not to be done. It is a complex process that begins in childhood and continues throughout life.

Moral theories provide different frameworks through which nurses can view and clarify disturbing client care situations. Nurses can use moral theories in developing explanations for their ethical decisions and actions and in discussing problem situations with others. Consequence-based (teleological) theories look to the outcomes of an action in judging whether that action is right or wrong. Principle-based theories (deontological) involve logical and formal processes and emphasize individual rights, duties, and obligations. The morality of an action is determined not by its consequences but by whether it is done according to an impartial, objective principle. Relationships-based (caring) theories stress courage, generosity, commitment, and the need to nurture and maintain relationships. Caring theories judge actions according to a perspective of caring and responsibility.

A moral framework guides moral decisions, but it does not determine the outcome. Imagine a situation in which a frail, older adult client has made it clear that he does not want further surgery, but the family and surgeon insist. Three nurses have each decided that they will not help with preparations for surgery and that they will work through proper channels to try to prevent it. Using consequence-based reasoning, Nurse A thinks, "Surgery will cause him more suffering; he probably will not survive it anyway, and the family may even feel guilty later." Using principles-based reasoning, Nurse B thinks, "This violates the principle of autonomy. This man has a right to decide what happens to his body." Using caring-based reasoning, Nurse C thinks, "My relationship to this client commits me to protecting him and meeting his needs, and I feel such compassion for him. I must try to help the family understand that he needs their support." Each of these perspectives is based on the nurse's moral framework.

Moral principles are statements about broad, general, philosophical concepts such as autonomy and justice. They provide the foundation for moral rules, which are specific prescriptions for actions. For example, the rule "People should not lie" is based on the moral principle of respect for persons (autonomy). Principles are useful in ethical discussions because even if people disagree about which action is right in a situation, they may be able to agree on the principles that apply. Such an agreement can serve as the basis for a solution that is acceptable to all parties.

Autonomy refers to the right to make one's own decisions. Nurses who follow this principle recognize that each client is unique, has the right to be what that person is, and has the right to choose personal goals. People have "inward autonomy" if they have the ability to make choices; they have "outward autonomy" if their choices are not limited or imposed by others.

Honoring the principle of autonomy means that the nurse respects a client's right to make decisions even when those choices seem to the nurse not to be in the client's best interest. It also means treating others with consideration. In a health care setting, this principle is violated, for example, when a nurse disregards clients' subjective accounts of their symptoms (e.g., pain). Finally, respect for autonomy means that people should not be treated as an impersonal source of knowledge or training. This principle comes into play, for example, in the requirement that clients provide informed consent before tests, procedures, or participating as a research subject can be carried out.

Nonmaleficence is the duty to "do no harm." Although this would seem to be a simple principle to follow, in reality it is complex. Harm can mean intentionally causing harm, placing someone at risk of harm, or unintentionally causing harm. In nursing, intentional harm is never acceptable. However, in health care a person may be at risk of harm such as when administering medications, since many drugs carry the potential for risk in addition to their beneficial effects. Unintentional harm occurs when a risk could not have been anticipated. Caregivers do not always agree on the degree of risk that is morally permissible in order to attempt the beneficial result.

Beneficence means "doing good." Nurses are obligated to do good, that is, to implement actions that benefit clients and their support persons. However, doing good can also pose a risk of doing harm. For example, a nurse may advise a client about a strenuous exercise program to improve general health, but should not do so if the client is at risk of a heart attack.

Justice is often referred to as fairness. Nurses often face decisions in which a sense of justice should prevail. For example, a nurse making home visits finds one client tearful and depressed, and knows she could help by staying for 30 more minutes to talk. However, that would take time from her next client, who is a diabetic who needs a great deal of teaching and observation. The nurse will need to weigh the facts carefully in order to divide her time justly among her clients.

Fidelity means to be faithful to agreements and promises. By virtue of their standing as professional caregivers, nurses have responsibilities to clients, employers, government, and society, as well as to themselves. Nurses often make promises such as "I'll be right back with your pain medication" or "I'll find out for you." Clients take such promises seriously, and so should nurses.

Veracity refers to telling the truth. Although this seems straightforward, in practice choices are not always clear. Should a nurse tell the truth when it is known that it will cause harm? Does a nurse tell a lie when it is known that the lie will relieve anxiety and fear? Lying to sick or dying people is rarely justified. The loss of trust in the nurse and the anxiety caused by not knowing the truth, for example, usually outweigh any benefits derived from lying.

Nurses must also have professional accountability and responsibility. According to the *Code of Ethics for Nurses* (ANA, 2001), **accountability** means "answerable to oneself and others for one's own actions," while *responsibility* refers to "the specific accountability or liability associated with the performance of duties of a particular role." Thus, the ethical nurse is able to explain the rationale behind every action and recognizes the standards to which he or she will be held.

NURSING ETHICS   In the past, nurses looked on ethical decision making as the physician's responsibility. However, no one profession is responsible for ethical decisions, nor does expertise in one discipline such as medicine or nursing necessarily make a person an expert in ethics. As situations become more complex, input from all caregivers becomes increasingly important.

Ethical standards of the Joint Commission on Accreditation of Healthcare Organizations (JCAHO) mandate that health care institutions provide ethics committees or a similar structure to write guidelines and policies and to provide education, counseling, and support on ethical issues (JCAHO, 2006). These multidisciplinary committees may include nurses and can be asked to review a case and provide guidance to a competent client, an incompetent client's family, or health care providers. They ensure that relevant facts of a case are brought out, provide a forum in which diverse views can be expressed, provide support for caregivers, and can reduce the institution's legal risks. In some settings, ethics rounds are held.

Nursing Code of Ethics   A **code of ethics** is a formal statement of a group's ideals and values. It is a set of ethical principles that (a) is shared by members of the group, (b) reflects their moral judgments over time, and (c) serves as a standard for their professional actions. Codes of ethics usually have higher requirements than legal standards, and they are never lower than the legal standards of the profession. Nurses are responsible for being familiar with the code that governs their practice.

International, national, and state nursing associations have established codes of ethics. The International Council of Nurses (ICN) first adopted a code of ethics in 1953, and the most recent revisions were printed in 2005. The ANA first adopted a *Code for Nurses* in 1950. The current version reflects several major changes in the code, now called the *Code of Ethics for Nurses* (Box 2–4). A statement on compassion has been added, and the duty to protect patients has been broadened to include all patient rights. Several previous provisions have been revised, and the provision on delegation has been significantly enhanced to reflect the increased use of unlicensed assistive personnel.

Nursing codes of ethics exist for many purposes. They inform the public about the minimum standards of the profession and help them understand professional nursing conduct, they provide a sign of the profession's commitment to the public it serves, outline the major ethical considerations of the profession, provide ethical standards for professional behavior, guide the profession in self-regulation, and remind nurses of the special responsibility they assume when caring for the sick.

BOX 2–4   ANA Code of Ethics for Nurses (Approved July 2001)

1. The nurse, in all professional relationships, practices with compassion and respect for the inherent dignity, worth, and uniqueness of every individual, unrestricted by considerations of social or economic status, personal attributes, or the nature of health problems.
2. The nurse's primary commitment is to the patient, whether an individual, family, group, or community.
3. The nurse promotes, advocates for, and strives to protect the health, safety, and rights of the patient.
4. The nurse is responsible and accountable for individual nursing practice and determines the appropriate delegation of tasks consistent with the nurse's obligation to provide optimum patient care.
5. The nurse owes the same duties to self as to others, including the responsibility to preserve integrity and safety, to maintain competence, and to continue personal and professional growth.
6. The nurse participates in establishing, maintaining, and improving health care environments and conditions of

employment conducive to the provision of quality health care and consistent with the values of the profession through individual and collective action.
7. The nurse participates in the advancement of the profession through contributions to practice, education, administration, and knowledge development.
8. The nurse collaborates with other health professionals and the public in promoting community, national, and international efforts to meet health needs.
9. The profession of nursing, as represented by associations and their members, is responsible for articulating nursing values, for maintaining the integrity of the profession and its practice, and for shaping social policy.

Note: Reprinted with permission from American Nurses Association, *Code of Ethics for Nurses with Interpretive Statements*, © 2001 Nursesbooks.org, Silver Spring, MD 20910.

Origins of Ethical Conflicts in Nursing   Nurses' growing awareness of ethical conflicts has occurred largely because of social and technological changes and nurses' conflicting loyalties and obligations. Current social issues include providing health care to all, despite ability to pay. Workplace redesign under managed care involves issues of fairness and allocation of resources. Technology creates new issues that did not exist in earlier times, such as organ transplantation, care of very small premature infants, and the ability to predict future illness based on genetic code. Because of their unique position in the health care system, nurses experience conflicts among their loyalties and obligations to clients, families, primary care providers, employing institutions, and licensing bodies. According to the nursing code of ethics, the nurse's first loyalty is to the client. However, it is not always easy to determine which action best serves the client's needs.

Making Ethical Decisions   Responsible ethical reasoning is rational and systematic. It should be based on ethical principles and codes rather than on emotions, intuition, fixed policies, or precedent (that is, an earlier similar occurrence). A good decision is one that is in the client's best interest and at the same time preserves the integrity of all involved. Nurses have ethical obligations to their clients, to the agency that employs them, and to primary care providers (Box 2–5). Therefore, nurses must weigh competing factors when making ethical decisions. Although ethical reasoning is principle based and has the client's well-being at the center, being involved in ethical problems and dilemmas is stressful for the nurse. The nurse may feel torn between obligations to the client, the family, and the employer. What is in the client's best interest may be contrary to the nurse's personal belief system. In settings in which ethical issues arise frequently, nurses should establish support systems

such as team conferences and use of counseling professionals to allow expression of their feelings.

Many nursing problems are not moral problems at all, but simply questions of good nursing practice. An important first step in ethical decision making is to determine whether a moral situation exists. The following criteria may be used:

- A difficult choice exists between actions that conflict with the needs of one or more persons.
- Moral principles or frameworks exist that can be used to provide some justification for the action.
- The choice is guided by a process of weighing reasons.
- The decision must be freely and consciously chosen.
- The choice is affected by personal feelings and by the particular context of the situation.

Although the nurse's input is important, in reality, several people are usually involved in making an ethical decision. The client, family, spiritual support persons, and other members of the health care team work together in reaching ethical decisions. Therefore, collaboration, communication, and compromise are important skills for health profession-

---

BOX 2–5   Examples of Nurses' Obligations in Ethical Decisions

- Maximize the client's well-being.
- Balance the client's need for autonomy with family members' responsibilities for the client's well-being.
- Support each family member and enhance the family support system.
- Carry out hospital policies.
- Protect other clients' well-being.
- Protect the nurse's own standards of care.

als. When nurses do not have the autonomy to act on their moral or ethical choices, compromise becomes essential.

Strategies to Enhance Ethical Decisions and Practice Several strategies help nurses overcome possible organizational and social constraints that may hinder the ethical practice of nursing and create moral distress for nurses. A nurse is advised to do the following:

- Become aware of one's own values and the ethical aspects of nursing.
- Be familiar with nursing codes of ethics.
- Seek continuing education opportunities to stay knowledgeable about ethical issues in nursing.
- Respect the values, opinions, and responsibilities of other health care professionals that may be different from one's own.
- Participate in or establish ethics rounds. Ethics rounds use hypothetical or real cases that focus on the ethical dimensions of client care rather than on the client's clinical diagnosis and treatment.
- Serve on institutional ethics committees.
- Strive for collaborative practice in which nurses function effectively in cooperation with other health care professionals.

SPECIFIC ETHICAL ISSUES Some of the ethical problems nurses encounter most frequently are issues in the care of HIV/AIDS clients, abortion, organ transplantation, end-of-life decisions, cost-containment issues that jeopardize client welfare and access to health care (resource allocation), and breaches of client confidentiality (e.g., computerized information management).

HIV/AIDS Because of its association with sexual behavior, illicit drug use, and physical decline and death, AIDS has developed a social stigma. Other ethical issues involve testing for HIV status and for the presence of AIDS in health professionals and clients. Questions arise as to whether testing of all providers and clients should be mandatory or voluntary and whether test results should be released to insurance companies, sexual partners, or caregivers. As with all ethical dilemmas, there are both positive and negative implications of each possibility for specific individuals.

Abortion Abortion is a highly publicized issue about which many people feel very strongly. Debate continues, pitting the principle of sanctity of life against the principle of autonomy and the woman's right to control her own body. This is an especially volatile issue because no public consensus has yet been reached. Most state and provincial laws have provisions known as conscience clauses that permit individual physicians and nurses, as well as institutions, to refuse to assist with an abortion if doing so violates their religious or moral principles. However, nurses have no right to impose their values on a client. Nursing codes of ethics support clients' rights to information and counseling in making decisions.

Organ Transplantation Ethical issues related to organ transplantation include allocation of organs, selling of body parts, involvement of children as potential donors, consent, clear definition of death, and conflicts of interest between potential donors and recipients. In some situations, a person's religious belief may also present conflict.

End-of-Life Issues The increase in technological advances and the growing number of older adults have expanded the ethical dilemmas faced by older adults and the health care professions. Providing them with information and professional assistance, as well as the highest quality of care and caring, is of the utmost importance during these times. Some of the most frequent disturbing ethical problems for nurses involve issues that arise around death and dying. These include euthanasia, assisted suicide, termination of life-sustaining treatment, and withdrawing or withholding of food and fluids.

Allocation of Scarce Health Resources Allocation of limited supplies of health care goods and services, including organ transplants, artificial joints, and the services of specialists, has become an especially urgent issue as medical costs continue to rise and more stringent cost-containment measures are implemented. Nursing care is also a health resource with a reducing supply and increasing demand, creating ethical issues requiring workplace redesign with fewer RNs and more unlicensed caregivers and short-staffing concerns. The moral principle of autonomy cannot be applied if it is not possible to give each client what he or she chooses. In this situation, health care providers may use the principle of justice—attempting to choose what is most fair to all. Nurses must continue to look for ways to balance economics and caring in the allocation of health resources.

Management of Personal Health Information In keeping with the principle of autonomy, nurses are obligated to respect clients' privacy and confidentiality. Privacy is both a legal and an ethical mandate. Clients must be able to trust that nurses will reveal details of their situations only as appropriate and will communicate only the information necessary to provide for their health care. Computerized client records make sensitive data accessible to more people, and create issues of confidentiality. Nurses should help develop and follow security measures and policies to ensure appropriate use of client data.

Advocacy

When people are ill, they are frequently unable to assert their rights as they would if they were healthy. An **advocate** is one who expresses and defends the cause of another. The health care system is complex, and many clients are too ill to deal with it. If they are to keep from "falling through the cracks," clients need an advocate to cut through the layers of bureaucracy and help them get what they require.

Values basic to client advocacy include seeing the client as a holistic autonomous being who has the right to make choices and decisions. Clients have the right to expect a nurse–client relationship based on respect, trust, collaboration in problem solving and consideration of their thoughts and feeling. It is the nurse's responsibility to ensure that the client has access to health care services that meet health needs. Clients may also advocate for themselves. Today, clients are seeking more self-determination and control over their own bodies when they are ill.

If a client lacks decision-making capacity, is legally incompetent, or is a minor, these rights can be exercised on the client's behalf by a designated surrogate or proxy decision maker. It is important, however, for the nurse to remember that client control over health decisions is a Western view. In other societies, such decisions may normally be made by the head of the family or another member of the community. The nurse must ascertain the client's and family's views and honor their traditions regarding the locus of decision making.

To help make clients' rights more explicit to both the client and the health care provider, several versions of a patient's bill of rights have been published by consumer organizations. A national bill, H.R. 4628 "Patients' Bill of Rights Act of 2004," is based on the 2001 bipartisan Senate-passed bill that was introduced in the House but never passed. Under the bill, clients would be guaranteed certain rights under their health insurance plans, including the following:

- Basic standards for access to care, including clinical trials
- The ability to gain access to their own physician, and the doctor's ability to communicate with the client without fear of insurance company retaliation
- The assurance that medical decisions about client care will be made by physicians according to sound medical principles

- A fair, independent external review process if needed care is denied by their insurance company
- The right to hold their health plan accountable if a negligent medical decision resulted in injury or harm

THE ADVOCATE'S ROLE   The overall goal of the client advocate is to protect clients' rights. An advocate informs clients about their rights and provides them with the information they need to make informed decisions. An advocate supports clients in their decisions, giving them full or at least mutual responsibility in decision making when they are capable of it. The advocate must be careful to remain objective and not convey approval or disapproval of the client's choices. Advocacy requires accepting and respecting the client's right to decide, even if the nurse believes the decision to be wrong. In mediating, the advocate directly intervenes on the client's behalf, often by influencing others.

Although the goals of advocacy remain the same, home care poses unique concerns for the nurse advocate. For example, while in the hospital, people may operate from the values of the nurses and primary care providers. When they are at home, they tend to operate from their own personal values and may revert to old habits and ways of doing things that may not be beneficial to their health. The nurse may see this as noncompliance; nevertheless, client autonomy must be respected. Limited resources and a lack of client care services may shift the focus from client welfare to concerns about resource allocation. Financial considerations can limit the availability of services and materials, making it difficult to ensure that client needs are met.

CHAPTER HIGHLIGHTS

- Accountability is an essential concept of professional nursing practice under the law.
- Nurses need to understand laws that regulate and affect nursing practice to ensure that their actions are consistent with current legal principles and to protect themselves from liability.
- Nurse practice acts legally define and describe the scope of nursing practice that the law seeks to regulate.
- Competence in nursing practice is determined and maintained by various credentialing methods, such as licensure, certification, and accreditation, that protect the public's welfare and safety.
- Standards of practice published by national and state nursing associations, agency policies and procedures, and job descriptions further delineate the scope of a nurse's practice.
- The nurse has specific legal obligations and responsibilities to clients and employers. As a citizen, the

nurse has the rights and responsibilities shared by all individuals in the society.
- Collective bargaining is one way nurses can improve their working conditions and economic welfare.
- Informed consent implies that (a) the consent was given voluntarily, (b) the client was of age and had the capacity and competency to understand, and (c) the client was given enough information on which to make an informed decision.
- The Americans with Disabilities Act of 1990 prohibits discrimination on the basis of disability in employment, public services, and public accommodations. Nurses need to know how the ADA affects nursing practice.
- Chemical dependence in health care workers is a problem, in part, because of the high levels of stress involved in many health care settings and the easy access to addictive drugs. Chemical impairment includes abuse of alcohol and addictive drugs. The nurse needs to know the proper

reporting of nursing colleagues whose practice is chemically impaired.

- Nurses must be knowledgeable of their responsibilities about legal issues surrounding death: advance directives, autopsies, certification of death, DNR orders, euthanasia, inquests, and organ donation.

- Nurse malpractice, an unintentional tort, can be established when the following criteria are met: (a) the nurse (defendant) owed a duty to the client, (b) the nurse failed to carry out that duty according to standards, (c) there was foreseeability of harm, (d) the client's injury was caused by the nurse's failure to follow the standard, and (e) the client (plaintiff) was injured. The nurse is liable for damages that may be compensated.

- Nurses can be held liable for intentional torts, such as assault and battery, false imprisonment, invasion of privacy, and defamation.

- The Health Insurance Portability and Accountability Act of 1996 (HIPAA) is the first nationwide legislation to protect privacy for health information. HIPAA includes four specific areas: a uniform standard for electronic transfer of information among organizations; standardized numbers for identifying providers, employers, and health plans; a security rule; and a privacy rule.

- Good Samaritan acts protect health professionals from claims of malpractice when they offer assistance at the scene of an emergency, provided that there is no willful wrongdoing or gross departure from normal standards of care.

- Nursing students and practicing nurses can obtain professional liability insurance through professional nursing associations.

- When a client is accidentally injured or involved in an unusual situation, the nurse's first responsibility is to take steps to protect the client and then to notify appropriate agency personnel.

- Nursing students are held to the same standard as licensed nurses and, therefore, need to make certain that they are prepared to provide the necessary care to assigned clients. It is important that students ask for help or supervision in situations for which they feel inadequately prepared.

- Values are enduring beliefs that give direction and meaning to life and guide a person's behavior.

- Values clarification is a process in which people identify, examine, and develop their own values.

- Nursing ethics refers to the moral problems that arise in nursing practice and to ethical decisions that nurses make.

- Morality refers to what is right and wrong in conduct, character, or attitude.

- Moral issues are those that arouse conscience, are concerned with important values and norms, and evoke words such as *good, bad, right, wrong, should*, and *ought*.

- Three common moral frameworks (approaches) are consequence-based (teleological), principles-based (deontological), and relationship-based (caring-based) theories.

- Moral principles (e.g., autonomy, beneficence, nonmaleficence, justice, fidelity, and veracity) are broad, general philosophical concepts that can be used to make and explain moral choices.

- A professional code of ethics is a formal statement of a group's ideals and values that serves as a standard and guideline for the group's professional actions and informs the public of its commitment.

- Ethical problems are created as a result of changes in society, advances in technology, conflicts within nursing itself, and nurses' conflicting loyalties and obligations (e.g., to clients, families, employers, primary care providers, and other nurses).

- Nurses' ethical decisions are influenced by their moral theories and principles, levels of cognitive development, personal and professional values, and nursing codes of ethics.

- The goal of ethical reasoning, in the context of nursing, is to reach a mutual, peaceful agreement that is in the best interests of the client; reaching the agreement may require compromise.

- Nurses are responsible for determining their own actions and for supporting clients who are making moral decisions or for whom decisions are being made by others.

- Nurses can enhance their ethical practice and client advocacy by clarifying their own values, understanding the values of other health care professionals, becoming familiar with nursing codes of ethics, and participating in ethics committees and rounds.

- Client advocacy involves concern for and actions on behalf of another person or organization in order to bring about change.

- The functions of the advocacy role are to inform, support, and mediate.

THINK ABOUT IT

Refer to the chapter-opening scenario and answer these questions.

1. Can Bakaar legally discuss what he did in the clinical area? Defend your answer, explaining how Bakaar can maintain the confidentiality of his clients.

2. What ethical obligation does Bakaar hold in regard to the client's confidentiality and other rights?

3. If licensure is required to work as a nurse, how is a student nurse's practice legally protected?

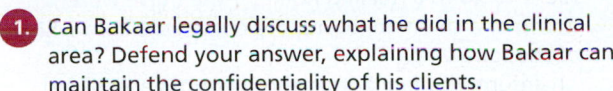 *See suggested responses to Think About It on MyNursingKit.*

TEST YOUR KNOWLEDGE

1. A primary care provider's orders indicate that a surgical consent form needs to be signed. Since the nurse was not present when the primary care provider discussed the surgical procedure, which statement best illustrates the nurse fulfilling the client advocate role?
   1. "The doctor has asked that you sign this consent form."
   2. "Do you have any questions about the procedure?"
   3. "What were you told about the procedure you are going to have?"
   4. "Remember that you can change your mind and cancel the procedure."

2. Although the client refused the procedure, the nurse insisted and inserted a nasogastric tube in the right nostril. The nurse has committed which of the following?
   1. An unintentional tort
   2. Assault
   3. Invasion of privacy
   4. Battery

3. A primary care provider prescribes one tablet, but the nurse accidently administers two. After notifying the primary care provider, the nurse monitors the client carefully for untoward effects of which there are none. Is the client likely to be successful in suing the nurse for malpractice?
   1. No, the client was not harmed.
   2. No, the nurse notified the physician.
   3. Yes, a breach of duty exists.
   4. Yes, foreseeability is present.

4. A nursing student is employed and working as an unlicensed assistive personnel (UAP) on a busy surgical unit. The nurses know that the UAP is enrolled in a nursing program and will be graduating soon. A nurse asks the UAP if he has performed a urinary catheterization on clients while in the nursing program. When the UAP says "Yes," the nurse asks him to help her out by doing a urinary catheterization on a postsurgical client. What is the best response by the UAP?
   1. "Let me get permission from the client first."
   2. "Sure. Which client is it?"
   3. "I can't do it unless you supervise me."
   4. "I can't do it. Is there something else I can help you with?"

5. The nurse's partner/spouse undergoes exploratory surgery at the hospital where the nurse is employed. Which of the following practices is most appropriate?
   1. Because the nurse is an employee, access to the chart is allowed.
   2. The relationship with the client provides the nurse special access to the chart.
   3. Access to the chart requires a signed release form from the client.
   4. The nurse can ask the surgeon to discuss the outcome of the surgery.

6. An ethical issue arises involving the nurse's assigned client. One of the most important nursing responsibilities in managing this client care situation would be which of the following:
   1. Be able to defend the morality of one's own actions.
   2. Remain neutral and detached when making ethical decisions.
   3. Ensure that a team is responsible for deciding ethical questions.
   4. Follow the client's and family's wishes exactly.

7. Which of the following situations most clearly demonstrates that the nurse is violating the underlying principles associated with professional nursing ethics?
   1. The nurse applies fetal monitoring, which the hospital policy permits despite literature that both supports and refutes the value of this practice.
   2. When asked about the purpose of a medication, a nurse colleague responds, "Oh, I never look them up. I just give what is prescribed."
   3. The nurses on the unit agree to sponsor a fund-raising event to support a labor strike proposed by fellow nurses at another facility.
   4. A client reports that he didn't quite tell the doctor the truth when asked if he was following his therapeutic diet at home.

8. Following a motor vehicle accident, the parents refuse to permit withdrawal of life support from the child who has no apparent brain function. Although the nurse believes the child should be allowed to die and organ donation should be considered, the nurse supports their decision. Which moral principle provides the basis for the nurse's actions?
   1. Respect for autonomy
   2. Nonmaleficence
   3. Beneficence
   4. Justice

9. Which of the following statements would be *most* helpful when a nurse is assisting clients in clarifying their values?
   1. "That was not a good decision. Why did you think it would work?"
   2. "The most important thing is to follow the plan of care. Did you follow all your doctor's orders?"
   3. "Some people might have made a different decision. What led you to make your decision?"
   4. "If you had asked me, I would have given you my opinion about what to do. Now, how do you feel about your choice?"

10. After recovering from her hip replacement, an older adult client wants to go home. The family wants the client to go to a nursing home. If the nurse were acting as a client advocate, the nurse would do which of the following:
    1. Inform the family that the client has a right to decide on her own.
    2. Ask the primary care provider to discharge the client to home.
    3. Suggest the client hire a lawyer to protect her rights.
    4. Help the client and family communicate their views to each other.

∞ *See answers to Test Your Knowledge in Appendix A.*

REFERENCES AND SELECTED BIBLIOGRAPHY

American Association of Colleges of Nursing. (1998). *The essentials of baccalaureate education for professional nursing practice*. Washington, DC: Author.

American Nurses Association. (2003). *Nursing: Scope and standards of practice*. Washington, DC: Author.

American Nurses Association. (2001). *Code of ethics for nurses with interpretive statements*. Washington, DC: Author.

American Nurses Association. (2007). *The American Nurses Association position statement on registered nurse utilization of unlicensed personnel*. Retrieved October 24, 2009, from http://www .nursingworld.org/ UnlicensedAssistivePersonnel

Blair, P. D. (2002). Report impaired practice-stat. *Nursing Management, 33*(1), 24–25.

Brent, N. J. (2001). *Nurses and the law* (2nd ed.). Philadelphia: W. B. Saunders.

Croke, E. M. (2003). Nurses, negligence, and malpractice. *American Journal of Nursing, 103*(9), 54–63.

Danis, S. J. (2004). The impaired nurse. *Nursing Spectrum*. Retrieved from http://www2.nursingspectrum.com/CE/ Self-Study_modules/syllabus.htm?ID=24

Equal Employment Opportunity Commission. (2009). *Guidelines on discrimination because of sex (Section 1604.11 Sexual harassment Code of Federal Regulations, Title 29, Vol. 4)*. Retrieved October 24, 2009, from http://www.eeoc.gov/types/sexual_harassment.html

Gallup Organization. (2007). *Nurses remain atop honesty and ethics list*. Princeton, NJ: Author. Retrieved October 24, 2009, from http://www.gallup.com/video/103117/ Nurses-Top-Ethics-Honesty.aspx#

Guido, G. W. (2009). *Legal and ethical issues in nursing* (5th ed.). Upper Saddle River, NJ: Prentice Hall.

Joint Commission on Accreditation of Healthcare Organizations. (2006). 2006 *Comprehensive accreditation manual for hospitals*. Oakbrook Terrace, IL: Author.

Quallich, S. A. (2005). Practice of informed consent, The. *AAACN Viewpoint, 17*(1), 49–51. Retrieved October 24, 2009, from http://findarticles.com/p/articles/ mi_qa4022/is_200507/ai_n15352129

Sheehan, J. P. (2001). Legally speaking: Delegating to UAPs—A practical guide. *RN, 64*(7), 65–66.

Trossman, S. (2003). Nurses' addictions. *American Journal of Nursing, 103*(9), 27–28.

U.S. Department of Health and Human Services. (2003). *Summary of the HIPAA privacy rule*. Retrieved October 24, 2009, from http://www.hhs.gov/ocr/ privacy/hippa/understanding/summary

Watson, P. G. (2000). The Americans with Disabilities Act: More rights for people with disabilities. *Rehabilitation Nursing, 25*(4), 145–147.

Zimmerman, P. G., & Jackson, M. (2004). Delegating to unlicensed assistive personnel. *Nursing Spectrum*. Retrieved August 12, 2008, from http://www2.nursingspectrum.com/CE/ Self-Study_modules/syllabus.htm?!D=42

Health Care Delivery Systems

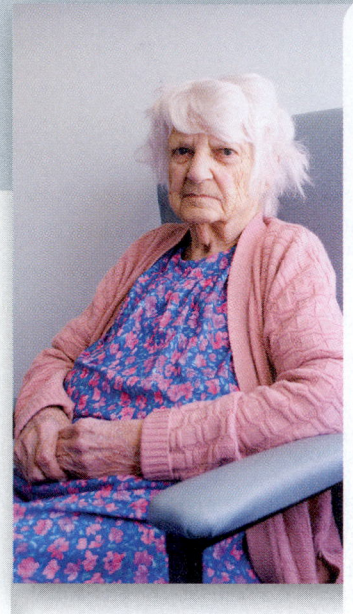

Martha Jones is a 93-year-old woman who lives alone in a three-story single-family home. When her husband died eight years ago, her four children tried to talk her into moving to an independent living facility for seniors, but she said she had lived in this home for more than 60 years and planned to die here. Two of her children live in the same state, but only one lives within 10 miles, so responsibility for helping Martha, who doesn't drive due to declining vision, has fallen on her second daughter, Bernice. Married with two teenage children and a full-time job, Bernice tries to drop by her mother's house at least twice a week and picks up groceries on the way. They speak on the phone every day. When Bernice doesn't get an answer one evening, she jumps in her car and drives to her mother's house and finds she has fallen down the stairs and has been lying there unable to get up for the past three hours. Bernice calls 911, and emergency workers respond quickly.

LEARNING OUTCOMES

After completing this chapter, you will be able to:

1. List three levels of prevention and give examples of each level.

2. List different types of health care agencies and describe the type of health care service each provides.

3. List the members of the health care team and describe each team member's role in providing client care.

4. List factors that influence the delivery of health care and explain how each factor impacts the delivery of care.

5. List different frameworks for delivering care and explain how each differs, including the advantages and disadvantages of each.

6. Define community-based health care and list settings for delivery of care in the community.

7. Define the importance of care continuity and describe six key components.

8. List unique aspects of home health nursing.

9. List the roles of home health nurses as they relate to the dimensions of home health nursing.

KEY TERMS

Caregiver role strain p70
Case management p58
Collaboration p64
Coinsurance p59

Community p62
Community-based health care (CBHC) p61
Continuity of care p65

Critical pathway p58
Discharge planning p65
Durable medical equipment (DME) p68

Health care system p51
Health maintenance organization (HMO) p60

HEALTH CARE DELIVERY

A **health care system** is the totality of services offered by all health disciplines. It is one of the largest industries in the United States. Previously, the major purpose of a health care system was to provide care to the ill and injured. However, with increasing awareness of health promotion, illness prevention, and levels of wellness, health care systems are changing, as are the roles of nurses in these areas. The services provided by a health care system are commonly categorized according to type and level.

Levels of Prevention

Health care services are often described in a way that correlates with levels of disease prevention: (a) primary prevention, which consists of health promotion and illness prevention, (b) secondary prevention, which consists of diagnosis and treatment, and (c) tertiary prevention, which consists of rehabilitation, health restoration, and palliative care.

PRIMARY PREVENTION: HEALTH PROMOTION AND ILLNESS PREVENTION
Based on the notion of maintaining an optimum level of wellness, the World Health Organization (WHO) developed a project called Healthy People. The U.S. Department of Health and Human Services (2000) project that evolved from the original work is called *Healthy People 2010* and has two primary goals: (a) increase quality and years of healthy life and (b) eliminate health disparities. *Healthy People 2010* is a national primary prevention program and, like all primary prevention programs, addresses such areas as adequate and proper nutrition, weight control, exercise, and stress reduction. Health promotion activities emphasize the important role clients play in maintaining their own health and encourage them to maintain the highest level of wellness they can achieve. Illness prevention programs may be directed at the client or the community and involve such practices as providing immunizations, identifying risk factors for illnesses, and helping people make good personal choices in order to prevent these illnesses from occurring. Illness prevention also includes environmental programs that can reduce the incidence of illness or disability.

CLINICAL ALERT

As insurance companies have realized that keeping people healthy is less expensive than treating illnesses, their health care insurance plans have begun to pay for preventive health care activities.

SECONDARY PREVENTION: DIAGNOSIS AND TREATMENT
Secondary prevention is aimed at diagnosing and treating existing health problems. In the past, the largest segment of health care services was dedicated to secondary prevention in both hospitals and physicians' offices. Within the last few decades, in an attempt to reduce health care costs, freestanding diagnostic and treatment facilities have evolved and serve an ever-growing numbers of clients. An important part of secondary prevention is the early detection of a disease. This can be accomplished through routine screening or by performing focused screenings that are aimed at those with increased risk for a specific disease. Community-based agencies such as the American Heart Association or the American Cancer Society have become instrumental in providing screenings and education regarding self-detection of high-risk symptoms.

TERTIARY PREVENTION: REHABILITATION, HEALTH RESTORATION, AND PALLIATIVE CARE
The goal of tertiary prevention is to help people return to their previous level of health after an illness or trauma. When full recovery is not possible, the goal is to help them attain the highest level they are capable of, given their current health status. Rehabilitative care emphasizes the importance of assisting clients to function in the physical, mental, social, economic, and vocational areas of their lives. If an injury is temporary, rehabilitation can assist the client to return to former functional levels. If the injury is permanent, rehabilitation helps the client adjust the way they perform activities in order to achieve maximum abilities. Tertiary services also include palliative care, which is care aimed at reducing symptoms versus providing a cure. One form of palliative care is end-of-life care that provides comfort and treatment of symptoms. Tertiary services can be provided in many settings, including the hospital, hospice, or the home.

Health Care Agencies and Services

Health care agencies and services in the United States and Canada are both varied and numerous. Some health care agencies or systems provide services in different settings; for example, a hospital may provide acute inpatient services, outpatient clinic or ambulatory care services, same-day surgery, and emergency room services (Figure 3–1). Hospice services may be provided in the hospital, the home, a long-term care facility, or another agency within the community. Because the array of health care agencies and services is so great, nurses often need to help clients choose that

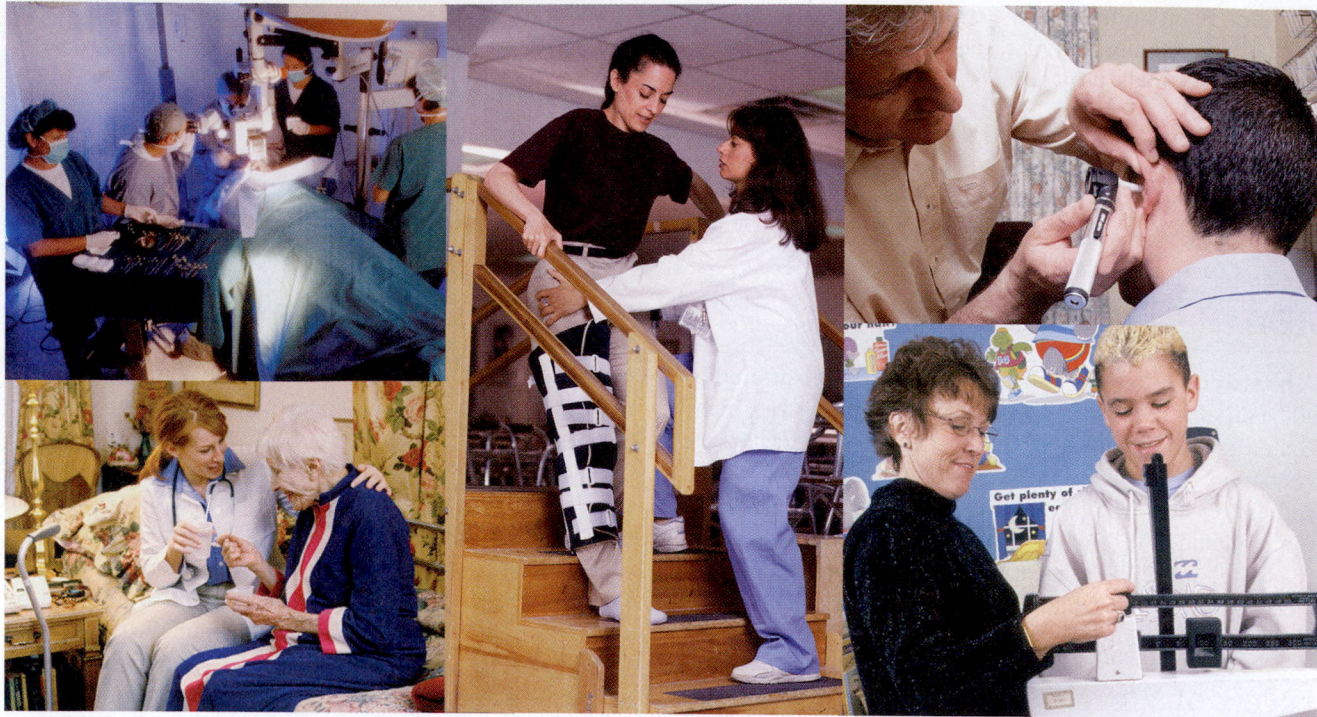

Figure 3–1 ● Various health care settings.

which best suits their needs. Clients may be seen by any number and types of nurses and other providers, depending on their care needs and ability to pay for services.

Public health services are provided by the government at local, state, and federal levels. Health agencies at the state, county, or city level vary according to the need of the area. Their funds, generally from taxes, are administered by elected or appointed officials. Local health departments have the responsibility for developing programs to meet the health needs of people, providing the necessary nursing and other staff and facilities to carry out these programs, continually evaluating the effectiveness of the programs, and monitoring the changing needs. State health organizations are responsible for assisting the local health departments. In some remote areas, state departments also provide direct services to people. The Public Health Service (PHS) of the U.S. Department of Health and Human Services is an official agency at the federal level with functions for research and providing training, assistance to communities in planning and developing health facilities, and assisting state and local communities through financing and provision of trained personnel. The National Institutes of Health (NIH), the Centers for Disease Control and Prevention, and the National Institute of Mental Health are just a few examples of federal public health services; each provides websites that are excellent resources for health care information.

Physicians' offices are a primary care setting, meaning they are the first source of care for meeting preventive, health promotion, treatment, and recovery needs of the client. Most physicians either have their own office or work with several other physicians in a group practice. Clients usually go to a physician's office for routine health screening, illness diag-

nosis, and treatment. Nurse practitioners often practice in these settings as well, sometimes alongside the physicians and other times in independent settings. LPN/LVNs and unlicensed assistive personnel are often hired to provide client care, although some physician's offices may hire RNs as well.

Ambulatory care centers may be found in many communities. Most ambulatory care centers have diagnostic and treatment facilities providing medical, nursing, laboratory, and radiological services, and they may or may not be associated with an acute care hospital. Some ambulatory care centers provide services to people who require minor surgical procedures that can be performed outside the hospital and do not require an overnight stay. These centers offer two advantages: They permit the client to live at home while obtaining necessary health care, and they free costly hospital beds for seriously ill clients. The term *ambulatory care center* has replaced the term *clinic* in many places.

Occupational health clinics, or industrial clinics, are gaining importance as a setting for employee health care. Employee health has long been recognized as important to productivity. Today, more companies recognize the value of healthy employees and encourage healthy lifestyles by providing exercise facilities and coordinating health promotion activities. Today, nursing functions in industrial health care include work safety, preventive health education, annual employee health screening for tuberculosis, and maintaining immunization information. Other functions may include screening for such health problems as hypertension, obesity, caring for employees following injury, and counseling.

Hospitals can be classified according to their ownership or control as governmental (public) or nongovernmental (private). The federal government provides hospital facilities for veterans and merchant mariners (VA hospitals). Military hospitals provide care to military personnel and their families. Private hospitals are often operated by churches, companies, communities, and charitable organizations. Private hospitals may be for-profit or not-for-profit. Although hospitals are chiefly viewed as institutions that provide care, they have other functions, such as providing sources for health-related research and teaching. The variety of health care services hospitals provide usually depends on their size and location. Large urban hospitals usually have inpatient beds, emergency services, diagnostic facilities, ambulatory surgery centers, pharmacy services, intensive and coronary care services, and multiple outpatient services provided by clinics. Some large hospitals have other specialized services such as spinal cord injury and burn units, oncology services, and infusion and dialysis units. In addition, some hospitals have substance abuse treatment units and health promotion units. Small rural hospitals are often limited to inpatient beds, radiology and laboratory services, and basic emergency services. The number of services a rural hospital provides is usually directly related to its size and its distance from an urban center.

Subacute care facilities are a variation of inpatient care designed for someone who has an acute illness, injury, or exacerbation of a disease process. Clients may be admitted after, or instead of, acute hospitalization or to administer one or more technically complex treatments. Generally, the individual's condition is such that the care does not depend heavily on high-technology monitoring or complex diagnostic procedures. Subacute care requires the coordinated services of an interdisciplinary team including physicians, nurses, and other relevant professional disciplines. Subacute care is generally more intensive than long-term care and less than acute care.

Extended care (long-term care) facilities, formerly called nursing homes, are often multilevel campuses that include independent living quarters for seniors, assisted living, skilled nursing (intermediate care), and extended care (long-term care) facilities. They provide differing levels of personal care for those who are chronically ill or are unable to care for themselves without assistance. Traditionally, extended care facilities provided care only for older adult clients, but they now provide care to clients of all ages who require rehabilitation or custodial care. Because clients are being discharged earlier from acute care hospitals, some clients may still require supplemental care in a skilled nursing or extended care facility before they return home.

CLINICAL ALERT

Older adults in extended care facilities may move among levels of care several times—from independent living, to a hospital, to a rehabilitation center, to long-term care, and hopefully back to independent or assisted living. The sequence varies as will the length of time in each setting.

Retirement or assisted living centers consist of separate houses, condominiums, or apartments for residents. Residents live relatively independently; however, many of these facilities offer meals, laundry services, nursing care, transportation, and social activities. Some centers have a separate hospital to care for residents with short-term or long-term illnesses. These centers often work collaboratively with other community services including case managers, social services, and hospice to meet the needs of the residents who live there. The retirement or assisted living center is intended to meet the needs of people who are unable to remain at home but do not require hospital or long-term care. Nurses in retirement and assisted living centers provide limited care to residents, usually related to the administration of medications and minor treatments, but conduct significant health promotion and health screening activities.

Rehabilitation centers are usually independent community centers or special units. However, because rehabilitation ideally starts the moment the client enters the health care system, nurses who are employed on pediatric, psychiatric, or surgical units of hospitals also help to rehabilitate clients. Rehabilitation centers play an important role in assisting clients to restore their health and to recuperate. Today, the concept of rehabilitation is applied to all illnesses and injuries (physical and mental). Nurses in the rehabilitation setting coordinate client activities and ensure that clients are complying with their treatments. This type of nursing often requires specialized skills and knowledge.

Home health care agencies have become an essential aspect of the health care delivery system because of the implementation of prospective payment and the resulting early discharge of clients from hospitals. As concerns about the cost of health care have escalated, the use of the home as a care delivery site has increased. In addition, the scope of services offered in the home has broadened. Home health care nurses and other staff offer education to clients and families and also provide comprehensive care to acute, chronic, and terminally ill clients.

Day-care centers serve many functions and many age groups. Some day-care centers provide care for infants and children while parents work. Elder care centers often provide care involving socializing, exercise programs, and stimulation. Some centers provide counseling and physical therapy. Nurses who are employed in day-care centers may provide medications, treatments, and counseling, thereby facilitating continuity between day care and home care.

Rural care hospitals were created as a result of the 1987 Omnibus Budget Reconciliation Act to provide emergency care to clients in rural areas. In 1997, the Balanced Budget Act authorized the Medicare Rural Hospital Flexibility Program to assist rural hospitals to continue to make available primary care access and improve emergency care for rural residents. This program established a new classification called critical access hospitals, which receive federal funding to remain open and provide the breadth of services needed for rural residents, including interfaces with regional tertiary care centers. Each state has an Office of Rural Health

Programs that assesses and identifies interventions for the health care needs of the local population. Nurses in rural settings must be generalists who are able to manage a wide variety of clients and health care problems. Due to their training in providing comprehensive primary care across the life span, nurse practitioners are particularly suited to these roles.

Hospice services has come to mean interdisciplinary health care service for the dying provided in the home or another health care setting. The central concept of the hospice movement, as distinct from the acute care model, is not saving life but improving or maintaining the quality of life until death. Hospice nurses serve primarily as case managers and supervise the delivery of direct care by other members of the team. The place of health care delivery may vary as the client's condition declines or the family's ability to care for the client changes. The hospice nurse does ongoing needs assessments of the client and family and then helps to find the appropriate resources for them to make their lives more comfortable.

Crisis centers provide emergency services to clients experiencing life crises. These centers may operate out of a hospital or in the community, and most provide 24-hour telephone service. Some also provide direct counseling to people at the center or in their homes. The primary purpose of the center is to help people cope with an immediate crisis as well as providing guidance and support for long-term therapy. Nurses working in crisis centers need well-developed communication and counseling skills in order to immediately identify the person's problems, determine their coping skills, and offer assistance to help the person locate needed resources for long-term support.

Mutual support and self-help groups arose largely because people felt their needs were not being met by the existing health care system. In North America today, there are more than 500 mutual support or self-help groups that focus on nearly every major health problem or life crisis people experience. Alcoholics Anonymous, which was formed in 1935, served as the model for many of these groups. The National Self-Help Clearinghouse provides information on current support groups and guidelines about how to start a self-help group. The nurse's role in self-help groups is discussed in Chapter 14 ∞ .

Providers of Health Care

The providers of health care, also referred to as the health care team or health professionals, are nurses and health personnel from different disciplines who coordinate their skills to assist clients and their support persons. Their mutual goal is to restore a client's health and promote wellness. The choice of personnel for a particular client depends on the needs of the client. Health teams commonly include the nurse and several different personnel. Nurses' roles are described in Chapter 1 ∞ and throughout this textbook. The providers that follow are not an all-inclusive list of the many potential members of a health care team.

- **Nurses'** roles vary with client needs, the nurse's credentials, and the type of employment setting.

- **Alternative or complementary health care providers** are practitioners who deliver health care not commonly considered part of Western medicine. See Chapter 5 ∞ for a detailed description of these.
- **Case managers** function to ensure that clients receive fiscally sound, appropriate care in the best setting and may include a nurse, social worker, occupational therapist, physical therapist, or any other member of the health care team.
- **Dentists** diagnose and treat problems of the teeth, gums, and oral structures and perform preventive measures to maintain healthy teeth and oral cavities.
- **Dietitians** have special knowledge about the diets required to maintain health and to treat disease.
- **Nutritionists** have special knowledge about nutrition and food and function to recommend healthy diets along with broad advisory services about the purchase and preparation of foods.
- **Occupational therapists** assist clients with impaired function to gain the skills to perform activities of daily living by teaching skills that are both therapeutic and fulfilling.
- **Paramedical technologists** include laboratory, radiological, and nuclear medicine technologists; these are just a few examples of paramedical technologists in the expanding field of medical technology.
- **Pharmacists** prepare and dispense pharmaceuticals in hospital and community settings while monitoring and evaluating the actions and effects of medications on clients.

CLINICAL ALERT

Significant overlap may occur among health care providers. For example, an anesthesiologist (MD), a neonatal care nurse, or a respiratory therapist may be responsible for assisting a newborn baby with breathing problems. All providers perform client teaching.

- **Physical therapists** assist clients with musculoskeletal problems, treating movement dysfunctions by means of heat, water, exercise, massage, and electric current while assessing client mobility and strength, providing therapeutic measures, and teaching new skills.
- **Physicians** are responsible for medical diagnoses, determining the therapy required, along with providing health promotion, and disease prevention in their practice.
- **Physician assistants** diagnose and treat certain conditions under the direction of a physician. Depending on state laws, nurses may not be legally permitted to follow a PA's orders unless they are cosigned by a physician.
- **Podiatrists** diagnose and treat foot conditions both medically and surgically.
- **Respiratory therapists** are skilled in therapeutic measures used in the care of clients with respiratory problems, including oxygen therapy devices, inter-

mittent positive pressure breathing respirators, artificial mechanical ventilators, and accessory devices used in inhalation therapy.

- **Social workers** counsel and support clients regarding problems of day-to-day living such as finances, marital difficulties, and adoption of children.
- **Spiritual support personnel** include chaplains, pastors, rabbis, priests, and other religious advisors who attend to the spiritual needs of clients.
- **Unlicensed assistive personnel** are staff members who assume delegated basic client care and may be called certified nurse assistants, hospital attendants, nurse technicians, patient care technicians, or orderlies.

Factors Affecting Health Care Delivery

Today's health care consumers have greater knowledge about health than in previous years, and they are increasingly influencing health care delivery. Formerly, people expected a physician to make decisions about their care; today, however, consumers expect to be involved in decision making. Consumers have also become aware of how lifestyle affects health. As a result, they desire more information and services related to health promotion and illness prevention. A number of other factors affect the health care delivery system.

INCREASING NUMBER OF OLDER ADULTS By 2020 it is estimated that the number of U.S. adults over the age of 65 will be more than 53 million (U.S. Census Bureau, 2004). Long-term illnesses are prevalent among this group, and they frequently require special housing, treatment services, financial support, and social networks. The frail elderly, considered to be people over age 85, are projected to be the fastest growing population in the United States and will number over 76.5 million by 2020 and almost 90 million by 2030 (U.S. Census Bureau, 2004). See Figure 3–2 for a breakdown of older adults by state. Because only 5% of older people are institutionalized with health problems, substantial home management and nursing support services are required to assist those living in their homes and communities. Older people like to feel they are part of a community. The feeling of being a useful, wanted, and productive citizen is essential to every person's health. Special programs are being designed in communities so that the talents and skills of this group will be used and not lost to society.

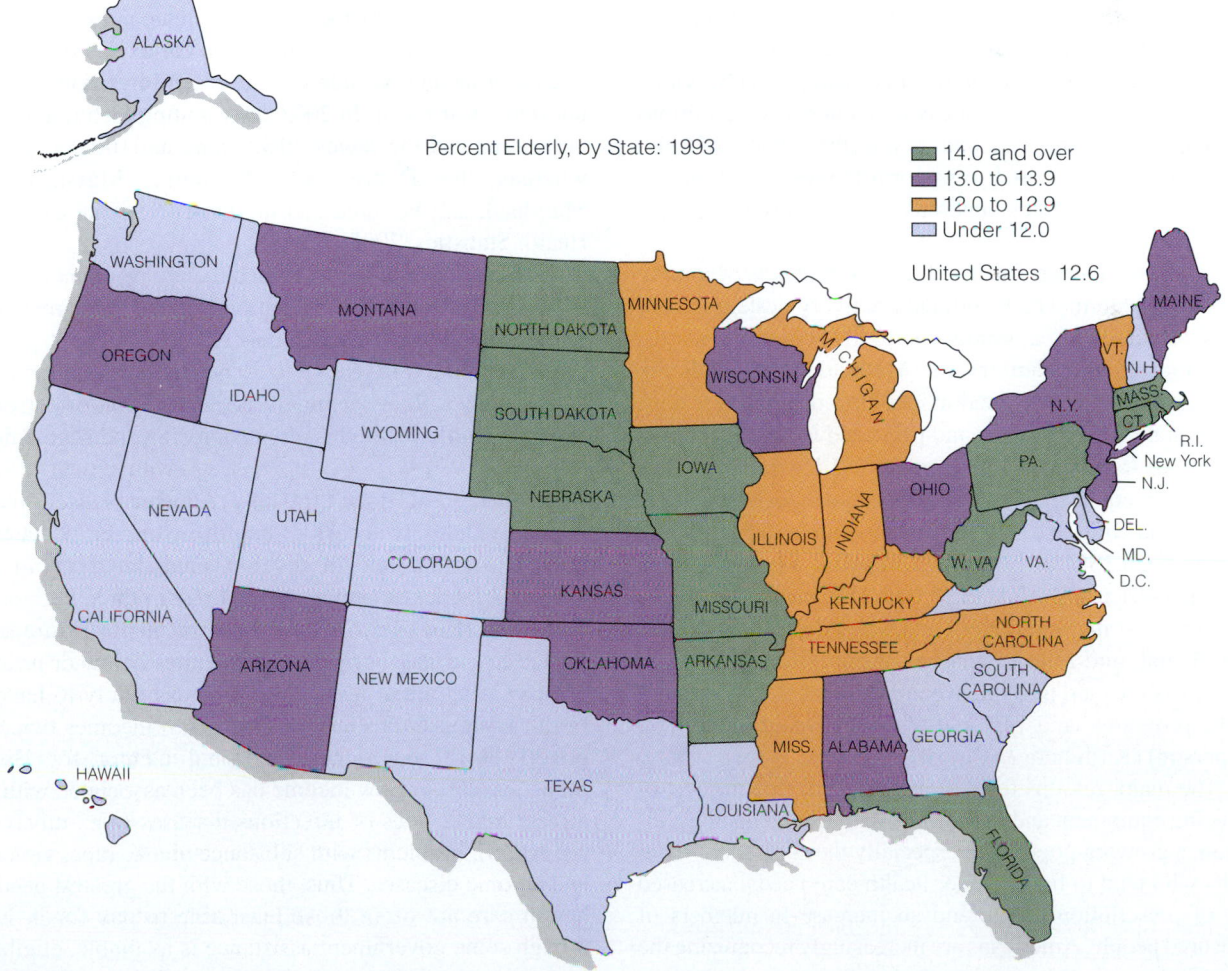

Percent Elderly, by State: 1993

■ 14.0 and over
■ 13.0 to 13.9
■ 12.0 to 12.9
□ Under 12.0

United States   12.6

Figure 3–2 ○ Numbers of older adults in U.S. regions.

Source: http://www.census.gov/population/www/pop-profile/elderpop.html

ADVANCES IN TECHNOLOGY Scientific knowledge and technology related to health care are changing and improving constantly. Improved diagnostic procedures and sophisticated equipment permit early recognition of diseases that might otherwise have remained undetected. New antibiotics and medications are continually being developed to treat infections and multiple drug-resistant organisms. Surgical procedures involving the heart, lungs, and liver that were nonexistent 20 years ago are common today. Laser and microscopic procedures streamline the treatment of diseases that required surgery in the past. As scientists learn more about human genetics, treatments and preventive strategies are becoming increasingly more effective.

Computers, bedside charting, and the ability to store and retrieve large volumes of information in databases are commonplace in health care organizations. In addition, as a result of the Internet and the World Wide Web access from numerous public and private locations, clients now have access to medical information similar to that of health care providers. It is important for nurses to help clients evaluate the reliability of information they find on the Internet because not all websites provide good information.

These discoveries have changed consumer access to health care. Clients are now more likely to be treated in the community, utilizing resources, technology, and treatments outside the hospital. Technological advances and specialized treatments and procedures may come, unfortunately, with a high price tag. Some diagnostic equipment may cost millions of dollars. Due to this expenditure plus the expense of training specialized personnel to perform the tests, each procedure can cost consumers hundreds or thousands of dollars.

ECONOMICS Paying for health care services is becoming a greater problem. The health care delivery system is very much affected by a country's total economic status. According to the Centers for Medicaid and Medicare Services (CMS, 2006), health spending in 2004 was $1.8 trillion in the United States and projected to reach $3.6 trillion by 2014, increasing an average of 7.1% per year. This is currently equal to over $5,000 per year for every man, woman, and child and will more than double to $11,000 by 2014. About 33% are inpatient hospital expenses, 21% physician office and clinic expenses, 15% prescription drug expenses, and the remainder emergency department, home care, dental, and related services. Approximately 42% of these costs are paid through private insurance, 45% through public programs, and 14% out-of-pocket (paid directly by the person) (Kashihara & Carper, 2005).

The major reasons for cost increases include the cost of replacing equipment and facilities with newer technology, inflation, a growing population especially the segment of older adults who tend to have greater health care needs, increased cost of prescription drugs, and an increase in numbers of uninsured people. Americans are increasingly recognizing the right of all people to have adequate health care so the number of people seeking health care, and the frequency of their interactions with health care providers, has increased.

WOMEN'S HEALTH The women's movement has been instrumental in changing health care practices. Examples are the provision of childbirth services in more relaxed settings such as birthing centers, and the provision of overnight facilities for parents in children's hospitals. Until recently, women's health issues focused on the reproductive aspects of health, disregarding many health care concerns that are unique to women. Investigators are beginning to recognize the need for research that examines women, and not just men, regarding health issues such as osteoporosis, heart disease, and responses to various treatment modalities. Current provision of health care shows an increased emphasis on the psychosocial aspects of women's health, including the impact of career, delayed childbearing, role of caregiver to older family members, and extended life span.

UNEVEN DISTRIBUTION OF SERVICES Serious problems in the distribution of health services exist in the United States. Two facets of this problem are (a) uneven distribution and (b) increased specialization. In some areas, particularly remote and rural locations, there are insufficient health care professionals and services available to meet the health care needs of individuals. Rural clients may need to drive long distances to obtain the services they require. Uneven distribution is evidenced by the relatively higher number of nurses per capita in the New England states versus the low number in California and Nevada (Figure 3–3). Physicians are also unevenly distributed: In 2003, Mississippi, Idaho, Iowa, and Oklahoma had the fewest physicians per 100,000 people, whereas the District of Columbia, Massachusetts, Maryland, and Vermont had the most (National Center for Health Statistics, 2005).

An increasing number of health care personnel provide specialized services. Specialization can lead to fragmentation of care and, often, increased cost of care. To clients, it may mean receiving care from 5 to 30 people during their hospital experience. This seemingly endless stream of personnel and paperwork required is often confusing and frightening.

ACCESS TO HEALTH INSURANCE Another problem plaguing individuals is access to health insurance. Data from 2004 show that one in seven Caucasians, one in five African Americans, and more than one in three Latinos are uninsured (Rhoades, 2006b). Lack of health insurance is related to income. Persons with incomes below or near the poverty level are at least three times as likely to have no health insurance coverage as those with incomes twice the poverty level or higher (National Center for Health Statistics, 2005). Low income has been associated with relatively higher rates of infectious diseases (e.g., tuberculosis, AIDS), problems with substance abuse, rape, violence, and chronic diseases. Thus, those with the greatest need for health care are often those least able to pay for it. Even though some government assistance is available, eligibility for government insurance programs and benefits varies considerably from state to state and is continually being reevaluated. Many more clients may be underinsured,

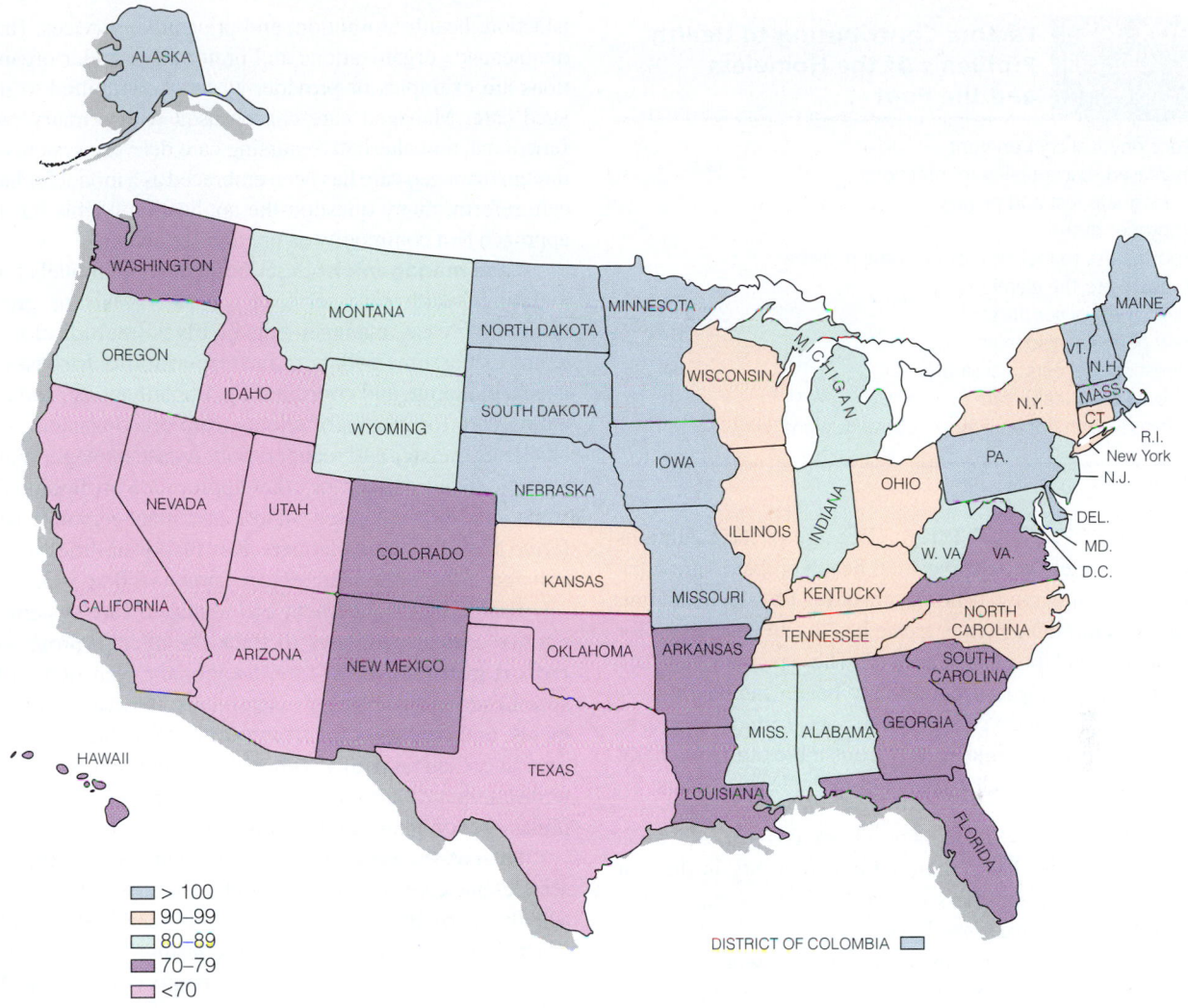

Figure 3–3 ● Number of nurses per 100,000 population map.

Source: Data from Department of Health & Human Services, Bureau of Health Professions, Division of Nursing. (2004). The registered nurse population: National sample survey of registered nurses March 2004. Preliminary findings. Retrieved January 11, 2006, from http://bhpr.hrsa.gov/healthworkforce/reports/rnpopulation/preliminaryfindings.htm

meaning they have some insurance for catastrophic events but must meet deductibles or copayments that keep them from seeking preventive care. For example, a common private insurance plan requires the client to pay $2,000 in deductible before the insurance company will cover 80% of costs. Only after the client has paid up to $10,000 out of pocket will the insurance company cover 100% of the cost.

Many clients cannot afford to pay for a doctor's visit and thus are unable to meet the initial $2,000 deductible; therefore they are unlikely to seek preventive care or even secondary care needed to treat an illness. See Box 3–1 to review "Nursing's Agenda for Health Care Reform." Other aspects of variations in health beliefs and practices among people of different cultures are found in Chapter 4 ∞.

BOX 3–1   Nursing's Agenda for Health Care Reform

- A restructured health care system that (a) enhances consumer access to services by delivering primary health care in community-based settings, (b) fosters consumer responsibility for personal health, self-care, and informed decision making in selecting health care services, and (c) facilitates using the most cost-effective providers and therapeutic options in the most appropriate settings.
- A federally defined standard package of essential health care services available to all citizens and residents of the United States provided and financed through an integration of public and private plans and sources.

- A phase-in of essential services.
- Planned change to anticipate health service needs that correlate with changing national demographics.
- Steps to reduce health care costs.
- Case management for those with continuing health care needs.
- Provisions for long-term care.
- Insurance reforms to improve access to coverage.

Note: Reprinted with permission from American Nurses Association, Nursing's Agenda for Health Care Reform, © 2001 Nursesbooks.org, Silver Spring, MD 20910.

| BOX 3–2 | Factors Contributing to Health Problems of the Homeless and the Poor |

- Poor physical environment
- Increased susceptibility to infections
- Inadequate rest and privacy
- Improper nutrition
- Poor access to facilities for personal hygiene
- Exposure to the elements
- Lack of social support
- Few personal resources
- Questionable personal safety
- Inconsistent health care
- Difficulty with adherence to treatment plans

THE HOMELESS AND THE POOR   Because of the conditions in which homeless people live, their health problems are often exacerbated and may become chronic. Physical, mental, social, and emotional factors create health care challenges for the homeless and the poor (Box 3–2). These persons may lack convenient or timely transportation to health care facilities—especially if repeated visits are necessary. Limited access to health care services significantly contributes to the general poor health of the homeless and poor in the United States.

DEMOGRAPHIC CHANGES   The characteristics of North American families have changed considerably in the last few decades. The numbers of single-parent families and alternative family structures have increased markedly. Most of the single-parent families are headed by women, many of whom work and require assistance with child care, whether the child is sick or healthy.

Recognition of the cultural and ethnic diversity of the United States and Canada is also increasing. Health care professionals and agencies are aware of this diversity and are employing strategies to meet the challenges presented.

Frameworks for Care

A number of configurations for the delivery of nursing care support continuity of care and cost effectiveness. These include managed care, case management, patient-focused care, differentiated practice, shared governance, the case method, the functional method, team nursing, and primary nursing. These have evolved, some from each other, for reasons such as the need to decrease health care costs and to improve the utilization of limited human and physical resources. A particular agency may use more than one configuration.

Managed care describes a health care system whose goals are to provide cost-effective, quality care that focuses on decreased costs and improved outcomes for groups of clients. The care of a client is carefully planned from initial contact to the conclusion of the specific health problem. In managed care, health care providers and agencies collaborate to render the most appropriate, fiscally responsible care possible. Managed care denotes an emphasis on cost controls, customer sat-

isfaction, health promotion, and preventive services. Health maintenance organizations and preferred provider organizations are examples of provider systems committed to managed care. Managed care can be used with primary, team, functional, and alternative nursing care delivery systems. Although managed care has been embraced as a model for health care reform, many question the application of this business approach to a commodity as precious as health.

Case management describes a range of models for integrating health care services for individuals or groups. Generally, case management involves multidisciplinary teams that assume collaborative responsibility for assessing needs, planning, and coordinating, implementing, and evaluating care for groups of clients from preadmission to discharge or transfer and recuperation. A case manager may be a nurse, social worker, or other appropriate professional. In some areas of the United States, case managers may be referred to as discharge planners. Key responsibilities for case managers/discharge planners are shown in Box 3–3.

Both case management and managed care systems often use critical pathways to track the client's progress. A **critical pathway** is an interdisciplinary plan or tool that specifies interdisciplinary assessments, interventions, treatments, and outcomes for health-related conditions across a time line. Critical pathways are also called critical paths, interdisciplinary plans, anticipated recovery plans, interdisciplinary action plans, and action plans.

Patient-focused care is a delivery model that brings all services and care providers to clients. The supposition is that if activities normally provided by auxiliary personnel (e.g., physical therapy, respiratory therapy, ECG testing, and phlebotomy) are moved closer to the client, the number of personnel involved and the number of steps involved to get the work done are decreased. Cross-training, the development of multiskilled workers who can perform tasks or functions in more than one discipline, is an essential element of patient-focused care.

Differentiated practice is a system in which the best possible use of nursing personnel is based on their educational preparation and resultant skill sets. Thus, differentiated practice models consist of specific job descriptions for nurses according to their education or training. The model is customized within each health care institution by the nurses employed there. The institution must first identify the nursing competencies required by the clients within the specific practice environment. This model further requires the delineation of roles between both licensed nursing personnel and UAPs. This enables nurses to progress and assume roles and

| BOX 3–3 | Responsibilities of Case Managers/Discharge Planners |

- Assessing clients and their homes and communities
- Coordinating and planning client care
- Collaborating with other health professionals
- Monitoring clients' progress
- Evaluating client outcomes

responsibilities appropriate to their level of experience, capability, and education. As with managed care and case management, differentiated nursing practice seeks to provide quality care at an affordable cost.

Shared governance models can be used in concert with other models of nursing delivery. It is an organizational model in which nursing staff are cooperative with administrative personnel in making, implementing, and evaluating client care policies. The focus of this model is to encourage participation of nurses in decision making at all levels of the organization. Individuals may participate either at their own request or as part of their job role criteria. More commonly, nurses participate through serving in decision-making groups, such as committees and task forces. The decisions made may also address employment conditions, cost-effectiveness, long-range planning, productivity, and wages and benefits. The underlying principle of shared governance is that employees will be more committed to the organizational goals if they have had input into planning and decision making.

The **case method**, also referred to as total care, is one of the earliest nursing models developed. In this client-centered method, one nurse is assigned to and responsible for the comprehensive care of a group of clients during an 8- or 12-hour shift. For each client, the nurse assesses needs, designs nursing plans, formulates diagnoses, implements care, and evaluates the effectiveness of care. In this method, a client has consistent contact with one nurse during a shift but may have different nurses on other shifts. The case method, considered the precursor of primary nursing, continues to be used in a variety of practice settings such as intensive care nursing.

The **functional nursing method** focuses on the jobs to be completed (e.g., bed making, temperature measurement). In this task-oriented approach, personnel with less preparation than the professional nurse perform less complex care requirements. It is based on a production and efficiency model that gives authority and responsibility to the person assigning the work, for example, the head nurse. Clearly defined job descriptions, procedures, policies, and lines of communication are required. The functional approach to nursing is economical and efficient and permits centralized direction and control. Its disadvantages are fragmentation of care and the possibility that nonquantifiable aspects of care, such as meeting the client's emotional needs, may be overlooked.

Team nursing is the delivery of individualized nursing care to clients by a team led by a professional nurse. A nursing team consists of registered nurses, licensed practical nurses, and unlicensed assistive personnel. This team is responsible for providing coordinated nursing care to a group of clients with each health care member providing care at a level consistent with their education while the registered nurse retains responsibility and authority for the client's overall care while delegating appropriate tasks to other team members. Proponents of this model believe the team approach increases the efficiency of the registered nurse. Opponents state that inpatients' high acuity of illness leaves little to be delegated.

Primary nursing is a system in which one nurse is responsible for overseeing the total care of a number of clients 24 hours a day, 7 days a week, even if he or she does not deliver all the care personally. It is a method of providing continuity of care that is comprehensive, individualized, and consistent. The primary nurse assesses and prioritizes each client's needs, identifies nursing diagnoses, develops a plan of care with the client, and evaluates the effectiveness of care. Associate nurses provide care when the primary nurse is not working, but the primary nurse coordinates and communicates information about the client's health to other nurses and other health professionals through the nursing care plan. Primary nursing encompasses all aspects of the professional role, including teaching, advocacy, decision making, and continuity of care. The primary nurse is the first-line manager of the client's care with all its inherent accountabilities and responsibilities.

Financing Health Care

Although efforts have been made to control the costs of health care, these costs continue to increase. Employers, legislators, insurers, and health care providers continue to collaborate in efforts to resolve the issues surrounding how to best finance health care costs. Among these efforts, the United States has implemented some cost-containment strategies including health promotion and illness prevention activities, managed care systems, and alternative insurance delivery systems. The U.S. Center for Outcomes and Effectiveness Research (COER) conducts and supports studies on the outcomes and effectiveness of diagnostic, therapeutic, and preventive health care services and procedures, including cost.

PAYMENT SOURCES IN THE UNITED STATES   In most situations, a health care agency receives funding from several of the available payment sources. Almost all insurance plans include a per-visit or per-prescription copayment.

Medicare is a federal insurance plan to cover older adults 65 years of age or older and those with permanent disabilities and their dependents who are eligible for disability insurance under Social Security. Medicare offers several options including hospital care, outpatient services, and prescription coverage. Part A provides insurance for hospitalization, home care, and hospice care. Part B is voluntary and provides partial coverage of outpatient and physician services to people eligible for Part A. Part D is the voluntary prescription drug plan begun in January 2006. Most clients pay a monthly premium for Part B or D coverage. All Medicare clients pay a deductible and **coinsurance** (the percentage share of an approved charge that is paid by the client). Medicare does not cover dental care, dentures, eyeglasses, hearing aids, or examinations to prescribe and fit hearing aids.

Medicaid is a federal public assistance program paid out of general taxes to people who require financial assistance for health care, such as people with low incomes. Medicaid is paid by federal and state governments. Each state program is distinct. Some states provide very limited coverage, whereas others pay for dental care, eyeglasses, and/or prescription drugs.

Persons with disabilities or those who are blind may be eligible for special payments called **Supplemental Security**

Income (SSI) benefits. These benefits are also available to people not eligible for Social Security, and payments are not restricted to health care costs. Clients often use this money to purchase medicines or to cover costs of extended health care.

State Children's Health Insurance Program (SCHIP) was established by the U.S. government in 1997 to provide insurance coverage for the children of poor and working-class individuals. The program expands coverage for children under Medicaid and subsidizes low-cost state insurance alternatives. Coverage includes visits to primary health care providers, prescription medicines, and hospitalization. State eligibility requirements vary, but generally, children 18 years and under who live in families earning less than $34,100 per year (for a family of four) are eligible.

The **Prospective Payment System** was initiated to curtail health care costs in the United States. This legislation limits the amount paid to hospitals that are reimbursed by Medicare. Reimbursement is made according to a classification system known as diagnosis-related groups (DRGs). The system has categories that establish pretreatment diagnosis billing categories and hospitals are paid a predetermined amount for a client with a specific diagnosis.

INSURANCE PLANS   A variety of plans has come into existence to finance health care in the United States. These include private insurance and group insurance. Each individual and group plan offers different options for consumers to consider when choosing a prepaid health care program.

Private insurance is provided by are numerous commercial health insurance carriers offering a wide range of coverage plans classified by either not-for-profit or for-profit. Private health insurance usually pays 80% of the costs of health care services. With private insurance health plans, the insurance company reimburses the health care provider a fee for each service provided (fee-for-service). The term *third-party reimbursement* refers to the insurance company that pays the client's (first party) bill to the provider (second party). These insurance plans may be purchased either as an individual plan or as part of a group plan through a person's employer, union, student association, or similar organization and often carry a monthly premium paid by the individual. Employers may pay part of the cost of the insurance if it is purchased as part of a group plan.

Health maintenance organizations (HMOs) are group health care agencies that provide health maintenance and treatment services to voluntary enrollees. A fee is set without regard to the amount or kind of services needed or provided. The HMO plan emphasizes client wellness; the better the health of the person, the fewer the HMO services that are needed and the greater the agency's profit. Members of HMOs choose a primary care provider (PCP): an internal medicine physician, general practitioner, or nurse practitioner who evaluates their health status and coordinates their care. The PCP can make a referral to a specialist if the need arises, but the cost of the specialist is not covered without this referral. Nurses working for HMOs focus on preventive and health promotion aspects of care.

The **preferred provider organization (PPO)** consists of a group of providers and perhaps a health care agency (often hospitals) that provide an insurance company or employer with health services at a discounted rate. One advantage of the PPO is that it provides clients with a choice of health care providers and services. Providers can belong to one or several PPOs, and the client can choose among the providers belonging to the PPO. A disadvantage of PPOs is that they tend to be slightly more expensive than HMO plans, and if individuals wish to join a PPO, they might have to pay more for the additional choices.

Preferred provider arrangements (PPAs) are similar to PPOs. The main difference is that the PPAs can be contracted with individual health care providers, whereas PPOs involve an organization of health care providers. A PPA plan can be limited or unlimited. A limited PPA restricts the client to using only preferred providers of health care; an unlimited PPA permits the client to use any health care provider in the area who accepts the contractual agreement of the plan. Again, with PPAs, more choices in health care providers may mean more cost to the enrollee.

Independent practice associations (IPAs) are somewhat like HMOs and PPOs. The IPA provides care in offices, just as the providers belonging to a PPO do. The difference is that clients pay a fixed prospective payment to the IPA, and the IPA pays the provider. In some instances, the health care provider bills the IPA for services; in others, the provider receives a fixed fee for services given. At the end of the fiscal year, any surplus money is divided among the providers; any loss is assumed by the IPA.

Physician/hospital organizations (PHOs) are joint ventures between a group of private practice physicians and a hospital. PHOs combine both resources and personnel to provide managed care alternatives and medical services. PHOs work with a variety of insurers to provide services. A typical PHO includes primary care providers and specialists.

An **integrated delivery system (IDS)** may include a PHO. Such a system incorporates acute care services, home health care, extended and skilled care facilities, and outpatient services. Most integrated delivery systems provide care throughout the life span. Insurers can contract with IDSs to provide all required services, rather than the insurer contracting with multiple agencies for the same services. Ideally, an IDS enhances continuity of care and communication between professionals and various agencies providing managed care.

COMMUNITY NURSING AND CARE CONTINUITY

The location of client care is expanding out of traditional settings into the community and neighborhoods. Many things influence whether clients select to receive their care in hospitals or in community settings. Some variables include clients' knowledge and awareness of community resources, cost, availability of home care, and perceived safety of home care.

Research is needed to show whether there are differences in health outcomes based on location of care. The most recent data show a decrease in the percent of total health care dollars that were spent in hospitals and an increase in dollars spent for home care (National Center for Health Statistics, 2005).

The Movement of Health Care to the Community

Consumers and health care professionals often express major dissatisfaction with the current health care system, which focuses on acute, hospital-based care. Although plans to reform the health care system have been proposed nationally and internationally, no single plan has been adopted. Drafts of legislative reform in the United States include initiatives directed at cost control through managed care competition, providing health insurance for the poor, and transforming the insurance industry. Nurses, professional organizations, and consumers influence health care reform. Nurses help to influence political decision making regarding health care by membership in their professional organizations.

Consumers are effecting major changes in health care delivery systems. Consumers are adopting health-related values that include the following:

- Health means more than the absence of disease; it encompasses well-being and quality of life.
- Quality of life is related to a healthy community that includes healthy families and a healthy environment.
- Individuals can actively participate in promoting and maintaining their health through behavior and lifestyle changes.
- Disease prevention is important.

These values indicate that consumers support an increased emphasis on health care services and programs that promote wellness and restoration and prevent disease.

Primary Health Care and Primary Care

Another major influence promoting health care reform has been the work on *Healthy People 2000* and *Healthy People 2010* (U.S. Department of Health and Human Services [USDHHS], 2000). These projects present health-related objectives that provide a framework for national health promotion, health protection, and disease prevention. Details of *Healthy People 2010* are discussed in Chapter 5 ∞.

The term *primary health care* (PHC) was coined in the World Health Assembly by WHO and the United Nations International Children's Emergency Fund (UNICEF). **Primary health care (PHC)** is defined as essential health care based on practical, scientifically sound, and socially acceptable methods and technology made universally accessible to individuals and families in the community through their full participation and at a cost that the community and country can afford to maintain at every stage of their development in the spirit of self-reliance and self-determination. (WHO, 1978, p. 35). The term *primary health care* is not to be confused with *primary prevention*, which includes inter-

ventions aimed at preventing illness or injury such as immunizations, or primary nursing, which is a means of delivering health care that places responsibility for the client's plan of care in the hands of the primary nurse.

Primary health care incorporates five principles:

- Equitable distribution
- Appropriate technology
- A focus on health promotion and disease prevention
- Community participation
- A multisectoral approach

Deep concern about health care for the majority of the world's population, specifically lower life expectancies and high mortality rates among children, led to the global health strategy of primary health care. The WHO declaration emphasized health or well-being as a fundamental right and a worldwide social goal. It attempted to address inequality in health status of persons in all countries and to target government responsibility for policies that would promote economic, social, and health development. Both economic and social development was considered basic to the achievement of health for all. Thus, primary health care (PHC) extends beyond the boundaries of traditional health care services. It involves issues of the environment, agriculture, housing, and other social, economic, and political issues such as poverty, transportation, unemployment, economic development to sustain the population, and so on. A major feature of PHC is that consumers, governments, and public institutions such as public health departments and city councils should be involved in the planning and delivery of health care.

PHC differs from primary care (PC). Primary care addresses personal health services and not population-based public health services. **Primary care (PC)**, according to the Institute of Medicine (IOM), is "the provision of integrated, accessible health care services by clinicians who are accountable for addressing a large majority of personal health services, developing a sustained partnership with patients, and practicing in the context of family and community" (IOM, 1994, p. 15).

PHC is community based and driven and requires active community involvement in making decisions to improve health. PC, on the other hand, is expert driven and involves health professionals who advise individuals and communities about what is best for their health. Other differences are shown in Table 3–1.

There are also similarities between PHC and PC. Both acknowledge the prevention and promotion components of health and well-being. Both strive for universal access to and affordability of health care, support empowerment of the client, and target those at risk for preventable health problems.

Community-Based Health Care

Community-based health care (CBHC) is a PHC system that provides health-related services within the context of people's daily lives—that is, in places where people spend their time, for example, in the home, in shelters, in long-term care

TABLE 3–1	Differences between Primary Care and Primary Health Care

PRIMARY CARE	PRIMARY HEALTH CARE
• Community participation is provider directed.	• Community participation is client directed.
• The professional's role is expert, provider, authority, and team leader.	• The professional's role is facilitator, consultant, and resource.
• Collaboration occurs among members of the health care team.	• Collaboration goes beyond the health care sector.
• The individual or family is the focus.	• The community or some aggregate is the focus.
• Access is limited.	• Access is universal.
• Health care is available within given health care institutions.	• Health care is available where people live and work.
• Empowerment is a provider-assisted process.	• Empowerment is a collaborative, enabling process.

Note: Reprinted from *Nursing Outlook, 43*(1), D. Barnes et al., "Primary Health Care and Primary Care: A Confusion of Philosophies," pp. 7–16. Copyright 1995, with permission of Elsevier.

residences, at work, in schools, in senior citizens' centers, in ambulatory settings, and in hospitals. The care is directed toward a specific group within the geographic neighborhood. In contrast to the traditional health care system that focuses primarily on the ill and the injured, community-based care is holistic. It involves a broad range of services designed not only to restore health but also to promote health, prevent illness, and protect the public. To be truly effective, a CBHC system needs to (a) provide easy access to care, (b) be flexible in responding to the care needs that individuals and families identify, (c) promote care between and among health care agencies through improved communication mechanisms, (d) provide appropriate support for family caregivers, and (e) be affordable.

Community Health

A **community** is a collection of people who share some attribute of their lives and interact with each other in some way. Groups that constitute a community because of common member interests are often referred to as *communities of interest*. A community can also be defined as a social system in which the members interact formally or informally and form networks that operate for the benefit of all people in the community. In community health, the community may be viewed as having a common health problem, such as a high incidence of infant mortality or of tuberculosis, HIV infection, or another communicable disease. A population is composed of people who share some common characteristic but who do not necessarily interact with each other. Community health nursing focuses on promoting and preserving the health of population groups.

Communities are living entities similar to individuals and families. As such, the nurse needs to carry out an assessment of this community as the client. Several community assessment frameworks have been devised. Students who enroll in a community health nursing course will study these in some detail. Box 3–4 shows major aspects of a community assessment.

Planning community health may be oriented toward improved crisis management, disease prevention, health maintenance, or health promotion. The responsibility for planning at the community level is usually broadly based on, and needs to include, as many of the community partners as possible. The exact resources and skills of members of the community often depend on the size of the community. A broadly based planning group is more likely to create a plan that is acceptable to members of the community. Also, people who are involved in planning become educated about the problems, the resources, and the interrelationships within the system.

In community health, evaluation determines whether the planned interventions have led to the achievement of the established goals and objectives; for example, was the immunization rate of preschool children improved? Because community health is usually a collaborative process between health providers, community leaders, politicians, and consumers, all may be involved in the evaluation process. Often the community health nurse is the agent of evaluation, collecting and assessing the data that determine the effectiveness of implemented programs.

Community-Based Settings

Traditionally, community nursing services have been provided in county and state health departments (public health nursing), in schools (school nursing), in workplaces (occupational nursing), and in homes (home health care and hospice nursing). Over the years, numerous other settings have been established, including day-care centers, senior centers, storefront clinics, homeless shelters, mental health centers, crisis centers, drug rehabilitation programs, and ambulatory care centers. More recent settings for community nursing practice include nurse-managed community nursing centers, parish nursing, and telehealth projects.

Community nursing centers provide primary care to specific populations and are staffed by nurse practitioners and community health nurses. Although the nurses are the primary providers of care to clients visiting the center, a physician's consultation is available as needed. Nursing centers may be located in schools, workplaces, or other community agencies, or be free standing. Nursing centers

BOX 3–4 Major Aspects of a Community Assessment

Physical Environment

Consider the natural boundaries, size, and population density; types of dwellings; and incidence of crime, vandalism, and substance abuse.

Education

Consider educational facilities; existing school health facilities; type and amount of health services handled by the school; school lunch programs; extracurricular sports, libraries, and counseling services; continuing education or extended education programs; and extent of parental involvement in the schools.

Safety and Transportation

Consider fire, police, and sanitation services; sources of water and its treatment; quality of the air; garbage disposal service; availability and safety of public transportation; and availability of ambulance services.

Politics and Government

Consider kind of government; organizations active in the community; influential people in the community; issues that have recently appeared on local ballots; and the average election turnout.

Health and Social Services

Consider existing hospitals, health care facilities, and health care services; number, type, and routine caseloads of community health professionals; geographic, economic, and cultural accessibility to health care services; sources of health information; level of immunization among children and adults; life expectancy in the community; availability of home health care and long-term care services; and availability of transportation service to all major health facilities.

Communication

Consider local newspapers; radio and TV stations, postal services, Internet access, and telephone services; frequency of public forums; and presence of informal bulletin boards.

Economics

Consider the main industries and occupations; percentage of the population employed or attending school; income levels and quality and type of housing; occupational health programs; and major employers in the community.

Recreation

Consider recreational facilities in the community and outside the community; theaters and movie houses; number and types of church and religious services; number and utilization of playgrounds, pools, parks, and sports facilities; level of participation in various church programs; and number and types of social committees, organizations, and clubs available.

Note: From *Community as Partner: Theory and Practice in Nursing*, 4th ed. (pp. 172–173), by E. T. Anderson and J. McFarlane, 2004, Philadelphia: Lippincott Williams & Wilkins. Adapted with permission.

---

must interface with nurse-managed services in other settings across the health care continuum, that is, services being provided to clients in their home, hospital, or long-term care facility. Various categories of community nursing centers include community outreach centers, institution-based centers, school-based centers, and wellness centers.

Parish nursing was founded in the United States in Illinois in the mid-1980s by Reverend Granger Westberg (Smith, 2003) and became a specialty recognized by the ANA in 1998. The roles of the parish nurse include counseling, educating, referring, and facilitating. Parish nurses help to integrate faith and health. An estimated 3,000 parish nurses serve churches, synagogues, and temples in the United States (Figure 3–4). Most are volunteers, but some are employees paid by the congregation or an affiliated institution such as a health system or community agency. Parish nursing is nondenominational, includes nurses of all religious faiths, and is one of the few community-based nursing roles found with a similar structure and focus in nations around the world.

Telehealth projects use communication and information technology to provide health information and health care services to people in rural, remote, or underserved areas. Video conferencing or "video clinics" enable health care workers to provide distant consultation to assess and treat ambulatory clients who have a variety of health care needs. These video conferences are similar to any outpatient clinic visit except that the client and health care specialist

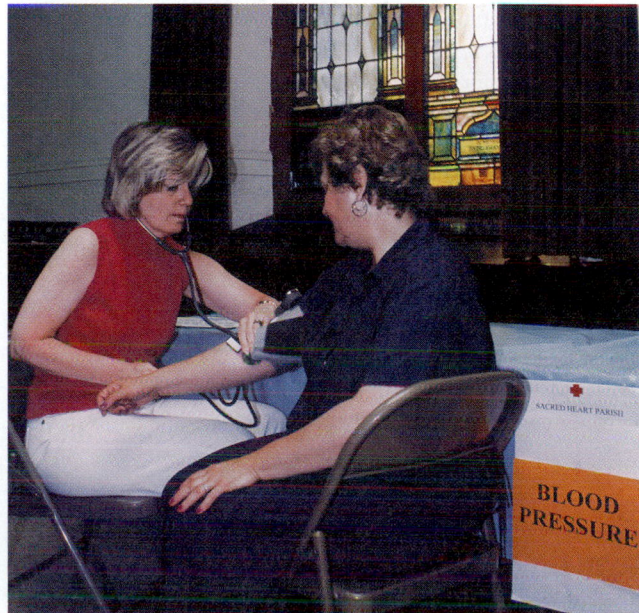

Figure 3–4 ● Some parish-based health services provide care to community residents in addition to members of the congregation.

are miles apart. A related development to telehealth is telenursing, in which nurses provide client teaching and health promotion to distant clients.

Community-Based Nursing

Community-based nursing (CBN) is nursing care directed toward specific individuals. However, community-based nursing involves nursing care that is not confined to one practice setting. It extends beyond institutional boundaries and involves a network of nursing services: nursing wellness centers, ambulatory care, acute care, long-term care nursing services, telephone advice, home health, school health, and hospice services. For example, a nurse case manager may be involved in (a) visiting a newly admitted client in the hospital to take a detailed nursing history, confer with the primary nurse, and begin discharge planning; (b) making several home visits to monitor a client recently transferred from a hospital to a long-term care agency to discuss the client's progress with the nursing staff; or (c) making consultative telephone calls to other health professionals (physicians, social workers, respiratory therapists, and so on) and to clients who are managing self-care independently but who may need support.

CLINICAL ALERT

Community-based nursing and community health nursing are not the same concept. Community-based nursing focuses on care of individuals in geographically local settings, whereas community health nursing emphasizes the promotion and preservation of the health of groups (populations or aggregates).

Other nurses who work in community-based settings, such as case managers, occupational health nurses, school nurses, and public health department nurses, need to be prepared to make home visits. Home visits can provide information that is not obtainable in other ways. Nurses practicing in community-based integrated health care systems need to have specific knowledge and skill including: (a) determinants of a healthy community; (b) primary and secondary preventive strategies for people of all ages; (c) health promotion strategies for individuals, families, and communities;

(d) how to participate in collaborative and interdisciplinary teamwork; (e) determinants of an accessible, cost-effective, integrated health care system; (f) decision-making processes that involve active participation by consumers and balance cost and quality care; and (g) concepts of information management. Community-based nurses also require up-to-date clinical skills and knowledge of complex technology, public health policy, and strategies to influence and effect change.

Collaboration among health care professionals becomes increasingly important as more practitioners specialize in progressively more narrow areas of expertise while others take on the generalist role. Over time, the boundaries and legal scope of practice of each health care profession may change. To deliver optimal health care for the client, nurses must work as a member of the team providing comprehensive health care whether they work in community health, acute care facilities, or in any other area of practice.

In 1992, the ANA Congress on Nursing Practice adopted the following operational definition of the concept of collaboration:

> Collaboration means a collegial working relationship with another health care provider in the provision of (to supply) patient care. Collaborative practice requires (may include) the discussion of patient diagnosis and cooperation in the management and delivery of care. Each collaborator is available to the other for consultation either in person or by communication device, but need not be physically present on the premises at the time the actions are performed. The patient-designated health care provider is responsible for the overall direction and management of patient care (ANA, 1992).

Nurses collaborate with nursing colleagues and other health care professionals. They frequently collaborate about client care but may also be involved, for example, in collaborating on bioethical issues, on legislation, on health-related research, and with professional organizations. Box 3–5 outlines selected aspects of the nurse's role as a collaborator.

BOX 3–5   The Nurse as a Collaborator

With Nurse Colleagues

- Shares personal expertise with other nurses and elicits the expertise of others to ensure quality client care.
- Develops a sense of trust and mutual respect with peers that recognizes their unique contributions.

With Other Health Care Professionals

- Recognizes the contribution that each member of the interdisciplinary team can make by virtue of his or her expertise and view of the situation.
- Listens to each individual's views.
- Shares health care responsibilities in exploring options, setting goals, and making decisions with clients and families.
- Participates in collaborative interdisciplinary research to increase knowledge of a clinical problem or situation.

With Professional Nursing Organizations

- Seeks opportunities to collaborate with and within professional organizations.
- Serves on committees in state (or provincial) and national nursing organizations or specialty groups.
- Supports professional organizations in political action to create solutions for professional and health care concerns.

With Legislators

- Offers expert opinions on legislative initiatives related to health care.
- Collaborates with other health care providers and consumers on health care legislation to best serve the needs of the public.

To fulfill a collaborative role, nurses need to assume accountability and increased authority in practice areas. Education is integral to ensuring that the members of each professional group understand the collaborative nature of their roles, specific contributions, and the importance of working together. Each professional needs to understand how an integrated delivery system centers on the client's health care needs rather than on the particular care given by one group. Key elements necessary for collaboration include effective communication skills, mutual respect, trust, and a decision-making process.

An important aspect of decision making is satisfied when the interdisciplinary team focuses on the client's priority needs and organizing interventions accordingly. The discipline best able to address the client's needs is given priority in planning and is responsible for providing its interventions in a timely manner. Nurses, by the nature of their holistic practice, are often able to help the team identify priorities and areas requiring further attention.

CONTINUITY OF CARE

A major responsibility of the nurse is to ensure **continuity of care**. Continuity of care is the coordination of health care services by health care providers for clients moving from one health care setting to another and between and among health care professionals. Continuity ensures uninterrupted and consistent services for the client from one level of care to another. When coordinated appropriately, it maintains client-focused individualized care and helps optimize the client's health status. To provide continuity of care, nurses needs to initiate discharge planning for all clients when they are admitted to any health care setting, to involve the client and family or support persons in the planning process, and to collaborate with other health care professionals to ensure that all client needs are met.

However, achieving continuity assumes that needed client data are shared with only those who have the right and need to acquire the information, while implementing strategies to protect client privacy. In the computer age, this has become a complex requirement since standards for coding and transmitting data are not universal and authentication of authority to access may be breached. The privacy aspect of HIPAA (discussed in Chapter 2 ∞) will result in a balance between protecting disclosure of confidential client information and the need for certain data to be released to specific agencies. Ultimately, clients will have increased control over their own information, and those who violate the rule face significant penalties. Case managers and public health nurses need to maintain vigilance to protect the privacy of client health care information when sending and receiving telephone messages, faxes, and electronic documentation when in field settings as well as within health care facilities in order to maintain compliance with HIPAA regulations.

Care across the Life Span

The majority of children and older adults receive their health care in their communities rather than in hospitals. Home births, school-based childhood immunization programs, sex education for teens, chronic disease management in adults, and hospice care are all opportunities for the nurse to work with clients within the wide variety of community health organizations in order to provide wellness and illness care. Research has shown that community-based programs can have substantial positive impact on self-care and well-being (see, for example, Farrell, Wicks, & Martin, 2004). A wide variety of initiatives focused on care provided in the community for children is found at the American Academy of Pediatrics website.

Discharge Planning

Discharge planning is the process of preparing a client to leave one level of care for another within or outside the current health care agency. Usually, discharge planning refers to the client leaving the hospital for home. However, discharges occur among many other settings. Within a facility it can occur from one unit to another. Clients may move from a hospital to a long-term care agency, from a rehabilitation center to home, or from a home health care setting to a hospital, and so on.

Each agency generally has its own policies and procedures related to discharge. Many agencies have case managers or discharge planners, a health or social services professional who coordinates the transition and acts as a link between the discharging agency and the receiving facility. Often, a nurse assumes this responsibility of providing continuity of care.

Discharge planning needs to begin when a client is admitted to an agency, especially in hospitals where stays are considerably shortened. Effective discharge planning involves ongoing assessment to obtain comprehensive information about the client's changing needs and nursing care plans to ensure the client's and caregivers' needs are met. In some situations discharge planning necessitates health team conferences and family conferences. At a health team conference, health care professionals focus on ways to individualize care for the client. At a family conference, both health professionals and the family discuss family issues related to the client. Both types of conferences give the client, family, and health care professionals the opportunity to mutually plan care and set goals.

Nurses preparing to send clients home from the hospital need to assess their clients' personal and health data; abilities to perform the activities of daily living; any physical, cognitive, or other functional limitations; caregivers' responses and abilities; adequacy of financial resources; community supports; hazards or barriers that the home environment presents; and need for health care assistance in the home. Box 3–6 outlines details about each of these parameters.

The data establish nursing activities that are required before the client is discharged. These activities most often

BOX 3–6	Discharge Planning: Home Assessment Parameters

Personal and Health Data

Age; sex; height and weight; cultural beliefs and practices; medical history; current health status; prognosis; surgery

Abilities to Perform Activities of Daily Living

Abilities for dressing; eating; toileting; bathing (tub, shower, sponge); ambulating (with or without aids such as a cane, crutches, walker, wheelchair); transferring (from bed to chair, in and out of bath, in and out of car); meal preparation; transportation; shopping

Disabilities/Limitations

Sensory losses (auditory, visual); motor losses (paralysis, amputation); communication disorders; mental confusion or depression; incontinence

Caregivers' Responses/Abilities

Principal caregiver's relationship to client; thoughts and feelings about client's discharge; expectations for recovery; health and coping abilities; comfort with performing needed care

Financial Resources

Financial resources and needs (note equipment, supplies, medications, special foods required)

Community Supports

Family members, friends, neighbors, volunteers; resources such as Medicaid; food stamps; nutrition services; health centers; community health nurses; day programs; legal assistance; home care; respite care

Home Hazard Appraisal

Safety precautions (stairs with or without handrails; lighting in rooms, hallways, stairways; night-lights in hallways or bathroom; grab bars near toilet and tub; firmly attached carpets and rugs); self-care barriers (lack of running water, lack of wheelchair access to bathroom or home, lack of space for required equipment, lack of elevator)

Need for Health Care Assistance

Home-delivered meals; special dietary needs; volunteers for telephone reassurance, friendly visiting, transportation, shopping; assistance with bathing; assistance with housekeeping; assistance with wound care, ostomies, tubes, intravenous medications

---

include (a) teaching the client to cope with continuing self-care at home and (b) a home care referral.

Clients need help to understand their situation, to make health care decisions, and to learn new health behaviors. Because of today's shortened hospital stays, it is often unrealistic to attempt to teach clients everything they need to know. Referral to a home health agency for follow-up teaching may be necessary. Essential information before discharge includes information about medications, dietary and activity restrictions, signs of complications that need to be reported to the primary care provider, follow-up appointments and telephone numbers, and where supplies can be obtained. Clients or caregivers also need to demonstrate safe performance of any necessary treatments. Information needs to be provided verbally and in writing. Details about effective teaching strategies are provided in Chapter 14∞. Reinforcement of acute care discharge information will often fall in the domain of the community-oriented nurse. Client issues related to health literacy, language barriers, and access to resources to carry out the provided health care instruction are major concerns to community nurses.

The referral process is a systematic problem-solving approach that helps clients to use resources that meet their health care needs. The process involves knowledge of community resources and an ability to solve problems, set priorities, coordinate, and collaborate. Home care referrals are often made before discharge. Referrals need to present as much information as possible about the client and the hospitalization to the agency. Most agencies have well-established protocols and detailed referral forms. The nurse caring for the hospital client is responsible for confirming and documenting that the relevant referrals have been made.

LIFESPAN CONSIDERATIONS
Health Care Delivery

Children

The Search Institute has identified evidence-based assets characteristic of healthy communities and of different age groups of children. The impact of these assets has been studied in children from birth through adolescence, and many communities across the United States are using them to structure programs for children and youth. Among the assets are such things as family support, family values of equality and social justice, involvement of children and youth with adults and community organizations, constructive use of young people's time, and engagement in learning. The institute also has five action strategies for transforming communities for the betterment of youth, which involve engaging adults, mobilizing youth, activating organizations, expanding programs, and influencing policy.

Older Adults

Older adults often require various levels of health care delivery. Clients may go back and forth between these levels as their needs fluctuate. At various times and situations, they might need care from hospitals, home care, extended care facilities, ambulatory care, and assisted living. Maintaining communications and providing continuity of care during these changes are essential.

Caregivers of older adults are often older themselves and may have health problems of their own. Attention should be given to signs of emotional and physical fatigue and other problems that might arise for them. Community health nurses have the opportunity to do ongoing assessments of this as they see clients and caregivers in their home environment. They can then provide support and resources as needed.

In order to identify and recommend referrals, the nurse must already be familiar with the resources that are available in the community. Using this knowledge, plus information regarding the client's previous awareness and choice of community resources, hospital nurses play a key role in maintaining effective continuity of health care.

To ensure appropriate reimbursement to the home health agency, the primary care provider must provide a written order for a home care referral and subsequent home visits. Clients must meet specific criteria to have Medicare or other third-party payers reimburse them for home care services.

HOME HEALTH NURSING

Historically, home care consisted primarily of nurses providing private duty care in clients' homes and care of the ill by their own family members. However, the delivery of professional nursing services in home settings has increased in frequency, scope, and complexity in the past two decades. Home care today involves a wide range of health care professionals providing services in the home setting to people recovering from an acute illness or injury, or who are disabled, or who have a chronic condition. A number of factors have contributed to this trend, among them rising health care costs, an aging population, and a growing emphasis on managing chronic illness and stress, preventing illness, and enhancing the quality of life. In the not-too-distant past, home health care occurred at the end of the client care continuum—that is, after discharge from an acute care facility. Today the trend is changing to use of home health care services to avoid hospitalization.

Hospice nursing, support and care of the dying person and family, is often considered a subspecialty of home health nursing because hospice services are frequently delivered to terminally ill clients in their residence. See Chapter 29 ∞ for further information about hospice care.

Home health nursing is one of the growing sectors of the health care system. Factors that have contributed to the growth of home health care include (1) the increase in the older population, who are frequent recipients of home care; (2) third-party payers who favor home care to control costs; (3) the ability of agencies and institutions to successfully deliver high-technology services in the home; and (4) consumers who prefer to receive care in the home rather than in an institution. A common misperception by the general public is that home health nursing is only custodial in its scope of practice. However, health promotion is one of the intentions for the home health nurse in order to promote client self-care. Home care nurses are actively engaged in providing support and education for family caregivers as well as clients.

Unique Aspects of Home Health Nursing

Home care nurses must function independently in a variety of unfamiliar home settings and situations. Because the home is the family's territory, power and control issues in delivering nursing care differ from those in the hospital. Due to the limited time for visits and the possibly lengthy interval between visits, this process does not always occur as quickly as it might when nursing within an acute care facility.

Health care that is provided in the home is often given with other family members present. Families may feel freer to question advice, to ignore directions, to do things differently, and to set their own priorities and schedules. Home care nurses implement every step of the nursing process, using critical-thinking skills in designing, implementing, and evaluating the plan of care.

Home health nurses have identified significant advantages in caring for individuals and families in the home. The home setting is intimate, which fosters familiarity, sharing, connections, and caring between clients, families, and their nurse. Behaviors are more natural, cultural beliefs and practices are more visible, and multigenerational interactions are more likely to occur. Nurses often get to know the client and family well, as they may care for clients over weeks or months.

Home health nurses have also identified issues that negatively affect care in the home. More than any other care providers, these nurses have firsthand knowledge of and experience related to the burden of caregiving and the role of family dynamics in health care practices. In the interest of cutting health care costs, policy makers, third-party payers, and medical providers are placing increasingly complex responsibilities on clients' families and significant other(s). Family caregiving demands may go on for months or years, placing the caregivers themselves (many of whom are older adults) at risk for physiologic and psychosocial problems. Additionally, nurses enter homes where the living conditions and support systems may be inadequate.

Nurses caring for clients in rural home settings have challenges different from those in urban or suburban environments. These include the need for flexibility since clients may live far distances from the nurse and require care in the evening or at night, creativity and the ability to practice independently since fewer resources (including other nurses) are available, and the ability to work in an environment over which there is little nurse control (Boucher, 2005). Thus, those nurses who require a high degree of certainty, structure, and consistency are less likely to be successful in rural home health locations.

The home health nurse practices a variety of roles when caring for clients. In addition to providing hands-on care, home health nurses serve as health educators to the client, caregivers, and families. Indirect care is provided by the home health nurse to the client each time the nurse consults with other health care providers about ways to improve nursing care for the client. This consultation about client care issues often manifests itself in multidisciplinary care conferences where the role of the home health nurse is as client advocate.

The Home Health Care System

The need for home health care may be identified by any person involved with the client. Clients are referred to a home health agency or private duty nursing agency. Individuals with extremely complex needs, beyond those that direct nursing care alone can provide, may benefit from the services of an agency with direct connections to a medical equipment company. Payment for home health is accomplished through private pay, third-party reimbursement, or a combination of sources.

After an initial set of physician's orders is obtained, a nursing evaluation visit is scheduled to enroll the client and identify the client's needs. The initial visit, often referred to as "opening the case," should include the client and the immediate family involved with the client's care. At this visit, the nurse develops a plan of care, which must be reviewed, approved, authorized, and signed by the attending physician before home health agency providers can continue with services.

Home health agencies offer coordinated professional, skilled, and paraprofessional services. Because clients often require the services of several professionals, case coordination (case management) is essential. This responsibility generally rests with the registered nurse. Depending on the agency, additional providers may include nurse practitioners, practical nurses, nursing assistants, home health care aides, physical therapists, occupational therapists, respiratory therapists, speech therapists, social workers, dietitians, and a pastoral care minister or chaplain. In addition, it is not unusual for home health agencies to offer the services of specialized nurses such as wound/ostomy/continence nurses or diabetes educators. The care plan implemented by the home health agency may require services once or twice a day, up to 7 days a week. The minimum time of each period of care, or visit, is usually 1 hour.

There are several different types of home health agencies. Official or public agencies are operated by state or local governments and financed primarily by tax funds. Voluntary or private not-for-profit agencies are supported by donations, endowments, charities, and third-party reimbursement. Private, proprietary agencies are for-profit organizations and are governed by either individual owners or national corporations. Institution-based agencies operate under a parent organization, such as a hospital, funded by the same sources as the parent. Regardless of the type of agency, all home health agencies must meet specific standards for licensing, certification, and accreditation.

Private duty agencies may be referred to as a registry that contracts with individual practitioners (e.g., nurses, home health aides) to care for the client in the home. The client may require care coverage from the agency for 4 to 24 hours a day. However, the agency is not focused uniquely on providing personnel for home care assignments but also supplies staff to hospitals, clinics, and other care settings. Thus, it does not afford the coordinated focus of a home care agency. Private duty care is expensive. Commercial insurance generally provides limited reimbursement. Otherwise, the client must pay privately.

A **durable medical equipment (DME)** company provides health care equipment for the client at home. The types of equipment can range from hospital beds and bedside commodes to ventilators and apnea monitors. Most DME companies today seek accreditation from the Joint Commission on Accreditation of Healthcare Organizations (JCAHO) to ensure compliance with quality standards for equipment and services.

Health care agencies in the United States receive reimbursement for services they provide from various sources: Medicare and Medicaid, private insurance companies, and private pay. The Medicare and Medicaid programs have strict guidelines governing reimbursement for home health care (Centers for Medicare & Medicaid Services, 2004). The agency must also meet specific conditions. Not-for-profit agencies, such as the Visiting Nurses Associations (VNAs), are reimbursed by public and private insurance plus charitable donations to the agency.

All health care agencies are expected to adhere to established guidelines and provide care within the predetermined reimbursement levels. Treatment plans (developed by the home health agency providers and authorized by the physician) are used by the reimbursement source. Only interventions identified on the treatment plan are paid for. Periodically the reimbursement source may request the home health provider's notes to substantiate what is being done in the home. This is a major reason why accurate documentation is critical.

Roles of the Home Health Nurse

Historically, nurses who provided direct services in the home were strong generalists who focused on long-term preventive, educational, and rehabilitative outcomes. Today many home health nurses possess high-technology skills that were formerly used only in acute care settings. Nurses collaborate with physicians and other health care professionals in providing care. They play a key role in facilitating an effective plan of care as clients move among hospitals, home, school, work, and other care settings such as clinics or long-term care. Major roles of the home health nurse are those of advocate, caregiver (provider of direct care), educator, and case manager or coordinator.

Dimensions of Home Health Nursing

PERSPECTIVES OF THE CLIENT   Home care clients include a diverse population that encompasses all ages, a variety of health problems, and families of different structures and cultural backgrounds. Home care clients have a wide range of health problems that include disabilities, perinatal problems, mental illnesses, and acute and chronic illnesses. The nurse should not assume that the client understands the various personnel and their roles in providing home health care.

Although the person receiving care is considered the primary client in home care, the client's family can be considered secondary clients because they are often associated with caregiving and have a major impact on the client's wellness status. The home health nurse will encounter many different family structures ranging from single families to extended families and dwellings that house multiple families. In the home setting, family members may include not only persons related by birth and marriage, but also friends, other significant individuals, and animals.

Various cultural influences also affect the client's health care beliefs and practices. The home health nurse needs to be culturally sensitive. See Chapter 4 ∞ for detailed information about making cultural assessments and providing culturally competent care.

CLIENT SAFETY   Hazards in the home are major causes of falls, fire, poisoning, and other accidents, such as those caused by improper use of household equipment. The appraisal of such hazards and suggestions for remedies is an essential nursing function. See the Client Teaching box for home hazards and Chapter 20 ∞ for a discussion of potential hazards and preventive actions for individuals of all ages.

Obviously home health nurses cannot expect to change a family's living space and lifestyle. However, they can express their concern and react appropriately when a situation suggests that an injury is imminent. Nurses must document information they provide and the family's response to instruction, and make ongoing assessments about the family's use of safety precautions.

Other aspects of client safety relate to emergency situations. The home health nurse can assist the client and caregivers by posting a list of all emergency telephone numbers, listing client medications with potential side effects, helping the client apply for a medical alert system, enrolling the client in a program that places all of the client's vital medical information in one place, and recommending that the client enroll in an emergency response system.

NURSE SAFETY   Some less desirable living locations pose additional personal safety concerns for the nurse. Many home health agencies have contracts with security firms to escort nurses needing to see clients in potentially unsafe neighborhoods. The nurse should avoid taking any personal belongings during these visits and have a preestablished mechanism to signal for help. Home health agencies provide training for nurses in ways to decrease personal risk. See the accompanying Research Note for one example.

INFECTION CONTROL   The goal of infection control in the home is to protect clients, caregivers, and the general

---

CLIENT TEACHING · Home Hazard Appraisal for Adults

Client and Environment

- *Walkways and stairways (inside and outside):* Note uneven sidewalks or paths, broken or loose steps, absence of handrails or placement on only one side of stairways, insecure handrails, congested hallways or other traffic areas, and adequacy of lighting at night.
- *Floors:* Note uneven and highly polished or slippery floors and any unanchored rugs or mats.
- *Furniture:* Note hazardous placement of furniture with sharp corners. Note chairs or stools that are too low to get into and out of or that provide inadequate support.
- *Bathroom(s):* Note presence of grab bars around tubs and toilets, nonslip surfaces in tubs and shower stalls, handheld showerhead, adequacy of night lighting, need for raised toilet seat or bath chair in tub or shower, ease of access to shelves, and water temperature regulated at a maximum of 49°C (120°F).
- *Kitchen:* Note pilot lights (gas stove) in need of repair, inaccessible storage areas, and hazardous furniture.
- *Bedrooms:* Note adequacy of lighting, in particular the availability of night-lights and accessibility of light switches; ease of access to commode, urinal, or bedpan; and need for hospital bed or bed rails.
- *Electrical:* Note unanchored or frayed electrical cords and outlets that are overloaded or near water.
- *Fire protection:* Note presence or absence of smoke detectors, fire extinguisher, and fire escape plan, and improper storage of combustibles (e.g., gasoline) or corrosives (e.g., rust remover).
- *Toxic substances:* Note improperly labeled cleaning solutions.
- *Communication devices:* Note presence of method to call for help, such as a telephone or intercom in the bedroom and elsewhere (e.g., kitchen), and access to emergency telephone numbers.
- *Medications:* Note medications kept beyond date of expiration, adequacy of lighting for medication cabinet or storage, and method of disposal of sharp objects such as needles used for injections.

RESEARCH NOTES · Do Nurses Making Home Visits Worry about Their Own Safety?

The researchers in this study surveyed 83 rehabilitation nurses who performed home visits. A common theme in the responses was concern for personal safety. Community issues related to poor communication systems, delayed notification of dangerous situations, weather conditions predisposing to automobile hazards, and difficulty in locating clients' homes due to unfamiliar and possibly dangerous neighborhoods. Home issues included poor sanitation, inadequate housing, uncontrolled pets, and client lifestyle. Authors proposed specific guidelines for nurses such as ensuring that cell phones functioned properly; having cars properly serviced, especially for hot or freezing weather; contacting family members for driving directions or meeting the nurse at a central location and guiding the nurse to the home; carrying a signal device such as a whistle or alarm; carrying cleaning supplies such as gloves, drapes, water, and paper towels; advising the family regarding cancellation of visits; and reporting to agencies if violence or abuse is detected.

Implications

Although safety issues for any nurse visiting the client's home will vary somewhat based on the location and client characteristics, nurses must be prepared with strategies to prevent and cope with issues if they arise. All home care nurses should be thoroughly trained by the agency and know both public and private resources for assistance. The nurse also has a role in educating and assisting clients to avoid and correct unsafe situations.

Note: From "Safety Concerns for Rehabilitation Nurses in Home Care," by B. Brillhart, B. Kruse, and L. Heard, 2004, *Rehabilitation Nursing, 29*, pp. 227–229.

community from the transmission of disease. This is particularly important for clients who are immunocompromised, who have infectious or communicable diseases, or who have draining wounds, drainage tubes, or other invasive access devices. The nurse's major role in infection control is health teaching. Clients and caregivers need to learn about effective hand washing, use of gloves, handling of linens, disposal of wastes and soiled dressings, and the practice of infection control (standard precautions). Infection control can present a challenge to the home health nurse, especially if the home care facilities are not conducive to basic aseptic requirements such as running water for hand washing.

An important aspect of infection control involves handling the home health nurse's equipment and supplies. Supplies may include materials for hand cleansing; assessment equipment such as stethoscope, blood pressure cuff and monitor, thermometer, and tape measure; infection control items such as gowns, goggles, masks, gloves, and blood spill kit; and antimicrobial cleaning agents.

The same organizations that accredit hospitals evaluate home health nurses' practice. Deficiencies in the use of appropriate infection control practices are common findings during these evaluations (Sturkey, Linker, Keith, & Comeau, 2005). Although some modifications in technique may be indicated in the home setting, such as the use of clean rather than sterile technique in caring for chronic wounds, all the basic principles still apply. Nurses need to follow agency protocol about aseptic practice in the home.

CAREGIVER SUPPORT   Caregiving may be directed to individuals of any age and varies from short term to long term according to the physical or mental disabilities of the care receivers. Others who are recovering from a surgical procedure require care only on a temporary basis. Most caregivers have close relationships with the care receiver. Many caregiving relationships represent changes from the caring and caregiving intrinsic to all close relationships to an extraordinary and unequal burden for the caregiver. Caregivers may experience **caregiver role strain** when they have physical, emotional, social, and financial burdens that can seriously jeopardize their own health and well-being.

The home health nurse needs to recognize signs of caregiver role strain and suggest ways to minimize or alleviate this problem. Signs of caregiver overload include difficulty performing routine tasks for the client, reports of declining physical energy and insufficient time for caregiving, concern that caregiving responsibilities interfere with other roles such as those of parent, spouse, worker, friend, anxiety about ability to meet future care needs of client, feelings of anger and depression, and dramatic changes in the home environment's appearance.

The nurse needs to encourage caregivers to express their feelings and at the same time convey understanding about the difficulties associated with caregiving and acknowledge the caregivers' competence. The nurse can obtain a realistic appraisal of the situation by asking a caregiver to describe a typical day and daily or weekly leisure and social activities. It is also helpful to identify activities for which assistance is desired.

Activities that are commonly done by nurses and aides, such as changing an occupied bed and transferring a client from bed to chair, may be overwhelming to a caregiver who has not performed them before. Demonstrating them in the home and allowing caregivers to perform them with the nurse's supervision increases their confidence and increases the likelihood of them asking for assistance in other situations.

When activities for which assistance is required are identified, the nurse and caregiver need to identify possible sources of help. Both volunteer and agency sources need to be explored. Volunteer sources of help may include family members, neighbors, friends, church associates, or caregiver support groups in the community. Other sources include, for example, a home health aide for light housekeeping and grocery shopping, Meals on Wheels, day care, transportation, and counseling and social services. Families with a chronically ill member may benefit from a weekend respite—a program some hospitals provide in which the client is admitted to a skilled unit for observation and care, enabling the caregiver a break from ongoing health care needs.

Caregivers need to be reminded of the importance of caring for themselves by getting adequate rest, eating nutritious meals, asking for help, delegating household chores, and making time for leisure activities or simply some time alone. Family members other than the caregiver also may need help to learn ways to support the caregiver. The nurse may discuss the importance to the caregiver of regular phone calls, cards, letters, and visits; offer encouragement to take day trips or a vacation; listen without giving advice; acknowledge the burden of caregiving and the need to feel appreciated; and so on.

A particular challenge exists when the nurse is in a position to be a caregiver to a family member. Although the nurse's clinical expertise and familiarity with the client and setting can be especially useful, negotiating the professional distancing that is sometimes needed when providing care to clients can be difficult with family. The nurse may feel obligated to provide care, even when this is over and above regular employment responsibilities. The nurse must have the opportunity to step back and experience the role and emotions of being a family member—not only those of being a nurse.

The Practice of Nursing in the Home

The home health nurse assesses the health care demands of the client and family and the home and community environment. This process actually begins when the nurse contacts the client for the initial home visit and reviews documents received from the referral agency. The goal of the initial visit is to obtain a comprehensive clinical picture of the client's needs.

Most agencies have a packet that includes forms for consent to treatment; physical, psychosocial, and spiritual assessment; medications; pain assessment; family data; financial assessment including insurance verification; client's bill of rights; care plan; and daily visit notes. During the initial home visit, the home health nurse obtains a health his-

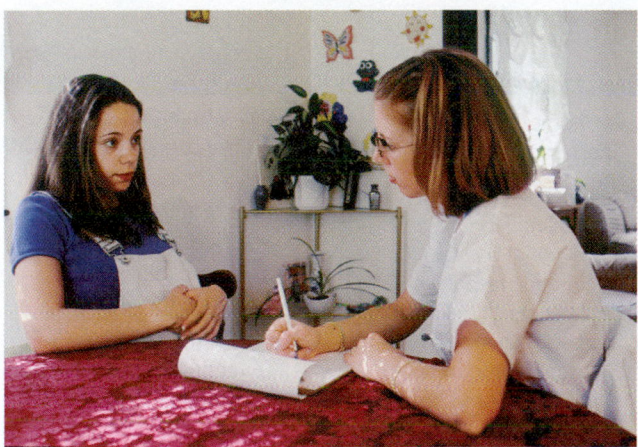

Figure 3–5 ⊙ Interviewing the home care client.

tory from the client (see Figure 3–5), examines the client, observes the relationship of the client and caregiver, and assesses the home and community environment. Parameters of assessment of the home environment include client and caregiver mobility, client ability to perform self-care, the cleanliness of the environment, the availability of caregiver support, safety, food preparation, financial supports, and the emotional status of the client and caregiver.

Following this initial client examination, the nurse determines whether further consults and support personnel are needed. Before completing the initial interview, the nurse also discusses what the client and family can expect from home care, what other health care providers may be needed to help the client achieve independence, and the frequency of home visits.

ESTABLISHING HEALTH ISSUES As in other care environments, the nurse identifies both actual and potential client problems. One of the most common examples of health issues that nurses address with clients in home care settings is lack of knowledge related to health conditions and self-care. Because client education is considered a skill reimbursed by Medicare and other commercial insurance carriers, it is important for the nurse to include knowledge deficits within the plan of care.

PLANNING AND DELIVERING CARE The nurse needs to encourage and permit clients to make their own health management decisions. Alternatives may need to be suggested for some decisions if the nurse identifies potential harm from a chosen course of action. Strategies to meet goals generally include teaching the client and family techniques of care and identifying appropriate resources to assist the client and family in maintaining self-sufficiency.

To implement the plan, the home health nurse performs nursing interventions, including teaching; coordinates and uses referrals and resources; provides and monitors all levels of technical care; collaborates with other disciplines and providers; identifies clinical problems and solutions from research and other health literature; supervises ancillary personnel; and advocates for the client's right to self-determination.

A large part of the nurse's role involves teaching the client and caregiver the necessary skills for self-care. Medication instruction about dosage, frequency of administration, and possible side effects is of particular concern for many clients. (See Chapter 22 ∞ for more information.) Clients who are receiving high-technology interventions are often anxious about their ability to manage such sophisticated equipment. The home health nurse is challenged to alleviate the client's fears and to provide thorough instruction, demonstration, and periodic evaluation of the client and family's performance of such skills. Members of the home care team specially trained in the skill generally make periodic visits to service the equipment and to monitor the client's skills.

Even though the client and family may become independent in self-care skills, the home health nurse still has the ultimate responsibility to ensure the client is receiving the prescribed therapy at the appropriate timed intervals. Ongoing communication with the primary care provider about the client's progress is critical, and the nurse must make ongoing assessments to ensure that all aspects of the care are being followed.

On subsequent home visits, the nurse observes the same parameters assessed on the initial home visit and relates findings to the expected outcomes or goals. The nurse can also teach caregivers parameters of evaluation so that they can obtain professional intervention if needed. Documentation of care given and the client's progress toward goal achievement at each visit is essential. Notes must also reflect plans for subsequent visits and when the client may be sufficiently prepared for self-care and discharge from the agency.

The Future of Home Health Care

What is the future for home health care? More studies are needed to determine the practicality, safety, effectiveness, cost, and satisfaction with home care—especially new models of "hospital-at-home" care. Trends in the home health care industry include:

1. Ethics committees to handle ethical issues that arise in the home. These committees may be necessary for agencies to receive accreditation.
2. Third-party reimbursement for community clinical nurse specialists and psychiatric nurse specialists. These advanced practice nurses can provide education, support, counseling, and therapy for clients and their families.
3. Third-party reimbursement for social workers. Social workers can assist clients and their families in the home with financial and household problems, freeing the nurse to focus on nursing care.
4. Nurse pain specialists to assess and manage pain in the home, thus avoiding costly hospitalizations and procedures.
5. Pet care for clients who may become too ill to care for them. Clients can make arrangements for the care of a pet if they are hospitalized or die.
6. Electronic home visits. A computerized system can obtain information, such as blood pressure readings, allowing case managers to review a client's progress from off-site.

LIFESPAN CONSIDERATIONS   Home Care

Children

One goal of *Healthy People 2010* is to reduce the number of children with disabilities living in care facilities from over 24,000 in 1997 to 0 by 2010 (U.S. Department of Health and Human Services, 2000). Ideally, all children with disabilities would live in a secure, "permanent" family environment. Such an environment is one that supports family strengths, connects families to their community, and fosters ongoing, secure relationships. At times, children with disabilities may need to be placed in adoptive or medical foster homes. Home health nurses can strengthen family functioning by:

- Providing information, advice, and instruction on care of the child.
- Identifying natural support systems (e.g., extended family, neighbors, friends).
- Helping families find community resources to meet their needs (e.g., respite care, technical and equipment services).
- Assisting families with alternative placement options as needed (e.g., medical foster care).
- Advocating for families with other health care providers and policy makers.

Older Adults

Clients who have been hospitalized are often discharged after short stays and may still be acutely ill. This becomes a challenge for home health nurses in planning and implementing care. Special areas of concern for older adults in this situation include the following:

- Healing time is slower due to changes that normally occur in aging, such as impaired circulation and alteration in immune response.
- Changes in medications or lingering traces of anesthesia may alter cognitive status, even though the effect is usually temporary.
- Weakness and fatigue create safety issues, such as risk for falling.
- Chronic diseases already present may have been complicated by other conditions acquired while hospitalized.
- Assessment should be initiated while the client is in the hospital to determine the need for assistive devices or environmental changes when the client returns home. Some examples of these devices are walkers, raised toilet seats, safety bars in the bathroom, and better lighting. Good planning eases the transition to home care for the client and caregiver.

In the future, although the number of older adults will increase, fewer family caregivers may be available. However, older adults appreciate receiving care from family members (Crist, 2005), and nurses should facilitate this when possible.

CHAPTER HIGHLIGHTS

- Health care delivery services can be categorized by the type of service: (1) primary prevention: health promotion and illness prevention, (2) secondary prevention: diagnosis and treatment, and (3) tertiary prevention: rehabilitation, health restoration, and palliative care.
- Hospitals provide a wide variety of services on an inpatient and outpatient basis. Hospitals can be categorized as for-profit or not-for-profit, public or private, acute care or long-term care. Many other settings, such as clinics, offices, and day-care centers, also provide care.
- Various providers of health care coordinate their skills to assist a client. Their mutual goal is to restore a client's health and promote wellness.

- The role of the nurse in providing care to clients varies depending on the employment setting, the nurse's credentials, and the needs of the client.
- The many factors affecting health care delivery include the increasing number of older adults, advances in knowledge and technology, economics, increased emphasis on women's health, uneven distribution of health services, access to health care, health care of the homeless and poor, HIPAA, and demographic changes.
- Delivery of nursing care that supports continuity of client-focused care and is cost effective may be implemented by any of the following methods: managed care, case management, patient-focused care, differentiated

- practice, shared governance, case method, functional method, team nursing, or primary care nursing.
- In the United States, health care is financed largely through government agencies and private organizations that provide health care insurance, prepaid plans, and federally funded programs. Government-financed plans include Medicare and Medicaid. Private plans include Blue Cross and Blue Shield. Prepaid group plans include HMOs, PPOs, PPAs, IPAs, and PHOs.
- Health care costs, access to health care, and the quality of health care are major areas of concern about the current health care system.
- A community is a collection of people who share some attribute of their lives.
- For community assessment, eight subsystems proposed by Anderson and McFarlane (2004) can be used: physical environment, education, safety and transportation, politics and government, health and social services, communication, economics, and recreation.
- *Nursing's Agenda for Health Care Reform* by the ANA (1991) and *Healthy People 2010* by the USDHHS (2000) have set forth recommendations for health care reform. These focus on accessibility of health care services, health promotion and disease prevention, and steps to consider how health care costs can be reduced.
- Consumers support an increased emphasis on health care measures that promote wellness.
- Community-based health care, akin to primary health care, provides health-related services in places where people spend their time—in homes, in shelters, in long-term care residences, at work, in schools, in senior citizen centers, and so on.
- Approaches are emerging to address community-based care. These include an integrated health care system, community initiatives, community coalitions, managed care, case management, and outreach programs using lay health workers.
- Numerous community settings have been established. More recent ones include nurse-managed community nursing centers, parish nursing, and telehealth projects.
- Community-based nursing directs nursing care toward specific individuals. It is not confined to one practice setting; it extends beyond institutional boundaries involving a network of nursing services: nursing wellness centers, ambulatory care, long-term care, home health, and hospice care.
- To practice in community health care systems, nurses need knowledge and competencies such as determinants of a healthy community, primary and secondary preventive strategies, health-promotion strategies, collaborative and interdisciplinary teamwork, determinants of an accessible and cost-effective health care system, a decision-making process that involves consumers, and information management. Education in public health policy and strategies to influence and effect change are essential.
- Collaboration among health care providers is key to maintaining continuity of care as clients move through the health care system.

- A major responsibility of the nurse is to ensure continuity of care as clients move from one level of care to another.
- Continuity of care involves (a) discharge planning that begins when clients are admitted to an agency, (b) cooperation with the client and support persons, and (c) interdisciplinary collaboration.
- Nurses need to ensure that clients have essential information and skills to manage self-care before being discharged to their homes. In some situations referral to a home health agency is necessary.
- Home health care is an alternative to acute and subacute health care facilities. The trend has changed from using home health care after hospitalization to using it to avoid hospitalization.
- Hospice nursing, often considered a subspecialty of home nursing, supports terminally ill clients and their families during the last stages of life and bereavement.
- Home health agencies offer skilled professional and paraprofessional services. Because clients often require the services of several professionals simultaneously, case coordination is essential.
- There are several types of home health agencies: official or public agencies, voluntary or private not-for-profit agencies, private proprietary agencies, and institution-based agencies. All home health agencies must meet specific standards for licensing, certification, and accreditation.
- Private duty agencies provide professional nursing and home health aide care for 4 to 24 hours per day.
- Health care agencies in the United States receive reimbursement for services they provide from various sources: Medicare and Medicaid, private insurance companies, and private pay. The Medicare and Medicaid programs have strict guidelines.
- Referrals for home health services may be made by the client's physician, a nurse, a social worker, a therapist, a discharge planner, or a family member. Home care requires, however, a physician's order and an approved treatment plan.
- Major roles of the home health nurse are those of advocate, caregiver, educator, and case manager.
- The home health nurse assesses the care needs of clients in their home; plans, implements, and supervises that care; teaches clients and their families self-care; and mobilizes the resources of hospitals, primary care providers, and community agencies in meeting the needs of the clients and their families.
- Home care clients include a diverse population that encompasses all ages, a variety of health problems, and families of different structures and cultural backgrounds. The home health nurse needs to be culturally sensitive, that is, become aware of the client's culture, and form a nursing care plan with the client that incorporates the client's culture.
- Important dimensions of home health nursing include the home visit in which the nurse assesses the client and they make plans for care, client and nurse safety, infection control, and caregiver support.

THINK ABOUT IT

Refer to the chapter-opening scenario and answer these questions.

Mrs. Jones is diagnosed with a fractured hip requiring surgery. After surgery she will need intensive therapy to help her regain strength, especially after a week of bed rest, in order to be able to walk again. Answer the following critical thinking questions:

1. Describe care that will be provided to Mrs. Jones at all three levels of prevention.

2. What method of payment can you be relatively certain Mrs. Jones uses to pay for her health care?

3. What community-based services might be available, based on those available in your area, that could help Bernice provide for her mother's needs if she returns to living independently in her home?

∞ *See suggested responses to Think About It on MyNursingKit.*

TEST YOUR KNOWLEDGE

1. The nurse would recognize which of the following activities as primary prevention?
   1. Antibiotic treatment for a suspected urinary tract infection
   2. Occupational therapy to assist a client in adapting his or her home environment following a stroke
   3. Nutrition counseling for young adults with a strong family history of high cholesterol
   4. Removal of tonsils for a client with recurrent tonsillitis

2. Which of the following statements is true regarding types of health care agencies?
   1. Hospitals provide only acute, inpatient services.
   2. Public health agencies are funded by governments to investigate and provide health programs.
   3. Surgery can be performed only inside a hospital setting.
   4. Skilled nursing, extended care, and long-term care facilities provide care for the older adults whose insurance no longer covers hospital stays.

3. *Nursing's Agenda for Health Care Reform* submitted by the American Nurses Association (ANA, 1991) included which of the following?
   1. Primary health care should be based in acute care hospitals.
   2. A minimum standard of health care for all persons should be paid for completely with public funds.
   3. Case management should be focused on clients with enduring health care needs.
   4. Essential services should be initiated simultaneously to avoid gaps.

4. Which of the following is characteristic of nursing care provided in community-based health?
   1. Clients are primarily those with identified illnesses.
   2. Clients are individuals in groups according to their geographic commonalities.
   3. Care is paid for by the community as a whole rather than by individuals.
   4. All clients are case managed.

5. When performing collaborative health care, the nurse must implement which of the following?
   1. Assume a leadership role in directing the health care team.
   2. Rely on the expertise of other health care team members.
   3. Be physically present for the implementation of all aspects of the care plan.
   4. Delegate decision-making authority to each health care provider.

6. The nurse concludes that effective discharge planning (hospital to home) has been conducted when the client states which of the following?
   1. "As soon as I get home, the nurse will come out, look at where I live, and see what kind of care I will need."
   2. "All I need are my medications and a ride home. Then I'm all ready for discharge."
   3. "When I visit my doctor in 10 days, they will show me how to change my bandages."
   4. "I have the phone numbers of the home care nurse and the therapist who will visit me at home tomorrow."

7. A large disaster in a community resulted in the destruction of many family homes, and many individuals were injured. The assistance of community health nurses and home health nurses are needed. The home health nurse is most likely to perform which of the following?
   1. Provide for a safe water supply.
   2. Monitor for communicable diseases.
   3. Establish communication and support systems.
   4. Assess and treat individual clients.

8. If a primary care provider prescribed the following, which could be delegated to the home health aide?
   1. Feeding and bathing the client
   2. Teaching the client about medications
   3. Assessing wound healing progress
   4. Adjusting oxygen flow

9. After the nurse instructed a client about the rationale for sitting with feet elevated to enhance venous return, the client refuses to perform the activity. Which statement by the nurse would be most useful?
1. "If you won't cooperate, I can't help you."
2. "Tell me the reasons you won't put your feet up."
3. "It is essential that you do this."
4. "I'll notify your doctor that you are unable to keep your feet up."

10. A home health nurse is providing care for a client who has paralysis on one side and whose spouse provides most of the care. Which of the following might the nurse evaluate as a possible sign of caregiver role strain?
1. The caregiver loses weight and has insomnia.
2. The caregiver asks other family and friends for help.
3. The caregiver asks the nurse what other ways he or she can help the client.
4. The caregiver seems sad whenever the client's prognosis is discussed.

∞ *See answers to Test Your Knowledge in Appendix A.*

EXPLORE PEARSON **mynursingkit™**

MyNursingKit is your one stop for online chapter review materials and resources. Prepare for success with additional NCLEX®-style practice questions, interactive assignments and activities, web links, animations and videos, and more!

Register your access code from the front of your book at
www.mynursingkit.com.

REFERENCES AND SELECTED BIBLIOGRAPHY

Abrams, S. E. (2004). From function to competency in public health nursing, 1931–2003. *Public Health Nursing, 21,* 507–510.

Agency for Health care Research and Quality. (2004). Hospital nurse staffing and quality of care. *Research in Action, Issue 14.* AHRQ Publication No. 04-0029. Retrieved June 9, 2006, from http://www.ahrq.gov/research/nursestaffing/nursestaff.htm

Agency for Health care Research and Quality. (2005). *Guide to health care quality.* Retrieved June 24, 2006, from http://www.ahrq.gov/consumer/guidetoq

Allan, J., Barwick, T. A., Cashman, S., Cawley, J. F., Day, C., Douglass, C. W., et al. (2004). Clinical prevention and population health: Curriculum framework for health professions. *American Journal of Preventive Medicine, 27,* 471–476.

Allender, J. A., & Spradley, B. W. (2004). *Community health nursing: Promoting and protecting the public's health.* Philadelphia: Lippincott Williams & Wilkins.

American Association of Colleges of Nursing. (1995). *A model for differentiated nursing practice.* Washington, DC: Author.

American Nurses Association. (1991). *Nursing's agenda for health care reform.* Kansas City, MO: Author.

American Nurses Association. (1992). *House of delegates report: 1992 convention,* *Las Vegas, Nevada* (pp. 104–120). Kansas City, MO: Author.

American Nurses Association. (1999). *Scope and standards of home health nursing practice.* Washington, DC: American Nurses Publishing.

American Public Health Association. (1996). *The definition and role of public health nursing: A Statement of APHA Public Health Nursing Section.* Washington, DC: Author.

Anderson, E. T., & McFarlane, J. (2004). *Community as partner: Theory and practice in nursing* (4th ed.). Philadelphia: Lippincott Williams & Wilkins.

Barnes, D., Eribes, C., Juarbe, T., Nelson, M., Proctor, S., Sawyer, L., et al. (1995). Primary health care and primary care: A confusion of philosophies. *Nursing Outlook, 43*(1), 7–16.

Bedard, M., Koivuranta, A., & Stuckey, A. (2004). Health impact on caregivers of providing informal care to a cognitively impaired older adult: Rural versus urban settings. *Canadian Journal of Rural Medicine, 9*(1), 15–34.

Boucher, M. A. (2005). Making it: Qualities needed for rural home care nursing. *Home Healthcare Nurse, 23,* 103–108.

Bradley, P. J. (2003). Family caregiver assessment: Essential for effective home health care. *Journal of Gerontological Nursing, 29*(2), 29–36.

Brillhart, B., Kruse, B., & Heard, L. (2004). Safety concerns for rehabilitation nurses in home care. *Rehabilitation Nursing, 29,* 227–229.

Brown, G. (2004). Nursing and its future status. *Minority Nurse Newsletter, 11*(1), 1.

Brudenell, I. (2003). Parish nursing: Nurturing body, mind, spirit, and community. *Public Health Nursing, 20*(2), 85–94.

Byrne, M. (2003). Culture-derived strategies of a pediatric home-care nursing specialty team. *International Nursing Review, 50*(1), 34–43.

Campbell, R., Sefl, T., Wasco, S. M., & Ahrens, C. E. (2004). Doing community research without a community: Creating safe space for rape survivors. *American Journal of Community Psychology, 33,* 253–261.

Caruso, J. T., Scala-Foley, M. A., Archer, D., & Reinhard, S. C. (2004). Making sense of Medicare: A Medicare house call. *American Journal of Nursing, 104*(7), 71–72.

Castleman, J., & Gailor, N. (2004). Informal caregiving burden: An overlooked aspect of the lives and health of women transitioning from welfare to employment? *Public Health Nursing, 21,* 24–31.

Cawley, J., & Simon, K. I. (2005). Health insurance coverage and the macroeconomy. *Journal of Health Economics, 24,* 299–315.

Centers for Medicaid and Medicare Services (CMS). (2006). *National health expenditure data.* Retrieved November 3, 2009, from http://www.cms.hhs.gov/ NationalHealthExpendData/

Centers for Medicare & Medicaid Services. (2001). *Medicare home health agency manual* (HCFA Publication No. 11, PB 98-955200). Retrieved June 12, 2006, from http://www.cms.hhs.gov/manuals/ downloads/pub_11.zip

Centers for Medicare & Medicaid Services. (2004). *Medicare and home health care* (CMS Publication 10969). Baltimore: U.S. Department of Health & Human Services.

Clark, M. J. (2003). *Community health nursing: Caring for populations* (4th ed.). Upper Saddle River, NJ: Prentice Hall.

Clark, N., & Buell, A. (2004). Community assessment: An innovative approach. *Nurse Educator, 29,* 203–207.

Cooper, L. A., Roter, D. L., Johnson, R. L., Ford, D. E., Steinwachs, D. M., & Powe, N. R. (2003). Patient-centered communication, ratings of care, and concordance of patient and physician race. *Annals of Internal Medicine, 13,* 907–915.

Crist, J. D. (2005). The meaning for elders of receiving family care. *Journal of Advanced Nursing, 49,* 485–493.

Cutler, D. M. (2004). *Your money or your life: Strong medicine for America's health care system.* New York: Oxford University Press.

Davis, R., Cook, D., & Cohen, L. (2005). A community resilience approach to reducing ethnic and racial disparities in health. *American Journal of Public Health, 95,* 2168–2173.

DeLenardo, C. (2004). Web-based tools steer patient-focused care. *Nursing Management, 35*(12), 60–64.

Department of Health & Human Services, Bureau of Health Professions, Division of Nursing. (2004). *Preliminary findings: 2004 national sample survey of registered nurses.* Retrieved November 3, 2009, from http://bhpr.hrsa.gov/ healthworkforce/rnsurvey04/default. htm

deTornyay, R. (1992). Reconsidering nursing education: The report of the Pew Health Professions Commission. *Journal of Nursing Education, 31,* 296–301.

Erickson, J. I., & Miller, S. (2005). Caring for patients while respecting their privacy: Renewing our commitment. *Online Journal of Issues in Nursing, 10*(2), Manuscript 2. Retrieved June 11, 2006, from http://www.nursingworld.org/ojin/ topic27/tpc27_1.htm

Ervin, N., Scrivener, K., & Simmons, T. (2004). Using the linkage model for integrating evidence into home care nursing practice. *Home Health Care Nurse, 22,* 606–611.

Farrell, K., Wicks, M. N., & Martin, J. C. (2004). Chronic disease self-management improved with enhanced self efficacy. *Clinical Nursing Research, 13,* 289–308.

Feuer, L. (2004). The growing population of uninsured: Are you prepared for the challenge? *Case Manager, 15,* 19–21.

Frist, W. H. (2005). Overcoming disparities in U.S. health care. *Health Affairs, 24,* 445–451.

Furaker, C., Hellstrom-Muhli, U., & Walldal, E. (2004). Quality of care in relation to a critical pathway from the staff's perspective. *Journal of Nursing Management, 12,* 309–316.

Gesler, W. M., Dougherty, M., Arcury, T. A., Skelly, A. H., & Nash, S. (2003). The importance of obtaining information from assessment of community service providers for a disease prevention program. *Journal of Multicultural Nursing & Health, 9*(2), 14–21.

Gordon, J. A., Emond, J. A., & Camargo, C. A. (2005). The State Children's Health Insurance Program: A multicenter trial of outreach through the emergency department. *American Journal of Public Health, 95,* 250–253.

Grant, J. S., Glandon, G. L., Elliott, T. R., Giger, J. N., & Weaver, M. (2004). Caregiving problems and feelings experienced by family caregivers of stroke survivors the first month after discharge. *International Journal of Rehabilitation Research, 27,* 105–111.

Grumbach, K., Miller, J., Mertz, E., & Finocchio, L. (2004). How much public health in public health nursing practice? *Public Health Nursing, 21,* 266–276.

Hall, L. M., Doran, D., & Pink, G. H. (2004). Nurse staffing models, nursing hours, and patient safety outcomes. *Journal of Nursing Administration, 34,* 41–45.

Harrington, C., & Estes, C. L. (Eds.). (2004). *Health policy and nursing: Crisis and reform in the U.S. health care delivery system* (4th ed.). Boston: Jones & Bartlett.

Hartung, S. Q. (2005). Choosing home health as a specialty and successfully transitioning into practice. *Home Health Care Management and Practice, 17,* 70–87.

Hing, E., Cherry, D. K., & Woodwell, D. A. (2005). National ambulatory medical care survey: 2003 summary. *Advance data from vital and health statistics;* No. 3645. Retrieved June 25, 2006, from http://www.cdc.gov/nchs/data/ad/ad365 .pdf

Hogue, E. (2003). Five crucial legal issues for home care providers. *Remington Report, 11*(1), 22–24.

Huttlinger, K., Schaller-Ayers, J. M., Kenny, B., & Ayers, J. W. (2004). Research and collaboration in rural community health. *Online Journal of Rural Nursing and Health Care, 4* (1). Retrieved November 3, 2009, from http://www.rno.org/journal/ index.php/online-journal/article/viewFile/ 126/124

Institute of Medicine. (1994). *Defining primary care: An interim report.* Washington, DC: National Academy Press.

Institute of Medicine. (2004). *Uninsured in America.* Retrieved June 6, 2006, from http://www.iom.edu/Object.File/Master/ 21/040/0.pdf

Jennings, C. P. (2004). Insuring America's health: Principles and recommendations: IOM report. *Policy, Politics, and Nursing Practice, 5,* 100–101.

Joint Commission on Accreditation of Healthcare Organizations. (2004). *2004–2005 Comprehensive accreditation manual for home care.* Oakbrook Terrace, IL: Author.

Kashihara, D., & Carper, K. (2005). *National health care expenses in the U.S. civilian noninstitutionalized population, 2003.* Statistical Brief No. 103. Rockville, MD: Agency for Healthcare Research and Quality. Retrieved June 25, 2006, from http://www.meps.ahrq. gov/papers/st103/ stat103.pdf

Keller, S., Hunter, D., & Shortt, S. (2004). The impact of hospital restructuring on home care nursing. *Canadian Journal of Nursing Leadership, 17*(2), 82–89.

Kovner, A. R., & Knickman, J. R. (2008). *Jonas & Kovner's health care delivery in the United States* (9th ed.). New York: Springer.

Kraus, M., Morgan, C., & Matteson, P. (2003). "Razoo Health": A community-based nursing education initiative. *Journal of Nursing Education, 42,* 304–310.

Langa, K., Valenstein, M., Fendrick, A., Kabeto, M., & Vijan, S. (2004). Extent and cost of informal caregiving for older Americans with symptoms of depression. *American Journal of Psychiatry, 161,* 857–863.

Mainous, A. G., Koopman, R. J., Gill, J. M., Baker, R., & Pearson, W. S. (2004). Relationship between continuity of care and diabetes control: Evidence from the Third National Health and Nutrition Examination Survey. *American Journal of Public Health, 94,* 66–70.

Maurer, F. A., & Smith, C. M. (2004). *Community/public health nursing practice: Health for families and populations.* St. Louis: Elsevier.

National Center for Health Statistics. (2005). *Health: United States, 2005.* Hyattsville, MD: Author.

Pew Health Professions Commission. (1991). *Healthy America: Practitioners for 2005. An agenda for action for U.S. health professional schools.* San Francisco: Author.

Porche, D. J. (2003). *Public and community health nursing practice: A population-based approach.* Thousand Oaks, CA: Sage.

Porter, E. J., & Ganong, L. H. (2005). Older widows' speculations and expectancies concerning professional home-care providers. *Nursing Ethics, 12,* 507–521.

Quad Council. (2003). *Quad Council PHN competencies.* Retrieved June 11, 2006, from http://www.achne.org/Documents/ Final_PHN_Competencies.pdf

Reinhart, E. (2005). *Infection control in home care.* Boston: Jones & Bartlett.

Rhoades, J. A. (2006a). *The uninsured in America, 1996–2005: Estimates for the U.S. civilian noninstitutionalized population under age 65.* Statistical Brief #130. Rockville, MD: Agency for Healthcare Research and Quality. Retrieved June 25, 2006, from http://www.meps.ahrq.gov/ papers/st130/stat130.pdf

Rhoades, J. A. (2006b). *The uninsured in America, First half of 2005: Estimates for the U.S. civilian noninstitutionalized population under age 65.* Statistical Brief No. 129. Rockville, MD: Agency for Healthcare Research and Quality. Retrieved June 25, 2006, from http:// www.meps.ahrq.gov/papers/st129/ stat129.pdf

Schumacher, K., & Marren, J. (2004). Home care nursing for older adults: State of the science. *Nursing Clinics of North America, 39,* 443–471.

Short, P. F., & Graefe, D. R. (2003). Battery-powered health insurance? Stability in coverage of the uninsured. *Health Affairs, 22,* 244–255.

Simpson, S. H., Majumdar, S. R., & Marrie, T. J. (2003). Physician-related barriers to the adoption of a critical pathway for community-acquired pneumonia: A qualitative analysis. *Journal of General Internal Medicine, 18* (Suppl. 1), 275–280.

Smith, C., Cowan, C., Sensing, A., & Catlin, A. (2005). Health spending growth slows in 2003. *Health Affairs, 24,* 185–194.

Smith, S. D. (Ed.). (2003). *Parish nursing: A handbook for the new millennium.* Binghamton, NY: Haworth Press.

Stanhope, M., & Lancaster, J. (2003). *Community and public health nursing* (6th ed.). St. Louis: Elsevier.

Sturkey, E. N., Linker, S., Keith, D. D., & Comeau, E. (2005). Improving wound care outcomes in the home setting. *Journal of Nursing Care Quality, 20,* 349–355.

Taft, S. H., Pierce, C. A., & Gallo, C. L. (2005). From hospital to home and back again: A study in hospital admissions and deaths for home care patients. *Home Health Care Management and Practice, 17,* 467–480.

U.S. Census Bureau. (2004). *U.S. interim projections by age, sex, race, and Hispanic origin.* Retrieved November 3, 2009, from http://www.census.gov/population/www/projections/pp147.html

U.S. Department of Health and Human Services. (2000). *Healthy people 2010: Understanding and improving health* (2nd ed.). Washington, DC: U.S. Government Printing Office.

Weisman, G. D., Kovach, D., & Cashin, S. E. (2004). Differences in dementia services and settings across place types and regions. *American Journal of Alzheimer's Disease and Other Dementias, 19,* 291–308.

World Health Organization. (1978). *Primary health care: Report of the international conference on primary health care.* Geneva: Author.

Culture and Heritage

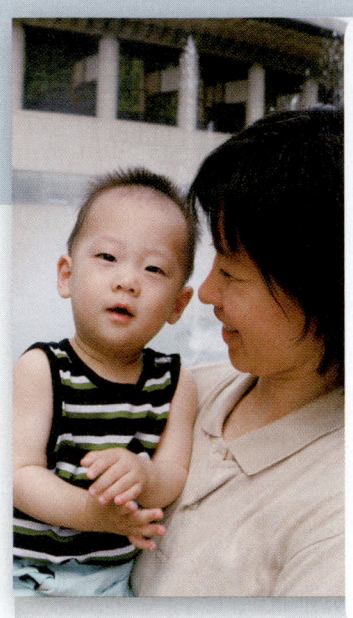

Michelle Sakong is a 26-year-old Korean American born to parents who moved to the United States from South Korea before she was born. Michelle vaguely remembers learning some words in Korean when she was a little girl but doesn't remember any of the language now. She often teases her parents about being "old world" and tells them to "enter the 21st century" in an attempt to get them to act in what she thinks of as the "American way." Despite the enjoyment she gets from teasing her Mom and Dad, she secretly enjoys the reliability of the customs and traditions she associates with being home. Her culture has become even more important to her now that she has a child of her own. She wants her children to know the culture of her grandparents and to also take comfort in traditions and customs.

LEARNING OUTCOMES

After completing this chapter, you will be able to:

1. List and describe six federal agencies, initiatives, and laws that influence the provision of cultural health care.

2. List and describe 11 components of culturally focused nursing and describe a strategy for conveying cultural sensitivity for each component.

3. List four components of heritage consistency and give examples for each behavior that would be considered consistent or inconsistent with heritage.

4. Differentiate biomedical care from folk healing, and magico-religious health beliefs from scientific or holistic health beliefs.

5. Identify factors related to communication with culturally diverse clients and colleagues.

6. Identify key questions to ask when conducting a heritage assessment.

7. List strategies for implementing nursing care using cultural preservation and maintenance and cultural accommodation and negotiation.

To provide quality care, nurses must be informed and sensitive to culturally diverse and subjective meanings of health, illness, caring, and healing practices. **Culture** can be defined as the nonphysical traits that are shared by a group of people and passed from generation to generation (Spector, 2008). Culture includes the "thoughts, communications, actions, customs, beliefs, values, and institutions of racial, ethnic, religious, or social groups" (Office of Minority Health, 2001, p. 131). Culture defines how health is perceived, how health care information is received, how rights and protections are exercised, what is considered to be a health problem, how symptoms and concerns about the health problem are expressed, who should provide treatment and how, and what kind of treatment should be given. While people from a given cultural group share certain beliefs, values, and experiences, nurses must be aware that there can be widespread diversity within a group and respect those differences. Factors such as age, education, socioeconomic status, gender, and area of origin influence these differences. Stereotyping must always be avoided.

The term "cultural mosaic" is replacing the term "melting pot" to describe people in the United States because a mosaic more accurately describes the ways people of many cultures maintain their cultural heritage for many generations. **Heritage** is defined as something that is handed down from generation to generation; it includes far more than material possessions, also including traditions and customs. In addition to the indigenous people of North America (Native Americans and Native Alaskans), a great deal of diversity is seen within and among those who have lived in the United States for many generations as well as immigrants who are new to the country.

CLINICAL ALERT

Culture and language are vital factors in how nursing care is delivered and received, and the diverse cultural needs of clients are expected to be met.

NATIONAL AGENCIES AND TRENDS

The demographic changes in the overall population of the United States and the influence of immigration on health services are major reasons for the immense need for culturally focused nursing care. The efforts described in the following list are evidence of increased emphasis on providing culturally appropriate health care.

- The U.S. Department of Health and Human Services (USDHHS) houses the Office of Minority Health "to improve and protect the health of racial and ethnic minority populations through the development of health policies and programs that will eliminate health disparities" (n.d.). In collaboration with other organizations, it developed the *National Standards for Culturally and Linguistically Appropriate Services in Health Care* (CLAS). Culture and language have a considerable impact on how clients access and respond to health care services.

- The Centers for Disease Control and Prevention (CDC) also has an Office of Minority Health to "promote health and quality of life by preventing and controlling the disproportionate burden of disease, injury and disability among racial and ethnic minority populations" (n.d.).

- The purpose of the National Center on Minority Health and Health Disparities (NCMHD) in the National Institutes of Health "is to promote minority health and to lead, coordinate, support, and assess the NIH effort to reduce and ultimately eliminate health disparities" (n.d.).

- The nursing profession plays a major role in REACH: Racial and Ethnic Approaches to Community Health, which strives to eliminate racial and ethnic disparities (inequalities) in infant mortality; in screening and management of breast and cervical cancer, cardiovascular diseases, diabetes, and HIV infections/AIDS; and in child and adult immunizations.

- One of the major goals of *Healthy People 2010* is to eliminate health disparities by gender, race or ethnicity, education, income, disability, geographic location, and sexual orientation (details of *Healthy People 2010* are discussed in Chapter 5 ∞). To achieve these goals, the Health Resources and Services Administration (HRSA) aims to increase the number of underrepresented racial and ethnic groups entering the nursing profession (Public Health Foundation, 2001).

- Current nursing practice has been largely influenced by the *National Healthcare Disparities Report*, which is a comprehensive overview of disparities in health care among racial, ethnic, and socioeconomic groups in the general U.S. population and among priority populations (Agency for Healthcare Research and Quality, 2005). This report indicates that, although the quality of health care has improved and differences in access and quality between whites and minorities have decreased overall, the quality and access disparity for Hispanics has widened.

Demographic Changes

The U.S. Census Bureau (2005a) revealed that in 2004, 98.5% of Americans identified themselves as belonging to a single race. Of the total, 80.4% identify themselves as white, 12.7% as black or African American, 4.2% as Asian, and 1% as American Indian or Alaska Native. Those Americans who indicated they were of Hispanic or Latino origin were 14.1% of the total American population. Census Bureau projections (2004) are that the U.S. population overall will continue to increase by approximately 27 million persons each decade, and that by 2050, Hispanics will increase by 70 million to represent 24% of the total while white non-Hispanics will decrease from 69% to 50% of the total.

Nurses are predominantly white in a percentage disproportionate to the demographic profile of the United States. Table 4–1 compares the percentages of American Indian, Asian/Pacific Islander, black non-Hispanic, Hispanic, and white non-Hispanic nurses in 2004 (USDHHS, 2004).

Immigration

According to the U.S. Census Bureau (2005b), the foreign-born population in the United States numbered 34.2 million in 2004, which corresponds to 12% of the total U.S. population. This is a 2.3% increase from 2003. Of these, 53% were born in Latin America (Central and South America), 25% in Asia, 14% in Europe, and the remaining 8% in other regions of the world. Second-generation Americans who were born in the United States but have one or both parents born in a foreign country accounted for 11% of the total U.S. population (30.4 million). Figure 4–1 demonstrates the cultural heritage of people in the United States in different areas.

TABLE 4–1	Percentages of American Indian, Asian/Pacific Islander, Black Non-Hispanic, Hispanic, and White Non-Hispanic Nurses in 2004

POPULATION	PERCENT
American Indian/Alaska Native	0.4
Asian/Pacific Islander and other	3.3
Black non-Hispanic	4.6
Hispanic	1.8
White non-Hispanic	88.4
Two or more races	1.5

Note: From "The Registered Nurse Population: Preliminary Findings from the National Sample Survey of Registered Nurses, March 2004," by U.S. Department of Health and Human Services Health Resources and Service Administration Bureau of Health Professions. Retrieved April 21, 2006, from http://bhpr.hrsa.gov/healthworkforce/reports/rnpopulation/preliminaryfindings.htm

---

LIFESPAN CONSIDERATIONS
International Adoption

Children

International adoption of children by families in the United States is increasing, with over 150,000 children adopted in the past 14 years. These children present many challenges, and the care given by pediatric health providers can strongly influence the success with which they are assimilated into their new families. Understanding and assessing adopted children's potential issues early and intervening appropriately can lead to stronger family bonds. Children who arrive in the United States should be evaluated within 10 to 14 days for the following:

- Immunization history (blood titers may be appropriate)
- Infectious disease, parasites, general health (CBC, thyroid, liver function, and other blood work)
- Tuberculosis exposure (PPD)
- Developmental history and status, including speech, language, motor, and social development
- Vision and hearing
- Dental health

Note: Adapted from "International adoption: A health and developmental prospective," by P. Mason & C. Narad, 2005, *Seminars in Speech and Language, 26*(1), 1–9.

CULTURAL NURSING CARE

Responsibility for cultural health care is shared among "individuals, professional associations, regulatory bodies, health services delivery and accreditation organizations, educational institutions, and governments" (Canadian Nurses Association, 2004, p. 1). Professional nursing care is culturally sensitive, culturally appropriate, and culturally competent. This type of nursing is critical to meeting the complex care needs of a given person, family, and community. Cultural nursing care is the provision of nursing care across cultural boundaries, taking into account the context in which the client lives as well as the situations in which the client's health problems arise.

- **Culturally sensitive** implies that nurses possess some basic knowledge of and constructive attitudes toward the health traditions observed among the diverse cultural groups found in the setting in which they are practicing.
- **Culturally appropriate** implies that nurses possess and apply the underlying background knowledge to provide a given client with the best possible health care.
- **Culturally competent** implies that, within the delivered care, nurses understand and attend to the total context of the client's situation and use a complex combination of knowledge, attitudes, and skills.

Transcultural nursing focuses on providing care within the differences and similarities of the beliefs, values,

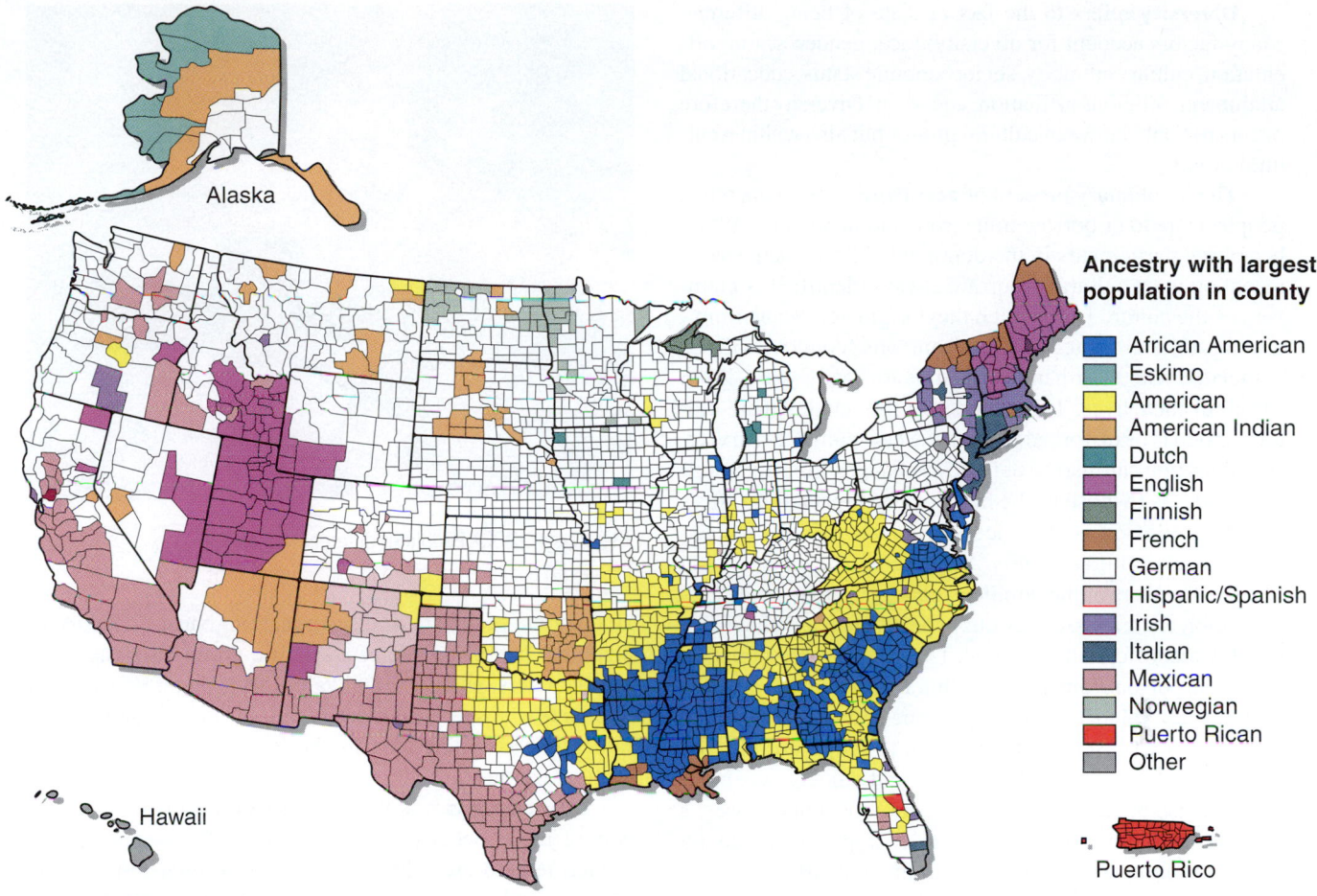

Alaska

Ancestry with largest population in county

- African American
- Eskimo
- American
- American Indian
- Dutch
- English
- Finnish
- French
- German
- Hispanic/Spanish
- Irish
- Italian
- Mexican
- Norwegian
- Puerto Rican
- Other

Hawaii

Puerto Rico

Figure 4–1 ⊙ Cultural heritages across the United States.
Source: U.S. Census data 2000.

and patterns of cultures (Leininger & McFarland, 2005). Countless conflicts in health care delivery arenas are predicated on cultural misunderstandings. Although many of these misunderstandings are related to universal situations, such as verbal and nonverbal language misunderstandings, the conventions of courtesy, sequencing of interactions, phasing of interactions, objectivity, and so forth, many cultural misunderstandings are unique to the delivery of nursing care. Cultural nursing care is essential and demands that nurses be able to assess and interpret a given client's health beliefs, practices, and cultural needs. Cultural nursing care alters the perspective of nursing care delivery because it enables the nurse to understand, from a cultural perspective, the manifestations of the client's health care beliefs and practices.

Concepts Related to Cultural Nursing Care

All groups of people face issues in adapting to their environment: providing nutrition and shelter, caring for and educating children, dividing labor, developing social organization, controlling disease, and maintaining health. Humans adapt

to varying environments by developing cultural solutions to meet these needs. Culture is a universal experience, but no two cultures are exactly alike. Cultural patterns are learned, and it is important for nurses to note that members of a particular group may not share identical cultural experiences. Thus, each member of a cultural group is somewhat different from his or her own cultural counterparts.

A **subculture** is usually composed of people who have a distinct identity and yet are related to a larger cultural group. Large cultural groups often have cultural subgroups or subsystems. A subcultural group generally shares ethnic origin or physical characteristics with the larger cultural group. Examples of cultural subgroups include occupational, societal, and ethnic groups.

Bicultural is used to describe a person who has dual patterns of identification and crosses two cultures, lifestyles, and sets of values (Spector, 2008). For example, a young man whose father is Cherokee and whose mother is European American may honor his traditional Cherokee heritage while also being influenced by his mother's cultural values. Another example exists in large areas of Canada where both British and French influences are strong.

Diversity refers to the fact or state of being different. Many factors account for diversity: race, gender, sexual orientation, culture, ethnicity, socioeconomic status, educational attainment, religious affiliation, and so on. Diversity therefore occurs not only between cultural groups but also within a cultural group.

The involuntary process of **acculturation** occurs when people adapt to or borrow traits from another culture. While becoming participants in the dominant culture, members of a nondominant cultural group are always identified as members of the culture from which they originate. People immigrating to the United States from any country will be associated with their native countries for many years, if not for all of their lives. The member of the nondominant cultural group is often forced to learn the new culture to survive. Acculturation can also be defined as changes from one's cultural patterns to those of the host society (Spector, 2008).

Assimilation is the process by which an individual develops a new cultural identity. Assimilation means becoming like the members of the dominant culture. The process of assimilation encompasses various aspects, such as behavioral, marital, identification, and civic. The underlying assumption is that the person from a given cultural group loses his or her original cultural identity to acquire the new one. In fact, because this is a conscious effort, it is not always possible, and the process may cause severe stress and anxiety. Assimilation can also be described as a collection of subprocesses: a process of inclusion through which a person gradually ceases to conform to any standard of life that differs from the dominant group standards and, at the same time, a process through which the person learns to conform to all the dominant group standards. The process of assimilation is considered complete when the foreigner is fully merged into the dominant cultural group (McLemore & Romo, 2005).

Race is the classification of people according to shared biologic characteristics, genetic markers, or features. People of the same race have common characteristics such as skin color, bone structure, facial features, hair texture, and blood type. Different ethnic groups can belong to the same race, and different cultures can be found within one ethnic group. It is important to understand that not all people of the same race have the same culture. Culture should not be confused with either race or ethnic group. People of Hispanic or Latino origin can be of any race (Figure 4–2).

Prejudice is a negative belief or preference that is generalized about a group and that leads to "prejudgment." Prejudice occurs because either the person making the judgment does not understand the particular person or his or her heritage, or the person making the judgment generalizes an experience with one individual from a culture to all members of that group. It may also be referred to as *racism*. A related concept is **xenophobia**—the fear or dislike of people different from oneself.

Stereotyping is assuming that all members of a culture or ethnic group are alike. Stereotyping may be based on generalizations founded in research, or it may be unrelated to reality. Stereotyping that is unrelated to reality is frequently

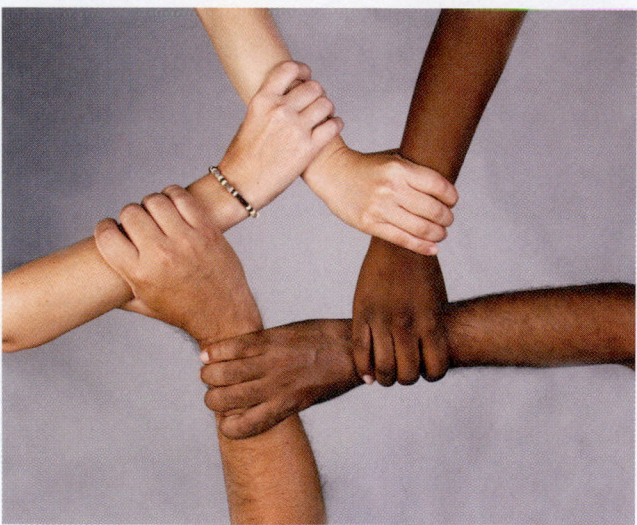

Figure 4–2 ● People of different races.

an outcome of racism or discrimination. Nurses need to realize that not all people of a specific group have the same health beliefs, practices, and values. It is therefore essential to identify a specific client's beliefs, needs, and values rather than assuming they are the same as those attributable to the larger group.

Ethnocentrism is the belief that one's own culture or way of life is better than that of others. Ethnocentric individuals tend to view the world from their own cultural perspective and may have difficulty recognizing that others view the same world differently. Other viewpoints are considered not only different, but wrong or of lesser importance.

Discrimination is the differential treatment of individuals or groups based on categories such as race, ethnicity, gender, social class, or exceptionality. This occurs when a person acts on prejudice and denies other persons one or more of their fundamental rights.

Culture shock occurs in response to transition from one cultural setting to another. A person's former behavior patterns are ineffective in such a setting, and basic cues for social behavior are absent (Spector, 2008). This phenomenon may occur when one moves from one geographic location to another or when a person immigrates to a new country. It may occur when a person is admitted into a hospital and has to adapt to a foreign situation. Expressions of culture shock may range from confusion and anxiety, to silence and immobility, to agitation, rage, or fury.

HERITAGE CONSISTENCY

Heritage consistency, a concept developed by Zitzow and Estes (1981), relates to the observance of beliefs and practices of a person's traditional cultural system (Spector, 2008). The concept has been expanded in an attempt to study the degree to which a person's lifestyle reflects his or her traditional culture. The values indicating heritage consistency exist on a continuum, and a person can possess characteristics of both heritage consistency (**traditional**), that is, observance of the beliefs and practices of one's traditional cultural belief system; and heritage inconsistency, the observance of the beliefs and practices of one's acculturated (or modern) belief system. The model of heritage consistency has four overlapping components: culture, ethnicity, religion, and socialization.

Culture is a complex whole in which each part is related to every other part. It is learned, and the capacity to learn culture is genetic, but the subject matter is not genetic and must be learned by each person in his or her family and social community. Culture also depends on an underlying social matrix, including knowledge, belief, art, law, morals, and custom. Nursing involves the identification of cultural traits and the integration of such cultural elements in the delivery of care (Turton, 2003).

Cultural background is a fundamental component of one's **ethnic** background or ethnicity, a group within the social system that claims to possess variable traits such as a common religion or language. There are at least 106 groups in the United States that meet many of the characteristics of an ethnic group. The percent of the total numbers coming from a specific area have remained relatively constant during the past 15 years for some groups (e.g., Europe and the Caribbean), while others have experienced greater increases (e.g., Africa) (U.S. Census Bureau, 2005b).

The third major component of a person's heritage is religion. Although the word has many definitions, religion may be considered a system of beliefs, practices, and ethical values about divine or superhuman power or powers worshipped as the creator(s) and ruler(s) of the universe. The practice of religion is revealed in numerous cults, sects, denominations, and churches. Ethnicity and religion are clearly related, and one's religion quite often is determined by one's ethnic group (Figures 4–3 and 4–4). Religion gives a person a frame of reference and a perspective with which to organize information. Religious teachings about health help to present a meaningful philosophy and system of practices within a system of social controls having specific val-

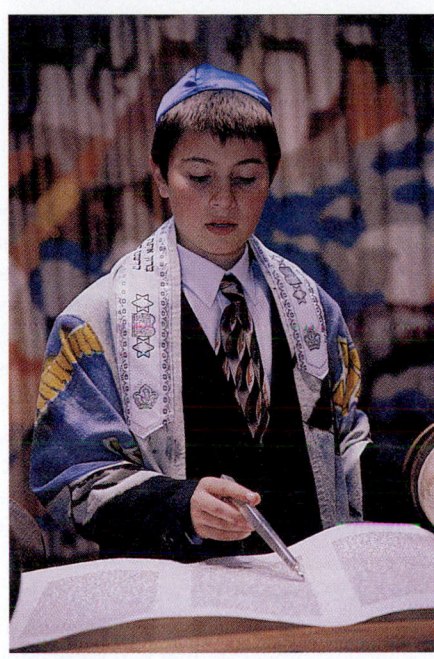

Figure 4–4 ○ Many religions celebrate the passage from child to adult, such as the Jewish bar mitzvah.

ues, norms, and ethics. Illness is sometimes seen as the punishment for the violation of religious codes and morals. It is not possible to isolate the aspects of culture, religion, and ethnicity that shape a person's world view. Each is part of the other, and all three are united within the person. See Chapter 28 ∞ for more information on spirituality.

Socialization is the process of being raised within a culture and acquiring the characteristics of that group. Education is a form of socialization. For many people who have been socialized within the boundaries of a traditional culture the modern "American" or Western culture becomes a second cultural identity. They may find socialization into the American culture to be an extremely difficult and painful process. They may prefer familiar alternative treatments as opposed to modern health care resources (more information is available on alternative medicine in Chapter 5 ∞). As time passes, many people experience biculturalism and divided loyalties.

SELECTED PARAMETERS OF CULTURAL NURSING CARE

HEALTH Traditions Model

The HEALTH traditions model (Spector, 2008) is predicated on the concept of holistic health and describes what people do from a traditional perspective to maintain, protect, and restore health. Health is seen as a balance between the body, mind, and spirit. These aspects are in constant flux and change over time, yet each is completely related to the others and also related to the context of the person. The context includes the person's family, culture, work, community, history, and environment

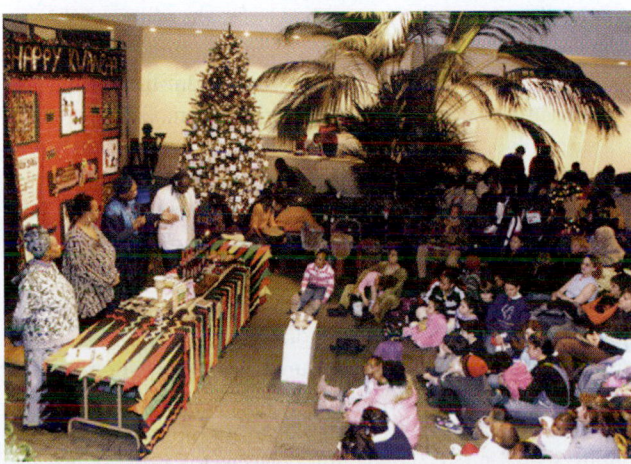

Figure 4–3 ○ A celebration of Kwanzaa.

(Spector, 2008). A major aspect of conducting the heritage assessment of a client is to determine what items are used by a specific person and its meaning to the person.

Health Beliefs and Practices

Three views of health beliefs include magico-religious, scientific, and holistic. In the **magico-religious health belief** view, health and illness are controlled by supernatural forces. The client may believe that illness is the result of "being bad" or opposing God's will. Getting well is also viewed as dependent on God's will. Some cultures believe that magic can cause illness. A sorcerer or witch may put a spell or hex on the client. Some people view illness as possession by an evil spirit. Although these beliefs are not supported by empirical evidence, clients who believe that such things can cause illness may in fact become ill as a result. Such illnesses may require magical treatments in addition to scientific treatments

The biomedical or **scientific health belief** is based on the belief that life and life processes are controlled by physical and biochemical processes that can be manipulated by humans. The client with this view will believe that illness is caused by germs, viruses, bacteria, or a breakdown of the body. This client will expect a pill, or treatment, or surgery to cure health problems.

The **holistic health belief** holds that the forces of nature must be maintained in balance or harmony. Human life is one aspect of nature that must be in harmony with the rest of nature, and illness will result when it is not. The medicine wheel is an ancient symbol used by Native Americans of North and South America to express many concepts. For health and wellness, the medicine wheel teaches the four aspects of the individual's nature: the physical, the mental, the emotional, and the spiritual. The four dimensions must be in balance to be healthy. The concept of yin and yang in the Chinese culture and the hot–cold theory of illness in many Spanish cultures are examples of holistic health beliefs. The nurse must keep in mind that a treatment strategy that is consistent with the client's beliefs may have a better chance of being successful.

Sociocultural forces, such as politics, economics, geography, religion, and the predominant health care system, influence the client's health status and health care behavior. For example, people who have limited access to scientific health care may turn to folk medicine or folk healing. **Folk medicine** is defined as those beliefs and practices relating to illness prevention and healing that derive from cultural traditions rather than from modern medicine's scientific base. Folk medicine is thought to be more humanistic than biomedical health care. The consultation and treatment takes place in the community of the recipient, frequently in the home of the healer. It may be less expensive than scientific or biomedical care. The healer often prepares the treatments, for example, herbs to be ingested, poultices to be applied, or charms or amulets to be worn. A frequent component of treatment is some ritual practice on the part of the healer or the client to cause healing to occur. Because folk healing is more culturally based, it is often more comfortable and less frightening for the client.

RESEARCH NOTES — Evidence-Based Practice

Treatments once considered to be folk treatments, including acupuncture, therapeutic touch, and massage, are now being investigated for their therapeutic effect. The National Center for Complementary and Alternative Medicine at the National Institutes of Health provides up-to-date information on this line of research: http://nccam.nih.gov.

It is important for the nurse to obtain information about folk or family healing practices that may have been used before or while the client used Western medical treatment. Often clients are reluctant to disclose the use of home remedies with health care professionals for fear of being laughed at or rebuked. However, a study on complementary and alternative medicine (CAM) used by adults in 2007 indicated that 38.3% of adults reported using CAM healing practices, up from 36% in 2002 (NCCAM). The increased use of alternative healing practices in the United States represents an opportunity for nurses to inform clients about what the nursing profession offers in this regard (Chapter 5 ∞). Figure 4–5 indicates CAM use by age.

Family Patterns

The family is the basic unit of society. Cultural values can determine communication within the family group, the norm for family size, and the roles of specific family members. In some families, the man is considered the provider and decision maker while other families are matriarchal with the mother or grandmother viewed as the leader of the family. The nurse needs to identify who has the "authority" to make decisions in a client's family and include that person in health care discussions.

The value placed on children and older adults within a society is culturally derived. In some cultures, children are not disciplined by spanking or other forms of physical punishment. Rather, children are allowed to interact with their environment while caregivers provide subtle direction to prevent harm or injury. In other cultures, older adults are considered the holders of the culture's wisdom and are therefore highly respected. Responsibility for caring for older relatives is determined by cultural practices. In many cultures, older relatives who cannot live independently live with a married son or daughter and family.

Cultural gender-role behavior may also affect nurse–client interactions. In some countries, men dominate and women have little status. Men from these countries may not accept instruction from a female nurse or primary care provider but will be receptive to the same instruction given by a male nurse or primary care provider. Some cultures have a prevailing concept of machismo, or male superiority. The positive aspects of machismo require that the adult man provide for and protect his family, including extended family members. The woman is expected to maintain the home and raise the children.

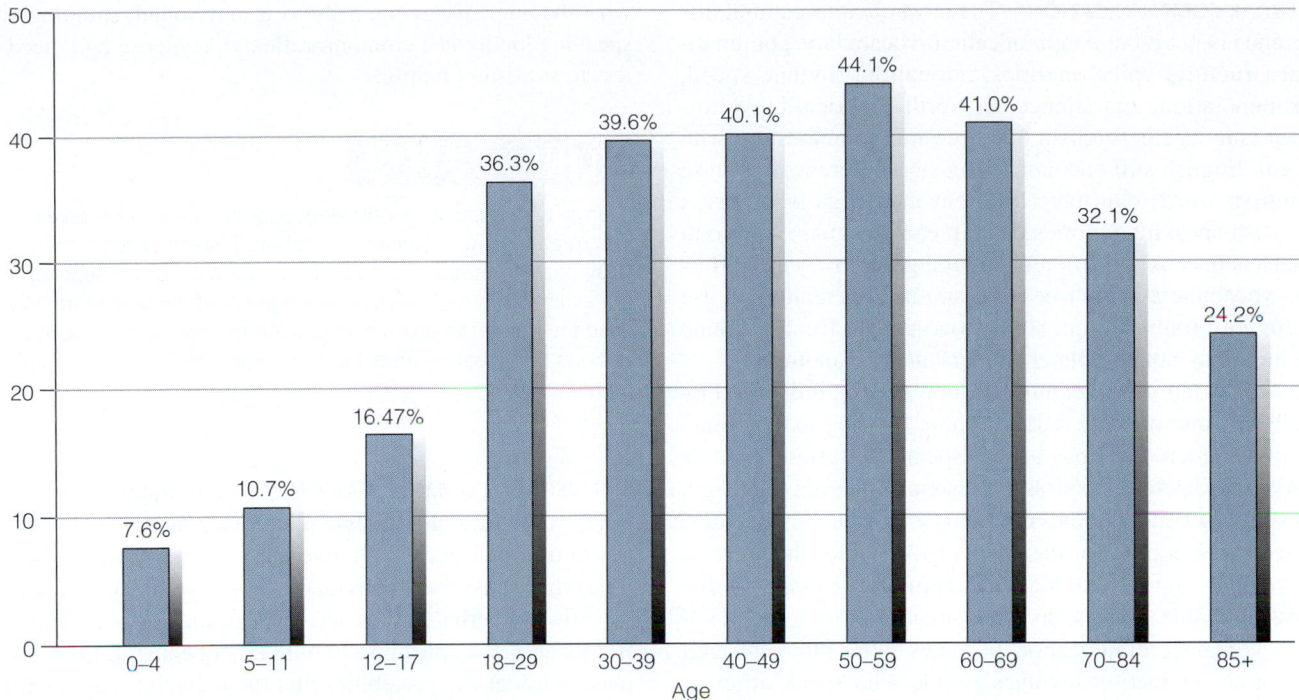

Figure 4–5 ○ Use of complementary and alternative medicine by age group.

Source: Barnes PM, Bloom B, Nahin R. *CDC National Health Statistics Report #12.* Complementary and Alternative Medicine Use Among Adults and Children: United States, 2007.

Cultural family values may also dictate the extent of the family's involvement in the hospitalized client's care. In some cultures, only the nuclear and the extended family will want to visit for long periods and participate in care. In other cultures, the entire community may want to visit and participate in the client's care. This can cause concern on nursing units with strict visiting policies. The nurse should evaluate the positive benefits of family participation in the client's care and modify visiting policies as appropriate.

Cultures that value the needs of the extended family as much as those of the individual may believe that personal and family information must stay within the family. Some cultural groups are very reluctant to disclose family information to outsiders, including health care professionals. This attitude can present difficulties for health care professionals who require knowledge of family interaction patterns to help clients with emotional problems.

Naming systems in many cultures differ from those in North America. In some cultures (e.g., Japanese and Vietnamese), the family name comes first and the given name second. One or two names may be added between the family and given names. Other nomenclature may be used to delineate gender, child, or adult status. For example, in traditional Japanese culture, adults address other adults by their surname followed by *san,* meaning *Mr., Mrs.,* or *Miss.* An example is Maurakami san. The children are referred to by their first names followed by *kun* for boys and *chan* for girls. Sikhs and Hindus traditionally have three names. Hindus have a personal name, a complimentary name, and then a family name. Sikhs have a personal name, then the title *Singh* for men and *Kaur* for women, and lastly the family

name. Names by marriage also vary. In Central America, a woman who marries retains her father's name and takes her husband's. For example, if Louisa Viccario marries Carlos Gonzales she becomes Louisa Viccario de Gonzales. The connecting *de* means "belonging to." Their son is Pedro Gonzales Viccario. Nurses need to become familiar with appropriate ways to address clients.

Communication Style

Communication and culture are closely interconnected. Through communication, the culture is transmitted from one generation to the next, and knowledge about the culture is transmitted within the group and to those outside the group. Communicating effectively with clients of various ethnic and cultural backgrounds is critical to providing culturally competent nursing care. There are cultural variations in both verbal and nonverbal communication.

BOX 4–1   Physician's Office Considerations

The physician's office or ambulatory care setting provides a unique opportunity to assess family interactions and function. The client is usually not as acutely ill as those requiring hospitalization, resulting in a family functioning under less stress and more normally. Who accompanies the client to the health care site? Do family members participate in health care discussions and decision making? Does the client bring family members into the examination room, or do family members stay in the waiting room? All of these assessment findings can help to demonstrate cultural beliefs of the family.

VERBAL COMMUNICATION The most obvious cultural difference is in verbal communication: vocabulary, grammatical structure, voice qualities, intonation, rhythm, speed, pronunciation, and silence. In North America, the dominant language is English; however, immigrant groups who speak English still encounter language differences because English words can have different meanings in different English-speaking cultures. Within each language, different dialects may exist. Different cultural groups may use different vocabulary, apply rules of grammar differently, and use different pronunciation, so that two people from the same culture may not completely understand one another.

Initiating verbal communication may be influenced by cultural values. Some cultures value "getting to the point" while other cultures may believe social courtesies should be established before business or personal topics are discussed. Discussing general topics can convey that the nurse is interested and has time for the client. This enables the nurse to develop a rapport with the client before progressing to discussion that is more personal.

Verbal communication becomes even more difficult when an interaction involves people who speak different languages. Both clients and health professionals experience frustration when they are unable to communicate verbally with each other. The objective of the professional interpreter is to transfer the words of the speaker into an utterance in a second language that conveys the same meaning (California Healthcare Interpreters Association, 2002, p. 70). Some states mandate hospitals to have certified interpreters available for clients who require them. Asking a family member or other nonprofessional to interpret can create difficulties. Cultural rules often dictate who can discuss what with whom. The use of interpreters is further discussed in Chapter 13 ∞.

CLINICAL ALERT

Professional interpreters are mandated in many states and should always be used whenever possible. The risk of miscommunication when using a family member as an interpreter has been well documented and should be avoided to maintain both the privacy and safety of the client.

Nurses and other health care providers must remember that clients for whom English is a second language may lose command of their English when they are in stressful situations. Clients who have used English comfortably for years in social and business communication may forget and revert back to their primary language when they are ill or distressed. It is important for the nurse to assure the client that this is normal and to promote behaviors to facilitate verbal communication. A nurse should avoid speaking to a client in the client's primary language if the nurse is not fluent in the language because an error could result in harm to the client. If the client has a limited knowledge of English, speaking slowly and clearly may help the client grasp the meaning of what the nurse is saying. Silly as it may sound, shouting or speaking loudly is a common reflexive response and, needless to say, is not helpful.

CLINICAL ALERT

Nurses who speak a second language fluently may be asked to interpret for others. Nursing schools and health care institutions may not permit nursing students to interpret for consent for a procedure because limited knowledge about the procedure may lead the student to give inaccurate information. Check the institution's policy before agreeing to interpret for institutional staff and physicians.

NONVERBAL COMMUNICATION To communicate effectively with culturally diverse clients, the nurse needs to be aware of two aspects of nonverbal communication behaviors: what nonverbal behaviors mean to the client and what specific nonverbal behaviors mean in the client's culture. Before assigning meaning to nonverbal behavior, the nurse must consider the possibility that the behavior may have a different meaning for the client and the family. To provide safe and effective care, nurses who work with specific cultural groups should learn more about cultural behavior and communication patterns within these cultures.

Nonverbal communication can include the use of silence, touch, eye movement, facial expressions, and body posture. Some cultures are quite comfortable with long periods of silence, whereas others consider it appropriate to speak before the other person has finished talking. Many people value silence and view it as essential to understanding a person's needs or use silence to preserve privacy. Some cultures view silence as a sign of respect, whereas to other people silence may indicate agreement.

Touching involves learned behaviors that can have both positive and negative meanings. In American culture, a firm handshake is a recognized form of greeting that conveys character and strength. In some European cultures, greetings may include a kiss on one or both cheeks. In some societies, touch is considered magical and, because of the belief that the soul can leave the body on physical contact, casual touching is forbidden. In some Asian cultures only certain older adults are permitted to touch the head of others, and children are never patted on the head. Nurses should therefore touch a client's head only with permission.

Cultures dictate what forms of touch are appropriate for individuals of the same and opposite gender. In many cultures, for example, a kiss is not appropriate for a public greeting between persons of the opposite sex, even those who are family members; however, a kiss on the cheek is acceptable as a greeting among individuals of the same sex. The nurse should watch interaction among clients and families for cues to the appropriate degree of touch in that culture. The nurse can also assess the client's response to touch when providing nursing care, for example, by noting the client's reaction to physical examination or a bath.

Facial expression can also vary between cultures. Italian, Jewish, African American, and Spanish-speaking persons are more likely to smile readily and use facial expression to communicate feelings, whereas Irish, English, and Northern European people tend to have less facial expression and are less open in their response, especially to strangers (Spector, 2008). Facial expressions can also convey a meaning opposite to what is felt or understood.

Eye movement during communication has cultural foundations. In Western cultures, direct eye contact is regarded as important and generally shows that the other is attentive and listening. It conveys self-confidence, openness, interest, and honesty. Lack of eye contact may be interpreted as secretiveness, shyness, guilt, lack of interest, or even a sign of mental illness. However, other cultures may view eye contact as impolite or an invasion of privacy. The nurse should not misinterpret the character of a client who avoids eye contact.

Body posture and hand gestures are also culturally learned. For example, the V sign means victory in some cultures, but it is an offensive gesture in other cultures. Tapping the index finger on one's temple may mean someone is intelligent in the United States but crazy in Holland.

Communication is an essential part of establishing a relationship with a client and his or her family. It is also important for developing effective working relationships with health care colleagues. To enhance their practice, nurses can observe the communication patterns of clients and colleagues and be aware of their own communication behaviors.

Space Orientation

Space is a relative concept that includes the individual, the body, the surrounding environment, and objects within that environment. The relationship between the individual's own body and objects and persons within space is learned and is influenced by culture. In Western cultures, spatial distances are defined as the intimate zone, the personal zone, and the social and public zones. The size of these areas may vary

with the specific culture. Nurses move through all three zones as they provide care for clients. The nurse needs to be aware of the client's response to movement toward them. The client may physically withdraw or back away if the nurse is perceived as being too close. The nurse will need to explain to the client why there is a need to be close. To assess the lungs with a stethoscope, for example, the nurse needs to move into the client's intimate space. The nurse should first explain the procedure and await permission to continue.

Clients who reside in long-term care facilities, or who are hospitalized for an extended time, may want to personalize their space. They may want to arrange their room differently or control the placement of objects on their bedside cabinet or over-bed table. The nurse should be responsive to clients' needs to have some control over their space. When there are no medical contraindications, clients should be permitted and encouraged to have objects of personal significance. Having personal and cultural items in one's environment can increase self-esteem by promoting not only one's individuality but also one's cultural identity. Of course, the nurse should caution the client about responsibility for loss of personal items.

Time Orientation

Time orientation refers to an individual's focus on the past, the present, or the future. Most cultures include all three time orientations, but one orientation is more likely to dominate. The American focus on time tends to be directed to the future, emphasizing time and schedules. Other cultures may have a different concept of time. For example, Navajos do not have a word for "late" and a Navajo mother may not become upset if her child does not achieve a specific developmental milestone, such as walking or toileting, on schedule.

Nursing and health care's culture places great value on time and following a schedule. Appointments are scheduled, and treatments are prescribed with time parameters. Medication orders include how often the medicine is to be taken and when (e.g., digoxin 0.25 mg, once a day, in the morning). Nurses need to be aware that time may have a different meaning for clients. When caring for clients who are "present oriented," it is important to avoid fixed schedules. The nurse can offer a time range for activities and treatments. For example, instead of telling the client to take digoxin every day at 10:00 AM, the nurse might tell the client to take it every day in the morning or every day after getting out of bed.

Nutritional Patterns

Most cultures have staple foods that are plentiful or readily accessible in their environment. Even clients who have been in the United States or Canada for several generations often continue to eat the foods of their cultural homeland. The way food is prepared and served is also related to cultural practices. Food-related cultural behaviors can include whether to breast-feed or bottle-feed infants and when to introduce solid foods to them. Food can also be considered part of the remedy for illness. Religious practice associated with specific cultures affects diet.

PROVIDING CULTURALLY COMPETENT NURSING CARE

All phases of the nursing process are affected by the client's and the nurse's cultural values, beliefs, and behaviors. As the client's culture and the nurse's culture come together in the nurse–client relationship, a unique cultural environment is created that can improve or impair the client's outcome. Self-awareness of personal biases can enable nurses to modify their behaviors or (if they are unable to do so) to remove themselves from situations where care may be compromised. Nurses can become more aware of their own culture through values clarification (see Chapter 2 ∞). The nurse must also consider the cultural values dominant in the health care setting because those may influence the client's outcome.

Campinha-Bacote's model of cultural competence (2003) is also of special relevance to understand the core practice competences of culturally appropriate nursing care. In this model, nurses are encouraged to integrate into their practice the following five constructs: (a) cultural awareness, (b) cultural knowledge, (c) cultural skills, (d) cultural encounters, and (e) cultural desires. According to this model, nurses need to have a desire to become culturally competent and sensitive, as well as actively look for opportunities and experiences that are cross-cultural.

NURSING MANAGEMENT

ASSESSING

To conduct a heritage assessment, the nurse asks certain questions in an assessment interview. This facilitates communication with clients and their families. The assessment interview is designed to determine if clients identify with their traditional cultural heritage (heritage consistent) or if they have acculturated into the dominant culture of the modern society they reside in (heritage inconsistent). The interview facilitates conversation and helps in the planning of cultural care. Once a conversation begins and the person describes aspects of his or her cultural heritage, the nurse can develop an understanding of the person's unique health and illness beliefs, practices, and cultural needs.

Examples of Heritage Consistency

The following factors and examples indicative of heritage consistency can be explored to determine the depth to which a person identifies with his or her traditional heritage, that is, the cultural beliefs and practices of his or her family heritage:

- The person's childhood development occurred in the person's country of origin or in an immigrant neighborhood of a similar ethnic group in the United States.
- Extended family members encouraged participation in traditional religious and cultural activities.
- The individual engages in frequent visits to the country of origin or returns to the "old neighborhood" in the United States if possible.
- The individual's family home is within the ethnic community of which he or she is a member.
- The individual participates in ethnic cultural events.
- The individual was raised in an extended family setting. The person's social frame of reference is the family.
- The individual maintains regular contact with the extended family.
- The individual's name has not been Americanized.
- The individual was educated in a parochial (nonpublic) school with a religious or ethnic philosophy similar to the family's background. The person's education plays an enormous role in socialization, and the major purpose of education is to socialize a given person into the dominant culture. Children learn English and the customs and norms of American life in the schools. In the parochial or private schools, they not only learn English but also are socialized in the culture and norms of the particular religious or ethnic group that is sponsoring the school.
- The individual engages in social activities primarily with others of the same religious or ethnic background.
- The individual has knowledge of the culture and language of origin.
- The individual expresses pride in his or her heritage.

Conveying Cultural Sensitivity

The process of heritage and health traditions assessment is important. How and when questions are asked requires sensitivity and clinical judgment. The timing and phrasing of questions need to be adapted to the individual. Timing is important in introducing questions. Sensitivity is needed in phrasing questions. Trust must be established before clients can be expected to volunteer and share sensitive information. The nurse therefore needs to spend time with clients, introduce some social conversation, and convey a genuine desire to understand their values and beliefs.

Before a heritage assessment begins, determine what language the client speaks and the client's degree of fluency in English. It is also important to learn about the client's communications patterns and space orientation. This is accomplished by observing both verbal and nonverbal communication. What nonverbal communication behaviors does the client exhibit? What significance do these behaviors have for the nurse–client interaction? What is the client's proximity to other people and objects within the environment? How does the client react to the nurse's movement toward the client? What cultural objects within the environment have importance for health promotion or health maintenance?

It is vital for nurses to be culturally sensitive and to convey this sensitivity to clients, support people, and other health care personnel. Some ways to do so follow:

- Always address clients, support people, and other health care personnel by their last names (e.g., Mrs. Aylia, Dr. Rush) until they give you permission to use other names. In some cultures, the more formal style of address is a sign of respect, whereas the informal use of first names may be considered disrespect. It is important to ask people how they wish to be addressed.
- When meeting a person for the first time, introduce yourself by your full name, and then explain your role (e.g., "My name is Alicia Bernett and I am a student nurse at Nightingale School of Nursing"). This helps establish a relationship and provides an opportunity for clients, others, and nurses to learn the pronunciation of one another's names and their roles.
- Be authentic with people, and be honest about the knowledge you lack about their culture. When you do not understand a person's actions, politely and respectfully seek information.
- Use language that is culturally sensitive; for example, say "gay," "lesbian," or "bisexual" rather than "homosexual"; do not use "man" or "mankind" when referring to a woman. Ask if the person prefers to be referred to as "Hispanic" or "Latino"; as an "African American" or "Black."
- Find out what the client thinks about his or her health problems, illness, and treatments. Assess whether this information is congruent with the dominant health care culture. If the beliefs and practices are incongruent, establish whether this will have a negative effect on the client's health.
- Do not make any assumptions about the client, and always ask about anything you do not understand.
- Show respect for the client's values, beliefs, and practices, even if they differ from your own or from those of the dominant culture. If you do not agree with them, it is important to respect the client's right to hold these beliefs (Table 4–2).
- Show respect for the client's support people. In some cultures, men in the family make decisions affecting the client, while in other cultures women make the decisions.
- Make a concerted effort to obtain the client's trust, but do not be surprised if it develops slowly or not at all. The heritage assessment takes time and usually needs to extend over several meetings.

DIAGNOSING

The nursing diagnoses developed by NANDA focus on nursing care provided in the United States and Canada and are based on Western cultural beliefs. It is essential to expand the understanding of nursing practice to include cultural beliefs of Eastern cultures as well. Nurses must provide appropriate care to clients of any culture. This is accomplished through developing cultural sensitivity and considering how a client's culture influences his or her responses to health conditions, much as the nurse considers how a client's age or gender influences a nursing diagnosis, plan, and delivery of nursing care.

Impaired verbal communication may be an appropriate nursing diagnosis for a client who does not speak or understand English. Deficient knowledge may be used when a client lacks knowledge of Western medical treatment options. Risk for compromised human dignity may be an appropriate nursing diagnosis if the client's cultural needs are not being met or are at risk for being overlooked.

PLANNING

Cultural competence in nursing involves delivering care that integrates the mind, the body, the spirit, and the cultural values of the individual (Fontaine, 2010). A potential outcome is that clients can "promote, maintain, and/or regain mutually desired and obtainable levels of health within the realities of their life circumstances" (Kagawa-Singer & Kassim-Lakha, 2010, p. 580). There are several steps involved in the process that lead to the development of cultural competency. The knowledge and skills necessary to incorporate cultural care into standard nursing require the acquisition of a broad base of knowledge about different heritages and social structures. It is an ongoing process, and the skills and knowledge base grow over time. As one's knowledge base grows, the ability to convey cultural sensitivity also grows.

The following are examples of the necessary steps:

1. Become aware of your own cultural heritage. Where were your parents and grandparents born? What are examples of their traditional health and illness beliefs and practices? Do they value stoic behavior in relation to pain, or is it permissible to state that you are in pain? Are the rights of the individual valued over and above the rights of the family? Only by knowing one's own culture (values, practices, and beliefs) can a person be ready to learn about another's.
2. Become aware of the client's heritage and health traditions as described by the client. It is important to avoid assuming that all people of one ethnic background have the same cultural beliefs and values. When the nurse has knowledge of the client's culture, mutual respect between client and nurse is more likely to develop.

TABLE 4–2	Cultural Beliefs			
	AFRICAN AMERICAN	**HISPANIC OR LATINO**	**ASIAN**	**NATIVE AMERICAN**
Medical Practices	Menstruation believed to rid body of dirty and excess blood Use of home remedies High incidence of lactose intolerance	Hot–cold balance Ice water only when requested Believe in postpartum rest Sponge baths after birth Tend not to complain of pain, especially men Family may attend to body after death	Coining and cupping traditional Fevers treated by wrapping in blankets and giving warm liquids No ice water unless requested Use of herbal remedies Chinese medicine taken differently May not report pain because it may seem they are accusing the professional of inadequate care	Focus on harmony within oneself, with others, and the environment to maintain health Medicine men (often older adults in the community) may use healing herbs, purification rituals, or assist in restoring balance between the person, the community, and the environment
Family	Strong family links Issues around gender identity, expected roles and independence Older adults held in high regard	Strong family links Allow family members to spend as much time as possible and provide non-technical care Family rather than individual makes decisions	Affection between family members is rarely exhibited in public Family may request client not be told of terminal diagnosis to avoid depressing client	Family structure varies within tribes—may be matriarchal or patriarchal Extended families with adopted relatives living in close proximity with high fertility rates, low percentage of out-of-wedlock births, strong roles for women Value traditional beliefs Deep respect for older adults
Religion	Primary religion is Baptist, other Protestant religions, or Muslim	Strong belief in fate and external control Primary religion is Roman Catholic	Combination of Buddhist and Christian religions are predominant	There is no word for religion because it is not seen as a separate thing but integral to all aspects of life, health, and well-being
Personal Space, Time	Focus on present time Open displays of emotion are acceptable and common	May avoid eye contact as sign of respect	Eye contact is avoided to award respect	Focus on present time

Note: Information for all but the last column came from Russell, S. S. (2005). *Cultural considerations at the end-of-life.* AACN viewpoint. Retrieved 3/3/08 from http://findarticles.com/p/articles/mi_qa4022/is_200503/ai_n13632953/pg_3. Information about Native Americans came from Tsai, G., & Alanis, L. (2004). *Journey to thinking multiculturally: The Native American culture: A historical and reflective perspective.* Retrieved April 14, 2009, from Communiqué website: http://www.nasponline.org/publications/cq/cq328native.aspx

3. Become aware of adaptations the client made to live in a North American culture. During this part of the interview, a nurse can also identify the client's preferences in health practices, diet, hygiene, and so on.

4. Form a nursing plan with the client that incorporates his or her cultural beliefs regarding the maintenance, protection, and restoration of health. In this way, cultural values, practices, and beliefs can be incorporated with the necessary nursing care.

IMPLEMENTING

The implementation of cultural nursing care includes (a) cultural preservation and maintenance and (b) cultural accommodation and negotiation. Cultural preservation may involve the use of cultural health care practices, such as giving herbal tea, chicken soup, or "hot foods" to the ill client. Accommodation of the client's viewpoint and negotiating appropriate care requires expert communication skills, such

CULTURALLY COMPETENT CARE — Families

- Include cultural assessment of the client and family as part of overall assessment.
- Learn the rituals, customs, and practices of the major cultural groups with whom you come into contact. Learn to appreciate the richness of diversity and consider it an asset rather than a hindrance in your practice.
- Don't make assumptions about beliefs or practices.
- Ask about the client's use of cultural or alternative approaches to healing.

- Identify your personal biases, attitudes, prejudices, and stereotypes.
- Recognize that it is the client's (or family's) right to make their own health care choices. Explain in detail the client's condition and the treatment plan if the client is willing for you to do this.
- Convey respect and cooperate with traditional helpers and caregivers.

as responding empathetically, validating information, and effectively summarizing content. Negotiation is a collaborative process. It acknowledges that the nurse–client relationship is reciprocal and that different views exist of health, illness, and treatment. The nurse attempts to bridge the gap between the nurse's scientific approach and the client's cultural perspectives. During the negotiation process, the client's views are explored and acknowledged. Relevant scientific information is then provided. If the client's views reveal that certain behaviors would not affect the client's condition adversely, then they are incorporated in planning care. If the client's views can lead to harmful behavior or outcomes, then an attempt is made to shift the client's perspectives to the scientific view.

Negotiation occurs when cultural treatment practices conflict with those of the health care system. It must be determined precisely how the client is managing the illness, what practices could be harmful, and which practices can be safely combined with Western medicine. Consider these examples of potential conflicts between cultural beliefs or practices and the dominant American health care system:

- Native American women value large body size and may be resistant to weight control.
- The decision to circumcise male infants is often made based on cultural and family beliefs and can occasionally conflict with medical advice.
- A Hispanic or Asian client may be unable to obtain hospice care if the family will not permit the client to be informed of the diagnosis or prognosis.
- Members of the Jehovah's Witness faith do not accept blood transfusions even in life-threatening situations.
- Orthodox Sikhs do not cut their hair. This can conflict with the need to shave the skin for medical procedures.

When a client chooses to follow only cultural practices and declines all prescribed medical or nursing interventions,

LONG-TERM CARE CONSIDERATIONS
Cultural Considerations

Clients in long-term care often reside in the facility for long periods of time and are, as such, inviting the health care provider into their home. Accommodating cultural differences in how they furnish their space is essential to the sense of home the client needs to feel comfortable in their space. Adding cultural considerations to the client's plan of care will improve client outcomes.

the nurse and client must adjust the client goals. Monitoring the client's condition to identify changes in health and to recognize impending crises before they become irreversible may be all that is realistically achievable. At a time of crisis, the opportunity may arise to renegotiate care.

Providing cultural nursing care is challenging. It requires discovery of the meaning of the client's behavior, flexibility, creativity, and knowledge to adapt nursing interventions. An effort must be made to learn from each experience. This knowledge will improve the delivery of culture-specific care to future clients. The accompanying box offers suggestions for providing such care to clients and families.

EVALUATING

Evaluating nursing care of clients that incorporates the concepts of heritage and ethnicity is performed in the same way as with any client. Client outcomes are compared with the goals and expected outcomes established following comprehensive assessment that includes sensitivity to cultural diversity. However, if the outcomes are not achieved, and the client and nurse are from different cultures, the nurse should be especially careful to consider whether the client's belief system has been adequately included as an influencing factor.

CHAPTER HIGHLIGHTS

- The Office of Minority Health is a major resource for nursing students when working with racial, ethnic, and cultural groups.
- *The National Standards for Culturally and Linguistically Appropriate Services in Health Care* (CLAS) should be understood by nurses and applied their professional practice.
- *Healthy People 2010* calls for nursing to contribute to eliminating health disparities by gender, race or ethnicity, education, income, disability, geographic location, and sexual orientation.
- Racial and Ethnic Approaches to Community Health (REACH 2010) is an initiative that motivates nurses and other health professionals to center their academic and research efforts on infant mortality, deficits in breast and cervical cancer screening/management, cardiovascular diseases, diabetes, HIV infections/AIDS, and child and adult immunizations.
- People in the United States come from a variety of backgrounds, and many retain at least some of their traditional values, including health beliefs and practices.

- People may live within their traditional heritage or they may embrace both their original ethnocultural traditional heritage(s) and the modern culture of the United States.
- An individual's heritage and cultural background can influence health beliefs and practices.
- Through acculturation, most groups in the United States modify some of their traditional cultural characteristics.
- Personal characteristics also modify an individual's cultural values, beliefs, and practices.
- Health beliefs and practices, family patterns, communication style, space and time orientation, and nutritional patterns may influence the relationship between the nurse and the client who have different cultural backgrounds.
- When assessing a client, the nurse considers the client's cultural values, beliefs, and practices related to health and health care.

THINK ABOUT IT

Refer to the chapter-opening scenario and answer these questions.

1. As the nurse caring for Michelle when she is admitted in labor with her second child, what questions would you ask when conducting a cultural assessment?

2. Michelle and her mother ask the nurse if a shaman can visit Michelle and perform a ceremony to prevent problems with the birth and the baby. The ceremony requires a small table on which a lit candle and holy water will be placed. How will you respond to this request?

3. To provide more culturally appropriate care for Michelle, where could you learn more information about Korean cultural beliefs?

∞ *See suggested responses to Think About It on MyNursingKit.*

TEST YOUR KNOWLEDGE

1. The major factor contributing to the increased emphasis on the need for proficiency in cultural nursing practice in the United States includes which of the following?
    1. An increasing birth rate
    2. Limited access to health care services
    3. Demographic changes
    4. A decreasing rate of immigration

2. Which of the following behaviors is most indicative of culturally sensitive nursing practice?
    1. Helping clients recognize the need to adapt health practices to fit commonly accepted practices
    2. Discussing the meaning of the medical regime to the client
    3. Informing clients that lack of adherence to medical regime may be detrimental
    4. Asking a person from the same culture to explain the relevance of the intervention

3. In initiating care for a client from a different culture than the nurse, which of the following would be an appropriate statement?
    1. "Since, in your culture, people don't drink ice water, I will bring you hot tea."
    2. "Do you have any books I could read about people from your culture?"
    3. "Please let me know if I do anything that is not acceptable in your culture."
    4. "You will need to set aside your usual customs and practices while you are in the hospital."

4. Which of the following behaviors is most representative of a *culturally competent* nurse?
    1. Helps clients of Native American heritage identify ways to relate more to their culture.
    2. Helps parents of Latino heritage recognize that their children need to speak English.

3. Interprets and validates beliefs of a client with African American heritage.
4. Asks a nurse of Japanese heritage to teach others dosage calculations since Asians are good at math.

5. Students ask the nurse to explain the differences between culture and race. Which of the following is the nurse's best response?
1. Culture is limited to a shared language or religion.
2. Race describes common characteristics within a specific heritage group.
3. Culture is socially oriented and race addresses shared physical traits.
4. Culture is the degree by which one's lifestyle matches one's heritage.

6. The nurse is caring for a client who is a second-generation American. His grandparents emigrated from Japan and both he and his parents were born in the United States. In order to provide culturally competent care the nurse would:
1. Anticipate that the client will have many Asian cultural beliefs.
2. Anticipate that this client will be completely acculturated.
3. Anticipate that this client may have shared beliefs from both the Asian culture and the American culture.
4. Assess the client's cultural beliefs.

7. The male nurse is caring for a female client from the Middle East who requests that a female nurse be assigned to her care. The male nurse's best response would be:
1. "I've been assigned to take care of you today but I will place a note on your chart to assign only female nurses in the future to your care."
2. "I am just as competent as a female nurse and will provide you with excellent care."
3. "I will talk to my charge nurse about changing the client assignment."
4. "Does your religion prevent you from being cared for by a male health care provider?"

8. The nurse is checking the dietary trays delivered to the unit this afternoon and finds a client who actively practices Orthodox Jewish beliefs has received a tray containing pot roast, skim milk, vegetables, and coffee. The nurse's best action would be to:
1. Instruct the nursing assistant to deliver the tray after removing the coffee.
2. Call the dietary department to send a tray without beef.
3. Have dietary replace the entire tray.
4. Ask the client if lactose-free milk would be preferable.

9. The home health nurse is caring for an Asian American who refuses to take the blood pressure medication prescribed and insists that acupuncture will resolve her health issues. How can the nurse best help this client?
1. Notify the physician of the client's choice and monitor her blood pressure for a possible crisis.
2. Ask the nurse's supervisor to assign an Asian American nurse to this client.
3. Act as a client advocate by insisting that the client take her medication.
4. Discharge the client and explain that the client should call if she changes her mind and agrees to follow the plan of care.

10. The nurse, caring for a Hispanic client, would use knowledge of which of the following practices to provide culturally sensitive care? Select all that apply.
1. Herbal medicines are used to treat illness.
2. The family might want to hire mourners if the client dies.
3. Staring at the client's child will be interpreted as preventing the "evil eye."
4. Use of hot and cold foods is important when treating the illness.
5. The client may prefer a caregiver of the same gender.

∞ *See answers to Test Your Knowledge in Appendix A.*

REFERENCES AND SELECTED BIBLIOGRAPHY

Agency for Healthcare Research and Quality. (2005). *2005 national healthcare quality and disparities report.* Rockville, MD: Author.

Alexander, R. (2006). Diversity, cultural competence, and the nursing student. *Imprint, 53*(2), 43–45.

Andrews, J. D. (2005). *Cultural, ethnic and religious reference manual for health care providers* (3rd ed.). Winston-Salem, NC: Jamarda Resources.

Betancourt, J. R., Green, A. R., Carrillo, J. E., & Park, E. R. (2005). Cultural competence and health care disparities: Key perspectives and trends. *Health Affairs, 24,* 499–505.

Buerhaus, P. I., Staiger, D. O., & Auerbach, D. I. (2004). New signs of a strengthening U.S. nurse labor market? *Health Affairs, 23,* 526–533.

California Healthcare Interpreters Association. (2002). *California standards for healthcare interpreters: Ethical principles, protocols, and guidance on roles and interventions.* Los Angeles: Author.

Campinha-Bacote, J. (2003). Many faces: Addressing diversity in health care. *Online Journal of Issues in Nursing, 8*(1), Manuscript 2. Retrieved October 14, 2009, from http://www.nursingworld.org/MainMenuCategories/ANAMarketplace/ANAPeriodicals/OJIN/TableofContents/Volume82003/No1Jan2003/AddressingDiversityinHealthCare.aspx

Campinha-Bacote, J. (2003). *The process of cultural competence in the delivery of healthcare services* (3rd ed.). Cincinnati, OH: Transcultural C.A.R.E. Associates.

Canadian Nurses Association. (2004). *Position statement: Promoting culturally competent care.* Retrieved October 14, 2009, from http://cna-aiic.ca/CNA/documents/pdf/publications/PS73_Promoting_Culturally_ Competent_CareMarch_2004_e.pdf

Centers for Disease Control and Prevention. (n.d.). *Mission.* Retrieved October 14, 2009, from http://www.cdc.gov/omh/AboutUs/aboutUs.htm

Collins, C. C., Decker, S. I., & Esquibel, K. A. (2004). Definitions of health: Comparison of Hispanic and African-American elders. *Journal of Multicultural Nursing & Health, 10*(3), 13–18.

Cook, C. (2003). The many faces of diversity: Overview and summary. *Online Journal of Issues in Nursing, 8*(1). Retrieved October 14, 2009, from http://nursingworld.org/ojin/topic20/tpc20ntr.htm

D'Avanzo, C., & Geissler, E. M. (2003). *Pocket guide to cultural health assessment* (3rd ed.). St. Louis: Mosby.

Dennis, B. P., & Small, E. B. (2003). Incorporating cultural diversity in nursing care: An action plan. *ABNF Journal, 14,* 17–26.

Fontaine, K. L. (2010). *Complementary and alternative therapies for nursing practice* (3rd ed.). Upper Saddle River, NJ: Pearson Education.

Frenn, M., Malin, S., Villarruel, A., Slaikeu, K., McCarthy, S., Freeman, J., et al. (2005). Determinants of physical activity and low-fat diet among low income African American and Hispanic middle school students. *Public Health Nursing, 22,* 89–97.

Galanti, G. A. (2008). *Caring for patients from different cultures* (4th ed.). Philadelphia: University of Pennsylvania Press.

Giger, J. N., & Davidhizar, R. E. (2004). *Transcultural nursing* (4th ed.). St. Louis: Mosby Year Book.

Giorgianni, S. J. (Ed.). (2004). Diversity in healthcare delivery. *Pfizer Journal. VIII*(2), 4–14.

Green-Hernandez, C., Quinn, A. A., Denman-Vitale, S., Falkenstern, S. K., & Judge-Ellis, T. (2004). Making nursing care culturally competent. *Holistic Nursing Practice, 18*(4), 215–218.

Hascup, V. A. (2004). Transcultural nursing. *Advance for Nurses, 2*(15), 28–29.

Jeffreys, M. (2006). Cultural competence in clinical practice. *Imprint, 53*(2), 37–41.

Jones, M. E., Cason, C. L., & Bond, M. L. (2004). Cultural attitudes, knowledge, and skills of a health workforce. *Journal of Transcultural Nursing, 15,* 283–290.

Kagawa-Singer, M., & Kassim-Lakha, S. (2003). A strategy to reduce cross-cultural miscommunication and increase the likelihood of improving health outcomes. *Academic Medicine, 78,* 577–587.

Kavanaugh, K. H., & Knowlden, V. (2004). *Many voices: Toward caring culture in healthcare and healing.* Madison: University of Wisconsin Press.

Leininger, M. M., & McFarland, M. R. (2005). *Culture care diversity & universality: A worldwide nursing theory* (2nd ed.). Boston: Jones & Bartlett.

Lipson, J. G., & Dibble, S. L. (Eds.). (2005). *Culture & clinical care.* San Francisco: UCSF Nursing Press.

Mason, P., & Narad, C. (2005). International adoption: A health and developmental prospective. *Seminars in Speech and Language 26*(1),1–9.

McLemore, S. D., & Romo, H. D. (2005). *Racial and ethnic relations in America* (7th ed.). Boston: Allyn & Bacon.

Muñoz, C., & Hilgenberg, C. (2005). Ethnopharmacology: Understanding how ethnicity can affect drug response is essential to providing culturally competent care. *American Journal of Nursing, 105*(8), 40–49.

Munoz, C. C., & Luckman, J. (2004). *Transcultural communication in nursing* (2nd ed.). Clifton Park, NY: Thomson Delmar.

National Center for Complementary and Alternative Medicine (NCCAM). (2009). *2007 Statistics on CAM use in the United States.* Retrieved October 14, 2009, from National Institute of Health website: http://nccam.nih.gov/news/camstats/2007/

National Center on Minority Health and Health Disparities. (n.d.). *Mission.* Retrieved October 14, 2009, from http://ncmhd.nih.gov/about_ncmhd/mission.asp

Norr, K. F., Crittenden, K. S., Lehrer, E. L., Reyes, O., Boyd, C. B., Nacion, K. W., et al. (2003). Maternal and infant outcomes at one year for a nurse-health advocate home visiting program serving African Americans and Mexican Americans. *Public Health Nursing, 20,* 190–203.

Office of Minority Health. (2001). *National standards for culturally and linguistically appropriate services in health care.* Washington, DC: U. S. Department of Health and Human Services.

Pinquart, M., & Sörenson, S. (2005). Ethnic differences in stressors, resources, and psychological outcomes of family caregiving: A meta-analysis. *Gerontologist, 45,* 90–106.

Purnell, L., & Paulanka, B. (2004). *A guide to culturally competent healthcare.* Philadelphia: Davis.

Public Health Foundation. (2001). *The key ingredient of the National Prevention Agenda: Workforce development—A companion document to Healthy People 2010.* Retrieved October 14, 2009, from ftp://ftp.hrsa.gov/bhpr/nationalcenter/hp2010.pdf

Rawlings-Anderson, K. (2004). Assessing the cultural and religious needs of older people. *Nursing Older People, 16*(8), 29–33.

Rhee, H. (2005). Racial/ethnic differences in adolescents' physical symptoms. *Journal of Pediatric Nursing, Nursing Care of Children and Families, 20,* 153–162.

Sensor, C. S. (2006). Culturally competent care in the workplace. *Imprint, 53*(2), 46–51.

Shen, Z. (2004). Cultural competence models in nursing: A selected annotated bibliography. *Journal of Transcultural Nursing, 15,* 317–322.

Spector, R. E. (2008). *Cultural diversity in health and illness* (7th ed.). Upper Saddle River, NJ: Pearson Education.

Tsai, G., & Alanis, L. (2004). *Journey to thinking multiculturally: the Native American culture: A historical and reflective perspective.* Retrieved October 14, 2009, from Communique website: http://www.nasponline.org/publications/cq/cq328native.aspx

Turton, P. (2003). Education for integration: A view from the bridge! *Complementary Therapies in Nursing and Midwifery, 9*(1), 20–22.

U.S. Bureau of Labor Statistics. (2004). *Table 3c. The 10 occupations with the largest job growth, 2002–12.* Retrieved October 14, 2009, from http://www.bls.gov/news.release/ecopro.t05.htm

U.S. Census Bureau. (2001). *Profiles of general demographic characteristics 2000.* Washington, DC: U.S. Department of Commerce.

U.S. Census Bureau. (2004). *U.S. interim projections by age, sex, race, and Hispanic origin.* Retrieved October 14, 2009, from http://www.census.gov/ipc/www/usinterimproj

U.S. Census Bureau. (2005a). *Annual estimates of the population by sex, race and Hispanic or Latino origin for the United States: April 1, 2000 to July 1, 2004* (NC-EST2004-03). Retrieved October 14, 2009, from http://www.census.gov/popest/national/asrh/NC-EST2004-srh.html

U.S. Census Bureau. (2005b). *Foreign born population tops 34 million.* Retrieved October 14, 2009, from http://www.census.gov/Press-Release/www/releases/archives/foreignborn_population/003969.html

U.S. Department of Health and Human Services Office of Minority Health, (n.d.). *Mission*. Retrieved October 14, 2009, from http://www.omhrc.gov/templates/browse .aspx?lvl=1&lvlID=7

U.S. Department of Health and Human Services Health Resources and Service Administration Bureau of Health Professions. (2004). *The registered nurse population: Findings from the 2004 National Sample Survey of Registered Nurses, March 2004*. Retrieved October 14, 2009, from http://bhpr.hrsa.gov/

healthworkforce/rnsurvey04/appendixb .htm

Vivian, C., & Dundes, L. (2004). The crossroads of culture and health among the Roma (Gypsies). *Journal of Nursing Scholarship, 36*, 86–91.

Waters, V. L. (2004). Cultivate corporate culture and diversity. *Nursing Management, 35*(1), 36–37.

Wittig, D. R. (2004). Knowledge, skills, and attitudes of nursing students regarding culturally congruent care of Native

Americans. *Journal of Transcultural Nursing, 15(1)*, 54–61.

Yeo, S. (2004). Language barriers and access to care. *Annual Review of Nursing Research, 22*, 59–73.

Zitzow, D., & Estes, G. (1981). The heritage consistency continuum in counseling Native American students. In *Contemporary American Indian issues in higher education*. Los Angeles: American Indian Studies Center, University of California.

Health Beliefs and Practices

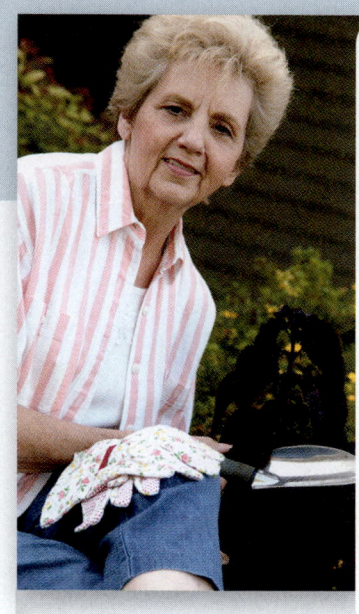

Betty Gracely, 66 years old, has always been healthy and is more than happy to tell anyone who will listen about her lack of trust in the health care system. She has lived alone since the death of her husband from lung cancer three years ago, smokes two to three packs of cigarettes a day, and is active in the community. She takes hormone supplements for hypothyroidism but has no other health problems. For the past few weeks she has noticed she becomes short of breath more easily and has developed a chronic cough. When friends or family tell her she should see a doctor, she just laughs and says, "If it's not broke, don't fix it" or "Doctors make more money if they can tell you there's something wrong, even if there isn't."

LEARNING OUTCOMES

After completing this chapter, you will be able to:

1. Differentiate health, wellness, and well-being.

2. Define the seven components of wellness and explain how they overlap.

3. Explain the relationship of individuality, holism, and homeostasis to nursing practice.

4. Compare the stages of Maslow's and Kalish's hierarchies and give examples of behaviors likely to be seen in a person seeking to meet each need.

5. List and define factors affecting health status, beliefs, practices, and health care adherence.

6. Explain Suchman's stages of illness.

7. Describe effects of illness on individuals' and family members' roles and functions.

8. Differentiate health promotion from health protection or illness prevention.

9. Identify various types and sites of health promotion programs.

10. Explain the stages of health behavior change.

11. List actions the nurse could take while developing, implementing, and evaluating plans of care for health promotion.

12. Describe six concepts basic to alternative practices.

13. Give examples of healing environments.

14. List four types of systematized health care, botanical healing, manual healing methods, mind body therapies, and miscellaneous therapies and describe the goal of each type of therapy.

15. Identify strategies you could use to incorporate nutrition and spiritual therapy into your nursing practice.

CONCEPTS OF HEALTH, WELLNESS, AND WELL-BEING

Nurses' understanding of health and wellness largely determines the scope and nature of their nursing practice. Clients' health beliefs also influence their health practices. Some people think of health and wellness (or well-being) as the same thing or, at the very least, as accompanying one another. However, health may not always accompany well-being. A person who has a terminal illness may have a sense of well-being; conversely, another person may lack a sense of well-being yet be in a state of good health. Today's health care providers are increasing their emphasis on promoting health and wellness in individuals, families, and communities.

Health

Traditionally **health** was defined in terms of the presence or absence of disease. The World Health Organization (WHO) takes a more holistic view of health. Its constitution defines health as "a state of complete physical, mental, and social well-being, and not merely the absence of disease or infirmity" (WHO, 1948). This definition:

- Reflects concern for the individual as a total person functioning physically, psychologically, and socially. Mental processes determine people's relationship with their physical and social surroundings, their attitudes about life, and their interaction with others.
- Places health in the context of environment. People's lives, and therefore their health, are affected by everything they interact with—not only environmental influences such as climate and the availability of food, shelter, clean air, and water to drink, but also other people, including family, lovers, employers, co-workers, friends, and associates.

Health has also been defined in terms of role and performance. Talcott Parsons (1951), an eminent American sociologist and creator of the concept "sick role," conceptualized health as the ability to maintain normal roles.

In 1980, the American Nurses Association (ANA) defined health in its social policy statement as "a dynamic state of being in which the developmental and behavioral potential of an individual is realized to the fullest extent possible" (ANA, 1980, p. 5). In this definition, health is more than a state or the absence of disease; it includes striving toward optimal functioning. In 2004, the ANA also stated that health is "An experience that is often expressed in terms of wellness and illness, and may occur in the presence or absence of disease or injury" (2004, p. 48).

PERSONAL DEFINITIONS OF HEALTH Health is a highly individual perception. Consider the following examples of individuals who would probably say they are healthy even though they have physical impairments that some would consider an **illness:**

- A 15-year-old with diabetes takes injectable insulin each morning. He plays on the school soccer team and is editor of the high school newspaper.
- A 32-year-old is paralyzed from the waist down and needs a wheelchair for mobility. He is taking accounting at a nearby college and uses a specially designed automobile for transportation.
- A 72-year-old takes antihypertensive medications to treat high blood pressure. She bowls once a week, is a member of the neighborhood golf club, makes handicrafts for a local charity, and travels two months each year.

Many people define and describe health as the following:

- Being free from symptoms of disease and pain as much as possible
- Being able to be active and to do what they want
- Being in good spirits most of the time

These characteristics indicate that health is not something that a person achieves suddenly at a specific time. It is an ongoing process—a way of life—through which a person develops and encourages every aspect of the body, mind, and feelings to interrelate harmoniously as much as possible. Many factors affect individual definitions of health. Definitions vary according to an individual's previous experiences, expectations of self, age, and sociocultural influences.

BOX 5–1	Developing a Personal Definition of Health

The following questions can help nurses develop a personal definition of health.

- Is a person more than a biophysiologic system?
- Is health more than the absence of disease symptoms?
- Is health the ability of an individual to perform work?
- Is health the ability of an individual to adapt to the environment?
- Is health a condition of a person's actualization?
- Is health a state or a process?

- Is health the effective functioning of self-care activities?
- Is health static or changing?
- Are health and wellness the same?
- Are disease and illness different?
- Are there levels of health?
- Is wellness, health, and illness separate entities or points along a continuum?
- Is health socially determined?
- How do you rate your health and why?

Nurses should be aware of their own personal definitions of health and appreciate that other people have their own individual definitions as well. A person's definition of health influences behavior related to health and illness. By understanding clients' perceptions of health and illness, nurses can provide more meaningful assistance to help them regain or attain a state of health by their own personal definitions. For aid in developing a personal definition of health, see Box 5–1.

Wellness and Well-Being

Wellness is a state of well-being. Basic aspects of wellness include self-responsibility; an ultimate goal; a dynamic, growing process; daily decision making in the areas of nutrition, stress management, physical fitness, preventive health care, and emotional health; and, most importantly, the whole being of the individual.

Anspaugh, Hamrick, and Rosato (2006) propose seven components of wellness (see Figure 5–1). To realize optimal health and wellness, people must deal with the factors within each component:

- *Physical.* The ability to carry out daily tasks, achieve fitness, maintain adequate nutrition and proper body fat, avoid abusing drugs and alcohol or using tobacco products, and generally practice positive lifestyle habits.
- *Social.* The ability to interact successfully with people and within the environment of which each person is a part, to develop and maintain intimacy with significant others, and to develop respect and tolerance for those with different opinions and beliefs.
- *Emotional.* The ability to manage stress and express emotions appropriately. Emotional wellness involves the ability to recognize, accept, and express feelings and to accept one's limitations.
- *Intellectual.* The ability to learn and use information effectively for personal, family, and career development. Intellectual wellness involves striving for continued growth and learning to deal with new challenges effectively.
- *Spiritual.* The belief in some force (nature, science, religion, or a higher power) that serves to unite human beings and provide meaning and purpose to life. It includes a person's own morals, values, and ethics.

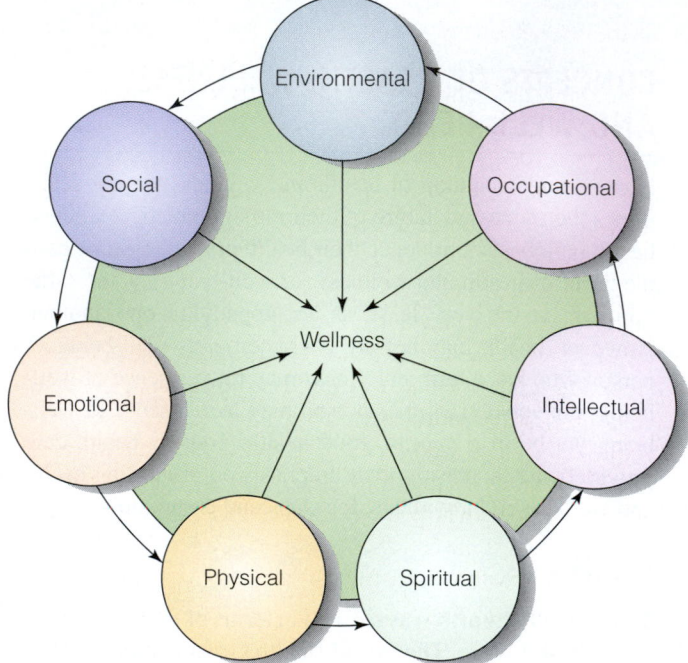

Figure 5–1 ⬤ The seven components of wellness.
(From *Wellness: Concepts and Applications,* 6th ed. (p. 4), by D. J. Anspaugh, M. H. Hamrick, and F. D. Rosato, copyright 2006. Reproduced with permission of the McGraw-Hill Companies.)

- *Occupational.* The ability to achieve a balance between work and leisure time. A person's beliefs about education, employment, and home influence personal satisfaction and relationships with others.
- *Environmental.* The ability to promote health measures that improve the standard of living and quality of life in the community. This includes influences such as food, water, and air.

The seven components overlap to some extent, and factors in one component often directly affect factors in another. For example, a person who learns to control daily stress levels from a physiologic perspective is also helping to maintain the emotional stamina needed to cope with a crisis. Wellness involves working on all aspects of the model.

It is important to remember that many aspects of well-being are subjective and the client is the best source of information. Clients may appear healthy, assessment findings may be within normal limits, and yet the client may feel pain, lethargy, or "not quite right." "Well-being is a subjective perception of vitality and feeling well . . . can be described objectively, experienced, and measured . . . and can be plotted on a continuum" (Hood & Leddy, 2003, p. 264). It is a component of health.

CONCEPT OF INDIVIDUALITY   To help clients attain, maintain, or regain an optimal level of health, nurses need to understand clients as individuals. Each individual is a unique being who is different from every other human being, with a different combination of genetics, life experiences, and environmental interactions.

Dimensions of individuality include the person's total character, self-identity, and perceptions. The person's total character encompasses behaviors, emotional state, attitudes, values, motives, abilities, habits, and appearances. The person's self-identity encompasses perception of self as a separate and distinct entity alone and in interactions with others. The person's perceptions encompass the way the person interprets the environment or situation, directly affecting how he or she thinks, feels, and acts in any given situation.

When providing care, nurses need to focus on the client within both a total care and an individualized care context. In the total care context, the nurse considers all the principles and areas that apply when taking care of any client of that age and condition. In the individualized care context, the nurse becomes acquainted with the client as an individual, using the total care principles that apply to this person at this time. For example, a nurse who is advising the mother of a preschooler understands that the child's desire to explore his or her world is a developmental stage that all preschoolers experience. However, a preschooler diagnosed with attention deficit/hyperactivity disorder may have an increased risk of accidents and injuries when interacting with the environment, due to his or her impulsivity and poor self-control. When instructing the mother, an understanding of how many children she has, what her parenting style is, and how she responds to stress would all contribute to individualizing care for this client and family.

CONCEPT OF HOLISM   Nurses are concerned with the individual as a whole, complete, or holistic person, not as an assembly of parts and processes. In nursing, the concept of **holism** emphasizes that nurses must keep the whole person in mind and strive to understand how one area of concern relates to the whole person. The nurse must also consider the relationship of the individual to the external environment and to others. For example, in helping a man who is grieving over the death of his spouse, the nurse explores the impact of the loss on the whole person (i.e., on the man's appetite, rest and sleep pattern, energy level, sense of well-being, mood, usual activities, family relationships, and relationships with others). Nursing interventions are directed toward restoring overall harmony, so they depend on the man's sense of purpose and meaning of his life.

CONCEPT OF HOMEOSTASIS   The concept of **homeostasis** was first introduced by Cannon (1939) to describe the relative

constancy of the internal processes of the body, such as blood oxygen and carbon dioxide levels, blood pressure, body temperature, blood glucose, and fluid and electrolyte balance. To Cannon, the word *homeostasis* did not imply something stagnant, set, or immobile; it meant a condition that might vary but remained relatively constant. Cannon viewed the human being as separate from the external environment and constantly endeavoring to maintain physiologic **equilibrium,** or balance, through adaptation to that environment. Homeostasis, then, is the tendency of the body to maintain a state of balance or equilibrium while continually changing.

Physiologic Homeostasis   Physiologic homeostasis means that the internal environment of the body is relatively stable and constant. All cells of the body require a relatively constant environment to function; thus the body's internal environment must be maintained within narrow limits. Homeostatic mechanisms have four main characteristics:

1. They are self-regulating.
2. They are compensatory.
3. They tend to be regulated by negative feedback systems.
4. They may require several feedback mechanisms to correct only one physiologic imbalance.

Homeostasis occurs within the physiologic **system,** a set of interacting identifiable parts or components. The fundamental components of a system are matter, energy, and communication. Without any one of these, a system does not exist. The individual is a human system with matter (the body), energy (chemical or thermal), and communication (e.g., the nervous system). The boundary of a system, such as the skin in the human system, is a real or imaginary line that differentiates one system from another system or a system from its environment.

There are two general types of systems: closed and open. A closed system does not exchange energy, matter, or information with its environment; it receives no input from the environment and gives no output to the environment. In an open system, energy, matter, and information move into and out of the system through the system boundary. All living systems, such as plants, animals, people, families, and communities, are open systems, since their survival depends on a continuous exchange of energy. They are, therefore, in a constant state of change. An open system depends on the quality and quantity of its input, output, and feedback. After the input is absorbed by the system, it is processed in a way useful to the system in a transformation known as *throughput.*

Feedback is the mechanism by which some of the output of a system is returned to the system as input. Feedback enables a system to regulate itself by redirecting the output back into the system, thus forming a feedback loop. This input influences the behavior of the system and its future output. Negative feedback inhibits change; positive feedback stimulates change. Most biologic systems are controlled by negative feedback to bring the system back to stability. This type of feedback system senses and counteracts any deviations from normal. The deviations may be greater or less than

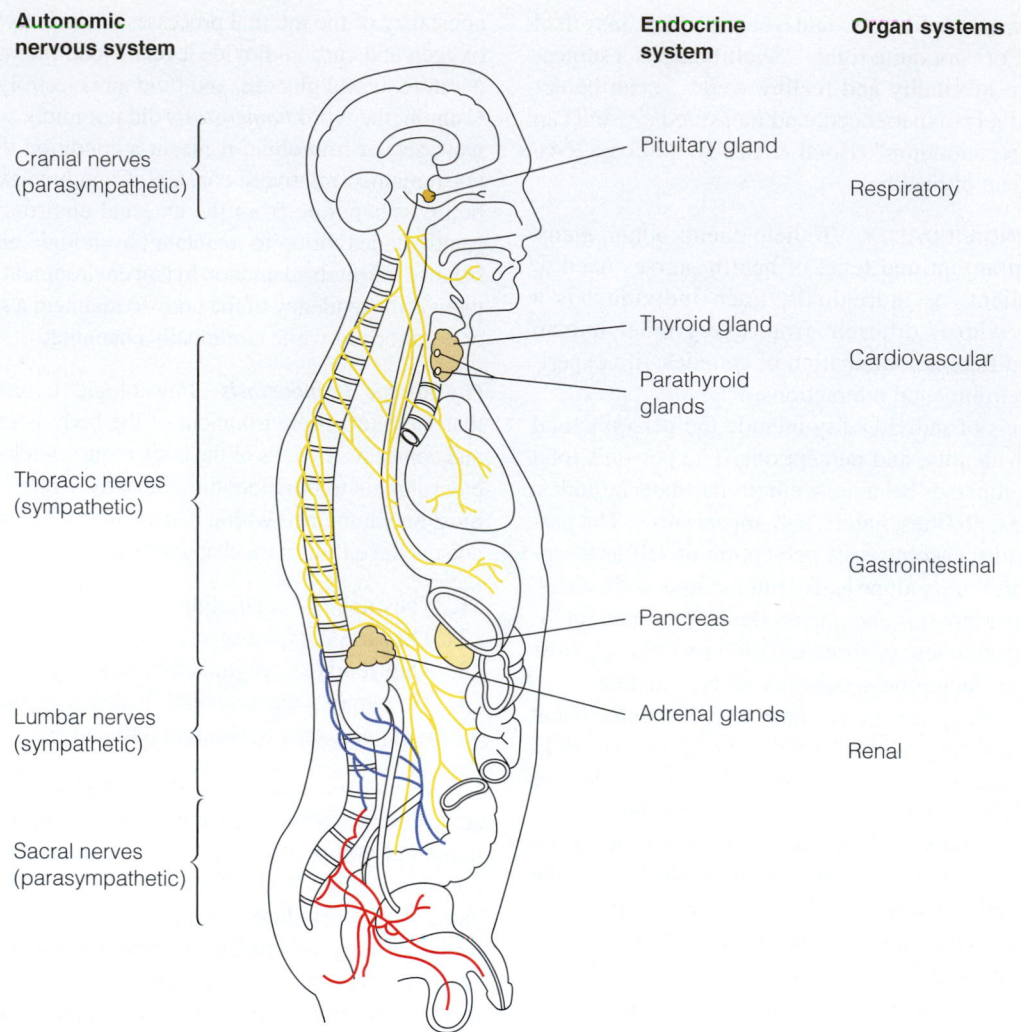

Figure 5–2 ⬤ The homeostatic regulators of the body: autonomic nervous system, endocrine system, and specific organ systems.

the normal level or range. For example, an increase in the production of parathyroid hormone is stimulated by a drop in blood calcium, but when additional parathyroid hormone raises the level of blood calcium, the hormone's production is then inhibited (see Figure 5–2). People interact with the environment by adjusting themselves to it or adjusting it to themselves. This premise directs the nurse to look at environmental factors influencing the system and to plan nursing interventions to help the client maintain homeostasis.

Psychologic Homeostasis   The term psychologic homeostasis refers to emotional or psychologic balance or a state of mental well-being. It is maintained by a variety of mechanisms. Each person has certain psychologic needs that must be met to maintain psychologic homeostasis. When one or more of these needs is not met or is threatened, certain coping mechanisms are activated to protect the person and provide psychologic homeostasis.

Psychologic homeostasis is acquired or learned through the experience of living and interacting with others. In addition, societal norms and culture influence behavior. Some

prerequisites for a person to develop psychologic homeostasis can be summarized as follows:

- A stable physical environment in which the person feels safe and secure.
- A stable psychologic environment from infancy onward, so that feelings of trust and love develop. Growing children and adolescents also need kind but firm and consistent discipline, encouragement, and support to be their own unique selves.
- A social environment that includes adults who are healthy role models. Children learn the customs and values of society from these individuals.
- A life experience that provides satisfactions. Throughout life, people encounter many frustrations. People deal with these better if enough satisfying experiences have occurred to counterbalance the frustrating ones.

Assessing the Health of Individuals

A thorough assessment of the individual's health status is basic to health promotion. Components of this assessment are the health history and physical examination, physical fitness assessment, lifestyle assessment, health risk appraisal, health beliefs review, and life-stress review. Details about these assessments are discussed in Chapters 7 and 17 ∞ .

MODELS OF HEALTH AND WELLNESS

Because health is such a complex concept, various researchers have developed models or paradigms to explain health and, in some instances, its relationship to illness or injury. Models can be helpful in assisting health professionals to meet the health and wellness needs of individuals. Nurses need to clarify their understanding of health, wellness, and illness for the following reasons:

- Nurses' definitions of health largely determine the scope and nature of nursing practice.
- People's health beliefs influence their health practices.

Models of health include the clinical model, the role performance model, the adaptive model, the eudemonistic model, the agent-host-environment model, and health–illness continua.

Clinical Model

The narrowest interpretation of health occurs in the clinical model. People are viewed as physiologic systems with related functions, and health is identified by the absence of signs and symptoms of disease or injury. It is considered the state of not being "sick." In this model the opposite of health is disease or injury.

Role Performance Model

Health is defined in terms of the individual's ability to fulfill societal roles, that is, to perform his or her work. People usually fulfill several roles, and certain individuals may consider non-work roles paramount in their lives. According to this model, people who can fulfill their roles are healthy even if they have clinical illness.

Adaptive Model

In the adaptive model, health is a creative process; disease is a failure in adaptation, or maladaptation. The aim of treatment is to restore the ability of the person to adapt, that is, to cope. According to this model, extreme good health is flexible adaptation to the environment and interaction with the environment to maximum advantage. Sister Callista Roy's adaptation model of nursing (Roy, 1999) views the person as an adaptive system. The focus of this model is stability, although there is also an element of growth and change.

Eudemonistic Model

The eudemonistic model incorporates a comprehensive view of health. Health is seen as a condition of actualization or realization of a person's potential. Actualization is the apex of the fully developed personality, described by Abraham Maslow. In this model the highest aspiration of people is fulfillment and complete development, which is actualization. Illness, in this model, is a condition that prevents self-actualization. Pender defines health as "the actualization of inherent and acquired human potential through goal-directed behavior, competent self-care, and satisfying relationships with others while adjustments are made as needed to maintain structural integrity and harmony with relevant environments" (Pender, Murdaugh, & Parsons, 2006, p. 23).

Agent-Host-Environment Model

The model is used primarily in predicting illness rather than in promoting wellness, although identification of risk factors that result from the interactions of agent, host, and environment are helpful in promoting and maintaining health. The model has three dynamic interactive elements including the agent (any environmental factor or stressor that can lead to illness or disease), host (person at risk of acquiring a disease), and environment (all factors external to the host that may or may not predispose the person to the development of disease). Because each of the agent-host-environment factors constantly interacts with the others, health is an ever-changing state. When the variables are in balance, health is maintained; when variables are not in balance, disease occurs.

Health–Illness Continua

Health–illness continua can be used to measure a person's perceived level of wellness. Health and illness or disease can be viewed as the opposite ends of a health continuum. From a high level of health a person's condition can move through good health, normal health, poor health, and extremely poor health, eventually to death. People move back and forth within this continuum day by day. There is no distinct boundary across which people move from health to illness or from illness back to health. How people perceive themselves and how others see them in terms of health and illness will also affect their placement on the continuum. The ranges in which people can be thought of as healthy or ill are considerable.

DUNN'S HIGH-LEVEL WELLNESS GRID Dunn (1959) described a health grid in which a health axis and an environmental axis intersect. The grid demonstrates the interaction of the environment with the illness–wellness continuum. The health axis extends from peak wellness to death, and the environmental axis extends from very favorable to very unfavorable. Family wellness enhances wellness in individuals. In a well family that offers trust, love, and support, the individual does not have to expend energy to meet basic needs and can move forward on the wellness continuum.

TRAVIS'S ILLNESS–WELLNESS CONTINUUM The illness–wellness continuum (Figure 5–3) developed by Travis ranges from high-level wellness to premature death (Travis & Ryan, 2001). The model illustrates two arrows pointing in opposite directions and joined at a neutral point. Movement to the right of the neutral point indicates

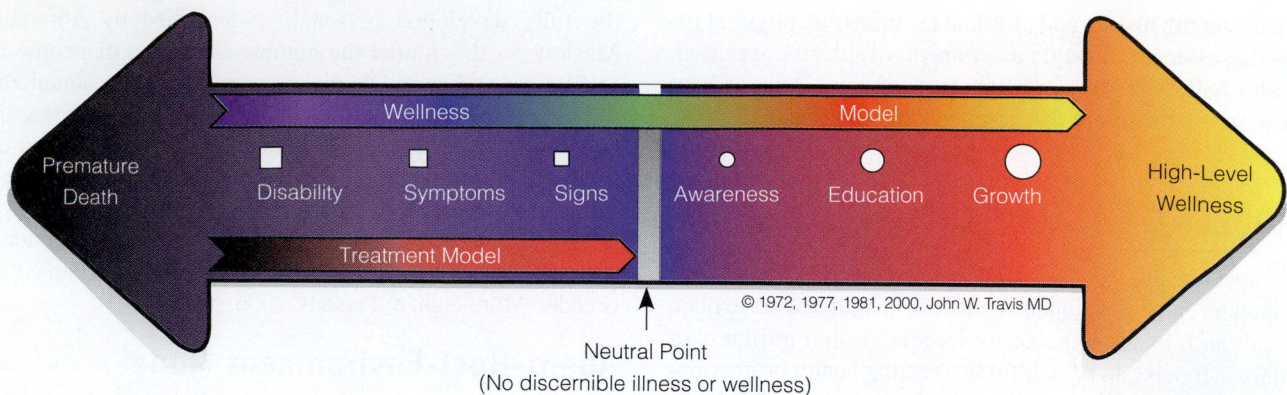

Figure 5–3 ● Illness-wellness continuum.
(Reprinted with permission, *Wellness Workbook*, Travis & Ryan, Ten Speed Press, Berkeley, CA. © 1981, 1988 by John W. Travis, MD. www.thewellspring.com.)

increasing levels of health and well-being for an individual. This is achieved in three steps: (a) awareness, (b) education, and (c) growth. In contrast, movement to the left of the neutral point indicates progressively decreasing levels of health. Travis and Ryan believe it is possible to be physically ill and at the same time oriented toward wellness, or be physically healthy and at the same time function from an illness mentality. The model also compares the traditional treatment model with the wellness model.

The 4+ Model of Wellness

A newer model, the 4+ model of wellness (Baldwin & Conger, 2001), consists of the four domains of the inner self—physical, spiritual, emotional, and intellectual—plus the elements of the outer systems (environment, culture, nutrition, safety, and many other elements). The nurse assesses the inner self for strengths and excesses, sources of nurturing and of depletion, and the interactions between the inner self and the outer systems. This model is useful when working with individuals, families, or communities.

Needs Theories

In needs theories, human needs are ranked on an ascending scale according to how essential the needs are for survival.

MASLOW'S HIERARCHY OF NEEDS   Abraham Maslow (1970), perhaps the most renowned needs theorist, ranks human needs on five levels (see Figure 5–4 and Box 5–2). The five levels in ascending order are as follows:

- *Physiologic needs.* Needs such as air, food, water, shelter, rest, sleep, activity, and temperature maintenance are crucial for survival.
- *Safety and security needs.* The need for safety has both physical and psychologic aspects. The person needs to feel safe, both in the physical environment and in relationships.
- *Love and belonging needs.* The third level of needs includes giving and receiving affection, attaining a place in a group, and maintaining the feeling of belonging.
- *Self-esteem needs.* The individual needs both self-esteem and esteem from others.

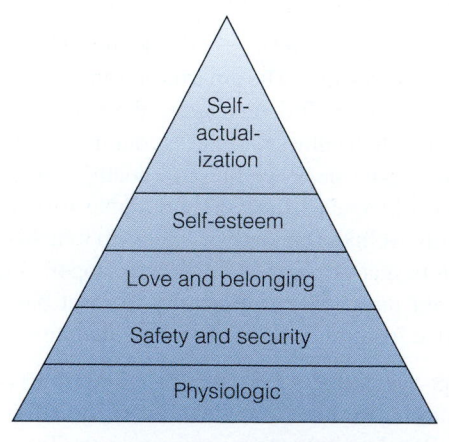

Maslow's hierarchy of needs

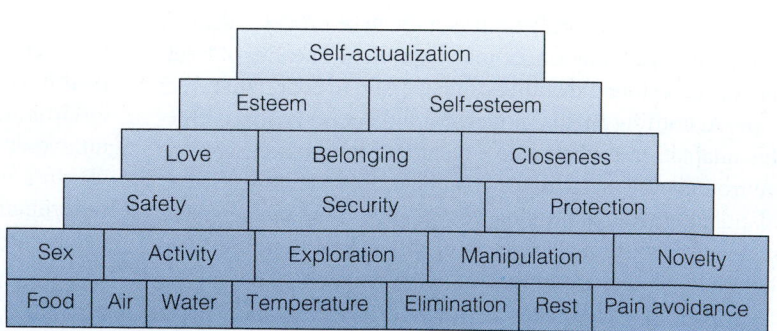

Maslow's hierarchy of needs, as adapted by Kalish

Figure 5–4 ● Maslow's needs.
From Abraham Maslow, *Motivation and Personality,* © 1954. Material was reprinted by permission of Pearson Education, Inc., Upper Saddle River, NJ.

| BOX 5–2 | Maslow's Characteristics of a Self-Actualized Person |

- Is realistic, sees life clearly, and is objective about his or her observations
- Judges people correctly
- Has superior perception, is more decisive
- Has clear notion of right and wrong
- Is usually accurate in predicting future events
- Understands art, music, politics, and philosophy
- Possesses humility, listens to others carefully
- Is dedicated to some work, task, duty, or vocation
- Is highly creative, flexible, spontaneous, courageous, and willing to make mistakes
- Is open to new ideas
- Is self-confident and has self-respect

- Has low degree of self-conflict; personality is integrated
- Respects self, does not need fame, possesses a feeling of self-control
- Is highly independent, desires privacy
- Can appear remote and detached
- Is friendly, loving, and governed more by inner directives than by society
- Can make decisions contrary to popular opinion
- Is problem centered rather than self-centered
- Accepts the world for what it is

Note: From *Toward a Psychology of Being,* 2nd ed., by A. H. Maslow, copyright 1968, New York: Van Nostrand Reinhold. Reprinted with permission of John Wiley & Sons, Inc.

- *Self-actualization.* When the need for self-esteem is satisfied, the individual strives for self-actualization, the innate need to develop one's maximum potential and realize one's abilities and qualities.

KALISH'S HIERARCHY OF NEEDS Richard Kalish (1983) adapted Maslow's hierarchy of needs into six levels rather than five. He suggests an additional category between the physiologic needs and the safety and security needs. This category, referred to as *stimulation needs,* includes sex, activity, exploration, manipulation, and novelty (see Figure 5–4). Kalish emphasizes that children need to explore and manipulate their environments to achieve optimal growth and development. He notes that adults, too, often seek novel adventures or stimulating experiences before considering their safety or security needs.

CHARACTERISTICS OF BASIC NEEDS All people have the same basic needs; however, each person's needs and reactions to those needs are influenced by the culture with which the person identifies.

- People meet their own needs relative to their own priorities.
- Although basic needs generally must be met, some needs can be deferred.
- Failure to meet needs results in one or more homeostatic imbalances, which can eventually result in illness.
- A need can make itself felt by either external or internal stimuli.
- A person who perceives a need can respond in several ways to meet it. The choice of response is largely a result of learned experiences, lifestyle, and the values of the culture.
- Needs are interrelated. Some needs cannot be met unless related needs are also met.

Needs can be satisfied in healthy and unhealthy ways. Ways of meeting basic needs are considered healthy when they are not harmful to others or to self, conform to the individual's sociocultural values, and are within the law. Conversely, unhealthy behavior may be harmful to others or to self, does not conform to the individual's sociocultural values, or is not within the law. People who satisfy their basic needs appropriately are healthier, happier, and more effective than those whose needs are frustrated.

Knowledge of the theoretical bases of human needs assists nurses in responding therapeutically to a client's behaviors and in understanding themselves and their own responses to needs. Human needs serve as a framework for assessing behaviors, assigning priorities to desired outcomes, and planning nursing interventions.

Developmental Stage Theories

Developmental stage theories categorize a person's behaviors or tasks into approximate age ranges or in terms that describe the features of an age group. The age ranges of the stages do not take into account individual differences; however, the categories do describe characteristics associated with the majority of individuals at periods when distinctive developmental changes occur and with the specific tasks that must be accomplished. See Chapter 9 ∞ for further information about developmental stages.

Developmental stage theories allow nurses to describe typical behaviors of an individual within a certain age group, explain the significance of those behaviors, predict behaviors that might occur in a given situation, and provide a rationale to control behavioral manifestations. Individuals can be compared with a representative group of people at the same point in time or compared at different points in time. The nurse's knowledge of developmental stage theories can be used in parental and client education, counseling, and anticipatory guidance.

HEALTH BELIEF MODELS

Several theories or models of health beliefs and behaviors have been developed to help determine whether an individual is likely to participate in disease prevention and health promotion activities. These models can be useful tools in developing programs for helping people change to healthier lifestyles and develop a more positive attitude toward preventive health measures.

Health Locus of Control Model

Locus of control (LOC) is a concept from social learning theory that nurses can use to determine whether clients are likely to take action regarding health, that is, whether clients believe that their health status is under their own or others' control. People who believe that they have a major influence on their own health status—that health is largely self-determined—are called *internals*. People who exercise internal control are more likely than others to take the initiative on their own health care, be more knowledgeable about their health, and adhere to prescribed health care regimens. By contrast, people who believe their health is largely controlled by outside forces are referred to as *externals*. Research has shown that locus of control plays a role in clients' choices about health behaviors.

Rosenstock's and Becker's Health Belief Models

In the 1950s Rosenstock (1974) proposed a health belief model intended to predict which individuals would or would not use preventive measures such as screening for early detection of cancer. Becker (1974) modified the health belief model to include these components: individual perceptions, modifying factors, and variables likely to affect initiating action. The health belief model is based on motivational theory. Rosenstock (1974) assumed that good health is an objective common to all people. Becker added "positive health motivation" as a consideration.

Individual perceptions include the following:

- *Perceived susceptibility*
- *Perceived seriousness*
- *Perceived threat*

Factors that modify a person's perceptions include the following:

- *Demographic variables.* Demographic variables include age, gender, race, and ethnicity.
- *Sociopsychological variables.* Social pressure or influence from peers or other reference groups may encourage preventive health behaviors even when individual motivation is low.
- *Structural variables.* Knowledge about the target disease and prior contact with it are structural variables that are presumed to influence preventive behavior.
- *Cues to action.* Cues can be either internal or external. Internal cues include feelings of fatigue, uncomfortable symptoms, or thoughts about the condition of an ill person who is close. External cues include mass media campaigns, advice from others, newspaper articles, or Internet pages.

The likelihood of a person's taking recommended preventive health action depends on the perceived benefits of the action minus the perceived barriers to the action.

Nurses play a major role in helping clients implement healthy behaviors. They help clients monitor health, they supply anticipatory guidance, and they impart knowledge about health. Nurses can reduce barriers to action and support positive actions.

In addition to applying these models, the nurse uses other resources to evaluate options in planning interventions to maximize wellness. Two very useful documents developed by federal agencies are the *Guide to Community Preventive Services* from the Centers for Disease Control and Prevention and the third edition of the *Guide to Clinical Preventive Services* from the U.S. Public Health Service. A major emphasis in both sets of documents is providing evidence-based recommendations for practices and policies aimed at improving health. Both documents are updated as the data become available and can be retrieved from their respective websites.

RESEARCH NOTES | How Can Nurses Help Prevent Childhood Obesity?

The prevalence rate of obesity among children in the United States has been rising in recent years. Crawford and colleagues' (2004) pilot study aimed to improve the self-efficacy of staff counseling clients enrolled in the Women, Infants, and Children (WIC) program about childhood obesity. The study compared a sample of 51 WIC employees split into an intervention group that received educational sessions to help them identify ways to make changes in eating habits, activity information, and pedometers to promote the 10,000-steps-per-day program, and a control group. The intervention group was more likely to make healthy food choices when supported by the environment, to make positive changes in counseling parents about their children's weight issues, and to feel more confident in encouraging the WIC clients to be physically active with their own children.

Implications

Evidence suggests that overweight children have at least one associated biochemical or cardiovascular risk factor. The need for effective programs to help control America's growing waistline among our youngest citizens is becoming imperative. Chronic health issues such as obesity require the establishment of long-term supportive relationships between the nurse and the client. Nurses can contribute and encourage lifestyle alterations to improve client health by modeling behaviors, providing educational materials, and counseling.

Note: From "Walking the Talk: Fit WIC Wellness Programs Improve Self-Efficacy in Pediatric Obesity Prevention Counseling," by P. B. Crawford, W. Gosliner, P. Strode, S. E. Samuels, L. Craypo, C. Burnett, et al., 2004, *American Journal of Public Health, 94,* pp. 1480–1485.

VARIABLES INFLUENCING HEALTH STATUS, BELIEFS, AND PRACTICES

Many variables influence a person's health status, beliefs, and behaviors or practices. These factors may or may not be under conscious control. People can usually control their health behaviors and can choose healthy or unhealthy activities. In contrast, people have little or no choice over their genetic makeup, age, sex, culture, and sometimes their geographic environments. Box 5–3 differentiates health status, beliefs, and behaviors or practices.

Health behavior is intended to prevent illness or disease or to provide for early detection of disease. Nurses preparing a plan of care with an individual need to consider the person's health beliefs before they suggest a change in health behaviors.

Internal Variables

Internal variables include biologic, psychologic, and cognitive dimensions. They are often described as nonmodifiable variables because, for the most part, they cannot be changed. However, when internal variables are linked to health problems, the nurse must be even more diligent about working with the client to influence external variables that may assist in health promotion and prevention of illness. Regular health exams and appropriate screening for early detection of health problems become even more important.

BIOLOGIC DIMENSION Genetic makeup, gender, age, and developmental level all significantly influence a person's health.

Genetic makeup influences biologic characteristics, innate temperament, activity level, and intellectual potential. It has been related to susceptibility to specific disease. In some cases, genetic predisposition for health or illness is enhanced when parents are from the same ethnic genetic pool.

Gender influences the distribution of disease. Certain acquired and genetic diseases are more common in one sex than in the other.

Age is also a significant factor. The distribution of disease varies with age.

Developmental level has a major impact on health status.

> **BOX 5–3 Health Status, Beliefs, and Behaviors**
>
> - *Health status.* State of health of an individual at a given time. A report of health status may include anxiety, depression, or acute illness and thus describe the individual's problem in general. Health status can also describe such specifics as pulse rate and body temperature.
> - *Health beliefs.* Concepts about health that an individual believes are true. Such beliefs may or may not be founded on fact. Some of these are influenced by culture.
> - *Health behaviors.* The actions people take to understand their health state, maintain an optimal state of health, prevent illness and injury, and reach their maximum physical and mental potential.

PSYCHOLOGIC DIMENSION Psychologic (emotional) factors influencing health include mind–body interactions and self-concept.

Mind–body interactions can affect health status positively or negatively. Emotional responses to stress affect body function. Prolonged emotional distress may increase susceptibility to organic disease or precipitate it. Emotional distress may influence the immune system through central nervous system and endocrine alterations. Alterations in the immune system are related to the incidence of infections, cancer, and autoimmune diseases. Increasing attention is being given to the mind's ability to direct the body's functioning. Relaxation, meditation, and biofeedback techniques are gaining wider recognition by individuals and health care professionals. Emotional reactions also occur in response to body conditions.

Self-concept is how a person feels about self (self-esteem) and perceives the physical self (body image), needs, roles, and abilities. Self-concept affects how people view and handle situations. Such attitudes can affect health practices, responses to stress and illness, and the times when treatment is sought.

COGNITIVE DIMENSION Cognitive, or intellectual, factors influencing health include lifestyle choices and spiritual and religious beliefs.

Lifestyle refers to a person's general way of living, including living conditions and individual patterns of behavior that are influenced by sociocultural factors and personal characteristics. In brief, lifestyle is often considered as behavior and activities over which people have control. Lifestyle choices may have positive or negative effects on health. Practices that have potentially negative effects on health are often referred to as **risk factors.**

Spiritual and religious beliefs can significantly affect health behavior. Religious beliefs may impact decisions regarding blood transfusions, diet, or health practices such as circumcision. The influence of spirituality and religion is discussed further in Chapter 28 ∞.

External Variables

External variables affecting health include the physical environment, standards of living, family and cultural beliefs, and social support networks.

ENVIRONMENT People are becoming increasingly aware of their environment and how it affects their health and level of wellness. Geographic location determines climate, and climate affects health. Pollution of the water, air, and soil affects the health of cells. Other substances in the environment, such as asbestos or smoke, are considered carcinogenic. Another environmental hazard is radiation. The improper use of x-rays or exposure to the sun can cause harm.

The main component of acid rain is sulfur dioxide, produced by ore smelters and related industries. The other components are nitrogen oxides. These emissions are thought by scientists to damage forests, lakes, and rivers.

Another environmental hazard is an increase in the "greenhouse effect." Carbon dioxide in the earth's atmosphere acts like the glass roof of a greenhouse holding in heat, and as carbon dioxide levels increase due to industrial and automobile emissions, the surface temperature of the earth may also be increasing.

Other sources of environmental contamination are pesticides and chemicals used to control weeds and plant diseases. These contaminants can be found in some animals and plants that are subsequently ingested by people. In excessive levels, they are harmful to health.

STANDARDS OF LIVING   An individual's standard of living is related to health, morbidity, and mortality. Hygiene, food habits, and the propensity to seek health care advice and follow health regimens vary among high-income and low-income groups.

Low-income families often define health in terms of work; if people can work they are healthy. They tend to be fatalistic and believe that illness is not preventable. Because their present problems are so great and all efforts are exerted toward survival, an orientation to the future may be lacking.

The environmental conditions of poverty-stricken areas also have a bearing on overall health. Slum neighborhoods are overcrowded and in a state of deterioration. Sanitation services tend to be inadequate. Many streets are strewn with garbage, and rodents are common. Fires and crime are constant threats. Recreational facilities are almost nonexistent, forcing children to play in streets and alleys.

Occupational roles also predispose people to certain illnesses. For instance, some industrial workers may be exposed to carcinogenic agents. More-affluent people may fulfill stressful social or occupational roles that predispose them to stress-related diseases. Such roles may also encourage overeating or social use of drugs or alcohol.

FAMILY AND CULTURAL BELIEFS   The family passes on patterns of daily living and lifestyles. Emotional health depends on a social environment that is free of excessive tension and does not isolate the person from others. A climate of open communication, sharing, and love fosters the fulfillment of the person's optimum potential.

Culture and social interactions also influence how a person perceives, experiences, and copes with health and illness. Each culture has ideas about health, and these are often transmitted from parents to children. People of certain cultures may perceive home remedies or tribal health customs as superior to, and more dependable than, the health care practices of North American society. Cultural rules, values, and beliefs give people a sense of being stable and able to predict outcomes. The challenging of old beliefs and values by second-generation cultural groups may give rise to conflict, instability, and insecurity, in turn contributing to illness.

SOCIAL SUPPORT NETWORKS   Having a support network and job satisfaction helps people avoid illness. Support people also help the person confirm that illness exists. People with inadequate support networks sometimes allow themselves to become increasingly ill before confirming the illness and seeking therapy. Support people also provide the stimulus for an ill person to become well again.

HEALTH CARE ADHERENCE

Adherence is the extent to which an individual's behavior coincides with medical or health advice. Degree of adherence may range from disregarding every aspect of the recommendations to following the total therapeutic plan. There are many reasons why some people adhere and others do not (see Box 5–4).

To enhance adherence, nurses need to ensure that the client is able to perform the prescribed therapy, understands the necessary instructions, is a willing participant in establishing goals of therapy, and values the planned outcomes of behavior changes. Examples of questions to be included in assessment are found in the Assessment Interview box.

When a nurse identifies nonadherence, it is important to take the following steps:

- *Establish why the client is not following the regimen.* Depending on the reason, the nurse can provide information, correct misconceptions, attempt to decrease expense, act as an advocate to alter the plan of care, or suggest counseling if psychologic problems are interfering with adherence.
- *Demonstrate caring.* Show sincere concern about the client's problems and decisions and at the same time accept the client's right to a course of action.
- *Encourage healthy behaviors through positive reinforcement.*
- *Use aids to reinforce teaching.*
- *Establish a therapeutic relationship of freedom, mutual understanding, and mutual responsibility with the client and support persons.* By providing knowledge, skills, and information, the nurse gives clients control over their health and establishes a cooperative relationship, which results in greater adherence.

BOX 5–4   Factors Influencing Adherence

- Client motivation to become well
- Degree of lifestyle change necessary
- Perceived severity of the health care problem
- Value placed on reducing the threat of illness
- Difficulty in understanding and performing specific behaviors
- Degree of inconvenience of the illness itself or of the regimens
- Beliefs that the prescribed therapy or regimen will or will not help
- Complexity, side effects, and duration of the proposed therapy
- Specific cultural heritage that may make adherence difficult
- Degree of satisfaction and quality and type of relationship with the health care providers
- Overall cost of prescribed therapy

ASSESSMENT INTERVIEW — Determining the Risk for Medication Nonadherence

- Are you having side effects from any of your medications?
- Do you think your medications are helping?
- Do you have "tools" to remind you to take your medication? Examples could be an alarm or environmental cues (e.g., 6:00 news).
- Is there someone at home who helps you with your medications?
- How many times per day are your medications prescribed?

- How many pills do you take every day?
- Are there any special storage requirements for your medications?
- How much do your medication requirements interfere with your lifestyle?
- How well are you able to follow special dosing requirements?
- How many doses of your medications have you missed over the last 3 days?

CLINICAL ALERT

Chronic illness often requires complicated treatment regimens for lengthy periods that may include significant adverse reactions and be very costly. Thus, clients with chronic illnesses may be at increased risk for treatment nonadherence.

Aspects influencing clients of varying ages are found in the Lifespan Considerations box.

ILLNESS AND DISEASE

Disease can be described as an alteration in body functions resulting in a reduction of capacities or a shortening of the normal life span. Traditionally intervention by primary care providers has the goal of eliminating or slowing disease processes. Multiple factors are considered to interact in causing disease and determining an individual's response to treatment. The causation of a disease is called its **etiology.**

LIFESPAN CONSIDERATIONS — Medication Nonadherence

Children

Microbial resistance to antibiotics has increased significantly in recent years, making it critical that antibiotics given to children are necessary, administered correctly by parents in the home, and taken as prescribed. Providers, parents, and children must work together in order to increase the adherence rate in taking antibiotics. Adherence is influenced by

- Attitudes toward medications; some parents may think that when their child is feeling better, the medication is no longer necessary.
- Past experience; children may remember a bad experience with taking a medication and resist parents' efforts to give an antibiotic.
- Cost of medication; generic drugs are less costly than brand-name drugs, and can be equally effective.
- Cultural issues; providers must work with families who have language or cultural differences to make sure they understand the family's needs and communicate the provider's recommendations.
- Number of doses necessary; adherence improves if there are fewer doses per day, and fewer days that the antibiotic will be taken.
- Taste and palatability; pharmaceutical companies continue to develop liquid medication that will be more acceptable to young children.

Adolescents

Several causes of nonadherence are specific to teenagers. It is important for the nurse to consider these when working with adolescents, because they

- Don't consider the consequences of their actions, living in the "here and now."
- Are in the early stages of problem solving and may regress during stressful periods.
- Assert independence by rejecting adult values.
- Conform to their peers and don't like being "different," focusing on self-concept and body image.
- May be unable to distinguish benefits from disadvantages.

Older Adults

Issues that influence adherence in older adults include the following:

- Lifestyle choices and individual responsibility for health maintenance
- Availability of home and community-based services to maximize independence
- Alternative/complementary therapies
- Housing and home modifications to accommodate the physical aspects of aging
- Affordable and accessible transportation
- Preventive nursing and medical care
- The caregiving crisis that overburdens some family and informal caregivers
- Forgetfulness or dementia
- Feeling that they have lived their life and it is time for life to end

A description of the etiology of a disease includes the identification of all causal factors that act together to bring about the particular disease. Nurses have traditionally taken a holistic view of people and base their practice on the multiple-causation theory of health problems.

There are many ways to classify illness and disease; one of the most common is as acute or chronic. **Acute** illness is typically characterized by severe symptoms of relatively short duration. The symptoms often appear abruptly and subside quickly and, depending on the cause, may or may not require intervention by health care professionals. Some acute illnesses are serious, but many subside without medical intervention or with the help of over-the-counter medications. Following an acute illness, most people return to their normal level of wellness. A **chronic** illness is one that lasts for an extended period, usually six months or longer, and often for the person's life. Chronic illnesses usually have a slow onset and often have periods of **remission,** when the symptoms disappear, and exacerbation, when the symptoms reappear.

Nurses are involved in caring for chronically ill individuals of all ages in all types of settings—homes, nursing homes, hospitals, clinics, and other institutions. Care needs to be focused on promoting the highest level possible of independence, sense of control, and wellness. Clients often need to modify their activities of daily living, social relationships, and perception of self and body image. In addition, many must learn how to live with increasing physical limitations and discomfort.

Illness Behaviors

When people become ill, they behave in certain ways that sociologists refer to as illness behavior. Illness behavior, a coping mechanism, involves ways individuals describe, monitor, and interpret their symptoms, take remedial actions, and use the health care system. How people behave when they are ill is highly individualized and affected by many variables, such as age, sex, occupation, socioeconomic status, religion, ethnic origin, psychologic stability, personality, education, and modes of coping.

Parsons (1979) described four aspects of the sick role:

1. Clients are not held responsible for their condition.
2. Clients are excused from certain social roles and tasks.
3. Clients are obliged to try to get well as quickly as possible.
4. Clients or their families are obliged to seek competent help.

Suchman (1979) described five stages of illness: symptoms, sick role, medical care contact, dependent client role, and recovery or rehabilitation. Not all clients progress through each stage. Other clients may progress through only the first two stages and then recover. Details of Suchman's five stages follow.

STAGE 1 SYMPTOM EXPERIENCES   At this stage the person comes to believe something is wrong. Stage 1 has three aspects: the physical experience of symptoms, the cognitive aspect of interpreting symptoms, and the emotional response. During this stage, the unwell person usually consults others about the symptoms or feelings.

STAGE 2 ASSUMPTION OF THE SICK ROLE   The individual now accepts the sick role and seeks confirmation from family and friends. Often people continue with self-treatment and delay contact with health care professionals as long as possible. During this stage people may be excused from normal duties and role expectations. Emotional responses such as withdrawal, anxiety, fear, and depression are not uncommon depending on the severity of the illness, perceived degree of disability, and anticipated duration of the illness. When symptoms of illness persist or increase, the person is motivated to seek professional help.

STAGE 3 MEDICAL CARE CONTACT   Sick people seek the advice of a health professional either on their own initiative or at the urging of significant others. When people seek professional advice they are really asking for three types of information: validation of real illness, explanation of symptoms in understandable form, and/or reassurance that they will recover or prediction of outcome. The client may accept or deny the diagnosis. If the diagnosis is accepted, the client usually follows the prescribed treatment plan. If the diagnosis is not accepted, the client may seek the advice of other health care professionals or quasi-practitioners who will provide a diagnosis that fits the client's perceptions.

STAGE 4 DEPENDENT CLIENT ROLE   After accepting the illness and seeking treatment, the client becomes dependent on the professional for help. People vary greatly in the degree of ease with which they can give up their independence, particularly in relation to life and death. Role obligations can complicate the decision to give up independence. Most people accept their dependence on the primary care provider, although they retain varying degrees of control over their own lives. For some clients illness may meet dependence needs that have never been met and thus provide satisfaction. Other people have minimal dependence needs and do everything possible to return to independent functioning. A few may even try to maintain independence to the detriment of their recovery.

STAGE 5 RECOVERY OR REHABILITATION   During this stage the client is expected to relinquish the dependent role and resume former roles and responsibilities. For people with acute illness, the time as an ill person is generally short and recovery is usually rapid, making it relatively easy to return to their former lifestyles. People who have long-term illnesses and must adjust their lifestyles may find recovery more difficult. For clients with a permanent disability, this final stage may require therapy to learn how to make major adjustments in functioning.

Effects of Illness

Illness brings about changes in both the involved individual and in the family. The changes vary depending on the nature, severity, and duration of the illness, attitudes associated with the illness by the client and others, the financial demands, the lifestyle changes incurred, adjustments to usual roles, and so on.

IMPACT ON THE CLIENT   Ill clients may experience behavioral and emotional changes, changes in self-concept and body image, and lifestyle changes. Behavioral and emotional changes associated with short-term illness are generally mild and short lived ranging from irritability to lack of energy or desire to interact. More acute responses are likely with severe, life-threatening, chronic, or disabling illness. Anxiety, fear, anger, withdrawal, denial, a sense of hopelessness, and feelings of powerlessness are all common responses to severe or disabling illness. Certain illnesses can also change the client's body image or physical appearance, especially if there is severe scarring or loss of a limb or special sense organ. The client's self-esteem and self-concept may also be affected. Many factors can play a part in low self-esteem and a disturbance in self-concept: loss of body parts and function, pain, disfigurement, dependence on others, unemployment, financial problems, inability to participate in social functions, strained relationships with others, and spiritual distress. Nurses need to help clients express their thoughts and feelings, and to provide care that helps the client effectively cope with change.

Ill individuals are also vulnerable to loss of autonomy, the state of being independent and self-directed without outside control. Family interactions may change so that clients may no longer be involved in making family decisions or even decisions about their own health care. Nurses need to support clients' right to self-determination and autonomy as much as possible by providing them with sufficient information to participate in decision-making processes and to maintain a feeling of being in control.

Illness also often necessitates a change in lifestyle. In addition to participating in treatments and taking medications, the ill person may need to change diet, activity and exercise, and rest and sleep patterns. Nurses can help clients adjust their lifestyles by providing explanations about necessary adjustments, making arrangements to accommodate lifestyle when possible, encouraging other health providers to become familiar with the client's lifestyle and support the healthy aspects, and reinforce desirable changes.

IMPACT ON THE FAMILY   A person's illness affects not only the person who is ill but also the family or significant others. The kind of effect and its extent depend chiefly on three factors: (a) the member of the family who is ill, (b) the seriousness and length of the illness, and (c) the cultural and social customs the family follows. The changes that can occur in the family include role changes, task reassignments, increased demands on time, increased stress secondary to anxiety, financial problems, loneliness resulting from separation or loss, and change in social customs.

See Chapter 11 ∞ for further information about the effects of illness on the family.

HEALTH PROMOTION

Health promotion is an important component of nursing practice. It is a way of thinking that revolves around a philosophy of wholeness, wellness, and well-being. In the past two decades, the public has become increasingly aware of and interested in health promotion. Many people are aware of the relationship between lifestyle and illness and are developing health-promoting habits, such as getting adequate exercise, rest, and relaxation; maintaining good nutrition; and controlling the use of tobacco, alcohol, and other drugs.

Defining Health Promotion

Considerable differences appear in the literature regarding the use of the terms *health promotion, primary prevention, health protection*, and *illness prevention*. Edelman and Mandle (2006) state that "prevention, in a narrow sense, means avoiding the development of disease in the future, and, in the broader sense, consists of all interventions to limit progression of a disease" (p. 13). The levels of prevention occur at various points of a course of disease progression.

Pender, Murdaugh, and Parsons (2006) consider health promotion to be different from disease prevention or health protection. They define **health promotion** as "behavior motivated by the desire to increase well-being and actualize human health potential," and **disease prevention** or **health protection** as "behavior motivated by a desire to actively avoid illness, detect it early, or maintain functioning within the constraints of illness" (p. 7). The individual's underlying motivation for the behavior is the major difference. Box 5–5 provides an overview of the differences between health promotion and health protection.

BOX 5–5	Differences between Health Promotion and Health Protection

Health Promotion	*Health Protection*
Not disease oriented	Illness or injury specific
Motivated by personal, positive "approach" to wellness	Motivated by "avoidance" of illness
Seeks to expand positive potential for health	Seeks to thwart the occurrence of insults to health and well-being

Note: From *Health Promotion in Nursing Practice*, 5th ed. (p. 8), by N. J. Pender, C. L. Murdaugh, and M. A. Parsons, 2006, Upper Saddle River, NJ: Pearson Education. Reprinted with permission.

The difficulty in separating the terms *health promotion* and *disease prevention/health protection* lies in the fact that an activity may be carried out for numerous reasons. For example, a 40-year-old male may begin a program of walking three miles each day. If the goal of his program were to "decrease the risk of cardiovascular disease," then the activity would be considered disease prevention or health protection. By contrast, if the motivation for his walking regimen were to "increase his overall health and feeling of well-being," then the activity would be considered a health promotion behavior. It is most helpful to think of health promotion and health protection as being complementary processes because both affect quality of health (Table 5–1).

Health promotion can be offered to all clients regardless of their health and illness status or age. For example, weight-control measures can benefit both overweight clients without disease and clients with cardiac or joint disease. Age-specific health promotion activities are discussed in Chapters 9 and 10 ∞. See Lifespan Considerations for examples of health promotion topics.

Healthy People 2010

The vision of health promotion was initially expressed in 1979 with the surgeon general's report *Healthy People*, which emphasized health promotion and disease prevention. *Healthy People 2000* followed in 1990 and provided a framework for national health promotion, health protection, and preventive service strategy. The current *Healthy People 2010: Understanding and Improving Health* (U.S. Department of Health and Human Services [USDHHS], 2000) presents a comprehensive 10-year strategy for promoting health and preventing illness, disability, and premature death. The two major goals of *Healthy People 2010* reflect the nation's changing demographics:

- "Increase quality and years of healthy life" indicates the aging or "graying" of the population.
- "Eliminate health disparities" reflects the diversity of the population.

To support these goals, *Healthy People 2010* is organized into 28 focus areas to improve health (Box 5–6). *Healthy People 2010* also establishes a set of leading health indicators that reflect the major public health concerns in the United States at the beginning of the 21st century (Box 5–7). Each indicator relates to a number of the health objectives. It is expected that these indicators will help develop action plans to improve the health of both individuals and communities.

TABLE 5–1 **Levels of Prevention**	
LEVEL AND DESCRIPTION	EXAMPLES
Primary prevention Generalized health promotion and specific protection against disease. It precedes disease or dysfunction and is applied to generally healthy individuals or groups.	• Health education about injury and poisoning prevention, standards of nutrition and of growth and development for each stage of life, exercise requirements, stress management, protection against occupational hazards, and so on • Immunizations • Risk assessments for specific disease • Family planning services • Environmental sanitation and provision of adequate housing, recreation, and work conditions
Secondary prevention Emphasizes early detection of disease, prompt intervention, and health maintenance for individuals experiencing health problems. Includes prevention of complications and disabilities.	• Screening surveys and procedures of any type (e.g., Denver Developmental Screening Test, hypertension screening) • Encouraging regular medical and dental checkups • Teaching self-examination for breast and testicular cancer • Assessing the growth and development of children • Nursing assessments and care provided in home, hospital, or other agency to prevent complications (e.g., maintaining skin integrity; turning, positioning, and exercising clients; ensuring adequate rest, food, and fluid intake; promoting fecal and urinary elimination; administering medical therapies such as medications; and so on)
Tertiary prevention Begins after an illness, when a defect or disability is fixed, stabilized, or determined to be irreversible. Its focus is to help rehabilitate individuals and restore them to an optimum level of functioning within the constraints of the disability.	• Referring a client who has had a colostomy to a support group • Teaching a client who has diabetes to identify and prevent complications • Referring a client with a spinal cord injury to a rehabilitation center to receive training that will maximize use of remaining abilities

LIFESPAN CONSIDERATIONS Health Promotion Topics

Infants

Infant–parent attachment/bonding

Breastfeeding

Sleep patterns

Playful activity to stimulate development

Immunizations

Safety promotion and injury control

Children

Nutrition

Dental checkups

Rest and exercise

Immunizations

Safety promotion and injury control

Adolescents

Communicating with the teen

Hormonal changes

Nutrition

Exercise and rest

Peer group influences

Self-concept and body image

Sexuality

Safety promotion and accident prevention

Older Adults

Adequate sleep

Appropriate use of alcohol

Dental/oral health

Drug management

Exercise

Foot health

Health screening recommendations

Hearing aid use

Immunizations

Medication instruction

Mental health

Nutrition

Physical fitness

Preventive health services

Safety precautions

Smoking cessation

Weight control

The foundation for *Healthy People 2010* is the belief that individual health is closely linked to community health and the reverse. Thus, the vision for *Healthy People 2010* is "Healthy People in Healthy Communities" (USDHHS, 2000, p. 3). Partnerships are important to improve individual and community health. Businesses, local government, and civic, professional, and religious organizations can all participate.

Sites for Health Promotion Activities

Health promotion programs are found in many settings. Programs and activities may be offered to individuals and families in the home or in the community setting and at schools, hospitals, or work sites. Some individuals may feel more comfortable having a nurse, diet counselor, or fitness expert

BOX 5–6 **The 28 Focus Areas in *Healthy People 2010***

- Access to quality health services
- Arthritis, osteoporosis, and chronic back conditions
- Cancer
- Chronic kidney disease
- Diabetes
- Disability and secondary conditions
- Educational and community-based programs
- Environmental health
- Family planning
- Food safety
- Health communication
- Heart disease and stroke
- HIV
- Immunization and infectious diseases
- Injury and violence prevention
- Maternal, infant, and child health
- Medical product safety
- Mental health and mental disorders
- Nutrition and overweight
- Occupational safety and health
- Oral health
- Physical activity and fitness
- Public health infrastructure
- Respiratory diseases
- Sexually transmitted diseases
- Substance abuse
- Tobacco use
- Vision and hearing

Note: U.S. Department of Health and Human Services, 2000.

BOX 5–7   **The Leading Health Indicators in** *Healthy People 2010*

- Physical Activity
  Regular physical activity throughout life is important for maintaining a healthy body, enhancing psychological well-being, and preventing premature death (p. 26).
- Overweight and Obesity
  Overweight and obesity are major contributors to many preventable causes of death. On average, higher body weights are associated with higher death rates. The number of overweight children, adolescents, and adults has risen over the past four decades (p. 28).
- Tobacco Use
  Cigarette smoking is the single most preventable cause of disease and death in the United States (p. 30).
- Substance Abuse
  Alcohol and illicit drug use are associated with many of this country's most serious problems, including violence, injury, and HIV infection (p. 32).
- Responsible Sexual Behavior
  Unintended pregnancies and sexually transmitted infections (STIs), including infection with the human immunodeficiency virus that causes AIDS, can result from unprotected sexual behaviors (p. 34).
- Mental Health
  Approximately 20% of the U.S. population is affected by mental illness during a given year; no one is immune. Of all

mental illnesses, depression is the most common disorder. Major depression is the leading cause of disability and is the cause of more than two-thirds of suicides each year (p. 36).
- Injury and Violence
  More than 400 Americans die each day from injuries due primarily to motor vehicle crashes, firearms, poisonings, suffocation, falls, fires, and drowning (p. 38).
- Environmental Quality
  An estimated 25% of preventable illnesses worldwide can be attributed to poor environmental quality. Two indicators of air quality are ozone (outdoor) and environmental tobacco smoke (indoor) (p. 40).
- Immunization
  Vaccines are among the greatest public health achievements of the 20th century. Immunizations can prevent disability and death from infectious diseases for individuals and can help control the spread of infections within communities (p. 42).
- Access to Health Care
  Strong predictors of access to quality health care include having health insurance, a higher income level, and a regular primary care provider or other source of ongoing health care. Use of clinical preventive services, such as early prenatal care, can serve as indicators of access to quality health care services (p. 44).

Note: U.S. Department of Health and Human Services, 2000.

---

come to their home for teaching and follow-up on individual needs. This type of program, however, is not cost effective for most individuals. Many people prefer the group approach, find it more motivating, and enjoy the socializing and support. Most programs offered in the community are group oriented.

Community programs are frequently offered by cities and towns. The type of program depends on the current concerns and the expertise of the sponsoring department or group. Program offerings may include health promotion, specific protection, and screening for early detection of disease. Hospitals began the emphasis on health promotion and prevention by focusing on the health of their employees. Programs offered by health care organizations initially began with a specific focus on prevention. Gradually, issues related to the health and lifestyle of the employee were addressed. Increasingly, hospitals have offered a variety of these programs and others to the community as well as to their employees. Such community activities enhance the public image of the hospital, increase the health of the surrounding population, and generate some additional income.

School health promotion programs may serve as a foundation for children of all ages to gain basic knowledge about personal hygiene and issues in the health sciences. Because school is the focus of a child's life for so many years, the school provides a cost-effective and convenient setting for health-focused programs. Worksite programs for health promotion have developed out of the need for businesses to control the rising cost of health care and employee absenteeism. Many industries feel that both employers and em-

ployees benefit from healthy lifestyles and behaviors. The convenience of the worksite setting makes these programs particularly attractive to many adults who would otherwise not be aware of them or motivated to attend them. Health promotion programs may be held in the company cafeteria so that employees can watch a film or attend a discussion group during their lunch break. Benefits to the worker may include an increased feeling of well-being, fitness, weight control, and decreased stress. Benefits to the employer may include an increase in employee motivation and productivity, an increase in employee morale, a decrease in absenteeism, and a lower rate of employee turnover, all of which may decrease business and health care costs.

Older adults who have retired often have more time for health promotion activities than they did before retirement. The nurse can inform older adults of available community resources such as walking groups. Nurses can address the need for health protection and health promotion through teaching classes at retirement communities and other community resource centers for older adults.

Health Promotion Model

The initial version of the Health Promotion Model (HPM) focused on health-promoting behaviors rather than health protection or illness prevention behaviors. The initial model has been replaced by the Health Promotion Model (Revised). The HPM is a competence- or approach-oriented model in which the motivational source for behavior change is based on the individual's subjective value of the change—that is, how the client perceives the benefits of changing the given health behavior. The HPM does not include "fear" or "threat" as a motivating source for changing health behavior (Pender, Murdaugh, & Parsons, 2006, p. 48). The variables in the revised HPM and their interrelationships are described next.

INDIVIDUAL CHARACTERISTICS AND EXPERIENCES The importance of an individual's unique personal factors or characteristics and experiences will depend on the target behavior for health promotion. There is flexibility in the HPM to select those characteristics that are relevant to the particular health behavior. Personal factors are categorized as biological, psychological, and sociocultural. Some personal factors that influence health behaviors can be changed whereas others, such as age, cannot. Health behaviors are based on previous experience, knowledge, and skill in health-promoting actions. Individuals who made a habit of a previous health-promoting behavior and received a positive benefit as a result will engage in future health-promoting behaviors. In contrast, a person with a history of barriers to achieving the behavior remembers the "hurdles," which creates a negative effect. The nurse can assist by focusing on the positive benefits of the behavior, teaching how to overcome the hurdles and providing positive feedback for the client's successes.

Nursing interventions usually focus on factors that can be modified. It is just as important, however, to also focus on factors that cannot be changed, such as family history. While a client may not be able to modify risks for a specific disease, such as family history, nurses must be aware of these risks and direct more support and information to this group, reinforcing the idea that even with a strong family history, early detection and treatment are especially important and often improve the client's outcome. Helping to transform fear into hope for early detection can make a difference in health attitudes and behaviors.

BEHAVIOR-SPECIFIC COGNITIONS AND AFFECT This set of variables is considered to be of major motivational significance for acquiring and maintaining health-promoting behaviors. Behavior-specific cognitions constitute a critical "core" for intervention because they can be modified through nursing interventions. They include perceived benefits of action, perceived barriers to action, perceived self-efficacy, activity-related affect, interpersonal influences, and situational influences.

COMMITMENT TO A PLAN OF ACTION Commitment to a plan of action involves two processes: commitment and identifying specific strategies for carrying out and reinforcing the behavior. Strategies are important because commitment alone often results in "good intentions" and not actual performance of the behavior.

IMMEDIATE COMPETING DEMANDS AND PREFERENCES Competing demands are those behaviors over which an individual has a low level of control. For example, an unexpected work or family responsibility may compete with a planned visit to the health club, and not responding to this

responsibility may cause a more negative outcome than missing the exercise routine. Competing preferences are behaviors over which an individual has a high level of control; however, this control depends on the individual's ability to be self-regulating or to not "give in."

BEHAVIORAL OUTCOME Health-promoting behavior, the outcome of the Health Promotion Model, is directed toward attaining positive health outcomes for the client. Health-promoting behaviors should result in improved health, enhanced functional ability, and better quality of life at all stages of development (Pender, Murdaugh, & Parsons, 2006, p. 57).

Stages of Health Behavior Change

One theory of health behavior change believes change is a cyclic phenomenon in which people progress through several stages. In the first stage, the person does not think seriously about changing a behavior; by the time the person reaches the final stage, he or she is successfully maintaining the change in behavior. Several behavior change models have been proposed. The Transtheoretical Model (TTM), proposed by Prochaska, Redding, and Evers (2002) is discussed here. As shown in Figure 5–5, the stages are (a) precontemplation, (b) contemplation, (c) preparation, (d) action, (e) maintenance, and (f) termination. If the person does not succeed in changing behavior, relapse occurs.

In the **precontemplation stage,** the person does not think about changing his or her behavior in the next six months. The person may be uninformed or underinformed about the consequences of the risk behavior(s). The person who has tried changing previously and was unsuccessful may now see the behavior as his or her "fate" or believe that change is hopeless. Individuals in this stage tend to avoid reading, talking, or thinking about their high-risk behaviors (Prochaska et al., 2002, p. 100).

During the **contemplation stage,** the person acknowledges having a problem, seriously considers changing a specific behavior, actively gathers information, and verbalizes plans to change the behavior in the near future (e.g., next six months). The person, however, may not be ready to commit to action. Some people may stay in the contemplative stage for months or years before taking action. When contemplators begin the transition to the preparation stage, their thinking is clearly marked by two changes: focusing on the solution rather than the problem and thinking more about the future than the past (Prochaska, Norcross, & DiClemente, 1994, p. 43).

The **preparation stage** occurs when the person intends to take action in the immediate future (e.g., within the next month). Some people in this stage may have already started making small behavioral changes, such as buying a self-help book. At this stage, the person makes the final specific plans to accomplish the change.

The **action stage** occurs when the person actively implements behavioral and cognitive strategies of the action plan to interrupt previous health risk behaviors and adopt new ones. This stage requires the greatest commitment of time and energy.

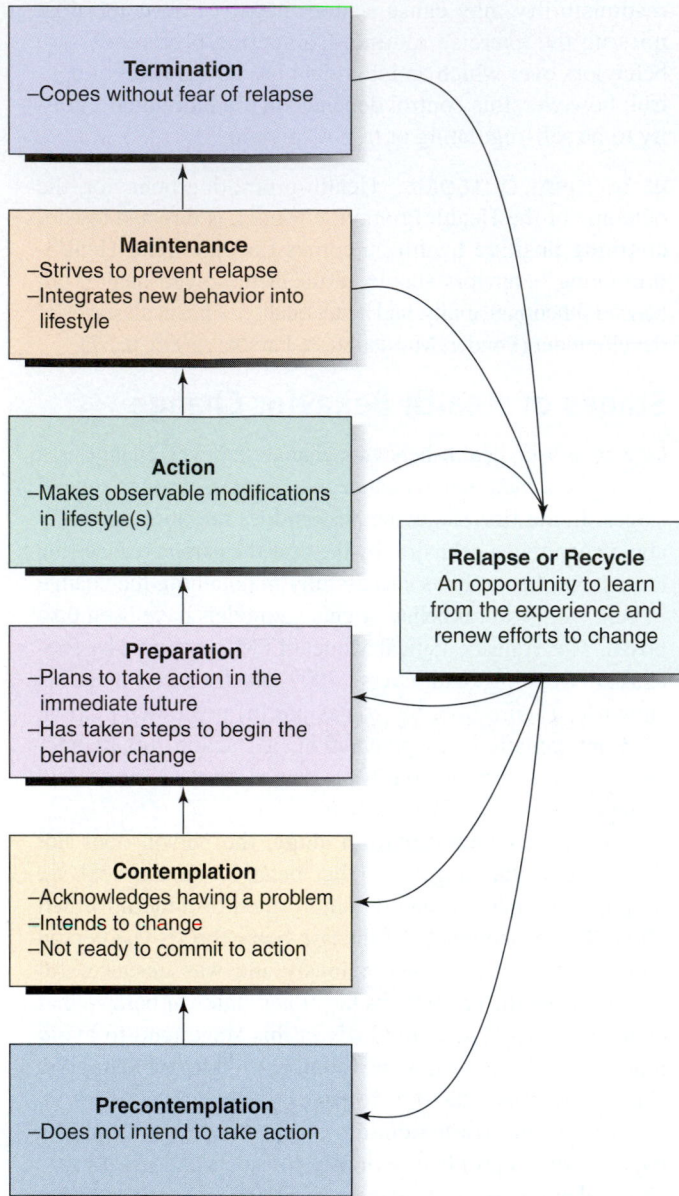

Figure 5–5 ⬤ The stages of change are rarely linear. It is more common for people to recycle several times through the stages. The person who takes action and has a relapse (recycles through some or all of the stages again) is more apt to be successful the next time than the individual who never takes action.

(Diagram based on content from *Changing for Good* by James O. Prochaska, John C. Norcross, and Carlo C. DiClemente. Copyright 1994 by James O. Prochaska, John C. Norcross, and Carlo C. DiClemente. Reprinted by permission of HarperCollins Publishers, Inc.; and "The Transtheoretical Model and Stages of Change" by James O. Prochaska, Colleen A. Redding, and Kerry E. Evers in *Health Behaviors and Health Education: Theory, Research, and Practice* (3rd ed.), 2002, by Karen Glanz, Barbara K. Rimer, and Frances Marcus Lewis, Eds.)

During the **maintenance stage,** the person strives to prevent relapse by integrating newly adopted behaviors into his or her lifestyle. This stage lasts until the person no longer experiences temptation to return to previous unhealthy behaviors. Without a strong commitment to maintenance, there will be a relapse, usually to the precontemplation or contemplation stage (Prochaska et al., 1994, p. 45).

The **termination stage** is the ultimate goal where the individual has complete confidence that the problem is no longer a temptation or threat. It is as if they never acquired the habit in the first place (Prochaska et al., 2002, p. 102). Experts debate whether some behaviors can be terminated versus requiring continual maintenance.

These six stages are cyclical; people generally move through one stage before progressing to the next. However, at any point a person may relapse or recycle to any previous stage. In fact, the average successful self-changer recycles through the stages several times before making it to the top and exiting the cycle (Prochaska et al., 1994, pp. 47–48). The majority of individuals who relapse return to the contemplation stage. During this time they can think about what they learned and plan for the next action attempt. Box 5–8 suggests a method to assess your stage of change for a health behavior.

The Nurse's Role in Health Promotion

Individuals and communities who seek to increase their responsibility for personal health and self-care require health education. The trend toward health promotion has created the opportunity for nurses to strengthen the profession's influence on health promotion, disseminate information that promotes an educated public, and assist individuals and communities to change long-standing health behaviors.

A variety of programs can be used for the promotion of health, including (a) information dissemination, (b) health risk appraisal and wellness assessment, (c) lifestyle and behavior change, and (d) environmental control programs.

Information dissemination is the most basic type of health promotion program. This method makes use of a variety of media to offer information to the public about the risk of particular lifestyle choices and personal behavior, as well as the

BOX 5–8	Assessing Stages of Health Behavior Change

Stages of change for positive health behaviors may be assessed with the following true-false questions:

1. I currently do not (specify exact behavior, e.g., exercise 30 minutes three times a week, eat two to four servings of fruit daily) and do not intend to start in the next six months. (Precontemplation)
2. I currently do not (specify behavior), but I am thinking about starting to do so in the next six months. (Contemplation)
3. I have tried several times to (specify behavior), but I am seriously thinking of trying again in the next month. (Planning)
4. I have (specify behavior) regularly for less than six months. (Action)
5. I have (specify behavior) regularly for more than six months. (Maintenance)

Note: From "A Transtheoretical Model of Behaviors and Change," by J. O. Prochaska, C. A. Redding, & K. E. Evers. In K. Glanz, B. K. Rimer, and F. M. Lewis (Eds.), *Health Behavior and Health Education: Theory, Research and Practice.* Copyright © 2002 Jossey-Bass. Reprinted with permission of John Wiley & Sons, Inc.

benefits of changing that behavior and improving the quality of life. Information dissemination is a useful strategy for raising the level of knowledge and awareness of individuals and groups about health habits. When planning information dissemination, it is important to consider factors such as cultural factors and different age groups. Knowing the best place and method to distribute information will increase the effectiveness. It is just as critical to know where people get "misinformation."

Health risk appraisal and wellness assessment programs are used to apprise individuals of the risk factors that are inherent in their lives in order to motivate them to reduce specific risks and develop positive health habits. Wellness assessment programs are focused on more positive methods of enhancement, in contrast to the risk factor approach used in the health appraisal. A variety of tools is available to facilitate these assessments. Some of these tools are computer based and can therefore be offered to educational institutions and industries at a reasonable cost.

Lifestyle and behavior change programs require the participation of the individual and are geared toward enhancing the quality of life and extending the life span. Individuals generally consider lifestyle changes after they have been informed of the need to change their health behavior and have become aware of the potential benefits of the process. Many programs are available to the public, both on a group and individual basis, some of which address stress management, nutrition awareness, weight control, smoking cessation, and exercise.

Environmental control programs have been developed in response to the continuing increase of contaminants of human origin that have been introduced into our environment. The most common concerns of community groups are toxic and nuclear wastes, nuclear power plants, air and water pollution, and herbicide and pesticide use.

Health promotion activities involve collaborative relationships with both clients and primary care providers. The role of the nurse is to work *with* people, not *for* them—that is, to act as a facilitator of the process of assessing, evaluating, and understanding health. The nurse may act as advocate, consultant, teacher, or coordinator of services. For examples of the nurse's role in health promotion, see Box 5–9. In these roles, the nurse may work with individuals of all age groups and diverse family units or concentrate on a specific population, such as new parents, school-age children, or older adults. In any case, the nursing process is a basic tool for the nurse in a health promotion role. Although the process is the same, the nurse emphasizes teaching the client (who can be either an individual or a family unit) self-care responsibility. Adult clients decide the goals, determine the health promotion plans, and take responsibility for the success of the plans.

THE NURSING PROCESS AND HEALTH PROMOTION

A thorough assessment of the individual's health status is basic to health promotion. As nurses move toward greater autonomy in providing client care, expanded assessment skills are essential to provide the meaningful data needed for health planning.

BOX 5–9   The Nurse's Role in Health Promotion

- Model healthy lifestyle behaviors and attitudes.
- Facilitate client involvement in the assessment, implementation, and evaluation of health goals.
- Teach clients self-care strategies to enhance fitness, improve nutrition, manage stress, and enhance relationships.
- Assist individuals, families, and communities to increase their levels of health.
- Educate clients to be effective health care consumers.
- Assist clients, families, and communities to develop and choose health-promoting options.
- Guide clients' development in effective problem solving and decision making.
- Reinforce clients' personal and family health-promoting behaviors.
- Advocate in the community for changes that promote a healthy environment.

ASSESSING

Components of this assessment are the health history and physical examination, physical fitness assessment, lifestyle assessment, spiritual assessment, social support systems review, health risk assessment, health beliefs review, and life-stress review.

Health History and Physical Examination

The health history and physical examination discussed in Chapter 17 ∞ provide a means for detecting any existing problems. The age of the individual must be considered when collecting data. A nutritional assessment is an important part of the health history. The nurse must consider both age and body build of the client when gathering information on dietary patterns. See Chapter 31 ∞ for more information about nutritional assessment.

Physical Fitness Assessment

During an evaluation of physical fitness, the nurse assesses several components of the body's physical functioning: muscle endurance, flexibility, body composition, and cardiorespiratory endurance. Specific guidelines for obtaining measurements and the optimal values for men, women, and children can be found in physical fitness texts. Older adults need to be monitored carefully for fatigue during strength and endurance tests. A common test for muscular endurance is performing sit-ups with knees bent (bent-knee sit-ups) for one minute. The number of sit-ups performed during that time is compared to standardized charts.

Flexibility of the joints and muscles greatly increases an individual's ability to move about with ease and comfort. Trunk flexion is one test used to measure the client's ability to stretch the back and thigh muscles. In this test the client sits on an examining table or the floor with the legs fully extended, the feet placed flat against a box, and the arms and hands stretched forward as far as possible, holding the position for a count of three. The distance the client can reach beyond the near edge of the box is measured in inches or, if the client is unable to reach the box, the distance between the fingertips and the box is measured and recorded as a negative number.

Body composition indicates the ratio of body fat to muscle and is estimated through skinfold measurements. Skinfold measurements are obtained by grasping the skinfold (skin layers and subcutaneous fat) between the thumb and forefinger and measuring the skinfold at subcutaneous sites (chest, midaxillary, triceps, subscapula, abdomen, suprailiac, and thigh) with special calipers. Generally three measurements are taken at each site and the average values summed. The technique for measuring skin folds is described in Chapter 31 ∞. One test for cardiorespiratory endurance is the step test. Individuals step up and down on a 16- to 17-inch step for 3 minutes at a prescribed rate (e.g., 22 to 24 steps per minute). After the test, the client sits in a chair while the nurse assesses the apical or carotid pulse rate from 5 to 20 seconds into recovery.

Lifestyle Assessment

Lifestyle assessment focuses on the personal lifestyle and habits of the client as they affect health. Categories of lifestyle generally assessed are physical activity, nutritional practices, stress management, and such habits as smoking, alcohol consumption, and drug use. Other categories may be included. Several tools are available to assess lifestyle. The goals of lifestyle assessment tools are to provide an opportunity for clients to assess the impact of their present lifestyle on their health and a basis for decisions related to desired behavior and lifestyle change.

Spiritual Health Assessment

Spiritual health is the ability to develop one's inner nature to its fullest potential, including the ability to discover and articulate one's basic purpose in life, to learn how to experience love, joy, peace, and fulfillment, and how to help ourselves and others achieve their fullest potential (Pender, Murdaugh, & Parsons, 2006, p. 108). Spiritual beliefs can affect a person's interpretation of events in his or her life and, therefore, an assessment of spiritual well-being is a part of evaluating the person's overall health. See Chapter 28 ∞ for more information.

Social Support Systems Review

Understanding the social context in which a person lives and works is important in health promotion. Individuals and groups, through interpersonal relationships, can provide comfort, assistance, encouragement, and information. Social support fosters successful coping and promotes satisfying and effective living. Social support systems contribute to health by creating an environment that encourages healthy behaviors, promotes self-esteem and wellness, and provides feedback that the person's actions will lead to desirable outcomes. The Culturally Competent Care feature addresses aspects of social support within the context of culture.

CULTURALLY COMPETENT CARE | **Cultural Aspects of Social Support**

It is important to understand how various subgroups of American society may define social support.

- In the African American community, the family and church have been major providers of social support.
- Hispanic-Latino Americans and Asian Americans view the family as being a major social support system.
- Asian Americans respect older adults and use shame and harmony in giving and receiving support.
- Native Americans live in social networks that foster mutual assistance and support.

Note: From *Health Promotion in Nursing Practice,* 5th ed. (pp. 239–240), by N. J. Pender, C. L. Murdaugh, and M. A. Parsons, 2006, Upper Saddle River, NJ: Pearson Education. Reprinted with permission.

According to Pender et al. (2002), the nurse begins a social support system review by asking the client to list individuals who provide personal support, indicate the relationship of each person, and identify which individuals have been a source of support for five or more years. This assessment allows the nurse and client to discuss and evaluate the adequacy of the client's support system together and, if necessary, plan options for enhancing the support system.

Health Risk Assessment

A health risk assessment (HRA) is an assessment and educational tool that indicates a client's risk for disease or injury during the next 10 years by comparing the client's risk with the mortality risk of the corresponding age, sex, and racial group. The client's general health, lifestyle behaviors, and demographic data are compared to data from a large national sample. Individual risk reports are based on statistics for the population group that matches the individual's surveyed characteristics. The HRA includes a summary of the person's health risks and lifestyle behaviors with educational suggestions on how to reduce the risk. Recently, HRAs have begun to reflect a broader approach to health as companies use the HRA as a means to begin a health promotion and risk reduction program. Occupational health nurses can identify risk factors and subsequently plan interventions aimed to decrease illness, absenteeism, and disability. HRAs are helpful for assessing individual and group health risks. They are not, however, substitutes for medical care and are not appropriate for all individuals.

Health Beliefs Review

Clients' health beliefs need to be clarified, particularly those beliefs that determine how they perceive control of their own health care status. Several instruments are available that assess a person's health-belief measures. Assessment of clients' health beliefs provides the nurse with an indication of how much the clients believe they can influence or con-

---

LIFESPAN CONSIDERATIONS Factors Affecting Health Promotion and Illness Prevention

Children

Childhood obesity is becoming a serious health problem. Data collected by the Centers for Disease Control and Prevention (CDC) show that nearly 16% of American children are overweight, up from 6.5% in 1980 (National Center for Health Statistics, 2004). Obesity and overweight in children contributes to long-term health problems such as heart disease and diabetes mellitus.

Although specific causes of obesity and appropriate management to reduce weight will vary from child to child, healthy eating habits and adequate exercise patterns form the basis for healthy growth and prevention of being overweight in children. It is the responsibility of parents and caregivers to provide children with healthy food choices and an environment that makes eating a pleasure. It is the responsibility of children to decide how much and what foods to eat. Adults must be role models for their children, eating well and exercising regularly themselves.

Older Adults

In older adults, health promotion and illness prevention are important, but often the focus is on learning to adapt to and live with increasing changes and limitations. Maximizing strengths continues to be of prime importance in maintaining optimal function and quality of life. Factors to be aware of that might indicate a need for additional information or resources include these:

- An increase in physical limitations
- Presence of one or more chronic illnesses
- Change in cognitive status
- Difficulty in accessing health care services due to transportation problems
- Poor support system
- Need for environmental modifications for safety and to maintain independence
- Attitude of hopelessness and depression, which decreases the motivation to use resources or learn new information

---

trol health through personal behaviors. Several cultures have a strong belief in fate. If people hold this belief, they do not feel that they can do anything to change the course of their disease. Being aware of these differences can provide a better indication of readiness and motivation on the part of the client to engage in healthy behaviors. See the Lifespan Considerations for factors that might indicate a need for additional information or resources for older adults.

Life Stress Review

There is abundant literature about the impact of stress on mental and physical well-being. A variety of stress-related instruments has been found in the literature. Studies have shown that a high score is associated with the increased possibility of illness in an individual.

Validating Assessment Data

Following the collection of assessment data, the nurse and client need to review, validate, and summarize the information. This step is carried out jointly by the nurse and the client. During this process, the nurse verbally reviews the current practices and attitudes of the client. This allows validation of the information by the client and may increase awareness of the need to change behavior. The nurse and client need to consider the following:

- Any existing health problems
- The client's perceived degree of control over health status
- Key health beliefs
- Level of physical fitness and nutritional status
- Illnesses for which the client is at risk
- Current positive health practices
- Spirituality

- Sources of life stress and ability to handle stress
- Social support systems
- Information needed to enhance health care practices

DIAGNOSING

Nursing diagnoses accepted by the North American Nursing Diagnosis Association (NANDA) have generally focused on impaired or imbalanced health patterns or problems. The definition, however, of the NANDA wellness diagnoses states: "Describes human responses to levels of wellness in an individual, family, or community that have a readiness for enhancement" (2005, p. 277). Wellness diagnoses can be applied at all levels of prevention but are particularly useful for healthy clients who require teaching for health promotion, disease prevention, and personal growth. When the nurse and client conclude that the client has positive function in a certain pattern area, such as adequate nutrition or effective coping, the nurse can use this information to help the client reach a higher level of functioning.

A wellness diagnosis is preceded by the modifier "readiness for enhanced." Wellness diagnoses provide a clear focus for planning interventions without indicating that a problem exists. The following examples are included in the NANDA taxonomy:

- *Readiness for Enhanced Spiritual Well-being*
- *Readiness for Enhanced Coping*
- *Readiness for Enhanced Nutrition*
- *Readiness for Enhanced Knowledge (Specify)*
- *Readiness for Enhanced Parenting*
- *Readiness for Enhanced Self-concept*
- *Readiness for Enhanced Immunization Status*
- *Readiness for Enhanced Self-care*

PLANNING

Health promotion plans need to be developed according to the needs, desires, and priorities of the client. The client decides on health promotion goals, the activities or interventions to achieve those goals, the frequency and duration of the activities, and the method of evaluation. During the planning process the nurse acts as a resource person rather than as an advisor or counselor. The nurse provides information when asked, emphasizes the importance of small steps to behavioral change, and reviews the client's goals and plans to make sure they are realistic, measurable, and acceptable to the client.

Pender, Murdaugh, & Parsons, (2006, pp. 127–141) outline several steps in the process of developing a joint health promotion-prevention plan. These steps actively involve both the nurse and the client:

1. *Review and summarize data from assessment.*
2. *Reinforce strengths and competencies of the client.*
3. *Identify health goals and related behavior-change options.*
4. *Identify behavioral or health outcomes.*
5. *Develop a behavior-change plan.*
6. *Reiterate benefits of change.*
7. *Address environmental and interpersonal facilitators and barriers to change.*
8. *Determine a time frame for implementation.*
9. *Formalize commitment to behavior-change plan.*
10. *Explore available resources.*

IMPLEMENTING

Implementing is the "doing" part of behavior change. Self-responsibility is emphasized for implementing the plan. Depending on the client's needs, the nursing interventions may include supporting, counseling, facilitating, teaching, consulting, enhancing the behavior change, and modeling.

A major nursing role is to support the client. A vital component of lifestyle change is ongoing support that focuses on the desired behavior change and is provided in a nonjudgmental manner. Support can be offered by the nurse on an individual basis or in a group setting. The nurse can also facilitate the development of support networks for the client, such as family members and friends.

Individual Counseling Sessions

Counseling sessions may be routinely scheduled as part of the plan or may be provided if the client encounters difficulty in carrying out interventions or meets insurmountable barriers to change. In a counseling relationship, the nurse and client share ideas. In this sharing relationship, the nurse acts as a facilitator, promoting the client's decision making in regard to the health promotion plan.

Telephone or Computer Counseling

Regular telephone sessions or computer interaction may be provided to the client to answer questions, review goals and strategies, and reinforce progress. The client may find that scheduling a weekly interaction is helpful or may wish to initiate a call if a problem occurs. The client is asked, "Is your plan working?" If the plan is not working, the nurse asks, "What would you like to do?" The client may wish to continue or may wish to change the plan to a more realistic one. Telephone or computer support is efficient for the busy client who may not have the time for regular, in-person sessions.

Group Support

Group sessions provide an opportunity for participants to learn the experiences of others in changing behavior. Group contact gives individuals a renewed commitment to their goals. Groups can be scheduled at monthly or less frequent intervals for over a year.

Facilitating Social Support

Social networks, such as family and friends, can facilitate or impede the efforts directed toward health promotion and prevention. The nurse's role is to assist the client to assess, modify, and develop the social support necessary to achieve the desired change. To provide the necessary support, families must communicate effectively, be aware of and support each other's needs and goals, and provide help and assistance to one another to achieve those goals. The client may wish the nurse to meet with the family or significant others and help enlist their understanding and support.

Providing Health Education

Health education programs on a variety of topics discussed earlier can be provided to groups, individuals, or communities. Group programs need to be planned carefully before they are implemented. The decision to establish a health promotion program must be based on the health needs of the people; also, specific health promotion goals must be set. After the program is implemented, outcomes must be evaluated.

Enhancing Behavior Change

Whether people will make and maintain changes to improve health or prevent disease depends on many interrelated factors. To help clients succeed in implementing behavior changes, the nurse needs to understand the stages of change and effective interventions that focus on progressing the individual through the stages of change. Guidelines for assisting the client toward behavior change are offered in the Practice Guidelines. Figure 5–6 provides suggested strategies to assist clients depending on their stage of change. As Saarmann, Daugherty, and Riegel (2000) point out, the nursing goal is not necessarily to change behavior but to advance the client to the next stage of change (p. 285).

Modeling

Through observing a model, the client acquires ideas for behavior and coping strategies that can be used with specific

PRACTICE GUIDELINES   **Enhancing Behavior Change**

Establish Rapport

- Provide privacy and a perception of a collaborative, equal-power relationship.
- If time allows, ask the client to describe a "typical" day. Usually the problematic behavior is described; however, even if it is not, the listening will strengthen rapport and the personal information may be helpful in understanding the client's current situation.

Set Agenda

- Allow the client to identify concerns. If there are multiple concerns (e.g., smoking, exercise, diet, stress), it is best to focus on one specific behavior at a time. Ask the client which behavior he or she feels most ready to *think* about changing.

Assess Importance, Confidence, and Readiness

- A client's readiness to change is often influenced by his or her perception of importance and confidence.
- Importance refers to the personal value of change. Questions that elicit this information can include: "How do you feel at the moment about [state the change]?" "How important is it to you to [state the change]?" "On a scale of 1 to 10, with 1 being not important and 10 very important, what number would you give yourself?"
- Confidence relates to mastering the skills needed to achieve the behavior and the situations in which behavior change will be challenging to the client. A potential question to use to assess confidence is "If you decided right now to change, how confident would you feel about succeeding?"

Exchange Information and Reduce Resistance

- Exchanging information and reducing resistance are performed throughout the various stages of behavior change.
- Ask clients if they would like information and about what.
- Present information in a neutral tone of voice, and avoid using the word "you" too much. Referring to other people (versus "you") and what happens to them makes the information less threatening to the client.
- After presenting the information, ask for the client's interpretation of the information.
- Three *traps* that increase resistance and *strategies to avoid the traps* include:
  - Taking control away. *Instead,* emphasize personal choice and control.
  - Misjudging importance, confidence, or readiness. Often this results in talking about action before the client is ready. It is important to *reexamine* the client's feelings about importance and confidence as they influence readiness to make a specific change.
  - Meeting force with force. Instead of attacking or defending through argument, sit back and use reflective listening. Try to understand how the client is feeling. The resistance usually subsides and the discussion can move in a different direction.

Note: From *Health Behavior Change: A Guide for Practitioners,* by S. Rollnick, P. Mason, and C. Butler. Copyright © 1999, with permission from Elsevier.

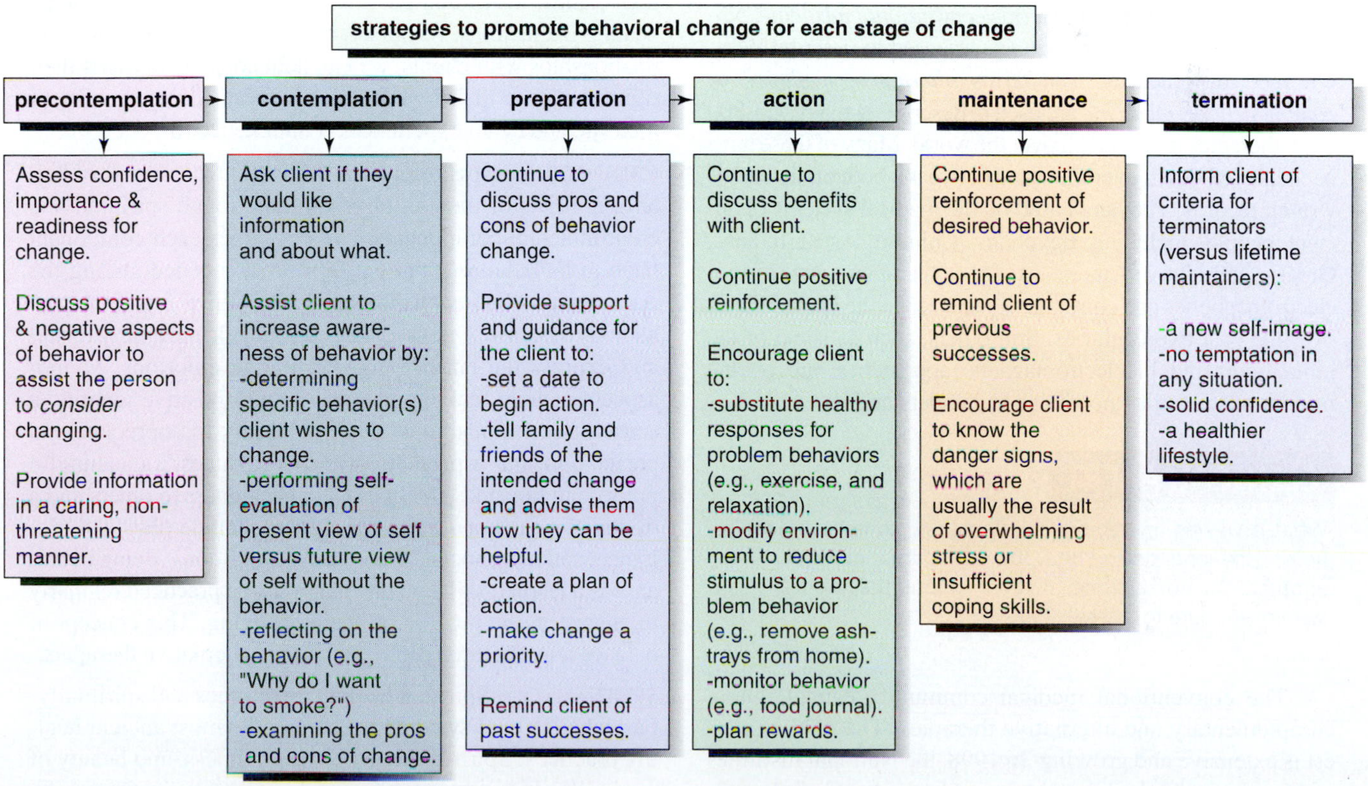

---

strategies to promote behavioral change for each stage of change

precontemplation	contemplation	preparation	action	maintenance	termination
Assess confidence, importance & readiness for change. Discuss positive & negative aspects of behavior to assist the person to *consider* changing. Provide information in a caring, non-threatening manner.	Ask client if they would like information and about what. Assist client to increase aware-ness of behavior by: -determining specific behavior(s) client wishes to change. -performing self-evaluation of present view of self versus future view of self without the behavior. -reflecting on the behavior (e.g., "Why do I want to smoke?") -examining the pros and cons of change.	Continue to discuss pros and cons of behavior change. Provide support and guidance for the client to: -set a date to begin action. -tell family and friends of the intended change and advise them how they can be helpful. -create a plan of action. -make change a priority. Remind client of past successes.	Continue to discuss benefits with client. Continue positive reinforcement. Encourage client to: -substitute healthy responses for problem behaviors (e.g., exercise, and relaxation). -modify environ-ment to reduce stimulus to a pro-blem behavior (e.g., remove ash-trays from home). -monitor behavior (e.g., food journal). -plan rewards.	Continue positive reinforcement of desired behavior. Continue to remind client of previous successes. Encourage client to know the danger signs, which are usually the result of overwhelming stress or insufficient coping skills.	Inform client of criteria for terminators (versus lifetime maintainers): -a new self-image. -no temptation in any situation. -solid confidence. -a healthier lifestyle.

Figure 5–6 ● Strategies to promote behavioral change for each stage of change.

problems. The client is not expected to mimic the sequence of actions or behavior patterns of the model. The nurse and client should mutually select models with whom the client can identify, since the cultural and ethnic backgrounds and age of the nurse and client often differ. Models should be people the client respects. Nurses should also serve as models of wellness. To model effectively, nurses need to have a philosophy and lifestyle that demonstrate good health habits.

EVALUATING

Evaluation takes place on an ongoing basis, both during the attainment of short-term goals and after the completion of long-term goals. Goals are written during the planning phase, and a date is determined for attaining the specific results or behaviors that are desired to promote health or prevent illness. During evaluation, the client may decide to continue with the plan, reorder priorities, change strategies, or revise the health protection promotion contract. Evaluation of the plan is a collaborative effort between the nurse and the client.

COMPLEMENTARY AND ALTERNATIVE HEALING MODALITIES

Most nursing education in the United States, Canada, Europe, and Australia has been under the umbrella of biomedicine. Thus, nurses from these parts of the world are familiar and comfortable with biomedical beliefs, theories, practices, strengths, and limitations. Fewer nurses have studied alternative medical theories and practices and as a result may lack information or even harbor misinformation about these healing practices. In this chapter the terms *conventional medicine, biomedicine,* and **allopathic** *medicine* are used to describe Western medical practices. The terms *alternative medicine* or *complementary medicine* are used to describe as many as 1,800 other therapies practiced all over the world. Many of these have been handed down over thousands of years, both orally and as written records. They are based on the medical systems of ancient people, including Egyptians, Chinese, Asian Indians, Greeks, and Native Americans. Other therapies, such as bioelectromagnetics and chiropractic, evolved in the United States over the past two centuries. Still others, such as some of the mind–body and bioelectromagnetic approaches, are on the frontier of scientific knowledge and understanding.

CLINICAL ALERT

What is viewed as traditional, alternative, complementary, or holistic by one person may be considered mainstream by another. Do not assume anything about the client's belief system—be sure to assess.

The conventional medical community cannot ignore complementary and alternative therapies. The public interest is extensive and growing. In 1998, the National Institutes of Health established the National Center for Complementary and Alternative Medicine to provide research, educa-

tional grants, and dissemination of information to the public. In March 2000, President Clinton ordered the establishment of the White House Commission on Complementary and Alternative Medicine Policy whose mission it is to make legislative and administrative recommendations for the integration of conventional and alternative medicine.

Basic Concepts

Several concepts are common to most alternative practices. These are holism, humanism, balance, spirituality, energy, and healing environments.

HOLISM   Although they represent diverse approaches, alternative therapies share certain attributes. They are based on the paradigm of whole systems and the belief that people are more than physical bodies with fixable and replaceable parts. Combined mental, emotional, spiritual, relationship, and environmental components, referred to as *holism,* are considered to play crucial and equal roles in a person's state of health. Interventions are individualized within the entire context of the person's life. The focus of the American Holistic Nurses Association (AHNA) is to enhance the healing of the whole person from birth to death.

HUMANISM   The **humanist** perspective includes propositions such as the following: the mind and body are indivisible, people have the power to solve their own problems, people are responsible for the patterns of their lives, and well-being is a combination of personal satisfaction and contributions to the larger community. Nursing is in a unique position to take a leadership role in integrating alternative healing methods into Western health care systems. Nurses have historically used their hands, heart, and head in more natural and traditional healing interactions. As nurses, by virtue of our education and relationships with clients, we can help consumers assert their right to choose their own healing journey and the quality of their life and death experiences (Fontaine, 2010).

BALANCE   In terms of optimal wellness, the concept of balance consists of mental, physical, emotional, spiritual, and environmental components. Not only does each component have to be balanced, but equilibrium is needed among the components. *Physical* aspects include optimal functioning of all body systems. *Emotional* aspects include the ability to feel and express the entire range of human emotions. *Mental* aspects include feelings of self-worth, a positive identity, a sense of accomplishment, and the ability to appreciate and create. *Spiritual* aspects involve moral values, a meaningful purpose in life, and a feeling of connectedness to others and a divine source. *Environmental* aspects include physical, biologic, economic, social, and political conditions. Being in balance is a learned skill and one that must be practiced regularly to engage in the process of healthful living. This concept of balance appears throughout the various alternative therapies.

SPIRITUALITY   Spiritual healing techniques and spiritually-based health care systems are among the most ancient healing practices. Spirit is the liveliness, richness, and beauty of one's life. It is who we are and how we are in the world. **Spirituality** (see Chapter 28 ∞) includes the drive to become all that one can be, and is bound to intuition, creativity, and motivation. It is the dimension that involves relationship with oneself, with others, and with a higher power. Spirituality is that which gives people meaning and purpose in their lives. It involves finding significant meaning in the entirety of life, including illness and death.

ENERGY The concept of energy has been recognized for centuries, and in most cultures. Energy is viewed as the force that integrates the body, mind, and spirit; it is that which connects everything. Chinese Taoist scholars believed that energy was the basic building material of the universe. Albert Einstein and other physicists proved that matter and energy are the same and that energy is not only the raw material of the cosmos but the glue that holds it together. Modern scientists now look at the universe in terms of forces of tiny particles of matter. Their experimental findings are similar to the intuitive observation of China's ancient scholars. Everything in the world—animate and inanimate—is made of energy. People are beings of energy, living in a universe composed of energy.

Two terms common in various healing practices and related to energy and balance are grounding and centering. *Grounding,* as its name suggests, relates to one's connection with the ground and, in a broader sense, to one's whole contact with reality. Being grounded suggests stability, security, independence, having a solid foundation, and living in the present rather than escaping into dreams. *Centering* refers to the process of bringing oneself to the center or middle. When people are centered, they are fully connected to the part of their bodies where all their energies meet. Centering is the process of focusing one's mind on the center of energy allowing one to operate intuitively, with awareness, and to channel energy throughout the body.

HEALING ENVIRONMENTS Nursing has always focused on creating healing environments for those who have been entrusted to our care. We create healing environments when we use our hands, heart, and mind to provide holistic nursing care. We create healing environments when we empower others by providing the knowledge, skills, and support that allow them to tap into their inner wisdom and make healthy decisions for themselves. Healing environments are a synthesis of the medical-curing approach and the nursing-healing approach. We need a healthy balance between technology and compassion.

Nurses must also create healing environments for themselves. Nurses need to learn how to restore their energy and replenish themselves. What happens to nurses who don't sincerely care for themselves or take the time to replenish themselves? It soon becomes obvious by their behavior that they are stagnant or depleted; they are less patient, less tolerant, more irritable, and unhappy. Their state of "burnout" contaminates all aspects of their professional and personal lives. Box 5–10 lists methods that can be useful to nurses working to foster their own health and well-being.

Healing Modalities

Ethnocentrism, the assumption that one's own cultural or ethnic group is superior to others, has often prevented Western health

---

BOX 5–10 **Self-Healing Methods for Nurses**

- Clarify values and beliefs. Identify those things that are important, meaningful, and valuable to you, and assess whether your actions are consistent with your beliefs. For example, do you value time spent with your children and time reading or listening to music?
- Set realistic goals. Identify long-term goals and then short-term goals that will help you meet the long-term goals. For example, a long-term goal might be to experience an increase in emotional and physical comfort. A short-term goal might be to take a 30-minute walk each evening.
- Challenge the belief that others always come first. Overinvolvement with clients leads to overwork and overly solicitous helping that neglects the client's responsibilities, autonomy, and resources. It leaves little time for fulfillment of personal needs. Identify behaviors that indicate overinvolvement, such as saying yes much too often, a tendency to avoid conflict whenever possible, feeling selfish when not responding to someone else's needs, and always listening to others who need emotional support but seldom asking anyone to pay attention to your emotional needs. Assess whether you need to adjust your perspective and behavior. Learn to ask for what you need, acknowledge that you are doing the best you can, and affirm that you can meet your own needs as well as care for others.

- Learn to manage stress. Stress management requires the following:
  - Acknowledge the mind–body connection, that is, the relationship among thoughts, feelings, behaviors, and the physiologic response to stress.
  - Monitor stress warning signals and invoke the relaxation response on a regular basis such as once a day for 20 minutes or twice a day for 10 minutes. "Mini-relaxations" (e.g., taking several deep breaths and thinking about something pleasant such as your favorite pet) throughout the day can also be used to counter the tension and anxiety associated with stress.
  - Develop the skill of personal presence (physically "being there" and psychologically "being with" a client or other person). To be available to others in this way requires practicing the skill of being present to yourself. Avoid allowing yourself to be hurried, distracted, or fragmented. Focus full attention on the activity you are doing at the moment.
  - Maintain and enhance physical health. Eat healthy, balanced meals, exercise regularly, and obtain adequate rest.
  - Develop a support network. Fellow nurses can often provide perspectives and insights to help cope with commonly shared experiences.

Note: From "Awakening the Healer Within," by C. L. Wells-Federman, 1996, *Holistic Nursing Practice, 10,* pp. 13–29. Adapted with permission.

care practitioners from learning new ways to promote health and prevent chronic illness. With consumer demand for a broader range of options, we must open our minds to the idea that other cultures and countries have valid ways of preventing and curing diseases. Although the information may be new to us, many of these traditions are hundreds or even thousands of years old and have long been part of the medical mainstream in other cultures. This information could be useful for Western countries. The nurse should inquire about healing modalities the client may have used previously (see Assessment Interview).

SYSTEMATIZED HEALTH CARE PRACTICES   A number of health care practices have been systematized throughout

ASSESSMENT INTERVIEW | **Complementary and Alternative Therapies**

- Tell me about your use of teas, herbs, vitamins, or other natural products to improve your health.
- What traditional or folk remedies are used in your family?
- Do you meditate, pray, or use relaxation techniques, music, or yoga for healing purposes?
- What alternative therapies have you used (acupuncture, touch therapies, magnets, hypnosis, etc.)?

TABLE 5–2   **Examples of Cultural Health Care Practices**

TYPE OF SYSTEM	VIEW OF ILLNESS	EMPHASIS	VIEW OF HEALTH	INTERVENTIONS
Ayurveda (India)	State of imbalance in body systems	Interdependence of health and quality of societal life	Mental health – good memory, comprehension, intelligence, and reasoning ability Emotional health – evenly balanced emotional state and sense of well-being Physical health – abundant energy and proper functioning of senses, digestion, and elimination	Lifestyle interventions are major preventive and therapeutic approach
Traditional Chinese Medicine	Imbalance or interruption in the flow of qi	Mind, body, spirit, and emotions are never separated	Balance of qi Body's organ systems have a physical, emotional, spiritual, and psychological function	Herbal medicine, acupuncture, acupressure, massage, heat therapy, qigong, t'ai chi, and nutritional lifestyle counseling
Native American Healing	Illness begins in the head; must get rid of ideas that predispose to illness. If the mind is negative, the body will be drained	Spirituality and medicine are inseparable	Balance or harmony of mind and body, requires being in harmony with all things	Medicine women and men act as channels through which Great Power helps others achieve well-being Health care often dispensed through a ritual or ceremony with healer entering into a loving and compassionate relationship with client and they join or merge as process unfolds Use of sweat lodge, singing, pipe ceremony, sun dance, and vision question
Curanderism (Latin American)	Disease is caused by social, psychological, physical, and spiritual factors that can come from natural or supernatural forces	Encompasses mind, body, spirit, and soul	Health is achieved by maintaining balance such as hot and cold or the spiritual and physical	Use of plant remedies, loving-touch massage, prayer, channeling of advice from helpful spirits, and heart-to-heart talks in addition to Western medical practices Practices are local, with different practices in different areas

TABLE 5–3	Botanical Healing

TYPE OF HEALING	DESCRIPTION
Herbal Medicine	Use of plants and their derivatives for treating disease. While many Western medications originated from herbs and plants, not all plant life is beneficial. Most present no danger if taken appropriately, but clients should be encouraged to inform health providers of what herbal supplements they are taking because they can interact with other medications or cause side effects if taken in excess or over a prolonged period of time. Practice Guidelines lists cautions and contraindications for popular herbal preparations.
Aromatherapy	Therapeutic use of essential oils of plants in which fragrance plays an important part. Chemicals found in the essential oils are absorbed into the body resulting in physiologic or psychologic benefits. Different oils may calm, stimulate, or boost the immune system. Table 5–4 lists helpful oils.
Homeopathy	Self-healing system assisted by small doses of remedies or medicines used for a variety of acute and chronic disorders, developed by Samuel Hahnemann. The law of similars claims a natural substance that produces a given symptom in a healthy person cures a sick person if taken in very small amounts. Natural healing compounds are prepared through a process of serial dilution.
Naturopathy	A system of medicine and way of life with emphasis on client responsibility, client education, health maintenance, and disease prevention. It may be the model of the future. Naturopathic physicians are educated in a manner similar to conventional medical education holding the same view of human physiology, body functions, and disease processes, but naturopathic physicians do not provide emergency care or perform surgery, rarely prescribing drugs and treating clients in private practice or outpatient clinics. The goal of treatment is restoration of health and normal body function using many different complementary and alternative medicine therapies, using the least invasive interventions possible, including dietetics, therapeutic nutrition, herbs, physical therapy, spinal manipulation, acupuncture, lifestyle counseling, stress management, exercise therapy, homeopathy, and hydrotherapy.

TABLE 5–4	Helpful Oils to Have at Home

OIL	USE
Chamomile	Soothes muscle aches, sprains, swollen joints; GI antispasmodic; rub on abdomen for colic, indigestion, gas; decreases anxiety, stress-related headaches; decreases insomnia; can be used with children
Eucalyptus	Feels cool to skin and warm to muscles; decreases fever; relieves pain; anti-inflammatory; antiseptic, antiviral, and expectorant to respiratory system in steam inhalation; boosts immune system
Ginger	Helps ward off colds; calms upset stomach, decreases nausea; soothes sprains, muscle spasms
Jasmine	Uplifting and stimulating, antidepressant; massage abdomen and lower back for menstrual cramps
Lavender	Calming, sedative for insomnia; massage around temples for headache; inhale to speed recovery from colds, flu; massage chest to decrease congestion; heals burns
Tea Tree	First-aid kit in a bottle; antifungal, good for athlete's foot; soothes insect bites, stings, cuts, wounds; in bath for yeast infection; drops on handkerchief for coughs, congestion

the centuries and throughout the world. These typically include an entire set of values, attitudes, and beliefs that generate a philosophy of life, not simply a group of remedies (Table 5–2).

BOTANICAL HEALING   Botanical (plant) healings are used by 80% of the world's population. These include herbs, aromatherapy, **homeopathy,** and **naturopathy** (see Tables 5–3 and 5–4 and Practice Guidelines).

NUTRITIONAL THERAPY   Nutritional therapy consists of the consumption of specific types of diets (see Chapter 31 ∞) or supplements, including vitamins, minerals, amino acids, herbs and other botanicals, and miscellaneous substances such as enzymes and fish oils for the purpose of preventing or treating illness. Supplements are not considered medications. The Dietary Supplement Health and Education Act of 1994 requires that the companies selling these products determine their safety, but they are not required to publicize this information or to inform the Food and Drug Administration of reports of adverse reactions.

There are three major concerns for clients' use of nutritional supplements: efficacy, consistency, and safety. Often, research conducted to determine the effectiveness of supplements has been flawed in design or produced conflicting results. Nurses should assist clients in gathering reliable information about supplements such as information available from the National Institutes of Health Office of Dietary Supplements website. Supplements are manufactured by many different companies and often contain a variety of substances in varying amounts. The specific amount of a substance needed to produce the desired effect may not be known, and there is no guarantee that each dose (pill, capsule, tablet, or

Cautions and Contraindications for Popular Herbal Preparations

- Feverfew, garlic, ginger, and ginkgo may increase the anticoagulant effects of aspirin and anticoagulant medications.
- Echinacea may reduce the effectiveness of immunosuppressants. It has not been found effective in treating colds in children ages 2 to 11 (Taylor et al., 2003).
- Garlic may cause a need for an increased dose of antihypertensives.
- Ginseng may interact with caffeine and cause irritability. It may decrease the effectiveness of glaucoma medications.

- Milk thistle reduces the effectiveness of oral contraceptives.
- St. John's wort may potentiate antidepressant medications, causing severe agitation, nausea, confusion, and possible cardiac problems.
- Saw palmetto may give false low prostate-specific antigen (PSA) levels, thereby delaying diagnosis of prostate cancer.
- Valerian may increase the sedative effects of antianxiety medication.

liquid) contains a consistent amount of the substance. There are no legal definitions of the words *standardized, certified,* or *verified* for supplements. As mentioned in the discussion of herbs, not all supplements are harmless. Some supplements cause adverse effects such as diarrhea or high blood pressure, while others become dangerous when taken in combination with certain medications (see Practice Guidelines). Another safety concern with supplements is that they may contain contamination with dangerous substances such as mold, bacteria, pesticides, and metals (Rolfes, Pinna, & Whitney, 2008). Nurses must assess clients for use of dietary supplements and include teaching about the known benefits and risks of supplements in the care planning.

MANUAL HEALING METHODS   Manual healing methods include chiropractic, massage, and other modalities (Table 5–5).

The three most prominent therapies using the hands to alter the biofield, or energy field, are therapeutic touch (TT), healing touch (HT), and Reiki. All three approaches could be simply defined as the use of the hands on or near the body with the intention to help or to heal. The goals are to accelerate the person's own healing process and to facilitate healing at all levels of body, mind, emotions, and spirit. All three are forms of treatment and are not designed to diagnose physical conditions. Nor are they meant to replace conventional surgery, medicine, or drugs in treating organic disease.

MIND–BODY THERAPIES   In mind–body therapies, individuals focus on realigning or creating balance in mental processes to bring about healing. These therapies include yoga, meditation, hypnotherapy, guided imagery, biofeedback, qigong, t'ai chi, and Pilates.

Yoga has been practiced for thousands of years in India, where it is a way of life that includes ethical models for behavior and mental and physical exercises aimed at producing spiritual enlightenment. It is a method for life that can complement and enhance any system of religion, or it can be practiced completely apart from religion. The Western approach to yoga tends to be more fitness oriented with the goal of managing stress, learning to relax, and increasing vitality and well-being. Even

for those who are inactive and out of shape, sick, or weak, sets of easy exercises can help to loosen the joints and stimulate circulation. If practiced regularly, these simple exercises alone make a great difference in people's health and well-being.

Beginning research indicates people with diabetes who practice yoga may increase the release of insulin from the pancreas (Manjunatha, Vempati, Ghosh, & Bijlani, 2005). Other research demonstrates that yoga as a lifestyle intervention reduces oxidative stress which is increased in a variety of chronic degenerative diseases (Yadav, Ray, Vempati, & Bijlani, 2005). People with exercise-induced bronchoconstriction experience a significant improvement after 40 days of 90 minutes of yoga in the morning and 60 minutes in the evening (Jaber, 2002).

Meditation is a general term for a wide range of practices that involve relaxing the body and easing the mind. Meditation is a process that anyone can use to calm themselves, cope with stress, and, for those with spiritual inclinations, feel as one with God or the universe. Meditation can be practiced individually or in groups and is easy to learn. It requires no change in belief system and is compatible with most religious practices. Meditation often involves progressive relaxation exercises (Box 5–11).

If practiced regularly, such as 20 minutes twice a day, meditation produces widespread positive effects on physical and psychologic functioning. The autonomic nervous system responds with a decrease in heart rate, lower blood pressure, decreased respiratory rate and oxygen consumption, and a lower arousal threshold. Meditation's residual effects—improved stress-coping abilities—are a protection against daily stress and anxiety. All other self-healing methods are improved with the practice of meditation.

Hypnotherapy is the application of hypnosis in a wide variety of medical and psychologic disorders. Hypnosis is a trance state or an altered state of consciousness in which an individual's concentration is focused and distraction is minimized. People in trances are aware of what is going on around them but choose not to focus on it and can return to normal awareness whenever they choose. Hypnosis is not a surrender of control; it is only an advanced form of relaxation. Hyp-

TABLE 5–5 Examples of Manual Healing Methods

TYPE OF HEALING METHOD	BELIEF REGARDING HEALTH	BELIEF REGARDING DISEASE	INTERVENTIONS TO TREAT DISEASE	OUTCOMES
Chiropractic	Health is a state of balance, especially of the nervous and musculoskeletal system. When the spine is aligned, energy flows freely to all body cells and organs, nurturing the body's innate ability to work effectively.	Range of motion is improved when fibrous adhesions within joints are broken or small tags from the joint capsule are released through manipulation. Mechanicoreceptors in the joint are stimulated through manipulation, resulting in relaxation of the paraspinal muscles.	Spinal adjustment	Reduce or eliminate pain. Correct spinal dysfunction. Preventive maintenance to reduce recurrence of problems
Massage	Massage is believed to: Relieve muscle tension. Reduce muscle spasm. Improve joint flexibility and range of motion. Improve posture. Lower blood pressure. Slow heart rate. Promote deeper and easier breathing. Improve the health of the skin. Reduce anxiety/relaxation	Massage speeds the removal of metabolic waste products from exercise or inactivity allowing more oxygen and nutrients to reach the cells and tissues. Release of muscle tension helps unblock and balance the overall flow of life energy throughout the body.	Massage – strong, sustained touch	In addition to the physical benefits, massage also satisfies the need for caring and nurturing touch, increasing feelings of well-being, decreasing depression, and enhancing self-image
Acupuncture, acupressure, reflexology	Rooted in the concept of qi, or life energy, that flows through the body along pathways known as meridians forming tiny whirlpools close to the skin surface at places called acupuncture points. These points function somewhat like a gate to moderate the flow of qi.	When the flow of energy becomes blocked or congested, people experience pain, frustration, irritability, or a sense of vulnerability. Applying pressure or stimulating specific points on the body, known as acupuncture points, relieves pain, cures certain diseases, and promotes wellness.	Acupuncture uses needles. Acupressure uses finger pressure. Reflexology is acupressure performed on the feet primarily but may also include manipulation of the hands or ears	Research has indicated acupuncture improves memory, orientation, and activities of daily living for those with certain types of dementia (Yu, Zhang, Liu, Meng, & Han, 2006). Clinical trials have demonstrated effectiveness for osteoarthritis (Novey, 2002), and fibromyalgia (Singh et al., 2006).

notherapy can be used to help people gain self-control, improve self-esteem, and become more autonomous. In some medical facilities, hypnosis is routinely used with a variety of conditions, usually in conjunction with other forms of medical, surgical, psychiatric, or psychologic treatment. It can be used with nonmedical clients as well, in working through problems of living or situations of performance anxiety, and in changing bad habits. Depending on the complexity and seriousness of the complaint, treatment typically runs from two to ten sessions.

Guided imagery is a state of focused attention, much like hypnosis, that encourages changes in attitudes, behavior, and physiologic reactions. Guided imagery can help us learn how to stop troublesome thoughts and focus on images that help us relax and decrease the negative impact of stressors. In guided imagery, the images may be created by the therapist based on the needs and desires of the client. Clients can also create the images as a way to understand the meaning of symptoms or to access inner resources. Imagery stimulates changes in many body functions such as heart rate, blood pressure, respiratory patterns, brain wave rhythms and patterns, electrical characteristics of the skin, local blood flow and temperature, gastrointestinal motility and secretions, sexual arousal, and levels of various hormones and

RESEARCH
NOTES

Can Massage Help Renal Clients' Sleep Disturbances?

It is common for persons living with end-stage renal disease (ESRD) to report occurrences of sleep disturbances. Due to this recurring problem, the purpose of this study was to test the effectiveness of acupoints massage for clients with ESRD experiencing sleep disturbances and diminished quality of life. Ninety-eight participants were recruited for this double-blind, randomized control trial. Participants were randomized into the treatment group (receiving acupressure per protocol plus usual care), placebo group (receiving sham acupressure plus usual care), or control group (usual care).

Results of the study indicated significant differences between the acupressure and control groups in subjective sleep quality, sleep duration, habitual sleep efficiency, and sleep sufficiency. The sham acupressure group did report improvements in subjective sleep quality but not as great compared with the participants in the acupressure group.

Implications

Nurses caring for persons living with ESRD may use the data from this study in addressing sleep problems with nonpharmacological interventions. Acupoints massage can be considered a rapid and effective intervention in promoting an enhanced quality of life for persons with ESRD.

Note: From "Acupoints massage in improving the quality of sleep and quality of life in patients with end-stage renal disease," by S. L. Tsay, J. R. Rong, and P. F. Lin, 2003, *Journal of Advanced Nursing, 42*(2), pp. 134–142. Contributed by Dolores Huffman, PhD, RN, Associate Professor of Nursing, Purdue University Calumet.

BOX 5–11   Guidelines for Progressive Relaxation

- Sit comfortably in a chair, with your feet flat on the ground.
- Tense and tighten your right fist. Focus on the feeling of tension as you do so.
- Allow the muscles in your right fist to relax. Contrast the difference in feeling from tension to relaxation.
- Repeat the preceding two steps for the left fist.
- Now tense and relax both your left and right fists.
- Focus on and relish the feeling of relaxation.
- Now tighten the muscles in both fists and both arms. Feel the tension, fully relax the muscles, and again focus on the sensation of relaxation.

- Progressively tighten and relax each muscle group in the body: toes, ankles, knees, buttocks and groin, stomach and lower back muscles, chest and upper back muscles, shoulders, forehead, jaw muscles.
- Couple deep breathing with progressive relaxation. While relaxing your muscles, inhale deeply, send the breath to the fist (or other muscle group), and exhale.

The entire exercise should last a minimum of 10 minutes.

---

neurotransmitters. The American Holistic Nurses Association and an organization called Beyond Ordinary Nursing offer a nurses' certificate program in imagery.

Biofeedback is a method for learned control of physiologic responses of the body. It is a relaxation technique that uses electronic equipment to amplify the electrochemical energy produced by body responses. Normally out of conscious awareness, biofeedback provides perceptible information that individuals can use to gain voluntary control over various physiologic processes such as blood flow in the hands, sweat gland activity, insomnia, muscle spasms, hyperventilation, gastrointestinal symptoms, and incontinence.

Qigong and t'ai chi are two of a number of therapies focus on movement, body awareness, and breathing; their purpose is to maintain health as well as to correct specific problems. Qigong (pronounced *chee goong*) is a Chinese discipline consisting of breathing and mental exercises combined with body movements. T'ai chi (pronounced *teye chee*) arose out of qigong and is a discipline that combines physical fitness, meditation, and self-defense. Both disciplines consist of soft, slow, continuous movements that are circular in nature. The softness of movements develops energy without nervousness. The slowness of movements requires attentive control that quiets the mind and develops one's powers of awareness and concentration. The continuous circular nature of the movements develops strength and endurance. Almost anyone can participate in movement-oriented therapies, which can be done alone, in pairs, or in large groups.

Pilates (pronounced *pih lah' tees*) is a method of physical movement and exercise designed to stretch, strengthen, and balance the body, in particular the core or center including the abdominal region. It is based in principles of yoga, Zen meditation, and ancient Greek and Roman physical regimens. Exercises, coupled with focused breathing patterns, are done on the floor or with simple types of equipment. Benefits include increased lung capacity, improved flexibility and joint health, muscular coordination, increased bone density, and better posture and balance. Pilates can help rehabilitate back, knee, hip, shoulder, and stress injuries, and relieve muscle aches.

SPIRITUAL THERAPY   Health care sciences have begun to demonstrate that spirituality, faith, and religious commitment may play a role in promoting health and reducing illness. For more information about spirituality, see Chapter 28 ∞.

Within the context of **faith and prayer,** faith refers to our beliefs and expectations about life, ourselves, and others. In a religious context, faith refers to a belief in a supreme being who listens and responds to people and who cares about their well-being. In a spiritual context, faith is thought of as the power to accept the nature of life as it is and live in the present moment. It is a sense of letting go of the need to control while trusting and waiting for the moment when answers come.

Prayer is most often defined simply as a form of communication and fellowship with the deity or creator. It is also defined as an "active process of appealing to a higher spiritual power, specifically for health reasons" when used within CAM (Barnes, Powell-Griner, McFann, & Nahin, 2004). The universality of prayer is evidenced by all cultures having some form of prayer. Prayer has been and continues to be used in times of difficulty and illness even in the most secular societies. Prayer is a self-care strategy that provides comfort, increases hope, and promotes healing and psychologic well-being (Dijoseph & Cavendish, 2005; Hampton & Weinert, 2006).

MISCELLANEOUS THERAPIES   There are some therapies that do not fit into any of the preceding categories. These include music therapy, humor and laughter, bioelectromagnetics, detoxifying therapies, and animal-assisted therapy.

Music Therapy   Using music to improve health recognizes the balance or harmony of body, mind, and spirit. In a state of optimal health, all frequencies are in harmony, like a finely tuned piano. In fact, music is often used in healing, from the ancient sounds of the drum, rattle, bone flute, and other primitive instruments to the use of current music as a prescription for health.

Music therapy can be used in a variety of practice settings. Quiet, soothing music without words is often used to induce relaxation. Music recordings are often used to relax and distract clients in operative settings, intensive care units, birthing rooms, rehabilitation and physical therapy units, and sleep induction units.

Humor and Laughter   Health care professionals recently have focused on the positive effects of humor and laughter on health and disease, although Florence Nightingale wrote about the therapeutic effects of laughing in 1860. Humor involves the ability to discover, express, or appreciate the comical or bizarre, to be amused by one's own imperfections or the whimsical aspects of life, and to see the funny side of an otherwise serious situation. Humor in nursing is defined as helping the client "to perceive, appreciate, and express what is funny, amusing, or ludicrous in order to establish relationships, relieve tension, release anger, facilitate learning, or cope with painful feelings" (Bulecheck, Butcher, & Dochterman,

2008, p. 409). Elaboration of these functions of humor in nursing situations follows:

- *Establishing relationships.* Humor decreases the social distance between persons and assists in putting persons at ease. When tension is decreased, people can focus on the message and on other people rather than on their own feelings. Use of humor helps the nurse establish rapport with clients, an important factor in achieving success in nursing interventions.
- *Relieving tension and anxiety.* The effective use of humor relieves the tension of emotionally charged events. The personal nature of humor, for example, helps clients deal with the impersonal nature of wearing a hospital gown and numbered ID band and with embarrassing questions and uncomfortable tests. People can also use humor prophylactically to decrease stress.
- *Releasing anger and aggression.* Humor helps individuals act out impulses or feelings in a safe and nonthreatening manner. It dissipates feelings of anger and aggression by focusing on the comic elements of a situation.
- *Facilitating learning.* Many lectures and presentations begin with a joke or cartoon. Humor not only reduces the presenter's anxiety but also gains the audience's attention. People learn more when humor is used and anxiety levels are reduced. People also recall more information when they associate information with a joke. Use of humor in instruction, however, needs to be carefully planned so that it will contribute to learning.
- *Coping with painful feelings.* People may use humor to blunt the immediate effect of situations that are too painful, such as the effect of a threatening diagnosis or treatment. Humor diminishes anxiety and fear and reduces tension, thus enabling the person to confront and deal with the situation (Christie & Moore, 2005).

Humor also has physiologic benefits that involve alternating states of stimulation and relaxation. Laughter stimulates increases in respiratory rate, heart rate, muscular tension, and oxygen exchange. A state of relaxation follows laughter, during which heart rate, blood pressure, respiration, and muscle tension decrease. Humor stimulates the production of catecholamines and hormones. It also releases endorphins, thereby increasing pain tolerance.

Humor brings out and integrates people's positive emotions: hope, faith, will to live, festivity, purpose, and determination. It therefore has healing properties. To use humor effectively, nurses need to be aware of their own feelings as well as the feelings of others and cultural variations in what people consider humorous.

Many health care settings are now interested in providing humor as a caring skill and have recognized that "laughter is the best medicine." "Humor rooms" are being created for clients and staff that are supplied with items such as games, funny audiotapes and videotapes, humorous books, and collections of cartoons.

Bioelectromagnetics   Bioelectromagnetics is the emerging science that studies how living organisms interact with electromagnetic fields. It works on the principle that every animal, plant, and mineral has an electromagnetic field that enables organic beings and inorganic objects, such as crystals, to communicate and interact as part of a single, unified energy system. Magnetic fields are able to penetrate the body and affect the functioning of cells, tissues, organs, and systems. These therapies work best in combination with other healing modalities and are considered to be adjunct treatments to conventional medicine. Magnets are used to relieve joint pain and headaches, to speed up healing of wounds by increasing blood flow, and to improve bone repair (Wolsko et al., 2004).

Contraindications for magnetic therapy include pregnancy, pacemakers, implanted defibrillators, aneurysm clips in the brain, cochlear implants, or other implanted electrical devices. They should not be used by people on anticoagulants, those with an actively bleeding or open wound, or those with a freshly torn muscle.

Infrared Photoenergy Therapy   Infrared photoenergy therapy is a safe and effective treatment to improve sensory impairment associated with peripheral neuropathy. The treatments are given with the Anodyne Therapy System three to five times a week for two weeks. It is believed that the treatment works by increasing energy inside cells, as well as by improving circulation. Research demonstrates improved sensation in the feet, less pain, and improved balance (Leonard, Farooqi, & Myers, 2004).

Detoxifying Therapies   Many cultures and religions, past and present, have rituals of purification. In Western cultures, some people are currently fascinated with the concept of detoxification, the belief that physical impurities and toxins must be cleared from the body to achieve better health. The use of water as a healing treatment is known as *hydrotherapy* used to decrease pain, decrease fever, reduce swelling, reduce cramps, induce sleep, and improve physical and mental tone. It must be used with great care in the very young or old who have poor heat regulation and also with people experiencing a prolonged illness or fatigue. *Colonics,* or colon therapy, is based on the idea that high-fat, Western diets lead to an accumulation of a thick, glue-like substance in the colon, which in turn produces toxins that lead to disease. Colonics is the procedure for washing the inner wall of the colon by filling it with water or herbal solutions and then draining it.

Chelation Therapy   Chelation therapy is the introduction of chemicals into the bloodstream that bind with heavy metals in the body. Ethylene diamine tetraacetic acid (EDTA) is a synthetic amino acid that readily binds to lead. The U.S. Federal Drug Administration has approved EDTA for the treatment of lead poisoning, hypercalcemia, and ventricular fibrillation secondary to digitalis toxicity.

Animal-Assisted Therapy   Animal-assisted therapy is the use of specifically selected animals as a treatment modality in health and human service settings. It has been shown to be a successful intervention for people with a variety of physical or psychologic conditions. Throwing an object for a dog to retrieve or brushing the animal increases upper extremity range of motion. Reaching for the object the dog has retrieved improves coordination. Ambulating with a dog improves mobility. Recalling the animal's name helps with memory. Using simple commands increases language production. Attending to the animal and the situation increases attention and concentration. Therapeutic horseback riding, or hippotherapy, is the use of the rhythmic movement of the horse to increase sensory processing and improve posture, balance, and mobility in people with movement dysfunctions. See the Long-Term Care Consideration box.

Horticultural Therapy   Horticultural therapy, also called gardening or a healing garden, is an adjunct therapy to occupational and physical therapy. People may view nature, visit a healing garden or a wander garden, or actually participate in gardening. When it is a communal activity, gardening decreases social isolation by fostering interactions with others. Horticultural therapy stimulates the five senses, provides leisure activities, improves motor function, provides a sense of achievement, and improves self-esteem (Detweiler & Warf, 2005; Milligan, Gatrell, & Bingley, 2004).

LONG-TERM CARE CONSIDERATION
Resident Animals

Resident animals live at long-term health care facilities. Species include fish, birds, hamsters, gerbils, guinea pigs, rabbits, cats, and dogs. Some staff report that full-time pets become so perceptive that they actually gravitate to the rooms of people who are the most isolated or depressed. Those residents who have regular visits are more receptive to treatment, have a greater incentive to recover, and have an increased will to live (*Animals in Residential Facilities*, 2003). The contributions companion animals (personal pets) make to the emotional well-being of people include providing unconditional love and opportunities for affection; achievement of trust, responsibility, and empathy toward others; a reason to get up in the morning; and a source of reassurance.

CHAPTER HIGHLIGHTS

- Nursing involves viewing the client as an individual in a holistic way.
- Homeostasis is the tendency of the body to maintain a state of relative balance or constancy in response to a changing internal and external environment. Physiologic homeostasis is maintained by coordinated functioning of the autonomic nervous, endocrine, respiratory, cardiovascular, renal, and gastrointestinal systems. Psychologic homeostasis, or emotional well-being, is acquired or learned through the experience of living and interacting with others.
- Although each individual has unique characteristics, certain needs are common to all people.
- Maslow's hierarchy of human needs consists of five categories: physiologic (survival) needs, safety needs, love and belonging needs, self-esteem needs, and self-actualization needs.
- *Healthy People 2010* (USDHHS, 2000) presents a comprehensive 10-year strategy for promoting health and preventing illness of both individuals and communities.
- Health promotion is defined as client behavior directed toward developing well-being and actualizing human health potential. Health protection is client behavior geared toward preventing illness, detecting it early, or maintaining function.
- The nurse's role in health promotion is to act as a facilitator of the process of assessing, evaluating, and understanding health. It is the opportunity for nurses to strengthen the profession's influence on health promotion, disseminate information that promotes an educated public, and assist individuals and communities to change long-standing adverse health behaviors.
- Nurses need to clarify their understanding of health because their definitions of health largely determine the scope and nature of nursing practice. Likewise, people's health beliefs influence their health practices.
- Wellness is an active, seven-dimensional process of becoming aware of and making choices toward a higher level of well-being. The seven dimensions of wellness are the physical, social, emotional, intellectual, spiritual, occupational, and environmental dimensions.
- Well-being is considered a subjective perception of balance, harmony, and vitality. It is a state rather than a process.
- Because notions of health are highly individual, the nurse must determine a client's perception of health in order to

provide meaningful assistance. This involves well-developed communication skills. Nurses need to be aware of their own personal definitions of health.
- Health belief and behavior models have been developed to help determine whether an individual is likely to participate in disease prevention and health promotion activities. Two of these are the locus of control model and Rosenstock's and Becker's health belief models.
- A person's decision to implement health behaviors or to take action to improve health depends on such factors as the importance of health to the person, perceived threat of a particular disease or severity of the health care problems, perceived benefits of preventive or therapeutic actions, inconvenience and unpleasantness involved, degree of lifestyle change necessary, cultural ramifications, and cost.
- Nurses can enhance health care adherence by identifying the reasons for nonadherence if it occurs, demonstrating caring, using positive reinforcement to encourage healthy behaviors, using aids to reinforce teaching, and establishing a therapeutic relationship of freedom, mutual understanding, and mutual responsibility with the client and support persons.
- An individual's usual pattern of behavior changes with illness and hospitalization, which disrupt a person's privacy, autonomy, lifestyle, roles, and finances.
- Nurses need to be aware that the illness of one member of a family affects all other members.
- The concepts common to most alternative practices include holism, humanism, balance, spirituality, energy, and healing environments.
- We create healing environments when we provide holistic nursing care, take time to be with clients in deeply caring ways, and balance technology and compassion.
- If we do not create healing environments for ourselves, we are in danger of nursing "burnout."
- Ancient health care practices typically include an entire set of values, attitudes, and beliefs that generate a philosophy of life, not simply a group of remedies. Biomedicine is reductionistic rather than holistic.
- Mind–body therapies such as yoga, meditation, hypnotherapy, guided imagery, biofeedback, qigong, t'ai chi, and Pilates all focus on realigning or creating balance in mental and physical processes to bring about healing.

THINK ABOUT IT

Refer to the chapter-opening scenario and answer these questions.

1. How do Mrs. Gracely's health care beliefs influence her health and health care behaviors?

2. When assessing Mrs. Gracely, what questions might you ask before attempting to discuss prevention and promotion strategies?

3. How might you overcome Mrs. Gracely's cynicism regarding health care providers in order to help her improve her lifestyle choices regarding health promotion?

4. What CAM therapies might you recommend for Mrs. Gracely?

∞ *See suggested responses to Think About It on MyNursingKit.*

TEST YOUR KNOWLEDGE

1. While hospitalized, a client is very worried about business activities. The client spends a great deal of time on the phone and with colleagues instead of resting. Which of the following principles of need therapy applies?
1. His higher level need cannot be met unless the lower level physiologic need is met.
2. His lower level physiologic needs are being deferred while higher needs are addressed.
3. The higher need takes precedence and the lower need no longer must be met.
4. It is necessary for someone else to meet his higher-level needs so he can focus on the lower-level need.

2. A client who is 46 pounds overweight tells you, "I was just born to be fat. I don't have the willpower." Although weight loss occurred while attending two previous programs that "guaranteed" weight loss, the weight returned along with extra pounds after each program. According to the Health Promotion Model, the nurse is most likely to focus on which of the following behavior-specific cognitions and affects variable for this client?
1. Perceived barriers to action
2. Perceived self-efficacy
3. Interpersonal influences
4. Situational influences

3. Which of the following individuals would have an increased possibility of illness in the near future?
1. A 25-year-old man who recently married his high school sweetheart
2. A 35-year-old man who broke up with the girl he had dated for six months
3. A 40-year-old woman who started a nursing program
4. A 50-year-old woman whose husband died a month ago

4. The nurse, assisting a client in the action stage of change, would use which of the following strategies?
1. Reinforce the importance of providing rewards for positive behavior.
2. Ask the client if he or she would like information.
3. Guide the client to create a plan of action.
4. Remind the client of previous successes.

5. If a client fails to follow the information or teaching provided, how should the nurse respond?
1. Give up, as the client doesn't want to change.
2. Develop a tough approach.
3. Reteach the information, as the nurse is the expert.
4. Reassess the client's importance given to the behavior and readiness to change it.

6. The nurse recognizes which of the following as an example of the emotional component of wellness?
1. The client chooses health foods.
2. A new father decides to take parenting classes.
3. A client expresses frustration with her partner's substance abuse.
4. A widow with no family decides to join a bowling league.

7. Which one of the following individuals appears to have "taken on" the sick role?
1. An obese client states, "I deserve to have a heart attack."
2. A mother is ill and says, "I won't be able to make your lunch today."
3. A man with low back pain misses several physical therapy appointments.
4. An older adult states, "My horoscope says I will be well again."

8. A client asks the nurse the differences between traditional therapies and alternative therapies. Which of the following is the best response?
1. Alternative therapies cost less than traditional therapies.
2. Alternative therapies are used if traditional therapies are ineffective.
3. Alternative therapies can be as effective as traditional therapies for some conditions.
4. Alternative therapies utilize products from nature but traditional therapies do not.

9. Before meeting with a client with a terminal illness, a new graduate nurse reviews information on spirituality. Which of the following is the *best* explanation of spirituality?
1. That which gives people purpose and meaning in their lives
2. A formalized religious dogma
3. A nondenominational community service
4. People being responsible for their life patterns

10. In which of the following ways do nurses create healing environments?
1. Use technology to prevent hospital-acquired infections.
2. Empower clients to make healthy decisions for themselves.
3. Place aquariums in day rooms of nursing homes.
4. Ensure that physicians' orders are carried out.

∞ *See answers to Test Your Knowledge in Appendix A.*

REFERENCES AND SELECTED BIBLIOGRAPHY

American Nurses Association. (1980). *Nursing: A social policy statement.* Kansas City, MO: Author.

American Nurses Association. (2003). *Nursing: A social policy statement* (2nd ed.). Kansas City, MO: Author.

American Nurses Association. (2004). *Nursing: Scope and standards of practice.* Washington, DC: Author.

Animals in residential facilities: Guidelines and resources for success. (2003). Renton, WA: Delta Society.

Anspaugh, D. J., Hamrick, M., & Rosato, F. D. (2006). *Wellness: Concepts and applications* (6th ed.). New York: McGraw-Hill.

Baldwin, J. H., & Conger, C. O. (2001). Health promotion and wellness. In K. S. Lundy & S. Janes (Eds.), *Community health nursing: Caring for the public's health* (pp. 286–307). Boston: Jones & Bartlett.

Barnes, P. M., Powell-Griner, E., McFann, K., & Nahin, R. L. (2004). Complementary and alternative medicine use among adults, United States, 2002. *Advance Data from Vital and Health Statistics*, no. 343. Hyattsville, MD: Anderson National Center for Health Statistics.

Becker, M. H. (Ed.). (1974). *The health belief model and personal health behavior.* Thorofare, NJ: Charles B. Slack.

Benson, H., Dusek, J. A., Sherwood, J. B., Lam, P., Bethea, C. F., Carpenter, W., et al. (2006). The Study of Therapeutic Effects of Intercessory Prayer (STEP) in cardiac bypass patients: A multicenter randomized trial of uncertainty and certainty of receiving intercessory prayer. *American Heart Journal, 151*, 934–942.

Brinkhaus, B., Witt, C. M., Jena, S., Linde, K., Streng, A., Wagenpfeil, S., et al. (2006). Acupuncture in patients with chronic low back pain. *Archives of Internal Medicine, 166*, 450–457.

Briss, P. A., Brownson, R. C., Fielding, J. E., & Zaza, S. (2004). Developing and using the Guide to Community Preventive Services: Lessons learned about evidence-based public health. *Annual Review of Public Health, 25*, 281–302.

Bulechek, G. M., Butcher, H. K., & Dochterman, J. M. (Eds.). (2008). *Nursing interventions classification (NIC)* (5th ed.). St. Louis, MO: Mosby.

Bulkeley, K. (2003). *Dreams of healing.* New York: Paulist Press.

Cannon, W. B. (1939). *The wisdom of the body* (2nd ed.). New York: Norton.

Chan, K., Qin, L., Lau, M., Woo, J., Au, S., Choy, W., et al. (2004). A randomized, prospective study of the effects of Tai Chi Chun exercise on bone mineral density in postmenopausal women. *Archives of Physical Medicine and Rehabilitation, 85*, 717–722.

Christie, W., & Moore, C. (2005). The impact of humor on patients with cancer. *Clinical Journal of Oncology Nursing, 9*, 211–218.

Coughlin, S. S., Uhler, R. J., Richards, T., & Wilson, K. M. (2003). Breast and cervical cancer screening practices among Hispanic and non-Hispanic women residing near the United States–Mexico border, 1999–2000. *Family & Community Health, 26*(2), 130–139.

Crawford, P. B., Gosliner, W., Strode, P., Samuels, S. E., Craypo, L., Burnett, C., et al. (2004). Walking the talk: Fit WIC wellness programs improve self-efficacy in pediatric obesity prevention counseling. *American Journal of Public Health, 94*, 1480–1485.

Cross, M. (2004). CDC begins to provide resources for workplace wellness programs. *Managed Care, 13*(6), 54–55.

Denison, B. (2004). Touch the pain away. *Holistic Nursing Practice, 18*(3), 142–151.

Detweiler, M. B., & Warf, C. (2005). Dementia wander garden aids post cerebrovascular stroke restorative therapy. *Alternative Therapies in Health and Medicine, 11*(4), 54–58.

Dijoseph, J., & Cavendish, R. (2005). Expanding the dialogue on prayer relevant to holistic care. *Holistic Nursing Practice, 19*, 147–154.

Dossey, B. M., Keegan, L., & Guzzetta, C. (2004). *Pocket guide for holistic nursing.* Boston: Jones & Bartlett.

Driessnack, M. (2004). Remember me: Mask making with chronically and terminally ill children. *Holistic Nursing Practice, 18*, 211–214.

Dunn, H. L. (1959). High-level wellness for man and society. *American Journal of Public Health, 49*, 786–792.

Edelman, C. L., & Mandle, C. L. (2006). *Health promotion throughout the lifespan* (6th ed.). St. Louis: Mosby.

Fontaine, K. L. (2010). *Complementary & alternative therapies for nursing practice* (3rd ed.). Upper Saddle River, NJ: Pearson Education.

Goode, M., Wales, S., & Crisp, J. (2004). The role of specialist nurses in improving treatment adherence in children with a chronic illness. *Australian Journal of Advanced Nursing, 21*(4), 41–45.

Grunbaum, J. A., Kann, L., Kinchen, S., Ross, J., Hawkings, J., Lowry, R., et al. (2004, May 21). Youth risk behavior surveillance— United States, 2003. *MMWR Surveillance Summaries, 53* (No. SS-2), 1–96.

Gunderson, A. J., & Tomkowiak, J. M. (2004). Dynamic health promotion for the geriatric population. *Rehabilitation Nursing, 29*(2), 45–48.

Hakim, R. M., Newton, R. A., Segal, J., & DuCette, J. P. (2004). A group intervention to reduce fall risk factors in community dwelling older adults. *Physical and Occupational Therapy in Geriatrics, 22*(1), 1–20.

Hampton, J. S., & Weinert, C. (2006). An exploration of spirituality in rural women with chronic illness. *Holistic Nursing Practice, 20*(1), 27–33.

Holmes, T. H., & Rahe, T. H. (1967). The social readjustment rating scale. *Journal of Psychosomatic Research, 11*(8), 213–218.

Hood, L., & Leddy, S. K. (2003). *Leddy & Pepper's conceptual bases of professional nursing* (5th ed.). Philadelphia: Lippincott Williams & Wilkins.

Irwin, M. R., Pike, J. L., Cole, J. C., & Oxman, M. N. (2003). Effects of a behavioral intervention, tai chi chih, on varicella-zoster virus specific immunity and health functioning in older adults. *Psychosomatic Medicine, 65*, 824–830.

Jaber, R. (2002). Respiratory and allergic diseases. *Primary Care, 29*, 231–261.

Johnson, J. L., Kalaw, C., Lovato, C. Y., Baillie, L., & Chambers, N. A. (2004). Crossing the line: Adolescents' experiences of controlling their tobacco use. *Qualitative Health Research, 14*(9), 1276–1291.

Kalish, R. A. (1983). *The psychology of human behavior* (5th ed.). Monterey, CA: Brooks/Cole.

Laverack, G. (2004). *Health promotion practice: Power & empowerment.* Thousand Oaks, CA: Sage.

Leavell, H. R., & Clark, E. G. (1965). *Preventive medicine for the doctor in his community* (3rd ed.). New York: McGraw-Hill.

Lenarz, M. (2003). *The chiropractic way.* New York: Bantam Books.

Leonard, D. R., Farooqi, M. H., & Myers, S. (2004). Restoration of sensation, reduced pain, and improved balance in subjects with diabetic peripheral neuropathy. *Diabetes Care, 27*(1), 168–172.

Leong, J., Molassiotis, A., & Marsh, H. (2004). Adherence to health recommendations after a cardiac rehabilitation programme in post-myocardial infarction patients: The role of health beliefs, locus of control and psychological status. *Clinical Effectiveness in Nursing, 8*(1), 26–38.

Li, F., Fisher, K. J., Harmer, P., Irbe, D., Tearse, R. G., & Weimer, C. (2004). Tai chi and self rated quality of sleep and daytime sleepiness in older adults: A randomized controlled trial. *Journal of the American Geriatrics Society, 52,* 892–900.

Manjunatha, S., Vempati, R. P., Ghosh, D., & Bijlani, R. L. (2005). An investigation into the acute and long-term effects of selected yogic postures on fasting and postprandial glycemia and insulinemia in healthy young subjects. *Indian Journal of Physiology and Pharmacology, 49,* 319–324.

Maslow, A. H. (1968). *Toward a psychology of being* (2nd ed.). New York: Wiley.

Maslow, A. H. (1970). *Motivation and personality* (2nd ed.). New York: Harper& Row.

Milligan, C., Gatrell, A., & Bingley, A. (2004). Cultivating health. *Social Science & Medicine, 58,* 1781–1793.

Moore, T. (2005). Best practice guidelines: An invitation to reflect on therapeutic touch practice. *Journal of Nursing Care Quality, 20*(1), 90–94.

Murray, R. B., & Zentner, J. P., & Yakimo, R. (2008). *Health promotion strategies through the life span* (8th ed.). Upper Saddle River, NJ: Pearson Education.

NANDA International. (2009). *NANDA nursing diagnoses: Definitions and classification 2009–2011.* West Sussex, U.K.: Wiley-Blackwell.

National Center for Complementary and Alternative Medicine. (2004). *Expanding horizons of health care: Strategic plan 2005–2009.* Washington, DC: U.S. Department of Health and Human Services.

National Center for Health Statistics. (2004). *Health, United States, 2004. With chartbook on trends in the health of Americans.* Hyattsville, MD: Author.

Nightingale, F. (1969). *Notes on nursing: What it is, and what it is not.* New York: Dover. (Original work published 1860)

North American Nursing Diagnosis Association. (2007). *Nursing diagnoses: Definitions & classification 2007–2008.* Philadelphia: Author.

Novey, D. W. (2002). Osteoarthritis. *Primary Care, 29,* 263–277.

Ornish, D. (2004). *Dr. Dean Ornish's program for reversing heart disease* (rev. ed.). New York: Ballantine.

Parsons, T. (1951). *The social system.* Glencoe, IL: Free Press.

Parsons, T. (1979). Definitions of health and illness in the light of American values and social structure. In E. G. Jaco (Ed.), *Patients, physicians, and illness* (3rd ed.). New York: Free Press.

Pender, N. J., Murdaugh, C. L., & Parsons, M. J. (2006). *Health promotion in nursing practice* (5th ed.). Upper Saddle River, NJ: Pearson Education.

Potter, P. (2003). What are the distinctions between Reiki and therapeutic touch? *Clinical Journal of Oncology Nursing, 7*(1), 1–3.

President's Commission on Health Needs of the Nation. (1953). *Building Americans'* *health* (Vol. 2). Washington, DC: U.S. Government Printing Office.

Prochaska, J. O., Norcross, J. C., & DiClemente, C. C. (1994). *Changing for good: A revolutionary six-stage program for overcoming bad habits and moving your life positively forward.* New York: Avon Books/Harper Collins.

Prochaska, J. O., Redding, C. A., & Evers, K. E. (2002). The transtheoretical model and stages of change. In *Health behavior and health education: Theory, research, and practice* (3rd ed., pp. 99–120). San Francisco: Jossey-Bass.

Rolfes, S. R., Pinna, K., & Whitney, E. (2008). Understanding normal and clinical nutrition (8th ed.). Belmont, CA: Thomson.

Rollnick, S., Mason, P., & Butler, C. (1999). *Health behavior change. A guide for practitioners.* Edinburgh: Churchill Livingstone.

Rosenstock, I. M. (1974). Historical origins of the health belief model. In M. H. Becker (Ed.), *The health belief model and personal health behavior.* Thorofare, NJ: Charles B. Slack.

Rosina, R., Crisp, J., & Steinbeck, K. (2003). Treatment adherence of youth and young adults with and without a chronic illness. *Nursing & Health Sciences, 5*(2), 139–147.

Roy, C. (1999). *The Roy adaptation model* (2nd ed.). Upper Saddle River, NJ: Prentice Hall.

Saarmann, L., Daugherty, J., & Riegel, B. (2000). Patient teaching to promote behavioral change. *Nursing Outlook, 48*(6), 281–287.

Schenk, S., & Hartley, K. (2002). Nurse coach: Healthcare resource for this millennium. *Nursing Forum, 37*(3), 14–20.

Singh, B. B., Wu, W. S., Hwang, S. H., Khorsan, R., Der-Martirosian, C., Vinjamury, S. P., et al. (2006). Effectiveness of acupuncture in the treatment of fibromyalgia. *Alternative Therapies in Health and Medicine, 12*(2), 34–41.

Stibich, M., & Wissow, L. (2006). Meaning shift: Findings from wellness acupuncture. *Alternative Therapies in Health and Medicine, 12*(2), 42–48.

Substance Abuse and Mental Health Services Administration. (2004). *Results from the 2003 national survey on drug use and health: National findings (Office of Applied Studies, NSDUH Series H-25, DHHS Publications No. SMA 04-3964).* Rockville, MD. U.S. Department of Health and Human Services, Substance Abuse and Mental Health Services Administration, Office of Applied Studies.

Suchman, E. A. (1979). Stages of illness and medical care. In E. G. Jaco (Ed.), *Patients, physicians, and illness* (3rd ed.). New York: Free Press.

Taylor, E. J. (2003). Prayer's clinical issues and implications. *Holistic Nursing Practice, 17,* 179–188.

Taylor, J. A., Weber, W., Standish, L., Quinn, H., Goesling, J., McGann, M., et al. (2003). Efficacy and safety of Echinacea in treating upper respiratory tract infections in children. *Journal of the American Medical Association, 290,* 2824–2830.

Toth, E., Mahumdar, S., Guirguis, L., Lawanczuk, R., Lee, T., & Johnson, J. (2003). Compliance with clinical practice guideline for type 2 diabetes in rural patients: Treatment gaps and opportunities for improvement. *Pharmacotherapy, 23,* 659–665.

Travis, J. W., & Ryan, R. S. (2001). *Simply well.* Berkeley, CA: Ten Speed Press.

Tsay, S. L., Rong, J. R., & Lin, P. F. (2003). Acupoints massage in improving the quality of sleep and quality of life in patients with end-stage renal disease. *Journal of Advanced Nursing, 42*(2), 134–142.

U.S. Department of Health and Human Services. (2000). *Healthy people 2010: Understanding and improving health* (2nd ed.). Washington, DC: U.S. Government Printing Office.

U.S. Surgeon General. (1979). *Healthy people: The surgeon general's report on health promotion and disease prevention* (DHHS Pub. No. 79-55071). Washington, DC: U.S. Government Printing Office.

Wallston, K. A., Stein, M. J., & Smith, C. A. (1994). Form C of the MHLC scales: A condition-specific measure of locus of control. *Journal of Personality Assessment, 63,* 534–553.

Wallston, K. A., Wallston, B. S., & DeVellis, R. (1978, Spring). Development of the Multidimensional Locus of Control (MHLC) scales. *Health Education Monographs, 6,* 160–170.

Wardell, D. W., & Weymouth, K. F. (2004). Review of studies of healing touch. *Journal of Nursing Scholarship, 36,* 147–154.

Wells-Federman, C. L. (1996). Awakening the healer within. *Holistic Nursing Practice, 10,* 13–29.

Wolsko, P. M., Eisenberg, D. M., Simon, L. S., Davis, R. B., Walleczek, J., Mayo Smith, M., et al. (2004). Double blind placebo controlled trial of static magnets for the treatment of osteoarthritis of the knee: Results of a pilot study. *Alternative Therapies in Health and Medicine, 10*(2), 36–43.

World Health Organization. (1948). *Preamble to the constitution of the World Health Organization as adopted by the International Health Conference.* New York, 19–22 June 1946; signed on 22 July 1946 by the representatives of 61 States (Official Records of the World Health Organization, no. 2, p. 100) and entered into force on 7 April 1948.

Wu, A. M., Tang, C. S., & Kwok, T. C. (2004). Self-efficacy, health locus of control, and psychological distress in elderly Chinese women with chronic illnesses. *Aging & Mental Health, 8*(1), 21–28.

Yadav, R. K., Ray, R. B., Vempati, R., & Bijlani, R. L. (2005). Effect of a comprehensive yoga-based lifestyle modification program on lipid peroxidation. *Indian Journal of Physiology and Pharmacology, 49,* 358–362.

Yu, J., Zhang, X., Liu, C., Meng, Y., & Han, J. (2006). Effect of acupuncture treatment on vascular dementia. *Neurological Research, 28,* 97–103.

The Nursing Process

Critical Thinking and Clinical Reasoning

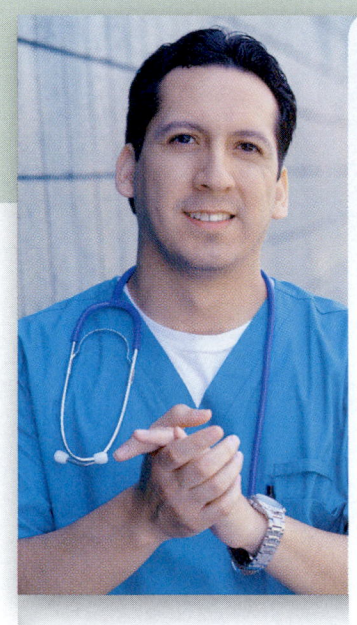

Upon graduating from nursing school Tom passed his NCLEX® examination and was granted a nursing license. Tom soon accepted a position working on a medical unit of an acute care hospital in his community. Many of the clients on the unit had multisystem problems, and most were very sick. After completing a three-month orientation to the facility and the unit, Tom began working night shift with staffing usually consisting of four RNs, two LPNs, and two unlicensed assistive personnel to care for a maximum of 36 clients.

Tonight, Tom entered an assigned client's room and found the client short of breath. Tom applied a pulse oximeter probe to a finger that was cold and mildly cyanotic and obtained a reading of 94%. Tom decided the client's shortness of breath was actually hyperventilation secondary to an invasive procedure scheduled for tomorrow morning, and administered a sedative to relax the client. Two hours later when Tom returned to the room, he found the client pulseless and not breathing. He immediately called for help and started CPR.

LEARNING OUTCOMES

After completing this chapter, you will be able to:

1. Define the key terms.

2. List and define the skills and attitudes of critical thinking.

3. Analyze the requirement for critical thinking in the delivery of safe, effective, and professional nursing practice.

4. Explore the need for critical thinking in the nursing process.

5. Explain how the skills of critical thinking can improve client outcomes.

6. Explore methods of demonstrating critical thinking as a student nurse.

7. Summarize how to use problem-solving, prioritizing, and decision-making skills when making clinical judgments.

8. Demonstrate clinical reasoning and the formation of accurate clinical judgments when caring for clients in the clinical facility or simulation lab.

9. Inventory your strengths and weaknesses as related to the attributes required for clinical success.

Although **critical thinking** has many definitions, one of the most useful for nursing is from the National League for Nursing (2000): "Critical thinking in nursing practice is a discipline specific, reflective **reasoning** process that guides a nurse in generating, implementing, and evaluating approaches for dealing with client care and professional concerns" (p. 2). Nurses are expected to use critical thinking to solve client problems and make better decisions. Thus, critical thinking, problem solving, and decision making are interrelated processes, with creativity enhancing the result. Critical thinking is an essential component to clinical decision making.

CRITICAL THINKING

Critical thinking is essential to safe, competent, skillful nursing practice. The amount of knowledge that nurses must use, and the continuing rapid growth of this knowledge, prevent nurses from being effective practitioners if they attempt to function with only the information acquired in school or outlined in books. Decisions that nurses must make about client care and about the distribution of limited resources force them to think and act in areas where there are neither clear answers nor standard procedures, and where conflicting forces turn decision making into a complex process. Nurses therefore need to embrace the attitudes that promote critical thinking and master critical-thinking skills in order to process and evaluate both previously learned and new information. Box 6–1 lists some reasons supporting the importance of critical thinking.

Nurses use critical-thinking skills in a variety of ways:

- *Nurses use knowledge from other subjects and fields.* Because nurses deal holistically with human responses, they must draw meaningful information from other subject areas in order to understand the meaning of client data and to plan effective interventions. Nursing students take courses in the biologic and social sciences and in the humanities to acquire a strong foundation on which to build their nursing knowledge and skill.
- *Nurses deal with change in stressful environments.* Nurses work in rapidly changing situations. Treatments, medications, and technology change constantly, and a client's condition may change from minute to minute. Routine actions may therefore not be adequate to deal with the situation at hand. Familiarity with the routine for giving medications, for example, does not help the nurse deal with a client who is frightened of injections or one who does not wish to take a medication. When unexpected situations arise, critical thinking enables the nurse to recognize important cues, respond quickly, and adapt interventions to meet specific client needs.
- *Nurses make important decisions.* During the course of a workday, nurses make vital decisions of many kinds. These decisions often determine the well-being of clients and even their very survival, so it is important that the decisions be sound. Nurses use critical thinking to collect and interpret the information

MyNursingKit | Thinking Critically

BOX 6–1   Top 10 Reasons to Improve Thinking

10. Things aren't what they used to be or what they will be.
9. Patients are sicker, with multiple problems.
8. More consumer involvement (patients and families).
7. Nurses must be able to move from one setting to another.
6. Rapid change and information explosion requires us to develop new learning and workplace skills.
5. Consumers and payers demand to see evidence of benefits, efficiency, and results.
4. Today's progress often creates new problems that can't be solved by old ways of thinking.

3. Redesigning care delivery and nursing curricula is useless if students and nurses don't have the thinking skills required to deal with today's world.
2. It can be done—it doesn't have to be that difficult.
1. Your ability to focus your thinking to get the results you need can make the difference between whether you succeed or fail in this fast-paced world.

Note: Reprinted from *Critical Thinking in Nursing: A Practical Approach,* 3rd ed., R. Alfaro-LeFevre, Copyright 2004, with permission from Elsevier.

needed to make decisions. Nurses must use good judgment, for example, to decide which observations must be reported to the primary care provider immediately and which can be noted in the client record for the primary care provider to address later, during a routine visit with the client.

- *Nurses work as part of a team.* In a team exist differing opinions, beliefs, and biases presented regarding clinical decisions. The nurse must be able to accept the information gathered from team members and sort through it using critical thinking in order to make sound decisions regarding client care and nursing practice. Determining who the nurse will use as a resource person when questions arise, who must be carefully supervised, and making appropriate nursing assignments are all situations requiring critical thinking.

Creativity is a major component of critical thinking. When nurses incorporate creativity into their thinking, they are able to find unique solutions to unique problems. **Creativity** is thinking that results in the development of new ideas and products. Creativity in problem solving and decision making is the ability to develop and implement new and better solutions.

Creativity is required when the nurse encounters a new situation or a client situation in which traditional interventions are not effective. For example, a pediatric home health nurse is caring for a 6-year-old girl who has ineffective respirations following abdominal surgery. The primary care provider has ordered incentive spirometry. The child is frightened by the equipment and tires quickly during the treatments. The nurse offers her a bottle of blow bubbles and a blowing wand. She is delighted with blowing bubbles. The nurse knows that the respiratory effort in blowing bubbles will promote alveolar expansion and suggests that she blow bubbles between incentive spirometry treatments.

Creative thinkers must have knowledge of the problem. They must have assessed the present problem and be knowledgeable about the underlying facts and principles that ap-

ply. For example, in the previous situation, the nurse knows the anatomy and physiology of respiratory function and is aware of the purpose of incentive spirometry. The nurse also understands pediatric growth and development. In trying to assist the child, the nurse builds on this knowledge and comes up with a creative solution. Using creativity, nurses:

- Generate many ideas rapidly.
- Are generally flexible and natural; that is, they are able to change viewpoints or directions in thinking.
- Create original solutions to problems.
- Tend to be independent and self-confident, even when under pressure.
- Demonstrate individuality.

Skills in Critical Thinking

Complex mental processes such as analysis, problem solving, and decision making require the use of cognitive critical-thinking skills. These skills include critical analysis, inductive and deductive reasoning, making valid **inferences**, differentiating facts from opinions, evaluating the credibility of information sources, clarifying **concepts**, and recognizing **assumptions**.

Critical analysis is the application of a set of questions to a particular situation or idea to determine essential information and ideas and discard superfluous information and ideas. The questions are not sequential steps; rather, they are a set of criteria for judging an idea. Not all questions must be applied in every situation, but one should be aware of all of the questions in order to choose those questions appropriate to a given situation. Socrates (born about 470 BC) was a Greek philosopher who developed the Socratic method of posing a question and seeking an answer. Box 6–2 lists Socratic questions to use in critical analysis. Socratic questioning is a technique one can use to look beneath the surface, recognize and examine assumptions, search for inconsistencies, examine multiple points of view, and differentiate what one knows from what one merely believes. Nurses should employ So-

---

BOX 6–2	Socratic Questions

Questions about the Question (or Problem)

- Is this question clear, understandable, and correctly identified?
- Is this question important?
- Could this question be broken down into smaller parts?
- How might _____ state this question?

Questions about Assumptions

- You seem to be assuming _____; is that so?
- What could you assume instead? Why?
- Does this assumption always hold true?

Questions about Point of View

- You seem to be using the perspective of _____. Why?
- What would someone who disagrees with your perspective say?
- Can you see this any other way?

Questions about Evidence and Reasons

- What evidence do you have for that?
- Is there any reason to doubt that evidence?
- How do you know?
- What would change your mind?

Questions about Implications and Consequences

- What effect would that have?
- What is the probability that will actually happen?
- What are the alternatives?
- What are the implications of that?

cratic questioning when listening to an end-of-shift report, reviewing a history or progress notes, planning care, assessing a client, or discussing a client's care with colleagues.

Two other critical-thinking skills are inductive and deductive reasoning. In **inductive reasoning**, generalizations are formed from a set of facts or observations. When viewed together, certain bits of information suggest a particular **interpretation**. Inductive reasoning moves from specific examples (premises) to a generalized **conclusion**—for example, after touching several hot flames (premise), we conclude that *all* flames are hot. A nurse who observes a client who has dry skin, poor turgor, sunken eyes, and dark amber urine and who is otherwise determined to be dehydrated (premise) concludes that the presence of those signs indicate that other clients are dehydrated.

Deductive reasoning, by contrast, is reasoning from the general premise to the specific conclusion. If you begin with the premise that the sum of the angles in any triangle is always 180 degrees, you can then conclude that the sum of the angles in the triangle you happen to have is also 180 degrees. A nurse might start with a premise that all children love peanut butter sandwiches. If the client is a child, then the child will love peanut butter sandwiches. This is an example in which the premise is not always valid and, thus, the conclusion also may not be valid. Nurses use critical thinking to help analyze situations and establish which premises are valid.

In critical thinking, the nurse also differentiates statements of fact, inference, judgment, and opinion. Table 6–1 shows how these may be applied to a client. Evaluating the credibility of information sources is an important step in critical thinking. Unfortunately, we cannot always believe what we read or are told. The nurse may need to ascertain the accuracy of information by checking other documents or validation data with other informants or sources.

To comprehend a client situation clearly, the nurse and the client must agree on the meaning of terms. For example, if the client says to the nurse "I think I have a tumor," the nurse needs to clarify what this word means to the client—the medical definition of tumor (a solid mass) or the common lay meaning of cancer—before responding. Persons also live their lives under certain assumptions. Some people view humans as having a basically generous nature whereas others believe that the human tendency is for people to act in their own best interest. The nurse may believe that life should be considered worth living no matter what the condition, whereas the client believes that quality of life is more important than quantity of life. If the difference in their beliefs is recognized and they understand that they make choices based on these assumptions, they can still work together toward an acceptable plan of care by respecting their difference in beliefs. Difficulty arises when people do not take the time to consider what assumptions underlie their beliefs and actions.

Attitudes That Foster Critical Thinking

Certain attitudes are crucial to critical thinking. These attitudes are based on the assumption that a rational person is motivated to develop, learn, and grow. A critical thinker works to develop the following attitudes or traits: independence, fair-mindedness, insight, intellectual humility, intellectual courage, integrity, perseverance, confidence, and curiosity.

INDEPENDENCE   Critical thinking requires that individuals think for themselves. People acquire many beliefs as children, not necessarily based on reason but in order to have an explanation they comprehend. As they mature and acquire knowledge and experience, critical thinkers examine their beliefs in the light of new evidence. Critical thinkers seriously consider a wide range of ideas, learn from them, and then make their own judgments about them. Nurses are open-minded about considering different methods of performing technical skills—not just the single way they may have been taught in school. They are not easily swayed by the opinions of others but take responsibility for their own views (Catalano, 2003).

FAIR-MINDEDNESS   Critical thinkers are fair-minded, assessing all viewpoints with the same standards and not basing their judgments on personal or group bias or prejudice (Catalano, 2003). Fair-mindedness helps one to consider opposing points of view and to try to understand new ideas fully before rejecting or accepting them. Critical thinkers strive to be open to the possibility that new evidence could change their minds.

INSIGHT INTO EGOCENTRICITY   Critical thinkers are open to the possibility that their personal biases or social pressures and customs could unduly affect their thinking. They

---

TABLE 6–1   **Differentiating Types of Statements**

STATEMENT	DESCRIPTION	EXAMPLE
Facts	Can be verified through investigation	Blood pressure reading is 124/80
Inferences	Conclusions drawn from the facts, going beyond facts to make a statement about something not currently known	Cardiac output is the result of heart rate and stroke volume so if stroke volume decreases heart rate must increase to compensate.
Judgments	Evaluation of facts or information that reflects values or other criteria; a type of opinion	It is harmful to the client's health if the blood pressure drops too low.
Opinions	Beliefs formed over time and include judgments that may fit facts or be in error	Nursing intervention can assist in maintaining the client's blood pressure within normal limits.

actively try to examine their own biases and bring them to awareness each time they think or make a decision.

INTELLECTUAL HUMILITY Intellectual humility means having an awareness of the limits of one's own knowledge. Critical thinkers are willing to admit what they do not know; they are willing to seek new information and to rethink their conclusions in light of new knowledge. They never assume that what everybody believes to be right will always be right, because new evidence may emerge.

INTELLECTUAL COURAGE TO CHALLENGE THE STATUS QUO AND RITUALS With an attitude of courage, one is willing to consider and examine fairly one's own ideas or views, especially those to which one may have a strongly negative reaction. This type of courage comes from recognizing that beliefs are sometimes false or misleading. Values and beliefs are not always acquired rationally. Rational beliefs are those that have been examined and found to be supported by solid reasons and data. After such examination, it is inevitable that some beliefs previously held to be true will be found to contain questionable elements and that some truth will emerge from ideas considered dangerous or false. Courage is needed to be true to new thinking in such cases, especially if social penalties for nonconformity are severe.

INTEGRITY Intellectual integrity requires that individuals apply the same rigorous standards of proof to their own knowledge and beliefs as they apply to the knowledge and beliefs of others. Critical thinkers question their own knowledge and beliefs as quickly and thoroughly as they challenge those of another. They are readily able to admit and evaluate inconsistencies within their own beliefs and between their own beliefs and those of another.

PERSEVERANCE Nurses who are critical thinkers show perseverance in finding effective solutions to client and nursing problems. This determination enables them to clarify concepts and sort out related issues, in spite of difficulties and frustrations. Confusion and frustration are uncomfortable, but critical thinkers resist the temptation to find a quick and easy answer. Important questions tend to be complex and confusing and therefore often require a great deal of thought and research to arrive at an answer. The nurse needs to continue to address the issue until it is resolved.

CONFIDENCE Critical thinkers believe that well-reasoned thinking will lead to trustworthy conclusions. Therefore, they cultivate an attitude of confidence in the reasoning process and examine emotion-laden arguments using the standards for evaluating thought, by asking questions such as these: Is that argument fair? Is it based on sufficient evidence? The critical thinker develops skill in both inductive reasoning and deductive reasoning. As the nurse gains greater awareness of the thinking process and more experience in improving such thinking, confidence in the process will grow. This nurse will not be afraid of disagreement and indeed will be concerned when others agree too quickly. Such a nurse can serve as a role model to colleagues, inspiring and encouraging them to think critically as well.

TABLE 6–2	Universal Intellectual Standards
STANDARD	SAMPLE QUESTION
Clarity	What is an example of this?
Accuracy	How can I find out if that is true?
Relevance	How does that help me with the issue?
Logic	Does that follow from the evidence?
Breadth	Do I need to consider another point of view?
Precision	Can I be more specific?
Significance	Which of these facts is most important?
Completeness	Have I missed any important aspects?
Fairness	Am I considering the thinking of others?
Depth	What makes this a difficult problem?

Note: From *A Guide for Educators to Critical Thinking Competency Standards* by R. Paul & L. Elder, Foundation for Critical Thinking, 2005. Adapted with permission. www.criticalthinking.org

CURIOSITY The mind of a critical thinker is filled with questions: Why do we believe this? What causes that? Does it have to be this way? Could something else work? What would happen if we did it another way? Who says that is so? The curious nurse may value tradition but is not afraid to examine traditions to be sure they are still valid.

Standards of Critical Thinking

How can one know whether one is thinking critically? Paul and Elder (2005) proposed that thinkers can use universal standards, shown in Table 6–2. Understanding the standards for critical thinking promotes the reliability and validity of the thinking process and makes appropriate reasoning more likely. Forneris (2004), building on the work of many modern educational theorists, described core attributes of critical thinking: reflection, context, dialogue, and time. Reflection involves determining what data are relevant and making connections between that data and the decisions reached. Context is an essential consideration in nursing since care must always be individualized, taking knowledge and applying it to real people. Dialogue, which need not involve other persons, refers to the process of serving as both teacher and student in learning from situations, questioning, making connections, and determining motivation. Finally, the attribute of time emphasizes the value of using past learning in current situations that then guide future actions.

APPLYING CRITICAL THINKING TO NURSING PRACTICE

Nurses function effectively some part of every day without thinking critically. Many small decisions are based primarily on habit with minimal thinking involved; examples include selecting what uniform to wear, choosing which route to take to work, and deciding what to eat for lunch. Psychomotor skills in nursing often involve minimal thinking, such as operating a familiar piece of equipment. However, the higher-order skills of critical thinking are put into play as soon as the nurse begins to use the nursing process to provide client care, which involves highly individualized people who do not all respond to a situation in the same way.

The nursing process is a systematic, rational method of planning and providing individualized nursing care. The phases of the nursing process—assessing, diagnosing, planning, implementing, and evaluating—are discussed in detail in the chapter that follows. The nursing process serves as a method of solving problems, guiding the critical thinking process through rational steps to improve clinical reasoning and clinical decision making.

A nurse employs critical thinking when setting priorities for the day. When analyzing a situation and planning strategies for conflict resolution or change, the nurse manager uses critical-thinking attitudes and skills. The nurse clinician and nurse manager seek awareness of their thinking as they are thinking, as they apply standards for thinking, and as their thinking progresses.

Problem Solving

In problem solving, the nurse obtains information that clarifies the nature of the problem and suggests possible solutions. The nurse then carefully evaluates the possible solutions and chooses the best one to implement. The situation is carefully monitored over time to ensure its initial and continued effectiveness. The nurse does not discard the other solutions but holds them in reserve in the event that the first solution is not effective. The nurse may also encounter a similar problem in a different client situation where an alternative solution is determined to be the most effective. Therefore, problem solving for one situation contributes to the nurse's body of knowledge for problem solving in similar situations. Commonly used approaches to problem solving include trial and error, intuition, the research process, and the scientific/modified scientific method.

Trial and error is one way to solve problems. In this manner a number of approaches are tried until a solution is found. This method is somewhat haphazard and does not control for possible harm that could result from one of the trials. It does not consider alternatives systematically, so one cannot know why the solution works. Trial-and-error methods in nursing care can be dangerous because the client might suffer harm if an approach is inappropriate. However, nurses often use trial and error in the home setting where, due to logistics, equipment, and client lifestyle, hospital procedures may not work as effectively and creative approaches are needed.

Intuition is the understanding or learning of things without the conscious use of reasoning. It is also known as sixth sense, hunch, instinct, feeling, or suspicion. As a problem-solving approach, intuition is viewed by some people as a form of guessing and, as such, an inappropriate basis for nursing decisions. However, others view intuition as an essential and legitimate aspect of clinical judgment acquired through knowledge and experience. The nurse must first have the knowledge base necessary to practice in the clinical area and

then use that knowledge in clinical practice. Clinical experience allows the nurse to recognize cues and patterns and begin to reach correct conclusions. Nurses may intuitively know that something is not right, but then use a more analytical approach to determine why and how to respond.

Although the intuitive method of problem solving is gaining recognition as part of nursing practice, it is not recommended for novices or students, because they usually lack the knowledge base and clinical experience on which to make a valid judgment. Experience is important in improving intuition because the rapidity of the judgment depends on the nurse having seen similar client situations many times before.

The research process and **scientific method**, discussed in Chapter 1 ∞, are formalized, logical, systematic approaches to solving problems. The classic scientific method is most useful when the researcher is working in a controlled situation. Health professionals, often working with people in uncontrolled situations, require a modified approach to the scientific method for solving problems. Critical thinking is important in all problem-solving processes as the nurse evaluates potential solutions to a given problem and makes a decision to select the most appropriate solution for that situation.

Clinical Decision Making

Decision making is a critical-thinking process for choosing the best actions to meet a desired goal. Decisions must be made whenever several mutually exclusive choices are available or when there is an option to act or not. Nurses make decisions in the course of solving problems. Decision making, however, is also used in situations that do not involve problem solving. Nurses make value decisions, time management decisions, scheduling decisions, and priority decisions.

Nurses must make decisions and assist clients to make decisions. When faced with several client needs at the same time, the nurse must prioritize and decide which client to assist first. The nurse may (a) look at advantages and disadvantages of each option, (b) apply Maslow's hierarchy of needs, (c) consider which tasks can be delegated to others, or (d) use another priority-setting framework. When a client is trying to make a decision about what course of treatment to follow, the nurse may need to provide information or resources the client can use in making a decision. Nurses must make decisions in their own personal and professional lives.

Here are sequential steps to the decision-making process:

1. *Identify the purpose.* The nurse identifies why a decision is needed and what needs to be determined.
2. *Set the criteria.* When the nurse sets the criteria for decision making, three questions must be answered: What is the desired outcome, what needs to be preserved, and what needs to be avoided? For example, for a client with pain, the criteria would be as follows:
   a. What is the desired outcome? Relief of pain.
   b. What needs to be preserved? Physical functioning, cognitive functioning, psychologic functioning.
   c. What needs to be avoided? Central nervous system depression, respiratory depression, nausea.

3. *Weight the criteria.* In this step, the decision maker sets priorities or ranks activities or services from least important to most important as they relate to the specific situation. Because the weighting is specific to the situation, an activity may be ranked as most important in one situation and of less importance in another situation. For example, the nurse avoids medication that can cause sedation of a client with a head injury, but for a client with terminal cancer, pain relief may be more important than avoiding the sedative side effects of the pain medication.

4. *Seek alternatives.* The decision maker identifies possible ways to meet the criteria. In clinical situations, the alternatives may be selected from a range of nursing interventions or client care strategies. Pain may be treated with oral or injectable medications, as needed (prn) or on a schedule, or without pharmacologic intervention at all, instead using complementary alternative modalities (CAM).

5. *Examine alternatives.* The nurse analyzes the alternatives to ensure that there is an objective rationale in relation to the established criteria for choosing one strategy over another. For pain that results from a procedure, CAM may not be strong enough relief, and oral medication may be effective but act too slowly, so an intravenous narcotic might be the better choice.

6. *Project.* The nurse applies creative thinking and skepticism to determine what might go wrong as a result of a decision and develops plans to prevent, minimize, or overcome any problems. If the intravenous narcotic is selected, what safety procedures need to be in place—for example, a narcotic antidote and supplemental oxygen?

7. *Implement.* The decision plan is placed into action. The pain treatment is begun.

8. *Evaluate the outcome.* As with all nursing care, in evaluating, the nurse determines the effectiveness of the plan and whether the initial purpose was achieved. How does the client rate the level of pain following the procedure?

The decision-making process is supported by the use of the nursing process, which share similarities, and the nurse uses decision making in all phases of the nursing process. It is essential that the nurse use critical thinking in each step or phase of these processes so that decisions and care are well considered and delivered with the highest possible quality.

DEVELOPING CRITICAL-THINKING ATTITUDES AND SKILLS

After gaining an idea of what it means to think critically, solve problems, and make decisions, nurses need to become aware of their own thinking style and abilities. Acquiring critical-thinking skills and a critical attitude then becomes a matter of practice. Critical thinking is not an "either-or" phenomenon; people develop and use it more or less effectively along a continuum. Some people make better evaluations than others do, some people believe information from nearly any source, and still others seldom believe anything without carefully evaluating the credibility of the information. Critical thinking is not easy. Solving problems and making decisions is risky. Sometimes the outcome is not what was desired. With effort, however, everyone can achieve some level of critical thinking to become an effective problem solver and clinical decision maker.

Self-Assessment

The nurse should consider some of the attitudes discussed earlier that facilitate critical thinking, such as curiosity, fair-mindedness, humility, courage, and perseverance. A nurse might benefit from a rigorous personal assessment to determine which attitudes he or she already possesses and which need to be cultivated. This could also be done with a partner or as a group. The nurse first determines which attitudes are held strongly and form a base for thinking and which are

---

RESEARCH NOTES | **Are Education, Experience, and Critical-Thinking Ability Related to Clinical Decision Making?**

This pilot study investigated the premise that there would be relationships between the education and experience of critical care nurses and their ability to make consistent clinical decisions. Critical-thinking ability, as measured by skills and dispositions tests, was also expected to correlate with decision making. Fifty-four nurses with a BSN or MSN working in adult critical care units in teaching hospitals were included in the study. Results showed that, overall, the more complex the clinical situation, the less consistent the nurses were in their decisions. Intuition, as a decision-making strategy, was most related to consistent decisions. No correlation was found between education or total years of experience and consistency in decision making. There was an association between years of experience in critical care and decision consistency.

Implications

This study reinforces that decision making and critical thinking are complex when applied in real clinical situations. That the results showed greater consistency in decisions when intuition was used and when the nurse had more years of critical care nursing experience (not just overall nursing experience) suggests that there is a type of nurse thinking in that clinical specialty that does not necessarily evolve with more global exposure to client care. It also suggests that the method of thinking used by nurses who choose critical care practice may be an inherent characteristic.

Note: From "Critical Thinking and Clinical Decision Making in Critical Care Nursing: A Pilot Study," by F. D. Hicks, S. L. Merritt, & A. S. Elstein, 2003, *Heart & Lung, 32,* pp. 169–180.

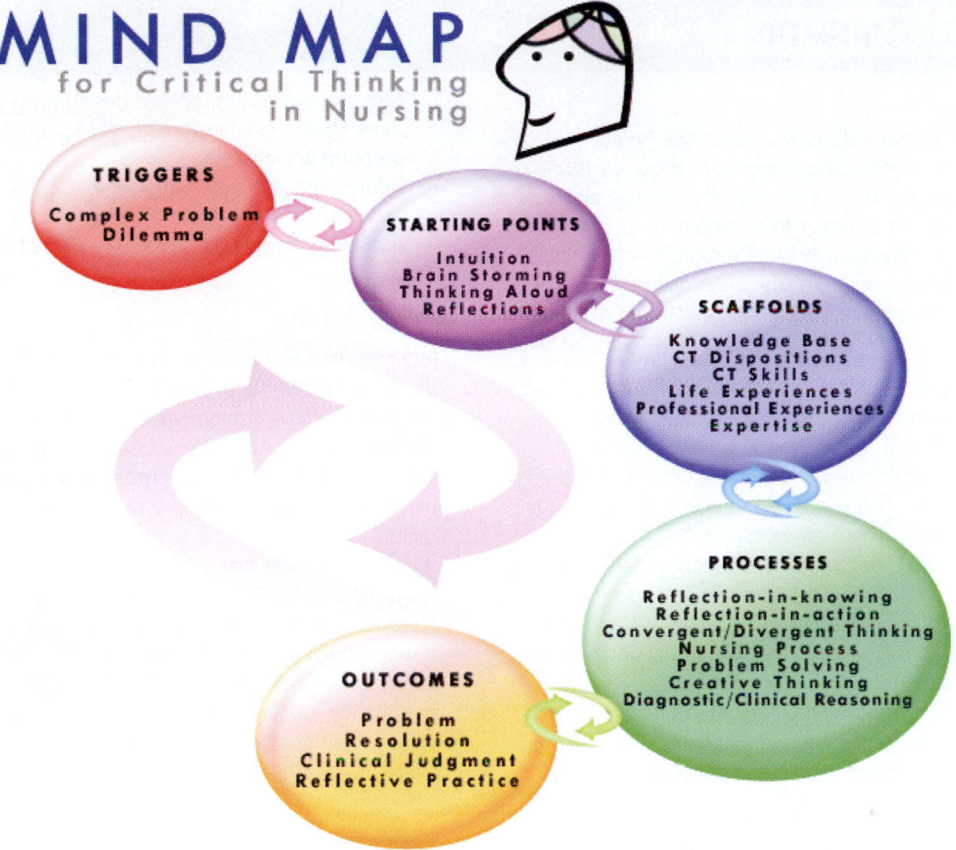

Figure 6–1 ● Mind map for critical thinking in nursing.

Note: Duphorne, P., & Giddens, J. (2004). Critical Thinking in Nursing Resource funded by intramural grant of College of Nursing, University of New Mexico.

held minimally or not at all. The nurse also needs to reflect on situations where he or she made decisions that were later regretted, and analyzes thinking processes and attitudes or asks a trusted colleague to assess them. Identifying weak or vulnerable skills and attitudes is also important.

Reflection, at every step of critical thinking and nursing care, helps examine the ways in which the nurse gathers and analyzes data, makes decisions, and determines the effectiveness of interventions. Reflection requires the nurse to pause in order to consider his or her beliefs, knowledge, values, and abilities in the particular situation at hand. The purpose of this reflection is to determine if the current course of action is the best one and to improve future actions. Figure 6–1, the Mind Map for Critical Thinking in Nursing, is a visual depiction of the interactive loops of concepts used in critical thinking. Note that the action of reflection appears as part of three of the steps shown: the starting points, processes, and outcomes.

Tolerating Dissonance and Ambiguity

The nurse needs to take deliberate efforts to cultivate critical-thinking attitudes. For example, to develop fair-mindedness, one could deliberately seek out information that is in opposition to one's own views; this provides practice in understanding and learning to be open to other viewpoints. It is a human tendency to seek out information that corresponds to one's previously held beliefs and to ignore evidence that may contradict cherished ideas. This perspective is true for both the nurse and the client. Older adults may have great difficulty accepting the pervasiveness of technology or that people don't stay in the hospital as long as they did in the 1970s or that having a diagnosis of cancer doesn't always mean that one is going to die. On the other hand, older adults have a wealth of knowledge and experience and often know better than the health care provider knows what will work well and be acceptable to them. Nurses should increase their tolerance for ideas that contradict previously held beliefs, and they should practice suspending judgment.

Suspending judgment means tolerating ambiguity for a time. If an issue is complex, it may not be resolved quickly or neatly, and judgment should be postponed. For a while, the nurse will need to say "I don't know" and be comfortable with that answer until more is known. Although postponing judgment may not be feasible in emergency situations where fast action is required, it is usually feasible in other situations.

Seeking Situations Where Good Thinking Is Practiced

Nurses will find it valuable to attend conferences in clinical or educational settings that support open examination of all

LIFESPAN CONSIDERATIONS   Health Care Decisions

Children

Parents most often make decisions about the health care of children. Growing children can participate in those decisions in age-appropriate ways. As described by Piaget, the ability of children to reason and critically think about themselves and their situation develops gradually (see Chapter 9 ∞). At each stage, nurses should be aware of the ways children think and sensitive to how they can be involved in health care decisions:

- Infants progress from reflexive behavior to simple, repetitive behavior and then to imitative behaviors, learning the concepts of cause and effect and object permanence. Though not involved in making decisions, they need to be comforted and secure as care is given.
- Toddlers and preschoolers are very egocentric and engage in magical thinking. They cannot reason out the implications of care, but need explanations in language they can understand. Play therapy and use of dolls and toys can help them adjust to care, and they can sometimes be given options (e.g., do you want your dressing changed before breakfast or after?).
- School-age children tend to be concrete thinkers. They benefit from simple, direct explanations; hands-on exploration of equipment and materials; and helping the

care provider as appropriate during procedures. Involving these children in care can increase cooperation and decrease anxiety.
- Adolescents are increasingly able to think abstractly and may make many of their own health care decisions. They should be actively consulted as a part of the family system.

Older Adults

It is important to include all adult clients in decision making and planning nursing care, but it is especially difficult to do this when working with older adults who have impaired cognitive abilities such as Alzheimer's disease. The nurse should allow them as much control and input as possible, keeping things simple and direct so they understand. Older adults with impairments are usually unable to perform multiple tasks or even to think of more than one step at a time. The nurse must have patience and be willing to calmly repeat instructions if necessary. Presenting and discussing issues in basic terms helps to maintain respect and dignity and allows older adults to participate in their own care for as long as possible. If the older adult is unable to perform self-care activities such as bathing or health-related activities such as a dressing change, the nurse seeks appropriate alternative methods for assisting the older adult with these.

---

sides of issues and respect for opposing viewpoints. Cultivating a questioning attitude, using either Socratic questioning or another technique, is vital. Nurses need to review the standards for evaluating thinking and apply them to their own thinking. If nurses are aware of their own thinking—while they are doing the thinking—they can detect thinking errors.

Creating Environments That Support Critical Thinking

A nurse cannot develop or maintain critical-thinking attitudes in a vacuum. Nurses in leadership positions must be particularly aware of the climate for thinking that they establish, and they must actively create a stimulating environment that encourages differences of opinion and fair examination of ideas and options. Nurses must embrace exploration of the perspectives of persons from different ages, cultures, religions, socioeconomic levels, and family structures. As leaders, nurses should encourage colleagues to examine evidence carefully before they come to conclusions, and to avoid "group think," the tendency to defer unthinkingly to the will of the group.

CLINICAL REASONING

Critical thinking is of profound importance because it allows the nurse to demonstrate effective clinical reasoning. **Clinical reasoning** is an active process by which nurses make judg-

ments, including both the deliberate process of generating alternatives, weighing them against the evidence, and choosing the most appropriate response, and those patterns that might be characterized as engaged, practical reasoning (Tanner, 2006). Clinical reasoning is logical thinking that links thoughts together in meaningful ways. It is reflective, concurrent, and creative thinking about clients and client care—the kind of reasoning used in the nursing process (Wilkinson, 2007).

Clinical Judgments

Clinical reasoning begins with clinical judgments. **Clinical judgments** are conclusions and opinions about clients' health drawn from patient data. They may or may not be the result of critical thinking although in most instances the client will benefit from the use of critical thinking. Clinical judgments are similar to decision making in that nurses make judgments about the meaning of client data and about nursing actions that should be taken on the client's behalf. Clinical judgments are part of the nursing process (Wilkinson, 2007). Clinical judgment is an interpretation or conclusion about a patient's needs, concerns, or health problems, along with the decision about whether or not to take action, use or modify standard approaches, or improvise new approaches as deemed appropriate by the client's response (Tanner, 2006). It uses values or other criteria to evaluate or draw conclusions about information.

Clinical reasoning requires sound judgments; otherwise the reasoning process is initiated on faulty data. These judgments are often based on objective data, the nurse's beliefs, knowledge of the client and his or her typical response patterns, the experience and knowledge level of the nurse, the context in which the situation occurs, the culture of both the client and the nurse, the reasoning pattern of the nurse, and past errors in judgment made by the nurse in similar situations (Tanner, 2006).

Reasoning Patterns

Nurses use a variety of reasoning patterns depending on the nurse's initial grasp of the situation, the demands of the situation, and the goals of the nurse's practice. The three interrelated patterns of reasoning used by experienced nurses include analytic processes, intuition, and narrative thinking. Analytic processes are used to break down a situation into its elements in order to generate alternative actions and the systematic and rational weighing of these alternatives against clinical data or the likelihood of achieving outcomes. It is useful when the nurse lacks essential knowledge or experience, there is a mismatch between what is expected and what actually happens, or there are many different possibilities to choose from. Intuition, as discussed earlier in this chapter, is often based on an undefinable feeling as the result of previous experience with a similar situation. Narrative thinking is the nurse's attempt to make sense of a given situation by interpreting concerns, intents and motives (Tanner, 2006). Narrative thinking uses talking about the events as a method of interpreting and decision making.

The nurse with strong clinical reasoning skills approaches each client situation from a moral engaged stance. The goal of client treatment is to individualize care to meet each client's unique needs in any given situation. Taking the time to gather all of the pertinent data, and learn what the client's goals of treatment are, what outcome they can reasonably expect, and how the client interprets the situation helps the nurse to make more appropriate clinical decisions for that client.

Requirements for Effective Clinical Reasoning

Requirements for effective clinical reasoning and decision making include cognitive ability, creativity, curiosity, interpersonal skills, cultural competence, psychomotor skills, and technological skills (Wilkinson, 2007). These requirements are used every day in almost every nursing situation.

Cognitive skills include decision making, problem solving, and critical thinking. Maintaining competence in the nurse's chosen field of expertise is an important component of maintaining cognitive skills and requires ongoing education long after graduating from your current nursing program. Nurses who do not participate in continuing education, whether advanced degrees, in-services, or webinars soon become dangerous care providers.

Creativity and curiosity allows the nurse to look at each event and question "Why am I doing this in this way?" "Is it an effective approach?" "Could I do this better, differ-

ently, with improved client outcomes, more cost effectively, or in a more efficient way?" Further, nurses should be motivated to understand the rationale for every nursing action and if no rationale exists, or does not have the desired outcome, should work to have the practice discontinued, changed, or evaluated for performance standards.

Interpersonal skills are those skills that improve relationships between the nurse and others, whether the client or other members of the health care team. This includes communication skills (written, spoken and nonverbal), knowledge of human behavior and social systems, and the ability to develop trusting relationships by listening and conveying compassion, interest, and information.

Cultural competence allows the nurse to work within the cultural belief system of the client to resolve health problems. Nurses must be aware of both similarities and differences among cultural groups and demonstrate cultural sensitivity in order to develop a trusting relationship with the client. Cultural care is discussed in more detail in Chapter 4 ∞.

Psychomotor skills are important to the implementation of nursing care, specifically skills of nursing. The nurse gains the client's trust and achieves the desired outcomes through proper performance of client care tasks.

Technological skills are becoming increasingly more important in the highly technical field of nursing. Nurses work with a great deal of computerized and technical equipment and must learn how to work with it properly as well as troubleshoot problems to prevent client injury (Wilkinson, 2007). The nurse who responds to a monitor alarm without first assessing the client to determine the validity of the identified problem is treating the machine instead of the client, which can reduce client outcomes.

CLINICAL SUCCESS

Critical thinking and clinical reasoning are important components of clinical success, for students as well as in future nursing practice as graduates. In order to care for your assigned clients, whose conditions often change quickly and sometimes without warning, the ability to analyze events accurately and determine the correct course of action will be very important to your success as both a student and a practicing nurse in the clinical area.

As you progress through your nursing program you will have multiple opportunities to care for clients in a variety of different health care settings. To succeed in the clinical facility it is important that you understand the expectations your instructors have for your performance. Most schools of nursing use an evaluation form that describes the behavior that you will be evaluated on with the goal of helping students recognize their strengths and weaknesses. Learning to accept an evaluation of your performance is an important aspect of improving your nursing practice, as a student and throughout your career. When you graduate and begin to work as a nurse you will be evaluated regularly by your nurse manager. While everyone loves to hear how well they are doing, growth and improvement comes from learning where there is need for improvement along with recommendations for changes in performance that will increase effectiveness and/or efficiency.

It would be unusual for a student to enter a nursing program with the goal of becoming a minimally competent nurse. Most students have the goal of graduating as an excellent nurse who provides safe client care that results in positive outcomes. Your instructors want to assist you in meeting your goal of becoming excellent nurses. To improve your clinical performance and help you move from beginner to entry-level nursing, they may provide you with constructive criticism. To get the most out of this criticism it is important that you understand they are not picking on you, and that the advice they offer is based on knowledge of the profession of nursing and the expectations you will face as a graduate functioning autonomously. Accept criticism in a thoughtful manner, use your critical thinking skills to determine why the instructor might be providing this input, weigh and think about what you are told, and discuss how you could change the way you are performing within your new role. Learning to accept recommendations for improvement, along with compliments about the things you are doing well, will move you toward improved nursing abilities both as students and throughout a lifetime of nursing practice.

Safety

The first key to clinical success is maintaining safety, both for yourself and your client. Whenever you are preparing to care for a client, use your critical thinking skills to question the safety of your considered action. Use clinical reasoning to analyze what will, or may, happen if you carry out your actions as you are currently planning to perform it. Using critical thinking to consider both the anticipated, and potentially unexpected, result of actions is important to achieving positive client outcomes. Before making clinical judgments about what is occurring, ascertain that you have gathered all the pertinent data you need to reach that judgment.

Never perform any procedure that you are not completely competent to perform. If you are not sure what to do, ask your instructor or someone who has been identified as a resource on the nursing unit. There is nothing more dangerous than a nurse who does what they guess may be right. Taking chances could cause injury, so always talk with your instructor when you aren't absolutely sure how to respond. Collaboration with peers is an important part of nursing practice. Observe the nurses on the unit and see how often they collaborate with one another. That old expression that two heads are better than one became a well-used expression because it is so true. Nurses work as a team, and as students your instructor will be the primary person you should collaborate with because your peers are also inexperienced like you. However, some nurses on the unit may be identified as good resources for students and can also be used for collaborative purposes.

Follow facility rules and policies. It is important to familiarize yourself with the facility policy. Remember that you are legally functioning as a nurse within the facility and your practice must fall within the scope as defined by your state board of nursing and the agency policies and procedures. If a policy or procedure doesn't seem to make sense to you, discuss it with your clinical instructor or nursing resource before proceeding. As graduate nurses, part of your nursing orientation will include a discussion of your facility's policies and procedures. It is important to use these resources as students to increase your familiarity with them.

Practice your skills until you feel confident in your ability to perform them. Learn about your client by reading their medical records and becoming familiar with the medications they are taking, their medical diagnoses (both primary and secondary), and the treatments your client will require while you are caring for them. Nurses never administer any medication or treatment without being familiar with the purpose, anticipated outcome, potential adverse effects, and care needs associated. Learning what your client may need will help you prepare for your clinical experience and perform safely. While change is expected in client care, and something unexpected often happen, at least you will be ready for the normal course of events. Maintaining currency is expected throughout your career. One thing nurses can count on in health care is that things change. Procedures will change, new information will be learned, treatment for diseases will differ as evidence demonstrates better ways to do things, and technological advances will bring about new and wonderful equipment. To remain current after your formal education is completed, you must continue to learn what is occurring in your field or you will quickly become outdated and obsolete.

Think about your own safety and protect yourself from harm. Use good techniques when lifting or moving clients, perform procedures properly, follow proper asepsis techniques, and use personal protective equipment appropriately. It is also important to consider your loved ones' safety. When you come home from clinical, change out of your uniform before greeting family members and wash your uniform separately from other family laundry to avoid cross-contamination. Never wear your used uniform to the grocery store, mall, or out to dinner because the uniform may be contaminated and you could potentially infect others.

Safety is always paramount to clinical success. No matter how much you know or how well you prepare, if you do not function safely your nursing care will be dangerous.

Professionalism

Professionalism will determine how others perceive you and what they conclude about your abilities as a nurse. This is true not only for clients but also with physicians, peers, managers/instructors, and other members of the health care team. Professionalism is a combination of many factors (Table 6–3).

Dress neatly in a clean uniform that is pressed and wrinkle free. Avoid excessive jewelry because it not only takes away from your professional appearance but can also harbor microbes that could infect the client. Tongue rings and artificial fingernails are particularly dangerous because they collect so many pathogens. Avoid perfumed gels, lotions, and hair products. Many people are allergic to perfumes, and it can be discomforting for the client who doesn't feel well when the health care worker is heavily scented. Keep shoes clean and polished. Hair should be restrained so that it does not fall on the client or into a wound. Can you imagine changing a client's surgical dressing and having your hair fall into the wound? That would not be very good for the client! Prior to leaving the house for clinical, look at yourself in the mirror and use your critical thinking skills to analyze your appearance. Do you portray the professional appearance you wish to demonstrate?

Professionalism isn't just how you dress. How you walk, or your carriage, can also indicate your degree of professionalism. Avoid slouching or drooping—it not only indicates lack of professionalism, but it also tends to indicate your lack of confidence in yourself. Professionals speak in well-modulated voices and do not shout, use profanity, or act in a threatening manner. While professionals may speak with passion and emphasis, they do so with the recognition that everyone has a right to his or her own opinion and a right to be heard.

How you interact with others is also an indication of your professionalism. Showing respect for others, being trustworthy and honest, and working well with others on the health care team are all aspects of professionalism. Learning to deal with conflict effectively, to handle emergencies calmly and communicating effectively will be part of what you learn in the clinical arena.

Another aspect of professionalism is portraying a confident image. Confidence can be hard to come by early in your nursing program, but will develop as you gain experience. Providing care for vulnerable populations can be intimidating at first. However, as you grow within your new role it will become easier. Clients look to you for answers and want to trust that what you tell them is true, realistic, and appropriate. How you respond will determine whether the client recognizes you as a knowledgeable and competent professional. Imagine asking a nurse a question about your health care regimen and having the nurse respond, stuttering and struggling to put words together, looking fearful and uncertain about how to respond, starting a sentence and then interrupting to start the sentence over again. How confident would you be in the information this nurse is providing, even if the nurse is very actually very knowledgeable and competent? Observe the nurses in the clinical facility and identify those who portray confidence and those who do not. Use those who do approach situations with confidence as role models.

Acting as a professional is essential to being perceived as a professional (Figure 6–2). As with all other aspects of your new role as a nurse, behaving professionally is a learned skill that you will carry throughout your nursing practice.

Responsibility and Accountability

In order to succeed in the clinical arena nurses must demonstrate responsibility and accountability. Responsibility differs from accountability because responsibility is the obligation to act, while accountability is the obligation to answer for the action (Human Resources and Social Development Canada, 2005). Responsibility involves trust, respect, and honesty in that nurses are answerable to the client, their employer, and themselves for providing care in a prescribed manner with an obligation to perform properly and in a timely manner. Accountability requires the ability to act honestly and build trust. When nurses accept responsibility, they are then accountable for the performance of this act.

The nurse demonstrates responsibility by arriving to the clinical facility a little early. If you need to be there by 7, arrive at 6:45 or 6:50 so you have time to prepare to begin work. Come prepared with your stethoscope, a working pen, and any other equipment you might need. Responsibility is also demonstrated by performing competently, knowledgeably, and honestly.

As a student nurse, one of your primary responsibilities is to take full advantage of your opportunity to work in the clinical agency by taking and looking for all learning opportunities. When you are not busy providing care to your assigned client, help others on the unit with their assignments. Look for things that you can observe or participate in that are occurring on the nursing unit. Ask the more experienced nurses to notify you if the need for a procedure arises so you can gain experience performing the skill. The more opportunities you find as a student, the more competent you will be as a graduate. As you observe and participate in

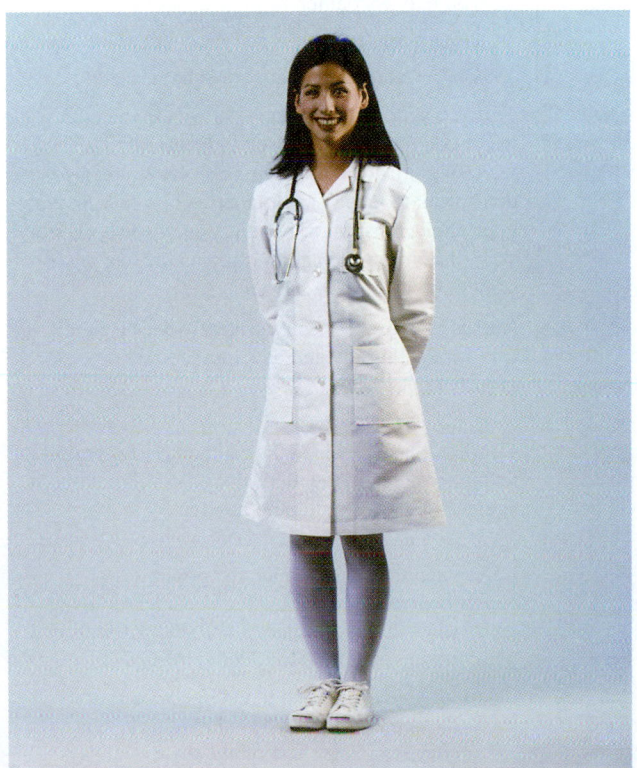

Figure 6–2 ○ Maintain a professional appearance.
(Phototake NYC.)

clinical care opportunities, remember to use your critical thinking skills. Ask yourself "Why are they doing that?" or "Is that the best way to do that?" If you see something you don't understand, have the intellectual curiosity and courage to question why it was done, or what caused them to decide to do that. All members of the health care team have something to share, but often will not do so unless you show interest and ask questions. These traits and skills will make you a valuable member of the nursing team when you graduate and begin to work within your field.

Accountability is demonstrated by doing what you have committed to do. If a client asks a question and you say you will find an answer and return, make sure you follow through. This builds trust. If you make a mistake, admit your error in order to reduce the consequences to the client. Accountability is also demonstrated by accurately documenting your actions in the client's medical records.

Communication

Good communication skills will improve your likelihood for success in the clinical facility. Remember that communication with clients should be therapeutic, not social. Keep your communications with clients focused on the client.

As a student nurse it is particularly important that you report any deviations from normal or baseline to your in-

TABLE 6–3	Inventory of Personal Attributes for Clinical Success	
QUESTIONS TO ASK	INTERPRETATION OF RESULTS	SUGGESTIONS
Ask your peers to describe what your appearance says about you.	Your peers, especially older peers, can give you some insight into how others see you if they are willing to answer honestly.	It can be almost impossible to see ourselves as others see us. Poll a number of people you trust to be honest with you and the combination of input you receive will provide you with a good idea of what type of persona you are displaying.
Do you normally arrive to appointments on time?	The past can be a good indicator of the future. If you are often late, time management skills may be needed.	Time management skills can be learned. • Leave the house 15 minutes earlier and plan your route. • Consider possible traffic or other time wasters you may encounter. • Get up earlier. • Use a calendar to plan your schedule.
How comfortable are you about admitting you don't know something or need help doing something?	If you are uncomfortable asking for help, or like to be thought of as the person who always knows the answer, you may be reluctant to ask for help.	This is a skill that requires practice. On the one hand, you don't always want to be afraid to act without guidance, but on the other hand you also don't want to take risks or chances. Try talking with your clinical instructor privately as this may reduce your discomfort with admitting you don't know something in front of a group.
What do your parents, grandparents, or other older people say about your style of dress?	How older adults see you is a good indicator of what your clients, who will often be older adults, will think when you introduce yourself.	Nurses tend to dress conservatively because they care for a culturally and developmentally diverse group of clients.
How do you deal with conflict? Is it effective in getting the results you want?	Finding yourself conflicting with others often, or that most conflicts end with a sense of dissatisfaction, may indicate poor conflict resolution skills.	Conflict management skills can be very helpful in helping you learn how to deal with conflict without aggression or becoming too passive.
Are you "accident prone"?	Accident-prone people tend to act without thinking and then suffer the results.	Before acting, think through the possible consequences of the action and consider alternate approaches that may reduce risk. This will improve your nursing practice by reducing mistakes.
When an emergency occurs, are you more likely to act first and think later or think first and then act?	Nurses encounter many situations that require rapid response. How to respond must be carefully considered to improve client outcomes.	Learning how to respond to emergencies is a learned response. When you find yourself in an emergency, no matter how acute, there is always time to stop and use your critical thinking attributes to come up with the best course of action.

structor or the nurse assigned to the client. As you gain experience and knowledge, knowing when to report deviations and who to report them to is an important component of your nursing practice. You are also responsible for reporting on your client whenever you leave the unit and at the end of the day. You should never leave the unit, even for two minutes, without informing your instructor and the nurse assigned to your client that you will be gone whether you are going to lunch, the restroom, or a postconference following clinical. As a graduate nurse, when leaving the unit, you will ask a peer to watch out for your assigned clients while you are gone.

CHAPTER HIGHLIGHTS

- Nurses need critical-thinking skills and attitudes to be safe, competent, skillful practitioners.
- Critical thinking is a process that guides a nurse in generating, implementing, and evaluating approaches for dealing with client care and professional concepts (NLN, 2000).
- Nurses use critical thinking as they apply knowledge from other subjects and fields to nursing practice, deal with change in stressful environments, and make important decisions related to client care. When nurses incorporate creativity into their thinking, they are able to find unique solutions to unique problems.
- Creativity enhances critical thinking. Creative nurses generate many ideas rapidly, are flexible and natural, create original solutions to problems, tend to be independent and self-confident, and demonstrate individuality.
- Critical-thinking skills include the ability to do critical analysis, perform inductive and deductive reasoning, make valid inferences, differentiate facts from opinions, evaluate the credibility of information sources, clarify concepts, and recognize assumptions.
- Critical thinkers have certain attitudes: independence, fair-mindedness, insight, intellectual humility, intellectual courage to challenge the status quo and rituals, integrity, perseverance, confidence, and curiosity.
- Critical thinking consists of high-level cognitive processes that include problem solving and decision making. There are several problem-solving methods: trial and error, intuition, the nursing process, the scientific method, and the modified scientific method. Nurses use the scientific method or research process when they participate in nursing and health research.

- The nursing process and critical thinking are interrelated and interdependent, but they are not identical. Both involve problem solving, decision making, and creativity.
- Nurses must make decisions in both their personal and professional lives. The steps of the decision-making process include identifying the purpose of the decision, setting the criteria, weighing the criteria, seeking alternatives, examining alternatives, projecting, implementing, and evaluating the action.
- Everyone has at least some level of critical-thinking skill, and that skill can be developed with practice. Some guidelines to enhance critical-thinking skills and attitudes include performing a self-assessment, tolerating dissonance and ambiguity, seeking situations where good thinking is productive, and creating environments that support critical thinking.
- Clinical reasoning is the process by which nurses make clinical judgments in an attempt to accurately analyze client data. Good clinical reasoning requires the use of critical thinking and sound reasoning processes.
- Nurses use a variety of reasoning patterns that are influenced by the situation, the level of understanding about the situation, and the goals of the nurse's practice.
- In order to succeed in the clinical area it is essential for students to understand the clinical instructor's expectations for success. Evaluation of performance involves identifying the nurse's strengths and weaknesses with a goal of improving performance. Components of the clinical evaluation include safety, professionalism, responsibility and accountability, and communication skills.

THINK ABOUT IT

Refer to the chapter-opening scenario and answer these questions.

1. What could Tom have done differently that may have improved the client's outcome?

2. Using critical thinking skills, rewrite the scenario, with Tom taking the proper steps from the beginning.

3. If you were his supervisor, what suggestions would you make to Tom to improve his performance the next time he was faced with a situation like this?

∞ *See suggested responses to Think About It on MyNursingKit.*

TEST YOUR KNOWLEDGE

1. A client with diarrhea has a physician's order for a bulk laxative daily. The nurse, not realizing that bulk laxatives can help solidify certain types of diarrhea, concludes, "The physician does not know the client has diarrhea." This statement is an example of:
   1. A fact.
   2. An inference.
   3. A judgment.
   4. An opinion.

2. A client reports feeling hungry but does not eat when food is served. Using critical-thinking skills, the nurse's priority action would be to:
   1. Assess why the client is not eating the food provided.
   2. Leave the food at the bedside until the client is hungry enough to eat.
   3. Notify the primary care provider that tube feeding may be indicated.
   4. Conclude that the client is not really hungry.

3. The nurse talks with the nurse manager to voice concern about the way the holiday schedule was prepared, believing it is unfair. The manager states that it is the same type of schedule used in the past and other nurses have no problems with it. The nurse remains concerned about the schedule and displays critical thinking with which of the following responses?
   1. Accepting the preferences of the other nurses since they are in the majority.
   2. Recognizing that the nurse's concerns were incorrect.
   3. Considering going to a higher authority than the manager for an explanation.
   4. Continuing to query the manager until the nurse understands the explanation.

4. The client who is short of breath benefits from the head of the bed being elevated. Because this position can result in skin breakdown in the sacral area, the nurse decides to study the amount of sacral pressure occurring in other positions. This decision is an example of which of the following?
   1. The scientific method.
   2. The trial-and-error method.
   3. Intuition.
   4. The nursing process.

5. In the decision-making process, the nurse sets and weighs the criteria, examines alternatives, and performs which of the following before implementing the plan?
   1. Reexamines the purpose for making the decision
   2. Consults the client and family members to determine their view of the criteria
   3. Identifies and considers various means for reaching the outcomes
   4. Determines the logical course of action should intervening problems arise

6. The client, who is preparing for discharge, tells the nurse she is feeling very anxious. The nurse would demonstrate critical thinking within the nursing process by:
   1. Calling the physician to report this symptom.
   2. Providing additional discharge teaching to reduce the client's anxiety.
   3. Assessing the client for the source of anxiety.
   4. Adding the nursing diagnosis of anxiety to the client's plan of care.

7. The nursing student is receiving the mid-term clinical evaluation from the instructor. The instructor advises the student to increase teamwork, helping other team members when they have free time. The student demonstrates critical thinking with which of the following responses?
   1. "I always help others when I'm at clinical. I don't know why you're saying that."
   2. "You just don't like me and you're always looking for ways to criticize me."
   3. "Oh, I'm sorry. I didn't realize I wasn't performing well. I'll do better next time."
   4. "Can you tell me what things I'm doing that leads you to feel I am not acting as a team player?"

8. The client, who had abdominal surgery yesterday, tells the nurse that he is feeling suddenly short of breath. Which of the following would be an appropriate clinical judgment for the nurse to make based on this data? Select all that apply.
   1. The client needs to perform deep breathing and coughing to clear the airway.
   2. The client is not effectively meeting oxygen needs.
   3. The nurse needs to assess the client.
   4. The nurse should apply oxygen and notify the physician.
   5. The client is receiving excessive narcotics for pain control, affecting oxygenation.

9. The student nurses will have their first clinical experience tomorrow. Which of the following actions would demonstrate responsibility?
   1. Buying the very best and most expensive stethoscope available.
   2. Going to bed early enough to allow for a good night's sleep tonight.
   3. Reviewing all of their class notes since the beginning of the program.
   4. Calling the nursing instructor to verify where and when to go to report as soon as they awaken in the morning tomorrow.

10. The student nurse is caring for a client whose condition suddenly deteriorates. The client becomes short of breath and then stops breathing and pulse ceases. The nurse prioritizes actions by performing which of the following actions first?
    1. Begin CPR.
    2. Call for help.
    3. Assess the client.
    4. Get the crash cart.

∞ *See answers to Test Your Knowledge in Appendix A.*

REFERENCES AND SELECTED BIBLIOGRAPHY

Alfaro-LeFevre, R. (2004). *Critical thinking in nursing: A practical approach* (3rd ed.). Philadelphia: Saunders.

Allen, G. D., Rubenfield, M. G., & Scheffer, B. K. (2004). Reliability assessment of critical thinking. *Journal of Professional Nursing, 20*(1), 15–22.

Benner, P. E., Hooper-Kyriakidis, P. L., & Stannard, D. (1999). *Clinical wisdom and in critical care: A thinking-in-action approach*. Philadelphia: Saunders.

Catalano, J. T. (2003). *Nursing now! Today's issues, tomorrow's trends* (3rd ed.). Philadelphia: Davis.

Elder, L., & Paul, R. (2003). *A miniature guide for students and faculty to the foundations of analytic thinking: How to take thinking apart and what to look for when you do*. Dillon Beach, CA: Foundation for Critical Thinking.

Forneris, S. G. (2004). Exploring the attributes of critical thinking: A conceptual basis. *International Journal of Nursing Education Scholarship, 1*(1), Article 9, 1–19. Retrieved June 18, 2006, from http://www.bepress.comlijnes/vol1/iss1/art9

Hicks, F. D., Merritt, S. L., & Elstein, A. S. (2003). Critical thinking and clinical decision making in critical care nursing: A pilot study. *Heart & Lung, 32,* 169–180.

Hood, L. J., & Leddy, S. K. (2003). *Leddy & Pepper's conceptual bases of nursing practice* (5th ed.). Philadelphia: Lippincott Williams & Wilkins.

Human Resources and Social Development Canada. (2005). *Appendix D: Glossary and acronyms*. Retrieved October 9, 2008, from http://www.hrsdc.gc.ca/en/cs/fas/as/sds/appd_sds03.shtml

Jackson, M., Ignatavicius, D. D., & Case, B. (2006). *Conversations in critical thinking and clinical judgment*. Boston: Jones & Bartlett.

Moore, B. N., & Parker, R. (2007). *Critical thinking* (8th ed.). Boston: McGraw-Hill.

National League for Nursing. (2000). *Think tank on critical thinking*. New York: Author.

Paul, R., & Elder, L. (2005). *A guide for educators to critical thinking competency standards*. Dillon Beach, CA: Foundation for Critical Thinking.

Rubenfeld, M. G., & Scheffer, B. (2006). *Critical thinking TACTICS for nurses*. Boston: Jones & Bartlett.

Staib, S. (2003). Teaching and measuring critical thinking. *Journal of Nursing Education, 42,* 498–507.

Tanner, C. A. (2006). Thinking like a nurse: A research-based model of clinical judgment in nursing. *Journal of Nursing Education, 45*(6), 204–211.

Wilkinson, J. M. (2007). *Nursing process and critical thinking* (4th ed.). Upper Saddle River, NJ: Pearson Education.

The Nursing Process

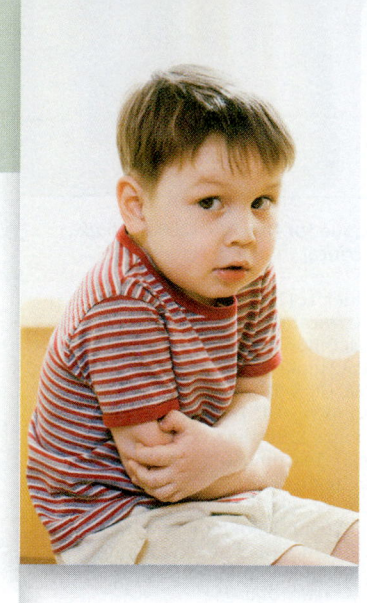

Mary Roth, RN, is the school nurse at McGhee Preschool. Her first client of the day is Jim Vance, a 4-year-old preschooler, who enters her office saying, "I don't feel well." When Mary asks him what's wrong, he says, "I just don't feel right." Mary helps him to lie down on the examination table and takes his vital signs. His temperature is slightly elevated at 100.8 oral, heart rate is on the high side of normal at 100, and his respiratory rate is 20. Mary asks him if he has pain, and Jim says yes, in his stomach. Mary asks him to point to where it hurts, and he points to his lower right quadrant. She then asks him if he feels like he might throw up, and he says yes, a little bit. He says he didn't eat breakfast this morning to keep from throwing up because he didn't want his mother to make him stay home from school. Mary examines his abdomen and finds rebound tenderness, and suspects he may have appendicitis. Mary calls Jim's mother and suggests she pick him up and take him to see his primary provider. While waiting for Mrs. Vance to arrive, Mary moves him from the examination room to a cot to lie down until his mother comes, and she sits with him and reads him a story. When Jim asks for a drink of water, Mary suggests he wait until after he sees the doctor. Mrs. Vance calls the school later that day to thank Mary and tell her that Jim had an appendectomy and was doing well.

LEARNING OUTCOMES

After completing this chapter, you will be able to:

1. Contrast the different components of the nursing process, identifying the purpose, major activities, and interaction of each phase.

2. Differentiate among objective, subjective, primary and secondary data, and identify how each type is collected.

3. Contrast various forms of interviewing styles, including directive and nondirective, using both open-ended and closed questions.

4. Identify the components of each type of nursing diagnosis.

5. Compare nursing diagnoses, medical diagnoses, and collaborative problems.

6. Prepare a nursing diagnosis statement following the basic steps.

7. Differentiate the three types of planning performed by the nurse and activities that occur within each.

8. Demonstrate how to individualize a standard or preprinted care plan to create a comprehensive nursing plan of care.

9. Develop a comprehensive nursing care plan for an assigned client.

10. Identify factors nurses should consider when setting priorities.

11. Establish goals, desired outcomes, and indicators related to nursing diagnoses using Nursing Outcome Classifications.

12. Describe the process of selecting and choosing nursing interventions, using the Nursing Interventions Classification, while planning client care.

13. List the three categories of skills used to implement nursing interventions and five activities performed during the implementation phase.

14. Detail the five components of the evaluation process and two components of an evaluation statement.

15. Demonstrate the steps involved in reviewing and modifying the client's care plan.

16. Contrast quality improvement and quality assurance, listing the three components of quality evaluation.

KEY TERMS

Assessing p151
Cephalocaudal p157
Collaborative care plan p169
Concept map p169
Critical pathway p169
Cues p159
Data p151
Defining characteristics p161
Desired outcomes p171
Diagnosis p160
Discharge planning p168

Etiology p160
Evaluating p179
Evaluation statement p181
Goals p171
Implementing p178
Indicator p172
Individualized care plan p168
Inference p159
Interview p155
Multidisciplinary care plan p169
Nursing diagnosis p160

Nursing Intervention p167
Nursing Interventions Classifications (NIC) p175
Nursing Outcomes Classification (NOC) p172
Planning p167
Policies p169
Priority setting p171
Procedures p169
Protocol p169
Qualifiers p161
Quality assurance (QA) p183

Quality improvement (QI) p183
Rapport p155
Rationale p169
Risk factors p161
Sentinel event p183
Sign p153
Standing order p169
Symptom p152
Taxonomy p160
Validation p159

OVERVIEW OF THE NURSING PROCESS

The nursing process is an organized approach to client care used as a means of problem solving. The purpose of the nursing process is to identify a client's health status and actual or potential health care problems or needs, to establish plans to meet the identified needs, and to deliver specific nursing interventions to meet those needs. The client may be an individual, a family, a group, or a community.

While the nursing process is divided into five phases, it is a fluid process that helps nurses to approach client care from an organized manner. It is closely related to problem solving and requires critical thinking at all stages.

Phases of the Nursing Process

The phases of the nursing process are not separate entities but overlapping, continuing subprocesses. Assessing, which may be considered the first phase of the nursing process, is also carried out during the implementing and evaluating phases. For example, while administering medications (implementing), the nurse continuously notes the client's skin color, level of consciousness, heart rate, and so on.

Each phase of the nursing process affects the others; they are closely interrelated (Figure 7–1). The quality of the data collected impacts the choice of nursing diagnosis and the plan of care created.

Characteristics of the Nursing Process

The nursing process has distinctive characteristics that enable the nurse to respond to the changing health status of the client. These characteristics include its cyclic and dynamic nature, client centeredness, focus on problem solving and decision making, interpersonal and collaborative style, universal applicability, and use of critical thinking (Table 7–1).

ASSESSING

Assessing is the systematic and continuous collection, organization, validation, and documentation of **data** (information). In effect, assessing is a continuous process carried out during all phases of the nursing process. All phases of the nursing process depend on the accurate and complete

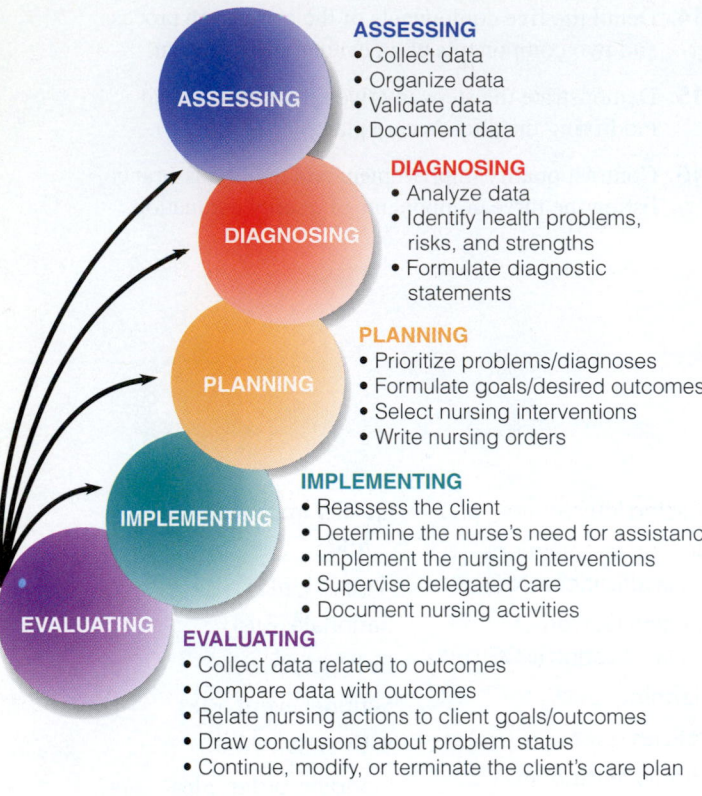

ASSESSING
- Collect data
- Organize data
- Validate data
- Document data

DIAGNOSING
- Analyze data
- Identify health problems, risks, and strengths
- Formulate diagnostic statements

PLANNING
- Prioritize problems/diagnoses
- Formulate goals/desired outcomes
- Select nursing interventions
- Write nursing orders

IMPLEMENTING
- Reassess the client
- Determine the nurse's need for assistance
- Implement the nursing interventions
- Supervise delegated care
- Document nursing activities

EVALUATING
- Collect data related to outcomes
- Compare data with outcomes
- Relate nursing actions to client goals/outcomes
- Draw conclusions about problem status
- Continue, modify, or terminate the client's care plan

Figure 7–1 ⬤ The nursing process in action.

TABLE 7–1	Examples of Critical Thinking in the Nursing Process
NURSING PROCESS PHASE	**CRITICAL-THINKING ACTIVITIES**
Assessing	Making reliable observations
	Distinguishing relevant from irrelevant data
	Distinguishing important from unimportant data
	Validating data
	Organizing data
	Categorizing data according to a framework
	Recognizing assumptions
	Identifying gaps in the data
Diagnosing	Finding patterns and relationships among cues
	Making inferences
	Suspending judgment when lacking data
	Stating the problem
	Examining assumptions
	Comparing patterns with norms
	Identifying factors contributing to the problem
Planning	Forming valid generalizations
	Transferring knowledge from one situation to another
	Developing evaluative criteria
	Hypothesizing
	Making interdisciplinary connections
	Prioritizing client problems
	Generalizing principles from other sciences
Implementing	Applying knowledge to perform interventions
	Testing hypotheses
Evaluating	Deciding whether hypotheses are correct
	Making criterion-based evaluations

Note: From *Nursing Process & Critical Thinking*, 4th ed. (pp. 66–69), by J. M. Wilkinson, 2007, Upper Saddle River, NJ: Pearson Prentice Hall. Adapted with permission.

collection of data. There are four different types of assessments: initial assessment, problem-focused assessment, emergency assessment, and time-lapsed reassessment (see Table 7–2). Assessments vary according to their purpose, timing, and client status.

Nursing assessments focus on a client's responses to a health problem. A nursing assessment should include the client's perceived needs, health problems, related experience, health practices, values, and lifestyles. To be most useful, the data collected should be relevant to a particular health problem. Therefore, nurses should think critically about what to assess. The Joint Commission on Accreditation of Healthcare Organizations (2005) requires that each client have an initial assessment consisting of a history and physical performed and documented within 24 hours of admission as an inpatient.

The assessment process involves four closely related activities: collecting data, organizing data, validating data, and documenting data (see Figure 7–2).

Collecting Data

Data collection is the process of gathering information about a client's health status. It must be both systematic and continuous to prevent the omission of significant data and reflect a client's changing health status.

A database is all the information about a client; it includes the nursing health history (see Box 7–1), physical assessment, primary care provider's history and physical examination, results of laboratory and diagnostic tests, and material contributed by other health personnel.

Client data should include past history as well as current problems. Past surgical procedures, folk healing practices, and chronic diseases are examples of historical data. Current data relate to present circumstances, such as pain, nausea, sleep patterns, and religious practices. To collect data accurately, both the client and nurse must actively participate. Data can be subjective or objective and of constant or variable types, and from a primary or secondary source.

TYPES OF DATA Subjective data, also referred to as **symptoms** or covert data, are apparent only to the person affected and can be described or verified only by that per-

TABLE 7–2	**Types of Assessment**		
TYPE	TIME PERFORMED	PURPOSE	EXAMPLE
Initial assessment	Performed within specified time after admission to a health care agency	To establish a complete database for problem identification, reference, and future comparison	Nursing admission assessment
Problem-focused assessment	Ongoing process integrated with nursing care	To determine the status of a specific problem identified in an earlier assessment	Hourly assessment of client's fluid intake and urinary output in an ICU Assessment of client's ability to perform self-care while assisting a client to bathe
Emergency assessment	During any physiologic or psychologic crisis of the client	To identify life-threatening problems To identify new or overlooked problems	Rapid assessment of a person's airway, breathing status, and circulation during a cardiac arrest Assessment of suicidal tendencies or potential for violence
Time-lapsed reassessment	Several months after initial assessment	To compare the client's current status to baseline data previously obtained	Reassessment of a client's functional health patterns in a home care or outpatient setting or, in a hospital, at shift change

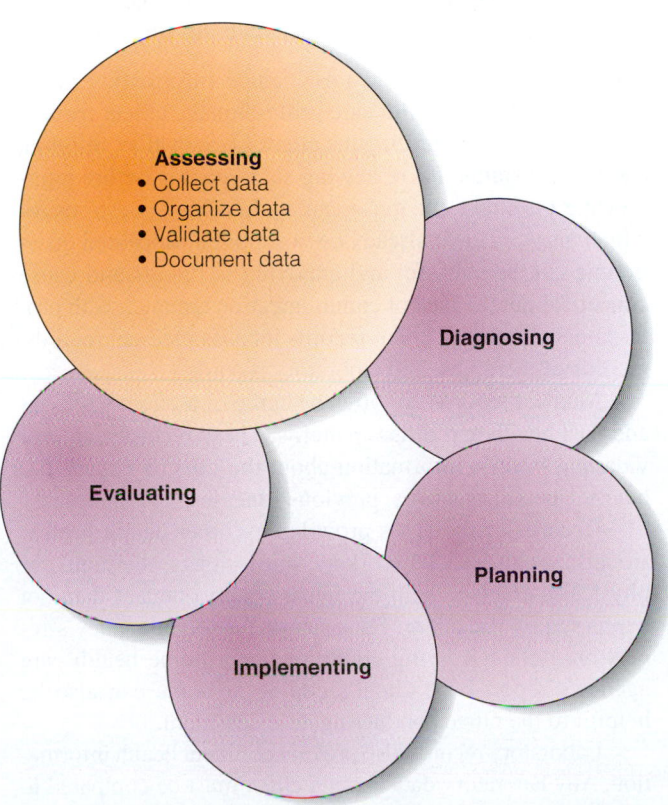

Figure 7–2 ○ Assessing. The assessment process involves four closely related activities.

son. Itching, pain, and feelings of worry are examples of subjective data. Subjective data include the client's sensations, feelings, values, beliefs, attitudes, and perception of personal health status and life situation.

Objective data, also referred to as **signs** or overt data, are detectable by an observer or can be measured or tested against an accepted standard. They can be seen, heard, felt, or smelled, and they are obtained by observation or physical examination. For example, a discoloration of the skin or a blood pressure reading is objective data. During the physical examination, the nurse obtains objective data to validate subjective data and to complete the assessment phase of the nursing process.

Constant data is information that does not change over time, such as race or blood type. Variable data can change quickly, frequently, or rarely and include such data as blood pressure, age, and level of pain.

A complete database provides a baseline for comparing the client's responses to nursing and medical interventions.

SOURCES OF DATA   Sources of data are primary or secondary. The client is the primary source of data. Family members or other support persons, other health professionals, records and reports, laboratory and diagnostic analyses, and relevant literature are secondary or indirect sources. In fact, all sources other than the client are considered secondary sources. All data from secondary sources should be validated if possible.

BOX 7–1	**Components of a Nursing Health History**

Biographic Data

Client's name, address, age, sex, marital status, occupation, religious preference, health care financing, and usual source of medical care.

Chief Complaint or Reason for Visit

The answer given to the question "What is troubling you?" or "Can you tell me the reason you came to the hospital or clinic today?" The chief complaint should be recorded in the client's own words.

History of Present Illness

- When and how the symptoms started
- How often the problem occurs, exact location, and activity when problem occurred
- Character of the complaint, symptoms associated, and factors that aggravate or alleviate the problem

Past History

Childhood illnesses, childhood immunizations, allergies, accidents and injuries, past hospitalizations, and medications currently taken.

Family History of Illness

To ascertain risk factors for certain diseases, the ages of siblings, parents, and grandparents and their current state of health or, if they are deceased, the cause of death are obtained. Particular attention should be given to disorders such as heart disease, cancer, diabetes, hypertension, obesity, allergies, arthritis, tuberculosis, bleeding, alcoholism, and any mental health disorders.

Lifestyle

Personal habits, diet, sleep/rest patterns, ADLs, and recreation/hobbies

Social Data

Family relationships/friendships, ethnic affiliations, education, occupational history, economic status, and home/neighborhood conditions

Psychologic Data

Major stressors, usual coping patterns, and communication style

Patterns of Health Care

All health care resources the client is currently using and has used in the past including primary care provider, specialists, dentist, folk practitioners, health clinic, or health center; whether the client considers the care being provided adequate; and whether access to health care is a problem.

Client The best source of data is usually the client, unless they are too ill, young, or confused to communicate clearly. The client can provide subjective data that no one else can offer. Most often, the term *primary data* refers to statements made by the client but also include those objective data that can be directly obtained by the nurse from the client such as gender. Some clients cannot or do not wish to provide accurate data. These include young children, and clients who are confused, afraid, embarrassed, or distrustful, or do not speak the nurse's language (D'Amico & Barbarito, 2007).

Support People Family members, friends, and caregivers who know the client well often can supplement or verify information provided by the client. They might convey information about the client's response to illness, the stresses the client was experiencing before the illness, family attitudes on illness and health, and the client's home environment.

Support people are an especially important source of data for a client who is very young, unconscious, or confused. In some cases—a client who is physically or emotionally abused, for example—the person giving information may wish to remain anonymous. Before eliciting data from support people, the nurse should ensure that the client, if mentally able, accepts such input. The nurse should also indicate on the nursing history that the data were obtained from a support person.

Information supplied by family members, significant others, or other health professionals is considered subjective if it is not based on fact. If the client's daughter says, "Dad is very confused today," that is secondary subjective data because it is an interpretation of the client's behavior by the daughter. The nurse should attempt to verify the reported confusion by interviewing the client directly. However, if the daughter says, "Dad said he thought it was the year 1941 today," that may be considered secondary objective data since the daughter heard her father state this directly.

Client Records Client records include information documented by various health care professionals. Client records also contain data regarding the client's occupation, religion, and marital status. By reviewing such records before interviewing the client, the nurse can avoid asking questions for which answers have already been supplied. Repeated questioning can be stressful and annoying to clients and cause concern about the lack of communication among health professionals. Types of client records include medical records, records of therapies, and laboratory records.

Medical records are often a source of a client's present and past health and illness patterns. These records can provide nurses with information about the client's coping behaviors, health practices, previous illnesses, and allergies.

Records of therapies provided by other health professionals, such as social workers, nutritionists, dietitians, or physical therapists, help the nurse obtain relevant data not expressed by the client. For example, a social agency's report on a client's living conditions or a home health care agency's report on a client's coping at home can also be helpful to the nurse conducting an assessment.

Laboratory records also provide pertinent health information. Any laboratory data about a client must be compared to the agency or performing laboratory's norms for that particular test and for the client's age, sex, and other significant client data. Diagnostic studies commonly ordered are discussed in

Chapter 20 ∞. The nurse must always consider the information in client records in light of the present situation.

Health Care Professionals   Because assessment is an ongoing process, verbal reports from other health care professionals serve as other potential sources of information about a client's health. Nurses, social workers, primary care providers, and physiotherapists, for example, may have information from either previous or current contact with the client. Sharing of information among professionals is especially important to ensure continuity of care when clients are transferred to and from home and health care agencies. However, information should always be shared considering confidentiality and the health care provider's need to know the information.

Literature   The review of nursing and related literature, such as professional journals and reference texts, can provide additional information for the database. A literature review includes, but is not limited to: standards or norms against which to compare findings, cultural and social health practices, spiritual beliefs, assessment data, nursing interventions and evaluation criteria relevant to a client's health problems, information about medical diagnosis, treatment and prognoses, and current methodologies and research findings.

DATA COLLECTION METHODS   The principal methods used to collect data are observing, interviewing, and examining. Observation occurs whenever the nurse is in contact with the client or support persons. Interviewing is used mainly while taking the nursing health history or questioning the client. Examining is the major method used in the physical health assessment. In reality, the nurse uses all three methods simultaneously when assessing clients.

Observing   To *observe* is to gather data by using the senses. Observation is a conscious, deliberate skill that is developed through effort and with an organized approach. Although nurses observe mainly through sight, most of the senses are engaged during careful observations.

Observation has two aspects: (a) noticing the data and (b) selecting, organizing, and interpreting the data. A nurse who observes that a client's face is flushed must relate that observation to findings such as body temperature, activity, environmental temperature, or blood pressure. Errors can occur in selecting, organizing, and interpreting data. For example, a nurse might not notice certain signs, either because they are unexpected or because they do not conform to preconceptions about a client's illness. Nurses often need to focus on specific data in order not to be overwhelmed by a multitude of data. Observing, therefore, involves distinguishing data in a meaningful manner.

The experienced nurse is often able to attend to an intervention and make important observations at the same time. The beginning student must learn to make observations and complete tasks simultaneously. Nursing observations must be organized so that nothing significant is missed.

Interviewing   An **interview** is planned communication or conversation with a purpose, such as to get or give informa-

tion, identify problems of mutual concern, evaluate change, teach, provide support, or provide counseling or therapy. Interviewing can be directive or nondirective. The directive interview is highly structured and elicits specific information. The nurse establishes the purpose of the interview and controls the interview, at least at the outset. The client responds to questions but may have limited opportunity to ask questions or discuss concerns. Nurses frequently use directive interviews to gather and to give information when time is limited. The purpose of a nondirective interview is to build **rapport**, an understanding between two or more people. During a nondirective interview, the nurse allows the client to control the purpose, subject matter, and pacing.

A combination of directive and nondirective approaches is usually appropriate during the information-gathering interview. The nurse begins by determining areas of concern for the client. If a client expresses worry about surgery, the nurse pauses to explore the client's worry and to provide support. Simply noting the worry, without dealing with it, can leave the impression that the nurse does not care about the client's concerns or dismisses them as unimportant.

TYPES OF INTERVIEW QUESTIONS   Questions are often classified as closed or open ended, and neutral or leading. Closed questions, used in the directive interview, are restrictive and generally require only short answers. Closed questions often begin with "when," "where," "who," "what," "do (did, does)," or "is (are, was)." A highly stressed person and someone who has difficulty communicating will find closed questions easier to answer than open-ended questions.

Open-ended questions, associated with the nondirective interview, invite clients to discover and explore, elaborate, clarify, or illustrate their thoughts or feelings. An open-ended question specifies only the broad topic to be discussed, and invites answers longer than one or two words. Such questions give clients the freedom to divulge only the information that they are ready to disclose. The open-ended question is useful at the beginning of an interview or to change topics and to elicit attitudes. Open-ended questions may begin with "what" or "how."

The type of question a nurse chooses depends on the needs of the client at the time. Nurses often find it necessary to use a combination of closed and open-ended questions throughout an interview to accomplish the goals of the interview and obtain needed information. See Box 7-2 for the advantages and disadvantages of open-ended and closed questions.

A neutral question is a question the client can answer without direction or pressure from the nurse, is open ended, and is used in nondirective interviews. A leading question, by contrast, is usually closed, used in a directive interview, and thus directs the client's answer. The leading question gives the client less opportunity to decide whether the answer is true or not. Leading questions create problems if the client, in an effort to please the nurse, gives inaccurate responses. This can result in inaccurate data.

PLANNING THE INTERVIEW AND SETTING   Before beginning an interview, the nurse reviews available information, for example, the operative report, information about the current illness, or literature about the client's health problem. The nurse also reviews the agency's data collection form to identify which data must be collected and which data are within the nurse's discretion to collect based on the specific client. If a form is not available, most nurses prepare an interview guide to help them remember areas of information and determine what questions to ask. The guide includes a list of topics and subtopics rather than a series of questions.

Both nurses and clients should be comfortable in order to encourage an effective interview by balancing several factors. Each interview is influenced by time, place, seating arrangement or distance, and language.

Time. Nurses need to plan interviews with clients when the client is physically comfortable and free of pain, and when interruptions by friends, family, and other health professionals are minimal. Nurses should schedule interviews with clients in their homes at a time selected by the client. The nurse should arrange the interview at a time when the nurse is not likely to be pulled away or interrupted.

Place. A well-lit, well-ventilated room that is relatively free of noise, movements, and distractions encourages communication. In addition, a place where others cannot overhear or see the client is desirable in order to encourage the client to feel free to share confidential information.

Seating Arrangement. A nurse who stands and looks down at a client in bed or a chair risks intimidating the client. Sitting opposite the client in a chair is less formal than sitting behind a table or standing at the foot of the bed. During an initial admission interview, a client may feel less confronted if there is an overbed table between the client and the nurse. Sitting on a client's bed may invade the client's personal space, making them feel hemmed in and making staring difficult to avoid.

A seating arrangement with the nurse behind a desk and the client seated across creates a formal setting that suggests a business meeting between a superior and a subordinate. In contrast, a seating arrangement in which the parties sit on two chairs placed at right angles to a desk or table or a few feet apart, with no table between, creates a less formal atmosphere, and the nurse and client tend to feel on equal terms. In groups, a horseshoe or circular chair arrangement can avoid a superior, or head-of-the-table, position.

Distance. The distance between the interviewer and interviewee should be neither too small nor too great, because people feel uncomfortable when talking to someone who is too close or too far away. Those who study the use of space (known as *proxemics*) find that, as a species, humans are highly territorial but we are rarely aware of it unless our space is somehow violated. Most people feel comfortable maintaining a distance of 2 to 3 feet during an interview. Some clients require more or less personal space, depending on their cultural and personal needs. For additional information, see Chapter 4 ∞.

Language. Failure to communicate in language the client can understand is a form of discrimination. The nurse must con-

---

BOX 7–2   Selected Advantages and Disadvantages of Open-Ended and Closed Questions

Open-Ended Questions

Advantages
1. They let the interviewee do the talking.
2. The interviewer is able to listen and observe.
3. They are easy to answer and nonthreatening.
4. They reveal what the interviewee thinks is important.
5. They may reveal the interviewee's lack of information, misunderstanding of words, frame of reference, prejudices, or stereotypes.
6. They can provide information the interviewer may not ask for.
7. They can reveal the interviewee's degree of feeling about an issue.
8. They can convey interest and trust because of the freedom they provide.

Disadvantages
1. They take more time.
2. Only brief answers may be given.
3. Valuable information may be withheld.
4. They often elicit more information than necessary.
5. Responses are difficult to document and require skill in recording.
6. The interviewer requires skill in controlling an open-ended interview.
7. Responses require psychologic insight and sensitivity from the interviewer.

Closed Questions

Advantages
1. Questions and answers can be controlled more effectively.
2. They require less effort from the interviewee.
3. They may be less threatening, since they do not require explanations or justifications.
4. They take less time.
5. Information can be asked for sooner than it would be volunteered.
6. Responses are easily documented.
7. Questions are easy to use and can be handled by unskilled interviewers.

Disadvantages
1. They may provide too little information and require follow-up questions.
2. They may not reveal how the interviewee feels.
3. They do not allow the interviewee to volunteer possibly valuable information.
4. They may inhibit communication and convey lack of interest by the interviewer.
5. The interviewer may dominate the interview with questions.

Note: From *Interviewing: Principles and Practices,* 11th ed. By C. J. Stewart and W. B. Cash, Jr., 2006, McGraw-Hill. Reprinted with permission from The McGraw-Hill Companies.

vert complicated medical terminology into common English usage, and interpreters or translators are needed if the client and the nurse do not speak the same language or dialect (a variation in a language spoken in a particular geographic region). Translating medical terminology is a specialized skill because not all persons fluent in the conversational form of the language are familiar with anatomic or other health terms. Interpreters, however, may make judgments about precise wording but also about subtle meanings that require additional explanation or clarification according to the specific language and ethnicity. They may edit the original source to make the meaning clearer or more culturally appropriate.

If giving written documents to clients, the nurse must determine that the client can read in his or her native language. Live translation is preferred since the client can then ask questions for clarification. Nurses must be cautious when asking family members, client visitors, or agency nonprofessional staff to assist with translation. Issues of confidentiality or gender mismatch can interfere with effective communication. Services such as AT&T Language Line are available 24 hours a day in about 140 languages, for a fee paid by the health care provider. Many large agencies create their own on-call translator services for the languages or dialects commonly spoken in their area.

Even among clients who speak English, there may be differences in understanding terminology. Clients from different parts of the country may have strong accents, or clients less well educated and teen clients may ascribe different meanings to words. For example, "cool" may imply something good to one client and something not warm to another. The nurse must always confirm accurate understandings.

STAGES OF AN INTERVIEW   An interview has three major stages: the opening, or introduction, the body, or development, and the closing.

The Opening.   The opening can be the most important part of the interview because what is said and done at that time sets the tone for the remainder of the interview. The purposes of the opening are to establish rapport and orient the interviewee. Establishing rapport is a process of creating goodwill and trust. The nurse must be careful not to overdo this stage; too much superficial talk can arouse anxiety about what is to follow and may appear insincere. In orientation, the nurse explains the purpose and nature of the interview. The nurse tells the client how the information will be used and usually states that the client has the right not to provide data.

The Body.   In the body of the interview, the client communicates what he or she thinks, feels, knows, and perceives in response to questions from the nurse. Effective development of the interview demands that the nurse use communication techniques that make both parties feel comfortable and serve the purpose of the interview (see Chapter 11 ∞). For communicating during an interview, see "Practice Guidelines."

The Closing.   The nurse terminates the interview when the needed information has been obtained although occasionally it may be the client who terminates, such as when de-

---

PRACTICE GUIDELINES   **Communication during an Interview**

- Listen attentively, using all your senses, and speak slowly and clearly.
- Use language the client understands, and clarify points that are not understood.
- Plan questions to follow a logical sequence.
- Ask only one question at a time. Multiple questions limit the client to one choice and may confuse the client.
- Acknowledge the client's right to look at things the way they appear to him or her and not the way they appear to the nurse or someone else.
- Do not impose your own values on the client.
- Avoid using personal examples, such as saying, "If I were you. . ."
- Nonverbally convey respect, concern, interest, and acceptance.
- Be aware of the client's and your own body language.
- Be conscious of the client's and your own voice inflection, tone, and affect.
- Sit down to talk with the client (be at an even level).
- Use and accept silence to help the client search for more thoughts or to organize them.
- Use eye contact and be calm, unhurried, and sympathetic.

---

ciding not to give any more information or when unable to offer more information for some other reason. The closing is important for maintaining rapport and trust and for facilitating future interactions. Techniques commonly used to close an interview include offering to answer questions, signaling the purpose of the communication has been met ("Well, those are all the questions I have for now"), thanking the client, expressing concern for the client's welfare and future, planning for the next meeting, and/or providing a summary to verify accuracy and agreement.

Examining   The physical examination or physical assessment is a systematic data collection method that uses observation to detect health problems. To conduct the examination, the nurse uses techniques of inspection, auscultation, palpation, and percussion (see Chapter 17 ∞).

The physical examination is carried out systematically. It may be organized, according to the examiner's preference, in a head-to-toe approach or a body systems approach. Usually, the nurse first records a general impression about the client's overall appearance and health status. Then the nurse takes such measurements as vital signs, height, and weight. The **cephalocaudal**, or head-to-toe, approach begins the examination at the head; progresses to the neck, thorax, abdomen, and extremities; and ends at the toes. The nurse, using a body systems approach, investigates each system individually. During the physical examination, the nurse assesses all body parts and compares findings on each side of the body. These techniques are discussed in detail in Chapters 16 and 17 ∞.

Instead of performing a complete examination, the nurse may focus on a specific problem area based on the client's needs. On occasion, the nurse may find it necessary to resolve a client complaint or problem before completing the examination. Alternatively, the nurse may perform a screening examination. A screening examination, also called a review of systems, is a brief review of essential functioning of various body parts or systems. Data obtained from this examination are measured against norms or standards, such as ideal height and weight standards or norms for body temperature or blood pressure levels.

Organizing Data

The nurse uses a written (or computerized) format that organizes the assessment data systematically. This is often referred to as a nursing health history, nursing assessment, or nursing database form. The format may be modified according to the client's physical status such as one focused on musculoskeletal data for orthopedic clients.

CONCEPTUAL MODELS/FRAMEWORKS Most schools of nursing and health care agencies have developed their own structured assessment format. Many of these are based on selected nursing models or frameworks (see Chapter 1 ∞). Three examples are Gordon's functional health pattern framework, Orem's self-care model, and Roy's adaptation model.

Gordon (2009) provides a framework of 11 functional health patterns. Gordon uses the word *pattern* to signify a sequence of recurring behavior. The nurse collects data about dysfunctional as well as functional behavior. Thus, by using Gordon's framework to organize data, nurses are able to discern emerging patterns.

Orem (2001) delineates eight universal self-care requisites of humans (Box 7–3). Roy (2009) outline the data to

---

BOX 7–3 Orem's Self-Care Model

Universal Self-Care Requisites

1. The maintenance of a sufficient intake of air.
2. The maintenance of a sufficient intake of water.
3. The maintenance of a sufficient intake of food.
4. The provision of care associated with elimination processes and excrement.
5. The maintenance of a balance between activity and rest.
6. The maintenance of a balance between solitude and social interaction.
7. The prevention of hazards to human life, human functioning, and human well-being.
8. The promotion of human functioning and development within social groups in accord with human potential, known human limitations, and human desire to be normal.
   (Normalcy is used in the sense of that which is essentially human and that which is in accord with the genetic and constitutional characteristics and the talents of individuals.)

Note: Adapted from *Nursing: Concepts of Practice*, 6th ed. D. E. Orem, p. 225, Copyright 2001, with permission from Elsevier.

BOX 7–4 Roy's Adaptation Model

Adaptive Modes

1. Physiologic needs
   - Activity and rest
   - Nutrition
   - Elimination
   - Fluid and electrolytes
   - Oxygenation
   - Protection
   - Regulation: temperature
   - Regulation: the senses
   - Regulation: endocrine system
2. Self-concept
   - Physical self
   - Personal self
3. Role function
4. Interdependence

Note: Adapted from *The Roy Adaptation Model*, 3rd ed., by C. Roy, 2009, Upper Saddle River, NJ: Pearson Education.

---

be collected according to the Roy adaptation model and classify observable behavior into four categories: physiologic, self-concept, role function, and interdependence (Box 7–4).

Data collection tools may be organized according to body systems and specific nursing concerns without using a particular nursing model. Others may be based on the functional health patterns. As a rule, the nurse organizes the data using the same model on which the data collection tool is based.

WELLNESS MODELS Nurses use wellness models to assist clients to identify health risks and to explore lifestyle habits and health behaviors, beliefs, values, and attitudes that influence levels of wellness. Such models generally include health history, physical fitness evaluation, nutritional assessment, life-stress analysis, lifestyle and health habits, health beliefs, sexual health, spiritual health, relationships, and health-risk appraisals. (See Chapter 5 ∞ for details.)

NON-NURSING MODELS Frameworks and models from other disciplines may also be helpful for organizing data. These frameworks are narrower than the model required in nursing; therefore, the nurse usually needs to combine these with other approaches to obtain a complete history.

The body systems model focuses on abnormalities of the integumentary, respiratory, cardiovascular, nervous, musculoskeletal, gastrointestinal, genitourinary, reproductive, and immune systems. Maslow's hierarchy of needs model clusters data pertaining to each of Maslow's needs including physiologic, safety and security, love and belongingness, self-esteem, and self-actualization needs. (See Chapter 5 ∞ for details.)

Developmental Theories Several physical, psychosocial, cognitive, and moral developmental theories may be used by nurses in specific situations. Examples include Havighurst's age periods and developmental tasks, Freud's psychosexual phases of development, Erikson's psychosocial stages of development, Piaget's phases of cognitive development, or Kohlberg's stages of moral development. (See Chapter 9 ∞ for additional information.)

Validating Data

The information gathered during the assessment phase must be complete, factual, and accurate because the nursing diagnoses and interventions are based on this information. **Validation** is the act of double-checking or verifying data to confirm that it is accurate and factual. Validating data helps the nurse ensure that assessment information is complete and that objective and subjective data agree, obtain additional information that may have been overlooked, avoid jumping to conclusions and focusing in the wrong direction to identify problems, and differentiate between cues and inferences. **Cues** are subjective or objective data that can be directly observed by the nurse while **inferences** are the nurse's interpretation or conclusions made based on the cues.

Not all data require validation. For example, data such as height, weight, birth date, and most laboratory studies that can be measured with an accurate scale can be accepted as factual. However, if a client's laboratory studies returned with values far different than anticipated or seen in the past, it may be necessary to perform the study again to validate results. As a rule, the nurse validates data when there are discrepancies between data obtained in the nursing interview (subjective data) and the physical examination (objective data), or when the client's statements differ at different times in the assessment. Guidelines for validating data are shown in Table 7–3. To collect data accurately, nurses need to be aware of their own biases, values, and beliefs and to separate fact from inference, interpretation, and assumption (see Chapter 6 ∞).

To build an accurate database, nurses must validate assumptions regarding the client's physical or emotional behavior. The client's response may validate the nurse's assumptions or prompt further questioning. Failure to validate assumptions can lead to an inaccurate or incomplete nursing assessment and could compromise client safety.

Documenting Data

To complete the assessment phase, the nurse records client data. Accurate documentation is essential and should include all data collected about the client's health status. Data are recorded in a factual manner and not interpreted by the nurse. A judgment or conclusion such as "appetite good" or "normal appetite" may have different meanings for different people. To increase accuracy, the nurse records subjective data in the client's own words, using quotation marks. Restating in other words what someone says increases the chance of changing the original meaning (see Chapter 8 ∞).

TABLE 7–3	Validating Assessment Data	
GUIDELINES	**EXAMPLE**
Compare subjective and objective data to verify the client's statements with your observations.	Client's perceptions of "feeling hot" need to be compared with measurement of the body temperature.
Clarify any ambiguous or vague statements.	*Client:* "I've felt sick on and off for 6 weeks."
	Nurse: "Describe what your sickness is like. Tell me what you mean by 'on and off.'"
Be sure your data consist of cues and not inferences.	*Observation:* Dry skin and reduced tissue turgor
	Inference: Dehydration
	Action: Collect additional data that are needed to make the inference in the diagnosing phase. For example, determine the client's fluid intake, amount and appearance of urine, and blood pressure.
Double-check data that are extremely abnormal.	*Observation:* A resting pulse of 30 beats per minute or a blood pressure of 210/95
	Action: Repeat the measurement. Use another piece of equipment as needed to confirm abnormalities, or ask someone else to collect the same data.
Determine the presence of factors that may interfere with accurate measurement.	A crying infant will have an abnormal respiratory rate and will need quieting before accurate assessment can be made.
Use references (textbooks, journals, research reports) to explain phenomena.	A nurse considers tiny purple or bluish black swollen areas under the tongue of an older adult client to be abnormal until reading about physical changes of aging. Such varicosities are common.

LIFESPAN CONSIDERATIONS
Assessment

Children

Consider this example: A 4-year-old girl is admitted following emergency surgery for a ruptured appendix. She is awake and alert, but refuses to talk. Her parents have had little sleep for over 24 hours and are extremely anxious.

- Gathering assessment data in this situation requires the nurse to be sensitive to the parents' needs for rest and assurance; at the same time, the nurse must collect information to compile an adequate database for appropriate nursing care decisions. Assessment will be problem focused, monitoring the condition of the child as she recovers from surgery and being alert to potential problems.
- The parents become the major source of subjective data, although the child should be encouraged to tell the nurse how she is feeling.
- Objective data collected include vital signs; level of and response to pain; bleeding or discharge from the incision; mobility; integrity of dressings, intravenous lines, catheters, nasogastric tubes, or other medical devices; and affect.
- Since children are a part of families, assessment will include observation of family dynamics and questions that could lead to care of the family system.

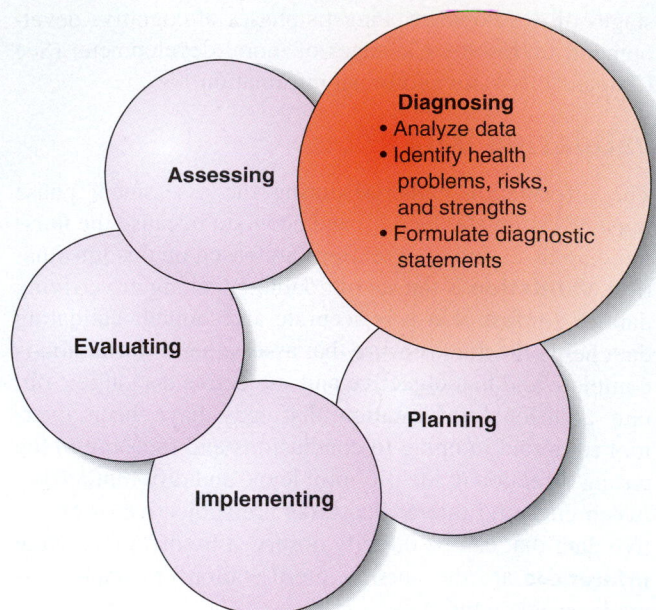

Figure 7–3 ⦿ Diagnosing. The pivotal second phase of the nursing process.

DIAGNOSING

Diagnosing is the second phase of the nursing process. In this phase, nurses use critical-thinking skills to interpret assessment data and identify client strengths and problems. Diagnosing is a pivotal step in the nursing process. Activities preceding this phase are directed toward formulating the nursing diagnoses; the care-planning activities following this phase are based on the nursing diagnoses (see Figure 7–3).

The purpose of the North American Nursing Diagnosis Association (NANDA) is to define, refine, and promote a taxonomy of nursing diagnostic terminology of general use to professional nurses. A **taxonomy** is a classification system or set of categories arranged based on a single principle or set of principles. The members of NANDA include staff nurses, clinical specialists, faculty, directors of nursing, deans, theorists, and researchers. The group has currently approved more than 170 nursing diagnosis labels for clinical use and testing. In 2000, Taxonomy I was revised and is now referred to as Taxonomy II.

NANDA Nursing Diagnoses

To use the concept of nursing diagnoses effectively in generating and completing a nursing care plan, nurses must be familiar with the definitions of terms used, the types, and the components of nursing diagnoses.

DEFINITIONS   The term *diagnosing* refers to the reasoning process, whereas the term **diagnosis** is a statement or conclusion regarding the nature of a phenomenon. The standardized NANDA names for the diagnoses are called diagnostic labels; and the client's problem statement, consisting of the diagnostic label plus **etiology** (causal relationship between a problem and its related or risk factors), is called a **nursing diagnosis**.

In 1990, NANDA adopted an official working definition of nursing diagnosis: ". . . a clinical judgment about individual, family, or community responses to actual and potential health problems/life processes. A nursing diagnosis provides the basis for selection of nursing interventions to achieve outcomes for which the nurse is accountable" (as cited in NANDA International, 2009, p. 419). This definition implies the following:

- Professional nurses (registered nurses) are responsible for making nursing diagnoses, even though other nursing personnel may contribute data to the process of diagnosing and may implement specified nursing care. The American Nurses Association *Nursing: Scope and Standards of Practice* (2004) states that professional nurses are accountable for this phase of the nursing process. The Joint Commission on Accreditation of Healthcare Organizations requires evidence of nursing diagnoses in clients' medical records as well (Joint Commission, 2005).
- The domain of nursing diagnosis includes only those health states that nurses are educated and licensed to treat. For example, generalist nurses are not educated to diagnose or treat diseases such as diabetes mellitus;

this task is defined legally as within the practice of medicine. Yet nurses can diagnose and treat *Deficient Knowledge, Ineffective Coping,* or *Imbalanced Nutrition,* all of which are the human responses to the medical diagnosis of diabetes mellitus.

- A nursing diagnosis is a judgment made only after thorough, systematic data collection.
- Nursing diagnoses describe a continuum of health states: deviations from health, presence of risk factors, and areas of enhanced personal growth.

TYPES OF NURSING DIAGNOSES The five types of nursing diagnoses are actual, risk, wellness, possible, and syndrome.

1. An *actual diagnosis* is a client problem that is present at the time of the nursing assessment. Examples are *Ineffective Breathing Pattern* and *Anxiety.* An actual nursing diagnosis is based on the presence of associated signs and symptoms.
2. A risk nursing diagnosis is a clinical judgment that a problem does not exist, but the presence of **risk factors** indicates that a problem is likely to develop unless nurses intervene.
3. A wellness diagnosis "describes human responses to levels of wellness in an individual, family or community." (NANDA International, 2009, p. 420).
4. A possible nursing diagnosis is one in which evidence about a health problem is incomplete or unclear. A possible diagnosis requires more data either to support or to refute it.
5. A syndrome diagnosis is a diagnosis that is associated with a cluster of other diagnoses.

COMPONENTS OF A NANDA NURSING DIAGNOSIS A nursing diagnosis has three components: (1) the problem and its definition, (2) the etiology, and (3) the defining characteristics. Each component serves a specific purpose.

Problem (Diagnostic Label) and Definition A diagnostic label describes the client's health problem or response for which nursing therapy is given. It describes the client's health status clearly and concisely in a few words. The purpose of the diagnostic label is to direct the formation of client goals and desired outcomes. It may also suggest some nursing interventions.

To be clinically useful, diagnostic labels need to be specific; when the word *Specify* follows a NANDA label, the nurse states the area in which the problem occurs, for example, *Deficient Knowledge* (*Medications*) or *Deficient Knowledge* (*Dietary Adjustments*).

Qualifiers are words that have been added to some NANDA labels to give additional meaning to the diagnostic statement. Common qualifiers include:

- *Deficient* (inadequate in amount, quality, or degree; not sufficient; incomplete)
- *Impaired* (made worse, weakened, damaged, reduced, deteriorated)
- *Decreased* (lesser in size, amount, or degree)

TABLE 7–4	Examples of Nursing Diagnoses with Different Etiologies	
DIAGNOSTIC LABEL (PROBLEM)	CLIENT	ETIOLOGY
Constipation	Al Martinez	Long-term laxative use
	Jerry Wong	Inactivity and insufficient fluid intake
Anxiety	Tanya Brown	Threat to physiologic integrity: possible cancer diagnosis
	Caitlin Shea	Effects of aging (reduced hearing, vision, mobility)

- *Ineffective* (not producing the desired effect)
- *Compromised* (to make vulnerable to threat)

Each diagnostic label approved by NANDA carries a definition that clarifies its meaning.

Etiology (Related Factors and Risk Factors) This component of a nursing diagnosis identifies one or more probable causes of the health problem, gives direction to the required nursing therapy, and enables the nurse to individualize the client's care. Differentiating among possible causes in the nursing diagnosis is essential because each may require different nursing interventions. Table 7–4 provides examples of problems that have different etiologies and therefore require different interventions.

Defining Characteristics **Defining characteristics** are the cluster of signs and symptoms that indicate the presence of a particular diagnostic label. For actual nursing diagnoses, the defining characteristics are the client's signs and symptoms. For risk nursing diagnoses, no subjective and objective signs are present. Thus, the factors that cause the client to be more vulnerable to the problem form the etiology of a risk nursing diagnosis.

The NANDA lists of defining characteristics are still being developed and refined. Characteristics are listed separately according to whether they are subjective or objective in nature.

DIFFERENTIATING NURSING DIAGNOSES FROM MEDICAL DIAGNOSES A nursing diagnosis is a statement of nursing judgment and refers to a condition that nurses, by virtue of their education, experience, and expertise, are licensed to treat. A medical diagnosis is made by a physician and refers to a condition that only a physician can treat. Medical diagnoses refer to disease processes—specific pathophysiologic responses that are fairly uniform from one client to another. In contrast, nursing diagnoses describe the human response, a client's physical, sociocultural, psychologic, and spiritual responses to an illness or a health problem. A client's medical diagnosis remains the same for as long as the disease process is present, but nursing diagnoses change as the client's responses change.

Nurses have responsibilities related to both medical and nursing diagnoses. Nursing diagnoses relate to the nurse's independent functions, that is, the areas of health care that are unique to nursing and separate and distinct from medical management.

It is possible that a nurse cannot prescribe all the care for a nursing diagnosis, but the nurse can prescribe most of the interventions needed for prevention or resolution. For example, most clients with a nursing diagnosis of *Pain* have medical orders for analgesics, but many independent nursing interventions can also alleviate pain. With regard to medical diagnoses, nurses are obligated to carry out physician-prescribed therapies and treatments, that is, dependent functions.

DIFFERENTIATING NURSING DIAGNOSES FROM COLLABORATIVE PROBLEMS A collaborative problem is a type of potential problem that nurses manage using both independent and physician-prescribed interventions. Independent nursing interventions for a collaborative problem focus mainly on monitoring the client's condition and preventing development of the potential complication. Definitive treatment of the condition requires both medical and nursing interventions.

Collaborative problems are present when a particular disease or treatment is present; that is, each disease or treatment has specific complications that are always associated with it. For example, a statement of collaborative problems is "Potential complication of pneumonia: atelectasis, respiratory failure, pleural effusion, pericarditis, and meningitis."

Nursing diagnoses, by contrast, involve human responses, which vary greatly from one person to the next. Therefore, the same set of nursing diagnoses cannot be expected to occur with all persons who have a particular disease or condition; moreover, a single nursing diagnosis may occur as a response to any number of diseases. Thus, the nurse uses nursing diagnoses rather than collaborative problems whenever possible, since nursing diagnoses are more individualized to a specific client and emphasize human responses to which the nurse can independently take action. Table 7–5 provides a comparison of nursing diagnoses, medical problems, and collaborative problems.

The Diagnostic Process

The diagnostic process uses the critical-thinking skills of analysis and synthesis. Critical thinking is a cognitive process during which a person reviews data and considers explanations before forming an opinion. Analysis is the separation into components, that is, the breaking down of the

TABLE 7–5 Comparison of Nursing Diagnoses, Medical Diagnoses, and Collaborative Problems

	NURSING DIAGNOSES	MEDICAL DIAGNOSES	COLLABORATIVE PROBLEMS
Example	*Activity Intolerance* related to decreased cardiac output	Myocardial infarction	Potential complication of myocardial infarction: congestive heart failure
Description	Describe human responses to disease process or health problem; consist of a one-, two-, or three-part statement, usually including problem and etiology	Describe disease and pathology; do not consider other human responses; usually consist of not more than three words	Involve human responses—mainly physiologic complications of disease, tests, or treatments; consist of a two-part statement of situation/pathophysiology and the potential complication
Orientation and responsibility for diagnosing	Oriented to the individual; nurses responsible for diagnosing	Oriented to pathology; physician responsible for diagnosing; diagnosis not within the scope of nursing practice	Oriented to pathophysiology; nurses responsible for diagnosing
Nursing focus	Treat and prevent	Implement medical orders for treatment and monitor status of condition	Prevent and monitor for onset or status of condition
Nursing actions	Independent	Dependent (primarily)	Some independent actions, but primarily for monitoring and preventing
Duration	Can change frequently	Remains the same while disease is present	Present when disease or situation is present
Classification system	Classification system is developed and being used but is not universally accepted	Well-developed classification system accepted by the medical profession	No universally accepted classification system

whole into its parts (deductive reasoning). Synthesis is the opposite, that is, the putting together of parts into the whole (inductive reasoning). See Chapter 6 ∞ to review the concepts of deductive and inductive reasoning.

The diagnostic process is used continuously by most nurses. The diagnostic process has three steps including analyzing data; identifying health problems, risks and strengths; and formulating diagnostic statements.

ANALYZING DATA   In order to analyze data the nurse compares data against standards looking for significant cues, clusters cues in order to generate tentative hypothesis, and identifies gaps and inconsistencies in data. For experienced nurses, these activities occur continuously rather than sequentially.

Comparing Data with Standards   Nurses draw on knowledge and experience to compare client data to standards and norms and identify significant and relevant cues. The nurse uses a wide range of standards, such as growth and development patterns, normal vital signs, and laboratory values. A cue is considered significant if it points to a negative or positive change in health status or pattern, varies from norms of the client population, or indicates a developmental delay.

Clustering Cues   Data clustering, or grouping cues, is a process of determining the relatedness of facts and determining whether any patterns are present, whether the data represent isolated incidents, and whether the data are significant. This is the beginning of synthesis. The nurse may cluster data inductively by combining data from different assessment areas to form a pattern. Or the nurse may begin with a framework, such as Gordon's functional health patterns, and organize the subjective and objective data into the appropriate categories. The latter is a deductive approach to data clustering (see Chapter 6 ∞). Data clustering involves making inferences about the data. The nurse interprets the possible meaning of the cues, and labels the cue clusters with tentative diagnostic hypotheses.

Identifying Gaps and Inconsistencies in Data   Skillful assessment minimizes gaps and inconsistencies in data. However, data analysis should include a final check to ensure that data are complete and correct. Inconsistencies may be conflicting data as a result of measurement error, expectations, and inconsistent or unreliable reports.

IDENTIFYING HEALTH PROBLEMS, RISKS, AND STRENGTHS After data are analyzed, the nurse and client can together identify strengths and problems. This is primarily a decision-making process (see Chapter 6 ∞). After grouping and clustering the data, the nurse and client together identify problems that support tentative actual, risk, and possible diagnoses. Note that some data may indicate a possible problem but when clustered with other data, the possible problem disappears. In addition the nurse must determine whether the client's problem is a nursing diagnosis, medical diagnosis, or collaborative problem. See Figure 7–4 and Table 7–5.

The nurse and client also establish the client's strengths, resources, and abilities to cope. Most people have a clearer

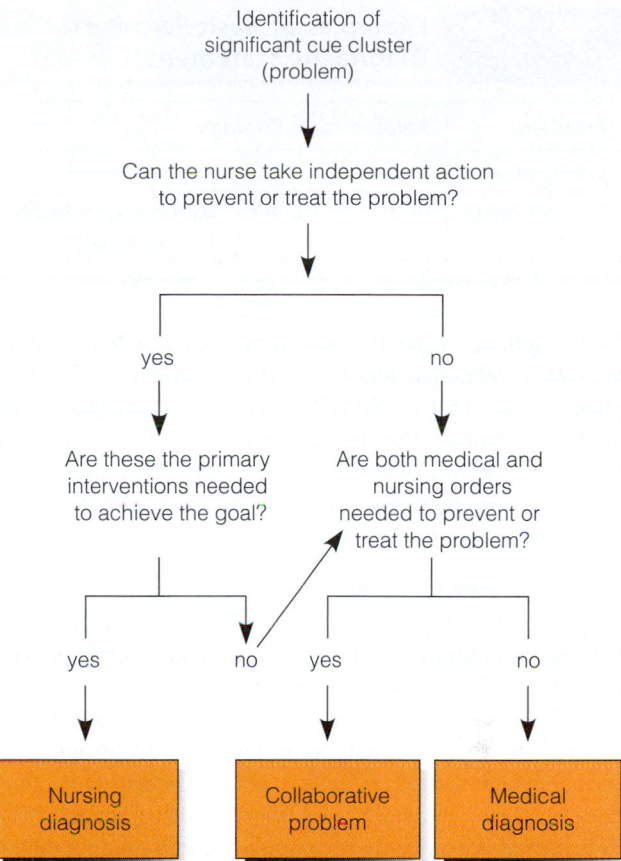

Figure 7–4 ○ Decision tree for differentiating among nursing diagnoses, collaborative problems, and medical diagnoses.

perception of their problems or weaknesses than of their strengths and assets, which they often take for granted. By taking an inventory of strengths, the client can develop a more well-rounded self-concept and self-image. Strengths can be an aid to mobilizing health and regenerative processes. A client's strengths can be found in the nursing assessment record, the health examination, and the client's records.

FORMULATING DIAGNOSTIC STATEMENTS   Most nursing diagnoses are written as two-part or three-part statements, but there are variations of these.

Basic Two-Part Statements   The basic two-part statement includes the following:

1. *Problem (P):* statement of the client's response (NANDA label)
2. *Etiology (E):* factors contributing to or probable causes of the responses

The two parts are joined by the words *related to* rather than *due to.* The phrase *due to* implies that one part causes or is responsible for the other part. By contrast, the phrase *related to* merely implies a relationship. Some examples of two-part nursing diagnoses are shown in Box 7–5.

For NANDA labels that contain the word *Specify,* the nurse must add words to indicate the problem more specifically. The format is still a two-part statement. For example,

---

BOX 7–5	Examples of Basic Two-Part Diagnostic Statement

Problem	Related to	Etiology
Constipation	related to	prolonged laxative use
Severe Anxiety	related to	threat to physiologic integrity: possible cancer diagnosis

---

Noncompliance (Specify) would be *Noncompliance (Diabetic Diet)* related to denial of having disease. For ease in alphabetizing, many NANDA lists are arranged with qualifying words after the main word (e.g., *Infection, Risk for*). Avoid writing diagnostic statements in that manner; instead, write them as they would be stated in normal conversation (e.g., *Risk for Infection*).

Basic Three-Part Statements   The basic three-part nursing diagnosis statement is called the PES format: P is for problem, E is for etiology, and S is for signs and symptoms manifested by the client. Actual nursing diagnoses can be documented by using the three-part statement (see Box 7–6) because the signs and symptoms have been identified. This format cannot be used for risk diagnoses because the client does not have signs and symptoms of the diagnosis. The PES format is especially recommended for beginning diagnosticians because the signs and symptoms validate why the diagnosis was chosen and make the problem statement more descriptive. The PES format can create very long problem statements, sometimes making the problem and etiology unclear. To minimize long problem statements, the nurse can record the signs and symptoms in the nursing notes instead of on the care plan. Another possibility, recommended for students, is to list the signs and symptoms on the care plan below the nursing diagnosis, grouping the subjective (S) and objective (O) data. The signs and symptoms are easily accessible, and the problem and etiology stand out clearly.

One-Part Statements   Some diagnostic statements, such as wellness diagnoses and syndrome nursing diagnoses, consist of a NANDA label only. As the diagnostic labels are refined, they tend to become more specific, so that nursing interventions can be derived from the label itself. Therefore, an etiology may not be needed. For example, adding an etiology to the label *Rape-Trauma Syndrome* does not make the label any more descriptive or useful.

NANDA has specified that any new wellness diagnoses will be developed as one-part statements beginning with the words *Readiness for Enhanced* followed by the desired higher level wellness. Currently the NANDA list includes several wellness diagnoses, including *Spiritual Well-Being, Effective Breastfeeding, Health-Seeking Behaviors*, and *Anticipatory Grieving*. These are usually accepted as one-part statements but may be made more explicit by adding a descriptor, for example, *Health-Seeking Behaviors (Low-Fat Diet)*.

Variations of Basic Formats   Variations of the basic one-, two-, and three-part statements include the following:

1. Writing *unknown etiology* when the defining characteristics are present but the nurse does not know the cause or contributing factors.
2. Using the phrase *complex factors* when there are too many etiologic factors or when they are too complex to state in a brief phrase.
3. Using the word *possible* to describe either the problem or the etiology. When the nurse believes more data are needed about the client's problem or the etiology, the word *possible* is inserted.
4. Using *secondary to* to divide the etiology into two parts, thereby making the statement more descriptive and useful. The part following *secondary to* is often a pathophysiologic or disease process or a medical diagnosis, as in *Risk for Impaired Skin Integrity* related to decreased peripheral circulation secondary to diabetes.
5. Adding a second part to the general response or NANDA label to make it more precise.

Collaborative Problems   Carpenito-Moyet (2009) has suggested that all collaborative (multidisciplinary) problems begin with the diagnostic label *Potential Complication* (PC). Nurses should include in the diagnostic statement both the possible complication they are monitoring and the disease or treatment that is present to produce it. When monitoring for a group of complications associated with a disease or pathology, the nurse states the disease and follows it with a list of the complications. In some situations, an etiology might be helpful in suggesting interventions. Nurses should write the etiology when (a) it clarifies the problem statement, (b) it can be concisely stated, and (c) it helps to suggest nursing actions. See the examples in Box 7–7.

Evaluating the Quality of the Diagnostic Statement   In addition to using the correct format, nurses must consider the con-

---

BOX 7–6	Examples of Basic Three-Part Diagnostic Statement

Problem	Related to	Etiology	As Manifested by	Signs and Symptoms
Situational Low Self-Esteem	related to (r/t)	feelings of rejection by husband	as manifested by (a.m.b.)	hypersensitivity to criticism; states "I don't know if I can manage by myself" and rejects positive feedback

BOX 7–7	Examples of Collaborative Problems

Disease/Situation	Complication	Related to	Etiology
Potential complication of childbirth:	hemorrhage	related to	uterine atony
			retained placental fragments
			bladder distention
Potential complication of diuretic therapy:	arrhythmia	related to	low serum potassium

tent of their diagnostic statements. The statements should be accurate, concise, descriptive, and specific. The nurse must always validate the diagnostic statements with the client and compare the client's signs and symptoms to the NANDA defining characteristics. For risk problems, the nurse compares the client's risk factors to NANDA risk factors. After writing nursing diagnoses, the nurse checks them against the criteria in Table 7–6.

AVOIDING ERRORS IN DIAGNOSTIC REASONING Some error is inherent in any human undertaking, and diagnosis is no exception. However, it is important that nurses make nursing diagnoses with a high level of accuracy. Nurses can avoid some common errors of reasoning by recognizing them and applying the appropriate critical-thinking skills. Error can occur at any point in the diag-

nostic process: data collection, data interpretation, and data clustering. The following suggestions help to minimize diagnostic error:

- *Verify.* Hypothesize possible explanations of the data, but realize that all diagnoses are only tentative until they are verified. Begin and end the diagnostic process by talking with the client and family. When collecting data, ask them what their health problems are and what they believe the causes to be. At the end of the process, ask them to confirm the accuracy and relevance of your diagnoses.
- *Build a good knowledge base and acquire clinical experience.* Nurses must apply knowledge from many different areas to recognize significant cues and patterns and generate hypotheses about the data.

TABLE 7–6	Guidelines for Writing a Nursing Diagnostic Statement

GUIDELINE	CORRECT STATEMENT	INCORRECT OR AMBIGUOUS STATEMENT
1. State in terms of a problem, not a need.	*Deficient Fluid Volume* (problem) related to fever	*Fluid Replacement* (need) related to fever
2. Word the statement so that it is legally advisable.	*Impaired Skin Integrity* related to immobility (legally acceptable)	*Impaired Skin Integrity* related to improper positioning (implies legal liability)
3. Use nonjudgmental statements.	*Spiritual Distress* related to inability to attend church services secondary to immobility (nonjudgmental)	*Spiritual Distress* related to strict rules necessitating church attendance (judgmental)
4. Make sure that both elements of the statement do not say the same thing.	*Risk for Impaired Skin Integrity* related to immobility	*Impaired Skin Integrity* related to ulceration of sacral area (response and probable cause are the same)
5. Be sure that cause and effect are correctly stated (i.e., the etiology causes the problem or puts the client at risk for the problem).	*Pain: Severe Headache* related to fear of addiction to narcotics	*Pain* related to severe headache
6. Word the diagnosis specifically and precisely to provide direction for planning nursing intervention.	*Impaired Oral Mucous Membrane* related to decreased salivation secondary to radiation of neck (specific)	*Impaired Oral Mucous Membrane* related to noxious agent (vague)
7. Use nursing terminology rather than medical terminology to describe the client's response.	*Risk for Ineffective Airway Clearance* related to accumulation of secretions in lungs (nursing terminology)	*Risk for Pneumonia* (medical terminology)
8. Use nursing terminology rather than medical terminology to describe the probable cause of the client's response.	*Risk for Ineffective Airway Clearance* related to accumulation of secretions in lungs (nursing terminology)	*Risk for Ineffective Airway Clearance* related to emphysema (medical terminology)

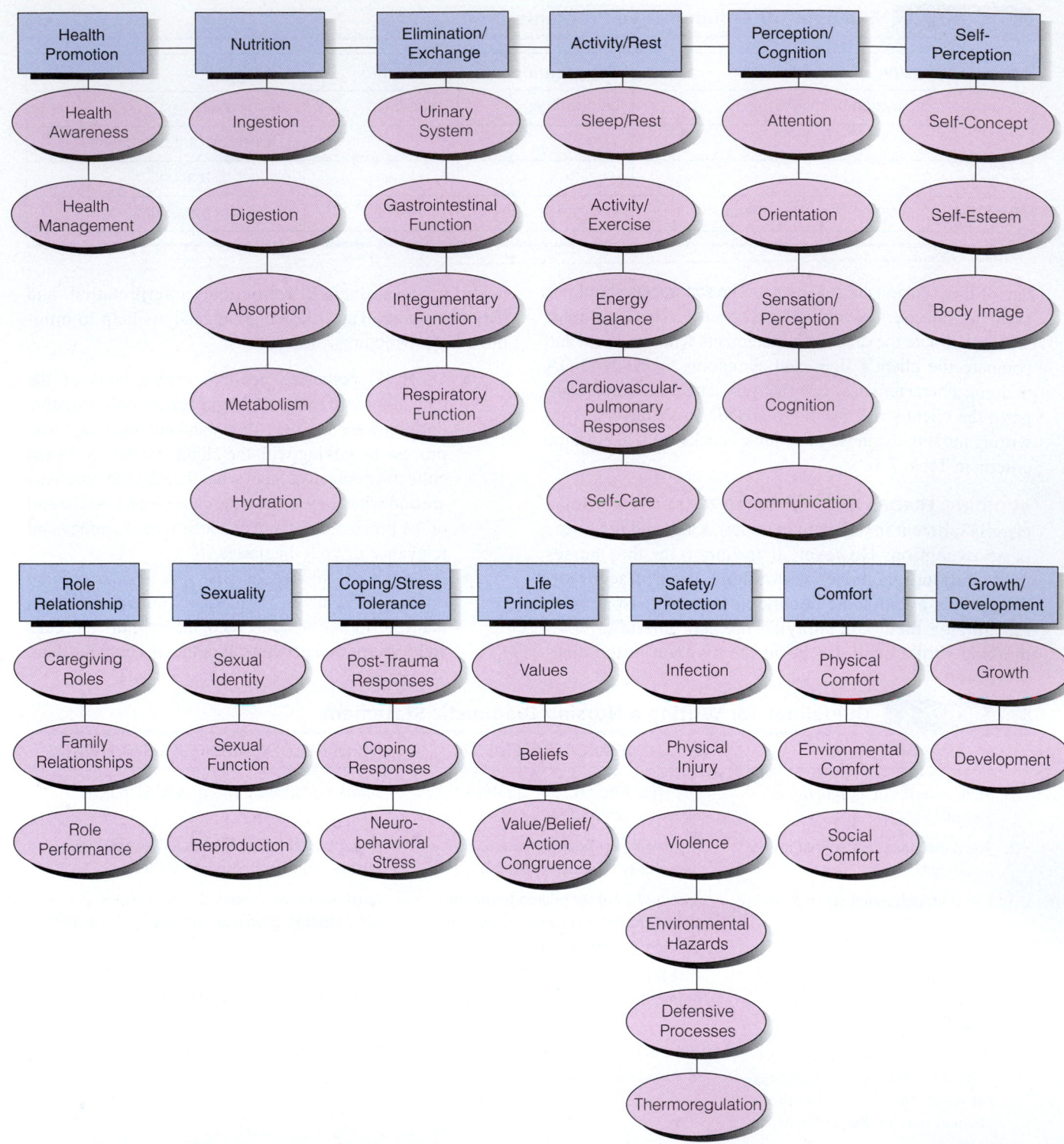

Figure 7–5 ⬤ Taxonomy II.

Source: From *Nursing Diagnoses: Definitions and Classifications*, 2009–2011 by NANDA International, 2009, West Sussex, U.K. Wiley-Blackwell. Adapted with permission.

- *Have a working knowledge of what is normal.* Nurses need to know the population norms for data measurement and determine what is usual for a particular person. The nurse should compare actual findings to the client's baseline when possible.
- *Consult resources.* Professional literature, nursing colleagues, and other professionals are all appro-

priate resources. The nurse should use a nursing diagnosis handbook to determine whether the client's signs and symptoms truly fit the NANDA label chosen.
- *Base diagnoses on patterns rather than on an isolated incident.*
- *Improve critical-thinking skills.* (See Chapter 6 ∞.)

Ongoing Development of Nursing Diagnoses

Having undergone refinements, revisions, and acceptance of new diagnoses, the NANDA taxonomy is now called Taxonomy II (NANDA International, 2009). Taxonomy II has three levels: domains, classes, and nursing diagnoses (Figure 7–5). The diagnoses are coded according to seven axes: diagnostic concept, time, unit of care, age, health status, descriptor, and topology. In addition, diagnoses are listed alphabetically by concept, not by first word. Review and refinement of diagnostic labels continue as new and modified labels are discussed at each biannual conference.

In 1997, NANDA changed the name of its official journal from *Nursing Diagnosis* to *Nursing Diagnosis: The International Journal of Nursing Language and Classification.* The subtitle emphasizes that nursing diagnosis is part of a larger, developing system of standardized nursing language. This system includes classifications of nursing interventions (NIC) and nursing outcomes (NOC) that are being developed by other research groups and linked to the NANDA diagnostic labels. Research groups are examining what nurses do from these three different perspectives (diagnoses, interventions, and outcomes) to clarify and communicate the role nurses play in the health care system. A standardized language will also enable nurses to implement a Nursing Minimum Data Set needed for computerized client records.

LIFESPAN CONSIDERATIONS
Diagnosing

Children

Many developmental issues in pediatrics are not considered problems or illnesses, yet can benefit from nursing intervention. When applied to children and families, nursing diagnoses may reflect a condition or state of health. Assessment of the family system might lead the nurse to conclude that the family is ready and able, even eager, to take on the new roles and responsibilities of being parents. An appropriate diagnosis for such a family could be *Readiness for Enhanced Family Processes*, and nursing care could be directed to educating and providing encouragement and support to the parents.

Older Adults

Older adults tend to have multiple problems with complex physical and psychosocial needs when they are ill. If the nurse has done a thorough, accurate assessment, nursing diagnoses can be selected to cover all problems and, at the same time, prioritize the special needs. As these conditions improve, then other nursing diagnoses might require more attention. Each nursing diagnosis has specific expected outcomes and nursing interventions. The client's strengths should be an essential consideration in all phases of the nursing process.

PLANNING

Planning is a deliberative, systematic phase of the nursing process that involves decision making and problem solving. In planning, the nurse refers to the client's assessment data and diagnostic statements for direction in formulating client goals and designing the nursing interventions required to prevent, reduce, or eliminate the client's health problems (see Figure 7–6). A **nursing intervention** is "any treatment, based upon clinical judgment and knowledge, that a nurse performs to enhance patient/client outcomes" (Bulechek, Butcher, & Dochterman, 2008, p. xxi). The end product of the planning phase is a client care plan.

Although planning is basically the nurse's responsibility, input from the client and support persons is essential if a plan is to be effective. Nurses do not plan for the client, but encourage the client to participate actively to the fullest extent possible.

Types of Planning

Planning begins with the first client contact and continues until the nurse–client relationship ends, usually when the client is discharged from the health care agency. All planning is multidisciplinary and includes the client and family to the fullest extent possible in every step.

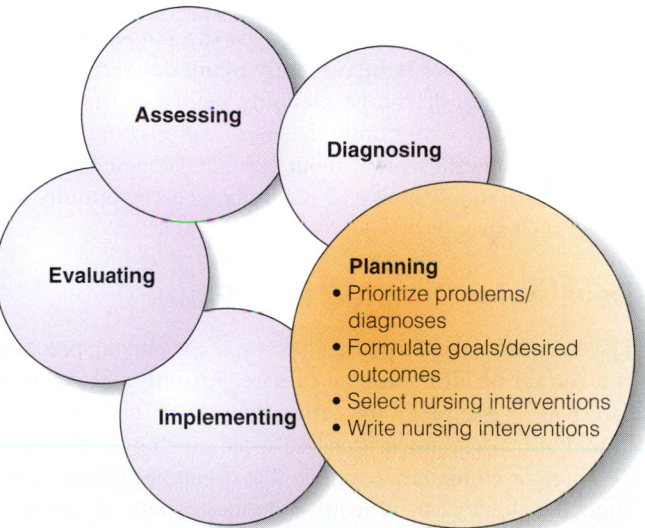

Figure 7–6 ○ Planning. The third phase of the nursing process, in which the nurse and client develop client goals/desired outcomes and nursing interventions to prevent, reduce, or alleviate the client's health problems.

HOME CARE CONSIDERATIONS

In a home setting, the client's support people and caregivers are the ones who implement the plan of care; thus, its effectiveness depends largely on them.

INITIAL PLANNING   The nurse who performs the admission assessment usually develops the initial comprehensive plan of care. This nurse has the benefit of the client's body language as well as some intuitive kinds of information that are not available solely from the written database. Planning should be initiated as soon as possible after the initial assessment.

ONGOING PLANNING   Ongoing planning is done by all nurses who work with the client. As nurses obtain new information and evaluate the client's responses to care, they can individualize the initial care plan further. Ongoing planning also occurs at the beginning of a shift as the nurse plans the care to be given that day. Using ongoing assessment data, the nurse carries out daily planning for the following purposes:

1. To determine whether the client's health status has changed
2. To set priorities for the client's care during the shift
3. To decide which problems to focus on during the shift
4. To coordinate the nurse's activities so that more than one problem can be addressed at each client contact

DISCHARGE PLANNING   **Discharge planning**, the process of anticipating and planning for needs after discharge, is a crucial part of comprehensive health care and should be addressed in each client's care plan. Because the average stay of clients in acute care hospitals has become shorter, people are sometimes discharged requiring complicated home care. Although clients may be discharged to other agencies, such care is increasingly being delivered in the home. Effective discharge planning begins at first client contact and involves comprehensive and ongoing assessment to obtain information about the client's ongoing needs. (For details about discharge planning, see "Continuity of Care" in Chapter 3 ∞.)

Developing Nursing Care Plans

The end product of the planning phase of the nursing process is a formal or informal plan of care. An informal nursing care plan is a strategy for action that exists in the nurse's mind but is often not written. A formal nursing care plan is a written or computerized guide that organizes information about the client's care. The most obvious benefit of a formal written care plan is that it provides for continuity of care.

LONG-TERM CARE CONSIDERATION
Care Plans

Nurses tend to learn more about clients in long-term care than clients in acute care settings because of the length of time they spend with both the client and family. It is important to revise care plans to reflect the gained information, as well as the client's changing condition and goal achievement. Alterations in the client's plan of care assure that care provided is current and individualized.

A standardized care plan is a formal plan that specifies the nursing care for groups of clients with common needs. An **individualized care plan** is tailored to meet the unique needs of a specific client—needs that are not addressed by the standardized plan. It is important that all caregivers work toward the same outcomes and, if available, use approaches shown to be effective with a particular client. Nurses also use the formal care plan for direction about what needs to be documented in client progress notes and as a guide for delegating and assigning staff to care for clients. Standardized care plans, or preprinted care plans, should be individualized to reflect the client's specific needs that may not apply to all clients with those diagnoses. When nurses use the client's nursing diagnoses to develop goals and nursing interventions, the result is a holistic, individualized plan of care that will meet the client's unique needs.

Care plans include the actions nurses must take to address the client's nursing diagnoses and produce the desired outcomes. The nurse begins the plan when the client is admitted to the agency and constantly updates it throughout the client's stay in response to changes in the client's condition and evaluations of goal achievement. During the planning phase, the nurse must (a) decide which of the client's problems need individualized plans and which problems can be addressed by standardized plans and routine care, and (b) write individualized desired outcomes and nursing interventions for client problems that require nursing attention beyond preplanned, routine care.

The complete plan of care for a client is made up of several different documents that (a) describe the routine care needed to meet basic needs, (b) address the client's nursing diagnoses and collaborative problems, and (c) specify nursing responsibilities in carrying out the medical plan of care. A complete plan of care integrates dependent and independent nursing functions into a meaningful whole and provides a central source of client information.

STANDARDIZED APPROACHES TO CARE PLANNING   Most health care agencies have devised a variety of preprinted, standardized plans for providing essential nursing care to specified groups of clients who have certain needs in common. Standards of care, standardized care plans, protocols, policies, and procedures are developed and accepted by the nursing staff in order to (a) ensure that minimally acceptable standards are met and (b) promote efficient use of nurses' time by removing the need to author common activities that are done over and over for many of the clients on a nursing unit.

Standards of care describe nursing actions for clients with similar medical conditions rather than individuals, and they describe achievable rather than ideal nursing care. They define the interventions for which nurses are held accountable; they do not contain medical interventions. Standards of care are usually agency records and not part of the client's care plan, but they may be referred to in the plan. Standards of care may or may not be organized according to problems or nursing diagnoses. They are written from the perspective of the nurse's responsibilities.

Standardized care plans are preprinted guides for the nursing care of a client who has a need that arises frequently in the agency. They are written from the perspective of what care the client can expect. They should not be confused with standards of care. Although the two have some similarities, they have important differences. The use of standardized care plans is supported by the Joint Commission on Accreditation of Healthcare Organizations standards for nursing care, which no longer require a handwritten care plan for every client.

Standardized care plans:

- Are kept with the client's individualized care plan on the nursing unit and become part of the permanent record.
- Provide detailed interventions and contain additions or deletions from the agency's standards of care.
- Typically are written in the nursing process format: Problem ➔ Goals/Desired Outcomes ➔ Nursing Interventions ➔ Evaluation
- Frequently include checklists, blank lines, or empty spaces to allow the nurse to individualize goals and nursing interventions.

Like standards of care and standardized care plans, **protocols** are preprinted to indicate the actions commonly required for a particular group of clients. Protocols may include both the physician's orders and nursing interventions. Depending on the agency, protocols may or may not be included in the client's permanent record.

Policies and **procedures** are developed to govern the handling of frequently occurring situations. Some policies and procedures are similar to protocols and specify what is to be done in a given situation. If a policy covers a situation pertinent to client care, it is usually noted on the care plan. Policies are institutional records and do not become a part of the care plan or permanent record.

A **standing order** is a written document about policies, rules, regulations, or orders regarding client care. Standing orders give nurses the authority to carry out specific actions under certain circumstances, often when a physician is not immediately available.

Regardless of whether care plans are handwritten, computerized, or standardized, nursing care must be individualized to fit the unique needs of each client. In practice, a care plan usually consists of both preprinted and nurse-created sections. The nurse uses standardized care plans for predictable, commonly occurring problems, and creates an individual plan for unique problems or approaches to problems that apply to a specific client. For example, a standardized care plan may indicate the need for dressing changes, but an individualized care plan would detail what type of dressing or when the client prefers to have dressing changes performed.

FORMATS FOR NURSING CARE PLANS Although formats differ from agency to agency, the care plan is often organized into four columns or categories: (a) nursing diagnoses, (b) goals/desired outcomes, (c) nursing interventions, and (d) evaluation. Some agencies use a three-column plan in which evaluation is done in the goals column or in the nurses' notes; others have a five-column plan that adds a column for assessment data preceding the nursing diagnosis column.

Student Care Plans Because student care plans are a learning activity as well as a plan of care, they may be more lengthy and detailed than care plans used by working nurses. To help students learn to write care plans, educators may require that more of the plan be handwritten. They may also modify the three-, four-, or five-column plan by adding a column for "Rationale" after the nursing interventions column. A **rationale** is the scientific principle given as the reason for selecting a particular nursing intervention. Students may also be required to cite supporting literature for their stated rationale. Another method of organizing and representing care plan information is the use of a concept map.

A **concept map** is a visual tool in which ideas or data are enclosed in circles or boxes of some shape and relationships between these are indicated by connecting lines or arrows. Concept maps are creative endeavors. They can take many different forms and encompass various categories of data, according to the creator's interpretation of the client or health condition. The concept map in this chapter is another way of depicting the nursing care plan and includes unique boxes that enclose assessment, nursing diagnosis, outcomes, and interventions. The arrows represent the flow of the phases of the nursing process. Concept maps other than care plans are often used to depict complex relationships among ideas, processes, actions, and so on. Students are often asked to complete pathophysiology flow sheets or concept maps as a method of learning and demonstrating the linkages among disease processes, laboratory data, medications, signs and symptoms, risk factors, and other relevant data (Figure 7–7).

Computerized Care Plans Computers are increasingly being used to create and store nursing care plans. The computer can generate both standardized and individualized care plans. Nurses access the client's stored care plan from a centrally located terminal at the nurses' station or from terminals in client rooms. For an individualized plan, the nurse chooses the appropriate diagnoses from a menu suggested by the computer. The computer then lists possible goals and nursing interventions for those diagnoses; the nurse chooses those appropriate for the client and types in any additional goals and interventions or nursing actions not listed on the menu. The nurse can read the plan on the computer screen or print out an updated working copy.

MULTIDISCIPLINARY (COLLABORATIVE) CARE PLANS A **multidisciplinary care plan** is a standardized plan that outlines the care required for clients with common, predictable—usually medical—conditions. Such plans, also referred to as **collaborative care plans** and **critical pathways**, sequence the care that must be given on each day during the projected length of stay for the specific type of condition. Like the traditional nursing care plan, a multidisciplinary care plan can specify outcomes and nursing interventions to address client problems (including nursing diagnoses).

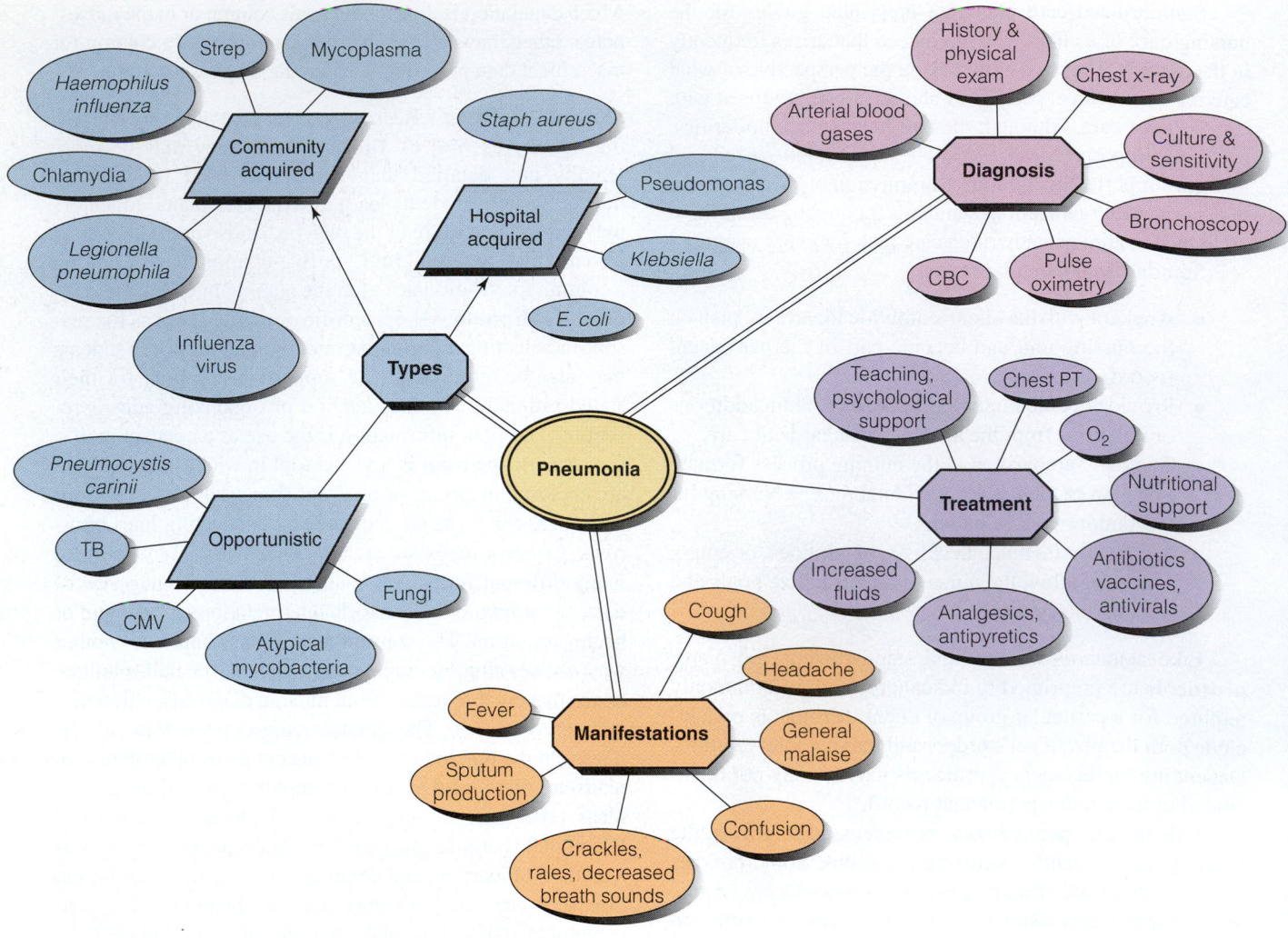

Figure 7–7 ● A sample pathophysiology concept map.

However, it includes medical treatments to be performed by other health care providers as well.

The plan is usually organized with a column for each day, listing the interventions that should be carried out and the client outcomes that should be achieved on that day. There are as many columns on the multidisciplinary care plan as the preset number of days allowed for the client's diagnosis-related group (DRG). (For further information, see Chapter 3 ∞.) Multidisciplinary care plans do not include detailed nursing activities. They should be drawn from but do not replace standards of care and nursing care plans.

GUIDELINES FOR WRITING NURSING CARE PLANS   The nurse should use the following guidelines when writing nursing care plans:

1. *Date and sign the plan.*
2. *Use category headings:* "Nursing Diagnoses," "Goals/Desired Outcomes," "Nursing Interventions," and "Evaluation." Include a date for the evaluation of each goal.

3. *Use standardized/approved medical or English symbols, abbreviations, and key words rather than complete sentences to communicate your ideas unless the agency policy dictates otherwise.*
4. *Be specific.*
5. *Refer to procedure books or other sources of information rather than including all the steps on a written plan.*
6. *Tailor the plan to the unique characteristics of the client by ensuring that the client's choices, such as preferences about the times of care and the methods used, are included.*
7. *Ensure that the nursing plan incorporates preventive and health maintenance aspects as well as restorative ones.*
8. *Ensure that the plan contains interventions for ongoing assessment of the client*
9. *Include collaborative and coordination activities in the plan.*
10. *Include plans for the client's discharge and home care needs.*

The Planning Process

In the process of developing client care plans, the nurse engages in the following activities:

- Setting priorities
- Establishing client goals/desired outcomes
- Selecting nursing interventions
- Writing individualized nursing interventions to be performed on care plans

SETTING PRIORITIES   **Priority setting** is the process of establishing a preferential sequence for addressing nursing diagnoses and interventions. The nurse and client begin planning by ranking nursing diagnosis in the order to be addressed. Instead of rank-ordering diagnoses, nurses can group them as having high, medium, or low priority. Life-threatening problems are designated as high priority. Health-threatening problems are assigned medium priority because they may result in delayed development or cause destructive physical or emotional changes. A low-priority problem is one that arises from normal developmental needs or that requires only minimal nursing support.

It is not necessary to resolve all high-priority diagnoses before addressing others. The nurse may partially address a high-priority diagnosis and then deal with a diagnosis of lesser priority. Furthermore, because the client may have several problems, the nurse often deals with more than one diagnosis at a time. Priorities change as the client's responses, problems, and therapies change. The nurse must consider a variety of factors when assigning priorities, including the following:

1. *Client's health values and beliefs:* Values concerning health may be more important to the nurse than to the client. When there is such a difference of opinion, the client and nurse should discuss it openly to resolve any conflict. However, in a life-threatening situation the nurse usually must take the initiative.
2. *Client's priorities:* Involving the client in prioritizing and care planning enhances cooperation. Sometimes, however, the client's perception of what is important conflicts with the nurse's knowledge of potential problems or complications. The nurse should share knowledge to help the client make an informed choice.
3. *Resources available to the nurse and client:* If money, equipment, or personnel are scarce in a health care agency, then a problem may be given a lower priority than usual. Nurses in a home setting do not have the resources of a hospital. If the necessary resources are not available, the solution for that problem might need to be postponed, or the client may need a referral. Client resources, such as finances or coping ability, may also influence the setting of priorities.
4. *Urgency of the health problem:* Regardless of the framework used, life-threatening situations require that the nurse assign them high priority. Situations that affect the integrity of the client have high priority. Such health problems as drug abuse and radical alteration of self-concept due to amputation can be destructive both to the individual and to the family.
5. *Medical treatment plan:* The priorities for treating health problems must be congruent with treatment by other health professionals.

ESTABLISHING CLIENT GOALS/DESIRED OUTCOMES   After establishing priorities, the nurse and client set goals for each nursing diagnosis. On a care plan, the **goals/desired outcomes** describe, in terms of observable client responses, what the nurse hopes to achieve by implementing the nursing interventions. The terms *goal* and *desired outcome* are used interchangeably in this text, except when discussing and using standardized language. Some references also use the terms *expected outcome, predicted outcome, outcome criterion,* or *objective.* Some nursing literature differentiates the terms by defining goals as broad statements about the client's status, and desired outcomes as the more specific, observable criteria used to evaluate whether the goals have been met. When goals are stated broadly, the care plan must include both goals and desired outcomes. They are sometimes combined into one statement linked by the words "as evidenced by."

Writing the broad, general goal first may help students to think of the specific outcomes that are needed, but the broad goal is just a starting point for planning. It is the specific, observable outcomes that must be written on the care plan and used to evaluate client progress. Table 7–7 shows examples of broad goals and specific outcomes.

TABLE 7–7   Examples of Deriving Desired Outcomes from Nursing Diagnoses

NURSING DIAGNOSIS	OPPOSITE HEALTHY RESPONSES (GOALS)	DESIRED OUTCOMES—THE CLIENT WILL
Impaired Physical Mobility: inability to bear weight on left leg, related to inflammation of knee joint	Improved mobility	Ambulate with crutches by end of the week.
	Ability to bear weight on left leg	Stand without assistance by end of the month.
Ineffective Airway Clearance related to poor cough effort, secondary to incision pain and fear of damaging sutures	Effective airway clearance	Have lungs clear to auscultation during entire postoperative period.
		Have no skin pallor or cyanosis by 12 hours postoperation.
		Within 24 hours after surgery, demonstrate good cough effort.

The Nursing Outcomes Classification Standardized or common nursing language is required in all phases of the nursing process if nursing data are to be included in computerized databases that are analyzed and used in nursing practice. The **Nursing Outcomes Classification (NOC)** describes client outcomes that respond to nursing interventions. In the taxonomy, over 330 outcomes belong to one of seven domains and a class within the domain. Each NOC is assigned a four-digit identifier, indicated in this text by square brackets, and a definition. Table 7–8 shows a NOC outcome associated with movement.

A NOC outcome is similar to a goal in traditional language. It is "[a]n individual, family, or community state, behavior, or perception that is measured along a continuum in response to a nursing intervention(s)" (Moorhead, Johnson, & Maas, 2008, p. xix). The NOC outcomes are broadly stated and conceptual. To be measured, an outcome must be made more specific by identifying the indicators that apply to a particular client. An **indicator** is "a more concrete individual, family, or community state, behavior, or perception that serves as a cue for measuring an outcome" (Moorhead, Johnson, Maas, p. xix) and is similar to desired outcomes in traditional language. Indicators are also stated in neutral terms, but each outcome includes a five-point scale (a measure) that is used to rate the client's status on each indicator. When using the NOC taxonomy to write a desired outcome on a care plan, the nurse writes the label, the indicators that apply to the particular client, and the location on the measuring scale that is desired for each indicator. For example, using the NOC outcome in Table 7–8 for the client diagnosed in Table 7–7, the individualized desired outcomes would read as follows:

> *Mobility Level:* Transfer performance (5, completely independent) Ambulation: walking (4, independent with assistive device)

Stated in traditional language, that goal would read: "Client will have improved mobility, as evidenced by ability to transfer independently and walk with assistive device (walker)."

Purpose of Desired Goals/Outcomes Desired outcomes/goals serve the following purposes:

1. Provide direction for planning nursing interventions.
2. Serve as criteria for evaluating client progress.
3. Enable the client and nurse to determine when the problem has been resolved.
4. Help motivate the client and nurse by providing a sense of achievement.

Long-Term and Short-Term Goals Goals may be short term or long term. A short-term goal might be "Client will raise right arm to shoulder height by Friday." In the same context, a long-term goal might be "Client will regain full use of right arm in 6 weeks." Short-term goals are useful (a) for clients who require health care for a short time and (b) for those who are frustrated by long-term goals that seem difficult to attain and who need the satisfaction of achieving a short-term goal.

Relationship of Desired Goals/Outcomes to Nursing Diagnoses Goals are derived from the client's nursing diagnoses—primarily from the diagnostic label. The diagnostic label con-

TABLE 7–8	Example of a Standardized Client Outcome (NOC)

Domain I: Functional Health

Class C: Mobility

Outcome: Mobility [0208]

Definition: Ability to move purposefully in own environment independently with or without assistive device

MOBILITY OVERALL RATING	SEVERELY COMPROMISED	SUBSTANTIALLY COMPROMISED	MODERATELY COMPROMISED	MILDLY COMPROMISED	NOT COMPROMISED
Indicators					
Balance	1	2	3	4	5
Coordination	1	2	3	4	5
Gait	1	2	3	4	5
Muscle movement	1	2	3	4	5
Joint movement	1	2	3	4	5
Body positioning performance	1	2	3	4	5
Transfer performance	1	2	3	4	5
Running	1	2	3	4	5
Jumping	1	2	3	4	5
Crawling	1	2	3	4	5
Walking	1	2	3	4	5
Moves with ease	1	2	3	4	5

Note: From *Nursing Outcomes and Classification (NOC),* (4th ed). (p. 502), by S. Moorhead, M. Johnson, M. L. Maas, and E. Swanson, Eds., St. Louis, MO: Mosby. Reprinted with permission.

<table>
<tr><td>

LONG-TERM CARE CONSIDERATION

Long Term Goals

While nursing care of clients in acute care settings may focus predominantly on short-term goals, nursing care of clients in long-term care often work to meet long-term goals. Long-term goal setting is best divided into short-term goals that motivate the client and help them track the small improvements they are making as they move toward meeting long-term goals. When long-term goals are met, they should be noted as resolved on the care plan and focus can move toward maintaining that goal and working toward another long-term goal.

</td></tr>
</table>

tains the unhealthy response; it states what should change. For example, if the nursing diagnosis is *Risk for Deficient Fluid Volume* related to diarrhea and inadequate intake secondary to nausea, the essential goal statement might be "The client will reestablish fluid balance, as evidenced by urinary and stool output in balance with fluid intake, normal skin turgor, and moist mucous membranes." In this example, a general goal (fluid balance) is stated as the opposite of the problem (*Deficient Fluid Volume*) and then followed by a list of observable desired outcomes. If achieved, the outcomes would be evidence that the problem, *Deficient Fluid Volume*, has been prevented.

For every nursing diagnosis, the nurse must write the desired outcome or outcomes that, when achieved, directly demonstrates resolution of the problem. When developing goals/desired outcomes, ask the following questions:

1. What is the client's problem?
2. What is the opposite, healthy response?
3. How will the client look or behave if the healthy response is achieved? (What will I be able to see, hear, measure, palpate, smell, or otherwise observe with my senses?)
4. What must the client do and how well must the client do it to demonstrate problem resolution or to demonstrate the capability of resolving the problem?

Components of Goal/Desired Outcome Statements Goal/desired outcome statements should usually have the following four components:

1. *Subject.* The subject, a noun, is the client, any part of the client, or some attribute of the client. The subject is often omitted in goals; it is assumed that the subject is the client unless indicated otherwise.
2. *Verb.* The verb specifies an action the client is to perform. Verbs that denote directly observable behaviors, such as *administer, show,* or *walk,* must be used.
3. *Conditions or modifiers.* Conditions or modifiers may be added to the verb to explain the circumstances under which the behavior is to be performed. They explain what, where, when, or how.
4. *Criterion of desired performance.* The criterion indicates the standard by which a performance is evaluated or the level at which the client will perform the specified behavior. These criteria may specify time or speed, accuracy, distance, and quality. To establish a time-achievement criterion, the nurse needs to ask "How long?" To establish an accuracy criterion, the nurse asks "How well?" Similarly, the nurse asks "How far?" and "What is the expected standard?" to establish distance and quality criteria, respectively.

Table 7–9 illustrates the format that should be used to write outcomes.

Guidelines for Writing Goals/Desired Outcomes The following guidelines can help nurses write useful goals and desired outcomes:

1. Write goals and outcomes in terms of client responses, not nurse activities. Beginning each goal statement with *the client will* may help focus the goal on client behaviors and responses. Avoid statements that start with *enable, facilitate, allow, let, permit,* or similar verbs followed by the word *client.* These verbs indicate what the nurse hopes to accomplish, not what the client will do.
2. Be sure that desired outcomes are realistic for the client's capabilities, limitations, and designated time

TABLE 7–9 **Examples of Components of Goals/Desired Outcomes**

SUBJECT	VERB	CONDITIONS/MODIFIERS	CRITERION OF DESIRED PERFORMANCE
Client	drinks	2500 mL of fluid	daily (time)
Client	administers	correct insulin dose	using aseptic technique (quality standard)
Client	lists	three hazards of smoking (after reading literature)	(accuracy indicated by "three hazards")
Client	recalls	five symptoms of diabetes before discharge	(accuracy indicated by "five symptoms")
Client	walks	the length of the hall without a cane	by date of discharge (time)
Client's ankle	measures	less than 10 inches in circumference	in 48 hours (time)
Client	performs	leg ROM exercises as taught	every 8 hours (time)
Client	identifies	foods high in salt from a prepared list	before discharge (time)
Client	states	the purposes of his medications	before discharge (time)

span, if it is indicated. The term *limitations* refers to finances, equipment, family support, social services, physical and mental condition, and time.

3. Ensure that the goals and desired outcomes are compatible with the therapies of other professionals.
4. Make sure that each goal is derived from only one nursing diagnosis. Keeping the goal statement related to only one diagnosis facilitates evaluation of care by ensuring that planned nursing interventions are clearly related to the diagnosis.
5. Use observable, measurable terms for outcomes. Avoid words that are vague and require interpretation or judgment by the observer. If used in outcomes, these phrases can lead to disagreements about whether the outcome was met. These phrases may be suitable for a broad client goal but are not sufficiently clear and specific to guide the nurse when evaluating client responses.
6. Make sure the client considers the goals/desired outcomes important and values them.

Some clients may know what they wish to accomplish with regard to their health problem; others may not know all the outcome possibilities. The nurse must actively listen to the client to determine personal values, goals, and desired outcomes in relation to current health concerns. Clients are usually motivated and expend the necessary energy to reach goals they consider important.

SELECTING NURSING INTERVENTIONS AND ACTIVITIES

Nursing interventions and activities are the actions that a nurse performs to achieve client goals. The specific interventions chosen should focus on eliminating or reducing the etiology of the nursing diagnosis, which is the second clause of the diagnostic statement. When it is not possible to change the etiologic factors, the nurse chooses interventions to treat the signs and symptoms or the defining characteristics in NANDA terminology. Interventions for risk nursing diagnoses should focus on measures to reduce the client's risk factors, which are also found in the second clause. Correct identification of the etiology during the diagnosing phase provides the framework for choosing successful nursing interventions.

Types of Nursing Interventions Nursing interventions are identified and written during the planning step of the nursing process; however, they are actually performed during the implementation stage. Nursing interventions include both direct and indirect care, as well as nurse-initiated, physician-initiated, and other provider-initiated treatments. Direct care is an intervention performed through interaction with the client. Indirect care is an intervention performed away from but on behalf of the client such as interdisciplinary collaboration or management of the care environment.

Independent interventions are those activities that nurses are licensed to initiate on the basis of their knowledge and skills. They include physical care, ongoing assessment, emotional support and comfort, teaching, counseling, environmental management, and making referrals to other health care professionals. In performing an autonomous activity, the nurse determines that the client requires certain nursing interventions, carries them out or delegates them to other nursing personnel to perform, and is accountable for the decision and the actions.

Dependent interventions are activities carried out under the physician's orders or supervision, or according to specified routines. Physicians' orders commonly direct the nurse to provide medications or intravenous therapy, facilitate diagnostic tests, perform treatments, provide diet therapy, and assist with activity. The nurse is responsible for assessing the need for, explaining, and carrying out the medical orders. Nursing interventions may be written to individualize the medical order based on the client's status. For example, for a medical order of "Progressive ambulation, as tolerated," a nurse might write the following:

1. Dangle for 5 min, 12 h postop.
2. Stand at bedside 24 h postop; observe for pallor, dizziness, and weakness.
3. Check pulse before and after ambulating. Do not progress if pulse > 110.

Collaborative interventions are actions the nurse carries out in collaboration with other health team members, such as physical therapists, social workers, dietitians, and physicians. Collaborative nursing activities reflect the overlapping responsibilities of, and collegial relationships between, health personnel.

The amount of time the nurse spends in an independent versus a collaborative or dependent role varies according to the clinical area, type of institution, and specific position of the nurse.

Considering the Consequences of Each Intervention Usually several possible interventions can be identified for each nursing goal. The nurse's task is to choose those that are most likely to achieve the desired client outcomes. The nurse begins by considering the risks and benefits of each intervention. An intervention may have more than one consequence. Determining the consequences of each intervention requires nursing knowledge and experience.

Criteria for Choosing Nursing Interventions After considering the consequences of the alternative nursing interventions, the nurse chooses one or more that are likely to be most effective. Although the nurse bases this decision on knowledge and experience, the client's input is important. The following criteria can help the nurse choose the best nursing interventions. The plan must be:

- Safe and appropriate for the individual's age, health, and condition.
- Achievable with the resources available.
- Congruent with the client's values, beliefs, and culture.
- Congruent with other therapies.
- Based on nursing knowledge and experience or knowledge from relevant sciences (i.e., based on a rationale).

- Within established standards of care as determined by state laws, professional associations, and the policies of the institution.

WRITING INDIVIDUALIZED NURSING INTERVENTIONS After choosing the appropriate nursing interventions, the nurse writes them on the care plan. Nursing interventions on the care plan are dated when they are written and reviewed regularly at intervals that depend on the individual's needs. The format of written interventions is similar to that of outcomes: verb, conditions, and modifiers, plus time element. The action verb starts the intervention and must be precise. The time element answers when, how long, or how often the nursing action is to occur. In some settings, the intervention (and other segments of the nursing care plan) is signed. The signature of the nurse prescribing the intervention shows the nurse's accountability and has legal significance.

Relationship of Nursing Interventions to Problem Status Depending on the type of client problem, the nurse writes interventions for observation, prevention, treatment, and health promotion. *Observations* include assessments made to determine whether a complication is developing, as well as observation of the client's responses to nursing and other therapies. The nurse should write observations for both real problems and those for which the client is at risk. *Prevention interventions* prescribe the care needed to avoid complications or reduce risk factors. They are needed mainly for potential nursing diagnoses and collaborative problems. *Treatments* include teaching, referrals, physical care, and other care needed for an actual nursing diagnosis. Some interventions may accomplish either prevention or treatment functions, depending on the status of the problem. *Health promotion interventions* are appropriate when the client has no health problems or when the nurse makes a wellness nursing diagnosis. Such nursing interventions focus on helping the client identify areas for improvement that will lead to a higher level of wellness and actualize the client's overall health potential.

Delegating Implementation Delegating is another activity that occurs during the planning phase of the nursing process. While choosing and writing nursing interventions on the client's care plan, the nurse must also determine who should actually perform the activity. The American Nurses Association defines delegation as "the transfer of responsibility for the performance of an activity from one person to another while retaining accountability for the outcome." This differs from assignment, which is a "downward or lateral transfer of both the responsibility *and accountability* [emphasis added] of an activity from one individual to another" (ANA, 1997, Attachment I, #5–6). The ability to delegate client care and assign tasks is a vital skill for registered nurses because many health care institutions use assistive personnel. To delegate appropriately, the nurse must match the needs of the client and family with the skills and knowledge of the available caregivers. This requires knowing the background, experience, knowledge, skills, and strengths of each person, and understanding which tasks are, and are not, within their legal scope of practice.

The nurse has two responsibilities in delegating and assigning: (1) appropriate delegation of duties and (2) adequate supervision of personnel to whom work is delegated or assigned. The nurse can delegate certain tasks to an unlicensed person but cannot assign responsibility for total nursing care. The nurse is responsible for seeing that delegated tasks are carried out properly. Assistive personnel may perform tasks such as measuring intake and output, but the RN is still responsible for analyzing data, planning care, and evaluating outcomes. Because there are no universal standards for the training of unlicensed personnel, nurses often must assume responsibility for supplementing the training those staff members have received (see also Chapter 15 ∞).

The Nursing Interventions Classification

In addition to the efforts of NANDA to standardize the language for describing problems that require nursing care and to create a taxonomy of standardized client outcome labels, nurse researchers also recognized the need for a standardized language to describe the interventions that nurses perform. A taxonomy of nursing interventions referred to as the **Nursing Interventions Classification (NIC)** taxonomy is updated every 4 years. This taxonomy consists of three levels: (a) level 1, domains; (b) level 2, classes; and (c) level 3, interventions. Table 7–10 shows the seven domains and 30 classes of interventions within the taxonomy.

More than 540 interventions (level 3) have been developed. Similar to NANDA diagnoses, each broadly stated intervention includes a label (name), a definition, and a list of activities that outline the key actions of nurses in carrying out the intervention.

All NIC interventions have been linked to NANDA nursing diagnostic labels. The nurse can look up a client's nursing diagnosis to see which nursing interventions are suggested. However, each nursing diagnosis contains suggestions for several interventions, so nurses need to select the appropriate interventions based on their judgment and knowledge of the client. For example, the nursing diagnostic label *Disturbed Sleep Pattern* has 10 NIC interventions listed for problem resolution and 18 additional optional interventions (see Box 7–8).

When planning and documenting care in an agency that uses the NIC taxonomy, the nurse chooses the broad intervention label and chooses the activities appropriate for the client and individualizes them to fit the supplies, equipment, and other resources available in the agency. When writing individualized nursing interventions on a care plan, the nurse should record customized activities rather than the broad intervention labels.

The NIC taxonomy provides many benefits to nurse practitioners, nurse educators, nurse administrators, and the nursing profession as a whole (see Box 7–9).

TABLE 7–10   NIC Taxonomy

LEVEL 1: DOMAINS	LEVEL 2: CLASSES (LETTERED FOR CROSS-REFERENCING)
Domain 1 Physiological: Basic Care that supports physical functioning	A. Activity and Exercise Management: Interventions to organize or assist with physical activity and energy conservation and expenditure B. Elimination Management: Interventions to establish and maintain regular bowel and urinary elimination patterns and manage complications due to altered patterns C. Immobility Management: Interventions to manage restricted body movement and the sequelae D. Nutrition Support: Interventions to modify or maintain nutritional status E. Physical Comfort Promotion: Interventions to promote comfort using physical techniques F. Self-Care Facilitation: Interventions to provide or assist with routine activities of daily living
Domain 2 Physiological: Complex Care that supports homeostatic regulation	G. Electrolyte and Acid–Base Management: Interventions to regulate electrolyte/acid–base balance and prevent complications H. Drug Management: Interventions to facilitate desired effects of pharmacological agents I. Neurologic Management: Interventions to optimize neurologic functions J. Perioperative Care: Interventions to provide care before, during, and immediately after surgery K. Respiratory Management: Interventions to promote airway patency and gas exchange L. Skin/Wound Management: Interventions to maintain or restore tissue integrity M. Thermoregulation: Interventions to maintain body temperature within a normal range N. Tissue Perfusion Management: Interventions to optimize circulation of blood and fluids to the tissue
Domain 3 Behavioral Care that supports psychosocial functioning and facilitates lifestyle changes	O. Behavior Therapy: Interventions to reinforce or promote desirable behaviors or alter undesirable behaviors P. Cognitive Therapy: Interventions to reinforce or promote desirable cognitive functioning or alter undesirable cognitive functioning Q. Communication Enhancement: Interventions to facilitate delivering and receiving verbal and nonverbal messages R. Coping Assistance: Interventions to assist another to build on own strengths, to adapt to a change in function, or to achieve a higher level of function S. Patient Education: Interventions to facilitate learning T. Psychological Comfort Promotion: Interventions to promote comforts using psychological techniques
Domain 4 Safety Care that supports protection against harm *Domain 5 Family* Care that supports the family unit	U. Crisis Management: Interventions to provide immediate short-term help in both psychological and physiological crises V. Risk Management: Interventions to initiate risk-reduction activities and continue monitoring risks over time W. Childbearing Care: Interventions to assist in understanding and coping with the psychological and physiological changes during the childbearing period X. Childrearing Care: Interventions to assist in child rearing Y. Lifespan Care: Interventions to facilitate family unit functioning and promote the health and welfare of family members throughout the lifespan
Domain 6 Health System Care that supports effective use of the health care delivery system *Domain 7 Community* Care that supports the health of the community	Z. Health System Mediation: Interventions to facilitate the interface between patient/family and the health care system a. Health System Management: Interventions to provide and enhance support services for the delivery of care b. Information Management: Interventions to facilitate communication among health care providers c. Community Health Promotion: Interventions that promote the health of the whole community d. Community Risk Management: Interventions that assist in detecting or preventing health risks to the whole community

Note: From *Nursing Interventions Classification (NIC),* 5th ed. (pp. 74–75), by G. M. Bulechek, H. K. Butcher, and J. M. Dochterman, Eds., 2008, St. Louis, MO: Mosby. Reprinted with permission.

BOX 7–8	Examples of NIC Interventions Linked to the NANDA Nursing Diagnosis of Disturbed Sleep Pattern

Disturbed Sleep Pattern

Definition: Time limited disruption of sleep (natural, periodic suspension of consciousness) amount and quality

Suggested Nursing Interventions for Problem Resolution

Dementia Management

Environmental Management

Environmental Management: Comfort

Medication Administration

Medication Management

Medication Prescribing

Security Enhancement

Simple Relaxation Therapy

Sleep Enhancement

Touch

Additional Optional Interventions

Anxiety Reduction

Autogenic Training

Bathing

Calming Technique

Coping Enhancement

Energy Management

Exercise Promotion

Exercise Therapy: Ambulation

Kangaroo Care

Meditation

Music Therapy

Nutrition Management

Pain Management

Positioning

Progressive Muscle Relaxation

Self-Care Assistance: Toileting

Simple Massage

Urinary Incontinence Care: Enuresis

Note: Adapted from *Nursing Interventions Classification (NIC)* 5th ed. (p. 877), by G. M. Bulechek, H. K. Butcher, J. M. Dochterman, Eds., 2008, St. Louis, MO: Mosby. Reprinted with permission.

BOX 7–9	Benefits of the Nursing Interventions Classification

- Helps demonstrate the impact that nurses have on the health care delivery system.
- Standardizes and defines the knowledge base for nursing curricula and practice.
- Facilitates the appropriate selection of a nursing intervention.
- Facilitates communication of nursing treatments to other nurses and other providers.
- Enables researchers to examine the effectiveness and cost of nursing care.
- Assists educators to develop curricula that better articulate with clinical practice.

- Facilitates the teaching of clinical decision making to novice nurses.
- Assists administrators in planning more effectively for staff and equipment needs.
- Promotes the development of a reimbursement system for nursing services.
- Facilitates the development and use of nursing information systems.
- Communicates the nature of nursing to the public.

Note: From *Nursing Interventions Classification (NIC)* 4th ed. (p. vi), by J. C. Dochterman and G. M. Bulechek, Eds., 2004, St. Louis, MO: Mosby. Reprinted with permission.

LONG-TERM CARE CONSIDERATIONS
Expected Outcomes

Older Adults

When a client is in an extended care facility or a long-term care facility, interventions and medications often remain the same day after day. It is important to review the care plan on a regular basis, because changes in the condition of older adults may be subtle and go unnoticed. This applies to both changes of improvement or deterioration. Either one should receive attention so that appropriate revisions can be made in expected outcomes and interventions. Outcomes need to be realistic with consideration given to the client's physical condition, emotional condition, support systems, and mental status. Outcomes often have to be stated and expected to be completed in very small steps. For instance, a client who has had a cerebrovascular accident may spend weeks learning to brush her own teeth or dress herself. When these small steps are successfully completed, it gives the client a sense of accomplishment and motivation to continue working toward increasing self-care. This particular example also demonstrates the need to work collaboratively with other departments, such as physical and occupational therapy, to develop the nursing care plan.

IMPLEMENTING

In the nursing process, implementing is the action phase in which the nurse performs the nursing interventions. Using NIC terminology, **implementing** consists of doing and documenting the activities that are specific nursing actions needed to carry out the interventions. The nurse performs or delegates the nursing activities for the interventions that were developed in the planning step and then concludes the implementing step by recording nursing activities and the resulting client responses.

Although the nurse may act on the client's behalf, professional standards support client and family participation in all phases of the nursing process. The degree of participation depends on the client's health status.

Relationship of Implementing to Other Nursing Process Phases

The first three nursing process phases—assessing, diagnosing, and planning—provide the basis for the nursing actions performed during the implementing step. In turn, the implementing phase provides the actual nursing activities and client responses that are examined in the final phase, the evaluating phase. Using data acquired during assessment, the nurse can individualize the care given in the implementing phase, tailoring the interventions to fit a specific client rather than applying them routinely to categories of clients.

While implementing nursing care, the nurse continues to reassess the client at every contact, gathering data about the client's responses to the nursing activities and about any new problems that may develop. Some routine nursing activities are assessments such as measuring vital signs.

Implementing Skills

To implement the care plan successfully, nurses need cognitive, interpersonal, and technical skills. These skills are distinct from one another; in practice nurses use them in various combinations and with different emphasis, depending on the activity.

The cognitive skills (intellectual skills) include problem solving, decision making, critical thinking, and creativity. They are crucial to safe, intelligent nursing care (see Chapter 6 ∞).

Interpersonal skills are all of the activities, verbal and nonverbal, people use when interacting directly with one another. The effectiveness of a nursing action often depends largely on the nurse's ability to communicate with others. The nurse uses therapeutic communication to understand the client and in turn be understood. A nurse also needs to work effectively with others as a member of the health care team.

Interpersonal skills are necessary for all nursing activities. Interpersonal skills include conveying knowledge, attitudes, feelings, interest, and appreciation of the client's cultural values and lifestyle. Before nurses can be highly skilled in interpersonal relations, they must have self-awareness and sensitivity to others (see Chapters 12 and 27 ∞).

Technical skills are purposeful "hands-on" skills such as manipulating equipment, giving injections, bandaging, moving, lifting, and repositioning clients. These skills are also called tasks, procedures, or psychomotor skills. The term *psychomotor* refers to physical actions that are controlled by the mind, not reflexive. Technical skills require knowledge and manual dexterity. The number of technical skills expected of a nurse has greatly increased in recent years because of the pervasive use of technology, especially in acute care hospitals.

Process of Implementing

The process of implementing (see Figure 7–8) normally includes the following:

- Reassessing the client
- Determining the nurse's need for assistance
- Implementing the nursing interventions
- Supervising the delegated care
- Documenting nursing activities

Reassessing the Client

Just before implementing an intervention, the nurse must reassess the client to make sure the intervention is still needed. Even though an order is written on the care plan, the client's condition may have changed. New data may indicate a need to change the priorities of care or the nursing activities.

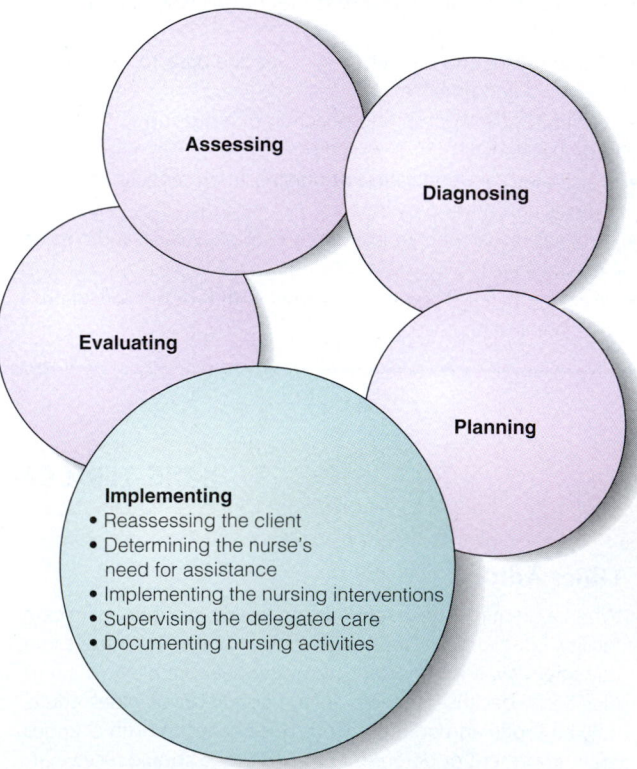

Figure 7–8 ○ Implementing. The fourth phase of the nursing process, in which the nurse implements the nursing interventions and documents the care provided.

DETERMINING THE NURSE'S NEED FOR ASSISTANCE When implementing some nursing interventions, the nurse may require assistance for one or more of the following reasons:

- The nurse is unable to implement the nursing activity safely or efficiently alone.
- Assistance would reduce stress on the client.
- The nurse lacks the knowledge or skills to implement a particular nursing activity.

IMPLEMENTING THE NURSING INTERVENTIONS It is important to explain to the client what interventions will be done, what sensations to expect, what the client is expected to do, and what the expected outcome is. For many nursing activities it is also important to ensure the client's privacy. The number and kind of direct nursing interventions are almost unlimited. Nurses also coordinate client care. This activity involves scheduling client contacts with other departments and serving as a liaison among the members of the health care team.

When implementing interventions, nurses should follow these guidelines:

- Base nursing interventions on scientific knowledge, nursing research, and professional standards of care (evidence-based practice) when these exist. The nurse must be aware of the scientific rationale, as well as possible side effects or complications, of all interventions.
- Clearly understand the interventions to be implemented and question any that are not understood. The nurse is responsible for intelligent implementation of medical and nursing plans of care. This requires knowledge of each intervention, its purpose in the client's plan of care, any contraindications, and changes in the client's condition that may affect the order.
- Adapt activities to the individual client. A client's beliefs, values, age, health status, and environment are factors that can affect the success of a nursing action.
- Implement safe care.
- Provide teaching, support, and comfort. See Chapter 14 ∞ for details on client teaching and Box 14–1 for examples of verbs used in writing learning outcomes. The nurse should always explain the purpose of interventions, what the client will experience, and how the client can participate. The client must have sufficient knowledge to agree to the plan of care and to be able to assume responsibility for as much self-care as possible. These independent nursing activities enhance the effectiveness of nursing care plans.
- Be holistic. The nurse must always view the client as a whole and consider the client's responses in that context.
- Respect the dignity of the client and enhance the client's self-esteem. Providing privacy and encouraging clients to make their own decisions are ways of respecting dignity and enhancing self-esteem.

- Encourage clients to participate actively in implementing the nursing interventions. Active participation enhances the client's sense of independence and control. However, clients vary in the degree of participation they desire. Some want total involvement in their care, whereas others prefer little involvement. The amount of desired involvement may be related to the severity of the illness; the client's culture; or the client's fear, understanding of the illness, and understanding of the intervention.

SUPERVISING DELEGATED CARE If care has been delegated to other health care personnel, the nurse responsible for the client's overall care must ensure that the activities have been implemented according to the care plan. Other caregivers may be required to communicate their activities to the nurse by documenting them on the client record, reporting verbally, or filling out a written form. The nurse validates and responds to any adverse findings or client responses. This may involve modifying the nursing care plan.

DOCUMENTING NURSING ACTIVITIES After carrying out the nursing activities, the nurse completes the implementing phase by recording the interventions and client responses in the nursing progress notes. These are a part of the agency's permanent record for the client. Nursing care must not be recorded in advance because the nurse may determine on reassessment of the client that the intervention should not or cannot be implemented.

The nurse may record routine or recurring activities in the client record at the end of a shift. In the meantime, the nurse maintains a personal record of these interventions on a worksheet. In some instances, it is important to record a nursing intervention immediately after it is implemented. This is particularly true of the administration of medications and treatments because recorded data about a client must be up to date, accurate, and available to other nurses and health care professionals. Immediate recording helps safeguard the client, for example, from receiving a duplicate dose of medication.

Nursing activities are communicated verbally as well as in writing. When a client's health is changing rapidly, the charge nurse and/or the physician may want to be kept up to date with verbal reports. Nurses also report client status at change of shift and on a client's discharge to another unit or health agency in person, via a voice recording, or in writing. For information on documenting and reporting, see Chapter 8 ∞.

EVALUATING

To evaluate is to judge or to appraise. Evaluating is the fifth and last phase of the nursing process. In this context, **evaluating** is a planned, ongoing, purposeful activity in which clients and health care professionals determine (a) the client's progress toward achievement of goals/outcomes and (b) the effectiveness of the nursing care plan. Evaluation is an important aspect of the nursing process because conclusions drawn from the evaluation determine whether further assessment is indicated, the plan of care should be revised or maintained, and the nursing interventions should be terminated, continued, or changed.

Evaluation is continuous. Evaluation done while, or immediately after, implementing a nursing order enables the nurse to make on-the-spot modifications to the intervention as indicated by the client's response. Evaluation performed at specified intervals shows the extent of progress toward goal achievement and enables the nurse to correct any deficiencies and modify the care plan as needed. Evaluation continues until the client achieves the health goals or is discharged from nursing care. Evaluation at discharge includes the status of goal achievement and the client's self-care abilities with regard to follow-up care. Most agencies have a special discharge record for this evaluation.

Through evaluating, nurses demonstrate responsibility and accountability for their actions, indicate interest in the results of the nursing activities, and demonstrate a desire not to perpetuate ineffective actions but to adopt more effective ones.

Relationship of Evaluating to Other Nursing Process Phases

Successful evaluation depends on the effectiveness of the steps that precede it. Assessment data must be accurate and complete so that the nurse can formulate appropriate nursing diagnoses and desired outcomes. Accurate assessment data also serves as a basis for comparison when evaluating the client's response. The desired outcomes must be stated concretely in behavioral terms if they are to be useful for evaluating client responses. And finally, without the implementing phase in which the plan is put into action, there would be nothing to evaluate.

The evaluating and assessing phases overlap. As previously stated, assessment (data collection) is ongoing and continuous at every client contact. However, data are collected for different purposes at different points in the nursing process. During the assessment phase the nurse collects data for the purpose of making diagnoses. During the evaluation step the nurse collects data for the purpose of comparing it to preselected goals and judging the effectiveness of the nursing care. The act of assessing (data collection) is the same; the differences lie in (a) when the data are collected and (b) how the data are used.

Process of Evaluating Client Responses

Before evaluation, the nurse identifies the desired outcomes (indicators) that will be used to measure client goal achievement. (This is done in the planning step.) Desired outcomes serve two purposes: They establish the kind of evaluative data that need to be collected and provide a standard against which the data are judged.

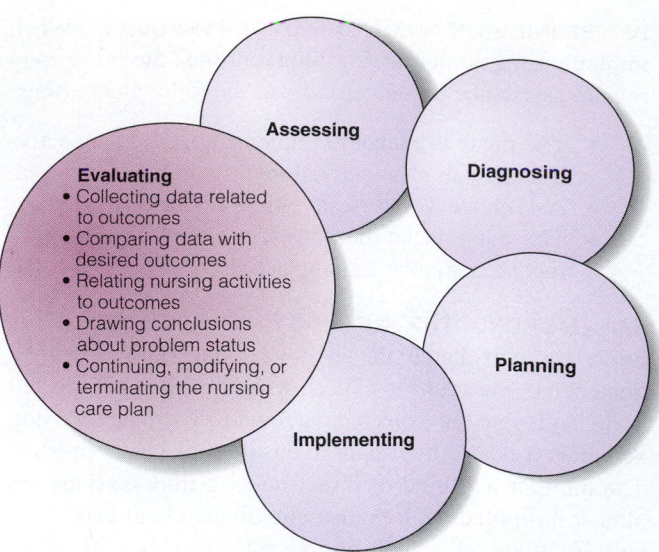

Figure 7–9 ○ Evaluating. The final phase of the nursing process, in which the nurse determines the client's progress toward goal achievement and the effectiveness of the nursing care plan. The plan may be continued, modified, or terminated.

The evaluation process has five components (see Figure 7–9):

- Collecting data related to the desired outcomes (NOC indicators)
- Comparing the data with outcomes
- Relating nursing activities to outcomes
- Drawing conclusions about problem status
- Continuing, modifying, or terminating the nursing care plan

COLLECTING DATA   Using the clearly stated, precise, and measurable desired outcomes as a guide, the nurse collects data so that conclusions can be drawn about whether goals have been met. It is usually necessary to collect both objective and subjective data.

Some data may require interpretation. Examples of objective data requiring interpretation are the degree of tissue turgor of a dehydrated client or the degree of restlessness of a client with pain. Examples of subjective data needing interpretation include complaints of nausea or pain by the client. When interpreting subjective data, the nurse must rely upon either (a) the client's statements or (b) objective indicators of the subjective data, even though these indicators may require further interpretation. Data must be recorded concisely and accurately to facilitate the next part of the evaluating process.

COMPARING DATA WITH OUTCOMES   If the first two parts of the evaluation process have been carried out effectively, it is relatively simple to determine whether a desired outcome has been met. Both the nurse and client play an active role in comparing the client's actual responses with the desired outcomes. When determining whether a goal has been achieved, the nurse can draw one of three possible conclusions:

1. The goal was met; that is, the client response is the same as the desired outcome.
2. The goal was partially met; that is, either a short-term goal was achieved but the long-term goal was not, or the desired outcome was only partially attained.
3. The goal was not met.

After determining whether a goal has been met, the nurse writes an evaluative statement either on the care plan or in the nurse's notes. An **evaluation statement** consists of two parts: a conclusion and supporting data. The conclusion is a statement that the goal/desired outcome was met, partially met, or not met. The supporting data are the list of client responses that support the conclusion.

Data in the Evaluation Statements column represent the client's responses to care as observed by the nurse. In practice, care plans usually do not have a column for evaluation statements; rather, these are recorded in the nurse's notes. If NOC indicators are being used with the outcomes, scores on the scales after intervention would be compared with those measured at baseline to determine improvement. The column explaining rationale for continuing or modifying the plan is often included in a student care plan.

RELATING NURSING ACTIVITIES TO OUTCOMES The fourth aspect of the evaluating process is determining whether the nursing activities had any relation to the outcomes. It should never be assumed that a nursing activity was the cause of or the only factor in meeting, partially meeting, or not meeting a goal.

DRAWING CONCLUSIONS ABOUT PROBLEM STATUS The nurse uses judgments about goal achievement to determine whether the care plan was effective in resolving, reducing, or preventing client problems. When goals have been met, the nurse can draw one of the following conclusions about the status of the client's problem:

- The actual problem stated in the nursing diagnosis has been resolved, or the potential problem is being prevented and the risk factors no longer exist. In these instances, the nurse documents that the goals have been met and discontinues the care for the problem.
- The potential problem stated in the nursing diagnosis is being prevented, but the risk factors are still present. In this case, the nurse keeps the problem on the care plan.
- The actual problem still exists even though some goals are being met. Therefore, the nursing interventions must be continued even though this one goal was met.

When goals have been partially met or when goals have not been met, two conclusions may be drawn:

- The care plan may need to be revised, since the problem is only partially resolved. The revisions may need to occur during the assessing, diagnosing, planning, or implementing phase.

OR

- The care plan does not need revision, because the client merely needs more time to achieve the previously established goal(s). To make this decision, the nurse must assess why the goals are being only partially achieved, including whether the evaluation was conducted too soon.

Continuing, Modifying, and Terminating the Nursing Care Plan

After drawing conclusions about the status of the client's problems, the nurse modifies the care plan as indicated. Depending on the agency, modifications may be made by drawing a line through portions of the care plan, or marking portions using a highlighting pen, or writing "Discontinued" (dc'd), "goal met," or "problem resolved" and the date.

Whether or not goals were met, a number of decisions need to be made about continuing, modifying, or terminating nursing care for each problem. See Table 7–11 for a checklist to use when reviewing a care plan. Although the checklist uses a closed-ended yes/no format, its only intent is to identify areas that require the nurse's further examination.

Before making modifications, the nurse must determine if the plan as a whole was not completely effective. This requires a review of the entire care plan and a critique of each step of the nursing process involved in its development using critical thinking.

ASSESSING An incomplete or incorrect database influences all subsequent steps of the nursing process and care plan. If data are incomplete, the nurse needs to reassess the client and record the new data. In some instances, new data may indicate the need for new nursing diagnoses, new goals, and/or new nursing interventions.

DIAGNOSING If the database was incomplete, new diagnostic statements may be required. If the database was complete, the nurse needs to analyze whether the problems were identified correctly and whether the nursing diagnoses were relevant to that database. After making judgments about problem status, the nurse revises or adds new diagnoses as needed to reflect the most recent client data.

PLANNING: DESIRED OUTCOMES If a nursing diagnosis was inaccurate, obviously the goal statement will need revision. If the nursing diagnosis was appropriate, the nurse then checks if the goals were realistic and attainable. Unrealistic goals require correction. The nurse should also determine whether priorities have changed and whether the client still agrees with the priorities. Goals must also be written for any new nursing diagnoses.

PLANNING: NURSING INTERVENTIONS The nurse investigates whether the nursing interventions were related to goal

TABLE 7–11 **Evaluation Checklist**

ASSESSING	DIAGNOSING	PLANNING	IMPLEMENTING
_____ Are data complete, accurate, and validated?	_____ Are nursing diagnoses relevant and accurate?	**Desired Outcomes**	_____ Was client input obtained at each step of the nursing process?
_____ Do new data require changes in the care plan?	_____ Are nursing diagnoses supported by the data?	_____ Do new nursing diagnoses require new goals?	_____ Were goals and nursing interventions acceptable to the client?
	_____ Has problem status changed (i.e., potential, actual, risk)?	_____ Are goals realistic?	_____ Did the caregivers have the knowledge and skill to perform the interventions correctly?
	_____ Are the diagnoses stated clearly and in correct format?	_____ Was enough time allowed for goal achievement?	_____ Were explanations given to the client prior to implementing?
	_____ Have any nursing diagnoses been resolved?	_____ Do the goals address all aspects of the problem?	
		_____ Does the client still concur with the goals?	
		_____ Have client priorities changed?	
		Nursing Interventions	
		_____ Do nursing interventions need to be written for new nursing diagnoses or new goals?	
		_____ Do the nursing interventions seem to be related to the stated goals?	
		_____ Is there a rationale to justify each nursing order?	
		_____ Are the nursing interventions clear, specific, and detailed?	
		_____ Are new resources available?	
		_____ Do the nursing interventions address all aspects of the client's goals?	
		_____ Were the nursing interventions actually carried out?	

achievement and whether the best nursing interventions were selected. Even when diagnoses and goals were appropriate, the nursing interventions selected may not have been the best ones to achieve the goal. New nursing interventions may reflect changes in the amount of nursing care the client needs, scheduling changes, or rearrangement of nursing activities to group similar activities or to permit longer rest or activity periods for the client. If new nursing diagnoses have been written, then new nursing interventions will also be necessary.

IMPLEMENTING Even if all sections of the care plan appear to be satisfactory, the manner in which the plan was imple-

mented may have interfered with goal achievement. Before selecting new interventions, the nurse should check whether they were carried out. Other personnel may not have carried them out, either because the interventions were unclear or because they were unreasonable in terms of external constraints such as money, staff, time, and equipment.

After making the necessary modifications to the care plan, the nurse implements the modified plan and begins the nursing process cycle again. Refer to the Nursing Care Plan at the end of this chapter to see how the plan was modified after evaluation of goal achievement and review of the nursing process. A line has been drawn through portions the nurse wished to delete; additions to the care plan are shown in italics.

Evaluating the Quality of Nursing Care

In addition to evaluating goal achievement for individual clients, nurses are also involved in evaluating and modifying the overall quality of care given to groups of clients. This is an essential part of professional accountability. In each of the processes described in this section, nurses and all other health care providers work together as an interdisciplinary team focused on improving client care. The activities both use and contribute to evidence-based practice.

A **quality-assurance (QA)** program is an ongoing, systematic process designed to evaluate and promote excellence in the health care provided to clients. Quality assurance frequently refers to evaluation of the level of care provided in a health care agency, but it may be limited to the evaluation of the performance of one nurse or more broadly involve the evaluation of the quality of the care in an agency, or even in a country. Quality assurance requires evaluation of three components of care: structure, process, and outcome. Each type of evaluation requires different criteria and methods, and each has a different focus.

Structure evaluation focuses on the setting in which care is given. It answers this question: What effect does the setting have on the quality of care? Structural standards describe desirable environmental and organizational characteristics that influence care, such as equipment and staffing.

Process evaluation focuses on how the care was given. It answers questions such as these: Is the care relevant to the client's needs? Is the care appropriate, complete, and timely? Process standards focus on the manner in which the nurse uses the nursing process. Some examples of process criteria are "Checks client's identification band before giving medication" and "Performs and records chest assessment, including auscultation, once per shift."

Outcome evaluation focuses on demonstrable changes in the client's health status as a result of nursing care. Outcome criteria are written in terms of client responses or health status, just as they are for evaluation within the nursing process. For example, "How many clients undergoing hip repairs develop pneumonia?" or "How many clients who have a colostomy experience an infection that delays discharge?"

QUALITY IMPROVEMENT   There are currently strong national efforts at evaluating and improving the quality of health care based on internal assessment by health care providers and increasing awareness by the public that medical errors are not uncommon and can be lethal. The Quality of Health Care in America Committee of the Institute of Medicine issued a landmark report: *To Err Is Human: Building a Safer Health System* in 2000. The entire report is available at the National Academies Press website. The emphases of the report are increasing knowledge related to medical errors and establishing systems for enhancing safe care. Since the report was issued, improved attention to these issues has come from a variety of sources. However, the complexity of the health care system, including methods of reimbursement, difficulties with leadership, and fear of threats to autonomy, have limited progress (Leape & Berwick, 2005).

CLINICAL ALERT

Bad systems—and not bad people—lead to most errors.

The Center for Quality Improvement and Patient Safety (CQuIPS) within the Agency for Healthcare Research and Quality (2004) has as its mission to "improve[s] the quality and safety of all Americans through strategic partnerships." Specifically, CQuIPS:

1. Conducts and supports user-driven research on patient safety and health care quality measurement, reporting, and improvement.
2. Develops and disseminates reports and information on health care quality measurement, reporting, and improvement.
3. Collaborates with stakeholders across the health care system to implement evidence-based practices, accelerating and amplifying improvements in quality and safety for patients.
4. Assesses our own practices to ensure continuous learning and improvement for the Center and its members."

In addition, the mission of the Joint Commission on Accreditation of Healthcare Organizations (Joint Commission, 2005a) is: "To continuously improve the safety and quality of care provided to the public through the provision of health care accreditation and related services that support performance improvement in health care organizations." The Joint Commission has put great emphasis on the importance of "sentinel events." Although each agency must define sentinel events for itself, the definition must be consistent with that given by The Joint Commission (2005b):

- A **sentinel event** is an unexpected occurrence involving death or serious physical or psychological injury, or the risk thereof. Serious injury specifically includes loss of limb or function. The phrase, "or the risk thereof" includes any process variation for which a recurrence would carry a significant chance of a serious adverse outcome.
- Such events are called "sentinel" because they signal the need for immediate investigation and response.

The organization must respond to the sentinel event by assessing the cause, identifying a plan for intervention, and evaluating the results of the plan. Often, assessment involves a root cause analysis. Root cause analysis is a process for identifying the factors that bring about deviations in practices that lead to the event. It focuses primarily on systems and processes, not individual performance. It begins with examination of the single event but with the goal of determining which organizational improvements are needed to decrease the likelihood of such events occurring again.

Unlike quality assurance, **quality improvement (QI)** follows client care rather than organizational structure, focuses on process rather than individuals, and uses a systematic approach with the intention of *improving* the quality of care rather than *ensuring* the quality of care. QI studies often focus on identifying and correcting a system's problems. QI is also known as continuous quality improvement (CQI), total quality management (TQM), performance improvement (PI), or persistent quality improvement (PQI).

NURSING AUDIT An audit means the examination or review of records. A retrospective audit (meaning one relating to past events) is the evaluation of a client's record after discharge from an agency. A concurrent audit is the evaluation of a client's health care while the client is still receiving care from the agency. These evaluations use interviewing, direct observation of nursing care, and review of clinical records to determine whether specific evaluative criteria have been met.

Another type of evaluation of care is the *peer review*. In nurse peer review, nurses functioning in the same capacity, or peers, appraise the quality of care or practice performed by other equally qualified nurses. The peer review is based on preestablished standards or criteria. There are two types of peer reviews: individual and nursing audits. The individual peer review focuses on the performance of an individual nurse. The nursing audit focuses on evaluating nursing care through the review of records. The success of these audits depends on accurate documentation.

LIFESPAN CONSIDERATIONS
Evaluating

Evaluation of goals, selected outcomes, and interventions needs to be continuous, with ongoing assessment and reassessment of the situation. Priority needs can change quickly and must be reprioritized when problems occur. Infants and young children are vulnerable to rapid change in their condition due to their small body size, disproportionate size of organs, and immaturity of body systems. Also, they may not be able to verbalize how they are feeling. Older adults may have conditions that impair communication, such as aphasia from a cerebrovascular accident, dementia, multiple sclerosis, or other neurological conditions. In such cases, the nurse needs to be even more astute in performing nonverbal assessments, being alert to potential problems, and detecting changes in the client's condition. If evaluations are done often and thoroughly, changes can be made quickly to intervene more effectively and improve outcomes. Constant assessment, communication, and interpersonal skills are as essential in the evaluation phase as they are in the initial assessment.

Nursing Care Plan   Fluid Volume Excess

Biographic Data: Gertrude Bellamy is an 80-year-old African American woman who lost her husband 3 years ago. She is a retired fifth-grade teacher, attends the Baptist church regularly, and carries both Medicare and Blue Cross Blue Shield supplemental insurance.

Chief Complaint: "I'm feeling a little bit short of breath, my ankles are all swollen, and I've gained 12 pounds in the last three days."

History of Present Illness: Reports that her children threw a surprise birthday party for her 3 days ago and served all of her favorite dishes, which she knew were high in salt but states, "I'm 80 years old. You don't reach that milestone every day so I thought it would be okay if I went off my diet for one day." Woke this morning feeling a little short of breath and noticed it improved when she sat in her recliner but even with her feet propped up her ankle edema continued to worsen.

Pertinent Past Medical History:
- Medical diagnosis of congestive heart failure, chronic renal failure, hypertension
- Allergies to penicillin, sulfa, and seafood
- Has been hospitalized three times in the past 2 years secondary to congestive heart failure exacerbations
- Surgical history includes appendectomy in 1952 and cholecystectomy in 1980
- Takes Digoxin 0.125 mg. PO daily, Lasix 40 mg. PO daily, potassium chloride 40 mEq. Bid, hydrochlorothiazide 75 mg. PO daily, aspirin 81 mg. PO daily, multivitamin 1 capsule daily, Tylenol 650 mg. PO PRN, and Ambien 5 mg. PRN

Family History: Parents died in a car accident when she was a teenager—they had no known medical conditions at the time, a brother died from a myocardial infarction at age 57, sister died from lung cancer at age 71, and two maternal uncles died from colon cancer.

Lifestyle: Ms. Bellamy has never smoked, drinks 1–2 alcoholic beverages per week, and denies use of any illegal medications or supplements. She drinks one cup of coffee in the morning and a cup of caffeine-free tea in the evening. Her beverage of choice is water. She follows a 2 g sodium diet and tries to limit fat and calories to prevent weight gain. She reports that she usually sleeps well at night but occasionally experiences a single night of insomnia and takes Ambien when that occurs, usually less than once per month. She takes a 1 hour nap most afternoons. She continues to drive and performs activities of daily living independently. She enjoys reading and music and is actively involved in her Baptist church.

Social Data: She lives alone in a single-family home in the suburbs of a large city where she has lived for 45 years. She describes her neighborhood as safe, pleasant, and consisting of a number of older adult friends she has known for many years. She has four children, three of whom live within 5 miles of her home. She describes a close family relationship with her children and their families, who visit frequently and help with home maintenance that she is no longer able to perform independently, such as mowing the grass, minor home repairs, and heavy lifting. One of her daughters usually accompanies her to doctor's appointments. She has a master's degree in early childhood education and continues to work with children through church programs since retiring from teaching.

Psychological Data: Mrs. Bellamy is a pleasant, alert, and oriented woman who denies any major stressors in her life. She communicates clearly and appropriately.

Patterns of Health Care: Mrs. Bellamy sees her family physician (Dr. B. Kamara) every 3 months and whenever she isn't feeling well. She also sees a nephrologist (Dr. R. Orr) twice a year and a cardiologist (Dr. A. Hawkins) two or three times per year. Visits with specialists result from referrals from her family physician. She is happy with the care she provides and reports that all of her doctors take good care of her.

Pertinent Nursing Assessment Data:
  Subjective:
  • Reports "mild shortness of breath" worse when supine, improves in Fowler's position
  • Reports recent increased sodium intake
  • Reports decrease in frequency of urination

Objective:
  • Vital signs: 97.8°F (36.5°C) oral – 96 – 22 128/92
  • Jugular vein distention
  • Hematocrit 28%
  • Oxygen saturation 90%
  • Breath sounds: fine rales in the bases bilaterally
  • Weight 128 lbs. – increase of 14 pounds from last physician's office visit
  • 4+ pitting edema to mid-calf
  • Skin turgor within normal limits for age

Nursing Diagnosis: Fluid volume excess

Definition: Increased isotonic fluid retention.

Defining Characteristics: Shortness of breath, abnormal breath sounds, change in respiratory pattern, edema, change in hematocrit, jugular vein distention, orthopnea, weight gain

Related factors: Excess sodium intake, renal dysfunction, heart failure

NURSING OUTCOMES CLASSIFICATION	NURSING INTERVENTIONS CLASSIFICATION	NURSING ACTIVITIES
Fluid balance will not be compromised (in excess) as evidenced by	Electrolyte monitoring Fluid management Fluid monitoring Urinary elimination management	• Maintain accurate intake and output • Monitor for indications of change in fluid status • Monitor laboratory results relevant to fluid retention • Instruct client and family on reduced sodium diet • Maintain and allocate fluid intake over 24 hours (1 liter per day allowed—500 on day shift, 350 on evening shift, 150 on night shift)
• Stable body weight		• Weigh daily and monitor trends • Elevate extremities to increase venous return
• Absence of edema		• Specify location and degree of edema on scale of 1+ to 4+ • Assess edematous legs for impaired circulation or altered skin integrity • Assess effects of medication and treatment on leg edema
• Absence of adventitious breath sounds		• Assess for pulmonary or cardiovascular complications as indicated by respiratory distress, increased pulse rate, increased blood pressure, abnormal heart sounds, or abnormal lung sounds
• Absence of jugular vein distention		• Assess and document jugular vein for distention
		Collaborative Activities: • Consult with primary physician about use of antiembolism stockings • Consult nutritionist to provide diet adequate in protein and limited sodium • Notify physician if signs and symptoms of fluid volume excess persist or worsen • Administer diuretics as prescribed **Home Care:** • Assist client and family to integrate diet and exercise restrictions into their lifestyle • Assess compliance with medical treatments and medications • Assist client and family to recognize signs and symptoms of worsening level of excess fluid volume • Instruct the client to weigh daily using the same scale and notify physician if there is more than a 3-pound weight change in 24 hours

(continued)

Nursing Care Plan *(continued)*

EVALUATION STATEMENTS	NURSING RE-ASSESSMENT DATA	CHANGE TO NURSING INTERVENTIONS	EXPLANATION FOR CONTINUING OR MODIFYING NURSING INTERVENTIONS
Fluid balance will not be compromised (in excess) as evidenced by	After 24 hours in the acute care facility:		
• Stable body weight	Weight now 118 pounds reflecting a 10-pound weight loss	Continue to monitor daily weight	No alteration to plan of care—outcome is partially met but has not regained normal body weight and will require continued monitoring to determine trend
• Absence of edema	Edema now 1+ in feet to ankles	Continue to monitor and document location and degree of edema 1+ to 4+ Continue to assess legs for impaired or altered skin integrity bid Continue to assess effects of medication and treatment for edema q4h Client should elevate legs several times per day but no longer needs to maintain continuous elevation	Outcome partially met—edema less severe Outcome partially met – edema less severe but requires monitoring Outcome partially met—edema less severe but requires monitoring Outcome partially met—with lessening severity of edema time spent with legs elevated can be reduced to comfort
• Absence of adventitious breath sounds	Breath sounds clear and equal, respirations easy and regular	Assessments should be continued but reduce frequency to q4h	Outcome met—while this aspect of the client's outcome has been met, the condition which created it still exists so the client should be routinely assessed for alteration in breath sounds
• Absence of jugular vein distention	Jugular vein no longer distended	Assess for jugular vein distention q4h	Outcome met—while this aspect of the client's outcome has been met, the condition which created it still exists so the client should be routinely assessed for recurrence of jugular vein distention

(Wilkinson, 2008)

CHAPTER HIGHLIGHTS

- The nursing process is a systematic, rational method of planning and providing individualized nursing care for individuals, families, groups, and communities with each phase building upon, and depending upon, other stages.
- The goals of the nursing process are to identify a client's actual or potential health care needs, to establish plans to meet the identified needs, and to deliver and evaluate specific nursing interventions to meet those needs.
- Assessing involves collecting, organizing, validating, and recording data.
- The nursing assessment must be complete and accurate because nursing diagnoses and interventions are based on this information.

- Data must be recorded in a factual manner, without interpretation or inferences.
- Diagnosing is the process of making a clinical judgment (nursing diagnosis) about a client's potential or actual health problems.
- The purpose of the North American Nursing Diagnosis Association (NANDA) is to define, refine, and promote a taxonomy of nursing diagnostic terminology.
- A nursing diagnosis is a clinical judgment about the client's responses to actual and potential health problems or life processes involving critical thinking that provides a basis for selecting nursing interventions to achieve outcomes for which the nurse is accountable.

- The three phases of the diagnostic process are data analysis; identification of the client's health problems, health risks, and strengths; and formulation of diagnostic statements.
- The organizing principles for the NANDA Taxonomy II are the seven axes: diagnostic concept, time, unit of care, age, potentiality, descriptor, and topology.
- Planning involves setting priorities, writing goals/desired outcomes, and establishing a written plan for nursing interventions with the goal of preventing, reducing, or eliminating a client's health problems.
- The planning process includes setting diagnostic priorities, establishing client goals/desired outcomes, selecting nursing interventions, and writing individualized nursing interventions on the care plan.
- A taxonomy of nursing outcome statements, the Nursing Outcomes Classification (NOC) has been developed to describe measurable states, behaviors, or perceptions that respond to nursing interventions. Each has a definition, a measuring scale, and indicators.
- Implementing is carrying out the nursing interventions that are focused on the etiology of the nursing diagnosis. It incorporates all the activities performed to promote health, prevent complications, treat present problems, and facilitate the client's coping with chronic alterations in health status.

- Projecting the consequences of each nursing strategy requires nursing knowledge and experience.
- A taxonomy of nursing interventions referred to as the Nursing Interventions Classification (NIC) taxonomy has been developed. These interventions have been linked to the NANDA nursing diagnostic labels. Similar to NANDA diagnoses, each broadly stated intervention includes a label (name), a definition, and a list of activities that outline the key actions of nurses in carrying out the intervention.
- Reassessing occurs simultaneously with the implementing phase of the nursing process and begins before implementing to assure the action is still necessary.
- The implementing phase terminates with the documentation of the nursing activities and client responses.
- Evaluating is the process of comparing client responses to preselected outcomes to determine whether goals have been met. It includes review and modification of the care plan based on decision making about problem status.
- Quality assurance evaluation includes consideration of the structures, processes, and outcomes of nursing care.
- Quality improvement is a philosophy and process internal to the institution, and does not rely on inspections by an external agency.

THINK ABOUT IT

Refer to the chapter-opening scenario and answer these questions.

1. List the information the nurse assessed and label each as objective or subjective information.

2. Why did the nurse need to ask Jim specific questions about pain and nausea? How did changing from general questions to specific questions help Mary gather better information?

3. Mary suspects the medical diagnosis of appendicitis. What nursing diagnosis would be appropriate for this client?

4. What implementations did the nurse initiate to care for Jim while waiting for his mother to arrive?

∞ *See suggested responses to Think About It on MyNursingKit.*

TEST YOUR KNOWLEDGE

1. Which of the following would the nurse best categorize as secondary subjective data?
   1. The nurse measures a weight loss of 10 pounds since the last clinic visit.
   2. Spouse states the client has lost all appetite.
   3. The nurse palpates edema in lower extremities.
   4. Client states severe pain when walking up stairs.

2. The nurse wishes to determine the client's feelings about a recent diagnosis. Which interview question is most likely to elicit this information?
   1. "What did the doctor tell you about your diagnosis?"
   2. "Are you worried about how the diagnosis will affect you in the future?"
   3. "Tell me about your reactions to the diagnosis."
   4. "How is your family responding to the diagnosis?"

3. In the diagnostic statement "Excess fluid volume related to decreased venous return as manifested by lower extremity edema (swelling)," the nurse would determine the etiology of the problem is which of the following?
   1. Excess fluid volume
   2. Decreased venous return
   3. Edema
   4. Unknown

4. The nurse would use a collaborative problem instead of a nursing or medical diagnosis:
   1. If both medical and nursing interventions are required to treat the problem.
   2. When independent nursing actions can be utilized to treat the problem.

3. In cases where nursing interventions are the primary actions required to treat the problem.
4. When no medical diagnosis (disease) can be determined.

5. The nurse assesses a postoperative client with an abdominal wound and finds the client drowsy when not stimulated. The client's pain is ranked 2 on a scale of 0 to 10, vital signs are within normal range, and extremities are warm with good pulses but very dry skin. The client declines oral fluids due to nausea, and reports no bowel movement in the past 2 days. Hip dressing is dry with drains intact. Which of the following elements is most likely to be considered of highest priority in the nursing care plan?
   1. Pain
   2. Nausea
   3. Inactivity
   4. Potential for wound infection

6. The nurse selects the nursing diagnosis of *Risk for Impaired Skin Integrity* related to immobility, dry skin, and surgical incision. Which of the following represents a properly stated outcome/goal? The client will:
   1. Turn in bed q2h.
   2. Report the importance of applying lotion to skin daily.
   3. Have intact skin during hospitalization.
   4. Use a pressure-reducing mattress.

7. The care plan includes a nursing intervention "4/2/09 Measure client's fluid intake and output. F. Jenkins, RN." What element of a proper nursing intervention has been omitted?
   1. Action verb
   2. Content
   3. Time
   4. None

8. When initiating the implementation phase of the nursing process, the nurse performs which of the following steps first?
   1. Carrying out nursing interventions
   2. Determining the need for assistance
   3. Reassessing the client
   4. Documenting interventions

9. The client has a high-priority nursing diagnosis of *Risk for Impaired Skin Integrity* related to the need for several weeks of imposed bed rest. The nurse evaluates the client after 1 week and finds the skin integrity is not impaired. When the care plan is reviewed, the nurse should perform which of the following?
   1. Delete the diagnosis since the problem has not occurred.
   2. Keep the diagnosis since the risk factors are still present.
   3. Modify the nursing diagnosis to *Impaired Mobility*.
   4. Demote the nursing diagnosis to a lower priority.

10. If the nurse planned to evaluate the length of time clients must wait for a nurse to respond to the client's call bell on each shift, it would reflect which of the following processes?
   1. Structure evaluation
   2. Process evaluation
   3. Outcome evaluation
   4. Audit

∞ See answers to Test Your Knowledge in Appendix A.

REFERENCES AND SELECTED BIBLIOGRAPHY

Ackley, B. J., & Ladewig, G. B. (2008). *Nursing diagnosis handbook: A guide to planning care* (8th ed.). St. Louis: Elsevier Health Sciences.

Agency for Healthcare Research and Quality. (2004). *Mission statement: Center for Quality Improvement and Patient Safety.* Rockville, MD. Retrieved April 16, 2006, from http://www.ahrq.gov/about/cquips/cquipsmiss.htm

Alfaro-LeFevre. R. A. (2005a). *Applying the nursing process: Promoting collaborative care* (6th ed.). Philadelphia: Lippincott Williams & Wilkins.

Alfaro-LeFevre, R. A. (2005b). *The nursing process made easy: Concept mapping and care planning for students.* Philadelphia: Lippincott Williams & Wilkins.

American Nurses Association. (1973). *Standards of nursing practice.* Kansas City, MO: Author.

American Nurses Association. (1997). *The American Nurses Association position statement on registered nurse utilization of unlicensed personnel.* Kansas City, MO: Author. Retrieved November 14, 2009, from http://www.nursingworld.org/UnlicensedAssistive Personnel

American Nurses Association. (1999). *Nursing quality indicators: Guide for implementation.* Washington, DC: Author.

American Nurses Association. (2000). *Nursing quality indicators beyond acute care: Literature review.* Washington, DC: Author.

American Nurses Association. (2004). *Nursing: Scope and standards of practice.* Kansas City, MO: Author.

Berlowitz, D. R., Young, G. J., Hickey, E. C., Saliba, D., Mittman, B. S., Czarnowski, E., et al. (2003). Quality improvement implementation in the nursing home. *Health Services Research, 38*(1 Part 1), 65–83.

Bulechek, G. M., Butcher, H. K., Dochterman, J. M. (Eds.). (2008). *Nursing interventions: classification (NIC)* (5th ed.). St. Louis, MO: Mosby.

Burkhart, L., Konicek, D., Moorhead, S., & Androwich, I. (2005). Mapping parish nurse documentation into the Nursing Interventions Classification: A research method. *CIN: Computers Informatics Nursing, 23*, 220–229.

Carpenito-Moyet, L. J. (2009). *Nursing diagnosis: Application to clinical practice* (13th ed.). Philadelphia: Lippincott Williams & Wilkins.

D'Amico, D., & Barbarito, C. (2007). *Health & physical assessment in nursing.* Upper Saddle River, NJ: Pearson Prentice Hall.

Doenges, M. E., & Moorhouse, M. F. (2008). *Application of nursing process and nursing diagnosis: An interactive text for diagnostic reasoning* (5th ed.). Philadelphia: Davis.

Doenges, M. E., Moorhouse, M. F., & Geissler-Murr, A. C. (2005). *Nursing diagnosis manual: Planning, individualizing, and documenting client care.* Philadelphia: Davis.

Gardner, P. (2003). *Nursing process in action.* Albany, NY: Delmar.

Gordon, M. (1982). Historical perspective: The National Group for Classification of Nursing Diagnoses. In M. J. Kim & D. A. Moritz (Eds.), *Classification of nursing diagnoses: Proceedings of the fourth national conference.* New York: McGraw-Hill.

Gordon, M. (2009). *Manual of nursing diagnosis* (12th ed.). St. Louis: Mosby.

Hall, L. (1955, June). Quality of nursing care. *Public Health News.* Newark, NJ: State Department of Health.

Johnson, D. E. (1959). A philosophy of nursing. *Nursing Outlook, 7*, 198–200.

Johnson, M., Bulechek, G. B., Butcher, H., Dochterman, J., Moorhead, S., Maas, M., et al. (Eds.). (2005). *NANDA, NOC and NIC linkages: Nursing diagnoses, outcomes, and intervention* (2nd ed.). St. Louis: Elsevier Health Sciences.

Joint Commission on Accreditation of Healthcare Organizations. (2005). *Accreditation manual for hospitals.* Chicago: Author.

Joint Commission on Accreditation of Healthcare Organizations. (2005). *2005 Comprehensive accreditation manual for hospitals.* Chicago: Author.

Joint Commission on Accreditation of Healthcare Organizations. (2005a). *Mission statement.* Retrieved November 14, 2009, from http://www.jointcommission.org/AboutUs/joint_commission_facts.htm

Joint Commission on Accreditation of Healthcare Organizations. (2005b). *Sentinel event policy and procedures.* Retrieved November 14, 2009, from http://www.jointcommission.org/AboutUs/Fact_Sheets/

Kim, M. J., McFarland, G. K., & McLane, A. M. (Eds.). (1984). *Classification of nursing diagnoses: Proceedings of the fifth national conference.* St. Louis: Mosby.

Kohn, L. T., Corrigan, J. M., & Donaldson, M. S. (Eds.). (2000). *To err is human: Building a safer health system.* Washington, DC: Committee on Quality of Health Care in America, Institute of Medicine National Academy Press. Retrieved June 21, 2006, from http://books.nap.edu/books/0309068371/html/index.html

Ladewig, G. B., & Ackley, B. J. (2005). *Mosby's guide to nursing diagnosis.* St. Louis: Elsevier Health Sciences.

Lamont, S. C. (2003). Discomfort as a potential nursing diagnosis: A concept analysis and literature review. *International Journal of Nursing Terminologies and Classifications, 14*(4 Suppl), 5.

Leape, L. L., & Berwick, D. M. (2005). Five years after To Err Is Human: What have we learned? *Journal of the American Medical Association, 293*, 2384–2390.

Lopes, M. H. B., & Higa, R. (2003). Mixed incontinence in women: A new nursing diagnosis. *International Journal of Nursing Terminologies and Classifications, 14*(4 Suppl), 49.

Martinez de Castillo, S. L. (2003). *Strategies, techniques, & approaches to thinking: Case studies in clinical nursing* (2nd ed.). St. Louis: Saunders.

Moorhead, S., Johnson, M., Maas, M. L. & Swanson, E. (Eds.). (2008). *Nursing outcomes classification (NOC)* (4th ed.). St. Louis: Mosby.

NANDA International. (2009). *NANDA nursing diagnoses: Definitions and classification 2009–20011.* West Sussex. U.K. Wiley-Blackwell.

Olenek, K., Skowronski, T., & Schmaltz, D. (2003). Geriatric nursing assessment. *Journal of Gerontological Nursing, 29*, 5–9.

Orem, D. E. (2001). *Nursing: Concepts of practice* (6th ed.). St. Louis: Mosby.

Orlando, I. (1961). *The dynamic nurse–patient relationship.* New York: Putnam.

Roy, C. (2009). *The Roy adaptation model* (3rd ed.). Upper Saddle River, NJ: Pearson Education.

Seaback, W. (2005). *Nursing process: Concept & application* (2nd ed.). Albany, NY: Delmar.

Stewart, C. J., & Cash, Jr., W. B. (2006). *Interviewing principles and practices* (11th ed.). New York: McGraw-Hill.

von Krogh, G., Dale, C., & Naden, D. (2005). A framework for integrating NANDA, NIC, and NOC terminology in electronic patient records. *Journal of Nursing Scholarship, 37*, 275–281.

Wiedenbach, E. (1963). The helping art of nursing. *American Journal of Nursing, 63*(11), 54–57.

Wilkinson, J. M. (2008). *Nursing diagnosis handbook: With NIC interventions and NOC outcomes* (9th ed.). Upper Saddle River, NJ: Prentice Hall.

Wilkinson, J. M. (2007). *Nursing process & critical thinking* (4th ed.). Upper Saddle River, NJ: Prentice Hall Health.

Informatics, Documentation, and Reporting

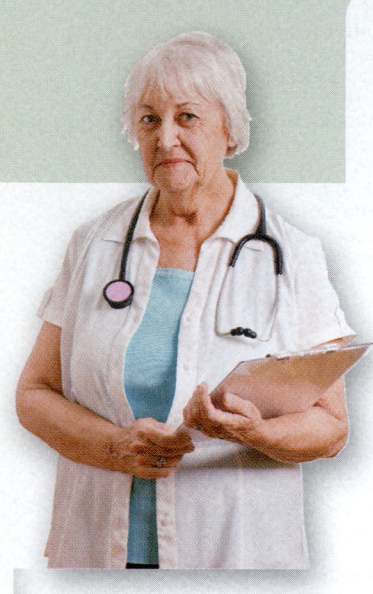

Felicia is an experienced nurse who frequently acts as a resource for other nurses because of her knowledge and attention to detail when providing care to her assigned clients. For the past few days Felicia has been caring for an older adult woman who experienced an acute CVA that left her hemiplegic and aphasic. Because the client was admitted in a malnourished and debilitated status, Felicia has been paying especially close attention to skin integrity, repositioning the client at least every two hours and often hourly as her assignment allows. On the third day Felecia notes that the client's skin is beginning to break down and there is a small open area on the sacrum. Felicia initiates treatment for the pressure ulcer immediately.

Six months later Felicia is notified that the family of this client has filed a lawsuit against the hospital and nurses claiming malpractice resulting in the formation of a pressure ulcer.

LEARNING OUTCOMES

After completing this chapter, you will be able to:

1. List strategies for maintaining client records using legal and ethical standards.

2. Describe the purposes for keeping client records.

3. Compare and contrast different documentation methods: source-oriented and problem-oriented medical records, PIE, focus charting, charting by exception, computerized records, and the case management model.

4. Analyze how various forms in the client record are used to document the nursing process.

5. Compare and contrast the documentation needs for clients in different types of facilities.

6. Demonstrate how to follow the guidelines for effective recording that meets legal and ethical standards.

7. Describe the use of computers for documenting client status.

8. List ways computers are used by nurses in addition to documentation.

9. Identify essential guidelines for reporting client data.

Effective communication among health professionals is vital to the quality of client care. Generally, health personnel communicate through discussion, reports, and records. A discussion is an informal oral consideration of a subject by two or more health care personnel to identify a problem or establish strategies to resolve a problem. A **report** is oral, written, or computer-based communication intended to convey information to others. For instance, nurses always report on clients at the end of a hospital work shift.

DOCUMENTATION

A record is written or computer based. The process of making an entry on a client record is called recording, **charting**, or **documenting**. A clinical record, also called a chart or **client record**, is a formal, legal document that provides evidence of a client's care. Although health care organizations use different systems and forms for documentation, all client records have similar information.

Each health care organization has policies about recording and reporting client data, and each nurse is accountable for practicing according to these standards. Agencies also indicate which nursing assessments and interventions can be recorded by nurses and which can be charted by unlicensed personnel. The Joint Commission on Accreditation of Healthcare Organizations (The Joint Commission) requires client record documentation to be timely, complete, accurate, confidential, and specific to the client.

Ethical and Legal Considerations

The American Nurses Association code of ethics (2001a) states that ". . . the nurse has a duty to maintain confidentiality of all patient information" (p. 12). The client's record is protected legally as a private record of the client's care. Access to the record is restricted to health professionals involved in giving care to the client on a need-to-know basis, meaning only those involved in caring for the client may access personal information. The institution or agency is the rightful owner of the client's record, but the client is the rightful owner of the information contained within the record.

As a result, the client may not remove the record but does have the right to read the information. Agency policy must be followed when the client requests access to the medical record.

Changes in the laws regarding client privacy became the official standard on April 14, 2003. HIPAA regulations maintain privacy and confidentiality of protected health information (PHI). Chapter 2 ∞ reviews HIPAA regulations.

CLINICAL ALERT

Take safety measures before faxing confidential information. A fax cover sheet should contain instruction that the faxed material is to be given only to the named recipient. Consent is needed from the client to fax information. Check that the fax number is correct, check the number on the display of the machine after dialing, and check a third time before pressing the "send" button. Follow up with the agency receiving the fax to assure that the private records are received and placed in a secure location as soon as the fax has been sent.

Because of the increased use of computerized client records, health care agencies have developed policies and procedures to ensure the privacy and confidentiality of client information stored in computers. Following are some suggestions for ensuring the confidentiality and security of computerized records:

1. A personal password is required to enter and sign off computer files. Do not share this password with anyone, including other health team members.
2. After logging on, never leave a computer terminal unattended without logging off.
3. Do not leave client information displayed on the monitor where others may see it.
4. Shred all unneeded computer-generated worksheets.
5. Know the facility's policy and procedure for correcting an entry error.
6. Follow agency procedures for documenting sensitive material.
7. Information technology (IT) personnel must install a firewall to protect the server from unauthorized access.

Purposes of Client Records

Client records are kept for a number of purposes.

COMMUNICATION   The record serves as the vehicle by which different health professionals who interact with a client communicate with each other. This prevents fragmentation, repetition, and delays in client care.

PLANNING CLIENT CARE   Each health professional uses data from the client's record to plan care for that client. Nurses use baseline and ongoing data to evaluate the effectiveness of the nursing care plan. The care plan is documented in the client's medical record to provide continuity of care.

AUDITING HEALTH AGENCIES   An audit is a review of client records for quality-assurance purposes (see Chapter 7 ∞). Accrediting agencies such as The Joint Commission may review client records to determine if a particular health agency is meeting its stated standards.

RESEARCH   The information contained in a record can be a valuable source of data for research. The treatment plans for a number of clients with the same health problems can yield information helpful in determining the effectiveness of a treatment.

EDUCATION   Students in health disciplines often use client records as educational tools. A record can frequently provide a comprehensive view of the client, the illness, effective treatment strategies, and factors that affect the outcome of the illness.

REIMBURSEMENT   Documentation helps a facility receive reimbursement from the federal government. For a facility to obtain payment through Medicare, the client's clinical record must support all charges. Codable diagnoses, such as DRGs, are supported by accurate, thorough recording by nurses. If additional care, treatment, or length of stay becomes necessary for the client's welfare, thorough charting will help justify these needs.

LEGAL DOCUMENTATION   The client's record is a legal document and is usually admissible in court as evidence. In some jurisdictions, however, the record is considered inadmissible as evidence when the client objects, because information the client gives to the physician is confidential.

HEALTH CARE ANALYSIS   Information from records may assist health care planners to identify agency needs, such as overutilized and underutilized hospital services. Records can be used to establish the costs of various services and to identify those services that cost the agency money versus those that generate revenue.

Documentation Systems

A number of documentation systems are in current use: the source-oriented record; the problem-oriented medical record; the problems, interventions, evaluation (PIE) model; focus charting; charting by exception (CBE); computerized documentation; and case management.

SOURCE-ORIENTED RECORD   The traditional client record is a **source-oriented record**. Each person or department makes notations in a separate section or sections of the client's chart. In this type of record, information about a particular problem is distributed throughout the record. Box 8–1 lists the components of a source-oriented record.

  Narrative charting is a traditional part of the source-oriented record. It consists of written notes that include routine care, normal findings, and client problems. There is no right or wrong order to the information, although chronological order is frequently used. Few institutions use only narrative charting today. Narrative recording is being replaced by other systems, such as charting by exception and focus charting. However, narrative charting is expedient in emergency situations (see Figure 8–1). Many agencies combine narrative charting with another system. For example, an agency using a charting-by-exception system (discussed later) may use narrative charting when describing abnormal

		NURSING NOTES	
Date	Time		
6/6/07	1400	Passive ROM exercises provided for R arm and leg.	
		Active assistive exercises to L arm and leg. Has scratch	
		marks on L and R forearms. States,?My skin on my back	
		and arms has been itchy for a week.? Rash not evident.	
		No previous history of pruritus. Is allergic to elastoplast	
		but has not been in contact. Dr. J. Wong notified.	
			T. Ritchie, RN
	1430	Applied calamine lotion to back and arms. Incontinent	
		of urine. Is restless.	T. Ritchie, RN

Figure 8–1 ● An example of narrative notes.

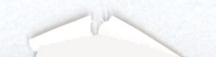

findings. When using narrative charting, it is important to organize the information in a clear, coherent manner. Using the nursing process as a framework is one way to do this.

Source-oriented records are convenient because care providers from each discipline can easily locate the forms on which to record data and it is easy to trace the information specific to one's discipline. The disadvantage is that information about a particular client problem is scattered throughout the chart, so it is difficult to find chronological information on a client's problems and progress. This can lead to decreased communication among the health team, an incomplete picture of the client's care, and a lack of coordination of care (Lippincott Williams & Wilkins, 2003, 2007).

PROBLEM-ORIENTED MEDICAL RECORD   In the problem-oriented medical record (POMR), or **problem-oriented record (POR)**, the data are arranged according to the problems the client has rather than the source of the information. Members of the health care team contribute to the problem list, plan of care, and progress notes. Plans for each active or potential problem are drawn up, and progress notes are recorded for each problem.

The advantages of POMR are that (a) it encourages collaboration and that (b) the problem list in the front of the chart alerts caregivers to the client's needs, making it easier to track the status of each problem. Its disadvantages are that (a) caregivers differ in their ability to use the required charting format, (b) it takes constant vigilance to maintain an up-to-date problem list, and (c) it is somewhat inefficient because assessments and interventions that apply to more than one problem must be repeated. The four basic components of the POMR are the database, the problem list, the plan of care,

BOX 8–1	Components of the Source-Oriented Record

Admission (face) sheet
Initial nursing assessment
Graphic record
Daily care record
Special flow sheets
Medication record
Nurses' notes
Medical history and physical examination
Physician's order sheet
Physician's progress notes
Consultation records
Diagnostic reports
Consultation reports
Client discharge plan and referral
Summary

and the progress notes (see Figure 8–2). In addition, flow sheets and discharge notes are added to the record as needed.

SOAP Format   Within the **progress note**, various formats may be used. The SOAP format is one of these formats. **SOAP** is an acronym for subjective data, objective data, assessment, and planning. Over the years, the SOAP format has been modified to SOAPIE or SOAPIER. The acronyms *SOAPIE* and *SOAPIER* refer to formats that add interventions, evaluation, and revision. Newer versions of this format eliminate the subjective and objective data and start with *assessment,* which

No.	Date Entered	Date Inactive	Client Problem
#1	3/9/07		CVA resulting in Rt hemiplegia and left-sided weakness
#1A	3/9/07		Self-care deficit (hygiene, toileting, grooming, feeding)
#1B	3/9/07		Impaired physical mobility (unable to turn and position self) Redefined 2/7/08
#1C	3/9/07		Total urinary incontinence Redefined 1/17/08
#1D	3/9/07		Progressive dysphasia
#2	3/9/07		Constipation r/t immobility Redefined 6/10/07
#3	3/9/07		History of depression
#4	3/9/07		Essential hypertension
~~#5~~	~~6/6/07~~	~~7/11/07~~	~~Pruritus~~
#2	6/10/07		Risk for constipation r/t insufficient fiber intake
#1C	1/17/08		Urge urinary incontinence at night
#1B	2/7/08		Impaired physical mobility (needs 2-person assistance to transfer and walk)

Figure 8–2 ⬤ A client's problem list in the POMR. Note that problems 1B, 1C, and 2 were redefined on the dates indicated and listed subsequently.

SOAP Format

6/6/07 #5 Generalized pruritus
1400 S— "My skin is itchy on my back and arms, and it's been like this for a week."
O— Skin appears clear—no rash or irritation noted. Marks where client has scratched noted on left and right forearms. Allergic to elastoplast but has not been in contact. No previous history of pruritus.
A— Altered comfort (pruritus): cause unknown.
P— Instructed not to scratch skin.
— Applied calamine lotion to back and arms at 1430 h.
— Cut fingernails.
— Assess further to determine whether recurrence associated with specific drugs or foods.
— Refer to physician and pharmacist for assessment.
T. Ritchie, RN

SOAPIER Format

6/6/07 #5 Generalized pruritus
1400 S— "My skin is itchy on my back and arms, and it's been like this for a week."
O— Skin appears clear—no rash or irritation noted. Marks where client has scratched noted on left and right forearms. Allergic to elastoplast but has not been in contact. No previous history of pruritus.
A— Altered comfort (pruritus): cause unknown.
P— Instruct to not scratch skin.
— Apply calamine lotion as necessary.
— Cut nails to avoid scratches.
— Assess further to determine whether recurrence associated with specific drugs or foods.
— Refer to physician and pharmacist for assessment.
I — Instructed not to scratch skin. Applied calamine lotion to back and arms at 1430 h. Assisted to cut fingernails. Notified physician and pharmacist of problem.
1600 E— States, "I'm still itchy. That lotion didn't help."
R— Remove calamine lotion and apply hydrocortisone cream as ordered.
T. Ritchie, RN

APIE Format

6/6/07 A— Generalized pruritus r/t unknown cause
1400 States, "My skin is itchy on my back and arms, and it's been like this for a week." Skin appears clear. No rash or irritations noted. Marks where client has scratched noted on left and right forearms. Allergic to elastoplast but has not been in contact. No previous history of pruritus.
P— Instruct to not scratch skin.
— Apply calamine lotion as necessary.
— Cut nails to avoid scratches.
— Assess further to determine whether recurrence associated with specific drugs or foods.
— Refer to physician and pharmacist for assessment.
I — Instructed not to scratch skin. Applied calamine lotion to back and arms at 1430 h. Assisted to cut fingernails. Notified physician and pharmacist of problem.
E— States, "I'm still itchy. That lotion didn't help."
T. Ritchie, RN

Figure 8–3 ● Examples of nursing progress notes using SOAP, SOAPIER, and APIE formats.

combines the subjective and objective data. The acronym then becomes *AP, APIE,* or *APIER.* See Figure 8–3.

PIE FORMAT The **PIE** documentation model groups information into three categories. PIE is an acronym for problems, interventions, and evaluation of nursing care. This system consists of a client care assessment flow sheet and progress notes. The **flow sheet** uses specific assessment criteria in a particular format, such as human needs or functional health patterns. The time parameters for a flow sheet can vary from minutes to months. After the assessment, the nurse establishes and records specific problems on the progress notes, often using North American Nursing Diagnosis Association (NANDA) diagnoses to word the problem. If there is no approved nursing diagnosis for a problem, the nurse develops a problem statement using NANDA's three-part format. The *problem statement* is labeled "P" and referred to by number (e.g., P #5). The

interventions employed to manage the problem are labeled "I" and numbered according to the problem (e.g., I #5). The *evaluation* of the effectiveness of the interventions is also labeled and numbered according to the problem (e.g., E #5).

The PIE system eliminates the traditional care plan and incorporates an ongoing care plan into the progress notes. Therefore, the nurse does not have to create and update a separate plan. A disadvantage is that the nurse must review all the nursing notes before giving care to determine which problems are current and which interventions were effective.

FOCUS CHARTING **Focus charting** is intended to make the client, and client concerns and strengths, the focus of care. Three columns for recording are usually used: date and time, focus, and progress notes. The *focus* may be a condition, a nursing diagnosis, a behavior, a sign or symptom, an acute change in the client's condition, or client strength. The progress notes are organized into (D) data, (A) action, and

(R) response, referred to as DAR. The *data* category reflects the assessment phase of the nursing process. The *action* category reflects planning and implementation and includes immediate and future nursing actions. It may also include any changes to the plan of care. The *response category* reflects the evaluation phase of the nursing process and describes the client's response to any nursing and medical care.

The focus charting system provides a holistic perspective of the client and the client's needs. It also provides a nursing process framework for the progress notes. The three components do not need to be recorded in order, and each note does not need to have all three categories. Flow sheets and checklists are frequently used on the client's chart to record routine nursing tasks and assessment data.

Date/Hour	Focus	Progress Notes
2/11/07 0900	Pain	**D:** Guarding abdominal incision. Facial grimacing. Rates pain at "8" on scale of 0–10.
		A: Administered morphine sulfate 4 mg IV.
0930		**R:** Rates pain at "1." States willing to ambulate.

CHARTING BY EXCEPTION   Charting by exception (CBE) is a documentation system in which only abnormal or significant findings or exceptions to norms are recorded. CBE incorporates three key elements (Guido, 2005) including flow sheets, standards of care, and bedside access to chart forms.

The advantages of this system are that it eliminates lengthy, repetitive notes and makes client changes in condition more obvious. Inherent in CBE is the presumption that the nurse did assess the client and determined what responses were normal and abnormal. Many nurses believe in the saying "not charted, not done" and subsequently may feel uncomfortable with the CBE documentation system. Sullivan (2004) suggests writing N/A on flow sheets where the items are not applicable and avoid blank spaces. This would then avoid the possible misinterpretation that the assessment or intervention was not done by the nurse.

CASE MANAGEMENT   The case management model emphasizes quality, cost-effective care delivered within an established length of stay. This model uses a multidisciplinary approach to planning and documenting client care, using *critical pathways*. These forms identify the outcomes that certain groups of clients are expected to achieve on each day of care, along with the interventions necessary for each day. See Figure 8–4 and Chapter 3 ∞ for more information about critical pathways.

Along with critical pathways, the case management model incorporates graphics and flow sheets. Progress notes typically use some type of charting by exception. A goal that is not met is called a **variance**. A variance is a deviation to what is planned on the critical pathway—unexpected occur-

CRITICAL PATHWAY: TOTAL HIP REPLACEMENT

	DOS/Day 1	Days 2–3
Pain Management	Outcome: • Verbalizes comfort or tolerance of pain Circle: V NV Variance:	Outcome: • Verbalizes comfort with pain control measures Circle: V NV Variance:
Respiratory	Outcomes: • Breath sounds clear to auscultation • Achieves 50% of volume goal on incentive spirometer Circle: V NV Variance:	Outcomes: • Breath sounds clear to auscultation • Achieves 100% of volume goal on incentive spirometer Circle: V NV Variance:
Key: V = Variance	NV = No Variance	
Signature:	Initials:	
Signature:	Initials:	

Figure 8–4 ◉ Excerpt from a critical pathway documentation form.

rences that affect the planned care or the client's responses to care. When a variance occurs, the nurse writes a note documenting the unexpected event, the cause, and actions taken to correct the situation or justify the actions taken. See Table 8–1 for an example of how a variance might be documented.

The case management model promotes collaboration and teamwork among caregivers, helps to decrease length of stay, and makes efficient use of time. Because care is goal focused, the quality may improve. However, critical pathways work best for clients with one or two diagnoses and few individualized needs. Clients with multiple diagnoses (e.g., a client with a hip fracture, pneumonia, diabetes, and pressure sore) or those with an unpredictable course of symptoms (e.g., a neurological client with seizures) are difficult to document on a critical path.

Documenting Nursing Activities

The client record should describe the client's ongoing status and reflect the full range of the nursing process. Regardless of the records system used in an agency, nurses document evidence of the nursing process on a variety of forms throughout the clinical record (Table 8–2).

A comprehensive admission assessment, also referred to as an initial database, nursing history, or nursing assessment, is completed when the client is admitted to the nursing unit (see Chapter 7 ∞). The nurse generally records ongoing assessments or reassessments on flow sheets or on nursing progress notes.

According to Smith and Dougherty (2001), The Joint Commission requires that the clinical record include evidence of client assessments, nursing diagnoses and/or client needs, nursing interventions, client outcomes, and evidence of a current nursing care plan. Depending on the records system being

TABLE 8–1	Example of Variance Documentation (Critical Pathway)

A client has had a below-the-knee amputation. On the third postoperative day he has a temperature of 38.8°C (102°F). Lung sounds are clear and he is not coughing. The nurse notices redness and skin breakdown over the client's sacrum. The critical pathway outcomes specified for Day 3 are "Oral temperature 37.7C (100F)" and "Skin intact over bony prominences." The nurse should chart the following variances:

DATE/TIME	VARIANCE	CAUSE	ACTION TAKEN/PLANS
4/16/07 0900	Elevated temperature (102F)	Possible sepsis	4/16—Blood cultures × 3 per order. Monitor temp. q1h. Monitor I&O, hydration, and mental status.
4/16/07 1130	Impaired skin integrity: Stage 1 redness, 2-inch circular area on sacrum	Client does not move about in bed unless reminded	4/16—Positioned on L side. Turn side-to-side q2h while awake. On every client contact, remind client to move about in bed. Apply Duoderm after bath.

TABLE 8–2	Documentation for the Nursing Process

STEP*	DOCUMENTATION FORMS
Assessment	Initial assessment form, various flow sheets
Nursing diagnosis	Nursing care plan, critical pathway, progress notes, problem list
Planning	Nursing care plan, critical pathway
Implementing	Progress notes, flow sheets
Evaluating	Progress notes

*All steps are recorded on discharge/referral summaries.

used, the nursing care plan may be separate from the client's chart, recorded in progress notes and other forms in the client record, or incorporated into a multidisciplinary plan of care. Care plans can be traditional or standardized. (See Chapter 7 ∞ for additional information.)

The **Kardex** is a widely used, concise method of organizing and recording data about a client, making information quickly accessible to all health professionals. The system consists of a series of cards kept in a portable index file or on computer-generated forms. The card for a particular client can be quickly accessed to reveal specific data. The Kardex may or may not become a part of the client's permanent record. In some organizations it is a temporary worksheet written in pencil for ease in recording frequent changes in details of a client's care. The information on Kardexes may be organized into sections including pertinent information, allergies, medications, intravenous fluids, daily treatments and procedures, diagnostic procedures, client needs, problem list, goals, or nursing approaches. It provides a quick visual guide that any nurse caring for the client may record on. Whether the Kardex is a written paper or computerized, it is important to have a place on it to record date and initials of the person reviewing or revising it.

A flow sheet enables nurses to record nursing data quickly and concisely and provides an easy-to-read record of the client's condition over time. Various flow sheets may be used such as graphic intake and output, medication administration, or skin assessment records, to name a few.

Progress notes written by nurses provide information about the progress a client is making toward achieving desired outcomes. Therefore, in addition to assessment and reassessment data, progress notes include information about client problems and nursing interventions. The format used depends on the documentation system used in the institution. Various kinds of nursing progress notes are discussed in the "Documentation Systems" section earlier in this chapter.

A discharge note and referral summary are completed when the client is being discharged or transferred to another institution or to a home setting where a visit by a community health nurse is required. See the discussion of discharge planning in Chapter 3 ∞, and the assessment parameters suggested when preparing clients to go home. Many institutions provide forms for these summaries. Some records combine the discharge plan, including instructions for care, and the final progress note. Many are designed with checklists to facilitate data recording. If the discharge plan is given directly to the client and family, it is imperative that instructions be written in terms that can be readily understood.

If a client is transferred within the facility or from a long-term facility to a hospital, a report needs to accompany the client to ensure continuity of care in the new area. It should include all components of the discharge instructions, but also describe the condition of the client before the transfer. Any teaching or client instruction that has been done should also be described and recorded.

If the client is being transferred to another institution or to a home setting where a visit by a home health nurse is required, the discharge note takes the form of a referral summary. Regardless of format, discharge and referral summaries usually include some or all of the following:

- Description of client's physical, mental, and emotional status at discharge or transfer
- Resolved health problems

- Unresolved continuing health problems and continuing care needs; may include a review-of-systems checklist
- Treatments that are to be continued
- Current medications
- Restrictions that relate to (a) activity such as lifting, stair climbing, walking, driving, work, (b) diet, and (c) bathing such as sponge bath, tub, or shower
- Functional/self-care abilities in terms of vision, hearing, speech, mobility with or without aids, meal preparation and eating, preparing and administering medications, and so on
- Comfort level
- Support networks
- Client education provided in relation to disease process, activities and exercise, special diet, medications, specialized care or treatments, follow-up appointments, and so on
- Discharge destination
- Referral services

DOCUMENTATION IN OTHER FACILITIES

Long-Term Care Documentation   Long-term facilities usually provide two types of care: skilled or intermediate. Clients needing skilled care require more extensive nursing care and specialized nursing skills. In contrast, an intermediate care focus is needed for clients who usually have chronic illnesses and may only need assistance with activities of daily living (such as bathing and dressing).

Requirements for documentation in long-term care settings are based on professional standards, federal and state regulations, and the policies of the health care agency. Laws influencing the kind and frequency of documentation required are the Health Care Financing Administration and the Omnibus Budget Reconciliation Act (OBRA) of 1987. The OBRA law, for example, requires that (a) a comprehensive assessment (the Minimum Data Set [MDS] for Resident Assessment and Care Screening) be performed within 4 days of a client's admission to a long-term care facility, (b) a formulated plan of care must be completed within 7 days of admission, and (c) the assessment and care screening process must be reviewed every 3 months.

LONG-TERM CARE CONSIDERATION
Documentation

Older adults in long-term care facilities tend to have chronic conditions and generally experience subtle, small changes in their condition. However, when problems do occur, such as a hip fracture, CVA, or pneumonia, they are serious and require prompt attention. This points out the importance of keeping Kardexes and charting in long-term facilities current and up to date in the event that the client needs to be transferred for more skilled care and further treatment. A thorough transfer summary will facilitate communication and promote continuity of care in these situations.

PRACTICE GUIDELINES
Long-Term Care Documentation

- Keep records of visits and phone calls received.
- Review and revise the plan of care every 3 months or whenever the client's health status changes.
- Document and report any change in the client's condition to the primary care provider and the client's family within 24 hours.
- Document all measures implemented in response to a change in the client's condition.
- Make sure that progress notes address the client's progress in relation to the goals or outcomes defined in the plan of care.

Documentation must also comply with requirements set by Medicare and Medicaid. These requirements vary with the level of service provided and other factors. For example, Medicare provides little reimbursement for services provided in long-term care facilities except for services that require skilled care such as chemotherapy, tube feedings, ventilators, and so on. For such Medicare clients, the nurse must provide daily documentation to verify the need for service and reimbursement.

Nurses need to familiarize themselves with regulations influencing the kind and frequency of documentation required in long-term care facilities. Usually the nurse completes a nursing care *summary* at least once a week for clients requiring skilled care and every 2 weeks for those requiring intermediate care. Summaries should address specific problems, mental status, ADLs, hydration and nutrition status, safety measures, medications, treatments, preventive measures, and behavioral modifications assessment as needed.

See the Practice Guidelines for documentation in long-term care facilities.

Home Care Documentation   In 1985 the Health Care Financing Administration mandated that home health care agencies standardize their documentation methods to meet requirements for Medicare and Medicaid and other third-party disbursements. Two records are required: (a) a home health certification and plan of treatment form and (b) a medical update and patient information form. The nurse assigned to the home care client usually completes the forms, which must be signed by both the nurse and the attending physician. See the Practice Guidelines for home health care documentation.

Some home health agencies provide nurses with laptop or handheld computers to make records available in multiple locations. With the use of a modem, the nurse can add new client information to records at the agency without traveling to the office.

General Guidelines for Recording

The client's record is a legal document and may be used to provide evidence in court. Many factors are considered in recording. Health care personnel must not only maintain the confidentiality of the client's record but also meet legal standards in the process of recording.

PRACTICE GUIDELINES **Home Health Care Documentation**

- Complete a comprehensive nursing assessment and develop a plan of care to meet Medicare and other third-party payer requirements. Some agencies use the certification and plan of treatment form as the client's official plan of care.
- Write a progress note at each client visit, noting any changes in the client condition; nursing interventions performed (including education and instructional brochures and materials provided to the client and home caregiver); client responses to nursing care; and vital signs as indicated.
- Provide a monthly progress nursing summary to the attending physician and to the reimburser to confirm the need to continue services.
- Keep a copy of the care plan in the client's home and update it as the client's condition changes.

- Report changes in the plan of care to the physician and document that these were reported. Medicare and Medicaid will reimburse only for the skilled services provided that are reported to the physician.
- Encourage the client or home caregiver to record data when appropriate.
- Write a discharge summary for the physician to approve the discharge and to notify the reimbursers that services have been discontinued. Include all services provided, the client's health status at discharge, outcomes achieved, and recommendations for further care.

TABLE 8–3 **Commonly Used Abbreviations***

ABBREVIATION	TERM	ABBREVIATION	TERM
Abd	Abdomen	meds	Medications
ABO	The main blood group system	mL (ml)	Milliliter
ac	Before meals	mod	Moderate
ADL	Activities of daily living	Neg	Negative
ad lib	As desired	Ø	None
Adm	Admitted or admission	#	Number or pounds
AM	Morning	NPO (NBM)	Nothing by mouth
amb	Ambulatory	NS (N/S)	Normal saline
amt	Amount	O_2	Oxygen
approx	Approximately	OD	Right eye or overdose
bid	Twice daily	OOB	Out of bed
BM (bm)	Bowel movement	OS	Left eye
BP	Blood pressure	pc	After meals
BRP	Bathroom privileges	PE (PX)	Physical examination
c̄	With	per	By or through
C	Celsius (centigrade)	PM	Afternoon
CBC	Complete blood count	PPO	By mouth
c/o	Complains of	postop	Postoperatively
DAT	Diet as tolerated	preop	Preoperatively
drsg	Dressing	prep	Preparation
Dx	Diagnosis	PRN	When necessary
ECG (EKG)	Electrocardiogram	qid	Four times a day
F	Fahrenheit	(R)	Right
fld	Fluid	s̄	Without
GI	Gastrointestinal	STAT	At once, immediately
gtt	Drop	tid	Three times a day
h (hr)	Hour	TO	Telephone order
H_2O	Water	TPR	Temperature, pulse, respirations
I&O	Intake and output	VO	Verbal order
IV	Intravenous	VS	Vital signs
LMP	Last menstrual period	WNL	Within normal limits
(L)	Left	wt	Weigh

*Institutions may elect to include some of these abbreviations on their "Do Not Use" list. Check the agency's policy.

Document the date and time of each recording. This is essential not only for legal reasons but also for client safety. Record the time in the conventional manner or according to the 24-hour clock, which avoids confusion about whether a time was AM or PM.

Follow the agency's policy about the frequency of documenting, and adjust the frequency as a client's condition indicates. As a rule, documenting should be done as soon as possible after an assessment or intervention. No recording should be done *before* providing nursing care.

All entries must be legible and easy to read to prevent interpretation errors. Hand printing or easily understood handwriting is usually permissible. Follow the agency's policies about handwritten recording. All entries on the client's record are made in dark ink so that the record is permanent and changes can be identified. Dark ink reproduces well on microfilm and in duplication processes. Follow the agency's policies about the type of pen and ink used for recording.

Use only commonly accepted abbreviations, symbols, and terms that are specified by the agency. Many abbreviations are standard and used universally; others are used only in certain geographic areas. Many health care facilities supply an approved list of abbreviations and symbols to prevent confusion. When in doubt about whether to use an abbreviation, write the term out in full until certain about the abbreviation. Table 8–3 lists some common abbreviations, and Table 8–4 lists abbreviations

TABLE 8–4	"Do Not Use" List—The Minimum Required List Established by The Joint Commission	
ABBREVIATION	**POTENTIAL PROBLEM**	**PREFERRED TERM**
U (for unit)	Mistaken as zero, four, or cc	Write "unit"
IU (for international unit)	Mistaken as IV (intravenous) or 10 (ten)	Write "international unit"
Q.D., Q.O.D. (Latin abbreviation for once daily and every other day)	Mistaken for each other. The period after the Q can be mistaken for an "I" and the "O" can be mistaken for "I".	Write "daily" and "every other day"
Trailing zero (X.0 mg) [Note: prohibited only for medication-related notations]; Lack of leading zero (.X mg)	Decimal point is missed.	Never write a zero by itself after a decimal point (X mg), and always use a zero before a decimal point (0.X mg)
MS MSO$_4$ MgSO$_4$	Confused for one another. Can mean morphine sulfate or magnesium sulfate.	Write "morphine sulfate" or "magnesium sulfate"
In addition to the "minimum required list" above, the following should be considered when expanding the "Do Not Use" list.		
µg (for microgram)	Mistaken for mg (milligrams) resulting in one thousand-fold dosing overdose.	Write "mcg"
H.S. (for half-strength or Latin abbreviation for bedtime)	Mistaken for either half-strength or hour of sleep (at bedtime). q.H.S. mistaken for every hour. All can result in a dosing error.	Write out "half-strength" or "at bedtime"
T.I.W. (for three times a week)	Mistaken for three times a day or twice weekly resulting in an overdose.	Write "3 times weekly" or "three times weekly"
S.C. or S.Q. (for subcutaneous)	Mistaken as SL for sublingual, or "5 every."	Write "Sub-Q," "subQ," or "subcutaneously"
D/C (for discharge)	Interpreted as discontinue whatever medications follow (typically discharge meds).	Write "discharge"
c.c. (for cubic centimeter)	Mistaken for U (units) when poorly written.	Write "mL" or "milliliters"
A.S., A.D., A.U. (Latin abbreviation for left, right, or both ears)	Mistaken for OS, OD, and OU, etc.	Write "left ear," "right ear" or "both ears"
< (less than) and > (greater than)	Misinterpreted as the number "7" or the letter "L"	Write "greater than" or "less than"
Abbreviations for drug names	Misinterpretation due to similar abbreviations for multiple drugs	Write drug names in full
Apothecary units	Unfamiliar to many practitioners, confused with metric units	Use metric units
@	Mistaken for the number "2" (two)	Write "at"

Note: © The Joint Commission, 2009. Reprinted with permission.

which The Joint Commission placed on the "Do Not Use" list to reduce errors. Correct spelling is also essential for accuracy in recording. If you are unsure how to spell a word, look it up in a dictionary or other resource book.

CLINICAL ALERT

Incorrect spelling makes a negative impression on the reader and thereby decreases the nurse's credibility.

Each recording on the nursing notes is signed by the nurse making it. The signature includes the name and title; for example, "Susan J. Green, RN" or "SJ Green, RN." Some agencies have a signature sheet, and after signing this signature sheet, nurses can use their initials. With computerized charting, each nurse has his or her own code, which allows the documentation to be identified. The following title abbreviations are often used, but nurses need to follow agency policy about how to sign their names.

RN	registered nurse
LVN	licensed vocational nurse
LPN	licensed practical nurse
NA	nursing assistant
CNA	certified nursing assistant
NS	nursing student
PCA	patient care associate/assistant
SN	student nurse

Notations on records must be accurate and correct. Accurate notations consist of facts or observations rather than opinions or interpretations. Similarly, when a client expresses worry about the diagnosis or problem, this should be quoted directly on the record. When describing something, avoid general words, such as *large, good,* or *normal,* which can be interpreted differently. The client's name and identifying information should be stamped or written on each page of the clinical record. Before making any entry, check that it is the correct chart. Do not identify charts by room number only; check the client's name. Special care is needed when caring for clients with the same last name. Write on every line but never between lines. If a blank appears in a notation, draw a line through the blank space so that no additional information can be recorded at any other time or by any other person, and sign the notation.

When a recording mistake is made, draw a line through it and write the words *mistaken entry* above or next to the original entry, with your initials or name (depending on agency policy). Do not erase, blot out, or use correction fluid. The original entry must remain visible. When using computerized charting, the nurse needs to be aware of the agency's policy and process for correcting documentation mistakes. (See Figure 8–5 for an example.)

CLINICAL ALERT

Avoid writing the word *error* when a recording mistake has been made. Some believe that the word error is a "red flag" for juries and can lead to the assumption that a clinical error has caused a client injury.

When charting, document all events in the order in which they occur. Nurses' notes need to reflect the nursing process. Update or delete problems as needed. Record only the information that pertains to the client's health problems and care. Any other personal information that the client conveys is inappropriate for the record. Recording irrelevant information may be considered an invasion of the client's privacy and/or libelous. However, the information that is recorded needs to be complete and helpful to the client and health care professionals. Care that is *omitted* because of the client's condition or refusal of treatment must also be recorded. Document what was omitted, why it was omitted, and who was notified. Recordings need to be brief as well as complete to save time in communication. The client's name and the word *client* are omitted.

CLINICAL ALERT

Do not assume that the person reading your charting will know that a common intervention has occurred because you believe it to be an "obvious" component of care.

Accurate, complete documentation should give legal protection to the nurse, the client's other caregivers, the health care facility, and the client. Admissible in court as a legal document, the clinical record provides proof of the quality of care given to a client. Documentation is usually viewed by juries and attorneys as the best evidence of what really happened to the client. For the best legal protection, the nurse should not only adhere to professional standards of nursing care but also follow agency policy and procedures for intervention and documentation in all situations—especially high-risk situations.

Date	Time	Progress Notes
9/12/2007	0800	~~Breath sounds diminished throughout all lung fields. C/O "shortness of breath".~~ N. Smith, RN.
9/12/2007	0805	Mistaken entry above, wrong client --N. Smith, RN.

Figure 8–5 ● Correcting a charting error.

PRACTICE GUIDELINES

Documentation

Do

- Chart a change in a client's condition *and* show that follow-up actions were taken.
- Read the nurses' notes prior to care to determine if there has been a change in the client's condition.
- Be timely. A late entry is better than no entry; however, the longer the period of time between actual care and charting, the greater the suspicion.
- Use objective, specific, and factual descriptions.
- Correct charting errors.
- Chart all teaching.
- Record the client's actual words by putting quotes around the words.

- Chart the client's response to interventions.
- Review your notes—are they clear and do they reflect what you want to say?

Don't

- Leave a blank space for a colleague to chart later.
- Chart in advance of the event.
- Use vague terms.
- Chart for someone else.
- Use "patient" or "client," as it is their chart.
- Alter a record even if requested by a superior or a physician.
- Record assumptions or words reflecting bias.

RESEARCH NOTES

Does Nursing Documentation Reflect Individualized Client Care?

Using qualitative metasynthesis, the researchers reviewed and analyzed qualitative research reports focusing on the documentation of nursing care published between 1996 and 2003. The aim of this study was to increase understanding of the content of documenting nursing care and to show how ethical principles relating to individualized care are visible in the documentation. Ethical care includes the value of respecting clients and, therefore, documenting what the clients believe to be important in their care.

Three themes emerged. One of the themes reflected the demands of the organization. That is, the organizations wanted the documentation to show measurable results of nursing care that could subsequently affect financial implications. The second theme reflected nurses' attitudes and duties. Nurses did not consider documentation to be important and viewed it negatively or with indifference. The third theme reflected clients' involvement in their care. It became clear that the client's views were seldom referred to in the documentation. Nurses mainly documented physical functions of the client.

Implications

This study reflected the small amount of documentation given to clients' wishes and needs. The researchers point out that the more structured the documentation system (e.g., computerized charting), the more the focus will be on nursing tasks rather than individualizing nursing care for the health of the client. Although nurses advocate the need for individualized client care, it is not visible in the nursing documentation. Is it time to clearly define the purpose of documentation? Who is the documentation for—the organization, the nurse, or the client?

Note: From "Documentation of Individualized Patient Care: A Qualitative Metasynthesis," by O. Karkkainen, T. Bondas, and K. Eriksson, 2005, *Nursing Ethics, 12*(2), pp. 123–132. Copyright © Sage Publications Ltd, 2005. Reproduced with permission of Sage Publications, London.

CLINICAL ALERT

Complete charting, for example, by using the steps of the nursing process as a framework, is the best defense against malpractice.

COMPUTERIZED DOCUMENTATION AND INFORMATICS

Computers have become a part of everyday life for many people, including nurses. Computers are used for educating nursing students and clients; assessing, documenting, and testing clients' health conditions; managing medical records; communicating among health care providers and with clients; and conducting nursing research. All nurses must have a basic level of computer literacy in order to perform their jobs.

General Computer Concepts

Informatics refers to the science of computer information systems. **Nursing informatics** is the science of using computer information systems in the practice of nursing. It is defined by the American Nurses Association (ANA, 2001b) as "A specialty that integrates nursing science, computer science, and information science to manage and communicate data, information, and knowledge in nursing practice . . . to support patients, nurses, and other providers in their decision-making in all roles and settings" (p. 46).

This is a relatively young science—the first Nursing Information Systems conference was held in the United States in 1977. Nurses have taken significant strides since then to design and adapt computer processes to enhance client care, education, administration and management, and nursing research. Advanced practice in nursing informatics is a growing specialty. The first ANA certification examination in nursing informatics was given in October 1995.

The terminology used to describe the parts and functions of computer systems can be confusing. New terms emerge daily and it is a challenge to keep up with them. This section describes the most common computer hardware and software nurses may come across in the work setting.

COMPUTER HARDWARE AND SOFTWARE

Hardware is the actual components of the computer that allow them to function. Microcomputers, faster and smaller versions of the old supercomputer or mainframe, are individual systems referred to as desktop or personal computers (PCs). These include portable laptops, notebooks, tablets, or personal digital assistants (PDAs). The basic components of computer hardware include the central processing unit and one or more types of data input and output devices.

The central processing unit (CPU) is in the box that contains the computer hardware necessary to process and store data. Also located with the CPU are the power supply, disk drives, chips, and connections for all the other computer hardware, referred to as **peripherals**. The speed of the computer is determined by three components: the CPU processor (measured in gigahertz), the amount of memory, and the speed of data location or transfer rate of the disk drives (seek time).

In order for data to be kept for later retrieval, the computer must store the information in an electronic form. Computer information is measured in bytes (usually 1 byte is one letter, digit, or character), kilobytes (1,000 bytes = 1 KB), megabytes (1 million bytes = 1 MB), or gigabytes (1 billion bytes = 1 GB).

While the computer is turned on, data and instructions for the computer are loaded into random-access memory (RAM). Storage in RAM is temporary and is lost when the computer is turned off. The more RAM a computer has, the faster it can process data and the more applications that can be used at the same time. To save their work, computer users store data on magnetic hard drives, CDs or DVDs, or portable data devices such as USB memory keys.

Input devices are used to put information into a computer. There are several ways to get information into a computer. The most common method is to use a keyboard. The mouse is a pointing device with buttons used to choose items or initiate an action. Some computer screens respond to touch from a finger, light pen, or wand. Print or cursive handwriting can be displayed directly on the computer screen or translated into typeface for storage. Many computers also have a microphone and can respond to voice commands. Other electronic devices used for entering data into a computer are scanners and analog-to-digital converters.

CLINICAL ALERT

Personal digital assistants (PDAs) are handheld computers that can interface with PCs, networks, or phone systems. Nurses increasingly use them as calendar/date books, address books, drug and disease database storage devices, and data entry and retrieval devices.

Output devices display data from the computer. The results of computer data entry are usually displayed first on the computer screen or monitor and then through a printer. Both monitors and printers display text and graphics. Computer data can also be output to audio and video displays.

Communication devices allow computers and people to interact from great distances. The term *online* refers to a computer being connected to other computers in a network. The network is often coordinated by one computer, the network server. PCs linked directly to other nearby PCs and servers by wires or wireless communications devices constitute a local-area network (LAN). Distant locations can be linked through a wide area network (WAN), virtual network, or private network. These larger distances can be covered by sending the data through standard telephone wires or a high-speed data connection, or integrated services digital network line. The technology for network connections and devices changes rapidly and continues to advance.

Computer software refers to programs, also called applications, that instruct the hardware to perform certain tasks. The most commonly used software programs are word processors, databases, spreadsheets, utilities such as communications, and presentation graphics programs.

COMPUTER SYSTEMS

The concept of a computer system—not in the sense of one machine but of a network of computers, users, programs, and procedures in an organization—implies that there is identifiable input, processing, output, and feedback. The two most common types of computer systems used by nurses are management information systems and hospital information systems.

Management Information Systems A management information system (MIS) is designed to facilitate the organization and application of data used to manage an organization or department. The system provides analyses used for strategic planning, decision making, and evaluation of management activities. All levels of management benefit from the ability to access the data.

Hospital Information Systems A **hospital information system (HIS)** is an MIS that focuses on the types of data needed to manage client care activities and health care organizations. As with any system, the goal is to provide people with the data they need to determine appropriate actions and control them. Typically an HIS will have subsystems in the areas of admissions, medical records, clinical laboratory, pharmacy, order entry, and finance. The personnel in these areas record the data needed to allow management of billing, quality assurance, scheduling, and inventory both within their own areas and across the institution. Increasingly, accrediting organizations mandate the use of an HIS and require that reports be submitted using computerized formats. Eventually, integrated HISs will form the center of all record keeping and analysis for interdisciplinary health care.

World Wide Web and the Internet The Internet is a worldwide network that connects other networks. Connections among networks and PCs via the Internet allow for almost instantaneous transmission among distant sites and can include text, audio, and video. The World Wide Web (WWW) refers to the complex links among web pages or websites, accessed through "addresses" called universal resource locators (URLs). URLs begin with the designation http://, often followed by www. URLs end with a designation that denotes the type of site. For example, .com is for commercial and personal sites, .org for organizations, .edu for educational institutions, and .gov for government sites.

Tens of thousands of health-related websites exist, many new ones appearing and others becoming "dead links" daily. No standardized controls exist to ensure that the information provided is current or accurate. Nurses should evaluate health websites as they access them and assist clients in doing the same. Tools for doing this include (as of this publication) *Evaluating Internet Resources* from the State University of New York at Albany and *Criteria for Assessing the Quality of Health Information on the Internet—Policy Paper* from the Health Information Technology Institute of Mitretek Systems Health Summit Working Group (Box 8–2).

Computers in Nursing Practice

Many activities of the registered nurse involve collecting, recording, and using data. Computers are well suited to assist the nurse in these functions. Specifically, the nurse records client information in computer records, accesses other departments' information on the client from centralized computers, uses computers to manage client scheduling, and uses programs for unique applications such as home health nursing and case management.

DOCUMENTATION OF CLIENT STATUS AND MEDICAL RECORD KEEPING Nurses need access to standardized forms, policies, and procedures. Also, nurses need to be able to gather broader client information such as length of stay for specific diagnoses. Computers can assist with each of these.

BEDSIDE DATA ENTRY There are several different types of computerized bedside data entry systems. These allow recording of client assessments, medication administration (Figure 8–6), progress notes, care plan updating, client acuity, and accrued charges. The terminal can be fixed or handheld, and hardwired to the central system, or cordless with the ability to transmit the data to distant sites, such as from the client's home to the agency office. A slightly different type of bedside terminal is the point-of-care or point-of-service computer. In this case the terminal is located near, but not necessarily by, the client.

Computer-Based Client Records **Electronic medical records (EMRs)** or **computer-based patient records (CPRs)** permit electronic client data retrieval by caregivers, administrators, accreditors, and other persons who require the data. The Computer-Based Patient Record Institute, established in 1992, identified four ways the EMR could improve health care: (a) constant availability of client health information across the life span, (b) ability to monitor quality, (c) access to warehoused (stored) data, and (d) ability for clients to share in knowledge and activities influencing their own health.

Because of the way computers provide access to the EMR, providers easily retrieve specific data such as trends in vital sign, immunization records, and current problems. The

BOX 8–2 | **Criteria for Evaluating Internet Health Information**

- *Credibility:* includes the source, currency, relevance/utility, and editorial review process for the information.
- *Content:* must be accurate and complete, and an appropriate disclaimer provided.
- *Disclosure:* includes informing the user of the purpose of the site, as well as any profiling or collection of information associated with using the site.
- *Links:* evaluated according to selection, architecture, content, and back linkages.
- *Design:* encompasses accessibility, logical organization (navigability), and internal search capability.
- *Interactivity:* includes feedback mechanisms and means for exchange of information among users.
- *Caveats:* clarification of whether site function is to market products and services or is a primary information content provider.

Note: Assessing the Quality of Internet Health Information. Summary. Agency for Health Care Policy and Research, Rockville, MD, and Mitretek Systems, McLean, VA. Accessed December 31, 2009 from http://www.ahrq.gov/data/infoqual.htm.

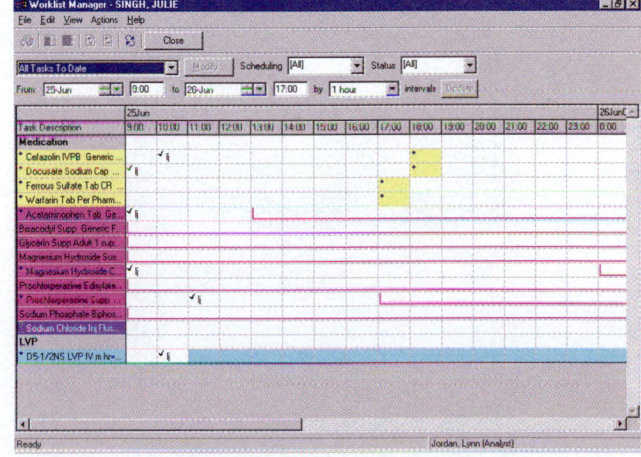

Figure 8–6 ⭘ This screen shows a MAR (medication administration record) for several regularly scheduled medications. The worksheet displays the next time the medications are scheduled to be administered.

(Courtesy of Sutter Health.)

RESEARCH NOTES

Does Point-of-Care Nursing Documentation Make a Difference?

This article reports on five research studies aimed at determining whether or not bedside electronic charting made a difference in quality of documentation and nurses' satisfaction. The studies were very diverse, ranging from a pilot examination of functionality, usefulness, and acceptability to a large chart review of compliance with accreditation charting standards. In each case, results indicated that electronic charting improved compliance with documentation standards. Time spent charting was decreased and nurse satisfaction increased. The authors recognized that these were early studies and resistance to change may influence reproducibility of the magnitude of the results in larger institutions.

Implications

Novel approaches to charting that reduce the time and effort of recording will likely be of broad interest to nurses. Anything that allows more time to be spent with clients and enhances the ease of documentation—especially the more routine and standard reports required—is a positive move. However, it is far too early to have complete confidence that satisfaction with electronic bedside charting will be maintained over time as the novelty wears off. Institutions are spending many dollars on new computer charting systems. At the minimum, the cost is well spent even if only for the consistency of charting and the ability to mine the data for outcomes assessment and quality improvement. However, much more research on the effects of online charting is needed.

Note: From "The Times They Are a Changing: Effects of Online Nursing Documentation Systems," by C. Langowski, 2005, *Quality Management in Health Care, 14,* pp. 121–125.

system can be designed to warn providers about conflicting medications or client parameters that indicate dangerous conditions (Figure 8–7). Sophisticated systems allow replay of audio, graphic, or video data for comparison with current status. All text is legible and can be searched for keywords.

There are several areas of concern with EMRs. Maintaining privacy and security of data is a significant issue (Olson, 2003). One way that computers can protect data is by user authentication via passwords or biometric identifiers—only those persons who have a legitimate need to access the data receive the password. Additional policies and procedures for protecting the confidentiality of EMRs are evolving as the use of computer systems becomes more widespread. One role of the nurse informaticist is to develop policies and procedures that promote effective and secure use of computerized records by nurses and other health care professionals.

Currently, there are no national standards for how data in EMRs should be organized or what specific data should be included. HIPAA regulations (also see Chapter 2 ∞) are playing a key role in establishing these. Nurses need to be involved in the design, implementation, and evaluation of EMRs to maximize their use and effectiveness.

Data Standardization and Classifications There are many reasons why nursing would benefit from standard classifications of terms used to describe and measure clinical, disease, procedure, and outcomes data. One reason is that, for nursing to be recognized for the value it adds to client well-being, research-based findings must show client improvement by accepted standards. This necessitates agreement to use common, consistent, clear, and rule-based standards.

Nursing classifications or taxonomies have been developed. The Nursing Minimum Data Set (NMDS) contains 16 elements of nursing data, along with their definitions, in three categories: nursing care, client demographics, and service. The NMDS can be used for data collection and documentation and allows sharing of information regarding the quality, cost, and effectiveness of nursing. In the United States, five classification systems are used: the North American Nursing Diagnosis Association (NANDA) taxonomy, the Omaha System, the Home Health Care Classification (HHCC), the Nursing Interventions Classification (NIC), and the Nursing Outcomes Classification (NOC). In addition, the International Council of Nurses has proposed an International Classification for Nursing Practice, a common language for describing nursing problems (or diagnoses), interventions, and outcomes. It may take years to determine which standards will allow optimal access to and manipulation of computerized records, and who will be the determining body.

Figure 8–7 ⬤ One of the strengths of an electronic medical record is its ability to alert the clinician to potential drug interactions using warnings like the one displayed. (Courtesy of Sutter Health.)

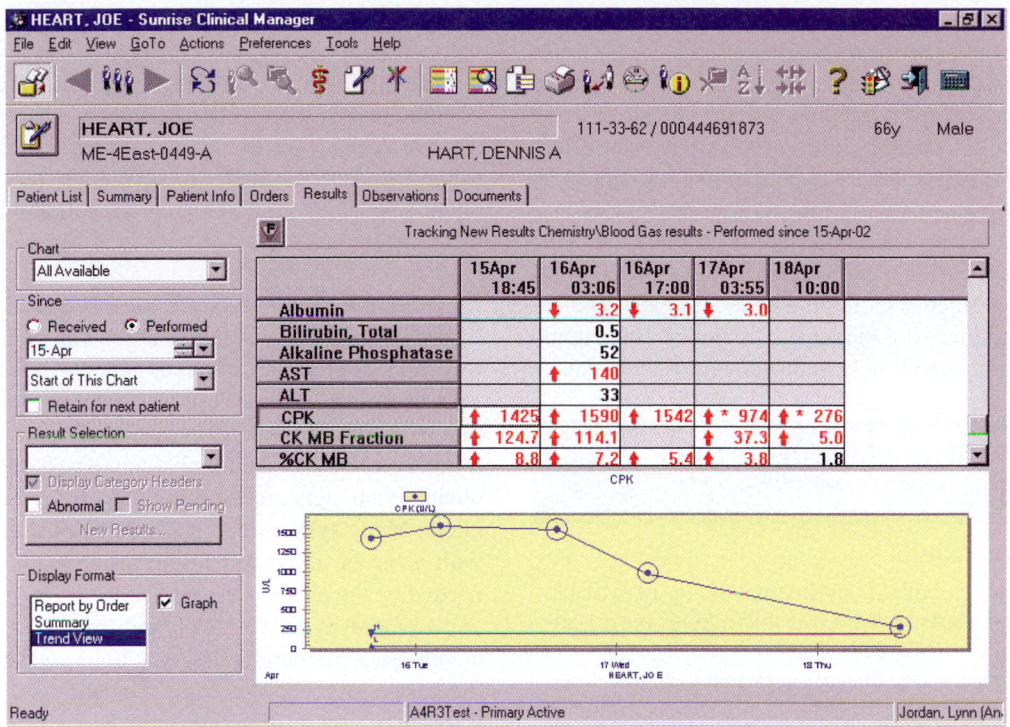

Figure 8–8 ○ Lab results are displayed in a trend view graph.
(Courtesy of Sutter Health.)

Tracking Client Status Once an EMR has been established, the nurse can retrieve and display a client's physiologic parameters across time (see Figure 8–8). In addition to the rather straightforward viewing of trends in vital signs, for example, the nurse can also track more global client progress. Standardized nursing care plans, care maps, critical pathways, or other prewritten treatment protocols can be stored in the computer and easily placed in the EMR electronically. Then the nurse and other health care personnel can examine progress toward and variance from the expected plan directly on the computer.

ELECTRONIC ACCESS TO CLIENT DATA Besides computers designed for record keeping, other computers are used extensively in health care to assess and monitor clients' conditions. The data accumulated from various electronic devices can be part of the EMR and also stored for research purposes. Electronic records take up much less space than paper records and may be stored more securely. Copies can be made easily onto different electronic media that are generally more compact and durable than paper. Data can also be transmitted to a consulting specialist in another location. Further, more than one health care provider can access records at the same time.

Client Monitoring and Computerized Diagnostics Nursing has benefited greatly from the myriad of client monitors. Although most of these monitors are applied externally, implanted electronic monitors are also proving to have great value. These instruments can be used in any care setting, from intensive care to the home. Most keep a record of the most recent values. Some can transmit their data to a more sophisticated computer or print out a paper record. Some have digital displays that "talk" to the user, giving instructions or results. Most also have error detection or alarms that indicate either that the instrument is malfunctioning or that the assessed value is outside predetermined parameters. These devices, with their minute but powerful computer chips, make it possible to extend the nurse's observations and provide valid and reliable data. In various specialty areas of health care, clients undergo diagnostic procedures in which computers play a major role.

Telemedicine/Telehealth One of the most exciting areas being developed in computer-assisted health care is telemedicine. Telemedicine uses technology to transmit electronic data about clients to persons at distant locations. Concerns regarding telehealth relate to legal and ethical issues. Who has responsibility for the client when a teleconsult is used? Does the care provider need to be licensed in the state or province where the client's primary care is given? The National Council of State Boards of Nursing has declared that the applicable regulations are those for where the client resides and not where the provider is located. This is also one of the reasons for the initiation of the Mutual Recognition Compact that boards of nursing are promulgating to facilitate nurses' licensure in several states.

PRACTICE MANAGEMENT Beyond direct client care, computers also assist nurses in many ways in the management of their work. In hospitals, data terminals are commonly used to order supplies, tests, meals, and services from other departments. Tracking of these orders allows the nursing service to determine the most frequent or most costly items used by a particular nursing unit. Computers are used extensively for scheduling. Each practice needs to keep track of procedures health care workers perform, client diagnoses, and time spent with clients so that billing can be accurate. With managed care, information tracking is also aimed at determining trends in health problems and the need for providers with specific skills. The use of computerized databases filled with unique codes for each medication, medical and nursing diagnosis, treatment, and supply allows for accurate and timely management of these data.

LIFESPAN CONSIDERATIONS
Computer Use

Children and Adults

Computer programs, both CD and Internet-based, are available for children and adults to learn everything from foreign language to algebra.

There are many issues of concern related to frequent and extended use of computers by all ages. In particular, repetitive motion injuries (especially of the hand) can occur with extensive typing and use of the computer mouse, eye strain can occur from computer monitor viewing, and musculoskeletal damage is related to inadequate ergonomic arrangement of desk chairs, surface height, and monitor placement. Students and adults who use computers daily should be thoroughly evaluated and instructed in the prevention of these conditions.

Parents need to be reminded of potential risks to children from Internet contact with strangers and adult-only websites. They also need to monitor schoolchildren's use of computers to ensure they are not being sidetracked from homework into computer games and messaging.

All persons should be wary to protect their financial and personal information when conducting business via computer.

Older Adults

Computer classes are being taught to increasing numbers of older adults. Use of the computer provides them with an avenue of communication and exposure to a vast amount of health care information. Although nurses have little control over what Internet sites will be accessed, it is important to teach clients and the general public to evaluate information from the site and to be aware that misinformation can also be presented. Important guidelines that increase the validity of a site are as follows:

- The article or information lists the author and credentials and/or the institution from which the information came.
- A date is listed that states when information was updated.
- If health care information is presented, a disclaimer should be included. The disclaimer presents limitations of the information and should say that it is not medical advice.

Computer-assisted programs can be very effective teaching aids for older adults. They may provide audio and visual instruction and may even be interactive. They are useful for teaching about medical conditions and medications and for providing information about procedures and surgeries to be performed.

Computerized clinical record systems are being developed as a way to manage the huge volume of information required in contemporary health care. Nurses use computers to store the client's database, add new data, create and revise care plans, and document client progress. Some institutions have a computer terminal at each client's bedside, or nurses carry a small handheld terminal, enabling the nurse to document care immediately after it is given.

Multiple flow sheets are not needed in computerized record systems because information can be easily retrieved in a variety of formats. For example, the nurse can obtain results of a client's blood test, a schedule of all clients on the unit who are to have surgery during the day, a suggested list of interventions for a nursing diagnosis, a graphic chart of a client's vital signs, or a printout of all progress notes for a client. Many systems can generate a work list for the shift, with a list of all treatments, procedures, and medications needed by the client.

Computers make care planning and documentation relatively easy. To record nursing actions and client responses, the nurse either chooses from standardized lists of terms or types narrative information into the computer. Automated speech-recognition technology now allows nurses to enter data by voice for conversion to written documentation. Again, according to HIPAA, if the spoken word is used to create PHI, the nurse must be alert and aware of others who might hear the dictation.

The computerization of clinical records has made it possible to transmit information from one care setting to another. The Nursing Minimum Data Set (NMDS) is an effort to establish standards for collecting standardized, essential nursing data for inclusion in computer databases. Selected pros and cons of computer documentation are shown in Box 8–3.

REPORTING

The purpose of reporting is to communicate specific information to a person or group of people. A report, whether oral or written, should be concise, including pertinent information but no extraneous detail. In addition to change-of-shift reports and telephone reports, reporting can also include the sharing of information or ideas with colleagues and other health professionals about some aspect of a client's care. Examples include the care plan conference and nursing rounds.

Change-of-Shift Reports

A change-of-shift report is given to all nurses on the next shift. Its purpose is to provide continuity of care for clients by providing the new caregivers a quick summary of client needs and details of care to be given. Change-of-shift reports may be written or given orally, either in a face-to-face exchange or by audiotape recording. Reports are sometimes

BOX 8–3	**Selected Pros and Cons of Computer Documentation**

Pros

- Computer records can facilitate a focus on client outcomes.
- Bedside terminals can synthesize information from monitoring equipment.
- It allows nurses to use their time more efficiently.
- The system links various sources of client information.
- Client information, requests, and results are sent and received quickly.
- Links to monitors improve accuracy of documentation.
- Bedside terminals eliminate the need to take notes on a worksheet before recording.
- Bedside terminals permit the nurse to check an order immediately before administering a treatment or medication.

- Information is legible.
- The system incorporates and reinforces standards of care.
- Standard terminology improves communication.

Cons

- Client's privacy may be infringed on if security measures are not used.
- Breakdowns make information temporarily unavailable.
- The system is expensive.
- Extended training periods may be required when a new or updated system is installed.

given at the bedside, and clients as well as nurses may participate in the exchange of information. Box 8–4 lists key elements of a change-of-shift report.

CLINICAL ALERT

Be aware of where the shift report takes place in order to maintain client confidentiality. An area that is private and free from interruption is best.

Telephone Reports

Health professionals frequently report about a client by telephone. Nurses inform primary care providers about a change in a client's condition; a radiologist reports the results of an x-ray study; a nurse may report to a nurse on another unit about a transferred client. The nurse receiving a telephone report should document the date and time, the name of the person giving the information, and the subject of the information received, and sign the notation. The person receiving the information should repeat it back to the sender to ensure accuracy.

BOX 8–4	**Key Elements of a Change-of-Shift Report**

- Follow a particular order (e.g., follow room numbers in a hospital).
- Provide basic identifying information for each client (e.g., name, room number, bed designation).
- For new clients, provide the reason for admission or medical diagnosis (or diagnoses), surgery (date), diagnostic tests, and therapies in past 24 hours.
- Include significant changes in client's condition and present information in order (i.e., assessment, nursing diagnoses, interventions, outcomes, and evaluation). For example, "Mr. Ronald Oakes said he had an aching pain in his left calf at 1400 hours. Inspection revealed no other signs. Calf pain is related to altered blood circulation. Rest and elevation of his legs on a footstool for 30 minutes provided relief."
- Provide exact information, such as "Ms. Jessie Jones received morphine 6 mg IV at 1500 hours," not "Ms. Jessie Jones received some morphine during the evening."
- Report clients' need for special emotional support. For example, a client who has just learned that his biopsy results revealed malignancy and who is now scheduled for a laryngectomy needs time to discuss his feelings before preoperative teaching is begun.

- Include current nurse-prescribed and primary care provider-prescribed orders.
- Provide a summary of newly admitted clients, including diagnosis, age, general condition, plan of therapy, and significant information about the client's support people.
- Report on clients who have been transferred or discharged from the unit.
- Clearly state priorities of care and care that is due after the shift begins. For example, in a 7 AM report the nurse might say, "Mr. Li's vital signs are due at 0730, and his IV bag will need to be replaced by 0800." Give this information at the end of that client's report, because memory is best for the first and last information given.
- Be concise. Don't elaborate on background data or routine care (e.g., do not report "Vital signs at 0800 and 1150" when that is the unit standard). Do not report coming and going of visitors unless there is a problem or concern, or visitors are involved in teaching and care.

Social support and visits are the norm.

When giving a telephone report to a primary care provider, it is important that the nurse be concise and accurate. Begin with name and relationship to the client. Telephone reports usually include the client's name and medical diagnosis, changes in nursing assessment, vital signs related to baseline vital signs, significant laboratory data, and related nursing interventions. The nurse should have the client's chart ready to give the primary care provider any further information. After reporting, the nurse should document the date, time, and content of the call.

Telephone Orders

Physicians often order a therapy for a client by telephone. Most agencies have specific policies about telephone orders. Many agencies allow only registered nurses to take telephone orders.

While the primary care provider gives the order, *write* the complete order down and *read* it back to the primary care provider to ensure accuracy. Question the primary care provider about any order that is ambiguous, unusual, or contraindicated by the client's condition. Then transcribe the order onto the physician's order sheet, indicating it as a verbal order (VO) or telephone order (TO). See Box 8–5 for selected guidelines. Once the order is transcribed on the physician's order sheet, the order must be countersigned by the primary care provider within a time period described by agency policy. Many acute care hospitals require that this be done within 24 hours.

Care Plan Conferences

A care plan conference is a meeting of a group of nurses to discuss possible solutions to certain problems of a client, such as inability to cope with an event or lack of progress toward goal attainment. The care plan conference allows each nurse an opportunity to offer an opinion about possible solutions to the problem. Other health professionals may be invited to attend the conference to offer their expertise; for example, a social worker may discuss the family problems of a severely burned child, or a dietitian may discuss the dietary problems of a client who has diabetes. Care plan conferences are most effective when there is a climate of respect.

Nursing Rounds

Nursing rounds are procedures in which two or more nurses visit selected clients at each client's bedside to obtain information that will help plan nursing care, provide clients the opportunity to discuss their care, and evaluate the nursing care a client has received. During rounds, the nurse assigned to the client provides a brief summary of the client's nursing needs and the interventions being implemented. Nursing rounds offer advantages to both clients and nurses: Clients can participate in the discussions, and nurses can see the client and the equipment being used. To facilitate client participation in nursing rounds, nurses need to use terms that the client can understand. Medical terminology excludes the client from discussion.

BOX 8–5 **Guidelines for Telephone and Verbal Orders**

1. Know the state nursing board's position on who can give and accept verbal and phone orders.
2. Know the agency's policy regarding phone orders (e.g., colleague listens on extension and cosigns order sheet).
3. Ask the prescriber to speak slowly and clearly.
4. Ask the prescriber to spell out the medication if you are not familiar with it.
5. Question the drug, dosage, or changes if they seem inappropriate for this client.
6. Write the order down or enter into a computer.
7. Read the order back to the prescriber. Use words instead of abbreviations (i.e., three times a day instead of tid).
8. Write the order on the physician's order sheet. Record date and time and indicate it was a telephone order (TO). Sign name and credentials.
9. When writing a dosage always put a zero before a decimal if the number is less than 1 (i.e., 0.3 mL) but never place unnecessary zeroes after a decimal (i.e., 6 mg is correct, but 6.0 mg can be misinterpreted as 60 mg).
10. Write out units (e.g., 15 units of insulin, not 15 u of insulin).
11. Transcribe the order.
12. Follow agency protocol about the prescriber's protocol for signing telephone orders (e.g., within 24 hours).

Other:
- Never follow a voice-mail order. Call the prescriber for a client order. Write it down and read it back for confirmation.

Note: Adapted from "JCAHO Says Watch Your P's and Q's," by editors of *Nursing 2004*, 2004, *Nursing, 34*(3), p. 55; and "FAQs for the 2006 National Patient Safety Goals" by Joint Commission on Accreditation of Healthcare Organizations, 2006. Retrieved April 30, 2006, from http://www .jointcommission.org/NR/rdonlyres/7C116D6D-AE82-449E-BA45-1DE49D2A0A34/0/06_npsg_faq.pdf

CHAPTER HIGHLIGHTS

- Client records are legal documents that provide evidence of a client's care. The nurse has a legal and ethical duty to maintain confidentiality of the client's record; this includes special measures to protect client information stored in computers.
- Client records are kept for a number of purposes, including communication, planning client care, auditing health agencies, research, education, reimbursement, legal documentation, and health care analysis.
- In source-oriented clinical records, each health care professional group provides its own record. Recording is oriented around the source of the information.
- In problem-oriented clinical records, recording is organized around client problems.
- Examples of documentation systems include PIE, focus charting, charting by exception (CBE), computerized documentation, and case management.
- Computers make care planning and documentation relatively easy. The use of computer terminals at the bedside allows immediate documentation of nursing actions.
- The Kardex is used to organize client data, making information quick to access for health professionals.
- Nursing progress notes provide information about the progress the client is making toward desired outcomes. The format for the progress note depends on the documentation system at the facility.
- Long-term documentation varies depending on the level of care provided and requirements set by Medicare and Medicaid.
- Home health agencies must standardize their documentation methods to meet requirements for Medicare and Medicaid and other third-party disbursements.
- Legal guidelines for the process of recording in a client record include documenting date and time, legible entries, using dark ink, using correct terminology and spelling, accuracy, appropriateness, completeness, conciseness, and including an appropriate signature.

- Computer hardware consists of the central processing unit, memory, the keyboard and other input devices, and the monitor and other output devices.
- Common computer software programs used in nursing are word processors, databases, spreadsheets, communications, computer-assisted instruction, and presentation graphics.
- A hospital information system (HIS) organizes data from various areas in the hospital such as admissions, medical records, clinical laboratory, pharmacy, and finance.
- Bedside entry of nursing data is becoming more prevalent. Studies on whether these systems save nursing time have conflicting results.
- Electronic medical records (EMRs) enable longitudinal data to be collected on a client and made available to all health care providers who require it. Such data warehousing also enables research to be conducted on quality of care, client outcomes, and a variety of other parameters. However, no national standards exist for the structure or contents of these records.
- Computer monitoring and diagnosing of client conditions is widespread.
- Telehealth, the conduction of the health care profession using electronic means of communication, is a growing area that generates both excitement and concerns.
- Data terminals in health care settings allow placing of order requests and retrieval of client data and accounts. Appointments can be scheduled on computer.
- Computers are used by home health nurses to record client data and to communicate with the central office. Clients can also have computers in the home that allow them to monitor their own health status and send information about their condition to the nurse.
- The purpose of reporting is to communicate specific information for the goal of improving quality of care. Examples include change-of-shift reports, telephone reports, telephone orders, care plan conferences, and nursing rounds.

THINK ABOUT IT

Refer to the chapter-opening scenario and answer these questions.

1. How would you document this client's skin care?

2. Other than documenting in the medical record, what other documentation and reporting is important for maintaining continuity of care for this client?

3. When Felicia reviews her notes in the client's medical record after learning of the lawsuit, she notices she did not do a very good job documenting all the care she had initiated in an attempt to prevent skin breakdown for this client. What can Felicia do now to improve this documentation?

∞ *See suggested responses to Think About It on MyNursingKit.*

TEST YOUR KNOWLEDGE

1. When documenting in the client's medical record the nurse recognizes which of the following as the greatest concern associated with the utilization of an electronic client record system?
1. Cost
2. Accuracy
3. Privacy
4. Durability

2. A client insists that the nurse use a treatment method discovered on an Internet website. Which of the following is the most appropriate nursing response?
1. "The treatment must be examined to see if it is appropriate."
2. "Most website treatments have not been studied or researched."
3. "The person establishing the website is the only one who can use it on clients."
4. "Websites are like advertising; they are biased and may not be legitimate."

3. Which of the following actions by a nurse ensures confidentiality of a client's computer record?
1. The nurse logs on to the client's file and leaves the computer to answer the client's call light.
2. The nurse shares her computer password with co-workers who assist with documentation.
3. The nurse closes a client's computer file and logs off when not directly in front of the computer.
4. The nurse leaves client computer worksheets at the computer workstation.

4. After making a documentation error, which action should the nurse take?
1. Use correcting liquid to cover the mistake and make a new entry.
2. Draw a line through it and write *error* above the entry.
3. Draw a line through it and write *mistaken entry* above it.
4. Draw a line through the mistake and write *mistaken entry* with initials above it.

5. Which charting entry would be the most defensible if the nurse is called to court?
1. Client fell out of bed.
2. Client drunk on admission.
3. Large bruise on left thigh.
4. Notified Dr. Jones of BP of 90/40.

6. The nurse is caring for a client who has been in the hospital for 2 days. The nurse thinks that the client's blood pressure (B/P) seems high. What is the next step?
1. Ask the client about past blood pressure ranges.
2. Review the graphic record on the client's record.
3. Examine the medication record for antihypertensive medications.
4. Review the progress notes included in the client's record.

7. A student nurse observes the change-of-shift report. Which of the following behaviors by the reporting nurse represent effective nursing practice? Select all that apply.
1. Provides the medical diagnosis or reason for admission.
2. States the time the client last received pain medication.
3. Speaks loudly when giving report.
4. States priorities of care due shortly after report.
5. Reports on number of visitors for each client.

8. Which nursing documentation entries are written correctly? Select all that apply.
1. MS 5 mg. given IV for c/o abdominal pain.
2. Lanoxin 0.25 mg given orally per Dr. Smith's stat order.
3. KCl 15cc's given orally for K+ level of 2.9.
4. Regular insulin 10.0 u given SQ for capillary blood glucose of 180.
5. Ambien 5 mg given orally at bedtime per request.

9. A 74-year-old female is brought to the E.D. c/o right hip pain. The right leg is shorter than the left and is externally rotated. During inspection, the nurse observes what appears to be cigarette burns on the client's inner thighs. Which of the following is the most appropriate documentation?
1. Six round skin lesions the size of a pencil eraser partially healed on the inner thighs bilaterally.
2. Several cigarette burns on both of the client's inner thighs at various stages of healing.
3. Multiple lesions on inner thighs possibly related to elder abuse.
4. Several lesions on inner thighs similar to cigarette burns.

10. The nurse overhears an unlicensed assistive personnel (UAP) make the following comment: "The nurses spend all their time at the desk writing in the medical record. Their time would be better spent providing care to the client." The nurse's best response would be:

1. "Documenting is an essential form of communicating the care provided to clients and contributes to how the client will be cared for in the future."
2. "Nurses have to document to avoid lawsuits, so that is why you see us sitting at the desk all the time. It's not our choice."
3. "Nurses would prefer to provide client care instead of documenting, but facility policy dictates that we have to chart as we provide care."
4. "Nurses document because the facility performs audits to make sure everything is recorded and we'll get in trouble if we miss something."

∞ *See answers to Test Your Knowledge in Appendix A.*

EXPLORE PEARSON **mynursingkit**™

MyNursingKit is your one stop for online chapter review materials and resources. Prepare for success with additional NCLEX®-style practice questions, interactive assignments and activities, web links, animations and videos, and more!

Register your access code from the front of your book at
www.mynursingkit.com.

REFERENCES AND SELECTED BIBLIOGRAPHY

American Nurses Association. (1999). *Position statement: Privacy and confidentiality.* Retrieved December 5, 2009, from http://www.nursingworld.org/EthicsHumanRightsRevised12/8/06.htm

American Nurses Association. (2001a). *Code of ethics for nurses with interpretive statements.* Washington, DC: Author.

American Nurses Association. (2001b). *Scope and standards of nursing informatics practice.* Washington, DC: American Nurses Publishing.

Bond, C. S. (2004). Web users' information retrieval methods and skills. *Online Information Review, 28,* 254–259.

Bowles, K. H. (2004). Sharpen decision making with computerized support tools. *Nursing Management, 35,* 19–20.

Burke, L., & Weill, B. (2008). *Information technology for the health professions* (3rd ed.). Upper Saddle River, NJ: Pearson Education.

Burt, C. W., & Jing, E. (2005). Use of computerized clinical support systems in medical settings: United States, 2001–03. *Advance Data from Vital and Health Statistics,* No. 353 (PHS) 2005-1250. Hyattsville, MD:

National Center for Health Statistics. Retrieved June 14, 2006, from http://www.cdc.gov/nchs/data/ad/ad353.pdf

Chastain, A. R. (2003). Nursing informatics: Past, present and future. *Tennessee Nurse, 66*(1), 8–10.

Clark, A. P. (2003). What's all the HIPAA hype? *Nurse Practitioner Supplement: The 2004 Sourcebook for Advanced Practice Nurses,* 6–11.

Computer-Based Patient Record Institute. (1992). *Newsletters and membership brochures.* Chicago: Author.

Couvillon, J. S. (2006). *Nursing informatics: Practical issues for today's nurse.* Sudbury, MA: Jones & Bartlett.

Dickerson, S. S., Boehmke, M., Ogle, C., & Brown, J. K. (2005). Out of necessity: Oncology nurses' experiences integrating the Internet into practice. *Oncology Nursing Forum, 32,* 355–362.

Editors of Nursing 2004. (2004). JCAHO says watch your p's and q's. *Nursing, 34*(3), 55.

Feeg, V. D. (2003). What's this HIPAA stuff. . . and does it affect me? *Pediatric Nursing, 29*(2), 93, 133.

Fernandez, R. D., & Spragley, F. (2004). Focus on streamlined documentation. *Nursing Management, 35*(10), 25–29.

Gallagher, P. M. (2004). Maintain privacy with electronic charting. *Nursing Management, 35*(2), 16–17.

Guido, G. W. (2009). *Legal and ethical issues in nursing* (5th ed.). Upper Saddle River, NJ: Pearson Education.

Hamilton, A. V., Coyle, G. A., & Heinen, M. G. (2004). Applied technology rounds out e-documentation. *Nursing Management, 35*(9), 44–47.

Health Summit Working Group. (1999). *Criteria for assessing the quality of health information on the Internet: Policy paper.* McLean, VA: Mitretek Systems. Retrieved March 5, 2006, from http://hitiweb.mitretek.org/docs/policy.html

Hendrix, L. (2004). Paging pointers: Here's how to make the most of your calls to health care providers. *Nursing, 34*(5), 32hn4–32hn6.

Hunt, E. C., Sproat, S. B., & Kitzmiller, R. R. (2004). *The nursing informatics implementation guide.* New York: Springer-Verlag.

Joos, I., Nelson, R., Whitman, N., & Smith, M. (2005). *Introduction to computers for healthcare professionals* (4th ed.). Sudbury, MA: Jones & Bartlett.

Joint Commission on Accreditation of Healthcare Organizations. (2006). *2006 National Patient Safety Goals—FAQs*. Retrieved December 5, 2009, from http://www.jointcommission.org/PatientSafety/NationalPatientSafetyGoals/default.htm

Kirkley, D., & Stein, M. (2004). Nurses and clinical technology: Sources of resistance and strategies for acceptance. *Nursing Economics, 22*(4), 216–222.

Kroll, M. (2003). What were you thinking? Charting rules to keep you legally safe. *Journal of Gerontological Nursing, 29*(3), 15–16.

Langowski, C. (2005). The times they are a changing: Effects of online nursing documentation systems. *Quality Management in Health Care, 14*, 121–125.

Lippincott Williams & Wilkins. (2003). *Complete guide to documentation*. Philadelphia: Author.

Lippincott Williams & Wilkins. (2007). *Chart smart* (2nd ed.). Philadelphia: Author.

Maddox, P. J. (2003). HIPAA: Update on rule revisions and compliance requirements. *Medsurg Nursing, 12*(1), 59–63.

Mascara, C. M., Czar, P., & Hebda, T. (2004). *Internet resource guide for nurses & health care professionals* (3rd ed.). Upper Saddle River, NJ: Prentice-Hall.

Miller, J., & Glusko, J. (2003). Standing up to the scrutiny of medical malpractice. *Nursing Management, 34*(10), 20–22.

Montgomery, K. S., & Fitzpatrick, J. J. (Eds.). (2005). *Internet for nursing research*. New York: Springer.

Murphy, E. K. (2003). Charting by exception. *AORN Journal, 78*(5), 821–823.

Olson, L. (2003). Privacy and confidentiality in an electronic age. *Chart, 100*, 9.

Rossel, C. L. (2003). HIPAA: An informatics system perspective. *Chart, 100*, 11.

Saba, V. K., & McCormick, K. A. (Eds.). (2006). *Essentials of nursing informatics* (4th ed.). New York: McGraw-Hill.

Seaver, M. (2005). A helping handheld computer: Technology at the point of care. *2005 Pathways to Success*, 46–50. Retrieved June 14, 2006, from http://www2.nursingspectrum.com/CE/Self-Study_modules/course.html?ID=202

Simpson, R. L. (2004). Information technology. Measuring change: How technology increases nursing's diversity. *Nursing Management, 35*, 12, 14.

Smith, C. M., & Dougherty, M. (2001). Practice brief: Requirements for the acute care record. *Journal of AHIMA, 72*(3), 56A–56G.

Smith, L. S. (2003). Chart smart: Handling documentation errors. *Nursing, 33*(10), 73.

Smith, L. S. (2004). Documenting refusal of treatment. *Nursing, 34*(4), 79.

Sullivan, G. H. (2004). Legally speaking: Does your charting measure up? *RN, 67*(3), 61–65.

Tanner, A., Pierce, S., & Pravikoff, D. (2004). Moving the nursing information agenda forward. *CIN, Computers Informatics Nursing, 22*, 300–302.

Thede, L. Q. (2003). *Informatics and nursing: Opportunities and challenges*. Philadelphia: Lippincott Williams & Wilkins.

Development and Family Health

Promoting Health Throughout the Lifespan

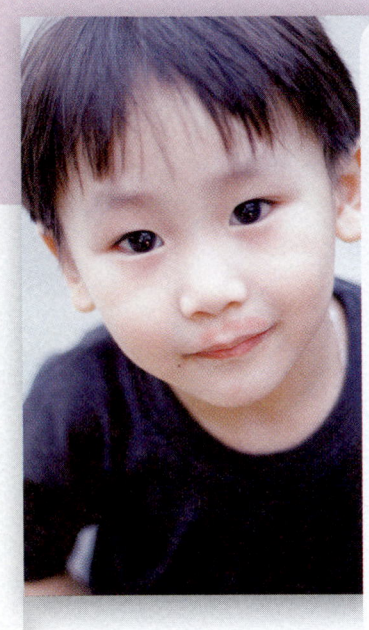

Mark Tien, of Chinese heritage, is almost 5 years old, and today is a very exciting day for him. His mother is taking him to register for kindergarten in the fall. He knows that his job will be to study hard and get good grades by learning as much as he can. He can't wait to learn all the new things his parents have told him will be taught. He didn't attend preschool because his family felt he was too young and that kindergarten was soon enough for him to start learning "the ways of the world."

In addition to enrolling him in school, Mark's mother is taking him to see the pediatrician for his annual examination and to make sure he has received all the immunizations required to start school. When the nurse weighs and measures him, she finds he has grown since his last visit, but the graph of his measurements shows he is in the bottom 25% in both height and weight. Nonetheless, he is considered to be developing as expected for his age. He receives his school immunizations and is told he is all set to start school.

LEARNING OUTCOMES

After completing this chapter, you will be able to:

1. Define the key terms.

2. Differentiate between growth and development.

3. List factors that influence growth and development.

4. List and describe the stages of growth and development according to Freud, Erikson, Havighurst, Vygotsky, Peck, and Gould.

5. List and describe the stages of cognitive development according to Piaget.

6. Compare Kohlberg's and Gilligan's theories of moral development.

7. Describe cognitive, psychosocial, moral, and spiritual development throughout the lifespan.

8. Describe usual growth throughout the lifespan.

9. List developmental assessment activities and expected findings throughout the lifespan.

10. Identify selected health risks and health promotion activities associated with different stages throughout the lifespan.

KEY TERMS

Accommodation p220

Adaptation p220

Assimilation p220

Baby boomer p241

Defense mechanism p216

Denver Developmental
    Screening Test
    (DDST-II) p227

Development p215

Developmental stage
    p217

Developmental task p219

Failure to thrive p227

Generation X p241

Generation Y p241

Growth p215

Menopause p244

Morality p221

Peer p231

Personality p216

Primary sexual
    characteristics p237

Puberty p236

Regression p230

Repression p233

Secondary sexual
    characteristics p237

Self-concept p229

Separation anxiety p230

CONCEPTS OF GROWTH AND DEVELOPMENT

The terms *growth* and *development* both refer to dynamic processes that are ongoing throughout the lifespan. **Growth** describes physical changes such as an increase in size. It is measured quantitatively and includes indicators such as height, weight, bone size, and dentition. The pattern of physiologic growth is similar for all people although growth rates vary during different stages of growth and development. The growth rate is rapid during the prenatal, neonatal, infant, and adolescent stages but slower during childhood. Physical growth is minimal during adulthood.

Development is an increase in the complexity of function and skill progression. It is the capacity and skill of a person to adapt to the environment. Development is the behavioral changes associated with aging and includes psychosocial, moral, spiritual, and cognitive advances.

Growth and development are independent, interrelated processes. For example, an infant's muscles, bones, and nervous system must grow to a certain point before the infant is able to sit up or walk, but growth does not assure development. Growth generally takes place during the first 20 years of life; development also takes place during that time but it continues throughout the lifespan even after growth has slowed or stopped. Principles of growth and development are shown in Box 9–1.

FACTORS INFLUENCING GROWTH AND DEVELOPMENT

Many factors can influence growth and development. Knowledge of these factors helps the nurse to intervene to promote growth and development of the individual.

- **Genetics** are established at conception and remain unchanged throughout life and determines such characteristics as gender, physical characteristics and, to some extent, temperament.
- **Temperament** determines the way individuals respond to their external and internal environment, setting the stage for the interactive dynamics of growth and development, and may persist throughout the lifespan of the individual.
- **Family** provides support and safety for the child, are a major constant in the child's life, and are involved in their children's physical and psychologic well-being and development, socializing the child through family dynamics (Ball & Bindler, 2006). Parents and caregivers set expected behaviors and model appropriate behavior.
- **Nutrition** is an essential component of growth and development determining if the child will reach his or her full potential or be at risk for health and developmental problems.

BOX 9–1   Principles of Growth and Development

- Growth and development are continuous, orderly, sequential processes influenced by maturational, environmental, and genetic factors.
- All humans follow the same pattern of growth and development.
- The sequence of each stage is predictable, although the time of onset, the length of the stage, and the effects of each stage vary with the person.
- Learning can either help or hinder the maturational process, depending on what is learned.
- Each developmental stage has its own characteristics.

- Growth and development occur in cephalocaudal and proximodistal directions (see Figure 9–1), which is particularly obvious at birth.
- Development proceeds from simple to complex.
- Development becomes increasingly differentiated, developing from a generalized response to a skilled specific response.
- Certain stages of growth and development are more critical than others.
- The pace of growth and development is uneven throughout the lifespan.

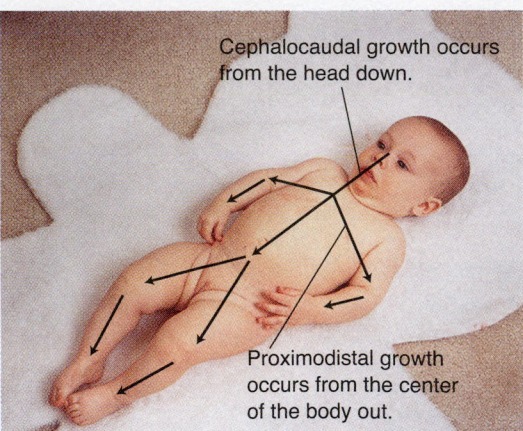

Cephalocaudal growth occurs from the head down.

Proximodistal growth occurs from the center of the body out.

Figure 9–1 ● Cephalocaudal and proximodistal growth.

- **Environmental** factors such as living conditions, socioeconomic status, climate, and community can influence growth and development.
- **Health** issues, such as illness, injury, or hospitalization can affect growth and development.
- **Cultural** customs can influence a child's growth and development including practices such as nutrition, child-rearing, and educational expectations.

Growth and development is divided into specific age ranges, or stages, as indicated by Table 9–1. Each stage carries significant characteristics of both growth and of development that will impact how nursing care is provided.

THEORIES OF GROWTH AND DEVELOPMENT

Numerous researchers have advanced theories about the stages and aspects of growth and development. Each theorist has considered a specific component of growth and development such as psychosocial, cognitive, moral, spiritual, and behavioral aspects.

Psychosocial Theories

Psychosocial development refers to the development of personality. **Personality**, a complex concept that is difficult to define, can be considered as the outward (interpersonal) expression of the inner (intrapersonal) self. It encompasses a person's temperament, feelings, character traits, independence, self-esteem, self-concept, behavior, ability to interact with others, and ability to adapt to life changes.

Many theorists attempt to account for psychosocial development in humans in order to explain the development of a person's personality and the causes of that person's behavior.

FREUD (1856–1939) While some of his theory has dropped out of popularity, Sigmund Freud introduced a number of concepts about development that are still used today, such as the concepts of the unconscious mind, defense mechanisms, and the id, ego, and superego. Freud defined the unconscious mind as the part of the mind the person is unaware exists that motivates behavior. He saw three parts of the unconscious mind: the id, the ego, and the superego. This concept of the unconscious is one of Freud's major contributions to the field of psychiatry. The id responds to pleasure seeking, desiring immediate gratification with no thoughts of long-term consequences, rules, or realism. The ego is the realistic part of the person's mind balancing the gratification demands of the id with the limitations of social and physical circumstances. The methods the ego uses to fulfill the needs of the id in a socially acceptable manner are called *defense mechanisms* or *adaptive mechanisms*. **Defense mechanisms**, or adaptive mechanisms as they are more commonly called today, are the result of conflicts between the id's impulses and the anxiety created by the conflicts due to social and environmental restrictions. The third aspect of the personality, according to Freud, is the superego. The superego contains the conscience and the ego ideal. The conscience consists of society's "do nots," usually as a result of parental and cultural teachings. The ego ideal comprises the standards of perfection toward which the individual strives. Freud proposed that the underlying motivation to human development is a dynamic, psychic energy, which he called libido.

According to Freud's theory of psychosexual development, the personality develops in five overlapping stages from birth to adulthood. The libido changes its location of emphasis within the body from one stage to another. Therefore, a particular body area has special significance to a client at a particular stage. Initially, the infant focuses on the oral area, demonstrated through need to suck and eat. The anal stage occurs during the toddler period when the child learns to control the bowel. The phallic stage occurs during the preschool period when children begin to recognize the difference between girls and boys, mothers and fathers. These stages are called *pregenital stages*. During the latency period, occurring during the school age stage, the child's energy is directed toward school and developing same-sex relationships, with a reduction in sexual impulses. Finally, during the genital stage, which begins in puberty and continues through the rest of the lifespan, energy is directed toward sexual maturity and developing skills to cope with the environment.

Freudian theory asserts that the individual must meet the needs of each stage in order to move successfully to the next developmental stage. If the person does not achieve a satisfactory progression at one stage, the personality becomes fixated at that stage. Fixation is immobilization, or the inability of the personality to proceed to the next stage because of anxiety. Ideally, an individual progresses through each stage with balance between the id, ego, and superego.

ERIKSON (1902–1996) Erik H. Erikson (1963, 1964) adapted and expanded Freud's theory of development to include the entire lifespan, believing that people continue to

TABLE 9–1	Stages of Growth and Development		
STAGE	**AGE**	**SIGNIFICANT CHARACTERISTICS**	**NURSING IMPLICATIONS**
Neonatal	Birth to 28 days	Behavior is largely reflexive and develops to more purposeful behavior.	Assist parents to identify and meet needs.
Infancy	1 month to 1 year	Physical growth is rapid.	Control the infant's environment so that physical and psychologic needs are met.
Toddlerhood	1 to 3 years	Motor development permits increased physical autonomy. Psychosocial skills increase.	Safety and risk-taking strategies must be balanced against the child's need to explore the environment in order to meet growth and development needs.
Preschool	3 to 6 years	The preschooler's world is expanding. New experiences allow the preschooler to practice social role during play. Physical growth slows.	Provide opportunities for play and social activity.
School age	6 to 12 years	Stage includes the preadolescent period (10 to 12 years). Peer group increasingly influences behavior. Physical, cognitive, social, and communication skills increase.	Allow time and energy for the school-age child to pursue hobbies and school activities. Recognize and support child's achievement.
Adolescence	12 to 20 years	Self-concept changes with biologic development. Values are tested. Physical growth accelerates. Stress increases, especially in the face of conflicts.	Assist adolescents to develop coping behaviors. Help adolescents develop strategies for resolving conflicts.
Young adulthood	20 to 40 years	A personal lifestyle develops. Person establishes a relationship with a significant other and a commitment to something.	Accept adult's chosen lifestyle and assist with necessary adjustments relating to health. Recognize the person's commitments. Support change as necessary for health.
Middle adulthood	40 to 65 years	Lifestyle changes due to other changes such as grown children leaving home, change in occupational goals, planning for retirement.	Assist clients to plan for anticipated changes in life, to recognize the risk factors related to health, need for health screening, and to focus on strengths rather than weaknesses.
Older adulthood			
Young-old	65 to 74 years	Adaptation to retirement and changing physical abilities is often necessary. Chronic illness may develop.	Assist clients to keep physically and socially active and to maintain peer group interactions.
Middle-old	75 to 84 years	Adaptation to decline in speed of movement, reaction time, and increasing dependence on others may be necessary.	Assist clients to cope with loss (e.g., hearing, sensory abilities, and eyesight; death of loved one). Provide necessary safety measures.
Old-old	85 and over	Increasing physical problems may develop.	Assist clients with self-care as required, and with maintaining as much independence as possible.

develop throughout life. He described eight stages of development (see Table 9–2).

Erikson's theory proposes that life is a sequence of **developmental stages** or levels of achievement. Each stage signals a task that must be accomplished. The resolution of the task can be complete, partial, or unsuccessful. Erikson believed that the more success an individual has at each developmental stage, the healthier the personality of the individual. Failure to complete any developmental stage influences the person's ability to progress to the next level and damages the ego.

When using Erikson's developmental framework, nurses should be aware of indicators of positive and negative resolution of each developmental stage. According to Erikson, the environment is highly influential in development. Nurses can enhance a client's development by being aware of the individual's developmental stage and assisting with the development of coping skills related to stressors experienced at that specific level. Nurses can strengthen a client's positive resolution of a developmental task by providing the individual with appropriate opportunities and encouragement. For example, a 10-year-old child (industry

| TABLE 9–2 | Erikson's Eight Stages of Development | | | | |

STAGE	AGE	CENTRAL TASK	INDICATORS OF POSITIVE RESOLUTION	INDICATORS OF NEGATIVE RESOLUTION	NURSING IMPLICATIONS
Infancy	Birth to 18 months	Trust versus mistrust	Learning to trust others	Mistrust, withdrawal, estrangement	Meet infant's needs such as feeding, warmth, touch, comfort.
Early childhood	18 months to 3 years	Autonomy versus shame and doubt	Self-control without loss of self-esteem Ability to cooperate and to express oneself	Compulsive self-restraint or compliance Willfulness and defiance	Encourage child's desire to explore the environment while maintaining safety.
Late childhood	3 to 5 years	Initiative versus guilt	Learning the degree to which assertiveness and purpose influence the environment Beginning ability to evaluate one's own behavior	Lack of self-confidence Pessimism, fear of wrongdoing Overcontrol and overrestriction of own activity	Recognize child's literal interpretation of what is said, desire to please, and need for a measure of control when possible.
School age	6 to 12 years	Industry versus inferiority	Beginning to create, develop, and manipulate Developing sense of competence and perseverance	Loss of hope, sense of being mediocre Withdrawal from school and peers	Support child's need to keep up with schoolwork, hobbies, and friends. Involve child in care as much as possible.
Adolescence	12 to 20 years	Identity versus role confusion	Coherent sense of self Plans to actualize one's abilities	Feelings of confusion, indecisiveness, and possible antisocial behavior	Recognize the need to be like peers and fear of body changes making them different. Allow peers to visit.
Young adulthood	18 to 25 years	Intimacy versus isolation	Intimate relationship with another person Commitment to work and relationships	Impersonal relationships Avoidance of relationship, career, or lifestyle commitments	Support need for involvement of significant other. Help to minimize impact of illness on work and relationships.
Adulthood	25 to 65 years	Generativity versus stagnation	Creativity, productivity, concern for others	Self-indulgence, self-concern, lack of interests and commitments	Teach need for health screenings. Support inclusion of family in decision making.
Maturity	65 years to death	Integrity versus despair	Acceptance of worth and uniqueness of one's own life Acceptance of death	Sense of loss, contempt for others	Respect need to be involved in care planning. Support social network. Show respect and do not talk down to them because they are older.

Note: Modified from "Figure of Erikson's Stages of Personality Development," from Childhood and Society by Erik H. Erikson. Copyright 1950, © 1963 by W. W. Norton & Company Inc., renewed © 1978, 1991 by Erik H. Erikson. Used by permission of W. W. Norton & Company, Inc.

versus inferiority) can be encouraged to be creative, to finish schoolwork, and to learn how to accomplish these tasks within the limitations imposed by health status.

Erikson emphasized that people must change and adapt their behavior to maintain control over their lives. He theorized that no one stage of personality development can be bypassed, and people may become fixated at one stage if they fail to meet the challenges required of them. It is not uncommon for people of all ages to regress to a previous stage under anxious or stressful conditions, especially children.

HAVIGHURST (1900–1991) Robert Havighurst believed that learning is basic to life and that people continue to learn throughout the lifespan. He described growth and

TABLE 9–3	Havighurst's Age Periods and Developmental Tasks

Infancy and Early Childhood

1. Learning to walk
2. Learning to take solid foods
3. Learning to talk
4. Learning to control the elimination of body wastes
5. Learning sex differences and sexual modesty
6. Achieving psychologic stability
7. Forming simple concepts of social and physical reality
8. Learning to relate emotionally to parents, siblings, and other people
9. Learning to distinguish right from wrong and developing a conscience

Middle Childhood

1. Learning physical skills necessary for ordinary games
2. Building wholesome attitudes toward oneself as a growing organism
3. Learning to get along with age-mates
4. Learning an appropriate masculine or feminine social role
5. Developing fundamental skills in reading, writing, and calculating
6. Developing concepts necessary for everyday living
7. Developing conscience, morality, and a scale of values
8. Achieving personal independence
9. Developing attitudes toward social groups and institutions

Adolescence

1. Achieving new and more mature relations with age-mates of both sexes
2. Achieving a masculine or feminine social role
3. Accepting one's physique and using the body effectively
4. Achieving emotional independence from parents and other adults
5. Achieving assurance of economic independence
6. Selecting and preparing for an occupation

7. Preparing for marriage and family life
8. Developing intellectual skills and concepts necessary for civic competence
9. Desiring and achieving socially responsible behavior
10. Acquiring a set of values and an ethical system as a guide to behavior

Early Adulthood

1. Selecting a mate
2. Learning to live with a partner
3. Starting a family
4. Rearing children
5. Managing a home
6. Getting started in an occupation
7. Taking on civic responsibility
8. Finding a congenial social group

Middle Age

1. Achieving adult civic and social responsibility
2. Establishing and maintaining an economic standard of living
3. Assisting teenage children to become responsible and happy adults
4. Developing adult leisure-time activities
5. Relating oneself to one's spouse as a person
6. Accepting and adjusting to the physiologic changes of middle age
7. Adjusting to aging parents

Later Maturity

1. Adjusting to decreasing physical strength and health
2. Adjusting to retirement and reduced income
3. Adjusting to death of a spouse
4. Establishing an explicit affiliation with one's age group
5. Meeting social and civil obligations
6. Establishing satisfactory physical living arrangements

Note: From Robert J. Havighurst, *Developmental Tasks and Education*, 3rd ed. Published by Allyn and Bacon, Boston, MA. Copyright © 1972 by Pearson Education. Reprinted by permission of the publisher.

development as occurring during six stages, each associated with six to ten tasks to be learned (see Table 9–3).

Havighurst promoted the concept of developmental tasks in the 1950s. A **developmental task** is "a task which arises at or about a certain period in the life of an individual, successful achievement of which leads to his happiness and to success with later tasks, while failure leads to unhappiness in the individual, disapproval by society, and difficulty with later tasks" (Havighurst, 1972, p. 2).

Havighurst's developmental tasks provide a framework that the nurse can use to evaluate a person's general accomplishments. However, some nurses find that the broad categories limit its usefulness as a tool in assessing specific accomplishments, particularly those of infancy and childhood. In a multicultural society, the definition of success of tasks may vary with values and belief systems as well (e.g., not all individuals may wish to marry or bear children), making these tasks less relevant for some.

CHESS AND THOMAS   Early research on temperament conducted in the 1950s by Stella Chess and Alexander Thomas identified nine temperamental qualities seen in children's behavior (see Table 9–4). The "goodness of fit" between children's temperamental qualities and the demands of their environment contributes to positive interaction and positive growth and development (Rothbart, 2004). Goodness of fit refers to whether parents' expectations of their child's behavior are consistent with the child's temperament type. When parents understand a child's temperament characteristics, they are better able to shape the environment to meet the child's needs (Ball & Bindler, 2006, p. 143).

VYGOTSKY (1896–1934)   Lev Vygotsky, referred to as a "social constructivist," explored the concept of cognitive development within a social, historical, and cultural context, arguing that adults guide children to learn and that development depends on the use of language, play, and

TABLE 9–4	Temperamental Qualities
CHARACTERISTIC	EXAMPLES OF BEHAVIOR STYLE
Activity level	Active, restless, always on the move versus quiet, inactive
Sensitivity	Apparently oblivious to stimuli versus reacts to minimal stimuli
Intensity	Minimal reaction to stimuli versus reacts strongly and intensely
Adaptability	Responds smoothly to unexpected events versus resists change
Distractibility	Focuses on tasks versus easily distracted by minimal stimuli
Approach/ Withdrawal	Jumps right into activities versus hesitant to engage
Mood	Cheerful
Persistence	Sticks to tasks versus easily gives up
Regularity	Demonstrates patterns of behavior versus random activity

extensive social interaction. These ideas have been used in treatment of children with learning disorders, autism, mental handicaps, and other disabilities (Edwards, 2002). These ideas also support the benefit of adult social learning opportunities via group interaction and observation. Vygotsky truly supported social learning and reinforcement through work, group discussion, and other means.

PECK Theories and models about adult development are relatively more recent than theories of infant and child development. Research into adult development has been stimulated by a number of factors, including increased longevity and healthier old age. In the past, development was viewed as complete by the time of physical maturity, and aging was considered a decline following maturity. The emphasis was on the negative aspects rather than the positive aspects of aging. However, Robert Peck (1968) believes that although physical capabilities and functions decrease with old age, mental and social capacities tend to increase in the latter part of life.

Peck proposes three developmental tasks during old age, in contrast to Erikson's one (integrity versus despair):

1. *Ego differentiation versus work-role preoccupation.* An adult's identity and feelings of worth are highly dependent on that person's work role. On retirement, people may experience feelings of worthlessness unless they derive their sense of identity from a number of roles so that one such role can replace the work role or occupation as a source of self-esteem. For example, a man who likes to garden or golf can obtain ego rewards from those activities, replacing rewards formerly obtained from his occupation.
2. *Body transcendence versus body preoccupation.* This task calls for the individual to adjust to decreasing physical capacities and at the same time maintain feel-

ings of well-being. Preoccupation with declining body functions reduces happiness and satisfaction with life.
3. *Ego transcendence versus ego preoccupation.* Ego transcendence is the acceptance without fear of one's death as inevitable. This acceptance includes being actively involved in one's own future beyond death. Ego preoccupation, by contrast, results in holding onto life and a preoccupation with self-gratification.

GOULD Roger Gould is another theorist who has studied adult development. He believes that transformation is a central theme during adulthood: "Adults continue to change over the period of time considered to be adulthood and developmental phases may be found during the adult span of life" (Gould, 1972, p. 33). According to Gould, the 20s is the time when a person assumes new roles; in the 30s, role confusion often occurs; in the 40s the person becomes aware of time limitations in relation to accomplishing life's goals; and in the 50s, the acceptance of each stage as a natural progression of life marks the path to adult maturity.

Cognitive Theory

Cognitive development refers to the manner in which people learn to think, reason, and use language. It involves a person's intelligence, perceptual ability, and ability to process information. Cognitive development represents a progression of mental abilities from illogical to logical thinking, from simple to complex problem solving, and from understanding concrete ideas to understanding abstract concepts.

The most widely known cognitive theorist is Jean Piaget (1896–1980). His theory of cognitive development has contributed to other theories, such as Kohlberg's theory of moral development and Fowler's theory of the development of faith, both discussed in this chapter. According to Piaget (1966), cognitive development is an orderly, sequential process in which a variety of new experiences (stimuli) must exist before intellectual abilities can develop. Piaget's cognitive developmental process is divided into five major phases: the sensorimotor phase, the preconceptual phase, the intuitive thought phase, the concrete operations phase, and the formal operations phase (Table 9–5).

In each phase, the person uses three primary abilities: assimilation, accommodation, and adaptation. **Assimilation** is the process through which humans encounter and react to new situations by using the mechanisms they already possess. In this way, people acquire knowledge and skills as well as insights into the world around them. **Accommodation** is a process of change whereby cognitive processes mature sufficiently to allow the person to solve problems that were unsolvable before. This adjustment is possible chiefly because new knowledge has been assimilated. **Adaptation**, or coping behavior, is the ability to handle the demands made by the environment.

Nurses can employ Piaget's theory of cognitive development when developing teaching strategies. Assessing the client for cognitive developmental level will allow the nurse to adjust the approach to the client's ability to comprehend

TABLE 9–5	Piaget's Phases of Cognitive Development	
PHASES AND STAGES	**AGE**	**SIGNIFICANT BEHAVIOR**
Sensorimotor phase	Birth to 2 years	
Stage 1 Use of reflexes	Birth to 1 month	Most action is reflexive.
Stage 2 Primary circular reaction	1 to 4 months	Perception of events is centered on the body. Objects are extension of self.
Stage 3 Secondary circular reaction	4 to 8 months	Acknowledges the external environment. Actively makes changes in the environment.
Stage 4 Coordination of secondary schemata	8 to 12 months	Can distinguish a goal from a means of attaining it.
Stage 5 Tertiary circular reaction	12 to 18 months	Tries and discovers new goals and ways to attain goals. Rituals are important.
Stage 6 Inventions of new means	18 to 24 months	Interprets the environment by mental image. Uses make-believe and pretend play.
Preconceptual phase	2 to 4 years	Uses an egocentric approach to accommodate the demands of an environment. Everything is significant and relates to "me." Explores the environment. Language development is rapid. Associates words with objects.
Intuitive thought phase	4 to 7 years	Egocentric thinking diminishes. Thinks of one idea at a time. Includes others in the environment. Words express thoughts.
Concrete operations phase	7 to 11 years	Solves concrete problems. Begins to understand relationships such as size. Understands right and left. Cognizant of viewpoints.
Formal operations phase	11 to 15 years	Uses rational thinking. Reasoning is deductive and futuristic.

Note: Adapted from *The Origin of Intelligence*, by J. Piaget, 1966, Copyright © 1966. International Universities Press, Inc. Reprinted with permission.

what is taught. When teaching adults, nurses may become aware that some adults are more comfortable with concrete thought and slower to acquire and apply new information than are other adults. Amending their teaching style will increase the success of the teaching plan.

Behaviorism

Behaviorist theory states that learning takes place when an individual's reaction to a stimulus is either positively or negatively reinforced. The more rapid, consistent, and positive the reinforcement is, the more likely a behavior is to be learned and retained.

B.F. Skinner (1904–1990) believed that organisms learn as they respond to or "operate on" their environment. His research led to the term "operant conditioning," in which he maintained that rewarded or reinforced behavior will be repeated; behavior that is punished will be suppressed. Skinner's theory is of particular use with clients diagnosed with mental health disorders, especially those with substance abuse problems.

Moral Theories

Moral development, a complex process not fully understood, involves learning what ought to be and what ought not to be done. It is more than imprinting parents' rules and virtues or values on children. The term *moral* means "relating to right and wrong." The terms *morality, moral behavior,* and *moral development* should be distinguished. **Morality** refers to the requirements necessary for people to live together in society; moral behavior is the way a person perceives those requirements and responds to them; moral development is the pattern of change in moral behavior with age (see Chapter 2 ∞).

KOHLBERG Lawrence Kohlberg's theory specifically addresses moral development in children and adults (Kohlberg, 1981, 1984). The morality of an individual's decision was not Kohlberg's concern; rather, he focused on the reasons an individual makes a decision. According to Kohlberg (1927–1987), moral development progresses through three levels and six stages. Levels and stages are not always linked to a certain developmental stage, because some people progress to a higher level of moral development than do others.

At Kohlberg's first level, called the *premoral* or *preconventional level*, children are responsive to cultural rules and labels of good and bad, right and wrong. However, children interpret these in terms of the physical consequences of their actions, that is, punishment or reward. At the second level, the *conventional level*, the individual is concerned about maintaining the expectations of the family, group, or nation and sees this as right. The emphasis at this level is conformity and loyalty to one's own expectations as well as society's. Level three is called the *postconventional, autonomous,* or *principled level*. At this level, people make an effort to define

TABLE 9–6	Kohlberg's Stages of Moral Development	
LEVEL	**STAGE**	**AVERAGE AGE**
I. PRECONVENTIONAL Person is responsive to cultural rules of labels of good and bad, right or wrong. Externally established rules determine right or wrong actions. Person reasons in terms of punishment, reward, or exchange of favors. **EGOCENTRIC FOCUS**	**1. Punishment and Obedient Orientation** Fear of punishment, not respect for authority, is the reason for decisions, behavior, and conformity.	Toddler to 7 years
	2. Instrumental Relativist Orientation Conformity is based on egocentricity and narcissistic needs. There is no feeling of justice, loyalty, or gratitude. "I'll do something if I get something for it or because it pleases you."	Preschooler through school age
II. CONVENTIONAL Person is concerned with maintaining expectations and rules of the family, group, nation, or society. A sense of guilt has developed and affects behavior. The person values conformity, loyalty, and active maintenance of social order and control. Conformity means good behavior or what pleases or helps another and is approved. **SOCIETAL FOCUS**	**3. Interpersonal Concordance Orientation** Decisions and behavior are based on concerns about others' reactions; the person wants others' approval or a reward. An empathic response, based on understanding of how another person feels, is a determinant for decisions and behavior. ("I can put myself in your shoes.")	School age through adulthood (Most American women are in this stage)
	4. Law-and-Order Orientation The person wants established rules from authorities, and the reason for decisions and behavior is that social and sexual rules and traditions demand the response. ("I'll do something because it's the law and my duty.")	Adolescence and adulthood (Most men are in this stage)
III. POSTCONVENTIONAL The person lives autonomously and defines moral values and principles that are distinct from personal identification with group values. He or she lives according to principles that are universally agreed on and that the person considers appropriate for life. **UNIVERSAL FOCUS**	**5. Social Contract Legalistic Orientation** The social rules are not the sole basis for decisions and behavior because the person believes a higher moral principle applies such as equality, justice, or due process.	Middle-age or older adult. Only 20% or less of Americans achieve this stage.
	6. Universal Ethical Principle Orientation Decisions and behaviors are based on internalized rules, on conscience rather than social laws, and on self-chosen ethical and abstract principles that are universal, comprehensive, and consistent.	Middle-age or older adult. Few people attain or maintain this stage. Examples of this stage are seen in times of crisis or extreme situations.

Note: From *Health Promotion Strategies Through the Life Span*, 8th ed. (pp. 232–233), by R. B. Murray, J. P. Zentner, and R. Yakimo, 2009, Upper Saddle River, NJ: Pearson Education. Adapted with permission.

valid values and principles without regard to outside authority or to the expectations of others (see Table 9–6).

GILLIGAN After more than 10 years of research with women subjects, Carol Gilligan (1982) reported that women often consider the dilemmas Kohlberg used in his research to be irrelevant. Women scored consistently lower on Kohlberg's scale of moral development in spite of the fact that they approached moral dilemmas with considerable sophistication. Gilligan believes that most frameworks for research in moral development do not include the concepts of caring and responsibility.

Gilligan found that moral development proceeds through three levels and two transitions, with each level rep-

resenting a more complex understanding of the relationship of self and others. Each transition results in a crucial reevaluation of the conflict between selfishness and responsibility (Murray, Zentner, & Yakimo, 2009, p. 233).

- *Stage 1: Caring for oneself.* In this first stage of development, the person is concerned only with caring for the self. The individual feels isolated, alone, and unconnected to others. There is no concern or conflict with the needs of others because the self is the most important. The focus of this stage is survival. The transition of this stage occurs when the individual begins to view this approach as selfish and moves toward responsibility. The person begins to realize a need for relationships and connections with other people.

- *Stage 2: Caring for others.* During this stage, the individual begins to understand the need for caring relationships with others and the responsibility that comes with them. The definition of responsibility includes self-sacrifice, where "good" is considered to be "caring for others." The individual now approaches relationships with a focus of not hurting others causing the individual to be more responsive and submissive to others' needs, excluding any thoughts of meeting one's own needs. A transition from goodness to truth occurs when the individual recognizes that this approach can cause difficulties with relationships because of the lack of balance between caring for oneself and caring for others. The woman makes decisions on personal intentions and consequences of actions rather than on how she thinks others will react (Murray, Zentner, & Yakimo, 2009, p. 234).
- *Stage 3: Caring for self and others.* During this last stage, a person sees the need for a balance between caring for others and caring for the self. Care remains the focus on which decisions are made. However, the person recognizes the interconnections between the self and others and realizes that if one's own needs are not met, other people may also suffer.

Gilligan (1982) believes women often see morality in the integrity of relationships and caring, so that the moral problems they encounter are different from those of men. Men tend to consider what is right to be what is just, whereas for women what is right is taking responsibility for others as a self-chosen decision (p. 140). The ethic of justice, or fairness, is based on the idea of equality: Everyone should receive the same treatment. This is the development path usually followed by men and widely accepted by moral theorists. By contrast, the ethic of care is based on the premise of nonviolence: No one should be harmed. This is the path typically followed by women but given little attention in the literature of moral theory.

Spiritual Theories

The spiritual component of growth and development refers to individuals' understanding of their relationship with the universe and their perceptions about the direction and meaning of life.

FOWLER James Fowler describes the development of faith as a force that gives meaning to a person's life. He uses the term *faith* as a form of knowing, a way of being in relation to "an ultimate environment." To Fowler, "faith is a relational phenomenon; it is an active 'mode-of-being-in-relation' to another or others in which we invest commitment, belief, love, risk and hope" (Fowler & Keen, 1985, p. 18). Fowler's stages in the development of faith are given in Table 9–7.

Fowler's theory and developmental stages were influenced by the work of Piaget, Kohlberg, and Erikson. Fowler believes that the development of faith is an interactive process between the person and the environment (Fowler, Streib, & Keller, 2004). In each of Fowler's stages, new patterns of thought, values, and beliefs are added to those already held by the individual; therefore the stages must follow in sequence. Faith stages, according to Fowler, are separate from the cognitive stages of Piaget: They evolve from a combination of knowledge and values.

WESTERHOFF Westerhoff describes faith as a way of being and behaving that evolves from an experienced faith guided by parents and others during a person's infancy and childhood to an owned faith that is internalized in adulthood and serves as a directive for personal action (see Table 9–8). For the client who is ill, faith—whether in a higher authority (e.g., God, Allah, Jehovah), in the client's own self, in the health care team, or in a combination of all—provides strength and trust.

TABLE 9–7 Fowler's Stages of Spiritual Development

STAGE	AGE	DESCRIPTION
0. Undifferentiated	0 to 3 years	Infant unable to formulate concepts about self or the environment
1. Intuitive-projective	4 to 6 years	A combination of images and beliefs given by trusted others, mixed with the child's own experience and imagination
2. Mythic-literal	7 to 12 years	Private world of fantasy and wonder; symbols refer to something specific; dramatic stories and myths used to communicate spiritual meanings
3. Synthetic-conventional	Adolescent or adult	World and ultimate environment structured by the expectations and judgments of others; interpersonal focus
4. Individuating-reflexive	After 18 years	Constructing one's own explicit system; high degree of self-consciousness
5. Paradoxical-consolidative	After 30 years	Awareness of truth from a variety of viewpoints
6. Universalizing	Maybe never	Becoming an incarnation of the principles of love and justice

Note: From *Life Maps: Conversations in the Journey of Faith,* by J. Fowler and S. Keen, 1985, Waco, TX: Word Books; and *How to Help Your Child Have a Spiritual Life: A Parents' Guide to Inner Development,* by A. Hollander, 1980, New York: A and W Publishers. Adapted with permission.

TABLE 9–8 Westerhoff's Four Stages of Faith

STAGE	AGE	BEHAVIOR
Experienced faith	Infancy/early adolescence	Experiences faith through interaction with others who are living a particular faith tradition.
Affiliative faith	Late adolescence	Actively participates in activities that characterize a particular faith tradition; experiences awe and wonderment; feels a sense of belonging.
Searching faith	Young adulthood	Through a process of questioning and doubting own faith, acquires a cognitive as well as an affective faith.
Owned faith	Middle adulthood/old age	Puts faith into personal and social action and is willing to stand up for what the individual believes even against the nurturing community.

Note: From *Will Our Children Have Faith?* (1976) By John Westerhoff. Reprinted with permission from the author.

DEVELOPMENT THROUGHOUT THE LIFESPAN

A thorough understanding of growth and development assists the nurse in individualizing care to meet the needs of each client. This section will take the concepts of growth and development and apply them to each stage of the lifespan, emphasizing the nursing considerations, health assessment, and promotion of health and wellness for each age group.

Conception and Prenatal Development

The fertilized ovum develops into an organism with most of the features of a human during the embryonic phase encompassing the first 8 weeks of pregnancy. Within the first 3 weeks the tissues differentiate into the ectoderm (outer layer), mesoderm (middle layer), and endoderm or entoderm (inner layer). From the beginning of the third week through the eighth week after conception, these layers form the basic structure of all of the body's complex organs and systems.

Traditionally, pregnancy has been divided into three periods called trimesters, each of which lasts about 3 months. Each trimester includes certain landmarks for developmental changes in the mother and the fetus. The two phases of intrauterine life can also be considered in trimesters. The embryonic phase is the first trimester, and the fetal phase includes the second and third trimesters. The embryonic phase is when the embryo's organs and tissues are developing. The fetal phase of development is characterized by a period of rapid growth in the size of the fetus. Both genetic and environmental factors affect its growth. The fetus gains most of its weight during the last 2 months in utero.

HEALTH PROMOTION During the intrauterine stage of development, the embryo or fetus relies on the maternal blood flow through the placenta to meet its basic survival needs. The health of the mother is essential for proper growth and development.

Oxygen To meet the fetal demands for oxygen, the pregnant mother gradually increases her normal blood flow by about one-third, peaking at about 8 months. Respiratory rate and cardiac output increase significantly during this period. Initially the heart of the embryo lies outside its body. It is then repositioned in the chest early in the second trimester. By 20 weeks the fetal heartbeat is audible through a fetoscope; the heartbeat is audible as early as the 10th week if a Doppler stethoscope with ultrasound is used.

Nutrition and Fluids The fetus obtains nourishment from the placental circulation and by swallowing amniotic fluid. Nutritional needs are met when the mother eats a well-balanced diet containing sufficient calories and nutrients to meet both her needs and those of the fetus. Adequate folic acid, one of the B vitamins, is important in order to prevent neural tube defects (e.g., spina bifida) in the fetus.

Rest and Activity The fetus sleeps most of the time and develops a pattern of sleep and wakefulness that usually persists after birth. Fetal activity can be felt by the mother at about the fifth lunar month of pregnancy.

Elimination Fetal feces are formed in the intestines from swallowed amniotic fluid throughout pregnancy, but are normally not excreted until after birth. Inadequate oxygenation of the fetus during the third trimester can result in relaxation of the anal sphincter and passage of feces into the amniotic fluid. Urine normally is excreted into the amniotic fluid when the kidneys mature (16 to 20 weeks).

Temperature Maintenance Amniotic fluid usually provides a safe and comfortable temperature for the fetus. Significant changes in maternal temperature can alter the temperature of the amniotic fluid and the fetus, resulting in birth defects.

Safety The embryo is particularly vulnerable to damage from a teratogen, which is anything that adversely affects normal cellular development in the embryo or fetus (Venes, 2005). It is important for the nurse to inquire about possible pregnancy when giving medications that are known teratogens and to also ask when the woman is scheduled for tests that involve radiography (x-ray). Box 9–2 lists some of the risk factors associated with abnormal fetal development.

Neonates and Infants (Birth to 1 Year)

Babies are considered neonates from birth to the end of the first month. Infants are babies from 1 month to 1 year of age.

PHYSICAL DEVELOPMENT A neonate's basic task is adjustment to the environment outside the uterus, which requires

BOX 9–2	Maternal Factors that Contribute to a Higher Risk of Low-Birth-Weight Babies

- Underweight before pregnancy, or less than 21 pounds gained during pregnancy
- Inadequate prenatal care
- Age of 17 years or younger, or over 40 years
- History of hypertension
- Low socioeconomic level
- Smoking cigarettes or use of addictive drugs or alcohol during pregnancy
- Exposure to toxic substances or chemicals
- Complications during pregnancy, poor health status, vaginal bleeding, or exposure to infections
- High stress levels, including physical or emotional abuse
- Previous low-birth-weight infants or multiple miscarriages
- Having given birth less than 6 months or 10 or more years before. A safe interval between pregnancies is a minimum of 18 to 23 months
- Many of these factors are interrelated and affected by low socioeconomic level

Note: From *Health Promotion Strategies Through the Life Span*, 8th ed. (p. 233), by R. B. Murray and J. P. Zentner, R. Yakimo, 2009. Reprinted by permission.

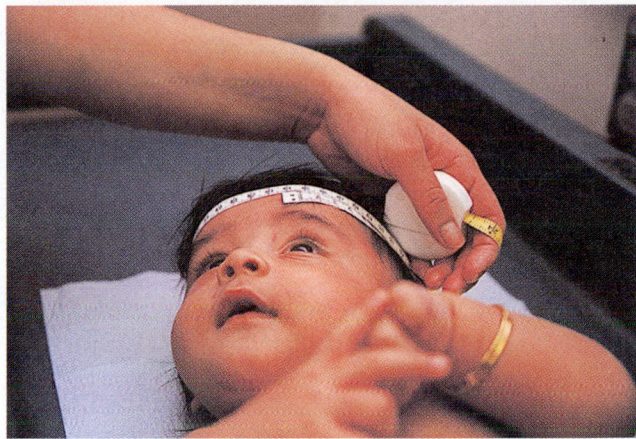

Figure 9–2 ⬤ An infant's head circumference is measured around the skull, above the eyebrows, and around the occiput.

breathing, sleeping, sucking, eating, swallowing, digesting, and eliminating. Infants continue to grow and develop rapidly during the first year, learning more skills as they interact with their world. Infants undergo significant physiologic change in weight, length, head growth, vision, and motor development. Some of these changes can be assessed using standardized growth charts based on growth of groups of American children (Centers for Disease Control [CDC], 2000).

Weight   Just after birth, most infants lose 5% to 10% of their birth weight because of fluid loss. This weight loss is normal, and infants usually regain that weight in about 1 week. After several days, babies usually gain weight at the rate of 150 to 210 g (5 to 7 oz) weekly for 6 months. By 5 months of age, infants usually reach twice their birth weight, and by age 12 months, three times their birth weight.

Length   Female babies on average are smaller than male babies. Babies from different ethnic groups may vary by height, weight, and head circumference, so ethnicity must be considered when determining what is "normal" for any particular infant. By 6 months infants gain another 13.75 cm (5.5 in.) of height. By 12 months they add another 7.5 cm (3 in.). The rate of increase in height is largely influenced by the baby's size at birth and by nutrition.

Head and Chest Circumference   Assessment of head circumference is of particular importance in infants and children to determine the growth rate of the skull and the brain. An infant's head should be measured at every visit to the primary care provider or nurse until the child is 2 years old (see Figure 9–2). The chest circumference of the newborn is usually less than the head circumference by about 2.5 cm (1 in.). As the infant grows, the chest circumference becomes larger than the head circumference. At about 9 or 10 months the head and chest circumferences are about the same, and after 1 year of age the chest circumference is larger.

Head Molding   The heads of many newborn babies are misshapen because of the molding of the head that occurs during vaginal deliveries. Molding of the head occurs due to fontanels and sutures in the skull. Fontanels are unossified membranous gaps in the bone structure of the skull. Sutures are junction lines of the skull bones that override to provide flexibility for molding of the head. Within a week, a newborn's head usually regains its symmetry, which is reassuring to the parents. The larger anterior fontanel can increase in size for several months after birth. After 6 months the size gradually decreases until closure occurs between 9 and 18 months. The posterior fontanel between the parietal bones and the occipital bone closes between 2 and 3 months after birth.

Vision   The newborn can follow large moving objects and blinks in response to bright light and sound. The pupils of the newborn respond slowly, and the eyes cannot focus on close objects. By 1 month the infant can focus his or her gaze on objects and follow moving ones. At 4 months the infant recognizes a parent's smile, although social smiles may appear as early as 2 months. The 4-month-old has almost complete color vision and follows objects through a 180-degree arc. A 5-month-old infant reaches for objects. Between 6 and 10 months the infant can fix on an object and follow it in all directions. By 12 months depth perception has fully developed, and the infant will consistently be able to recognize where a change in level occurs, such as at the edge of the bed.

Hearing   Newborns with intact hearing will react with a startle to a loud noise, a reaction called the *Moro reflex.* Within a few days, they are able to distinguish different sounds. By 2 to 3 months they will actively coo, smile, or gurgle to sounds and voices. Between 3 and 6 months the infant will look for sounds, pausing an activity to listen and responding with distress or pleasure to angry or happy voices. Between 6 and 9 months individual words begin to take on meaning and the infant may look at named objects or people.

The 9- to 12-month-old infant understands many words, uses gestures, may articulate one or two words with a specific reference, and, by 1 year of age, responds to simple commands.

Smell and Taste   The senses of smell and taste are functional shortly after birth. Newborns prefer sweet tastes and tend to decrease their sucking in response to liquids with a salty content. They are able to recognize the smell of their mother's milk and respond to this smell by turning toward the mother.

Touch   The sense of touch is well developed at birth. Skin-to-skin touching is important for an infant's development. The infant responds positively to the warmth, love, and security it perceives when touched, held, and cuddled. The newborn is sensitive to temperature extremes and has poor self-regulation of body temperature. In response to pain, young babies react diffusely and cannot isolate the discomfort.

Reflexes   Reflexes of the newborn are unconscious, involuntary responses of the nervous system to external and internal stimuli. Reflexes normally present at birth are the rooting, sucking, Moro, palmar grasp, plantar, tonic neck, stepping, and Babinski reflexes. Infant reflexes disappear during the first year of life in an ordered sequence, a process that allows the infant to develop voluntary movements. In addition, the abilities to yawn, stretch, sneeze, burp, and hiccup are all present at birth.

Motor Development   Motor development is the development of the baby's abilities to control movements. Initially, body movement is uncoordinated. Table 9–9 outlines some of the motor and social development milestones.

PSYCHOSOCIAL DEVELOPMENT   According to Erikson (1963), the central crisis at this stage is trust versus mistrust. Resolution of this stage determines how the person approaches subsequent developmental stages. During the first year of life, infants depend on adults for all their physiologic and psychologic needs. Fulfillment of these needs is required for the infant to develop a basic sense of trust. Parents and caregivers can enhance this sense of trust by (a) being sensitive to the infant's needs and meeting these needs promptly and skillfully; (b) responding consistently to an infant's needs; and (c) providing a predictable environment in which routines are established. Mothering or nurturing behavior, such as consistent care, handling, stroking, and cuddling, is essential for healthy psychosocial development. By 8 months, most infants exhibit attachment to their parents or caregivers and may show displeasure when left with strangers.

The newborn reacts socially to caregivers by paying attention to the face or voice and by cuddling when held. The baby is able to interact with the environment by responding to various stimuli such as touch and sound. Table 9–9 provides examples of motor and social development.

Crying is the infant's initial reaction to stress, and the major way they communicate stress. Infants learn gradually to tolerate stress. According to Freud, infants have an oral focus, many of their activities and pleasures are mouth-centered, and they reduce tension by sucking and chewing on objects. Nurses and family members can reduce the stress of an infant by maintaining the infant's routine as much as possible and providing a consistent, predictable environment.

COGNITIVE DEVELOPMENT   Piaget referred to the initial period of cognitive development as the sensorimotor phase. This phase has six stages, three of which take place during the first year. From 4 to 8 months infants begin to have perceptual recognition. By 6 months they respond to new stimuli, and they remember certain objects and look for them for a short time. By 12 months infants have a concept of both space and time. They experiment to reach a goal, such as a toy on a chair. An infant's cognitive development proceeds from reflexive ability of the newborn to using one or two actions to attain a goal by the age of 1 year.

MORAL DEVELOPMENT   Infants associate right and wrong with pleasure and pain. What gives them pleasure is right, since they are too young to reason otherwise. When infants receive abundant positive responses from parents and care-

| | TABLE 9–9 | **Examples of Motor and Social Development in Infancy** |

AGE	MOTOR DEVELOPMENT	SOCIAL DEVELOPMENT
Newborn	Turns head from side to side when in a prone position. Grasps by reflex when object is placed in palm of hand.	Displays displeasure by crying and satisfaction by soft vocalizations. Attends to adult face and voice by eye contact and quieting.
4 months	Rolls over. Sits with support, holds head steady when sitting.	Babbles, laughs, and increased response to verbal play.
6 months	Lifts chest and shoulders off table when prone, bearing weight on hands. Manipulates small objects.	Starts to imitate sounds. Vocalizes one-syllable sounds: "ma ma," "da da."
9 months	Creeps and crawls. Uses pincer grasp with thumb and forefinger.	Complies with simple verbal commands. Displays fear of being left alone (e.g., going to bed). Waves "bye-bye."
12 months	Walks alone with help. Uses spoon to feed self.	Clings to mother in unfamiliar situations. Demonstrates emotions such as anger and affection.

givers such as smiles, caresses, and voice tones of approval in these early months, they learn that certain behaviors are wrong or good and that pain or pleasure is the consequence.

HEALTH RISKS   A number of health problems of neonates and infants require interventions from health care personnel. Safety concerns are of particular importance.

Failure to Thrive   **Failure to thrive** is a unique syndrome in which an infant falls below the fifth percentile for weight and height on a standard growth chart or is falling in percentiles on a growth chart (Pillitteri, 2010). The two categories for this syndrome are organic causes (e.g., cardiac disease) and inorganic causes, which usually involve the parent–child relationship. Infants deprived of mothering, especially from months 3 to 15, will not learn to form significant relationships or to trust others. Touch, cuddling, and visual and auditory stimulation are all critical for the infant. It is through these mechanisms that the infant comes to know self and the environment. Infants who fail to establish a loving, responsive relationship with a caregiver often fail to develop normally. Infants with inorganic failure to thrive show delayed development without any physical cause. They are often malnourished and fail to gain weight and grow normally.

Infant Colic   Colic is acute abdominal pain caused by periodic contractions of the intestines. It occurs in infants as young as 2 weeks of age and for most infants disappears by 3 months of age. Although the direct cause is not known, colic tends to occur in infants with sensitive temperaments. Factors such as swallowing air, feeding too rapidly, allergies, taking excessive amounts of carbohydrates, infant emotional distress, and anxiety of the caregiver may be associated with colic.

   To help relieve the colic, the nurse can assess the infant during feeding and suggest possible changes. Suggestions may include cuddling the infant, swaddling, rocking, and finding the position that provides the infant with the most comfort (Karp, 2003; Schmitt, 2006).

Crying   Crying is often of great concern to parents. When an infant's crying lasts up to 10 to 12 hours a day, it is described as colicky (see the preceding section). A crying or fussy period lasting 1 to 2 hours a day is usually considered normal for infants.

Child Abuse   Reports of child abuse have increased in recent years, and the stress of having a baby with colic or excessive crying can put some parents or caregivers at risk for child abuse. It can take various forms, including physical abuse, physical neglect, sexual abuse, and emotional abuse and neglect. Shaken baby syndrome (SBS) is violent shaking of the infant, causing whiplash. The shaking, combined with impact, often against a soft surface, can lead to severe brain injury in infants. These injuries often occur without external evidence of head injury. Subdural and retinal hemorrhages accompanied by the absence of external signs of trauma are hallmarks of the syndrome (Geddes, 2004). Nurses should teach parents and caregivers about the dangers associated with shaking infants and the need to seek help if they feel they could harm their baby.

Sudden Infant Death Syndrome   The sudden and unexpected death of an infant may be a case of sudden infant death syndrome (SIDS). A postmortem examination usually fails to reveal a cause. The highest incidence of SIDS occurs in the second to fourth month of life, and boys are more susceptible than girls. Babies born prematurely are at increased risk of SIDS. Research has shown that sleeping on the back, not prone, greatly decreases the risk of SIDS. *Healthy People 2010* includes an objective to increase the percentage of healthy full-term infants who are put down to sleep on their backs (USDHHS, 2000).

HEALTH ASSESSMENT AND PROMOTION   Newborns require thorough physical assessments because of the risk of congenital anomalies. Health promotion is important throughout the lifespan.

Apgar Scoring   Newborn babies can be assessed immediately by the Apgar scoring system. This provides a numeric indicator of the baby's physiologic capacities to adapt to extrauterine life. Each of five signs is assigned a maximum score of 2, so that the maximum score achievable is 10. A score under 7 suggests that the baby is having difficulty, and a score under 4 indicates that the baby's condition is critical requiring immediate neonatal resuscitation. Apgar scoring is usually carried out 60 seconds after birth and is repeated in 5 minutes. Those with very low scores will be reassessed at 10 minutes.

Developmental Screening Tests   Development can be assessed by observing the infant's behavior and by using standardized tests such as the **Denver Developmental Screening Test (DDST-II)**. The DDST-II is used to screen children from birth to 6 years of age. The test is intended to estimate the abilities of a child compared to those of an average group of children of the same age. Four main areas of development are screened: personal-social, fine-motor adaptive, language, and gross motor.

Ongoing Nursing Assessments   During ongoing assessments, the nurse examines and observes the infant, taking into account variations that occur with developmental age and activity. Failure to meet a developmental milestone at an average age may be normal for that infant, but it is important to provide follow-up assessment to determine developmental trends. In addition, the nurse actively listens to the caregiver for possible problems or areas of concern and reviews with caregivers the expected behavior or characteristics for the particular age group. It is important for the caregiver to know that certain behaviors, responses, and activities of the infant are normal and expected. It is also important to discuss the many individual differences that can, quite normally, occur. The assessment interview is also a time to be supportive of the parent's role, to assess the attachment of the mother to the infant, and to observe the interactions between the infant and caregivers.

   The first month of life is critical for physical adjustments to extrauterine life and for the psychosocial adjustment of the parents. From 1 month to 1 year, infants experience rapid change, with advances in physical growth

---

BOX 9–3   Health Promotion Guidelines for Infants

Health Examinations

- Screening of newborns for hearing loss; follow-up at 3 months and early intervention by 6 months if appropriate
- At 2 weeks and at 2, 4, 6, and 12 months

Protective Measures

- Immunizations: diphtheria, tetanus, acellular pertussis (DTaP), inactivated poliovirus vaccine (IPV), pneumococcal, measles-mumps-rubella (MMR), *Haemophilus influenzae* type B (HIB), hepatitis B (HepB), varicella and influenza vaccines as recommended
- Fluoride supplements if there is inadequate water fluoridation (less than 0.7 part per million)
- Screening for tuberculosis
- Screening for phenylketonuria (PKU) and other metabolic conditions
- Prompt attention for illnesses
- Appropriate skin hygiene and clothing

Infant Safety

- Importance of supervision
- Car seat, crib, playpen, bath, and home environment safety measures
- Feeding measures (e.g., avoid propping bottle)
- Provide toys with no small parts or sharp edges

- Eliminate toxins in the environment (e.g., chemicals, radon, lead, mercury)
- Use smoke and carbon monoxide (CO) detectors in home

Nutrition

- Breastfeeding to age 12 months
- Breastfeeding and bottle-feeding techniques
- Formula preparation
- Feeding schedule
- Introduction of solid foods
- Need for iron supplements at 4 to 6 months

Elimination

- Characteristics and frequency of stool and urine elimination
- Diarrhea and its effects

Rest/Sleep

- Establish routine for sleep and rest patterns

Sensory Stimulation

- Touch: holding, cuddling, rocking
- Vision: colorful, moving toys
- Hearing: soothing voice tones, music, singing
- Play: toys appropriate for development

---

and psychosocial development. For a summary of health and wellness promotion, see Box 9–3.

Toddlers (1 to 3 Years)

Toddlers develop from having no voluntary control to being able to walk and speak. They also learn to control their bladder and bowels, and they acquire a wide variety of information about their environment.

PHYSICAL DEVELOPMENT   Toddlers are usually chubby, with relatively short legs and a large head. The face appears small when compared to the skull, but as the toddler grows, the face seems to grow from under the skull and appears better proportioned. Toddlers normally have a pronounced lumbar lordosis and a protruding abdomen. The abdominal muscles develop gradually with growth, and the abdomen flattens.

DEVELOPMENTAL ASSESSMENT GUIDELINES
The Infant

In these five developmental areas, does the infant do the following?

Physical Development

- Demonstrate physical growth (weight, length, head and chest circumference) within the normal range.
- Manifest appropriately sized fontanels for age.
- Exhibit vital signs within normal range for age.
- Display ability to habituate to stimuli and to calm self.

Motor Development

- Perform gross and fine motor milestones within the normal range for age.
- Exhibit reflexes appropriate for age.
- Display symmetric movements.
- Exhibit no hyper- or hypotonia.

Sensory Development

- Follow a moving object within normal range for age.
- Respond to sounds, such as talking or clapping hands.
- Coo, babble, laugh, vocalize, and imitate sounds as expected for age.

Psychosocial Development

- Interact appropriately with parent through body movements and vocalizations.

Development in Activities of Daily Living

- Eat and drink appropriate amounts of breast milk, formula, and/or solid foods.
- Exhibit an elimination pattern within normal range for age.
- Exhibit a rest and sleep pattern appropriate for age.

Weight   Two-year-olds can be expected to weigh approximately four times their birth weight. The weight gain is about 2 kg (5 lb) between ages 1 and 2 years and about 1 to 2 kg (2 to 5 lb) between 2 and 3 years. The 3-year-old weighs about 13.6 kg (30 lb).

Height   A toddler's height can be measured as height or length. Height is measured while the toddler stands, and length is measured while the toddler is in a recumbent position. Although the measurements differ slightly, nurses must specify which measurement is used to avoid confusion. Between ages 1 and 2 years, the average growth in height is 10 to 12 cm (4 to 5 in.), and between 2 and 3 years it slows to 6 to 8 cm (2 1/2 to 3 1/2 in.).

Head Circumference   The head circumference of the toddler increases about 2.5 cm (1 in.) on average each year. By 24 months the head is 80% of the average adult size, and the brain is 70% of its adult size.

Sensory Abilities   Visual acuity is fairly well established by 1 year of age; average estimates of acuity for the toddler are 20/70 at 18 months and 20/40 at 2 years of age. Accommodation to near and far objects is fairly well developed by 18 months and continues to mature with age. At 3 years of age, the toddler can look away from a toy prior to reaching out and picking it up. This ability requires the integration of visual and neuromuscular mechanisms.

The senses of hearing, taste, smell, and touch become increasingly developed and associated with each other. Hearing in the 3-year-old is at adult levels. The taste buds of the toddler are sensitive to the natural flavors of food, and the 3-year-old prefers familiar odors and tastes. Touch is a very important sense, and a distressed toddler is often soothed by tactile sensations.

Motor Abilities   Fine muscle coordination and gross motor skills improve during toddlerhood. At the age of 18 months toddlers can pick up raisins or cereal pieces and place them in a receptacle. They can also hold a spoon and a cup and can walk upstairs with assistance. They will probably crawl down the stairs.

At 2 years, toddlers can hold a spoon and put it into the mouth correctly. They are able to run, their gait is steady, and they can balance on one foot and ride a tricycle (Figure 9–3). By 3 years most children are toilet trained, although they still may have the occasional accident when intent on play or during the night.

PSYCHOSOCIAL DEVELOPMENT   According to Freud, the ages of 2 and 3 years represent the anal phase of development, when the rectum and anus are the especially significant areas of the body. Erikson viewed the period from 18 months to 3 years as the time when the central developmental task is autonomy versus shame and doubt.

Toddlers begin to develop their sense of autonomy by asserting themselves with the frequent use of the word "no." They are often frustrated by restraints to their behavior and between ages 1 and 3 may have temper tantrums. However,

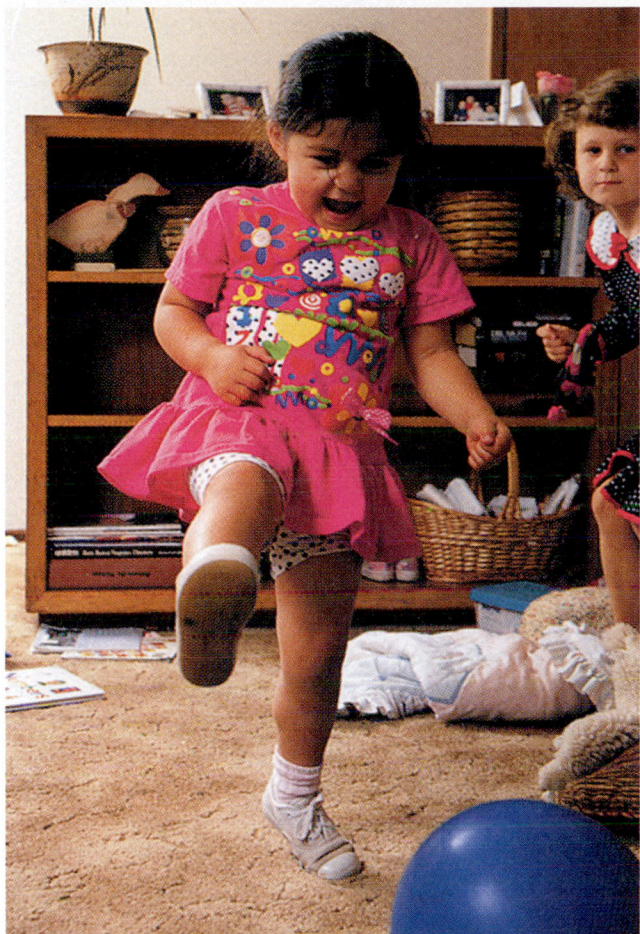

Figure 9–3 ⦿ A toddler has enough gross and fine motor ability to jump and kick a ball.

with the guidance of their caregivers they slowly gain control over their emotions. Parents need to have a great deal of patience coupled with an understanding of the importance of this developmental milestone. To be effective, caregivers need to give the child some measure of control and at the same time be consistent in setting limits so that the child learns the results of misbehavior. The nurse can also assist the parents and caregivers in promoting the toddler's development by suggesting the activities summarized in Box 9–4.

Self-concept is made up of body image development, feelings about self, adaptive and defensive mechanisms, reactions from others, and one's perceptions of these reactions, attitudes, values, and many of life's experiences (Starr, 2004). Children learn to develop a sense of self-concept through their immediate social environment, in which their parents or caregivers play a significant role. If the children's social interactions with their parents are negative, the children may begin to see themselves as bad. This perception is the basis of a negative self-concept. Parents need to give toddlers positive input so that they can develop a positive and healthy self-concept. With a healthy sense of self-esteem and security, the toddler is able to deal with periodic failures later in life without damage to self-esteem.

| BOX 9–4 | **Fostering the Toddler's Psychosocial Development** |

- Provide toys suitable for the toddler, including some toys challenging enough to motivate but not so difficult that the toddler will fail. (Failure will intensify feelings of self-doubt and shame.)
- Make positive suggestions rather than commands. Avoid an emotional climate of negativism, blame, and punishment.
- Give the toddler choices, all of which are safe; however, limit number to two or three.
- When toddler has a temper tantrum, make sure the child is safe, and then leave.
- Help the toddler to develop inner control by setting and enforcing consistent, reasonable limits.
- Praise the toddler's accomplishments; give random and spontaneous feedback for positive behavior.

Although toddlers like to explore the environment, they always need to have a significant person nearby. Parents need to know that young children experience acute **separation anxiety**, the fear and frustration that come with parental absences. Abandonment is their greatest fear. Experience with separation helps the child cope with parental absences. Children need room for exploration and interaction with other children and adults. At the same time, they need to know that the parental bond of a loving and close relationship remains secure.

Regression or reverting to an earlier development stage may be indicated by bed-wetting or using baby talk. Nurses can assist parents by helping them understand that this behavior is normal and indicates that these toddlers are trying to establish their position in the family.

During the toddler stage, receptive and expressive language skills are developing quickly. Children can understand words and follow directions long before they can actually form them into sentences.

COGNITIVE DEVELOPMENT   According to Piaget, the toddler completes the fifth and sixth stages of the sensorimotor phase and starts the preconceptual phase at about 2 years of age. In the fifth stage, the toddler solves problems by a trial-and-error process. By stage 6, toddlers can solve problems mentally. During Piaget's preconceptual phase, toddlers develop considerable cognitive and intellectual skills. They learn about the sequence of time. They have some symbolic thought; for example, a chair may represent a place of safety, and a blanket may symbolize comfort. Concepts start to form in late toddlerhood. A concept develops when the child learns words to represent classes of objects or thoughts.

MORAL DEVELOPMENT   According to Kohlberg, the first level of moral development is the preconventional stage when children respond to punishment and reward. During the second year of life, children begin to know that some activities elicit affection and approval. They also recognize that certain rituals, such as repeating phrases from prayers,

also elicit approval. This provides children with feelings of security. By 2 years of age, toddlers are learning what attitudes their parents or caregivers hold about moral matters.

SPIRITUAL DEVELOPMENT   According to Fowler (1981), the toddler's stage of spiritual development is undifferentiated. Toddlers may be aware of some religious practices, but they are primarily involved in learning information and determining emotional reactions rather than establishing spiritual beliefs. A toddler may repeat short prayers at bedtime, conforming to a ritual, because praise and affection result. The parent's or caregiver's response enhances the toddler's sense of security.

HEALTH RISKS   Toddlers experience significant health problems due to injuries, visual problems, dental caries, and respiratory and ear infections. As they seek autonomy, they are prone to accidents as they explore new things.

Injuries   Injuries are the leading cause of mortality of toddlers. They are curious and like to feel and taste everything. The most common causes of fatal injuries are automobile crashes, drowning, burns, poisoning, and falls. Parents or other caregivers need to take the appropriate preventive measures to guard against these health threats (Figure 9–4).

Visual Problems   During this period, the toddler should be screened for amblyopia. Amblyopia (reduced visual acuity in one eye) is usually the result of strabismus (cross-eye) but can be caused by refractive errors (e.g., myopia) or opacities in the lens. Initially the child with amblyopia has straight eyes, but the condition can lead to deviation of the "lazy" eye and loss of vision.

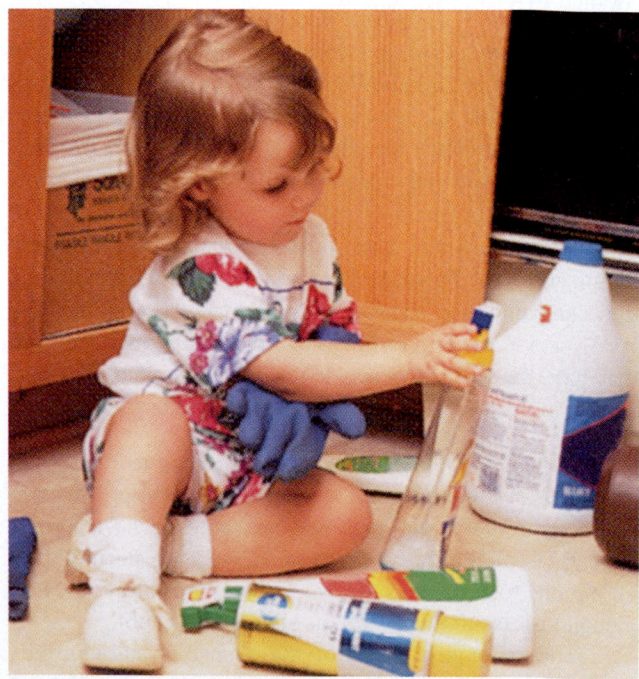

Figure 9–4 Keep medicines and other poisonous materials locked away.

Dental Caries Dental caries occur frequently during the toddler period, resulting from the interaction between the tooth surface, the *Streptococcus mutans* bacterium, and carbohydrates, especially sugar, in the diet. Prolonged exposure of teeth to carbohydrates can cause caries.

Respiratory Tract and Ear Infections Respiratory and middle ear infections are common during toddlerhood; their incidence increases with exposure to other children, with use of a bottle during naps or at bedtime, or if bottles are propped for feedings. Respiratory infections contribute significantly to visits to the pediatric primary care provider in the toddler years.

HEALTH ASSESSMENT AND PROMOTION Growth and development in the toddler and preschool years provide the basis for a child's future health and well-being. It is essential that nurses do accurate and timely assessments to promote health and detect problems early, thus allowing for early interventions. Providing health education, information about growth and development, and anticipatory guidance to parents or caregivers is also an important nursing role. Assessment activities for the toddler are similar to those for the infant in terms of measuring weight, length (height), and vital signs (see the Developmental Assessment Guidelines).

Promoting health and wellness includes such areas as accident prevention, toilet training, and good dental hygiene. For a summary of health promotion for toddlers, see Box 9–5.

Preschoolers (4 to 5 Years)

During the preschool period physical growth slows, but control of the body and coordination increase greatly. The preschoolers' world gets larger as they meet relatives, friends, **peers**, and neighbors.

PHYSICAL DEVELOPMENT By the time children are 4 or 5 years old, they become taller and thinner than toddlers because children tend to grow more in height than in weight. The preschooler's brain reaches almost its adult size by age 5. The extremities of the body grow more quickly than the body trunk, making the child's body appear somewhat out of proportion. The posture of preschoolers gradually changes as the pelvis is straightened and the abdominal muscles become stronger. Thus the preschooler appears slender with erect posture.

Weight Weight gain in preschool children is generally slow. By 5 years they have added only another 3 to 5 kg (7 to 12 lb) to their 3-year-old weight, increasing it to somewhere between 18 and 20 kg (40 and 45 lb).

Height Preschool children grow about 5 to 6.25 cm (2.0 to 2.5 in.) each year. Thus by 4 years of age they double the birth length and measure about 102 cm (41 in.).

Vision Preschool children are generally hyperopic (farsighted), that is, unable to focus on near objects. As the eye grows in length, it becomes emmetropic (it refracts light normally). If the eyes become too long, the child becomes myopic (nearsighted). In severe cases of hyperopia or myopia, glasses may be prescribed. By the end of the preschool years, visual ability has improved; normal vision for the 5-year-old is approximately 20/30. The Snellen E chart can be used to assess the preschooler's vision.

Hearing and Taste The hearing of the preschool child has reached optimal levels, and the ability to listen has matured

---

DEVELOPMENTAL ASSESSMENT GUIDELINES
The Toddler

In these four developmental areas, does the toddler do the following?

Physical Development

- Demonstrate physical growth (weight, height, and head circumference) within normal range.
- Manifest vital signs within normal range for age.
- Exhibit vision and hearing abilities within normal range.

Motor Development

- Perform gross and fine motor milestones within the normal range for age. For example, by 3 years of age is the toddler able to do the following?
  - Walk up steps without assistance.
  - Balance on one foot, jump, and walk on toes.
  - Copy a circle.
  - Build a bridge from blocks.
  - Ride a tricycle.

Psychosocial Development

- Perform psychosocial developmental milestones for age. For example, by 3 years of age is the toddler able to do the following?
  - Express likes and dislikes.
  - Display curiosity and ask questions.
  - Accept separation from mother for short periods of time.
  - Begin to play and communicate with children and others outside the immediate family.
  - Understand words such as *up, down, cold,* and *hungry.*
  - Speak in sentences of three to four words.
  - Imitate religious rituals of the family.

Development in Activities of Daily Living

- Feed self.
- Eat and drink a variety of foods.
- Begin to develop bowel and bladder control.
- Exhibit a sleep pattern appropriate for age.
- Dress self.

BOX 9–5   **Health Promotion Guidelines for Toddlers**

Health Examinations

- At 15 and 18 months and then as recommended by the primary care provider
- Dental visit starting at age 3 or earlier

Protective Measures

- Immunizations: continuing DTaP, IPV series, pneumococcal, MMR, *Haemophilus influenzae* type B, hepatitis B, hepatitis A, and influenza vaccines as recommended
- Screenings for tuberculosis and lead poisoning
- Fluoride supplements if there is inadequate water fluoridation (less than 0.7 part per million)

Toddler Safety

- Importance of constant supervision and teaching child to obey commands
- Home environment safety measures (e.g., lock medicine cabinet)
- Outdoor safety measures (e.g., close supervision near water)
- Appropriate toys

- Eliminate toxins in environment (e.g., pesticides, herbicides, mercury, lead, arsenic in playground materials)
- Use smoke and carbon monoxide (CO) detectors in home

Nutrition

- Importance of nutritious meals and snacks
- Teaching simple mealtime manners
- Dental care

Elimination

- Toilet training techniques

Rest/Sleep

- Dealing with sleep disturbances

Play

- Providing adequate space and a variety of activities
- Toys that allow "acting on" behaviors and provide motor and sensory stimulation

---

since the toddler age. As for the sense of taste, preschoolers show their preferences by asking for something "yummy," and may refuse something they consider "yucky." At about age 3, children may display food "jags," refusing to eat some foods or only eating a few particular foods. It is important that parents not engage the child in a "battle of wills" over food. If parents provide healthful foods in an environment that is pleasant and comfortable, the child will eat what is needed.

Motor Abilities   By 5 years of age, children are able to wash their hands and face and brush their teeth. They are self-conscious about exposing their bodies and go to the bathroom without telling others. Typically, preschool children run with increasing skill each year. By age 5, they run skillfully and can jump three steps. Preschoolers can balance on their toes and dress themselves without assistance.

PSYCHOSOCIAL DEVELOPMENT   Erikson wrote that the major developmental crisis of the preschooler is initiative versus guilt. Preschoolers must solve problems in accordance with their consciences. Their personalities continue to develop. Erikson viewed the success of this milestone as determining the individual's self-concept. According to Erikson, preschoolers must learn what they can do. As a result, preschoolers imitate behavior, and their imaginations and creativity become lively.

Parents and caregivers can enhance the self-concept of the preschooler by providing opportunities for new achievements where the child can learn, repeat, and master. The self-concept of the preschooler is also based on gender identification (see Figure 9–5). Parents need to be aware that preschoolers are curious about their own bodies and sexual

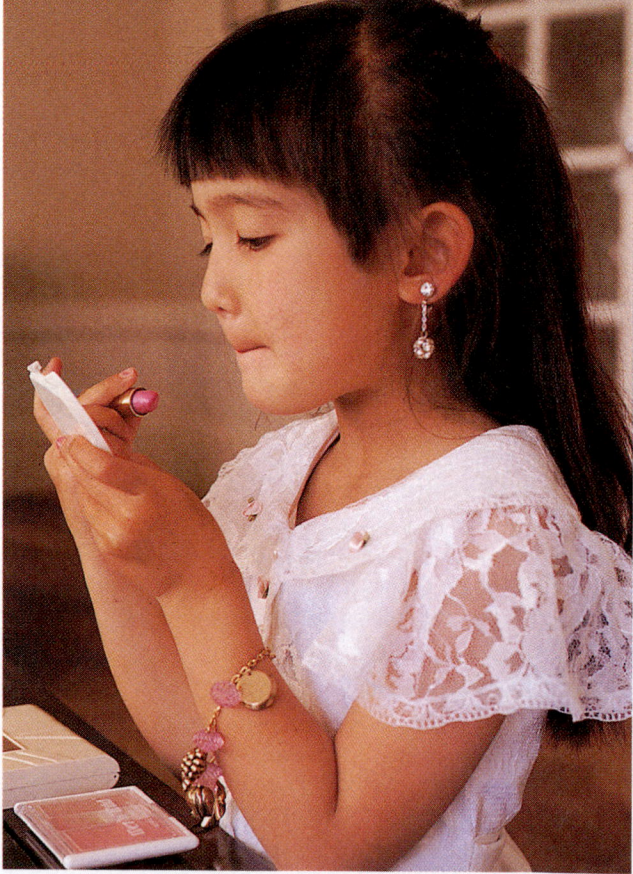

Figure 9–5 ⦿ Preschoolers often identify with the parent of the same sex and like to mimic behavior.

functions, as well as those of others, and will often ask questions. Freud theorized that the preschooler is in the phallic stage of development. The biologic focus of the child during this stage is the genital area, and masturbation is common. The phase of close emotional relationships with both parents change to the phase Freud referred to as the Electra (girls' sexual attraction to their fathers) or Oedipus (boys' sexual attraction to their mothers) complexes.

Four adaptive mechanisms are learned: identification, introjection, imagination, and repression. Identification occurs when the child perceives the self as similar to another person and behaves like that person. Introjection is similar to identification. It is the assimilation of the attributes of others. When preschoolers observe their parents, they assimilate many of their values and attitudes. Imagination is an important part of preschoolers' lives, helping children make sense of the world and giving them a sense of control and mastery. The preschooler has an active imagination and fantasizes in play. **Repression** is removing experiences, thoughts, and impulses from awareness. The child who is exposed to an emotional trauma may remove it from his or her awareness.

Preschool children gradually emerge as social beings. At the age of 3 or 4, they learn to play with a small number of peers. Preschoolers participate more in the family than they did previously. Children of 4 years are often dogmatic in their speech; they tend to believe that what they know is right. Four-year-olds love nonsense words and can string them together much to an adult's exasperation. At 4, children are aggressive in their speech and capable of long conversations, often mixing fact and fiction. By 5 years of age, speaking skills are well developed. Children use words purposefully and ask questions to acquire information. They do not merely practice speaking as 3- and 4-year-olds do, but speak as a means of social interaction. Exaggeration is common among 4- and 5-year-olds.

Preschoolers also become increasingly aware of themselves. They know where their body begins and ends as well as the correct names for different parts. Preschoolers also learn about their feelings, and know and understand the words *cry*, *sad*, *laugh* and the feelings related to them. They also begin to learn how to control their feelings and behavior. Preschoolers need to feel that they are loved and that they are an important part of the family. The child who has to compete with siblings for parental attention will often display jealousy, called sibling rivalry. Guidance and discipline are important parts of the parental role during the preschool years.

COGNITIVE DEVELOPMENT   The preschooler's cognitive development, according to Piaget, is the phase of intuitive thought. Children are still egocentric, but egocentrism gradually subsides as they experience their expanding world. Preschoolers learn through trial and error, and they think of only one idea at a time. They do not understand relationships such as those between mother and father or sister and brother. Children start to understand that words are associated with objects in late toddlerhood or the early preschool years. Preschoolers become concerned about death as something inevitable, but they do not explain it.

They also associate death with others rather than themselves. Most children at the age of 5 years can count pennies; however, the opportunity to spend money usually does not occur until they attend school. Reading skills also start to develop at this age. Young children like fairy tales and books about animals and other children.

MORAL DEVELOPMENT   Preschoolers are capable of prosocial behavior, that is, any action that a person takes to benefit someone else. The term *prosocial* is synonymous with *kind* and connotes sharing, helping, protecting, giving aid, befriending, showing affection, and giving encouragement. At this stage of development, preschoolers do not have a fully formed conscience; however, they do develop some internal controls. Moral behavior is learned largely by modeling, initially after parents and later caregivers. The preschooler usually behaves well in social settings.

Children who perceive their parents as strict may become resentful or overly obedient. Preschoolers usually control their behavior because they want love and approval from their parents. Moral behavior to a preschooler may mean taking turns at play or sharing. Nurses can assist parents or caregivers by discussing moral development and encouraging them to give preschoolers recognition for actions such as sharing. It is also important for parents to answer preschoolers' "why" questions and discuss values with them.

SPIRITUAL DEVELOPMENT   Many preschoolers enroll in Sunday school or faith-oriented classes. According to Fowler, children from the ages of 4 to 6 years are at the intuitive-projective stage of spiritual development. Faith at this stage is primarily a result of the teaching of significant others. Children learn to imitate religious behavior, although they don't understand the meaning of the behavior. Preschoolers require simple explanations of spiritual matters. Children at this age use their imaginations to envision such ideas as angels or the devil.

HEALTH RISKS   Preschoolers often have health problems similar to those they had in toddlerhood. Respiratory tract problems and communicable diseases frequently occur as the preschooler interacts with other children. Accidents and dental caries continue to be problems during this age.

HEALTH ASSESSMENT AND PROMOTION   During assessment, the preschooler can often participate in answering questions with assistance from parents or caregivers. Preschoolers can also describe the types of activities they enjoy. Guidelines for the preschooler are shown in the Developmental Assessment Guidelines.

Promoting health and wellness includes such areas as accident prevention, dental health, good nutrition, cognitive stimulation, and sufficient sleep. For a summary of health promotion, see Box 9–6.

School-Age Children (6 to 12 Years)

The school-age period starts when children are about 6 years of age, when the deciduous teeth are shed. This period includes the preadolescent (prepuberty) period. It ends at about 12 years,

DEVELOPMENTAL ASSESSMENT GUIDELINES
The Preschooler

In these four developmental areas, does the preschooler do the following?

Physical Development

- Demonstrate physical growth (weight, height) within normal range.
- Manifest vital signs within normal range for age.
- Exhibit vision and hearing abilities within normal range.

Motor Development

- Perform gross and fine motor milestones within the normal range for age. For example, by 5 years of age is the preschooler able to do the following?
  - Jump rope and skip.
  - Climb playground equipment.
  - Ride a bicycle with training wheels.
  - Print letters and numbers.

Psychosocial Development

- Perform psychosocial developmental milestones for age. For example, by 5 years of age is the preschooler able to do the following?
  - Separate easily from parents.

- Display imagination and creativity.
- Enjoy playing with peers in cooperative activities.
- Understand right from wrong and respond to others' expectations of behavior.
- Identify four colors.
- Exhibit increasing vocabulary using complete sentences and all parts of speech.
- Cooperate in doing simple chores (e.g., putting away toys).
- Demonstrate awareness of sexual differences.

Development in Activities of Daily Living

- Demonstrate development of toilet training.
- Perform simple hygiene measures.
- Dress and undress self.
- Engage in bedtime rituals and demonstrate ability to put self to sleep.

---

with the onset of puberty. Puberty is the age when the reproductive organs become functional and secondary sex characteristics develop. Because the average age of onset of puberty is 10 for girls and 12 for boys, some people define the school-age years as 6 to 10 for girls and 6 to 12 for boys. Skills learned during this stage are particularly important in relation to work later in life and willingness to try new tasks.

PHYSICAL DEVELOPMENT   The school-age child gains weight rapidly and thus appears less thin than previously.

Individual differences due to both genetic and environmental factors are obvious at this time.

Weight   At 6 years boys tend to weigh about 21 kg (46 lb), about 1 kg (2 lb) more than girls. The weight gain of school children from 6 to 12 years of age averages about 3.2 kg (7 lb) per year, but the major weight gains occur from age 10 to 12 for boys and from 9 to 12 for girls. By 12 years of age boys and girls weigh on the average 40 to 42 kg (88 to 95 lb); girls are usually heavier.

BOX 9–6   Health Promotion Guidelines for Preschoolers

Health Examinations

- Every 1 to 2 years

Protective Measures

- Immunizations: continuing DTaP, IPV series, MMR, hepatitis, pneumococcal, influenza, and other immunizations as recommended
- Screenings for tuberculosis
- Vision and hearing screening
- Regular dental screenings and fluoride treatment

Preschooler Safety

- Educating child about simple safety rules (e.g., crossing the street)
- Teaching child to play safely (e.g., bicycle and playground safety)
- Educating to prevent poisoning; exposure to toxic materials

Nutrition

- Importance of nutritious meals and snacks

Elimination

- Teaching proper hygiene (e.g., washing hands after using bathroom)

Rest/Sleep

- Dealing with sleep disturbances (e.g., night terrors, sleepwalking)

Play

- Providing times for group play activities
- Teaching child simple games that require cooperation and interaction
- Providing toys and dress-ups for role-playing

Height   At 6 years both boys and girls are about the same height, 115 cm (46 in.). They are about 150 cm (60 in.) by 12 years. Around puberty, children of both sexes have a growth spurt, girls between 10 and 12 years and boys between 12 and 14 years. Thus girls may be taller than boys at 12 years.

The extremities tend to grow more quickly than the trunk; thus school-age children's bodies appear somewhat ill proportioned. By 6 years of age the thoracic curvature starts to develop and lordosis disappears.

Vision   The depth and distance perception of children 6 to 8 years of age is accurate. By age 6 children have full binocular vision. The eye muscles are well developed and coordinated, and both eyes can focus on one object at the same time.

Hearing and Touch   Auditory perception is fully developed in school-age children, who are able to identify fine differences in voices, both in sound and in pitch. At this stage, children also have a well-developed sense of touch and are able to locate points of heat and cold on all body surfaces. They are also able to identify an unseen object, such as a pencil or a book, simply by touch (called stereognosis).

Prepubertal Changes   Little change takes place in the reproductive and endocrine systems until the prepuberty period. During prepuberty, at about ages 9 to 13, endocrine functions slowly increase. This change in endocrine function can result in increased perspiration and more active sebaceous glands. Girls may have a sticky vaginal discharge (leukorrhea) prior to puberty.

Motor Abilities   During the middle years (6 to 10), children perfect their muscular skills and coordination. By 9 years most children are becoming skilled in games of interest, such as football or baseball. By 9 years most children have sufficient fine motor control for such activities as drawing, building models, or playing musical instruments.

PSYCHOSOCIAL DEVELOPMENT   According to Erikson, the central task of school-age children is industry versus inferiority. At this time children begin to create and develop a sense of competence and perseverance. School-age children are motivated by activities that provide a sense of worth. Failure to achieve industry can lead to a sense of inferiority. If children have been successful in previous stages, they are motivated to be industrious and to cooperate with others toward a common goal.

Freud described the period from 6 through 12 years of age as the latency stage. During this time the focus is on physical and intellectual activities, while sexual tendencies seem to be repressed.

In school, children have the restraints of the school system imposed on their behavior, and they learn to develop internal controls. Children tend to compare their skills with those of their peers in a number of areas, including motor development, social development, and language, resulting in maturation of self-concept. This comparison assists in the development of self-concept. The typical 6- and 7-year-old is a member of a peer group that is usually informal and transitory, with leadership changing from time to time. Children gradually become less self-centered and more cooperative within a group. Peers can have a greater influence than the family. During middle to late childhood, children may join a more formalized group of peers, which is often structured around common interests. Although the focus of interest for this age group has moved to school, peers, and other activities, the home remains the crucial place for the child's development of high self-esteem.

COGNITIVE DEVELOPMENT   According to Piaget, the ages 7 to 11 years mark the phase of concrete operations. During this stage the child changes from egocentric interactions to cooperative interactions (see Figure 9–6). Children at this time develop logical reasoning from intuitive reasoning. Children also learn about cause-and-effect relationships at this age. The concept of money gains meaning for children when they start school. The concept of time is also learned at this age.

Reading skills are usually well developed later in childhood, and what a child reads is largely influenced by the family. By 9 years of age most children are self-motivated. They compete with themselves, and they like to plan in advance. By 12 years they are motivated by inner drive rather than by competition with peers. They like to talk, to discuss different subjects, and to debate.

MORAL DEVELOPMENT   Some school-age children are at Kohlberg's stage 1 of the preconventional level, acting to avoid punishment. Other school-age children may be in stage 2 with an instrumental–relativist orientation, doing things to benefit themselves. Fairness, that is, everyone getting a fair share or chance, becomes important. Later in childhood, most children progress to the conventional level. This level has two stages: Stage 3 is the "good boy–nice girl" stage, and stage 4 is the law and order orientation. Children usually reach the conventional level between the ages of 10 and 13. The child shifts from the concrete interests of individuals to the interests of groups.

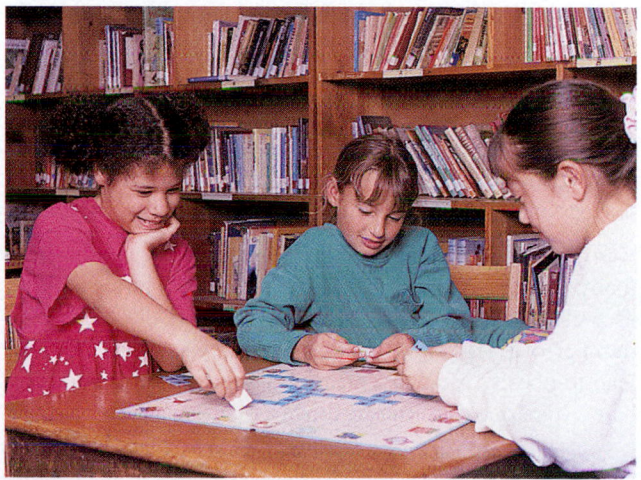

Figure 9–6 ⬤ Expanding cognitive skills enables school-age children to interact cooperatively in activities of an increasingly complex nature, as shown by the children playing this board game.

BOX 9–7	Health Promotion Guidelines for School-Age Children

Health Examinations

- Annual physical examination or as recommended

Protective Measures

- Immunizations as recommended (e.g., MMR, meningococcal, tetanus-diphtheria, adult preparation [Td])
- Screening for tuberculosis
- Periodic vision, speech, and hearing screenings
- Regular dental screenings and fluoride treatment
- Providing accurate information about sexual issues (e.g., reproduction, AIDS)

School-Age Child Safety

- Using proper equipment when participating in sports and other physical activities (e.g., helmets, pads)
- Encouraging child to take responsibility for own safety (e.g., participating in bicycle and water safety courses)

Nutrition

- Importance of child not skipping meals and eating a balanced diet
- Experiences with food that may lead to obesity

Elimination

- Utilizing positive approaches for elimination problems (e.g., enuresis)

Play and Social Interactions

- Providing opportunities for a variety of organized group activities
- Accepting realistic expectations of child's abilities
- Acting as role models in acceptance of other persons who may be different
- Providing a home environment that limits TV viewing and video games and encourages completion of homework and healthy exercise

---

The motivation for moral action at this stage is to live up to what significant others think of the child.

SPIRITUAL DEVELOPMENT According to Fowler, the school-age child is at stage 2 in spiritual development, the mythic–literal stage. Children learn to distinguish fantasy from fact. Spiritual facts are those beliefs that are accepted by a religious group, whereas fantasy is thoughts and images formed in the child's mind. Parents and the minister, rabbi, or priest help the child distinguish fact from fantasy. These people still influence the child more than do peers in spiritual matters. When children do not understand such events as the creation of the world, they use fantasy to explain them. The school-age child needs to have concepts such as prayer presented in concrete terms.

School-age children may ask many questions about God and religion in these years and will generally believe that God is good and always present to help. Just before puberty, children become aware that their prayers are not always answered and become disappointed. At this age, some children reject religion, whereas others continue to accept it. This decision is largely influenced by the parents or caregivers. If a child continues religious training, the child is ready to apply reason rather than blind belief in most situations.

HEALTH RISKS School-age children continue to have as many communicable diseases, dental caries, and accidents as preschoolers. Another health concern is the increasing number of overweight children. Obesity in childhood can lead to obesity as adults, creating an increased risk for diabetes, hypertension, and cardiovascular disease.

HEALTH ASSESSMENT AND PROMOTION During the assessment interview the nurse responds to questions from the parent or other caregiver, gives appropriate feedback, and lends encouragement and support. The nurse also demonstrates interest in the child and enthusiasm for the

child's strengths. Guidelines for the school-age child are shown in the Developmental Assessment Guidelines.

Promoting health and wellness includes dental hygiene and regular dental examinations, safety measures to prevent accidents, promoting a healthy diet and physical fitness, supporting autonomy and self-esteem, and hygiene measures to prevent infections. Box 9–7 provides health promotion guidelines for this age group.

Adolescents (12 to 18 Years)

Adolescence is the period during which the person becomes physically and psychologically mature and acquires a personal identity, preparing to enter adulthood and take on the associated responsibilities. The length of adolescence is culturally determined to some extent. In North America, adolescence is longer than in some cultures, extending to 18 or 20 years of age.

Puberty is the first stage of adolescence, starting between ages 10 and 14 in girls and 12 and 16 in boys, defined by sexual organs beginning to grow and mature. Menarche (onset of menstruation) occurs in girls. Ejaculation (expulsion of semen) occurs in boys. The adolescent period is often subdivided into three stages: early adolescence lasts from ages 12 to 13; middle adolescence extends from 14 to 16 years; and late adolescence extends from 17 to 18 or 20 years. Late adolescence is a more stable stage than the other two. In the late period, adolescents are involved mostly with planning their future and gaining economic independence.

PHYSICAL DEVELOPMENT During puberty, growth is markedly accelerated compared to the slow, steady growth of the child. This period, marked by sudden and dramatic physical changes, is referred to as the adolescent growth spurt. In boys, the growth spurt usually begins

---

DEVELOPMENTAL ASSESSMENT GUIDELINES

The School-Age Child

In these four developmental areas, does the school-age child do the following?

Physical Development

- Demonstrate physical growth (weight, height) within normal range.
- Manifest vital signs within normal range for age.
- Exhibit vision and hearing abilities within normal range.
- Demonstrate male or female prepubertal changes within normal range.

Motor Development

- Possess coordinated motor skills for age. For example, by 12 years of age, is the child able to do the following?
  - Do tricks on a bike, climb a tree, shimmy up a rope.
  - Throw and catch a small ball.
  - Play a musical instrument.

Psychosocial Development

- Perform psychosocial developmental milestones for age. For example, by 12 years of age is the child able to do the following?
  - Make friends of the same sex and establish a peer group.

- Become less dependent on family and venture away from them.
- Interact well with parents.
- Control strong and impulsive feelings.
- Articulate an understanding of right and wrong.
- Participate in organized competitions.
- Read, print, and manipulate numbers and letters easily.
- Express positive feelings about school and school activities.
- Exhibit a concept of money and make change for small amounts of money.
- Express self in a logical manner and talk through problems.
- Enjoy riddles and read and understand comics.
- Invest in a hobby or collection.
- Like to help others.
- Think of self as likable and healthy.

Development in Activities of Daily Living

- Demonstrate concern for personal cleanliness and appearance.
- Express need for privacy.

---

between ages 12 and 16; in girls, it begins earlier, usually between ages 10 and 14. Because the growth spurt begins earlier in girls, girls may be taller than boys during this time frame.

Physical Growth   Physical growth continues throughout adolescence. Growth is fastest for boys at about 14 years, and the maximum height is often reached at about 18 or 19 years. Some men add another 1 or 2 cm to their height during their 20s as the vertebral column gradually continues to grow. During the period of 10 to 18 years of age, the average American male doubles his weight, gaining about 32 kg (72 lb), and grows about 41 cm (16 in.). The fastest rate of growth in girls occurs at about age 12; they reach their maximum height at about 15 to 16 years. During ages 10 to 18, the average American female gains about 25 kg (55 lb) and grows about 24 cm (9 in.). Physical growth during adolescence is greatly influenced by a number of factors, such as heredity, nutrition, medical care, illness, physical and emotional environment, family size, and culture.

Glandular Changes   The eccrine and apocrine glands increase their secretions and become fully functional during puberty. The eccrine glands, found over most of the body, produce sweat. The apocrine glands develop in the axillae, anal and genital areas, in external auditory canals, and around the umbilicus and areola of the breasts. Apocrine sweat is released onto the skin in response to emotional stimuli only. Sebaceous glands also become active under the influence of androgens, becoming most active on the face, neck, shoulder, upper back, and chest, often causing acne.

Sexual Characteristics   During puberty, both primary and secondary sex characteristics develop. **Primary sexual characteristics** relate to the organs necessary for reproduction while **secondary sexual characteristics** differentiate the male from the female but do not relate directly to reproduction.

PSYCHOSOCIAL DEVELOPMENT   According to Erikson (1963), the psychosocial task of the adolescent is the establishment of identity. The danger of this stage is role confusion. The inability to settle on an occupational identity commonly disturbs the adolescent. Less commonly, doubts about sexual identity arise. Because of the adolescent's dramatic body changes, the development of a stable identity is difficult. Erikson says that adolescents help one another through this identity crisis by forming cliques and a separate youth culture, often excluding those who are considered "different." Adolescent cliques can be excessively clannish and cruel in excluding out-groupers; this intolerance is a temporary defense against identity confusion (Erikson, 1963, p. 236) (see Figure 9–7).

In their search for a new identity, adolescents have to reprocess many of the previous stages of development. The task of developing trust in self and others is again encountered when adolescents look for ideal persons whom they can trust and with whom they can prove trustworthy. Development of autonomy is restaged in their search for ways to express the right to choose freely. Free choice and autonomy present conflicts arising between behaving well in the eyes of the parents and behaving in a manner that may expose

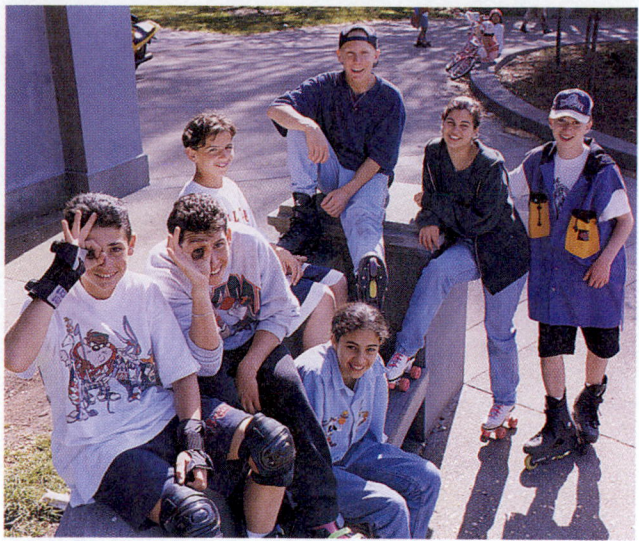

Figure 9–7 ● Adolescent peer group relationships enhance a sense of belonging, self-esteem, and self-identity.

them to the ridicule of peers. The sense of initiative is also restaged. The adolescent has unlimited imagination and ambition and aspires to great accomplishments. The sense of industry is reenacted when the adolescent chooses a career. The extent to which these tasks were successfully achieved earlier influences the adolescent's ability to develop a healthy self-concept and self-identity.

The adolescent needs to establish a self-concept that accepts both personal strengths and weaknesses. Many adolescents experience temporary difficulty in developing a positive self-image due to dramatic changes in body structure and

function as well as greater expectations to assume responsibilities. Adolescents who are accepted, loved, and valued by family and peers generally tend to gain confidence and feel good about themselves, developing a more positive self-image. Teenagers with physical disabilities or illnesses are particularly vulnerable to peer rejection. Nurses and educators can promote peer understanding and acceptance by leading discussions within the peer group, explaining the problems an individual with a particular disability or condition might face. Establishing groups of peers who have similar problems can provide an opportunity for the individual to develop close relationships with others and feel valued and accepted.

Although sexual identification begins at about 3 or 4 years of age, it is a significant part of adolescence. Establishing a sense of sexual identity and clarifying one's sexual orientation occurs during late adolescence. Later, adolescents begin to establish intimacy with a partner or partners. This intimacy lays the groundwork for the commitments of adulthood. Sexual experimentation is not part of true intimacy, but once intimacy is achieved, sexual activity is often included. Homosexual youth may experience a great deal of confusion during this process, since homosexuality is not openly accepted in all groups and their questions about self and identity may go unanswered. Sexual exploration increases the risk for sexually transmitted infections (STIs) and pregnancy.

From the age of 15 years, many adolescents gradually draw away from the family and gain independence. This need for independence combined with the need for family support sometimes creates conflict within the adolescent and between the adolescent and the family. Adolescents also have to resolve their ambivalent feelings toward the parent of the opposite sex. As part of the resolution, adolescents may develop

---

RESEARCH NOTES

What Effect Does Mandated Parental Notification Have on Adolescent Contraceptive Use?

Jones and her colleagues (2005) surveyed 1,526 adolescent girls younger than 18 years who were seeking reproductive health services to determine what effect notifying their parents would have on their choices about contraception and sexual activity.

Sixty percent of the sample stated that their parents were aware of the adolescent's visit to the clinic, and many parents had encouraged their daughters to seek reproductive health care services at the clinic. Characteristics of the girls who were most likely to have parents aware of their clinic visit included: younger than 15 years, non-Hispanic blacks, used a hormonal method of contraception, had made two or more clinic visits for prescription contraceptives in the past year, and lived with their mothers.

Of those who had not told their parents of their visit to the clinic, 25% stated they did not want their parents to know they were sexually active. Another 22% said they were responsible for their own health care and made decisions independently.

When asked what contraceptive or sexual activity choices they would make if parental notification were required, respondents indicated several strategies. Fifty-nine percent said they would continue to access care in the clinic; most of these were girls whose parents were already aware of their visit. Over 45% said they

would use over-the-counter (OTC) methods such as condoms. Seven percent said they would stop having sex, but only 1% listed this as their only option.

Teenagers whose parents were not aware of their clinic visit said they would be less likely to continue to visit the clinic and more likely to use OTC methods. Overall, nearly 20% of the sample said they would engage in risky sexual behavior (including no protection or withdrawal) if parental notification were mandated, and 5% indicated they would not seek care for STDs.

Implications

This research suggests that, although the parents of many adolescent girls are aware of their daughters' reproductive health care, mandating providers to notify parents could lead to increased risky sexual behavior and subsequent increases in adolescent pregnancy and sexually transmitted disease.

Note: From "Adolescents' Reports of Parental Knowledge of Adolescents' Use of Sexual Health Services and Their Reactions to Mandated Parental Notification for Prescription Contraception," by R. K. Jones, A. Purcell, S. Singh, L. B. Finder, 2005, *Journal of the American Medical Association* 293(3), pp. 340–348. Reprinted with permission.

brief crushes on adults outside the family. Some of the discord in the family at this time is due to the generation gap.

COGNITIVE DEVELOPMENT   Cognitive abilities mature during adolescence. Between the ages of 11 and 15, the adolescent begins Piaget's formal operations stage of cognitive development. The main feature of this stage is that people can think beyond the present and beyond the world of reality. This type of thinking requires logic, organization, and consistency. In social interactions, adolescents often practice this increasing ability to think abstractly, and parents may misunderstand their child's intent, seeing the teen as arguing or being contrary, which can lead to unnecessary confusion and conflict.

The adolescent becomes more informed about the world and environment. Adolescents use new information to solve everyday problems and can communicate with adults on most subjects. The adolescent's capacity to absorb and use knowledge is great. Adolescents usually select their own areas for learning; they explore interests from which they may evolve a career plan. Study habits and learning skills developed in adolescence are used throughout life.

MORAL DEVELOPMENT   According to Kohlberg, the young adolescent is usually at the conventional level of moral development. Most still accept the Golden Rule and want to abide by social order and existing laws. Adolescents examine their values, standards, and morals. They may discard the values they have adopted from parents in favor of values they consider more suitable.

When adolescents move into the postconventional or principled level, they start to question the rules and laws of society. Right thinking and right action become a matter of personal values and opinions, which may conflict with societal laws. Adolescents consider the possibility of rationally changing the law and emphasize individual rights. Not all adolescents or even adults proceed to this postconventional level.

SPIRITUAL DEVELOPMENT   According to Fowler, the adolescent or young adult reaches the synthetic-conventional stage of spiritual development. As adolescents encounter different groups in society, they are exposed to a wide variety of opinions, beliefs, and behaviors regarding religious matters. The adolescent may reconcile the differences in one of the following ways:

- Deciding any differences are wrong
- Compartmentalizing the differences
- Obtaining advice from a significant other

Often the adolescent believes that various religious beliefs and practices have more similarities than differences. At this stage, the adolescent's focus is on interpersonal rather than conceptual matters.

Nursing activities relative to this stage of spiritual development include the following:

- Presenting an open, accepting attitude to adolescents' questions and statements regarding spiritual matters and their implications for health.

- Arranging for adolescents to see a member of their religious faith if so desired, or to talk with members of their church peer group for support.
- Providing a comfortable environment in which adolescents can practice the rituals of their faith.

HEALTH RISKS   Principal adolescent health risks are the consequences of risky behavior, such as injury related to accidents, sexually transmitted disease, drug experimentation, and teen pregnancy. Psychologic and emotional challenges of adolescence may lead to psychologic problems. The developing brain is susceptible to addiction; and the first manifestation of schizophrenia may appear in late adolescence (Toga, Thompson, & Sowell, 2006). In late adolescence, with communal living, as in college dormitories, adolescents are at increased risk for infectious diseases such as measles and pneumococcal meningitis.

The 2003 Youth Risk Behavior Surveillance reported the following health-risk behaviors for youth and young adults (Grunbaum et al., 2004): 70.8% of all deaths in the 10 to 24 age group resulted from four causes:

- Motor vehicle crashes (see Figure 9–8)
- Other unintentional injuries (e.g., falls, drowning, poisoning)
- Homicides
- Suicide

During the month prior to the survey, high school students engaged in the following risk behaviors:

- 18.2% never wore a seat belt
- 30% had ridden with a driver who had been drinking alcohol
- 17% had carried a weapon
- 44.9% had drunk alcohol
- 22.4% had used marijuana
- 8.5% had attempted suicide at some time in the previous 12 months

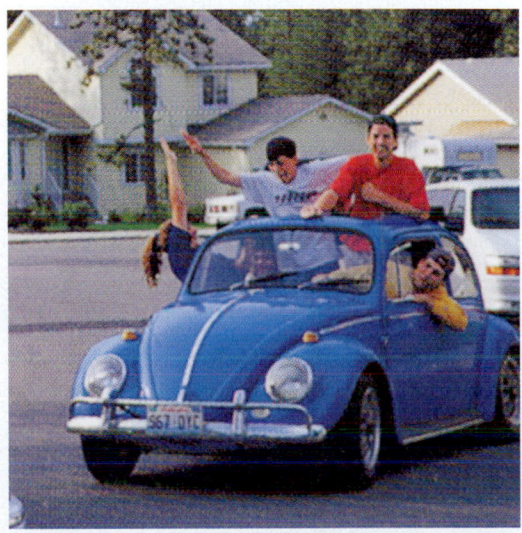

Figure 9–8 ● To prevent motor vehicle crashes, insist on driver's education classes and enforce rules about safe driving.

DEVELOPMENTAL ASSESSMENT GUIDELINES
The Adolescent

In these three developmental areas, does the adolescent do the following?

Physical Development

- Exhibit physical growth (weight, height) within normal range for age and sex.
- Demonstrate male or female sexual development consistent with standards.
- Manifest vital signs within normal range for age and sex.
- Exhibit vision and hearing abilities within normal range.

Psychosocial Development

- Interact well with parents, teachers, peers, siblings, and persons in authority.
- Like self.
- Think and plan for the future, such as college or a career.
- Choose a lifestyle and interests that fit own identity.
- Determine own beliefs and values.
- Begin to establish a sense of identity in the family.
- Seek help from appropriate persons about problems.

Development in Activities of Daily Living

- Demonstrate knowledge of physical development, menstruation, reproduction, and birth control.
- Exhibit healthy lifestyle practices in nutrition, exercise, recreation, sleep patterns, and personal habits.
- Demonstrate concern for personal cleanliness and appearance.

Suicide in adolescents has declined in recent years but continues to be a significant problem. Older adolescents, males, and non-Hispanic American Indians and Alaskan Natives have the highest rates of suicides among adolescents (National Adolescent Health Information Center, 2006). Psychologic, social, and physiologic stressors are apparent causes for the number of suicides; recent research indicates that use of antidepressant drugs in children is associated with a slight increase of suicide risk (Hammad, Laughren, & Racoosin, 2006). Other adolescent health problems are cardiovascular disease, depression, tooth decay, gingivitis, malalignment of teeth, neglect, and abuse.

Eating Disorders The desire to "fit in" often leads to unhealthy dietary practices (Edelman & Mandle, 2010). As discussed in Chapter 32 ∞, common problems related to nutrition and self-esteem among adolescents include obesity, anorexia nervosa, and bulimia. Nurses need to help adolescents create a wellness plan that addresses body image, diet, weight concerns, and exercise.

HEALTH ASSESSMENT AND PROMOTION Guidelines for growth and development of the adolescent are shown in the Developmental Assessment Guidelines.

Adolescents are usually self-directed in meeting their health needs. Because of maturation changes, however, they need teaching and guidance in a number of health care areas. Promoting health and wellness includes screening for tobacco, alcohol, and drug use; screening for sexual practices; checking blood pressure, height, and weight; and ensuring that immunizations are current. For a summary of health promotion, see Box 9–8.

BOX 9–8   Health Promotion Guidelines for Adolescents

Health Examinations

- As recommended by the primary care provider

Protective Measures

- Immunizations as recommended, such as adult tetanus-diphtheria vaccine, MMR, pneumococcal, and hepatitis B vaccine
- Screening for tuberculosis
- Periodic vision and hearing screenings
- Regular dental assessments
- Obtaining and providing accurate information about sexual issues

Adolescent Safety

- Adolescent's taking responsibility for using motor vehicles safely (e.g., completing a driver's education course, wearing seat belt and helmet)
- Making certain that proper precautions are taken during all athletic activities (e.g., medical supervision, proper equipment)
- Parents' keeping lines of communication open and being alert to signs of substance abuse and emotional disturbances in the adolescent

Nutrition and Exercise

- Importance of healthy snacks and appropriate patterns of food intake and exercise
- Factors that may lead to nutritional problems (e.g., obesity, anorexia nervosa, bulimia)
- Balancing sedentary activities with regular exercise

Social Interactions

- Encouraging and facilitating adolescent success in school
- Encouraging adolescent to establish relationships that promote discussion of feelings, concerns, and fears
- Parents' encouraging adolescent peer group activities that promote appropriate moral and spiritual values
- Parents' acting as role models for appropriate social interactions
- Parents' providing a comfortable home environment for appropriate adolescent peer group activities
- Parents' expecting adolescents to participate in and contribute to family activities

RESEARCH NOTES

What Workforce Differences Exist between Nursing Staff of Different Generations?

Difficulties in understanding differences in work habits and communication styles of those in another age group are now common in the workplace. This descriptive research study examined the generational profiles of two groups (the Silent Generation [born in years 1925–1942] and **Baby Boomers** versus **Generation X** and **Generation Y**) regarding communication styles and significance of tasks to help nurse managers maximize their department's effectiveness.

One of the authors developed a survey tool to examine the generational profiles of staff members of two departments (medical–surgical and critical care) and the communication styles of the participants. The survey consisted of 22 questions asking about the characteristics of the respondent's generation, the significance of tasks, and their communication styles.

There were no statistically significant differences between the generational groups in the area of communication styles and significance of tasks. Other findings were consistent with generational profiles revealed in other studies. For example:

- The Silent Generation and Baby Boomer group identified themselves as principled, idealistic, experts, caring, savvy, and diverse. However, they viewed computers as frightening and complicated.
- Generations X and Y perceived themselves as idealistic. They wanted freedom and flexibility plus immediate feedback in terms of job completion and performance.

Implications

Nurse managers need to understand each generation's different values and expectations. Knowing this information will help the nurse manager to facilitate a positive work environment. It can also mean that different orientations, training, opportunities for advancement, benefits, and perks may need to be implemented.

Note: From J. Hu, C. Herrick, and K. A. Hodgin, "Managing the Multigenerational Nursing Team," *Health Care Manager, 23*(4), pp. 334–341. Copyright © 2004 Lippincott, Williams & Wilkins. Reprinted with permission.

Young Adults (20 to 40 Years)

The age at which a person is considered an adult depends on how adulthood is described in the person's social and cultural context, and this defining age is changing. Legally, a person in the United States can vote at 18. The legal age for alcohol consumption outside the home varies among states from 18 to 21. Another criterion of adulthood is financial independence, which is also highly variable. Some adolescents support themselves as early as 16 years of age. In contrast, some young adults are financially dependent on their families for many years longer.

Adulthood may also be indicated by moving away from home and establishing one's own living arrangements, which occurs at different ages for individuals. Some adolescents leave home because of family problems. In recent years, however, "boomerang kids" have become more common as young adults have moved back into their parents' homes after an initial period of independent living. The factors contributing to this trend include high housing costs, high divorce rates, high unemployment rates, and the problems resulting from substance abuse and maladaptive behaviors.

PHYSICAL DEVELOPMENT   The human body is at its most efficient functioning at about age 25 years. The musculoskeletal system is well developed and coordinated. This is the period when athletic endeavors reach their peak. All other systems of the body are also functioning at peak efficiency. Emerging adults tend to be high-risk takers (Nelson & Barry, 2005), placing their high-functioning bodies at substantial risk of serious injury.

Although physical changes are minimal during this stage, weight and muscle mass may change as a result of diet and exercise. Health outcomes in older adulthood may have their genesis in younger adult behaviors and choices (Hartman-Stein & Potkanowicz, 2003). Extensive physical and psychosocial changes occur in pregnant and lactating women, as discussed in maternity nursing textbooks.

PSYCHOSOCIAL DEVELOPMENT   In contrast to the minimal physical changes, psychosocial development of the young adult is extensive. Box 9–9 reviews this psychosocial development according to the theories of Freud, Erikson, and Havighurst.

BOX 9–9   Psychosocial Development: Young Adult

The young adult
- Is in the genital stage in which energy is directed toward attaining a mature sexual relationship, according to Freud's theory.
- Is in the intimacy versus isolation phase of Erikson's stages of development.
- Has the following developmental tasks, according to Havighurst:
  - Selecting a mate
  - Learning to live with a partner
  - Starting a family

- Rearing children
- Managing a home
- Getting started in an occupation
- Taking on civic responsibility
- Finding a congenial social group
- Has the following characteristics, according to Nelson and Barry (2005):
  - Separation from parents
  - Exploration of new identities for self
  - Personal discovery and self-discovery
  - High-risk behavior

Young adults face a number of new experiences and changes in lifestyle as they progress toward maturity. They make choices about education and employment, whether to marry or remain single, starting a home, and rearing children. Social responsibilities include forming new friendships and assuming some community activities.

Occupational choice and education are largely inseparable. Education influences occupational opportunities; conversely, an occupation, once chosen, can determine the education needed and sought. As the role of women has changed, many women now choose to assume active careers and civic roles in society in addition to their roles as mother and/or wife. Some women work out of necessity, rather than choice (Figure 9–9).

Although nontraditional lifestyles are becoming more acceptable in society, attitudes toward these various lifestyles can contribute social pressures that lead to stress responses. The multiple roles of adulthood may also create stress as a result of role conflict.

COGNITIVE DEVELOPMENT   Young adults are able to use formal operations, characterized by the ability to think abstractly and employ logic. Most adults identify strongly with the values and norms of their social group and will act in ways that are consistent with those norms (Pfaffenberger, 2005).

Recently, researchers in the field of psychology have suggested that Piaget's formal operational stage is not the last stage of human development. Some have proposed a concept of postformal thought. *Postformal thought* includes creativity, intuition, and the ability to consider information in relationship to other ideas (Murray & Zentner, 2001). Postformal thinkers possess an understanding of the temporary or relative nature of knowledge. They are able to comprehend and balance arguments created by both logic and emotion. Few adults reach this stage (only about 10%), but these adults are marked by greater tolerance and the skills of noticing and resolving complex problems (Pfaffenberger, 2005).

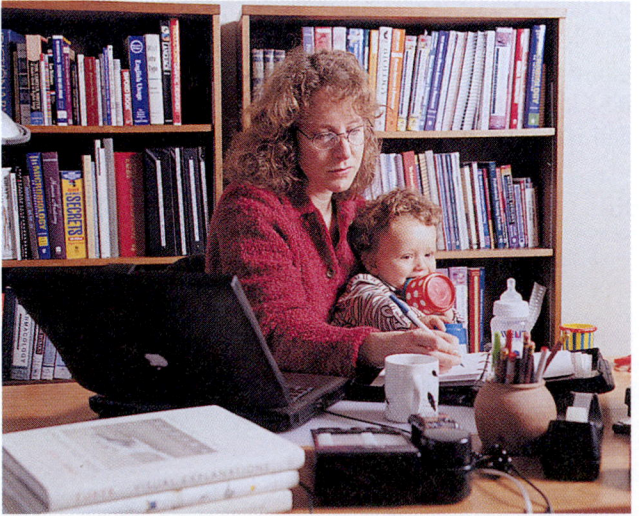

Figure 9–9 ○ Many young women combine active careers with motherhood.

MORAL DEVELOPMENT   Young adults who have mastered the previous stages of Kohlberg's theory of moral development enter the postconventional level. At this time, the person is able to separate self from the expectations and rules of others and to define morality in terms of personal principles. When individuals perceive a conflict with society's rules or laws, they judge according to their own principles. This type of reasoning is called *principled reasoning*. Gilligan argues that as individuals approach young adulthood, men and women tend to define moral problems somewhat differently. Men often use an "ethic of justice" and define moral problems in terms of rules and rights. Women, by contrast, often define moral problems in terms of obligation to care and to avoid hurt.

SPIRITUAL DEVELOPMENT   According to Fowler, the individual enters the individuating-reflective period sometime after 18 years of age. During this period, the individual focuses on reality. A 27-year-old adult may ask philosophical questions regarding spirituality and may be self-conscious about spiritual matters. The religious teaching that the young adult had as a child may now be accepted or redefined. Cavendish, Luise, Bauer, et al. (2001) demonstrated that young adults may depend on spirituality and seek guidance from a higher power, but do so privately.

HEALTH RISKS   Young adulthood is generally a healthy time of life. Health risks that do occur and are common in this age group include injuries, suicide, substance abuse, hypertension, sexually transmitted infection (STI), abuse of women, and certain malignancies. Some of the problems such as injuries, substance abuse, and STIs are related to behaviors that could possibly be prevented through appropriate education and other primary prevention strategies. Suicide is the third leading cause of death among adolescents and the leading cause of death among young adults in the United States (Edelman & Mandle, 2010). The nurse's role in the prevention of suicide includes identifying behaviors that may indicate potential problems. Hypertension is a major problem for young African American adults, particularly men. Substance abuse is a major threat to the health of young adults. Nursing strategies related to drug abuse include teaching about the complications of their use, changing individual attitudes toward drug abuse, and counseling regarding problems that lead to drug abuse. In addition, assessment of the young adult for substance abuse may help the nurse identify a problem early on, and assist the young adult client to access intervention services. Testicular cancer is the most common neoplasm in men aged 20 to 34 (USDHHS, 2004). Cancer of the breast is a leading cause of death among young adult women. Young adult women should also be screened for cervical cancer.

HEALTH ASSESSMENT AND PROMOTION   Assessment guidelines for the growth and development of the young adult are shown in the accompanying Developmental Assessment Guidelines.

Young adults are usually interested in meeting their health needs. However, because of the many stresses and

BOX 9–10	Health Promotion Guidelines for Young Adults

Health Tests and Screenings

- Routine physical examination (every 1 to 3 years for females; every 5 years for males)
- Immunizations as recommended, such as tetanus-diphtheria boosters every 10 years, meningococcal vaccine if not given in early adolescence (Bilukha & Rosenstein, 2005), and hepatitis B vaccine
- Regular dental assessments (every 6 months)
- Periodic vision and hearing screenings
- Professional breast examination every 1 to 3 years
- Papanicolaou smear annually within 3 years of onset of sexual activity
- Testicular examination every year
- Screening for cardiovascular disease (e.g., cholesterol test every 5 years if results are normal; blood pressure to detect hypertension; baseline electrocardiogram at age 35)
- Tuberculosis skin test every 2 years
- Smoking: history and counseling, if needed

Safety

- Motor vehicle safety reinforcement (e.g., using designated drivers when drinking, maintaining brakes and tires)
- Sun protection measures
- Workplace safety measures
- Water safety reinforcement (e.g., no diving in shallow water)

Nutrition and Exercise

- Importance of adequate iron intake in diet
- Nutritional and exercise factors that may lead to cardiovascular disease (e.g., obesity, cholesterol and fat intake, lack of vigorous exercise)

Social Interactions

- Encouraging personal relationships that promote discussion of feelings, concerns, and fears
- Setting short- and long-term goals for work and career choices

---

changes that occur throughout this 20-year period, the nurse needs to offer teaching and guidance in several health care areas. The nurse may wish to discuss some or all of the health promotion topics outlined in Box 9–10. These topics are discussed in detail in subsequent chapters throughout the book.

DEVELOPMENTAL ASSESSMENT GUIDELINES
The Young Adult

In these three developmental areas, does the young adult do the following?

Physical Development

- Exhibit weight within normal range for age and sex.
- Manifest vital signs (e.g., blood pressure) within normal range for age and sex.
- Demonstrate visual and hearing abilities within normal range.
- Exhibit appropriate knowledge (e.g., about sexually transmitted infections) and attitudes about sexuality.

Psychosocial Development

- Feel independent from parents.
- Have a realistic self-concept.
- Like self and direction life is going.
- Interact well with family.
- Cope with the stresses of change and growth.
- Have well-established bonds with significant others, such as marriage partner or close friends.
- Have a meaningful social life.
- Demonstrate emotional, social, and economic responsibility for own life.
- Have a set of values that guide behavior.

Development in Activities of Daily Living

- Have a healthy lifestyle.

Middle-Aged Adults (40 to 65 Years)

The middle years, from 40 to 65, have been called the years of stability and consolidation. For most people, it is a time when children have grown and moved away or are moving away from home. Thus partners generally have more time for and with each other and time to pursue interests they may have deferred for years (see Figure 9–10).

Middle adults often reach full maturity. Maturity is the state of maximal function and integration, or the state of being

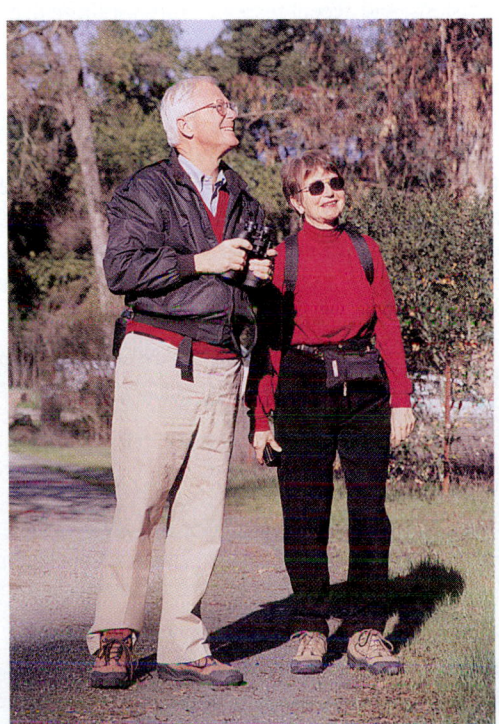

Figure 9–10 ⬤ Middle-aged adults have time to pursue interests that may have been put aside for child care.

TABLE 9–10	Physical Changes of the Middle-Aged Adult
CATEGORY	**DESCRIPTION**
Appearance	Hair begins to thin, and gray hair appears. Skin turgor and moisture decrease, subcutaneous fat decreases, and wrinkling occurs. Fatty tissue is redistributed, resulting in fat deposits in the abdominal area.
Musculoskeletal system	Skeletal muscle bulk decreases at about age 60. Thinning of the intervertebral discs causes a decrease in height of about 1 inch. Calcium loss from bone tissue is more common among postmenopausal women. Muscle growth continues in proportion to use.
Cardiovascular system	Blood vessels lose elasticity and become thicker.
Sensory perception	Visual acuity declines, often by the late 40s, especially for near vision (presbyopia). Auditory acuity for high-frequency sounds also decreases (presbycusis), particularly in men. Taste sensations also diminish.
Metabolism	Metabolism slows and may result in weight gain.
Gastrointestinal system	Gradual decrease in tone of large intestine may predispose the individual to constipation.
Urinary system	Nephron units are lost during this time, and glomerular filtration rate decreases.
Sexuality	Hormonal changes take place in both men and women.

fully developed. Many other characteristics are generally recognized as representative of maturity. Mature individuals are guided by an underlying philosophy of life. They take many perspectives into account and are tolerant of the views of others. A comprehensive philosophy allows a person to make sense out of life and thus helps that person maintain a sense of purpose and hope in the face of human tragedies. Mature persons are open to new experiences and continued growth; they can tolerate ambiguity, are flexible, and can adapt to change. In addition, mature people have the quality of self-acceptance; they are able to be reflective and insightful about life and to see themselves as others see them. Mature persons also assume responsibility for themselves and expect others to do the same. They confront the tasks of life in a realistic and mature manner, make decisions, and accept responsibility for those decisions.

PHYSICAL DEVELOPMENT   A number of changes that start when young adults are in their mid-20s become noticeable as the fifth decade approaches. At 40, most adults can function as effectively as they did in their 20s. However, during ages 40 to 65 many physical changes take place. These are summarized in Table 9–10.

Both men and women experience decreasing hormonal production during the middle years. **Menopause** refers to the cessation of menstruation, occurring when 12 months pass without a menstrual period. Menopause usually occurs sometime between ages 40 and 55. At this time, ovarian activity declines until ovulation ceases. Common symptoms, related to a decline in estrogen, are hot flashes, chilliness, a tendency of the breasts to become smaller and less dense, and a decrease in metabolic rate that may lead to weight gain. Insomnia and headaches may also occur. Psychologically, menopause can be an anxiety-producing time, especially if the ability to bear children is an integral part of the woman's self-concept. For other women, menopause may produce few symptoms, physically or psychologically (Banister, 2000).

Sexual arousal in both men and women takes longer after midlife than in younger adulthood. In men there is no change comparable to menopause in women, although the term climacteric (andropause) has been used to denote the change in sexual response in men. Androgen levels decrease very slowly. Some men may have difficulties achieving sexual arousal for psychologic or physical reasons. See Chapter 28 ∞ for further details about sexual health.

PSYCHOSOCIAL DEVELOPMENT   Havighurst outlined seven tasks for this age group (see Box 9–11). Erikson (1963, p. 266) viewed the developmental chore of the middle-aged adult as

BOX 9–11	Psychosocial Development: Middle-Aged Adult

The middle-aged adult
- Is in the generativity versus stagnation phase of Erikson's stages of development.
- According to Havighurst, has the following developmental tasks:
  - Achieving adult civic and social responsibility
  - Establishing and maintaining an economic standard of living
  - Assisting teenage children to become responsible and happy adults
  - Developing adult leisure-time activities
  - Relating oneself to one's spouse as a person
  - Accepting and adjusting to the physiologic changes of middle age
  - Adjusting to aging parents

- Balances the needs of multiple constituencies (children, parents, work, etc.)
- Has work as a central theme
- According to Slater (2003), has the additional developmental tasks of:
  - Inclusivity versus exclusivity
  - Pride versus embarrassment (in children, work, or creativity)
  - Responsibility versus ambivalence (making choices about commitments)
  - Career productivity versus inadequacy
  - Parenthood versus self-absorption
  - Being needed versus alienation
  - Honesty versus denial (with oneself)

generativity versus stagnation. Generativity is defined as concern for establishing and guiding the next generation. People in their 20s and 30s tend to be self- and family-centered. In middle age, the individual is "linked to the welfare of others" (Lachman, 2004, p. 306). Marriage partners have more time for companionship and recreation. Generative middle-aged persons are able to feel a sense of comfort in their lifestyle and receive gratification from charitable endeavors. Erikson wrote that people who are unable to expand their interests at this time and who do not assume the responsibilities of middle age suffer a sense of boredom and impoverishment, or stagnation resulting in difficulty accepting their aging bodies becoming withdrawn and isolated, preoccupied with self. Some may regress to younger patterns of behavior.

A new freedom to be independent and follow one's individual interests arises. Prior to this period, the marriage partner or significant other was crucial to a definition of self. Now the middle-aged person does not make comparisons with others, often no longer fears aging or death, relaxes the sense of competitiveness, and enjoys the independence and freedom of middle age. Other people's opinions become less important, and the earlier habit of trying to please everyone is overcome. The person establishes ethical and moral standards that are independent of the standards of others. Religious and philosophical concerns become important.

The "midlife crisis" occurs when individuals recognize that they have reached the halfway mark of life. The universality of midlife crisis is disputed by some who suggest that some mid-lifers may experience a crisis that promotes further development, while some may have consistently functioned in a crisis mode from early life (Lachman, 2004). Mid-lifers begin to recognize that time is at a premium and that life is finite. Youthfulness and physical strength can no longer be taken for granted.

COGNITIVE DEVELOPMENT   The middle-aged adult's cognitive and intellectual abilities change very little. Cognitive processes include reaction time, memory, perception, learning, problem solving, and creativity. Reaction time during the middle years stays much the same or diminishes during the later part of the middle years. Memory and problem solving are maintained through middle adulthood. Learning continues and can be enhanced by increased motivation at this time in life. Genetic, environmental, and personality factors in early and middle adulthood account for the large difference in the ways in which individuals maintain mental abilities (Edelman & Mandle, 2010). The experiences of the professional, social, and personal life of middle-aged persons will be reflected in their cognitive performance. Thus, approaches to problem solving and task completion will vary considerably in a middle-aged group.

MORAL DEVELOPMENT   According to Kohlberg, the adult can move beyond the conventional level to the postconventional level. Kohlberg believed that extensive experience of personal moral choice and responsibility is required before people can reach the postconventional level. Kohlberg found that few of his subjects achieved the highest level of moral reasoning. To move from stage 4, a law and order orientation, to stage 5, a social contract orientation, requires that the individual move to a stage in which rights of others take precedence. Recent research demonstrates that moral development continues through adulthood, and that few individuals attain stage 5 before age 40 (Dawson, 2002).

SPIRITUAL DEVELOPMENT   Not all adults progress through Fowler's stages to the fifth, called the paradoxical–consolidative stage. At this stage, the individual can view "truth" from a number of viewpoints. Fowler's fifth stage corresponds to Kohlberg's fifth stage of moral development. Fowler believes that only some individuals after the age of 30 years reach this stage. In middle age, people tend to be less dogmatic about religious beliefs, and religion often offers more comfort to the middle-aged person than it did previously. People in this age group often rely on spiritual beliefs to help them deal with illness, death, and tragedy.

HEALTH PROBLEMS   Many middle-aged adults remain healthy; however, the risk of developing a health problem is greater than that of the young adult. Leading causes of death in this age group include motor vehicle and occupational injuries, chronic disease, and cardiovascular disease. Lifestyle patterns in combination with aging, family history, and developmental stressors and situational stressors are often related to health problems. The nurse can play an

---

DEVELOPMENTAL ASSESSMENT GUIDELINES
The Middle-Aged Adult

In these three developmental areas, does the middle-aged adult do the following?

Physical Development

- Exhibit weight within normal range for age and sex.
- Manifest vital signs (e.g., blood pressure) within normal range for age and sex.
- Manifest visual and hearing abilities within normal range.
- Exhibit appropriate knowledge and attitudes about sexuality (e.g., about menopause).
- Verbalize any changes in eating, elimination, or exercise.

Psychosocial Development

- Accept aging body.
- Feel comfortable and respect self.
- Enjoy new freedom to be independent.
- Accept changes in family roles (e.g., having teenage children and aging parents).
- Interact effectively and share companionable activities with life partner.
- Expand and renew previous interests.
- Pursue charitable and altruistic activities.
- Have a meaningful philosophy of life.

Development in Activities of Daily Living

- Follow preventive health practice.

BOX 9–12	Health Promotion Guidelines for Middle-Aged Adults

Health Tests and Screening

- Physical examination (every 3 to 5 years until age 40, then annually)
- Immunizations as recommended, such as a tetanus booster every 10 years, and current recommendations for influenza vaccine
- Regular dental assessments (e.g., every 6 months)
- Tonometry for signs of glaucoma and other eye diseases every 2 to 3 years or annually if indicated
- Breast examination annually by primary care provider
- Testicular examination annually by primary care provider
- Screenings for cardiovascular disease (e.g., blood pressure measurement; electrocardiogram and cholesterol test as directed by the primary care provider)
- Screenings for colorectal, breast, cervical, uterine, and prostate cancer (see cancer screening guidelines in Chapter 17 ∞)
- Screening for tuberculosis every 2 years
- Smoking: history and counseling, if needed

Safety

- Motor vehicle safety reinforcement, especially when driving at night
- Workplace safety measures
- Home safety measures: keeping hallways and stairways lighted and uncluttered, using smoke detectors, using nonskid mats and handrails in the bathrooms

Nutrition and Exercise

- Importance of adequate protein, calcium, and vitamin D in diet
- Nutritional and exercise factors that may lead to cardiovascular disease (e.g., obesity, cholesterol and fat intake, lack of vigorous exercise)
- An exercise program that emphasizes skill and coordination

Social Interactions

- The possibility of a midlife crisis: encourage discussion of feelings, concerns, and fears
- Providing time to expand and review previous interests
- Retirement planning (financial and possible diversional activities), with partner if appropriate

---

important role in teaching middle-aged clients about preventive health care to avoid or minimize the risk of such health problems.

Mental Health Alterations   Developmental stressors, such as menopause, climacteric, aging, and impending retirement, and situational stressors, such as divorce, unemployment, and death of a spouse, can precipitate increased anxiety and depression in middle-aged adults. Clients may benefit from support groups or individual therapy to help them cope with specific crises.

HEALTH ASSESSMENT AND PROMOTION   Assessment guidelines for the growth and development of the middle-aged adult are shown in the Developmental Assessment Guidelines on page 245. Middle-aged adults usually take care of their health needs and are interested in maintaining health and preventing the acceleration of the aging process (Acton & Malathum, 2000).

The nurse may choose to discuss some or all of the health promotion topics with the middle-aged adult client (see Box 9–12). These topics are discussed in detail in subsequent chapters throughout the book.

CHAPTER HIGHLIGHTS

- The terms *growth* and *development* represent independent, interrelated, and dynamic processes. Growth is physical change and is similar for all people, while development is a change in the complexity of function and skill that varies among individuals as they adapt in a unique manner to their own environment. Both growth and development are influenced by genetic and environmental factors.
- Components of growth and development are generally categorized as physiologic, psychosocial, cognitive, moral, and spiritual. Psychological theorists have contributed to understanding how each individual progresses through the developmental stages: Erikson developed theories about psychosocial development, Freud about psychosexual development, Piaget about cognitive development, Kohlberg about moral development, and Fowler and Westerhoff about spiritual development.
- Throughout the lifespan, individuals grow and develop to meet anticipated milestones.

- While growth generally stops during young adulthood, development continues throughout the lifespan. Each stage of development is marked by specific responsibilities, challenges, and milestones that must be reached in order to have success in future stages.
- Milestones of childhood development are based on average age of achievement. A child's failure to meet a milestone does not indicate developmental delay but must be assessed as one part of the child's development and compared with their progress in meeting other milestones.
- The nurse uses knowledge of growth and development when caring for all clients throughout the lifespan to determine developmental needs, safety needs, approach to care and client teaching, and health promotion needs.
- Clients who fail to meet the goals of one stage of development will find it difficult, if not impossible, to meet successive stages of development.

THINK ABOUT IT

Refer to the chapter-opening scenario and answer these questions.

1. What factors may contribute to Mark's height and weight falling into the 25th percentile? What observations or questions might help the nurse further determine if this child is at risk for lagging growth?

2. What milestones might the nurse have noted Mark had met in order to determine he was developing appropriately?

3. What milestones will Mark need to achieve in order to be successful in school this fall?

∞ *See suggested responses to Think About It on MyNursingKit.*

TEST YOUR KNOWLEDGE

1. The nurse knows that the study of growth and development is exploration of the:
   1. Physical changes of the growing child.
   2. Increasing complexity of function and skill progression of the aging child.
   3. Environmental factors such as family, religion, and culture of the growing child.
   4. Physical developments and the increasing level and progression of function and skill of the growing child.

2. A 5-year-old boy arrives for the preadmission work-up for a surgical procedure. When the nurse brings in the intravenous (IV) control pump, the child states: "I am afraid that it will bite me because I have been bad." Using knowledge of Piaget, Erikson, and Fowler, which of the following is the best nursing action?
   1. Reassure the child by providing opportunities for touching and exploring the machine, as well as explaining how it works.
   2. Understand that his imagination is out of control. Tell him that his fears are unfounded and that he needs to be a "big boy."
   3. Recognize that he is too young to understand and that he needs to be quickly distracted.
   4. Acknowledge his need for fantasy by reassuring him that if he is a "good boy" the bad machine will not bite him.

3. The nurse is caring for a 2-year-old child who was relinquished to a hospital emergency department anonymously at a few hours of age. The child has lived in a number of foster families and is displaying developmental delays. The nurse anticipates that factors influencing this child's growth and development are:
   1. Genetics.
   2. Nutrition.
   3. Health.
   4. Environment.

4. The nurse is assessing a school-age child and determines the child is in the concrete operations phase, using logical reasoning, when the parent informs the nurse the child has been involved in which of the following activities?
   1. A science-fair project comparing how fast different objects fall from a set height
   2. Taking responsibility for wishing a sibling would go away causing the child to become ill
   3. Understanding how geometric figures might fit into a futuristic and idealistic world
   4. Learning to ride a bike

5. Which statement about moral development in adults does the nurse consider most accurate? Select all that apply.
   1. Moral development is completed during adolescence.
   2. Moral development continues throughout adulthood.
   3. Moral development is highly individualized.
   4. Moral development correlates to spiritual development.
   5. Moral development occurs in specific stages at specific ages.

6. A 14-year-old is scheduled to have surgical repair of a spinal curvature (scoliosis). The adolescent will be hospitalized for about 2 weeks. What nursing intervention will be most helpful during her hospital stay?
   1. Encourage peer visits.
   2. Instruct parents to room-in with her.
   3. Encourage her to go to the recreation room.
   4. Encourage her to arrange for her teachers to provide her with homework.

7. Which of the following statements made by the nurse most accurately describes physical development during the school-age years?
   1. A child's weight almost triples.
   2. A child begins shedding deciduous teeth.
   3. Few physical changes occur during middle childhood.
   4. Fat gradually increases, which contributes to a child's heavier appearance.

8. The nurse is caring for a 3-year-old child admitted to the hospital following a motor vehicle crash. The mother is shocked when the child wets the bed, explaining to the nurse that the child has been completely toilet trained for more than 6 months. The nurse's priority response would explain that:
   1. The child's bladder may have been damaged by the incident.
   2. The child's behavior indicates attention seeking.
   3. It is normal for a child to regress in development when hospitalized.
   4. It is important to seek a psychiatric consultation because the child may have been traumatized by the incident resulting in this behavior.

9. The nurse is caring for an adolescent who recently began menstruation. The teen's mother expresses concern about the client's increased weight and fat deposits. The adolescent's weight and height are within normal range. The most appropriate nursing action would be to:
   1. Give reassurance that these changes are normal.
   2. Suggest dietary measures to control weight gain.
   3. Recommend increased exercise to control weight gain.
   4. Encourage low-fat diet to prevent fat deposition.

10. A nurse working in a pediatrician's office is performing a routine physical exam on a preschooler when the mother says they are looking forward to opening the swimming pool in their backyard. Which of the

following would be a priority teaching point for the nurse to discuss with this parent?

1. Supervise children at all times when near any water.
2. Enroll children in swimming classes at an early age to ensure water safety.
3. Emphasize the danger inherent in swimming and caution child to never go near the water.
4. Allow unsupervised play only in "kiddy pools" designated for young children.

∞ *See answers to Test Your Knowledge in Appendix A.*

EXPLORE PEARSON **mynursingkit™**

MyNursingKit is your one stop for online chapter review materials and resources. Prepare for success with additional NCLEX®-style practice questions, interactive assignments and activities, web links, animations and videos, and more!

Register your access code from the front of your book at
www.mynursingkit.com.

REFERENCES AND SELECTED BIBLIOGRAPHY

Acton, G. J., & Malathum, P. (2000). Basic need status and health-promoting self-care behaviors in adults. *Western Journal of Nursing Research 22*(7), 796–811.

Afifi, T. D. (2003). "Feeling caught" in stepfamilies: Managing boundary turbulence through appropriate communication privacy rules. *Journal of Social and Personal Relationships, 20*, 729–755.

Albrecht, S. A., Maloni, J. A., Thomas, K. K., Jones, R., Halleran, J., & Osborne, J. (2004). Smoking cessation counseling for pregnant women who smoke: Scientific basis for practice for AWHONN's SUCCESS project. *Journal of Obstetric, Gynecologic & Neonatal Nursing, 33*(3), 298–305.

American Cancer Society. (2005). *Cancer facts and figures, 2005.* Retrieved December 5, 2009, from http://www.cancer.org/docroot/STT/content/STT_1x_Cancer_Facts_Figures_2005.asp

Anderson, M. E., Johnson, D.C., & Batal, H. A. (2005). Sudden infant death syndrome and prenatal maternal smoking: Rising attributed risk in the back to sleep era. *BMC Medicine, 3*(1), 4.

Armstrong, T. D., & Crowther, M. R. (2002). Spirituality among older African Americans. *Journal of Adult Development, 9*(1), 3–12.

Ball, J. W., & Bindler, R. C. (2006). *Child health nursing.* Upper Saddle River, NJ: Pearson Education.

Ball, R. S. (1977). The Gesell developmental schedules: Arnold Gesell (1880–1961). *Journal of Abnormal Child Psychology, 5*(3), 233–239.

Banister, E. M. (2000). Women's midlife confusion: "Why am I feeling this way?" *Issues in Mental Health Nursing, 21*, 745–764.

Bauer, J. J., & McAdams, D. P. (2004). Personal growth in adults' stories of life transitions. *Journal of Personality, 72*(3), 573–602.

Berger, L. M. (2005). Income, family characteristics, and physical violence toward children. *Child Abuse and Neglect, 29*(2), 107–133.

Bilukha, O. O., & Rosenstein, N. (2005). Prevention and control of meningococcal disease. Recommendations of the Advisory Committee on Immunization Practices (ACIP). *Morbidity and Mortality Weekly Report, 54* (RR-7), 1–21.

Bostwick, J. M., & Seaman, J. S. (2004). Hospitalized patients and alcohol: Who is being missed? *General Hospital Psychiatry, 26*(1), 59–62.

Brown, C. G. (2004). Testicular cancer: An overview. *Urologic Nursing, 24*(2), 83–93.

Burns, C. E., Dunn, A. M., Brady, M. A., Starr, N. B., & Blosser, C. G. (2004). *Pediatric primary care: A handbook for nurse practitioners* (3rd ed.). Philadelphia: Saunders.

Callahan, S. T., & Cooper, W. O. (2005). Uninsurance and health care access among young adults in the United States. *Pediatrics, 116*(1), 88–95.

Cavendish, R., Luise, B. K., Bauer, M., et al. (2001). Recognizing opportunities for spiritual enhancement in young adults. *Nursing Diagnosis, 12*(3), 77–92.

Centers for Disease Control. (2000). *2000 growth charts: United States.* Retrieved October 28, 2009, from http://www.cdc.gov/growthcharts

Centers for Disease Control and Prevention. (2004). *Trends in reportable sexually transmitted diseases in the United States, 2003.* Atlanta, GA: Author.

Chang, F., & Burns, B. M. (2005). Attention in preschoolers: Associations with effortful control and motivation. *Child Development, 76*(1), 247–263.

Cook, J. T., Frank, D. A., Berkowitz, C., Black, M. M., Casey, P. H., Cutts, D. B., et al. (2004). Food insecurity is associated with adverse health outcomes among human infants and toddlers. *Journal of Nutrition, 134*(6), 1432–1438.

Dawson, T. L. (2002). New tools, new insights: Kohlberg's moral judgement stages revisited. *International Journal of Behavioral Development, 26*(2), 154–166.

Doswell, W. M., Portis, S., Jemison, T., Kaufmann, J., Braxter, B., & Green, L. (2004). The NIA Group. Building a sense of purpose in preadolescent African American girls: A novel approach to nursing leadership in community health. *Nursing Leadership Forum, 8*(3), 95–100.

Dubowitz, L. M. S., & Dubowitz, V. (1977). *Gestational age of the newborn.* Menlo Park, CA: Addison-Wesley.

Edelman, C. L., & Mandle, C. L. (2010). Health promotion throughout the life span (7th ed.). St. Louis: Mosby.

Edwards, M. E. (2002). Attachment, mastery, and interdependence: A model of parenting processes. *Family Process, 41*(3), 389–404.

Ehrenreich, B. (2002). *Nickled and dimed: On (not) getting by in America.* New York: Owl Books.

Elkins, M., & Cavendish, R. (2004). Developing a plan for pediatric spiritual care. *Holistic Nursing Practice, 18*(4), 179–184.

Erikson, E. H. (1963). *Childhood and society* (2nd ed.). New York: Norton.

Erikson, E. H. (1964). *Insight and responsibility: Lectures on the ethical implications of psychoanalytic insight.* New York: Norton.

Erikson, E. H. (1985). *The life cycle completed: A review.* New York: Norton.

Fields, J. (2004). America's families and living arrangements: 2003. *Current population reports* (U.S. Census Bureau Report No. P20–553). Washington, DC: Author.

Forman, D. R., Aksan, N., & Kochanska, G. (2004). Toddler's responsive imitation predicts preschool-age conscience. *Psychological Science, 15*(10), 699–704.

Fowler, J. W. (1981). *Stages of faith: The psychology of human development and the quest for meaning.* New York: Harper & Row.

Fowler, J. W. (1982). *Stages of faith.* San Francisco: Harper Collins.

Fowler, J. W., & Keen, S. (1985). *Life maps: Conversations in the journey of faith.* Waco, TX: Word Books.

Fowler, J. W., Streib, H., & Keller, B. (2004). *Manual for faith development research* (3rd ed.). Bielefeld, Atlanta, Research Center for Biographical Studies in Contemporary Religion; Center for Research in Faith and Moral Development, Emory University, Atlanta, GA.

Freud, S. (1923). *The ego and the id.* London: Hogarth Press.

Freud, S. (1961). *The ego and the id and other works* (Vol. 19). J. Strachey, Trans. London: Hogarth Press and the Institute of Psychoanalysis.

Geddes, J. F. (2004). The evidence base for shaken baby syndrome. *BMJ, 328*, 719–720.

Gesell, A. (1934). *An atlas of infant behavior: A systematic delineation of the forms and early growth of human behavior patterns.* New Haven, CT: Yale University Press.

Gesell, A. (2006). *Britannica student encyclopedia.* Retrieved May 14, 2006, from http://www.britannica.com/ebi/article-927-4541

Gilligan, C. (1982). *In a different voice: Psychological theory and women's development.* Cambridge, MA: Harvard University Press.

Glanz, K., Rimer, B. K., & Lewis, F. M. (2008). *Health behavior and health education: Theory, research, and practice* (4th ed.). San Francisco: Jossey-Bass.

Gould, R. L. (1972). The phases of adult life: A study in developmental psychology. *American Journal of Psychiatry, 129*, 33–43.

Grunbaum, J. A., Kann, L., Kinchen, S. A., Ross, J., Hawkins, J., Lowry, R., et al. (2004). Youth risk behavior surveillance—United States, 2003. *Morbidity and Mortality Weekly Report, 53*(SS-2), 1–96.

Hammad, T. A., Laughren, T., & Racoosin, J. (2006). Suicidality in pediatric patients treated with antidepressant drugs. *Archives of General Psychiatry, 63*(3), 246–248.

Hartman-Stein, P. E., & Potkanowicz, E. S. (2003). Behavioral determinants of healthy aging: Good news for the baby boomer generation. *Online Journal of Issues in Nursing, 8*(2), Manuscript #5. Retrieved December 5, 2009, from http://www.nursingworld.org/MainMenuCategories/ANAMarketplace/ANAPeriodicals/OJIN/TableofContents/Vol142009/No3Sept09/Articles-Previous-Topics/Update-and-Baby-Boomer-Generation.aspx

Havighurst, R. J. (1972). *Developmental tasks and education* (3rd ed.). Boston: Allyn & Bacon.

Hill, K. S. (2004). Defy the decades with multigenerational teams. *Nursing Management, 35*(1), 32–35.

Hollander, A. (1980). *How to help your child have a spiritual life: A parent's guide to inner development.* New York: A and W Publishers.

Hu, J., Herrick, C., & Hodgin, K. A. (2004). Managing the multigenerational nursing team. *Health Care Manager, 22*, 334–341.

Jack, S. M., Bouck, L. M. S., Beynon, C. E., Ciliska, D. K., & Mitchell, M. J. L. (2005). Marketing a hard-to-swallow message. Recommendations for the design of media campaigns to increase awareness about the risks of binge drinking. *Canadian Journal of Public Health, 96*(3), 189–193.

Jones, R. K., Purcell, A., Singh, S., & Finer, L. B. (2005). Adolescents' reports of parental knowledge of adolescents' use of sexual health services and their reactions for mandated parental notification for prescription contraception. *Journal of the American Medical Association, 293*(3), 340–348.

Karp, H. (2003). *The happiest baby on the block.* New York: Bantam Books.

Kohlberg, L. (1971). *Recent research in moral development.* New York: Holt, Rinehart & Winston.

Kohlberg, L. (1981). *Essays on moral development: Vol. 1. The philosophy of moral development.* San Francisco: Harper & Row.

Kohlberg, L. (1981). *The psychology of moral development: Moral stages and the idea of justice.* San Francisco: Harper & Row.

Kohlberg, L. (1984). *Essays on moral development: Vol. 2. The psychology of moral development.* San Francisco: Harper & Row.

Kohlberg, L. (1984). *The psychology of moral development: The nature and validity of moral stages.* San Francisco: Harper & Row.

Kvigne, V. L., Leonardo, G. R., Neff-Smith, M., Brock, E., Borzelleca, J., & Welty, T. K. (2004). Characteristics of children who have full or incomplete fetal alcohol syndrome. *Journal of Pediatrics, 145*(5), 635–640.

Lachman, M. E. (2004). Development in midlife. *Annual Review of Psychology, 55*, 305–31.

Landenburger, K. M., & Campbell, J. C. (2003). Violence and human abuse. In M. Stanhope & J. Lancaster (Eds.), *Community and public health nursing* (6th ed., pp. 874–901). St. Louis: Mosby.

Ling, P. M., & Glantz, S. A. (2002). Why and how the tobacco industry sells cigarettes to young adults: Evidence from industry documents. *American Journal of Public Health, 92*, 908–916.

Malloy, M. H., & Freeman, D. H. (2004). Age at death, season, and day of death as indicators of the effect of the back to sleep program on sudden infant death syndrome in the United States, 1992–1999. *Archives of Pediatric and Adolescent Medicine, 158*(4), 359–365.

Manners, J., Durkin, K., & Nesdale, A. (2004). Promoting advanced ego development among adults. *Journal of Adult Development, 11*(1), 19–28.

Maslow, A. H. (1970). *Motivation and personality.* New York: Harper & Row.

Mathre, M. L. (2004). Alcohol, tobacco, and other drug problems in the community. In

M. Stanhope & J. Lancaster (Eds.), *Community and public health nursing* (6th ed., pp. 848–873). St. Louis: Mosby.

Mattson, S. (2000). Providing culturally competent care strategies and approaches for perinatal clients. *AWHONN Lifelines, 4*(5), 37–39.

McKinney, E. S. (2005). *Maternal-child nursing* (2nd ed.). Philadelphia: Saunders.

Mitchell, K. (2002). Women's morality: A test of Carol Gilligan's theory. *Journal of Social Distress and the Homeless, 11*(1), 81–110.

Morrone, M., & Rathbun, A. (2003). Health education and food safety behavior in the university setting. *Journal of Environmental Health, 65*(7), 9–15.

Murray, R. B., Zentner, J. P., & Yakimo, R. (2009). *Health promotion strategies through the life span* (8th ed.). Upper Saddle River, NJ: Pearson Education.

National Adolescent Health Information Center. (2006). Fact sheet on suicide: Adolescents & young adults. Retrieved October 28, 2009, from http://nahic.ucsf.edu/downloads/Suicide.pdf.

Nelson, L. J., & Barry, C. M. (2005). Distinguishing features of emerging adulthood: The role of self-classification as an adult. *Journal of Adolescent Research, 20*, 242–262.

Oman, R. F., Vesely, S., Aspy, C. B., McLeroy, K. R., Rodine, S., & Marshall, L. (2004). The potential protective effect of youth assets on adolescent alcohol and drug use. *American Journal of Public Health, 94*(8), 1425–1430.

Paludi, M. A. (2002). *Human development in multicultural contexts. A book of readings.* Upper Saddle River, NJ: Prentice Hall.

Peck, R. (1968). Psychological developments in the second half of life. In B. L. Neugarten (Ed.), *Middle age and aging.* Chicago: University of Chicago Press.

Pfaffenberger, A. H. (2005). Optimal adult development: An inquiry into the dynamics of growth. *Journal of Humanistic Psychology, 45*(3), 279–301.

Piaget, J. (1966). *Origins of intelligence in children.* New York: Norton.

Pillitteri, A. (2010). *Maternal & child health nursing: Care of the childbearing & childrearing family* (5th ed.). Philadelphia: Lippincott Williams & Wilkins.

Polan, E., & Taylor, D. (2007). *Journey across the life span. Human development and health promotion* (3rd ed.). Philadelphia: FA Davis.

Roberts, K. S. (2003). Providing culturally sensitive care to the childbearing Islamic family: Part II. *Advances in Neonatal Care, 3*(5), 250–255.

Rothbart, M. K. (2004). Commentary: Differentiated measures of temperament and multiple pathways to childhood disorders. *Journal of Clinical Child and Adolescent Psychology, 33*(1), 82–87.

Sanots, S. R., & Cox, K. (2000). Workplace adjustment and intergenerational differences between Matures, Boomers, and Xers. *Nursing Economics, 18*(1), 7–13.

Schmidt, M. I., Duncan, B. B., Bang, H., Pankow, J. S., Ballantyne, C. M., Golden, S.H., et al. (2005). Identifying individuals at high risk for diabetes: The atherosclerosis risk in communities study. *Diabetes Care, 28*(8), 2013–2018.

Schmitt, B. D. (2006). *Pediatric telephone protocols: Office version* (11th ed.). Elk Grove Village, IL: American Academy of Pediatrics.

Sheehy, G. (1995). *New passages. Mapping your life across time.* New York: Ballantine Books.

Simpson, K. R., & Creehan, P. A. (2007). *AWHONN'S perinatal nursing* (3rd ed.). Philadelphia: Lippincott.

Slater, C. L. (2003). Generativity versus stagnation: An elaboration of Erikson's adult stage of human development. *Journal of Adult Development, 10*, 53–65.

Society for Adolescent Medicine. (2003). *Health guide for America's teens.* Germantown, WI: Securitec Publications.

Starr, N. B. (2004). Self-perception. In C. E. Burns et al., *Pediatric primary care: A handbook for nurse practitioners.* Philadelphia: Saunders.

Stevenson, J. S. (1977). *Issues and crises during middlescence.* New York: Appleton-Century-Crofts.

Stewart, S. H., Conrod, P. J., Marlatt, G. A., Comeau, M. N., Thush, C., & Krank, M. (2005). New developments in prevention and early intervention for alcohol abuse in youths. *Alcoholism, Clinical and Experimental Research, 29*(2), 278–286.

Strock, G. A., Cottrell, E. R., Abang, A. E., Buschbacher, R. M., & Hannon, T. S. (2005). Childhood obesity: A simple equation with complex variables. *Journal of Long Term Effects of Medical Implants, 15*(1), 15–32.

Swearingen, S., & Liberman, A. (2004). Nursing generations: An expanded look at the emergence of conflict and its resolution. *Health Care Manager, 23*(1), 54–65.

Stuart-Hamilton, I. (2006). *The psychology of ageing. An introduction* (4th ed.). London and Philadelphia: Jessica Kingsley Publishers.

Thornton, E. W., Sykes, K. S., & Tang, W. K. (2004). Health benefits of tai chi exercise: Improved balance and blood pressure in middle-aged women. *Health Promotion International, 19*(1), 33–36.

Toga, A. W., Thompson, P. M., & Sowell, E. R. (2006). Mapping brain maturation. *Trends in Neurosciences, 29*(3), 148–159.

Tucker, J. S., Klein, D. J., & Elliott, M. N. (2004). Social control of health behaviors: A comparison of young, middle-aged, and older adults. *Journal of Gerontology, 59B*(4), 147–150.

U.S. Department of Health and Human Services. (2000a). *Healthy people 2010: Objectives for improving health. Part B: Focus area 16. Maternal, infant, and child health. Understanding and improving health* (2nd ed.) [Electronic version]. Washington, DC: Author. Retrieved March 14, 2005, from http://www.healthypeople.gov/document/html/volume2/16mich.htm

U.S. Department of Health and Human Services (USDHHS). (2000b). *Healthy people 2010* (2nd ed.). Washington, DC: Government Printing Office.

U.S. Department of Health and Human Services. (2004). *Summary health statistics for U. S. adults: National Health Interview Survey, 2002.* DHHS Publication No. (PHS) 2004-1550. Hyattsville, MD: Author.

U. S. Preventive Services Task Force. (2003). *Guide to clinical preventive services, 3rd edition: Periodic updates.* Rockville, MD: Agency for Health Care Research and Quality. Retrieved June 6, 2006, from http:// www.ahrq.gov/clinic/gcpspu.htm

U. S. Preventive Services Task Force. (2004). *Screening for testicular cancer: Recommendation statement.* Rockville, MD: Agency for Health Care Research and Quality. Retrieved June 6, 2006, from http://www.ahrq.gov/clinic/uspstf/uspstest.htm

Venes, D. (Ed.). (2005). *Taber's cyclopedic medical dictionary* (20th ed.). Philadelphia: Davis.

Ventura, J. J., Abrna, J. C., Mosher, W. D., & Hanshaw, S. (2004). Estimated Pregnancy rates for the United States, 1990–2000: An update. *National Vital Statistics Report, 52*(23), 1–10. Centers for Disease Control. USDHHS.

Westerhoff, J. (1976). *Will our children have faith?* New York: Seabury Press.

Wolfe, E. L., Davis, T., Guydish, J., & Delucchi, K. L. (2005). Mortality risk associated with perinatal drug and alcohol use in California. *Journal of Perinatology, 25*(2), 93–100.

WHO Multicentre Growth Reference Study Group. (2006). WHO Child Growth Standards based on length/height, weight and age. *Acta Pædiatrica,* Suppl. 450, 76–85.

Promoting Health in Elders

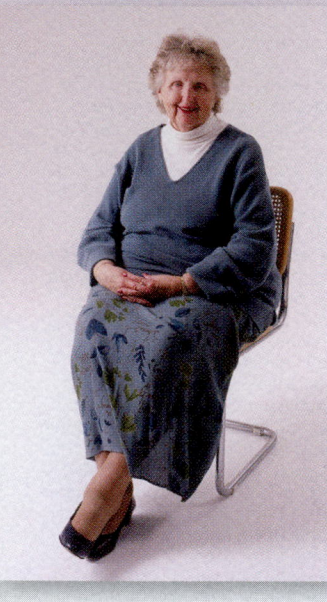

Florence Robinson, 84 years old, enjoys looking through her photograph album. When she looks in the mirror she hardly recognizes the face looking back. She compares the face she sees today with the pictures of herself as a young mother, and she wonders where the time went. Florence lives alone in a suburb of a large city. Her husband died 6 years ago from amyotrophic lateral sclerosis. They have two grown children who live in another state and try to visit their mother at least once a year. Florence has a large group of friends who get together several times a week to play cards, go to the movies, or go out to dinner. Once a month they attend the senior center square dance and then go out for pancakes.

Occasionally Florence worries about what will happen if she is unable to live alone and take care of herself. She shares her concerns with her friends, who admit they have the same worry. Recently Florence has noticed she gets tired easily and becomes short of breath while climbing the stairs to her bedroom. Last night she had to stop halfway up the stairs and catch her breath. She calls her doctor and talks with the triage nurse about her new symptoms.

LEARNING OUTCOMES

After completing this chapter, you will be able to:

1. Identify the different categories of older adults from 65 to 100 years of age.

2. Describe demographic, socioeconomic, ethnicity, and health characteristics of older adults in the United States.

3. Describe ageism and its contribution to the development of negative stereotypes about older adults.

4. Compare and contrast gerontology and geriatrics.

5. Describe the development of gerontological nursing and the roles of the gerontological nurse.

6. Describe different care settings for older adults.

7. List the common biologic theories of aging.

8. Describe the usual physical changes that occur during older adulthood.

9. Review common psychosocial theories about aging, developmental tasks of the older adult, and psychosocial changes that the older adult adjusts to during the aging process.

10. Explain changes in cognitive abilities while aging.

11. Compare Kohlberg's and Gilligan's theories of moral reasoning in older adults.

12. Describe spirituality and aging.

13. Describe health problems common in older adults.

14. Identify health promotion topics for older adulthood.

adult day care p255	dementia p267	gerontology p252	sensory memory p265
ageism p252	disengagement theory p261	long-term memory p265	short-term memory p265
assisted living p254		perception p264	
continuity theory p261	geriatrics p252	recent memory p265	

The United States is experiencing a "graying of America" as the older adult population steadily grows. By the mid-21st century, older adults are projected to outnumber young people (Mauk, 2006, p. 30).

CHARACTERISTICS OF OLDER ADULTS IN THE UNITED STATES

Older adults represent an increasingly diverse population in the United States. A review of the major characteristics of the older adult population includes demographic, socioeconomic, ethnicity, and health characteristics.

Demographic

At one time, all individuals over the age of 65 were considered old. With advancements in disease control, living conditions, and health technology, people are living longer. A 65-year-old American woman may expect to live another 19 years, and a 65-year-old American man may expect to reach the age of 81 (Federal Interagency Forum on Age-Related Statistics [FIFAS], 2008). People 85 years and older are the fastest growing of all age groups in the country, numbering 5.3 million in 2002, but projected to reach 21 million by the year 2050 (FIFAS, 2008). The older adult population are as heterogeneous as any other age group that spans 40 years or more. As a result, the categories of aging have expanded from one to four with each one having a distinct set of interests and health care needs. See Box 10–1.

Socioeconomic

Socioeconomic characteristics such as gender, marital status, education, income, and living arrangements vary among the young-old and old-old groups (Miller, 2004). Women outnumber men. For example, the young-old and old-old groups have nearly 2 million more women than men (Mauk, 2006, p. 31). Women have a longer life expectancy than men. In addition, women are more likely than men to be widowed and there are higher remarriage rates for older men.

The level of education can affect the socioeconomic status of the older adult. Higher education is usually associated with higher incomes. According to Miller (2004), educational levels for older adults are gradually increasing as indicated by the increasing percentage rates of people 65 years and older who have completed high school. However, there is significant variation among racial and ethnic groups. Usually, older adults have lower incomes than younger adults, and people 85 years and older have the lowest median income (Miller, 2004, p. 14).

Living arrangements of older adults are linked not only to income, but also to health status. Most live in a variety of community settings with only 4.3% living in nursing homes (FIFAS, 2008). Older people who live alone are more likely to live in poverty than people in the same age category who are married (Mauk, 2006). Older women are twice as likely to be living alone. Living arrangements vary by race and ethnicity. The rate of living alone increases as age increases.

Ethnicity

The growing population of older adults consists of increasing numbers of minority members. Projected to 2050, the higher proportion of the older adult white population will continue. However, the nonwhite older adult population is expected to increase with Hispanics being the fastest growing subpopulation group (Meiner & Lueckenotte, 2006). These numbers emphasize the importance of nurses being culturally sensitive and competent. See Table 10–1 for a comparison of the older adult population growth.

BOX 10–1 **Categorizing the Aging Population**

- Young-old: 65 to 74 years
- Old: 75 to 84 years
- Old-old: 85+

Note: From C. Eliopoulos, *Gerontological Nursing*, 6th ed. Copyright © Lippincott Williams & Wilkins, 2005. Reprinted with permission.

TABLE 10–1 **Comparison of Older Adult Population for 2003 Census and Projected Population for 2050 Census Ethnicity**

ETHNICITY	2003 CENSUS	2050 PROJECTION
White	83%	61%
Black	8%	12%
Asian	3%	8%
Hispanic	6%	18%

Note: K. L. Mauk, *Gerontological Nursing* 2006: Jones and Bartlett Publishers, Sudbury, MA. www.jbpub.com. Reprinted with permission.

BOX 10–2	Focus Areas in *Healthy People 2010* That Are Relevant to Older Adults

- Access to quality health services
- Arthritis, osteoporosis, and chronic back conditions
- Cancer
- Chronic kidney disease
- Diabetes
- Disability and secondary conditions
- Educational and community-based programs
- Food safety
- Health communication
- Heart disease and stroke
- Immunization and infectious diseases

- Injury and violence prevention
- Mental health and mental conditions
- Nutrition and obesity
- Oral health
- Physical activity and fitness
- Respiratory diseases
- Substance abuse
- Tobacco use
- Vision and hearing

Note: U.S. Department of Health and Human Services.

Health

Chronic health problems and disabilities increase as age increases. However, disease is *not* a normal outcome of aging. The vast majority (73%) of older Americans rated their health as good, very good, or excellent (National Center for Health Statistics [NCHS], 2003), even though most have chronic health conditions, and 20% report a disability (FIFAS, 2008). Nurses need to be aware that promoting health and wellness and assessing and promoting functional abilities for activities of daily living continue to be valid and important for 65-year-old clients who have 16 to 19 more years to enjoy life. In fact, the goals of *Healthy People 2010* include focus areas relevant to older adults. See Box 10–2.

ATTITUDES TOWARD AGING

Because older adult numbers are increasing, nurses will be caring for older adults at some point. It is important for nurses to be aware of their own values and attitudes toward aging and the older adult, and examine whether myths or stereotypes influence those attitudes.

Ageism

American society values youth. See the Culturally Competent Care box to see how different cultures view older adults. **Ageism** is a term to describe the deep and profound prejudice in American society against older adults (Meiner & Lueckenotte, 2006, p. 13). It is a discrimination based solely on age. Unfortunately, this negative attitude toward aging or older adults exists among some health care professionals (Ebersole, Hess, Touhy, & Jett, 2009; Mauk, 2006). This attitude is another reason for nurses to self-reflect personal beliefs and values toward older adults.

Myths and Stereotypes

Ageism contributes to the development of negative stereotypes about older adults. Stereotypes occur when younger people do not understand or identify with older adults as unique human beings. Instead, they generalize undesirable characteristics (e.g., senile, old-fashioned, unproductive, inflexible) to all

older adults. Many negative attitudes about aging are based on myths and incorrect information. See Table 10–2. As a result, it is important for nurses to provide accurate information about aging. This has been found to be an effective intervention for reducing negative stereotypes and improving attitudes about aging (Miller, 2004, p. 11).

GERONTOLOGICAL NURSING

The growth of the older adult population is characterized by unique and diverse individuals who may require a variety of health care professionals to meet their health care needs. **Gerontology** is a term used to define the study of aging from a biological, psychological, and sociological perspective. Gerontology is multidisciplinary and is a specialized area within various disciplines such as nursing, psychology, and social work. **Geriatrics** is associated with the medical care (e.g., diseases and disabilities) of the older adult.

Development

Gerontological nursing involves advocating for the health of older persons at all levels of prevention (Mauk, 2006, p. 9). In the 1960s, gerontological nursing became a subspecialty of nursing. In the 1980s, gerontological nursing leaders stated that most practicing nurses did not have sufficient knowledge about gerontology. This prompted discussion of how to prepare nurses for gerontological nursing. Since the late 1990s, the nursing profession has recognized the importance of preparing all practicing nurses with basic gerontological knowledge. As a result, schools of nursing provide classes or courses about nursing care of the older adult. Practicing gerontological nurses can obtain gerontological nursing certification through the American Nurses Association. Advanced practice in gerontological nursing requires a master's degree in nursing, of which there are two options: the gerontological clinical nurse specialist and the gerontological nurse practitioner.

Roles

The gerontological nurse has many roles: provider of care, teacher, manager, advocate, and research consumer. As

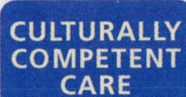

How Different Cultures View Older Adults

Chinese

- Traditional Chinese values place the family and society over the individual. Many American-born Chinese may not be as traditional but still hold values of respect for elders and authority.
- The oldest son has obligations toward the family and is expected to respect and care for parents.
- The tradition of "filial piety" is the value of total respect for the family, especially the older adults. This respect for older adults was advocated by Confucius, the famous Chinese philosopher, and many Chinese and Chinese-American families choose to follow these ancient principles.

Native American

- Traditionally, older adults are respected for their wisdom, experience, and knowledge.
- Older adults, regardless of tribe, assume significant roles as teachers and caretakers of the young.

Vietnamese

- Older adults are given high respect in Vietnamese society. They are considered the carriers of tradition, knowledge, and wisdom. Age is considered an asset, not a liability.
- Older grandparents and parents stay with the family for support and care.
- Older adults may prepare meals and care for grandchildren if both the husband and wife work.
- In Vietnam, older adults are the leaders and decision makers in the family and are often sought for advice. When these older adults move to the United States, they can become socially and culturally isolated for many reasons (e.g., lack of English, age, lack of training for work). In contrast, the younger family members become more Americanized and may behave in ways their older adults do not approve. This can create tension in families where older adults feel ignored and not respected.

Black/African American

- Older adults are respected, obeyed, and considered a source of wisdom.
- To survive to old age is often considered an accomplishment reflecting personal strength, resourcefulness, and faith.

Hispanic/Latino

- Older adults are held in high esteem.
- Old age is viewed as a positive time in the life of the older adult.
- Care for older adults is provided by the extended family. It is expected that children will care for their aging parents.

Korean

- Traditional Koreans value filial piety and respect for older adults.
- In Korean culture, children are taught to respect older adults whether the adults are right or wrong.
- There is the expectation that the children will take care of their parents in old age.
- Two important family holidays that are celebrated with feasts include the 60th birthday and the 70th birthday.

TABLE 10–2 Myths and Realities of Aging

MYTH	REALITY
People are old at 65.	Perception of age is based on health and functional ability, rather than their chronological age.
In today's society, families no longer care for older people.	In the United States, 80% of the care of older adults is provided by their families.
As people grow older, it is natural for them to want to withdraw from society.	Because older people are unique individuals, each of them responds differently to society.
In old age, there is an inevitable decline in all intellectual abilities.	A few areas of cognitive ability decline in older adulthood, but other areas show improvement.
Older adults cannot learn complex new skills.	Older adults are capable of learning new things, but the speed with which they process information slows with age.
Older people are not interested in sexual activity because they are less able to perform.	Older adults not only remain sexually interested and active, they are one of the most at risk for sexually transmitted diseases. If sexual activity in older people declines, it is because of social reasons or risk factors.
Most old people are depressed and should be allowed to withdraw from society.	About one-third of older people exhibit depressive symptoms; however, depression is a very treatable condition at any age.
Most older people have incontinence of urine or bowel and require the use of adult diapers.	Incontinence does not occur in all older adults and is always considered abnormal requiring intervention when it occurs.

Note: Adapted from C. A. Miller, *Nursing for Wellness in Older Adults*, 4th ed. Copyright © Lippincott, Williams & Wilkins, 2004. Reprinted with permission.

provider of care, the nurse gives direct care to older adults in a variety of settings. The teaching of gerontological nurses often focuses on modifiable risk factors (e.g., healthy diet, physical activity, stress management). Gerontological nurse managers balance the concerns of the older adult, family, and nurses and other interdisciplinary team members. As an advocate, the gerontological nurse empowers older adults by helping them remain independent and strengthen their autonomy and decision making. Being a research consumer requires nurses to read the latest professional literature for evidence-based practice to improve the quality of nursing care for the older adult.

CARE SETTINGS FOR OLDER ADULTS

Gerontological nurses practice in many settings. Older adults are the primary users of health care services from acute care facilities to rehabilitation, long-term care, and the community (Stanley, Blair, & Beare, 2005). No matter the setting, older adults require health assessment and promotion.

Acute Care Facilities

Older adults are the majority of clients cared for in acute care. For example, people who are 65 and older use the emergency department (ED) at a higher rate than any other age group (Capezuti & Harrington, 2004). Nearly half of the clients who die in hospitals spend part or all of their last 3 days in critical care (Seery, 2004).

Nurses in an acute care setting focus on protecting the health of the older adult, with the goal of the older adult returning to his or her prior level of independence. Examples include:

- Preventing nosocomial infections (e.g., urinary tract infections, pneumonia).
- Preventing therapy-related problems (e.g., confusion, sleeplessness, dehydration, decreased nutrition).
- Treating the health problem that resulted in the older adult's admission plus assessing for potential undiagnosed health problems (e.g., depression, drug and/or alcohol abuse).
- Preventing complications (e.g., decubitus ulcer).

Older adults often perceive that being in the hospital could change their ability to be autonomous and independent. As a result, nurses need to assess the older adult's stage or perception of need for control and autonomy during hospitalization and his or her fears and hopes about being discharged from the hospital setting.

Long-Term Care Facilities

The objective of long-term care is to provide a place of safety and care to attain optimal wellness and independence for each individual (Stanley et al., 2005, p. 94). In the long-term care setting, the individual is referred to as a resident. Long-term care includes many different levels of care. These may

include assisted living, intermediate care, skilled care, and Alzheimer's units. Older adults who do not feel safe living alone or require additional help with activities of daily living (ADLs) may desire **assisted living**. They usually have their own apartment. The assisted living facility provides meals, weekly activities, and a pleasant environment to socialize with other residents. Some assisted living units are part of a larger facility. When residents require additional assistance, they may enter intermediate care. Residents of intermediate care are no longer able to live independently. This level of care provides 24-hour direct nursing contact (Mauk, 2006).

Skilled care units or skilled nursing facilities (SNFs) are for older adults who require a higher level of nursing care because the acuity level of the client requires a greater nurse-to-client ratio. Gerontological nurses working in SNFs often care for clients with tube feedings, IVs, chronic wounds, and ventilators.

Many long-term care facilities offer specialized units for clients with Alzheimer's disease (AD), which involves progressive dementia, memory loss, and inability to care for themselves. The gerontological nurses working in Alzheimer's units have specialized knowledge and help family members understand and cope with the disease process affecting their loved one.

Hospice

Gerontological nurses may also work in hospice and care for dying persons and their families. The majority of hospice clients are older adults. Hospice requires a great deal of patience, expertise, understanding, interdisciplinary communication, and compassion skills on the part of gerontology nurses (Mauk, 2006, p. 23).

Rehabilitation

Rehabilitation may be found in several settings: acute care hospital, subacute or transitional care, and long-term care facilities. Many older adults benefit from a rehabilitation program where the goal is to maintain physical independence (e.g., after orthopedic surgery, stroke, or amputation). The nurse is an important member of the interdisciplinary rehabilitation team. The role of the nurse is often as a health care coordinator, manager, and counselor for older adults and their families (Stanley et al., 2005). For example, nurses monitor the client's health care, assist with ADLs, and facilitate the client's adjustment and coping with the disability.

Community

Gerontological nurses provide nursing care in many types of community settings. Nurses often assess the older adult's needs and then try to match the need with a community resource. A few of the different community areas for gerontological nurses to practice include:

- *Home health care.* Home care is designed for those who are homebound due to severity of illness or disability (Mauk, 2006). Research has shown that home

RESEARCH NOTES

How Do Older Adults Manage Personal Integrity during Hospitalization?

For this grounded theory research study the researcher collected in-depth interviews of five older adults ranging from 77 to 85 years of age. These older adults, who lived independently in the community prior to hospitalization, were admitted for medical reasons related to a chronic underlying health problem. The researcher also interviewed family members of each older adult and an RN who provided nursing care for them. In addition to the interviews, the researcher observed each older adult for at least 2 hours each day.

The research findings resulted in a theory entitled Managing Personal Integrity. Jacelon, the researcher, defines personal integrity as a dynamic, intrinsic quality of the self with the properties of health, dignity, and autonomy. The findings indicated that each property was a focus of the older adults during their hospitalization.

Hospital routine was strange and different for the older adult. All of their prior routines were taken away and they felt a loss of control. According to this research, the older adult progressed through three stages of independence and autonomy. First, they willingly gave up their autonomy and sense of control when they were admitted to the hospital because they wanted to get better. They focused primarily on their health. As they started to improve, the older adults wanted to increase their autonomy and sense of control, focusing on their dignity. For example, they accomplished more by themselves and took more responsibility for self-care. They also participated more in the plan of care by asking questions about their medications and tests.

Before discharge, with the reasons for the hospitalization resolving, the older adults felt more of a sense of control and began to reassert their autonomy. They took more responsibility for both their activities of daily living and their health by preparing for discharge and resuming independent functioning at home.

Implications

This study reflects the importance of autonomy to the older adult. According to Jacelon, autonomy has two components: independence (the physical ability to act) and control (the ability to make decisions on one's own behalf). As nurses work with more and more older adults in the acute care hospital setting, it is important to remember the stages of independence and autonomy experienced by older adults during the different phases of hospitalization as reflected in this study. Strategies to enhance an increased sense of control and autonomy by the older adult include providing adequate information in a timely manner, allowing participation in the scheduling of activities, explaining any changes in the plan of care, and viewing hospitalized older adults as individuals who wish to regain their autonomy and dignity.

Note: Based on "Older Adults and Autonomy in Acute Care: Increasing Patients' Independence and Control During Hospitalization," by C. S. Jacelon, 2004, *Journal of Gerontological Nursing, 30*(11), pp. 29–36. Copyright © 2004 SLACK, Inc.

health for older adults prevents hospital readmissions (Stanley et al., 2005).

- *Nurse-run clinics.* The clinics focus on managing chronic illness. Nurses follow up with either telephone contacts or home visits within a week after discharge from a hospital. Again, this often helps decrease hospital readmissions.
- *Adult day care.* The older adult may receive **adult day care** where the focus is on social activities or health care where the level of nursing care can vary (e.g., bathing, medication administration, wound dressing). Some adult day-care centers provide both social and health care. Family members who care for older parents but may need to work during the day or need some respite from the continual care often use these services. This is an alternative to institutionalizing the older adult.

PHYSIOLOGICAL AGING

There are nearly 40 different theories of aging in the biologic, psychologic, and social sciences, and many in gerontological nursing. Clearly, there are more questions as to how people age than there are answers. At this point, it is helpful to distinguish between normal aging and successful aging. The most promising theories for explaining physical aging include genetics (Kirkwood & Austad, 2000), oxidative stress (Finkel & Holbrook, 2000), and cellular changes (DePinto,

2000). These theories may be generally grouped into (a) theories that hypothesize aging as a consequence of accumulated damage to informational molecules, and (b) theories that hypothesize aging as a consequence of regulation by specific genes (Kane, Ouslander, & Abrass, 2009).

As the person ages, a number of physical changes occur. In general, lean body mass is reduced, fat tissue increases, and bone mass decreases. Extracellular fluid remains constant; however, intracellular fluid decreases and leads to reduced total body fluid. Thus, older adults are at risk for developing dehydration (Eliopoulos, 2009). Table 10–3 provides a summary of the normal physical changes associated with aging.

Integument

Obvious changes occur in the integumentary system (skin, hair, nails) with age. The skin becomes drier, less elastic, and more fragile, making the older person more susceptible to skin tears and shearing injuries. The hair loses color, the fingernails and toenails become thickened and brittle, and in women over 60, facial hair increases.

Responses to these changes vary among individuals and cultures. For example, one person may feel distinguished with gray hair, whereas another may feel embarrassed or depressed, interpreting gray hair as a sign of losing one's youth.

These integumentary changes accompany progressive losses of subcutaneous fat and muscle tissue, muscle atrophy, and loss of elastic fiber, resulting in a "double" chin, sagging of eyelids and earlobes, and wrinkling of skin, especially in

TABLE 10–3 Normal Physical Changes Associated with Aging

PHYSICAL CHANGES	RATIONALE	HEALTH PROMOTION
Integumentary		
Increased skin dryness	Decrease in sebaceous gland activity and tissue fluid	Increase fluid intake, apply emollients to moisten
Increased skin pallor	Decreased vascularity	Adequate iron intake, exercise to increase cardiac output and perfusion
Increased skin fragility	Reduced thickness and vascularity of the dermis; loss of subcutaneous fat	Care to prevent friction and skin damage
Progressive wrinkling and sagging of the skin	Loss of skin elasticity, increased dryness, and decreased subcutaneous fat	Assist the client to express feelings related to changes in body image and accept changes associated with aging
Brown "age spots" (lentigo senilis) on exposed body parts (e.g., face, hands, arms)	Clustering of melanocytes (pigment-producing cells)	Assist the client to express feelings related to changes in body image and accept changes associated with aging
Decreased perspiration	Reduced number and function of sweat glands	Caution when exposed to high temperatures to include adequate fluid intake and avoid extremes of temperature
Thinning and graying of scalp, pubic, and axillary hair	Progressive loss of pigment cells from the hair bulbs	Assist client to express feelings related to changes in body image and accept changes associated with aging
Slower nail growth and increased thickening with ridges	Increased calcium deposition	Assist client to express feelings related to changes in body image and accept changes associated with aging
Neuromuscular		
Decreased speed and power of skeletal muscle contractions	Decrease in muscle fibers	Teach fall prevention
Slowed reaction time	Diminished conduction speed of nerve fibers and decreased muscle tone	Testing to determine driver safety
Loss of height (stature)	Atrophy of intervertebral discs, increased flexion at hips and knees	Assist client to express feelings related to changes in body image and accept changes associated with aging
Loss of bone mass	Bone reabsorption outpaces bone reformation	Promote adequate intake of calcium, vitamin D, and phosphorous, especially in women
Joint stiffness	Drying and loss of elasticity in joint cartilage	Promote exercises that do not place undue stress on joints such as swimming
Impaired balance	Decreased muscle strength, reaction time, and coordination, change in center of gravity	Teach fall prevention activities
Greater difficulty in complex learning and abstraction	Fewer cells in cerebral cortex	Teach older adults about changes in cognitive processes, and recommend exercises to promote cognitive abilities
Sensory/Perceptual		
Loss of visual acuity	Degeneration leading to lens opacity (cataracts), thickening, and inelasticity (presbyopia)	Assess for visual changes and promote improved lighting to prevent injury
Increased sensitivity to glare and decreased ability to adjust to darkness	Changes in the ciliary muscles; rigid pupil sphincter; decrease in pupil size	Test for driver safety at night
Partial or complete glossy white circle around the periphery of the cornea (arcus senilis)	Fatty deposits	Assess for peripheral vision and promote safety related to change in vision
Progressive loss of hearing (presbycusis)	Changes in the structures and nerve tissues in the inner ear; thickening of the eardrum	Promote hearing testing and use of hearing aids when needed

TABLE 10–3   **Normal Physical Changes Associated with Aging—continued**

PHYSICAL CHANGES	RATIONALE	HEALTH PROMOTION
Decreased sense of taste, especially the sweet sensations at the tip of the tongue	Decreased number of taste buds in the tongue because of tongue atrophy	Teach about anticipated changes in sense of taste
Decreased sense of smell	Atrophy of the olfactory bulb at the base of the brain (responsible for smell perception)	Teach about anticipated changes in sense of smell
Increased threshold for sensations of pain, touch, and temperature	Possible nerve conduction and neuron changes	Promote care in preventing injury related to diminished sensation preventing client from feeling pain related to pressure or temperature
Pulmonary		
Decreased ability to expel foreign or accumulated matter	Decreased elasticity and ciliary activity	Teach coughing exercises to promote airway clearance
Decreased lung expansion, less effective exhalation, reduced vital capacity, and increased residual volume	Weakened thoracic muscles; calcification of costal cartilage, making the rib cage more rigid with increased anterior-posterior diameter; dilation from inelasticity of alveoli	Teach deep breathing exercises to promote lung excursion
Difficult, short, heavy, rapid breathing (dyspnea) following intense exercise	Diminished delivery and diffusion of oxygen to the tissues to repay the normal oxygen debt because of exertion or changes in both respiratory and vascular tissues	Promote periods of rest during intense exercise to allow for adequate oxygenation
Cardiovascular		
Reduced cardiac output and stroke volume, particularly during increased activity or unusual demands; may result in shortness of breath on exertion and pooling of blood in the extremities	Increased rigidity and thickness of heart valves (hence decreased filling/emptying abilities); decreased contractile strength	Promote vascular return through use of antiemboli stockings and/or positioning, and awareness of need for rest periods during exercise to promote tissue oxygenation
Reduced elasticity and increased rigidity of arteries	Increased calcium deposits in the muscular layer	Promote blood pressure and cholesterol screening to maintain adequate tissue perfusion
Increase in diastolic and systolic blood pressure	Inelasticity of systemic arteries and increased peripheral resistance	Promote blood pressure screenings to monitor for changes
Orthostatic hypertension	Reduced sensitivity of the blood pressure–regulating baroreceptors	Teach clients to stand slowly in order to prevent falling
Gastrointestinal		
Delayed swallowing time	Alterations in the swallowing mechanism	Teach client to chew food thoroughly and take small bites
Increased tendency for indigestion	Gradual decrease in digestive enzymes, reduction in gastric pH, and slower absorption rate	Promote upright positioning after meals, small frequent meals, and avoidance of tight waist bands on clothing
Increased tendency for constipation	Decreased muscle tone of the intestines; decreased peristalsis; decreased free body fluid	Promote adequate intake of fluids and fiber, avoid reliance on enemas or laxatives
Urinary		
Reduced filtering ability of the kidney and impaired renal function	Decreased number of functioning nephrons (basic functional units of the kidney) and arteriosclerotic changes in blood flow	Promote screening for kidney function
Less effective concentration of urine	Decreased tubular function	Promote healthy diet and electrolyte screening, teach symptoms of dehydration
Urinary urgency and urinary frequency	Enlarged prostate gland in men; weakened muscles supporting the bladder or weakness of the urinary sphincter in women	Teach Kegel exercises to strengthen perineal muscles

(continued)

TABLE 10–3	Normal Physical Changes Associated with Aging—continued	
PHYSICAL CHANGES	**RATIONALE**	**HEALTH PROMOTION**
Tendency for nocturnal frequency and retention of residual urine	Decreased bladder capacity and tone	Promote fall prevention when getting up at night to void, teach importance of bladder emptying
Genitals		
Prostate enlargement (benign) in men	Exact mechanism is unclear; possible endocrine changes	Promote routine prostate screening
Multiple changes in women (shrinkage and atrophy of the vulva, cervix, uterus, fallopian tubes, and ovaries; reduction in secretions; and changes in vaginal flora)	Diminished secretion of female hormones and more alkaline vaginal pH	Promote annual pelvic examinations and monthly breast self-exams for early cancer detection
Increased time to sexual arousal	Changes in blood supply to penis, clitoris	Suggest alternative positions to reduce energy expenditure to allow more time for arousal
Decreased firmness of erection, increased refractory period (men)	Changes in blood supply	Explain normal changes in physiology
Decreased vaginal lubrication and elasticity (women)	Loss of estrogen effects	Promote use of lubricants to prevent vaginal tearing
Immunological		
Decreased immune response; lowered resistance to infections	T cells less responsive to antigens; B cells produce fewer antibodies	Promote infection control measures
Poor response to immunization	Immune system changes may precipitate insulin resistance	Encourage annual immunizations as recommended by the CDC, and regular screening for diabetes mellitus
Decreased stress response		
Endocrine		
Increased insulin resistance	Unclear mechanism	
Decreased thyroid function		

areas exposed to sun. Bony prominences may become visible. In older women, the breasts become less firm and may sag. Loss of subcutaneous fat also decreases older adults' tolerance of cold.

Health promotion teaching about skin care for older adults can include the following:

- Maintaining healthy skin
  - Ensure optimal nutrition.
  - Maintain adequate hydration.
  - Prevent skin dryness by using emollient lotions after bathing or showering, when the skin is still moist.
  - Avoid skin products that contain perfume or alcohol.
  - Assess the frequency of bathing/showering.
- Avoiding sun damage
  - Use sun-screening lotions with sun protection factor (SPF) of 15 or higher.
  - Wear wide-brimmed hats, sun visors, and sunglasses when exposed to the sun.
  - Observe for any skin changes (e.g., new lesions, change in mole size or color) and seek medical evaluation.

- Preventing skin injury
  - Do not use strong detergent to launder clothes.
  - Avoid rough texture in clothing.
  - Avoid highly starched linens.
  - Use soft washcloths, towels, and bed linens.

Neuromusculoskeletal

With aging comes gradual reduction in the speed and power of skeletal or voluntary muscle contractions and sustained muscular effort. Exercise can strengthen weakened muscles, and up to about age 50 the skeletal muscles can increase in bulk and density. After that time there is a steady decrease in muscle fibers (sarcopenia), even in older master athletes (Taylor et al., 2004), ultimately leading to the typical wasted appearance of the very old person. The mechanism of age-related sarcopenia appears to be related to denervation of the muscle. Thus older adults often complain about their lack of strength and how quickly they tire. Activities can still be carried out, but at a slower pace, and with greater expenditure of energy (Taylor et al., 2004). Often balance is impaired with age, and is related to loss of muscle strength. Muscle endurance diminishes with age, resulting in muscle fatigue after short periods of exercise for the older adult.

There is substantial evidence, however, that the muscles that do remain in the older adult can be strengthened through exercise and training, with resulting improvements in functional status.

The person's reaction time slows with age. Reaction time can be delayed further by decreased muscle tone as a result of diminished physical activity. Older adults compensate for this reaction difference by being exceptionally cautious, for instance, in their driving habits, which exasperates some impatient younger drivers.

Loss in overall stature occurs with age. This can be exaggerated by muscular weakness resulting in a stooping posture and kyphosis (humpback of the upper spine). Imbalance in the rates of absorption and formation of bone tissue occurs with aging, so that older adults have more porous and fragile bones than do younger adults, making older adults prone to serious fractures. Osteoporosis, a pathologic decrease in bone density that is more common in older than younger adults, may lead to spontaneous (i.e., without a fall or other trauma to the bone) fractures that are called pathologic fractures. Osteoporosis occurs more frequently in people with insufficient intake of dietary calcium, in women after menopause, in Caucasians and Asians, and in individuals who are immobilized or physically inactive. Often considered a woman's disease, it is important to remember that osteoporosis affects men also (Curry & Hogstel, 2002).

Joints and their supporting structures change with age, including decreased elasticity, strength, and hydration of the tendons and ligaments, making movement stiffer and more restricted. Stiffness is aggravated by inactivity; for example, if a person sits too long, the joints become stiff, and the person has difficulty standing and walking. These changes may be compounded by osteoarthritis. A continual program of physical activity and proper nutrition will slow bone density loss and decrease muscle atrophy and stiffness (see Figure 10–1).

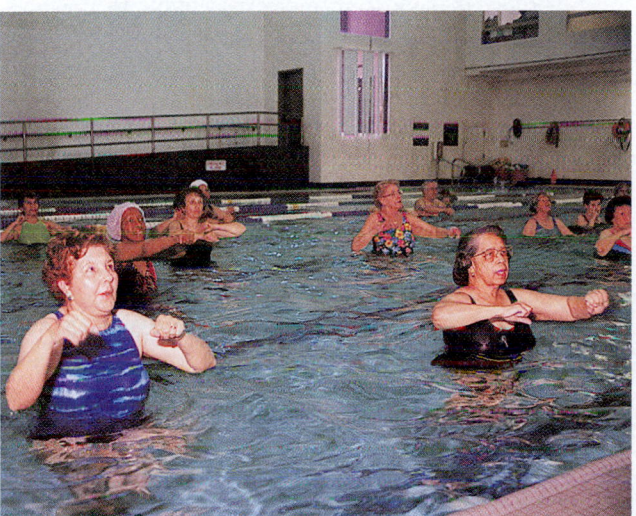

Figure 10–1 ⬤ A regular program of exercise is important for maintenance of joint mobility and muscle tone and can promote socialization.

As indicated, these age-related changes may affect the mobility and safety of the older adult, putting them at risk for falls and fractures. For health promotion, the nurse assesses the musculoskeletal functioning of the older adult and identifies any risk factors that may contribute to falls or the ability to perform ADLs. Health promotion interventions often include providing information about the risk factors for osteoporosis and the importance of adequate intake of calcium and vitamin D.

Sensory/Perceptual

Each of the five senses becomes less efficient in older adulthood. Changes in vision associated with aging include the obvious changes around the eye, such as the shrunken appearance of the eyes due to loss of orbital fat, the slowed blink reflex, and the looseness of the eyelids, particularly the lower lid, due to poorer muscle tone. Other changes result in loss of visual acuity, less power of adaptation to darkness and dim light, a decrease in accommodation to near and far objects, loss of peripheral vision, atrophy of lacrimal glands resulting in dry eyes, and difficulty in discriminating similar colors, especially blues, greens, and purples.

Presbyopia, the inability to focus or accommodate due to a loss of flexibility of the lens, causes a decrease in near vision. This generally starts around age 40. Visual acuity lessens gradually after age 50 and more rapidly after age 70 (Tabloski, 2010).

By the age of 80, nearly all older adults have some lens opacity (cataracts) that reduces visual acuity and causes glare to be a problem. In addition to cataracts, three other conditions result in visual impairment and blindness: age-related macular degeneration (ARMD), glaucoma, and diabetic retinopathy (Tabloski, 2010). It is important for the nurse to promote health by informing older adults to schedule routine eye examinations to maintain and protect their vision. Also, wearing sunglasses will help avoid the damaging effect of ultraviolet light.

The loss of hearing ability related to aging, called presbycusis, affects people over age 65. Gradual loss of hearing is more common among men than women, perhaps because men are more frequently in noisy work environments. Hearing loss is greater in the higher frequencies than the lower. Thus older adults with hearing loss usually hear speakers with low, distinct voices best. Hard consonants (e.g., *k, d, t*) and long vowel sounds (e.g., *ay, ee*) are more easily recognized, and sibilant sounds (*s, th, f*) are the most difficult to hear. Older adults may have more difficulty compensating for hearing loss than the young, who pay closer attention to the lip movements of the speaker.

If family members notice communication problems or social withdrawal of the older adult, the nurse should provide health promotion teaching by suggesting a referral for hearing screening. Also, the ears should be checked for impacted earwax. If hearing has diminished, assistive listening devices are available and the nurse can provide information to the client and family. To help avoid increased hearing loss, inform the older adult to use ear protection devices when working in or around activities that give off loud noise.

Older people have a poorer sense of taste and smell and are less stimulated by food than the young. It is common for the sense of smell to decline more than the sense of taste. These changes significantly affect appetite in the older adult, contributing to poor nutrition. Decreased or absent sense of smell and taste also add to the health hazard of increased salt usage and safety issues (e.g., being unable to smell a gas leak). It is important for the nurse to teach the older adult and family about the safety issues involved with a decreased sense of taste and smell and what strategies can be implemented to promote safety (e.g., dating and labeling foods, using smoke alarms).

Loss of skin receptors takes place gradually, producing an increased threshold for sensations of pain, touch, and temperature. The older person may not be able to distinguish hot from cold or the intensity of heat. Stimuli causing severe pain in a younger person may cause only minor sensation or pressure in older adults. This places the older adult at higher risk for burns and other injuries. Again, it is important for the nurse to teach about the involved safety risks and subsequent interventions (e.g., setting the temperature of the water heater to 110°F to prevent scalding).

Pulmonary

Respiratory efficiency is reduced with age. Tidal volume (the amount of air moved in and out during normal respiration) remains the same, but the older adult has a decreased vital capacity. This means the older adult is unable to compensate for increased oxygen need by significantly increasing the amount of air inspired. Dyspnea (difficult breathing) occurs frequently with increased activity, such as running for a bus or carrying heavy parcels upstairs. A greater volume of residual air is left in the lungs after expiration, and the capacity to cough efficiently decreases because of weaker expiratory muscles. Mucous secretions tend to collect more readily in the respiratory tree. Thus susceptibility to respiratory infections increases with age.

Health promotion teaching includes information about the following:

- Cessation of smoking, if appropriate
- Preventing respiratory infections by washing hands
- Ensuring the influenza and pneumonia vaccinations are up to date

Cardiovascular

The working capacity of the heart diminishes with age. This is particularly evident when increased demands are made on the heart, such as during periods of exercise or emotional stress. The heart rate at normal rest may decrease with age. However, the heart rate of the older person is slower to respond to stress and slower to return to normal after periods of physical activity.

Changes in the arteries occur concurrently. Reduced arterial elasticity may result in diminished blood supply to, for instance, the legs and the brain, resulting in pain on exertion in the calf muscles and dizziness, respectively. In addition, there may be a delay in the circulatory adjustments required when a person quickly stands up from a lying or sitting position. The delay results in an abrupt drop in systolic blood pressure known as *orthostatic hypotension*.

For blood pressure measurements, it is not unusual to have a slight increase in the systolic pressure while the diastolic pressure remains the same. For many years, isolated systolic hypertension was considered to be "normal" in older adults, and was frequently not treated. Newer evidence indicates that a systolic pressure of greater than 140 mm Hg is as problematic in older adults as in younger ones, and should be as aggressively treated (Joint National Committee on Prevention, Detection, Evaluation, and Treatment of High Blood Pressure [JNC 7], 2003). A significant increase in blood pressure is more likely the result of other factors such as diet, weight, or stress rather than age (Polan & Taylor, 2007).

Health promotion activities involve detecting and reducing risks for cardiovascular disease. To detect risks, the older adult should have his or her blood pressure checked annually. The older adult should be aware of his or her cholesterol level and have it rechecked at appropriate intervals, depending on the results of the blood test (e.g., the higher the level, the more frequently it should be rechecked). To reduce risks of cardiovascular disease, the nurse should inform the client about the importance of the following: smoking cessation (if applicable), maintaining ideal body weight, exercising daily, avoiding foods high in sodium and fat and eating fruits and vegetables, and discussing the use of low-dose aspirin therapy with the primary provider (Miller, 2004).

Gastrointestinal

Age-related changes in the gastrointestinal system include:

- Periodontal disease, which can lead to tooth loss. With age, tooth enamel becomes harder and more brittle, making teeth more susceptible to fractures. The root of the tooth shrinks and the gingival retracts. The bones that support the teeth decrease in density and height, all leading to tooth loss (Eliopoulos, 2009).
- Reduced saliva which may lead to xerostomia (dry mouth) and make the oral mucosa of the older adult more susceptible to infection.
- Decreased esophageal motility slowing the esophageal emptying process.
- Decreased stomach motility and emptying time. Also, a higher pH of the stomach contributes to increased incidence of gastric irritation in the older adult.
- Decreased production of intrinsic factor leading to pernicious anemia.
- Decreased intestinal absorption, motility, and blood flow.

Health promotion teaching for older adults includes effective oral hygiene and preventive dental care (e.g., semiannual teeth cleaning). Nutrition is important including appropriate diet and sufficient fluid intake. Maintenance of a regular bowel routine is helpful, and screening for colorectal cancer is important (e.g., annual fecal occult blood test, sigmoidoscopy every 5 years, and colonoscopy every 10 years) (Meiner & Lueckenotte, 2006, p. 563).

Urinary

The excretory function of the kidney diminishes with age, but usually not significantly below normal levels unless a disease process intervenes. The kidney's filtering abilities may also be impaired; thus waste products may be filtered and excreted more slowly. For this reason, the nurse should be aware of whether medications that are administered are excreted via the kidney or liver. Drugs that are metabolized predominantly in the kidney may accumulate in the older adult, and the nurse needs to watch for signs of toxicity.

More noticeable changes are those related to the bladder. Complaints of urinary urgency and urinary frequency are common. The capacity of the bladder and its ability to completely empty diminish with age. Many older adults need to arise during the night to void (nocturia) and may experience retention of residual urine, predisposing them to bladder infections.

Although susceptible to urinary incontinence (UI) because of changes in the kidney and bladder, UI is *never* normal. The nurse must promptly investigate UI, particularly when of new onset. Urinary incontinence has many ill effects on older adults, including social isolation, falls, and skin breakdown.

The nurse can teach the following health promotion activities for good urinary function in the older adult:

- Drink sufficient fluids daily (e.g., 8 to 10 glasses of noncaffeinated liquid).
- Drink fluids even if you do not feel thirsty. (The thirst mechanism in older adults is diminished.)
- Avoid foods that can irritate the bladder (e.g., sugar, caffeine, alcohol, chocolate, artificial sweeteners, and spicy and acidic foods).
- Practice pelvic muscle exercises to stop or control stress incontinence.

The nurse should explain that incontinence is not a normal change related to aging.

Genitals

Degenerative changes in the gonads are gradual in men. Production of testosterone continues, and the testes can produce sperm well into old age although there is a gradual decrease in the number of sperm produced. In women the degenerative changes in the ovaries are noticed by the cessation of menses in middle age during the menopause.

Changes in the gonads of older women result from diminished secretion of the ovarian hormones. Some changes, such as the shrinking of the uterus and ovaries, go unnoticed. Other changes are obvious. The breasts atrophy, and lubricating vaginal secretions are reduced. Reduced natural lubrication may be the cause of painful intercourse, which may be addressed through the use of lubricating jellies.

The older man will notice several age-related changes in his sexual response and performance, but it is important for both the client and nurse to know that sexual response and performance should be present in the older adult. For both men and women, the major age-related change in sexual response is timing: it takes longer to become sexually aroused, longer to complete intercourse, and longer before sexual arousal can occur again (Butler & Lewis, 2003). In general, the man's libido may decrease, but not disappear. If the man reports a loss in sexual interest, the nurse should be as concerned as when a younger man reports a loss of interest in sexual activity. Older men achieve an erection that is less firm than in younger men, but still capable of penetration. Ejaculation may take longer to occur, and the older man may have difficulty anticipating or delaying ejaculation.

Older women also experience changes in their sexual responses. It takes longer for the woman to become sexually aroused and produce vaginal lubrication, and the labia and uterus do not fully elevate, making penetration slightly more difficult (Butler & Lewis, 2003). The clitoris remains an important part of orgasm, but may become irritated more easily because the clitoral hood is less protective than in younger women. During orgasm, the uterus will contract less frequently, but the contractions remain vigorous, and orgasm is as intense as in younger women.

The nurse needs excellent communication skills when providing health education about sexual function. A survey of older adults found that they prefer that the health care professional use open, respectful, nonjudgmental, and plain English when discussing sexuality (Miller, 2004, p. 488). Older adults are fully capable of enjoying sexual activity. If they experience problems with sexual function, they should seek professional advice from their primary care provider or other appropriate health care professional.

PSYCHOSOCIAL AGING

A number of theories have attempted to explain psychosocial aging. These theories focus on behavior and attitude changes during the aging process. One of the earliest, **disengagement theories**, developed in the early 1960s by Cumming and Henry, proposed that aging involves mutual withdrawal (disengagement) between the older person and others in their environment. It has been widely criticized for the assumptions that disengagement is appropriate for the older adult. According to Havighurst's activity theory, the best way to age is to stay active physically and mentally, and according to Atchley's **continuity theory**, people maintain their values, habits, and behavior in old age. A person who is accustomed to having people around will continue to do so, and the person who prefers not to be involved with others is more likely to disengage. This theory accounts for the great variety of behavior seen in older people.

According to Erikson, the developmental task at this time is ego integrity versus despair. People who attain ego integrity view life with a sense of wholeness and derive satisfaction from past accomplishments. They view death as an acceptable completion of life. People who develop integrity accept "one's one and only life cycle" (Erikson, 1963, p. 263). By contrast, people who despair often believe they have made poor choices during life and wish they could live life over.

Acknowledging that the "young-old" and "old-old" differ not only in physical characteristics but also in psychosocial responses, many people have difficulty with Erikson's singular developmental task. Peck (1968) proposed the following three developmental tasks of the older adult in contrast to Erikson's task of ego integrity versus despair:

1. Ego differentiation versus work-role preoccupation
2. Body transcendence versus body preoccupation
3. Ego transcendence versus ego preoccupation

For details about these tasks see Chapter 9 ∞. See Box 10–3 for further developmental tasks of the older adult.

Retirement

A majority of the people in the United States over age 65 are unemployed (FIFAS, 2008). However, many who are healthy continue to work on a full- or part-time basis. Work offers these people a better income, a sense of self-worth, and the chance to continue long-established routines. It is important to remember that setting the retirement age at 65 is arbitrary and has no relationship to the abilities of the worker. Also, some older adults need to work for economic reasons. Retirement usually causes income to decrease by 35% or more (Meiner & Lueckenotte, 2006, p. 143). Older

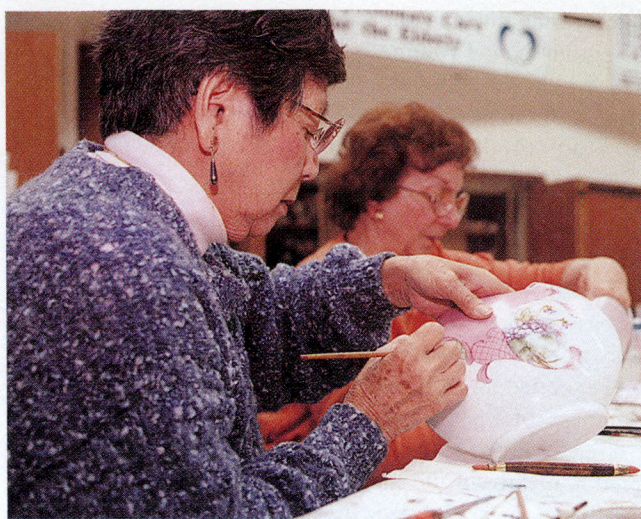

Figure 10–2 ● Many older adults find creative outlets during retirement.

adults may find that their retirement income has not kept up with inflation. They may also realize that they need to continue working to meet medical and insurance costs.

Retirement can be a time when projects or recreational activities deferred for a long time can be pursued, or it can be a difficult time of adjustment. Either way, retirement requires a process of adaptation (see Figure 10–2). Retired people are no longer governed by an alarm clock and can get up when they please. The enjoyment of staying up later is another luxury. Few older adults, however, spend much time resting or sleeping. Being accustomed to activity most of their lives, most find many outlets, including jobs, community projects, travel, volunteer services, intellectual or recreational pursuits, or hobbies (Figure 10–3).

The lifestyle of later years is to a large degree formulated in youth. This fact was recognized by the poet Robert Browning: "Grow old along with me! / The best is yet to be, / The last of life, for which the first was made." People who attempt suddenly to refocus and enrich their lives at retirement usually have difficulty. Those who learned early in life to live well-balanced and fulfilling lives are generally more successful in retirement. The woman who has been concerned only with the accomplishments of her children or the man who has been concerned only with the paycheck and his job status can be left with a feeling of emptiness when children leave and the job no longer exists. The later years can foster a sense of integrity and continuity, or they can be years of despair.

Economic Change

The financial needs of older adults vary considerably (FIFAS, 2008). Though most need less money for clothing, entertainment, and work, and although some own their homes outright, costs continue to rise, making it difficult for some to manage. Food and medical costs alone are often a financial burden. Adequate financial resources enable the older person to remain independent.

BOX 10–3	Developmental Tasks of the Older Adult

65 to 74 Years

- Adjusting to decreasing physical strength and health
- Adjusting to retirement and lower and fixed income
- Adjusting to the death of parents, spouses, and friends
- Adjusting to new relationships with adult children
- Adjusting to leisure time
- Adjusting to slower physical and cognitive responses
- Keeping active and involved
- Making satisfying living arrangements as aging progresses

75 Years and Older

- Adapting to living alone
- Safeguarding physical and mental health
- Adjusting to the possibility of moving into a nursing home
- Remaining in touch with other family members
- Finding meaning in life
- Adjusting to one's own death

Note: Modified from *Health Promotion Strategies Through the Life Span,* 8th ed., by R. B. Murray, J. P. Zentner, & R. Yakimo, 2009, Upper Saddle River, NJ: Pearson Education.

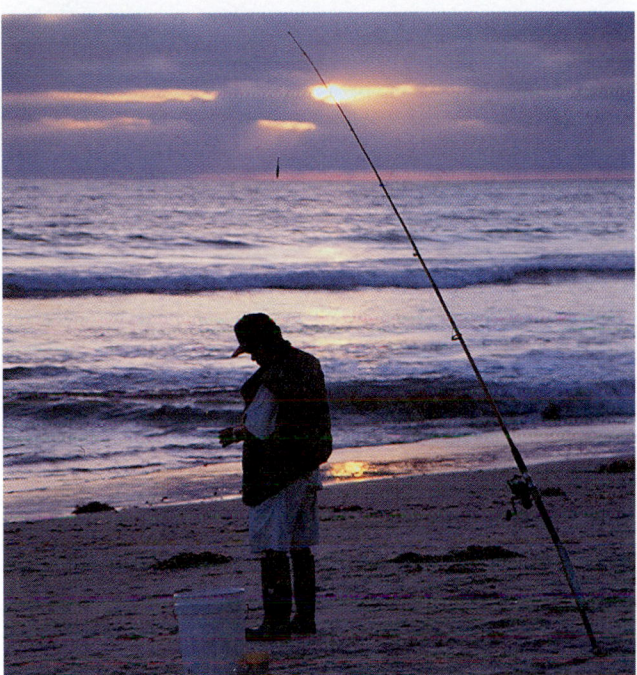

Figure 10–3 ● Retirement provides time for enjoying hobbies.

Problems with income are often related to low retirement benefits, lack of pension plans for many workers, and the increased length of the retirement years. Older members of minority groups often have greater financial problems than older whites (FIFAS, 2008). Older women of all ages usually have lower incomes than men, and the oldest women may be the poorest.

Nurses should be aware of the costs of health care. For example, while assisting a client to plan a diet, the nurse must consider which foods the client can afford to buy. The nurse or the client can request the physician to order lower priced medications, or assist the older client to apply for medication assistance programs operated by pharmaceutical companies. In addition, the supplies used in a client's care should be as economical as possible.

Grandparenting

Grandparents traditionally provide gifts, money, and other forms of support (e.g., baby-sitting) for younger family members. They also provide a sense of continuity, family heritage, rituals, and folklore (Ebersole, Hess, Touhy, & Jett, 2009). However, the rate of grandparents being the primary caregiver for their grandchildren is increasing. The major reasons for grandparents raising grandchildren include substance abuse, incarceration, teen pregnancy, emotional problems, and parental death (Butler & Zakari, 2005).

While loving their grandchildren, the grandparents often experience stress, anxiety, financial hardships, and potential deteriorating health. For example, they must cope with their own chronic health problems while caring for their grandchildren. It is important for nurses to assess and help maintain the health of the grandparents.

Relocation

During late adulthood, many people experience relocation. A variety of factors may lead to this decision. The house or apartment may be too large or too expensive. The work involved in maintaining the house may become burdensome or impossible for the aged person or couple. Some older adults with decreased mobility want living arrangements that are all on one floor or need more accessible bathroom facilities.

Making the decision to move is stressful. Moving to an apartment may mean leaving the comfort of the family home and the neighbors and friends of several decades. Some older adults need to move nearer to their children for general support and supervision. For many, this decision is difficult and stressful. For others, relocation is voluntary. The person may be seeking a more moderate climate with better recreational facilities geared to a more leisurely lifestyle. Adjustment will be much easier for the older adult making a voluntary move.

More living choices and options are available for the older adult today. Depending on their needs, examples include:

- *Assisted living.* This is a facility that meets the needs of the older person (e.g., wide doorways, grab bars in the bathroom, a call light). Various degrees of personal care assistance may be provided.
- *Adult day care.* The older adult who lives at home can attend a day-care center that provides health and social services to the older person. While the older adult is at day care, the caregiver has a respite from the daily care.
- *Adult foster care and group homes.* These programs offer services to individuals who can care for themselves but require some form of supervision for safety purposes.

Some older adults, however, must relocate to long-term care facilities or nursing homes. The decision to enter a nursing home is frequently made when they can no longer care for themselves, often because of problems of mobility and memory impairment. The facilities in nursing homes differ in many ways and offer varying degrees of independence to the residents. All provide meals but vary in giving other services, such as assistance with hygiene and dressing, physical therapy or exercise, recreational activities, transportation services, and medical and nursing supervision.

Nurses in hospitals should find out whether a client is being discharged to a nursing home or to a private home. Nursing homes require appropriate information to provide for continuity of care, and the older adult often requires emotional support when they are unable to return to their home. Clients returning home, however, may require the assistance of a home care nurse.

Maintaining Independence and Self-Esteem

Most American older adults thrive on independence. It is important to them to be able to look after themselves even if they have to struggle to do so. Although it may be difficult for younger family members to watch an older person completing tasks in a slow, determined way, older adults need this sense of accomplishment. Children might notice that the aging father or mother with failing vision cannot keep the kitchen as clean as before. The aging parent may be slower and less meticulous in carpentry tasks or gardening. To maintain the older adult's sense of self-respect, nurses and family members need to encourage them to do as much as possible for themselves, provided that safety is maintained. Many young people, including nurses, mistakenly think that they are helpful to older adults when they take over for them and do the job much faster and more efficiently.

Nurses need to acknowledge the older adult's ability to think, reason, and make decisions. Most are willing to listen to suggestions and advice, but they do not want to be ordered around. The nurse can support a decision by an older adult even if eventually the decision is reversed because of failing health.

Older adults appreciate the same thoughtfulness, consideration, and acceptance of their abilities as younger people do. They are not "wrinkled babies," and certainly do not represent a homogeneous group. There is as much diversity among older adults as there is in any other population group, and the nurse should be just as wary of stereotyping older adults as with stereotyping any other group. The values and standards held by older people need to be accepted, whether they are related to ethical, religious, or household matters. For example, the nurse should respect an older person's decision to hang the laundry outside rather than to use a dryer, or to cook on a conventional stove rather than in a microwave oven.

Facing Death and Grieving

Well-adjusted aging couples usually thrive on companionship. Many couples rely increasingly on their partners for this company and may have few outside friends. Great bonds of affection and closeness can develop during this period of aging together and nurturing each other. When a mate dies, the remaining partner inevitably experiences feelings of loss, emptiness, and loneliness. Many are capable of living alone and can manage to do so; however, reliance on younger family members may increase as age advances and ill health occurs. Some widows and widowers remarry, particularly the latter because most widowers are less inclined than widows to maintain a household.

More women than men face bereavement and solitude because women usually live longer (FIFAS, 2008). Older adults are often reminded of the brevity of life by the death of friends. It is a time when they review their life with happiness or regret. Feelings of serenity or guilt and inadequacy can arise. Independence established prior to loss of a partner makes this adjustment period easier. A person who has some meaningful friendships, economic security, ongoing interests in the community, private hobbies, and a peaceful philosophy of life copes more easily with bereavement.

Successful relationships with children and grandchildren are also of inestimable value. See Chapter 30 ∞ for a discussion about facing death.

Nurses help clients who are alone a great deal to adjust to their living arrangements or lifestyle so that they have more companionship. Moving to a retirement home that has other people in similar circumstances and organized social activities is one example. Many communities provide social centers for the older adults, for example, drop-in centers or community centers that offer day trips for seniors. Nurses refer clients to services and encourage them to obtain companionship.

COGNITIVE ABILITIES AND AGING

Piaget's phases of cognitive development end with the formal operations phase. However, considerable research on cognitive abilities and aging is currently being conducted. Intellectual capacity includes perception, cognitive agility, memory, and learning.

Perception

Perception, or the ability to interpret the environment, depends on the acuteness of the senses. If the aging person's senses are impaired, the ability to perceive the environment and react appropriately is diminished. Changes in the nervous system may also affect perceptual capacity.

Changes in the cognitive structures occur as a person ages. The brain loses mass with aging. In addition, blood flow to the brain decreases, the meninges thicken, and brain metabolism slows. As yet, little is known about the effect of these physical changes on the cognitive functioning of the older adult. Lifelong mental activity, particularly verbal activity, helps the older adult retain a high level of cognitive function and helps maintain long-term memory.

Cognitive Ability

In older adults, changes in cognitive abilities are more often a difference in speed than in ability. Overall the older adult maintains intelligence, problem solving, judgment, creativity, and other well-practiced cognitive skills. Intellectual loss generally reflects a disease process such as atherosclerosis, which causes the blood vessels to narrow and diminishes perfusion of nutrients to the brain. Most older adults do not experience cognitive impairments, with only 15% of older men and 11% of older women manifesting moderate or severe memory impairment (FIFAS, 2008). It is important to note, however, that memory impairment is more prevalent in persons over age 85 than persons between the ages of 65 and 69. Cognitive impairment that interferes with normal life is not considered part of normal aging. A decline in intellectual abilities that interferes with social or occupational functions should always be regarded as abnormal. Family members should be advised to seek prompt medical evaluation.

Memory

Memory is also a component of intellectual capacity that involves the following steps:

1. Momentary perception of stimuli from the environment referred to as **sensory memory**.
2. Storage in **short-term memory** (information held in the brain for immediate use or what one has in mind at a given moment). An example of this type of memory is when you call information for a telephone number and remember the number only for the brief time needed to dial the number. Short-term memory also deals with activities or the recent past of minutes to a few hours that is often referred to as **recent memory**.
3. Encoding in which the information leaves short-term memory and enters **long-term memory**, the repository for information stored for periods longer than 72 hours and usually weeks and years. Memories of childhood friends, teachers, and events are stored in long-term memory. Older people who remember the flowers in their wedding bouquet or the names of the boys on their dance card are drawing from long-term memory.

In older adults, retrieval of information from long-term memory can be slower, especially if the information is not frequently used. Most age-related differences, however, occur in short-term memory. Older adults tend to forget the recent past. This forgetfulness can be improved by the use of memory aids, making notes or lists, and placing objects in consistent locations.

Learning

Older people need additional time for learning, largely because of the problem of retrieving information. Motivation is also important. Older adults have more difficulty than younger ones in learning information they do not consider meaningful; therefore, the nurse should be particularly careful to discover what is meaningful to the older adult before attempting client education. See Chapter 14 ∞.

MORAL REASONING

Much of the theoretical and empirical work related to moral development in older adults was conducted in the 1980s, and few current studies can be found. According to Kohlberg (1984), moral development is completed in the early adult years. Kohlberg hypothesized that an older person at the preconventional level obeys rules to avoid pain and the displeasure of others. At stage 1, a person defines good and bad in relation to self, whereas older people at stage 2 may act to meet another's needs as well as their own. Older adults at the conventional level follow society's rules of conduct in response to the expectations of others. Pratt, Diessner, Pratt, Hunsberger, and Pancer (1996) found that moral reasoning does not decline in old age.

Gilligan (1982), however, challenged Kohlberg's stages as not being applicable to women. She developed a theory of moral reasoning based on the concept of caring. She believed that women base moral judgments on connectedness to others and the value of relationships, while Kohlberg based his stages on concepts of justice, objectivity, and preservation of rights. Subsequent research has demonstrated that men and women do make moral decisions differently, and represent Kohlberg (men) and Gilligan (women) along gender lines. Older adults, however, begin to make moral decisions that are consistent with *both* Kohlberg and Gilligan (Pinch & Parsons, 1997). Older men consider relationships, as well as justice, in moral decisions, and older women add justice to the factors they consider in moral situations.

The value and belief patterns that are important to older adults may be different from those held by younger people because they developed during a time that was very different from today. In addition, a large number of today's older adults are either foreign-born or first-generation citizens. Cultural background, life experiences, gender, religion, and socioeconomic status all influence one's values. The nurse must identify and consider the specific values of the older client when nursing care is planned.

SPIRITUALITY AND AGING

Older adults can contemplate new religious and philosophical views and try to understand ideas missed previously or interpreted differently. The older person may derive a sense of worth by sharing experiences or views. In contrast, the older adult who has not matured spiritually may feel impoverishment or despair as the drive for economic and professional success lessens.

Many older adults take their faith and religious practice very seriously, and display a high level of spirituality. It would be a mistake, however, to assume that religiosity increases with age. Today's older adults grew up in a time when religion was much more important than it is for younger people today. The participation of older adults in religious organizations, therefore, is more likely to be a continuation of lifelong habits than a correlate of aging (McFadden, 1996). Many older people have strong religious convictions and continue to attend religious meetings or services. Involvement in religion often helps the older adult to resolve issues related to the meaning of life, to adversity, or to good fortune. Religion may also be an important coping resource, leading to enhanced well-being. The "old-old" person who cannot attend formal services often continues religious participation in a more private manner. Assisting the older person to participate in religious and spiritual practices is an important nursing responsibility.

HEALTH PROBLEMS

Health problems that older adults may experience include injuries, chronic disabling diseases such as hypertension and arthritis, drug abuse and misuse, alcoholism, dementia, and abuse. Leading causes of death in people ages 65 and over are heart disease, cancer, cerebrovascular disease (stroke), lower respiratory disease, pneumonia/influenza, and diabetes mellitus (FIFAS, 2008).

Injuries

Injury prevention is a major concern for older people. *Healthy People 2010* (USDHHS, 2000) reports that falls account for 87% of all fractures among adults 65 years and older (pp. 13–15). Because vision is limited, reflexes are slowed, and bones are brittle, caution is required in climbing stairs, driving a car, and even walking. Driving, particularly night driving, requires caution because accommodation of the eye to light is impaired and peripheral vision is diminished. Older persons need to learn to turn the head before changing lanes and should not rely on side vision, for example, when crossing a street. Driving in fog or other hazardous conditions should be avoided.

Fires are a hazard for the older adult with a failing memory. They may forget that the iron or stove is left on or may not extinguish a cigarette completely. Because of reduced sensitivity to pain and heat, care must be taken to prevent burns when the person bathes or uses heating devices.

Many older adults suffer and die each year from hypothermia. Hypothermia is a body temperature below normal. A lowered metabolism and loss of normal insulation from thinning subcutaneous tissue decrease the older client's ability to retain heat. The older adult who spends time outdoors in cold weather, or who does not turn on the heat in the home is at significant risk for hypothermia.

Nurses can help older adults make the home environment safe by identifying and correcting specific hazards; for example, installing handrails on staircases. The nurse teaches the importance of taking only prescribed medications and contacting a health professional at the first indication of intolerance to them.

Persons with Alzheimer's disease or other types of dementia experience increasing safety needs as their condition deteriorates. Judgment becomes impaired as the disease progresses, and some environmental modification is needed to help the older adult remain safe. Some of these are keeping poisons and medications out of reach (preferably locked up), taking knobs off kitchen stoves to prevent burns and fires, and putting special locks on doors for persons who tend to wander. Attention should be given to these potential problems whether the client lives at home or is in a health facility.

Guidelines for injury prevention for the older adult are detailed in Chapter 21 ∞.

Chronic Disabling Illness

Many older adults function well within the community without impairments; others are afflicted with one or more chronic illnesses that may seriously impair their functioning. Examples of these are arthritis, osteoporosis, heart disease, stroke, obstructive lung disease, hearing and visual alterations, and cognitive dysfunctions. In addition, acute illnesses such as pneumonia, fractures, trauma from falls, motor vehicle crashes, or other incidents may create chronic health problems. Chronic illness brings many changes to the client and the family members. The client, for example, may need increasing help with the activities of daily living such as ambulation, feeding, hygiene, and so on; health care expenses often escalate and may become an economic concern; family roles may need to be altered; and family members may need to change their lifestyle to meet caregiving needs.

Drug Use and Misuse

The average older adult in the United States takes four to five prescription drugs and two over-the-counter (OTC) medicines every day. Episodes of acute illness may require additional medications. Clients may purchase OTC drugs to remedy common discomforts related to aging, such as constipation, sleep disturbance, and joint pain. Over the last few years, the use of vitamins, food supplements, and herbal remedies has increased. These agents fall under the category of OTC drugs and are often not reported by clients as part of their medicine regimen. An accurate assessment should include a listing of all these agents. Many of these agents have not had adequate testing for effectiveness, side effects, or interactions with other medications.

The complexities involved in the self-administration of medication may lead to a variety of misuse situations, including taking too much or too little medication, combining alcohol and medication, combining prescribed medications with OTC drugs, taking medications at the wrong time, or taking someone else's medication. Other potential misuse situations occur when more than one primary care provider prescribes medications and the client fails to tell each primary care provider what has been previously prescribed.

Additionally, the pharmacodynamics of drugs are altered in older adults. The variations in absorption, distribution, metabolism, and excretion of drugs are related to physiologic changes associated with aging. These variations are discussed in Chapter 23 ∞.

Most older adults living independently in the community take their medications with no supervision. Therefore, education about medications is important for safe medication-taking behaviors (Miller, 2004). The following strategies, taught by the nurse, can promote safe medication use by the older adult:

- Write a list of all the medications you are taking, including over-the-counter drugs and herbal supplements. Include any medication allergies on the list. Keep the list current and carry it in your purse or billfold.
- Know the reason you are taking each medication. Ask your primary care practitioner the reason for any new medication.
- Consider using a "pill organizer" system to help you remember to take your medications. This is helpful if you have many medications to take each day.
- Ask your pharmacist for easy-to-open containers if you have difficulty opening the medications.

RESEARCH
NOTES How Do You Take Away the Car Keys?

The issue of older drivers is a troublesome one. Driving is an important aspect of autonomy, and cherished by many older adults; yet there are concerns for the safety of the older driver as well as for others on the road. Nurses may be asked to assist family members to convince an older adult to stop driving.

The researchers studied interventions used to stop cognitively impaired older adults from driving. Older adults with mild cognitive impairment, family members of such adults, and professionals in geriatric care (n = 216) were interviewed about the decision to stop an older adult from driving, and the ways used to enforce the decision. The data were qualitatively analyzed using a grounded theory methodology. There was more agreement than disagreement among those interviewed. Unsafe behaviors that the participants identified included getting lost easily, being less aware of other drivers and pedestrians, and forgetting how to use equipment, such as brakes, in the car. Themes related to an increased likelihood that cognitively impaired older adults continued to drive included a desire to drive, availability of a car, lack of alternative transportation, and the willingness of someone to ride with the impaired older adult and "co-pilot." Strategies to keep the impaired older adult from driving fell into two main categories: those that included the older adult in the decision-making process, and those that were imposed by professionals or significant others. Involving the older adult in the decision making is an important nursing goal, but a restriction may need to be imposed for safety reasons. Factors that facilitate a successful intervention include a strong relationship between the older adult, primary care provider, and family members, and the obviousness of the driving impairment including "near misses."

Participants in the study identified the following strategies that family members can initiate, with coaching by the primary care provider:

- Begin to discuss the possibility of giving up driving before safety is a concern.
- Observe the older adult's driving abilities, and point out specific driving errors in a nonjudgmental way.
- Acknowledge that giving up driving is a loss for the older adult.
- Develop a feasible plan for alternative transportation.
- Point out the possibility of harming someone, or of possible legal action and financial repercussions.
- Have the older adult tested for driving safety. State and local agencies may be helpful in identifying sites that will specifically test for driving safety in relation to cognitive impairment.

Implications

Both the autonomy and the safety of the older adult and others are nursing concerns. Anticipatory guidance may help ease the transition from independent mobility to collaborative mobility with alternative transportation. Many rehabilitation facilities will test older adults for driver safety.

Note: Reprinted from *Geriatric Nursing*, vol. 26, by K. Jett, R. M. Tappen, and M. Rosselli, "Imposed Versus Involved: Different Strategies to Effect Driving Cessation in Cognitively Impaired Older Adults," pp. 111–116. Copyright 2005, with permission from Elsevier.

- If possible, obtain all medications from the same pharmacy. This allows the pharmacist to monitor for drug duplications and interactions.

Alcoholism

There are two types of older alcoholics: those who began drinking alcohol in their youth and those who began excessive alcohol use later in life to help them cope with the changes and problems of their older years. Many late-onset alcoholics are widowers.

Chronic drinking has major effects on all body systems, causes progressive liver and kidney damage, damages the stomach and related organs, and slows mental response, frequently leading to injuries and death. Alcohol interacts with various drugs, altering the normal effect of the medication on the body. Some medications have an increased effect when taken with alcohol (e.g., anticoagulants and narcotics), whereas the action of other medications (e.g., antibiotics) is inhibited. For the older adult who has a chronic illness and takes many medications, the combination of drugs and alcohol can lead to serious drug overdose.

Clients who are alcoholics should not be stereotyped or prejudged by the nurse. Rather, they should be accepted, listened to, and offered help. The nurse should assess the number and type of alcoholic beverages consumed as well as the pattern and frequency of consumption. It is important that the nurse discuss any medications the client is taking and review the side effects and interaction effects of alcohol and medication. The role of the nurse is to act as a client advocate and facilitate the treatment of the drinking problem in addition to the prevention of possible complications.

Dementia

Dementia is a progressive loss of cognitive function. It is critical that dementia be differentiated from delirium, an acute and reversible syndrome. Both may be characterized by changes in memory, judgment, language, mathematic calculation, abstract reasoning, and problem-solving ability. The most common causes of delirium are infection, medications, and dehydration. The most common type of dementia is Alzheimer's disease (AD), although there are other dementias. The cause of Alzheimer's disease is unknown, and the course is slow and insidious. Alzheimer's disease affects about 4.5 million people in the United States. Unless a prevention or cure is found, 14 million Americans will have Alzheimer's disease by the year 2050 (Agency on Aging, 2009).

The symptoms of AD may vary somewhat from client to client. The most prominent symptoms are cognitive

MyNursingKit | Alzheimer's Disease

dysfunctions, including decline in memory, learning, attention, judgment, orientation, and language skills. The symptoms are progressive and exhibit a steady decline in cognitive and physical abilities, lasting between 7 and 15 years and ending in death. In the last stage, the client requires total assistance, is unable to communicate, is incontinent, and may be unable to walk. There is no cure or specific treatment for AD. Several drugs have been developed, but none has been shown consistently to reverse the progression of the disease.

It is estimated that about 1 million people with AD are cared for in the home. The burden of care is frequently on women—wives and daughters—who are themselves aging. AD is devastating for the families and caregivers of its victims. The caregivers may experience physical and emotional exhaustion while they render continuous care. Caregiving is complicated when the client no longer recognizes family members or close friends. The nurse's responsibility is to provide supportive nursing care, accurate information, and referral assistance, if placement in a nursing care facility becomes necessary. Respite services may also be very helpful to the caregiver. It is important for the nurse to do an ongoing assessment of both the client and the caregiver, because changes will occur as the client's condition deteriorates.

Older Adult Mistreatment

Approximately 1 million to 2 million Americans over the age of 65 have been abused, neglected, or exploited (National Research Council Panel to Review Risk and Prevalence of Elder Abuse and Neglect, 2003). Older adult mistreatment may affect either sex; however, the victims most often are women over 75 years of age, physically or mentally impaired, and dependent for care on the abuser. The abuse may involve physical, psychologic, or emotional abuse; sexual abuse; financial abuse; violation of human or civil rights; and active or passive neglect.

When older adult mistreatment involves physical neglect, victims may suffer from dehydration, malnutrition, and oversedation. The victim may be deprived of necessary articles, such as glasses, hearing aids, or walkers. Psychologically, the person may suffer verbal assaults, threats, humiliation, or harassment. Abuse may also include failure to provide appropriate medications or medical treatment, isolation, unreasonable confinement, lack of privacy, an unsafe environment, and involuntary servitude. Some are financially exploited by relatives who steal from them or misuse their property or funds. Others are beaten and even raped by family members. Most victims experience two or more forms of abuse.

Older adult abuse or neglect may occur in private homes, senior citizens' homes, nursing homes, hospitals, and long-term care facilities. Many of the abusers are either sons or daughters; others include spouses, relatives (grandchildren, siblings, nieces, and nephews), and in some instances health care providers.

Older adults at home may fail to report abuse or neglect for many reasons. They may be ashamed to admit that their children have mistreated them or fear retaliation if they seek help. They may fear being sent to an institution. They frequently lack financial resources or lack the mental capacity to be aware of abuse or neglect and to report the situation. Examples of crimes are assault and financial abuse of an older person who is physically or mentally incompetent and has no trustworthy friend or relative to help. In some instances, nurses can intervene by educating caregivers about the needs of older adults and available resources to provide increased home support. They should also report the situation to the appropriate person in the health care agency.

Nurses should be familiar with the laws of their particular state regarding the reporting of suspected or known abuse. The legally competent adult cannot be forced, however, to leave the abusive situation and in many cases may decide to stay. If the client is not legally competent, court proceedings to attain guardianship can be initiated.

HEALTH ASSESSMENT AND PROMOTION

Assessment guidelines for the development of the older adult are shown in the accompanying Developmental Assessment Guidelines. Assessment activities include measurement of weight, height, and vital signs; observation of the skin for hydration status or presence of lesions; examination of visual acuity using the Snellen chart; examination of hearing acuity using the Weber and Rinne tests (see Chapter 17 ∞); and questions about the following:

- Usual dietary pattern
- Any problems with bowel or urinary elimination
- Activity/exercise and sleep/rest patterns
- Family and social activities and interests
- Any problems with reading, writing, or problem solving
- Adjustment to retirement or loss of partner

Health care professionals should also be alert for these signs:

- Symptoms of depression
- Risk factors for suicide
- Signs of abnormal bereavement
- Changes in cognitive function
- Medications that increase risk of falls
- Signs of physical abuse or neglect
- Skin lesions (malignant and peripheral)
- Tooth decay, gingivitis, loose teeth
- Peripheral arterial disease

Older persons are usually concerned about their health and interested in information and behavioral strategies directed toward improving it. The nurse may wish to discuss some or all of the health promotion topics outlined in Box 10–4. These topics are discussed in detail in subsequent chapters throughout the book.

DEVELOPMENTAL ASSESSMENT GUIDELINES
The Older Adult

In these three developmental areas, does the older adult do the following?

Physical Development

- Adjust to physiologic changes (e.g., appearance, sensory/perceptual, musculoskeletal, neurologic, cardiovascular).
- Adapt lifestyle to diminishing energy and ability.
- Maintain vital signs (especially blood pressure) within normal range for age and sex.

Psychosocial Development

- Manage retirement years in a satisfying manner.
- Participate in social and leisure activities.

- Have a social network of friends and support persons.
- View life as worthwhile.
- Have high self-esteem.
- Gain support from value system and/or spiritual philosophy.
- Accept and adjust to the death of significant others.

Development in Activities of Daily Living

- Exhibit healthy practices in nutrition, exercise, recreation, sleep patterns, and personal habits.
- Have the ability to care for self or to secure appropriate help with activities of daily living.
- Have satisfactory living arrangements and income to meet changing needs.

BOX 10–4 | **Health Promotion Guidelines for Older Adults**

Health Tests and Screening

- Total cholesterol and high-density lipid protein measurement every 3 to 5 years until age 75
- Aspirin, 81 mg, daily, if in high-risk group
- Diabetes mellitus screen every 3 years, if in high-risk group
- Smoking cessation
- Screening mammogram every 1 to 2 years (women)
- Clinical breast exam annually (women)
- Pap smear annually if there is a history of abnormal smears or previous hysterectomy for malignancy (United States Preventive Services Task Force, 2003)
  - Older women who have regular, normal Pap smears or hysterectomy for nonmalignant causes do NOT need Pap smears beyond the age of 65 (United States Preventive Services Task Force, 2003).
- Annual digital rectal exam
- Annual prostate-specific antigen (PSA)
- Annual fecal occult blood test (FOBT)
- Sigmoidoscopy every 5 years; colonoscopy every 10 years
- Visual acuity screen annually
- Hearing screen annually
- Depression screen periodically
- Family violence screen periodically
- Height and weight measurements annually
- Sexually transmitted disease testing, if in high-risk group
- Annual flu vaccine if over 65 or in high-risk group
- Pneumococcal vaccine at 65 and every 10 years thereafter
- Tetanus diptheria (Td) vaccine every 10 years

Safety

- Home safety measures to prevent falls, fire, burns, scalds, and electrocution

- Working smoke detectors and carbon monoxide detectors in the home
- Motor vehicle safety reinforcement, especially when driving at night
- Older adult driver skills evaluation (some states require for license renewal)
- Precautions to prevent pedestrian accidents

Nutrition and Exercise

- Importance of a well-balanced diet with fewer calories to accommodate lower metabolic rate and decreased physical activity
- Importance of sufficient amounts of vitamin D and calcium to prevent osteoporosis
- Nutritional and exercise factors that may lead to cardiovascular disease (e.g., obesity, cholesterol and fat intake, lack of exercise)
- Importance of 30 minutes of moderate physical activity daily; 20 minutes of vigorous physical activity 3 times per week

Elimination

- Importance of adequate roughage in the diet, adequate exercise, and at least six 8-ounce glasses of fluid daily to prevent constipation

Social Interactions

- Encouraging intellectual and recreational pursuits
- Encouraging personal relationships that promote discussion of feelings, concerns, and fears
- Assessment of risk factors for maltreatment
- Availability of social community centers and programs for seniors

CHAPTER HIGHLIGHTS

- The older adult population is steadily growing and projected to outnumber young people by the middle of the 21st century.
- Older adults are categorized into young-old (65 to 74 years), old (75 to 85 years), and old-old (85+).
- Older adults represent a diverse population in the United States. For example, women outnumber men, Hispanics are the fastest growing subpopulation group, and the majority of older adults rate their health as good even though most have chronic health conditions.
- It is important for nurses to be aware of their own values and attitudes toward aging and the older client, to avoid ageism, and to examine whether myths or stereotypes influence their personal attitudes and beliefs.
- The gerontological nurse has many roles: provider of care, teacher, manager, advocate, and research consumer.
- Older adults are primary users of health care services in different types of care settings, including acute care, rehabilitation, long-term care, and the community. No matter the setting, the older adult requires health assessment and health promotion.
- Several theories have been proposed to account for the biologic aging process: wear-and-tear, free-radical, genetic, cross-linking, and immunity theories.
- Older adults experience many physical changes associated with aging. All body systems undergo change: integumentary, neuromuscular, sensory/perceptual, pulmonary, cardiovascular, gastrointestinal, and genitourinary.

- Psychosocial theories about aging include the disengagement, activity, and continuity theories.
- The older adult has to adjust to possible psychosocial changes, including retirement (which necessitates financial and social adjustments), grandparenting, relocation, increasing dependence on others, and coping with losses and death.
- The cognitive abilities of the healthy older adult undergo some changes in perception, cognitive agility, memory, and learning.
- In the realm of moral reasoning, most older adults begin to blend concepts of justice and caring relationships into their moral decision making.
- Many older adults take their faith and religious practice seriously and display a high level of spirituality.
- Health problems of older adults include injuries, chronic disabling disease, drug use and misuse, alcoholism, dementia, and older adult mistreatment.
- Health promotion information for all adults needs to include positive health practices that can promote health and wellness. These include (a) recommended physical, visual, hearing, and dental assessments; (b) screenings for cardiovascular disease and tuberculosis; (c) breast and testicular self-examinations; (d) immunizations; (e) Papanicolaou smears for some older women; (f) safety precautions to prevent injuries; (g) the importance of appropriate nutrition and exercise; and (h) the importance of measures to prevent constipation.

THINK ABOUT IT

Refer to the chapter-opening scenario and answer these questions.

1. When Mrs. Robinson calls to describe the new symptoms she has been experiencing, you are the nurse who answers the phone. What would you say to Mrs. Robinson? Explain your answer.

2. When Mrs. Robinson is next seen at the provider's office, she asks you, the nurse, what she can do to reduce her concerns about lack of autonomy as she

ages. What information would you provide to reduce her anxiety?

3. While caring for Mrs. Robinson, you learn that she has been seeing several different specialists and is taking a number of medications her primary provider was unaware of. What information can you provide her to reduce the risk of pharmacologic complications?

∞ *See suggested responses to Think About It on MyNursingKit.*

TEST YOUR KNOWLEDGE

1. The nurse provides care for an older adult whose husband died 8 months ago. Which of the following behaviors indicates that the client is experiencing ineffective coping?
   1. She always shows the nurse photographs of her family.
   2. She no longer has her hair done at the beauty shop.
   3. She visits the cemetery and her husband's grave every 2 weeks.
   4. She is Catholic and goes to mass on a daily basis.

2. A nurse in a long-term care facility is caring for several older adults with noticeable hearing loss. The best way to communicate with the clients includes which of the following?
   1. Speak slowly using the proper volume and as few words as possible.
   2. Write the information using large lettering.
   3. Speak in a low and distinct voice tone.
   4. Have the client increase the volume in the hearing aid.

3. The nurse notices that an 85-year-old man at an adult day-care center frequently tells stories about when he was younger and how he came from New York City on the "orphan trains" and was adopted by a Swedish family in Nebraska. His stories are told in a very positive manner. The nurse assesses the client as:
   1. Requiring a geriatric psychiatric evaluation for further assessment.
   2. Displaying normal behavior for his developmental level.
   3. Requiring distraction to change the subject.
   4. Needing to become involved in more social activities.

4. A 70-year-old woman with Alzheimer's disease becomes agitated every evening, pacing and insisting on leaving to go "home." Which nursing interventions would be most appropriate for this client? Select all that apply.
   1. Take her to her room, turn the lights out, and leave her alone.
   2. Allow her to pace and inform her that she is at home.
   3. Turn on the television and encourage her to watch it with you.
   4. Touch her in a gentle way.
   5. Tell her that this is her new home and she will never be able to return to her old home because of her disease which makes it dangerous for her to live alone.

5. While being admitted to a rehabilitation unit, an 82-year-old woman mentions to the nurse that she "has trouble holding her water" and adds "if I could have that tube back in me like I had in the hospital, I wouldn't have so many accidents." What is the nurse's best response to this client?
   1. "Don't worry, the staff will bring plenty of pads to keep you dry."
   2. "Sounds like a good idea. I'll put the tube back in so you will stay dry."
   3. "Tell me more about your 'leaking' problem."
   4. "Just call the staff and we'll help you to the bathroom in time."

6. The nurse notices that when an 80-year-old man rises from a seated position, the client uses both arms to push himself up, and "rocks" back and forth before finally standing. What is the most appropriate nursing intervention for this client?
   1. Suggest a referral to physical therapy for strengthening exercises.

   2. Suggest a waist restraint to remind the client not to stand by himself.
   3. Praise the client for his attempts to remain independent.
   4. Assist the client to rise by grasping him under the axilla and pulling forward.

7. A healthy 78-year-old woman who is considering marriage to a healthy 79-year-old neighbor tells the nurse she wonders if they will be able to have sexual intercourse. Which of the following is the most appropriate nursing response?
   1. Sexual activity may be too demanding for the cardiac system.
   2. Older women maintain sexual function, but many older men are impotent.
   3. Most older people are not interested in sexual activity.
   4. Older men and women may have slower responses to sexual stimulation.

8. The client informs the nurse that he has difficulty clearly seeing the words in the newspaper unless he places the newspaper an arm's length away. The nurse documents this age-related change as:
   1. Presbycusis.
   2. Xerostomia.
   3. Presbyopia.
   4. Presbyesophagus.

9. The nurse integrates the theories of psychosocial aging into nursing care of older adults by applying which of the following principles? Older adults:
   1. Experience physical changes at a predictable rate.
   2. Are as individual as younger adults.
   3. Are best supported in long-term care facilities.
   4. Cause an economic drain on society.

10. The nurse, planning care for an 80-year-old client who underwent surgery three days ago for repair of an inguinal hernia, meets the client's developmental needs by:
    1. Assisting the client with all activities of daily living.
    2. Placing incontinence pads under the client to prevent skin damage.
    3. Arranging for a minister to speak with the client.
    4. Encouraging autonomy in providing self-care.

∞ *See answers to Test Your Knowledge in Appendix A.*

REFERENCES AND SELECTED BIBLIOGRAPHY

Abrams, A. C. (2009). *Clinical drug therapy* (9th ed.). Philadelphia: Lippincott Williams & Wilkins.

Agency on Aging. (2004). *Alzheimer's resource room: Professionals and providers.* Retrieved December 5, 2009, from http://www.aoa.gov

Amella, E. J. (2004). Presentation of illness in older adults. *American Journal of Nursing, 104*(10), 40–51.

Arnold, E. (2004). Sorting out the 3 D's: Delirium, dementia, depression. *Nursing, 34*(6), 36–42.

Atchley, R. C. (1989). A continuity theory of normal aging. *Gerontologist, 29,* 183–190.

Averill, J. B. (2005). Studies of rural elderly individuals: Merging critical ethnography with community-based action research. *Journal of Gerontological Nursing, 31*(12), 11–18.

Baier, F. (2006). The Medicare prescription drug benefit: Understanding the benefits and the gaps in this new coverage. *American Journal of Nursing, 106*(6), 66–72.

Butler, F. R., & Zakari, N. (2005). Grandparents parenting grandchildren: Assessing health status, parental stress, and social supports. *Journal of Gerontological Nursing, 31*(3), 43–54.

Butler, R. N., & Lewis, M. I. (2003). Sexuality and aging. In W. R. Hazzard, J. P. Blass, J. B. Halter, J. G. Ouslander, & M. E. Tinetti (Eds.), *Principles of geriatric medicine and gerontology* (5th ed., pp. 1277–1282). New York: McGraw-Hill.

Capezuti, E., & Harrington, C. (2004). Older adults in the ED. *American Journal of Nursing, 104*(5), 73.

Cataldo, J. K. (2003). Smoking and aging. Clinical implications part 1: Health and consequence. *Journal of Gerontological Nursing, 29*(3), 15–20.

Centers for Disease Control and Prevention (CDC). (2004). *Healthy aging: Preventing disease and improving quality of life among older Americans.* Retrieved December 5, 2009, from http://www.cdc.gov/aging/publications/reports.htm

Clark, M. J. (2003). *Community health nursing. Caring for populations* (4th ed.). Upper Saddle River, NJ: Prentice Hall.

Cumming, E., & Henry, W. E. (1961). *Growing old: The process of disengagement.* New York: Basic Books.

Curry, L., & Hogstel, M. (2002). Osteoporosis: Education and awareness can make a difference. *American Journal of Nursing, 102*(1), 26–33.

Danter, J. H. (2003). Put a realistic spin on geriatric assessment. *Nursing, 33*(12), 52–55.

De Pinto, R. A. (2000). The age of cancer. *Nature, 408*(9), 248–255.

Ebersole, P., Hess, P., & Luggen, A. S. (2004). *Toward healthy aging: Human needs and nursing response* (6th ed.). St. Louis: Mosby.

Ebersole, P., Hess, P., Touhy, T., & Jett, K. (2009). *Gerontological nursing & healthy aging* (3rd ed.). Philadelphia: Elsevier Mosby.

Edelman, C. L., & Mandle, C. L. (2010). *Health promotion throughout the life span* (7th ed.). St. Louis: Mosby Elsevier.

Edwards, H., & Chapman, H. (2004). Contemplating, caring, coping, conversing. A model for promoting mental wellness in later life. *Journal of Gerontological Nursing, 30*(5), 16–21.

Eliopoulos, C. (2009). *Gerontological nursing* (7th ed.). Philadelphia: Lippincott.

Erikson, E. H. (1963). *Childhood and society* (2nd ed.). New York: Norton.

Erikson, E. H. (1982). *The life cycle completed: A review.* New York: Norton.

Federal Interagency Forum on Aging-Related Statistics (FIFAS). (2008). *Older Americans 2008: Key indicators of well-being.* Washington, DC: U.S. Government Printing Office.

Finkel, T., & Holbrook, N. J. (2000). Oxidants, oxidative stress and the biology of aging. *Nature, 408*(9), 239–247.

Fowler, J. W. (1981). *Stages of faith: The psychology of human development and the quest for meaning.* New York: Harper & Row.

Freud, S. (1923). *The ego and the id.* London: Hogarth Press.

Gilligan, C. (1982). *In a different voice: Psychological theory and women's development.* Cambridge, MA: Harvard University Press.

Graf, C. (2006). Functional decline in hospitalized older adults. *American Journal of Nursing, 106*(1), 58–67.

Gray-Vickrey, P. (2004). Combating elder abuse. *Nursing, 34*(10), 47–51.

Haber, D. (2007). *Health promotion and aging: Practical applications for health professionals* (4th ed.). New York: Springer.

Havighurst, R. J. (1963). Successful aging. In R. H. Williams, C. Tibbitts, & W. Donohue (Eds.), *Processes of aging: Social and psychological perspectives* (Vol. 1, pp. 299–320). New York: Atherton.

Havighurst, R. J. (1972). *Developmental tasks and education* (3rd ed.). New York: Longman.

Hetzel, L., & Smith, A. (2001). *The 65 years and over population: 2000. Census 2000 brief.* Washington, DC: U.S. Census Bureau.

Jacelon, C. S. (2004). Older adults and autonomy in acute care. Increasing patients' independence and control during hospitalization. *Journal of Gerontological Nursing, 30*(11), 29–36.

Jett, K., Tappen, R. M., & Rosselli, M. (2005). Imposed versus involved: Different strategies to effect driving cessation in cognitively impaired older adults. *Geriatric Nursing, 26*(2), 111–116.

Joint National Committee on Prevention, Detection, Evaluation, and Treatment of High Blood Pressure [JNC 7]. (2003). *Seventh report* (NIH Publication No. 03–5233). Rockville, MD: Author.

Kane, R. L., Ouslander, J. G., & Abrass, I. B. (2009). *Essentials of clinical geriatrics* (6th ed.). New York: McGraw-Hill Medical Publishing Division.

Kirkwood, T. B. L., & Austad, S. N. (2000). Why do we age? *Nature, 408*(9), 233–238.

Kohlberg, L. (1971). *Recent research in moral development.* New York: Holt, Rinehart & Winston.

Kohlberg, L. (1981). *The psychology of moral development: Moral stages and the idea of justice.* San Francisco: Harper & Row.

Kohlberg, L. (1984). *The psychology of moral development: The nature and validity of moral stages.* San Francisco: Harper & Row.

Mauk, K. L. (2006). *Gerontological nursing: Competencies for care.* Boston: Jones & Bartlett.

McFadden, S. H. (1996). Religion and spirituality. In J. E. Birren (Ed.), *Encyclopedia of gerontology: Age, aging, and the aged* (pp. 387–397). San Diego: Academic Press.

Meiner, S. E., & Lueckenotte, A. G. (2006). *Gerontologic nursing* (3rd ed.). Philadelphia: Mosby Elsevier.

Mezey, M. D. (2001). *The encyclopedia of elder care.* New York: Springer.

Miller, C. A. (2004). *Nursing for wellness in older adults: Theory and practice* (4th ed.). Philadelphia: Lippincott Williams & Wilkins.

Murray, R. B., Zentner, J. P., & Yakimo, R. (2009). *Health promotion strategies through the life span* (8th ed.). Upper Saddle River, NJ: Pearson Education.

National Center for Health Statistics. (2003). *Health, United States, 2003.* Hyattsville, MD: Author.

National Research Council Panel to Review Risk and Prevalence of Elder Abuse and Neglect. (2003). *Elder mistreatment: Abuse, neglect, and exploitation in an aging America.* Washington, DC: Author.

Neugarten, B. (1974). Age groups in American society and the rise of the young-old. *Annals of the American Academy of Political and Social Science, 415,* 187–198.

Oeppen, J., & Vaupel, J. W. (2002). Broken limits to life expectancy. *Science, 296,* 1029–1031.

Paludi, M. A. (2002). *Human development in multicultural contexts. A book of readings.* Upper Saddle River, NJ: Prentice Hall.

Peck, R. (1955). Psychological developments in the second half of life. In J. Anderson (Ed.), *Psychological aspects of aging.* Washington, DC: American Psychological Association.

Peck, R. (1968). Psychological development in the second half of life. In B. L. Neugarten (Ed.), *Middle age and aging.* Chicago: University of Chicago Press.

Piaget, J. (1966). *Origins of intelligence in children.* New York: Norton.

Pinch, W. J. E., & Parsons, M. E. (1997). Moral orientation of elderly persons: Considering ethical dilemmas in health care. *Nursing Ethics, 4*(5), 380–393.

Polan, E., & Taylor, D. (2007). *Journey across the life span. Human development and health promotion* (3rd ed.). Philadelphia: Davis.

Pratt, M. W., Diessner, R., Pratt, A., Hunsberger, B., & Pancer, S. M. (1996). Moral and social reasoning and perspective taking in later life: A longitudinal study. *Psychology and Aging, 11*(1), 66–73.

Purnell, L. D., & Paulanka, B. J. (2008). *Transcultural health care: A culturally competent approach* (3rd ed.). Philadelphia: Davis.

Resnick, B. (2003). Health promotion practices of older adults: Model testing. *Public Health Nursing, 2*(1), 2–12.

Ross-Kerr, J. C., Warren, S., Schalm, C., Smith, D. L., & Godkin, M. D. (2003). Adult day programs: Who needs them? *Journal of Gerontological Nursing, 29*(12), 11–17.

Schneider, J. K., Eveker, A., Bronder, D. R., Meiner, S. E., & Binder, E. F. (2003). Exercise training program for older adults. Incentives and disincentives for participation. *Journal of Gerontological Nursing, 30*(4), 21–31.

Schneider, J. K., Mercer, G. T., Herning, M., Smith, C. A., & Prysak, M. D. (2004). Promoting exercise behavior in older adults: Using a cognitive behavioral intervention. *Journal of Gerontological Nursing, 30*(4), 45–53.

Seery, D. H. (2004). Shifting gears: From cure to comfort. *RN, 67*(11), 52–57.

Sheehy, G. (1995). *New passages. Mapping your life across time.* New York: Ballantine Books.

Stanley, M., Blair, K. A., & Beare, P. G. (2005). *Gerontological nursing: Promoting successful aging with older adults* (3rd ed.). Philadelphia: Davis.

Stotts, N. A., & Deitrich, C. E. (2004). The challenge to come: The care of older adults. *American Journal of Nursing, 104*(8), 40–47.

Substance Abuse and Mental Health Services Administration (SAMHSA). (2005, April 22). Substance abuse among older adults: 2002 and 2003 update. *NDSUH Report.* Retrieved June 11, 2006, from http://oas.samhsa.gov/2k5/olderadults/olderadults.htm

Tabloski, P. A. (2010). *Gerontological nursing.* (2nd ed.). Upper Saddle River, NJ: Pearson Prentice Hall.

Taylor, A. H., Cable, N. T., Faulkner, G., Hillsdon, M., Narici, M., & Van Der Bij, A. K. (2004). Physical activity and older adults: A review of health benefits and the effectiveness of interventions. *Journal of Sports Science, 22*(8), 703–723.

U.S. Department of Health and Human Services. (2000). *Healthy people 2010: Understanding and improving health* (2nd ed.). *Goal 15: Injury and violence prevention.* Washington, DC: Author.

U.S. Department of Health and Human Services. (2003). *A profile of older Americans: 2003.* Washington, DC: Administration on Aging.

U.S. Department of Health and Human Services. (2005). *28 focus areas of healthy people 2010.* Retrieved June 11, 2006, from http://www.healthypeople.gov/lhi/touch_fact.htm

U.S. Preventive Services Task Force. (2003). *Screening for Cervical Cancer. Recommendations and Rationale.* AHRQ Publication No. 03-515A. January 2003. Agency for Healthcare Research and Quality, Rockville, MD. Retrieved June 30, 2006, from, http://www.ahrq.gov/clinic/3rduspstf/cervcan/cervcanrr.htm

Wagnild, G. (2003). Resilience and successful aging: Comparison among low and high income older adults. *Journal of Gerontological Nursing, 29*(12), 42–49.

Wikstrom, B. M. (2004). Older adults and the arts. The importance of aesthetic forms of expression in later life. *Journal of Gerontological Nursing, 30*(9), 30–36.

Promoting Health in the Family

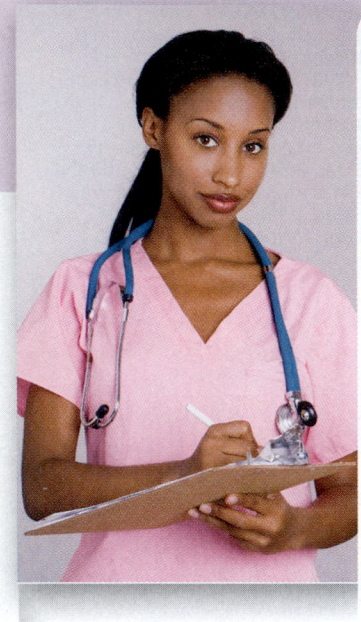

While working in a community health clinic, Keisha Smith, a senior nursing student, met the DuKayne family. Alex and April DuKayne have three children ages 8, 12, and 16 years of age. They report their favorite activities include playing on the computer, watching television and movies, and playing video games. Everyone in the family is overweight, and April and their 12-year-old son are obese. April talks with the nursing student about how she can change the family's diet to help them lose weight. She reports a strong family history in both her own family and Alex's for obesity, heart disease, high cholesterol, and hypertension. April says her mother was an excellent cook, and she uses many of her mother's recipes when making meals, including stews, pasta, and numerous beef entrees.

While talking with Mrs. DuKayne, the nurse notices the 16-year-old daughter rolling her eyes when her mother speaks, and she overhears Mr. DuKayne yelling at their 8-year-old son, who is curiously touching medical equipment on the table. Mrs. DuKayne matter-of-factly says, "Don't mind my husband. He's the disciplinarian in the family and he's always yelling at someone." She reports he is very strict and expects the children to "toe the line" when he tells them to do something.

LEARNING OUTCOMES

After completing this chapter, you will be able to:

1. Describe the roles and functions of the family.

2. Describe different types of families.

3. Identify theoretical frameworks used in family health promotion.

4. Identify the components of a family health assessment.

5. Identify common risk factors regarding family health.

6. Develop nursing diagnoses, outcomes, and interventions pertaining to family functioning.

7. Develop outcome criteria for specific nursing diagnoses related to family functioning.

Nurses assess and plan health care for three types of clients: the individual, the family, and the community. The beliefs and values of each person and the support received come in large part from the family and are reinforced by the community. Thus an understanding of family dynamics and the context of the community assists the nurse in planning care. When a family is the client, the nurse determines the health status of the family and its individual members, the level of family functioning, family interaction patterns, and family strengths and weaknesses.

FAMILY HEALTH

The **family** is a basic unit of society. It consists of those individuals, male or female, youth or adult, legally or not legally related, genetically or not genetically related, who are considered by the others to represent their significant persons. In the nursing profession, interest in the family unit and its impact on the health, values, and productivity of individual family members is expressed by **family-centered nursing**: nursing that considers the health of the family as a unit in addition to the health of individual family members. Many of the leading health indicators from *Healthy People 2010* will be achieved only through family behaviors, including physical activity, weight management, abstinence from substance abuse, responsible sexual behaviors, and maintaining immunization status (Healthy People 2010, 2001).

Functions of the Family

The economic resources needed by the family are secured by adult members. The family protects the physical health of its members by providing adequate nutrition and health care services. Nutritional and lifestyle practices of the family also directly affect the developing health attitudes and lifestyle practices of the children.

In addition to providing an environment conducive to physical growth and health, the family creates an atmosphere that influences the cognitive and the psychosocial growth of its members. Children and adults in healthy, functional families receive support, understanding, and encouragement as they progress through predictable developmental stages, as they move in or out of the family unit, and as they establish new family units. In families where members are physically and emotionally nurtured, individuals are challenged to achieve their potential in the family unit. As individual needs are met, family members are able to reach out to others in the family and the community, and to society.

Families from different cultures are an integral part of North America's rich heritage. Each family has values and beliefs that are unique to their culture of origin and that shape the family's structure, methods of interaction, health care practices, and coping mechanisms. These factors interact to influence the health of families. Families of a particular culture may cluster to form mutual support systems and to preserve their heritage; however, this practice may isolate them from the larger society (see Figure 11–1).

Becoming acculturated is a slow, stressful process of learning the language and customs of a new country. Children in cultural clusters often have greater contact with the world around them than do adults; through school, children become more proficient in language and more comfortable with new customs and behaviors. Sometimes children create conflict in the family when they bring home new ideas and

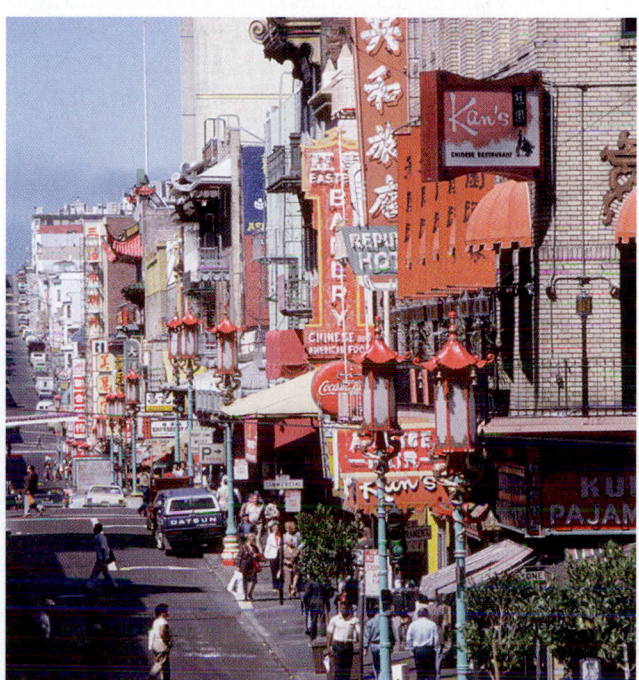

Figure 11–1 ● Cultural separation.
(Courtesy of Morton Beebe/Corbis.)

values. For more information about cultural aspects of health of individuals and families, see Chapter 4∞ .

Types of Families in Today's Society

Families consist of persons (structure) and their responsibilities within the family (roles). Government data are grouped by types of *households*: married couples with children, married couples without children, other family households (single-parent families), men living alone, women living alone, and other nonfamily households. A family structure of parents and their offspring is known as the **nuclear family**. The relatives of nuclear families, such as grandparents or aunts and uncles, compose the **extended family**. In some families, members of the extended family live with the nuclear family. Although members of the extended family may live in different areas, they may be a source of emotional or financial support for the family.

Some families live in houses, some in apartments; some live in urban areas, some in rural towns; and some are homeless. In cities, 40% of the homeless population may consist of families with children (U.S. Conference of Mayors, 2007).

TRADITIONAL FAMILY   The traditional family is viewed as an autonomous unit in which both parents reside in the home with their children, the mother often assuming the nurturing role and the father providing the necessary economic resources. In today's society both males and females are less bound to traditional role patterns. For example, fathers are more likely to be involved with the household chores, their children, and family life. The U.S. Census Bureau reported 26.5 million fathers in married-couple families, 98,000 of whom were stay-at-home fathers (caring for 336,000 children) in 2004. This was the first time the number of stay-at-home parents was analyzed in the census. Of all the families with children, the percentage consisting of married couples declined between 1980 and 1996 and has remained constant since then at about 68% (Fields, 2003).

TWO-CAREER FAMILY   In two-career (or dual-career) families, both partners are employed. They may or may not have children. Two-career families have steadily increased since the 1960s because of increased career opportunities for women, a desire to increase their standard of living, and economic necessity. Finding good-quality, affordable child care is one of the greatest stresses faced by working parents.

SINGLE-PARENT FAMILY   Of all types of households, about 9% (12 million) are single-parent families and the number continues to increase (Fields, 2003). Of these families, 10 million are headed by women and 2 million by men. There are many reasons for single parenthood, including death of a spouse, separation, divorce, birth of a child to an unmarried woman, or adoption of a child by a single man or woman. The stresses of single parenthood are many: child-

care concerns, financial concerns, role overload and fatigue in managing daily tasks, and social isolation.

ADOLESCENT FAMILY   Birth rates among teenagers peaked in 1991 and have decreased progressively since then to 47.7 births per 1000 women aged 15 to 19 in 2000 (Alan Guttmacher Institute, 2004). Rates are highest among black teens, followed by Hispanic and then white women. These young parents are often developmentally, physically, emotionally, and financially ill prepared to undertake the responsibility of parenthood. Adolescent pregnancies frequently interrupt or stop formal education. Children born to an adolescent are often at greater risk for health and social problems, and they have few role models to assist in breaking out of the cycle of poverty.

FOSTER FAMILY   Children who can no longer live with their birth parents may require placement with a family that has agreed to include them temporarily. The legal agreement between the foster family and the court to care for the child includes the expectations of the foster parents and the financial compensation they will receive. A family (with or without their own children) may house more than one foster child at a time or different children over many years. Hopefully, at some time the fostered child can return to the birth parent(s) or be legally and permanently adopted by other parents.

BLENDED FAMILY   Existing family units who join together to form new families are known as *blended, step,* or *reconstituted families.* There are no official statistics on the number of blended families, but a commonly accepted view is that about one of every three Americans is a member of a stepfamily. Family integration requires time and effort. Stresses occur as blended families get acquainted with each other, respect differences, and establish new patterns of behavior. When blended families with children form following the divorce or death of a parent, adjustment can be particularly challenged by the normal processes of grief and loss (see Chapter 30∞).

INTRAGENERATIONAL FAMILY   In some cultures, and as people live longer, more than two generations may live together. Children may continue to live with their parents even after having their own children, or the grandparents may move in with their grown children's families after some years of living apart. In other situations, a generation is skipped or missing; that is, grandparents live with and care for their grandchildren but the children's parents are not a part of this family. Many life events and choices can lead to this type of family.

COHABITING FAMILY   Cohabiting (or communal) families consist of unrelated individuals or families who live under one roof. Reasons for cohabiting may be a need for companionship, a desire to achieve a sense of family, testing a relationship or commitment, or sharing expenses and household management. Cohabiting families illustrate the flexibility and creativity of the family unit in adapting to individual challenges and changing societal needs.

GAY AND LESBIAN FAMILY   Homosexual adults form gay and lesbian families based on the same goals of caring and commitment seen in heterosexual relationships. In addition, the structure of gay and lesbian families is as diverse as that of heterosexual families—including stepfamilies and single-parent families. Children raised in these family units develop sex role orientations and behaviors similar to children in the general population.

Legal issues for same-sex couples are significant and constantly changing. *Domestic partner* policies extend the same rights and privileges to the partner of a nonmarried employee of the same or opposite gender as would be offered to spouses. California Family Code Section 297–297.5 defines domestic partners as "two adults who have chosen to share one another's lives in an intimate and committed relationship of mutual caring." Numerous state and federal legislation has been introduced in the United States to either allow or prohibit same-sex marriages or civil unions. It can be a challenge for the nurse to keep current on how such legislation affects health care issues such as insurance coverage and the right to consent for health care.

SINGLE ADULTS LIVING ALONE   Individuals who live by themselves represent a significant portion of today's society. In younger adults 18 to 34 years of age, about 10% live alone with little variation between males and females. However, among adults 65 years and older, about 20% of men live alone while about 40% of women live alone (Fields, 2003). Singles include young self-supporting adults who have recently left the nuclear family as well as older adults living alone. Young adults typically move in and out of living situations and may have membership in family, nonfamily household, and living alone categories at several different times. Older adults may find themselves single through divorce, separation, or the death of a spouse but generally remain living alone for the remainder of their lives.

APPLYING THEORETICAL FRAMEWORKS TO FAMILIES

A variety of theoretical frameworks provide the nurse with a holistic overview of health promotion for families across the life span. Major theoretical frameworks that nurses use in promoting the health of families are systems theory and structural–functional theory.

Systems Theory

A **system** is a set of interacting identifiable parts or components. The basic concepts of general systems theory were proposed in the 1950s. One of its major proponents, Ludwig von Bertalanffy (1980) introduced systems theory as a universal theory that could be applied to many fields of study. Nurses are increasingly using systems theory to understand not only biologic systems but also systems in families, communities, and nursing and health care. General systems theory provides a way of examining interrelationships and deriving principles.

Systems may be complex and the systems components are often studied as **subsystems**. For family systems, the subsystems would be individuals. Looking back up the hierarchy, the systems above other systems are referred to as **suprasystems**—the family is the suprasystem of the individual.

A system depends on the quality and quantity of its input, throughput, output, and feedback. Input consists of information, material, or energy that enters the system. After the input is absorbed by the system, it is processed in a way useful to the system. This transformation is called throughput. For example, food is input to the digestive system; it is digested (throughput) so that it can be used by the body. Output from

---

RESEARCH NOTES   **Are Adolescent Mothers Able to Promote a Healthy Life for Their Families?**

Much of the research on families headed by adolescent mothers has focused on the negative health aspects of these family units. Yet family and community theory suggests that no unit, family, or community will continue to exist with only negative factors. Black and Ford-Gilboe conducted a study with 41 adolescent mothers to test the families' resilience and ability to promote healthy lifestyles. The young mothers were asked to provide verbal responses to items on three questionnaires designed to gather information on the mother's health-promoting lifestyle practices and demographic background. The results validated the theoretical relationships between increased family resilience and the teenage mother's ability to promote healthy lifestyles for herself and her children.

Implications

Nursing focuses on the complete individual by assessing for both positive and negative health behaviors and risks. In the past, families headed by young single mothers tended to be viewed only in negative terms. By conducting research to examine the positive strengths of these types of family units, nursing is helping to place these families in a more positive light.

Note: From "Adolescent Mothers: Resilience, Family Health, Work, and Health Promoting Practices," by C. Black and M. Ford-Gilboe, 2004, *Journal of Advanced Nursing, 48*, pp. 351–360.

a system is energy, matter, or information given out by the system as a result of its processes. Output from the digestive system includes caloric energy, nutrients, urine, and feces.

Feedback is the mechanism by which some of the output of a system is returned to the system as input. Feedback enables a system to regulate itself by redirecting the output of a system back into the system as input, thus forming a feedback loop. This input influences the behavior of the system and its future output. **Negative feedback** inhibits change; **positive feedback** stimulates change.

The biologic system can be subdivided into the neurologic, musculoskeletal, respiratory, circulatory, gastrointestinal, and urinary subsystems, among others. Each subsystem can in turn be subdivided. For example, the urinary system consists of the kidneys, the ureters, and the bladder; the circulatory system consists of the heart and the blood vessels; the neurologic system consists of the brain, the spinal cord, and the nerves. The biologic system can also be subdivided into categories of needs or functional health patterns or activities of daily living, such as nutrition and hydration, sleep/rest, activity/exercise, elimination, and so on.

The psychologic and social systems consist of subsystems that include thinking, feeling, and interaction patterns. Names of the psychologic and social subsystems vary considerably according to individual nurse theorists. For example, Dorothy Johnson (as cited in Wilkerson & Loveland-Cherry, 2004), who describes the human system in terms of behaviors, lists the psychologic subsystems of attachment—affiliative, dependence, achievement, and aggressive.

The interrelatedness of all the parts of a system is the basis for nursing's holistic view of the client. A tumor of the liver affects the whole individual, that is, the person may be nauseated, tired, anxious, and so on. A psychologic problem such as stress or anxiety may also manifest itself by physiologic symptoms, such as sleeplessness, nausea, or changes in cardiac function.

The family unit can also be viewed as a system. Its members are interdependent, working toward specific purposes and goals. Families, as open systems, are continually interacting with and influenced by other systems in the community. Boundaries regulate the input from other systems that interact with the family system; they also regulate output from the family system to the community or to society. Boundaries protect the family from the demands and influences of other systems. Families are likely to accept input from outside sources, encourage individual members to adapt beliefs and practices to meet the changing demands of society, seek out health care information, and use community resources.

Structural–Functional Theory

The structural–functional theory, as the name implies, focuses on family structure and function. The structural component of the theory addresses the membership of the family and the relationships among family members. Intrafamily relationships are complex because of the numerous relationships that exist within the family structure—mother–daughter, brother–sister, spouse–partner, and so on. These relationships are constantly evolving as children mature and leave the family nest and adults age and become more dependent on others to meet their daily needs.

The functional aspect of the theory examines the effects of intrafamily relationships on the family system, as well as their effects on other systems. Some of the main functions of the family include developing a sense of family purpose and affiliation, adding and socializing new members, and providing and distributing care and services to members. A healthy family organizes its members and resources in meeting family goals; it functions in harmony, working toward shared goals.

Nurses generally use a combination of theoretical frameworks in promoting the health of individuals and families. For example, the nurse may provide education for the mother of a toddler who is struggling to accomplish the developmental stage of autonomy described by Erikson (1963). Simultaneously, the nurse may provide guidance for the same family in its stressful transition period between developmental stages as their older school-age child becomes an adolescent.

NURSING MANAGEMENT

ASSESSING

The purpose of family assessment is to determine the level of family functioning, clarify family interaction patterns, identify family strengths and weaknesses, and describe the health status of the family and its individual members. Also important are family living patterns, including communication, child rearing, coping strategies, and health practices. Family assessment gives an overview of the family process and helps the nurse identify areas that need further investigation. Nurses carry out a detailed assessment in specific target areas as they become more acquainted with the family and begin to understand family needs and strengths more fully. In planning interventions, nurses need to focus not only on problems but also on family strengths and resources as part of the nursing care plan (see Box 11–1).

The assessment begins with a complete health history. The nurse focuses first on the family unit and then on the individuals in that family. The health history is one of the most effective ways of identifying existing or potential health problems. Employment of a genogram will aid the nurse to visualize how all family members are genetically related to each other and to grasp how patterns of chronic conditions are present within the family unit. Genograms are composed of visual representations of gender and lines of birth descent through the generations (Figure 11–2). The history is followed by physical assessment of family members. If further evaluation is indicated, a referral is made to the appropriate health care professional.

The nurse should also develop an ecomap for family members individually and as a group to document the family unit's energy expenditures within the community setting.

BOX 11–1	Family Assessment Guide

Family Structure

- Size and type: nuclear, extended, or other type of family
- Age and gender of family members

Family Roles and Functions

- Family members working outside the home; type of work and satisfaction with it
- Household roles and responsibilities and how tasks are distributed
- Ways child-rearing responsibilities are shared
- Major decision maker and methods of decision making
- Family members' satisfaction with roles, the way tasks are divided, and the way decisions are made

Physical Health Status

- Current physical health status of each member
- Perceptions of own and other family members' health
- Preventive health practices (e.g., status of immunizations, oral hygiene practices, regularity of visual examinations)
- Routine health care, when and why primary care provider last seen

Interaction Patterns

- Ways of expressing affection, love, sorrow, anger, and so on
- Most significant family member in person's life
- Openness of communication with all family members

Family Values

- Cultural and religious orientations; degree to which cultural practices are followed
- Use of leisure time and whether leisure time is shared with total family unit
- Family's view of education, teachers, and the school system
- Health values: how much emphasis is put on exercise, diet, preventive health care

Coping Resources

- Degree of emotional support offered to one another
- Availability of support persons and affiliations outside the family (e.g., friends, church memberships)
- Sources of stress
- Methods of handling stressful situations and conflicting goals of family members
- Financial ability to meet current and future needs

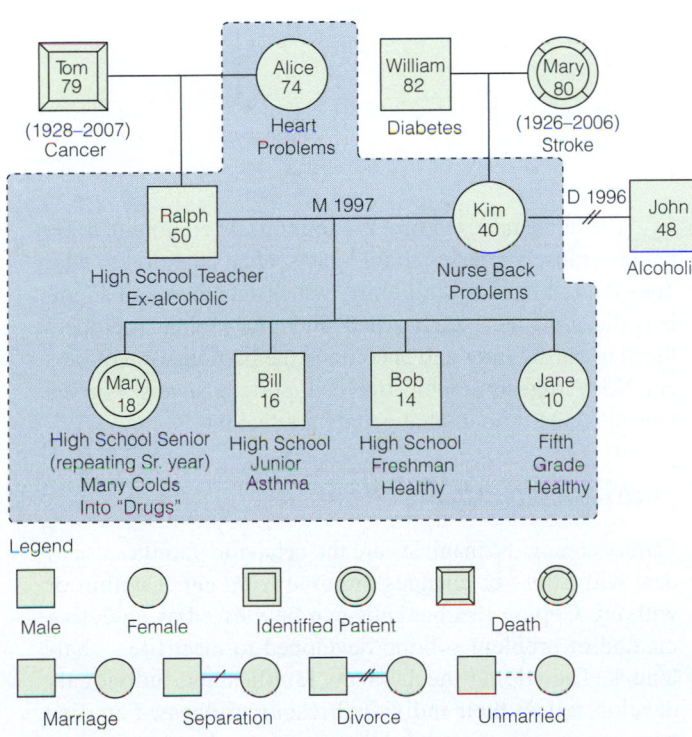

Legend

Figure 11–2 ◯ Example of a family genogram with accompanying legend (symbols used in genograms).

Ecomaps provide a visualization of how the family unit interacts with the external community environment such as schools, religious commitments, occupational duties, and recreational pursuits (see Figure 11–3). When the focus is on health, the appraisal includes information on lifestyle behaviors and health beliefs. The nurse uses data from the health appraisal to formulate a health profile. The health profile provides the data necessary to determine wellness or to establish a nursing diagnosis and to plan appropriate nursing interventions to promote optimal health through lifestyle modification.

Health Beliefs

To promote health, the nurse must understand the health beliefs of individuals and families. Health beliefs may reflect a lack of information or misinformation about health or disease. They may also include folklore and practices from different cultures. Because of the many advances in medicine and health care during the last few decades, clients may have outdated information about health, illness, treatment, and prevention. The nurse is frequently in a position to give information or correct misconceptions. This function is an important component of the nursing care plan. For additional information on health beliefs, see Chapter 5 ∞.

Family Communication Patterns

The effectiveness of family communication determines the family's ability to function as a cooperative, growth-producing unit. Messages are constantly being communicated among

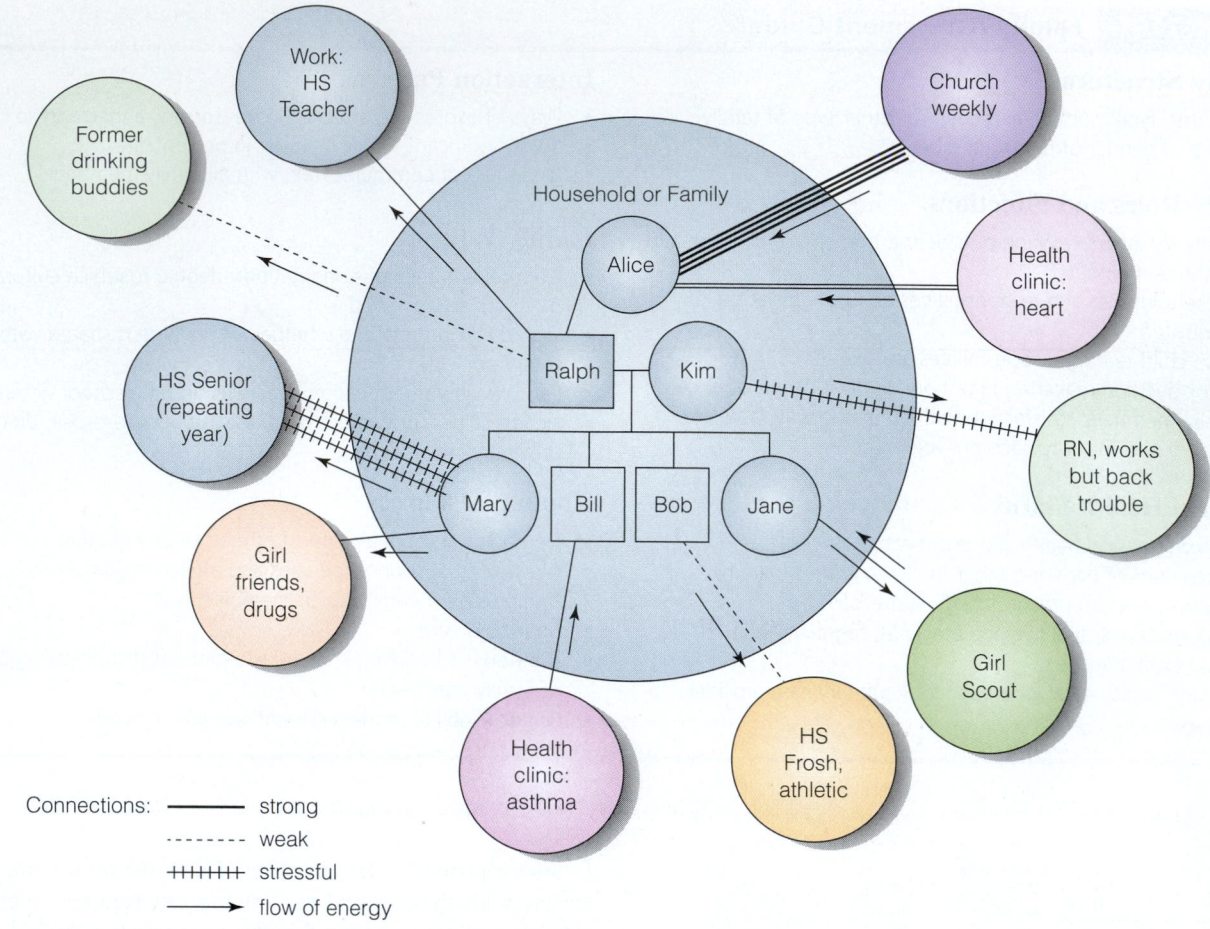

Figure 11–3 Example of a family ecomap. Many more components may be added to the map.

family members, both verbally and nonverbally. The information transmitted influences how members work together, fulfill their assigned roles in the family, incorporate family values, and develop skills to function in society. Intrafamily communication plays a significant role in the development of self-esteem, which is necessary for the growth of personality.

Families that communicate effectively transmit messages clearly. Members are free to express their feelings without fear of jeopardizing their standing in the family. Family members support one another and have the ability to listen, empathize, and reach out to one another in times of crisis. When the needs of family members are met, they are more able to reach out to meet the needs of others in society.

When patterns of communication among family members are dysfunctional, messages are often communicated unclearly. Verbal communication may be incongruent with nonverbal messages. Power struggles may be evidenced by hostility, anger, or silence. Members may be cautious in expressing their feelings because they cannot predict how others in the family will respond. When family communication is impaired, the growth of individual members is stunted. Members often turn to other systems to seek personal validation and gratification.

The nurse needs to observe intrafamily communication patterns closely. Nurses should pay special attention to who does the talking for the family, which members are silent, how disagreements are handled, and how well the members listen to one another and encourage the participation of others. Nonverbal communication is important because it gives valuable clues about what people are feeling.

Family Coping Mechanisms

Family coping mechanisms are the behaviors families use to deal with stress or changes imposed from either within or without. Coping mechanisms can be viewed as an active method of problem solving developed to meet life's challenges. The coping mechanisms families and individuals develop reflect their individual resourcefulness. Families may use coping patterns rather consistently over time or may change their coping strategies when new demands are made on the family. The success of a family largely depends on how well it copes with the stresses it experiences.

Nurses working with families realize the importance of assessing coping mechanisms as a way of determining how families relate to stress. Also important are the resources available to the family. Internal resources, such as knowledge, skills, effective communication patterns, and a sense of mutuality and purpose within the family, assist in the problem-solving process. In addition, external support systems promote coping and adaptation. These external systems may be extended family, friends, religious affiliations, health care professionals, or social services. The development of social support systems is particularly valuable today because many families, due to stress, mobility, or poverty, are isolated from the resources that would traditionally have helped them cope.

FAMILY VIOLENCE The incidence of family violence has increased in recent years. Statistics are not accurate, because many cases remain unreported, but a leading health indicator of Healthy People 2010 is to reduce injury and violence because of the prevalence of violence, much of which occurs within the family unit (Healthy People 2010, 2001). Family violence includes abuse between intimate partners, child abuse, and elder abuse, and may include physical, mental, and verbal abuse, as well as neglect. Early symptoms are evident in burns, cuts, fractures, and even death. Other manifestations often seen are depression, alcohol and substance abuse, and suicide attempts. Nurses should be alert to the symptoms of family violence and take appropriate measures to report it and obtain resources for the family.

Risk for Health Problems

Risk assessment helps the nurse identify individuals and groups at higher risk than the general population of developing specific health problems, such as stroke, diabetes, and lung cancer. The vulnerability of family units to health problems may be based on the maturity level of individual family members, heredity or genetic factors, sex or race, sociologic factors, and lifestyle practices.

MATURITY FACTORS Families with members at both ends of the age continuum are at risk of developing health problems. Families entering childbearing and child-rearing phases experience many changes in roles, responsibilities, and expectations. The many, often conflicting, demands on the family cause stress and fatigue, which may impede growth of individual family members and the functioning of the group as a unit. Adolescent mothers, because of their developmental level and lack of knowledge about parenthood, and single-parent families, because of role overload experienced by the head of the household, are more likely to develop health problems. Many older adults feel a lack of purpose and decreased self-esteem. These feelings in turn reduce their motivation to engage in health-promoting behaviors, such as exercise or community and family involvement.

HEREDITARY FACTORS Persons born into families with a history of certain diseases, such as diabetes or cardiovascular disease, are at greater risk of developing these conditions. A detailed family health history, including genetically transmitted disorders, is crucial to the identification of persons and families at risk. These data are used not only to monitor the health of individual family members but also to recommend modifications in health practices that poten-

tially reduce the risk, minimize the consequences, or postpone the development of genetically related conditions.

GENDER OR RACE Some family units or family members may be at risk of developing a disease by reason of gender or race. Males, for example, are at greater risk of having cardiovascular disease at an earlier age than females, and females are at greater risk of developing osteoporosis, particularly after menopause. Although it is sometimes difficult to separate genetic factors from cultural factors, certain risk factors seem to be related to race. Sickle-cell anemia, for example, is a hereditary disease limited to people of African descent, and Tay-Sachs is a neurodegenerative disease that occurs primarily in descendants of Eastern European Jews.

SOCIOLOGIC FACTORS Poverty is a major problem that affects not only the family but also the community and society. Poverty is a real concern among the rising number of single-parent families. As the number of these families increases, poverty will affect a large number of growing children.

When ill, the poor are likely to put off seeking services until the illness reaches an advanced state and requires longer or more complex treatment. Although the health of the people of industrialized nations has improved significantly during the past century, this progress has not benefited all segments of society, particularly the poor.

LIFESTYLE FACTORS Many diseases are preventable, the effects of some diseases can be minimized, or the onset of disease can be delayed through lifestyle modifications. Certain cancers, cardiovascular disease, adult-onset diabetes, and tooth decay are among the lifestyle diseases. The incidence of lung cancer, for example, would be greatly reduced if people stopped smoking. Good nutrition, dental hygiene, and use of fluoride—in the water supply, in toothpaste, as a topical application, or as supplements—have been shown to reduce dental decay or caries, one of America's most prevalent health problems.

Other important lifestyle considerations are exercise, stress management, and rest. Today health professionals have the knowledge to prevent or minimize the effects of some of the main causes of disease, disability, and death. The challenge is to disseminate information about prevention and to motivate families to make lifestyle changes prior to the onset of illness.

DIAGNOSING AND PLANNING

Data gathered during a family assessment may lead to the following nursing diagnoses:

- *Interrupted Family Processes,* a change in family relationships
- *Readiness for Enhanced Family Coping,* effective management of adaptive tasks by family member involved with the client's health challenge, who now exhibits desire and readiness for enhanced health and growth in regard to self and in relation to the client

- *Disabled Family Coping,* behavior of significant person (family member or other primary person) that disables his/her capacities to effectively address tasks essential to either person's adaptation to the health challenge
- *Impaired Parenting,* inability of the primary caretaker to create, maintain, or regain an environment that promotes the optimum growth and development of the child
- *Impaired Home Maintenance,* inability to independently maintain a safe, growth-promoting, immediate environment
- *Caregiver Role Strain,* difficulty in performing family caregiver role

Examples of contributing factors for one selected diagnosis, desired outcomes to evaluate the achievement of client goals, and the effectiveness of nursing interventions are listed in Identifying Nursing Diagnoses, Outcomes, and Interventions.

Being sensitive to cultural differences is important in assessment and planning care. Knowing who makes most of the decisions in the family, especially in health care, helps the nurse know to whom to direct questions in order to obtain information and also to whom to give instructions. The extended family unit is found in many cultures and there may be a difference in health beliefs and health practices within the family. Older members of the family may use their traditional practices, while younger members may have had more exposure to modern practices. Building a trusting relationship with these families is the first step toward planning more effective care by being able to talk to them about their beliefs and practices.

Nursing needs to focus on assisting the family to plan realistic goals/outcomes and strategies that enhance family functioning, such as improving communication skills, identifying and utilizing support systems, and developing and rehearsing parenting skills. Anticipatory guidance may assist well-functioning families in preparing for predictable developmental transitions that occur in the life of families.

IDENTIFYING NURSING DIAGNOSES, OUTCOMES, AND INTERVENTIONS — Clients with Disruption in Family Health

Data Cluster Mr. & Mrs. G's 6-year-old son has just been diagnosed with acute leukemia. They also have a 9-year-old daughter and a 4-year-old son.

NURSING DIAGNOSIS/DEFINITION	SAMPLE DESIRED OUTCOMES*/*DEFINITION*	NOC INDICATORS	SELECTED INTERVENTIONS*/*DEFINITION*	SAMPLE NIC ACTIVITIES
Interrupted Family Processes/Change in family relationships	Family Coping [2600]/*Family actions to manage stressors that tax family resources.*	Often demonstrated • Involves family members in decision making • Uses stress reduction strategies • Arranges for respite care	Family Integrity Promotion [7100]/*Promotion of family cohesion and unity* Normalization Promotion [7200]/*Assisting parents and other family members of children with chronic illness or disabilities in providing normal life experiences for their children and families*	• Determine family understanding of illness • Tell family members it is safe and acceptable to use typical expressions of affection • Refer for family therapy, as indicated • De-emphasize uniqueness of child's condition • Involve siblings in care and activities of child as appropriate
	Psychosocial Adjustment: Life Change [1305]/Adaptive *psychosocial response of an individual to a significant life change.*	Sometimes demonstrated • Sets realistic goals • Reports of feeling empowered	Family Process Maintenance [7130]/*Minimization of family process disruption effects*	• Determine typical family processes • Discuss strategies for normalizing family life with family members

*The NOC# for desired outcomes and the NIC# for nursing interventions are listed in brackets following the appropriate outcome or intervention. Outcomes, indicators, interventions, and activities are only a sample of those suggested by NOC and NIC and should be further individualized for each client.

BOX 11–2	Factors Determining the Impact of Illness on the Family

- The nature of the illness, which can range from minor to life threatening
- The duration of the illness, which ranges from short term to long term
- The residual effects of the illness, including none to permanent disability
- The meaning of the illness to the family and its significance to family systems
- The financial impact of the illness, which is influenced by factors such as insurance and ability of the ill member to return to work
- The effect of the illness on future family functioning (for instance, previous patterns may be restored or new patterns may be established)

The Family Experiencing a Health Crisis

Illness of a family member is a crisis that affects the entire family system. The family is disrupted as members abandon their usual activities and focus their energy on restoring family equilibrium. Roles and responsibilities previously assumed by the ill person are delegated to other family members, or those functions may remain undone for the duration of the illness. The family experiences anxiety because members are concerned about the sick person and the resolution of the illness. This anxiety is compounded by additional responsibilities when there is less time or motivation to complete the normal tasks of daily living. See Box 11–2 for some factors that determine the impact of illness on the family unit.

The family's ability to deal with the stress of illness depends on the members' coping skills. Families with good communication skills are better able to discuss how they feel about the illness and how it affects family functioning. They can plan for the future and are flexible in adapting these plans as the situation changes. An established social support network provides strength, encouragement, and services to the family during the illness. During health crises, families need to realize that it is a strength, not a sign of weakness, to turn to others for support. Nurses can be part of the support system for families, or they can identify other sources of support in the community.

During a crisis, families are often drawn together by a common purpose. In this time of closeness, family members have the opportunity to reaffirm personal and family values and their commitment to one another. Indeed, illness may provide a unique opportunity for family growth.

The Nurse's Role with Families Experiencing Illness

Nurses committed to family-centered care involve both the ailing individual and the family in the nursing process. Through their interaction with families, nurses can give support and information. Nurses make sure that not only the individual but also each family member understands the disease, its management, and the effect of these two factors on family functioning. The nurse also assesses the family's readiness and ability to provide continued care and supervision at home when warranted. After carefully planned instruction and practice, families are given an opportunity to demonstrate their ability to provide care under the supportive guidance of the nurse. When the care indicated is beyond the capability of the family, nurses work with families to identify available resources that are socially and financially acceptable.

In helping families reintegrate the ill person into the home, nurses use data gathered during family assessment to identify family resources and deficits. By formulating mutually acceptable goals for reintegration, nurses help families cope with the realities of the illness and the changes it may have brought about, which may include new roles and functions of family members or the need to provide continued medical care to the ill or recovering person. Working together, nurses and families can create environments that restore or reorganize family functioning during illness and throughout the recovery process.

Death of a Family Member

The death of a family member often has a profound effect on the family. The structure of the family is altered, and this change may in turn affect how it functions as a unit. Individual members experience a sense of loss. They grieve for the lost person, and they grieve for the family that once was. Family disorganization may occur. However, as the family begins to recover, a new sense of normalcy develops, the family reintegrates its roles and functions, and it comes to grips with the reality of the situation. This painful blow takes time to heal.

After the death of a member, families may need counseling to deal with their feelings and to talk about the person who died. They may also want to talk about their fears and hopes for the future. At this time, families often derive comfort from their religious beliefs and their spiritual advisers. Support groups are also available for families experiencing the pain of death. It is often difficult for nurses to deal with grieving families because the nurses also feel the loss and feel inadequate in knowing what to say or do. By understanding the effect death has on families, nurses can help families resolve their grief and move ahead with life. (See Chapter 30 ∞ for a discussion of loss and grieving.)

IMPLEMENTING AND EVALUATING

Nursing interventions are based on the medical diagnoses, nursing diagnoses, and selected goals or outcomes (see Identifying Nursing Diagnoses, Outcomes, and Interventions). In evaluating the success of the family care plan, the nurse assesses for the presence of the indicators identified for the chosen outcomes. If the indicators are present, it is likely that the outcome has been achieved. If the indicators or outcomes are partially or not met, all aspects of the family situation must be reexamined: Have the intervention activities been carried out? Are the indicators and outcomes appropriate? Is the nursing diagnosis proper? Has the medical condition or diagnosis changed?

Recognition of individual and family strengths helps to maintain wellness and also directs behavior in crises situations. If a plan of care has to be modified to be more effective, these strengths should be identified and utilized.

CHAPTER HIGHLIGHTS

- The family is the basic unit of society.
- The family plays an important role in forming the health beliefs and practices of its members.
- Information on how family members are genetically related is gathered via a genogram, while an ecomap allows the nurse to see where the family's energy is being expended.
- Family-centered nursing addresses the health of the family as a unit, as well as the health of family members.
- In today's society, many types of families exist: traditional, two-career, single-parent, those headed by one or more adolescent parents, foster, blended, intragenerational, cohabiting, and gay and lesbian. In addition, many single adults live alone.
- The purpose of family assessment is to determine the level of family functioning, to clarify family interaction patterns, to identify family strengths and weaknesses, and to describe the health status of the family and its individual members.
- Families at risk for health problems may be considered on the basis of family maturity level, presence of hereditary factors, sex or race, lifestyle practices, and sociologic factors such as poverty.
- Nursing diagnoses that relate to family health needs and problems include *Interrupted Family Processes; Readiness for Enhanced Family Coping; Disabled Family Coping; Impaired Parenting; Impaired Home Maintenance;* and *Caregiver Role Strain.*
- Nurses must examine their own values about family, health, illness, and death to be effective in supporting families in crisis.
- A variety of nursing theoretical frameworks provide the nurse with a holistic overview of health promotion of families across the life span.

THINK ABOUT IT

Refer to the chapter-opening scenario and answer these questions.

1. What factors may contribute to the family's weight problem? Explain your answer.

2. What recommendations would you make for this family for health promotion and illness prevention?

3. What health problems would you anticipate if this family does not change their lifestyle choices?

∞ *See suggested responses to Think About It on MyNursingKit.*

TEST YOUR KNOWLEDGE

1. Because a severely injured middle-aged client informed the nurse that he did not have any immediate family members, the nurse receives permission from the client to contact extended family members. Which of the following is most representative of extended family members whom the nurse will contact?
   1. Grandparents, aunts, and uncles
   2. Parents and spouse
   3. Children who no longer live at home
   4. Roommates and close family friends

2. When a father prepares to leave for work in the morning, his 3-year-old son starts to cry and scream. The father picks him up and delays leaving for a while. The father's behavior most reflects which part of a system?
   1. Input
   2. Throughput
   3. Output
   4. Feedback

3. A nurse should instruct a client who identifies "the family" as two college roommates, a dog, and a cat to perform which of the following when completing a family health history form?

1. Include all information about blood relatives and the animals and roommates that might influence his health.
2. Include only information about genetic/hereditary and environmental illnesses of blood relatives.
3. Leave the area blank since the client does not live with blood relatives.
4. Use the client's own judgment in completing the area since the physical exam is more important than the history.

4. A visual representation of family members by gender, age, health status, and lines of relationships through the generations is referred to as a _____.

5. In order to assess the impact of illness on the family as a unit it is essential that the nurse assess which of the following factors? Select all that apply.

1. The duration of the illness
2. The meaning of the illness to the family and its significance to family systems
3. The coping mechanisms used by other families with similar illnesses
4. The financial impact of the illness (including factors such as insurance and ability of the ill member to work)
5. The incidence of the illness in the community at large

6. An adult child brings a parent to an agency with signs and symptoms of potential fluid retention possibly related to excessive sodium intake. Further nursing assessment indicates inadequate food storage and preparation techniques in the home. Which of the following would be the most appropriate nursing diagnosis?

1. *Readiness for enhanced family coping*
2. *Disabled family coping*
3. *Impaired parenting*
4. *Caregiver role strain*

7. Prior to finalizing a family-oriented nursing care plan and implementing interventions, it is essential for the nurse to perform which of the following?

1. Meet with all family members simultaneously.
2. Confirm that the family health insurance covers all family members.
3. Establish a trusting relationship with the family as a group.
4. Complete a thorough history and physical examination of each family member.

8. When the nurse is utilizing a systems theory to assess family units, which of the examples listed below best illustrates a family unit that *does not* meet the criteria of a well-functioning system?

1. The family members allow input from outside the family unit.
2. The family members are interdependent.
3. Each member's personal boundaries are well-defined.
4. The primary activities of each member focus on personal purposes.

9. The nurse is assessing a pregnant 12-year-old girl at the neighborhood free clinic. The client reports a number of health and social problems for which she has been treated in the past. The nurse anticipates learning the client is a member of what type of family?

1. Gay or lesbian family
2. Blended family
3. Adolescent family
4. Intragenerational family

10. The nurse is using a structural–functional theory to assess the family. After learning the members of the family, the nurse's next step is to determine:

1. The relationship among family members.
2. The role of individual family members.
3. Family goals.
4. Family harmony.

∞ *See answers to Test Your Knowledge in Appendix A.*

REFERENCES AND SELECTED BIBLIOGRAPHY

Alan Guttmacher Institute. (2004). *U.S. teenage pregnancy statistics: Overall trends, trends by race and ethnicity and state-by-state information*. New York: Author.

American Nurses Association. (1998). *Culturally competent assessment for family violence*. Washington, DC: American Nurses Publishing.

Black, C., & Ford-Gilboe, M. (2004). Adolescent mothers: Resilience, family health, work and health-promoting practices. *Journal of Advanced Nursing, 48*, 351–360.

Bulechek, G. M., Butcher, H. K., Dochterman, J. M. (Eds.). (2008). *Nursing interventions: classification (NIC)* (5th ed.). St. Louis: Mosby.

Doane, G. H., & Varcoe, C. (2004). *Family nursing as relational inquiry*. Philadelphia: Lippincott Williams & Wilkins.

Erikson, E. (1963). *Childhood and society* (2nd ed.). New York: Norton.

Fields, J. (2003). *America's families and living arrangements: 2003*. Current Population Reports, P20–553. Washington, DC: U.S. Census Bureau.

Friedman, M. M., Bowden, V. R., & Jones, E. G. (2003). *Family nursing: Research, theory and practice* (5th ed.). Upper Saddle River, NJ: Prentice Hall.

Healthy People 2010. (2001). *Leading Health Indicators*. http://www.healthypeople.gov/LHI/lhiwhat.htm Accessed June 9, 2009

Locsin, R. C. (2003). Culture perspectives. The integration of family health, culture, and nursing: Prescriptions and practices. *Holistic Nursing Practice, 17*(1), 8–10.

Moorhead, S., Johnson, M., Maas, M. L., & Swanson, E. (Eds.). (2008). *Nursing outcomes classification (NOC)* (4th ed.). St. Louis: Mosby.

NANDA International. (2009). *NANDA nursing diagnoses: Definitions and classification 2009–2010*. West Sussex, U.K.: Wiley-Blackwell.

Rigazio-DiGilio, S. A. (2005). *Community genograms: Using individual, family, and cultural narratives with clients*. New York: Teachers College Press.

U.S. Census Bureau. (2004). *"Stay-at-home" parents top 5 million*. Washington, DC: Author. Retrieved May 5, 2006, from http://www.census.gov/Press-Release/www/releases/archives/families_households/003118.html

U.S. Conference of Mayors. (2007). *A status report on hunger and homelessness in America's cities: 2007*. Retrieved October 28, 2009, from http://usmayors.org/HHSurvey2007/hhsurvey07.pdf

von Bertalanffy, L. (1980). *General system theory* (revised from original 1969). New York: George Braziller.

Wilkerson, S. A., & Loveland-Cherry, C. J. (2004). Johnson's behavioral system model. In J. J. Fitzpatrick & A. L. Whall (Eds.), *Conceptual models of nursing: Analysis and application* (4th ed., pp. 83–103). Upper Saddle River, NJ: Prentice Hall Health.

Integral Aspects of Nursing

Caring

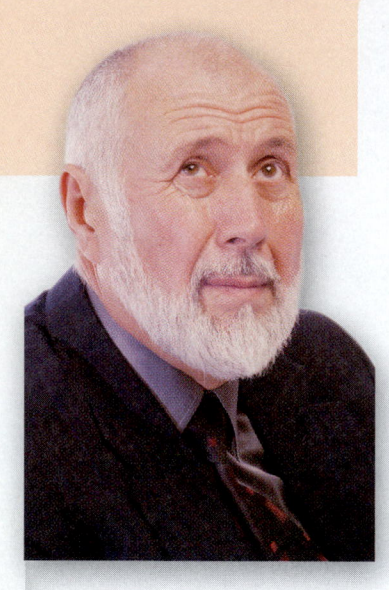

Franklin Fielder, 76 years old, is married with three grown children who are married and live in another state. He has seven grandchildren and two great grandchildren. His wife has never worked outside the home, and Franklin has supported his family as an attorney who is well known and respected within his community. Franklin began feeling short of breath with mild activity and visited his family doctor. Testing revealed lung cancer with metastasis to the liver. Franklin was referred to an oncologist and the treatment plan was decided upon, but he was told the mortality rate for this type of cancer is very high.

While receiving chemotherapy in the outpatient center, Franklin talks with the nurse administering his medications. He tells the nurse he looks forward to coming to the center because it is the only place where he can honestly discuss his feelings. He admits he tries hard to maintain optimism and feels a need to be positive and upbeat, and avoids discussing his fears with his family because his wife begins to cry if he mentions the possibility of his death. He says he feels like an actor and wishes he could be more truthful with those he loves, but he reveals that he actually feels guilty about leaving his family behind if he should die.

LEARNING OUTCOMES

After completing this chapter, you will be able to:

1. Define the key terms for this chapter.

2. Discuss the meaning of caring.

3. Identify nursing theories focusing on caring.

4. Analyze the importance of different types of knowledge in nursing.

5. Describe how nurses demonstrate caring in practice.

6. Evaluate the importance of self-care for the professional nurse.

7. Identify the value of reflective practice in nursing.

KEY TERMS

aesthetic knowing p292

caring p289

caring practice p289

empirical knowing p291

ethical knowing p292

personal knowing p292

reflection p296

In this age of technological competence and efficiency, the knowledge and skills embedded in caring practices are often overlooked. Phillips and Benner (1994) identified a "crisis in caring" across our society, especially involving members of the helping professions, such as nursing. Caring is central to all helping professions, and enables persons to create meaning in their lives. **Caring** means that people, relationships, and things matter.

PROFESSIONALIZATION OF CARING

Caring practice involves connection, mutual recognition, and involvement. Consider the following examples of caring, emerging from nursing situations:

- A client experiencing postoperative pain is given medication to control her symptoms, and then the nurse talks quietly and holds her hand for a few minutes as the pain resolves. The nurse's presence, in itself, provides comfort for the client.
- After the student nurse washes the client's hair and applies makeup, the immobilized older woman is helped to sit up in a wheelchair to greet her daughter and grandchildren. She is extremely grateful just to be able to sit up after weeks in bed. Her sense of dignity is enhanced by this personal care.

Just as clients benefit from caring practices, the nurses involved in these situations experience caring through knowing that they have made a difference in their clients' lives. Consider, for example, one nurse's feeling of satisfaction: "It is not something that can be defined but, you know . . . the feeling that you've made a difference to an individual, and had I not been there at that time, that would never have occurred" (Pask, 2003, p. 169).

As nurses feel free to concentrate their attention upon the other, they can make a positive difference to clients. The ability to give focused attention to clients means leaving the egocentric self behind. Students of nursing can develop this ability by studying the meaning of caring in nursing.

Caring as "Helping the Other Grow"

Milton Mayeroff (1990), a noted philosopher, has proposed that to care for another person is to help the caregiver grow and actualize himself. Caring is a process that develops over time, resulting in a deepening and transformation of the relationship. Recognizing the other as having potential and the need to grow, the caregiver does not impose direction, but allows the direction of the other person's growth to help determine how to respond.

Major ingredients of caring provide structure and further description of this process: (a) *knowing* means understanding the other's needs and how to respond to these needs; (b) *alternating rhythms* signifies moving back and forth between the immediate and long-term meanings of behavior, considering the past; (c) *patience* enables the other to grow in his own way and time; (d) *honesty* includes

awareness and openness to one's own feelings and a genuineness in caring for the other; (e) *trust* involves letting go, to allow the other to grow in his own way and own time; (f) *humility* means acknowledging that there is always more to learn, and that learning may come from any source; (g) *hope* is belief in the possibilities of the other's growth; and (h) *courage* is the sense of going into the unknown, informed by insight from past experiences.

Mayeroff proposes that the caring process has benefits for the one giving care. By helping the other grow, the caregiver moves toward self-actualization. By caring and being cared for, each person "finds his place" in the world. Through serving others through caring, persons live the meaning of their own lives.

NURSING THEORIES ON CARING

Caring is a multidimensional concept. In a comprehensive review of the concept of caring, Morse, Solberg, Neander, Battorff, and Johnson (1990) identified different definitions of caring, which were summarized as the following five viewpoints:

- Caring as a moral imperative
- Caring as an affect
- Caring as a human trait
- Caring as an interpersonal relationship
- Caring as a therapeutic intervention

Nurse scholars have reviewed the literature, conducted research, and analyzed nurses' experiences, resulting in the development of theories and models of caring. These theories and models are grounded in humanism and the idea that caring is the basis for human science. Several nursing theorists focus on caring: Leininger, Ray, Roach, Boykin and Schoenhofer, Watson, Swanson, and Benner and Wrubel.

Based on studies in nursing and anthropology, Leininger noted that caring, as nurturing behavior, has been present throughout history and is one of the most critical factors in helping people maintain or regain health. Leininger proposes that "caring is the essence of nursing, and the distinct, dominant, central, and unifying focus of nursing" (Leininger, 2001, p. 35). Her theory of culture care diversity and universality is based on the assumption that nurses must understand different cultures in order to function effectively.

Ray's theory of bureaucratic caring focuses on caring in organizations (e.g., hospitals) as cultures. The theory suggests that caring in nursing is contextual and is influenced by the organizational structure. In Ray's research, the meaning of caring varied in the emergency department, intensive care unit, oncology unit, and other areas of the hospital. For example, an intensive care unit had a dominant value of technological caring, and an oncology unit had a value of a more intimate, spiritual caring. Furthermore, the meaning of caring was further influenced by the role and position a person held. Staff nurses valued caring in terms of its relatedness to clients, while administrators valued caring as more system-related,

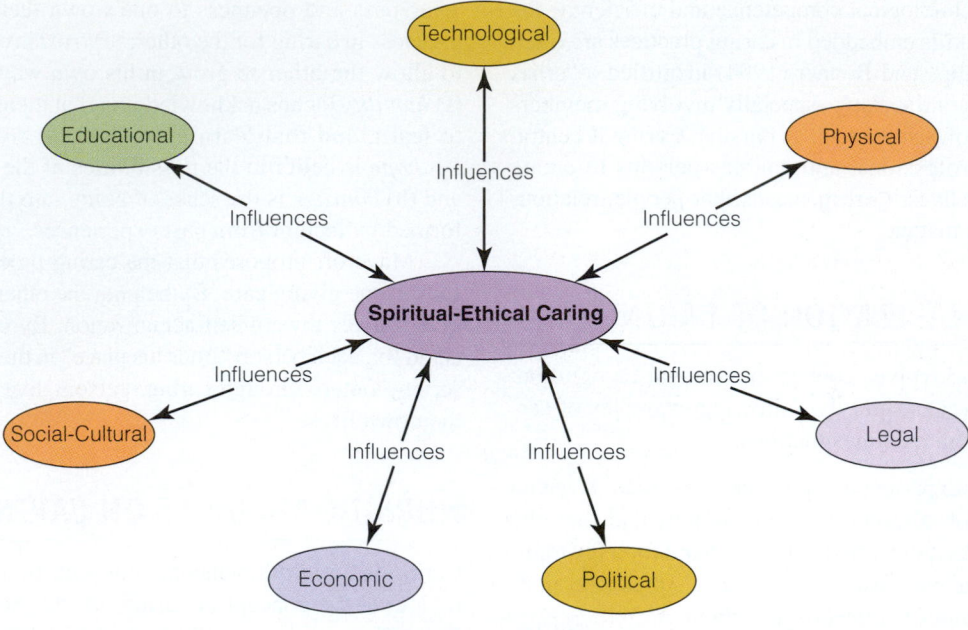

Figure 12–1 ● Concept map reflecting the theory of bureaucratic caring.

such as safeguarding the economic well-being of the hospital (Coffman, 2006). As depicted in Figure 12–1, spiritual-ethical caring influences each of the aspects of the bureaucratic system (political, legal, economic, educational, physiologic, social-cultural, and technological). Each of these aspects is different, but they make up a whole bureaucratic system (e.g., a hospital). Nurses influence client care by making choices about each of these aspects (Ray, 2001). Nurses make these choices with the interest of the client at heart and use ethical principles as the foundation for the basis of professional decision making. According to Ray (2001), "Spiritual-ethical caring for nursing does not question whether or not to care in complex systems, but intimates how sincere deliberations and ultimately the facilitation of choices for the good of others can or should be accomplished" (p. 429).

M. Simone Roach focuses on caring as a philosophical concept and proposes that caring is the human mode of being, or the "most common, authentic criterion of humanness" (Roach, 2002, p. 28). All persons are caring, and develop their caring abilities by being true to self, being real, and being who they truly are. Thus, caring is not unique to nursing. Roach considers caring to be unique in nursing, however, because caring is the center of all attributes used to describe nursing. Roach defines these attributes as the six Cs of caring: compassion, competence, confidence, conscience, commitment, and comportment. See Box 12–1 for definitions of each characteristic. The six Cs are used as a broad framework, suggesting categories of behavior that describe professional caring. Each category reflects specific values and includes virtuous actions by which a nurse can demonstrate caring.

BOX 12–1   The Six Cs of Caring in Nursing

Compassion

Awareness of one's relationship to others, sharing their joys, sorrows, pain, and accomplishments. Participation in the experience of another.

Competence

Having the knowledge, judgment, skills, energy, experience, and motivation to respond adequately to others within the demands of professional responsibilities.

Confidence

The quality that fosters trusting relationships. Comfort with self, client, and family.

Conscience

Morals, ethics, and an informed sense of right and wrong. Awareness of personal responsibility.

Commitment

Convergence between one's desires and obligations and the deliberate choice to act in accordance with them.

Comportment

Appropriate bearing, demeanor, dress, and language, that are in harmony with a caring presence. Presenting oneself as someone who respects others and demands respect.

Note: Adapted from *Caring, the Human Mode of Being,* 2nd ed. by M. S. Roach. Copyright © 2002 CHA Press. Reprinted with permission.

Boykin and Schoenhofer suggest that the purpose of the discipline and profession of nursing is to know persons and nurture them as persons living in caring and growing in caring (Purnell, 2006). Respect for persons as caring individuals and respect for what matters to them are assumptions underlying the theory of nursing as caring. Similar to Roach's idea that all persons are caring, Boykin and Schoenhofer emphasize the importance of the nurse knowing self as a caring person. Maintaining this approach may be difficult in practice environments that may depersonalize the nurse and view nursing care only as tasks that need to be completed. However, caring is a lifetime process, lived moment to moment by the nurse, and constantly unfolding. Through knowing self as a caring person, the nurse can be authentic to self, freeing oneself to truly be with others. This awareness of self allows the nurse to authentically care for others in nursing practice.

Watson's theory of human care views caring as the essence and the moral ideal of nursing. Human care is the basis for nursing's role in society; indeed, nursing's contribution to society lies in its moral commitment to human care. Nursing as human care goes beyond the realm of ethics, as described by Watson (1999, p. 29):

> Human caring in nursing, therefore, is not just an emotion, concern, attitude, or benevolent desire. Caring is the moral ideal of nursing whereby the end is protection, enhancement, and preservation of human dignity. Human caring involves values, a will and a commitment to care, knowledge, caring action, and consequences. All of human caring is related to intersubjective human responses to health-illness conditions; a knowledge of health-illness, environmental-personal interactions; a knowledge of the nurse caring process; self-knowledge, knowledge of one's power and transaction limitations.

Watson emphasizes nursing's commitment to care of the whole person as well as a concern for the health of individuals and groups. The nurse and client are co-participants in the client's movement toward health and wholeness. Watson labels this process transpersonal human caring, through which the nurse enters into the experience of the client, and the client can enter into the nurse's experience. By identifying with each other, the nurse and client gain self-knowledge and keep alive their common humanity, avoiding reducing the other to an object.

As Benner and Wrubel listened to expert nurses' stories and analyzed their meanings, caring emerged as the essence of excellence in nursing. Nursing is described as a relationship in which caring is primary because it sets up the possibility of giving and receiving help (Benner & Wrubel, 1989). As nurses gain expertise, they are more effective in focusing on what the client brings to the health care encounter. Caring facilitates the nurse's ability to problem solve and to implement individualized solutions. Caring is interactive, in that the strengths and abilities of the person who is cared for are as important as the skills of the nurse. A caring relationship requires a certain amount of client openness and capacity to respond to care. In caring practice, being with someone may be just as important as doing something for that person, if not more so. Caring practice involves client advocacy and provides the necessary conditions to help the client grow and develop (Gordon, Benner, & Noddings, 1996).

TYPES OF KNOWLEDGE IN NURSING

Nursing involves different types of knowledge that are integrated to guide nursing practice. Nurses require scientific competence (empirical knowledge), therapeutic use of self (personal knowing), moral/ethical awareness (ethical knowing), and creative action (aesthetic knowing). These four types of knowledge were identified by Carper (1978) from her observations of nurses' activities. An understanding of each type of knowledge is important for the student of nursing because only by integrating all ways of knowing can the nurse develop a professional practice. Figure 12–2 illustrates the interconnection of these different types of knowledge.

Empirical Knowing: The Science of Nursing

Knowledge about the empirical world is systematically organized into laws and theories for the purpose of describing, explaining, and predicting phenomena of special concern to the discipline of nursing. **Empirical knowing** ranges from factual, observable phenomena (e.g., anatomy, physiology, chemistry) to theoretical analysis (e.g., developmental theory, adaptation theory).

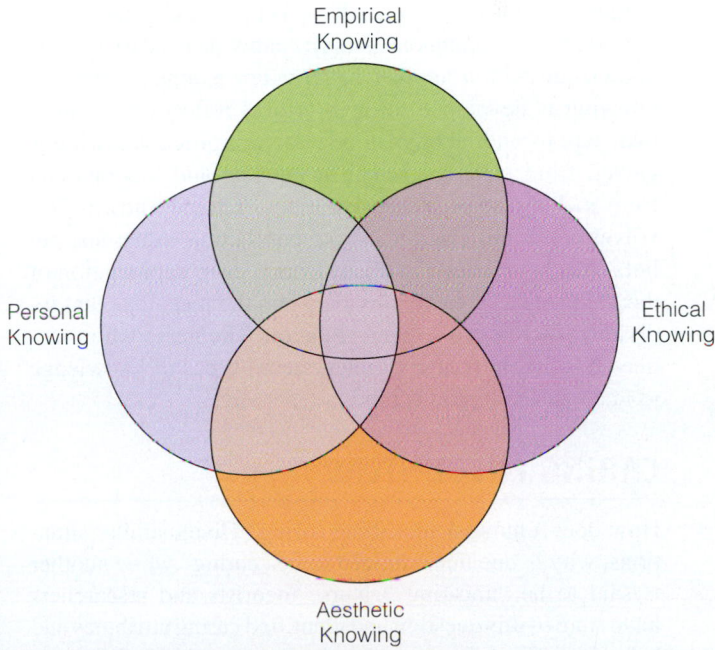

Figure 12–2 The four ways of knowing.

Aesthetic Knowing: The Art of Nursing

Aesthetic knowing is the art of nursing and is expressed by the individual nurse through his or her creativity and style in meeting the needs of clients. The nurse uses aesthetic knowing to provide care that is both effective and satisfying. Empathy, compassion, holism, and sensitivity are important modes in the aesthetic pattern of knowing.

Personal Knowing: The Therapeutic Use of Self

Personal knowledge is concerned with the knowing, encountering, and actualizing of the concrete, individual self. Because nursing is an interpersonal process, the way in which nurses view their own selves and the client is of primary concern in any therapeutic relationship. **Personal knowing** promotes wholeness and integrity in the personal encounter, achieves engagement rather than detachment, and denies the manipulative or impersonal approach.

Ethical Knowing: The Moral Component

Goals of nursing include the conservation of life, alleviation of suffering, and promotion of health. **Ethical knowing** focuses on matters of obligation or what ought to be done, and goes beyond simply following the ethical codes of the discipline. Nursing care involves a series of deliberate actions or choices that are subject to the judgment of right or wrong. Occasionally, the principles and norms that guide choices may be in conflict. The more sensitive and knowledgeable the nurse is to these issues, the more "ethical" he or she will be.

Developing Ways of Knowing

The methods for developing each type of knowledge are unique (Chinn & Kramer, 2005). The methods that are required for developing one pattern cannot be used to develop knowledge within another pattern. For example, personal knowing is developed through critical reflection on one's own actions and feelings in practice. Empirical knowing is gained from studying scientific models and theories and from making objective observations. Ethical knowing involves confronting and resolving conflicting values and beliefs. Aesthetic knowing arises from a deep appreciation of the uniqueness of each individual and the meanings that individual ascribes to a given situation. The nurse who practices effectively is able to integrate all types of knowledge to understand situations more holistically.

CARING ENCOUNTERS

How does a nurse demonstrate caring? Given similar situations, why is one nurse judged to be "caring" while another is said to be "uncaring"? Nurse theorists and researchers have studied this question and identified caring attributes and behaviors. Consider, for example, Roach's six Cs, Watson's carative factors (Chapter 1 ∞), and Swanson's structure of

TABLE 12–1	Caring Processes and Subdimensions from Swanson's Theory of Caring	
PROCESS AND DEFINITION	**SUBDIMENSIONS**
Knowing Striving to understand an event as it has meaning in the life of the other	Avoiding assumptions; centering on the one cared; assessing thoroughly; seeing cues; engaging the self of both
Being with Being emotionally present to the other	Being there; conveying ability; sharing feelings; not burdening
Doing for Doing for the other as he/she would do for the self if it were at all possible	Comforting; anticipating; performing competently/ skillfully; protecting; preserving dignity
Enabling Facilitating the other's passage through life transitions and unfamiliar events	Informing/explaining; supporting/allowing; focusing; generating alternatives/ thinking it through; validating/giving feedback
Maintaining Belief Sustaining faith in the other's capacity to get through an event or transition and face a future with meaning	Believing in/holding in esteem; maintaining a hope-filled attitude; offering realistic optimism; "going the distance"

Note: From K. Swanson, "Empirical Development of a Middle Range Theory of Caring," *Nursing Research, 40*(3), pp. 162–163. Copyright © 1991 Lippincott, Williams & Wilkins. Reprinted with permission.

caring (Table 12–1). Because caring is contextual, a nursing approach used with a client in one situation may be ineffective in another. Caring responses are as varied as clients' needs, environmental resources, and nurses' imaginations. Caring encounters are influenced by the diversity of human responses, the nurse's workload, and the preferences of the nurse and client (Cooper, 2001). When clients perceive the encounter to be caring, their sense of dignity and self-worth is increased, and feelings of connectedness are expressed.

Knowing the Client

Caring attends to the totality of the client's experience. The nurse asks: Who is this person? What is his or her history? Needs? Desires? Dreams? Spiritual beliefs? Who loves and cares for this person at home? Where is home and what resources are there? What does this person need today, from me, right now? Can he or she tell me what is needed? Personal knowledge of the client is a key in the caring relationship between nurse and client. The nurse aims to know who the client is, in his or her *uniqueness*. This knowledge is gained by observing and talking with the client and family, using listening and communication skills. The nurse cannot remain detached, but is actively engaged with the client.

Take, for example, an older man experiencing postoperative pain after removal of a cancerous prostate. The nurse

RESEARCH NOTES

Believing That I Make a Difference

The development of the nurse's moral agency, or sense of what should be done in a nursing situation, is a critical concept for caring practitioners. The purpose of this analysis was to describe the nature of moral agency in nursing by revealing how and why nurses see value in the work they do. The researcher analyzed interviews that had been transcribed and coded to draw out analytical themes. The analysis was based on the philosophy of Iris Murdoch, who drew attention to how individuals examine their responses to events in their lives, and in so doing develop how they see the world and themselves in relation to others.

When asked what sustained them in their work, nurses in the study often pointed to moments when their personal presence made a difference in clients' lives. For example:

- "When someone says you have really helped me, all the other things about it are invisible, it doesn't make any difference [speaking of the stress that she had to sustain]." (p. 166)
- "After a while things become a little bit routine. . . . And when I end up feeling like that something always seems to happen that makes you re-evaluate what you are doing, and that always tends to be very patient focused . . . it's where

you get feedback from a patient and you realize, well no one else, unless they were in this position, could have actually achieved that." (p. 168)

When nurses achieved their expectations and desires to make a positive difference to their clients, the nurses saw value in their work that was affirming to them. There is, then, a positive connection between nurses' view of themselves and what they achieve for their clients.

Implications

Students and developing practitioners of nursing need guidance and support in order to feel free to concentrate their attention upon the client. By knowing the client, nurses learn how they can make a positive difference in that person's life. Nurses who perceive this difference are able to embrace the goals of nursing as their own goals, and to better recognize the good that they do.

Note: Reprinted with permission from Sage Publications Ltd., from E. Pask, "Moral Agency in Nursing: Seeing Value in the Work and Believing That I Make a Difference." Copyright © 2003 Sage Publications Ltd., 2003.

---

assesses the client's pain, using an appropriate pain scale. The client's positioning, hygiene, amount of rest, and other physiologic variables are assessed for their effect on pain. In addition, there are a multitude of other factors that affect the client's perception of pain. Is this surgery likely to cure the cancer, or is it primarily palliative? The meaning of the diagnosis and surgery to this client affects his pain experience. The nurse discovers that this man lost his wife to cancer 2 years ago. His daughter, at the bedside, is his primary support. The nurse discusses with his daughter how she can make her father more comfortable.

Knowing the client and family ultimately involves the nurse and client in a caring transaction. By attending broadly to personal, ethical, aesthetic, and empirical knowledge, the nurse understands events as they have meaning in the life of the client. The nurse's *knowing the client* ultimately increases the possibilities for therapeutic interventions to be perceived as relevant.

Nursing Presence

Caring in nursing always takes place in a relationship. Watson (2002) describes the transpersonal caring relationship, in which the nurse enters into the life space of another person. Establishment of a caring relationship depends on a moral commitment by the nurse and the nurse's ability to assess and realize another person's state of being. Mutuality within this relationship involves a partnership between the nurse and client.

Swanson's category *being with* (Table 12–1) provides a description of nursing presence. By being emotionally present to the client and family, the nurse conveys that they and their experiences matter. Being present is a way of sharing in

the meanings, feelings, and lived experiences of the client. Physical presence is combined with the promise of availability, especially during a time of need. This may be as simple as responding promptly to a call bell on a hospital unit, or as complex as sitting with a parent who has just lost a child in a neonatal intensive care unit. In an account by the parent of a newborn with a serious heart defect, Schroeder (1998) described how a nurse periodically sat with her. "Her words and presence began to fill some of the emptiness inside me," (p. 19) she said. Quietly talking with the nurse helped this mother find meaning in her experience, as she "began to see that perhaps this experience wasn't just meaningless destruction, torture and death: regardless of outcome, we were all growing in ways denied ordinary people" (p. 20).

Covington (2003) defines caring presence as an "interpersonal, intersubjective human experience of connection within a nurse–client relationship that makes it safe for sharing oneself with another" (p. 312). The nurse brings conscious awareness (intentionality), and is open to opportunities for connection with the client. Through this sharing, both client and nurse attempt to discover meaning in the experience of health and illness. A possible outcome is transformation and growth of both client and nurse.

Empowering the Client

Through knowing the client and engaging in a mutual relationship, the nurse is able to identify and build upon client/family strengths. This empowering relationship includes mutual respect, trust, and confidence in the other's abilities and motives. According to Swanson (1993), the caring behavior of *enabling* is defined as "facilitating the other's passage through life transitions and unfamiliar events" (p. 356). Enabling also includes coaching, informing, explaining, supporting, assisting, guiding, focusing, and validating. There are times when enabling involves substitutive care (doing for the client who is unable to do for oneself), but doing no more than is needed at the time. At other times, enabling involves providing an environment in which the client can function safely and effectively. The nurse should remain mindful of professional boundaries and responsibilities, to avoid enabling pathologic choices by the client. The goal is always to facilitate growth and development.

Nurses both *advocate for* (verb) and are *advocates* (noun) for clients and families. Knowlden (1998) explored the meaning of caring in nursing and identified four dimensions of advocacy: (a) being a client advocate, (b) following through or following up, (c) providing resources, and (d) going above and beyond. A client in Knowlden's study described how his nurse was an advocate for him: "She keeps in touch with [my practitioner] to find out what's to be done. She gets through right away. They give us the run-around and get back 5 days later. . . . She has been instrumental in getting the tube changed" (p. 37). Through advocacy, nurses are champions for their clients. They empower clients and families through activities that enhance well-being, understanding, and self-care.

Compassion

Universally, clients equate compassion with caring. The caring nurse is described as warm and empathic, compassionate and concerned. In order to demonstrate empathy, the nurse must be able to identify with the client, appreciating the pain and discomfort of illness, or imagining "walking in his shoes," in regard to some part of the client's life experience.

Roach (2002) defines compassion as "a way of living born out of an awareness of one's relationship to all living creatures" (p. 50). Like empathy, compassion involves participating in the client's experience, with sensitivity to the person's pain or discomfort, and a willingness to share in their experience. Compassion is given as part of the caring relationship, as the nurse shares the client's joys, sorrows, pain, and accomplishments. Compassion is a gift from the heart, rather than an advanced skill or technique.

Attention to spiritual needs is part of compassionate care, particularly in the face of death and bereavement. The nurse is aware that spiritual and religious beliefs are important coping mechanisms in dealing with issues of mortality (see Chapter 29 ∞). The nurse does not impose his or her own spiritual beliefs, but rather assists the client and family in drawing upon their own beliefs as spiritual resources.

Comfort is often associated with compassionate care, and many nursing interventions are carried out to provide comfort. For example, bathing, positioning, talking, touching, and listening are often performed to increase the client's comfort level. Just like pain or discomfort, comfort is subjective and is defined as "whatever the client says it is," based on the individual's perceptions. Despite this subjectivity, comfort care is often the basis for nursing in settings ranging from intensive care to hospice, and serves as a motivator for nursing interventions. Nurses are challenged to be creative and innovative, basing interventions on knowledge of the client's preferences, in order to provide comfort care.

Competence

The competent nurse employs the necessary knowledge, judgment, skills, and motivation to respond adequately to the client's needs. Just as competence without compassion is cold and inhumane, compassion without competence is meaningless and dangerous. The competent nurse, as described by Roach (2002), understands the client's condition, its treatment, and associated care. The nurse is able to provide the necessary care, while guiding the client and family through the process. The nurse's abilities to assess, plan, implement, and evaluate a plan of care are focused on meeting the client's and family's needs. Practice of these skills requires a high level of cognitive, affective, technical, and administrative skills.

MAINTAINING CARING PRACTICE

The concept of caring for self seems almost foreign to many nurses and students of nursing, because of the professional emphasis on meeting others' needs. Yet, as nurses take on multiple commitments to family, work, school, and community, they risk exhaustion, burnout, and stress. Obstacles to self-care may be professional, related to the demands of a particular work setting, or may be personal, such as poor health habits or unrealistic expectations of self (see Chapter 30 ∞ for more information on stress and coping). Despite these challenges, it is imperative that nurses attend to their own needs, because caring for self is central to caring for others.

Caring for Self

Mayeroff (1990) describes caring for self as helping oneself grow and actualize one's possibilities. Self-care, when defined as responding to one's own needs to grow, is the opposite of the self-complacency that often accompanies egocentricity. Caring for self means taking the time to nurture oneself. This involves initiating and maintaining behaviors that promote healthy living and well-being. Although different activities may be helpful to different people, some examples of these activities are the following:

- A balanced diet
- Regular exercise
- Adequate rest and sleep
- Recreational activities
- Meditation and prayer

Self-care focuses on care of the self in the deepest sense. Self-awareness and self-esteem are intimately connected to self-care. Each person is unique and possesses individual strengths and weaknesses. Self-care practices are intentionally created by the self and vigilantly maintained. This is a lifelong unfolding process, leading to wholeness that comes from and contributes to self-esteem. In its code of ethics, the American Holistic Nurses Association states that "the nurse has a responsibility to model healthy behaviors. Holistic nurses strive to achieve harmony in their own lives and to assist others who are striving to do the same" (American Holistic Nurses Association, 1992, p. 275). Individuals with high self-esteem can critically problem solve and tackle obstacles more effectively. Self-care practices build self-esteem, leading to feelings of comfort and accomplishment.

A HEALTHY LIFESTYLE   Everyone needs to pay attention to nutrition and exercise, and to avoid unhealthy lifestyle practices. Key words for a healthy lifestyle are *balance* and *moderation*. These lifestyle practices are supplemented by regular physical examinations and health screenings.

Nutrition   Healthy eating is important for everyone. A nutritionally balanced eating plan provides more energy, builds endurance to carry out daily activities, and reduces the risk for certain health problems. Healthy eating means learning to make good choices in the foods eaten, preparing foods appropriately, and eating in moderation. It is important to select a variety of foods, to eat regular meals, and to eat the correct amount to maintain a healthy weight. Determining a healthy weight depends on several factors, including age, activity level, and the presence of weight-related medical problems such as high blood pressure. Dietary guidelines and standards for a healthy diet are included in Chapter 32 ∞.

Activity and Exercise   Exercise is recognized as a lifetime endeavor that is essential for energetic, active, and healthy living (see Figure 12–3). The benefits of exercise have been linked to many physiologic and psychologic responses, from a reduced feeling of stress to an increased sense of well-being. Exercise strengthens the heart, lungs, and blood vessels to prevent heart disease, keeps the joints flexible, and helps many people deal with sad or unhappy feelings. For persons who are overweight, exercise has the added benefit of burning calories, resulting in weight loss or maintenance. Whatever the exercise, whether walking or working out in a gym, 20 minutes of exercise two to three times a week is recommended (Maville & Huerta, 2002).

Nurses participate in strenuous activities that call for specialized knowledge of body mechanics and movement techniques to prevent self-injuries. Self-care practices are based on competence and compliance with these specialized techniques and knowledge of how to use assistive devices such as hydraulic lifts, belts, and sliding boards. An in-depth discussion of these techniques is included in Chapter 21 ∞.

Recreation   Self-care also includes taking time to do the things that bring joy and stimulate creativity. Nurses need to reward themselves, to experience spontaneity, and even to take downtime or time to do nothing. Defending the right to this time may take courage and conviction in the face of others' demands.

Avoiding Unhealthy Patterns   Part of staying healthy is avoiding unhealthy life patterns. This means avoiding activities or thought patterns that contribute to negative health outcomes. Negative thinking can create a stress response, with all its physiological, mental, and emotional outcomes. It is not what happens, but how events are perceived, that determines an individual's reaction. Practices such as identifying negative feelings, refocusing on the positive, and using humor are helpful to avert the stress response by changing thought patterns. Using positive affirmations can lead to greater self-esteem and control self-doubt. It is also important to avoid destructive lifestyle choices such as smoking, abuse of alcohol or drugs, and misusing medications.

MIND–BODY THERAPIES   The interconnectedness of the mind and body is the basis for the complementary therapies. Imagery, meditation, storytelling, music therapy, and yoga are complementary therapies that bring balance to thoughts and emotions. Practice of one or more mind–body therapies is an effective self-care strategy to help restore peace and balance. More in-depth information on different types of complementary therapies is included in Chapter 5 ∞.

Guided Imagery   Imagery is a mind–body intervention that uses the power of the imagination as a therapeutic tool. Imagery is used to promote relaxation, decrease anxiety, and enhance psychologic or spiritual insight. Through forming mental images of an object, event, or situation, the individual can reframe negative responses into positive images, enhancing healing and emotional well-being.

Meditation   Through quieting the mind and focusing it on the present, meditation assists the individual in releasing fears, worries, and doubts. The technique involves both relaxation and focused attention. Guidelines for mindfulness meditation include choosing a quiet space, sitting comfortably, achieving progressive relaxation through deep breathing, and focusing attention on breathing or a mental image.

Storytelling   Telling stories is a natural component of everyday conversation that can be utilized as a powerful tool

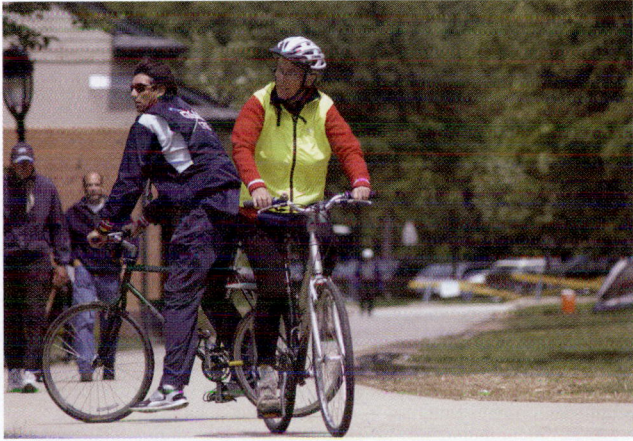

Figure 12–3 ⬤ Regular activity and exercise is an effective self-care practice.

to communicate with others (Struthers, 2002). As expressions of human consciousness, stories help individuals move toward wholeness. Indigenous groups conducted storytelling sessions with the participants sitting in a talking circle, a shape that assists the intuition in discerning that things occur in the manner they are intended to happen.

Music Therapy   Using music as therapy includes listening, singing, rhythm, and body movement. Quiet, soothing music is often used to induce relaxation. Active rhythms can awaken feelings of power and control. Familiar music allows the listener to recall past events or feelings. Music can also serve as an effective distraction technique. Each person's likes and dislikes are taken into account in order to achieve the desired emotional response.

Yoga   The practice of yoga unites the body, mind, and spirit. Through daily practice of the various postures and breathing practices of yoga, an individual can achieve increased balance and flexibility, mental alertness, and calmness. The bending, stretching, and holding properties of the postures help to relax and tone the muscles and improve function of the internal organs. Breath control is designed to still the mind and enhance awareness.

Reflection on Practice

Critical thinking, self-analysis, and reflection are required in order to learn from one's experience. The student matures as a practitioner by thinking about how values and standards guide practical experience. **Reflection** is thinking from a critical point of view, analyzing why one acted in a certain way, and assessing the results of one's actions. In order to develop oneself as a caring practitioner, reflection on practice must be personal and meaningful.

Reflective practice is a method of self-examination that involves thinking back over what happened in a nursing situation. It involves the whole person, including his or her emotions. Reflectivity includes becoming aware of how one feels about oneself and recognizing how one thinks and acts. This exploration of experiences leads to new understandings and appreciations. Through reflection, nurses can become more comfortable with an authentic way of being-in-the-world and can participate more fully in caring-healing relationships (Cumbie, 2001).

USING FOUR WAYS OF KNOWING   Reflection provides a method to explore alternative forms of nursing knowledge, including empirical, aesthetic, personal, and ethical types. Johns suggests the following questions for exploration of different ways of knowing (2000, p. 47):

- *Empirical knowing:* What knowledge informed me in this situation? What additional information did I need? Was I prepared to deal with this situation?
- *Personal knowing:* What were my thoughts and emotions in this situation? Why did I feel the way I did? To what extent was I concerned for the person? To what extent was I preoccupied with self?
- *Aesthetic knowing:* What was I trying to achieve? Why did I respond as I did? What were the consequences for the client/family? How were others feeling and how did I know this?

BOX 12–2   **Guidelines for Reflective Journaling**

Reflection is a window through which the student can view and focus on self, in ways that enable him or her to understand, confront, and work toward resolving the contradictions between actual and desirable practice. Reflection facilitates learning through everyday lived experiences. This guideline focuses on the concept of *being available*, which is the essence of effective holistic practice (Johns, 2000). The following outline can be used as a guide for journaling after each clinical experience:

1. Knowing what is desirable (ethical knowing)
   - What are your beliefs and values in relation to the situation?
   - Describe the contradictions between your values and the reality of the situation.
2. Knowing the person/family
   - What is the meaning of the health event to each person?
   - What are each person's values and needs?
   - What behaviors did you assess to reveal these meanings and needs?
   - How did your relationship (trust) with each person influence your knowing?
3. Concern for the person/family
   - Evaluate your level of concern for the person/family.
   - How easy or difficult was it to care about each person?
   - How did your personal reactions influence your concern?

4. The aesthetic response to the person (aesthetic knowing)
   - Assess the extent to which you were able to interpret the situation, envision what needed to be done, and respond appropriately to the person/family.
   - Were you able to expand on your ability to be available to the person and respond effectively?
5. Knowing and managing self's involvement with the person (personal knowing)
   - In what ways did you feel vulnerable in the situation?
   - How did you manage negative influences such as anxiety, stress, prejudice, loss of concern, preoccupation with self?
   - What did you feel you did well, or improved upon from previous experiences?
6. Creating and sustaining an environment where being available is possible
   - Were there environmental factors that constrained your availability to work with the client and family (norms, ways of relating, lack of resources, time, etc.)?

Note: From *"Becoming a Reflective Practitioner,"* by Chris Johns, 2000, pp. 69–70, Blackwell Science. Copyright © 2000 Blackwell Publishing. Reprinted with permission.

- *Ethical knowing:* Did I act for the best? What standards were relevant in this situation? Was there conflict of values between different persons' perspectives?

Reflective practice requires discipline, action, openness, and trust. It is a form of self-evaluation. Reflective journaling, as a tool for learning, is usually shared with a mentor or teacher, who works in partnership with the student. A guideline, such as the one in Box 12–2, provides structure for the journaling process. Writing reflections in a journal provides a space for the student to look at and acknowledge the deeper self. Guidance from a mentor or teacher can help the student view a nursing situation from many different perspectives. It helps the student find meaning in the event, understand and learn through it, and emerge at a higher level of understanding.

CHAPTER HIGHLIGHTS

- Caring practice involves connection, mutual recognition, and involvement between nurse and client. Caring is central to nursing practice.
- To care for another person is to help the person grow and actualize him or herself. By helping the other grow, the caregiver moves toward self-actualization. Caring behaviors described by Mayeroff include knowing, alternating rhythms, patience, honesty, trust, humility, hope, and courage.
- Caring is a multidimensional concept, summarized by Morse et al. as five viewpoints: (a) moral imperative, (b) affect, (c) human trait, (d) interpersonal relationship, and (e) therapeutic intervention.
- Various theorists have focused on caring as the essence of nursing. Each theory develops different aspects of caring, describing how caring is unique in nursing.
- Nursing involves different types of knowledge that are integrated to guide nursing practice. Empirical knowing includes scientific competence, personal knowing focuses on the self, ethical knowing requires moral/ethical awareness, and aesthetic knowing is the creative art of nursing.
- Caring encounters are influenced by the diversity of human responses. Common caring patterns include knowing the client, nursing presence, empowering the client, compassion, and competence.
- Caring for self is central to caring for others. Nurse self-care includes a balanced diet, regular exercise, adequate rest and sleep, recreational activities, and mind–body therapies.
- The nurse matures as a practitioner by reflecting on practice. Through reflection, nurses can grow and participate more fully in caring-healing relationships.

THINK ABOUT IT

Refer to the chapter-opening scenario and answer these questions.

1. How does the nurse care for Franklin?

2. How can the nurse advocate for the client by talking with Mrs. Fielder?

3. With a client like Franklin, who most likely has a terminal illness, how does psychologically supportive care compare to physically supportive caring?

∞ *See suggested responses to Think About It on MyNursingKit.*

TEST YOUR KNOWLEDGE

1. Which of the following examples illustrates that the nurse "knows" the client?
   1. The nurse provides a back rub to help the client relax, and then makes the bed with clean linen.
   2. The nurse listens as the client describes how he has been caring for his diabetes at home.
   3. The nurse administers a piggyback antibiotic for a client with pneumonia.
   4. The nurse explains the reason a specimen is required, collects it, and sends it to the lab.

2. The nurse teaches a client with diabetes how to make decisions about insulin management after discharge. This teaching most clearly reflects which caring activity?
   1. Empowering the client
   2. Compassion
   3. Knowing the client
   4. Nursing presence

3. The nurse allows the client to grow in his own way and time. According to Mayeroff, this behavior most clearly reflects which major ingredient of caring?
1. Humility
2. Knowing
3. Patience
4. Courage

4. Leininger's theory would provide the best framework for assessing which of the following nursing situations?
1. Because the Indonesian parents of an infant preferred to use hot/cold therapies to prevent seizures, they withheld the prescribed phenobarbital medication.
2. Staff nurses on a hospital unit discuss how to reorganize client care to provide more continuity of staff with clients.
3. Nurses in a community agency search for learning resources about intravenous therapy in the home setting.
4. A nurse manager explores ways to assist new nursing graduates to develop clinical skills on the hospital unit.

5. In a reflective journal, a nursing student writes this statement about a comatose client on the hospice unit: "The do-not-resuscitate order was not on the chart, and none of the nurses knew what measures should be taken if the client stopped breathing." This statement most clearly reflects which of the four ways of knowing?
1. Empirical
2. Personal
3. Ethical
4. Aesthetic

6. The nurse sits with the client and holds the client's hand as his pain decreases. This situation is an example of the following caring practice:
1. Nursing presence
2. Assessment
3. Knowing the client
4. Empowering

7. Which nursing theory is depicted by a model with spiritual-ethical caring in the center, surrounded by political, legal, economic, educational, physiologic, social-cultural, and technological systems?
1. Nursing as caring
2. Theory of bureaucratic caring
3. Caring, the human mode of being
4. Theory of human care

8. The nursing student reviews the pathophysiology of myocardial infarction, in preparation for the next day's clinical experience. This activity is an example of which type of knowledge development?
1. Empirical knowing
2. Aesthetic knowing
3. Personal knowing
4. Ethical knowing

9. The nurse documents which type of mind–body therapy described by the following activity: "The person sits quietly in a chair, breathing deeply and focusing on the mental image of a crystal"?
1. Storytelling
2. Yoga
3. Music therapy
4. Meditation

10. A 40-year-old client who comes to the clinic for a routine physical exam asks the nurse how much exercise is recommended for a healthy lifestyle. Which answer is most appropriate?
1. 10 minutes daily
2. 30 minutes daily
3. 20 minutes two to three times a week
4. 1 hour every other day

∞ *See answers to Test Your Knowledge in Appendix A.*

REFERENCES AND SELECTED BIBLIOGRAPHY

American Holistic Nurses Association. (1992). Code of ethics for holistic nurses. *Journal of Holistic Nursing, 10*(3), 275–276.

Benner, P. (2002). *From novice to expert: Excellence and power in clinical nursing practice.* Upper Saddle River, NJ: Prentice Hall Health.

Benner, P., & Wrubel, J. (1989). *The primacy of caring: Stress and coping in health and illness.* Menlo Park, CA: Addison-Wesley.

Boykin, A., & Schoenhofer, S. (2001). Nursing as caring: An overview of a general theory of nursing. In M. Parker (Ed.), *Nursing theories and nursing practice* (pp. 391–402). Philadelphia: Davis.

Cameron, J. (2002). *The artist's way.* New York: Tarcher/Putnam.

Canfield, J., Hansen, M. V., Mitchell-Autoio, N., & Thieman, L. (2001). *Chicken soup for the nurse's soul: 101 stories to celebrate, honor, and inspire the nursing profession.* Deerfield Beach, FL: Health Communications.

Carper, B. (1978). Fundamental patterns of knowing in nursing. *Advances in Nursing Science, 1*(1), 13–23.

Chenevert, M. (2006). *Mosby's tour guide to nursing school: A student's road survival kit* (6th ed.). St. Louis: Mosby.

Chinn, P., & Kramer, M. (2005). *Integrated knowledge development in nursing* (7th ed.). St. Louis: Mosby.

Coffman, S. (2006). Marilyn Anne Ray: Theory of bureaucratic caring. In A. Tomey & M. Alligood (Eds.), *Nursing theorists and their work* (6th ed., pp. 116–139). St. Louis: Mosby.

Cooper, C. (2001). *The art of nursing.* Philadelphia: Saunders.

Covington, H. (2003). Caring presence. *Journal of Holistic Nursing, 21*(3), 301–317.

Cumbie, S. (2001). The integration of mind-body-soul and the practice of humanistic nursing. *Holistic Nursing Practice, 15*(3), 56–62.

Dowling, M. (2004). Exploring the relationship between caring, love and intimacy in nursing. *British Journal of Nursing, 13*(21), 1289–1292.

Fink, J. (2005). Burned out? Here's help. *Nursing, 35*(4), 53.

Freshwater, D. (2002). *Therapeutic nursing.* London: Sage.

Gaydos, H. (2004). "Making special": A framework for understanding the art of holistic nursing. *Journal of Holistic Nursing, 22*(2), 152–163.

Godkin, J., & Godkin, L. (2004). Caring behaviors among nurses: Fostering a conversation of gestures. *Health Care Management Review, 29*(3), 258–267.

Gordon, S., Benner, P., & Noddings, N. (1996). *Caregiving.* Philadelphia: University of Pennsylvania Press.

Graber, D., & Mitcham, M. (2004). Compassionate clinicians take patient care beyond the ordinary. *Holistic Nursing Practice, 18*(2), 87–94.

Henry, L. G., & Henry, J. D. (2004). *The soul of the caring nurse. Stories & resources for revitalizing professional passion.* Washington, DC: American Nurses Association.

Hudacek, S. (2004). *Making a difference: Stories from the point of care* (Vol. II). Indianapolis, IN: Sigma Theta Tau International.

Hunter, L. (2002). Being with women: A guiding concept for the care of laboring women. *Journal of Obstetric, Gynecologic, and Neonatal Nursing, 31*(31), 555–562.

Jackson, C. (2004). Healing ourselves, healing others. *Holistic Nursing Practice, 18*(3), 127–141.

Johns, C. (2000). *Becoming a reflective practitioner.* Oxford, England: Blackwell Science.

Johns, C. (2002). *Guided reflection: Advancing practice.* Oxford, England: Blackwell Science.

Kapborg, I., & Bertero, C. (2003). The phenomenon of caring from the novice student nurse's perspective: A qualitative content analysis. *International Nursing Review, 50,* 183–192.

Knowlden, V. (1998). *The communication of caring in nursing.* Indianapolis, IN: Center Nursing Press.

Leininger, M. M. (2001). *Culture care diversity & universality: A theory of nursing.* Sudbury, MA: Jones & Bartlett.

Maville, J., & Huerta, C. (2002). *Health promotion in nursing.* Albany, NY: Delmar.

Mayeroff, M. (1990). *On caring.* New York: Harper Collins.

Miller, J., & Cutshall, S. (2001). *The art of being a healing presence: A guide for those in caring relationships.* Ft. Wayne, IN: Willowgreen.

Morse, J., Solberg, S., Neander, W., Battorff, J., & Johnson, J. (1990). Concepts of caring and caring as a concept. *Advances in Nursing Science, 13*(1), 1–14.

Parker, M. (2006). *Nursing theories and nursing practice* (2nd ed.). Philadelphia: F. A. Davis.

Pask, E. (2003). Moral agency in nursing: Seeing value in the work and believing that I make a difference. *Nursing Ethics, 10*(2), 165–174.

Phillips, S., & Benner, P. (1994). *The crisis of care: Affirming and restoring caring practices in the helping professions.* Washington, DC: Georgetown University Press.

Poirier, S., & Ayres, L. (2002). *Stories of family caregiving.* Indianapolis, IN: Center Nursing Publishing.

Purnell, M. (2006). Nursing as caring: A model for transforming practice. In A. Tomey & M. Alligood (Eds.), *Nursing theorists and their work* (6th ed.). St. Louis: Mosby.

Ray, M. (2001). The theory of bureaucratic caring. In M. Parker (Ed.), *Nursing theories and nursing practice* (pp. 422–431). Philadelphia: Davis.

Ray, M., Turkel, M., & Marino, F. (2002). The transformative process for nursing in workforce redevelopment. *Nursing Administration Quarterly, 26*(2), 1–14.

Roach, M. S. (2002). *Caring, the human mode of being* (2nd ed.). Ottawa, Ontario, Canada: CHA Press.

Ruth-Sahd, L. (2003). Reflective practice: A critical analysis of data-based studies and implications for nursing education. *Journal of Nursing Education, 42*(11), 488–497.

Schroeder, C. (1998). So this is what it's like: Struggling to survive in pediatric intensive care. *Advances in Nursing Science, 10*(4), 13–22.

Snyder, M., & Lindquist, R. (2010). *Complementary/alternative therapies in nursing* (6th ed.) New York: Springer.

Struthers, R. (2002). Storytelling as a healing tool. In M. Snyder & R. Lindquist (Eds.), *Complementary/alternative therapies in nursing* (4th ed., pp. 124–134). New York: Springer.

Swanson, K. (1991). Empirical development of a middle range theory of caring. *Nursing Research, 40*(3), 161–166.

Swanson, K. (1993). Nursing as informed caring for the well-being of others. *IMAGE: Journal of Nursing Scholarship, 25*(4), 352–357.

Swanson, K. (2001). A program of research on caring. In M. Parker (Ed.), *Nursing theories and nursing practice* (pp. 411–420). Philadelphia: Davis.

The Positive Way. (2006) Self-esteem questionnaire. Retrieved June 7, 2006, from http://www.positive-way.com/self-est1.htm

Tomey, A. M., & Alligood, M. (2006). *Nursing theorists and their work* (6th ed.). St. Louis: Mosby.

Turkel, M. (2003). A journey into caring as experienced by nurse managers. *International Journal for Human Caring, 7*(1), 20–26.

Tutton, E., & Seers, K. (2003). An exploration of the concept of comfort. *Journal of Clinical Nursing, 12,* 689–696.

Watson, J. (1999). *Nursing: Human science and human care. A theory of nursing.* Boston: Jones & Bartlett.

Watson, J. (2002). Intentionality and caring-healing consciousness: A practice of transpersonal nursing. *Holistic Nursing Practice, 16*(4), 12–19.

Watson, J., & Foster, R. (2003). The attending nurse caring model: Integrating theory, evidence and advanced caring-healing therapeutics for transforming professional practice. *Journal of Clinical Nursing, 12*(3), 360–365.

Wendler, M. C. (2002). *The heart of nursing: Expressions of creative art in nursing.* Indianapolis, IN: Sigma Theta Tau International.

Wieck, K. L. (2003). *Stories for nurses. Acts of caring.* St. Louis: Mosby.

Wilkin, K. (2003). The meaning of caring in the practice of intensive care nursing. *British Journal of Nursing, 12*(20), 1178–1292.

Wilt, D., & Smucker, C. (2001). *Nursing the spirit: The art and science of applying spiritual care.* Washington, DC: American Nurses Association.

Wiman, E., & Wikbland, K. (2004). Caring and uncaring encounters in nursing in an emergency department. *Journal of Clinical Nursing, 13,* 422–429.

Communication

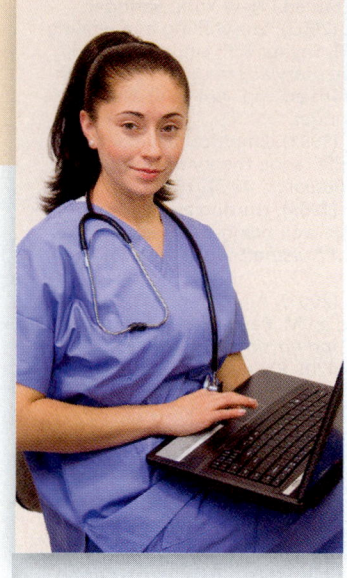

Barbara is a nurse in a long-term care facility that is planning to convert from paper documentation to computerized documentation, with the goal of being paperless within two years. The nurse administrator is assembling a group of nurses, including those in management and at the bedside, to advise the technology experts about nurses' needs for the new software system to be chosen. Barbara joins the committee and looks forward to sharing ideas at the first meeting.

When Barbara enters the conference room for the first meeting, she is surprised to find that there is no leader in charge. People are talking at the same time, some suggestions made by members of the committee are ridiculed, and no one seems to be listening to what others are saying. Barbara decides that she will notify her nurse manager that she will be unable to continue her membership on this committee.

LEARNING OUTCOMES

After completing this chapter, you will be able to:

1. Identify factors influencing the communication process.
2. Discuss nurse–client communication as a dynamic process.
3. Describe four phases of the helping relationship.
4. Identify features of effective groups.
5. Identify types of groups helpful in promoting health and comfort.
6. Discuss how nurses use communication skills in each phase of the nursing process.
7. State why effective communication is imperative among health professionals.
8. Differentiate major characteristics between assertive and nonassertive communication.

KEY TERMS

attentive listening p308
congruent
    communication p307
decode p301
elderspeak p308

empathy p314
encoding p301
feedback p302
group p316
group dynamics p316

helping relationships
    p313
personal space p306
process recording p321

proxemics p306
territoriality p307
therapeutic
    communication p308

Communication is a critical skill for nursing. It is the process by which humans meet their survival needs, build relationships, and experience emotions. In nursing, communication is a dynamic process used to gather assessment data, to teach and persuade, and to express caring and comfort. It is an integral part of the helping relationship.

COMMUNICATING

The term *communication* has various meanings, depending on the context in which it is used. To some, communication is the interchange of information between two or more people; in other words, the exchange of ideas or thoughts. This kind of communication uses methods such as talking and listening or writing and reading. However, painting, dancing, and storytelling are also methods of communication. In addition, thoughts are conveyed to others not only by spoken or written words but also by gestures or body actions.

Communication may have a more personal connotation than the interchange of ideas or thoughts. It can be a transmission of feelings or a more personal and social interaction between people. Frequently, one member of a couple comments that the other is not communicating. Some teenagers complain about a generation gap—being unable to communicate with understanding or feeling to a parent or authority figure. Sometimes a nurse is said to be efficient but lacking in something called *bedside manner*. For the purpose of this text, communication is any means of exchanging information or feelings between two or more people. It is a basic component of human relationships, including nursing.

The intent of any communication is to elicit a response. Thus, communication is a process. It has two main purposes: to influence others and to obtain information. Communication can be described as helpful or unhelpful. The former encourages a sharing of information, thoughts, or feelings between two or more people. The latter hinders or blocks the transfer of information and feelings.

Nurses who communicate effectively are better able to collect assessment data, initiate interventions, evaluate outcomes of interventions, initiate change that promotes health, and prevent legal problems associated with nursing practice. The communication process is built on a trusting relationship with a client and support persons. Effective communication is essential for the establishment of a nurse–client relationship.

Communication can occur on an intrapersonal level within a single individual as well as on interpersonal and group levels. Intrapersonal communication is the communication that you have with yourself; another name is *self-talk*. Both the sender and the receiver of a message usually engage in self-talk. It involves thinking about the message before it is sent, while it is being sent, and after it is sent, and it occurs constantly. Consequently, intrapersonal communication can interfere with a person's ability to hear a message as the sender intended.

The Communication Process

Face-to-face communication involves a sender, a message, a receiver, and a response, or feedback. In its simplest form, communication is a two-way process involving the sending and the receiving of a message. Because the intent of communication is to elicit a response, the process is ongoing; the receiver of the message then becomes the sender of a response, and the original sender then becomes the receiver.

SENDER The *sender,* a person or group who wishes to convey a message to another, can be considered the *source-encoder.* This term suggests that the person or group sending the message must have an idea or reason for communicating (source) and must put the idea or feeling into a form that can be transmitted. **Encoding** involves the selection of specific signs or symbols (codes) to transmit the message, such as which language and words to use, how to arrange the words, and what tone of voice and gestures to use. For example, if the receiver speaks English, the sender usually selects English words. If the message is "Mr. Johnson, you have to wait another hour for your pain medication," the tone of voice selected and a shake of the head can reinforce it. The nurse must not only deal with dialects and foreign languages but also cope with two language levels—the layperson's and the health professional's.

MESSAGE The second component of the communication process is the *message* itself—what is actually said or written, the body language that accompanies the words, and how the message is transmitted. The medium used to convey the message is the channel, and it can target any of the receiver's senses. It is important for the channel to be appropriate for the message and it should help make the intent of the message clearer.

Talking face to face with a person may be more effective in some instances than telephoning or writing a message. Recording messages on tape or communicating by radio or television may be more appropriate for larger audiences. Written communication is often appropriate for long explanations or for a communication that needs to be preserved. The nonverbal channel of touch is often highly effective.

RECEIVER The *receiver,* the third component of the communication process, is the listener, who must listen, observe, and attend. This person is the *decoder,* who must perceive what the sender intended (interpretation). Perception uses all of the senses to receive verbal and nonverbal messages. To **decode** means to relate the message perceived to the receiver's storehouse of knowledge and experience and to sort out the meaning of the message. Whether the message is decoded accurately by the receiver, according to the sender's intent, depends largely on their similarities in knowledge and experience and sociocultural background. If the meaning of the decoded message matches the intent of the sender, then the communication has been effective. Ineffective communication occurs when the message sent is misinterpreted by the receiver. For example, Mr. Johnson may perceive the message accurately—"No pain medication for another hour."

However, if experience has taught him that he can receive the pain medication early if a certain nurse is on duty, he will interpret the intent of the message differently.

RESPONSE   The fourth component of the communication process, the response, is the message that the receiver returns to the sender. It is also called **feedback**. Feedback can be either verbal, nonverbal, or both. Nonverbal examples are a nod of the head or a yawn. Either way, feedback allows the sender to correct or reword a message. In the case of Mr. Johnson, the receiver may appear irritated or say, "Well, the nurse on the other shift gives me my pain medication early if I need it." The sender then knows the message was interpreted accurately. However, now the original sender becomes the receiver, who is required to decode and respond.

Modes of Communication

Communication is generally carried out in two different modes: verbal and nonverbal. Verbal communication uses the spoken or written word; nonverbal communication uses other forms, such as gestures or facial expressions, and touch. Although both kinds of communication occur concurrently, the majority of communication is nonverbal. Learning about nonverbal communication is important for nurses in developing effective communication patterns and relationships with clients. Another form of communication has evolved with technology—electronic communication. The most common form of electronic communication is e-mail where an individual can send a message, by computer, to another person or group of people. It is important for nurses to know when it is appropriate and not appropriate to use e-mail when communicating with clients.

VERBAL COMMUNICATION   Verbal communication is largely conscious because people choose the words they use. The words used vary among individuals according to culture, socioeconomic background, age, and education. As a result, countless possibilities exist for the way ideas are exchanged. An abundance of words can be used to form messages. In addition, a wide variety of feelings can be conveyed when people talk.

When choosing words to say or write, nurses need to consider pace and intonation, simplicity, clarity and brevity, timing and relevance, adaptability, credibility, and humor.

Pace and Intonation   The manner of speech, as in the pace or rhythm and intonation, will modify the feeling and impact of the message. The intonation can express enthusiasm, sadness, anger, or amusement. The pace of speech may indicate interest, anxiety, boredom, or fear. For example, speaking slowly and softly to an excited client may help calm the client.

Simplicity   Simplicity includes the use of commonly understood words, brevity, and completeness. Many complex technical terms become natural to nurses. However, laypersons often misunderstand these terms. Words such as *vasoconstriction* or *cholecystectomy* are meaningful to the nurse

and easy to use but are ill advised when communicating with clients. Nurses need to learn to select appropriate, understandable terms based on the age, knowledge, culture, and education of the client. For example, instead of saying to a client, "The nurses will be catheterizing you tomorrow for a urine analysis," it may be more appropriate and understandable to say, "Tomorrow we need to get a sample of your urine, so we will collect it by putting a small tube into your bladder." The latter statement is more likely to elicit a response from the client as to why it is needed and whether it will be uncomfortable, because the person understands the message being conveyed by the nurse.

Clarity and Brevity   A message that is direct and simple will be more effective. Clarity is saying precisely what is meant, and brevity is using the fewest words necessary. The result is a message that is simple and clear. An aspect of this is congruence, or consistency, where the nurse's behavior or nonverbal communication matches the words spoken. When the nurse tells the client, "I am interested in hearing what you have to say," the nonverbal behavior would include the nurse facing the client, making eye contact, and leaning forward. The goal is to communicate clearly so that all aspects of a situation or circumstance are understood. To ensure clarity in communication, nurses also need to speak slowly and enunciate carefully.

Timing and Relevance   Nurses need to be aware of both relevance and timing when communicating with clients. No matter how clearly or simply words are stated or written, the timing needs to be appropriate to ensure that words are heard. Moreover, the messages need to relate to the person or to the person's interests and concerns.

This involves sensitivity to the client's needs and concerns. For example, a client who is enmeshed in fear of cancer may not hear the nurse's explanations about the expected procedures before and after gallbladder surgery. In this situation it is better for the nurse first to encourage the client to express concerns, and then to deal with those concerns. The necessary explanations can be provided at another time when the client is able to listen.

Another problem in timing is asking several questions at once. For example, a nurse enters a client's room and says in one breath, "Good morning, Mrs. Brody. How are you this morning? Did you sleep well last night? Your husband is coming to see you before your surgery, isn't he?" The client no doubt wonders which question to answer first, if any. A related pattern of poor timing is to ask a question and then not wait for an answer before making another comment. On the other hand, research shows that by allowing the client to respond to the social talk or chat, the nurse develops a rapport with the client (Fenwick, Barclay, & Schmeid, 2001). This rapport can help facilitate effective therapeutic communication.

Adaptability   Spoken messages need to be altered in accordance with behavioral cues from the client. This adjustment is referred to as *adaptability*. What the nurse says and how it is said must be individualized and carefully considered. This requires astute assessment and sensitivity on the part of the nurse. For example, a nurse who usually smiles, appears cheerful, and greets his client with an enthusiastic "Hi, Mrs. Brown!" notices that the client is not smiling and appears distressed. It is important for the nurse to then modify his tone of speech and express concern in his facial expression while moving toward the client.

Credibility   *Credibility* means worthiness of belief, trustworthiness, and reliability. Credibility may be the most important criterion of effective communication. Nurses foster credibility by being consistent, dependable, and honest. The nurse needs to be knowledgeable about what is being discussed and to have accurate information. Nurses should convey confidence and certainty in what they are saying, while being able to acknowledge their limitations (e.g., "I don't know the answer to that, but I will find someone who does").

Humor   The use of humor can be a positive and powerful tool in the nurse–client relationship, but it must be used with care. Humor can be used to help clients adjust to difficult and painful situations. The physical act of laughter can be an emotional and physical release, reducing tension by providing a different perspective and promoting a sense of well-being.

When using humor, it is important to consider the client's perception of what is considered humorous. Timing is also important to consider. MacDonald (2004) states that while humor and laughter can help reduce stress and anxiety in the early and recovery stages of a crisis, it may be considered offensive or distracting at a peak crisis period (p. 23).

NONVERBAL COMMUNICATION   Nonverbal communication is sometimes called *body language.* It includes gestures, body movements, use of touch, and physical appearance, including adornment. Nonverbal communication often tells others more about what a person is feeling than what is actually said, because nonverbal behavior is controlled less consciously than verbal behavior (see Figure 13–1). Nonverbal communication either reinforces or contradicts what is said verbally. For example, if a nurse says to a client, "I'd be happy to sit here and talk to you for a while," yet glances nervously at a watch every few seconds, the actions contradict the verbal message. The client is more likely to believe the nonverbal behavior, which conveys "I am very busy and need to leave."

Observing and interpreting the client's nonverbal behavior is an essential skill for nurses to develop. To observe nonverbal behavior efficiently requires a systematic assessment of the person's overall physical appearance, posture, gait, facial expressions, and gestures. Whatever is observed, the nurse needs to exercise caution in interpretation, always clarifying any observation with the client.

Clients who have altered thought processes, such as in schizophrenia or dementia, may experience times when expressing themselves verbally is difficult or impossible. During these times, the nurse needs to be able to interpret the feeling or emotion that the client is expressing nonverbally. An attentive nurse who clarifies observations very often portrays caring and acceptance to the client. This can be a

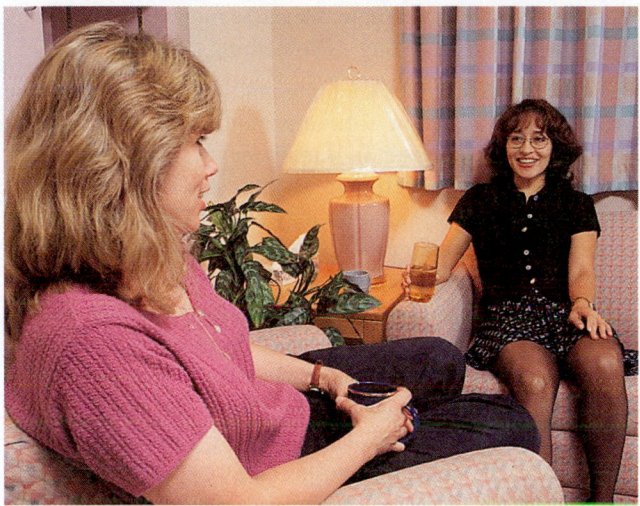

A

B

Figure 13–1 ● Nonverbal communication sometimes conveys meaning more effectively than words. **A,** The postures of these women indicate openness to communication. **B,** The listener's posture suggests resistance to communication.

beginning for establishing a trusting relationship between the nurse and the client, even in clients who have difficulty communicating appropriately.

Transculturally, nonverbal communication varies widely. Even for behaviors such as smiling and handshaking, cultures differ. For example, to many Hispanics smiling and handshaking are an integral part of an interaction and essential to establishing trust. The same behavior might be perceived by a Russian as insolent and frivolous.

The nurse cannot always be sure of the correct interpretation of the feelings expressed nonverbally. The same feeling can be expressed nonverbally in more than one way, even within the same cultural group. For example, anger may be communicated by aggressive or excessive body motion, or it may be communicated by frozen stillness. In some cultures, a smile may be used to conceal anger. Therefore, the interpretation of such observations requires validation with the client. For example, the nurse might say, "You look like you have been crying. Is something upsetting you?"

Personal Appearance   Clothing and adornments can be sources of information about a person. Although choice of apparel is highly personal, it may convey social and financial status, culture, religion, group association, and self-concept. Charms and amulets may be worn for decorative or for health protection purposes. When the symbolic meaning of an object is unfamiliar the nurse can inquire about its significance, which may foster rapport with the client.

How a person dresses is often an indicator of how the person feels. Someone who is tired or ill may not have the energy or the desire to maintain their normal grooming. When a person known for immaculate grooming becomes lax about appearance, the nurse may suspect a loss of self-esteem or a physical illness. The nurse must validate these observed nonverbal data by asking the client. For acutely ill clients in hospital or home care settings, a change in grooming habits may signal that the client is feeling better. A man may request a shave, or a woman may request a shampoo and some makeup.

Posture and Gait   The ways people walk and carry themselves are often reliable indicators of self-concept, current mood, and health. Erect posture and an active, purposeful stride suggest a feeling of well-being. Slouched posture and a slow, shuffling gait suggest depression or physical discomfort. Tense posture and a rapid, determined gait suggest anxiety or anger. The posture of people when they are sitting or lying can also indicate feelings or mood. Again, the nurse clarifies the meaning of the observed behavior by describing to the client what the nurse sees and then asking what it means or whether the nurse's interpretation is correct. For example, "You look like it really hurts you to move. I'm wondering how your pain is and if you might need something to make you more comfortable?"

Facial Expression   No part of the body is as expressive as the face (see Figure 13–2). Feelings of surprise, fear, anger, disgust, happiness, and sadness can be conveyed by facial expressions. Although the face may express the person's genuine emotions, it is also possible to control these muscles so the emotion expressed does not reflect what the person is feeling. When the message is not clear, it is important to get feedback to be sure of the intent of the expression. Many facial expressions convey a universal meaning. The smile expresses happiness. Contempt is conveyed by the mouth turned down, the head tilted back, and the eyes directed down the nose. No single expression can be interpreted accurately, however, without considering other reinforcing physical cues, the setting in which it occurs, the expression of others in the same setting, and the cultural background of the client.

Nurses need to be aware of their own expressions and what they are communicating to others. Clients are quick to notice the nurse's facial expression, particularly when the client feels unsure or uncomfortable. The client who questions the nurse about a feared diagnostic result will watch whether the nurse maintains eye contact or looks away when answering. The client who has had disfiguring surgery will examine the nurse's face for signs of disgust. It is impossible to control all facial expression, but the nurse must learn to control expressions of feelings such as fear or disgust in some circumstances.

Eye contact is another essential element of facial communication. In many cultures, mutual eye contact acknowledges recognition of the other person and a willingness to maintain communication. Often a person initiates contact with another person with a glance, capturing the person's attention prior to communicating. A person who feels weak or defenseless often averts the eyes or avoids eye contact; the communication received may be too embarrassing or too dominating.

Gestures   Hand and body gestures may emphasize and clarify the spoken word, or they may occur without words to indicate a particular feeling or to give a sign. A father awaiting information about his daughter in surgery may wring his hands, tap his foot, pick at his nails, or pace back and forth. A gesture may more clearly indicate the size or shape of an object. A wave good-bye and the motioning of a visitor toward a chair are gestures that have relatively universal meanings. Some gestures, however, are culture specific. The Anglo American gesture meaning "shoo" or "go away" means "come here" or "come back" in some Asian cultures. In the Hmong culture it is considered rude to point at something with your toe.

For people with special communication problems, such as the deaf, the hands are invaluable in communication. Many people who are deaf learn sign language. Ill persons who are unable to reply verbally can similarly devise a communication system using the hands. The client may be able to raise an index finger once for "yes" and twice for "no." Other signals can often be devised by the client and the nurse to denote other meanings.

ELECTRONIC COMMUNICATION   Computers are increasingly playing a big role in nursing practice. Many health care agencies are moving toward electronic medical records where nurses document their assessments and nursing care. Electronic mail (e-mail) can be used in health care facilities

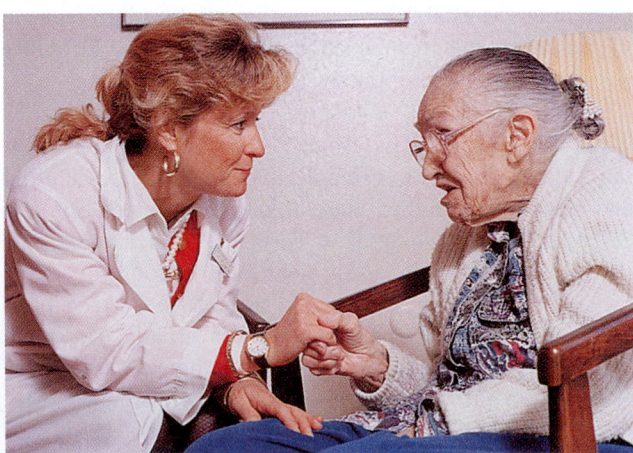

Figure 13–2 ○ The nurse's facial expression communicates warmth and caring.

for many purposes: schedule and confirm appointments, report normal lab results, conduct client education, and follow up with discharged clients (Austin, 2006, p. 76).

E-mail E-mail is the most common form of electronic communication. It is important for the nurse to know the advantages and disadvantages of e-mail and also other guidelines to ensure client confidentiality.

E-mail has many advantages. It is a fast, efficient way to communicate and it is legible. It provides a record of the date and time of the message that was sent or received. Some health facilities provide information to their clients on how they can reach, via e-mail, specified staff members. This improves communication and continuity of client care. E-mail promises better access, and one research study indicated that half of Internet users would like to communicate with a doctor online (Delbanco & Sands, 2004).

The disadvantage or negative aspect of e-mail is the risk to client confidentiality. The Health Insurance Portability and Accountability Act (HIPAA) requires organizations to apply "reasonable and appropriate safeguards" when e-mailing protected health information (PHI) (Anonymous, 2005). The health care agency needs to have an e-mail en-cryption system to ensure security. An agency may have its own system or outsource an encryption service.

Another disadvantage is one of socioeconomics. Not everyone has a computer. While there may be available access to a computer, not everyone has the necessary computer skills. E-mail may enhance communication with some clients but not all clients. Other forms of communication will be needed for clients who have limited abilities with speaking English, reading, writing, or using a computer.

Austin (2006) lists the following situations when it is best to avoid using e-mail:

- When the information is urgent and the client's health could be in jeopardy if he or she doesn't read it immediately.
- Highly confidential information (e.g., HIV status, mental health, chemical dependency).
- Abnormal lab data. If the information is confusing and could prompt many questions by the client, it is better to either see or telephone the person.

Agencies usually develop standards and guidelines for the use of e-mail in health care. It is important to know, per

---

LIFESPAN CONSIDERATIONS   Communication

The ability to communicate is directly related to the development of thought processes, the presence of intact sensory and motor systems, and the extent and nature of an individual's opportunities to practice communication skills. As children grow, their communication abilities change markedly.

Infants

- Infants communicate nonverbally, often in response to body feelings rather than in a conscious effort to be expressive.
- Infants' perceptions are related to sensory stimuli, so a gentle voice is soothing, for example, while tension and anger around them creates distress.

Toddlers and Preschoolers

- Toddlers and young children gain skills in both expressive (i.e., telling others what they feel, think, want, care about) and receptive (hearing and understanding what others are communicating to them) language.
- Allow time for them to complete verbalizing their thoughts without interruption.
- Provide a simple response to questions because they have short attention spans.
- Drawing a picture can provide another way for the child to communicate.

School-Age Children

- Talk to the child at his or her eye level to help decrease intimidation.
- Include the child in the conversation when communicating with the parents.

Adolescents

- Take time to build rapport with the adolescent.
- Use active listening skills.
- Project a nonjudgmental attitude and nonreactive behaviors, even when the adolescent says disturbing remarks.

Family Centered Care

Nurses can use the following communication techniques to work effectively with children and their families:

- Play, the universal language, allows children to use other symbols, not just words, to express themselves.
- Drawing, painting, and other art forms can be used by even nonverbal children.
- Storytelling, in which the nurse and child take turns adding to a story or putting words to pictures, can help the child feel safer in expressing emotions and feelings.
- Word games that pose hypothetical situations or put the child in control, such as "What if . . . ?" "If you could . . . ," "If a genie came and gave you a wish . . . ," can help a child feel more powerful or explore ideas about how to manage the illness.
- Read books with a theme similar to the child's condition or problem, then discuss the meaning, characters, and feelings generated by the book. Movies or videos can also be used in this way.
- Writing can be used by older children to reflect on their situation, develop meaning, and gain a sense of control.

In all interactions with children, it is important to give them opportunities to be expressive, listen openly, and respond honestly, using words and concepts they understand.

the agency's guidelines, what can be e-mailed to clients. Usually there is an e-mail consent form that the client signs. This form provides information about the risks of e-mail and authorizes the health agency to communicate with the client at a specified e-mail address.

Austin (2006) cautions the nurse to be sure to identify that the e-mail is "confidential" in the subject line. She advises including a disclaimer that the message is to be read only by the person to whom it is addressed and that no one else is authorized to read the message. Additionally, the disclaimer should state that if the e-mail is sent to anyone else by mistake, the recipient should contact the sender.

Information sent to a client via e-mail is considered part of the client's medical record. Therefore, a copy of the e-mail needs to be put in the client's chart. E-mails, like other documentation in the client's record, may be used as evidence during litigation.

E-mail is another form of communication that can enhance effective relationships with clients. It is not, however, a substitute for effective verbal and nonverbal communication. Nurses need to use their professional judgment about what form of communication(s) will best meet their client's health needs.

Factors Influencing the Communication Process

Many factors influence the communication process. Some of these are development, gender, values and perceptions, personal space, territoriality, roles and relationships, environment, congruence, and attitudes.

DEVELOPMENT   Language, psychosocial, and intellectual development move through stages across the life span. Knowledge of a client's developmental stage will allow the nurse to modify the message accordingly. The use of dolls and games with simple language may help explain a procedure to an 8-year-old. With adolescents who have developed more abstract thinking skills, a more detailed explanation can be given, whereas a well-educated, middle-aged business executive may wish to have detailed technical information provided. Older clients are apt to have had a wider range of experiences with the health care system, which may influence their response or understanding. With aging also come changes in vision and hearing acuity that can affect nurse–client interactions.

GENDER   From an early age, females and males communicate differently. Girls tend to use language to seek confirmation, minimize differences, and establish intimacy. Boys use language to establish independence and negotiate status within a group. These differences can continue into adulthood so that the same communication may be interpreted differently by a man and a woman.

VALUES AND PERCEPTIONS   *Values* are the standards that influence behavior, and *perceptions* are the personal view of an event. Because each person has unique personality traits, values, and life experiences, each will perceive and

interpret messages and experiences differently. For example, if the nurse draws the curtains around a crying woman and leaves her alone, the woman may interpret this as "The nurse thinks that I will upset others and that I shouldn't cry" or "The nurse respects my need to be alone." It is important for the nurse to be aware of a client's values and to validate or correct perceptions to avoid creating barriers in the nurse–client relationship.

PERSONAL SPACE   **Personal space** is the distance people prefer in interactions with others. **Proxemics** is the study of distance between people in their interactions. Middle-class North Americans use definite distances in various interpersonal relationships, along with specific voice tones and body language. Communication thus alters in accordance with four distances, each with a close and a far phase. Tamparo and Lindh (2007) list the following examples:

1. *Intimate:* Touching to 1½ feet
2. *Personal:* 1½ to 4 feet
3. *Social:* 4 to 12 feet
4. *Public:* 12 to 15 feet

Intimate distance communication is characterized by body contact, heightened sensations of body heat and smell, and vocalizations that are low. Vision is intense, is restricted to a small body part, and may be distorted. Intimate distance is frequently used by nurses. Examples include cuddling a baby, touching the sightless client, positioning clients, observing an incision, and restraining a toddler for an injection. It is a natural protective instinct for people to maintain a certain amount of space immediately around them, and the amount varies with individuals and cultures. When someone who wants to communicate steps too close, the receiver automatically steps back a pace or two. In their therapeutic roles, nurses often are required to violate this personal space. However, it is important for them to be aware when this will occur and to forewarn the client. In many instances, the nurse can respect (not come as close as) a person's intimate distance. In other instances, the nurse may come within intimate distance to communicate warmth and caring.

Personal distance is less overwhelming than intimate distance. Voice tones are moderate, and body heat and smell are noticed less. Physical contact such as a handshake or touching a shoulder is possible. More of the person is perceived at a personal distance, so that nonverbal behaviors such as body stance or full facial expressions are seen with less distortion. Much communication between nurses and clients occurs at this distance. Examples occur when nurses are sitting with a client, giving medications, or establishing an intravenous infusion. Communication at a close personal distance can convey involvement by facilitating the sharing of thoughts and feelings. On the other hand, it can also create tension if the distance encroaches upon the other's personal space (Figure 13–3). At the outer extreme of 4 feet, however, less involvement is conveyed.

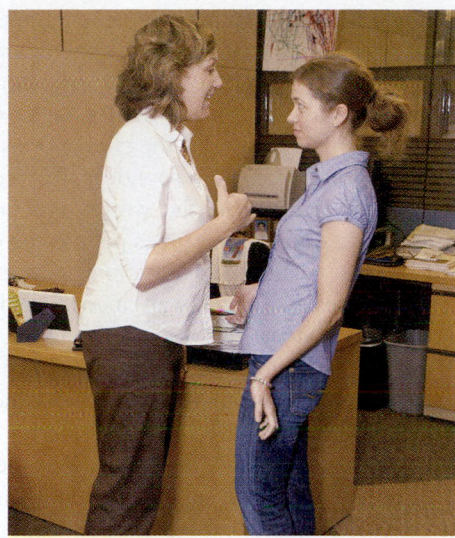

Figure 13–3 ● Personal space influences communication in social and professional interactions. Encroachment into another individual's personal space creates tension.

Bantering and some social conversations usually take place at this distance.

Social distance is characterized by a clear visual perception of the whole person. Body heat and odor are imperceptible, eye contact is increased, and vocalizations are loud enough to be overheard by others. Communication is therefore more formal and is limited to seeing and hearing. The person is protected and out of reach for touch or personal sharing of thoughts or feelings. Social distance allows more activity and movement back and forth. It is expedient in communicating with several people at the same time or within a short time. Examples occur when nurses make rounds or wave a greeting to someone. Social distance is important in accomplishing the business of the day. However, it is frequently misused. For example, the nurse who stands in the doorway and asks a client, "How are you today?" will receive a more noncommittal reply than the nurse who moves to a personal distance to make the same inquiry.

Public distance requires loud, clear vocalizations with careful enunciation. Although the faces and forms of people are seen at public distance, individuality is lost. Instead, the perception is of the group of people or the community.

TERRITORIALITY   **Territoriality** is a concept of the space and things that an individual considers as belonging to the self. Territories marked off by people may be visible to others. For example, clients in a hospital often consider their territory as bounded by the curtains around the bed unit or by the walls of a private room. This human tendency to claim territory must be recognized by all health care workers. Clients often feel the need to defend their territory when it is invaded by others; for example, when a visitor or nurse removes a chair to use at another bed, the visitor has inadvertently violated the territoriality of the client whose chair was

removed. Nurses need to obtain permission from clients to remove, rearrange, or borrow objects in their hospital area.

ROLES AND RELATIONSHIPS   The roles and the relationships between sender and receiver affect the communication process. Roles such as nursing student and instructor, client and primary care provider, or parent and child affect the content and responses in the communication process. Choice of words, sentence structure, and tone of voice vary considerably from role to role. In addition, the specific relationship between the communicators is significant. The nurse who meets with a client for the first time communicates differently from the nurse who has previously developed a relationship with that client.

ENVIRONMENT   People usually communicate most effectively in a comfortable environment. Temperature extremes, excessive noise, and a poorly ventilated environment can all interfere with communication. Also, lack of privacy may interfere with a client's communication about matters the client considers private. For example, a client who is worried about the ability of his wife to care for him after discharge from the hospital may not wish to discuss this concern with a nurse within hearing of other clients in the room. Environmental distraction can impair and distort communication.

CONGRUENCE   In **congruent communication**, the verbal and nonverbal aspects of the message match. Clients more readily trust the nurse when they perceive the nurse's communication as congruent. This will also help to prevent miscommunication. Congruence between verbal expression and nonverbal expression is easily seen by the nurse and the client. Nurses are taught to assess clients, but clients are often just as adept at reading a nurse's expression or body language. If there is an incongruence, the body language or nonverbal communication is usually the one with the true meaning. For example, when teaching a client how to care for a colostomy, the nurse might say, "You won't have any problem with this." However, if the nurse looks worried or disgusted while saying this, the client is less likely to trust the nurse's words.

INTERPERSONAL ATTITUDES   Attitudes convey beliefs, thoughts, and feelings about people and events. Attitudes are communicated convincingly and rapidly to others. Attitudes such as caring, warmth, respect, and acceptance facilitate communication, whereas condescension, lack of interest, and coldness inhibit communication.

Caring and *warmth* convey a feeling of emotional closeness, in contrast to an impersonal approach. Caring is more enduring and intense than warmth. It conveys deep and genuine concern for the person, whereas warmth conveys friendliness and consideration, shown by acts of smiling and attention to physical comforts (Brammer, 2003). Caring involves giving feelings, thoughts, skill, and knowledge. It requires psychologic energy and poses the risk of gaining little in return, yet by caring, people usually reap the benefits of greater communication and understanding.

Respect is an attitude that emphasizes the other person's worth and individuality. It conveys that the person's hopes and feelings are special and unique even though similar to others in many ways. People have a need to be different from—and at the same time similar to—others. Being too different can be isolating and threatening. A nurse conveys respect by listening open-mindedly to what the other person is saying, even if the nurse disagrees. Nurses can learn new ways of approaching situations when they conscientiously listen to another person's perspective.

Health care providers may unknowingly use speech that they believe shows caring but the client perceives as demeaning or patronizing. This frequently happens in settings that provide health care to older adults and/or individuals with obvious physical or mental disabilities (Williams, Kemper, & Hummert, 2004). **Elderspeak** is a speech style similar to babytalk, that gives the message of dependence and incompetence to older adults. It does not communicate respect. Many health care providers are not aware that they use elderspeak or that it can have negative meanings to the client. The characteristics of elderspeak include diminutives (inappropriate terms of endearment), inappropriate plural pronoun use, tag questions, and slow, loud speech (Williams et al., 2004, p. 22). See Table 13–1 for features of elderspeak and alternative strategies to use.

Acceptance emphasizes neither approval nor disapproval. The nurse willingly receives the client's honest feelings. An accepting attitude allows clients to express personal feelings freely and to be themselves. The nurse may need to restrict acceptance in situations where clients' behaviors are harmful to themselves or to others. Helping the client to find appropriate behaviors for feelings is often part of client teaching.

Therapeutic Communication

Therapeutic communication promotes understanding and can help establish a constructive relationship between the nurse and the client. Unlike the social relationship, where there may not be a specific purpose or direction, the therapeutic helping relationship is client and goal directed.

Nurses need to respond not only to the content of a client's verbal message but also to the feelings expressed. It is important to understand how the client views the situation and feels about it before responding. The content of the client's communication is the words or thoughts, as distinct from the feelings. Sometimes people can convey a thought in words while their emotions contradict the words; that is, words and feelings are incongruent. For example, a client says, "I am glad he has left me; he was very cruel." However, the nurse observes that the client has tears in her eyes as she says this. To respond to the client's *words,* the nurse might simply rephrase, saying, "You are pleased that he has left you." To respond to the client's *feelings,* the nurse would need to acknowledge the tears in the client's eyes, saying, for example, "You seem saddened by all this." Such a response helps the client to focus on her feelings. In some instances, the nurse may need to know more about the client and her resources for coping with these feelings.

Sometimes clients need time to deal with their feelings. Strong emotions are often draining. People usually need to deal with feelings before they can cope with other matters, such as learning new skills or planning for the future. This is most evident in hospitals when clients learn that they have a terminal illness. Some require hours, days, or even weeks before they are ready to start other tasks. Some need only time to themselves, others need someone to listen, others need assistance identifying and verbalizing feelings, and others need assistance making decisions about future courses of action.

ATTENTIVE LISTENING **Attentive listening** is listening actively, using all the senses, as opposed to listening passively with just the ear. It is probably the most important technique in nursing and is basic to all other techniques. Attentive listening is an active process that requires energy

---

TABLE 13–1 **Features of Elderspeak and Alternative Strategies**

ELDERSPEAK	ALTERNATIVE STRATEGY
Diminutives (inappropriately intimate terms of endearment, imply parent–child relationship). Examples: honey, sweetie, dearie, grandma	Refer to clients by their full name (e.g., Mrs. Robinson) or by their preferred name.
Inappropriate plural pronouns (substituting a collective pronoun, such as *we,* when referring to an independent older adult). Example: "Are *we* ready for *our* medicine?"	"Are *you* ready for *your* medicine?"
Tag questions (prompts the answer to the questions and implies the older adult can't act alone). Example: "You would rather wear the blue socks, *wouldn't you?*"	"Would you like to wear the blue socks?"
Shortened sentences, slow speech rate, and simple vocabulary (sounds like baby talk)	Use usual sentence structure, speech rate, and vocabulary.

Note: From "Enhancing Communication with Older Adults: Overcoming Elderspeak," by K. Williams, S. Kemper, & M. L. Hummert, 2004, *Journal of Gerontological Nursing.* Copyright © 2004 *SLACK,* Inc. Reprinted with permission.

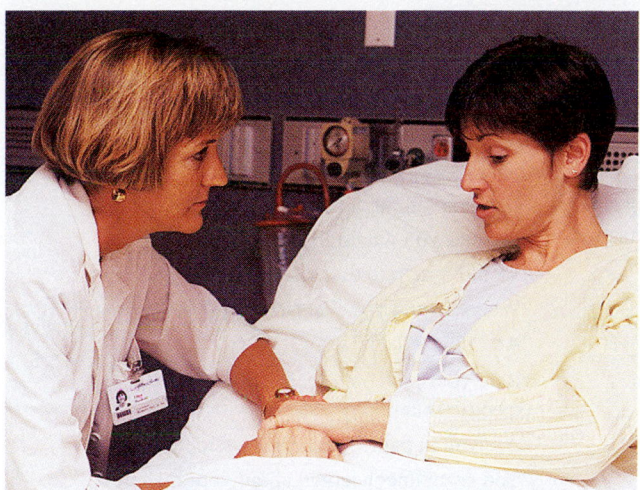

Figure 13–4 ⬤ The nurse conveys attentive listening through a posture of involvement.

and concentration. It involves paying attention to the total message, both verbal and nonverbal, and noting whether these communications are congruent. Attentive listening means absorbing both the content and the feeling the person is conveying, without selectivity. The listener does not select or listen solely to what the listener wants to hear; the nurse focuses not on the nurse's own needs but rather on the client's needs. Attentive listening conveys an attitude of caring and interest, thereby encouraging the client to talk (see Figure 13–4).

Attentive listening also involves listening for key themes in the communication. The nurse must be careful not to react quickly to the message. The speaker should not be interrupted and the nurse (the responder) should take time to think about the message before responding. As a listener, the nurse also should ask questions either to obtain additional information or to clarify.

Nurses need to be aware of their own biases. A message that reflects different values or beliefs should not be discredited for that reason. According to Rondeau (1992), the message sender (i.e., the client) should decide when to close a conversation. When the nurse closes the conversation, the client may assume that the nurse considers the message unimportant.

In summary, attentive listening is a highly developed skill, but fortunately it can be learned with practice. A nurse can convey attentiveness in listening to clients in various ways. Common responses are nodding the head, uttering "uh huh" or "mmm," repeating the words that the client has used, or saying "I see what you mean." Each nurse has characteristic ways of responding, and the nurse must take care not to sound insincere or phony.

PHYSICAL ATTENDING   Egan (2009) has outlined five specific ways to convey physical attending, which he defines as the manner of being present to another or being with another. Listening, in his frame of reference, is what a person does while attending. The five actions of physical attending, which convey a "posture of involvement," are described in Box 13–1.

Therapeutic communication techniques facilitate communication and focus on the client's concerns (see Table 13–2).

Barriers to Communication

Nurses need to recognize barriers or nontherapeutic responses to effective communication (see Table 13–3). Failure to listen, improperly decoding the client's intended message, and placing the nurse's needs above the client's needs are major barriers to communication.

BOX 13–1	Actions of Physical Attending

- Face the other person squarely. This position says, "I am available to you." Moving to the side lessens the degree of involvement.
- Adopt an open posture. The nondefensive position is one in which neither arms nor legs are crossed. It conveys that the person wishes to encourage the passage of communication, as the open door of a home or an office does.
- Lean toward the person. People move naturally toward one another when they want to say or hear something—by moving to the front of a class, by moving a chair nearer a friend, or by leaning across a table with arms propped in front. The nurse conveys involvement by leaning forward, closer to the client.
- Maintain good eye contact. Mutual eye contact, preferably at the same level, recognizes the other person and denotes

willingness to maintain communication. Eye contact neither glares at nor stares down another but is natural.
- Try to be relatively relaxed. Total relaxation is not feasible when the nurse is listening with intensity, but the nurse can show relaxation by taking time in responding, allowing pauses as needed, balancing periods of tension with relaxation, and using gestures that are natural.

These five attending postures need to be adapted to the specific needs of clients in a given situation. For example, leaning forward may not be appropriate at the beginning of an interview. It may be reserved until a closer relationship grows between the nurse and the client. The same applies to eye contact, which is generally uninterrupted when the communicators are very involved in the interaction.

TABLE 13–2   **Therapeutic Communication Techniques**

TECHNIQUE	DESCRIPTION	EXAMPLES
Using silence	Accepting pauses or silences that may extend for several seconds or minutes without interjecting any verbal response.	Sitting quietly (or walking with the client) and waiting attentively until the client is able to put thoughts and feelings into words.
Providing general leads	Using statements or questions that (a) encourage the client to verbalize, (b) choose a topic of conversation, and (c) facilitate continued verbalization.	"Can you tell me how it is for you?" "Perhaps you would like to talk about. . . ." "Would it help to discuss your feelings?" "Where would you like to begin?" "And then what?"
Being specific and tentative	Making statements that are specific rather than general, and tentative rather than absolute.	"Rate your pain on a scale of 0 to 10." (specific statement) "Are you in pain?" (general statement) "You seem unconcerned about your diabetes." (tentative statement) "You don't care about your diabetes and you never will." (absolute statement)
Using open-ended questions	Asking broad questions that lead or invite the client to explore (elaborate, clarify, describe, compare, or illustrate) thoughts or feelings. Open-ended questions specify only the topic to be discussed and invite answers that are longer than one or two words.	"I'd like to hear more about that." "Tell me about. . . ." "How have you been feeling lately?" "What brought you to the hospital?" "What is your opinion?" "You said you were frightened yesterday. How do you feel now?"
Using touch	Providing appropriate forms of touch to reinforce caring feelings. Because tactile contacts vary considerably among individuals, families, and cultures, the nurse must be sensitive to the differences in attitudes and practices of clients and self.	Putting an arm over the client's shoulder. Placing your hand over the client's hand.
Restating or paraphrasing	Actively listening for the client's basic message and then repeating those thoughts and/or feelings in similar words. This conveys that the nurse has listened and understood the client's basic message and also offers clients a clearer idea of what they have said.	*Client:* "I couldn't manage to eat any dinner last night—not even the dessert." *Nurse:* "You had difficulty eating yesterday." *Client:* "Yes, I was very upset after my family left." *Client:* "I have trouble talking to strangers." *Nurse:* "You find it difficult talking to people you do not know?"
Seeking clarification	A method of making the client's broad overall meaning of the message more understandable. It is used when paraphrasing is difficult or when the communication is rambling or garbled. To clarify the message, the nurse can restate the basic message or confess confusion and ask the client to repeat or restate the message. Nurses can also clarify their own message with statements.	"I'm puzzled." "I'm not sure I understand that." "Would you please say that again?" "Would you tell me more?" "I meant this rather than that." "I'm sorry that wasn't very clear. Let me try to explain another way."
Perception checking or seeking consensual validation	A method similar to clarifying that verifies the meaning of specific words rather than the overall meaning of a message.	*Client:* "My husband never gives me any presents." *Nurse:* "You mean he has never given you a present for your birthday or Christmas?" *Client:* "Well—not never. He does get me something for my birthday and Christmas, but he never thinks of giving me anything at any other time."

TABLE 13–2	Therapeutic Communication Techniques—continued	
TECHNIQUE	**DESCRIPTION**	**EXAMPLES**
Offering self	Suggesting one's presence, interest, or wish to understand the client without making any demands or attaching conditions that the client must comply with to receive the nurse's attention.	"I'll stay with you until your daughter arrives." "We can sit here quietly for a while; we don't need to talk unless you would like to." "I'll help you to dress to go home, if you like."
Giving information	Providing, in a simple and direct manner, specific factual information the client may or may not request. When information is not known, the nurse states this and indicates who has it or when the nurse will obtain it.	"Your surgery is scheduled for 11 AM tomorrow." "You will feel a pulling sensation when the tube is removed from your abdomen." "I do not know the answer to that, but I will find out from Mrs. King, the nurse in charge."
Acknowledging	Giving recognition, in a nonjudgmental way, of a change in behavior, an effort the client has made, or a contribution to a communication. Acknowledgment may be with or without understanding, verbal or nonverbal.	"You trimmed your beard and mustache and washed your hair." "I notice you keep squinting your eyes. Are you having difficulty seeing?" "You walked twice as far today with your walker."
Clarifying time or sequence	Helping the client clarify an event, situation, or happening in relationship to time.	*Client:* "I vomited this morning." *Nurse:* "Was that after breakfast?" *Client:* "I feel that I have been asleep for weeks." *Nurse:* "You had your operation Monday, and today is Tuesday."
Presenting reality	Helping the client to differentiate the real from the unreal.	"That telephone ring came from the program on television." "I see shadows from the window coverings." "Your magazine is here in the drawer. It has not been stolen."
Focusing	Helping the client expand on and develop a topic of importance. It is important for the nurse to wait until the client finishes stating the main concerns before attempting to focus. The focus may be an idea or a feeling; however, the nurse often emphasizes a feeling to help the client recognize an emotion disguised behind words.	*Client:* "My wife says she will look after me, but I don't think she can, what with the children to take care of, and they're always after her about something—clothes, homework, what's for dinner that night." *Nurse:* "Sounds like you are worried about how well she can manage."
Reflecting	Directing ideas, feelings, questions, or content back to clients to enable them to explore their own ideas and feelings about a situation.	*Client:* "What can I do?" *Nurse:* "What do you think would be helpful?" *Client:* "Do you think I should tell my husband?" *Nurse:* "You seem unsure about telling your husband."
Summarizing and planning	Stating the main points of a discussion to clarify the relevant points discussed. This technique is useful at the end of an interview or to review a health teaching session. It often acts as an introduction to future care planning.	"During the past half hour we have talked about. . . ." "Tomorrow afternoon we may explore this further." "In a few days I'll review what you have learned about the actions and effects of your insulin." "Tomorrow, I will look at your feeling journal."

TABLE 13–3	Barriers to Communication	
TECHNIQUE	**DESCRIPTION**	**EXAMPLES**
Stereotyping	Offering generalized and oversimplified beliefs about groups of people that are based on experiences too limited to be valid. These responses categorize clients and negate their uniqueness as individuals.	"Two-year-olds are brats." "Women are complainers." "Men don't cry." "Most people don't have any pain after this type of surgery."
Agreeing and disagreeing	Akin to judgmental responses, agreeing and disagreeing imply that the client is either right or wrong and that the nurse is in a position to judge this. These responses deter clients from thinking through their position and may cause a client to become defensive.	*Client:* "I don't think Dr. Broad is a very good doctor. He doesn't seem interested in his patients." *Nurse:* "Dr. Broad is head of the department of surgery and is an excellent surgeon."
Being defensive	Attempting to protect a person or health care services from negative comments. These responses prevent the client from expressing true concerns. The nurse is saying, "You have no right to complain." Defensive responses protect the nurse from admitting weaknesses in the health care services, including personal weaknesses.	*Client:* "Those night nurses must just sit around and talk all night. They didn't answer my light for over an hour." *Nurse:* "I'll have you know we literally run around on nights. You're not the only client, you know."
Challenging	Giving a response that makes clients prove their statement or point of view. These responses indicate that the nurse is failing to consider the client's feelings, making the client feel it necessary to defend a position.	*Client:* "I felt nauseated after that red pill." *Nurse:* "Surely you don't think I gave you the wrong pill?" *Client:* "I feel as if I am dying." *Nurse:* "How can you feel that way when your pulse is 60?" *Client:* "I believe my husband doesn't love me." *Nurse:* "You can't say that; why, he visits you every day."
Probing	Asking for information chiefly out of curiosity rather than with the intent to assist the client. These responses are considered prying and violate the client's privacy. Asking "why" is often probing and places the client in a defensive position.	*Client:* "I was speeding along the street and didn't see the stop sign." *Nurse:* "Why were you speeding?" *Client:* "I didn't ask the doctor when he was here." Nurse: *"Why didn't you?"*
Testing	Asking questions that make the client admit to something. These responses permit the client only limited answers and often meet the nurse's need rather than the client's.	"Who do you think you are?" (forces people to admit their status is only that of client) "Do you think I am not busy?" (forces the client to admit that the nurse really is busy)
Rejecting	Refusing to discuss certain topics with the client. These responses often make clients feel that the nurse is rejecting not only their communication but also the clients themselves.	"I don't want to discuss that. Let's talk about. . . ." "Let's discuss other areas of interest to you rather than the two problems you keep mentioning." "I can't talk now. I'm on my way for coffee break."
Changing topics and subjects	Directing the communication into areas of self-interest rather than considering the client's concerns is often a self-protective response to a topic that causes anxiety. These responses imply that what the nurse considers important will be discussed and that clients should not discuss certain topics.	*Client:* "I'm separated from my wife. Do you think I should have sexual relations with another woman?" *Nurse:* "I see that you're 36 and that you like gardening. This sunshine is good for my roses. I have a beautiful rose garden."
Unwarranted reassurance	Using clichés or comforting statements of advice as a means to reassure the client. These responses block the fears, feelings, and other thoughts of the client.	"You'll feel better soon." "I'm sure everything will turn out all right." "Don't worry."
Passing judgment	Giving opinions and approving or disapproving responses, moralizing, or implying one's own values. These responses imply that the client must think as the nurse thinks, fostering client dependence.	"That's good (bad)." "You shouldn't do that." "That's not good enough." "What you did was wrong (right)."
Giving common advice	Telling the client what to do. These responses deny the client's right to be an equal partner. Note that giving expert rather than common advice is therapeutic.	*Client:* "Should I move from my home to a nursing home?" *Nurse:* "If I were you, I'd go to a nursing home, where you'll get your meals cooked for you."

THE HELPING RELATIONSHIP

Nurse–client relationships are referred to by some as *interpersonal relationships,* by others as *therapeutic relationships,* and by still others as **helping relationships**. Helping is a growth-facilitating process that strives to achieve two basic goals (Egan, 2009):

1. Help clients manage their problems in living more effectively and develop unused or underused opportunities more fully.
2. Help clients become better at helping themselves in their everyday lives.

A helping relationship may develop over weeks of working with a client, or within minutes. The keys to the helping relationship are (a) the development of trust and acceptance between the nurse and the client and (b) an underlying belief that the nurse cares about and wants to help the client.

The helping relationship is influenced by the personal and professional characteristics of the nurse and the client. Age, sex, appearance, diagnosis, education, values, ethnic and cultural background, personality, expectations, and setting can all affect the development of the nurse–client relationship. Consideration of all of these factors, combined with good communication skills and sincere interest in the client's welfare, will enable the nurse to create a helping relationship.

Phases of the Helping Relationship

The helping relationship process can be described in terms of four sequential phases, each characterized by identifiable tasks and skills. The relationship must progress through the stages in succession because each builds on the one before. Nurses can identify the progress of a relationship by understanding these phases: preinteraction phase, introductory phase, working (maintaining) phase, and termination phase. Table 13–4 summarizes the tasks and skills required.

PREINTERACTION PHASE The preinteraction phase is similar to the planning stage before an interview. In most situations, the nurse has information about the client before the first face-to-face meeting. Such information may include the client's name, address, age, medical history, and/or social history. Planning for the initial visit may generate some anxious feelings in the nurse. If the nurse recognizes these feelings and identifies specific information to be discussed, positive outcomes can evolve.

INTRODUCTORY PHASE The introductory phase, also referred to as the *orientation phase* or the *prehelping phase,* is important because it sets the tone for the rest of the relationship. During this initial encounter, the client and the nurse closely observe each other and form judgments about the other's behavior. The three stages of this introductory phase are opening the relationship, clarifying the problem, and structuring and formulating the contract (Brammer, 2003). Other important tasks of the introduc-

tory phase include getting to know each other and developing a degree of trust.

After introductions, the nurse may initially engage in some social interaction to put the client at ease. For example, the nurse and client may talk about what a nice day it is and what they would like to do if at home.

During the initial parts of the introductory phase, the client may display some resistive behaviors. *Resistive behaviors* are those that inhibit involvement, cooperation, or change. They may be due to difficulty in acknowledging the need for help and thus a dependent role, fear of exposing and facing feelings, anxiety about the discomfort involved in changing problem-causing behavior patterns, and fear or anxiety in response to the nurse's approach, which may, in the client's opinion, be inappropriate.

Resistive behaviors can be overcome by conveying a caring attitude, genuine interest in the client, and competence. These behaviors of the nurse also foster the development of trust in the relationship. Trust can be described as a reliance on someone without doubt or question, or the belief that the other person is capable of assisting in times of distress and in all likelihood will do so. To trust another person involves risk; clients become vulnerable when they share thoughts, feelings, and attitudes with the nurse. Trust, however, enables the client to express thoughts and feelings openly.

By the end of the introductory phase, clients should begin to:

- Develop trust in the nurse.
- View the nurse as a competent professional capable of helping.
- View the nurse as honest, open, and concerned about their welfare.
- Believe the nurse will try to understand and respect their cultural values and beliefs.
- Believe the nurse will respect client confidentiality.
- Feel comfortable talking with the nurse about feelings and other sensitive issues.
- Understand the purpose of the relationship and the roles.
- Feel that they are active participants in developing a mutually agreeable plan of care.

WORKING PHASE During the working phase of a helping relationship, the nurse and the client begin to view each other as unique individuals. They begin to appreciate this uniqueness and care about each other. Caring is sharing deep and genuine concern about the welfare of another person. Once caring develops, the potential for empathy increases.

The working phase has two major stages: exploring and understanding thoughts and feelings, and facilitating and taking action. The nurse helps the client to explore thoughts, feelings, and actions and helps the client plan a program of action to meet preestablished goals.

TABLE 13–4 Tasks and Skills for Each Phase of the Helping Relationship

PHASE	TASKS	SKILLS
Preinteraction Phase	The nurse reviews pertinent assessment data and knowledge, considers potential areas of concern, and develops plans for interaction.	Organized data gathering; recognizing limitations and seeking assistance as required.
Introductory Phase		
1. Opening the relationship	Both client and nurse identify each other by name. When the nurse initiates the relationship, it is important to explain the nurse's role to give the client an idea of what to expect. When the client initiates the relationship, the nurse needs to help the client express concerns and reasons for seeking help. Vague, open-ended questions, such as "What's on your mind today?" are helpful at this stage.	A relaxed, attending attitude to put the client at ease. It is not easy for all clients to receive help.
2. Clarifying the problem	Because the client initially may not see the problem clearly, the nurse's major task is to help clarify the problem.	Attentive listening, paraphrasing, clarifying, and other effective communication techniques discussed in this chapter. A common error at this stage is to ask too many questions of the client. Instead, focus on priorities.
3. Structuring and formulating the contract (obligations to be met by both the nurse and client)	Nurse and client develop a degree of trust and verbally agree about (a) location, frequency, and length of meetings, (b) overall purpose of the relationship, (c) how confidential material will be handled, (d) tasks to be accomplished, and (e) duration and indications for termination of the relationship.	Communication skills listed above and ability to overcome resistive behaviors if they occur.
Working Phase	Nurse and client accomplish the tasks outlined in the introductory phase, enhance trust and rapport, and develop caring.	Listening and attending skills, empathy, respect, genuineness, concreteness, self-disclosure, and confrontation. Skills acquired by the client are nondefensive listening and self-understanding.
1. Exploring and understanding thoughts and feelings	The nurse assists the client to explore thoughts and feelings and acquires an understanding of the client. The client explores thoughts and feelings associated with problems, develops the skill of listening, and gains insight into personal behavior.	
2. Facilitating and taking action	The nurse plans programs within the client's capabilities and considers long- and short-term goals. The client needs to learn to take risks (i.e., accept that either failure or success may be the outcome). The nurse needs to reinforce successes and help the client recognize failures realistically.	Decision-making and goal-setting skills. Also, for the nurse: reinforcement skills; for the client: risk taking.
Termination Phase	Nurse and client accept feelings of loss. The client accepts the end of the relationship without feelings of anxiety or dependence.	For the nurse: summarizing skills; for the client: ability to handle problems independently.

Exploring and Understanding Thoughts and Feelings The nurse requires the following skills for this phase of the helping relationship:

- *Empathetic listening and responding.* Nurses must listen attentively and communicate (respond) in ways that indicate they have listened to what was said and understand how the client feels. The nurse responds to content or feelings or both, as appropriate. The

nurse's nonverbal behaviors are also important. Nonverbal behaviors indicating empathy include moderate head nodding, a steady gaze, moderate gesturing, and little activity or body movement. According to Egan (2009), **empathy** "can be seen as an intellectual process that involves understanding correctly another person's emotional state and point of view" and also as an emotional response experienced by the helper (p. 73). Empathetic listening focuses on a kind of "be-

BOX 13–2   **Components of Genuineness**

- The genuine helper does not take refuge in or overemphasize the role of counselor.
- The genuine person is spontaneous.
- The genuine person is nondefensive.
- The genuine person displays few discrepancies—that is, the person is consistent and does not think or feel one thing but say another.
- The genuine person is capable of deep self-disclosure (self-sharing) when it is appropriate.

ing with" clients to develop an understanding of them and their world. This understanding, however, must also be communicated effectively to the client— empathetic response. The end result of empathy is comforting and caring for the client and a helping, healing relationship.

- *Respect.* The nurse must show respect for the client's willingness to be available, desire to work with the client, and a manner that conveys the idea of taking the client's point of view seriously.
- *Genuineness.* Personal statements can be helpful in solidifying the rapport between the nurse and the client. The nurse might offer such comments as "I recall when I was in (a similar situation), and I felt angry about being put down." Egan (2009) has outlined five behaviors that are components of genuineness (see Box 13–2). Nurses need to exercise caution when making references about themselves. These statements must be used with discretion. The extreme of matching each of the client's problems with a better story of the nurse's own is of little value to the client.
- *Concreteness.* The nurse must assist the client to be concrete and specific rather than to speak in generalities. When the client says, "I'm stupid and clumsy," the nurse narrows the topic to the specific by pointing out, "You tripped on the rug."
- *Confrontation.* The nurse points out discrepancies between thoughts, feelings, and actions that inhibit the client's self-understanding or exploration of specific areas. This is done empathetically, not judgmentally.

During this first stage of the working phase, the intensity of interaction increases, and feelings such as anger, shame, or self-consciousness may be expressed. If the nurse is skilled in this stage and if the client is willing to pursue self-exploration, the outcome is a beginning understanding on the part of the client about behavior and feelings.

Facilitating Taking Action   Ultimately the client must make decisions and take action to become more effective. The responsibility for action belongs to the client. The nurse, however, collaborates in these decisions, provides support, and may offer options or information.

TERMINATION PHASE   The termination phase of the relationship is often expected to be difficult and filled with ambivalence. However, if the previous phases have evolved effectively, the client generally has a positive outlook and feels able to handle problems independently. On the other hand, because caring attitudes have developed, it is natural to expect some feelings of loss, and each person needs to develop a way of saying good-bye.

Many methods can be used to terminate relationships. Summarizing or reviewing the process can produce a sense of accomplishment. This may include sharing reminiscences of how things were at the beginning of the relationship and comparing them to how they are now. It is also helpful for both the nurse and the client to express their feelings about termination openly and honestly. Thus termination discussions need to start in advance of the termination interview. This allows time for the client to adjust to independence. In some situations referrals are necessary, or it may be appropriate to offer an occasional standby meeting to give support as needed. Follow-up phone calls or e-mails are other interventions that ease the client's transition to independence.

Developing Helping Relationships

Whatever the practice setting, the nurse establishes some type of helping relationship in which mutual goals (outcomes) are set with the client or, if the client is unable to participate, with support persons. Although special training in counseling techniques is advantageous, there are many ways of helping clients that do not require special training.

- Listen actively.
- Help to identify what the person is feeling. Often clients who are troubled are unable to identify or to label their feelings and consequently have difficulty working them out or talking about them. Responses such as "You seem angry about taking orders from your boss" or "You sound as if you've been lonely since your wife died" can help clients recognize what they are feeling and talk about it.
- Put yourself in the other person's shoes (i.e., empathize). Communicate to the client in a way that shows an understanding of the client's feelings and the behavior and experience underlying these feelings.
- Be honest. In effective relationships nurses honestly recognize any lack of knowledge by saying "I don't know the answer to that right now"; openly discuss their own discomfort by saying, for example, "I feel uncomfortable about this discussion"; and admit tactfully that problems do exist, for instance, when a client says "I'm a mess, aren't I?"
- Be genuine and credible. Clients will sense whether the nurse is truly concerned.
- Use your ingenuity. There are always many courses of action to consider in handling problems. Whatever course is chosen needs to further the achievement of the client's goals (outcomes), be compatible

with the client's value system, and offer the probability of success.

- Be aware of cultural differences that may affect meaning and understanding (see Chapter 4 ∞). To facilitate nurse–client interaction, recognize the language(s) and/or dialect(s) the client uses. Provide a bilingual interpreter as needed for clients limited in the English language.
- Maintain client confidentiality. To maintain the client's right to privacy, share information only with other health care professionals as needed for effective care and treatment.
- Know your role and your limitations. Every person has unique strengths and problems. When you feel unable to handle some problems, the client should be informed and referred to the appropriate health professional. Clarify functions and roles, specifically what is expected of the client, the nurse, and the primary care provider.

GROUP COMMUNICATION

People are born into a group (i.e., a family) and interact with others at all stages of life in various groups: peer groups, work groups, recreational groups, religious groups, and so on. A **group** is two or more people who have shared needs and goals, who take each other into account in their actions, and who thus are held together and set apart from others by virtue of their interactions. Groups exist to help people achieve goals (outcomes) that would be unattainable by individual effort alone. For example, groups can often solve problems more effectively than one person by pooling the ideas and expertise of several individuals; in addition, information can be disseminated to groups more quickly than to individuals.

Group Dynamics

The communication that takes place between members of any group is known as **group dynamics**. The manner of this communication will be determined by a number of interrelated factors and variables. Each member of the group will have an effect on the group dynamics, based on their motivation for participating, their similarity to other group members, the maturity of the group members in expressing their feelings, and the goal of the group.

The unique dynamics of each group will influence its maturation or group process, as well as the effectiveness of the group. Three main functions are required for any group to be effective. It must maintain a degree of group unity or cohesion. It needs to develop and modify its structure to improve its effectiveness. And it must accomplish its goals. The characteristics of an effectively functioning group are shown in Table 13–5.

Types of Health Care Groups

Much of a nurse's professional life is spent in a wide variety of groups, ranging from dyads (two-person groups) to large

professional organizations. As a participant in a group, the nurse may be required to fulfill different roles: member or leader, teacher or learner, adviser or advisee, and so on.

Common types of health care groups include task groups, teaching groups, self-help groups, self-awareness/growth groups, therapy groups, and work-related social support groups. There are similarities and differences among the characteristics of these various types of groups and the nurse's role.

TASK GROUPS The task group is one of the most common types of work-related groups to which nurses belong. Examples are health care planning committees, nursing service committees, nursing team meetings, nursing care conference groups, and hospital staff meetings. The focus of such groups is the completion of a specific task, and the format is defined at the outset by the leader and/or members. The methods vary according to the task to be performed.

The leader of a task group, usually called the chairperson, must be accepted by the members as an appropriate leader and therefore should be an expert in the area of task emphasis. The chairperson's role is to identify the specific task, clarify communication, and assist in expressing opinions and offering solutions. Committee members are generally selected in terms of their individual functional role and employment status, rather than in terms of their personal characteristics. Member participation is determined by the task. A target date for termination of the group is usually set in advance.

TEACHING GROUPS Teaching groups exist to impart information to the participants. Examples of teaching groups include continuing education and client health care groups. Numerous subjects are often handled via the group teaching format: childbirth techniques, birth control methods, effective parenting, nutrition, management of chronic illness such as diabetes, exercise for middle-aged and older adults, and instructions to family members about follow-up care for discharged clients. A nurse who leads a group in which the primary purpose is to teach or learn must be skilled in the teaching-learning process (see Chapter 14 ∞).

SELF-HELP GROUPS These are usually small, voluntary organization composed of individuals who share a similar health, social, or daily living problem. One of the central beliefs of the self-help movement is that people who experience a particular social or health problem have an understanding of that condition that those without it do not.

Self-help groups are available for a range of problems (e.g., stillbirth, parenting, pregnant adolescents, divorce, drug abuse, cancer, menopause, mental illness, diabetes, AIDS, women's health, caregivers of older adults, and grief). Alcoholics Anonymous was the first self-help group. Positive aspects of self-help groups are outlined in Box 13–3.

The major functions of the nurse's role in self-help groups include the following:

- Help clients form such groups by identifying key people who can act as facilitators.
- Share expertise with clients and help them gain appropriate knowledge and skills.

TABLE 13–5 Comparative Features of Effective and Ineffective Groups

FACTOR	EFFECTIVE GROUPS	INEFFECTIVE GROUPS
Atmosphere	Comfortable and relaxed; a working atmosphere in which people demonstrate their interest and involvement.	Tense; lacks privacy or voluntary commitment to the group.
Purpose	Goals, tasks, and outcomes are clarified, understood, and modified so that members of the group can commit themselves to purposes through cooperation.	Purposes are unclear, misunderstood, or imposed.
Leadership and member participation	Leadership is democratic with a shift in leadership from time to time depending on knowledge or experience.	Authoritarian; leader may dominate the group, or the members may defer unduly. Member participation is unequal, with some members dominating.
Communication	Open; ideas and feelings are encouraged.	Closed; only idea production is encouraged. Feelings are ignored. Members may have "hidden agendas" (personal goals at cross-purposes with group goals).
Decision making	By the group, although various decision-making procedures appropriate to the situation may be instituted.	By the highest authority in the group, or one or two strong members of the group, with minimal involvement by members. Disagreements are ignored.
Cohesion	Facilitated through valuing other group members, open expression of feelings, trust, and support.	Leader claims full credit for achievements. Comments are critical and focus on personal characteristics.
Conflict tolerance	The reasons for disagreements or conflicts are carefully examined, and the group seeks to resolve them.	Fear of conflict prevents decisions and growth.
Power	Determined by the members' abilities and the information they possess. Power is shared.	Determined by position in the group. Obedience to authority is strong. The issue is who controls, based on individual emotional needs of members.
Problem solving	High; constructive criticism is frequent, frank, relatively comfortable, and oriented toward problem solving.	Low; criticism may be destructive, taking the form of either overt or covert personal attacks.
Creativity	Encouraged.	Discouraged.

- Inform clients and support persons about existing self-help groups available to them.
- Participate as a member of a self-help group when this is appropriate. The nurse's role is that of a resource person, that is, of being "on tap, but not on top."
- Help out in times of crisis.

SELF-AWARENESS/GROWTH GROUPS These groups exist to develop or use interpersonal strengths. The overall aim is to improve the person's functioning in the group to which they return, whether job, family, or community. From the beginning, broad goals are usually apparent, for example, to study communication patterns, group process, or problem solving. Because the focus of these groups is interpersonal concerns around current situations, the work of the group is oriented to reality testing with a here-and-now emphasis. Members are responsible for correcting inefficient patterns of relating and communicating with each other. They learn group process through participation and involvement and guided exercises.

THERAPY GROUPS Therapy groups work toward self-understanding, more satisfactory ways of relating or handling stress, and changing patterns of behavior toward

BOX 13–3 Positive Aspects of Self-Help Groups

- Members can experience almost instant kinship because the essence of the group is the idea that "you are not alone."
- Members can talk about their feelings and listen to the concerns of others, knowing they all share this experience.
- The group atmosphere is generally one of acceptance, support, encouragement, and caring.
- Many members act as role models for newer members and can inspire them to attempt tasks they might consider impossible.
- The group provides the opportunity for people to help as well as to be helped—a critical component in restoring self-esteem after significant losses.

health. Members of the therapy group are referred to as clients or, in some settings, as patients. They are selected by health professionals after extensive selection interviews that consider the pattern of personalities, behaviors, needs, and identification of group therapy as the treatment of choice. Duration of therapy groups is not usually set. A termination date is usually mutually determined by the therapist and members.

WORK-RELATED SOCIAL SUPPORT GROUPS Many nurses experience high levels of vocational stress. Various types of group support can buffer such stress. Group members who know about the work of others can encourage and challenge members to be more creative and enthusiastic about their work and to achieve more. Members also can share the joys of success and the frustration of failure through active listening without giving advice or making judgments. This type of social support is best given outside of the work environment.

COMMUNICATION AND THE NURSING PROCESS

Communication is an integral part of the nursing process. Nurses use communication skills in each phase of the nursing process. Communication is also important when caring for clients who have communication problems. Communication skills are even more important when the client has sensory, language, or cognitive deficits.

NURSING MANAGEMENT

ASSESSING

To assess the client's communication, the nurse determines communication impairments or barriers and communication style. Remember that culture may influence when and how a client speaks. Obviously, language varies according to age and development. With children, the nurse observes sounds, gestures, and vocabulary.

Impairments to Communication

Various barriers may alter a client's ability to send, receive, or comprehend messages. These include language deficits, sensory deficits, cognitive impairments, structural deficits, and paralysis. The nurse must assess each to determine their presence.

LANGUAGE DEFICITS Determine the client's primary language for communicating and whether a fluent interpreter is required. Some clients who use English as a second language may have language skills that are inadequate to meet their needs.

SENSORY DEFICITS The ability to hear, see, feel, and smell are important adjuncts to communication. Deafness can significantly alter the message the client receives; impaired vision alters the ability to observe nonverbal behavior, such as a smile or a gesture; inability to feel and smell can impair the client's capabilities to report injuries or detect the smoke from a fire. For clients with severe hearing impairments, follow these steps:

- Look for a medical alert bracelet, necklace, or tag indicating hearing loss.
- Determine whether the client wears a hearing aid and whether it is functioning.

- Observe whether the client is attempting to see your face to read lips.
- Observe whether the client is attempting to use hands to communicate with sign language.

COGNITIVE IMPAIRMENTS Any disorder that impairs cognitive functioning (e.g., cerebrovascular disease, Alzheimer's disease, and brain tumors or injuries) may affect a client's ability to use and understand language. These clients may develop total loss of speech, impaired articulation, or the inability to find or name words. Certain medications such as sedatives, antidepressants, and neuroleptics may also impair speech, causing the client to use incomplete sentences or to slur words.

The nurse assesses whether these clients respond when asked a question and, if so, assesses the following: Is the client's speech fluent or hesitant? Does the client use words correctly? Can the client comprehend instructions as evidenced by following directions? Can the client repeat words or phrases? In addition, the nurse assesses the client's ability to understand written words: Can the client follow written directions? Can the client respond correctly by pointing to a written word? Can the client read aloud? Can the client recognize words or letters if unable to read whole sentences? The nurse uses large, clearly written words when trying to establish abilities in this area.

When the client is unconscious, the nurse looks for any indication that suggests comprehension of what is communicated (e.g., tries to arouse the client verbally and through touch). Ask a closed question like "Can you hear me?" and watch for a nonverbal response such as a nod of the head for yes or a shake for no; or ask for a hand squeeze or blink of the eye once for yes or twice for no.

STRUCTURAL DEFICITS Structural deficits of the oral and nasal cavities and respiratory system can alter a person's ability to speak clearly and spontaneously. Examples include cleft palate, artificial airways such as an endotracheal tube or tracheostomy, and laryngectomy (removal of the larynx). Extreme dyspnea (shortness of breath) can also impair speech patterns.

PARALYSIS If verbal impairment is combined with paralysis of the upper extremities that impairs the client's ability to write, the nurse should determine whether the client can point, nod, shrug, blink, or squeeze a hand. Any of these could be used to devise a beginning communication system.

Style of Communication

In assessing communication style, the nurse considers both verbal and nonverbal communication. In addition to physical barriers, some psychologic illnesses (e.g., depression or psychosis) influence the ability to communicate. The client may demonstrate constant verbalization of the same words or phrases, a loose association of ideas, or flight of ideas.

VERBAL COMMUNICATION When assessing verbal communication, the nurse focuses on three areas: the content of the

LIFESPAN CONSIDERATIONS
Communication with Older Adults

Older adults may have physical or cognitive problems that necessitate nursing interventions for improvement of communication skills. Some of the common ones are as follows:

- Sensory deficits, such as vision and hearing
- Cognitive impairment, as in dementia
- Neurological deficits from strokes or other neurological conditions, such as aphasia (expressive and/or receptive) and lack of movement
- Psychosocial problems, such as depression

Recognition of specific needs and obtaining appropriate resources for clients can greatly increase their socialization and quality of life. Interventions directed toward improving communication in clients with these special needs are as follows:

- Make sure that assistive devices, glasses, and hearing aids are being used and are in good working order.
- Make referrals to appropriate resources, such as speech therapy.

- Make use of communications aids, such as communication boards, computers, or pictures, when possible.
- Keep environmental distractions to a minimum.
- Speak in short, simple sentences, one subject at a time—reinforce or repeat what is said when necessary.
- Always face the person when speaking—coming up behind someone may be frightening.
- Include family and friends in conversation.
- Use reminiscing, either in individual conversations or in groups, to maintain memory connections and to enhance self-identity and self-esteem in the older adult.
- When verbal expression and nonverbal expression are incongruent, believe the nonverbal. Clarification of this and attentiveness to their feelings will help promote a feeling of caring and acceptance.
- Find out what has been important and has meaning to the person and try to maintain these things as much as possible. Even simple things such as bedtime rituals become important if they are lost in a hospital or extended care setting.

message, the themes, and verbalized emotions. In addition, the nurse considers the following:

- Whether the communication pattern is slow, rapid, quiet, spontaneous, hesitant, evasive, and so on
- The vocabulary of the individual, particularly any changes from the vocabulary normally used (for example, a person who normally never swears may indicate increased stress or illness by an uncharacteristic use of profanity.)
- The presence of hostility, aggression, assertiveness, reticence, hesitance, anxiety, or loquaciousness (incessant verbalization) in communication

- Difficulties with verbal communication, such as slurring, stuttering, inability to pronounce a particular sound, lack of clarity in enunciation, inability to speak in sentences, loose association of ideas, flight of ideas, or the inability to find or name words or identify objects
- Refusal or inability to speak

NONVERBAL COMMUNICATION Consider nonverbal communication in relation to the client's culture. Pay particular attention to facial expression, gestures, body movements, affect, tone of voice, posture, and eye contact.

RESEARCH NOTES
Can Clients with Advanced Dementia Participate in a Social Conversation?

The nursing literature provides general principles to use when communicating with clients with dementia. However, there is little research that documents the effectiveness of the principles or strategies. The purpose of this study by Perry, Galloway, Bottorff, and Nixon (2005) was to describe the communication strategies used by expert nurses in communicating with residents with advanced dementia and to assess the effectiveness of the strategies in supporting participation in social conversations.

The researchers used a descriptive study design. Two of the researchers led a weekly socialization group over a 10-week period for eight women with dementia. The socialization group sessions were audiotaped and transcribed verbatim. These data resulted in the formation of two taxonomies: one represented the nurses' communication and the other represented the participants' communication repertoire.

The research supported the use of a greater number of conversational strategies than what is often stated in the nursing literature. The findings also suggested that clients with advanced dementia are able to engage in social conversation beyond what was expected given their Mini-Mental State Examination (MMSE) score.

Implications

This study suggests that individuals with advanced dementia are able to participate in a conversation when nurses use a broad range of conversational strategies. Moreover, the use of socialization groups to allow clients with advanced dementia to interact with others is a cost-effective way of enhancing their quality of life.

Note: Adapted from "Nurse–Patient Communication in Dementia. Improving the Odds," by J. Perry, S. Galloway, J. Bottorff, and S. Nixon, 2005, *Journal of Gerontological Nursing,* Copyright © 2005 *SLACK,* Inc. Reprinted with permission.

DIAGNOSING

Impaired verbal communication may be used as a nursing diagnosis when "an individual experiences a decreased, delayed, or absent ability to receive, process, transmit, and use a system of symbols—anything that has meaning (i.e., transmits meaning)" (Wilkinson, 2009). Communication problems may be *receptive* (e.g., difficulty hearing) or *expressive* (e.g., difficulty speaking).

Wilkinson (2009) points out that the *Impaired Verbal Communication* diagnosis may not be useful when an individual's communication problems are caused by a psychiatric illness or a coping problem. In those instances, the diagnoses of *Fear* or *Anxiety* may be more appropriate. Other nursing diagnoses (NANDA International, 2009) used for clients experiencing communication problems that involve impaired verbal communication as the *etiology* could include the following:

- *Anxiety* related to impaired verbal communication
- *Powerlessness* related to impaired verbal communication
- *Situational Low Self-Esteem* related to impaired verbal communication
- *Social Isolation* related to impaired verbal communication
- *Impaired Social Interaction* related to impaired verbal communication.

PLANNING

When a nursing diagnosis related to impaired verbal communication has been made, the nurse and client determine outcomes and begin planning ways to promote effective communication. The overall client outcome for persons with *Impaired Verbal Communication* is to reduce or resolve the factors impairing the communication. Specific nursing interventions will be planned from the stated etiology. Examples of outcome criteria to evaluate the effectiveness of nursing interventions and achievement of client goals follow.

The client:

- Communicates that needs are being met.
- Begins to establish a method of communication:
  - Signals yes/no to direct questions using vocalization or agreed-on physical cue (e.g., eye blink, hand squeeze).
  - Uses verbal or nonverbal techniques to indicate needs.
- Perceives the message accurately, as evidenced by appropriate verbal and/or nonverbal responses.
- Communicates effectively:
  - Using dominant language
  - Using translator/interpreter
  - Using sign language
  - Using word board or picture board
  - Using a computer

- Regains maximum communication abilities.
- Expresses minimum fear, anxiety, frustration, and depression.
- Uses resources appropriately.

IMPLEMENTING

Nursing interventions to facilitate communication with clients who have problems with speech or language include manipulating the environment, providing support, employing measures to enhance communication, and educating the client and support person.

Manipulate the Environment

A quiet environment with limited distractions will make the most of the communication efforts of both the client and the nurse and increase the possibility of effective communication. Sufficient light will help in conveying nonverbal messages, which is especially important if visual or auditory acuity is impaired. Initially, the nurse needs to provide a calm, relaxed environment, which will help reduce any anxiety the client may have. Remember that any factor that affects communication can create feelings of frustration, anxiety, depression, or hostility in the client. Communication normally contributes to a client's sense of security and feelings that he or she is not alone, so communication problems may cause some clients to feel isolated and confused. To further reduce these emotions, the nurse should acknowledge and praise the client's attempts at communication.

Provide Support

The nurse should convey encouragement to the client and provide nonverbal reassurance, perhaps by touch if appropriate. If the nurse does not understand, it is critical to let the client know so that he or she can provide clarification with other words or through some other means of communication. When speaking with a client who will have difficulty understanding, the nurse should check frequently to determine what the client has heard and understood. Using open-ended questions will assist the nurse in obtaining accurate information about the effectiveness of communication. For example, Maria Perez, who has limited English skills, is being taught about diet related to her Crohn's disease. If the nurse asks, "Do you understand what to eat?" Maria may nod her head yes. However, this does not give the nurse confirmation that the message given has been received. Rather the nurse needs to say, "What do you think will be good for you to eat when you go home?" The nurse's body language (e.g., gestures, posture, facial expression, and eye contact) should convey acceptance and approval.

Employ Measures to Enhance Communication

First determine how the client can best receive messages: by listening, by looking, through touch, or through an interpreter. Ways to help communication include keeping words simple and concrete and discussing topics of interest to the client. It is often helpful to use alternative communication strategies such as word boards, pictures, or paper and pencil.

Often interpreters can assist a client and nurse to communicate when the client lacks fluency in the dominant language. Some hospitals have a list of interpreters for various languages who can assist at the bedside. While family members may agree to act as an interpreter, it is always best if the translator is objective and trained in medical interpreting. Family members should only be used as a last resort and require the client's permission for the sake of confidentiality. Family members may not translate as accurately as a professional interpreter because of their concern for the client's feelings, misunderstanding of medical terminology, or a desire to keep upsetting news from the client.

Educate the Client and Support Persons

Sometimes clients and support people can be prepared in advance for communication problems, for example, before an intubation or throat surgery. By explaining anticipated problems, the client is often less anxious when problems arise.

EVALUATING

Evaluation is useful for both client and nurse communication.

Client Communication

To establish whether client outcomes have been met in relation to communication, the nurse must listen actively, observe nonverbal cues, and use therapeutic communication skills to determine that communication was effective. Examples of statements indicating outcome achievement include "Using picture board effectively to indicate needs" or "The client stated, 'I listened more closely to my daughter yesterday and found out how she feels about our divorce.'"

Nurse Communication

For nurses to evaluate the effectiveness of their own communication with clients, process recordings are frequently used. A **process recording** is a verbatim (word-for-word) account of a conversation. It can be taped or written and includes all verbal and nonverbal interactions of both the client and nurse.

One method of writing a process recording is to make two columns on a page. The first column lists what the nurse and the client said along with the associated nonverbal behavior. The second column contains an analysis about the nurse's responses.

Once a process recording has been completed, it should be analyzed in terms of the content and meaning of the interaction based on communication theory. Each of the nurse's statements is interpreted in terms of the communication skill used, with the rationale for and effectiveness of its use. Any barriers to effective communication can be identified with a possible alternative response noted. The

outcome for nurses should be increased awareness and insight regarding their communication strengths, as well as identification of areas for future skills development.

COMMUNICATION AMONG HEALTH PROFESSIONALS

Effective communication among the health professions is as important as the promotion of therapeutic communication between the nurse and the client. For example, past studies show that more than 60% of medication errors are caused by mistakes in interpersonal communication (Maxfield, Grenny, McMillan, Patterson, & Switzler, 2005, p. 2).

A 2004 research study collected survey data from over 17,000 nurses, physicians, clinical-care staff, and administrators. This study explored their concerns of difficulty in communicating that may then cause errors and poor health outcomes. The findings resulted in a compelling report entitled *Silence Kills*. As Maxfield et al. (2005) reported, the study identified the categories of conversations that were especially difficult and, at the same time, especially essential for people in health care to master. How effective their conversations were related strongly to medical errors, client safety, quality of care, staff satisfaction, and turnover. The seven areas of concern were broken rules, mistakes, lack of support, incompetence, poor teamwork, disrespect, and micromanagement (p. 3). The report indicates, for example, that many of the health care workers observed colleagues taking dangerous shortcuts, showing poor clinical judgment, and exhibiting verbal abuse and/or intimidating behaviors. Despite their concerns, very few discussed their concerns with the co-worker. This silence strongly related to poorer health outcomes for clients.

On the other hand, the study also showed that those health care workers who were confident in their communication abilities to discuss their concerns with their co-workers were more satisfied and committed to staying in health care. Moreover, better client outcomes (i.e., fewer errors) were observed.

In response to the findings of this study, the American Association of Critical-Care Nurses (AACN) developed a set of national standards. One of their six standards for establishing and sustaining healthy work environments is skilled communication. Skilled communication states that nurses must be as proficient in communication skills as they are in clinical skills. See Box 13–4, which lists the critical elements for skilled communication that preserves a nurse's professional integrity while ensuring a client's safety (AACN, 2005).

Nurse and Physician Communication

There are guidelines for written documentation and for nurses communicating with clients. However, few guidelines exist for the frequent verbal communication that occurs between nurses and doctors. This lack of guidelines or format may contribute to medical errors as a result of communication problems.

AACN Communication Standard for Establishing and Sustaining Healthy Work Environments

Standard: Skilled Communication: Nurses must be as proficient in communication skills as they are in clinical skills.

Critical Elements for the Nurse

- Skilled communicators focus on finding solutions and achieving desirable outcomes.
- Skilled communicators seek to protect and advance collaborative relationships among colleagues.
- Skilled communicators invite and hear all relevant perspectives.
- Skilled communicators call upon goodwill and mutual respect to build consensus and arrive at common understanding.
- Skilled communicators demonstrate congruence between words and actions, holding others accountable for doing the same.
- Skilled communicators have access to appropriate communication technologies and are proficient in their use.

Note: From *AACN standards for establishing and sustaining healthy work environments: A journey to excellence* by American Association of Critical-Care Nurses, 2005. Aliso Viejo, CA. Adapted with permission. The six behaviors above have been identified as critical elements for the individual nurse to achieve skilled communication as part of creating a healthy work environment. Because communication involves at least two individuals and does not occur in a vacuum, the nurse should be aware that every health care organization shares responsibility for supporting skilled communication, based on identified critical elements for the organization.

COMMUNICATION STYLES   A few authors describe differences between nurse and physician communication. For example, Lindeke and Sieckert (2005) state that nurses usually strive for consensus whereas physicians focus on ruling out alternatives. These differences can make collaboration more difficult. Beyea (2004) describes nurses' communication style as narrative and descriptive versus the physician's style being focused on a need or problem. One model, called the situational briefing model, addresses these differences and provides a framework for nurses when communicating with a physician. See Box 13–5 for more details on this communication framework.

ASSERTIVE COMMUNICATION   Assertive communication promotes client safety by minimizing miscommunication with colleagues. People who use assertive communication are honest, direct, and appropriate while being open to ideas and respecting the rights of others.

An important characteristic of assertive communication includes the use of "I" statements versus "you" statements. The "you" statement places blame and puts the listener in a defensive position. On the other hand, the "I" statement encourages discussion. For example, a nurse who states "I am concerned about . . ." to a physician will be gaining the attention of the doctor while also giving the message of the importance to work together for the benefit of the client. It is then important for the nurse to be clear, concise, organized, and fully informed when verbally presenting the client concern.

NONASSERTIVE COMMUNICATION   Two types of interpersonal behaviors are considered nonassertive: submissive and aggressive.

When people use a submissive communication style they allow their rights to be violated by others (Catalano, 2008). They meet the demands and requests of others without regard to their own feelings and needs as they believe their own feelings are not important. Some experts believe that people who use the submissive behaviors or communication style are insecure and try to maintain their self-esteem by avoiding conflict (e.g., negative criticism and disagreement from others).

There is a fine line between assertive and aggressive communication. Assertive communication is an open ex-

---

RESEARCH NOTES   **What Are Effects of Disruptive Behavior?**

The goals of this study by Rosenstein and O'Daniel (2005) were to assess perceptions of the impact of disruptive behavior of both physicians and nurses and its effects on both providers and clinical outcomes. Disruptive behavior was defined as any inappropriate behavior, confrontation, or conflict, ranging from verbal abuse to physical and sexual harassment.

The researchers distributed surveys to over 1,500 RNs (72%), physicians (27%), and executive administrators (1%) in 50 hospitals across the country. The research revealed a high prevalence of disruptive behavior among nurses and physicians. This behavior affected nurse–physician relationships and also nurse–nurse and physician–physician relationships, indicating a problem within and across disciplines. All respondents reported that the disruptive behavior had a significant negative impact on their level of stress, frustration, concentration, collaboration, communication, and re-

lationships. The research results also showed a strong perception of an association between disruptive behavior and medical errors, which affected client safety, quality of care, and satisfaction.

Implications

This study confirms that disruptive behavior is associated with decreased psychologic well-being of health care providers. This impacts job satisfaction and retention of nurses, which affects the current nursing shortage. Disruptive behavior also affects client safety and clinical outcomes. Health care organizations must develop strategies, policies, and an organizational culture that reinforces acceptable codes of behavior.

Note: Based on "Disruptive Behavior & Clinical Outcomes: Perceptions of Nurses & Physicians," by A. Rosenstein and M. O'Daniel, 2005, *American Journal of Nursing, 105*(1), pp. 54–64.

| BOX 13–5 | Situational Briefing or SBAR (Situation, Background, Assessment, Recommendation) Model |

A Framework for Nurse–Physician Communication

Provide the following:

- Information about the client's current situation
- Background for the current clinical situation
- Assessment of the current problem
- Recommendation that addresses the client's need

Note: Reprinted from *AORN Journal,* vol. 790, S. Beyea, "Improving Verbal Communication in Clinical Care" pp. 1053–1057, Copyright 2004, with permission from AORN, Inc.

pression of ideas and opinions while respecting the rights, opinions, and ideas of others. Aggressive communication strongly asserts the person's legitimate rights and opinions with little regard or respect for the rights and opinions of others (Catalano, 2008). Aggressive communication is often perceived as a personal attack by the other person because aggressive communication humiliates, dominates, controls, or embarrasses the other person. By lowering the other person's self-esteem, the person using aggressive communication may feel superior, which helps increase his or her self-esteem. Catalano (2006) states that aggressive communication can take several different forms, including screaming, sarcasm, rudeness, belittling jokes, and even direct personal insults (p. 278).

CHAPTER HIGHLIGHTS

- Communication is a critical nursing skill used to gather assessment data for nursing diagnoses, to teach and persuade, and to express caring and comfort.
- Communication is a two-way interpersonal process involving the sender of the message and the receiver of the message. It also involves intrapersonal messages, or self-talk, which can affect the message, the interpretation of the message, and the response.
- Because the sender must encode the message and determine the appropriate channels for conveying it, and because the receiver must perceive the message, decode it, and then respond, the communication process includes four elements: sender, message, receiver, and feedback.
- Verbal communication is effective when the criteria of pace and intonation, simplicity, clarity and brevity, timing, relevance, adaptability, and credibility are met.
- Nonverbal communication often reveals more about a person's thoughts and feelings than verbal communication; it includes personal appearance, posture and gait, facial expressions, and gestures.
- When assessing verbal and nonverbal behaviors, the nurse needs to consider cultural influences and be aware that a single nonverbal expression can indicate any of a variety of feelings and that words can have various meanings.
- When communication is effective, verbal and nonverbal expressions are congruent.
- Electronic communication, particularly e-mail, is evolving into nursing practice. While e-mail provides positive advantages for improving communication and continuity of client care, the nurse needs to be aware of the risk to client confidentiality.
- Many factors influence the communication process: development, gender, values and perceptions, personal space (intimate, personal, social, and public distance), territoriality, roles and relationships, environment, congruence, and interpersonal attitudes.
- Many techniques facilitate therapeutic communication: using silence, providing general leads, being specific and tentative, using open-ended questions, using touch, restating or paraphrasing, seeking clarification, perception checking or seeking consensual validation, offering self, giving information, acknowledging, clarifying time or sequence, presenting reality, focusing, reflecting, summarizing, and planning.

- Techniques that inhibit communication include stereotyping, being defensive, challenging, testing, rejecting, changing topics and subjects, unwarranted reassurance, passing judgment, and giving common advice.
- The effective nurse–client relationship is a helping relationship that facilitates growth of the individual.
- Four phases of the helping relationship include the preinteraction phase, the introductory phase, the working phase, and the termination phase; each has a specific purpose or goal and requires specific skills of the nurse.
- Nurses interact with groups of clients and colleagues in a wide variety of settings. To use groups rationally and effectively, nurses must understand the features of effective groups.
- To help clients with communication problems the nurse manipulates the environment, provides support, employs measures to enhance communication, and educates the client and support persons.
- Process recordings are frequently made by nurses to evaluate their own communication. With them, nurses can analyze both the process and the content of the communication.
- Effective communication between health professionals is vital for client safety. A compelling research report entitled *Silence Kills* indicated that many health care workers observed concerning behaviors of their co-workers (e.g., poor clinical judgment, dangerous shortcuts, disrespectful communication). However, they did not discuss their concerns with the co-worker. As a result, this silence strongly related to poorer health outcomes for clients.
- Communication styles can differ between nurses and physicians. Nurses tend to be more narrative and descriptive and strive for consensus. Physicians focus on a need or problem and rule out alternatives. The situational briefing model is one approach to addressing these differences in communication style and approach.
- Assertive communication promotes client safety by minimizing miscommunication with colleagues. An important characteristic of assertive communication is to use "I" statements.
- Nonassertive communication includes two types of interpersonal behaviors: submissive and aggressive.

THINK ABOUT IT

Refer to the chapter-opening scenario and answer these questions.

1. In the task meeting Barbara attends, how could the group dynamics have been changed by an effective chairperson?

2. What features of this group tasked to prepare for computerized documentation were ineffective for helping the group to meet their goals?

3. If you were appointed as the chairperson for the group, what changes would you make to improve the group's effectiveness?

∞ *See suggested responses to Think About It on MyNursingKit.*

TEST YOUR KNOWLEDGE

1. A student nurse is caring for a 72-year-old client with Alzheimer's disease who is very confused. The most appropriate communication strategy should include which of the following?
  1. Written directions for bathing
  2. Speaking very loudly
  3. Gentle touch while providing ADLs
  4. Flat facial expression

2. The nurse forms a helping relationship with clients in order to achieve the goal of: (Select all that apply.)
  1. Resolving all of the client's problems.
  2. Increasing clients' autonomy to help themselves.
  3. Developing unused or underused opportunities more fully.
  4. Helping clients manage their problems in living more effectively.
  5. Creating a strong friendship between the client and the nurse.

3. The nurse who uses appropriate therapeutic listening skills will display which of the following behaviors? Select all that apply.
  1. Absorb both the content and the feeling the client is conveying.
  2. Presume an understanding of the client needs.
  3. Adopt an open professional posture.
  4. React quickly to the message.
  5. Encourage compliance with the treatment regimen.

4. A nurse tells a client who is struggling with cancer pain, "It is normal to feel frustrated about the discomfort." Which of the following is most representative of the skills associated with the working phase of the helping relationship?
  1. Respect
  2. Genuineness
  3. Concreteness
  4. Confrontation

5. A depressed client who has not bathed or dressed in clean clothes today is reading the lunch menu but is unable to make a decision. Which of the following would be the most appropriate nursing diagnosis for this client?
  1. Anxiety
  2. Powerlessness
  3. Chronic Low Self-Esteem
  4. Social Isolation

6. After being admitted for emergency surgery, an 80-year-old client has just returned to the room from the post-anesthesia room (PAR). Which nursing interventions are most likely to facilitate effective communication with this client? Select all that apply.
  1. Ask the client, "Do you know where you are?"
  2. Ask the client or support person about visual or learning problems.
  3. Inform the client and support person(s) about events likely to occur during the next 2 hours.
  4. Provide the client with instructions about discharge.
  5. Speak loudly and enunciate every syllable.

7. The nurse is communicating with a well-oriented older adult client in a long-term care setting. Which statement best reflects respectful and caring communication?
  1. "Are we ready for our shower?"
  2. "It's time to go to the dining room, honey."
  3. "Are you comfortable, Mrs. Smith?"
  4. "You would rather wear the slacks, wouldn't you?"

8. The client made the following statement to the nurse, "My doctor just told me that he cannot save my leg and that I need to have an above-the-knee amputation." Which of the following responses by the nurse is most appropriate?
  1. "Dr. Jones is an excellent surgeon."
  2. "Are you in pain?"
  3. "If I were you, I'd get a second opinion."
  4. "Tell me more. . . ."

9. The nurse is communicating with a primary care provider about medical interventions prescribed for a client. Which of the following statements is most representative of a collaborative nurse–physician relationship?
  1. "That new medication you prescribed for Mr. Black is ineffective."
  2. "I am worried about Mr. Black's blood pressure. It is not decreasing even with the new antihypertensive medication."
  3. "Can we talk about Mr. Black?"
  4. "Excuse me, doctor. I think we need to talk about Mr. Black's blood pressure."

10. The nurse asks the client, "What do you fear most about your surgery tomorrow?" This is an example of which of the following communication techniques?
  1. Providing general leads
  2. Seeking clarification
  3. Presenting reality
  4. Summarizing

∞ *See answers to Test Your Knowledge in Appendix A.*

REFERENCES AND SELECTED BIBLIOGRAPHY

Adubato, S. (2004). Making the communication connection. *Nursing Management, 35*(9), 33–35.

American Association of Critical-Care Nurses (AACN). (2005). *AACN standards for establishing and sustaining healthy work environment: A journey to excellence.* Aliso Viejo, CA: Author.

Anonymous. (2005). Meeting security regulations for e-mail. *Health Management Technology, 26*(10), 52–54.

Arford, P. H. (2005). Nurse–physician communication: An organizational accountability. *Nursing Economics, 23*(2), 72–77.

Austin, S. (2006). E-mail: So fast, so convenient, so . . . risky? *Nursing, 36*(2), 76–77.

Beyea, S. C. (2004). Improving verbal communication in clinical care. *AORN Journal, 79*(5), 1053–1057.

Brammer, L. M. (2003). *The helping relationship: Process and skills* (8th ed.). Upper Saddle River, NJ: Prentice Hall.

Bulechek, G. M., Butcher, H. K., & Dochterman, J. M. (Eds.). (2008). *Nursing interventions classification (NIC)* (5th ed.). St. Louis, MO: Mosby.

Burke, M., Boal, J., & Mitchell, R. (2004). Communicating for better care. Improving nurse–physician communication. *American Journal of Nursing, 104*(12), 40–47.

Catalano, J. T. (2008). *Nursing now! Today's issues, tomorrow's trends* (5th ed.). Philadelphia: Davis.

Delbanco, T., & Sands, D. Z. (2004). Electrons in flight—E-mail between doctors and patients. *New England Journal of Medicine, 350*(17), 1705–1708.

Egan, G. (2009). *The skilled helper: A problem-management approach to helping* (9th ed.). Pacific Grove, CA: Brooks/Cole.

Fenwick, J., Barclay, L., & Schmeid, V. (2001). Chatting: An important clinical tool in facilitating mothering in neonatal nurseries. *Advances in Nursing Science, 24,* 34–49.

Jonas-Simpson, C. M., Mitchell, G. J., Fisher, A., Jones, G., & Linscott, J. (2006). The experience of being listened to: A qualitative study of older adults in long-term settings. *Journal of Gerontological Nursing, 32*(1), 46–53.

Leonard, M., Frankel, A., Simmonds, T., & Vega, K. (2004). *Achieving safe and reliable healthcare: Strategies and solutions.* Chicago: Health Administration Press.

Lindeke, L. L., & Sieckert, A. M. (2005). Nurse–physician workplace collaboration. *Online Journal of Issues in Nursing, 10*(1), manuscript 4. Retrieved December 5, 2009, from http://www.nursingworld.org/MainMenuCategories/ANAMarketplace/ANAPeriodicals/OJIN/TableofContents/Volume102005/No1Jan05/tpc26_416011.aspx

MacDonald, C. M. (2004). A chuckle a day keeps the doctor away: Therapeutic humor & laughter. *Journal of Psychosocial Nursing & Mental Health Services, 42*(3), 18–25.

Mathew, F. M. (2003). Laughter is the best medicine: The value of humour in current nursing practice. *Nursing Journal of India, 94*(7), 146–147.

Maxfield, D., Grenny, J., McMillan, R., Patterson, K., & Switzler, A. (2005). *Silence kills. The seven crucial conversations for healthcare.* VitalSmarts, L.C.

Maxfield, D., Grenny, J., McMillan, R., Patterson, K., & Switzler, A. (2005). *Silence kills. The seven crucial conversations for healthcare.* VitalSmarts, L.C.

Mikanowicz, C. K. (2005). *Strategies for developing communication between nurses and physicians.* Retrieved May 29, 2005, from http://www.nursece.com/onlinecourses/957.html

Moorhead, S., Johnson, M., Maas, M. L., & Swanson, E. (Eds.). (2008). *Nursing Outcomes Classification (NOC).* (4th ed.). St. Louis: Mosby.

NANDA International. (2009). *NANDA nursing diagnosis: Definitions & classification 2009–2011.* West Sussex, U.K.: Wiley-Blackwell.

Perry, J., Galloway, S., Bottorff, J. L., & Nixon, S. (2005). Nurse–patient communication in dementia: Improving the odds. *Journal of Gerontological Nursing, 31*(4), 43–52.

Preston, P. (2005). Nonverbal communication: Do you really say what you mean? *Journal of Healthcare Management, 50*(2), 83–86.

Rondeau, K. V. (1992). Effective communication means really listening. *Canadian Journal of Medical Technology, 52*(2), 78–80.

Rosenstein, A. H., & O'Daniel, M. (2005). Disruptive behavior & clinical outcomes: Perceptions of nurses & physicians. *American Journal of Nursing, 105*(1), 54–64.

Slaven, A. (2003). Communication and the hearing-impaired patient. *Nursing Standard, 18*(1), 39–41.

Stiles, A. S., & Raney, T. J. (2004). Relationships among personal space boundaries, peer acceptance, and peer reputation in adolescents. *Journal of Child and Adolescent Psychiatric Nursing, 16*(4), 29–40.

Tamparo, C. T., & Lindh, W. Q. (2007). *Therapeutic communications for health professionals* (3rd ed.). Albany, NY: Delmar.

Utley-Smith, Q. (2004). Nursing competencies needed by new baccalaureate graduates. *Nursing Education Perspectives, 25*(4), 166–170.

Vazirani, S., Hays, R. D., Shapiro, M. F., & Cowan, M. (2005). Effect of a multidisciplinary intervention on communication and collaboration among physicians and nurses. *American Journal of Critical Care, 14*(1), 71–76.

Weeks, M. B. (2004). Nurse–physician communication—Discourse analysis. *Canadian Operating Room Nursing Journal, 22*(4), 33–37.

Weeks, M. B. (2005). Nurse-physician communication. *Canadian Operating Room Nursing Journal, 23*(1), 48–56.

Wilkinson, J. M., & Ahern, N. R. (2009). *Prentice Hall Nursing Diagnosis Handbook* (9th ed.). Upper Saddle River, NJ: Pearson Education.

Williams, K., Kemper, S., & Hummert, M. L. (2004). Enhancing communication with older adults: Overcoming elderspeak. *Journal of Gerontological Nursing, 30*(10), 17–25.

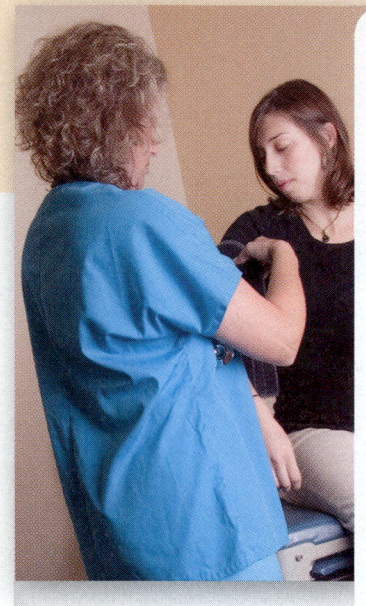

Frangelica Orleans, 43 years old, has not been feeling well lately, but she really can't put her finger on exactly what is bothering her. At work this morning she fainted, and her boss insisted she go to the employee clinic to be examined. After drawing blood and examining her, the provider told Ms. Orleans she has developed diabetes mellitus and referred her to her family provider for care. Ms. Orleans is to meet with the provider this afternoon. The provider examines her further, checks another blood glucose, and confirms the diagnosis of diabetes mellitus. Ms. Orleans is surprised and can't believe she's going to have to inject herself with insulin. She keeps saying to the nurse, "Are you sure? Could there be a mistake?" The nurse assures her there is no mistake. The nurse plans to teach her about diet modification, blood glucose monitoring, preventing common complications, follow-up care requirements, and medication administration.

LEARNING OUTCOMES

After completing this chapter, you will be able to:

1. Discuss the importance of the teaching role of the nurse.

2. Describe the attributes of learning.

3. Compare and contrast andragogy, pedagogy, and geragogy.

4. Discuss the learning theories of behaviorism, cognitivism, and humanism and how nurses can use each of these theories.

5. Describe the three domains of learning.

6. Identify factors that affect learning.

7. Discuss the implications of using the Internet as a source of health information.

8. Assess the learning needs of clients and the learning environment.

9. Identify nursing diagnoses, outcomes, and interventions that reflect the learning needs of clients.

10. Describe the essential aspects of a teaching plan.

11. Identify guidelines for effective teaching.

12. Discuss strategies to use when teaching clients of different cultures.

13. Identify methods to evaluate learning.

14. Demonstrate effective documentation of teaching–learning activities.

Teaching client education is a major aspect of nursing practice and an important independent nursing function. In 1992, the American Hospital Association passed *A Patient's Bill of Rights* mandating client education as a right of all clients. State nurse practice acts include client teaching as a function of nursing, thereby making teaching a legal and professional responsibility. In addition, the Joint Commission on Accreditation of Healthcare Organizations (The Joint Commission) recently expanded its standards of client education by nurses to include "evidence that patients and their significant others understand what they have been taught. This requirement means that providers must consider the literacy level, educational background, language skills, and culture of every client during the education process" (Bastable, 2008).

Client education is multifaceted, involving promoting, protecting, and maintaining health. It involves teaching about reducing health risk factors, increasing a person's level of wellness, and taking specific protective health measures.

TEACHING

Teaching is a system of activities intended to produce learning. The teaching process is intentionally designed to produce specific learning.

The teaching–learning process involves dynamic interaction between teacher and learner. Each participant in the process communicates information, emotions, perceptions, and attitudes to the other. The teaching process and the nursing process are much alike (see Table 14–1).

Nurses teach a variety of learners in various settings. They teach clients and their families or significant others in the hospital, primary care clinics, urgent care, managed care, the home, and assisted living and long-term care facilities. Nurses teach large and small groups of learners in community health education programs.

Nurses also teach professional colleagues and other health care personnel in academic institutions such as vocational schools, colleges, and universities, and in health care facilities such as hospitals or nursing homes.

Teaching Clients and Their Families

Nurses may teach individual clients in one-to-one teaching episodes. For example, the nurse may teach about wound care while changing a client's dressing or may teach about diet, exercise, and other lifestyle behaviors that minimize the risk of a heart attack for a client who has a cardiac problem. The nurse may also be involved in teaching family members or other support people who are caring for the client. Nurses working in obstetric and pediatric areas teach parents and sometimes grandparents or other family members how to care for children.

Because of the decreased length of hospital stays, time constraints on client education may occur. Nurses need to provide client education that will ensure the client's safe transition from one level of care to another and make appropriate plans for follow-up education in the client's home. Discharge plans must include information about what the client has been taught before transfer or discharge and what

TABLE 14–1	Comparison of the Teaching Process and the Nursing Process	
STEP	**TEACHING PROCESS**	**NURSING PROCESS**
1	Collect data; analyze client's learning strengths and deficits.	Collect data; analyze client's strengths and deficits.
2	Make educational diagnoses.	Make nursing diagnoses.
3	Prepare teaching plan: • Write learning outcomes. • Select content and time frame. • Select teaching strategies.	Plan nursing goals/desired outcomes and select interventions.
4	Implement teaching plan.	Implement nursing strategies.
5	Evaluate client learning based on achievement of learning outcomes.	Evaluate client outcomes based on achievement of goal criteria.

remains for the client to learn to perform self-care in the home or other residence (see Chapter 3 ∞).

Teaching in the Community

Nurses are often involved in community health education programs. Such teaching activities may be voluntary as part of the nurse's involvement in an organization such as the Red Cross or Planned Parenthood, or they may be compensated as part of the nurse's work role, such as school nurses. Community teaching activities may be aimed at large groups of people who have an interest in some aspect of health, such as nutrition classes, CPR or cardiac risk factor reduction classes, and bicycle or swimming safety programs. Community education programs can also be designed for small groups or individual learners, such as childbirth classes or family planning classes.

Teaching Health Personnel

Nurses are also involved in the instruction of professional colleagues through continuing education, in-service programs, and staff development. For example, experienced nurses may function as preceptors for new graduate nurses or for newly employed nurses. Nurses with specialized knowledge and experience share that knowledge and experience with nurses who are new to that practice area. Examples of such specialized courses include critical-care nursing, perioperative nursing, and quality improvement/quality assurance. In addition, nurses in nursing practice settings are often involved in the clinical instruction of nursing students.

Nurses are also involved in teaching other health professionals. Nurses may participate in the education of medical students or allied health students. In this capacity, the nurse educator clarifies the role of the nurse for other health professionals or how nurses can assist them in their care of the client.

LEARNING

Like all people, clients have a variety of learning needs. A **learning need** is a desire or a requirement to know something that is presently unknown to the learner. Learning needs include new knowledge or information but can also include a new or different skill or physical ability, or a new behavior or a need to change an old behavior. **Learning** is a change in human disposition or capability that persists and that cannot be solely accounted for by growth. Learning is represented by a change in behavior. See the Client Teaching box for attributes of learning.

An important aspect of learning is the individual's desire to learn and to act on the learning, referred to as **compliance**. In the health care context, compliance is the extent to which a person's behavior coincides with medical or health advice. Compliance is best illustrated when the person recognizes and accepts the need to learn, and then follows through with the appropriate behaviors that reflect the learning. For example, a person diagnosed as having diabetes willingly learns about the

---

> **CLIENT TEACHING**   **Attributes of Learning**
>
> Learning is:
>
> - An experience that occurs inside the learner.
> - The discovery of the personal meaning and relevance of ideas.
> - A consequence of experience.
> - A collaborative and cooperative process.
> - An evolutionary process that builds on past learning and experiences.
> - A process that is both intellectual and emotional.

needed special diet and then plans and follows the learned diet. Many people, however, view the term *compliance* in a negative perspective because the term implies the learner is submissive and this is in conflict with the learner's right to determine his or her own health care decisions rather than be told what to do by a health care professional. In addition, it is important not to label a client as noncompliant without obtaining further information. For example, the client intended to comply but was unable to do so because he could not afford the cost of the medications.

Another term seen in health care literature is **adherence**, which is commitment or attachment to a regimen. Bastable (2003) explains that both compliance and adherence refer to the "ability to maintain health-promoting regimens, which are determined largely by a health care provider" (p. 169).

Andragogy is the art and science of teaching adults, in contrast to **pedagogy**, the discipline concerned with helping children learn. **Geragogy** is the term used to describe the process involved in stimulating and helping older adults to learn (Hayes, 2005; John, 1988).

Nurses can use the following andragogic concepts about adult learners as a guide for client teaching (Hayes, 2005; Knowles, 1984):

- As people mature, they move from dependence to independence.
- An adult's previous experiences can be used as a resource for learning.
- An adult's readiness to learn is often related to a developmental task or social role (i.e., perceive a need in their life situation).
- An adult is more oriented to learning when the material is useful immediately, not sometime in the future.

Learning Theories

Three main theoretical constructs are behaviorism, cognitivism, and humanism.

BEHAVIORISM   Thorndike originally advanced behaviorism. His major contribution that applied to teaching is that learning should be based on the learner's behavior. In addition to Thorndike, major behaviorist theorists include Pavlov, Skinner, and Bandura.

In the behaviorist school of thought, an act is called a *response* when it can be traced to the effects of a stimulus. Behaviorists closely observe responses and then manipulate the environment to bring about the intended change. Thus, to modify a person's attitude and response, a behaviorist would either alter the stimulus condition in the environment or change what happens after a response occurs (Bastable, 2003, p. 45).

Skinner's and Pavlov's work focused on conditioning behavioral responses to a stimulus that causes the response or behavior. To increase the probability of a response, Skinner introduced the importance of positive reinforcement (e.g., a pleasant experience such as praise and encouragement) in fostering repetition of an action. Bandura, however, claims that most learning comes from observational learning and instruction rather than trial-and-error behavior. Bandura's research focuses on **imitation**, the process by which individuals copy or reproduce what they have observed, and **modeling**, the process by which a person learns by observing the behavior of others.

Nurses applying behavioristic theory will:

- Provide sufficient practice time and both immediate and repeat testing and redemonstration.
- Provide opportunities for learners to solve problems by trial and error.
- Select teaching strategies that avoid distracting information and that evoke the desired response.
- Praise the learner for correct behavior and provide positive feedback at intervals throughout the learning experience.
- Provide role models of desired behavior.

COGNITIVISM Cognitivism depicts learning as a complex cognitive activity. In other words, learning is largely a mental or intellectual or thinking process. The learner structures and processes information. Perceptions are selectively chosen by the individual, and personal characteristics have an impact on how a cue is perceived. Cognitivists also emphasize the importance of social, emotional, and physical contexts in which learning occurs, such as the teacher–learner relationship and the environment. Developmental readiness and individual readiness (expressed as motivation) are other key factors associated with cognitive approaches.

Major cognitive theorists include Piaget, Lewin, and Bloom. Piaget's five major phases of cognitive development include the sensorimotor phase, the preconceptual phase, the intuitive phase, the concrete operations phase, and the formal operations phase. Each phase is discussed in Chapter 9 ∞. According to Lewin, learning involves four different types of changes: change in cognitive structure, change in motivation, change in one's sense of belonging to the group, and gain in voluntary muscle control. His widely known theory of change has three basic stages: unfreezing, moving, and refreezing. These stages are discussed in detail in Chapter 15 ∞.

Bloom (1956) identified three domains or areas of learning: cognitive, affective, and psychomotor. The **cognitive domain**, the "thinking" domain, includes six intellectual abilities and thinking processes beginning with knowing, comprehending, and applying to analysis, synthesis, and evaluation. The **affective domain**, known as the "feeling" domain, is divided into categories that specify the degree of a "person's depth of emotional response to tasks" (Bastable, 2003, p. 330). It includes feelings, emotions, interests, attitudes, and appreciations. The **psychomotor domain**, the "skill" domain, includes motor skills such as giving an injection.

Nurses should include each of Bloom's three domains in client teaching plans. For example, teaching a client how to self-administer insulin is in the psychomotor domain. But an important part of a teaching plan for a client with diabetes is to teach why insulin is needed and what to do when not feeling well; this is in the cognitive domain. Helping the client accept the chronic implications of diabetes and maintain self-esteem is in the affective domain.

Nurses applying cognitive theory will:

- Provide a social, emotional, and physical environment conducive to learning.
- Encourage a positive teacher–learner relationship.
- Select multisensory teaching strategies since perception is influenced by the senses.
- Recognize that personal characteristics have an impact on how cues are perceived and develop appropriate teaching approaches to target different learning styles.
- Assess a person's developmental and individual readiness to learn and adapt teaching strategies to the learner's developmental level.
- Select behavioral objectives and teaching strategies that encompass the cognitive, affective, and psychomotor domains of learning.

HUMANISM Humanistic learning theory focuses on both cognitive and affective qualities of the learner. Prominent members of this school of thought include Abraham Maslow and Carl Rogers. According to humanistic theory, learning is believed to be self-motivated, self-initiated, and self-evaluated. Each individual is viewed as a unique composite of biologic, psychologic, social, cultural, and spiritual factors. Learning focuses on self-development and achieving full potential; it is best when it is relevant to the learner. Autonomy and self-determination are important; the learner identifies the learning needs and takes the initiative to meet these needs. The learner is an active participant and takes responsibility for meeting individual learning needs.

Nurses applying humanistic theory will:

- Convey empathy in the nurse–client relationship.
- Encourage the learner to establish goals and promote self-directed learning.
- Encourage active learning by serving as a facilitator, mentor, or resource for the learner.
- Use active learning strategies to assist the client's adoption of new behavior.
- Expose the learner to new relevant information and ask appropriate questions to encourage the learner to seek answers.

Using Learning Theories

Nurses using the **behaviorist theory** identify what is to be taught, and they immediately identify and reward correct responses. However, the theory is not easily applied to complex learning situations and limits the learner's role in the teaching process.

Users of **cognitive theory** recognize the developmental level of the learner and acknowledge the learner's motivation and environment. However, some or many of the motivational and environmental factors may be beyond the teacher's control.

Using **humanism**, the nurse focuses on the feelings and attitudes of learners, on the importance of the individual in identifying learning needs and in taking responsibility for them, and on the self-motivation of the learners to work toward self-reliance and independence.

Being aware of the focus and limitations of the various learning theories allows the nurse to use one or more of them when developing a teaching plan for a client. Knowing what is important (e.g., knowledge, motivation, feelings, attitudes) assists the nurse in choosing the appropriate learning theory or theories. The nurse also needs to be aware of the different factors that can affect the client's learning.

Factors Affecting Learning

Many factors can facilitate or hinder learning by a client. The nurse should be aware of these factors, particularly when teaching time is limited.

MOTIVATION   **Motivation** to learn is the desire to learn. It greatly influences how quickly and how much a person learns. Motivation is generally greatest when a person recognizes a need and believes the need will be met through learning. It is not enough for the need to be identified and verbalized by the nurse; it must be experienced by the client. Often the nurse's task is to help the client personally work through the problem and identify the need. Sometimes clients or support people need help identifying information relevant to their situation before they can see a need. For instance, clients with heart disease may need to know the effects of smoking before they recognize the need to stop smoking. Or adolescents may need to know the consequences of an untreated sexually transmitted disease before they see the need for treatment.

READINESS   **Readiness** to learn is the demonstration of behaviors or cues that reflect the learner's motivation to learn at a specific time. Readiness reflects not only the desire or willingness to learn but also the ability to learn at a specific time. For example, a client may want to learn self-care during a dressing change, but if the client experiences pain or discomfort he or she may not be able to learn. The nurse can provide pain medication to make the client more comfortable and more able to learn. The nurse's role is often to encourage the development of readiness.

ACTIVE INVOLVEMENT   When the learner is actively involved in the process of learning, learning becomes more

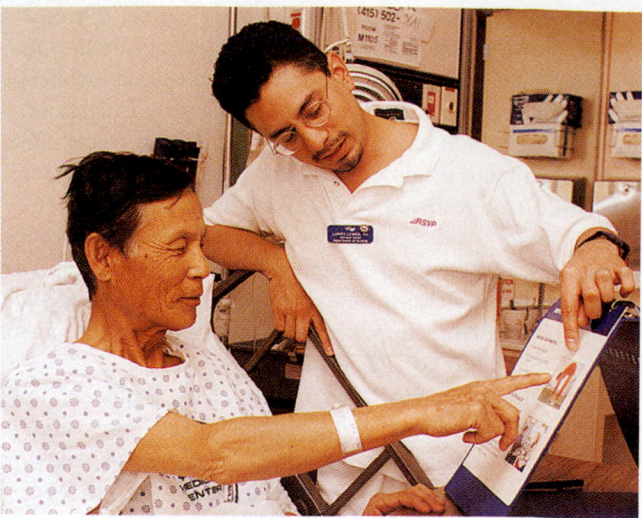

Figure 14–1 ⊙ Learning is facilitated when the client is interested and actively involved.

meaningful. If the learner actively participates in planning and discussion, learning is faster and retention is better (Figure 14–1). Active learning promotes critical thinking, enabling learners to problem solve more effectively. Clients who are actively involved in learning about their health care may be more able to apply the learning to their own situation. For example, clients who are actively involved in learning about their therapeutic diets may be more able to apply the principles being taught to their cultural food preferences and their usual eating habits. Passive learning, such as listening to a lecture or watching a film, does not foster optimal learning.

RELEVANCE   The knowledge or skill to be learned must be personally relevant to the learner. Clients learn more easily if they can connect the new knowledge to that which they already know or have experienced. For example, if a client is diagnosed with hypertension, is overweight, and has symptoms of headaches and fatigue, he is more likely to understand the need to lose weight if he remembers having more energy when he weighed less. The nurse needs to validate the relevance of learning with the client throughout the learning process.

FEEDBACK   *Feedback* is information regarding a person's performance to a desired goal. It has to be meaningful to the learner. Feedback that accompanies the practice of psychomotor skills helps the person to learn those skills. Support of desired behavior through praise, positively worded corrections, and suggestions of alternative methods are ways of providing positive feedback. Negative feedback such as ridicule, anger, or sarcasm can lead people to withdraw from learning. Such feedback, viewed as a type of punishment, may cause the client to avoid the teacher in order to avoid punishment.

NONJUDGMENTAL SUPPORT   People learn best when they believe they are accepted and will not be judged. The person who expects to be judged as a "poor" or "good" client will not learn as well as the person who feels no such threat. Once learners have succeeded in accomplishing a task or understanding a concept, they gain self-confidence in their ability to learn. This reduces their anxiety about failure and can motivate greater learning. Successful learners have increased confidence with which to accept failure.

SIMPLE TO COMPLEX Learning is facilitated by material that is logically organized and proceeds from the simple to the complex. Such organization enables the learner to comprehend new information, assimilate it with previous learning, and form new understandings. Of course, *simple* and *complex* are relative terms, depending on the level at which the person is learning. What is simple for one person may be complex for another.

REPETITION Repetition of key concepts and facts facilitates retention of newly learned material. Practice of psychomotor skills, particularly with feedback from the nurse, improves performance of those skills and facilitates their transfer to another setting.

TIMING People retain information and psychomotor skills best when the time between learning and active use of the learning is short; the longer the time interval, the easier it is to forget the learning. For example, a client who is only shown literature and videotapes about administering insulin but is not permitted to administer his or her own insulin until discharge from the hospital is unlikely to remember what was learned. However, giving his or her own injections while in the hospital enhances the client's learning.

ENVIRONMENT An optimal learning environment facilitates learning by reducing distraction and providing physical and psychologic comfort. It has adequate lighting that is free from glare, a comfortable room temperature, and good ventilation. Most students know what it is like to try to learn in a hot, stuffy room; the consequent drowsiness interferes with concentration. Noise can also distract the student and interfere with listening and thinking. To facilitate learning in a hospital setting, nurses should choose a time when no visitors are present and interruptions are unlikely.

Privacy is essential for some learning. For example, when a client is learning to change a colostomy bag, the presence of others can be embarrassing and thus interfere with learning. However, when a client is particularly anxious, having a support person present may give the client confidence.

Many factors inhibit learning. Some of the most common barriers to learning are described next and in Table 14–2.

TABLE 14–2 Barriers to Learning

BARRIER	EXPLANATION	NURSING IMPLICATIONS
Acute illness	Client requires all resources and energy to cope with illness.	Defer teaching until client is less ill.
Pain	Pain decreases ability to concentrate.	Conduct pain assessment before teaching.
Prognosis	Client can be preoccupied with illness and unable to concentrate on new information.	Defer teaching to a better time.
Biorhythms	Mental and physical performances have a circadian rhythm.	Adapt time of teaching to suit client.
Emotion (e.g., anxiety, denial, depression, grief)	Emotions require energy and distract from learning.	Deal with emotions and possible misinformation first.
Language	Client may not be fluent in the nurse's language.	Obtain services of an interpreter or nurse with appropriate language skills.
Age		
• Older adults	Vision, hearing, and motor control can be impaired in older adults.	Consider sensory and motor deficits and adapt in teaching plan.
• Children	Children have a shorter attention span and vocabulary differences.	Plan shorter and more active learning episodes.
Culture/religion	There may be cultural or religious restrictions on certain types of knowledge, for example, birth control information.	Assess the client's cultural/religious needs when planning learning activities.
Physical disability	Visual, hearing, sensory, or motor impairments may interfere with a client's ability to learn.	Plan teaching activities appropriate to learner's physical abilities. For example, provide audio learning tools for the client who is blind, or large-print materials for the client whose vision is impaired.
Mental disability	Impaired cognitive ability may affect the client's capacity for learning.	Assess client's capacity for learning and plan teaching activities to complement the client's ability while planning more complex learning for the client's caregivers.

EMOTIONS Emotions such as fear, anger, and depression can impede learning. A high level of anxiety resulting in agitation and the inability to focus or concentrate can also inhibit learning. Clients or families who are experiencing extreme emotional states may not hear spoken words or may retain only part of the communication. Emotional responses such as fear and anxiety decrease with information that relieves uncertainty. Medications may be prescribed for extremely distraught clients or families to reduce their anxiety and put them in an emotional state in which understanding or learning can occur.

PHYSIOLOGIC EVENTS Physiologic events such as a critical illness, pain, or sensory deficits inhibit learning. Because the client cannot concentrate and apply energy to learning, the learning itself is impaired. The nurse should try to reduce the physiologic barriers to learning as much as possible before teaching. For example, providing analgesics and rest before teaching is often helpful.

CULTURAL ASPECTS There are also cultural barriers to learning, such as language or values. The client who does not understand the nurse's language may learn little. Western medicine may conflict with a client's cultural healing beliefs and practices. To be effective, nurses must be culturally sensitive and competent; otherwise the client may be partially or totally noncompliant with recommended treatments. Another impediment to learning is differing values held by the client and the health team. For example, if a client comes from a culture that views being overweight or "plump" as positive, the nurse negotiates with the client to determine an acceptable weight and they develop a plan together (Purnell & Paulanka, 2005).

PSYCHOMOTOR ABILITY It is important that the nurse be aware of a client's psychomotor skills when planning teaching. Psychomotor skills can be affected by health. For example, an older client who has severe osteoarthritis of the hands may not be able to wrap a bandage. The following physical abilities are important for learning psychomotor skills:

1. *Muscle strength.* For example, an older client who cannot rise from a chair because of insufficient leg and muscle strength cannot be expected to learn to lift herself out of a bathtub.
2. *Motor coordination.* Gross motor coordination is required for movements such as walking, and fine motor coordination is needed when using utensils such as a fork for eating. For example, a client who has advanced amyotrophic lateral sclerosis (ALS) involving the lower limbs will probably be unable to use a walker.
3. *Energy.* Energy is required for most psychomotor skills, and learning these skills uses more energy. People who are ill or older adults often have limited energy resources; learning and carrying out these skills must be timed for when the client's energy sources are at their peak.
4. *Sensory acuity.* Sight is used for most learning (e.g., walking with crutches, changing a dressing, drawing a

medication into a syringe). Clients who have a visual impairment often need the assistance of a support person to carry out such tasks.

THE INTERNET AND HEALTH INFORMATION

The Internet has become a part of the lives of many Americans, allowing them to communicate and obtain information quickly. Internet technology has dramatically changed the activities of business, including health care. The term *e-health* is defined as "the application of Internet and other related technologies in the health care industry to improve the access, efficiency, effectiveness, and quality of clinical and business processes utilized by health care organizations, practitioners, patients, and consumers in an effort to improve the health status of patients" (Healthcare Information and Management Systems Society E-Health Special Interest Group, 2003, p. 4). E-health includes many aspects such as online appointment access, billing review, e-mail access between the client and health care provider, and online health information.

Online Health Information

The Pew Internet & American Life Project (2006) reports that 73% of American adults use the Internet. Using the Internet to locate health information is common. Health care online usage is growing twice as fast as any other online type of usage (Curran & Curran, 2005, p. 496). Eight out of 10 American Internet users have searched for information on at least one major health topic online. Certain groups of users are more likely to search the Internet for health information: women, adults younger than 65, college graduates, people with online experience, and those with broadband (high-speed) access (Pew Internet & American Life Project, 2005a, p. 1).

Access

The Pew Internet & American Life Project (2005b, p. 7) reported that there are three groups of adults in the United States: those who do not use the Internet, those with a modest connection, and those highly engaged with the Internet. Each group has its distinct characteristics.

Twenty-two percent of American adults have never used the Internet. They tend to have a high school or less education and to be over the age of 65. Forty percent of adults have a loose connection to the Internet. That is, they have access (usually dial-up) but do not use the Internet regularly. They are younger and more educated than the previous group. Thirty-three percent of American adults are highly engaged by using the Internet daily. They tend to have attended college and be under age 50; however, there are "pockets" of older adults who are also highly engaged in Internet use.

Older Adults and Use of the Internet

The Kaiser Family Foundation (2005, pp. 3–10) conducted a survey research study that provided the first close look at how older adults use the Internet for health information. Key findings of the report included:

- Only four in 10 older adults age 65 and over have used a computer.
- Seventy percent of "baby boomers" (age 50–64) use the Internet. Thus, the number of older adults using the Internet will increase over the next decade.
- There is a "digital divide" among older adults. Those older adults whose annual income is under $20,000, those who have a high school degree or less, those who are older (e.g., 75 and above), and older adult women are less likely to use the Internet.
- One in five older adults (65 and over) use the Internet for health information. These older adults are more likely to use TV and books for their health information.
- Many older adults do not trust the Internet as a source for health information except for the 50 to 64 age group who trust the Internet "a lot."
- Information on prescription drugs is the top reason for using the Internet for health information.
- Of those older adults who have used the Internet for health information, about half say it helped them and the other half say it wasn't helpful.
- Most older adults do not check the source of health information they find online.

Implications

The Internet is an important source of health information for many adult clients in the United States. Therefore, nurses need to know and be able to integrate this technology into the teaching plans for those clients who use the Internet. On the other hand, nurses also need to apply effective teaching strategies for those clients who do not use the Internet.

NURSE AS EDUCATOR

Being an educator or teacher is an important and primary role for the nurse. Clients and families have the right to health education in order to make informed decisions about their health. The nurse is in a position to promote healthy lifestyles through the application of health knowledge, the change process, learning theories, and the nursing and teaching process when teaching clients and their families.

NURSING MANAGEMENT

ASSESSING

A comprehensive assessment of learning needs incorporates data from the nursing history and physical assessment and addresses the client's support system. It also considers client characteristics that may influence the learning process: readiness to learn, motivation to learn, and reading and comprehension level, for example. Assessing a person's stage of change and any barriers to change is also important and often overlooked (see Chapter 5 ∞).

The nurse's knowledge of common learning needs required by clients experiencing similar health problems is another source of information. Learning needs change as the client's health status changes, so nurses must constantly reassess them.

Nursing History

Several elements in the nursing history provide clues to learning needs. These elements include (a) age, (b) the client's understanding and perceptions of the health problem, (c) health beliefs and practices, (d) cultural factors, (e) economic factors, (f) learning style, and (g) the client's support systems. Examples of interview questions to elicit this information are shown in the accompanying Assessment Interview. Note the number of open-ended questions.

AGE Age provides information on the person's developmental status that may indicate distinctive health teaching content and teaching approaches. Simple questions to school-age children and adolescents will elicit information on what they know. Observing children at play provides information about their motor and intellectual development as well as relationships with other children. For older people, conversation and questioning may reveal slow recall or limited psychomotor skills, sensory deficits, and learning difficulties (see Lifespan Considerations on p. 335).

CLIENTS' UNDERSTANDING OF HEALTH PROBLEM Clients' perceptions of their current health problems and concerns may indicate deficient knowledge or misinformation. In addition, the effects of the problem on the client's usual activities can alert the nurse to other areas requiring instruction. For example, people who cannot manage self-care at home often need information about community resources and services.

HEALTH BELIEFS AND PRACTICES A client's health beliefs and practices are important to consider in any teaching plan. The health belief model described in Chapter 5 ∞ provides a predictor of preventive health behavior. However, even if a nurse is convinced that a particular client's health beliefs should be changed, doing so may not be possible because so many factors are involved in a person's health beliefs.

CULTURAL FACTORS Many cultural groups have their own folk beliefs and practices, with a number of them related to diet, health, illness, and lifestyle. It is therefore important to discuss the client's cultural perspective on illness and therapy. The cultural practices and values held by clients will affect their learning needs. For example, the client may understand the health care information being taught but this

ASSESSMENT INTERVIEW — Learning Needs and Characteristics

Primary Health Problem

- Tell me what you know about your current health problem. What do you think caused it?
- What concerns do you have about it?
- How has the problem affected what you can or cannot do during your usual activities (e.g., work, recreation, shopping, housework)?
- What do you or did you do at home to relieve the problem? How helpful was it?
- How have the treatments you have started helped your problem?
- What, if any, difficulties have the treatments caused you (e.g., inconvenience, cost, discomfort)?
- Tell me about the tests (surgery, treatments) you are going to have.

Health Beliefs

- How would you describe your health generally?
- What things do you usually do to keep healthy?
- What health problems do you think you may be at risk for because of family history, age, diet, occupation, inadequate exercise, or other habits, such as smoking?
- What changes would you be willing to make to decrease your risk for these problems or to improve your health?

Cultural Factors

- What language do you use most often when speaking and writing?

- Do you seek the advice of another health practitioner?
- Do you use herbs or other medications or treatments commonly used in your cultural group?
- Does your current primary care provider know about these?
- What advice or treatments given previously by your primary care provider conflicted with values or beliefs you consider important?
- When a conflict arose, what did you do?

Learning Style

- Note the client's age and developmental level.
- What level of education have you received?
- Do you like to read?
- Where do you obtain health information (e.g., primary care provider, nurse, magazines, books, pharmacist, and so on)?
- How do you best learn new things?
  a. By reading about them
  b. By talking about them
  c. By watching a movie or demonstration
  d. By computer
  e. By listening to the teacher
  f. By first being shown how something works and then doing it
  g. On your own or in a group

Client Support System

- Would you like a family member or friend to help you learn about things you need to do to take care of yourself?
- Who do you think would be interested in learning with you?

---

learning may not be used if the client primarily believes in folk medical practices (see Chapter 4 ∞).

ECONOMIC FACTORS Economic factors can also affect a client's learning. For example, a client who cannot afford to obtain a new sterile syringe for each injection of insulin may find it difficult to learn to administer the insulin when the nurse teaches that a new syringe should be used each time.

LEARNING STYLE Considerable research has been done on people's learning styles. The best way to learn varies with the individual. Some people are visual learners and learn best by watching. Other people do not visualize an activity well; they learn best by actually manipulating equipment and discovering how it works. Other people can learn well from reading things presented in an orderly fashion. Still other people learn best in groups where they can relate to other people. For some, stressing the thinking part of a skill and its logic will promote learning. For other people, stressing the feeling part or interpersonal aspect motivates and promotes learning.

A client's learning style may be based in his or her cultural background. For example, clients from cultures that have a strong oral tradition may prefer educational videos presented in their language (Munoz & Luckmann, 2005).

The nurse seldom has the time or skills to assess each learner, identify the person's particular learning style, and then adapt teaching accordingly. What the nurse can do, however, is ask clients how they have learned things best in the past or how they like to learn. Many people know what helps them learn, and the nurse can use this information in planning the teaching. Using a variety of teaching techniques and varying activities during teaching are good ways to match learners with learning styles. One technique will be most effective for some clients, whereas other techniques will be suited to clients with different learning styles.

CLIENT SUPPORT SYSTEM The nurse explores the client's support system to determine the extent to which others may enhance learning and offer support. Family members or a close friend may help the client perform required skills at home and maintain required lifestyle changes.

Physical Examination

The general survey part of the physical examination provides useful clues to the client's learning needs, such as mental status, energy level, and nutritional status. Other parts of the physical examination reveal data about the

LIFESPAN CONSIDERATIONS   Special Teaching Considerations

Older Adults

Older adults often have chronic illnesses that require multiple treatments and/or medications. Health teaching will focus on the same areas as with other ages—health and wellness promotion and prevention of illness and accidents—but often the needs are greatest in learning to manage their lives in order to live with their chronic health conditions and to maintain optimal health and functioning. For older adults to be motivated to learn, the material must be practical and have meaning for them individually, especially if the information is new to them. Special considerations in teaching older adults include the following:

- Health promotion is a priority need and should include these areas:
  - Exercise
  - Nutrition
  - Safety habits
  - Having regular health checkups
  - Understanding medications
- Set achievable goals—involve the client and family in doing this.
- If developing written materials:
  - Use large print (e.g., at least 14-point font) in bulleted format.
  - Use buff-colored paper (avoids the glare of white paper).
  - Present the information at a fifth- to sixth-grade reading level.
- Increase time for teaching and allow for rest periods as processing of information is slower.
  - Verbal presentation of material should be well organized. Ensure that there is minimal distraction.
- Repeat information if necessary.
- Use return demonstrations with psychomotor skills, such as teaching someone to learn to do insulin injections.
- Determine where clients obtain most of their health information (e.g., newspapers, magazines, television).
- Use examples that they can relate to in their daily lives.
- Be aware of sensory deficits, such as hearing and vision.
- Use the setting with which the individual is most comfortable—either a group or one-on-one setting.
- If noncompliance is a problem, investigate the cause. It could be due to lack of finances, transportation problems, poor access to medical care, and so on.

Older adults come with a lifetime of experiences and learned knowledge of their own. Respect this and always have them use their strengths to work with any problems. Positive reinforcement and ongoing evaluation of what has been taught are important factors in effective health teaching with older adults.

Children

It has often been said that the parent is a child's first and most important teacher. Every interaction between a child and parent (or other adults and children) is a moment in which teaching and learning occurs, often unconsciously. Sometimes the results are ones parents desire and strive for; sometimes they are not what the parent would have wished.

In order to make parents more aware of the teaching they are doing, nurses can point out how the parent is using the concept of a "teaching loop" and how that "formal" teaching strategy can be applied more consciously to many parent–child interactions.

The teaching loop consists of four specific teaching behaviors that give children verbal instruction, role modeling, and positive feedback. These include:

- *Alerting:* Get children's attention by calling their name, touching them, or making a noise.
- *Instructing:* Give the child a short, specific instruction about what is to be done; modeling or demonstrating behavior can also be done (e.g., "Try it like this . . .").
- *Performing:* Give the child opportunity to practice the task, play with the toy, and explore the materials being used. Provide "enough" time, but with some structure or direction.
- *Reinforcing:* Give the child feedback; a positive or negative comment (e.g., "You poured the milk very well" or "No, that's not quite right; try turning it this way") that is specific to the task lets children know how they have done and encourages them to continue to learn.

Note: Adapted from *Gerontological Nursing: Promoting Successful Aging with Older Adults,* 3rd ed. (pp. 67–75) by M. Stanley, K. Blair, and P. G. Beare, 2005, Philadelphia: F. A. Davis; "Designing Written Medication Instructions: Effective Ways to Help Older Adults Self-Medicate" by K. Hayes, 2005, *Journal of Gerontological Nursing, 31*(5), 5–10. Adapted with permission; and "The Observation of Anglo-Mexican and Chinese-American Mothers Teaching Their Young Sons," by D. Steward and M. Steward, 1973, *Child Development, 44*, 329–337.

client's physical capacity to learn and to perform self-care activities. For example, visual ability, hearing ability, and muscle coordination affect the selection of content and approaches to teaching.

Readiness to Learn

Clients who are ready to learn often behave differently from those who are not. A client who is ready may search out information, for instance, by asking questions, reading books or articles, talking to others, and generally showing interest. The person who is not ready to learn is more likely to avoid the subject or situation. In addition, the unready client may change the subject when it is brought up by the nurse. For example, the nurse might say, "I was wondering about a good time to show you how to change your dressing," and the client responds, "Oh, my wife will take care of everything."

The nurse assesses for these readiness characteristics:

- *Physical readiness.* Is the client able to focus on things other than physical status, or are pain, fatigue, and immobility using up all of the client's time and energy?
- *Emotional readiness.* Is the client emotionally ready to learn self-care activities? Clients who are extremely

anxious, depressed, or grieving over their health status are not ready.

- *Cognitive readiness.* Can the client think clearly at this point? Are the effects of anesthesia and analgesia altering the client's level of consciousness?

Nurses can promote readiness to learn by providing physical and emotional support during the critical stage of recovery. As the client stabilizes physically and emotionally, the nurse can provide opportunities to learn.

Motivation

Motivation relates to whether the client wants to learn and is usually greatest when the client is ready, the learning need is recognized, and the information being offered is meaningful to the client. Assessment of motivation, however, may be difficult. Communication skills used by the nurse can obtain helpful information indicating a readiness for change such as "I'm really ready to lose weight this time." On the other hand, nonverbal behaviors such as disinterest, lack of attention, and missed appointments can indicate a decreased motivation to learn.

Nurses can increase a client's motivation in several ways:

- By relating the learning to something the client values and helping the client see the relevance of the learning
- By helping the client make the learning situation pleasant and nonthreatening
- By encouraging self-direction and independence
- By demonstrating a positive attitude about the client's ability to learn
- By offering continuing support and encouragement as the client attempts to learn (i.e., positive reinforcement)
- By creating a learning situation in which the client is likely to succeed (Succeeding in small tasks motivates the client to continue learning.)
- By assisting the client to identify the benefits of changing behavior

Health Literacy

A 1993 National Adult Literacy Study reported that the average reading ability of many American adults is at the fifth-grade level (Edmunds, 2005). A report from the Institute of Medicine (IOM, 2004) titled *Health Literacy: A Prescription to End Confusion* states that nearly half of all Americans—90 million people—have difficulty understanding and acting upon health information (p. 1). Moreover, studies that assessed a variety of health-related materials found that the reading level exceeded the twelfth-grade level.

Health literacy is the ability to read, understand, and act on health information, including such tasks as comprehending prescription labels, interpreting appointment slips, completing health insurance forms, and following instructions for diagnostic tests (Redman, 2004, pp. 30–31). Limited health literacy skills are often greater among certain groups: older adults, people with limited education, poor people, minority populations, and people with limited English proficiency.

Low health literacy skills are associated with poor health outcomes and higher health care costs (IOM, 2004). For example, a client may not be able to read a prescription to know how many pills to take or may take the wrong number of pills (e.g., "once" means eleven in Spanish). Clients with low literacy skills have less information about health promotion and/or management of a disease process for themselves and their families because they are unable to read the educational materials. As a result, they have higher rates of hospitalization than people with adequate health literacy.

It is a challenge for the nurse to teach clients with low or no reading and writing skills. However, such teaching is vitally important because clients with low literacy skills need learning opportunities to improve their health practices.

CLINICAL ALERT

The majority of people at the lowest reading levels will report that they "read well."

It is difficult, however, to assess a client's literacy skills because the shame and stigma associated with limited health literacy skills are major barriers. Clients may be too embarrassed to admit they cannot read. The following client behaviors may cause a nurse to suspect a literacy problem:

- Pattern of noncompliance
- Insisting that they already know the information
- Having a friend or family member read the document for them
- Pattern of excuses for not reading the instructions (e.g., glasses broken, stating they will read it later or when they get home)

There are many formulas for assessing reading level of written material. Most word processing programs have a feature that will calculate the readability for you. Nurses involved in developing written health teaching materials should write for lower reading levels (see Client Teaching). The goal is to have the education materials at a fifth- or sixth-grade level (Aldridge, 2004). People with good reading skills are not offended by simple reading material and prefer easy-to-read information. Even the simplest written directions, however, won't be helpful for the client with low or no reading skills. See the Client Teaching box for suggestions on how to teach clients with low literacy levels.

DIAGNOSING

Nursing diagnoses for clients with learning needs can be designated in two ways: as the client's primary concern or problem, or as the etiology of a nursing diagnosis associated with the client's response to health alterations or dysfunction (see Identifying Nursing Diagnoses, Outcomes, and Interventions).

- Keep language level at or below the fifth-grade level.
- Use active, not passive, voice.
- Use easy, common words of one or two syllables (e.g., *use* instead of *utilize,* or *give* instead of *administer*).
- Use the second person (*you*) rather than the third person (*the client*).
- Use a large type size (14 to 16 point).
- Write short sentences.
- Avoid using all capital letters.
- Place priority information first and repeat more than once.
- Use bold for emphasis.
- Use simple pictures, drawings, or cartoons, if appropriate.
- Leave plenty of white space.
- Obtain feedback from nurses and clients.

Learning Need as the Diagnostic Label

The North American Nursing Diagnosis Association (NANDA) includes the following diagnostic labels appropriate to a client's learning needs when the learning need is the primary concern:

- *Deficient Knowledge:* absence or deficiency of cognitive information related to a specific topic (NANDA, 2009, p. 171)

Whenever the diagnostic label *Deficient Knowledge* is used, either the client is seeking health information or the nurse has identified a learning need. The area of deficiency should always be included in the diagnosis. Following are

- Use multiple teaching methods: Show pictures. Read important information. Lead a small group discussion. Role-play. Demonstrate a skill. Provide hands-on practice.
- Emphasize key points in simple terms and provide examples.
- Limit the amount of information in a single teaching session. Instead of one long session with a great deal of information, it is better to have more frequent sessions with a major point at each session.
- Associate new information with something the client already knows and/or associates with his or her job or lifestyle.
- Reinforce information through repetition.
- Involve the client in the teaching.
- Obtain feedback: Ask the client specific questions about the information presented or ask the client to repeat it in his or her own words.
- Avoid handouts with many pages and classroom lecture format with a large group.

examples using the NANDA label *Deficient Knowledge* as the primary concern:

- *Deficient Knowledge (Low-Calorie Diet)* related to inexperience with newly ordered therapy
- *Deficient Knowledge (Home Safety Hazards)* related to denial of declining health and living alone

Wilkinson (2009) stresses that if *Deficient Knowledge* is used as the primary concern, one client goal must be "client will acquire knowledge about." The nurse needs to provide information that has the potential to change the client's behavior rather than focus on the behaviors caused by the client's lack of knowledge.

A second nursing diagnostic label where a learning need may be the primary concern is

- *Health-Seeking Behavior:* active seeking (by a person in stable health) of ways to alter personal health habits and/or the environment in order to move toward a higher level of health (Wilkinson, 2009, p. 310).

When this diagnostic label is used, the client is seeking health information; the client may or may not have an altered response or dysfunction at the time but may be seeking information to improve health or prevent illness. This diagnosis is especially appropriate for clients attending community health education programs. The following are examples using the NANDA label *Health-Seeking Behavior* as the primary concern:

- *Health-Seeking Behavior (Exercise and Activity)* related to desire to improve health behaviors and decrease risk of heart disease. This diagnosis may be appropriate for the client who has identified a personal health risk for a cardiac condition and wants to minimize that risk through exercise.
- *Health-Seeking Behavior (Home Safety Hazards)* related to desire to minimize risk of injury. This diagnosis may be appropriate for parents of a toddler who are seeking information to ensure that their home is safe for their child. The diagnosis might also be used when an adult child seeks information to ensure that the home of an older adult parent is free of risk factors for falls or other injuries common to older adults.

A third nursing diagnostic label where a learning need may be the primary concern is

- *Noncompliance:* behavior of person and/or caregiver that fails to coincide with a health-promoting or therapeutic plan agreed on by the person (and/or family and/or community) and health-care professional. In the presence of an agreed-on, health-promoting or therapeutic plan, person's or caregiver's behavior is fully or partially nonadherent and may lead to clinically ineffective or partially ineffective outcomes (NANDA, 2009, p. 297).

The diagnostic label *Noncompliance* should be used with caution. In general, the diagnosis *Noncompliance* is associated with the *intent* to comply, but situational factors make it difficult (Wilkinson, 2009, p. 424). Factors that influence a client's compliance with health teaching include understanding or comprehension of the teaching, the experienced negative side effects of the treatment, financial inability to carry out the treatment plan, language barriers, or poor teaching on the part of the health care team. *Noncompliance* should *not* be used for a client who is unable to follow instructions (e.g., cognitive disability) or for a client who makes an informed decision to refuse or not follow the medical treatment (Wilkinson, 2009, p. 424).

CLINICAL ALERT

The term *noncompliance* is often perceived as a negative label. Be sure to state the etiology in neutral, nonjudgmental words.

Deficient Knowledge as the Etiology

Another way to deal with identified learning needs of clients is to write deficient knowledge as the etiology, or second part, of the diagnosis statement. Such nursing diagnoses are written in the following format:

- *Risk for (Specify)* related to deficient knowledge (specify).

Examples include the following:

- *Risk for Impaired Parenting* related to deficient knowledge (skills in infant care and feeding)
- *Risk for Infection* related to deficient knowledge (sexually transmitted infections and their prevention)
- *Anxiety* related to deficient knowledge (bone marrow aspiration)

Other nursing diagnoses in which a knowledge deficit can be associated include the following etiologies:

- *Risk for Injury*
- *Ineffective Breastfeeding*
- *Impaired Adjustment*
- *Ineffective Coping*
- *Ineffective Health Maintenance.*

Note also that most NANDA-approved nursing diagnoses imply a teaching–learning need. For example, the nursing diagnosis *Constipation* suggests the need for a review of bowel hygiene practices including diet, hydration, and exercise/activity.

PLANNING

Developing a teaching plan is accomplished in a series of steps. Involving the client at this time promotes the formation of a meaningful plan and stimulates client motivation. The client who helps develop the teaching plan is more likely to achieve the desired outcomes.

CLINICAL ALERT

Knowing the client's stage of change helps determine which interventions will be useful to help the client change.

Determining Teaching Priorities

The client's learning needs must be ranked according to priority. The client and the nurse should do this together, with the client's priorities always being considered. Once a client's priorities have been addressed, the client is generally more motivated to concentrate on other identified learning needs. For example, a man who wants to know all about coronary artery disease may not be ready to learn how to change his lifestyle until he meets his own need to learn more about the disease. Nurses can also use theoretical frameworks, such as Maslow's hierarchy of needs, to establish priorities (see Chapter 3 ∞).

Setting Learning Outcomes

Learning outcomes can be considered the same as desired outcomes for other nursing diagnoses. They are written in the same way. Like client outcomes, learning outcomes:

- State the client (learner) behavior or performance, not nurse behavior. For example, "Identify personal risk factors for heart disease" (client behavior), *not* "Teach the client about cardiac risk factors" (nurse behavior).
- Reflect an observable, measurable activity. The performance may be visible (e.g., walking) or invisible (e.g., adding a column of figures). It is necessary, however, to be able to evaluate whether an unobservable activity has been mastered from some performance that represents the activity. For example, the performance of an outcome might be written: "Selects low-fat foods from a menu" (observable), *not* "understands low-fat diet" (unobservable). Examples of measurable verbs used for learning outcomes are shown in Box 14–1. Avoid using words such as *knows, understands, believes,* and *appreciates* because they are neither observable nor measurable.
- May add conditions or modifiers as required to clarify what, where, when, or how the behavior will be performed. Examples are "Demonstrates four-point crutch gait *correctly*" (condition), "Administers own insulin *independently* (condition) as taught," or "States *three* (condition) factors that affect blood sugar level."
- Include criteria specifying the time by which learning should have occurred. For example, "The client will state three things that affect blood sugar level *by end of second diabetic class.*"

Learning outcomes can reflect the learner's command of simple to complex concepts. For example, the learning outcome "The client will list cardiac risk factors" is a low-level knowledge outcome that simply requires the learner to identify all cardiac risk factors; it does not suggest applica-

BOX 14–1 Examples of Verbs for Writing Learning Outcomes

Cognitive Domain	Affective Domain	Psychomotor Domain
Compares	Accepts	Assembles
Describes	Attends	Calculates
Evaluates	Chooses	Changes
Explains	Discusses	Demonstrates
Identifies	Displays	Measures
Labels	Initiates	Moves
Lists	Joins	Organizes
Names	Participates	Shows
Plans	Shares	
Selects	Uses	
States		
Writes		

tion of the knowledge to the learner's own behaviors. The learning outcome "The client will list personal cardiac risk factors" requires that the learner not only know cardiac risk factors in general but also know his own behaviors that place him at risk for cardiac disease.

In writing learning outcomes, the nurse must be specific about what behaviors and knowledge (cognitive, psychomotor, and affective) learners must have to be able to positively influence their health state. In most cases, the learning needs are more complex than simple acquisition of knowledge and include the application of that knowledge to oneself (see Identifying Nursing Diagnoses, Outcomes, and Interventions).

Choosing Content

The content, or what is to be taught, is determined by learning outcomes. For instance, "Identify appropriate sites for insulin injection" means the nurse must include content about the body sites suitable for insulin injections. Nurses can select among many sources of information including books, nursing journals, Internet, and other nurses and primary care providers. Whatever sources the nurse chooses, content should be:

- Accurate.
- Current.
- Based on learning outcomes.
- Adjusted for the learner's age, culture, and ability.
- Consistent with information the nurse is teaching.
- Selected with consideration of how much time and what resources are available for teaching.

IDENTIFYING NURSING DIAGNOSES, OUTCOMES, AND INTERVENTIONS — Clients Requiring Teaching

DATA CLUSTER The nurse brings Mr. Steinberg the first dose of a medication ordered by his physician. The nurse asks whether anyone has explained what this medication is and why he is taking it. He says no.

NURSING DIAGNOSIS/DEFINITION	SAMPLE DESIRED OUTCOME*/DEFINITION	INDICATORS	SELECTED INTERVENTIONS*/DEFINITION	SAMPLE NIC ACTIVITIES
Deficient Knowledge (Medication Information) related to lack of exposure to newly prescribed medication/*Absence or deficiency of cognitive information related to specific topic*	Knowledge: Medication [1808]/*Extent of understanding conveyed about the safe use of medication*	Substantial: • Identification of correct medication name • Description of action of medication • Description of side effects of medication • Description of medication precautions	Teaching, Prescribed Medication [5616]/*Preparing a client to safely take prescribed medications and monitor for their effects*	• Inform the client of both the generic and brand names of the medication • Instruct the client on the purpose and action of the medication • Instruct the client on the dosage, route, and duration of the medication • Instruct the client on specific precautions to observe when taking the medication (e.g., no driving) as appropriate

(continued)

DATA CLUSTER George Evans is a 45-year-old man who has come to the clinic for his annual physical examination. He expresses concern about his family history of heart disease and requests information about activities to decrease his risk of heart disease.

Health-Seeking Behavior (Nutrition, Activity and Exercise Information) to reduce risk of heart disease/Active seeking (by a person in stable health) of ways to alter personal health habits and/or the environment in order to move toward a higher level of health	Adherence Behavior [1600]/*Self-initiated action taken to promote wellness, recovery, and rehabilitation*	Often demonstrated: • Asks health-related questions when indicated • Seeks health-related information from a variety of sources • Uses strategies to eliminate unhealthy behavior	Self-Modification Assistance [4470]/*Reinforcement of self-directed change initiated by the client to achieve personally important goals*	• Assist the client in identifying a specific goal for change • Assist the client in identifying target behaviors that need to change to achieve the desired goal • Appraise the client's present knowledge and skill level in relationship to the desired change • Explore with the client potential barriers to change behavior

DATA CLUSTER Mildred Cumming is a 74-year-old widow with a history of hypertension. Her blood pressure is 150/96. She is on daily antihypertensive therapy. When asked if she is taking her medication as prescribed, she tells the nurse that she is taking her medication every other day because it is expensive and she cannot afford to take it every day.

Noncompliance (With Medication Plan) related to insufficient finances/Behavior of person and/or caregiver that fails to coincide with a health-promoting or therapeutic plan agreed on by the person (and/or family and/or community) and health-care professional. In the presence of an agreed-on, health-promoting or therapeutic plan, person's or caregiver's behavior is fully or partially nonadherent and may lead to clinically ineffective or partially ineffective outcomes	Compliance Behavior [1601]/*Personal actions to promote wellness, recovery, and rehabilitation based on professional advice*	Consistently demonstrated: • Discusses prescribed treatment regimen with health care professional • Modifies treatment regimen as directed by a health care professional	Financial Resource Assistance [7380]/*Assisting an individual/family to secure and manage finances to meet health care needs*	• Determine if client is eligible for waiver programs • Inform client of available resources and assist in accessing resources (e.g., medication assistance program)

*The NOC # for desired outcomes and the NIC # for nursing interventions are listed in brackets following the appropriate outcome or intervention. Outcomes, indicators, interventions, and activities selected are only a sample of those suggested by NOC and NIC and should be further individualized for each client.

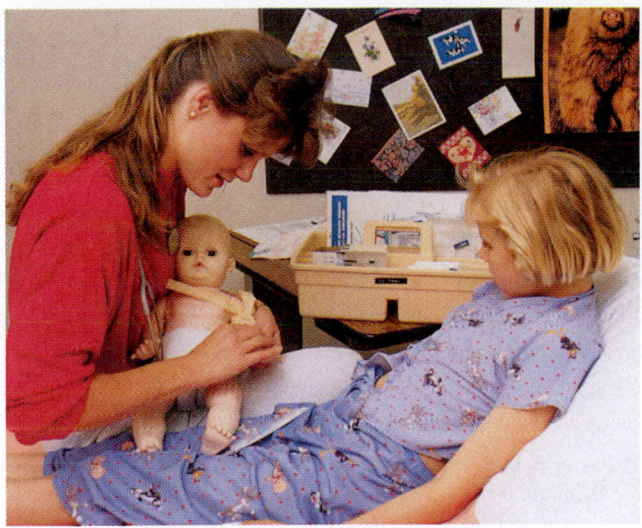

Figure 14–2 ● Teaching materials and strategies should be suited to the client's age and learning abilities.

Selecting Teaching Strategies

The method of teaching that the nurse chooses should be suited to the individual and to the material to be learned (Figure 14–2). For example, the person who cannot read needs material presented in other ways; a discussion is usually not the best strategy for teaching how to give an injection; and a nurse using group discussion for teaching should be a competent group leader. As stated earlier, some people are visually oriented and learn best through seeing; others learn best through hearing and having the skill explained. Table 14–3 lists selected teaching strategies.

Organizing Learning Experiences

To save nurses time in constructing their own teaching guides, some health agencies have developed teaching guides for teaching sessions that nurses commonly give. These guides standardize content and teaching methods and make it easier for the nurse to plan and implement client teaching. Standardized teaching plans also ensure consistency of content for the learner, thereby decreasing the risk of confusion if different practices are taught. For example, when teaching infant bathing, the nurse on the unit should be consistent about which soaps are appropriate for the infant's bath and distinguish those that are not. Whether the nurse is implementing a plan devised by another or developing an individualized teaching plan, some guidelines can help the nurse sequence the learning experience:

- Start with something the learner is concerned about; for example, before learning how to administer insulin to himself, an adolescent wants to know how to adjust his lifestyle and yet still play football.

> **CLINICAL ALERT**
>
> Leave a note pad and pen at the client's bedside and encourage him to write down his questions for the nurse or the primary care provider.

- Discover what the learner knows, and then proceed to the unknown. This gives the learner confidence. Sometimes you will not know the client's knowledge or skill base and will need to elicit this information either by asking questions or by having the client fill out a form, such as a pretest.
- Address early on any area that is causing the client anxiety. A high level of anxiety can impair concentration in other areas. For example, a woman highly anxious about her fear of the needle breaking off into the skin may not be able to learn how to self-administer an insulin injection until her fear is resolved.
- Teach the basics before proceeding to the variations or adjustments (e.g., simple to complex). It is confusing to learners to have to consider possible adjustments and variations before they master the basic concepts. For example, when teaching a female client how to insert a retention catheter, it is best to teach the basic procedure before teaching any adjustments that might be needed if the catheter stops draining after insertion.
- Schedule time for review of content and questions the client(s) may have to clarify information.

> **CLINICAL ALERT**
>
> If the client has no questions, you can help introduce questions by saying, "A few frequently asked questions are . . ."

IMPLEMENTING

The nurse needs to be flexible in implementing any teaching plan because the plan may need revising. The client may tire sooner than anticipated or be faced with too much information too quickly, the client's needs may change, or external factors may intervene. For instance, the nurse and the client plan to change his dressing at 10 AM, but when the time comes, the client wants to observe the nurse once more before actually doing it himself.

In this case, the nurse alters the teaching plan and discusses any desired information, provides another demonstration, and defers teaching the psychomotor skill until the next day. It is also important for nurses to use teaching techniques that enhance learning and reduce or eliminate any barrier to learning such as pain or fatigue (see Table 14–2 earlier in this chapter).

> **CLINICAL ALERT**
>
> Many nurses find that they teach while performing nursing care (e.g., giving medication). Remember to document this informal teaching also.

TABLE 14–3	Selected Teaching Strategies	

STRATEGY	MAJOR TYPE OF LEARNING	CHARACTERISTICS
Explanation or description (e.g., lecture)	Cognitive	Teacher controls content and pace.
		Learner is passive; therefore retains less information than when actively participating.
		Feedback is determined by teacher.
		May be given to individual or group.
One-to-one discussion	Affective, cognitive	Encourages participation by learner.
		Permits reinforcement and repetition at learner's level.
		Permits introduction of sensitive subjects.
Answering questions	Cognitive	Teacher controls most of content and pace.
		Learner may need to overcome cultural perception that asking questions is impolite and may embarrass the teacher.
		Can be used with individuals and groups.
		Teacher sometimes needs to confirm whether question has been answered by asking learner, for example, "Does that answer your question?"
Demonstration	Psychomotor	Often used with explanation.
		Can be used with individuals, small or large groups.
		Does not permit use of equipment by learner; learner is passive.
Discovery	Cognitive, affective	Teacher guides problem-solving situation.
		Learner is active participant; therefore, retention of information is high.
Group discussions	Affective, cognitive	Learner can obtain assistance from supportive group.
		Group members learn from one another.
		Teacher needs to keep the discussion focused and prevent monopolization by one or two learners.
Practice	Psychomotor	Allows repetition and immediate feedback.
		Permits hands-on experience.
Printed and audiovisual materials	Cognitive	Forms include books, pamphlets, films, programmed instruction, and computer learning.
		Learners can proceed at their own speed.
		Nurse can act as resource person, need not be present during learning.
		Potentially ineffective if reading level is too high.
		Teacher needs to select language of materials that meets learner needs if English is a second language (e.g., Spanish).
Role-playing	Affective, cognitive	Permits expression of attitudes, values, and emotions.
		Can assist in development of communication skills.
		Involves active participation by learner.
		Teacher must create supportive, safe environment for learners to minimize anxiety.
Modeling	Affective, psychomotor	Nurse sets example by attitude, psychomotor skill.
Computer-assisted learning programs	All types of learning	Learner is active.
		Learner controls pace.
		Provides immediate reinforcement and review.
		Use with individuals or groups.

Guidelines for Teaching

Knowledge alone is not enough to motivate a person to change a behavior. Do not assume that providing information will automatically result in clients changing their behavior. Learning what needs to be done to change behavior and acting on that knowledge are two different processes (Saarmann, Daugherty, & Riegel, 2000, p. 281). The stages of change, the person's willingness and perceived need to change, and barriers to change are important elements to reflect on when implementing a teaching plan (see Chapter 5 ∞). When a client is ready to change a health behavior and when implementing a teaching plan, the nurse may find the following guidelines helpful:

- Rapport between teacher and learner is essential. A relationship that is both accepting and constructive will best assist learning. Knowing the learner and the previously described factors that affect learning should be established before planning the teaching.

- The teacher who uses the client's previous learning in the present situation encourages the client and facilitates learning new skills. For instance, a person who already knows how to cook can use this knowledge when learning to prepare food for a special diet.

- The optimal time for each session depends largely on the learner. Whenever possible, ask the client for help to choose the best time, for example, when she feels most rested or when no other activities are scheduled. Look for "teachable moments" that may occur during normal routine care (Hohler, 2004). For example, if a client asks you why he needs a certain medication (e.g., Coumadin), this is an opportunity to explain the reason for the medication, signs to watch for, and if follow-up laboratory work is needed.

- The nurse teacher must be able to communicate clearly and concisely. The words used need to have the same meaning to the client as to the teacher. A client who is taught not to put water on an area of skin may think a wet washcloth is permissible for washing the area. In effect, the nurse needs to explain that no water or moisture should touch the area.

- Using a layperson's vocabulary enhances communication. Often nurses use terms and abbreviations that have meaning to other health professionals but make little sense to clients. Even words such as *urine* or *feces* may be unfamiliar to clients, and abbreviations such as ICU (intensive care unit) or PACU (post-anesthesia care unit) are often misunderstood.

- The pace of each teaching session also affects learning. Nurses should be sensitive to any signs that the pace is too fast or too slow. A client who appears confused or does not comprehend material when questioned may be finding the pace too fast. When the client appears bored and loses interest, the pace may be too slow, the learning period may be too long, or the client may be tired.

- An environment can detract from or assist learning; for example, noise or interruptions usually interfere with concentration, whereas a comfortable environment promotes learning. If possible, the client should be out of bed for learning activities. Most people associate their bed with rest and sleep, not with learning. Placing the client in a position and location associated with activity or learning may influence the amount of learning that takes place. For instance, a client who is shown a videotape while in bed may be more likely to become drowsy during instruction than a client who is sitting in a bedside chair.

- Teaching aids can foster learning and help focus a learner's attention. To ensure the transfer of learning, the nurse should use the type of supplies or equipment the client will eventually use. Before the teaching session, the nurse needs to assemble all equipment and visual aids and ensure that all audiovisual equipment is functioning effectively. See the Client Teaching box for teaching tools for children.

- Teaching that involves a number of the learner's senses often enhances learning. For instance, when teaching about changing a surgical dressing, the nurse can tell the client about the procedure (hearing), show how to change the dressing (sight), and show how to manipulate the equipment (touch).

- Learning is more effective when the learners discover the content for themselves. Ways to increase

---

CLIENT TEACHING — **Teaching Tools for Children**

- *Visits.* Visiting the hospital and treatment rooms; seeing people dressed in uniforms, scrub suits, protective gear.
- *Dress-up.* Touching and dressing up in the clothing they will see and wear.
- *Coloring books.* Using coloring books to prepare for treatments, surgery, or hospitalization; shows what rooms, people, and equipment will look like.
- *Storybooks.* Storybooks describe how the child will feel, what will be done, and what the place will look like. Parents can read these stories to children several times before the experience. Younger children like this repetition.
- *Dolls.* Practicing procedures on dolls or teddy bears that they will later experience; gives a sense of mastery of the situation. Custom dolls are often available for inserting tubes and giving injections, for example.
- *Puppet play.* Puppets can be used in role-play situations to provide information and show the child what the experience will be like; they help the child express emotions.
- *Health fairs.* Health fairs can educate children about their bodies and ways to stay healthy. Fairs can focus on high-risk problems children face, such as accident prevention, poison control, and other topics identified in the community as a concern.

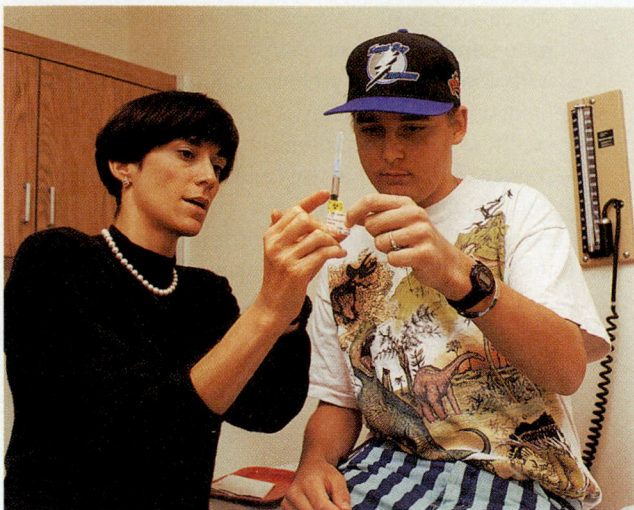

Figure 14–3 ○ Teaching activities may need to include hands-on client participation.

learning include stimulating motivation and self-direction, for example, (a) by providing specific, realistic, achievable outcomes; (b) by giving feedback; and (c) by helping the learner derive satisfaction from learning. The nurse may also encourage self-directed independent learning by encouraging the client to explore sources of information required. If certain activities do not assist the learner to attain outcomes, these need to be reassessed; perhaps other activities can replace them. Explanation alone may not be able to teach a client to handle a syringe. Actually handling the syringe may be more effective (Figure 14–3).

- Repetition reinforces learning. Summarizing content, rephrasing (using other words), and approaching the material from another point of view are ways of repeating and clarifying content. For instance, after discussing the kinds of foods that can be included in a diet, the nurse describes the foods again, but in the context of the three meals eaten during one day.

- It is helpful to employ "organizers" to introduce material to be learned. Advanced organizers provide a means of connecting unknown material to known material and generating logical relationships. The following statement can be an advanced organizer: "You understand how urine flows down a catheter from the bladder. Now I will show you how to inject fluid so that it flows up the catheter into the bladder." The details that follow are then seen within a framework that adds meaning.

- The anticipated behavioral changes that indicate learning has taken place must always be within the context of the client's lifestyle and resources. It would be unreasonable to expect a woman to soak in a tub of hot water two times a day if she did not have a bathtub or had to heat water on a stove.

Special Teaching Strategies

One-on-one discussion is the most common method of teaching used by nurses. However, nurses can choose from a number of special teaching strategies: client contracting, group teaching, computer-assisted instruction, discovery/problem solving, and behavior modification. Any strategy the nurse selects must be appropriate for the learner and the learning objectives.

CLIENT CONTRACTING Client contracting involves establishing a learning contract with a client that specifies certain outcomes and when they are to be met. Here is an example of a self-contract:

> I, Amy Martin, will exercise strenuously for
> 20 minutes three times per week for a period of
> 2 weeks and will then buy myself six yellow roses.
>
> Amy Martin   A. Ward, RN
>   January 12, 2010

The contract, drawn up and signed by the client and the nurse, may specify the learning outcomes, the responsibilities of the client and the nurse, and the methods of follow-up and evaluation. The contract can be changed in two ways: if the client meets the contract outcomes and wants to negotiate new learning outcomes, and if the client decides that he or she is unable to meet the existing learning outcomes and wants to revise them (Rankin, Stallings, & London, 2005, pp. 207–209). The learning contract allows for freedom, mutual respect, and mutual responsibility.

GROUP TEACHING Group instruction is economical, and it provides members with an opportunity to share with and learn from others. A small group allows for discussion in which everyone can participate. A large group often necessitates a lecture technique or use of films, videos, slides, or role playing by teachers.

It is important that all members involved in group instruction have a common need (e.g., prenatal health or preoperative instruction). It is also important that sociocultural factors be considered in the formation of a group.

COMPUTER-ASSISTED INSTRUCTION (CAI) Computer-assisted instruction is popular. Initially, the primary use of computer educational methods was cognitive learning of facts. Now, however, computers can also be used to teach the following:

- Application of information (e.g., answering questions after reading the information about a health subject)
- Psychomotor skills (e.g., filling a syringe on the computer screen to the correct dosage line on the syringe)
- Complex problem-solving skills (e.g., responding to questions based on a client situation)

Computers can be used in a variety of ways:

- Individual health care professionals or clients using one computer

- Families or small groups of three to five clients gathered around one computer taking turns running the program and answering questions together
- Large groups with the computer display screen projected onto an overhead screen and a teacher or one learner using the keyboard
- Individuals or small groups at computers using programs through shared network platforms or through Internet websites

Individuals using a computer are able to set the pace that meets their particular learning needs. Small groups are less able to do this, and large groups progress through the program at a pace that may be too slow for some learners and too fast for others. It is therefore helpful to group learners of similar needs and abilities together. Whether using the computer alone or in large groups, learners read and view informational material, answer questions, and receive immediate feedback. The correct answer is usually indicated by the use of colors, flashing signs, or written praise. When the learner selects an incorrect answer, the computer may respond with an explanation of why that was not the best answer and encouragement to try again. Many programs ask learners whether they want to review material on which the question and answer were based. Some computer programs feature simulated situations that allow learners to manipulate objects on the screen to learn psychomotor skills. When used to teach such skills, CAI must be followed up with practice on actual equipment supervised by the teacher.

Some clients may have a negative attitude about computers that could act as a barrier to learning. The nurse helps these clients by explaining how the computer can help meet their needs. Matching a computer program or website to the client's individual health circumstances may encourage computer use. Providing a resource list of free available community sites for training and access may also help. For clients who use the Internet, it is important for the nurse to teach the client how to evaluate if the site is a relevant and credible source for health information.

Most media catalogs, professional journals, and health care libraries contain information about computer software programs available to the nurse for client education. The media specialist or librarian in a health care facility or college is an excellent resource to help the nurse locate appropriate computer programs. Computer educational material is also available for clients with different language needs, for clients with special visual needs, and for clients at different growth and development levels.

DISCOVERY/PROBLEM SOLVING In using the discovery/problem-solving technique, the nurse presents some initial information and then asks the learners a question or presents a situation related to the information. The learner applies the new information to the situation and decides what to do. Learners can work alone or in groups. This technique is well suited to family learning. The teacher guides the learners through the thinking process necessary to reach the best solution to the question or the best action

to take in the situation. This may also be referred to as *anticipatory problem solving*. For example, the nurse educator might present information on diabetes and glucose management. Then the nurse might ask the learners how they think their insulin and/or diet should be adjusted if their morning glucose was too low. In this way, clients learn what critical components they need to consider to reach the best solution to the problem.

BEHAVIOR MODIFICATION The behavior modification system for changing behavior has as its basic assumptions (a) that human behaviors are learned and can be selectively strengthened, weakened, eliminated, or replaced; and (b) that a person's behavior is under conscious control. Under this system, desirable behavior is rewarded and undesirable behavior is ignored. The client's response is the key to behavior change. For example, clients trying to quit smoking are not criticized when they smoke, but they are praised or rewarded when they go without a cigarette for a certain period of time. For some people, a learning contract is combined with behavior modification, and includes the following pertinent features:

- Positive reinforcement (e.g., praise) is used.
- The client participates in the development of the learning plan.
- Undesirable behavior is ignored, not criticized.
- The expectation of the client and the nurse is that the task will be mastered (i.e., the behavior will change).

Transcultural Teaching

The nurse and clients of different cultural and ethnic backgrounds have additional barriers to overcome in the teaching–learning process. These barriers include language and communication problems, differing concepts of time, conflicting cultural healing practices, beliefs that may positively or negatively influence compliance with health teaching, and unique high-risk or high-frequency health problems that can be addressed with health promotion instruction (see Chapter 7 ∞). Nurses should consider the following guidelines when teaching clients from various ethnic backgrounds:

- *Obtain teaching materials, pamphlets, and instructions in languages used by clients.* Nurses who are unable to read the foreign language material for themselves can have the translator read the material to them. The nurse can then evaluate the quality of the information and update it with the translator's help as needed.
- *Use visual aids, such as pictures, charts, or diagrams, to communicate meaning.* Audiovisual material may be helpful if the English is spoken clearly and slowly. Even if understanding the verbal message is a problem for the client, seeing a skill or procedure may be helpful. In some instances, a translator can be asked to clarify the video. Alternatively the video may be available in several languages, and the nurse can request the necessary version from the company.

- *Use concrete rather than abstract words.* Use simple language (short sentences, short words), and present only one idea at a time.
- *Allow time for questions.* This helps the client mentally separate one idea or skill from another.
- *Avoid the use of medical terminology or health care language,* such as "taking your vital signs" or "apical pulse." Rather, nurses should say they are going to take a blood pressure or listen to the client's heart.
- *If understanding another's pronunciation is a problem, validate brief information in writing.* For example, during assessments, write down numbers, words, or phrases and have the client read them to verify accuracy.
- *Use humor very cautiously.* Meaning can change in the translation process.
- *Do not use slang words or colloquialisms.* These may be interpreted literally.
- *Do not assume that a client who nods, uses eye contact, or smiles is indicating an understanding of what is being taught.* These responses may simply be the client's way of indicating respect. The client may feel that asking the nurse questions or stating a lack of understanding is inappropriate because it might embarrass the nurse or cause the nurse to "lose face."
- *Invite and encourage questions during teaching.* Let clients know they are urged to ask questions and be involved in making information clearer. When asking questions to evaluate client understanding, avoid asking negative questions. These can be interpreted differently by people for whom English is a second language. "Do you understand how far you can bend your hip after surgery?" is better than the negative question "You don't understand how far you can bend your hip after surgery, do you?" With particularly difficult information or skills teaching, the nurse might say, "Most people have some trouble with this. May I please help you go through this one more time?" In some cultures, expressing a need is not appropriate, and expressing confusion or asking to be shown something again is considered rude.
- *When explaining procedures or functioning related to personal areas of the body, it may be appropriate to have a nurse of the same sex do the teaching.* Because of modesty concerns in many cultures and beliefs about what is considered appropriate and inappropriate male–female interaction, it is wise to have a female nurse teach a female client about personal care, birth control, sexually transmitted infections, and other potentially sensitive areas. If a translator is needed during explanation of procedures or teaching, the translator should also be female.
- *Include the family in planning and teaching. This promotes trust and mutual respect.* Identify the authoritative family member and incorporate that person into the planning and teaching to promote compliance and support of health teaching. In some cultures, the male head of household is the critical family member to include in health teaching; in other cultures, it is the eldest female member. See the Culturally Competent Care box.

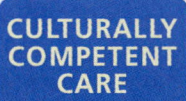
CULTURALLY COMPETENT CARE

Examples of Cultures That Value Family Inclusion in Client Teaching

Hispanic Americans

- Because of the value of family, it is important for the nurse to direct teaching to include all interested family members. Hispanic families provide support to each other and decision-making is usually made by the male and older adult figures in the family.
- Ensure adequate space when teaching to allow for all of the family members who may accompany the client seeking health information and care.

Black Americans

- The family structure has traditionally been matriarchal.
- It is important to recognize the dominant role that black women have in decision making and to share health information with them.
- Grandmothers play a central role in the Black American family and are often involved in support and care of their grandchildren.

Asian/Pacific Islanders

- Decision making is often a family matter. Therefore, it is important to include the family, especially the male authority figure, in the process of decision making for a situation.
- Respect is automatically given to health care professionals as they are viewed as knowledgeable.
- Asians often want to "save face" for themselves and others. As a result, they may agree to what is being said or nod their heads in agreement to avoid being considered offensive or disruptive by disagreeing with the nurse or doctor. They may need to be given permission to ask questions.

Note: From *Nurse as Educator: Principles of Teaching and Learning for Nursing Practice*, 3rd ed., by S. B. Bastable, 2008, Sudbury, MA: Jones and Bartlett.

- *Consider the client's time orientation.* The client may be more oriented to the present than the nurse. Cultures with a predominant orientation to the present include the Mexican American, Navajo Native American, Appalachian, Eskimo, and Filipino American cultures. Preventing future problems may be less significant for these clients than for others, so teaching prevention may be more difficult. For example, teaching a client why and when to take medications may be more difficult if the client is oriented to the present. In such instances, the nurse can emphasize preventing short-term problems rather than long-term problems. Failure to keep clinic appointments or to arrive on time is common in clients who have a present-time orientation. The nurse can help by accommodating these clients when they arrive for their appointment.
- *Schedules may be very flexible in present-oriented societies, with sleeping and eating patterns varying greatly.* Teaching clients to take medications at bedtime or with a meal does not necessarily mean that these activities will occur at the same time each day. For this reason, the nurse should assess the client's daily routine before teaching the client to pair a treatment or medication with an event the nurse assumes occurs at the same time every day. When teaching a client when to take medication, the nurse should determine whether a clock or watch is available to the client and whether the client can tell time.
- *Identify cultural health practices and beliefs.* Noncompliance with health teaching may be related to conflict with folk medicine beliefs. Noncompliance may also be related to lack of understanding or fatalism, a belief system in which life events are held to be predestined or fixed in advance and the individual is powerless to change them. To encourage compliance, the nurse needs to learn the client's explanation of why the illness developed and how it might be treated (Munoz & Luckmann, 2005).

The nurse should treat the client's cultural healing beliefs with respect and try to identify whether any are in agreement or in conflict with what is being taught. The nurse can then focus on the ones in agreement to promote the integration of new learning with the familiar health practices. The goal is to arrive at a mutually agreeable plan: Decide which instructions must be followed for client safety and negotiate less crucial folk healing practices.

EVALUATING

Evaluating is both an ongoing and a final process in which the client, the nurse, and often the support people determine what has been learned.

Evaluating Learning

The process of evaluating learning is the same as evaluating client achievement of desired outcomes for other nursing diagnoses. Learning is measured against the predetermined learning outcomes selected in the planning phase of the teaching process. Thus the outcomes serve not only to direct the teaching plan but also to provide outcome criteria for evaluation. For example, the outcome "Selects foods that are low in carbohydrates" can be evaluated by asking the client to name such foods or to select low-carbohydrate foods from a list.

The best method for evaluating depends on the type of learning. In *cognitive learning,* the client demonstrates acquisition of knowledge. Examples of the evaluation tools for cognitive learning include the following:

- Direct observation of behavior (e.g., observing the client selecting the solution to a problem using the new knowledge)
- Written measurements (e.g., tests)
- Oral questioning (e.g., asking the client to restate information or correct verbal responses to questions)
- Self-reports and self-monitoring. These can be useful during follow-up phone calls and home visits. Evaluating individual self-paced learning, as might occur with computer-assisted instruction, often incorporates self-monitoring.

The acquisition of *psychomotor skills* is best evaluated by observing how well the client carries out a procedure such as self-administration of insulin.

Affective learning is more difficult to evaluate. Whether attitudes or values have been learned may be inferred by listening to the client's responses to questions, noting how the client speaks about relevant subjects, and observing the client's behavior that expresses feelings and values. For example, have parents learned to value health sufficiently to have their children immunized? Do clients who state that they value health actually use condoms every time they have sex with a new partner?

Following evaluation, the nurse may find it necessary to modify or repeat the teaching plan if the objectives have not been met or have been met only partially. Follow-up teaching in the home or by phone may be needed for the client discharged from a health facility.

Behavior change does not always take place immediately after learning. Often individuals accept change intellectually first and then change their behavior only periodically (for example, a client who knows that she must lose weight, diets and exercises off and on). If the new behavior is to replace the old behavior, it must emerge gradually; otherwise, the old behavior may prevail. The nurse can assist clients with behavior change by allowing for client vacillation and by providing encouragement.

Evaluating Teaching

It is important for nurses to evaluate their own teaching and the content of the teaching program, just as they evaluate the effectiveness of nursing interventions for other nursing diagnoses. Evaluation should include a consideration of all factors—the timing, the teaching strategies, the amount of information, whether the teaching was helpful, and so on. The nurse may find, for example, that the client was overwhelmed with too much information, was bored, or was motivated to learn more.

Both the client and the nurse should evaluate the learning experience. The client may tell the nurse what was helpful, interesting, and so on. Feedback questionnaires and videotapes of the learning sessions can also be helpful.

The nurse should not feel ineffective as a teacher if the client forgets some of what is taught. Forgetting is normal and should be anticipated. Having the client write down information, repeating it during teaching, giving handouts on the information, and having the client be active in the learning process all promote retention.

DOCUMENTING

Documentation of the teaching process is essential because it provides a legal record that the teaching took place and communicates the teaching to other health professionals. If teaching is not documented, legally it did not occur.

It is also important to document the responses of the client and support people to teaching activities. What did the client or support person say or do to indicate that learning occurred? Has the client demonstrated mastery of a skill or the acquisition of knowledge? The nurse records this in the client's chart as evidence of learning. A sample documentation of charting follows:

1/8/2010 1130 Learning to use glucometer to check her own capillary blood glucose levels. Noted a slight hesitation with each step. Demonstrated correct technique. Stated that she is "feeling more comfortable" each time she does it but still "needs to stop and think about the process." Will continue to monitor client's progress.
— S. Brown, RN

Many agencies have multiple-copy client teaching forms that include the medical and nursing diagnoses, the treatment plan, and the client education. After the teaching session is completed, the client and the nurse sign the form and a copy of the form is given to the client as a record of teaching and as reinforcement of the content taught. A second copy of the completed and signed form is placed in the client's chart. The parts of the teaching process that should be documented in the client's chart include the following:

- Diagnosed learning needs
- Learning outcomes
- Topics taught
- Client outcomes
- Need for additional teaching
- Resources provided

The written teaching plan that the nurse uses as a resource to guide future teaching sessions might also include these elements:

- Actual information and skills taught
- Teaching strategies used
- Time framework and content for each class
- Teaching outcomes and methods of evaluation

CHAPTER HIGHLIGHTS

- Teaching clients and families about their health needs is a major role of the nurse. Nurses also teach colleagues, subordinates, nursing and other health care students, and groups in community education programs.
- Learning is represented by a change in behavior.
- Three main theories of learning are behaviorism, cognitivism, and humanism.
- Bloom identified three learning domains: cognitive, affective, and psychomotor.
- A number of factors affect learning, including motivation, readiness, active involvement, relevance, feedback, nonjudgmental support, repetition, timing, environment, emotions, physiologic events, psychomotor ability, and cultural aspects.

- Many adults in the United States use the Internet to access health information. The 22% of adults who have never used the Internet tend to have less education and to be over age 65. The current "baby boomers" (ages 50–64), however, use the Internet. As a result, it is projected that Internet use among older adults will increase as the baby boomers age.
- Teaching, like the nursing process, consists of six activities: assessing the learner, diagnosing learning needs, developing a teaching plan, implementing the plan, evaluating learning outcomes and teaching effectiveness, and documenting instructional activities.
- Teaching strategies chosen by the nurse should be suited to the client and to the material to be learned.

- A teaching plan is a written plan consisting of learning outcomes, content to teach, and strategies to use in teaching the content. The plan must be revised when the client's needs change or the teaching strategies prove ineffective.
- Evaluating the teaching–learning process is both an ongoing and a final process in which the client, nurse, and support people determine what has been learned.
- Documentation of client teaching is essential to communicate the teaching to other health professionals and to provide a record for legal and accreditation purposes.

THINK ABOUT IT

Refer to the chapter-opening scenario and answer these questions.

1. What barriers may the nurse face if an attempt is made to teach Ms. Orleans about diabetes mellitus at this time?

2. Before beginning to teach Ms. Orleans about how to care for her newly diagnosed medical condition, what assessments should the nurse make to improve the client's ability to understand?

3. How can the nurse determine if Ms. Orleans understands the information she is taught about her diet and administering insulin by subcutaneous injection?

∞ *See suggested responses to Think About It on MyNursingKit.*

TEST YOUR KNOWLEDGE

1. Which of the following activities would be classified as the affective domain of Bloom's taxonomy?
1. Teaching how to administer an injection
2. Learning to accept the loss of a limb
3. Learning to insert a catheter
4. Teaching how to read

2. Which of the following is the best method of helping a newly diagnosed diabetic client to learn the dietary requirements associated with the disease?
1. Provide a videotape that addresses the dietary requirements associated with the disease.
2. Ask a nutritionist to visit the client to present information and handouts about the diabetic diet.
3. Ask the client to make a list of her favorite foods and explain how they could work them into the diet.
4. Have the client attend a group meeting for diabetic clients to discuss their adaptation to this chronic health condition.

3. A nurse is scheduling a teaching situation. Which of the following clients is most ready to learn?
1. A 45-year-old man whose doctor just informed him that he has cancer
2. A 3-year-old child whose parents are reading a storybook about going to the hospital
3. A 60-year-old female who received medication 5 minutes ago for relief of abdominal pain
4. A 70-year-old man, recovering from a stroke, who has returned from physical therapy

4. How can the nurse best assess a client's style of learning?
1. Ask the client how he or she learns best.
2. Use a variety of teaching strategies.
3. Observe the client's interactions with others.
4. Ask family members.

5. A 74-year-old client who takes multiple medications tells the nurse, "I have no idea what that little yellow pill is for." What is the best nursing diagnosis for this client?
1. *Knowledge Deficit*
2. *Health-Seeking Behavior*
3. *Deficient Knowledge (Medication Information)*
4. *Noncompliance*

6. A client is scheduled to have a diagnostic procedure. Which questions by the nurse will most likely produce a "teachable moment"? Select all that apply.
1. "Have you ever had this procedure before?"
2. "What are your concerns about this procedure?"
3. "What would you like to know about the procedure?"
4. "Are you prepared for this procedure?"
5. "Don't worry, this procedure doesn't hurt at all."

7. A client needs to learn to self-administer insulin injections. Which statements reflect possible low literacy skills? Select all that apply.
1. "I will read the information later—I'm too tired right now."
2. "I've watched my brother give his own shots. I know how to do it."
3. "Just show my wife."
4. "Do you have a video showing how I should give myself the shot?"
5. "Let me read that brochure and then I'd like to discuss it."

8. A primary care provider admitted a client experiencing a hypertensive crisis because of failure to take prescribed medications. To determine learning needs, which assessment would have the highest priority?
1. Client's age
2. Client's perception of the effects of hypertension
3. Client's ability to purchase needed medications
4. Client's support system

9. A client has a learning outcome of: "Select foods that are low in fat content." Which of the following statements reflect that the client has met this learning outcome?
   1. "I understand the importance of maintaining a low-fat diet."
   2. "I feel better about myself now."
   3. "See how I revised my favorite recipe to be lower in fat."
   4. "Since changing my diet, my husband is also losing weight."

10. A client's learning outcome is: "Client will verbalize medication name, purpose, and appropriate precautions." Which of the following documented statements reflect evidence of learning?
   1. Taught name, purpose, and precautions for the new cardiac medication; seemed to understand.
   2. Written information about the medication provided and reviewed; correct responses were given to follow-up questions.
   3. Written information read to client; stated he would read it when he got home.
   4. Asked questions about the new cardiac medication; satisfied with the information.

∞ *See answers to Test Your Knowledge in Appendix A.*

EXPLORE **PEARSON mynursingkit™**

MyNursingKit is your one stop for online chapter review materials and resources. Prepare for success with additional NCLEX®-style practice questions, interactive assignments and activities, web links, animations and videos, and more!

Register your access code from the front of your book at
www.mynursingkit.com.

REFERENCES AND SELECTED BIBLIOGRAPHY

Aldridge, M. D. (2004). Writing and designing readable patient education materials. *Nephrology Nursing Journal, 31*(4), 373–377.

Bandura, A. (1971). Analysis of modeling processes. In A. Bandura (Ed.), *Psychological modeling.* Chicago: Aldine.

Bastable, S. (2008). *Nurse as educator: Principles of teaching and learning for nursing practice* (3rd ed.). Boston: Jones & Bartlett.

Bloom, B. S. (Ed.). (1956). *Taxonomy of education objectives. Book 1, Cognitive domain.* New York: Longman.

Brownson, K. (n.d.). *Improving patient education for poor readers.* Retrieved June 26, 2006, from http://www.nursingspectrum.com/ce/self-study_modules/syllabus.html?CCID=3121

Bulechek, G. M., Butcher, H. K., & Dochterman, J. M. (2008). *Nursing interventions classification (NIC)* (5th ed.). St. Louis, MO: Mosby.

Curran, M. A., & Curran, K. E. (2005). The e-health revolution: Competitive options for nurse practitioners as local providers. *Journal of the American Academy of Nurse Practitioners, 17*(12), 495–498.

Edmunds, M. (2005). Health literacy a barrier to patient education. *Nurse Practitioner, 30*(3), 54.

Escoffery, C., Miner, K. R., Adame, D.D., Butler, S., McCormick, L., & Mendell, E. (2005). Internet use for health information among college students. *Journal of American College Health, 53*(4), 183–188.

Hayes, K. (2005). Designing written medication instructions: Effective ways to help older adults self-medicate. *Journal of Gerontological Nursing, 31*(5), 5–10.

Healthcare Information and Management Systems Society E-Health Special Interest Group (SIG). (2003). *HIMSS e-health SIG white paper.* Retrieved June 9, 2006, from http://www.himss.org/content/files/ehealth_whitepaper.pdf

Hohler, S. E. (2004). Tips for better patient teaching. *Nursing, 34*(7), 32hn7–32hn8.

Hsu, J., Huang, J., Kinsman, J., Fireman, B., Miller, R., Selby, J., et al. (2005). Use of e-health services between 1999 and 2002: A growing digital divide. *Journal of the American Medical Informatics Association, 12*(2), 164–171.

Institute of Medicine. (2004). *Health literacy: A prescription to end confusion.* Washington, DC: National Academies Press.

John, M. T. (1988). *Geragogy: A theory for teaching the elderly.* New York: Haworth Press.

Kaiser Family Foundation. (2005). *E-health and the elderly: How seniors use the Internet for health information. Key findings from a national survey of older Americans.* Menlo Park, CA: Author.

Knowles, M. S. (1984). *Andragogy in action.* San Francisco: Jossey-Bass.

Leiner, M., Handal, G., & Williams, D. (2004). Patient communication: A multidisciplinary approach using animated cartoons. *Health Education Research, 19*(5), 591–595.

London, F. (2004). How to prepare families for discharge in the limited time available. *Pediatric Nursing, 30*(3), 212–227.

Lorig, K. R. (2003). Taking patient ed to the next level. *RN, 66*(12), 35–38.

Mauk, K. L. (2006). Reaching and teaching older adults. *Nursing, 36*(2), 17.

McCray, A. T. (2005). Promoting health literacy. *Journal of the American Medical Informatics Association, 12*(2), 152–163.

Monsivais, D., & Reynolds, A. (2003). Developing and evaluating patient education materials. *Journal of Continuing Education in Nursing, 34*(4), 172–176.

Moorhead, S., Johnson, M., Maas, M., & Swanson, E. (2008). *Nursing outcomes classification (NOC)* (4th ed.). St. Louis, MO: Mosby.

Munoz, C., & Luckmann, J. (2005). *Transcultural communication in nursing* (2nd ed.). Clifton Park, NY: Delmar Learning.

NANDA International. (2009). *NANDA nursing diagnoses: Definitions and classification 2009–2011.* West Sussex, U.K.: Wiley-Blackwell.

Pavlov, I. P. (1927). *Conditioned reflexes* (G. V. Anrep, trans.). London: Oxford University Press.

Pew Internet & American Life Project. (2005a). *Health information online.* Retrieved June 9, 2006, from http://www.pewinternet.org/PPF/r/165/report_display.asp

Pew Internet & American Life Project. (2005b). *Digital divisions.* Retrieved June 9, 2006, from http://www.pewinternet.org/PPF/r/165/report_display.asp

Pew Internet & American Life Project. (2006). *Demographics of Internet users.* Retrieved June 9, 2006, from http://www.pewinternet.org/trends.asp

Piaget, J. (1966). *Origins of intelligence in children.* New York: Norton.

Purnell, L. D., & Paulanka, B. J. (2005). *Guide to culturally competent health care.* Philadelphia: Davis.

Rankin, S. H., Stallings, K. D., & London, F. (2005). *Patient education in health and illness* (5th ed.). Philadelphia: Lippincott Williams & Wilkins.

Redman, B. K. (2004). *Advances in patient education.* New York: Springer.

Rogers, C. R. (1961). *On becoming a person.* Boston: Houghton-Mifflin.

Rogers, C. R. (1969). *Freedom to learn.* Columbus, OH: Merrill.

Saarmann, L., Daugherty, J., & Riegel, B. (2000). Patient teaching to promote behavioral change. *Nursing Outlook, 48,* 281–287.

Schultz, M. (2002). Low literacy skills needn't hinder care. *RN, 65*(4), 45–48.

Skinner, B. F. (1953). *Science and human behavior.* New York: Macmillan.

Smith, L. S. (2003). Help! My patient's illiterate. *Nursing, 33*(11), 32hn6–32hn8.

Stanley, M., Blair, K. A., & Beare, P. G. (2005). *Gerontological nursing: Promoting successful aging with older adults* (3rd ed.). Philadelphia: Davis.

Steward, D., & Steward, M. (1973). The observation of Anglo-Mexican and Chinese-American mothers teaching their young sons. *Child Development, 44,* 329–337.

Thomas, C., & Wolfe, H. (2005). Bulletin boards: Not just for kids anymore. *Nursing, 35*(7), 68.

Using technology to transform patient education. (2004). *RN, 67*(2), 26nm1–26nm4.

Wilkinson, J. M. (2009). *Nursing diagnosis handbook with NIC interventions and NOC outcomes* (9th ed.). Upper Saddle River, NJ: Prentice Hall Health.

Wilson, E. V., & Lankton, N. K. (2004). Modeling patients' acceptance of provider-delivered e-health. *Journal of the American Medical Informatics Association, 11*(4), 241–248.

Wingard, R. (2005). Patient education and the nursing process: Meeting the patient's needs. *Nephrology Nursing Journal, 32*(2), 211–214.

Leading, Managing, and Delegating

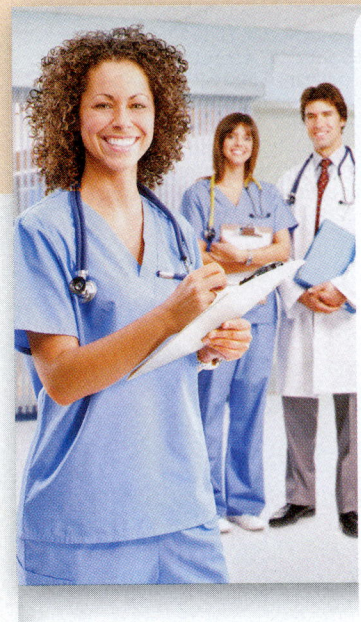

Majel is a nurse working the night shift on a normally busy pediatric unit. However, tonight the unit is quiet, with fewer clients than normal, and the clients are of lower acuity than normal. After checking on all of her clients, Majel returns to the nurse's station to find the staff in a spirited discussion about the facility's decision to group vacation time, sick time, and personal time into one bank called leave time. One staff nurse is concerned that now her vacation time will be limited if she calls in sick. The charge nurse is concerned that the new total number of leave days is less than the sum of the different days they had in the old plan. An unlicensed assistive personnel (UAP) says, "This place is always trying to save money at our expense." Majel listens for a while and then mentions the rising costs of operating an acute care facility and describes the benefits of the new policy for staff, including being able to use sick time for vacation if they remain healthy. She then leads a discussion of how they can promote healthful activity among the staff. Soon everyone is discussing ideas for how they can promote staff health.

LEARNING OUTCOMES

After completing this chapter, you will be able to:

1. Compare and contrast leadership and management.
2. Differentiate formal from informal leaders.
3. Compare and contrast different leadership styles.
4. Identify characteristics of an effective leader.
5. Compare and contrast the levels of management.
6. Describe the four functions of management.
7. Discuss the roles and functions of nurse managers.
8. Identify the skills and competencies needed by a nurse manager.
9. Describe the characteristics of tasks appropriate to delegate to unlicensed and licensed assistive personnel.
10. List the five rights of delegation.
11. Describe the role of the leader/manager in planning for and implementing change.

Although aspects of the individual nurse's role vary according to practice location and type, leadership, management, delegation, and change are consistent components of the role. Nurses function within health care systems, working with multiple clients and other health care providers. As a part of multidisciplinary teams, the nurse is often in a leadership position and frequently delegates aspects of care to others. There are opportunities in nursing to become leaders at various levels and also many situations in which the nurse functions as a manager and as a change agent.

THE NURSE AS LEADER AND MANAGER

The professional nurse frequently assumes the roles of leader and manager. These two roles are linked; that is, managers must have leadership abilities, and leaders often manage, but the two roles differ.

A **leader** influences others to work together to accomplish a specific goal. Leaders are often visionary; they are informed, articulate, confident, and self-aware. Leaders also usually have outstanding interpersonal skills and are excellent listeners and communicators. They have initiative and the ability and confidence to innovate change, motivate, facilitate, and mentor others. Within their organizations, nurse leaders participate in and guide teams that assess the effectiveness of care, implement evidence-based practice, and construct process improvement strategies. They may be employed in a variety of positions—from shift team leader to institutional president. Leaders may also hold volunteer positions such as chairperson of a professional organization or a community board of directors.

A **manager** is an employee of an organization who is given authority, power, and responsibility for planning, organizing, coordinating, and directing the work of others, and for establishing and evaluating standards. Managers understand organizational structure and culture. They control human, financial, and material resources. Managers set goals, make decisions, and solve problems. They initiate and implement change.

The purposes of nursing leadership include (a) improving the health status of individuals or families, (b) increasing the effectiveness and level of satisfaction among professional colleagues, and (c) improving the attitudes of citizens and legislators toward the nursing profession and their expectations of it.

As managers, nurses are responsible for managing client care. Some nurses assume a position within the organization as nurse manager, supervisor, or executive. As a manager, the nurse is responsible for (a) efficiently accomplishing the goals of the organization, (b) efficiently using the organization's resources, (c) ensuring effective client care, and (d) ensuring compliance with institutional, professional, regulatory, and governmental standards. Managers are also responsible for development of licensed and unlicensed personnel within their work group. Table 15–1 further compares the leader and manager roles. Figure 15–1 illustrates some of the leading and managing roles.

LEADERSHIP

Leadership may be formal or informal. The **formal leader**, or appointed leader, is selected by an organization and given official authority to make decisions and act. An **informal leader** is not officially appointed to direct the activities of others, but because of seniority, age, or special abilities, is recognized by the group as its leader and plays an important role in influencing colleagues, co-workers, or other group members to achieve the group's goals.

For there to be a leader of a group, there must also be followers. How many followers a leader has may be determined by organizational structure, charisma of the leader, or the leader's power. **Power** is the person's ability to control the environment. Power is sometimes referred to as "authority," which is seen as a more legitimate power conferred by a higher power authorizing the leader to make decisions.

TABLE 15–1	Comparison of Leader and Manager Roles	
LEADERS	**MANAGERS**
May or may not be officially appointed to the position	Are appointed officially to the position
Have power and authority to enforce decisions only as long as followers are willing to be led	Have power and authority to enforce decisions
Influence others toward goal setting, either formally or informally	Carry out predetermined policies, rules, and regulations
Are interested in risk taking and exploring new ideas	Maintain an orderly, controlled, rational, and equitable structure
Relate to people personally in an intuitive and empathetic manner	Relate to people according to their roles
Feel rewarded by personal achievements	Feel rewarded when fulfilling organizational mission or goals
May or may not be successful as managers	Are managers as long as the appointment holds
Manage relationships	Manage resources
Focus on people	Focus on systems

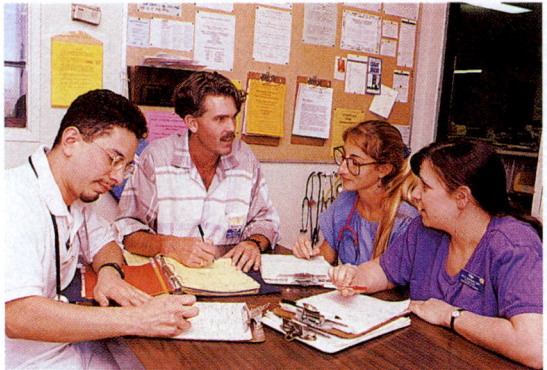

Figure 15–1 ● Nurses as leaders and managers.

Leadership Theory

Early leadership theories focused on what leaders are (trait theories), what leaders do (behavioral theories), and how leaders adapt their leadership style according to the situation (contingency theories). Theories about **leadership style** describe traits, behaviors, motivations, and choices used by individuals to effectively influence others.

CLASSIC LEADERSHIP THEORIES   The trait theorists found that leaders often possess specific traits and abilities, including good judgment, decisiveness, knowledge, adaptability, integrity, tact, self-confidence, and cooperativeness. The behaviorists believed that through education, training, and life experiences, leaders develop a particular leadership style. These styles have been characterized as autocratic, democratic, laissez-faire, and bureaucratic.

An **autocratic (authoritarian) leader** makes decisions for the group. The leader believes individuals are externally motivated (their driving force is extrinsic, they desire rewards from others) and are incapable of independent decision making. Likened to a dictator, the autocratic leader determines policies, giving orders and directions to the group. Under this leadership style, the group may feel secure because procedures are well defined and activities are pre-

dictable. Productivity may also be high. However, the group's needs for creativity, autonomy, and self-motivation are not met, and the degree of openness and trust between the leader and the group members is minimal or absent. Members are often dissatisfied with this leadership style; however, at times an autocratic style is the most effective. When urgent decisions are necessary (e.g., a cardiac arrest, a unit fire, or a terrorist attack), one person must assume the responsibility for making decisions without being challenged by other team members. When group members are unable or do not wish to participate in making a decision, the authoritarian style solves the problem and enables the individual or group to move on. This style can also be effective when a project must be completed quickly and efficiently.

A **democratic (participative, consultative) leader** encourages group discussion and decision making. This type of leader acts as a catalyst or facilitator, actively guiding the group toward achieving the group goals. Group productivity and satisfaction are high as group members contribute to the work effort. The democratic leader assumes individuals are internally motivated (their driving force is intrinsic, they desire self-satisfaction), are capable of making decisions, and value independence. Providing constructive feedback, offering information, making suggestions, and asking questions become the focus of the participative leader. This leadership style demands that the leader have faith in the group members to accomplish the goals. Although democratic leadership has been shown to be less efficient and more cumbersome than authoritarian leadership, it allows more self-motivation and more creativity among group members. It also calls for a great deal of cooperation and coordination among group members. This leadership style can be extremely effective in the health care setting.

The **laissez-faire (nondirective, permissive) leader** recognizes the group's need for autonomy and self-regulation. The leader assumes a "hands-off" approach. The leader presupposes the group is internally motivated. However, group members may act independently and at cross purposes because of a lack of cooperation and coordination. A laissez-faire style is most effective for groups whose members have

TABLE 15–2	**Comparison of Authoritarian, Democratic, and Laissez-Faire Leadership Styles**		
	AUTHORITARIAN (AUTOCRATIC)	DEMOCRATIC (PARTICIPATIVE)	LAISSEZ-FAIRE (PERMISSIVE)
Degree of control	Makes decisions alone	Collaborative	No control
Leader activity level	High	High	Minimal
Assumption of responsibility	Primarily the leader	Shared	Relinquished
Output of the group	High quantity, good quality	Creative, high quality	Variable, may be of poor quality
Efficiency	Very efficient	Less efficient than authoritarian	Inefficient

both personal and professional maturity, so that once the group has made a decision, the members become committed to it and have the required expertise to implement it. Individual group members then perform tasks in their area of expertise while the leader acts as resource person. Table 15–2 compares the authoritarian, democratic, and laissez-faire leadership styles.

The **bureaucratic leader** does not trust self or others to make decisions and instead relies on the organization's rules, policies, and procedures to direct the group's work efforts. Group members are usually dissatisfied with the leader's inflexibility and impersonal relations with them.

According to contingency theorists, effective leaders adapt their leadership style to the situation. A popular contingency theory describes the situational leader. The **situational leader** (a) flexes task and relationship behaviors, (b) considers the staff members' abilities, (c) knows the nature of the task to be done, and (d) is sensitive to the context or environment in which the task takes place. The task-orientation style focuses the leader on activities that encourage group productivity to get the work done. The relationship-orientation style is concerned with interpersonal relationships and focuses on activities that meet group members' needs.

Situational leaders adapt their leadership style to the readiness and willingness of the individual or group to perform the assigned task. When employees are insecure or unable or unwilling to perform the task, the leader uses a highly directive style, providing specific instructions and close supervision. If the group is motivated and willing but unable to perform the task, the leader again uses a highly directive style, but in this case, explains decisions and provides the opportunity for clarification. When the group is able but unwilling or lacking in confidence, the leader shares ideas and facilitates decision making. For a group that is willing, able, and confident to perform the task, the leader delegates, turning responsibility for decision making and implementation over to the group.

CONTEMPORARY LEADERSHIP THEORIES   Contemporary theorists have described charismatic leaders, transactional leaders, transformational leaders, and shared leadership.

A **charismatic leader** is rare and is characterized by an emotional relationship between the leader and the group members. The charming personality of the leader evokes strong feelings of commitment to both the leader and the leader's cause and beliefs. The followers of a charismatic leader often overcome extreme hardship to achieve the group's goals because of faith in the leader.

The **transactional leader** has a relationship with followers based on an exchange for some resource valued by the follower. These incentives are used to promote loyalty and performance. For example, in order to ensure adequate staffing on the night shift, the nurse manager entices a staff nurse to work the night shift in exchange for a weekend shift off. The transactional leader represents the traditional manager, focused on the day-to-day tasks of achieving organizational goals, and understanding and meeting the needs of the group.

In contrast, a **transformational leader** fosters creativity, risk taking, commitment, and collaboration by empowering the group to share in the organization's vision. The leader inspires others with a clear, attractive, and attainable goal and enlists them to participate in attaining the goal. Through shared values, honesty, trust, and continual learning the leader empowers the group. Independence, individual growth, and change are facilitated.

Shared leadership recognizes that a professional workforce is made up of many leaders. No one person is considered to have knowledge or ability beyond that of other members of the work group. Appropriate leadership is thought to emerge in relation to the challenges that confront the work group. Examples of shared leadership in nursing are self-directed work teams, coleadership, and shared governance. **Shared governance** is a method that aims to distribute decision making among a group of people.

Effective Leadership

Much has been written about effective leadership and style; some descriptive statements about effective leaders are listed in Box 15–1. Leadership is a learned process. To be an effective leader requires an understanding of factors such as needs, goals, and rewards that motivate people; knowledge of leadership skills and of the group's activities; and possession of the interpersonal skills to influence others. Principles of effective leadership include vision, influence, and acting as a role model.

Vision is a mental image of a possible and desirable future state. Leaders transform visions into realistic goals and communicate their visions to others who accept them as their own.

BOX 15–1	**Characteristics of Effective Leaders**

Effective leaders:

- Use a leadership style that is natural to them.
- Use a leadership style appropriate to the task and the members.
- Assess the effects of their behavior on others and the effects of others' behavior on themselves.
- Are sensitive to forces acting for and against change.
- Express an optimistic view about human nature.
- Are energetic.
- Are open and encourage openness, so that real issues are confronted.

- Facilitate personal relationships.
- Plan and organize activities of the group.
- Are consistent in behavior toward group members.
- Delegate tasks and responsibilities to develop members' abilities, not merely to get tasks performed.
- Involve members in all decisions.
- Value and use group members' contributions.
- Encourage creativity.
- Encourage feedback about their leadership style.
- Assess for and promote use of current technology.

Influence is an informal strategy used to gain the cooperation of others without exercising formal authority. Influence is exercised through persuasion and excellent communication skills; it is based on a trusting relationship with the followers.

An effective leader needs to show sensitivity to being a positive **role model**, demonstrating caring toward co-workers and clients. As is appropriate for any health and caring profession, leadership can also be humanistic, that is, acting in a way that stresses individuals' dignity and worth. Being a good leader takes thought, care, insight, commitment, and energy. In this way, the leader sets the example for others to follow.

CLINICAL ALERT

Nurses generally move from first- to middle- to upper-level management positions through promotion. In addition, nursing administration graduate academic programs are available at some nursing schools.

MANAGEMENT

The manager's job is to accomplish the work of the organization. To this end, managers perform roles and functions that vary with the type of organization and the level of management.

Levels of Management

Traditional management is divided into three levels of responsibility. **First-level managers** are responsible for managing the work of nonmanagerial personnel and the day-to-day activities of a specific work group or groups. Their primary responsibility is to motivate staff to achieve the organization's goals. This level of manager communicates staff issues to upper administration and reports administrative messages back to staff. Titles may include primary care nurse, team leader, nurse case manager, or charge nurse.

Middle-level managers supervise a number of first-level managers and are responsible for the activities in the departments they supervise. Middle-level managers serve as liaisons between first-level managers and upper-level man-

agers. They may be called supervisors, nurse managers, or head nurses.

Upper-level (top-level) managers are organizational executives who are primarily responsible for establishing goals and developing strategic plans. Nurse executives are registered nurses who are responsible for the management of nursing within the organization and the practice of nursing. Some nurse executives are also responsible for auxiliary units such as the pharmacy, laboratory, and dietary departments. Nurses in these positions may be called vice president for client care services, vice president for nursing, director of nursing, or chief nurse.

Management Functions

Four management functions are planning, organizing, directing, and coordinating. These four functions help to achieve the broad goal of quality client care.

PLANNING   Planning is an ongoing process that involves (a) assessing a situation, (b) establishing goals and objectives based on assessment of a situation or future trends, and (c) developing a plan of action that identifies priorities, delineates who is responsible, determines deadlines, and describes how the intended outcome is to be achieved and evaluated. In short, it involves deciding what, when, where, and how to do it, by whom, and with what resources. Distribution of money, personnel, equipment, and physical space are included in resource allocation. An upper-level manager spends considerable time planning the department's goals and services, determining numbers and types of nurses and other personnel needed to provide these services. On the other hand, a first-level manager such as a staff nurse spends less time planning but manages individual clients by use of the nursing process.

An example of the planning function is **risk management**, having in place a system to reduce danger to clients and staff. The steps of risk management include anticipating and seeking sources of risk; analyzing, classifying, and prioritizing risks; developing a plan to avoid and manage risk; gathering data that indicate success at avoiding or minimizing risk; and evaluating and modifying risk reduction programs. Central to the process of risk management is communication among all involved persons.

ORGANIZING   Organizing is also an ongoing process. After identifying the work and evaluating human and material resources, the manager arranges the work into smaller units. Organizing involves determining responsibilities, communicating expectations, and establishing the chain of command for authority and communication. Although upper-level managers delegate much of the work and responsibility and accountability for the work to others, they need to ensure that department objectives, priorities, job descriptions, lines of communication, nursing standards, procedures, and policies clearly describe the expectations.

DIRECTING   Directing is the process of getting the organization's work accomplished. Directing involves assigning and communicating expectations about the task to be completed, providing instruction and guidance, and ongoing decision making. Upper-level managers devote less time to directing than to planning, organizing, and controlling. Directing at this level of management generally involves supervision of the next level of managers such as those in middle management. Unit managers (charge nurses) and staff nurses devote more time to directing. For example, charge nurses direct shift work by assigning clients and scheduling meal and break times. Staff nurses direct the care of clients by ordering nursing care, communicating care in written care plans and shift reports, and supervising care that is given by others.

COORDINATING   Coordinating is the process of ensuring that plans are carried out and evaluating outcomes. The manager measures results or actions against standards or desired outcomes and then reinforces effective actions or changes ineffective ones. For example, an upper-level manager evaluates the effectiveness of recruitment, staff turnover, and budget performance. The charge nurse appraises staff performance. The staff nurse determines whether nursing interventions have helped the client achieve desired outcomes.

Principles of Management

A manager has authority, accountability, and responsibility. Authority is defined as the legitimate right to direct the work of others. It is an integral component of managing. Authority is conveyed through leadership actions; it is determined largely by the situation, and it is always associated with responsibility and accountability. The manager must accept the authority granted.

Accountability is the ability and willingness to assume responsibility for one's actions and to accept the consequences of one's behavior. Accountability can be viewed as hierarchic, starting at the individual level, then the institutional or professional level, and finally the societal level. At the individual or client level, accountability is reflected in the nurse's ethical integrity. At the institutional level, it is reflected in the statement of philosophy and objectives of the nursing department and nursing audits. At the professional level, it is reflected in standards of practice developed by national or provincial nursing associations. At the societal level, it is reflected in legislated nurse practice acts.

Responsibility is an obligation to complete a task. Managers are responsible for utilization of resources, communication to subordinates, and implementation of organizational goals and objectives.

Skills and Competencies of Nurse Managers

To be effective managers, nurses need to think critically, communicate well, manage resources effectively and efficiently, enhance employee performance, build and manage teams, manage conflict, manage time, and initiate and manage change. Change is discussed on pages 360–361.

CRITICAL THINKING   Critical thinking is a creative cognitive process that includes problem solving and decision making. The nurse manager reasons with logic, exploring assumptions, alternatives, and the consequences of actions. See Chapter 6 ∞ for further discussion of critical thinking.

COMMUNICATING   Managers report spending much of their day communicating. Good communication is essential and often determines the manager's success as a leader. Managers use both verbal and written communication. Effective managers communicate assertively, expressing their ideas clearly, accurately, and honestly.

Managers use networking, a process whereby professional links are established through which people can share ideas, knowledge, and information, offer support and direction to each other, and facilitate accomplishment of professional goals.

MANAGING RESOURCES   One of the greatest responsibilities of managers is their accountability for human, fiscal, and material resources. Budgeting and determining variances between the actual and budgeted expenses are crucial skills for any manager.

ENHANCING EMPLOYEE PERFORMANCE   Several ways of enhancing employee performance are available to managers. Managers are responsible for ensuring that employees develop through appropriate learning opportunities, whether through in-service education, facilitating attendance at professional workshops and conventions, or encouraging achievement of advanced education such as higher degrees or certifications. The nurse manager who empowers the staff by providing information, support, resources, and opportunities to participate will find that employees have greater commitment to the institution, are more effective in their role, have increased self-esteem, and are better able to meet their goals.

In addition, the manager may provide day-to-day coaching or serve as a mentor or preceptor. **Mentors** "give their time, energy, and material support to teach, guide, assist, counsel, and inspire a younger nurse. It is a nurturing relationship . . ." (Tomey, 2004, p. 365). Having a mentor is recognized as important for career development.

In the clinical area, the term **preceptor** is used to describe relationships in which the experienced nurse assists the "new" nurse in improving clinical nursing skill and judgment. The preceptor also instills understanding of the routines, policies, and procedures of the institution and the unit.

BUILDING AND MANAGING TEAMS   In addition to personnel development, the manager is responsible for building and managing the work team. Familiarity with group processes facilitates the manager's ability to lead the group and enhances development of the group into a work team. Groups develop in stages, during which roles and relationships are established. The purposes of the team as a whole and the role of each member must be clear. Each member must feel that the manager and the other members recognize his or her contributions. In health care, the team may consist of any health care providers: nurses, therapists, unlicensed personnel, clergy, and so on. All members of the team need to use effective communication skills.

Evaluating the group's work is another responsibility of the manager. Effectiveness, efficiency, and productivity are three outcome measures that are frequently used. In health care, effectiveness is a measure of the quality or quantity of services provided. Efficiency is a measure of the resources used in the provision of nursing services. In nursing, productivity is a performance measure of both the effectiveness and efficiency of nursing care. Productivity is frequently measured by the amount of nursing resources used per client or in terms of required versus actual hours of care provided.

MANAGING CONFLICT   Nurse managers are frequently in a position to manage conflict among people, groups, or teams. The conflict may arise from differing values, philosophies, or personalities. In health care, it can also arise due to competition for resources.

There are many methods the nurse can use to manage conflict and each has its advantages and disadvantages. Among the most common are compromise, negotiation, and collaboration. The new nurse manager may require training to become proficient in the use of these methods. Basic principles for all types of conflict management include demonstrating respect for all parties, avoiding blame, allowing full discussion, using ground rules during meetings to promote fairness, encouraging active listening, identifying the themes in the discussion, and exploring alternative solutions (Carroll, 2006).

MANAGING TIME   The effective nurse manager uses time effectively and assists others to do the same. Many factors inhibit good use of time, such as preference for doing things the nurse likes to do before things the nurse prefers not to have to do, emergencies or crises that divert one's attention, and unrealistic demands from others. Strategies that the manager, and all nurses, can use in order to use time well involve setting goals and priorities, delegating appropriately, examining how time is used, minimizing paperwork (automating whenever possible), and using regular schedules that avoid interruptions and set time limits on activities (Sullivan & Decker, 2009).

THE NURSE AS DELEGATOR

Delegation is the transference of responsibility and authority for an activity to a competent individual. The delegate assumes responsibility for the actual performance of the task or procedure. The delegator retains accountability for the outcome. Delegation is a tool that allows the delegator to devote more time to tasks that cannot be delegated. It also enhances the skills and abilities of the delegate, which builds self-esteem, promotes morale, and enhances teamwork and attainment of the organization's goals. In nursing, delegation refers to indirect care—the intended outcome is achieved through the work of someone supervised by the nurse—and involves defining the task, determining who can perform the task, describing the expectation, seeking agreement, monitoring performance, and providing feedback to the delegate regarding performance.

(margin, vertical) **MyNursingKit** | Delegating Successfully

---

RESEARCH NOTES   **Does One's Generation Influence How Nurses Prefer to Be Managed?**

In this study, 62 nurses, technicians, and secretaries from hospital units completed a survey to assess characteristics of the respondents' generation, significance of tasks, and their communication style. About half the respondents belonged to the baby boomers (born 1943–1960) and the other half belonged to generation X or generation Y (born 1961–1980). Respondents varied in their views regarding their preferred method of recognition. For example, older respondents preferred personal recognition while younger ones preferred public affirmation. Communication styles were similar between the groups. Not surprisingly, older respondents viewed technology as more complicated than younger ones. Baby boomers reported good commitment to remaining in a particular job for a long time, while generation Xers felt loyalty to their manager was of greater importance than length of employment. Based on the findings, the authors suggest areas in which nurse managers should consider approaching the generations differently.

Implications

All nurses interact with persons of the same and different generations, and information such as this can help us work together effectively. Understanding the viewpoint of others is a common and important role of the nurse in any position—leader, manager, or neither. In your work setting, it will be necessary to consider how the workforce is distributed among different generations with their unique perspectives.

Note: Based on "Managing the Multigenerational Nursing Team," by J. Hu, C. Herrick, and K. Allard Hodgin, 2004, *Health Care Manager, 23,* pp. 334–340.

BOX 15–2	Examples of Tasks That May and May Not Be Delegated to Unlicensed Assistive Personnel

Tasks that **May** Be Delegated to Unlicensed Assistive Personnel	Tasks that **May Not** Be Delegated to Unlicensed Assistive Personnel
• Taking of vital signs	• Assessment
• Measuring and recording intake and output	• Interpretation of data
• Client transfers and ambulation	• Making a nursing diagnosis
• Postmortem care	• Creation of a nursing care plan
• Bathing	• Evaluation of care effectiveness
• Feeding	• Care of invasive lines
• Gastrostomy feedings in established systems	• Administering parenteral medications
• Attending to safety	• Insertion of nasogastric tubes
• Weighing	• Client education
• Performing simple dressing changes	• Performing triage
• Suctioning of chronic tracheostomies	• Giving telephone advice
• Performing basic life support (CPR)	

Registered nurses increasingly delegate components of nursing care to other health care workers, especially unlicensed assistive personnel (UAP). An RN who delegates a task to another health care worker is accountable for selecting an appropriately skilled caregiver and for continued evaluation of the client's care. These "nurse extenders" may be identified by a variety of titles, including certified nursing aides/assistants, home health aides, patient care technicians, orderlies, or surgical technicians. They have had diverse degrees of training and experience. They are employees and do not include family members or friends who provide some client care.

Each state nurse practice act specifies which actions constitute the legal practice of nursing, which actions are the purview only of nurses, and which may be delegated to others. The National Council of State Boards of Nursing (NCSBN) published five "rights" of delegation: The nurse delegates the *right task*, under the *right circumstances*, to the *right person*, with the *right direction and communication*, and the *right supervision and evaluation* (1995).

It is not possible to generate an exhaustive list of exactly which actions may or may not be delegated to unlicensed personnel. Examples of tasks that may and may not be delegated are given in Box 15–2. A statement regarding delegation is included with the steps for each procedure in this book.

The unlicensed person may not delegate tasks to another person. Principles guiding the nurse's decision to delegate ensure the safety and quality of outcomes. These principles are listed in Box 15–3. Even if the task is one that may legally be delegated, the individual nurse must still determine if the task can be delegated to a particular UAP for a specific client. The NCSBN has created a grid to assist in this decision. Once the decision has been made to delegate, the nurse must communicate clearly to the UAP and verify that the UAP understands:

- The specific tasks to be done for each client.
- When each task is to be done.
- The expected outcomes for each task, including parameters outside of which the unlicensed person

BOX 15–3	Three Principles Used by the Nurse to Determine Delegation to Unlicensed Assistive Personnel

1. The nurse must assess the individual client prior to delegating tasks.
2. The client must be medically stable or in a chronic condition and not fragile.
3. The task must be considered routine for this client.
4. The task must not require a substantial amount of scientific knowledge or technical skill.
5. The task must be considered safe for this client.
6. The task must have a predictable outcome.
7. Learn the agency's procedures and policies about delegation.
8. Know the scope of practice and the customary knowledge, skills, and job description for each health care discipline represented on your team.
9. Be aware of individual variations in work abilities. Along with different categories of caregivers are individual

variations. Each individual has different experiences and may not be capable of performing every task cited in the job description.

10. When unsure about an assistant's abilities to perform a task, observe while the person performs it, or demonstrate it to the person and get a return demonstration before allowing the person to perform it independently.
11. Clarify reporting expectations to ensure the task is accomplished.
12. Create an atmosphere that fosters communication, teaching, and learning. For example, encourage staff to ask questions, listen carefully to their concerns, and make use of every opportunity to teach.

must immediately report to the nurse (and any action that must urgently be taken).

- Who is available to serve as a resource if needed.
- When and in what format (written or verbal) a report on the tasks is expected.

A specific task that can be delegated to one UAP may not be appropriate for a different UAP, depending on each UAP's experience and individual skill sets. Also, a task that is appropriate for the UAP to perform with one client may not be appropriate with a different client or the same client under altered circumstances. For example, the taking of routine vital signs may be delegated to the UAP for a client in stable condition but would not be delegated for the same client who has become unstable.

CLINICAL ALERT

Each nurse or other licensed or unlicensed health care provider is responsible for his or her own actions. Anyone who feels unqualified to perform a delegated task must decline to perform it.

The registered nurse delegates to licensed vocational/practical nurses (LVN/LPNs) and other RNs in additional to UAPs. The nurse must know the state-specific scope of practice for other licensed personnel in order to delegate effectively. LVN/LPNs require less direct supervision than UAPs. In some regions and some agencies, LVN/LPNs may perform tasks generally considered the role of the registered nurse if they have received special training (e.g., administration of intravenous fluids).

It is important to note that the nurse is not held legally responsible for the acts of the unlicensed person, but is accountable for the quality of the act of delegation and has ultimate responsibility to ensure that proper care is provided. Delegation can be an extremely useful strategy in providing thorough and effective nursing care. Skill in delegation, however, must be learned and developed over time. The nurse should not hesitate to consult with others regarding the appropriateness of delegation.

CHANGE

Change is the process of making something different from what it was. Change can involve gaining new knowledge or adapting what is currently known in the light of new information. It can also involve obtaining new skills. Change is an integral aspect of nursing, and nurses are often **change agents**, that is, individuals who initiate, motivate, and implement change. Change agents:

- Have excellent communication and interpersonal skills with individuals, groups, administration, and all levels of the organization involved in change.

- Have knowledge of available resources and how to use them: people, time, money, facilities, and information.
- Are skilled in problem solving.
- Are skilled in teaching.
- Are respected by those involved in the change.
- Have the ability to encourage and nurture those going through change.
- Are self-confident, are able to take risks, and inspire trust in themselves and others.
- Are able to make decisions.
- Have a broad base of knowledge.
- Have a good sense of timing.

CLINICAL ALERT

Change that is viewed as a threat by one nurse may be viewed as an opportunity by another nurse.

Types of Change

Planned change is an intended, purposeful attempt by an individual, group, organization, or larger social system to influence its own current status. Problem-solving skills, decision-making skills, and interpersonal skills are important factors in planned change.

Change may be considered covert or overt. A covert change is hidden or occurs without the individual's awareness. An example is the gradual, subtle increase in the severity of an illness. Overt change is change of which a person is aware. An example might be that a piece of equipment will no longer be available since the agency has changed vendors. People who experience overt change may also experience anxiety. Overt change often necessitates behavioral changes that are in conflict with the person's needs or goals.

Unplanned change is an alteration imposed by external events or persons. It occurs when unexpected events force a reaction. It is usually haphazard, and the results can be unpredictable. Drift is a type of unplanned change in which change occurs without effort on anyone's part. Situational, or natural, change also may be considered unplanned and occurs without any control by the person or group impacted. An example is the change that occurs because of a war or a natural disaster. Not all situational changes are negative. For example, as agencies open or close units, the nurse may have the opportunity to change to a new workplace.

Models of Change

In his classic work, Lewin (1951) describes that change involves three stages: unfreezing, moving, and refreezing. During the unfreezing stage, the need for change is recognized, driving and restraining forces are identified, alternative solutions are generated, and participants are motivated to change. In the second stage, moving, participants agree the status quo is undesirable and the actual change is planned in detail and implemented. In the final stage, refreezing, the change is integrated and stabilized.

An important aspect of planning change is establishing the likelihood of the acceptance of the change and then determining the criteria by which that acceptance can be identified. Accepting change often takes time, particularly when it does not fit into a person's attitudinal framework. The course of acceptance is easier for people if they are involved in the process. If possible, change should be instituted on a small or pilot scale before full implementation. To facilitate acceptance of the change, the change agent needs to identify common driving and restraining forces (see Box 15–4). Guidelines for dealing with resistance to change are found in Box 15–5.

All nurses are affected by change; nobody can avoid it. Nurses knowledgeable about the historical and current trends in nursing and present political, social, technological, and economic issues make rational plans to deal with opportunities to initiate and guide needed change and to respond to change that affects them in the workplace, government, organizations, and the community.

BOX 15–4	**Four Common Driving and Restraining Forces**

Driving Forces
- Perception that the change is challenging
- Economic gain
- Perception that the change will improve the situation
- Visualization of the future impact of change
- Potential for self-growth, recognition, achievement, and improved relationships

Restraining Forces
- Fear that something of personal value will be lost (e.g., threat to job security or self-esteem)
- Misunderstanding of the change and its implications
- Low tolerance for change related to intellectual or emotional insecurity
- Perception that the change will not achieve goals; failure to see the big picture
- Lack of time or energy
- Perceived loss of freedom to engage in particular behaviors

---

BOX 15–5	**Guidelines for Dealing with Resistance to Change**

1. Communicate with those who oppose the change. Get to the root of their reasons for opposition.
2. Clarify information and provide accurate information.
3. Be open to revisions but clear about what must remain.
4. Present the negative consequences of resistance (threats to organizational survival, compromised client care, and so on).
5. Emphasize the positive consequences of the change and how the individual or group will benefit. However, do not spend too much energy on rational analysis of why the change is good and why the arguments against it do not hold up. People's resistance frequently flows from feelings that are not rational.
6. Keep resisters involved in face-to-face contact with supporters. Encourage proponents to empathize with opponents, recognize valid objections, and relieve unnecessary fears.
7. Maintain a climate of trust, support, and confidence.
8. Follow the "politics of change." (a) Analyze the organizational chart; know the formal lines of authority.

Identify informal lines as well. (b) Identify key persons who will be affected by the change. Pay attention to those immediately above and below the point of change. (c) Find out as much as possible about these key people. What interests them, gets them excited, turns them off? What is on their personal and organizational agendas? Who typically aligns with whom on important decisions? (d) Begin to build a coalition of support before you start the change process. Identify the key people who will most likely support your idea and those who are most likely to be persuaded easily. Talk informally with them to flush out possible objections to your idea and potential opponents. What will the costs and benefits be to them—especially in political terms? Can your idea be modified in ways that retain your objectives but appeal to more key people?

Note: From *Effective Leadership and Management in Nursing*, 7th ed., by E. J. Sullivan and P. J. Decker, 2009, Upper Saddle River, NJ: Pearson Education. Adapted with permission.

CHAPTER HIGHLIGHTS

- Delegation is a tool that a nurse can use to improve productivity. The nurse transfers responsibility and authority to another but retains accountability for the task.

- The professional nurse frequently assumes the roles of leader and manager. Leaders, as employees or volunteers, influence others to accomplish a specific goal, whereas managers have responsibility and accountability for accomplishing the tasks of an organization.

- Managers plan, organize, direct, and coordinate in order to accomplish the work of the organization.
- Several leadership styles have been described, including autocratic, democratic, laissez-faire, and bureaucratic. These styles are often blended to fit the situation. Nurses need to know which style is most consistent with their behavior and learn to incorporate aspects of other styles into their practice.
- Nurse managers work in the organizational framework of the employing agency. Principles of

management include authority, accountability, and responsibility.
- Four major management functions are planning, organizing, directing, and coordinating.
- Effective managers need to be skilled at critical thinking, communication, resource management, enhancing employee performance, and managing teams, conflict, time, and change.
- Nurses function as change agents to initiate, motivate, and implement the change process.

THINK ABOUT IT

Refer to the chapter-opening scenario and answer these questions.

1. Did Majel act in a leadership role? Explain your answer.

2. What type of leadership role did Majel perform?

3. What impact did Majel have on the staff discussion?

∞ *See suggested responses to Think About It on MyNursingKit.*

TEST YOUR KNOWLEDGE

1. The nurse leader informs the staff of a local emergency and instructs them to stay at the hospital to prepare for major casualties. The staff display high levels of anxiety and disorganization. The most appropriate leadership style at this time is which of the following?
  1. Authoritarian
  2. Democratic
  3. Laissez-faire
  4. Bureaucratic

2. Which of the following approaches best illustrates transformational leadership?
  1. The leader stimulates group interest in establishing unit goals that contribute to the agency mission.
  2. The leader forms subgroups or task forces that make decisions about unit problems.
  3. The leader provides funding for continuing education conferences to staff who have not used any sick leave.
  4. The leader adjusts his/her strategies to fit the current situation.

3. Which of the following examples is reflective of a nurse manager with accountability but not authority?
  1. To reduce costs, administrators instruct the manager to inform the staff to reduce overtime.

  2. The manager evaluates the unit staff but cannot promote or terminate staff.
  3. The manager is to recommend a new staffing procedure to the institution's nurse manager group.
  4. The manager prepares a monthly budget variance report that includes plans to correct overspending.

4. An unlicensed assistive person (UAP) has previously performed client transfers safely (bed to chair) on many occasions. It would be inappropriate to delegate this unsupervised task to the UAP under which of the following conditions?
  1. The unit had a new wheelchair.
  2. This was an older adult client.
  3. It was the client's first time out of bed after surgery.
  4. The UAP has just returned from an extended leave of absence.

5. The nurse manager plans to implement a new method for scheduling staff vacations. Senior staff members oppose the change while newer staff members are more accepting. Which of the following would be the most effective strategy for resolving this difference?
  1. Provide extensive and detailed rationale for the proposed change, then implement.

2. Explain that the change will occur as designed, regardless of the staff's preference.
3. Withdraw the proposal to prevent a decrease in staff morale.
4. Encourage interaction between the opposing sides to attempt resolution.

6. Which of the following nurses displays leadership skills?
1. The nurse who can frequently be found talking with a group of staff members about the negative aspects of employment at this facility, resulting in poor staff morale
2. The nurse who is always cheerful and upbeat, showing up for work on time and providing excellent client care to assigned clients
3. The nurse who begins a program of continuing education for staff members, but classes are held at inconvenient times so attendance is low
4. The nurse manager who is perceived by staff as being involved only in budgetary matters and having little understanding of the work performed on the unit

7. Which of the following nurses is functioning as an informal nurse leader?
1. The unit manager
2. The charge nurse
3. The assistant unit manager
4. The nurse staff identify as a good resource

8. The nurse takes a staff position working in a magnet hospital that has established committees to meet unit needs such as the Standards and Practice Committee, the Staff Education Committee, and the Quality Assurance Committee. The nurse anticipates this facility will promote what type of leadership style?
1. Autocratic
2. Democratic
3. Laissez-faire
4. Bureaucratic

9. The charge nurse on the oncology unit receives a promotion to unit manager after completing her graduate degree and will now supervise the charge nurses and assistant unit manager. This position is best described as:
1. First level manager.
2. Middle manager.
3. Upper level manager.
4. Organizing manager.

10. The staff nurse, as a manager of client care, has which of the following management responsibilities? Select all that apply.
1. Authority
2. Accountability
3. Responsibility
4. Entitlement
5. Obligation

∞ *See answers to Test Your Knowledge in Appendix A.*

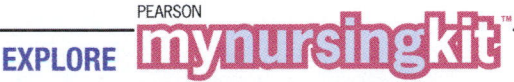

EXPLORE PEARSON mynursingkit™

MyNursingKit is your one stop for online chapter review materials and resources. Prepare for success with additional NCLEX®-style practice questions, interactive assignments and activities, web links, animations and videos, and more!

Register your access code from the front of your book at
www.mynursingkit.com.

REFERENCES AND SELECTED BIBLIOGRAPHY

Bower, F. (2000). *Nurses taking the lead: Personal qualities of effective leadership*. St. Louis: Mosby.

Carroll, P. (2006). *Nursing leadership and management: A practical guide*. Clifton Park, NY: Thomson Delmar Learning.

Carroll, P. L. (2006). *Nursing leadership and management: A practical guide*. Clifton Park, NY: Thomson Delmar Learning.

Hansten, R. I., & Jackson, M. (2009). *Clinical delegation skills: A handbook for professional practice* (4th ed.). Philadelphia: Jones & Bartlett.

Hu, J., Herrick, C., & Allard Hodgin, K. (2004). Managing the multigenerational nursing team. *Health Care Manager, 23*, 334–340.

Kelly-Heidenthal, P., & Marthaler, M. T. (2004). *Nursing delegation and priority setting*. Clifton Park, NY: Thomson Delmar.

Lewin, K. (1951). *Field theory in social science*. New York: Harper & Row.

Marquis, B. L., & Huston, C. J. (2005). *Leading roles and management functions in nursing* (5th ed.). Philadelphia: Lippincott Williams & Wilkins.

National Council of State Boards of Nursing. (1997). *Delegation: decision-making grid*. Chicago: Author. Retrieved December 5, 2009, from http://www.ncsbn.org/delegation_grid_NEW.pdf.

National Council of State Boards of Nursing. (1997). *Delegation decision-making grid*.

Chicago: Author. Retrieved May 12, 2006, from http://www.ncsbn.org/regulation/uap_delegation_documents.asp

Sullivan, E. J., & Decker, P. J. (2009). *Effective leadership and management in nursing* (7th ed.). Upper Saddle River, NJ: Pearson Education.

Tappen, R. M., Weiss, S. A., & Whitehead, D. K. (2010). *Essentials of nursing leadership and management* (4th ed.). Philadelphia: Davis.

Tomey, A. M. (2004). *Guide to nursing management and leadership* (7th ed.). St. Louis: Mosby.

Yoder-Wise, P. S. (2007). *Leading and managing in nursing* (4th ed.). St. Louis: Mosby.

Assessing Health

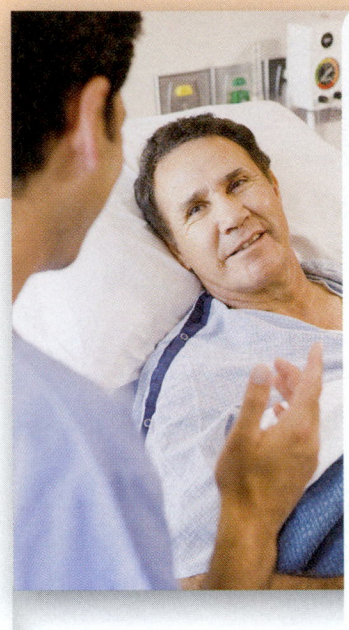

Martin Wiekolvich, 52 years old, was admitted to the medical unit with uncontrolled hypertension believed to be secondary to pheochromocytoma. He is scheduled for further testing tomorrow morning. The nurse enters his room to discuss the procedures to be performed and sees that Martin is breathing rapidly and is massaging his chest. Martin tells the nurse he feels like there is an elephant sitting on his chest and he is having trouble catching his breath. In response to the nurse's questions, Martin says the pain radiates down the left arm and he feels slightly nauseated. The nurse notices he is diaphoretic and has cyanotic fingertips.

The first thing the nurse does is measure his vital signs, which reveal a temperature of 97.2 axillary; radial pulse of 92 beats per minute that is weak, thready, and irregular with an apical rate of 112 per minute; respirations 28 per minute with full excursion, regular. Martin's blood pressure in his left arm is 108/56 and 96/48 in his right arm. Martin is transferred to the coronary care unit where he is diagnosed as having a myocardial infarction.

LEARNING OUTCOMES

After completing this chapter, you will be able to:

1. Explain how various factors impact temperature, pulse, respiration, blood pressure, and oxygen saturation.

2. Identify normal ranges for temperature, pulse, respiration, blood pressure, and oxygen saturation across the lifespan.

3. Compare different sites for obtaining temperature, pulse, blood pressure, and oxygen saturation, explaining why one site may be preferable in specific situations.

4. Demonstrate proper technique when obtaining measurement of temperature, pulse, respirations, blood pressure, and oxygen saturation, including appropriate characteristic assessment data for each measurement.

5. Describe each of the five phases of Korotkoff's sounds.

6. Identify nursing strategies appropriate for alterations in temperature, pulse, respiration, blood pressure, and oxygen saturation.

7. Identify when it is appropriate to delegate measurement of vital signs to unlicensed assistive personnel.

KEY TERMS

Afebrile p369

Apnea p383

Arrhythmia p377

Basal metabolic rate (BMR) p367

Blood pressure p385

Bradycardia p377

Bradypnea p383

Cardiac output p374

Compliance p374

Conduction p368

Convection p368

Diastolic pressure p385

Dysrhythmia p377

Exhalation p382

Expiration p382

Febrile p369

Hypertension p386

Hypotension p386

Hypothermia p370

Inhalation p382

Insensible heat loss p368

Insensible water loss p368

Inspiration p382

Korotkoff's sounds p388

Orthostatic hypotension p386

Point of maximal impulse p374

Pulse p374

Pulse oximeter p391

Pulse pressure p385

Pyrexia p369

Radiation p368

Respiration p382

Systolic pressure p385

Tachycardia p377

Tachypnea p383

Tidal volume p383

Ventilation p382

The vital signs are body temperature, pulse, respirations, and blood pressure. Recently, many agencies such as the Veterans Administration have designated pain as a fifth vital sign, to be assessed at the same time as each of the other four. Pain assessment is covered in Chapter 18 ∞. Pulse oximetry is also commonly measured at the same time as the traditional vital signs. They are called vital because, when looked at in total, they reflect changes in function that otherwise might not be observed. Monitoring a client's vital signs should never be an automatic or routine procedure; it should be a thoughtful, scientific assessment. Vital signs should be evaluated with reference to the client's present and prior health status, and compared to the client's usual and accepted normal standards.

When and how often to assess a specific client's vital signs are chiefly nursing judgments, depending on the client's health status. Some agencies have policies about frequency of assessing vital signs, and physicians may write orders specifying how often specific vital signs should be measured. However, ordered vital signs only set the minimum frequency; a nurse should measure vital signs more often if the client's health status requires it. Examples of times to assess vital signs are listed in Box 16–1.

Often, someone other than the nurse measures the client's vital signs. Prior to delegating this task to unlicensed assistive personnel (UAP), the nurse must have assessed the individual client and determined that the client is medically stable and that the vital sign measurement is considered routine for this client. Under those circumstances, the UAP may measure, record, and report vital signs, but interpretation of the measurements rests with the nurse. Vital signs of an unstable or fragile client should always be assessed by the nurse.

BODY TEMPERATURE

Body temperature reflects the balance between the heat produced and the heat lost from the body, and is measured in heat units called degrees. There are two kinds of body temperature: core temperature and surface temperature. Core temperature is the temperature of the deep tissues of the body, such as the abdominal cavity and pelvic cavity. It remains relatively constant. The normal core body temperature is a range of temperatures (Figure 16–1). The surface temperature is the temperature of the skin, the subcutaneous tissue, and fat. It, by contrast, rises and falls in response to the environment.

The body continually produces heat as a by-product of metabolism. When the amount of heat produced by the body equals the amount of heat lost, the person is in heat balance. A number of factors affect the body's heat production. The most important are these five:

1. *Basal metabolic rate (BMR).* The **basal metabolic rate (BMR)** is the rate of energy utilization in the body required to maintain essential activities such as breathing. Metabolic rates decrease with age. In general, the younger the person, the higher the BMR.
2. *Muscle activity.* Muscle activity, including shivering, increases the metabolic rate.
3. *Thyroxine output.* Increased thyroxine output increases the rate of cellular metabolism throughout the body. This effect is called chemical thermogenesis, the stimulation of heat production in the body through increased cellular metabolism.

BOX 16–1   Times to Assess Vital Signs

- On admission to a health care agency to obtain baseline data
- When a client has a change in health status or reports symptoms such as chest pain or feeling hot or faint
- Before and after surgery or an invasive procedure
- Before and/or after the administration of a medication that could affect the respiratory or cardiovascular systems, for example, before giving a digitalis preparation
- Before and after any nursing intervention that could affect the vital signs (e.g., ambulating a client who has been on bed rest)

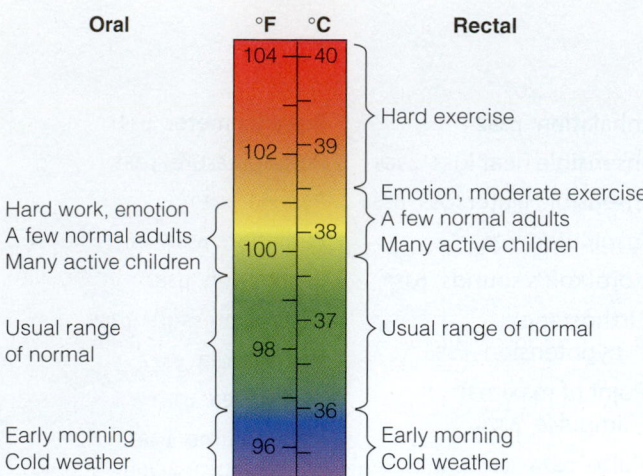

Figure 16–1 ○ Estimated ranges of body temperatures in normal persons.

Note: From Fever and the Regulation of Body Temperature, by E. F. DuBois, 1948, Springfield, IL: Charles C. Thomas. Reprinted with permission.

4. *Epinephrine, norepinephrine, and sympathetic stimulation/stress response.* These hormones immediately increase the rate of cellular metabolism in many body tissues. Epinephrine and norepinephrine directly affect liver and muscle cells, thereby increasing cellular metabolism.

5. *Fever.* Fever increases the cellular metabolic rate and thus increases the body's temperature further.

Heat is lost from the body through radiation, conduction, convection, and vaporization. **Radiation** is the transfer of heat from the surface of one object to the surface of another without contact between the two objects, mostly in the form of infrared rays. **Conduction** is the transfer of heat from one molecule to a molecule of lower temperature. Conduction normally accounts for minimal heat loss except, for example, when a body is immersed in cold water. The amount of heat transferred depends on the temperature difference and the amount and duration of the contact. **Convection** is the dispersion of heat by air currents. The body usually has a small amount of warm air adjacent to it. This warm air rises and is replaced by cooler air, and so people always lose a small amount of heat through convection. Vaporization is continuous evaporation of moisture from the respiratory tract and from the mucosa of the mouth and from the skin. This continuous and unnoticed water loss is called **insensible water loss**, and the accompanying heat loss is called **insensible heat loss**. Insensible heat loss accounts for about 10% of basal heat loss. When the body temperature increases, vaporization accounts for greater heat loss.

Regulation of Body Temperature

The system that regulates body temperature has three main parts: sensors in the shell and in the core, an integrator in the hypothalamus, and an effector system that adjusts the production and loss of heat. Most sensors or sensory receptors

are in the skin. The skin has more receptors for cold than warmth. Therefore, skin sensors detect cold more efficiently than warmth.

When the skin becomes chilled over the entire body, three physiologic processes to increase the body temperature take place: shivering increases heat production, sweating is inhibited to decrease heat loss, and vasoconstriction decreases heat loss.

The hypothalamic integrator, the center that controls the core temperature, is located in the preoptic area of the hypothalamus. When the sensors in the hypothalamus detect heat, they send out signals intended to reduce the temperature, that is, to decrease heat production and increase heat loss. In contrast, when the cold sensors are stimulated, signals are sent out to increase heat production and decrease heat loss.

The signals from the cold-sensitive receptors of the hypothalamus initiate effectors, such as vasoconstriction, shivering, and the release of epinephrine, which increases cellular metabolism and hence heat production. When the warmth-sensitive receptors in the hypothalamus are stimulated, the effector system sends out signals that initiate sweating and peripheral vasodilatation. Also, when this system is stimulated, the person consciously makes appropriate adjustments, such as putting on additional clothing.

Factors Affecting Body Temperature

Understanding the factors that affect body temperature helps nurses recognize normal temperature variations and understand the significance of body temperature measurements that deviate from normal. These factors include age, diurnal variations, exercise, hormones, stress, and environment.

1. *Age.* The infant is greatly influenced by the temperature of the environment and must be protected from extreme changes because they generate heat by burning brown fat located around the kidney. Hypothermia, with rapid burning of brown fat, can result in damage to the kidney. Children's temperatures continue to be more variable than those of adults until puberty. Many older people, particularly those over 75 years, are at risk of hypothermia (temperatures below 36°C, or 96.8°F) for a variety of reasons, such as inadequate diet, loss of subcutaneous fat, lack of activity, and reduced thermoregulatory efficiency. Older adults are also particularly sensitive to extremes in the environmental temperature due to decreased thermoregulatory controls.

2. *Diurnal variations (circadian rhythms).* Body temperatures normally change throughout the day, varying as much as 1.0°C (1.8°F) between the early morning and the late afternoon. The point of highest body temperature is usually reached between 1600 and 1800 hours (4:00 PM and 6:00 PM) (Mackowiak, Wasserman, & Levine, 1992), and the lowest point is reached during sleep between 0400 and 0600 hours (4:00 AM and 6:00 AM). (See Figure 16–2.)

3. *Exercise.* Hard work or strenuous exercise can increase body temperature to as high as 38.3°C to 40°C (101°F

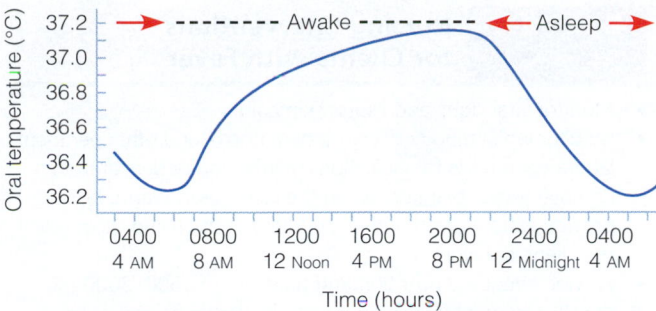

Figure 16–2 ● Range of oral temperatures during 24 hours for a healthy young adult.

to 104°F) measured rectally due to the increased heat from muscle action.

4. *Hormones.* Women usually experience more hormone fluctuations than men. In women, progesterone secretion at the time of ovulation raises body temperature by about 0.3°C to 0.6°C (0.5°F to 1.0°F) above basal temperature.

5. *Stress.* Stimulation of the sympathetic nervous system can increase the production of epinephrine and norepinephrine, thereby increasing metabolic activity and heat production. Nurses may anticipate that a highly stressed or anxious client could have an elevated body temperature for that reason.

6. *Environment.* Extremes in environmental temperatures can affect a person's temperature regulatory systems.

Alterations in Body Temperature

There are two primary alterations in body temperature: pyrexia and hypothermia.

PYREXIA A body temperature above the usual range is called **pyrexia**, hyperthermia, or (in lay terms) fever. A very high fever, such as 41°C (105.8°F), is called hyperpyrexia. The client who has a fever is referred to as **febrile**; the one who does not is **afebrile**.

Four common types of fevers are intermittent, remittent, relapsing, and constant. During an intermittent fever, the body temperature alternates at regular intervals between periods of fever and periods of normal or subnormal temperatures. During a remittent fever a wide range of temperature fluctuations (more than 2°C [3.6°F]) occurs over the 24-hour period, all of which are above normal. In a relapsing fever, short febrile periods of a few days are interspersed with periods of 1 or 2 days of normal temperature. During a constant fever, the body temperature fluctuates minimally but always remains above normal. A temperature that rises to fever level rapidly following a normal temperature and then returns to normal within a few hours is called a fever spike.

In some conditions, an elevated temperature is not a true fever. Two examples are heat exhaustion and heat stroke. Heat exhaustion is a result of excessive heat and dehydration. Signs of heat exhaustion include paleness, dizziness, nausea, vomiting, fainting, and a moderately increased temperature (101°F–102°F). Persons experiencing heat stroke generally have been exercising in hot weather, have warm, flushed skin, and often do not sweat. They usually have a temperature of 106°F or higher, and may be delirious, unconscious, or having seizures.

The clinical signs of fever vary with the onset, course, and abatement stages of the fever (see Clinical Manifestations). These signs occur as a result of changes in the set point of the temperature control mechanism regulated by the hypothalamus. Under normal conditions, whenever the core temperature rises, the rate of heat loss is increased, resulting in a fall in temperature toward the set-point level. Conversely, when the core temperature falls, the rate of heat production is increased, resulting in a rise in temperature toward the set point.

With a fever, the set point of the hypothalamic thermostat changes suddenly from the normal level to a higher than normal value as a result of the effects of tissue destruction, pyrogenic substances, or dehydration. Although the set point changes rapidly, the core body temperature reaches this new set point only after several hours. During this interval, the usual heat production responses that cause elevation of the body temperature occur: chills, feeling of coldness, cold skin due to vasoconstriction, and shivering. This is referred to as the chill phase.

CLINICAL MANIFESTATIONS   Fever

Onset (Cold or Chill Phase)
- Increased heart rate
- Increased respiratory rate and depth
- Shivering
- Pallid, cold skin
- Complaints of feeling cold
- Cyanotic nail beds
- "Gooseflesh" appearance of the skin
- Cessation of sweating

Course (Plateau Phase)
- Absence of chills
- Skin that feels warm
- Photosensitivity
- Glassy-eyed appearance
- Increased pulse and respiratory rates
- Increased thirst
- Mild to severe dehydration
- Drowsiness, restlessness, delirium, or convulsions
- Herpetic lesions of the mouth
- Loss of appetite (if the fever is prolonged)
- Malaise, weakness, and aching muscles

Defervescence (Fever Abatement/Flush Phase)
- Skin that appears flushed and feels warm
- Sweating
- Decreased shivering
- Possible dehydration

When the core temperature reaches the new set point, the person feels neither cold nor hot and no longer experiences chills (the plateau phase). Depending on the degree of temperature elevation, other signs may occur during the course of the fever. Very high temperatures, such as 41°C to 42°C (106°F to 108°F), damage the parenchyma of cells throughout the body, particularly in the brain where destruction of neuronal cells is irreversible. Damage to the liver, kidneys, and other body organs can also be great enough to disrupt functioning and eventually cause death.

When the cause of the high temperature is suddenly removed, the set point of the hypothalamic thermostat is suddenly reduced to a lower value, perhaps even back to the original normal level. In this instance, the hypothalamus now attempts to lower the temperature, and the usual heat loss responses causing a reduction of the body temperature occur: excessive sweating and a hot, flushed skin due to sudden vasodilatation. This is referred to as the flush phase. Nursing interventions for a client who has a fever are designed to support the body's normal physiologic processes, provide comfort, and prevent complications. During the course of fever and for at least 24 hours after the temperature returns to normal, the nurse needs to monitor the client's vital signs closely.

Nursing measures during the chill phase are designed to help the client decrease heat loss. At this time, the body's physiologic processes are attempting to raise the core temperature to the new set-point temperature. During the flush or crisis phase, the body processes are attempting to lower the core temperature to the reduced or normal set-point temperature. At this time, the nurse takes measures to increase heat loss and decrease heat production. Nursing interventions for a client with fever are shown in Box 16–2.

HYPOTHERMIA **Hypothermia** is a core body temperature below the lower limit of normal. The three physiologic mechanisms of hypothermia are (a) excessive heat loss, (b) inadequate heat production to counteract heat loss, and (c) impaired hypothalamic thermoregulation. The clinical signs of hypothermia are listed in the Clinical Manifestations box.

Hypothermia may be induced or accidental. Induced hypothermia is the deliberate lowering of the body temperature to decrease the need for oxygen by the body tissues such as

---

BOX 16–2 Nursing Interventions for Clients with Fever

- Monitor vital signs and assess skin color.
- Monitor white blood cell count, hematocrit, and other pertinent laboratory reports for indications of infection or dehydration.
- Remove excess blankets when the client feels warm, but provide extra warmth when the client feels chilled especially if the client is shivering.
- Provide adequate nutrition and fluids (e.g., 2500–3000 mL per day) to meet increased metabolic demands and prevent dehydration. Measure intake and output.
- Reduce physical activity to limit heat production, especially during the flush stage.
- Administer antipyretics (drugs that reduce the level of fever) as ordered.
- Provide oral hygiene to keep the mucous membranes moist.
- Provide a tepid sponge bath to increase heat loss through conduction.
- Provide dry clothing and bed linens.

---

during certain surgeries. Accidental hypothermia can occur as a result of (a) exposure to a cold environment, (b) immersion in cold water, and (c) lack of adequate clothing, shelter, or heat. In older adults the problem can be compounded by a decreased metabolic rate and the use of sedatives. If skin and underlying tissues are damaged by freezing cold frostbite will result especially in the hands, feet, nose, and ears.

Managing hypothermia involves removing the client from the cold and rewarming the client's body. For the client with mild hypothermia, the body is rewarmed by applying blankets; for the client with severe hypothermia, a hyperthermia blanket (an electronically controlled blanket that provides a specified temperature) is applied, and warm intravenous fluids are given. Wet clothing, which increases heat loss because of the high conductivity of water, should be replaced with dry clothing. See Box 16–3 for nursing interventions for clients who have hypothermia.

See Identifying Nursing Diagnoses, Outcomes, and Interventions for examples of applying the nursing process to clients with temperature alterations.

Assessing Body Temperature

The most common sites for measuring body temperature are oral, rectal, axillary, tympanic membrane, and skin/temporal

---

CLINICAL MANIFESTATIONS Hypothermia

- Decreased body temperature, pulse, and respirations
- Severe shivering (initially)
- Feelings of cold and chills
- Pale, cool, waxy skin
- Frostbite (nose, fingers, toes)
- Hypotension
- Decreased urinary output
- Lack of muscle coordination
- Disorientation
- Drowsiness progressing to coma

BOX 16–3 Nursing Interventions for Clients with Hypothermia

- Provide a warm environment.
- Provide dry clothing.
- Apply warm blankets.
- Keep limbs close to body.
- Cover the client's scalp with a cap or turban.
- Supply warm oral or intravenous fluids.
- Apply warming pads.

artery. Each of the sites has advantages and disadvantages (see Table 16–1).

The body temperature may be measured *orally*. For an accurate reading the nurse should delay measuring the oral temperature if the client has smoked or eaten food or fluids.

Oral temperature readings are contraindicated for clients who are confused because they may bite the thermometer.

Rectal temperature readings are considered to be the most accurate, second only to core temperature measurement, which requires more invasive instruments. In some agencies, taking

TABLE 16–1 Advantages and Disadvantages of Sites for Body Temperature Measurement

SITE AND TYPE OF THERMOMETER	ADVANTAGES	DISADVANTAGES
Oral – using glass nonmercury thermometer or digital thermometer	Accessible and convenient	Thermometers can break if bitten. Inaccurate if client has just ingested hot or cold food or fluid or smoked. Could injure the mouth following oral surgery.
Rectal – using glass nonmercury thermometer or digital thermometer	Reliable measurement	Inconvenient and more unpleasant for clients; difficult for client who cannot turn to the side. May be embarrassing for the adult or older child. Could injure the rectum following rectal surgery. Presence of stool may interfere with thermometer placement. If the stool is soft, the thermometer may be embedded in stool rather than against the wall of the rectum.
Axillary – using glass nonmercury thermometer or digital thermometer	Safe and noninvasive	The thermometer must be left in place a long time to obtain an accurate measurement.
Tympanic membrane – electronic tympanic thermometer	Readily accessible; reflects the core temperature. Very fast.	Can be uncomfortable and involves risk of injuring the membrane if the probe is inserted too far. Repeated measurements may vary. Right and left measurements can differ. Presence of cerumen can affect the reading.
Temporal artery – temporal artery thermometer	Safe and noninvasive; very fast.	Requires electronic equipment that may be expensive or unavailable; variation in technique needed if the client has perspiration on the forehead.
Skin – temperature-sensitive tape	Convenient, quick, noninvasive, useful for home and infants requiring frequent monitoring	Indicates surface, not core, temperature, effected by environmental temperature, only useful for indicating general surface temperature.

IDENTIFYING NURSING DIAGNOSES, OUTCOMES, AND INTERVENTIONS   **Imbalanced Body Temperature**

NURSING DIAGNOSIS/DEFINITION	SAMPLE DESIRED OUTCOMES*/DEFINITION	INDICATORS†	SELECTED INTERVENTIONS*/DEFINITION	SAMPLE ACTIVITIES (ALSO SEE BOXES 16–2 & 16–3)
Risk for Imbalanced Body Temperature/At risk for failure to maintain body temperature within normal range	Hydration [0602]/Adequate water in the intracellular and extracellular compartments of the body	• Moist mucous membranes • Urine output	Temperature Regulation [3900]/Attaining and/or maintaining body temperature within a normal range	Monitor temperature every 2 hours, as appropriate Promote adequate fluid and nutritional intake
Hyperthermia/Body temperature elevated above normal range	Thermoregulation [0800]/Balance among heat production, heat gain, and heat loss	• Skin temperature in expected range • Body temperature in expected range • Sweating when hot	Fever Treatment [3740]/Management of a patient with hyperpyrexia caused by nonenvironmental factors	Monitor intake and output Apply ice bag covered with a towel to groin Cover the patient with only a sheet

*The NOC # for desired outcomes and the NIC # for nursing interventions are listed in brackets following the appropriate outcome or intervention. Outcomes, indicators, interventions, and activities selected are only a sample of those suggested by NOC and NIC and should be further individualized for each client.

†The measurement scale for these indicators ranges from Extremely compromised to Not compromised. See MyNursingKit.

temperatures rectally is contraindicated for clients with myocardial infarction because it is believed that inserting a rectal thermometer can produce vagal stimulation, which in turn can cause abnormal heart rhythms. Rectal temperatures are contraindicated for clients who are undergoing rectal surgery, have diarrhea or diseases of the rectum, are immunosuppressed, have a clotting disorder, or have significant hemorrhoids.

The *axilla* is the preferred site for measuring temperature in newborns because it is accessible and safe. However, some research indicates that the axillary method is inaccurate when assessing a fever (Bindler & Ball, 2007). Nurses should check agency protocol when taking the temperature of newborns, infants, toddlers, and children. Adult clients for whom the axillary method of temperature assessment is appropriate include those for whom other temperature sites are contraindicated.

The *tympanic membrane*, or nearby tissue in the ear canal, is a frequent site for estimating core body temperature. Like the sublingual oral site, the tympanic membrane has an abundant arterial blood supply, primarily from branches of the external carotid artery. Because temperature sensors applied directly to the tympanic membrane can be uncomfortable and involve risk of membrane injury or perforation, noninvasive infrared thermometers are used.

The temperature may also be measured on the forehead using a chemical thermometer or a temporal artery thermometer. Forehead temperature measurements are most useful for infants and children when a more invasive measurement is not necessary.

TYPES OF THERMOMETERS   Traditionally, body temperatures were measured using mercury-in-glass thermometers. However, risk of mercury exposure has led to the use of nonmercury thermometers. In some cases, plastics have replaced glass and safer chemicals have replaced mercury in modern versions of the thermometer. However, the nurse may still encounter this type of thermometer. Although the amount of mercury in a thermometer (or in a fluorescent lightbulb) is minimal, should it break, cleanup must follow agency policy because the mercury is treated as a hazardous substance.

Electronic thermometers can provide a reading in only 2 to 60 seconds, depending on the model. The equipment consists of a battery-operated portable electronic unit, a probe that the nurse attaches to the unit, and a probe cover, which is usually disposable. Some models have a different circuit and probe for oral and rectal measurement.

Two specific types of oral thermometers that can be glass or electronic are basal and hypothermia. A basal thermometer is calibrated with 0.1°F intervals and is for fertility purposes, indicating the temperature rise that is associated with ovulation. Hypothermia thermometers have a greater low range than everyday thermometers, usually measuring temperatures from 81°F to 108°F.

Chemical disposable thermometers use liquid crystal in the shape of dots or bars that change color to indicate temperature. Heat sensitive tape or patches serve the same purpose. They may either single use disposable or reusable. To read the temperature, the nurse notes the highest reading among the dots that have changed color.

Temperature-sensitive tape may also be used to obtain a general indication of body surface temperature. It does not indicate the core temperature. The tape contains liquid crystals that change color according to temperature. When applied to the skin, usually of the forehead or abdomen, the temperature digits on the tape respond by changing color. The skin area should be dry. After the length of time specified by the manufacturer, a color appears on the tape. This method is particularly useful at home and for infants whose temperatures are to be monitored.

Infrared thermometers sense body heat in the form of infrared energy given off by a heat source, which in the ear canal is primarily the tympanic membrane. The infrared thermometer makes no contact with the tympanic membrane.

Temporal artery thermometers determine temperature using a scanning infrared thermometer that compares arterial temperature in the temporal artery of the forehead to the temperature in the room and calculates the heat balance to approximate the core temperature of the blood in the pulmonary artery (Roy, Powell, & Gerson, 2003). The probe is placed in the middle of the forehead and then drawn laterally to the hairline (Figure 16–3). If the client has perspiration on the forehead, the probe is also touched behind the earlobe so the thermometer can compensate for evaporative cooling.

TEMPERATURE SCALES   The body temperature is measured in degrees on two scales: Celsius (centigrade) and Fahrenheit. Sometimes a nurse needs to convert a Celsius reading to Fahrenheit, or vice versa. Although the conver-

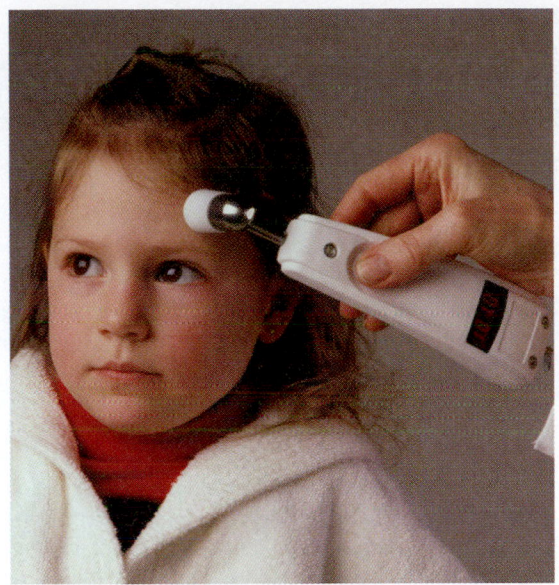

Figure 16–3 ○ A temporal artery thermometer.

sion can be accomplished using several different formulas, the most common is described here. To convert from Fahrenheit to Celsius, deduct 32 from the Fahrenheit reading and then multiply by the fraction 5/9. To convert from Celsius to Fahrenheit, multiply the Celsius reading by the fraction 9/5 and then add 32.

Skill 16–1 explains how to measure body temperature.

SKILL 16–1

ASSESSING BODY TEMPERATURE

PURPOSES
- To establish baseline data for subsequent evaluation and identify current temperature

ASSESSMENT
Assess
- Clinical signs of fever or hypothermia
- Site most appropriate for measurement
- Factors impacting the client that may alter core body temperature

PLANNING

Delegation

Routine measurement of the client's temperature can be delegated to unlicensed assistive personnel (UAP)—or to family members/caregivers in nonhospital settings. The nurse must explain the appropriate type of thermometer and site to be used and ensure that the person knows when to report an abnormal temperature and how to record the finding. The interpretation of an abnormal temperature and determination of appropriate responses are done by the nurse.

EQUIPMENT
- Thermometer
- Thermometer sheath or cover
- Water-soluble lubricant for a rectal temperature
- Clean gloves for a rectal temperature
- Towel for axillary temperature
- Tissues/wipes

(continued)

SKILL 16–1

ASSESSING BODY TEMPERATURE *(continued)*

IMPLEMENTATION

Preparation
Check that all equipment is functioning normally.

Performance
1. Prior to performing the procedure, introduce self and verify the client's identity using agency protocol. Explain to the client what you are going to do, why it is necessary, and how he or she can participate. Discuss how the results will be used in planning further care or treatments. **Rationale:** *Assure procedure is performed on correct client and reduce client anxiety.*
2. Perform hand hygiene and observe appropriate infection control procedures. Don gloves if performing a rectal temperature. **Rationale:** *Protects both the client and the nurse from infection.*
3. Provide for client privacy. **Rationale:** *Reduces client embarrassment and increase client comfort.*
4. Place the client in the appropriate position. **Rationale:** *Reduces risk of injury and improve accuracy of reading.*
5. Place the thermometer (see Box 16–4).
   - Apply a protective sheath or probe cover if appropriate. **Rationale:** *Prevents cross contamination of using device on multiple clients.*
   - Lubricate a rectal thermometer. **Rationale:** *Prevents tissue trauma when inserting the thermometer.*
6. Wait the appropriate amount of time. Electronic and tympanic thermometers will indicate that the reading is complete through a light or tone. Check package instructions for length of time to wait prior to reading chemical dot or tape thermometers. **Rationale:** *Improves accuracy of measurement.*

CLINICAL ALERT

Be sure to record the temperature from an electronic thermometer before replacing the probe into the charging unit. With many models, replacing the probe erases the temperature from the display.

7. Remove the thermometer and discard the cover or wipe with a tissue if necessary. If gloves were applied, remove and discard gloves. Perform hand hygiene.
8. Read the temperature and record it on your worksheet. If the temperature is obviously too high, too low, or inconsistent with the client's condition, recheck it with a different thermometer. **Rationale:** *Equipment can fail and it is important to treat the client, not the equipment. Rechecking with another thermometer assures the client receives appropriate treatment.*
9. Wash the thermometer if necessary and return it to the storage location. **Rationale:** *Wiping the thermometer prevents or reduces the risk of spreading pathogens to other clients. Returning it to the normal storage location makes multi-use thermometers available for other care providers.*
10. Document the temperature in the client record. A rectal temperature may be recorded with an "R" next to the value or with the mark on a graphic sheet circled. An axillary temperature may be recorded with "AX" or marked on a graphic sheet with an X. **Rationale:** *The site where the temperature is measured impacts the interpretation of the measurement.*

EVALUATION
- Compare the temperature measurement to baseline data, normal range for age of client, and client's previous temperatures. Analyze considering time of day and any additional influencing factors and other vital signs.
- Conduct appropriate follow-up such as notifying the primary care provider, giving a medication, or altering the client's environment. Teach the client how to lower an elevated temperature through actions such as increasing fluid intake, coughing and deep breathing, or removing heavy coverings or elevate a low temperature through proper attire, blankets, or a warming blanket.

PULSE

The **pulse** is a wave of blood created by contraction of the left ventricle of the heart generally representing the stroke volume output or the amount of blood that enters the arteries with each ventricular contraction. **Compliance** of the arteries is their ability to contract and expand. When a person's arteries lose their distensibility, as can happen in old age, greater pressure is required to pump blood into the arteries. **Cardiac output** is the volume of blood pumped into the arteries by the heart and equals the result of the stroke volume (SV) times the heart rate (HR) per minute.

In a healthy person, the pulse reflects the heartbeat; that is, the pulse rate is the same as the rate of the ventricular contractions of the heart. However, in some types of cardiovascular disease, the heartbeat and pulse rates can differ because the client's heart may produce very weak or small pulse waves that are not detectable in a peripheral pulse far from the heart. In these instances, the nurse should assess the heartbeat and the peripheral pulse. A peripheral pulse is a pulse located away from the heart. The apical pulse is a central pulse located at the apex of the heart. It is also referred to as the **point of maximal impulse (PMI).**

Factors Affecting the Pulse

The rate of the pulse is expressed in beats per minute (BPM). A pulse rate varies according to a number of factors.

LIFESPAN CONSIDERATIONS   Temperature

Infants

- The body temperature of newborns is extremely labile, and newborns must be kept warm and dry to prevent hypothermia.
- Using the axillary site, you need to hold the infant's arm against the chest. The axillary route may not be as accurate as other routes for detecting fevers in children (Bindler & Ball, 2007).
- The tympanic route is fast and convenient. Place the infant supine and stabilize the head. Pull the pinna straight back and slightly downward. Direct the probe tip anteriorly and insert far enough to seal the canal. The tip will not touch the tympanic membrane. Avoid the tympanic route in a child with active ear infections or tympanic membrane drainage tubes. The tympanic membrane route may be more accurate in determining temperature in febrile infants (Liu, Chang, & Chang, 2004; Nimah, Bshesh, Callahan, & Jacobs, 2006).
- When using a temporal artery thermometer, touching only the forehead or behind the ear is needed.
- The rectal route is least desirable in infants due to the risk of rectal perforation if the thermometer is inserted too far or the infant is not adequately restrained from moving.

Children

- Tympanic or temporal artery sites are preferred. For the tympanic route, have the child held on an adult's lap with the child's head held gently against the adult for support. Pull the pinna straight back and upward for children over age 3. Avoid the tympanic route in a child with active ear infections or tympanic membrane drainage tubes.
- The oral route may be used for children over age 3, but nonbreakable, electronic thermometers are recommended.
- For a rectal temperature, place the child prone across the lap of a parent or in a side-lying position with the knees flexed. Insert the thermometer 1 inch into the rectum.

Older Adults

- Older adults' temperatures tend to be lower than those of middle-aged adults.
- Older adults' temperatures are strongly influenced by both environmental and internal temperature changes. Their thermoregulation control processes are not as efficient as when they are younger, and they are at higher risk for both hypothermia and hyperthermia.
- Older adults can develop significant buildup of ear cerumen that may interfere with tympanic thermometer readings.
- Older adults are more likely to have hemorrhoids. Inspect the anus before taking a rectal temperature.
- Older adults' temperatures may not be a valid indication of the seriousness of the pathology of a disease. They may have pneumonia or a urinary tract infection and have only a slight temperature elevation. Other symptoms, such as confusion and restlessness, may be displayed and need follow-up to determine if there is an underlying process.
- Older adult client's conditions can change rapidly. Assess prior to measuring temperature to determine the best site.

BOX 16–4	Thermometer Placement
Oral	Place the bulb on either side of the frenulum.
Rectal	Apply clean gloves.
	Instruct the client to take a slow, deep breath during insertion.
	Never force the thermometer if resistance is felt.
	Insert 3.5 cm (1 1/2 in.) in adults.
Axillary	Pat the axilla dry if very moist.
	The bulb is placed in the center of the axilla.
Tympanic	Pull the pinna slightly upward and backward.
	Point the probe slightly anteriorly, toward the eardrum.
	Insert the probe slowly using a circular motion until snug.
Temporal artery	Brush hair aside if covering the TA area. With the probe flush on the center of the forehead, depress the red button; keep depressed. Slowly slide the probe midline across the forehead to the hair line, not down the side of the face. Lift the probe from the forehead and touch on the neck just behind the earlobe. Release the button.

The nurse should consider each of the following factors when assessing a client's pulse:

- *Age.* As age increases, the pulse rate gradually decreases overall. See Table 16–2 for specific variations in pulse rates from birth to adulthood.
- *Gender.* After puberty, the average male's pulse rate is slightly lower than the female's.
- *Exercise.* The pulse rate normally increases with activity. The rate of increase in the professional athlete is often less than in the average person because of greater cardiac size, strength, and efficiency.
- *Fever.* The pulse rate increases (a) in response to the lowered blood pressure that results from peripheral vasodilatation associated with elevated body temperature and (b) because of the increased metabolic rate.
- *Medications.* Some medications decrease the pulse rate, and others increase it.
- *Hypovolemia.* Loss of blood from the vascular system normally increases pulse rate. In adults the loss of circulating volume results in an adjustment of the heart rate to increase blood pressure as the body compensates for the lost blood volume. Adults can usually lose up to 10% of their normal circulating volume without adverse effects.

TABLE 16–2	Variations in Pulse and Respirations by Age	
AGE	PULSE AVERAGE (AND RANGES)	RESPIRATIONS AVERAGE (AND RANGES)
Newborn	130 (80–180)	35 (30–80)
1 year	120 (80–140)	30 (20–40)
5–8 years	100 (75–120)	20 (15–25)
10 years	70 (50–90)	19 (15–25)
Teen	75 (50–90)	18 (15–20)
Adult	80 (60–100)	16 (12–20)
Older adult	70 (60–100)	16 (15–20)

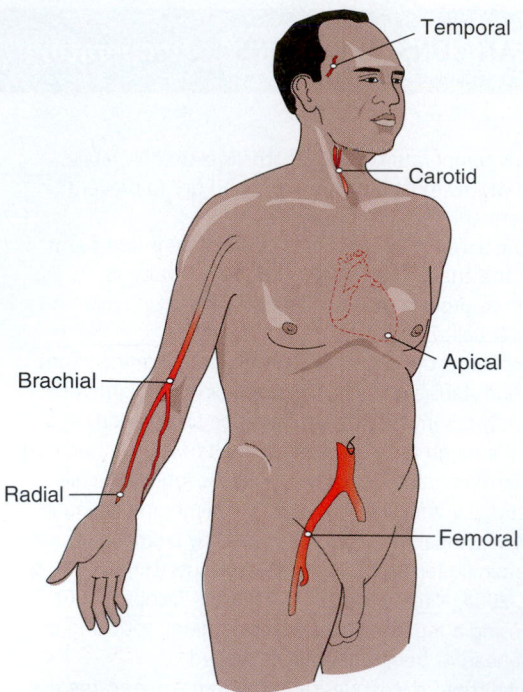

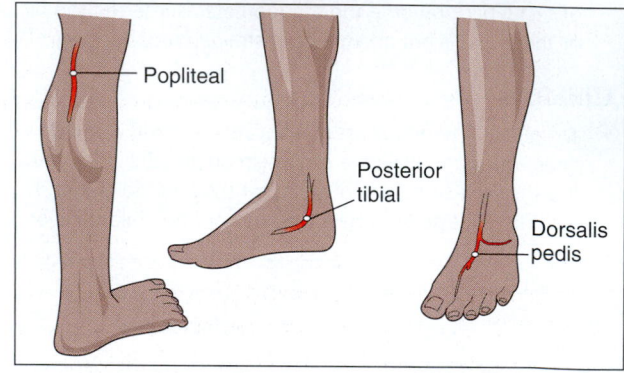

Figure 16–4 ◯ Nine sites for assessing pulse.

- *Stress.* In response to stress, sympathetic nervous stimulation increases the overall activity of the heart. Stress increases the rate as well as the force of the heartbeat. Fear and anxiety as well as the perception of severe pain stimulate the sympathetic system.
- *Position changes.* When a person is sitting or standing, blood usually pools in dependent vessels of the venous system. Pooling results in a transient decrease in the venous blood return to the heart and a subsequent reduction in blood pressure and increase in heart rate.
- *Pathology.* Certain diseases such as some heart conditions or those that impair oxygenation can alter the resting pulse rate.

Pulse Sites

A pulse may be measured in nine sites (see Figure 16–4).

1. Temporal, where the temporal artery passes over the temporal bone of the head. The site is superior (above) and lateral to (away from the midline of) the eye.
2. Carotid, at the side of the neck where the carotid artery runs between the trachea and the sternocleidomastoid muscle.

CLINICAL ALERT

Never press both carotids at the same time because this can cause a reflex drop in blood pressure or pulse rate.

3. Apical, at the apex of the heart. In an adult this is located on the left side of the chest, about 8 cm (3 in.) to the left of the sternum (breastbone) and at the fourth, fifth, or sixth intercostal space (area between the ribs). In older adults, the apex may be further left if there are conditions that have led to an enlarged heart. Before 4 years of age the apex is left of the midclavicular line (MCL); between 4 and 6 years, it is at the MCL. For a

child 7 to 9 years of age, the apical pulse is located at the fourth or fifth intercostal space.

4. Brachial, at the inner aspect of the biceps muscle of the arm or medially in the antecubital space.
5. Radial, where the radial artery runs along the radial bone, on the thumb side of the inner aspect of the wrist.
6. Femoral, where the femoral artery passes alongside the inguinal ligament.
7. Popliteal, where the popliteal artery passes behind the knee.
8. Posterior tibial, on the medial surface of the ankle where the posterior tibial artery passes behind the medial malleolus.
9. Pedal (dorsalis pedis), where the dorsalis pedis artery passes over the bones of the foot, on an imaginary line drawn from the middle of the ankle to the space between the big and second toes. The radial site is most commonly used in adults. It is easily found in most people and read-

IDENTIFYING NURSING DIAGNOSES, OUTCOMES, AND INTERVENTIONS — Ineffective Peripheral Tissue Perfusion

NURSING DIAGNOSIS/DEFINITION	SAMPLE DESIRED OUTCOMES*/DEFINITION	INDICATORS†	SELECTED INTERVENTIONS*/DEFINITION	SAMPLE ACTIVITIES
Ineffective Peripheral Tissue Perfusion/Decrease in oxygen resulting in the failure to nourish the tissues at the capillary level	Tissue Perfusion: Peripheral [0407]/Adequacy of blood flow through the small vessels of the extremities to maintain tissue function	• Distal peripheral pulses strong • Distal peripheral pulses symmetrical	Vital Signs Monitoring [6680]/Collection and analysis of cardiovascular, respiratory, and body temperature data to determine and prevent complications	Monitor presence and quality of pulses Take apical and radial pulses simultaneously and note the difference Monitor cardiac rhythm and rate

*The NOC # for desired outcomes and the NIC # for nursing interventions are listed in brackets following the appropriate outcome or intervention. Outcomes, indicators, interventions, and activities selected are only a sample of those suggested by NOC and NIC and should be further individualized for each client.

† The measurement scale for these indicators ranges from Extremely compromised to Not compromised. See MyNursingKit.

ily accessible. See Identifying Nursing Diagnoses, Outcomes, and Interventions for examples of applying the nursing process to clients with pulse alterations.

Assessing the Pulse

A pulse is commonly assessed by palpation (feeling) or auscultation (hearing). The pads of the middle three fingertips are used for palpating all pulse sites except the apex of the heart, applying moderate pressure. Excessive pressure can obliterate the pulse. A stethoscope is used for assessing apical pulses. A Doppler ultrasound stethoscope is used for pulses that are difficult to palpate. The DUS headset has earpieces similar to standard stethoscope earpieces, but it has a long cord attached to a volume-controlled audio unit and an ultrasound transducer. The DUS detects movement of red blood cells through a blood vessel. In contrast to the conventional stethoscope, it excludes environmental sounds and amplifies the pulsation.

Prior to assessing the pulse, the nurse should also be aware of factors that could influence pulse rate, including mediations, activity, or the need to place the client in a specific position. The nurse should be aware of baseline data about the client's normal and recent heart rate in order to determine significant variations.

When assessing the pulse, the nurse collects the following data: the rate, rhythm, volume, arerial wall elasticity, and presence or absence of bilateral equality. A fast heart rate (e.g., over 100 BPM in an adult) is referred to as **tachycardia**. A heart rate in an adult of less than 60 BPM is called **bradycardia**. If a client has either tachycardia or bradycardia, the apical pulse should be assessed.

The pulse rhythm is the pattern of the beats and the intervals between the beats. A normal pulse should be regular with equal time between beats. A pulse with an irregular rhythm is referred to as a **dysrhythmia** or **arrhythmia**. It may consist of random, irregular beats or a predictable pattern of irregular beats (documented as "regularly irregular"). When a dysrhythmia is detected, the apical pulse should be assessed. An electrocardiogram (ECG or EKG) is necessary to define the dysrhythmia further.

Pulse volume, also called the pulse strength or amplitude, refers to the force of blood with each beat. Usually, the pulse volume is the same with each beat. It can range from absent to bounding. A normal pulse can be felt with moderate pressure of the fingers and can be obliterated with greater pressure. A forceful or full blood volume that is obliterated only with difficulty is called a full or bounding pulse. A pulse that is readily obliterated with pressure from the fingers is referred to as weak, feeble, or thready.

The elasticity of the arterial wall reflects its expansibility or its deformities. A healthy, normal artery feels straight, smooth, soft, and pliable. Older adults often have inelastic arteries that feel twisted (tortuous) and irregular upon palpation.

When assessing a peripheral pulse to determine the adequacy of blood flow to a particular area of the body (perfusion), the nurse should also assess the corresponding pulse on the other side of the body. The second assessment gives the nurse data with which to compare the pulses. The pulse rate does not need to be counted when assessing for perfusion and equality.

When a peripheral pulse is located, it indicates that pulses more proximal to that location will also be present. For example, if the dorsalis pedis, the most distal pulse of the lower extremity, cannot be felt, the nurse next palpates for the posterior tibial pulse. If it is not felt, the popliteal pulse must be assessed. If the popliteal pulse is found, it is not necessary to assess the femoral pulse since it must also be present in order for the more distal pulse to exist.

Skill 16–2 provides guidelines for assessing a peripheral pulse.

SKILL 16-2

ASSESSING A PERIPHERAL PULSE

PURPOSES

- To identify whether the pulse rate is within normal range and establish baseline data for subsequent evaluation
- To determine whether the pulse rhythm is regular and the pulse volume is appropriate

- To determine equality of corresponding peripheral pulses on each side of the body and to evaluate blood perfusion to the extremities
- To monitor and assess changes in the client's health status
- To monitor clients at risk for pulse alterations

ASSESSMENT

Assess

- Clinical signs of cardiovascular alterations such as dyspnea, fatigue, pallor, cyanosis, palpitations, syncope, or impaired peripheral tissue perfusion

- Factors that may alter pulse rate
- Site that is most appropriate for assessment based on the purpose of the exam

PLANNING

> **Delegation**
>
> Measurement of the client's radial or brachial pulse can be delegated to UAP—or family members/caregivers in nonhospital settings. Reports of abnormal pulse rates or rhythms require reassessment by the nurse, who also determines appropriate action if the abnormality is confirmed. Examination of other peripheral pulses or use of a Doppler are generally not delegated to the UAP due to the skill required in locating and interpreting peripheral pulses other than the radial or brachial artery and in using Doppler ultrasound devices.

EQUIPMENT

- Watch with a second hand or indicator
- If using a DUS: transducer probe, stethoscope headset, transmission gel, and tissues/wipes

IMPLEMENTATION

Preparation

If using a DUS, check that the equipment is functioning normally.

Performance

1. Prior to performing the procedure, introduce self and verify the client's identity using agency protocol. Explain to the client what you are going to do, why it is necessary, and how he or she can participate. Discuss how the results will be used in planning further care or treatments. **Rationale:** *Assures procedure is performed on correct client and reduce client anxiety.*
2. Perform hand hygiene and observe appropriate infection control procedures. **Rationale:** *Protects both the client and the nurse from infection.*
3. Provide for client privacy. **Rationale:** *Reduces client embarrassment and increase client comfort.*
4. Select the pulse point. Normally, the radial pulse is taken, unless it cannot be exposed or circulation to another body area is to be assessed. **Rationale:** *Selection of pulse site can have an effect on the accuracy of the assessment.*
5. Assist the client to a comfortable resting position. When the radial pulse is assessed, with the palm facing downward, the client's arm can rest alongside the body or the forearm can rest at a 90-degree angle across the chest. For the client who can sit, the forearm can rest across the thigh, with the palm of the hand facing downward or inward. **Rationale:** *Reduces risk of injury and improve accuracy of reading.*
6. Palpate and count the pulse. Place two or three middle fingertips lightly and squarely over the pulse point. **Rationale:** *Using the thumb is contraindicated because the nurse's thumb has a pulse that could be mistaken for the client's pulse.*
   - Count for 15 seconds and multiply by 4. Record the pulse in beats per minute on your worksheet. If taking

a client's pulse for the first time, when obtaining baseline data, or if the pulse is irregular, count for a full minute. If an irregular pulse is found, also take the apical pulse. **Rationale:** *Experienced nurses can obtain a pulse measurement quickly by counting for only 15 seconds and multiplying by 4. However, if the pulse is irregular or it is the first time measuring the client's pulse rate a full minute is required to obtain an accurate reading.*

7. Assess the pulse rhythm and volume.
   - Assess the pulse rhythm by noting the pattern of the intervals between the beats. A normal pulse has equal time periods between beats. If this is an initial assessment, assess for 1 minute. **Rationale:** *Pulse assessment includes determining not only the rate but the regularity of the client's heart beat.*
   - Assess the pulse volume. A normal pulse can be felt with moderate pressure, and the pressure is equal with each beat. A forceful pulse volume is full; an easily obliterated pulse is weak. Record the rhythm and volume on your worksheet. **Rationale:** *Alterations in pulse volume can impact future treatment decisions.*
8. Document the pulse rate, rhythm, and volume and your actions in the client record. Also record pertinent related data such as variation in pulse rate compared to normal for the client and abnormal skin color and skin temperature in the nurse's notes. **Rationale:** *Documenting findings communicates information to other members of the health care team and provides a baseline for comparison of later trends. Documenting rhythm and volume demonstrates that you have assessed these factors.*

VARIATION: USING A DUS

- If used, plug the stethoscope headset into one of the two output jacks located next to the volume control. DUS units may have two jacks so that a second person can listen to the signals.
- Apply transmission gel either to the probe at the narrow end of the plastic case housing the transducer, or to the client's skin. **Rationale:** *Ultrasound beams do not travel well through air. The gel makes an airtight seal, which then promotes optimal ultrasound wave transmission.*
- Press the "on" button and hold the probe against the skin over the pulse site. Use a light pressure, and keep the probe in contact with the skin. **Rationale:** *Too much pressure can stop the blood flow and obliterate the signal.*

EVALUATION

- Compare the pulse rate to baseline data or normal range for age of client.
- Relate pulse rate and volume to other vital signs; pulse rhythm and volume to baseline data and health status.

- Adjust the volume if necessary. Distinguish artery sounds from vein sounds. The artery sound is distinctively pulsating and has a pumping quality. The venous sound is intermittent and varies with respirations. If arterial sounds cannot be easily heard, reposition the probe. **Rationale:** *Both artery and vein sounds are heard simultaneously through the DUS because major arteries and veins are situated close together throughout the body.*
- After assessing the pulse, remove all gel from the probe to prevent damage to the surface. Clean the transducer with water-based solution. **Rationale:** *Alcohol or other disinfectants may damage the face of the transducer.* Remove all gel from the client.

- If assessing peripheral pulses, evaluate equality, rate, and volume in corresponding extremities.
- Conduct appropriate follow-up such as notifying the primary care provider or giving medication.

APICAL PULSE ASSESSMENT   Assessment of the apical pulse is indicated for clients whose peripheral pulse is irregular or unavailable as well as for clients with known cardiovascular, pulmonary, and renal diseases. It is commonly assessed prior to administering medications that affect heart rate. The apical site is also used to assess the pulse for newborns, infants, and children up to 2 to 3 years old. Skill 16–3 presents guidelines for assessing the apical pulse.

SKILL 16–3

ASSESSING AN APICAL PULSE

PURPOSES

- To obtain the heart rate of infants and children until 3 years of age or of an adult with an irregular peripheral pulse or with cardiac, pulmonary, or renal disease and those receiving medications to improve heart action

- To establish baseline data for subsequent evaluation and determine whether the cardiac rate is within normal range and the rhythm is regular

ASSESSMENT

Assess

- Clinical signs of cardiovascular alterations
- Factors that may alter pulse rate

EQUIPMENT

- Watch with a second hand or indicator
- Stethoscope

PLANNING

Delegation
Due to the degree of skill and knowledge required, UAP are generally not responsible for assessing apical pulses.

- Antiseptic wipes

IMPLEMENTATION

Preparation
Clean the earpieces of the stethoscope prior to using them, especially if it is not a personal stethoscope.

Test stethoscope to determine that it is functioning properly.

Performance

1. Prior to performing the procedure, introduce self and verify the client's identity using agency protocol. Explain to the client what you are going to do, why it is necessary, and how he or she can cooperate. Discuss how the results will be used in planning further care or treatments. **Rationale:** *Assure procedure is performed on correct client and reduce client anxiety.*
2. Perform hand hygiene and observe appropriate infection control procedures. **Rationale:** *Protect both the client and the nurse from infection.*

3. Provide for client privacy. **Rationale:** *Reduce client embarrassment and increase client comfort.*
4. Position the client appropriately in a comfortable supine position or in a sitting position. Expose the area of the chest over the apex of the heart. **Rationale:** *Reduce risk of injury and improve accuracy of reading.*
5. Locate the apical impulse. This is the point over the apex of the heart where the apical pulse can be most clearly heard.
   - Palpate the angle of Louis (the angle between the manubrium, the top of the sternum, and the body of the sternum). It is palpated just below the suprasternal notch and is felt as a prominence.
   - Slide your index finger just to the left of the sternum, and palpate the second intercostal space.

(continued)

ASSESSING AN APICAL PULSE *(continued)*

- Place your middle or next finger in the third intercostal space, and continue palpating downward until you locate the fifth intercostal space.
- Move your index finger laterally along the fifth intercostal space toward the midclavicular line (MCL). Normally, the apical impulse is palpable at or just medial to the MCL. **Rationale:** *Proper location of the PMI will improve the accuracy of the assessment.*

6. Auscultate and count heartbeats.
   - Warm the diaphragm of the stethoscope by holding it in the palm of the hand for a moment. **Rationale:** *The metal of the diaphragm is usually cold and can startle the client when placed immediately on the chest.*
   - Insert the earpieces of the stethoscope into your ears in the direction of the ear canals, or slightly forward, *to facilitate hearing.*
   - Tap your finger lightly on the diaphragm *to be sure it is the active side of the stethoscope's head.* If necessary, rotate the head to select the diaphragm side.

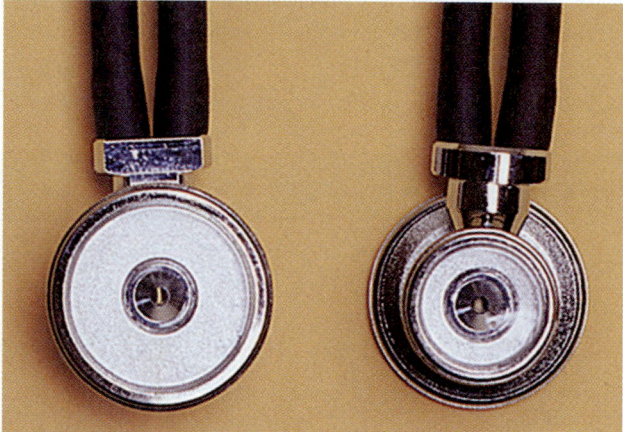

- Place the diaphragm of the stethoscope over the apical impulse and listen for the normal S_1 and S_2 heart sounds, which are heard as "lub-dub." **Rationale:** *The heartbeat is normally loudest over the apex of the heart.* Each lub-dub is counted as one heartbeat.
- If you have difficulty hearing the apical pulse, ask the supine client to roll onto his or her left side or the sitting client to lean slightly forward. **Rationale:** *This positioning moves the apex of the heart closer to the chest wall.*
- If the rhythm is regular, count the heartbeats for 30 seconds and multiply by 2. If the rhythm is irregular or when administering medications impacting heart rate, count the beats for 60 seconds. **Rationale:** *A 60-second count provides a more accurate assessment of an irregular pulse than a 30-second count.*

7. Assess the rhythm and the strength of the heartbeat.
   - Assess the rhythm of the heartbeat by noting the pattern of intervals between the beats. A normal pulse has equal time periods between beats.
   - Assess the strength (volume) of the heartbeat. Normally, the heartbeats are equal in strength and can be described as strong or weak.

8. Document the pulse site, rate, rhythm, and volume and nursing actions in the client record. Also record pertinent related data such as variation in pulse rate compared to normal for the client and abnormal skin color and skin temperature.

EVALUATION

- Relate the pulse rate to other vital signs. Relate the pulse rhythm to baseline data and health status.
- Report to the primary care provider any abnormal findings such as irregular rhythm, and reduced ability to hear the heartbeat, pallor, cyanosis, dyspnea, tachycardia, or bradycardia.
- Conduct appropriate follow-up such as administering medication ordered based on apical heart rate.

APICAL-RADIAL PULSE ASSESSMENT   An apical-radial pulse may need to be assessed for clients with certain cardiovascular disorders. Normally, the apical and radial rates are identical. An apical pulse rate greater than a radial pulse rate can indicate that the thrust of the blood from the heart is too weak for the wave to be felt at the peripheral pulse site, or it can indicate that vascular disease is preventing impulses from being trans-mitted. Any discrepancy between the two pulse rates is called a pulse deficit and needs to be reported promptly. In no instance is the radial pulse greater than the apical pulse.

An apical-radial pulse can be taken by two nurses or one nurse, although the two-nurse technique may be more accurate. Skill 16–4 outlines the steps for assessing an apical-radial pulse.

SKILL 16–4

ASSESSING AN APICAL-RADIAL PULSE

PURPOSE
- To determine adequacy of peripheral circulation or presence of pulse deficit

ASSESSMENT
Assess
- Clinical signs of hypovolemic shock

PLANNING

> **Delegation**
> UAP are generally not responsible for assessing apical-radial pulses.

EQUIPMENT
- Watch with a second hand or indicator
- Stethoscope
- Antiseptic wipes

IMPLEMENTATION

Preparation
If using the two-nurse technique, ensure that the other nurse is available at this time.

Performance
1. Prior to performing the procedure, introduce self and verify the client's identity using agency protocol. Explain to the client what you are going to do, why it is necessary, and how he or she can participate. Discuss how the results will be used in planning further care or treatments. **Rationale:** *Assures procedure is performed on correct client and reduces client anxiety.*
2. Perform hand hygiene and observe appropriate infection control procedures. **Rationale:** *Protects both the client and the nurse from infection.*
3. Provide for client privacy. **Rationale:** *Reduces client embarrassment and increases client comfort.*
4. Position the client appropriately. Assist the client to a comfortable supine or sitting position. Expose the area of the chest over the apex of the heart. If previous measurements were taken, determine what position the client assumed, and use the same position. **Rationale:** *This ensures an accurate comparative measurement.*
5. Locate the apical and radial pulse sites. In the two-nurse technique, one nurse locates the apical pulse by palpation or with the stethoscope while the other nurse palpates the radial pulse site (see Skills 16–2 and 16–3).
6. Count the apical and radial pulse rates.

Two-Nurse Technique
- Place the watch where both nurses can see it. The nurse who is taking the radial pulse may hold the watch.

- Decide on a time to begin counting. A time when the second hand is on 12, 3, 6, or 9 or an even number on digital clocks is usually selected. The nurse taking the radial pulse says "Start." **Rationale:** *This ensures that simultaneous counts are taken.*
- Each nurse counts the pulse rate for 60 seconds. Both nurses end the count when the nurse taking the radial pulse says "Stop." **Rationale:** *A full 60-second count is necessary for accurate assessment of any discrepancies between the two pulse sites.*
- The nurse who assesses the apical rate also assesses the apical pulse rhythm and volume. If the pulse is irregular, note whether the irregular beats come at random or at predictable times.
- The nurse assessing the radial pulse rate also assesses the radial pulse rhythm and volume.

One-Nurse Technique
- Assess the apical pulse for 60 seconds.
- Assess the radial pulse for 60 seconds.
Note: *If the client is connected to a cardiorespiratory monitor, the nurse can run a 60-second rhythm strip while counting the radial pulse in place of counting the apical pulse. However, the apical pulse should still be assessed for rhythm and volume.*

7. Document the apical and radial (AR) pulse rates, rhythm, volume, and any pulse deficit in the client record. Also record related data such as variation in pulse rate compared to normal for the client and other pertinent observations, such as pallor, cyanosis, or dyspnea.

EVALUATION
- Relate pulse rate and rhythm to other vital signs, to baseline data, and to general health status.
- Report to the primary care provider any changes from previous measurements or any discrepancy between the two pulses.

- Conduct appropriate follow-up such as administering medication or other actions to be taken for a discrepancy in the AR pulse rates.

LIFESPAN CONSIDERATIONS Pulse

Infants

- Use the apical pulse for the heart rate of newborns, infants, and children until 3 years of age to establish baseline data for subsequent evaluation, to determine whether the cardiac rate is within normal range, and to determine if the rhythm is regular.
- Place a baby in a supine position, and offer a pacifier if the baby is crying or restless. Crying and physical activity will increase the pulse rate. For this reason, take the apical pulse rate of infants and small children before assessing body temperatures. When possible, calm the child and allow time for the heart rate to return to normal rate before assessing the pulse.
- Locate the apical pulse in the fourth intercostal space, lateral to the midclavicular line during infancy.
- Brachial, popliteal, and femoral pulses may be palpated. Due to a normally low blood pressure and rapid heart rate, infants' other distal pulses may be hard to feel and may require use of a Doppler if indicated.
- Newborn infants may have heart murmurs that are not pathological, but reflect functional incomplete closure of fetal heart structures.

Children

- To take a peripheral pulse, position the child comfortably in the adult's arms, or have the adult remain close by. This may decrease anxiety and yield more accurate results.

- To assess the apical pulse, assist a young child to a comfortable supine or sitting position.
- Demonstrate the procedure to the child using a stuffed animal or doll, and allow the child to handle the stethoscope before beginning the procedure. This will decrease anxiety and promote cooperation.
- The apex of the heart is normally located in the fourth intercostal space in young children; fifth intercostal space in children 7 years of age and over.
  - Locate the apical impulse along the fourth intercostal space, between the MCL and the anterior axillary line.
- Count the pulse prior to other uncomfortable procedures so that the rate is not artificially elevated by the discomfort.

Older Adults

- If the client has severe hand or arm tremors, the radial pulse may be difficult to count.
- Cardiac changes in older adults, such as decrease in cardiac output, sclerotic changes to heart valves, and dysrhythmias often indicate that obtaining an apical pulse will be more accurate.
- Older adults often have decreased peripheral circulation, so pedal pulses should also be checked for regularity, volume, and symmetry.
- The pulse returns to baseline after exercise more slowly than with other age groups.

RESPIRATIONS

Respiration is the act of breathing. **Inhalation**, or **inspiration**, refers to the intake of air into the lungs. **Exhalation**, or **expiration**, refers to breathing out or the movement of gases from the lungs to the atmosphere. **Ventilation** is also used to refer to the movement of air in and out of the lungs.

There are basically two types of breathing: costal (thoracic) breathing and diaphragmatic (abdominal) breathing. Costal breathing involves the external intercostal muscles and other accessory muscles, such as the sternocleidomastoid muscles. It can be observed by the movement of the chest upward and outward. By contrast, diaphragmatic breathing involves the contraction and relaxation of the diaphragm, and it is observed by the movement of the abdomen, which occurs as a result of the diaphragm's contraction and downward movement.

Mechanics and Regulation of Breathing

During inhalation the diaphragm contracts (flattens), the ribs move upward and outward, and the sternum moves outward, thus enlarging the thorax and permitting the lungs to expand. During exhalation, the diaphragm relaxes, the ribs move downward and inward, and the sternum moves inward, thus decreasing the size of the thorax as the lungs are compressed. Inspiration is an active process requiring effort, while exhalation is a passive process that occurs without energy simply by allowing the chest and diaphragm to relax. Normally breathing is carried out automatically and effortlessly. A normal adult's inspiratory phase lasts 1 to 1.5 seconds, and the expiratory phase lasts 2 to 3 seconds.

Respiration is controlled by (a) respiratory centers in the medulla oblongata and the pons of the brain and (b) chemoreceptors located centrally in the medulla and peripherally in the carotid and aortic bodies. These centers and receptors respond to changes in the concentrations of oxygen (O_2), carbon dioxide (CO_2), and hydrogen (H^+) in the arterial blood. See Chapter 35 ∞ for details.

Factors Affecting Respirations

Several factors influence respiratory rate. Those that increase the rate include exercise (increases metabolism), stress (readies the body for "fight or flight"), increased environmental temperature, and lowered oxygen concentration at increased altitudes. Factors that may decrease the respiratory rate include decreased environmental temperature, certain medications (e.g., narcotics), and increased intracranial pressure.

CLINICAL ALERT

A sleeping adult's respirations can fall to fewer than 10 shallow breaths per minute. Use other vital signs to validate the client's condition.

The depth of a person's respirations can be established by watching the movement of the chest. Respiratory depth is generally described as normal, deep, or shallow. Deep respirations are those in which a large volume of air is inhaled and exhaled, inflating most of the lungs. Shallow respirations involve the exchange of a small volume of air and often the minimal use of lung tissue. During a normal inspiration and expiration, an adult takes in about 500 mL of air. This volume is called the **tidal volume**. For further information about pulmonary volumes and pulmonary capacities, see Chapter 35 ∞.

Body position also affects the amount of air that can be inhaled. People in a supine position experience two physiologic processes that suppress respiration: an increase in the volume of blood inside the thoracic cavity and compression of the chest. Consequently, clients lying on their back have poorer lung aeration, which predisposes them to the stasis of fluids and subsequent infection. Medications such as narcotics also affect the respiratory depth by depressing the respiratory centers in the brain. Hyperventilation refers to very deep, rapid respirations; hypoventilation refers to very shallow respirations. Breath sound assessment is described in Chapter 17 ∞.

Assessing Respirations

Resting respirations should be assessed when the client is relaxed. Respirations may need to be assessed after exercise to identify the client's tolerance to activity. Before assessing a client's respirations, a nurse should be aware of the client's normal breathing pattern, influence of health problems on respirations, medications affecting respirations, and the relationship of the client's respirations to cardiovascular function.

The rate, depth, rhythm, quality, and effectiveness of respirations should be assessed. The respiratory rate is normally described in breaths per minute. Breathing that is normal in rate and depth is called eupnea. For the respiratory rates for different age groups, see Table 16–2.

Respiratory rhythm refers to the regularity of the expirations and the inspirations. Normally, respirations are evenly spaced. Respiratory rhythm can be described as regular or irregular. An infant's respiratory rhythm may be less regular than an adult's. See Chapter 35 ∞ for details about abnormal respiratory rhythms.

Respiratory quality or character refers to those aspects of breathing that are different from normal, effortless breathing. Two of these aspects are the amount of effort a client must exert to breathe and the sound of breathing. Usually, breathing does not require noticeable effort. Sometimes, however, clients can breathe only with substantial effort—this is referred to as labored breathing.

The sound of breathing is also significant. Normal breathing is silent, but a number of abnormal sounds are obvious to the nurse's ear. Many sounds occur as a result of the presence of fluid in the lungs and are most clearly heard with a stethoscope. See Chapter 17 ∞ for methods used to assess lung sounds. For details about altered breathing patterns and terms used to describe various patterns and sounds, see Box 16–5.

The effectiveness of respirations is measured in part by the uptake of oxygen from the air into the blood and the release of carbon dioxide from the blood into expired air. The

---

| BOX 16–5 | Altered Breathing Patterns and Sounds |

Breathing Patterns

Rate

- **Tachypnea**—quick, shallow breaths
- **Bradypnea**—abnormally slow breathing
- **Apnea**—cessation of breathing

Volume

- *Hyperventilation*—overexpansion of the lungs characterized by rapid and deep breaths
- *Hypoventilation*—underexpansion of the lungs, characterized by shallow respirations

Rhythm

- *Cheyne-Stokes breathing*—rhythmic waxing and waning of respirations, from very deep to very shallow breathing and temporary apnea

Ease or Effort

- *Dyspnea*—difficult and labored breathing, during which the individual has a persistent, unsatisfied need for air and feels distressed
- *Orthopnea*—ability to breathe only in upright sitting or standing positions

Breath Sounds

Audible without Amplification

- *Stridor*—a shrill, harsh sound heard during inspiration with laryngeal obstruction
- *Stertor*—snoring or sonorous respiration, usually due to a partial obstruction of the upper airway
- *Wheeze*—continuous, high-pitched musical squeak or whistling sound occurring on expiration and sometimes on inspiration when air moves through a narrowed or partially obstructed airway. Fine wheezes may be audible only with a stethoscope.
- *Bubbling*—gurgling sounds heard as air passes through moist secretions in the respiratory tract

Chest Movements

- *Intercostal retraction*—indrawing between the ribs
- *Substernal retraction*—indrawing beneath the breastbone
- *Suprasternal retraction*—indrawing above the clavicles

Secretions and Coughing

- *Hemoptysis*—the presence of blood in the sputum
- *Productive cough*—a cough accompanied by expectorated secretions
- *Nonproductive cough*—a dry, harsh cough without secretions

amount of hemoglobin in arterial blood that is saturated with oxygen can be measured indirectly through pulse oximetry. A pulse oximeter provides a digital readout of both the client's pulse rate and the oxygen saturation. See the Identi-

fying Nursing Diagnoses, Outcomes, and Interventions for an example of applying the nursing process to a client with a breathing disorder.

Skill 16–5 outlines the steps for assessing respirations.

SKILL 16–5

ASSESSING RESPIRATIONS

PURPOSES
- To acquire baseline data against which future measurements can be compared and monitor respiratory rate and patterns in order to identify changes or monitor abnormalities

- To monitor respirations before or following the administration of a general anesthetic or any medication that influences respirations
- To monitor clients at risk for respiratory alterations

ASSESSMENT
Assess
- Skin and mucous membrane color
- Position assumed for breathing and chest movements

- Signs of inadequate ventilation such as dyspnea or activity intolerance
- Activity tolerance
- Chest pain
- Medications affecting respiratory rate

PLANNING

> **Delegation**
> Counting and observing respirations may be delegated to UAP. The follow-up assessment, interpretation of abnormal respirations, and determination of appropriate responses are done by the nurse.

EQUIPMENT
- Watch with a second hand or indicator

IMPLEMENTATION
Preparation
For a routine assessment of respirations, determine the client's activity schedule and choose a suitable time to monitor the respirations. A client who has been exercising will need to rest for 10–15 minutes to permit the accelerated respiratory rate to return to normal.

Performance
1. Prior to performing the procedure, introduce self and verify the client's identity using agency protocol. Explain to the client what you are going to do, why it is necessary, and how he or she can participate. Discuss how the results will be used in planning further care or treatments. **Rationale:** *Assures procedure is performed on correct client and reduces client anxiety.*
2. Perform hand hygiene and observe appropriate infection control procedures. **Rationale:** *Protects both the client and the nurse from infection.*
3. Provide for client privacy. **Rationale:** *Reduces client embarrassment and increases client comfort.*
4. Observe or palpate and count the respiratory rate.
   - Place a hand against the client's chest to feel the chest movements with breathing, or place the client's arm across the chest and observe the chest movements while supposedly taking the radial pulse. **Rationale:** *The client's awareness that the nurse is counting the respiratory rate*

could cause the client to purposefully alter the respiratory pattern.
   - Count the respiratory rate for 30 seconds if the respirations are regular. Count for 60 seconds if they are irregular. An inhalation and an exhalation count as one respiration. **Rationale:** *While counting for 30 seconds is more efficient, irregular respirations should be counted for 1 minute in order to obtain an accurate respiratory rate.*
5. Observe the depth, rhythm, and character of respirations.
   - Observe the respirations for depth by watching the movement of the chest. **Rationale:** *During deep respirations, a large volume of air is exchanged; during shallow respirations, a small volume is exchanged.*
   - Observe the respirations for regular or irregular rhythm. **Rationale:** *Normally, respirations are evenly spaced.*
   - Observe the character of respirations—the sound they produce and the effort they require. **Rationale:** *Normally, respirations are silent and effortless.*
6. Document the respiratory rate, depth, rhythm, and character on the appropriate record.

SAMPLE DOCUMENTATION
1/10/2010 1320 Respirations irregular, varying from 18–34/min. in past hour. Respiration shallower during tachypneic periods. Slight wheezing noted. Resp. therapist called to provide treatment. _____ D. Katano, RN

EVALUATION
- Relate respiratory rate to other vital signs, in particular pulse rate; relate respiratory rhythm and depth to baseline data and health status.
- Report to the primary care provider a respiratory rate significantly above or below the normal range and any notable change in respirations from previous assessments; irregular respiratory rhythm; inadequate respiratory depth;

abnormal character of breathing—orthopnea, wheezing, stridor, or bubbling; and any complaints of dyspnea.
- Conduct appropriate follow-up such as administering oxygen or other appropriate medications or treatments, positioning the client to ease breathing, and requesting involvement of other members of the health care team such as the respiratory therapist.

IDENTIFYING NURSING DIAGNOSES, OUTCOMES, AND INTERVENTIONS — Ineffective Breathing Pattern

NURSING DIAGNOSIS/DEFINITION	SAMPLE DESIRED OUTCOMES*/DEFINITION	INDICATORS†	SELECTED INTERVENTIONS*/DEFINITION	SAMPLE ACTIVITIES
Ineffective Breathing Pattern/Inspiration and/or expiration that does not provide adequate ventilation	Respiratory Status: Ventilation [0403]/Movement of air in and out of the lungs	• Respiratory rate IER (in expected range) • Ease of breathing	Respiratory Monitoring [3350]/Collection and analysis of respiratory data to ensure airway patency and adequate gas exchange	• Monitor for noisy respirations such as snoring • Monitor rate, rhythm, depth, and effort of respirations

*The NOC # for desired outcomes and the NIC # for nursing interventions are listed in brackets following the appropriate outcome or intervention. Outcomes, indicators, interventions, and activities selected are only a sample of those suggested by NOC and NIC and should be further individualized for each client.
†The measurement scale ranges from Extremely compromised to Not compromised. See MyNursingKit.

LIFESPAN CONSIDERATIONS   Respirations

Infants

- An infant or child who is crying will have an abnormal respiratory rate and rhythm and needs to be quieted before respirations can be accurately assessed.
- Infants and young children use their diaphragms for inhalation and exhalation. If necessary, place your hand gently on the infant's abdomen to feel the rapid rise and fall during respirations.
- Most newborns are complete nose breathers, and nasal obstruction can be life-threatening.
- Some newborns display "periodic breathing" in which they pause for a few seconds between respirations. This condition can be normal, but parents should be alert to prolonged or frequent pauses (apnea) that require medical attention.
- Compared to adults, infants have fewer alveoli and their airways have a smaller diameter. As a result, infants' respiratory rate and effort of breathing will increase with respiratory infections.

Children

- Because young children are diaphragmatic breathers, observe the rise and fall of the abdomen. If necessary, place your hand gently on the abdomen to feel the rapid rise and fall during respirations.
- Count respirations prior to other uncomfortable procedures so that the respiratory rate is not artificially elevated by the discomfort.

Older Adults

- Ask the client to remain quiet, or count respirations after taking the pulse.
- Older adults experience anatomic and physiologic changes that cause the respiratory system to be less efficient. Any changes in rate or type of breathing should be reported immediately.
- If the client has just come in from another room, allow the client to rest a minute or two before counting respirations.

BLOOD PRESSURE

Arterial **blood pressure** is a measure of the pressure exerted by the blood as it flows through the arteries. Because the blood moves in waves, there are two blood pressure measures. The **systolic pressure** is the pressure of the blood as a result of cardiac contraction of the ventricles. The **diastolic pressure** is the pressure when the ventricles are at rest. Diastolic pressure, then, is the lower pressure, present at all times within the arteries. The difference between the diastolic and the systolic pressures is called the **pulse pressure**. A normal pulse pressure is about 40 mm Hg but can be as high as 100 mm Hg during exercise. A consistently elevated pulse pressure occurs in arteriosclerosis. A low pulse pressure of less than 25 mm Hg occurs in conditions such as severe heart failure.

Blood pressure is measured in millimeters of mercury (mm Hg) and recorded as a fraction: systolic pressure over the dias-tolic pressure. A typical blood pressure for a healthy adult is 120/80 mm Hg (pulse pressure of 40). A number of conditions are reflected by changes in blood pressure. Because blood pressure can vary considerably among individuals, it is important for the nurse to know a specific client's baseline blood pressure.

Determinants of Blood Pressure

Arterial blood pressure is the result of several factors: the pumping action of the heart, the peripheral vascular resistance, and the blood volume and viscosity.

When the pumping action of the heart is weak, less blood is pumped into arteries (lower cardiac output), and the blood pressure decreases. When the heart's pumping action is strong and the volume of blood pumped into the circulation increases (higher cardiac output), the blood pressure increases.

Peripheral resistance is the resistance supplied by the blood vessels through which the blood flows. Increased peripheral vascular resistance can increase blood pressure impacting the diastolic pressure most. Some factors that create resistance in the arterial system are the capacity of the arterioles and capillaries, the compliance of the arteries, and the viscosity of the blood. The internal diameter, or capacity, of the arterioles and the capillaries determines in great part the peripheral resistance to the blood in the body. The smaller the space within a vessel, the greater the resistance found within that vessel. Normally, the arterioles are in a state of partial constriction. Increased vasoconstriction, such as occurs with smoking, raises the blood pressure, whereas decreased vasoconstriction lowers the blood pressure. If the elastic and muscular tissues of the arteries are replaced with fibrous tissue, the arteries lose much of their ability to constrict and dilate. This condition, most common in middle-aged and older adults, is known as arteriosclerosis.

When the blood volume decreases, the blood pressure decreases because of decreased fluid in the arteries. Conversely, when the volume increases, the blood pressure increases because of the greater fluid volume within the circulatory system.

Blood pressure is higher when the blood is highly viscous, that is, when the proportion of red blood cells to the blood plasma is high causing a thicker fluid. This proportion is referred to as the hematocrit. The viscosity increases markedly when the hematocrit is more than 60% to 65%.

Factors Affecting Blood Pressure

Among the factors influencing blood pressure are age, exercise, stress, race, obesity, sex, medications, diurnal variations, and disease processes.

- *Age.* Newborns have a mean systolic pressure of about 75 mm Hg. The pressure rises with age, reaching a peak at the onset of puberty, and then tends to decline somewhat. In older adults, elasticity of the arteries is decreased producing an elevated systolic pressure. Because the walls no longer retract as flexibly with decreased pressure, the diastolic pressure may also be high.
- *Exercise.* Physical activity increases the cardiac output and hence the blood pressure; thus 20 to 30 minutes of rest following exercise is indicated before the resting blood pressure can be reliably assessed.
- *Stress.* Stimulation of the sympathetic nervous system increases cardiac output and vasoconstriction of the arterioles, thus increasing the blood pressure. Severe pain can decrease blood pressure greatly by inhibiting the vasomotor center and producing vasodilatation.
- *Race.* African American males over 35 years have higher blood pressures than European American males of the same age.
- *Gender.* After puberty, females usually have lower blood pressures than males of the same age, thought to be due to hormonal variations. After menopause, women generally have higher blood pressures than before.
- *Medications.* Many medications, including caffeine, may increase or decrease the blood pressure.
- *Obesity.* Both childhood and adult obesity predispose to hypertension.
- *Diurnal variations.* Pressure is usually lowest early in the morning, when the metabolic rate is lowest, then rises throughout the day and peaks in the late afternoon or early evening.
- *Disease process.* Any condition affecting the cardiac output, blood volume, blood viscosity, and/or compliance of the arteries has a direct effect on the blood pressure.

A blood pressure that is persistently above normal is called **hypertension**. A single elevated blood pressure reading indicates the need for reassessment. Hypertension cannot be diagnosed unless an elevated blood pressure is found when measured twice at different times. It is usually asymptomatic and is often a contributing factor to myocardial infarctions. An elevated blood pressure of unknown cause is called *primary hypertension.* An elevated blood pressure of known cause is called *secondary hypertension.* Individuals with diastolic blood pressures of 80 to 89 mm Hg or systolic blood pressures of 120 to 139 mm Hg should be considered prehypertensive and, without intervention, may develop cardiac disease. Hypertension is diagnosed when either the diastolic blood pressure is 90 mm Hg or higher or when the systolic blood pressure is higher than 140 mm Hg (see Table 16–3). Factors associated with hypertension include thickening of the arterial walls, which reduces the size of the arterial lumen, and inelasticity of the arteries as well as such lifestyle factors as cigarette smoking, obesity, heavy alcohol consumption, lack of physical exercise, high blood cholesterol levels, and continued exposure to stress. Follow-up care should include lifestyle changes conducive to lowering the blood pressure as well as monitoring the pressure itself.

Hypotension is a blood pressure that is below normal, that is, a systolic reading consistently between 85 and 110 mm Hg in an adult whose normal pressure is higher than this. Clients whose blood pressure falls within this range and are asymptomatic may not require treatment. Symptoms of hypotension include dizziness, shortness of breath, confusion, or fainting.

Orthostatic hypotension is a blood pressure that falls when the client sits or stands. It is usually the result of peripheral vasodilatation in which blood leaves the central body or-

TABLE 16–3	Classification of Blood Pressure		
CATEGORY	SYSTOLIC BP MM HG		DIASTOLIC BP MM HG
Normal	<120	and	<80
Prehypertension	120–139	or	80–89
Hypertension, stage 1	140–159	or	90–99
Hypertension, stage 2	>160	or	>100

Note: From the "Seventh Report of the Joint National Committee for the Detection, Evaluation, and Treatment of High Blood Pressure," by National Institutes of Health, National Heart, Lung, and Blood Institute, 2004.

gans, especially the brain, and moves to the periphery, often causing the person to feel faint. Hypotension can also be caused by analgesics, bleeding, severe burns, and dehydration. It is important to monitor hypotensive clients carefully to prevent falls. When assessing for orthostatic hypotension record the client's pulse and blood pressure while supine and then again in the same spot when assisted to sit or stand. It is important to support the client in case of faintness to prevent injury. Repeat the sitting or standing blood pressure 3 minutes after standing. Record all three pressures indicating when each was taken. A rise in pulse of 15 to 30 beats per minute or a drop in blood pressure of 20 mm Hg systolic or 10 mm Hg diastolic indicates orthostatic hypotension (Irvin & White, 2004).

Assessing Blood Pressure

Blood pressure is measured with a blood pressure cuff, a sphygmomanometer, and a stethoscope. The blood pressure cuff consists of a rubber bag that can be inflated with air called the bladder (Figure 16–5). It is covered with cloth and has two tubes attached to it. One tube connects to a rubber bulb that inflates the bladder. A small valve on the side of this bulb traps and releases the air in the bladder. The other tube is attached to a sphygmomanometer. The sphygmomanometer indicates the pressure of the air within the bladder. There are two types of sphygmomanometers: aneroid and digital. The aneroid sphygmomanometer is a calibrated dial with a needle that points to the calibrations.

Many agencies use digital (electronic) sphygmomanometers (Figure 16–6), which eliminate the need to listen for the sounds of the client's systolic and diastolic blood pressures through a stethoscope. Electronic blood pressure devices should be calibrated periodically to

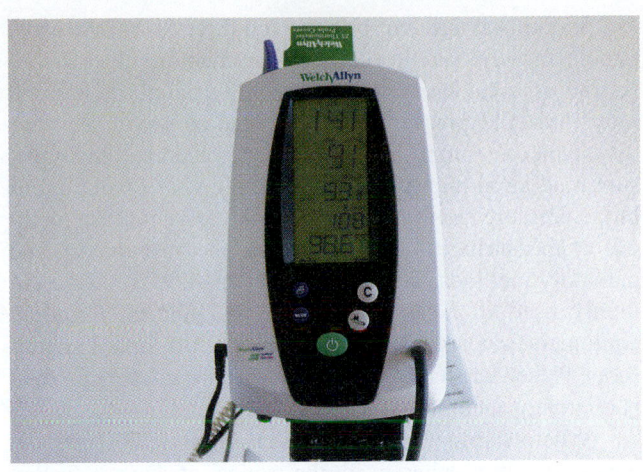

Figure 16–6 ○ Blood pressure monitors register systolic and diastolic blood pressures and often other vital signs.

check accuracy. All health care facilities should have manual blood pressure equipment available as backup. When a reading from the electronic device is inconsistent with the client's previous blood pressure readings it is important to check the blood pressure manually to assure accuracy of the reading.

Doppler ultrasound stethoscopes are also used to assess blood pressure. These are of particular value when blood pressure sounds are difficult to hear, such as in infants, obese clients, and clients in shock. If diastolic pressure cannot be heard using a Doppler ultrasound stethoscope it may be necessary to palpate blood pressure.

Blood pressure cuffs come in various sizes because the bladder must be the correct width and length for the client's arm. If the bladder is too narrow, the blood pressure reading will be erroneously elevated; if it is too wide, the reading will be erroneously low. The width should be 40% of the circumference, or 20% wider than the diameter of the midpoint, of the limb on which it is used. The arm circumference, not the age of the client, should always be used to determine bladder size. The nurse can determine whether the width of a blood pressure cuff is appropriate: Lay the cuff lengthwise at the midpoint of the upper arm, and hold the outermost side of the bladder edge laterally on the arm. With the other hand, wrap the width of the cuff around the arm, and ensure that the width is 40% of the arm circumference. The length of the bladder also affects the accuracy of measurement. The bladder should be sufficiently long to cover at least two-thirds of the limb's circumference.

The blood pressure is usually assessed in the client's upper arm using the brachial artery and a standard stethoscope. Assessing the blood pressure on a client's thigh is indicated when the arms cannot be used or when a thigh reading is needed. Blood pressure is not measured on a particular client's limb if the extremity is injured or diseased; a cast is in place; there has been surgical removal of lymph nodes proximal to the site; there is an intravenous infusion in that limb; or there is an arteriovenous fistula in that limb.

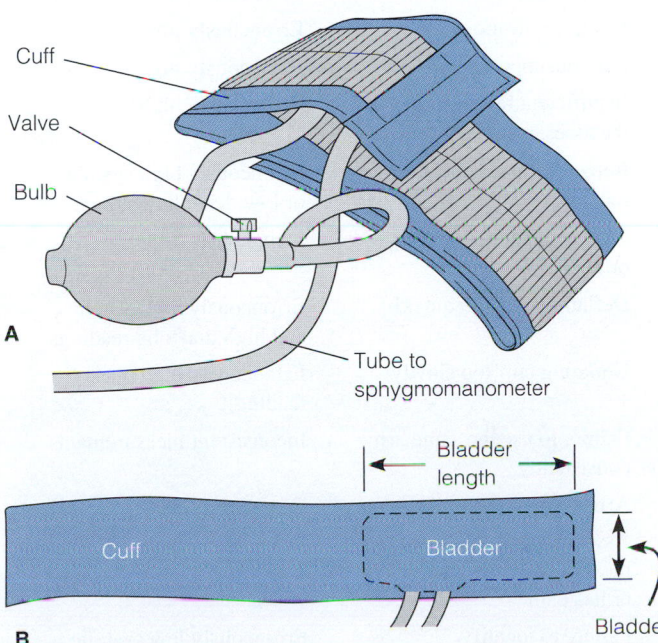

A

Cuff
Valve
Bulb

Tube to sphygmomanometer

Bladder length

Cuff

Bladder

Bladder width

B

Figure 16–5 ○ **A,** A blood pressure cuff and bulb; **B,** the bladder inside the cuff.

Blood pressure can be assessed directly or indirectly. Direct (invasive monitoring) measurement involves the insertion of a catheter into the brachial, radial, or femoral artery. Arterial pressure is represented as wavelike forms displayed on a monitor. With correct placement, this pressure reading is highly accurate and allows for continuous blood pressure monitoring. Two noninvasive indirect methods of measuring blood pressure are the auscultatory and palpatory methods. The auscultatory method is most commonly used in hospitals, clinics, and homes. Required equipment is a sphygmomanometer, a cuff, and a stethoscope. When carried out correctly, the auscultatory method is relatively accurate.

When taking a blood pressure using a stethoscope, the nurse identifies phases in the series of sounds called **Korotkoff's sounds**. First the nurse pumps the cuff up to about 30 mm Hg above the point where the pulse is no longer felt; that is the point when the blood flow in the artery is stopped. Then the pressure is released slowly (2 to 3 mm Hg per second) while the nurse observes the readings on the manometer and relates them to the sounds heard through the stethoscope. Five phases occur but may not always be audible (see Box 16–6).

The palpatory method is sometimes used when Korotkoff's sounds cannot be heard and electronic equipment to amplify the sounds is not available, or to prevent misdirection from the presence of an auscultatory gap. An auscultatory gap, which occurs particularly in hypertensive clients, is the temporary disappearance of sounds normally heard over the brachial artery when the cuff pressure is high followed by the reappearance of the sounds at a lower level.

This temporary disappearance of sounds may cover a range of 40 mm Hg. If a palpated estimation of the systolic pressure is not made prior to auscultation, the nurse may begin listening in the middle of this range and underestimate the systolic pressure. In the palpatory method of blood pressure determination, instead of listening for the blood flow sounds, the nurse uses light to moderate pressure to palpate the pulsations of the artery as the pressure in the cuff is released. The pressure is read from the sphygmomanometer when the first pulsation is felt.

Improving Accuracy of Blood Pressure Measurements

The importance of the accuracy of blood pressure assessments cannot be overemphasized. Many judgments about a client's health are made on the basis of blood pressure. It is an important indicator of the client's condition and is used extensively as a basis for nursing interventions and medical treatment. Two possible reasons for blood pressure errors are haste on the part of the nurse and subconscious bias. For example, a nurse may be influenced by the client's previous blood pressure measurements or diagnosis and "hear" a value consistent with the practitioner's expectations. Strategies for improving the accuracy of blood pressure readings are given in Table 16–4.

Skill 16–6 provides guidelines for assessing blood pressure.

BOX 16–6 Korotkoff's Sounds

- *Phase 1* The pressure level at which the first faint, clear tapping or thumping sounds are heard. These sounds gradually become more intense. To ensure that they are not extraneous sounds, the nurse should identify at least two consecutive tapping sounds. The first tapping sound heard during deflation of the cuff is the systolic blood pressure.
- *Phase 2* The period during deflation when the sounds have a muffled, whooshing, or swishing quality.
- *Phase 3* The period during which the blood flows freely through an increasingly open artery and the sounds become crisper and more intense and again assume a thumping quality but softer than in phase 1.
- *Phase 4* The time when the sounds become muffled and have a soft, blowing quality.
- *Phase 5* The pressure level when the last sound is heard. This is followed by a period of silence. The pressure at which the last sound is heard is the diastolic blood pressure in adults.*

*In agencies where the fourth phase is considered the diastolic pressure, three measures are recommended (systolic pressure, diastolic pressure, and phase 5). These may be referred to as systolic, first diastolic, and second diastolic pressures. The phase 5 (second diastolic pressure) reading may be zero; that is, the muffled sounds are heard even when there is no air pressure in the blood pressure cuff. In some instances, muffled sounds are never heard, in which case a dash is inserted where the reading would normally be recorded (e.g., /–/110).

TABLE 16–4 Impact of Procedural Alterations on Blood Pressure Assessment

ERROR	EFFECT
Bladder cuff too narrow	Erroneously high
Bladder cuff too wide	Erroneously low
Arm unsupported	Erroneously high
Insufficient rest before the assessment	Erroneously high
Repeating assessment too quickly	Erroneously high systolic or low diastolic readings
Cuff wrapped too loosely or unevenly	Erroneously high
Deflating cuff too quickly	Erroneously low systolic and high diastolic readings
Deflating cuff too slowly	Erroneously high diastolic reading
Failure to use the same arm consistently	Inconsistent measurements
Arm above level of the heart	Erroneously low
Assessing immediately after a meal or while client smokes or has pain	Erroneously high
Failure to identify auscultatory gap	Erroneously low systolic pressure and erroneously low diastolic pressure

SKILL 16–6

ASSESSING BLOOD PRESSURE

PURPOSES
- To obtain a baseline measure of arterial blood pressure for subsequent evaluation and determination of client's hemodynamic status
- To identify and monitor changes in blood pressure resulting from a disease process or medical therapy

ASSESSMENT
Assess for
- Signs and symptoms of hypertension
- Signs and symptoms of hypotension
- Factors affecting blood pressure
- Latex allergy and obtain a latex-free cuff and stethoscope if indicated

PLANNING

Delegation
Blood pressure measurement may be delegated to UAP for the stable client. The interpretation of abnormal blood pressure readings and determination of appropriate responses are done by the nurse.

EQUIPMENT
- Stethoscope or DUS
- Blood pressure cuff of the appropriate size
- Sphygmomanometer

IMPLEMENTATION
Preparation
1. Ensure that the equipment is intact and functioning properly. Check for leaks in the tubing of the sphygmomanometer.
2. Make sure that the client has not smoked or ingested caffeine within 30 minutes prior to measurement. **Rationale:** *Smoking constricts blood vessels, and caffeine increases the pulse rate. Both of these cause a temporary increase in blood pressure.*

Performance
1. Prior to performing the procedure, introduce self and verify the client's identity using agency protocol. Explain to the client what you are going to do, why it is necessary, and how he or she can participate. Discuss how the results will be used in planning further care or treatments. **Rationale:** *Assures procedure is performed on correct client and reduces client anxiety.*
2. Perform hand hygiene and observe appropriate infection control procedures. **Rationale:** *Protects both the client and the nurse from infection.*
3. Provide for client privacy. **Rationale:** *Reduces client embarrassment and increases client comfort.*
4. Position the client appropriately. **Rationale:** *Improve accuracy of reading.*
   - The adult client should be sitting unless otherwise specified. Both feet should be flat on the floor. **Rationale:** *Legs crossed at the knee result in elevated systolic and diastolic blood pressures* (Pickering et al., 2005).
   - The elbow should be slightly flexed with the palm of the hand facing up and the forearm supported at heart level. Readings in any other position should be specified. The blood pressure is normally similar in sitting, standing, and lying positions, but it can vary significantly by position in certain persons. **Rationale:** *The blood pressure increases when the arm is below heart level and decreases when the arm is above heart level.*
   - Expose the upper arm. **Rationale:** *The cuff is more likely to be placed properly if landmarks can be visualized.*
5. Wrap the deflated cuff evenly around the upper arm. Locate the brachial artery (see Figure 16–4). Apply the center of the bladder directly over the artery. **Rationale:** *The bladder inside the cuff must be directly over the artery to be compressed if the reading is to be accurate.*
   - For an adult, place the lower border of the cuff approximately 2.5 cm (1 in.) above the antecubital space. **Rationale:** *This location allows placement of the stethoscope directly over the artery without noise interference from the movement of the cuff.*
6. If this is the client's initial examination, perform a preliminary palpatory determination of systolic pressure. **Rationale:** *The initial estimate tells the nurse the maximal pressure to which the manometer needs to be elevated in subsequent determinations. It also prevents underestimation of the systolic pressure or overestimation of the diastolic pressure should an auscultatory gap occur.*
   - Palpate the brachial artery with the fingertips.
   - Close the valve on the bulb.
   - Pump up the cuff until you no longer feel the brachial pulse. At that pressure the blood cannot flow through the artery. Note the pressure on the sphygmomanometer at which pulse is no longer felt. **Rationale:** *This gives an estimate of the systolic pressure.*
   - Release the pressure completely in the cuff, and wait 1 to 2 minutes before making further measurements. **Rationale:** *A waiting period gives the blood trapped in the veins time to be released. Otherwise, false high systolic readings will occur.*
7. Position the stethoscope appropriately.
   - Cleanse the earpieces with antiseptic wipe. **Rationale:** *Earpieces collect pathogens and cerumen. Cleansing the earpieces will reduce the risk of infecting the nurse's ear canal, especially if the stethoscope is shared by others.*
   - Insert the ear attachments of the stethoscope in your ears so that they tilt slightly forward. **Rationale:** *Sounds are heard more clearly when the ear attachments follow the direction of the ear canal.*
   - Ensure that the stethoscope hangs freely from the ears to the diaphragm. **Rationale:** *If the stethoscope tubing rubs against an object, the noise can block the sounds of the blood within the artery.*

(continued)

SKILL 16–6

ASSESSING BLOOD PRESSURE *(continued)*

- Place the bell side of the amplifier of the stethoscope over the brachial pulse site. **Rationale:** *Because the blood pressure is a low-frequency sound, it is best heard with the bell-shaped diaphragm.*
- Place the stethoscope directly on the skin, not on clothing over the site. **Rationale:** *This is to avoid noise made from rubbing the amplifier against cloth.*
- Hold the diaphragm with the thumb and index finger. **Rationale:** *Creating a seal between the skin and the diaphragm reduces external sounds from being amplified by the stethoscope.*

8. Auscultate the client's blood pressure.
- Pump up the cuff until the sphygmomanometer reads 30 mm Hg above the point where the brachial pulse disappeared. **Rationale:** *If the cuff is not pumped to a high enough level the systolic pressure may be assessed erroneously.*
- Release the valve on the cuff carefully so that the pressure decreases at the rate of 2 to 3 mm Hg per second. **Rationale:** *If the rate is faster or slower, an error in measurement may occur.*
- As the pressure falls, identify the manometer reading at Korotkoff phases I, IV, and V. **Rationale:** *There is no clinical significance to phases II and III* (Pickering et al., 2005).
- Deflate the cuff rapidly and completely. **Rationale:** *Once the diastolic reading is identified the cuff can be deflated and the measurement recorded.*
- Wait 1 to 2 minutes before making further determinations. **Rationale:** *This permits blood trapped in the veins to be released.*
- Repeat the above steps to confirm the accuracy of the reading—especially if it falls outside the normal range. If there is more than a 5 mm Hg difference between the two readings, additional measurements may be taken and the results averaged (Pickering et al., 2005).

9. If this is the client's initial examination, repeat the procedure on the client's other arm. There should be a difference of no more than 10 mm Hg between the arms. The arm found to have the higher pressure should be used for subsequent examinations.

Variation: Obtaining a Blood Pressure by the Palpation Method

If it is not possible to use a stethoscope to obtain the blood pressure or if the Korotkoff's sounds cannot be heard, palpate the radial or brachial pulse site as the cuff pressure is released. The manometer reading at the point where the pulse reappears represents a value between auscultated systolic and diastolic values. When blood pressure is obtained by palpation, it is important to document that this method was used to allow for proper analysis of data. It may be documented as the reading over P (84/P) or as reading (palpated) such as 84 Palpated.

Variation: Taking a Thigh Blood Pressure

- Help the client to assume a prone position. If the client cannot assume this position, measure the blood pressure while the client is in a supine position with the knee slightly flexed. **Rationale:** *Slight flexing of the knee will facilitate placing the stethoscope on the popliteal space.*

- Expose the thigh, taking care not to expose the client unduly. **Rationale:** *Reduces client embarrassment and decreases client anxiety.*
- Locate the popliteal artery.
- Wrap the cuff evenly around the midthigh with the compression bladder over the posterior aspect of the thigh and the bottom edge above the knee. **Rationale:** *The bladder must be directly over the posterior popliteal artery if the reading is to be accurate.*
- If this is the client's initial examination, perform a preliminary palpatory determination of systolic pressure by palpating the popliteal artery.
- In adults, the systolic pressure in the popliteal artery is usually 20 to 30 mm Hg higher than that in the brachial artery because of use of a larger bladder; the diastolic pressure is usually the same.

Variation: Using an Electronic Indirect Blood Pressure Monitoring Device (Figure 16–6)

- Place the blood pressure cuff on the extremity according to the manufacturer's guidelines.
- Turn on the blood pressure switch.
- If appropriate, set the device for the desired number of minutes between blood pressure determinations.
- When the device has determined the blood pressure reading, note the digital results.

CLINICAL ALERT

Electronic/automatic blood pressure cuffs can be left in place for many hours. Remove the cuff and check skin condition periodically.

10. Remove the cuff.
11. Wipe the cuff with an approved disinfectant. **Rationale:** *Cuffs can become significantly contaminated.* Many institutions use disposable blood pressure cuffs. The client uses it for the length of stay and then it is discarded. This decreases the risk of spreading infection by sharing cuffs.
12. Document and report pertinent assessment data according to agency policy. Record two pressures in the form "130/80" where "130" is the systolic (phase 1) and "80" is the diastolic (phase 5) pressure. Record three pressures in the form "130/90/0," where "130" is the systolic, "90" is the first diastolic (phase 4), and sounds are audible even after the cuff is completely deflated (Pickering et al., 2005). Use the abbreviations RA or RL for right arm or right leg and LA or LL for left arm or left leg. Record a difference of greater than 10 mm Hg between the two arms or legs.

EVALUATION

- Relate blood pressure to other vital signs, to baseline data, and to health status.
- Report any significant change in the client's blood pressure.
- Conduct appropriate follow-up such as administration of medication. If the blood pressure is significantly higher or lower than usual, implement appropriate safety precautions.

Infants

- Use a pediatric stethoscope with a small diaphragm.
- The lower edge of the blood pressure cuff can be closer to the antecubital space of an infant.
- Use the palpation method if auscultation with a stethoscope or DUS is unsuccessful.
- Arm and thigh pressures are equivalent in children under 1 year of age.
- One quick way to determine the normal systolic blood pressure of a child is to use the following formula: Normal systolic BP = 80 + (2 × child's age in years)

Children

- Blood pressure should be measured in all children over 3 years of age and in children under 3 years of age with chronic medical conditions that impact blood pressure.
- Explain each step of the process and what it will feel like. Demonstrate on a doll.
- Use the palpation technique or electronic blood pressure devices for children under 3 years old.
- Cuff bladder width should be 40% and length should be 80% to 100% of the arm circumference.
- Perform procedures that are unlikely to make the child cry first and then take the blood pressure prior to other uncomfortable procedures so that the blood pressure is not artificially elevated by the discomfort. Blood pressure measurements will often make very young children cry.
- In children, the diastolic pressure is considered to be the onset of phase 4, where the sounds become muffled.
- In children, the thigh pressure is about 10 mm Hg higher than the arm.

Older Adults

- Skin may be very fragile. Do not allow cuff pressure to remain high any longer than necessary. If the cuff is to remain in place for an extended period of time, placing a soft cloth under the cuff may prevent tissue trauma from friction.
- Determine if the client is taking antihypertensives and, if so, when the last dose was taken.
- Medications that cause vasodilation along with the loss of baroreceptor efficiency in older adults place them at increased risk for having orthostatic hypotension. Measuring blood pressure while the client is in the lying, sitting, and standing positions, and noting any changes can determine this.
- If the client has arm contractures, assess the blood pressure by palpation, with the arm in a relaxed position. If this is not possible, take a thigh blood pressure.
- If the client is in a chair or low bed, position yourself so that you maintain the client's arm at heart level and you can read the sphygmomanometer at eye level.

OXYGEN SATURATION

A **pulse oximeter** is a noninvasive device that estimates a client's arterial blood oxygen saturation by means of a sensor attached to the client's finger (Figure 16–7), toe, nose, earlobe, or forehead (or around the hand or foot of a neonate). The pulse oximeter can detect hypoxemia before clinical signs and symptoms develop.

The pulse oximeter's sensor has two parts: (a) two light-emitting diodes (LEDs)—one red, the other infrared—that transmit light through nails, tissue, venous blood, and arterial blood; and (b) a photodetector placed directly opposite the LEDs. The photodetector measures the amount of red and infrared light absorbed by oxygenated and deoxygenated hemoglobin in peripheral arterial blood and reports it as SpO_2. Normal SpO_2 is 95% to 100%, and a SpO_2 below 70% is life threatening.

Pulse oximeters with various types of sensors are available from several manufacturers. The oximeter unit consists of an inlet connection for the sensor cable, and a faceplate that indicates (a) the oxygen saturation measurement (expressed as a percentage) and (b) the pulse rate. Cordless units are also available. The alarm limits can be preset and will signal high and low SpO_2 measurements and a high and low pulse rate. The high and low SpO_2 levels are generally preset at 100% and 85%, respectively, for adults. The high and low pulse rate alarms are usually preset at 140 and 50 BPM for

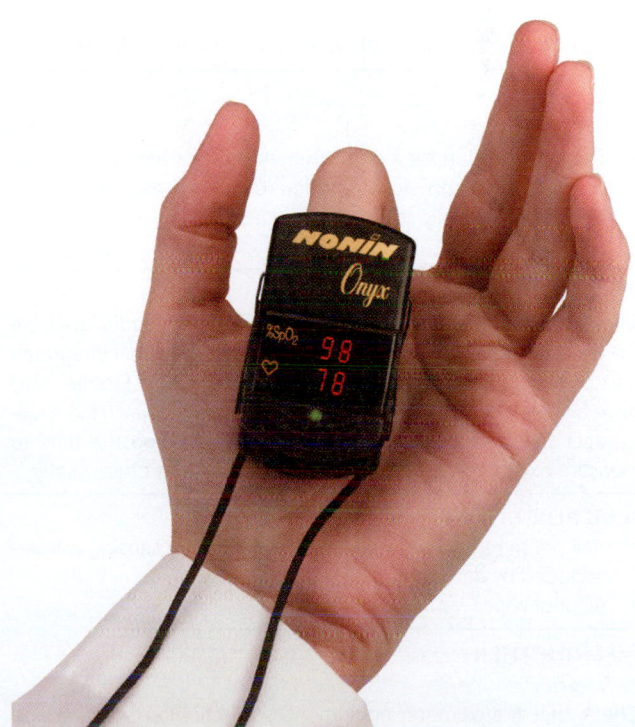

Figure 16–7 ○ Fingertip oximeter sensor (adult).

adults. These alarm limits can, however, be changed according to the manufacturer's directions or the client's needs.

Factors Affecting Oxygen Saturation Readings

- *Hemoglobin.* If the hemoglobin is fully saturated with oxygen, the SpO_2 will appear normal even if the total hemoglobin level is low. Thus, the client could be severely anemic and have inadequate oxygen to supply the tissues but the pulse oximeter would return a normal value.
- *Circulation.* The oximeter will not return an accurate reading if the area under the sensor has impaired circulation as indicated by cold or pale skin. The oximeter probe should always be placed in an area with good circulation in order to get an accurate reading.
- *Activity.* Shivering or excessive movement of the sensor site may interfere with accurate readings. A pulsation reading on the monitor should correspond to the client's heartbeat to help assure when an accurate and trustworthy reading is being obtained.
- *Carbon monoxide poisoning.* Pulse oximeters cannot discriminate between hemoglobin saturated with carbon monoxide versus oxygen. In this case, other measures of oxygenation are needed.

Assessing Oxygen Saturation

Skill 16–7 outlines the steps in measuring oxygen saturation.

LIFESPAN CONSIDERATIONS
Pulse Oximetry

Infants

- If an appropriate-sized finger or toe sensor is not available, consider using an earlobe or forehead sensor or one that can be wrapped around the palm of the hand or middle of the foot.
- The high and low SpO_2 levels are generally preset at 95% and 80% for neonates because administration of excessive oxygen to obtain a higher reading can be toxic and cause eye and lung tissue damage.
- The high and low pulse rate alarms are usually preset at 200 and 100 for neonates.
- The oximeter may need to be taped, wrapped with an elastic bandage, or covered by a stocking to keep it in place.

Children

- Instruct the child that the sensor does not hurt. Disconnect the probe whenever possible to allow for movement.
- Allow the child to measure your oxygen saturation before placing it on the child to reduce fear or anxiety.

Older Adults

- Use of vasoconstrictive medications, poor circulation, or thickened nails may make finger or toe sensors inaccurate.

SKILL 16–7

MEASURING OXYGEN SATURATION

PURPOSES
- To estimate the arterial blood oxygen saturation (SpO_2)
- To detect the presence of hypoxemia before visible signs develop

ASSESSMENT

Assess
- The best location for a pulse oximeter sensor based on the client's age and physical condition (Unless contraindicated, the finger is usually selected for adults.)
- The client's overall condition including risk factors for development of hypoxemia and hemoglobin level
- Vital signs, skin color and temperature, nail bed color, and tissue perfusion of extremities as baseline data
- Adhesive or latex allergy as many sensors contain one or both of these

PLANNING

Many hospitals and clinics have pulse oximeters readily available for use with other vital signs equipment (or even as an integrated part of the electronic blood pressure device). Other facilities may have a limited supply of oximeters, and the nurse may need to request it from the central supply department. Choose a time to measure oxygen saturation when the client can sit or lie quietly.

Delegation
Application of the pulse oximeter sensor and recording of the SpO_2 value may be delegated to UAP. The interpretation of the oxygen saturation value and determination of appropriate responses are performed by the nurse.

EQUIPMENT
- Nail polish remover as needed (pulse oximetry sensing will be occluded by dark nail polish)
- Alcohol wipe
- Sheet or towel
- Pulse oximeter

IMPLEMENTATION

Preparation
Check that the oximeter equipment is functioning normally and that the probe cord is intact.

Performance

1. Prior to performing the procedure, introduce self and verify the client's identity using agency protocol. Explain to the client what you are going to do, why it is necessary, and

how he or she can participate. Discuss how the results will be used in planning further care or treatments. **Rationale:** *Assures procedure is performed on the correct client and reduces client anxiety by introducing yourself and explaining the procedure before beginning.*

2. Perform hand hygiene and observe appropriate infection control procedures. **Rationale:** *Protects both the client and the nurse from infection.*

3. Provide for client privacy. **Rationale:** *Reduces client embarrassment and increases client comfort.*

4. Choose a sensor and site appropriate for the client's weight, size, condition, and desired location. Because weight limits of sensors overlap, a pediatric sensor could be used for a small adult.
   - If the client is allergic to adhesive, use a clip or sensor without adhesive. If using an extremity, assess the proximal pulse and capillary refill at the point closest to the site. **Rationale:** *Some sensors are wrapped around the finger using adhesive tape to hold them in place. This could create an allergic response.*
   - If the client has low tissue perfusion due to peripheral vascular disease or therapy using vasoconstrictive medications, use a nasal sensor or a reflectance sensor on the forehead. Avoid using lower extremities that have a compromised circulation and extremities that are used for infusions or other invasive monitoring. **Rationale:** *Proper selection of site is essential to obtaining an accurate reading. Choose a site that is well perfused and can be held steady. The ear may be a better choice for a client who has poor peripheral perfusion or a continuous twitch in the hands.*

5. Prepare the site.
   - Clean the site with an alcohol wipe before applying the sensor. **Rationale:** *Cleaning the site will reduce the risk of inaccurate measurements.*
   - It may be necessary to remove a female client's dark nail polish. **Rationale:** *Dark polish will reduce light sensing resulting in inaccurate results.*
   - Alternatively, position the sensor on the side of the finger rather than perpendicular to the nail bed (Rajkumar, Karmarkar, & Knot, 2006). **Rationale:** *The light will go through the tissue without having to pass through the nail as well.*

6. Apply the sensor, and connect it to the pulse oximeter.
   - Make sure the LED and photodetector are accurately aligned, that is, opposite each other on either side of the finger, toe, nose, or earlobe. Many sensors have markings to facilitate correct alignment of the LEDs and photodetector. **Rationale:** *Accuracy is improved if the LED and photodetector are in direct alignment with one another because the light moves through the tissue directly into the sensor.*
   - Attach the sensor cable to the connection outlet on the oximeter. Turn on the machine according to the manufacturer's directions. Appropriate connection will be confirmed by an audible beep indicating each arterial

pulsation. Some devices have a wheel that can be turned clockwise to increase the pulse volume and counterclockwise to decrease it. **Rationale:** *Increasing pulse volume will increase the sensitivity of the sensor to detect lower volume pulsations such as in a client with reduced peripheral perfusion.*
   - Ensure that the bar of light or waveform on the face of the oximeter fluctuates with each pulsation. **Rationale:** *When the machine is able to detect each pulsation it indicates that proper reading of oxygen saturation is also likely.*

7. Set and turn on the alarm when using continuous monitoring.
   - Check the preset alarm limits for high and low oxygen saturation and high and low pulse rates. Change these alarm limits according to the manufacturer's directions and client needs as indicated. Ensure that the audio and visual alarms are on before you leave the client. A tone will be heard and a number will blink on the faceplate. **Rationale:** *Different clients require different limits. Check the machine to make sure the limits are set appropriately for the client and set limits based on client's condition and needs.*
   - Test the volume of the alarm. **Rationale:** *Testing the volume of the alarm will assure that the alarm can be heard should it sound as well as protecting the client from an alarm set excessively high.*

8. Ensure client safety.
   - Inspect and/or move or change the location of an adhesive toe or finger sensor every 4 hours and a spring-tension sensor every 2 hours. **Rationale:** *The pressure from the sensor can cause tissue damage if allowed to remain in the same place for an extended period of time. Assure that the sensor is not too tight in order to prevent diminishing circulation to the site.*
   - Inspect the sensor site tissues for irritation from adhesive sensors. **Rationale:** *Clients with fragile tissue or reduced perfusion to the site can experience tissue injury even when the site is changed frequently.*

9. Ensure the accuracy of measurement.
   - Minimize motion artifacts by using an adhesive sensor, or immobilize the client's monitoring site. **Rationale:** *Movement of the client's finger or toe may be misinterpreted by the oximeter as arterial pulsations.*
   - If indicated, cover the sensor with a sheet or towel to block large amounts of light from external sources (e.g., sunlight, procedure lamps, or bilirubin lights in the nursery). **Rationale:** *Bright room light may be sensed by the photodetector and alter the SpO_2 value* (Popovich, Richiuso, & Danek, 2004).
   - Compare the pulse rate indicated by the oximeter to the radial pulse periodically. **Rationale:** *A large discrepancy between the two values may indicate oximeter malfunction and inaccurate readings.*

10. Document the oxygen saturation on the appropriate record at designated intervals.

EVALUATION
- Compare the oxygen saturation to the client's previous oxygen saturation level. Relate to pulse rate and other vital signs.
- Conduct appropriate follow-up such as notifying the primary care provider, adjusting oxygen therapy, or providing breathing treatments.

CHAPTER HIGHLIGHTS

- Vital signs reflect changes in body function that otherwise might not be observed and can frequently be the first indication of a change in the client's condition.
- Body temperature is the balance between heat produced by the body and heat lost from the body. Factors affecting body temperature include age, diurnal variations, exercise, hormones, stress, and environmental temperatures.
- Four common types of fever are intermittent, remittent, relapsing, and constant.
- During a fever, the set point of the hypothalamic thermostat changes suddenly from the normal level to a higher than normal level, but several hours elapse before the core temperature reaches the new set point.
- Hypothermia involves three mechanisms: excessive heat loss, inadequate heat production by body cells, and increasing impairment of hypothalamic thermoregulation.
- The nurse selects the most appropriate site to measure temperature according to the client's age and condition.
- Pulse rate and volume reflect the stroke volume output, the compliance of the client's arteries, and the adequacy of blood flow.
- Normally a peripheral pulse reflects the client's heartbeat, but it may differ from the heartbeat in clients with certain cardiovascular diseases; in these instances, the nurse takes an apical pulse and compares it to the peripheral pulse.

- Many factors may affect a person's pulse rate: age, gender, exercise, presence of fever, certain medications, hypovolemia, stress (in some situations), position changes, and pathology.
- Although the radial pulse is the site most commonly used, eight other sites may be used in certain situations.
- The difference between the apical and radial pulses is called pulse deficit.
- Respirations are normally quiet, effortless, and automatic and are assessed by observing respiratory rate, depth, rhythm, quality, and effectiveness.
- Blood pressure reflects cardiac output, peripheral vascular resistance, blood volume, and blood viscosity.
- Among the factors influencing blood pressure are age, exercise, stress, race, gender, medications, obesity, diurnal variations, and disease processes.
- Orthostatic hypotension occurs when the blood pressure falls as the client assumes an upright position.
- A blood pressure cuff that is improperly sized will give false readings.
- During blood pressure measurement, the artery must be held at heart level.
- A pulse oximeter measures the percent of hemoglobin saturated with oxygen. A normal result is 95% to 100%. Pulse oximeter sensors may be placed on the finger, hand, foot, or nose.

THINK ABOUT IT

Refer to the chapter-opening scenario and answer these questions.

1. Why would the nurse obtain Martin's vital signs before calling the doctor, administering oxygen, or performing any other intervention to help the client?

2. Why might Martin's apical pulse rate differ from his radial pulse rate?

3. How would hypertension complicate a client's cardiac function following a myocardial infarction?

4. Why is the client's axillary temperature so low?

∞ *See suggested responses to Think About It on MyNursingKit.*

TEST YOUR KNOWLEDGE

1. The client's temperature at 8:00 AM using an oral electronic thermometer is 36.1°C (97.2°F). If the respiration, pulse, and blood pressure are within normal range, what would the nurse do *next*?
   1. Wait 15 minutes and retake it
   2. Check what the client's temperature was last time
   3. Retake it using a different thermometer
   4. Document the temperature

2. Which of the following clients meets the criteria for selection of the apical site for assessment of the pulse rather than the radial pulse?
   1. A client in shock
   2. A client whose pulse changes with body position changes
   3. A client with an arrhythmia
   4. A client who underwent surgery less than 24 hours ago

3. When the nurse enters the room to measure vital signs in preparing the client for a diagnostic test, the client is on the phone. What technique should the nurse use to determine the respiratory rate?
   1. Count the respirations during conversational pauses.
   2. Ask the client to end the phone call now and resume it at a later time.
   3. Wait at the client's bedside until the phone call is completed and then count respirations.
   4. Since there is no evidence of distress or urgency, defer the measurement.

4. For a client with a previous blood pressure of 138/74 and pulse of 64, approximately how long should the nurse take to release the blood pressure cuff in order to obtain an accurate reading?
   1. 10–20 seconds
   2. 30–45 seconds
   3. 1–1.5 minutes
   4. 3–3.5 minutes

5. It would be appropriate for the nurse to delegate measuring of vital signs to a UAP for which of the following clients?
   1. A client being prepared for elective facial surgery with a history of stable hypertension
   2. A client receiving a blood transfusion with a history of transfusion reactions
   3. A client recently started on a new antiarrhythmic agent
   4. A client who has been repeatedly admitted secondary to asthma exacerbations

6. An 85-year-old client has had a stroke resulting in right-sided facial drooping, difficulty swallowing, and is unable to move or maintain position independently. The nurse determines that which of the following are appropriate sites for measuring body temperature? Select all that apply.
   1. Oral
   2. Rectal
   3. Axillary
   4. Tympanic
   5. Temporal artery

7. A nursing diagnosis of *Ineffective Peripheral Tissue Perfusion* would be validated by which one of the following?
   1. Bounding radial pulse
   2. Irregular apical pulse
   3. Carotid pulse stronger on the left side than the right
   4. Absent posterior tibial and pedal pulses

8. The nurse reports that the client has dyspnea when ambulating. The nurse is most likely to have assessed which of the following while the client was walking?
   1. Shallow respirations
   2. Wheezing
   3. Shortness of breath
   4. Coughing up blood

9. When auscultating the blood pressure, the nurse hears the following: From 200 mm Hg to 180 mm Hg: silence; then a thumping sound from 178 to 150 mm Hg: muffled sounds from 148 to 130 mm Hg; soft thumping sounds from 128 to 104 mm Hg; muffled sounds continuing down to 94 mm Hg; then silence
The nurse records the blood pressure as _____.

10. In Figure 16–8, which number indicates the client's oxygen saturation as measured by pulse oximetry? ____

∞ *See answers to Test Your Knowledge in Appendix A.*

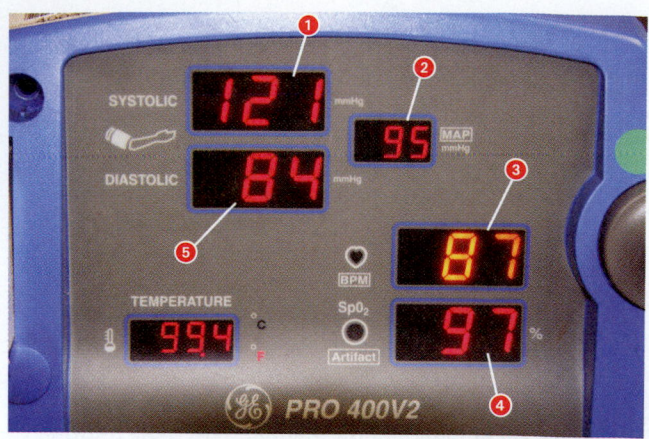

Figure 16–8 ● Vital signs monitor.

REFERENCES AND SELECTED BIBLIOGRAPHY

Artinian, N. T. (2004). Innovations in blood pressure monitoring, new, automated devices provide in home or around the clock readings. *American Journal of Nursing, 104*(8), 52–60.

Bindler, R. C., & Ball, J. W. (2007). *Clinical skills manual for pediatric nursing: Caring for children* (4th ed.). Upper Saddle River, NJ: Prentice Hall Health.

Bobrie, G., Chatellier, G., Genes, N., Clerson, P., Vaur, L., Vaisse, B., et al. (2004). Cardiovascular prognosis of "masked hypertension" detected by blood pressure self-measurement in elderly treated hypertensive patients. *Journal of the American Medical Association, 291*, 1342–1349.

Chan, M. M., Chan, M. D., & Chan, E. D. (2003). What is the effect of nail polish on pulse oximetry? *Chest, 123*, 2163–2164.

Davidhizar, R., & Shearer, R. (2004). Assisting patients to maintain a healthy blood pressure. *Journal of Practical Nursing, 54*(3), 5–8.

DuBois, E. F. (1948). *Fever and the regulation of body temperature.* Springfield, IL: Charles C. Thomas.

Irvin, D. J., & White, M. (2004). The importance of accurately assessing orthostatic hypotension. *Geriatric Nursing, 25*, 99–101.

Kempainen, R. R., & Brunette, D. D. (2004). The evaluation and management of accidental hypothermia. *Respiratory Care, 49*, 192–205.

Liu, C. C., Chang, R. E., & Chang, W. C. (2004). Limitations of forehead infrared body temperature detection for fever screening for severe acute respiratory syndrome. *Infection Control Hospital Epidemiology, 25*, 1109–1111.

Mackowiak, P. A., Wasserman, S. S., & Levine, M. M. (1992). A critical appraisal of 98.6 degrees F, the upper limit of the normal body temperature, and other legacies of Carl Reinhold August Wunderlich. *Journal of the American Medical Association, 268*, 1578–1580.

Marieb, E. N. & Hoehn, K. (2009). *Human anatomy and physiology* (8th ed.). San Francisco: Benjamin Cummings.

National Institutes of Health, National Heart, Lung, and Blood Institute. (2004). *The seventh report of the Joint National Committee on Prevention, Detection, Evaluation, and Treatment of High Blood Pressure* (NIH Publication No. 04–5230). Retrieved May 19, 2006, from http://www.nhlbi.nih.gov/guidelines/hypertension/jnc7full.htm

Nimah, M. M., Bshesh, K., Callahan, J., & Jacobs, B. R. (2006). Infrared tympanic thermometry in comparison with other temperature measurement techniques in febrile children. *Pediatric Critical Care Medicine, 7,* 48–55.

Pickering, T. G., Hall, J. E., Appel, L. J., Falkner, B. E., Graves, J., Hill, M. N., et al. (2005). Recommendations for blood pressure measurement in humans and experimental animals: Part 1: Blood pressure measurement in humans: A statement for professionals from the Subcommittee of Professional and Public Education of the American Heart Association Council on High Blood Pressure Research. *Circulation, 111,* 697–716.

Pinar, R., Sabuncu, N., & Oksay, A. (2004). Effects of crossed leg on blood pressure. *Blood Pressure, 13,* 252–254.

Popovich, D. M., Richiuso, N., & Danek, G. (2004). Pediatric health care providers' knowledge of pulse oximetry. *Pediatric Nursing, 30*(1), 14–20.

Rajkumar, A., Karmarkar, A., & Knott, J. (2006). Pulse oximetry: An Overview. *Journal of Perioperative Practice, 16,* 502–504.

Roy, S., Powell, K., & Gerson, L. W. (2003). Temporal artery temperature measurements in healthy infants, children, and adolescents. *Clinical Pediatrics, 42,* 433–437.

Rushing, J. (2004). Clinical do's & don'ts. Taking blood pressure accurately. *Nursing, 34*(11), 26.

Rushing, J. (2005). Clinical do's & don'ts. Assessing for orthostatic hypotension. *Nursing, 35*(1), 30.

Sclater, A., & Kannayiram. A. (2004). Orthostatic hypotension: A primary care primer for assessment and treatment. *Geriatrics, 59*(8), 22–27.

Smith, L. S. (2004). Temperature monitoring in newborns, a comparison of thermometry and measurement sites. *Journal of Neonatal Nursing, 10,* 157–165.

Viverais-Dresler, G., & Bakker, D. A. (2004). Blood pressure monitoring: Older adults' perceptions. *Journal of Gerontological Nursing, 30,* 44–52.

Woods, A. (2004). Loosening the grip of hypertension. *Nursing, 34*(12), 36–43.

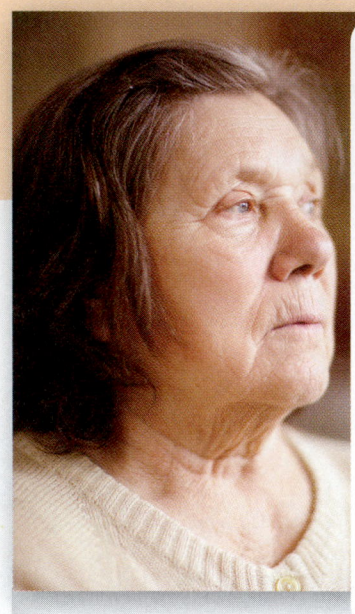

Mark Widmark, a nurse working in the emergency department, admits a 75-year-old female client with multiple traumatic injuries brought to the facility by ambulance. When asked how the injuries occurred, the client reports that she fell down the steps at her home. The paramedics who brought the client to the facility report that the home where she was found, and supposedly lives, is a ranch home with no steps to fall down. The nurse begins his assessment by measuring vital signs and notes several bruises in various stages of healing over the client's chest and abdomen, leading Mark to suspect the client may have been abused. Her medical records indicate she lives with her unmarried son, who has a substance abuse problem.

LEARNING OUTCOMES

After completing this chapter, you will be able to:

1. Define the key terms for the chapter.

2. Describe the purposes of the physical examination.

3. Contrast the four methods of examining the client and explain why one method may be more useful than another for specific purposes.

4. Contrast acceptable from atypical findings during the physical examination including the significance of atypical findings.

5. Compare various sequences for conducting a complete physical examination in an orderly fashion.

6. Differentiate variations in examination techniques appropriate for clients at different stages of the lifespan.

7. Demonstrate the performance of a physical examination.

KEY TERMS

Adventitious breath sounds p440	Dullness p403	Normocephalic p418	S₁ p447
Auscultation p403	Flatness p403	Otoscope p427	S₂ p447
Blanch test p411	Goniometer p464	Palpation p402	Thrill p448
Bruit p448	Hyperresonance p403	Percussion p403	Tympanic membrane p427
Cerumen p428	Inspection p402	Pitch p403	
Clubbing p411	Intensity p404	Pleximeter p403	Tympany p403
Crepitations p440	Jaundice p407	Reflex p413	Visual acuity p420
	Lift p447	Resonance p403	Visual fields p420

Adventitious breath sounds p440

Assessing a client's health status is a major component of nursing care and has two aspects: the nursing health history discussed in Chapter 7 ∞ and the physical examination discussed in this chapter. A physical examination can be any of three types: (a) a complete assessment (e.g., when a client is admitted to a health care agency); (b) examination of a body system (e.g., the cardiovascular system); or (c) examination of a body area (e.g., the lungs, when difficulty with breathing is observed). *Note:* Some nurses consider *assessment* to be the broad term used in applying the nursing process to health data and *examination* to be the physical process used to gather the data. In this text, the terms *assessment* and *examination* are sometimes used interchangeably—both referring to a critical investigation and evaluation of client status.

PHYSICAL HEALTH ASSESSMENT

A complete health assessment may be conducted starting at the head and proceeding in a systematic manner downward (head-to-toe assessment). However, the procedure can vary according to the age of the individual, the severity of the illness, the preferences of the nurse, the location of the examination, and the agency's priorities and procedures. The usual order of head-to-toe assessment is given in Box 17–1. Regardless of the procedure used, the client's energy and time need to be considered. The health assessment is therefore conducted in a systematic and efficient manner that results in the fewest position changes for the client.

Frequently, nurses assess a specific body area instead of the entire body. These specific assessments are made in relation to client complaints, the nurse's own observation of problems, the client's presenting problem, nursing interventions provided, and medical therapies.

The physical examination serves a number of purposes. It helps to obtain baseline data, verify data obtained in the nursing history, obtain data that will contribute to the nursing diagnosis and plan of care, evaluate client outcomes and response to treatment, make clinical judgments about health status, and identify areas for health promotion and prevention.

Preparing the Client

Most people need an explanation of the physical examination. Often clients are anxious about what the nurse will find and what will be done. They can be reassured during the examination by explanations at each step. The nurse should explain when and where the examination will take place, why it is important, and what will happen. Instruct the client that all information gathered and documented during the assessment is kept confidential in accordance with the Health Insurance Portability and Accountability Act (HIPAA). This means that only those health care providers who have a legitimate need to know the client's information will have access to it.

Health examinations are usually painless; however, it is important to determine in advance any positions that are contraindicated for a particular client. The nurse assists the client as needed to undress and put on a gown. Clients should empty their bladders before the examination. Doing so helps them feel more relaxed and facilitates palpation of the abdomen and pubic area. If a urinalysis is required, the urine should be collected in a container for that purpose.

When assessing adults it is important to recognize that people of the same age differ markedly. Box 17–2 provides special considerations for assessing adults, especially older adults.

BOX 17–1   Head-to-Toe Framework

- General survey
- Vital signs
- Head
  - Hair, scalp, cranium, face
  - Eyes and vision
  - Ears and hearing
  - Nose and sinuses
  - Mouth and oropharynx
  - Cranial nerves
- Neck
  - Muscles
  - Lymph nodes
  - Trachea
  - Thyroid gland
  - Carotid arteries
  - Neck veins
- Upper extremities
  - Skin and nails
  - Muscle strength and tone
  - Joint range of motion
  - Brachial and radial pulses
  - Biceps tendon reflexes
  - Tendon reflexes
  - Sensation
- Chest and back
  - Skin
- Chest shape and size
- Lungs
- Heart
- Spinal column
- Breasts and axillae
- Abdomen
  - Skin
  - Abdominal sounds
  - Specific organs (e.g., liver, bladder)
  - Femoral pulses
- Genitals
  - Testicles
  - Vagina
  - Urethra
- Anus and rectum
- Lower extremities
  - Skin and toenails
  - Gait and balance
  - Joint range of motion
  - Popliteal, posterior tibial, and pedal pulses
  - Tendon and plantar reflexes

BOX 17–2   Health Assessment of the Adult

- Be aware of normal physiologic changes that occur with age.
- Be aware of stiffness of muscles and joints from aging changes or history of orthopedic surgery. The client may need modification of the usual positioning necessary for examination and assessment.
- Expose only areas of the body to be examined in order to avoid chilling.
- Permit ample time for the client to answer your questions and assume the required positions.
- Be aware of cultural differences. The client may want a family member present during disrobing.
- Arrange for an interpreter if the client's language differs from that of the nurse.
- Ask clients how they wish to be addressed, such as Mrs. or Miss.
- Adapt assessment techniques to any sensory impairment; for example, make sure eyeglasses or hearing aids are nearby.
- If clients are older and/or frail it is wise to plan several assessment times in order to not overtire them.

The sequence of the assessment differs with children and adults. With children, always proceed from the least invasive or uncomfortable to the more invasive. Examination of the head and neck, heart and lungs, and range of motion can be done early in the process, while the ears, mouth, abdomen, and genitals should be left for the end of the exam.

Preparing the Environment

It is important to prepare the environment before starting the assessment. The time for the physical assessment should be convenient to both the client and the nurse. The environment needs to be well lighted and the equipment should be organized for efficient use. A client who is physically relaxed will usually experience little discomfort. The room should be warm enough to be comfortable for the client.

Providing privacy is important. Most people are embarrassed if their bodies are exposed or if others can overhear or view them during the assessment. Culture, age, and gender of both the client and the nurse influence how comfortable the client will be and what special arrangements might be needed. Family and friends should not be present unless the client asks for someone.

Positioning

Several positions are frequently required during the physical assessment. It is important to consider the client's ability to assume a position. The client's physical condition, energy level, and age should also be taken into consideration. Some positions are embarrassing and uncomfortable and therefore should not be maintained for long. The

TABLE 17–1	Client Positions and Body Areas Assessed		
POSITION	**DESCRIPTION**	**AREAS ASSESSED**	**CAUTIONS**
Dorsal recumbent	Back-lying position with knees flexed and hips externally rotated; small pillow under the head; soles of feet on the surface	Female genitals, rectum, and female reproductive tract	May be contraindicated for clients who have cardiopulmonary problems.
Supine (horizontal recumbent)	Back-lying position with legs extended; with or without pillow under the head	Head, neck, axillae, anterior thorax, lungs, breasts, heart, vital signs, abdomen, extremities, peripheral pulses	Tolerated poorly by clients with cardiovascular and respiratory problems.
Sitting	A seated position, back unsupported and legs hanging freely	Head, neck, posterior and anterior thorax, lungs, breasts, axillae, heart, vital signs, upper and lower extremities, reflexes	Older adults and weak clients may require support.
Lithotomy	Back-lying position with feet supported in stirrups; the hips should be in line with the edge of the table	Female genitals, rectum, and female reproductive tract	May be uncomfortable and tiring for older adults and often embarrassing.
Sims'	Side-lying position with lowermost arm behind the body, uppermost leg flexed at hip and knee, upper arm flexed at shoulder and elbow	Rectum, vagina	Difficult for older adults and people with limited joint movement.
Prone	Lies on abdomen with head turned to the side, with or without a small pillow	Posterior thorax, hip joint movement	Often not tolerated by older adults and people with cardiovascular and respiratory problems.

assessment is organized so that several body areas can be assessed in one position, thus minimizing the number of position changes needed (see Table 17–1).

Draping

Drapes should be arranged so that the area to be assessed is exposed and other body areas are covered. Exposure of the body is frequently embarrassing to clients. Drapes provide not only a degree of privacy but also warmth. Drapes are made of paper, cloth, or bed linen.

Instrumentation

All equipment required for the health assessment should be clean, in good working order, and readily accessible. Equipment is frequently set up on trays, ready for use. Various instruments are shown in Table 17–2.

Methods of Examining

Four primary techniques are used in the physical examination: inspection, palpation, percussion, and auscultation.

TABLE 17–2   Equipment and Supplies Used for a Health Examination

SUPPLIES		PURPOSE
Flashlight or penlight		To assist viewing of the pharynx and cervix or to determine the reactions of the pupils of the eye
Nasal speculum		To permit visualization of the lower and middle turbinates; usually, a penlight is used for illumination
Ophthalmoscope		A lighted instrument to visualize the interior of the eye
Otoscope		A lighted instrument to visualize the eardrum and external auditory canal (a nasal speculum may be attached to the otoscope to inspect the nasal cavities)
Percussion (reflex) hammer		An instrument with a rubber head to test reflexes
Tuning fork		A two-pronged metal instrument used to test hearing acuity and vibratory sense
Vaginal speculum		To assess the cervix and the vagina
Cotton applicators		To obtain specimens
Gloves		To protect the nurse
Lubricant		To ease insertion of instruments (e.g., vaginal speculum)
Tongue blades (depressors)		To depress the tongue during assessment of the mouth and pharynx

These techniques are discussed throughout this chapter as they apply to each body system.

Inspection is the visual examination, assessing by using the sense of sight. It should be deliberate, purposeful, and systematic. The nurse inspects with the naked eye and with instruments such as an otoscope (used to view the ear). In addition to visual observations, olfactory (smell) and auditory (hearing) cues are noted. Nurses frequently use visual inspection to assess moisture, color, and texture of body surfaces, as well as shape, position, size, color, and symmetry of the body. Lighting must be sufficient for the nurse to see clearly using either natural or artificial light. When using the auditory senses it is important to have a quiet environment for accurate hearing. Observation can be combined with the other assessment techniques.

Palpation is the examination of the body using the sense of touch. The pads of the fingers are used because their concentration of nerve endings makes them highly sensitive to tactile discrimination. Palpation is used to determine (a) texture; (b) temperature; (c) vibration; (d) position, size, consistency, and mobility of organs or masses (Box 17–3); (e) distention; (f) pulsation; and (g) the presence of pain upon pressure.

There are two types of palpation: light and deep. *Light* (superficial) *palpation* should always precede *deep palpation* because heavy pressure on the fingertips can dull the sense of touch. For light palpation, the nurse extends the dominant hand's fingers parallel to the skin surface and presses gently while moving the hand in a circle (see Figure 17–1). With light palpation, the skin is slightly depressed. If it is necessary to determine the details of a mass, the nurse presses lightly several times rather than holding the pressure.

Deep palpation is done with one or two hands (bimanually). In deep bimanual palpation, the nurse extends the dominant hand as for light palpation, placing the finger pads of the nondominant hand on the dorsal surface of the distal interphalangeal joint of the middle three fingers of the dominant hand (Figure 17–2). The top hand applies pressure while the lower hand remains relaxed to perceive the tactile sensations. When performing deep palpation using one hand, the finger pads of the dominant hand press over the area to be palpated. Often the other hand is used to support a mass or organ from below (Figure 17–3). *Deep palpation is usually not done during a routine examination and re-*

quires significant practitioner skill. It is performed with extreme caution because pressure can damage internal organs. It is usually not indicated in clients who have acute abdominal pain or pain that is not yet diagnosed.

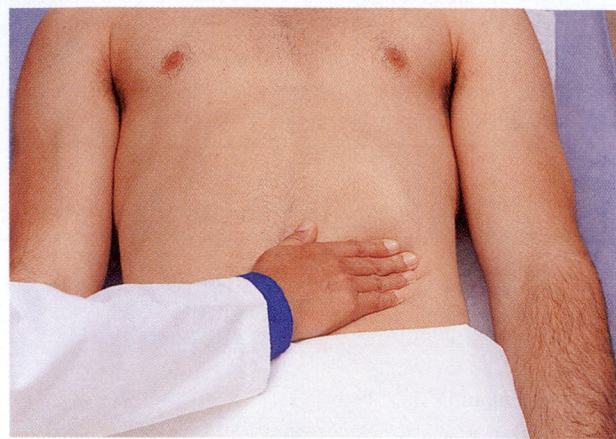

Figure 17–1 ● The position of the hand for light palpation.

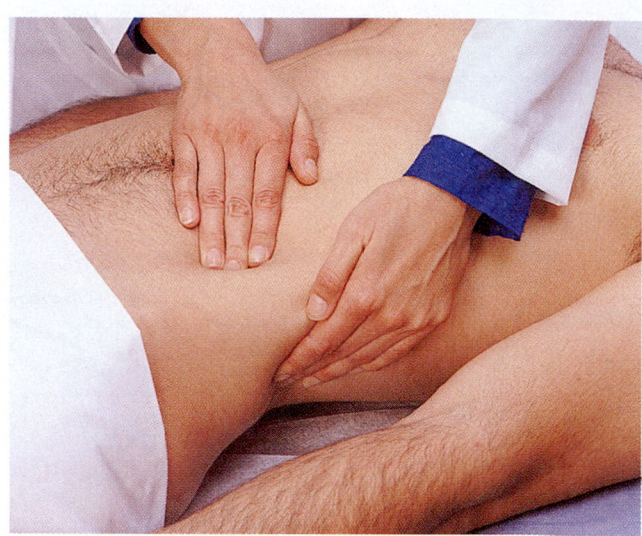

Figure 17–2 ● The position of the hands for deep bimanual palpation.

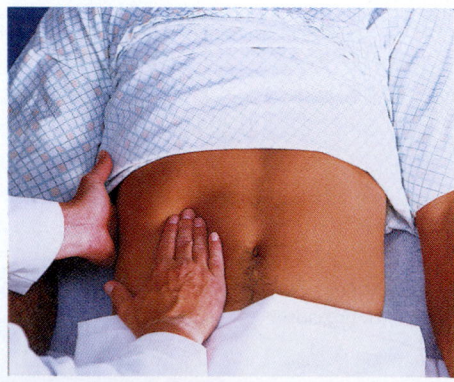

Figure 17–3 ● Deep palpation using the lower hand to support the body while the upper hand palpates the organ.

BOX 17–3	**Characteristics of Masses**

Location—Site on the body, dorsal/ventral surface

Size—Length and width in centimeters

Shape—Oval, round, elongated, irregular

Consistency—Soft, firm, hard

Surface—Smooth, nodular

Mobility—Fixed, mobile

Pulsatility—Present or absent

Tenderness—Degree of tenderness to palpation

To test skin temperature, it is best to use the dorsum or back of the hand and fingers, where the examiner's skin is thinnest. To test for vibration, the nurse should use the palmar surface of the hand. When performing palpation the nurse's hands should be warm and clean with short fingernails. Areas of tenderness should be palpated last and superficial palpation should precede deep palpation.

The effectiveness of palpation depends largely on the client's relaxation. Nurses can assist a client to relax by (a) gowning and/or draping the client appropriately, (b) positioning the client comfortably, and (c) ensuring that their own hands are warm before beginning. During palpation, the nurse should be sensitive to the client's verbal and facial expressions indicating discomfort.

Percussion is the act of striking the body surface to elicit sounds that can be heard or vibrations that can be felt. There are two types of percussion: direct and indirect. In *direct percussion,* the nurse strikes the area to be percussed directly with the pads of two, three, or four fingers or with the pad of the middle finger. The strikes are rapid, and the movement is from the wrist. This technique is not generally used to percuss the thorax but is useful in percussing an adult's sinuses.

Indirect percussion is the striking of an object held against the body area to be examined. In this technique, the middle finger of the nondominant hand, referred to as the **pleximeter**, is placed firmly on the client's skin. Only the distal phalanx and joint of this finger should be in contact with the skin. Using the tip of the flexed middle finger of the other hand, called the plexor, the nurse strikes the pleximeter, usually at the distal interphalangeal joint (see Figure 17–4). Some nurses may find a point between the distal and proximal joints to be a more comfortable pleximeter point. The motion comes from the wrist; the forearm remains stationary. The angle between the plexor and the pleximeter should be 90 degrees, and the blows must be firm, rapid, and short to obtain a clear sound.

Percussion is used to determine the size and shape of internal organs by establishing their borders. It indicates whether tissue is fluid filled, air filled, or solid. Percussion elicits five types of sound: flatness, dullness, resonance, hyperresonance, and tympany. **Flatness** is an extremely dull sound produced by very dense tissue, such as muscle or bone. **Dullness** is a thudlike sound produced by dense tissue such as the liver, spleen, or heart. **Resonance** is a hollow sound such as that produced by lungs filled with air. **Hyperresonance** is not an anticipated finding. It is described as booming and can be heard over an emphysema-

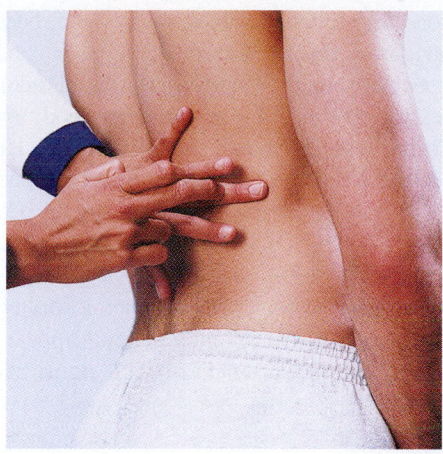

Figure 17–4 ● Indirect percussion. Using the finger of one hand to tap the finger of the other hand.

tous lung. **Tympany** is a musical or drumlike sound produced from an air-filled stomach. On a continuum, flatness reflects the most dense tissue and tympany the least dense tissue. A percussion sound is described according to its intensity, pitch, duration, and quality (see Table 17–3).

Auscultation is the process of listening to sounds produced within the body. Auscultation may be direct or indirect. *Direct auscultation* is the use of the unaided ear, for example, to listen to a respiratory wheeze or the grating of a moving joint. *Indirect auscultation* is the use of a stethoscope, which transmits the sounds to the nurse's ears. A stethoscope is used primarily to listen to sounds from within the body, such as bowel sounds or valve sounds of the heart and blood pressure.

The stethoscope tubing should be 30 to 35 cm (12 to 14 in.) long, with an internal diameter of about 0.3 cm (1/8 in.). It should have both a flat disc diaphragm and a bell-shaped amplifier (see figure in Skill 16–5 in Chapter 16 ∞). The diaphragm best transmits high-pitched sounds, and the bell best transmits low-pitched sounds such as some heart sounds. The earpieces of the stethoscope should fit comfortably into the nurse's ears, facing forward. The amplifier of the stethoscope is placed firmly but lightly against the client's skin. If the client has excessive hair, it may be necessary to dampen the hairs with a moist cloth so that they will lie flat against the skin and not interfere with clear sound transmission.

Auscultated sounds are described according to their pitch, intensity, duration, and quality. The **pitch** is the frequency of

TABLE 17–3	Percussion Sounds and Tones				
SOUND	INTENSITY	PITCH	DURATION	QUALITY	EXAMPLE OF LOCATION
Flatness	Soft	High	Short	Extremely dull	Muscle, bone
Dullness	Medium	Medium	Moderate	Thudlike	Liver, heart
Resonance	Loud	Low	Long	Hollow	Healthy lung
Hyperresonance	Very loud	Very low	Very long	Booming	Emphysematous lung
Tympany	Loud	High (distinguished mainly by musical timbre)	Moderate	Musical	Stomach filled with gas (air)

the vibrations. Low-pitched sounds, such as some heart sounds, have fewer vibrations per second than high-pitched sounds, such as bronchial sounds. The **intensity** (amplitude) refers to the loudness or softness of a sound. Some body sounds are loud, others are soft. The duration of a sound is its length. The quality of sound is a subjective description of a sound.

GENERAL SURVEY

Health assessment begins with a general survey that involves observation of the client's general appearance and mental status, and measurement of vital signs, height, and weight. Many components of the general survey are assessed while taking the client's health history, such as the client's body build, posture, hygiene, and mental status.

Appearance and Mental Status

The general appearance and behavior of an individual must be assessed in relationship to culture, educational level, socioeconomic status, and current circumstances. The client's age, sex, and race are also useful factors in interpreting findings that suggest increased risk for known conditions. Skill 17–1 describes how to assess general appearance and mental status.

SKILL 17–1

ASSESSING APPEARANCE AND MENTAL STATUS

PLANNING

Delegation
Due to the substantial knowledge and skill required, assessment of general appearance and mental status is not delegated to unlicensed assistive personnel (UAP). However, many aspects are observed during usual care and may be recorded by persons other than the nurse. Atypical findings must be validated and interpreted by the nurse.

EQUIPMENT
None

IMPLEMENTATION

Performance

1. Prior to performing the procedure, introduce self and verify the client's identity using agency protocol. Explain to the client what you are going to do, why it is necessary, and how he or she can cooperate. Discuss how the results will be used in planning further care or treatments.
2. Perform hand hygiene and observe appropriate infection control procedures.
3. Provide for client privacy.

ASSESSMENT	TYPICAL FINDINGS	ATYPICAL FINDINGS
4. Observe body build, height, and weight in relation to the client's age, lifestyle, and health.	Proportionate, varies with lifestyle	Excessively thin or obese
5. Observe client's posture and gait, standing, sitting, and walking.	Relaxed, erect posture; coordinated movement	Tense, slouched, bent posture; uncoordinated movement; tremors
6. Observe client's overall hygiene and grooming. Relate these to the person's activities prior to the assessment.	Clean, neat	Dirty, unkempt
7. Note body and breath odor in relation to activity level.	No body odor or minor body odor relative to recent activity level; no breath odor	Foul body odor; ammonia odor; acetone breath odor; foul breath
8. Observe for signs of distress in posture or facial expression.	No distress noted	Bending over because of abdominal pain, wincing, frowning, or labored breathing
9. Note obvious signs of health or illness.	Healthy appearance	Pallor; weakness; lesions
10. Assess the client's attitude.	Cooperative, able to follow instructions	Negative, hostile, withdrawn
11. Note the client's affect/mood; assess the appropriateness of the client's responses.	Appropriate to situation	Inappropriate to situation
12. Listen for quantity of speech, quality, and organization.	Understandable, moderate pace; clear tone and inflection; exhibits thought association	Rapid or slow pace; overly loud or soft; uses generalizations; lacks association
13. Listen for relevance and organization of thoughts.	Logical sequence; makes sense; has sense of reality	Illogical sequence; flight of ideas; confusion; vague
14. Document findings in the client record following facility policy.		

EVALUATION

• Perform a detailed follow-up examination of individual systems based on findings that deviated from expected for the client. Relate findings to previous assessment data if available.

• Report significant deviations to the primary care provider.

Vital Signs

Vital signs are measured (a) to establish baseline data against which to compare future measurements and (b) to detect actual and potential health problems. See Chapter 16 ∞ for measurements of temperature, pulse, respirations, blood pressure, and oxygen saturation. See Chapter 18 ∞ for pain assessment.

Height and Weight

In adults, the ratio of weight to height provides a general measure of health. By asking clients about their height and weight before actually measuring them, the nurse obtains some idea of the person's self-image. Excessive discrepancies between the client's responses and the measurements may provide clues to actual or potential problems in self-concept. Be aware of any significant unintentional weight gain or loss.

The nurse measures height with a measuring stick attached to weight scales or to a wall. The client should remove the shoes and stand erect, with heels together, and the heels, buttocks, and back of the head against the measuring stick; eyes should be looking straight ahead. The nurse raises the L-shaped sliding arm on the weight scale until it rests on top of the client's head, or places a small flat object such as a ruler or book on the client's head. The edge of the flat object should abut the measuring guide.

Weight is usually measured when a client is admitted to a health agency and may be repeated regularly. Scales measure in pounds (lb) or kilograms (kg), and the nurse may need to convert between the two systems. One kilogram is equal to 2.2 pounds. When accuracy is essential, the nurse should use the same scale each time (because every scale weighs slightly differently), take the measurements at the same time each day, and make sure the client has on a similar kind of clothing and no footwear. The client stands on a platform, and the weight is read from a digital display panel or a balancing arm. Clients who cannot stand are weighed on chair or bed scales. The bed scales have canvas straps or a stretcher-like apparatus. A machine lifts the client above the bed, and the weight is reflected either on a digital display panel or on a balance arm like that of a standing scale. Some agencies may have beds with built-in scales.

CLINICAL ALERT

Review the agency charting form before beginning your assessment to ensure that you have all of the equipment you need and know how to perform the assessment in a systematic approach.

THE INTEGUMENT

The integument includes the skin, hair, and nails. The examination begins with a generalized inspection using a good source of lighting, preferably indirect natural daylight.

Skin

Assessment of the skin involves inspection and palpation. The entire skin surface may be assessed at one time or as each aspect of the body is assessed. In some instances, the nurse may also use the olfactory sense to detect unusual skin odors; these are usually most evident in the skinfolds or in the axillae. Pungent body odor is frequently related to poor hygiene, hyperhidrosis (excessive perspiration), or bromhidrosis (foul-smelling perspiration).

Pallor is the result of inadequate circulating blood or hemoglobin and subsequent reduction in tissue oxygenation. In clients with dark skin, it is usually characterized by the absence of underlying red tones in the skin and may be most readily seen in the buccal mucosa. In brown-skinned clients, pallor may appear as a yellowish brown tinge; in black-skinned clients, the skin may appear ashen gray. Pallor in all people is usually most evident in areas with the least pigmentation such as the conjunctiva, oral mucous membranes, nail beds, palms of the hand, and soles of the feet.

LIFESPAN CONSIDERATIONS
General Survey

Infants

- Observation of children's behavior can provide important data for the general survey, including physical development, neuromuscular function, and social and interactional skills.
- It may be helpful to have parents hold older infants and very young children for part of the assessment.
- Measure height of children under age 2 in the supine position with knees fully extended.
- Weigh without clothing.
- Include measurement of head circumference until age 2. Standardized growth charts include head circumference up to age 3.

Children

- Anxiety in preschool-age children can be decreased by letting them handle and become familiar with examination equipment.
- School-age children may be very modest and shy about exposing parts of the body.
- Adolescents should be examined without parents present.
- Weigh children without shoes and with as little clothing as possible.

Older Adults

- Allow extra time for clients to answer questions.
- Adapt questioning techniques as appropriate for clients with hearing or visual limitations.
- Older adults with osteoporosis can lose several inches in height. Be sure to document height and ask if they are aware of becoming shorter in height.
- When asking about weight loss, be specific about amount and time frame, e.g., "Have you lost more than five pounds in the last two months?"

Macule, Patch Flat, unelevated change in color. Macules are 1 mm to 1 cm in size and circumscribed. Examples: freckles, measles, petechiae, flat moles. Patches are larger than 1 cm and may have an irregular shape. Examples: port wine birthmark, vitiligo (white patches), rubella. ❶

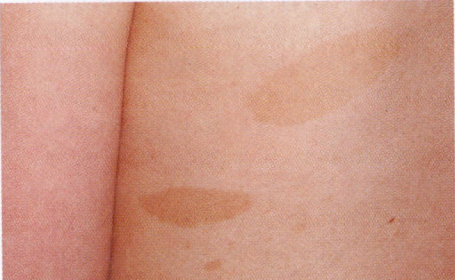

❶ **Multiple café-au-lait macules**

Nodule, Tumor Elevated, solid, hard mass that extends deeper into the dermis than a papule. Nodules have a circumscribed border and are 0.5 to 2 cm. Examples: squamous cell carcinoma, fibroma. Tumors are larger than 2 cm and may have an irregular border. Examples: malignant melanoma, hemangioma. ❹

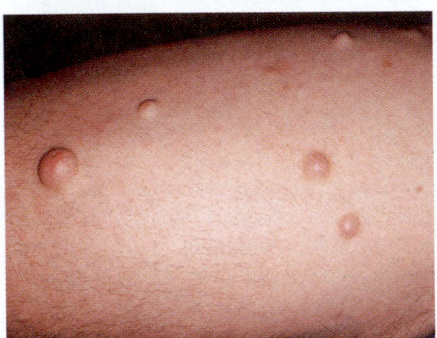

❹ **Peripheral neurofibromas**

Papule Circumscribed, solid elevation of skin. Papules are less than 1 cm. Examples: warts, acne, pimples, elevated moles. ❷

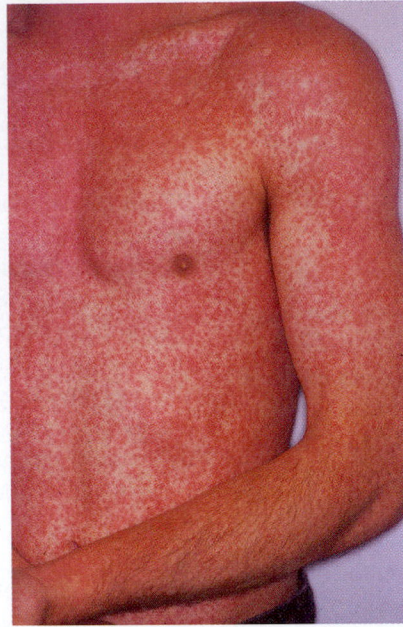

❷ **Papular drug eruption** (Courtesy Scott D. Bennion, MD)

Pustule Vesicle or bulla filled with pus. Examples: acne vulgaris, impetigo. ❺

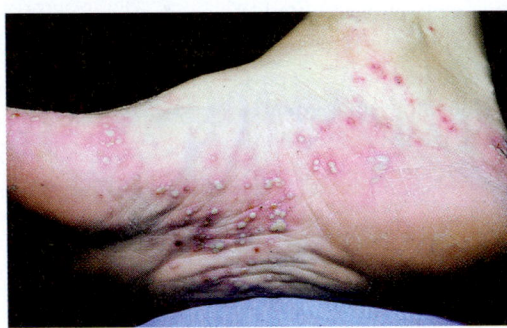

❺ **Chronic pustular psoriasis**

Plaque Plaques are larger than 1 cm. Examples: psoriasis, rubeola. ❸

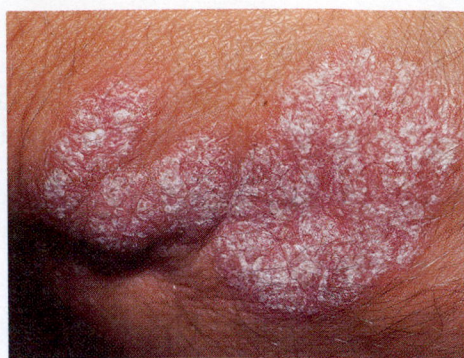

❸ **Psoriasis vulgaris**

Vesicle, Bulla A circumscribed, round or oval, thin translucent mass filled with serous fluid or blood.
Vesicles are less than 0.5 cm. Examples: herpes simplex, early chicken pox, small burn blister. Bullae are larger than 0.5 cm. Examples: large blister, second-degree burn, herpes simplex. ❻

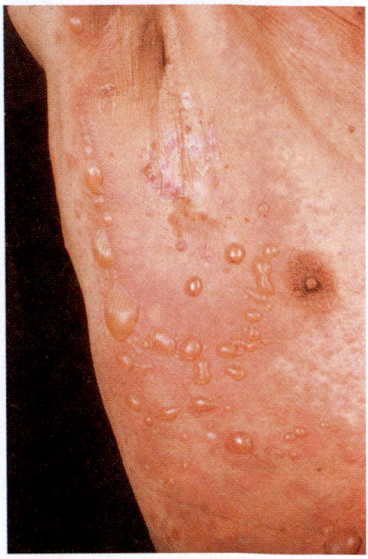

❻ **Bullous pemphigoid**

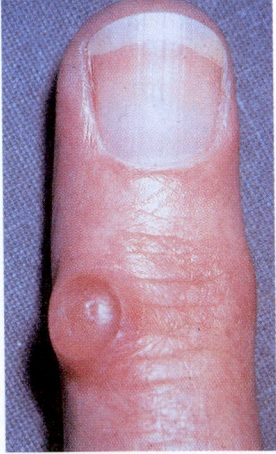

Cyst A 1-cm or larger, elevated, encapsulated, fluid-filled or semisolid mass arising from the subcutaneous tissue or dermis. Examples: sebaceous and epidermoid cysts, chalazion of the eyelid. ❼

❼ **Digital mucous cyst**

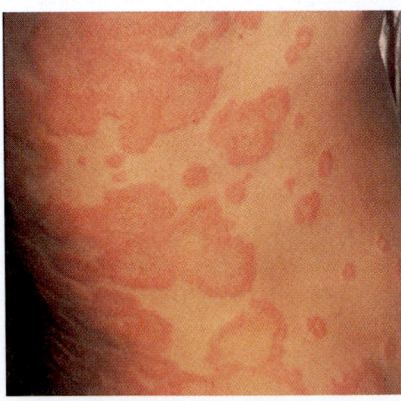

Wheal A reddened, localized collection of edema fluid; irregular in shape. Size varies. Examples: hives, mosquito bites. ❽

❽ **Allergic wheals, urticaria**

Figure 17–5 ⬤ Primary skin lesions.

Cyanosis (a bluish tinge) is most evident in the nail beds, lips, and buccal mucosa. In dark-skinned clients, close inspection of the palpebral conjunctiva (the lining of the eyelids) and palms and soles may also show evidence of cyanosis. **Jaundice** (a yellowish tinge) may first be evident in the sclera of the eyes and then in the mucous membranes and the skin. Nurses should take care not to confuse jaundice with the typical yellow pigmentation in the sclera of a dark-skinned client. If jaundice is suspected, the posterior part of the hard palate should also be inspected for a yellowish color tone. Erythema is a redness associated with a variety of rashes.

Dark-skinned clients have areas of lighter pigmentation, such as the palms, lips, and nail beds. Localized areas of hyperpigmentation (increased pigmentation) and hypopigmentation (decreased pigmentation) may also occur as a result of changes in the distribution of melanin (the dark pigment) or in the function of the melanocytes in the epidermis. An example of hyperpigmentation in a defined area is a birthmark. Other localized color changes may indicate a problem such as edema or a localized infection. Edema is the presence of excess interstitial fluid. An area of edema appears swollen, shiny, and taut and tends to blanch the skin color or, if accompanied by inflammation, may redden the skin. Generalized edema is most often an indication of impaired venous circulation and in some cases reflects cardiac dysfunction or venous abnormalities.

A skin lesion is an alteration in a client's skin appearance. Primary skin lesions are those that appear initially in response to some change in the external or internal environment of the skin (see Figure 17–5, *1–8*). Secondary skin lesions are those that do not appear initially but result from modifications such as chronicity, trauma, or infection of the primary lesion. Table 17–4

TABLE 17–4	**Secondary Skin Lesions**				
Atrophy	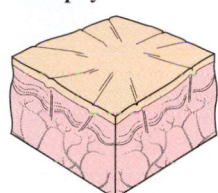	A translucent, dry, paperlike, sometimes wrinkled skin surface resulting from thinning or wasting of the skin due to loss of collagen and elastin. **Examples:** Striae, aged skin	**Ulcer**	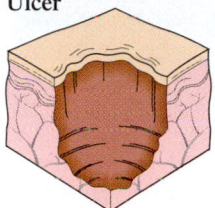	Deep, irregularly shaped area of skin loss extending into the dermis or subcutaneous tissue. May bleed. May leave scar. **Examples:** Decubitus ulcers (pressure sores), stasis ulcers, chancres
Erosion	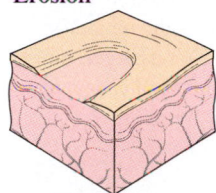	Wearing away of the superficial epidermis causing a moist, shallow depression. Because erosions do not extend into the dermis, they heal without scarring. **Examples:** Scratch marks, ruptured vesicles	**Fissure**	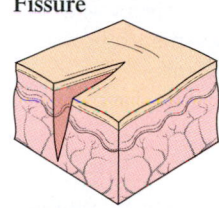	Linear crack with sharp edges, extending into the dermis. **Examples:** Cracks at the corners of the mouth or in the hands, athlete's foot
Lichenification	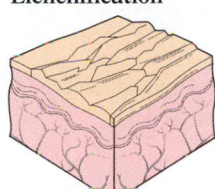	Rough, thickened, hardened area of epidermis resulting from chronic irritation such as scratching or rubbing. **Example:** Chronic dermatitis	**Scar**	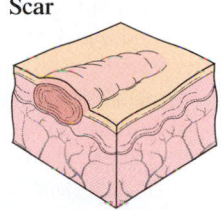	Flat, irregular area of connective tissue left after a lesion or wound has healed. New scars may be red or purple; older scars may be silvery or white. **Examples:** Healed surgical wound or injury, healed acne
Scales	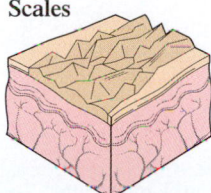	Shedding flakes of greasy, keratinized skin tissue. Color may be white, gray, or silver. Texture may vary from fine to thick. **Examples:** Dry skin, dandruff, psoriasis, and eczema	**Keloid**	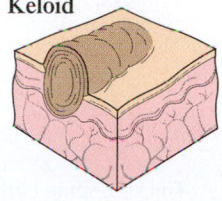	Elevated, irregular, darkened area of excess scar tissue caused by excessive collagen formation during healing. Extends beyond the site of the original injury. Higher incidence in people of African descent. **Examples:** Keloid from ear piercing or surgery
Crust	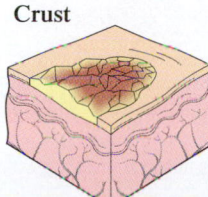	Dry blood, serum, or pus left on the skin surface when vesicles or pustules burst. Can be red-brown, orange, or yellow. Large crusts that adhere to the skin surface are called scabs. **Examples:** Eczema, impetigo, herpes, or scabs following abrasion	**Excoriation**	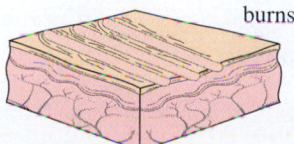	Linear erosion. **Examples:** Scratches, some chemical burns

illustrates secondary lesions. Nurses are responsible for describing skin lesions accurately in terms of location, distribution, and configuration as well as color, shape, size, firmness, texture, and characteristics of individual lesions.

CLINICAL ALERT

If possible and the client agrees, take a digital or instant photograph of significant skin lesions for the client record. Include a measuring guide (ruler or tape) in the picture to demonstrate lesion size. Clients must sign a release before any photograph can be taken.

Skill 17–2 describes how to assess the skin.

SKILL 17–2

ASSESSING THE SKIN

PLANNING
- Review characteristics of primary and secondary skin lesions if necessary (see Figure 17–5 and Table 17–4).
- Ensure that adequate lighting is available.

Delegation
Due to the substantial knowledge and skill required, assessment of the skin is not delegated to UAP. However, the skin is observed during usual care and these persons should record their findings. Atypical findings must be validated and interpreted by the nurse.

EQUIPMENT
- Millimeter ruler
- Clean gloves
- Magnifying glass

IMPLEMENTATION
Performance

1. Prior to performing the procedure, introduce self and verify the client's identity using agency protocol. Explain to the client what you are going to do, why it is necessary, and how he or she can cooperate. Discuss how the results will be used in planning further care or treatments.
2. Perform hand hygiene and observe appropriate infection control procedures.
3. Provide for client privacy.

4. Inquire if the client has any history of the following: pain or itching; presence and spread of lesions, bruises, abrasions, pigmented spots; previous experience with skin problems; associated clinical signs; family history; presence of problems in other family members; related systemic conditions; use of medications, lotions, home remedies; excessively dry or moist feel to the skin; tendency to bruise easily; association of the problem to season of year, stress, occupation, medications, recent travel, housing, and so on; recent contact with allergens, e.g., metal paint.

ASSESSMENT	TYPICAL FINDINGS	ATYPICAL FINDINGS
5. Inspect skin color (best assessed under natural light and on areas not exposed to the sun).	Varies from light to deep brown; from ruddy pink to light pink; from yellow overtones to olive	Pallor, cyanosis, jaundice, erythema
6. Inspect uniformity of skin color.	Generally uniform except in areas exposed to the sun; areas of lighter pigmentation (palms, lips, nail beds) in dark-skinned people	Areas of either hyperpigmentation or hypopigmentation
7. Assess edema, if present (i.e., location, color, temperature, shape, and the degree to which the skin remains indented or pitted when pressed by a finger). Measuring the circumference of the extremity with a millimeter tape may be useful for future comparison.	No edema	See the scale for describing edema. ❶
8. Inspect, palpate, and describe skin lesions. Apply gloves if lesions are open or draining. Palpate lesions to determine shape and texture. Describe lesions according to location, distribution, color, configuration, size, shape, type, or structure (see Box 17–4).	Freckles, some birthmarks, some flat and raised nevi; no abrasions or other lesions	Various interruptions in skin integrity; irregular, multicolored, or raised nevi

ASSESSMENT	**TYPICAL FINDINGS**	**ATYPICAL FINDINGS**
9. Observe and palpate skin moisture.	Moisture in skin folds and the axillae (varies with environmental temperature and humidity, body temperature, and activity)	Excessive moisture (e.g., in hyperthermia); excessive dryness (e.g., in dehydration)
10. Palpate skin temperature. Compare the two feet and the two hands, using the backs of your fingers.	Uniform; within acceptable range	Generalized hyperthermia (e.g., in fever); generalized hypothermia (e.g., in shock); localized hyperthermia (e.g., in infection); localized hypothermia (e.g., in arteriosclerosis)

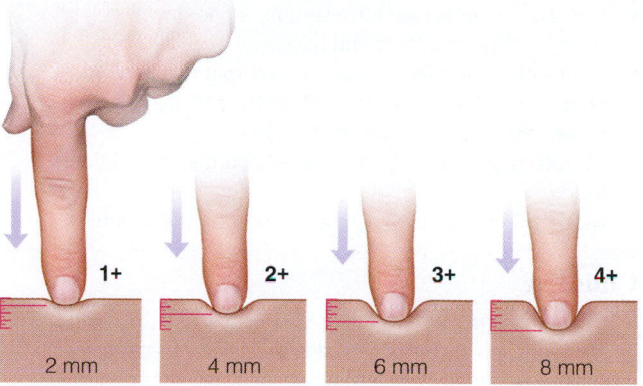

❶ Scale for grading edema.

11. Note skin turgor (fullness or elasticity) by lifting and pinching the skin on an extremity.	When pinched, skin springs back to previous state; may be slower in older adults	Skins stays pinched or tented or moves back slowly (e.g., in dehydration)

12. Document findings in the client record using forms or checklists supplemented by narrative notes when appropriate. Draw location of skin lesions on body surface diagrams. ❷

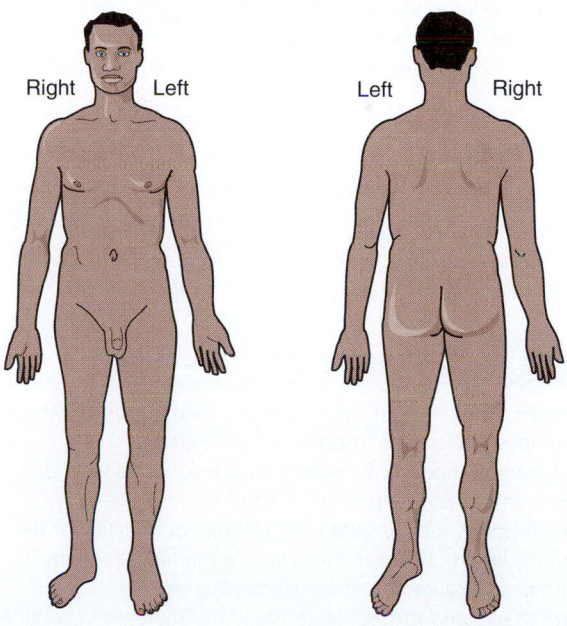

❷ Diagram for charting skin lesions.

EVALUATION

- Compare findings to previous skin assessment data if available to determine if lesions or abnormalities are changing.

- Report significant deviations from anticipated findings to the primary care provider.

LIFESPAN CONSIDERATIONS   Assessing the Skin

Infants

- Physiologic jaundice may appear in newborns 2 to 3 days after birth and usually lasts about 1 week. Pathologic jaundice, or that which indicates a disease, appears within 24 hours of birth and may last more than 8 days.
- Newborns may have milia (whiteheads), small white nodules over the nose and face, and vernix caseosa (white cheesy, greasy material on the skin).
- Premature infants may have lanugo, a fine downy hair covering their shoulders and back.
- In dark-skinned infants, areas of hyperpigmentation may be found on the back, especially in the sacral area.
- Diaper dermatitis may be seen in infants.
- If a rash is present, inquire in detail about immunization history.
- Assess skin turgor by pinching the skin on the abdomen.

Children

- Children normally have minor skin lesions (e.g., bruising or abrasions) on arms and legs due to their high activity level. Lesions on other parts of the body may be signs of disease or abuse, and a thorough history should be taken.
- Secondary skin lesions may occur frequently as children scratch or expose a primary lesion to microbes.
- With puberty, oil glands become more productive, and children may develop acne. Most persons 12 to 24 years have some acne.
- In dark-skinned children, areas of hyperpigmentation may be found on the back, especially in the sacral area.
- If a rash is present, inquire in detail about immunization history.

Older Adults

- Changes in white skin occur at an earlier age than in black skin.

- The skin loses its elasticity, and wrinkles. Wrinkles first appear on the skin of the face and neck, which are abundant in collagen and elastic fibers.
- The skin appears thin and translucent because of loss of dermis and subcutaneous fat.
- The skin is dry and flaky because sebaceous and sweat glands are less active. Dry skin is more prominent over the extremities.
- The skin takes longer to return to its natural shape after being tented between the thumb and finger.
- Due to the normal loss of peripheral skin turgor in older adults, assess for hydration by checking skin turgor over the sternum or clavicle.
- Flat tan to brown-colored macules, referred to as *senile lentigines* or *melanotic freckles,* are normally apparent on the back of the hand and other skin areas that are exposed to the sun. These macules may be as large as 1 to 2 cm.
- Warty lesions (*seborrheic keratosis*) with irregularly shaped borders and a scaly surface often occur on the face, shoulders, and trunk. These benign lesions begin as yellowish to tan and progress to a dark brown or black.
- *Vitiligo* tends to increase with age and is thought to result from an autoimmune response.
- Cutaneous tags (*acrochordons*) are most commonly seen in the neck and axillary regions. These skin lesions vary in size and are soft, often flesh colored, and pedicled.
- Visible, bright red, fine dilated blood vessels (*telangiectasias*) commonly occur as a result of the thinning of the dermis and the loss of support for the blood vessel walls.
- Pink to slightly red lesions with indistinct borders (*actinic keratoses*) may appear at about age 50, often on the face, ears, backs of the hands, and arms. They may become malignant if untreated.

BOX 17–4   Describing Skin Lesions

- *Type or structure.* Skin lesions are classified as *primary* (those that appear initially in response to some change in the external or internal environment of the skin) and *secondary* (those that do not appear initially but result from modifications such as chronicity, trauma, or infection of the primary lesion). For example, a vesicle (primary lesion) may rupture and cause an erosion (secondary lesion).
- *Size, shape, and texture.* Note size in millimeters and whether the lesion is circumscribed or irregular; round or oval shaped; flat, elevated, or depressed; solid, soft, or hard; rough or thickened; fluid filled or has flakes.
- *Color.* There may be no discoloration, one discrete color (e.g., red, brown, or black), several colors, as with *ecchymosis* (a bruise), in which an initial dark red or blue color fades to a

yellow color. When color changes are limited to the edges of a lesion, they are described as *circumscribed;* when spread over a large area, they are described as *diffuse.*
- *Distribution.* Distribution is described according to the location of the lesions on the body and symmetry or asymmetry of findings in comparable body areas.
- *Configuration.* Configuration refers to the arrangement of lesions in relation to each other. Configurations of lesions may be annular (arranged in a circle), may be clustered together or grouped, may be linear (arranged in a line), may be arc or bow shaped, may be merged together or indiscrete, may follow the course of cutaneous nerves, or may be meshed in the form of a network.

Hair

Assessing a client's hair includes inspecting the hair, considering developmental changes and ethnic differences, and determining the individual's hair care practices and factors influencing them. Much of the information about hair can be obtained by questioning the client.

Typically, hair is resilient and evenly distributed. In people with severe protein deficiency (kwashiorkor), the hair color is faded and appears reddish or bleached, and the texture is coarse and dry. Some therapies cause alopecia (hair loss), and some disease conditions and medications affect the coarseness of hair. For example, hypothyroidism can cause very thin and brittle hair.

Nails

Nails are inspected for nail plate shape, angle between the nail and the nail bed (fingernails), nail texture, nail bed color, and the intactness of the tissues around the nails. The nail plate is typically colorless and has a convex curve. The angle between the fingernail and the nail bed is typically 160 degrees (Figure 17–6, *A*). One nail abnormality is the spoon shape, in which the nail curves upward from the nail bed (Figure 17–6, *B*). This condition, called koilonychia, may be seen in clients with iron deficiency anemia. **Clubbing** is a condition in which the angle between the nail and the nail bed is 180 degrees or greater (Figure 17–6, *C* and *D*). Clubbing may be caused by a long-term lack of oxygen.

Nail texture is typically smooth. Excessively thick nails can appear in older adults, in the presence of poor circulation, or in relation to a chronic fungal infection. Excessively thin nails or the presence of grooves or furrows can reflect prolonged iron deficiency anemia. Beau's lines are horizontal depressions in the nail that can result from injury or severe illness (Figure 17–6, *E*).The nail bed is highly vascular, a characteristic that accounts for its color. A bluish or purplish tint to the nail bed may reflect cyanosis, and pallor may reflect poor arterial circulation. Should the client report a history of nail fungus (onychomycosis), a referral to a podiatrist or dermatologist for treatment of nail fungus may be appropriate. Symptoms of nail fungus include brittleness, discoloration, thickening, distortion of nail shape, crumbling of the nail, and loosening (detaching) of the nail.

The tissue surrounding the nails is typically intact epidermis. Paronychia is an inflammation of the tissues surrounding a nail (often referred to as an "ingrown nail"). The tissues appear inflamed and swollen, and tenderness is usually present. A **blanch test** can be carried out to test the capillary refill, that is, peripheral circulation. Nail bed capillaries typically blanch when pressed but quickly turn pink or their usual color when pressure is released. A slow rate of capillary refill may indicate circulatory problems.

Skill 17–3 describes how to assess the nails.

LIFESPAN CONSIDERATIONS
Assessing the Hair

Infants

- It is acceptable for infants to have either very little or a great deal of body and scalp hair.

Children

- As puberty approaches, axillary and pubic hair will appear.

Older Adults

- There may be loss of scalp, pubic, and axillary hair.
- Hairs of the eyebrows, ears, and nostrils become bristle-like and coarse.

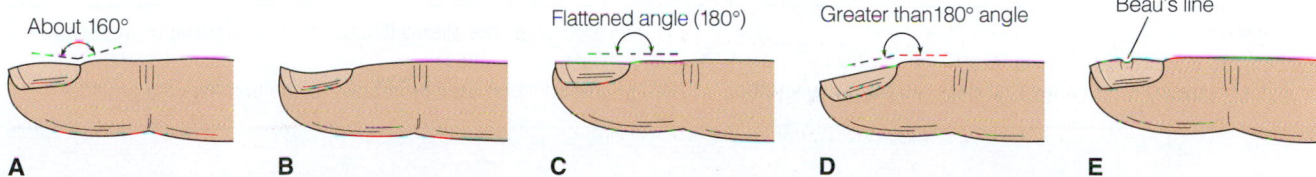

A   B   C   D   E

Figure 17–6 ● **A,** A normal nail, showing the convex shape and the nail plate angle of about 160 degrees; **B,** a spoon-shaped nail, which may be seen in clients with iron deficiency anemia; **C,** early clubbing; **D,** late clubbing (may be caused by long-term oxygen lack); **E,** Beau's line on nail (may result from severe injury or illness).

SKILL 17–3

ASSESSING THE NAILS

PLANNING

Delegation
Assessment of the nails is not delegated to UAP. However, many aspects are observed during usual care and may be recorded by persons other than the nurse. Atypical findings must be validated and interpreted by the nurse.

EQUIPMENT
None

IMPLEMENTATION

Performance
1. Prior to performing the procedure, introduce self and verify the client's identity using agency protocol. Explain to the client what you are going to do, why it is necessary, and how he or she can cooperate. Discuss how the results will be used in planning further care or treatments. In most situations, clients with artificial nails or polish on fingernails or toenails are not required to remove these for assessment. If the assessment cannot be conducted due to the presence of polish or artificial nails, document this in the record.
2. Observe appropriate infection control procedures.
3. Provide for client privacy.
4. Inquire if the client has any history of the following: presence of diabetes mellitus, peripheral circulatory disease, previous injury, or severe illness.

ASSESSMENT	TYPICAL FINDINGS	ATYPICAL FINDINGS
5. Inspect fingernail plate shape to determine its curvature and angle.	Convex curvature; angle of nail plate about 160° (Figure 17–6, A)	Spoon nail (Figure 17–6, B); clubbing (180° or greater) (Figure 17–6, C and D)
6. Inspect fingernail and toenail texture.	Smooth texture	Excessive thickness or thinness or presence of grooves or furrows; Beau's lines (Figure 17–6, E); discolored or detached nail—often due to fungus
7. Inspect fingernail and toenail bed color.	Highly vascular and pink in light-skinned clients; dark-skinned clients may have brown or black pigmentation in longitudinal streaks	Bluish or purplish tint (may reflect cyanosis); pallor (may reflect poor arterial circulation)
8. Inspect tissues surrounding nails.	Intact epidermis	Hangnails; paronychia (inflammation)
9. Perform blanch test of capillary refill. Press two or more nails between your thumb and index finger; look for blanching and return of pink color to nail bed.	Prompt return of pink or usual color (generally less than 4 seconds)	Delayed return of pink or usual color (may indicate circulatory impairment)
10. Document findings in the client record using forms or checklists supplemented by narrative notes when appropriate.		

EVALUATION
- Perform a detailed follow-up examination of other individual systems based on findings that deviated from expected or normal for the client. Relate findings to previous assessment data if available.
- Report significant deviations to the primary care provider.

LIFESPAN CONSIDERATIONS   Assessing the Nails

Infants
- Newborn nails grow very quickly, are extremely thin, and tear easily.

Children
- Bent, bruised, or ingrown toenails may indicate shoes that are too tight.
- Nail biting should be discussed with a family member.

Older Adults
- The nails grow more slowly and thicken.
- Longitudinal bands commonly develop, and the nails tend to split.
- Bands across the nails may indicate protein deficiency; white spots, zinc deficiency; and spoon-shaped nails, iron deficiency.
- Toenail fungus is more common and difficult to eliminate (although not dangerous to health).

THE NEUROLOGIC SYSTEM

A thorough neurologic examination may take 1 to 3 hours; however, routine screening tests are usually done first. If the results of these tests raise questions, more extensive evaluations are made. Three major considerations determine the extent of a neurologic exam: (a) the client's chief complaints, (b) the client's physical condition, because many parts of the examination require movement and coordination of the extremities, and (c) the client's willingness to participate and cooperate.

Examination of the neurologic system includes assessment of (a) mental status including level of consciousness, (b) the cranial nerves, (c) reflexes, (d) motor function, and (e) sensory function. Parts of the neurologic assessment are performed throughout the health examination.

General Cerebral Function

Assessment of mental status reveals the client's general cerebral function. These functions include intellectual (cognitive) as well as emotional (affective) functions. If problems with use of language, memory, concentration, or thought processes are noted during the nursing history, a more extensive examination is required during neurologic assessment.

LANGUAGE   Any defects in or loss of the power to express oneself by speech, writing, or signs, or to comprehend spoken or written language due to disease or injury of the cerebral cortex, is called aphasia. Aphasias can be categorized as sensory or receptive aphasia, and motor or expressive aphasia. Sensory or receptive aphasia is the loss of the ability to comprehend written or spoken words. Two types of sensory aphasia are auditory (or acoustic) aphasia and visual aphasia. Clients with auditory aphasia have lost the ability to understand the symbolic content associated with sounds. Clients with visual aphasia have lost the ability to understand printed or written figures. Motor or expressive aphasia involves loss of the power to express oneself by writing, making signs, or speaking. Clients may find that even though they can recall words, they have lost the ability to combine speech sounds into words.

ORIENTATION   This aspect of the assessment determines the client's ability to recognize other persons (*person*), awareness of when and where they presently are (*time* and *place*), and who they, themselves, are (*self*).

> ### CLINICAL ALERT
>
> Nurses often chart that the client is "awake, alert, & oriented x3 (or times three)." This refers to accurate awareness of person, time, and place. Remember, "person" indicates that the client recognizes others, not that the client can state what his or her own name is.

MEMORY   The nurse assesses the client's recall of information presented seconds previously (immediate recall), events or information from earlier in the day or examination (recent memory), and knowledge recalled from months or years ago (remote or long-term memory).

ATTENTION SPAN AND CALCULATION   This component determines the client's ability to focus on a mental task that is expected from a person whose intelligence is within normal range.

Level of Consciousness

Level of consciousness (LOC) can lie anywhere along a continuum from a state of alertness to coma. A fully alert client responds to questions spontaneously; a comatose client may not respond to verbal stimuli. The Glasgow Coma Scale was originally developed to predict recovery from a head injury; however, it is used by many professionals to assess LOC. It tests in three major areas: eye response, motor response, and verbal response. An assessment totaling 15 points indicates the client is alert and completely oriented. A comatose client scores 7 or less.

Cranial Nerves

The nurse needs to be aware of specific nerve functions and assessment methods for each cranial nerve to detect abnormalities. In some cases, each nerve is assessed; in other cases only selected nerve functions are evaluated. Routine examinations do not usually assess the cranial nerves unless involvement is suspected.

Reflexes

A **reflex** is an automatic response of the body to a stimulus. It is not voluntarily learned or conscious. The deep tendon reflex (DTR) is activated when a tendon is stimulated (tapped) and its associated muscle contracts. The quality of a reflex response varies among individuals and by age. As a person ages, reflex responses may become less intense.

Reflexes are tested using a percussion hammer. The response is described on a scale of 0 to 14. Experience is necessary to determine appropriate scoring for an individual. Several reflexes may be tested during the physical examination: (a) the biceps reflex, (b) the triceps reflex, (c) the brachioradialis reflex, (d) the patellar reflex, (e) the Achilles reflex, and (f) the plantar (Babinski) reflex.

Motor Function

Neurologic assessment of the motor system evaluates proprioception and cerebellar function. Structures involved in proprioception are the proprioceptors, the posterior columns of the spinal cord, the cerebellum, and the vestibular apparatus (which is innervated by cranial nerve VIII) in the labyrinth of the internal ear.

Proprioceptors are sensory nerve terminals, occurring chiefly in the muscles, tendons, joints, and the internal ear, that give information about movements and the position of the body. Stimuli from the proprioceptors travel through the posterior columns of the spinal cord. Deficits of function of the posterior columns of the spinal cord result in impairment of muscle and position sense. Clients with such impairment often must watch their own arm and leg movements to ascertain the position of the limbs.

The cerebellum (a) helps to control posture, (b) acts with the cerebral cortex to make body movements smooth and coordinated, and (c) controls skeletal muscles to maintain equilibrium.

Sensory Function

Sensory functions include touch, pain, temperature, position, and tactile discrimination. The first three are routinely tested. Generally, the face, arms, legs, hands, and feet are tested for touch and pain, although all parts of the body can be tested. If the client complains of numbness, peculiar sensations, or paralysis, the practitioner should check sensation more carefully over flexor and extensor surfaces of limbs, mapping out clearly any abnormality of touch or pain by examining responses in the area about every 2 cm (1 in.). This is a lengthy procedure and may be performed by a specialist. Abnormal responses to touch stimuli include loss of sensation (anesthesia); more than normal sensation (hyperesthesia); less than normal sensation (hypoesthesia); or an abnormal sensation such as burning, pain, or an electric shock (paresthesia).

A variety of common health conditions, including diabetes and arteriosclerotic heart disease, result in loss of the protective sensation in the lower extremities. This loss can lead to severe tissue damage. In efforts to identify clients at increased risk for damage to the feet, the Bureau of Primary Health Care of the U.S. government has established the Lower Extremity Amputation Prevention (LEAP) program. The most important aspect of LEAP is assessment of sensation using a special monofilament that delivers 10 grams of force. Health care providers should perform an initial foot screen on all clients with diabetes and at least annually thereafter. Clients who are at risk should have their feet and shoes evaluated at least four times a year to help prevent foot problems from occurring.

A detailed neurologic examination includes position sense, temperature sense, and tactile discrimination. Three types of tactile discrimination are generally tested: one- and two-point discrimination, the ability to sense whether one or two areas of the skin are being stimulated by pressure; stereognosis, the act of recognizing objects by touching and manipulating them; and extinction, the failure to perceive touch on one side of the body when two symmetric areas of the body are touched simultaneously.

Skill 17–4 describes how to assess the neurologic system.

SKILL 17–4

ASSESSING THE NEUROLOGIC SYSTEM

PLANNING

If possible, determine whether a screening or full neurologic examination is indicated. This will impact preparation of the client, equipment, and timing.

Delegation

Due to the substantial knowledge and skill required, assessment of the neurologic system is not delegated to UAP. However, many aspects of neurologic behavior are observed during usual care and may be recorded by persons other than the nurse. Atypical findings must be validated and interpreted by the nurse.

EQUIPMENT (DEPENDING ON COMPONENTS OF EXAMINATION)

- Sugar, salt, lemon juice, quinine flavors
- Percussion hammer
- Tongue depressors (one broken diagonally for testing pain sensation)
- Wisps of cotton to assess light-touch sensation
- Test tubes of hot and cold water for skin temperature assessment (optional)
- Pins or needles for tactile discrimination

IMPLEMENTATION

Performance

1. Prior to performing the procedure, introduce self and verify the client's identity using agency protocol. Explain to the client what you are going to do, why it is necessary, and how he or she can cooperate. Discuss how the results will be used in planning further care or treatments.
2. Perform hand hygiene and observe appropriate infection control procedures.
3. Provide for client privacy.
4. Inquire if the client has any history of the following: presence of pain in the head, back, or extremities, as well as onset and aggravating and alleviating factors; disorientation to time, place, or person; speech disorder; history of loss of consciousness, fainting, convulsions, trauma, tingling or numbness, tremors or tics, limping, paralysis, uncontrolled

muscle movements, loss of memory, mood swings, or problems with smell, vision, taste, touch, or hearing.

CLINICAL ALERT

All questions and tests used in a neurologic examination must be age, language, education level, and culturally appropriate. Individualize questions and tests before using them.

Language

5. If the client displays difficulty speaking:
   - Point to common objects, and ask the client to name them.
   - Ask the client to read some words and to match the printed and written words with pictures.

• Ask the client to respond to simple verbal and written commands, e.g., "point to your toes" or "raise your left arm."

Orientation

6. Determine the client's orientation to *person, time,* and *place* by tactful questioning. Ask the client the city and state of residence, time of day, date, day of the week, duration of illness, and names of family members. To evaluate the response, you must know the correct answer. More direct questioning may be necessary for some people. Most people readily accept these questions if initially the nurse asks, "Do you get confused at times?" If the client cannot answer these questions accurately, also include assessment of the *self* by asking the client to state his or her full name.

Memory

7. Listen for lapses in memory. Ask the client about difficulty with memory. If problems are apparent, three categories of memory are tested: immediate recall, recent memory, and remote memory.

   To assess immediate recall:

   • Ask the client to repeat a series of three digits, e.g., 7–4–3, spoken slowly.
   • Gradually increase the number of digits until the client fails to repeat the series correctly.
   • Start again with a series of three digits, but this time ask the client to repeat them backward. The average person can repeat a series of five to eight digits in sequence and four to six digits in reverse order.

   To assess recent memory:

   • Ask the client to recall the recent events of the day, such as how the client got to the clinic. This information must be validated, however.
   • Ask the client to recall information given early in the interview, e.g., the name of a doctor.
   • Provide the client with three facts to recall, e.g., a color, an object, and an address; or a three-digit number, and ask the client to repeat all three. Later in the interview, ask the client to recall all three items.

   To assess remote memory, ask the client to describe a previous illness or surgery, e.g., 5 years ago, or a birthday or anniversary.

Attention Span and Calculation

8. Test the ability to concentrate or maintain *attention span* by asking the client to recite the alphabet or to count backward from 100. Test the ability to calculate by asking the client to subtract 7 or 3 progressively from 100, i.e., 100, 93, 86, 79, or 100, 97, 94, 91 (referred to as *serial sevens* or *serial threes*). Normally, an adult can complete the serial sevens test in about 90 seconds with three or fewer errors. Because educational level, language, or cultural differences affect calculating ability, this test may be inappropriate for some people.

Level of Consciousness

9. Apply the Glasgow Coma Scale: eye response, motor response, and verbal response. An assessment totaling 15 points indicates the client is alert and completely oriented. A comatose client scores 7 or less (see Table 17–5).

Cranial Nerves

10. For the specific functions and assessment methods of each cranial nerve, see Table 17–6. Test each nerve not already evaluated in another component of the health assessment.

CLINICAL ALERT

The names and order of the cranial nerves can be recalled by a mnemonic device: "On old Olympus's treeless top, a Finn and German viewed a hop." The first letter of each word in the sentence is the same as the first letter of the name of the cranial nerve, in order.

Reflexes

11. Test reflexes using a percussion hammer, comparing one side of the body with the other to evaluate the symmetry of response.

0	No reflex response
+1	Minimal activity (hypoactive)
+2	Typical response
+3	More active than typical
+4	Maximal activity (hyperactive)

Patellar Reflex The patellar reflex tests the spinal cord level L-2, L-3, L-4.

   • Ask the client to sit on the edge of the examining table so that the legs hang freely.
   • Locate the patellar tendon directly below the patella (kneecap).
   • Deliver a blow with the percussion hammer directly to the tendon. **❶**

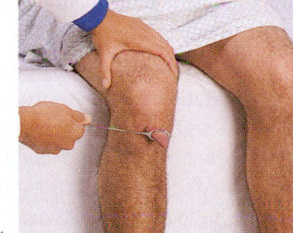

❶ The patellar reflex.

   • Observe the extension or kicking out of the leg as the quadriceps muscle contracts.
   • If no response occurs and you suspect the client is not relaxed, ask the client to interlock the fingers and pull. **Rationale:** *This action often enhances relaxation so that a more accurate response is obtained.*

Plantar (Babinski) Reflex The plantar, or Babinski, reflex is superficial. It may be absent in adults without pathology or overridden by voluntary control.

   • Use a moderately sharp object, such as the handle of the percussion hammer, a key, or an applicator stick.
   • Stroke the lateral border of the sole of the client's foot, starting at the heel, continuing to the ball of the foot, and then proceeding across the ball of the foot toward the big toe. **❷**

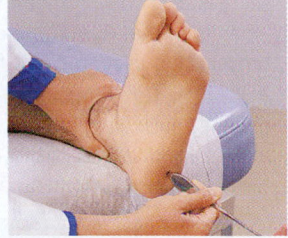

❷ The plantar (Babinski) reflex.

   • Observe the response. Normally, all five toes bend downward; this reaction is negative Babinski. In an abnormal (positive) Babinski response the toes spread outward and the big toe moves upward.

(continued)

ASSESSING THE NEUROLOGIC SYSTEM (continued)

Motor Function

ASSESSMENT	TYPICAL FINDINGS	ATYPICAL FINDINGS
12. Walking Gait Ask the client to walk across the room and back, and assess the client's gait.	Has upright posture and steady gait with opposing arm swing; walks unaided, maintaining balance	Has poor posture and unsteady, irregular, staggering gait with wide stance; bends legs only from hips; has rigid or no arm movements
13. Light-Touch Sensation Compare the light-touch sensation of symmetric areas of the body. **Rationale:** *Sensitivity to touch varies among different skin areas.*	Light tickling or touch sensation	Anesthesia, hyperesthesia, hypoesthesia, or paresthesia

- Ask the client to close the eyes and to respond by saying "yes" or "now" whenever the client feels the cotton wisp touching the skin.
- With a wisp of cotton, lightly touch one specific spot and then the same spot on the other side of the body. ❸
- Test areas on the forehead, cheek, hand, lower arm, abdomen, foot, and lower leg. Check a distal area of the limb first (i.e., the hand before the arm and the foot before the leg). **Rationale:** *The sensory nerve may be assumed to be intact if sensation is felt at its most distal part.*
- Ask the client to point to the spot where the touch was felt. **Rationale:** *This demonstrates whether the client is able to determine tactile location (point localization), i.e., can accurately perceive where the client was touched.*
- If areas of sensory dysfunction are found, determine the boundaries of sensation by testing responses about every 2.5 cm (1 in.) in the area. Make a sketch of the sensory loss area for recording purposes.

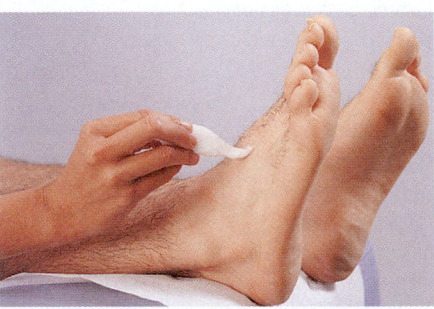

❸ Assessing light-touch sensation.

ASSESSMENT	TYPICAL FINDINGS	ATYPICAL FINDINGS
14. Pain Sensation	Able to discriminate "sharp" and "dull" sensations	Areas of reduced, heightened, or absent sensation (map them out for recording purposes)

Assess pain sensation as follows:
- Ask the client to close the eyes and to say "sharp," "dull," or "don't know" when the sharp or dull end of the broken tongue depressor is felt.
- Alternately, use the sharp and dull end to lightly prick designated anatomic areas at random, e.g., hand, forearm, foot, lower leg, abdomen. ❹ The face is not tested in this manner.

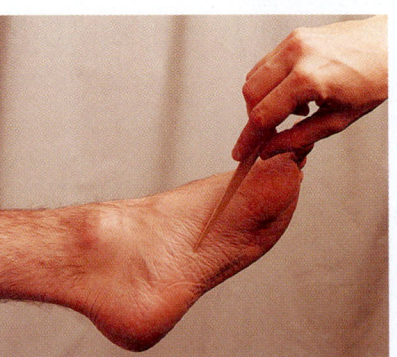

❹ Assessing pain sensation using a broken tongue depressor.

ASSESSMENT	TYPICAL FINDINGS	ATYPICAL FINDINGS

• Allow at least 2 seconds between each test to prevent summation effects of stimuli, i.e., several successive stimuli perceived as one stimulus.

15. Document findings in the client record using forms or checklists supplemented by narrative notes when appropriate. Describe any abnormal findings in objective terms, e.g., "When asked to count backward by threes, client made seven errors and completed the task in 4 minutes."

EVALUATION

• Perform a detailed follow-up examination of other systems based on findings that deviated from expected or normal for the client. Relate findings to previous assessment data if available.

• Report significant deviations to the primary care provider.

LIFESPAN CONSIDERATIONS Assessing the Neurologic System

Infants

• Reflexes commonly tested in newborns include:
  • Rooting: Stroke the side of the face near mouth; infant opens mouth and turns to the side that is stroked.
  • Sucking: Place nipple or finger 3 to 4 cm into mouth; infant sucks vigorously.
  • Tonic neck: Place infant supine, turn head to one side; arm on side to which head is turned extends; on opposite side, arm curls up (fencer's pose).
  • Palmar grasp: Place finger in infant's palm and press; infant curls fingers around.
  • Stepping: Hold infant as if weight bearing on surface; infant steps along, one foot at a time.
  • Moro: Present loud noise or unexpected movement; infant spreads arms and legs, extends fingers, then flexes and brings hands together; may cry.
• Most of these reflexes disappear between 4 and 6 months of age.

Children

• Present the procedures as games whenever possible.
• Positive Babinski reflex is abnormal after the child ambulates or at age 2.
• For children under age 5, the Denver Developmental Screening Test II provides a comprehensive neurologic evaluation— particularly for motor function.
• Note the child's ability to understand and follow directions.

• Assess immediate recall or recent memory by using names of cartoon characters. Normal recall in children is one less than age in years.
• Assess for signs of hyperactivity or abnormally short attention span.
• Children should be able to walk backward by age 2, balance on one foot for 5 seconds by age 4, heel-toe walk by age 5, and heel-toe walk backward by age 6.
• The Romberg test is appropriate over age 3.

Older Adults

• A full neurologic assessment can be lengthy. Conduct in several sessions if indicated, and cease the tests if the client is noticeably fatigued.
• A decline in mental status is not a normal result of aging. Changes are more the result of physical or psychologic disorders (e.g., fever, fluid and electrolyte imbalances, medications). Acute, abrupt-onset mental status changes are usually caused by delirium. These changes are often reversible with treatment. Chronic subtle insidious mental health changes are usually caused by dementia and are usually irreversible.
• Intelligence and learning ability are unaltered with age. Many factors, however, inhibit learning (e.g., anxiety, illness, pain, cultural barrier).
• Short-term memory is often less efficient. Long-term memory is usually unaltered.

(continued)

LIFESPAN CONSIDERATIONS   Assessing the Neurologic System *(continued)*

- Because old age is often associated with loss of support persons, depression is a common disorder. Mood changes, weight loss, anorexia, constipation, and early morning awakening may manifest it.
- The stress of being in unfamiliar situations can cause confusion in older adults.
- As a person ages, reflex responses may become less intense.
- Because older adults tire more easily than younger clients, a total neurologic assessment is often done at a different time than the other parts of the physical assessment.
- Although there is a progressive decrease in the number of functioning neurons in the central nervous system and in the sense organs, older adults usually function well because of the abundant reserves in the number of brain cells.
- Impulse transmission and reaction to stimuli are slower.

- Many older adults have some impairment of hearing, vision, smell, temperature and pain sensation, memory, and mental endurance.
- Coordination changes, including a reduced speed of fine finger movements. Standing balance remains intact, and Romberg's test remains negative.
- Reflex responses may slightly increase or decrease. Many show loss of Achilles reflex, and the plantar reflex may be difficult to elicit.
- When testing sensory function, the nurse needs to give older adults time to respond. Typically, older adults have unaltered perception of light touch and superficial pain, decreased perception of deep pain, and decreased perception of temperature stimuli. Many also reveal a decrease or absence of position sense in the large toes.

TABLE 17–5   **Levels of Consciousness: Glasgow Coma Scale**

FACULTY MEASURED	RESPONSE	SCORE
Eye opening	Spontaneous	4
	To verbal command	3
	To pain	2
	No response	1
Motor response	To verbal command	6
	To localized pain	5
	Flexes and withdraws	4
	Flexes abnormally	3
	Extends abnormally	2
	No response	1
Verbal response	Oriented, converses	5
	Disoriented, converses	4
	Uses inappropriate words	3
	Makes incomprehensible sounds	2
	No response	1

THE HEAD

During assessment of the head, the nurse inspects and palpates simultaneously and also auscultates. The nurse examines the skull, face, eyes, ears, nose, sinuses, mouth, and pharynx.

Skull and Face

The skull can take many shapes and still be considered normal. A normal head size is referred to as **normocephalic**. Names of areas of the head are derived from names of the underlying bones: frontal, parietal, occipital, mastoid process, mandible, maxilla, and zygomatic. Many disorders cause a change in facial shape or condition. Skill 17–5 describes how to assess the skull and face.

TABLE 17–6 **Cranial Nerve Functions and Assessment Methods**

CRANIAL NERVE	NAME	TYPE	FUNCTION	ASSESSMENT METHOD
I	Olfactory	Sensory	Smell	Ask client to close eyes and identify different mild aromas, such as coffee, vanilla, peanut butter, orange/lemon, chocolate.
II	Optic	Sensory	Vision and visual fields	Ask client to read Snellen-type chart; check visual fields by confrontation; and conduct an ophthalmoscopic examination (see Skill 17–6).
III	Oculomotor	Motor	Extraocular eye movement (EOM); movement of sphincter of pupil; movement of ciliary muscles of lens	Assess six ocular movements and pupil reaction (see Skill 17–6).
IV	Trochlear	Motor	EOM; specifically, moves eyeball downward and laterally	Assess six ocular movements (see Skill 17–6).
V	Trigeminal Ophthalmic branch	Sensory	Sensation of cornea, skin of face, and nasal mucosa	While client looks upward, lightly touch the lateral sclera of the eye with sterile gauze to elicit blink reflex. To test light sensation, have client close eyes, wipe a wisp of cotton over client's forehead and paranasal sinuses. To test deep sensation, use alternating blunt and sharp ends of a safety pin over same areas.
	Maxillary branch	Sensory	Sensation of skin of face and anterior oral cavity (tongue and teeth)	Assess skin sensation as for ophthalmic branch above.
	Mandibular branch	Motor and sensory	Muscles of mastication; sensation of skin of face	Ask client to clench teeth.
VI	Abducens	Motor	EOM; moves eyeball laterally	Assess directions of gaze.
VII	Facial	Motor and sensory	Facial expression; taste (anterior two-thirds of tongue)	Ask client to smile, raise the eyebrows, frown, puff out cheeks, close eyes tightly. Ask client to identify various tastes placed on tip and sides of tongue: sugar (sweet), salt, lemon juice (sour), and quinine (bitter); identify areas of taste.
VIII	Auditory Vestibular branch	Sensory	Equilibrium	Romberg test.
	Cochlear branch	Sensory	Hearing	Assess client's ability to hear spoken word and vibrations of tuning fork.
IX	Glossopharyngeal	Motor and sensory	Swallowing ability, tongue movement, taste (posterior tongue)	Apply tastes on posterior tongue for identification. Ask client to move tongue from side to side and up and down.
X	Vagus	Motor and sensory	Sensation of pharynx and larynx; swallowing; vocal cord movement	Assessed with cranial nerve IX; assess client's speech for hoarseness.
XI	Accessory	Motor	Head movement; shrugging of shoulders	Ask client to shrug shoulders against resistance from your hands and turn head to side against resistance from your hand (repeat for other side).
XII	Hypoglossal	Motor	Protrusion of tongue; moves tongue up and down and side to side	Ask client to protrude tongue at midline, then move it side to side.

SKILL 17–5

ASSESSING THE SKULL AND FACE

PLANNING

Delegation

Assessment of the skull and face is not delegated to UAP. However, many aspects are observed during usual care and may be recorded by persons other than the nurse. Atypical findings must be validated and interpreted by the nurse.

EQUIPMENT

None

IMPLEMENTATION

Performance

1. Prior to performing the procedure, introduce self and verify the client's identity using agency protocol. Explain to the client what you are going to do, why it is necessary, and how he or she can cooperate. Discuss how the results will be used in planning further care or treatments.
2. Perform hand hygiene and observe appropriate infection control procedures.
3. Provide for client privacy.
4. Inquire if the client has any history of the following: past problems with lumps or bumps, itching, scaling, or dandruff; history of loss of consciousness, dizziness, seizures, headache, facial pain, or injury; when and how any lumps occurred; length of time any other problem existed; any known cause of problem; associated symptoms, treatment, and recurrences.

ASSESSMENT	TYPICAL FINDINGS	ATYPICAL FINDINGS
5. Inspect the skull for size, shape, and symmetry.	Rounded (normocephalic and symmetric, with frontal, parietal, and occipital prominences); smooth skull contour	Lack of symmetry; increased skull size with more prominent nose and forehead; longer mandible (may indicate excessive growth hormone or increased bone thickness)
6. Palpate the skull for nodules or masses and depressions.	Smooth, uniform consistency; absence of nodules or masses	Sebaceous cysts; local deformities from trauma; masses, nodules
7. Inspect the facial features.	Symmetric or slightly asymmetric facial features; palpebral fissures equal in size; symmetric nasolabial folds	Increased facial hair; thinning of eyebrows; asymmetric features; exophthalmos; myxedema facies; moon face
8. Inspect the eyes for edema and hollowness.		Periorbital edema; sunken eyes
9. Note symmetry of facial movements. See Skill 17–4, Assessing the Neurologic System.	Symmetric facial movements	Asymmetric facial movements; drooping of lower eyelid and mouth; involuntary facial movements

10. Document findings in the client record using forms or checklists supplemented by narrative notes when appropriate.

EVALUATION

- Perform a detailed follow-up examination of other systems based on findings that deviated from expected or normal for the client. Relate findings to previous assessment data if available.
- Report significant deviations to the primary care provider.

LIFESPAN CONSIDERATIONS
Assessing the Skull and Face

Infants

- Newborns delivered vaginally can have elongated, molded heads, which take on more rounded shapes after a week or two. Infants born by cesarean section tend to have smooth, rounded heads.
- The posterior fontanel (soft spot) is about 1 cm in size and usually closes by 8 weeks. The anterior fontanel is larger, about 2 to 3 cm in size. It closes by 18 months.
- Newborns can lift their heads slightly and turn them from side to side. Voluntary head control is well established by 4 to 6 months.

Eyes and Vision

To maintain optimum vision, people need to have their eyes examined regularly throughout life. It is recommended that people under age 40 have their eyes tested every 3 to 5 years, or more frequently if there is a family history of diabetes, hypertension, blood dyscrasia, or eye disorders. After age 40, an eye examination is recommended every 2 years to rule out the possibility of glaucoma.

An eye assessment should be carried out as part of the client's initial physical examination; periodic reassessments need to be made for clients in long-term care. Examination of the eyes includes assessment of the external structures, **visual acuity** (the degree of detail the eye can discern in an image), ocular movement, and **visual fields** (the area an individual can see when looking straight ahead). Most eye assessment procedures involve inspection. Consideration is also given to developmental changes and to individual hygienic practices, if the client wears contact lenses or has an artificial eye.

Many people wear eyeglasses or contact lenses to correct common refractive errors of the lens of the eye. These errors include myopia (nearsightedness), hyperopia (farsightedness), and presbyopia (loss of elasticity of the lens and thus loss of ability to see close objects). Presbyopia begins at about 45 years of age. People notice that they have difficulty reading newsprint. When both far and near vision require correction, two lenses (bifocals) are required. Astigmatism, an uneven curvature of the cornea that prevents horizontal and vertical rays from focusing on the retina, is a common problem that may occur in conjunction with myopia and hyperopia. Astigmatism may be corrected with glasses or surgery.

Three types of eye charts are available to test visual acuity (see Figure 17–7). People with denominators of 40 or more on the Snellen chart with or without corrective lenses need to be referred to an ophthalmologist.

Common inflammatory visual problems that nurses may encounter in clients include conjunctivitis, dacry-

ocystitis, hordeolum, iritis, and contusions or hematomas of the eyelids and surrounding structures. Conjunctivitis (inflammation of the bulbar and palpebral conjunctiva) may result from foreign bodies, chemicals, allergenic agents, bacteria, or viruses. Redness, itching, tearing, and discharge occur. During sleep, the eyelids may become encrusted and matted together. Dacryocystitis (inflammation of the lacrimal sac) is manifested by tearing and a discharge from the nasolacrimal duct. Hordeolum (sty) is a redness, swelling, and tenderness of the hair follicle and glands that empty at the edge of the eyelids. *Iritis* (inflammation of the iris) may be caused by local or systemic infections and results in pain, tearing, and photophobia (sensitivity to light). Contusions or hematomas are "black eyes" resulting from injury.

Cataracts tend to occur in persons over 65 years old. This opacity of the lens or its capsule, which blocks light rays, is frequently removed and replaced by a lens implant. Cataracts may also occur in infants due to a malformation of the lens if the mother contracted rubella in the first trimester of pregnancy. Glaucoma (a disturbance in the circulation of aqueous fluid, which causes an increase in intraocular pressure) is the most frequent cause of blindness

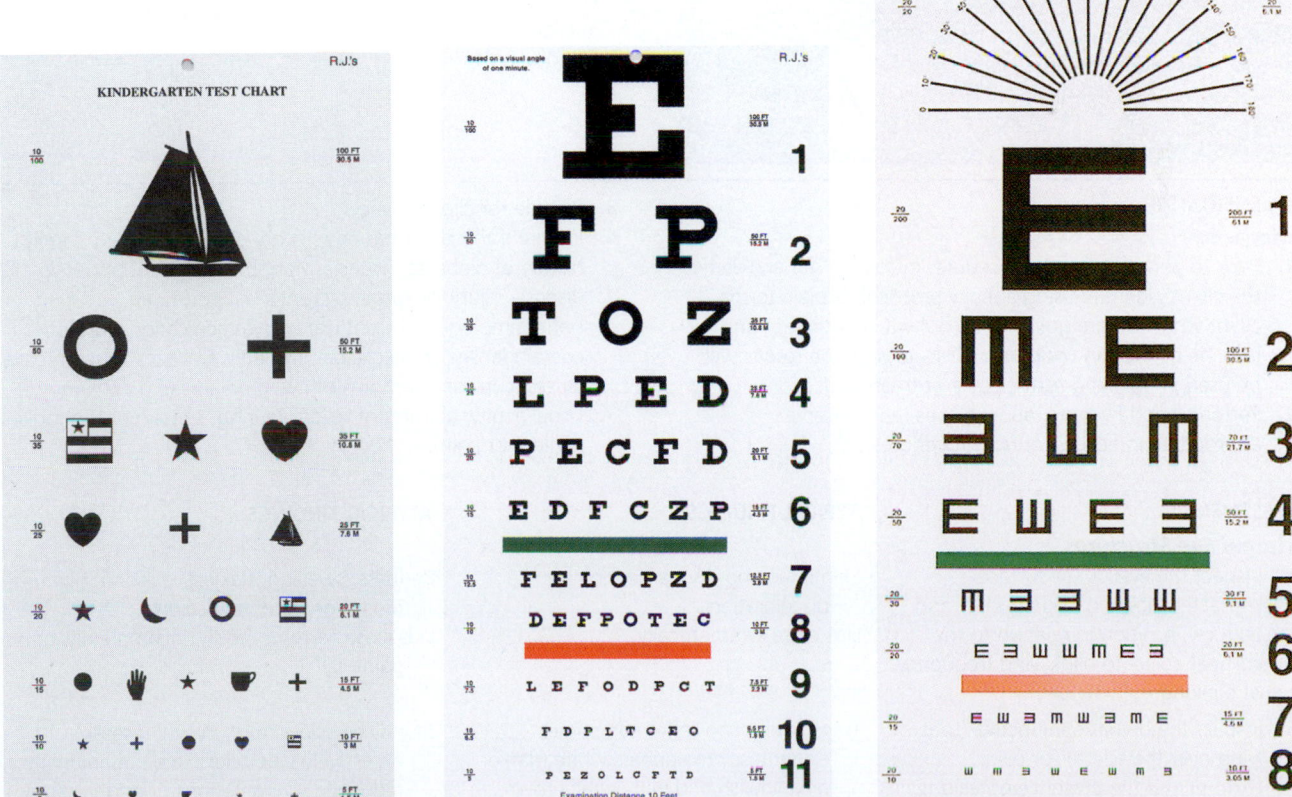

Figure 17–7 ● Three types of eye charts: the preschool children's chart (*left*), the Snellen standard chart (*center*), and the Snellen E chart for clients unable to read (*right*).

in people over 40. It can be controlled if diagnosed early. Danger signs of glaucoma include blurred or foggy vision, loss of peripheral vision, difficulty focusing on close objects, difficulty adjusting to dark rooms, and seeing rainbow-colored rings around lights.

Eyelids that lie at or below the pupil margin are referred to as ptosis and are usually associated with aging, edema from drug allergy or systemic disease (e.g., kidney disease), congenital lid muscle dysfunction, neuromuscular disease (e.g., myasthenia gravis), and third cranial nerve impairment. Eversion, an outturning of the eyelid, is called ectropion; inversion, an inturning of the lid, is called entropion. These abnormalities are often associated with scarring injuries or the aging process.

Pupils are normally black, are equal in size (about 3 to 7 mm in diameter), and have round, smooth borders. Cloudy pupils are often indicative of cataracts. Mydriasis (enlarged pupils) may indicate injury or glaucoma, or result from certain drugs. Miosis (constricted pupils) may indicate an inflammation of the iris or result from such drugs as morphine or pilocarpine. It is also an age-related change in older adults. Anisocoria (unequal pupils) may result from a central nervous system disorder; however, slight variations may be acceptable. The iris is typically flat and round. A bulging toward the cornea can indicate increased intraocular pressure.

Skill 17–6 describes how to assess a client's eye structures and visual acuity.

SKILL 17–6

ASSESSING THE EYE STRUCTURES AND VISUAL ACUITY

PLANNING
Place the client in an appropriate room for assessing the eyes and vision. The nurse must be able to control natural and overhead lighting during some portions of the examination.

Delegation
Due to the substantial knowledge and skill required, assessment of the eyes and vision is not delegated to UAP. However, many aspects are observed during usual care and may be recorded by persons other than the nurse. Atypical findings must be validated and interpreted by the nurse.

EQUIPMENT
- Cotton tip applicator
- Gauze square
- Clean gloves
- Millimeter ruler
- Penlight
- Snellen's or E chart
- Opaque card

IMPLEMENTATION
Performance

1. Prior to performing the procedure, introduce self and verify the client's identity using agency protocol. Explain to the client what you are going to do, why it is necessary, and how he or she can cooperate. Discuss how the results will be used in planning further care or treatments.
2. Perform hand hygiene, apply gloves, and observe appropriate infection control procedures.

3. Provide for client privacy.
4. Inquire if the client has any history of the following: family history of diabetes, hypertension, blood dyscrasia, or eye disease, injury, or surgery; client's last visit to an ophthalmologist; current use of eye medications; use of contact lenses or eyeglasses; hygienic practices for corrective lenses; current symptoms of eye problems (e.g., changes in visual acuity, blurring of vision, tearing, spots, photophobia, itching, or pain).

ASSESSMENT	TYPICAL FINDINGS	ATYPICAL FINDINGS
External Eye Structures		
5. Inspect the eyelids for surface characteristics (e.g., skin quality and texture), position in relation to the cornea, ability to blink, and frequency of blinking.	Skin intact; no discharge; no discoloration Lids close symmetrically	Redness, swelling, flaking, crusting, plaques, discharge, nodules, lesions Lids close asymmetrically, incompletely, or painfully
6. Inspect the bulbar conjunctiva (that lying over the sclera) for color, texture, and the presence of lesions.	Transparent; capillaries sometimes evident; sclera appears white (darker or yellowish and with small brown macules in dark-skinned clients)	Jaundiced sclera (e.g., in liver disease); excessively pale sclera (e.g., in anemia); reddened sclera; lesions or nodules (may indicate damage by mechanical, chemical, allergenic, or bacterial agents)

ASSESSMENT	TYPICAL FINDINGS	ATYPICAL FINDINGS
7. Inspect and palpate the lacrimal gland. • Using the tip of your index finger, palpate the lacrimal gland. ❶ • Observe for edema between the lower lid and the nose.	No edema or tenderness over lacrimal gland	Swelling or tenderness over lacrimal gland

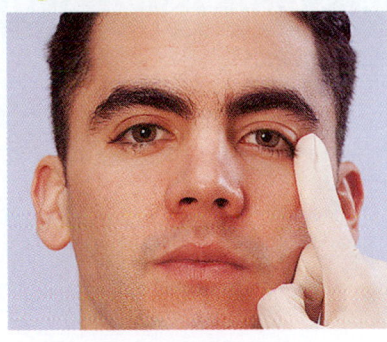

❶ Palpating the lacrimal gland.

ASSESSMENT	TYPICAL FINDINGS	ATYPICAL FINDINGS
8. Inspect the cornea for clarity and texture. Ask the client to look straight ahead. Hold a penlight at an oblique angle to the eye, and move the light slowly across the corneal surface.	Transparent, shiny, and smooth; details of the iris are visible In older people, a thin, grayish white ring around the margin, called arcus senilis, may be evident	Opaque; surface not smooth (may be the result of trauma or abrasion) Arcus senilis in clients under age 40
9. Inspect the pupils for color, shape, and symmetry of size. Pupil charts are available in some agencies. See ❷ for variations in pupil diameters.	Black in color; equal in size; typically 3 to 7 mm in diameter; round, smooth border, iris flat and round	Cloudiness, mydriasis, miosis, anisocoria; bulging of iris toward cornea

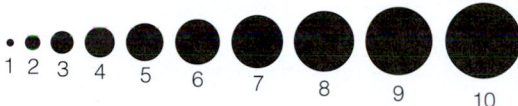

1 2 3 4 5 6 7 8 9 10

❷ Variations in pupil diameters in millimeters.

ASSESSMENT	TYPICAL FINDINGS	ATYPICAL FINDINGS
10. Assess each pupil's direct and consensual reaction to light to determine the function of the third (oculomotor) and fourth (trochlear) cranial nerves. • Partially darken the room. • Ask the client to look straight ahead. • Using a penlight and approaching from the side, shine a light on the pupil. • Observe the response of the illuminated pupil. It should constrict (direct response). • Shine the light on the pupil again, and observe the response of the other pupil. It should also constrict (consensual response).	Illuminated pupil constricts (direct response) Nonilluminated pupil constricts (consensual response)	Neither pupil constricts Unequal responses Absent responses
11. Assess each pupil's reaction to accommodation. • Hold an object (a penlight or pencil) about 10 cm (4 in.) from the bridge of the client's nose. • Ask the client to look first at the top of the object and then at a distant object (e.g., the far wall) behind the penlight. Alternate the gaze from the near to the far object.	Pupils constrict when looking at near object; pupils dilate when looking at far object; pupils converge when near object is moved toward nose	One or both pupils fail to constrict, dilate, or converge

(continued)

ASSESSING THE EYE STRUCTURES AND VISUAL ACUITY *(continued)*

ASSESSMENT	TYPICAL FINDINGS	ATYPICAL FINDINGS
• Observe the pupil response. The pupils should constrict when looking at the near object and dilate when looking at the far object. • Next, move the penlight or pencil toward the client's nose. The pupils should converge. To record normal assessment of the pupils, use the abbreviation PERRLA (pupils equally round and react to light and accommodation).		

Visual Fields

12. Assess peripheral visual fields to determine function of the retina and neuronal visual pathways to the brain and second (optic) cranial nerve.	When looking straight ahead, client can see objects in the periphery	Visual field smaller than typical (possible glaucoma); one-half vision in one or both eyes (possible nerve damage)

- Have the client sit directly facing you at a distance of 60 to 90 cm (2 to 3 ft).
- Ask the client to cover the right eye with a card and look directly at your nose.
- Cover or close your eye directly opposite the client's covered eye (i.e., your left eye), and look directly at the client's nose.
- Hold an object (e.g., a penlight or pencil) in your fingers, extend your arm, and move the object into the visual field from various points in the periphery. ❸ The object should be at an equal distance from the client and yourself. Ask the client to tell you when the moving object is first spotted.

  a. To test the temporal field of the left eye, extend and move your right arm in from the client's right periphery. Temporally, peripheral objects can be seen at right angles (90 degrees) to the central point of vision.

  b. To test the upward field of the left eye, extend and move the right arm down from the upward periphery. The upward field of vision is typically 50 degrees because the orbital ridge is in the way.

  c. To test the downward field of the left eye, extend and move the right arm up from the lower periphery. The downward field of vision is typically 70 degrees because the cheekbone is in the way.

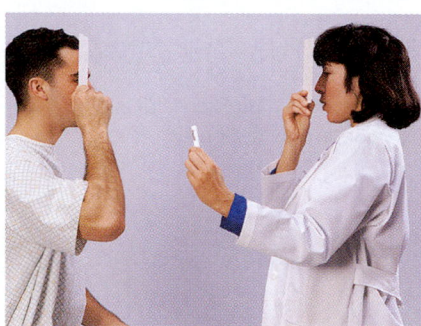

❸ Assessing the client's left peripheral visual field.

ASSESSMENT	TYPICAL FINDINGS	ATYPICAL FINDINGS
d. To test the nasal field of the left eye, extend and move your left arm in from the periphery. The nasal field of vision is typically 50 degrees away from the central point of vision because the nose is in the way.		
• Repeat the above steps for the right eye, reversing the process.		

Visual Acuity

13. Assess near vision by providing adequate lighting and asking the client to read from a magazine or newspaper held at a distance of 36 cm (14 in.). If the client normally wears corrective lenses, the glasses or lenses should be worn during the test.	Able to read newsprint	Difficulty reading newsprint unless due to aging process

CLINICAL ALERT

A Rosenbaum eye chart may be used to test near vision. It consists of paragraphs of text or characters in different sizes on a 3½ × 6½ inch card. Be sure the client has a literacy level appropriate for the text used.

14. Assess distance vision by asking the client to wear corrective lenses, unless they are used for reading only, i.e., for distances of only 36 cm (12 to 14 in.).	20/20 vision on Snellen-type chart	Denominator of 40 or more on Snellen-type chart with corrective lenses

- Ask the client to stand or sit 6 m (20 ft) from a Snellen or character chart, cover the eye not being tested, and identify the letters or characters on the chart.
- Take three readings: right eye, left eye, both eyes.
- Record the readings of each eye and both eyes (i.e., the smallest line from which the person is able to read one-half or more of the letters).

At the end of each line of the chart are standardized numbers (fractions). The top line is 20/200. The numerator (top number) is always 20, the distance the person stands from the chart. The denominator (bottom number) is the distance from which the eye can read the chart. Therefore, a person who has 20/40 vision can see at 20 feet from the chart what a normal-sighted person can see at 40 feet from the chart. Visual acuity is recorded as "$\overline{s}$−c" (without correction), or "$\overline{c}$−c" (with correction). You can also indicate how many letters were misread in the line, e.g., "visual acuity 20/40−2 $\overline{c}$−c" indicates that two letters were misread in the 20/40 line by a client wearing corrective lenses.

15. Document findings in the client record using forms or checklists supplemented by narrative notes when appropriate.

(continued)

ASSESSING THE EYE STRUCTURES AND VISUAL ACUITY *(continued)*

EVALUATION

- Perform a detailed follow-up examination of other systems based on findings that deviated from expected or normal for the client. Relate findings to previous assessment data if available.

- Report significant deviations to the primary care provider. Persons with denominators of 40 or more on the Snellen or character chart, with or without corrective lenses, may need to be referred to an optometrist or ophthalmologist.

LIFESPAN CONSIDERATIONS   Assessing the Eyes and Vision

Infants

- Infants 4 weeks of age should gaze at and follow objects.
- Ability to focus with both eyes should be present by 6 months of age.
- Infants do not have tears until about 3 months of age.
- A cover test and the corneal light reflex (Hirschberg) test should be conducted on infants to detect misalignment early and prevent amblyopia.
- Visual acuity is about 20/300 at 4 months and progressively improves.

Children

- Epicanthal folds, common in persons of Asian cultures, may cover the medial canthus and cause eyes to appear misaligned. Epicanthal folds may also be seen in young children of any race before the bridge of the nose begins to elevate.
- Preschool children's acuity can be checked with picture cards or the E chart. Acuity should approach 20/20 by 6 years of age.
- A cover test and the corneal light reflex (Hirschberg) test should be conducted on young children to detect misalignment early and prevent amblyopia.
- Always perform the acuity test with glasses on if a child has a prescription to wear lenses.
- Children should be tested for color vision deficit. From 8% to 10% of Caucasian males and from 0.5% to 1% of Caucasian females have this deficit; it is much less common in non-Caucasian children. The Ishihara or Hardy-Rand-Rittler test can be used.

Older Adults

Visual Acuity

- Visual acuity decreases as the lens of the eye ages and becomes more opaque and loses elasticity.

- The ability of the iris to accommodate to darkness and dim light diminishes.
- Peripheral vision diminishes.
- The adaptation to light (glare) and dark decreases.
- Accommodation to far objects often improves, but accommodation to near objects decreases.
- Color vision declines; older people are less able to perceive purple colors and to discriminate pastel colors.
- Many older adults wear corrective lenses; they are most likely to have hyperopia. Visual changes are due to loss of elasticity (presbyopia) and transparency of the lens.

External Eye Structures

- The skin around the orbit of the eye may darken.
- The eyeball may appear sunken because of the decrease in orbital fat.
- Skin folds of the upper lids may seem more prominent, and the lower lids may sag.
- The eyes may appear dry and lusterless because of the decrease in tear production from the lacrimal glands.
- A thin, grayish white arc or ring (*arcus senilis*) appears around part or all of the cornea. It results from an accumulation of a lipid substance on the cornea. The cornea tends to cloud with age.
- The iris may appear pale with brown discolorations as a result of pigment degeneration.
- The conjunctiva of the eye may appear paler than that of younger adults and may take on a slightly yellow appearance because of the deposition of fat.
- Pupil reaction to light and accommodation is typically symmetrically equal but may be less brisk.
- The pupils can appear smaller in size, unequal, and irregular in shape because of sclerotic changes in the iris.

Ears and Hearing

Assessment of the ear includes direct inspection and palpation of the external ear, inspection of the remaining parts of the ear by an **otoscope** (instrument for examining the interior of the ear, especially the eardrum, consisting essentially of a magnifying lens and a light), and determination of auditory acuity. The ear is usually assessed during an initial physical examination; periodic reassessments may be necessary for long-term clients or those with hearing problems. In some practice settings, only advanced practice nurses perform otoscopic examinations.

Audiometric evaluations, which measure hearing at various decibels, are recommended for children and older adults. A common hearing deficit with age is loss of ability to hear high-frequency sounds, such as *f, s, sh,* and *ph.* This neurosensory hearing deficit does not respond well to use of a hearing aid.

Conduction hearing loss is the result of interrupted transmission of sound waves through the outer and middle ear structures. Possible causes are a tear in the **tympanic membrane** or an obstruction, due to swelling or other causes, in the auditory canal. Sensorineural hearing loss is the result of damage to the inner ear, the auditory nerve, or the hearing center in the brain. Mixed hearing loss is a combination of conduction and sensorineural loss. Skill 17–7 describes how to assess the ears and hearing.

SKILL 17–7

ASSESSING THE EARS AND HEARING

PLANNING

It is important to conduct the ear and hearing examination in an area that is quiet. In addition, the location should allow the client to be positioned sitting or standing at the same level as the nurse.

Delegation

Assessment of the ears and hearing is not delegated to UAP. However, many aspects are observed during usual care and may be recorded by persons other than the nurse. Atypical findings must be validated and interpreted by the nurse.

EQUIPMENT

• Otoscope with several sizes of ear specula

IMPLEMENTATION

Performance

1. Prior to performing the procedure, introduce self and verify the client's identity using agency protocol. Explain to the client what you are going to do, why it is necessary, and how he or she can cooperate. Discuss how the results will be used in planning further care or treatments.
2. Perform hand hygiene and observe appropriate infection control procedures.

3. Provide for client privacy.
4. Inquire if the client has any history of the following: family history of hearing problems or loss; presence of ear problems or pain; medication history, especially if there are complaints of ringing in ears; hearing difficulty: its onset, factors contributing to it, and how it interferes with activities of daily living; use of a corrective hearing device: when and from whom it was obtained.
5. Position the client comfortably, seated if possible.

ASSESSMENT	TYPICAL FINDINGS	ATYPICAL FINDINGS
Auricles		
6. Inspect the auricles for color, symmetry of size, and position. To inspect position, note the level at which the superior aspect of the auricle attaches to the head in relation to the eye.	Color same as facial skin Symmetrical Auricle aligned with outer canthus of eye, about 10° from vertical. ❶	Bluish color of earlobes (e.g., cyanosis); pallor (e.g., frostbite); excessive redness (inflammation or fever) Asymmetry Low-set ears (associated with a congenital abnormality, such as Down syndrome)

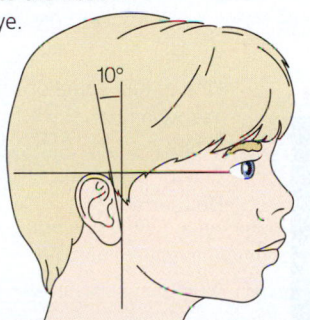

Normal alignment

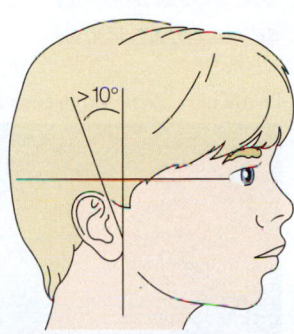

Low-set ears and deviation in alignment

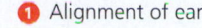 ❶ Alignment of ears.

(continued)

ASSESSING THE EARS AND HEARING *(continued)*

ASSESSMENT	TYPICAL FINDINGS	ATYPICAL FINDINGS
7. Palpate the auricles for texture, elasticity, and areas of tenderness. • Gently pull the auricle upward, downward, and backward. • Fold the pinna forward (it should recoil). • Push in on the tragus. • Apply pressure to the mastoid process.	Mobile, firm, and not tender; pinna recoils after it is folded	Lesions (e.g., cysts); flaky, scaly skin (e.g., seborrhea); tenderness when moved or pressed (may indicate inflammation or infection of external ear)

External Ear Canal and Tympanic Membrane

8. Using an otoscope, inspect the external ear canal for **cerumen**, skin lesions, pus, and blood.

- Attach a speculum to the otoscope. Use the largest diameter that will fit the ear canal without causing discomfort. **Rationale:** *This achieves maximum vision of the entire ear canal and tympanic membrane.*
- Tip the client's head away from you, and straighten the ear canal. For an adult, straighten the ear canal by pulling the pinna up and back. ❷ **Rationale:** *Straightening the ear canal facilitates vision of the ear canal and the tympanic membrane.*
- Hold the otoscope either (a) right side up, with your fingers between the otoscope handle and the client's head or (b) upside down, with your fingers and the ulnar surface of your hand against the client's head. ❸ **Rationale:** *This stabilizes the head and protects the eardrum and canal from injury if a quick head movement occurs.*
- Gently insert the tip of the otoscope into the ear canal, avoiding pressure by the speculum against either side of the ear canal. **Rationale:** *The inner two-thirds of the ear canal is bony; if the speculum is pressed against either side, the client will experience discomfort.*

9. Inspect the tympanic membrane for color and gloss.

Typical findings (item 8): Distal third contains hair follicles and glands
Dry cerumen, grayish-tan color; or sticky, wet cerumen in various shades of brown

Atypical findings (item 8): Redness and discharge
Scaling
Excessive cerumen obstructing canal

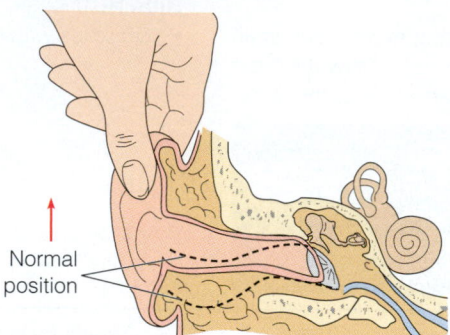

❷ Straightening the ear canal of an adult by pulling the pinna up and back.

Normal position

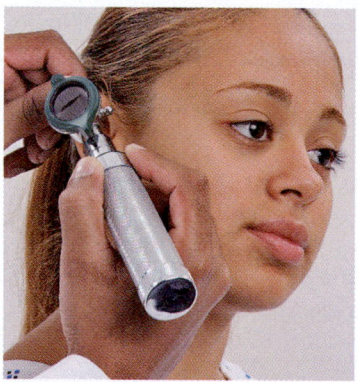 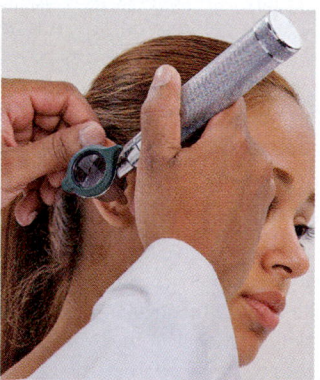

❸ Inserting an otoscope.

Typical findings (item 9): Pearly gray color, semitransparent ❹

Atypical findings (item 9): Pink to red, some opacity
Yellow-amber
White
Blue or deep red
Dull surface

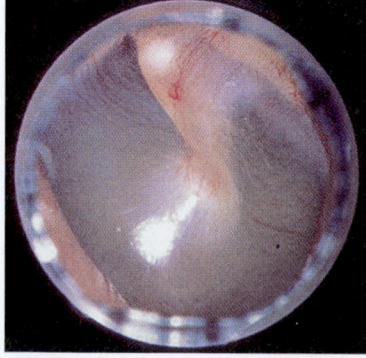

❹ Normal tympanic membrane.

ASSESSMENT	TYPICAL FINDINGS	ATYPICAL FINDINGS
Gross Hearing Acuity Tests		
10. Assess client's response to normal voice tones. If client has difficulty hearing the normal voice, proceed with the following test.	Normal voice tones audible	Normal voice tones not audible (e.g., requests nurse to repeat words or statements, leans toward the speaker, turns the head, cups the ears, or speaks in loud tone of voice)
11. Perform the watch tick test. The ticking of a watch has a higher pitch than the human voice. • Have the client occlude one ear. Out of the client's sight, place a ticking watch 2 to 3 cm (1 to 2 in.) from the unoccluded ear. • Ask what the client can hear. Repeat with the other ear.	Able to hear ticking in both ears	Unable to hear ticking in one or both ears
12. Document findings in the client record using forms or checklists supplemented by narrative notes when appropriate.		

EVALUATION

- Perform a detailed follow-up examination of the neurologic system based on findings that deviated from expected or

normal for the client. Relate findings to previous assessment data if available.

- Report significant deviations to the primary care provider.

LIFESPAN CONSIDERATIONS   Assessing the Ears and Hearing

Infants

To assess gross hearing, ring a bell from behind the infant or have the parent call the child's name to check for a response. Newborns will quiet to the sound and may open their eyes wider. By 3 to 4 months of age, the child will turn head and eyes toward the sound.

- All newborns should be assessed for hearing using auditory brain response testing prior to discharge from the hospital.

Children

- To inspect the external canal and tympanic membrane in children less than 3 years old, pull the pinna down and back. Insert the speculum only 1/4 to 1/2 inch.
- Hearing loss is becoming more common in adolescents and young adults, probably as a result of exposure to loud music and prolonged use of headsets at loud volumes.

Older Adults

- The skin of the ear may appear dry and be less resilient because of the loss of connective tissue.
- Increased coarse and wire-like hair growth occurs along the helix, antihelix, and tragus.
- The pinna increases in both width and length, and the earlobe elongates.
- Earwax is drier.
- The tympanic membrane is more translucent and less flexible. The intensity of the light reflex may diminish slightly.
- Sensorineural hearing loss occurs.
- Generalized hearing loss (presbycusis) occurs in all frequencies, although the first symptom is the loss of high-frequency sounds: the *f, s, sh,* and *ph* sounds. To such persons, conversation can be distorted and result in what appears to be inappropriate or confused behavior.

Nose and Sinuses

A nurse can inspect the nasal passages very simply with a flashlight. However, a nasal *speculum* and a penlight or an otoscope with a nasal attachment facilitates examination of the nasal cavity.

Assessment of the nose includes inspection and palpation of the external nose (the upper third of the nose is bone; the remainder is cartilage); patency of the nasal cavities; and inspection of the nasal cavities.

If the client reports difficulty or abnormality in smell, the nurse may test the client's olfactory sense by asking the client to identify common odors such as coffee or mint. This is done by asking the client to close the eyes and placing vials containing the scent under the client's nose.

The nurse also inspects and palpates the facial sinuses (Figure 17–8).

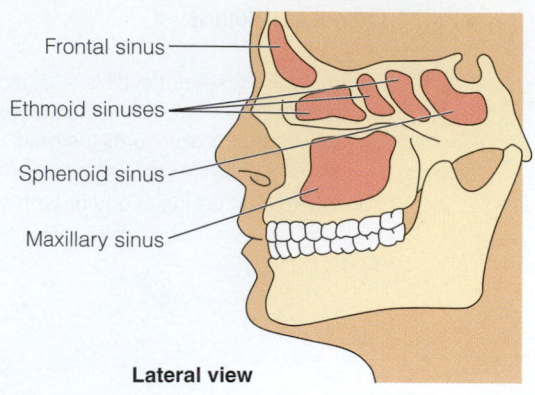

Lateral view

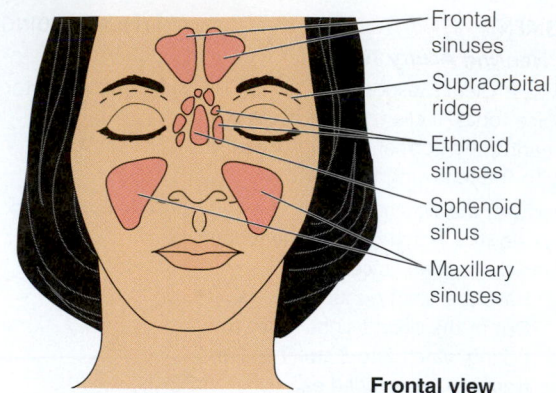

Frontal view

Figure 17–8 ○ The facial sinuses.

Mouth and Oropharynx

The mouth and oropharynx are composed of a number of structures: lips, inner and buccal mucosa, the tongue and floor of the mouth, teeth and gums, hard and soft palate, uvula, salivary glands, tonsillar pillars, and tonsils. By age 25, most people have all their permanent teeth. For information about structures of the teeth, see Chapter 22 ∞.

Dental caries (cavities) and periodontal disease (pyorrhea) are the two problems that most frequently affect the teeth. Both problems are commonly associated with plaque and tartar deposits. Plaque is an invisible soft film that adheres to the enamel surface of teeth; it consists of bacteria, molecules of saliva, and remnants of epithelial cells and leukocytes. When plaque is unchecked, tartar (dental calculus) forms. Tartar is a visible, hard deposit of plaque and dead bacteria that forms at the gum lines. Tartar buildup can alter the fibers that attach the teeth to the gum and eventually disrupt bone tissue. Periodontal disease is characterized by gingivitis (red, swollen gingiva, i.e., gum), bleeding, receding gum lines, and the formation of pockets between the teeth and gums. In advanced periodontal disease, the teeth are loose and pus is evident when the gums are pressed.

Other problems nurses may see are glossitis (inflammation of the tongue), stomatitis (inflammation of the oral mucosa), and parotitis (inflammation of the parotid salivary gland). The accumulation of foul matter (food, microorganisms, and epithelial elements) on the teeth and gums is referred to as sordes.

Skill 17–8 describes assessment of the mouth and oropharynx.

SKILL 17–8

ASSESSING THE MOUTH AND OROPHARYNX

PLANNING

If possible, arrange for the client to sit with the head against a firm surface such as a headrest or examination table. This makes it easier for the client to hold the head still during the examination.

Delegation

Assessment of the mouth and oropharynx is not delegated to UAP. However, many aspects are observed during usual care and may be recorded by persons other than the nurse. Atypical findings must be validated and interpreted by the nurse.

EQUIPMENT

- Clean gloves
- Tongue depressor
- 2×2 gauze pads
- Penlight

IMPLEMENTATION

Performance

1. Prior to performing the procedure, introduce self and verify the client's identity using agency protocol. Explain to the client what you are going to do, why it is necessary, and how he or she can cooperate. Discuss how the results will be used in planning further care or treatments.

2. Perform hand hygiene and observe appropriate infection control procedures.
3. Provide for client privacy.
4. Inquire if the client has any history of the following: routine pattern of dental care, last visit to dentist; length of time ulcers or other lesions have been present; denture discomfort; medications client is receiving.
5. Position the client comfortably, seated if possible.

ASSESSMENT	TYPICAL FINDINGS	ATYPICAL FINDINGS
Lips and Buccal Mucosa		
6. Inspect the outer lips for symmetry of contour, color, and texture. Ask the client to purse the lips as if to whistle.	Uniform pink color (darker, e.g., bluish hue, in Mediterranean groups and dark-skinned clients) Soft, moist, smooth texture Symmetry of contour Ability to purse lips	Pallor; cyanosis Blisters; generalized or localized swelling; fissures, crusts, or scales (may result from excessive moisture, nutritional deficiency, or fluid deficit) Inability to purse lips (may indicate facial nerve damage)
7. Inspect and palpate the inner lips and buccal mucosa for color, moisture, texture, and the presence of lesions. • Apply clean gloves. • Ask the client to relax the mouth, and, for better visualization, pull the lip outward and away from the teeth. • Grasp the lip on each side between the thumb and index finger. ❶ • Palpate any lesions for size, tenderness, and consistency. • Inspect the front teeth and gums.	Uniform pink color (freckled brown pigmentation in dark-skinned clients) Moist, smooth, soft, glistening, and elastic texture (drier oral mucosa in older adult due to decreased salivation)	Pallor; leukoplakia (white patches), red, bleeding Excessive dryness Mucosal cysts; irritations from dentures; abrasions, ulcerations; nodules

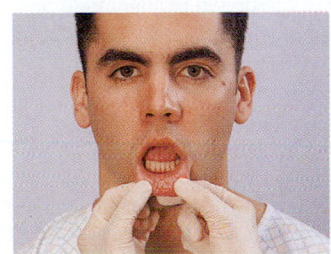

❶ Inspecting the mucosa of the lower lip.

Teeth and Gums		
8. Inspect the teeth and gums while examining the inner lips and buccal mucosa. • Ask the client to open the mouth again. Using a tongue depressor, retract the cheek. ❷ View the surface buccal mucosa from top to bottom and back to front. A flashlight or penlight will help illuminate the surface. Repeat the procedure for the other side.	32 adult teeth Smooth, white, shiny tooth enamel Pink gums (bluish or brown patches in dark-skinned clients) Moist, firm texture to gums No retraction of gums (pulling away from the teeth)	Missing teeth; ill-fitting dentures Brown or black discoloration of the enamel (may indicate staining or the presence of caries) Excessively red gums Spongy texture; bleeding; tenderness (may indicate periodontal disease) Receding, atrophied gums; swelling that partially covers the teeth

(continued)

SKILL 17–8

ASSESSING THE MOUTH AND OROPHARYNX *(continued)*

ASSESSMENT	TYPICAL FINDINGS	ATYPICAL FINDINGS

ASSESSMENT

- Ask the client to open the mouth again. Using a penlight to assist visualization, move a finger along the inside cheek. Another finger may be moved outside the cheek.
- Examine the back teeth. For proper vision of the molars, use the index fingers of both hands to retract the cheek. ❸ Ask the client to relax the lips and first close, then open, the jaw. **Rationale:** *Closing the jaw assists in observation of tooth alignment and loss of teeth; opening the jaw assists in observation of dental fillings and caries.* Observe the number of teeth, tooth color, the state of fillings, dental caries, and tartar along the base of the teeth. Note the presence and fit of partial or complete dentures.
- Inspect the gums around the molars. Observe for bleeding, color, retraction (pulling away from the teeth), edema, and lesions.
- Assess the texture of the gums by gently pressing the gum tissue with a tongue depressor.

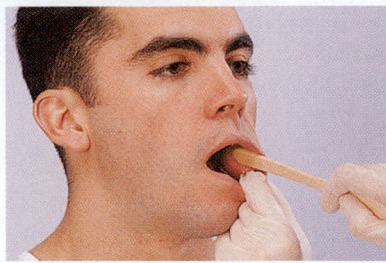
❷ Inspecting the buccal mucosa using a tongue depressor.

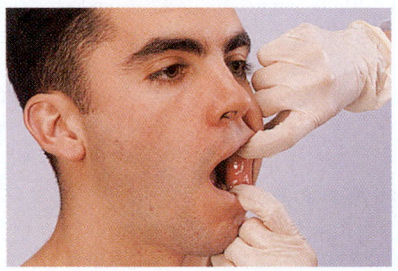
❸ Inspecting the back teeth.

ASSESSMENT	TYPICAL FINDINGS	ATYPICAL FINDINGS
9. Inspect the dentures. Ask the client to remove complete or partial dentures. Inspect their condition, noting in particular broken or worn areas.	Smooth, intact dentures	Ill-fitting dentures; irritated and excoriated area under dentures

Tongue/Floor of the Mouth

ASSESSMENT	TYPICAL FINDINGS	ATYPICAL FINDINGS
10. Inspect the surface of the tongue for position, color, and texture. Ask the client to protrude the tongue.	Central position Pink color (some brown pigmentation on tongue borders in dark-skinned clients); moist; slightly rough; thin whitish coating Smooth, lateral margins; no lesions Raised papillae (taste buds)	Deviated from center (may indicate damage to hypoglossal [twelfth cranial] nerve); excessive trembling Smooth red tongue (may indicate iron, vitamin B_{12}, or vitamin B_3 deficiency) Dry, furry tongue (associated with fluid deficit), white coating (may be oral yeast infection) Nodes, ulcerations, discolorations (white or red areas); areas of tenderness
11. Inspect tongue movement. Ask the client to roll the tongue upward and move it from side to side.	Moves freely; no tenderness	Restricted mobility
12. Inspect the base of the tongue, the mouth floor, and the frenulum. Ask the client to place the tip of the tongue against the roof of the mouth.	Smooth tongue base with prominent veins	Swelling, ulceration

ASSESSMENT	TYPICAL FINDINGS	ATYPICAL FINDINGS
13. Palpate the tongue and floor of the mouth for any nodules, lumps, or excoriated areas. To palpate the tongue, use a piece of gauze to grasp its tip (stabilize it), and with the index finger of your other hand, palpate the back of the tongue, its borders, and its base. ❹	Smooth with no palpable nodules	Swelling, nodules

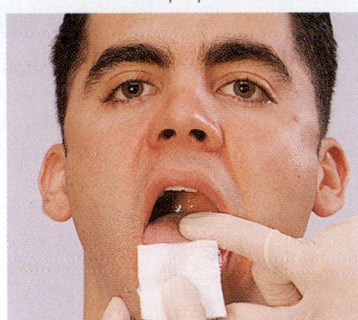

❹ Palpating the tongue.

ASSESSMENT	TYPICAL FINDINGS	ATYPICAL FINDINGS
14. To assess function of the glossopharyngeal and hypoglossal nerves, see the neurologic assessment, later in this chapter.		
Palates and Uvula		
15. Inspect the hard and soft palate for color, shape, texture, and the presence of bony prominences. Ask the client to open the mouth wide and tilt the head backward. Then, depress tongue with a tongue depressor as necessary, and use a penlight for appropriate visualization.	Light pink, smooth, soft palate Lighter pink hard palate, more irregular texture	Discoloration (e.g., jaundice or pallor) Palates the same color Irritations Exostoses (bony growths) growing from the hard palate
16. Inspect the uvula for position and mobility while examining the palates. To observe the uvula, ask the client to say "ah" so that the soft palate rises.	Positioned in midline of soft palate	Deviation to one side from tumor or trauma; immobility (may indicate damage to trigeminal [fifth cranial] nerve or vagus [tenth cranial] nerve)
Oropharynx and Tonsils		
17. Inspect the oropharynx for color and texture. Inspect one side at a time to avoid eliciting the gag reflex. To expose one side of the oropharynx, press a tongue depressor against the tongue on the same side about halfway back while the client tilts the head back and opens the mouth wide. Use a penlight for illumination, if needed.	Pink and smooth posterior wall	Reddened or edematous; presence of lesions, plaques, or drainage
18. Inspect the tonsils (behind the fauces) for color, discharge, and size.	Pink and smooth No discharge Of typical size or not visible • *Grade 1 (typical):* The tonsils are behind the tonsillar pillars (the soft structures supporting the soft palate).	Inflamed Presence of discharge Swollen • *Grade 2:* The tonsils are between the pillars and the uvula. • *Grade 3:* The tonsils touch the uvula. • *Grade 4:* One or both tonsils extend to the midline of the oropharynx.
19. Elicit the gag reflex by pressing the posterior tongue with a tongue depressor.	Present	Absent—may indicate problems with glossopharyngeal (ninth cranial) or vagus (tenth cranial) nerves
20. Document findings in the client record using forms or checklists supplemented by narrative notes when appropriate.		

EVALUATION
- Perform a detailed follow-up examination of neurological and other systems based on findings that deviated from expected or normal for the client. Relate findings to previous assessment data if available.
- Report significant deviations to the primary care provider.

LIFESPAN CONSIDERATIONS   Assessing the Mouth and Oropharynx

Infants

- Inspect the palate and uvula for a cleft. A bifid (forked) uvula may indicate an unsuspected cleft palate (i.e., a cleft in the cartilage that is covered by skin).
- Newborns may have a pearly white nodule on their gums, which resolves without treatment.
- The first teeth erupt at about 6 to 7 months of age. Assess for dental hygiene; parents should cleanse the infant's teeth daily with a soft cloth or soft toothbrush.
- Fluoride supplements should be given by 6 months if the child's drinking water contains less than 0.3 parts per million (ppm) fluoride.
- Children should see a dentist by 1 year of age.

Children

- Tooth development should be appropriate for age.
- White spots on the teeth may indicate excessive fluoride ingestion.
- Drooling is common up to 2 years of age.
- The tonsils are normally larger in children than in adults and commonly extend beyond the palatine arch until the age of 11 or 12 years.

Older Adults

- The oral mucosa may be drier than that of younger persons because of decreased salivary gland activity. Decreased salivation occurs in older adult people taking prescribed medications such as antidepressants, antihistamines, decongestants, diuretics, antihypertensives, tranquilizers, antispasmodics, and antineoplastics. Extreme dryness is associated with dehydration.
- Some receding of the gums occurs, giving an appearance of increased toothiness.
- Taste sensations diminish. Sweet and salty tastes are lost first. Older adult persons may add more salt and sugar to food than they did when they were younger. Diminished taste sensation is due to atrophy of the taste buds and a decreased sense of smell. It indicates diminished function of the fifth and seventh cranial nerves.
- Tiny purple or bluish-black swollen areas (varicosities) under the tongue, known as *caviar spots,* are not uncommon.
- The teeth may show signs of staining, erosion, chipping, and abrasions due to loss of dentin.
- Tooth loss occurs as a result of dental disease but is preventable with good dental hygiene.
- The gag reflex may be slightly sluggish.
- Older adults who are homebound or are in long-term care facilities often have teeth or dentures in need of repair, due to the difficulty of obtaining dental care in these situations. Do a thorough assessment of missing teeth and those in need of repair, whether they are natural teeth or dentures.

THE NECK

Examination of the neck includes the muscles, lymph nodes, trachea, thyroid gland, carotid arteries, and jugular veins. Areas of the neck are defined by the sternocleido-mastoid muscles, which divide each side of the neck into two triangles: the anterior and posterior. The trachea, thyroid gland, anterior cervical nodes, and carotid artery lie within the anterior triangle; the carotid artery runs parallel and anterior to the muscle (Figure 17–9). The posterior lymph nodes lie within the posterior triangle. Lymph nodes in the neck that collect lymph from the head and neck structures are grouped serially and referred to as *chains.* See Table 17–7.

Skill 17–9 describes how to assess the neck.

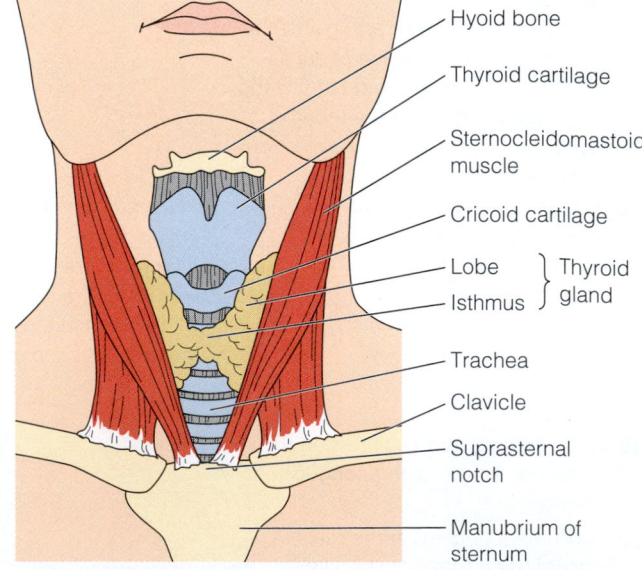

Figure 17–9 ⚪ Structures of the neck.

Hyoid bone

Thyroid cartilage

Sternocleidomastoid muscle

Cricoid cartilage

Lobe } Thyroid gland
Isthmus

Trachea

Clavicle

Suprasternal notch

Manubrium of sternum

TABLE 17–7   Lymph Nodes of the Head and Neck

NODE CENTER	LOCATION	AREA DRAINED
Head		
Occipital	At the posterior base of the skull	The occipital region of the scalp and the deep structures of the back of the neck
Postauricular (mastoid)	Behind the auricle of the ear or in front of the mastoid process	The parietal region of the head and part of the ear
Preauricular	In front of the tragus of the ear	The forehead and upper face
Floor of Mouth		
Submandibular (submaxillary)	Along the medial border of the mandible, halfway between the angle of the jaw and the chin	The chin, upper lip, cheek, nose, teeth, eyelids, part of the tongue and of the floor of the mouth
Submental	Behind the tip of the mandible in the midline, under the chin	The anterior third of the tongue, gums, and floor of the mouth
Neck		
Superficial anterior cervical (tonsillar)	Along the mandible, anterior to the sternocleidomastoid muscle	The skin and neck
Posterior cervical	Along the anterior aspect of the trapezius muscle	The posterior and lateral regions of the neck, occiput, and mastoid
Deep cervical	Under the sternocleidomastoid muscle	The larynx, thyroid gland, trachea, and upper part of the esophagus
Supraclavicular	Above the clavicle, in the angle between the clavicle and the sternocleidomastoid muscle	The lateral regions of the neck and lungs

SKILL 17–9

ASSESSING THE NECK

PLANNING

Delegation
Assessment of the neck is not delegated to UAP. However, many aspects are observed during usual care and may be recorded by persons other than the nurse. Atypical findings must be validated and interpreted by the nurse.

EQUIPMENT
None

IMPLEMENTATION
Performance
1. Prior to performing the procedure, introduce self and verify the client's identity using agency protocol. Explain to the client what you are going to do, why it is necessary, and how he or she can cooperate. Discuss how the results will be used in planning further care or treatments.

2. Perform hand hygiene and observe appropriate infection control procedures.
3. Provide for client privacy.
4. Inquire if the client has any history of the following: problems with neck lumps; neck pain or stiffness; when and how any lumps occurred; previous diagnoses of thyroid problems; and other treatments provided (e.g., surgery, radiation).

ASSESSMENT	TYPICAL FINDINGS	ATYPICAL FINDINGS
Neck Muscles		
5. Inspect the neck muscles for abnormal swellings or masses. Ask the client to hold the head erect.	Muscles equal in size; head centered	Unilateral neck swelling; head tilted to one side (indicates presence of masses, injury, muscle weakness, shortening of sternocleidomastoid muscle, scars)

(continued)

ASSESSING THE NECK *(continued)*

ASSESSMENT	TYPICAL FINDINGS	ATYPICAL FINDINGS
6. Observe head movement. Ask client to:	Coordinated, smooth movements with no discomfort	Muscle tremor, spasm, or stiffness
• Move the chin to the chest. **Rationale:** *This determines function of the sternocleidomastoid muscle.*	Head flexes 45°	Limited range of motion; painful movements; involuntary movements (e.g., up-and-down nodding movements associated with Parkinson's disease)
• Move the head back so that the chin points upward. **Rationale:** *This determines function of the trapezius muscle.*	Head hyperextends 60°	Head hyperextends less than 60°
• Move the head so that the ear is moved toward the shoulder on each side. **Rationale:** *This determines function of the sternocleidomastoid muscle.*	Head laterally flexes 40°	Head laterally flexes less than 40°
• Turn the head to the right and to the left. **Rationale:** *This determines function of the sternocleidomastoid muscle.*	Head laterally rotates 70°	Head laterally rotates less than 70°
7. Assess muscle strength.		
• Ask the client to turn the head to one side against the resistance of your hand. Repeat with the other side. **Rationale:** *This determines the strength of the sternocleidomastoid muscle.*	Equal strength	Unequal strength
• Ask the client to shrug the shoulders against the resistance of your hands. **Rationale:** *This determines the strength of the trapezius muscles.*	Equal strength	Unequal strength
Lymph Nodes		
8. Palpate the entire neck for enlarged lymph nodes.	Not palpable	Enlarged, palpable, possibly tender (associated with infection and tumors)
• Face the client, and bend the client's head forward slightly or toward the side being examined. **Rationale:** *This relaxes the soft tissue and muscles.*		
• Palpate the nodes using the pads of the fingers. Move the fingertips in a gentle rotating motion.		
• When examining the submental and submandibular nodes, place the fingertips under the mandible on the side nearest the palpating hand, and pull the skin and subcutaneous tissue laterally over the mandibular surface so that the tissue rolls over the nodes.		

ASSESSMENT	**TYPICAL FINDINGS**	**ATYPICAL FINDINGS**

- When palpating the supraclavicular nodes, have the client bend the head forward to relax the tissues of the anterior neck and to relax the shoulders so that the clavicles drop. Use your hand nearest the side to be examined when facing the client (i.e., your left hand for the client's right nodes). Use your free hand to flex the client's head forward if necessary. Hook your index and third fingers over the clavicle lateral to the sternocleidomastoid muscle. ❶
- When palpating the anterior cervical nodes and posterior cervical nodes, move your fingertips slowly in a forward circular motion against the sternocleidomastoid and trapezius muscles, respectively.
- To palpate the deep cervical nodes, bend or hook your fingers around the sternocleidomastoid muscle.

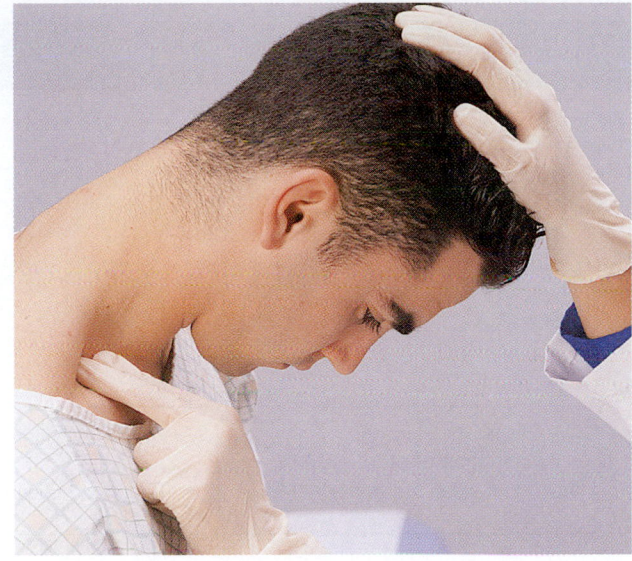

❶ Palpating the supraclavicular lymph nodes.

Trachea

9. Palpate the trachea for lateral deviation. Place your fingertip or thumb on the trachea in the suprasternal notch (Figure 17–9), and then move your finger laterally to the left and the right in spaces bordered by the clavicle, the anterior aspect of the sternocleidomastoid muscle, and the trachea.

Central placement in midline of neck; spaces are equal on both sides

Deviation to one side, indicating possible neck tumor; thyroid enlargement; enlarged lymph nodes

Thyroid Gland

10. Inspect the thyroid gland.
    - Stand in front of the client.
    - Observe the lower half of the neck overlying the thyroid gland for symmetry and visible masses.

    Not visible on inspection

    Visible diffuseness or local enlargement

    - Ask the client to extend the head and swallow. If necessary, offer a glass of water to make it easier for the client to swallow. **Rationale:** *This action determines how the thyroid and cricoid cartilages move and whether swallowing causes a bulging of the gland.*

    Gland ascends during swallowing but is not visible

    Gland is not fully movable with swallowing

11. Palpate the thyroid gland for smoothness. Note any areas of enlargement, masses, or nodules.
    Stand in front of or behind the client, and ask the client to lower the chin slightly. **Rationale:** *Lowering the chin relaxes the neck muscles, facilitating palpation.*

    Lobes may not be palpated
    If palpated, lobes are small, smooth, centrally located, painless, and rise freely with swallowing

    Solitary nodules

(continued)

ASSESSING THE NECK (continued)

	Absence of bruit	Presence of bruit
12. If enlargement of the gland is suspected, auscultate over the thyroid area for a bruit (a soft rushing sound created by turbulent blood flow). Use the bell of the stethoscope. **Rationale:** *The bell transmits this low-frequency sound better than the diaphragm does.*		
13. Document findings in the client record using forms or checklists supplemented by narrative notes when appropriate.		

EVALUATION

* Perform a detailed follow-up examination of other systems based on findings that deviated from expected or normal for the client. Relate findings to previous assessment data if available.
* Report significant deviations to the primary care provider.

LIFESPAN CONSIDERATIONS
Assessing the Neck

Infants and Children

* Examine the neck while the infant or child is lying supine. Lift the head and turn it from side to side to determine neck mobility.
* An infant's neck is normally short, lengthening by about age 3 years. This makes palpation of the trachea difficult.

THE THORAX AND LUNGS

Assessing the thorax and lungs is frequently critical to assessing the client's oxygenation status. Changes in the respiratory system can come about slowly or quickly. In clients with chronic obstructive pulmonary disease (COPD), such as chronic bronchitis, emphysema, and asthma, changes are frequently gradual. The onset of conditions such as pneumonia or pulmonary embolus is generally more acute or sudden.

Chest Landmarks

Locating the position of each rib and certain spinous processes is essential for identifying underlying lobes of the lung. Figure 17–10, *A*, shows an anterior view of the chest and underlying lungs; Figure 17–10, *B*, a posterior view; and Figure 17–10, *C*, right and left lateral views. Each lung is first divided into the upper and lower lobes by an oblique fissure that runs from the level of the spinous process of the third thoracic vertebra (T-3) to the level of the sixth rib at the midclavicular line. The right upper lobe is abbreviated RUL; the right lower lobe, RLL. Similarly, the left upper lobe is abbreviated LUL; the left lower lobe, LLL. The right lung is further divided by a minor fissure into the right upper lobe and right middle lobe (RML). This fissure runs an-

teriorly from the right midaxillary line at the level of the fifth rib to the level of the fourth rib.

These specific landmarks, that is, T-3 and the fourth, fifth, and sixth ribs, are located as follows. The starting point for locating the ribs anteriorly is the angle of Louis, the junction between the body of the sternum (breastbone) and the manubrium (the handlelike superior part of the sternum that joins with the clavicles). The superior border of the second rib attaches to the sternum at this manubriosternal junction (Figure 17–11). The nurse can identify the manubrium by first palpating the clavicle and following its course to its attachment at the manubrium. The nurse then palpates and counts distal ribs and intercostal spaces (ICSs) from the second rib. It is important to note that an ICS is numbered according to the number of the rib immediately *above* the space. When palpating for rib identification, the nurse should palpate along the midclavicular line rather than the sternal border because the rib cartilages are very close at the sternum. Only the first seven ribs attach directly to the sternum.

The counting of ribs is more difficult on the posterior than on the anterior thorax. For identifying underlying lung lobes, the pertinent landmark is T-3. The starting point for locating T-3 is the spinous process of the seventh cervical vertebra (C-7) (Figure 17–12). When the client flexes the neck anteriorly, a prominent process can be observed and palpated. This is the spinous process of the seventh cervical vertebra. If two spinous processes are observed, the superior one is C-7, and the inferior one is the spinous process of the first thoracic vertebra (T-1). The nurse then palpates and counts the spinous processes from C-7 to T-3. Each spinous process up to T-4 is adjacent to the corresponding rib number; for example, T-3 is adjacent to the third rib. After T-4, however, the spinous processes project obliquely, causing the spinous process of the vertebra to lie, not over its correspondingly numbered rib, but over the rib below. Thus, the spinous process of T-5 lies over the body of T-6 and is adjacent to the sixth rib.

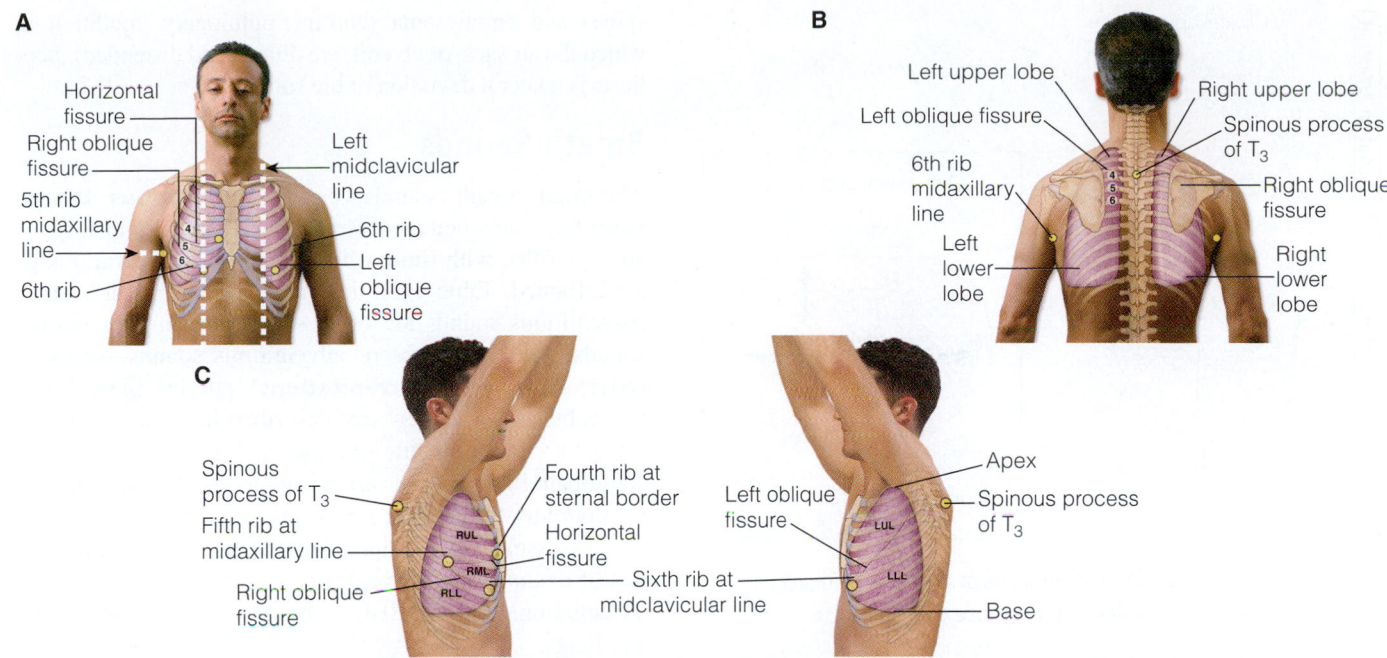

Figure 17–10 ⬤ Chest landmarks: **A,** anterior chest landmarks and underlying lungs; **B,** posterior chest landmarks and underlying lungs; **C,** lateral chest landmarks and underlying lungs.

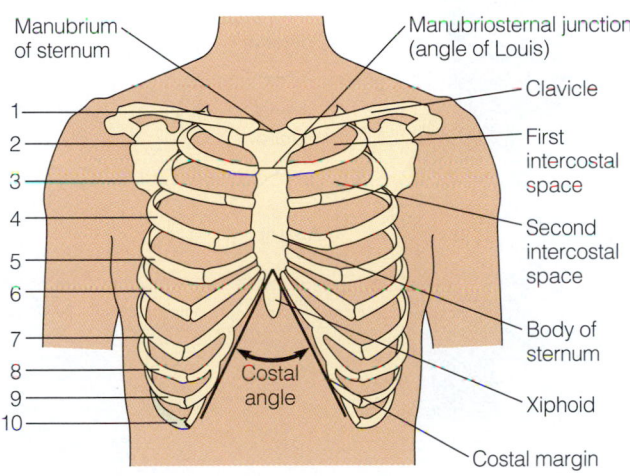

Figure 17–11 ⬤ Location of the anterior ribs, the angle of Louis, and the sternum.

Figure 17–12 ⬤ Location of the posterior ribs in relation to the spinous processes.

Chest Shape and Size

In adults, the thorax is oval. Its anteroposterior diameter is half its transverse diameter (Figure 17–13). The overall shape of the thorax is elliptical; that is, its diameter is smaller at the top than at the base. In older adults, kyphosis and osteoporosis alter the size of the chest cavity as the ribs move downward and forward.

There are several deformities of the chest (Figure 17–14). Pigeon chest (*pectus carinatum*), a permanent deformity, may be caused by rickets. A narrow transverse diameter, an increased anteroposterior diameter, and a protruding sternum

characterize pigeon chest. A funnel chest (*pectus excavatum*), a congenital defect, is the opposite of pigeon chest in that the sternum is depressed, narrowing the anteroposterior diameter. Because the sternum points posteriorly in clients with a funnel chest, abnormal pressure on the heart may result in altered function. A barrel chest, in which the ratio of the anteroposterior to transverse diameter is 1 to 1, is seen in clients with thoracic kyphosis (excessive convex curvature of the thoracic

Clinical appearance

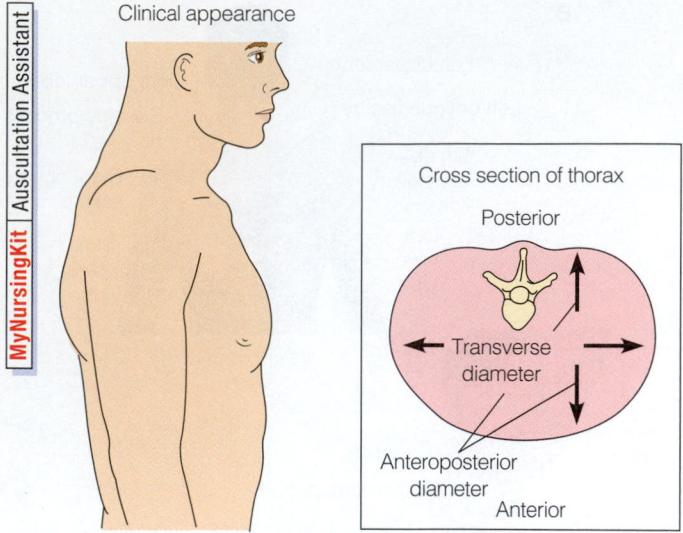

Cross section of thorax

Posterior

Transverse diameter

Anteroposterior diameter

Anterior

Figure 17–13 ◯ Configurations of the thorax showing anteroposterior diameter and transverse diameter.

spine) and emphysema (chronic pulmonary condition in which the air sacs, or alveoli, are dilated and distended). Scoliosis is a lateral deviation of the spine.

Breath Sounds

Abnormal breath sounds, called **adventitious breath sounds**, occur when air passes through narrowed airways or airways filled with fluid or mucus, or when pleural linings are inflamed. Table 17–8 describes normal breath sounds. Adventitious sounds are often superimposed over normal sounds. The four types of adventitious sounds—crackles (referred to as rales or **crepitations**), gurgles, pleural friction rubs, and wheezes—are described in Table 17–9. Absence of breath sounds over some lung areas is also a significant finding that is associated with collapsed and surgically removed lobes or severe pneumonia.

Assessment of the lungs and thorax includes all methods of examination: inspection, palpation, percussion, and auscultation. Skill 17–10 describes how to assess the thorax and lungs.

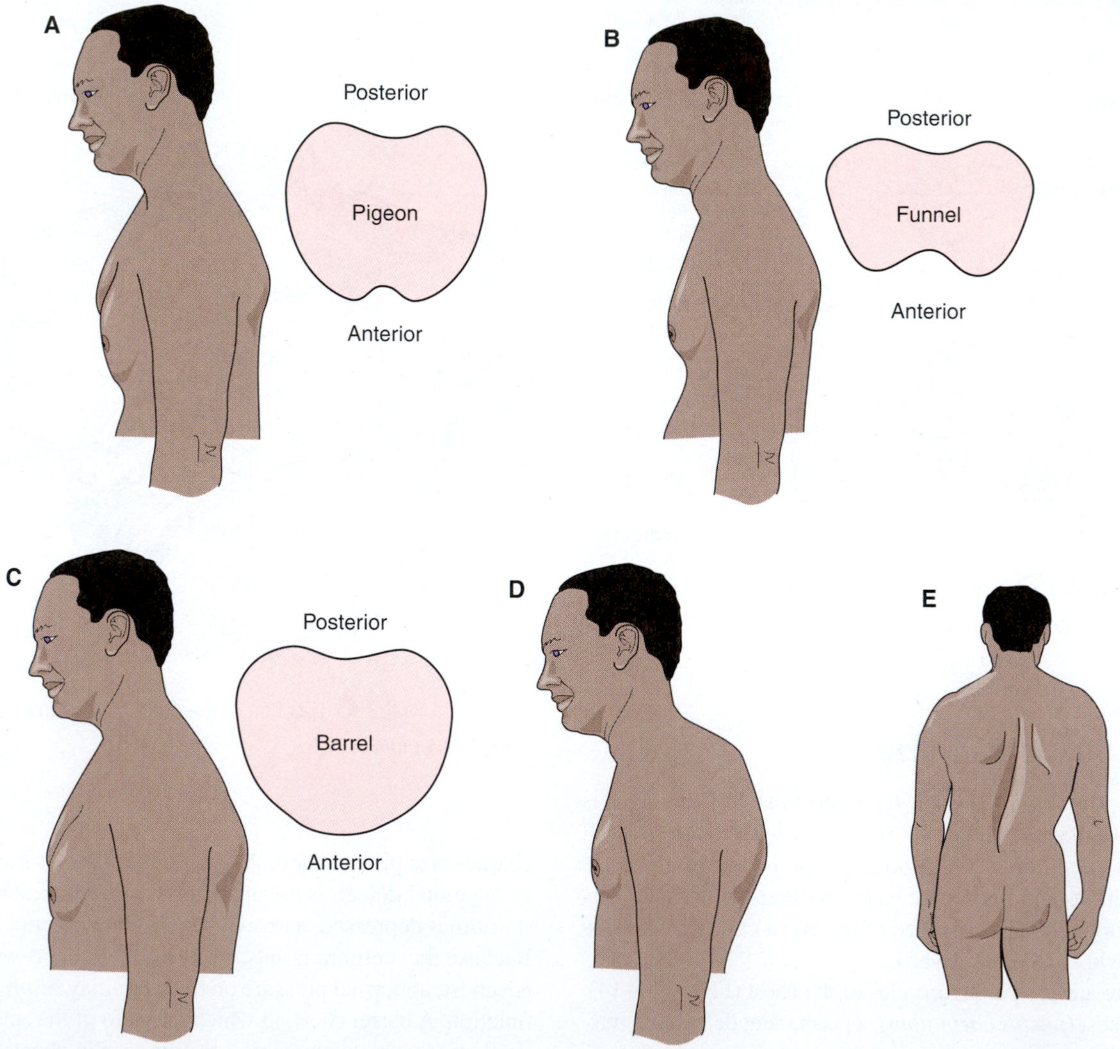

A

Posterior

Pigeon

Anterior

B

Posterior

Funnel

Anterior

C

Posterior

Barrel

Anterior

D

E

Figure 17–14 ◯ Chest deformities: *A,* pigeon chest; *B,* funnel chest; *C,* barrel chest; *D,* kyphosis; *E,* scoliosis.

TABLE 17–8 **Normal Breath Sounds**

TYPE	DESCRIPTION	LOCATION	CHARACTERISTICS
Vesicular	Soft-intensity, low-pitched, "gentle sighing" sounds created by air moving through smaller airways (bronchioles and alveoli)	Over peripheral lung; best heard at base of lungs	Best heard on inspiration, which is about 2.5 times longer than the expiratory phase (5:2 ratio)
Broncho-vesicular	Moderate-intensity and moderate-pitched "blowing" sounds created by air moving through larger airway (bronchi)	Between the scapulae and lateral to the sternum at the first and second intercostal spaces	Equal inspiratory and expiratory phases (1:1 ratio)
Bronchial (tubular)	High-pitched, loud, "harsh" sounds created by air moving through the trachea	Anteriorly over the trachea; not typically heard over lung tissue	Louder than vesicular sounds; have a short inspiratory phase and long expiratory phase (1:2 ratio)

TABLE 17–9 **Adventitious Breath Sounds**

NAME	DESCRIPTION	CAUSE	LOCATION
Crackles (rales)	Fine, short, interrupted crackling sounds; alveolar rales are high pitched. Sound can be simulated by rolling a lock of hair near the ear. Best heard on inspiration but can be heard on both inspiration and expiration. May not be cleared by coughing.	Air passing through fluid or mucus in any air passage	Most commonly heard in the bases of the lower lung lobes
Gurgles (rhonchi)	Continuous, low-pitched, coarse, gurgling, harsh, louder sounds with a moaning or snoring quality. Best heard on expiration but can be heard on both inspiration and expiration. May be altered by coughing.	Air passing through narrowed air passages as a result of secretions, swelling, tumors	Loud sounds can be heard over most lung areas but predominate over the trachea and bronchi
Friction rub	Superficial grating or creaking sounds heard during inspiration and expiration. Not relieved by coughing.	Rubbing together of inflamed pleural surfaces	Heard most often in areas of greatest thoracic expansion (e.g., lower anterior and lateral chest)
Wheeze	Continuous, high-pitched, squeaky musical sounds. Best heard on expiration. Not usually altered by coughing.	Air passing through a constricted bronchus as a result of secretions, swelling, tumors	Heard over all lung fields

SKILL 17–10

ASSESSING THE THORAX AND LUNGS

PLANNING

For efficiency, the nurse usually examines the posterior chest first, then the anterior chest. For posterior and lateral chest examinations, the client is uncovered to the waist and in a sitting position. A sitting or lying position may be used for anterior chest examination. The sitting position is preferred because it maximizes chest expansion. Good lighting is essential, especially for chest inspection.

Delegation

Assessment of the thorax and lungs is not delegated to UAP. However, many aspects of breathing are observed during usual care and may be recorded by persons other than the nurse. Atypical findings must be validated and interpreted by the nurse.

EQUIPMENT

- Stethoscope
- Skin marker/pencil
- Centimeter ruler

IMPLEMENTATION

Performance

1. Prior to performing the procedure, introduce self and verify the client's identity using agency protocol. Explain to the client what you are going to do, why it is necessary, and how he or she can cooperate. Discuss how the results will be used in planning further care or treatments.
2. Perform hand hygiene and observe appropriate infection control procedures.
3. Provide for client privacy. In women, drape the anterior chest when it is not being examined.
4. Inquire if the client has any history of the following: family history of illness, including cancer, allergies, tuberculosis; lifestyle habits such as smoking and occupational hazards (e.g., inhaling fumes); medications being taken; current problems (e.g., swellings, coughs, wheezing, pain).

ASSESSMENT	TYPICAL FINDINGS	ATYPICAL FINDINGS
Posterior Thorax		
5. Inspect the shape and symmetry of the thorax from posterior and lateral views. Compare the anteroposterior diameter to the transverse diameter.	Anteroposterior to transverse diameter in ratio of 1:2 Chest symmetric	Barrel chest; increased anteroposterior to transverse diameter Chest asymmetric
6. Inspect the spinal alignment for deformities. Have the client stand. From a lateral position, observe the three normal curvatures: cervical, thoracic, and lumbar.	Spine vertically aligned	Exaggerated spinal curvatures (kyphosis, lordosis)
• To assess for lateral deviation of spine (scoliosis), observe the standing client from the rear. Have the client bend forward at the waist and observe from behind.	Spinal column is straight, right and left shoulders and hips are at same height.	Spinal column deviates to one side, often accentuated when bending over. Shoulders or hips not even.
7. Palpate the posterior thorax.		
• For clients who have no respiratory complaints, rapidly assess the temperature and integrity of all chest skin.	Skin intact; uniform temperature	Skin lesions; areas of hyperthermia
• For clients who do have respiratory complaints, palpate all chest areas for bulges, tenderness, or abnormal movements. Avoid deep palpation for painful areas, especially if a fractured rib is suspected. In such a case, deep palpation could lead to displacement of the bone fragment against the lungs.	Chest wall intact; no tenderness; no masses	Lumps, bulges; depressions; areas of tenderness; movable structures (e.g., rib)

ASSESSMENT	TYPICAL FINDINGS	ATYPICAL FINDINGS
8. Palpate the posterior chest for respiratory excursion (thoracic expansion). Place the palms of both your hands over the lower thorax with your thumbs adjacent to the spine and your fingers stretched laterally. ❶ Ask the client to take a deep breath while you observe the movement of your hands and any lag in movement.	Full and symmetric chest expansion (i.e., when the client takes a deep breath, your thumbs should move apart an equal distance and at the same time; normally the thumbs separate 3 to 5 cm [1 1/2 to 2 in.] during deep inspiration)	Asymmetric and/or decreased chest expansion

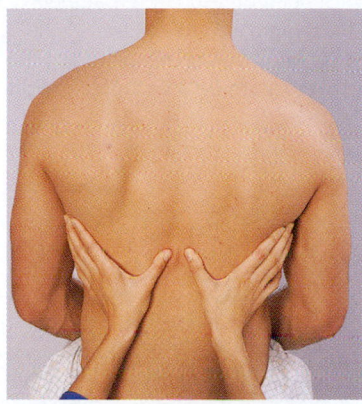

❶ Position of the nurse's hands when assessing respiratory excursion on the posterior thorax.

ASSESSMENT	TYPICAL FINDINGS	ATYPICAL FINDINGS
9. Palpate the chest for vocal (tactile) fremitus, the faintly perceptible vibration felt through the chest wall when the client speaks. • Place the palmar surfaces of your fingertips or the ulnar aspect of your hand or closed fist on the posterior chest, starting near the apex of the lungs (see ❷, position A). • Ask the client to repeat such words as "blue moon" or "one, two, three." • Repeat the two steps, moving your hands sequentially to the base of the lungs, through positions B–E in ❷. • Compare the fremitus on both lungs and between the apex and the base of each lung, using either one hand and moving it from one side of the client to the corresponding area on the other side *or* using two hands that are placed simultaneously on the corresponding areas of each side of the chest.	Bilateral symmetry of vocal fremitus Fremitus is heard most clearly at the apex of the lungs Low-pitched voices of males are more readily palpated than higher pitched voices of females	Decreased or absent fremitus (associated with pneumothorax) Increased fremitus (associated with consolidated lung tissue, as in pneumonia)

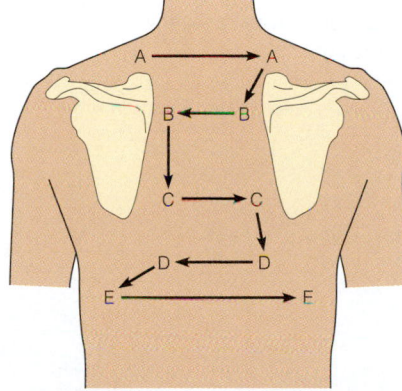

❷ Areas and sequence for palpating tactile fremitus on the posterior chest.

(continued)

SKILL 17–10

ASSESSING THE THORAX AND LUNGS *(continued)*

ASSESSMENT	TYPICAL FINDINGS	ATYPICAL FINDINGS

ASSESSMENT

10. Percuss the thorax.
Percussion of the thorax is performed to determine whether underlying lung tissue is filled with air, liquid, or solid material and to determine the positions and boundaries of certain organs. Because percussion penetrates to a depth of 5 to 7 cm (2 to 3 in.), it detects superficial rather than deep lesions. Percussion sounds and tones are described in Table 17–3, earlier. **3**

- Ask the client to bend the head and fold the arms forward across the chest. **Rationale:** *This separates the scapula and exposes more lung tissue to percussion.*
- Percuss in the intercostal spaces at about 5 cm (2 in.) intervals in a systematic sequence. **4**
- Compare one side of the lung with the other.
- Percuss the lateral thorax every few inches, starting at the axilla and working down to the eighth rib.

11. Percuss for diaphragmatic excursion (movement of the diaphragm during maximal inspiration and expiration).

- Ask the client to take a deep breath and hold it while you percuss downward along the scapular line until dullness is produced at the level of the diaphragm. Mark this point with a marking pencil, and repeat the procedure on the other side of the chest.
- Ask the client to take a few normal breaths and then expel the last breath completely and hold it while you percuss upward from the marked point to assess and mark the diaphragmatic excursion during deep expiration on each side.
- Measure the distance between the two marks.

12. Auscultate the chest using the flat-disc diaphragm of the stethoscope (*best for transmitting the high-pitched breath sounds*).

- Use the systematic zigzag procedure used in percussion
- Ask the client to take slow, deep breaths through the mouth. Listen at each point to the breath sounds during a complete inspiration and expiration.

TYPICAL FINDINGS

Percussion notes resonate, except over scapula
Lowest point of resonance is at the diaphragm (i.e., at the level of the eighth to tenth rib posteriorly)
Note: Percussion on a rib typically elicits dullness.

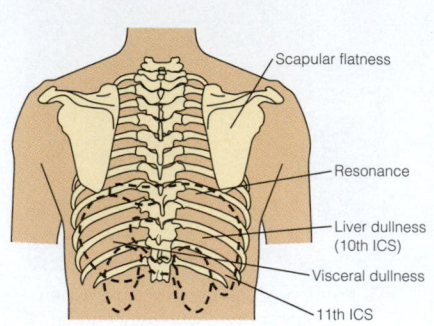

3 Normal percussion sounds on the anterior chest.

Scapular flatness
Resonance
Liver dullness (10th ICS)
Visceral dullness
11th ICS

Excursion is 3 to 5 cm (1 1/2 to 2 in.) bilaterally in women and 5 to 6 cm (2 to 3 in.) in men
Diaphragm is usually slightly higher on the right side

Vesicular and bronchovesicular breath sounds (see Table 17–8)

ATYPICAL FINDINGS

Asymmetry in percussion
Areas of dullness or flatness over lung tissue (associated with consolidation of lung tissue or a mass)

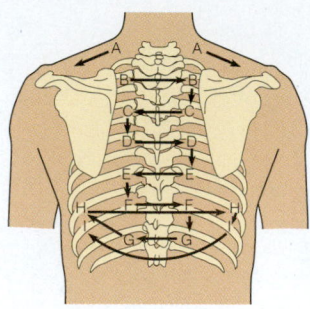

4 Sequence for posterior chest percussion.

Restricted excursion (associated with lung disorder)

Adventitious breath sounds (e.g., crackles, gurgles, wheeze, friction rub; see Table 17–8)

Absence of breath sounds

ASSESSMENT	TYPICAL FINDINGS	ATYPICAL FINDINGS
• Compare findings at each point with the corresponding point on the opposite side of the chest.		
13. Inspect breathing patterns (e.g., respiratory rate and rhythm).	Quiet, rhythmic, and effortless respirations (see Chapter 16 ∞)	See Chapter 16 ∞ , Box 16–5 for abnormal breathing patterns and sounds
14. Inspect the costal angle (angle formed by the intersection of the costal margins) and the angle at which the ribs enter the spine.	Costal angle is less than 90°, and the ribs insert into the spine at approximately a 45° angle (see Figure 17–11, earlier)	Costal angle is widened (associated with chronic obstructive pulmonary disease)
15. Palpate the anterior chest (see posterior chest palpation).		
16. Palpate the anterior chest for respiratory excursion. • Place the palms of both your hands on the lower thorax, with your fingers laterally along the lower rib cage and your thumbs along the costal margins. ❺ • Ask the client to take a deep breath while you observe the movement of your hands.	Full symmetric excursion; thumbs normally separate 3 to 5 cm (1 1/2 to 2 in.)	Asymmetric and/or decreased respiratory excursion

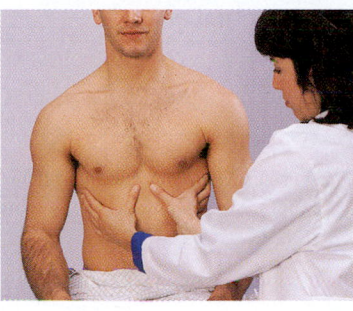

❺ Position of nurse's hands when assessing respiratory excursion on the anterior thorax.

17. Palpate tactile fremitus in the same manner as for the posterior chest and using the sequence shown in ❻. If the breasts are large and cannot be retracted adequately for palpation, this part of the examination is usually omitted.	Same as posterior vocal fremitus; fremitus is normally decreased over heart and breast tissue	Same as posterior fremitus

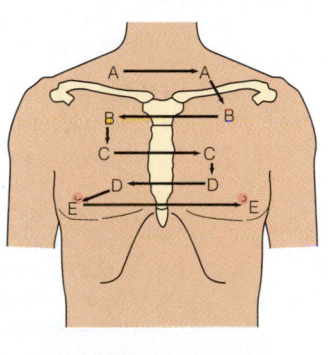

❻ Areas and sequence for palpating tactile fremitus on the anterior chest.

18. Percuss the anterior chest systematically. • Begin above the clavicles in the supraclavicular space, and proceed downward to the diaphragm. ❼ • Compare one side of the lung to the other. • Displace female breasts for proper examination.	Percussion notes resonate down to the sixth rib at the level of the diaphragm but are flat over areas of heavy muscle and bone, dull on areas over the heart and the liver, and tympanic over the underlying stomach. ❽	Asymmetry in percussion notes Areas of dullness or flatness over lung tissue

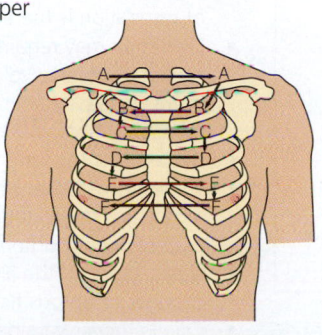

❼ Sequence for anterior chest percussion.

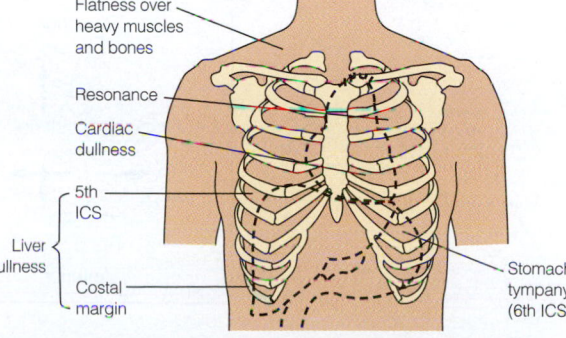

❽ Normal percussion sounds on the posterior chest.

(continued)

SKILL 17–10

ASSESSING THE THORAX AND LUNGS *(continued)*

ASSESSMENT	TYPICAL FINDINGS	ATYPICAL FINDINGS
19. Auscultate the trachea.	Bronchial and tubular breath sounds (see Table 17–8)	Adventitious breath sounds (see Table 17–9)
20. Auscultate the anterior chest. Use the sequence used in percussion ❼, beginning over the bronchi between the sternum and the clavicles.	Bronchovesicular and vesicular breath sounds (see Table 17–8)	Adventitious breath sounds (see Table 17–9)

21. Document findings in the client record using forms or checklists supplemented by narrative notes when appropriate.

SAMPLE DOCUMENTATION

1/21/10 0830 Lungs clear to auscultation except for fine crackles both lower lobes, lessened p coughing. Rarely moves in bed. Assisted to a chair and reviewed deep breathing exercises. Effective return demonstration. _____ N. Schmidt, RN

EVALUATION

- Relate findings to previous assessment data if available. Report significant deviations to the primary care provider.

LIFESPAN CONSIDERATIONS   Assessing the Thorax and Lungs

Infants

- The thorax is rounded; that is, the diameter from the front to the back (anteroposterior) is equal to the transverse diameter. See Figure 17–15. It is also cylindrical, having a nearly equal diameter at the top and the base. This makes it harder for infants to expand their thoracic space.
- To assess tactile fremitus, place the hand over the crying infant's chest.
- Infants tend to breathe using their diaphragm; assess rate and rhythm by watching the abdomen, rather than the thorax, rise and fall.
- The right bronchial branch is short and angles down as it leaves the trachea, making it easy for small objects to be inhaled. Sudden onset of cough or other signs of respiratory distress may indicate the infant has inhaled a foreign object.

Children

- By about 6 years of age, the anteroposterior diameter has decreased in proportion to the transverse diameter, with a 1:2 ratio present.

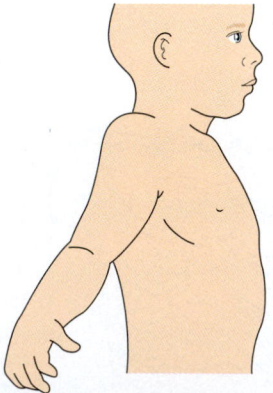
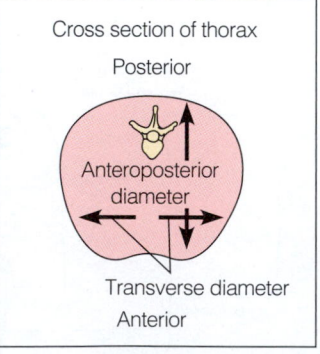

Clinical appearance

Cross section of thorax

Posterior

Anteroposterior diameter

Transverse diameter

Anterior

Figure 17–15 ● Configurations of the child's thorax showing anteroposterior diameter and transverse diameter.

- Children tend to breathe more abdominally than thoracically up to age 6.
- During the rapid growth spurts of adolescence, spinal curvature and rotation (scoliosis) may appear. Children should be assessed for scoliosis by age 12 and annually until their growth slows. Curvature greater than 10% should be referred for further medical evaluation.

Older Adults

- The thoracic curvature may be accentuated (kyphosis) because of osteoporosis and changes in cartilage, resulting in collapse of the vertebrae. This can also compromise and decrease normal respiratory effort.
- Kyphosis and osteoporosis alter the size of the chest cavity as the ribs move downward and forward.
- The anteroposterior diameter of the chest widens, giving the person a barrel-chested appearance. This is due to loss of skeletal muscle strength in the thorax and diaphragm and constant lung inflation from excessive expiratory pressure on the alveoli.
- Breathing rate and rhythm are unchanged at rest; the rate normally increases with exercise but may take longer to return to the preexercise rate.
- Inspiratory muscles become less powerful, and the inspiration reserve volume decreases. A decrease in depth of respiration is therefore apparent.
- Expiration may require the use of accessory muscles. The expiratory reserve volume significantly increases because of the increased amount of air remaining in the lungs at the end of a normal breath.
- Deflation of the lung is incomplete.
- Small airways lose their cartilaginous support and elastic recoil; as a result, they tend to close, particularly in basal or dependent portions of the lung.
- Elastic tissue of the alveoli loses its stretchability and changes to fibrous tissue. Exertional capacity decreases.
- Cilia in the airways decrease in number and are less effective in removing mucus; older adult clients are therefore at greater risk for pulmonary infections.

THE CARDIOVASCULAR AND PERIPHERAL VASCULAR SYSTEMS

Heart

Nurses assess the heart through inspection, palpation, and auscultation, in that sequence. Auscultation is more meaningful when other data are obtained first. The heart is usually assessed during an initial physical assessment; periodic reassessments may be necessary for long-term or at-risk clients or those with cardiac problems. Heart examinations are usually performed while the client is in a semireclined position.

In the average adult, most of the heart lies behind and to the left of the sternum. A small portion (the right atrium) extends to the right of the sternum. The upper portion of the heart (both atria), referred to as its *base*, lies toward the back. The lower portion (the ventricles), referred to as its *apex*, points anteriorly. The apex of the left ventricle actually touches the chest wall at or medial to the left midclavicular line (MCL) and at or near the fifth left intercostal space (LICS), which is slightly below the left nipple. This point is the point of maximal impulse (PMI).

> ### CLINICAL ALERT
>
> Remember that the base of the lungs is the lower (inferior) portion, and the base of the heart is the upper (superior) portion.

The precordium, the area of the chest overlying the heart, is inspected and palpated for the presence of abnormal pulsations or lifts or heaves. The terms **lift** and *heave,* often used interchangeably, refer to a rising along the sternal border with each heartbeat. A lift occurs when cardiac action is very forceful. It should be confirmed by palpation with the palm of the hand. Enlargement or overactivity of the left ventricle produces a heave lateral to the apex, whereas enlargement of the right ventricle produces a heave at or near the sternum.

Heart sounds can be heard by auscultation. The normal first two heart sounds are produced by closure of the valves of the heart. The first heart sound, **S₁**, occurs when the atrioventricular (A-V) valves close. These valves close when the ventricles have been sufficiently filled. Although the A-V valves do not close simultaneously, the closure occurs closely enough to be heard as one sound. S_1 is a dull, low-pitched sound described as "lub." After the ventricles empty the blood into the aorta and pulmonary arteries, the semilunar valves close, producing the second heart sound, **S₂**, described as "dub." S_2 has a higher pitch than S_1 and is shorter in duration. These two sounds, S_1 and S_2 ("lub-dub"), occur within 1 second or less, depending on the heart rate.

The two heart sounds are audible anywhere on the precordial area, but they are best heard over the aortic, pulmonic, tricuspid, and apical areas. Each area is associated with the closure of heart valves: the aortic area with the aortic valve (inside the aorta as it arises from the left ventricle); the pulmonic area with the pulmonic valve (inside the pulmonary artery as it arises from the right ventricle); the tricuspid area with the tricuspid valve (between the right atrium and ventricle); and the apical area with the mitral valve (between the left atrium and ventricle).

Associated with these sounds are systole and diastole. Systole is the period in which the ventricles contract. It begins with S_1 and ends at S_2. Systole is normally shorter than diastole. Diastole is the period in which the ventricles relax. It starts with S_2 and ends at the subsequent S_1. Normally no sounds are audible during these periods. The experienced nurse, however, may perceive extra heart sounds (S_3 and S_4) during diastole. Both sounds are low in pitch and heard best at the apex, with the bell of the stethoscope, and with the client lying on the left side. S_3 occurs early in diastole right after S_2 and sounds like "lub-dub-*ee*" (S_1, S_2, S_3) or "Kentuc-*ky*." It often disappears when the client sits up. S_3 is normal in children and young adults. In older adults, it may indicate heart failure. S_4 occurs near the very end of diastole just before S_1 and creates the sound of "*dee*-lub-dub" (S_4, S_1, S_2) or "*Ten*-nessee." S_4 is rarely heard in healthy young adults. S_4 may be heard in many older adult clients and can be a sign of hypertension.

Normal heart sounds are summarized in Table 17–10. The nurse may also hear abnormal heart sounds, such as clicks, rubs, and murmurs. These are caused by valve disorders or impaired blood flow within the heart and require advanced training to diagnose.

TABLE 17–10 Normal Heart Sounds

SOUND OR PHASE	DESCRIPTION	AREA			
		AORTIC	PULMONIC	TRICUSPID	APICAL
S_1	Dull, low pitched, and longer than S_2; sounds like "lub"	Less intensity than S_2	Less intensity than S_2	Louder than or equal to S_2	Louder than or equal to S_2
Systole	Normally silent interval between S_1 and S_2				
S_2	Higher pitch than S_1; sounds like "dub"	Louder than S_1	Louder than S_1; abnormal if louder than the aortic S_2 in adults over 40 years of age	Less intensity than or equal to S_1	Less intensity than or equal to S_1
Diastole	Normally silent interval between S_2 and next S_1				

Central Vessels

The carotid arteries supply oxygenated blood to the head and neck. Because they are the only source of blood to the brain, prolonged occlusion of these arteries can result in serious brain damage. The carotid pulses correlate with central aortic pressure, thus reflecting cardiac function better than the peripheral pulses. When cardiac output is diminished, the peripheral pulses may be difficult or impossible to feel, but the carotid pulse should be felt easily.

The carotid is also auscultated for a bruit. A **bruit** (a blowing or swishing sound) is created by turbulence of blood flow due either to a narrowed arterial lumen (a common development in older people) or to a condition, such as anemia or hyperthyroidism, which elevates cardiac output. If a bruit is found, the carotid artery is then palpated for a thrill. A **thrill**, which frequently accompanies a bruit, is a vibrating sensation like the purring of a cat or water running through a hose. It, too, indicates turbulent blood flow due to arterial obstruction.

The jugular veins drain blood from the head and neck directly into the superior vena cava and right side of the heart. The external jugular veins are superficial and may be visible above the clavicle. The internal jugular veins lie deeper along the carotid artery and may transmit pulsations onto the skin of the neck. External neck veins are typically distended and visible when a person lies down; they are flat and not as visible when a person stands up, because gravity encourages venous drainage. By inspecting the jugular veins for pulsations and distention, the nurse can assess the adequacy of function of the right side of the heart and venous pressure. Bilateral jugular vein distention (JVD) may indicate right-sided heart failure.

Skill 17–11 describes how to assess the heart and central vessels.

SKILL 17–11

ASSESSING THE HEART AND CENTRAL VESSELS

PLANNING

Heart examinations are usually performed while the client is in a semireclined position. The practitioner stands at the client's right side, where palpation of the cardiac area is facilitated and optimal inspection allowed.

Delegation

Assessment of the heart and central vessels is not delegated to UAP. However, many aspects of cardiac function are observed during usual care and may be recorded by persons other than the nurse. Atypical findings must be validated and interpreted by the nurse.

EQUIPMENT
- Stethoscope
- Centimeter ruler

IMPLEMENTATION

Performance

1. Prior to performing the procedure, introduce self and verify the client's identity using agency protocol. Explain to the client what you are going to do, why it is necessary, and how he or she can cooperate. Discuss how the results will be used in planning further care or treatments.
2. Perform hand hygiene and observe appropriate infection control procedures.
3. Provide for client privacy.
4. Inquire if the client has any history of the following: family history of incidence and age of heart disease, high cholesterol levels, high blood pressure, stroke, obesity, congenital heart disease, arterial disease, hypertension, and rheumatic fever; client's past history of rheumatic fever, heart murmur, heart attack, varicosities, or heart failure; present symptoms indicative of heart disease, e.g., fatigue, dyspnea, orthopnea, edema, cough, chest pain, palpitations, syncope, hypertension, wheezing, hemoptysis; presence of diseases that affect heart, e.g., obesity, diabetes, lung disease, endocrine disorders; lifestyle habits that are risk factors for cardiac disease, e.g., smoking, alcohol intake, eating and exercise patterns, areas and degree of stress perceived.

ASSESSMENT	TYPICAL FINDINGS	ATYPICAL FINDINGS
5. Simultaneously inspect and palpate the precordium for the presence of abnormal pulsations, lifts, or heaves.		
6. Auscultate the heart in all four anatomic sites: aortic, pulmonic, tricuspid, and apical (mitral). Auscultation need not be limited to these areas; however, the nurse may need to move the stethoscope to find the most audible sounds for each client.	S_1: Usually heard at all sites Usually louder at apical area S_2: Usually heard at all sites Usually louder at base of heart Systole: silent interval; slightly shorter duration than diastole at normal heart rate (60 to 90 beats/min) Diastole: silent interval; slightly longer duration than systole at normal heart rates S_3 in children and young adults S_4 in many older adults	Increased or decreased intensity Varying intensity with different beats Increased intensity at aortic area Increased intensity at pulmonic area Sharp-sounding ejection clicks S_3 in older adults S_4 may be a sign of hypertension
• Eliminate all sources of room noise. **Rationale:** *Heart sounds are of low intensity, and other noise hinders the nurse's ability to hear them.*		
• Keep the client in a supine position with head elevated 30° to 45°.		
• Use both the diaphragm and the bell to listen to all areas.		
• In every area of auscultation, distinguish both S_1 and S_2 sounds.		
• When auscultating, concentrate on one particular sound at a time in each area: the first heart sound, followed by systole, then the second heart sound, then diastole. Systole and diastole are normally silent intervals.		
• Later, reexamine the heart while the client is in the upright sitting position. **Rationale:** *Certain sounds are more audible in certain positions.*		
Carotid Arteries		
7. Palpate the carotid artery, using extreme caution.	Symmetric pulse volumes Full pulsations, thrusting quality Quality remains same when client breathes, turns head, and changes from sitting to supine position Elastic arterial wall	Asymmetric volumes (possible stenosis or thrombosis) Decreased pulsations (may indicate impaired left cardiac output) Increased pulsations Thickening, hard, rigid, beaded, inelastic walls (indicate arteriosclerosis)
• Palpate only one carotid artery at a time. **Rationale:** *This ensures adequate blood flow through the other artery to the brain.*		
• Avoid exerting too much pressure and massaging the area. **Rationale:** *Pressure can occlude the artery, and carotid sinus massage can precipitate bradycardia.* The carotid sinus is a small dilation at the beginning of the internal carotid artery just above the bifurcation of the common carotid artery, in the upper third of the neck.		
• Ask the client to turn the head slightly toward the side being examined. **Rationale:** *This makes the carotid artery more accessible.*		

(continued)

SKILL 17–11

ASSESSING THE HEART AND CENTRAL VESSELS *(continued)*

ASSESSMENT	TYPICAL FINDINGS	ATYPICAL FINDINGS

8. Auscultate the carotid artery.
  • Turn the client's head slightly away from the side being examined. **Rationale:** *This facilitates the placement of the stethoscope.*
  • Auscultate the carotid artery on one side and then the other.
  • Listen for the presence of a bruit. If you hear a bruit, gently palpate the artery to determine the presence of a thrill.
	No sound heard on auscultation	Presence of bruit in one or both arteries (suggests occlusive artery disease)

Jugular Veins

9. Inspect the jugular veins for distention while the client is placed in a semi-Fowler's position (30° to 45° angle), with the head supported on a small pillow.	Veins not visible (indicating right side of heart is functioning normally)	Veins visibly distended (indicating advanced cardiopulmonary disease)

10. If jugular distention is present, assess the jugular venous pressure (JVP).
  • Locate the highest visible point of distention of the internal jugular vein. Although either the internal or the external jugular vein can be used, the internal jugular vein is more reliable. **Rationale:** *The external jugular vein is more easily affected by obstruction or kinking at the base of the neck.*
  • Measure the vertical height of this point in centimeters from the sternal angle, the point at which the clavicles meet. ❶
  • Repeat the preceding steps on the other side.
		Bilateral measurements above 3 to 4 cm are considered elevated (may indicate right-sided heart failure)
		Unilateral distention (may be caused by local obstruction)

11. Document findings in the client record using forms or checklists supplemented by narrative notes when appropriate.		

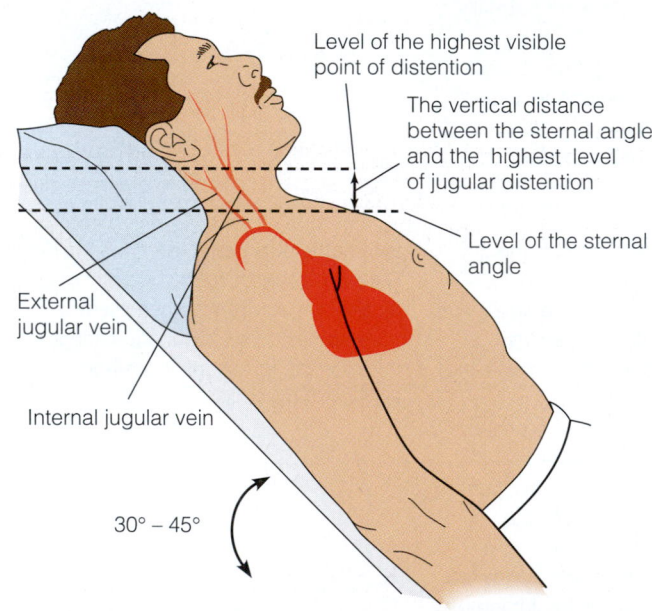

Level of the highest visible point of distention

The vertical distance between the sternal angle and the highest level of jugular distention

Level of the sternal angle

External jugular vein

Internal jugular vein

30° – 45°

❶ Assessing the highest point of distention of the jugular vein.

EVALUATION
- Perform a detailed follow-up examination based on findings that deviated from expected or normal for the client. Relate findings to previous assessment data if available.
- Report significant deviations to the primary care provider.

LIFESPAN CONSIDERATIONS   Assessing the Heart and Central Vessels

Infants

- Physiologic splitting of the second heart sound (S_2) may be heard when the child takes a deep breath and the aortic valve closes a split second before the pulmonic valve. If splitting of S_2 is heard during normal respirations, it is abnormal and may indicate an atrial-septal defect, pulmonary stenosis, or another heart problem.
- Infants may normally have sinus arrhythmia that is related to respiration. The heart rate slows during expiration and increases when the child breathes in.
- Murmurs may be heard in newborns as the structures of fetal circulation, especially the ductus arteriosus, close.

Children

- Heart sounds may be louder because of the thinner chest wall.

- A third heart sound (S_3), caused as the ventricles fill, is best heard at the apex and is present in about one-third of all children.
- The PMI is higher and more medial in children under 8 years old.

Older Adults

- If no disease is present, heart size remains the same size throughout life.
- Cardiac output and strength of contraction decrease, thus lessening the older person's activity tolerance.
- The heart rate returns to its resting rate more slowly after exertion than it did when the individual was younger.
- S_4 heart sound is considered typical in older adults.
- Extra systoles commonly occur. Ten or more systoles per minute are considered abnormal.
- Sudden emotional and physical stresses may result in cardiac arrhythmias and heart failure.

Peripheral Vascular System

Assessing the peripheral vascular system includes measuring the blood pressure, palpating peripheral pulses, and inspecting the skin and tissues to determine perfusion (blood supply to an area) to the extremities. Certain aspects of peripheral vascular assessment are often incorporated into other parts of the assessment procedure.

Skill 17–12 describes how to assess the peripheral vascular system.

SKILL 17–12

ASSESSING THE PERIPHERAL VASCULAR SYSTEM

PLANNING

Delegation
Due to the substantial knowledge and skill required, assessment of the peripheral vascular system is not delegated to UAP. However, many aspects of the vascular system are observed during usual care and may be recorded by persons other than the nurse. Atypical findings must be validated and interpreted by the nurse.

EQUIPMENT
None

IMPLEMENTATION
Performance
1. Prior to performing the procedure, introduce self and verify the client's identity using agency protocol. Explain to the client what you are going to do, why it is necessary, and how he or she can cooperate. Discuss how the results will be used in planning further care or treatments.

2. Perform hand hygiene and observe appropriate infection control procedures.
3. Provide for client privacy.
4. Inquire if the client has any history of the following: past history of heart disorders, varicosities, arterial disease, and hypertension; lifestyle habits such as exercise patterns, activity patterns and tolerance, smoking, and use of alcohol.

(continued)

SKILL 17–12

ASSESSING THE PERIPHERAL VASCULAR SYSTEM *(continued)*

ASSESSMENT	TYPICAL FINDINGS	ATYPICAL FINDINGS
Peripheral Pulses		
5. Palpate the peripheral pulses on both sides of the client's body individually, simultaneously (except the carotid pulse), and systematically to determine the symmetry of pulse volume. If you have difficulty palpating some of the peripheral pulses, use a Doppler ultrasound probe.	Symmetric pulse volumes Full pulsations	Asymmetric volumes (indicate impaired circulation) Absence of pulsation (indicates arterial spasm or occlusion) Decreased, weak, thready pulsations (indicate impaired cardiac output) Increased pulse volume (may indicate hypertension, high cardiac output, or circulatory overload)
Peripheral Veins		
6. Inspect the peripheral veins in the arms and legs for the presence and/or appearance of superficial veins when limbs are dependent and when limbs are elevated.	In dependent position, presence of distention and nodular bulges at calves When limbs elevated, veins collapse (veins may appear tortuous or distended in older people)	Distended veins in the thigh and/or lower leg or on posterolateral part of calf from knee to ankle
7. Assess the peripheral leg veins for signs of phlebitis. • Inspect the calves for redness and swelling over vein sites. • Palpate the calves for firmness or tension of the muscles, the presence of edema over the dorsum of the foot, and areas of localized warmth. **Rationale:** *Palpation augments inspection findings, particularly in greater pigmented people in whom redness may not be visible.* • Push the calves from side to side to test for tenderness. • Firmly dorsiflex the client's foot while supporting the entire leg in extension (Homans' test), or have the person stand or walk.	Limbs not tender Symmetric in size	Tenderness on palpation Pain in calf muscles with forceful dorsiflexion of the foot (positive Homans' test) Warmth and redness over vein Swelling of one calf or leg
Peripheral Perfusion		
8. Inspect the skin of the hands and feet for color, temperature, edema, and skin changes.	Skin color pink Skin temperature not excessively warm or cold No edema Skin texture resilient and moist	Cyanotic (venous insufficiency) Pallor that increases with limb elevation Dependent rubor, a dusky red color when limb is lowered (arterial insufficiency) Brown pigmentation around ankles (arterial or chronic venous insufficiency) Skin cool (arterial insufficiency) Marked edema (venous insufficiency) Mild edema (arterial insufficiency) Skin thin and shiny or thick, waxy, shiny, and fragile, with reduced hair and ulceration (venous or arterial insufficiency)
9. Assess the adequacy of arterial flow if arterial insufficiency is suspected.		

ASSESSMENT	TYPICAL FINDINGS	ATYPICAL FINDINGS
Capillary Refill Test		
• Squeeze the client's fingernail and toenail between your fingers sufficiently to cause blanching (about 5 seconds).	Capillary refill test: Immediate return of color	Delayed return of color (arterial insufficiency)
• Release the pressure, and observe how quickly normal color returns. Color normally returns immediately (less than 2 seconds).		

SAMPLE DOCUMENTATION

1/21/10 0830 Legs mottled red bilaterally toes to mid-calf. States "actually looks a bit better." Capillary refill 4–5 seconds in toes on both feet. Pedal pulses present but weak. Homans' test negative. c/o pain in calves after walking 100 feet.

_____ N. Schmidt, RN

10. Document findings in the client record using forms or checklists supplemented by narrative notes when appropriate.

EVALUATION

- Perform a detailed follow-up examination of the heart or central vessels, integument, or other systems based on findings that deviated from expected or normal for the client. Relate findings to previous assessment data if available.
- Report significant deviations to the primary care provider.

LIFESPAN CONSIDERATIONS | Assessing the Peripheral Vascular System

Infants

- Screen for coarctation of the aorta by palpating the peripheral pulses and comparing the strength of the femoral pulses with the radial pulses and apical pulse. If coarctation is present, femoral pulses will be diminished and radial pulses will be stronger.

Children

- Changes in the peripheral vasculature, such as bruising, petechiae, and purpura, can indicate serious systemic diseases in children (e.g., leukemia, meningococcemia).

Older Adults

- The overall effectiveness of blood vessels decreases as smooth muscle cells are replaced by connective tissue. The lower extremities are more likely to show signs of arterial and venous impairment because of the more distal and dependent position.
- Peripheral vascular assessment should always include upper and lower extremities' temperature, color, pulses, edema, skin integrity, and sensation. Any differences in symmetry of these findings should be noted.
- Proximal arteries become thinner and dilate.
- Peripheral arteries become thicker and dilate less effectively because of arteriosclerotic changes in the vessel walls.
- Blood vessels lengthen and become more tortuous and prominent. Varicosities occur more frequently.
- In some instances, arteries may be palpated more easily because of the loss of supportive surrounding tissues. Often, however, the most distal pulses of the lower extremities are more difficult to palpate because of decreased arterial perfusion.
- Systolic and diastolic blood pressures increase, but the increase in the systolic pressure is greater. As a result, the pulse pressure widens. Any client with a blood pressure reading above 140/90 should be referred for follow-up assessments.
- Peripheral edema is frequently observed and is most commonly the result of chronic venous insufficiency or low protein levels in the blood (hypoproteinemia).

THE BREASTS AND AXILLAE

The breasts of men and women are inspected and palpated. Men have some glandular tissue beneath each nipple, a potential site for malignancy, whereas mature women have glandular tissue throughout the breast. In females, the largest portion of glandular breast tissue is located in the upper outer quadrant of each breast. A projection of breast tissue from this quadrant extends into the axilla, called the *axillary tail of Spence*. The majority of breast tumors are located in this upper outer breast quadrant including the tail of Spence. During assessment, the nurse can localize specific findings by using this division of the breast into quadrants and the axillary tail. Skill 17–13 describes how to assess the breasts and axillae.

ASSESSING THE BREASTS AND AXILLAE

PLANNING

Delegation
Assessment of the breasts and axillae is not delegated to UAP. However, persons other than the nurse may record aspects observed during usual care. Atypical findings must be validated and interpreted by the nurse.

EQUIPMENT
- Centimeter ruler

IMPLEMENTATION

Performance

1. Prior to performing the procedure, introduce self and verify the client's identity using agency protocol. Explain to the client what you are going to do, why it is necessary, and how he or she can cooperate. Inquire whether the client has ever had a clinical breast exam previously. Discuss how the results will be used in planning further care or treatments.
2. Perform hand hygiene and observe appropriate infection control procedures.
3. Provide for client privacy.
4. Inquire if the client has a history of breast masses and what was done about them; pain or tenderness in the breasts and relation to the woman's menstrual cycle; discharge from the nipple; medication; risk factors that may be associated with development of breast cancer. Inquire if the client performs breast self-examination; technique used and when performed in relation to the menstrual cycle.

ASSESSMENT	TYPICAL FINDINGS	ATYPICAL FINDINGS
5. Inspect the breasts for size, symmetry, and contour or shape while the client is in a sitting position.	*Females:* Rounded shape; slightly unequal in size; generally symmetric *Males:* Breasts even with the chest wall; if obese, may be similar in shape to female breasts	Recent change in breast size; swellings; marked asymmetry
6. Inspect the skin of the breast for localized discolorations or hyperpigmentation, retraction or dimpling, localized hypervascular areas, swelling or edema. ❶	Skin uniform in color (same in appearance as skin of abdomen or back) Skin smooth and intact Diffuse symmetric horizontal or vertical vascular pattern in light-skinned people Striae (stretch marks); moles and nevi	Localized discolorations or hyperpigmentation Retraction or dimpling (result of scar tissue or an invasive tumor) Unilateral, localized hypervascular areas (associated with increased blood flow) Swelling or edema appearing as pig skin or orange peel due to exaggeration of the pores

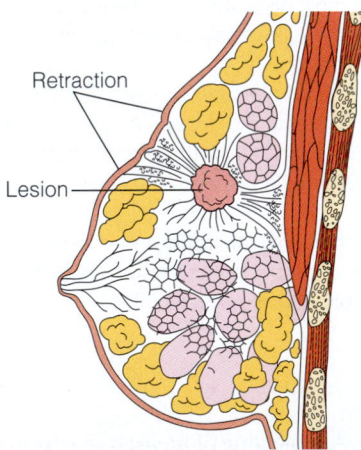

Retraction

Lesion

❶ A lesion causing retraction of the skin.

7. Emphasize any retraction by having the client
   - Raise the arms above the head.
   - Push the hands together, with elbows flexed. ❷
   - Press the hands down on the hips. ❸

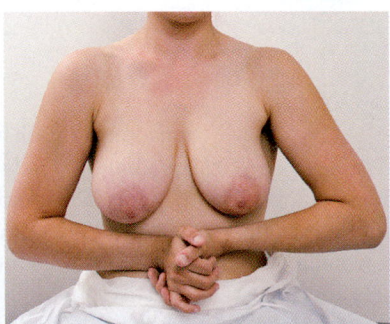

❷ Pushing the hands together to accentuate retraction of the breast tissue.

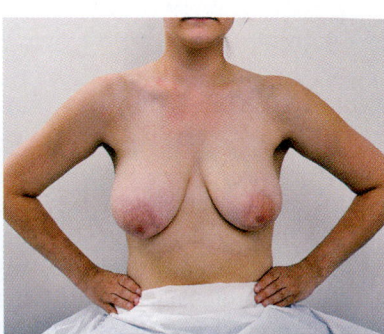

❸ Pressing the hands down on the hips to accentuate retraction of the breast tissue.

ASSESSMENT	TYPICAL FINDINGS	ATYPICAL FINDINGS
8. Inspect the areola area for size, shape, symmetry, color, surface characteristics, and any masses or lesions.	Round or oval and bilaterally the same Color varies widely, from light pink to dark brown Irregular placement of sebaceous glands on the surface of the areola (Montgomery's tubercles)	Any asymmetry, mass, or lesion
9. Inspect the nipples for size, shape, position, color, discharge, and lesions.	Round, everted, and equal in size; similar in color; soft and smooth; both nipples point in same direction (out in young women and men, downward in older women) No discharge, except from pregnant or breast-feeding females Inversion of one or both nipples that is present from puberty	Asymmetrical size and color Presence of discharge, crusts, or cracks Recent inversion of one or both nipples
10. Palpate the axillary, subclavicular, and supraclavicular lymph nodes ❹ while the client sits with the arms abducted and supported on the nurse's forearm. For palpation of clavicular lymph nodes, see page 437. Use the flat surfaces of all fingertips to palpate the four areas of the axilla: • the edge of the greater pectoral muscle (musculus pectoralis major) along the anterior axillary line • the thoracic wall in the midaxillary area • the upper part of the humerus, and • the anterior edge of the latissimus dorsi muscle along the posterior axillary line.	No tenderness, masses, or nodules	Tenderness, masses, or nodules

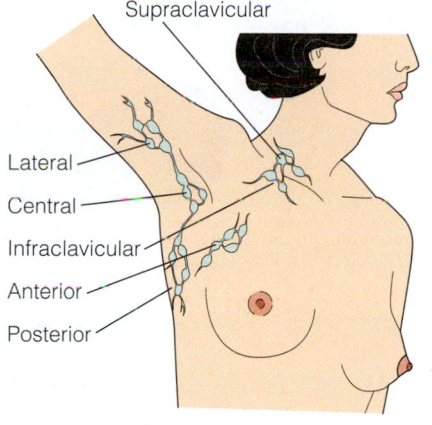
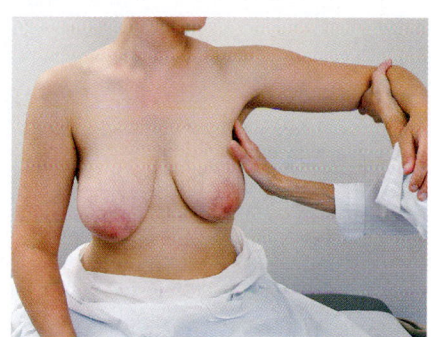

❹ Location and palpation of the lymph nodes that drain the lateral breast. **A,** Lymph nodes; **B,** Palpating the axilla.

ASSESSMENT	TYPICAL FINDINGS	ATYPICAL FINDINGS

11. Palpate the breast for masses, tenderness, and any discharge from the nipples. Palpation of the breast is generally performed while the client is supine. **Rationale:** *In the supine position, the breasts flatten evenly against the chest wall, facilitating palpation.* For clients who have a past history of breast masses, who are at high risk for breast cancer, or who have pendulous breasts, examination in both a supine and a sitting position is recommended.
• If the client reports a breast lump, start with the uninvolved breast to obtain baseline data that will serve as a comparison to the reportedly involved breast.
• To enhance flattening of the breast, instruct the client to abduct the arm and place her hand behind her head. Then place a small pillow or rolled towel under the client's shoulder.
• For palpation, use the palmar surface of the middle three fingertips (held together) and make a gentle rotary motion on the breast.
	No tenderness, masses, nodules, or nipple discharge	Tenderness, masses, nodules, or nipple discharge
		• If you detect a mass, record the following data:
		  a. **Location:** the exact location relative to the quadrants and axillary tail, or the clock and the distance from the nipple in centimeters.
		  b. **Size:** the length, width, and thickness of the mass in centimeters. If you are able to determine the discrete edges, record this fact.
		  c. **Shape:** whether the mass is round, oval, lobulated, indistinct, or irregular.
		  d. **Consistency:** whether the mass is hard or soft.
		  e. **Mobility:** whether the mass is movable or fixed.
		  f. **Skin over the lump:** whether it is reddened, dimpled, or retracted.
		  g. **Nipple:** whether it is displaced or retracted.
		  h. **Tenderness:** whether palpation is painful.

(continued)

SKILL 17–13

ASSESSING THE BREASTS AND AXILLAE *(continued)*

ASSESSMENT	TYPICAL FINDINGS	ATYPICAL FINDINGS

ASSESSMENT

- Choose one of three patterns for palpation:
  - a. Hands-of-the-clock or spokes-on-a-wheel ⑤
  - b. Concentric circles ⑥
  - c. Vertical strips pattern ⑦
- Start at one point for palpation, and move systematically to the end point to ensure that all breast surfaces are assessed.
- Pay particular attention to the upper outer quadrant area and the tail of Spence.

TYPICAL FINDINGS

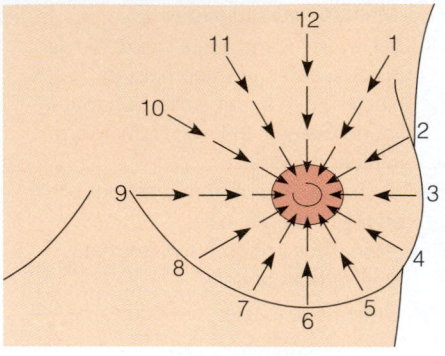

⑤ Hands-of-the-clock or spokes-on-a-wheel pattern of breast palpation.

ATYPICAL FINDINGS

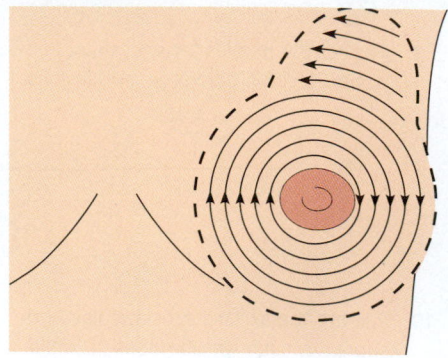

⑥ Concentric circles pattern for breast palpation.

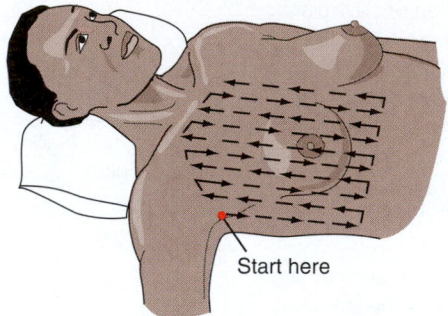

Start here

⑦ Vertical strips pattern of breast palpation.

12. Palpate the areola and the nipples for masses. Compress each nipple to determine the presence of any discharge. If discharge is present, milk the breast along its radius to identify the discharge-producing lobe. Assess any discharge for amount, color, consistency, and odor. Note also any tenderness on palpation.

No tenderness, masses, nodules, or nipple discharge

Tenderness, masses, nodules, or nipple discharge

13. Teach the client the technique of breast self-examination (see Chapter 28 ∞).

14. Document findings in the client record using forms or checklists supplemented by narrative notes when appropriate.

EVALUATION

- Perform a detailed follow-up examination based on findings that deviated from expected or normal for the client. Relate findings to previous assessment data if available.

- Report significant deviations to the primary care provider.

LIFESPAN CONSIDERATIONS   Assessing the Breasts and Axillae

Infants

- Newborns, both boys and girls, up to 2 weeks of age may have breast enlargement and white discharge from the nipples (witch's milk).
- Supernumerary ("extra") nipples infrequently are present as small dimples along the mammary chain; these may be associated with renal anomalies.

Children

- Female breast development begins between 9 and 13 years of age and occurs in five stages (Tanner stages). One breast may develop more rapidly than the other, but at the end of development, they are more or less the same size.
  Stage 1 Prepubertal with no noticeable change
  Stage 2 Breast bud with elevation of nipple and enlargement of the areola
  Stage 3 Enlargement of the breast and areola with no separation of contour
  Stage 4 Projection of the areola and nipple
  Stage 5 Recession of the areola by about age 14 or 15, leaving only the nipple projecting
- Boys may develop breast buds and have slight enlargement of the areola in early adolescence. Further enlargement of breast tissue (gynecomastia) can occur.

This growth is transient, usually lasting about 2 years, resolving completely by late puberty.
- Axillary hair usually appears in Tanner stages 3 or 4 and is related to adrenal rather than gonadal changes.

Pregnant Females

- Breast, areola, and nipple size increase.
- The areolae and nipples darken; nipples may become more erect; areolae contain small, scattered, elevated Montgomery's glands.
- Superficial veins become more prominent, and jagged linear stretch marks may develop.
- A thick yellow fluid (colostrum) may be expressed from the nipples after the first trimester.

Older Adults

- In the postmenopausal female, breasts change in shape and often appear pendulous or flaccid; they lack the firmness they had in younger years.
- The presence of breast lesions may be detected more readily because of the decrease in connective tissue.
- General breast size remains the same. Although glandular tissue atrophies, the amount of fat in breasts (predominantly in the lower quadrants) increases in most women.

THE ABDOMEN

The nurse locates and describes abdominal findings using two common methods of subdividing the abdomen: quadrants and regions. To divide the abdomen into quadrants, the nurse imagines two lines: a vertical line from the xiphoid process to the pubic symphysis, and a horizontal line across the umbilicus (see Figure 17–16). These quadrants are labeled right upper quadrant (*1*), left upper quadrant (*2*), right lower quadrant (*3*), and left lower quadrant (*4*). Using the second method, division into nine regions, the nurse imagines two vertical lines that extend superiorly from the midpoints of the inguinal ligaments, and two horizontal lines, one at the level of the edge of the lower ribs and the other at the level of the iliac crests (see Figure 17–17). Specific organs or parts of organs lie in each abdominal region (see Boxes 17–5 and 17–6).

In addition, practitioners often use certain landmarks to locate abdominal signs and symptoms. These are the xiphoid process of the sternum, the costal margins, the anterosuperior iliac spine, the inguinal ligaments (Poupart's ligaments), and the superior margin of the pubic symphysis (see Figure 17–18).

Assessment of the abdomen involves all four methods of examination. When assessing the abdomen, the nurse performs inspection first, followed by auscultation,

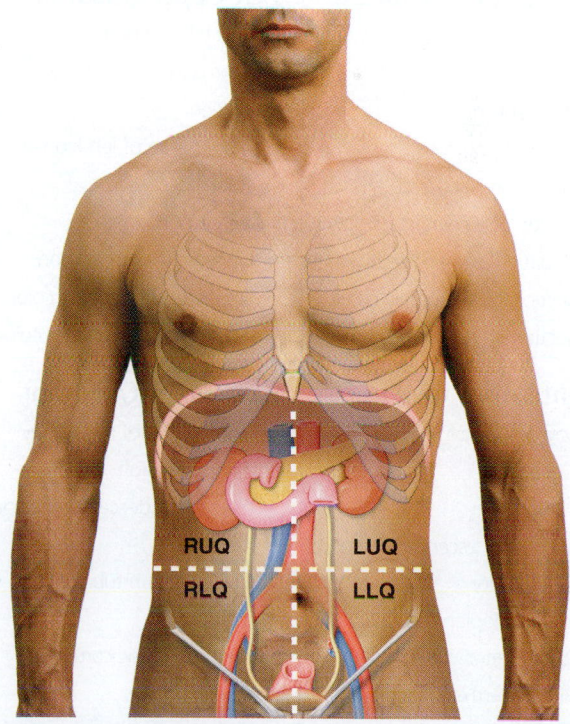

Figure 17–16 ⊙ The four abdominal quadrants and the underlying organs: *RUQ*, right upper quadrant; *LUQ*, left upper quadrant; *RLQ*, right lower quadrant; *LLQ*, left lower quadrant.

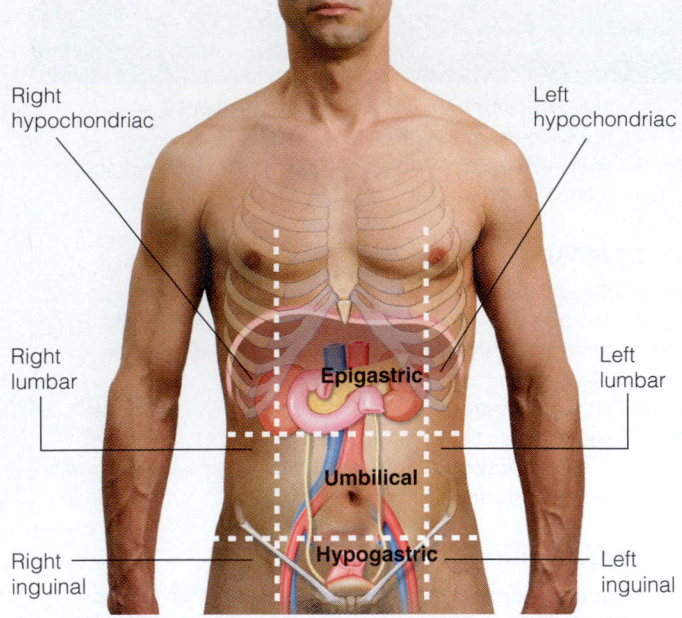

Figure 17–17 ⚬ The nine abdominal regions: epigastric; left and right hypochondriac; umbilical; left and right lumbar; suprapubic and hypogastric; left and right inguinal or iliac.

BOX 17–5	Organs in the Four Abdominal Quadrants

Right Upper Quadrant
Liver
Gallbladder
Duodenum
Head of pancreas
Right adrenal gland
Upper lobe of right kidney
Hepatic flexure of colon
Section of ascending colon
Section of transverse colon

Left Upper Quadrant
Left lobe of liver
Stomach
Spleen
Upper lobe of left kidney
Pancreas
Left adrenal gland
Splenic flexure of colon
Section of transverse colon
Section of descending colon

Right Lower Quadrant
Lower lobe of right kidney
Cecum
Appendix
Section of ascending colon
Right ovary
Right fallopian tube
Right ureter
Right spermatic cord
Part of uterus

Left Lower Quadrant
Lower lobe of left kidney
Sigmoid colon
Section of descending colon
Left ovary
Left fallopian tube
Left ureter
Left spermatic cord
Part of uterus

BOX 17–6	Organs in the Nine Abdominal Regions

Right Hypochondriac
Right lobe of liver
Gallbladder
Part of duodenum
Hepatic flexure of colon
Upper half of right kidney
Suprarenal gland

Right Lumbar
Ascending colon
Lower half of right kidney
Part of duodenum and jejunum

Right Inguinal
Cecum
Appendix
Lower end of ileum
Right ureter
Right spermatic cord
Right ovary

Epigastric
Aorta
Pyloric end of stomach
Part of duodenum
Pancreas
Part of liver

Umbilical
Omentum
Mesentery
Lower part of duodenum
Part of jejunum and ileum

Hypogastric (Pubic)
Ileum
Bladder
Uterus

Left Hypochondriac
Stomach
Spleen
Tail of pancreas
Splenic flexure of colon
Upper half of left kidney
Suprarenal gland

Left Lumbar
Descending colon
Lower half of left kidney
Part of jejunum and ileum

Left Inguinal
Sigmoid colon
Left ureter
Left spermatic cord
Left ovary

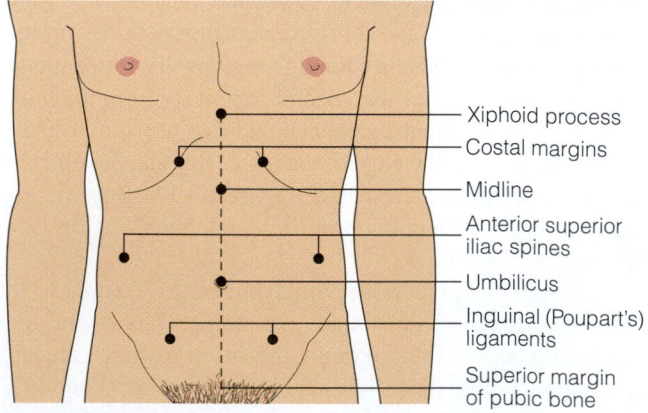

Xiphoid process
Costal margins
Midline
Anterior superior iliac spines
Umbilicus
Inguinal (Poupart's) ligaments
Superior margin of pubic bone

Figure 17–18 ⚬ Landmarks commonly used to identify abdominal areas.

percussion, and/or palpation. Auscultation is done before palpation and percussion because palpation and percussion cause movement or stimulation of the bowel, which can increase bowel motility and thus heighten bowel sounds, creating false results. Skill 17–14 describes how to assess the abdomen.

ASSESSING THE ABDOMEN

PLANNING
- Ask the client to urinate since an empty bladder makes the assessment more comfortable.
- Ensure that the room is warm since the client will be exposed.

Delegation
Assessment of the abdomen is not delegated to UAP. However, signs and symptoms of problems may be observed during usual care and should be recorded by those persons. Atypical findings must be validated and interpreted by the nurse.

EQUIPMENT
- Examining light
- Tape measure (metal or unstretchable cloth)
- Water-soluble skin-marking pencil
- Stethoscope

IMPLEMENTATION
Performance
1. Prior to performing the procedure, introduce self and verify the client's identity using agency protocol. Explain to the client what you are going to do, why it is necessary, and how he or she can cooperate. Discuss how the results will be used in planning further care or treatments.
2. Perform hand hygiene and observe appropriate infection control procedures.
3. Provide for client privacy.

4. Inquire if the client has any history of the following: incidence of abdominal pain; associated symptoms; change in appetite, food intolerances, and foods ingested in last 24 hours; specific signs and symptoms; previous problems and treatment.
5. Assist the client to a supine position, with the arms placed comfortably at the sides. Place small pillows beneath the knees and the head to reduce tension in the abdominal muscles. Expose the client's abdomen only from the chest line to the pubic area to avoid chilling and shivering, which can tense the abdominal muscles.

ASSESSMENT	TYPICAL FINDINGS	ATYPICAL FINDINGS
Inspection of the Abdomen		
6. Inspect the abdomen for skin integrity.	Unblemished skin Uniform color Silver-white striae (stretch marks) or surgical scars	Presence of rash or other lesions Tense, glistening skin (may indicate ascites, edema) Purple striae (associated with Cushing's disease or rapid weight gain and loss)
7. Inspect the abdomen for contour and symmetry:		
• Observe the abdominal contour while standing at the client's side when the client is supine.	Flat, rounded (convex), or scaphoid (concave)	Distended
• Ask the client to take a deep breath and to hold it. **Rationale:** *This makes an enlarged liver or spleen more obvious.*	No evidence of enlargement of liver or spleen	Evidence of enlargement of liver or spleen
• Assess the symmetry of contour while standing at the foot of the bed.	Symmetric contour	Asymmetric contour, e.g., localized protrusions around umbilicus, inguinal ligaments, or scars (possible hernia or tumor)

(continued)

ASSESSING THE ABDOMEN *(continued)*

ASSESSMENT	TYPICAL FINDINGS	ATYPICAL FINDINGS
• If distention is present, measure the abdominal girth by placing a tape around the abdomen at the level of the umbilicus. ❶		

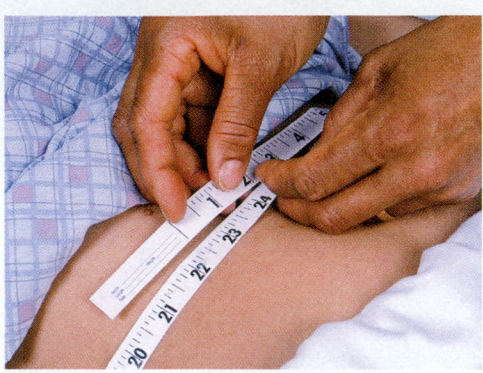

❶ Measuring abdominal girth.

ASSESSMENT	TYPICAL FINDINGS	ATYPICAL FINDINGS
8. Observe abdominal movements associated with respiration, peristalsis, or aortic pulsations.	Symmetric movements caused by respiration Visible peristalsis in very lean people Aortic pulsations in thin persons at epigastric area	Limited movement due to pain or disease process Visible peristalsis in non-lean clients (possible bowel obstruction) Marked aortic pulsations
9. Observe the vascular pattern.	No visible vascular pattern	Visible venous pattern (dilated veins) is associated with liver disease, ascites, and venocaval obstruction
Auscultation of the Abdomen		
10. Auscultate the abdomen for bowel sounds, vascular sounds, and peritoneal friction rubs. Warm the hands and the stethoscope diaphragms. **Rationale:** *Cold hands and a cold stethoscope may cause the client to contract the abdominal muscles, and these contractions may be heard during auscultation.*	Audible bowel sounds Absence of arterial bruits Absence of friction rub	Hypoactive, i.e., extremely soft and infrequent (e.g., one per minute). Hypoactive sounds indicate decreased motility and are usually associated with manipulation of the bowel during surgery, inflammation, paralytic ileus, or late bowel obstruction. Hyperactive/increased, i.e., high-pitched, loud, rushing sounds that occur frequently (e.g., every 3 seconds) also known as borborygmi.
For Bowel Sounds		
• Use the flat-disc diaphragm. **Rationale:** *Intestinal sounds are relatively high pitched and best accentuated by the diaphragm.* Light pressure with the stethoscope is adequate.		Hyperactive sounds indicate increased intestinal motility and are usually associated with diarrhea, an early bowel obstruction, or the use of laxatives. True absence of sounds (none heard in 3 to 5 minutes) indicates a cessation of intestinal motility.

ASSESSMENT	TYPICAL FINDINGS	ATYPICAL FINDINGS

- Ask when the client last ate. **Rationale:** *Shortly after or long after eating, bowel sounds may typically increase. They are loudest when a meal is long overdue. Four to 7 hours after a meal, bowel sounds may be heard continuously over the ileocecal valve area while the digestive contents from the small intestine empty through the valve into the large intestine.*

- Place diaphragm of the stethoscope in each of the four quadrants of the abdomen over all of the auscultatory sites shown in ❷.

- Listen for active bowel sounds—irregular gurgling noises occurring about every 5 to 20 seconds. The duration of a single sound may range from less than a second to more than several seconds.

For Vascular Sounds

- Use the bell of the stethoscope over the aorta, renal arteries, iliac arteries, and femoral arteries. ❸
- Listen for bruits.

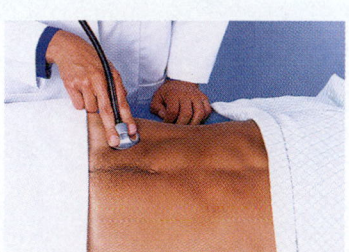

❷ Auscultating the abdomen for bowel sounds.

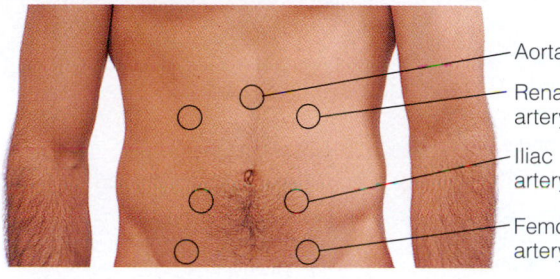

Aorta
Renal artery
Iliac artery
Femoral artery

❸ Sites for auscultating the abdomen.

Percussion of the Abdomen

11. Percuss several areas in each of the four quadrants to determine presence of tympany (gas in stomach and intestines) and dullness (decrease, absence, or flatness of resonance over solid masses or fluid). Use a systematic pattern: Begin in the lower right quadrant, proceed to the upper right quadrant, the upper left quadrant, and the lower left quadrant. ❹

Tympany over the stomach and gas-filled bowels; dullness, especially over the liver and spleen, or a full bladder

Large dull areas (associated with presence of fluid or a tumor)

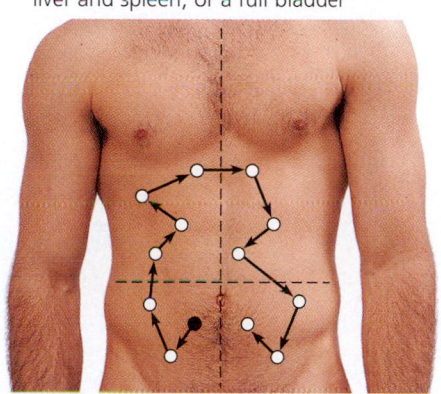

❹ Systematic percussion sites for all four quadrants.

Palpation of the Abdomen

12. Perform light palpation first to detect areas of tenderness and/or muscle guarding. Systematically explore all four quadrants. Ensure that the client's position is appropriate for relaxation of the abdominal muscles, and warm the hands. **Rationale:** *Cold hands can elicit muscle tension and thus impede palpatory evaluation.*

No tenderness; relaxed abdomen with smooth, consistent tension

Tenderness and hypersensitivity
Superficial masses
Localized areas of increased tension

(continued)

SKILL 17–14

ASSESSING THE ABDOMEN *(continued)*

| ASSESSMENT | TYPICAL FINDINGS | ATYPICAL FINDINGS |

Light Palpation

- Hold the palm of your hand slightly above the client's abdomen, with your fingers parallel to the abdomen.
- Depress the abdominal wall lightly, about 1 cm or to the depth of the subcutaneous tissue, with the pads of your fingers. ❺
- Move the finger pads in a slight circular motion.
- Note areas of tenderness or superficial pain, masses, and muscle guarding. To determine areas of tenderness, ask the client to tell you about them and watch for changes in the client's facial expressions.
- If the client is excessively ticklish, begin by pressing your hand on top of the client's hand while pressing lightly. Then slide your hand off the client's and onto the abdomen to continue the examination.

13. Perform deep palpation over all four quadrants.
    - Palpate sensitive areas last.
    - Press the distal half of the palmar surface of the fingers of one hand into the abdominal wall.

    or

    Use the bimanual method of palpation discussed earlier in this chapter.

- Depress the abdominal wall about 4 to 5 cm (1 1/2 to 2 in.). ❻
- Note masses and the structure of underlying contents. If a mass is present, determine its size, location, mobility, contour, consistency, and tenderness. Normal abdominal structures that may be mistaken for masses include the lateral borders of the rectus abdominis muscles, the feces-filled colon, the aorta, and the uterus.
- Check for rebound tenderness in areas where the client complains of pain. With one hand, press slowly and deeply over the area indicated and then lift the hand quickly. If the client does not complain of pain during the deep pressure but indicates pain at the release of the pressure, rebound tenderness is present. This can indicate peritoneal inflammation and should be reported to the primary care provider immediately.

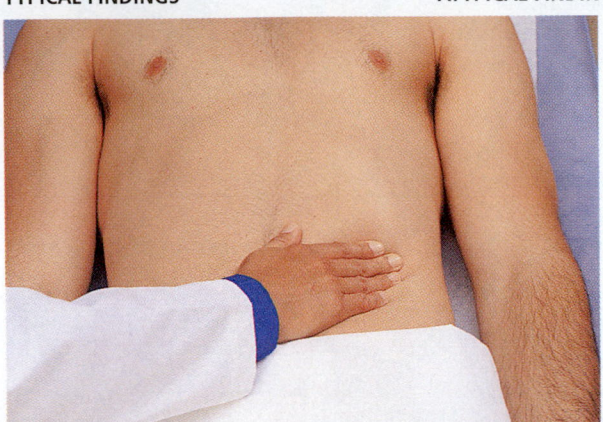

❺ Light palpation of the abdomen.

Tenderness may be present near xiphoid process, over cecum, and over sigmoid colon

Generalized or localized areas of tenderness
Mobile or fixed masses

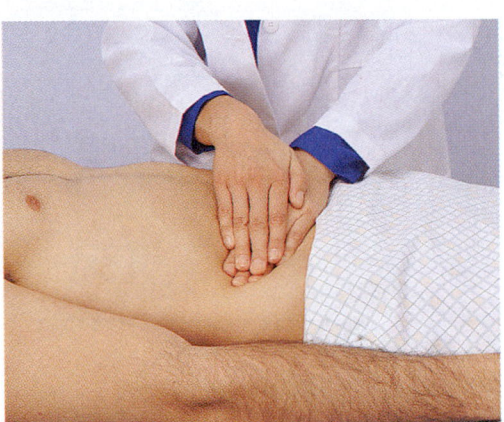

❻ Deep palpation of the abdomen.

ASSESSMENT	TYPICAL FINDINGS	ATYPICAL FINDINGS
Palpation of the Bladder		
14. Palpate the area above the pubic symphysis if the client's history indicates possible urinary retention. **7**	Not palpable	Distended and palpable as smooth, round, tense mass (indicates urinary retention)

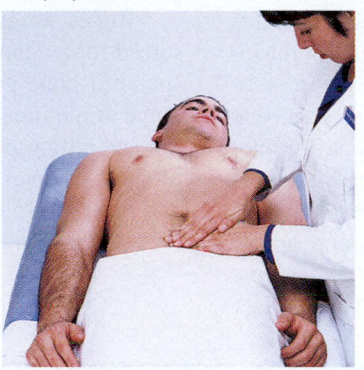

7 Palpating the bladder.

15. Document findings in the client record using forms or checklists supplemented by narrative notes when appropriate.

SAMPLE DOCUMENTATION

1/21/10 0945 c/o "gassy" pain LRQ. No BM x 48 hrs. Ate 75% regular diet yesterday. Abd flat. Active bowels sounds all 4 quadrants. Tympany above umbilicus, dull below. Liver 7 cm @ MCL. No masses palpated. 30 mL MOM given.————————N. Schmidt, RN

EVALUATION

- Perform a detailed follow-up examination of other systems based on findings that deviated from expected or normal for the client. Relate findings to previous assessment data if available.
- Report significant deviations to the primary care provider.

LIFESPAN CONSIDERATIONS   Assessing the Abdomen

Infants

- Internal organs of newborns and infants are proportionately larger than those of older children and adults, so their abdomens are rounded and tend to protrude.
- The infant's liver may be palpable 1 to 2 cm below the right costal margin.
- Umbilical hernias may be present at birth.

Children

- Toddlers have a characteristic "pot belly" appearance, which can persist until age 3 to 4 years.
- Late preschool and school-age children are leaner and have a flat abdomen.
- Peristaltic waves may be more visible than in adults.
- Children may not be able to pinpoint areas of tenderness; by observing facial expressions the examiner can determine areas of maximum tenderness.
- The liver is relatively larger than in adults. It can be palpated 1 to 2 cm below the right costal margin.
- If the child is ticklish, guarding, or fearful, use a task that requires concentration (such as squeezing the hands together) to distract the child, or have the child place his or her hands on yours as you palpate the abdomen, "helping" you to do the exam.

Older Adults

- The rounded abdomens of older adults are due to an increase in adipose tissue and a decrease in muscle tone.
- The abdominal wall is slacker and thinner, making palpation easier and more accurate than in younger clients. Muscle wasting and loss of fibroconnective tissue occur.

- The pain threshold in older adults is often higher; major abdominal problems such as appendicitis or other acute emergencies may therefore go undetected.
- Gastrointestinal pain needs to be differentiated from cardiac pain. Gastrointestinal pain may be located in the chest or abdomen, whereas cardiac pain is usually located in the chest. Factors aggravating gastrointestinal pain are usually related to either ingestion or lack of food intake; gastrointestinal pain is usually relieved by antacids, food, or assuming an upright position. Common factors that can aggravate cardiac pain are activity or anxiety; rest or nitroglycerin relieves cardiac pain.
- Stool passes through the intestines at a slower rate in older adults, and the perception of stimuli that produce the urge to defecate often diminishes.
- Fecal incontinence may occur in confused or neurologically impaired older adults.
- Many older adults erroneously believe that the absence of a daily bowel movement signifies constipation. When assessing for constipation, the nurse must consider the client's diet, activity, medications, and characteristics and ease of passage of feces as well as the frequency of bowel movements.
- The incidence of colon cancer is higher among older adults than younger adults. Symptoms include a change in bowel function, rectal bleeding, and weight loss. Changes in bowel function, however, are associated with many factors, such as diet, exercise, and medications.
- Decreased absorption of oral medications often occurs with aging.
- In the liver, impaired metabolism of some drugs may occur with aging.

THE MUSCULOSKELETAL SYSTEM

The musculoskeletal system encompasses the muscles, bones, and joints. The completeness of an assessment of this system depends largely on the needs and problems of the individual client. The nurse usually assesses the musculoskeletal system for muscle strength, tone, size, and symmetry of muscle development, and for tremors. A tremor is an involuntary trembling of a limb or body part. Tremors may involve large groups of muscle fibers or small bundles of muscle fibers. An intention tremor becomes more apparent when an individual attempts a voluntary movement, such as holding a cup of coffee. A resting tremor is more apparent when the client is at rest and diminishes with activity.

Bones are assessed for acceptable form. Joints are assessed for tenderness, swelling, thickening, crepitation (the sound of bone grating on bone), presence of nodules, and range of motion. Body posture is assessed for typical standing and sitting positions. For information about body posture, see Chapter 31 ∞ .

Skill 17–15 describes how to assess the musculoskeletal system.

SKILL 17–15

ASSESSING THE MUSCULOSKELETAL SYSTEM

PLANNING

Delegation
Assessment of the musculoskeletal system is not delegated to UAP. However, many aspects of its functioning are observed during usual care and may be recorded by persons other than the nurse. Atypical findings must be validated and interpreted by the nurse.

EQUIPMENT
• **Goniometer**

IMPLEMENTATION

Performance

1. Prior to performing the procedure, introduce self and verify the client's identity using agency protocol. Explain to the client what you are going to do, why it is necessary, and how he or she can cooperate. Discuss how the results will be used in planning further care or treatments.
2. Perform hand hygiene and observe appropriate infection control procedures.
3. Provide for client privacy.
4. Inquire if the client has any history of the following: presence of muscle pain: onset, location, character, associated phenomena (e.g., redness and swelling of joints), and aggravating and alleviating factors; limitations to movement or inability to perform activities of daily living; previous sports injuries; loss of function without pain.

ASSESSMENT	TYPICAL FINDINGS	ATYPICAL FINDINGS
Muscles		
5. Inspect the muscles for size. Compare the muscles on one side of the body to the same muscle on the other side. Measure discrepancies.	Equal size on both sides of body	Atrophy (a decrease in size) or hypertrophy (an increase in size), asymmetry
6. Inspect the muscles and tendons for contractures.	No contractures	Malposition of body part
7. Inspect the muscles for tremors.	No tremors	Presence of tremor
8. Palpate muscles at rest to determine muscle tonicity.	Normally firm	Atonic (lacking tone)
9. Palpate muscles while the client is active and passive for flaccidity, spasticity, and smoothness of movement.	Smooth coordinated movements	Flaccidity (weakness or laxness) or spasticity (sudden involuntary muscle contraction)
10. Test muscle strength. Compare the right side with the left side.	Equal strength on each body side	25% or less of typical strength
Bones		
11. Inspect the skeleton for structure.	No deformities	Bones misaligned
12. Palpate the bones to locate any areas of edema or tenderness.	No tenderness or swelling	Presence of tenderness or swelling (may indicate fracture, neoplasms, or osteoporosis)

ASSESSMENT	TYPICAL FINDINGS	ATYPICAL FINDINGS
Joints		
13. Inspect the joint for swelling. Palpate each joint for tenderness, smoothness of movement, swelling, crepitation, and presence of nodules.	No swelling No tenderness, swelling, crepitation, or nodules Joints move smoothly	One or more swollen joints Presence of tenderness, swelling, crepitation, or nodules
14. Assess joint range of motion. See Chapter 31 ∞ for the types of joint movements.	Varies to some degree in accordance with person's genetic makeup and degree of physical activity	Limited range of motion in one or more joints
15. Document findings in the client record using forms or checklists supplemented by narrative notes when appropriate.		

EVALUATION

- Perform a detailed follow-up examination of other systems based on findings that deviated from expected or normal for the client. Relate findings to previous assessment data if available.
- Report significant deviations to the primary care provider.

LIFESPAN CONSIDERATIONS   Assessing the Musculoskeletal System

Infants

- Palpate the clavicles of newborns. A mass and crepitus may indicate a fracture experienced during vaginal delivery. The newborn may also have limited movement of the arm and shoulder on the affected side.
- When the arms and legs of newborns are pulled to extension and released, newborns naturally return to the flexed fetal position.
- Check muscle strength by holding the infant lightly under the arms with feet placed lightly on a table. Infants should not fall through the hands and should be able to bear body weight on their legs if typical muscle strength is present.
- Check infants for developmental dysplasia of the hip (congenital dislocation) by examining for asymmetric gluteal folds, asymmetric abduction of the legs (Ortolani and Barlow tests), or apparent shortening of the femur.
- Infants should be able to sit without support by 8 months of age, crawl by 7 to 10 months, and walk by 12 to 15 months.
- Observe for symmetry of muscle mass, strength, and function.

Children

- Pronation and "toeing in" of the feet is common in children between 12 and 30 months of age.
- Genu varum (bowleg) is anticipated in children for about 1 year after beginning to walk.
- Genu valgus (knock-knee) is anticipated in preschool and early school-age children.
- Lordosis (swayback) is common in children before age 5.

- Observe the child in normal activities to determine motor function.
- During the rapid growth spurts of adolescence, spinal curvature and rotation (scoliosis) may appear. Children should be assessed for scoliosis by age 12 and annually until their growth slows. Curvature greater than 10% should be referred for further medical evaluation.
- Muscle mass increases in adolescence, especially as children engage in strenuous physical activity, and requires increased nutritional intake.
- Children are at risk for injury related to physical activity and should be assessed for nutritional status, physical conditioning, and safety precautions in order to prevent injury.
- Adolescent girls who participate in strenuous athletic activities are at risk for delayed menses, osteoporosis, and eating disorders; assessment should include a history of these factors.

Older Adults

- Muscle mass decreases progressively with age, but there are wide variations among different individuals.
- The decrease in speed, strength, resistance to fatigue, reaction time, and coordination in the older person is due to a decrease in nerve conduction and muscle tone.
- The bones become more fragile and osteoporosis leads to a loss of total bone mass. As a result, older adults are predisposed to fractures and compressed vertebrae.
- In most older adults, osteoarthritic changes in the joints can be observed.
- Note any surgical scars from joint replacement surgeries.

THE FEMALE GENITALS AND INGUINAL AREA

The examination of the genitals and reproductive tract of women includes assessment of the inguinal lymph nodes and inspection and palpation of the external genitals. Completeness of the assessment of the genitals and reproductive tract depends on the needs and problems of the individual client. In most practice settings, generalist nurses perform only inspection of the external genitals and palpation of the inguinal lymph nodes.

For sexually active adolescent and adult women, a Papanicolaou test (Pap test) is used to detect cancer of the cervix. If there is an increased or abnormal vaginal discharge, specimens should be taken to check for sexually transmitted disease.

Examination of the genitals usually creates uncertainty and apprehension in women, and the lithotomy position required can cause embarrassment. The nurse must explain each part of the examination in advance and perform the examination in an objective, supportive, and efficient manner. Not all agencies permit male practitioners to examine the female genitals. Some agencies may require the presence of another woman during the examination so that there is no question of unprofessional behavior. Most female clients accept examination by a male, especially if he is emotionally comfortable about performing it and does so in a matter-of-fact and competent manner. If the male nurse does not feel comfortable about this part of the examination or if the client is reluctant to be examined by a man, the nurse should refer this part of the examination to a female practitioner.

Skill 17–16 describes how to assess the female genitals and inguinal area.

SKILL 17–16

ASSESSING THE FEMALE GENITALS AND INGUINAL AREA

PLANNING

Delegation

Due to the substantial knowledge and skill required, assessment of the female genitals and inguinal lymph nodes is not delegated to UAP. However, persons other than the nurse may record any aspect that is observed during usual care. Atypical findings must be validated and interpreted by the nurse.

EQUIPMENT

- Clean gloves
- Drape
- Supplemental lighting, if needed

IMPLEMENTATION

Performance

1. Prior to performing the procedure, introduce self and verify the client's identity using agency protocol. Explain to the client what you are going to do, why it is necessary, and how she can cooperate. Discuss how the results will be used in planning further care or treatments.
2. Perform hand hygiene, apply gloves, and observe appropriate infection control procedures.
3. Provide for client privacy. Request the presence of another woman if desired, required by agency policy, or requested by the client.
4. Inquire regarding the following: age of onset of menstruation, last menstrual period (LMP), regularity of cycle, duration, amount of daily flow, and whether menstruation is painful; incidence of pain during intercourse; vaginal discharge; number of pregnancies, number of live births, labor or delivery complications; urgency and frequency of urination at night; blood in urine, painful urination, incontinence; history of sexually transmitted disease, past and present.
5. Cover the pelvic area with a sheet or drape at all times when not actually being examined. Position the client supine with feet elevated on the stirrups of an examination table. Alternatively, assist the client into the dorsal recumbent position with knees flexed and thighs externally rotated.

ASSESSMENT	TYPICAL FINDINGS	ATYPICAL FINDINGS
6. Inspect the distribution, amount, and characteristics of pubic hair.	There are wide variations; generally kinky in the menstruating adult, thinner and straighter after menopause Distributed in the shape of an inverse triangle	Scant pubic hair (may indicate hormonal problem) Hair growth should not extend over the abdomen
7. Inspect the skin of the pubic area for parasites, inflammation, swelling, and lesions. To assess pubic skin adequately, separate the labia majora and labia minora.	Pubic skin intact, no lesions Skin of vulva area slightly darker than the rest of the body Labia round, full, and relatively symmetric in adult females	Lice, lesions, scars, fissures, swelling, erythema, excoriations, varicosities, or leukoplakia

ASSESSMENT	TYPICAL FINDINGS	ATYPICAL FINDINGS
8. Inspect the clitoris, urethral orifice, and vaginal orifice when separating the labia minora.	Clitoris does not exceed 1 cm in width and 2 cm in length Urethral orifice appears as a small slit and is the same color as surrounding tissues No inflammation, swelling, or discharge	Presence of lesions Presence of inflammation, swelling, or discharge
9. Palpate the inguinal lymph nodes. ❶ Use the pads of the fingers in a rotary motion, noting any enlargement or tenderness.	No enlargement or tenderness	Enlargement and tenderness

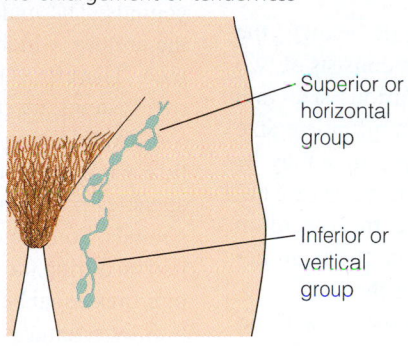

— Superior or horizontal group

— Inferior or vertical group

❶ Lymph nodes of the groin area.

10. Document findings in the client record using forms or checklists supplemented by narrative notes when appropriate.

EVALUATION

- Perform a detailed follow-up examination based on findings that deviated from expected or normal for the client. Relate findings to previous assessment data if available.

- Significant deviations indicate the need for an internal vaginal examination.

LIFESPAN CONSIDERATIONS   Assessing the Female Genitals and Inguinal Lymph Nodes

Infants

- Infants can be held in a supine position on the parent's lap with the knees supported in a flexed position and separated.
- In newborns, because of maternal estrogen, the labia and clitoris may be edematous and enlarged, and there may be a small amount of white or bloody vaginal discharge.
- Assess the mons and inguinal area for swelling or tenderness that may indicate presence of an inguinal hernia.

Children

- Ensure that you have the parent or guardian's approval to perform the examination and then tell the child what you are going to do. Preschool children are taught not to allow others to touch their "private parts."
- Assessment of adolescent girls is limited to inspection of the external genitals, unless the girl is sexually active. The exam should be conducted with the parent out of the room.
- Girls should be assessed for Tanner staging of pubertal development.
- Girls should have a Papanicolaou (Pap) test done if sexually active, or by age 18 years.
- Sexually active girls with abnormal vaginal discharge should be tested for sexually transmitted disease.

- The clitoris is a common site for syphilitic chancres in younger females.

Older Adults

- Labia are atrophied and flatter in older females.
- The clitoris is a potential site for cancerous lesions in older females.
- The vulva atrophies as a result of a reduction in vascularity, elasticity, adipose tissue, and estrogen levels. Because the vulva is more fragile, it is more easily irritated.
- The vaginal environment becomes drier and more alkaline, resulting in an alteration of the type of flora present and a predisposition to vaginitis. Dyspareunia (difficult or painful intercourse) is also a common occurrence.
- The cervix and uterus decrease in size.
- The fallopian tubes and ovaries atrophy.
- Ovulation and estrogen production cease.
- Vaginal bleeding unrelated to estrogen therapy is abnormal in older women.
- Prolapse of the uterus can occur in older females, especially those who have had multiple pregnancies.
- Older females may be arthritic and find the examination position uncomfortable.

In many agencies only nurse practitioners examine the internal genitals. However, generalist nurses often assist with this examination and need to be familiar with the procedure. Examination of the internal genitals involves (a) palpating Skene's and Bartholin's glands, (b) assessing the pelvic musculature, (c) inserting a vaginal speculum to inspect the cervix and vagina, and (d) obtaining a Papanicolaou smear.

The speculum examination of the vagina involves the insertion of a plastic or metal speculum that consists of two blades and an adjustable thumb screw. Various sizes are available (small, medium, and large); the appropriate size needs to be selected for each client. The speculum may be lubricated with water-soluble lubricant if specimens are not being collected. Most examiners lubricate the speculum with warm water. After visualizing the cervix, the examiner takes smear specimens from one or more of the sites.

The nurse's responsibilities when assisting with an examination of the internal female genitals include the following:

1. *Assembling equipment.* These include drapes, gloves, vaginal speculum, warm water or lubricant, and supplies for cytology and culture studies.
2. *Preparing the client.* Advise the client not to douche prior to the procedure. Explain the procedure. It should take only 5 minutes and is typically not painful. Assist the client to a lithotomy position as needed, and drape her appropriately.
3. *Supporting the client during the procedure.* This involves explaining the procedure as needed, and encouraging the client to take deep breaths that will help the pelvic muscles relax.
4. *Monitoring and assisting the client after the procedure.* Assist the client from the lithotomy position and with perineal care as needed.
5. *Documenting the procedure.* Include the date and time it was performed, the name of the examiner, and any nursing assessments and interventions.

THE MALE GENITALS AND INGUINAL AREA

In adult men, a complete examination includes assessment of the external genitals, the presence of any hernias, and the prostate gland. Nurses in some practice settings performing routine assessment of clients may assess only the external genitals. The male reproductive and urinary systems share the urethra, which is the passageway for both urine and semen. Therefore, in physical assessment of the male these two systems are frequently assessed together.

Examination of the male genitals by a female practitioner is becoming increasingly common, although not all agencies permit a female practitioner to examine the male genitals. Some agencies may require the presence of another person during the examination so that there is no question of unprofessional behavior. Most male clients accept examination by a female, especially if she is emotionally comfortable about performing it and does so in a matter-of-fact and competent manner. If the female nurse does not feel comfortable about this part of the examination or if the client is reluctant to be examined by a woman, the nurse should refer this part of the examination to a male practitioner. Development of secondary sex characteristics is assessed in relationship to the client's age.

All male clients should be screened for the presence of inguinal or femoral hernias. A hernia is a protrusion of the intestine through the inguinal wall or canal. Cancer of the prostate gland is the most common cancer in adult men and occurs primarily in men over age 50. Examination of the prostate gland is performed with the examination of the rectum and anus (see Skill 17–18).

Testicular cancer is much rarer than prostate cancer and occurs primarily in young men ages 15 to 35. Testicular cancer is most commonly found on the anterior and lateral surfaces of the testes. Testicular self-examination should be conducted monthly (see Chapter 28 ∞).

The techniques of inspection and palpation are used to examine the male genitals. Skill 17–17 describes how the nurse can conduct an assessment of the male genitals and inguinal area.

SKILL 17–17

ASSESSING THE MALE GENITALS AND INGUINAL AREA

PLANNING

Delegation
Due to the substantial knowledge and skill required, assessment of the male genitals and inguinal area is not delegated to UAP. However, persons other than the nurse may record any aspect that is observed during usual care. Atypical findings must be validated and interpreted by the nurse.

EQUIPMENT
• Clean gloves

IMPLEMENTATION

Performance

1. Prior to performing the procedure, introduce self and verify the client's identity using agency protocol. Explain to the client what you are going to do, why it is necessary, and how he can cooperate. Discuss how the results will be used in planning further care or treatments.
2. Perform hand hygiene, apply gloves, and observe appropriate infection control procedures.
3. Provide for client privacy. Request the presence of another person if desired, required by agency policy, or requested by the client.

4. Inquire if the client has any history of the following: usual voiding patterns and changes, bladder control, urinary incontinence, frequency, urgency, abdominal pain; symptoms of sexually transmitted infection; swellings that could indicate presence of hernia; family history of nephritis, malignancy of the prostate, or malignancy of the kidney.
5. Cover the pelvic area with a sheet or drape at all times when not actually being examined.

ASSESSMENT	TYPICAL FINDINGS	ATYPICAL FINDINGS
Pubic Hair		
6. Inspect the distribution, amount, and characteristics of pubic hair.	Triangular distribution, often spreading up the abdomen	Scant amount or absence of hair
Penis		
7. Inspect the penile shaft and glans penis for lesions, nodules, swellings, and inflammation.	Penile skin intact Appears slightly wrinkled and varies in color as widely as other body skin Foreskin easily retractable from the glans penis Small amount of thick white smegma between the glans and foreskin	Presence of lesions, nodules, swellings, or inflammation
8. Inspect the urethral meatus for swelling, inflammation, and discharge. • Compress or ask the client to compress the glans slightly to open the urethral meatus to inspect it for discharge.	Pink and slitlike appearance Positioned at the tip of the penis	Inflammation; discharge Variation in meatal locations (e.g., hypospadias, on the underside of the penile shaft, and epispadias, on the upper side of the penile shaft)
9. Palpate the penis for tenderness, thickening, and nodules. Use your thumb and first two fingers.	Smooth and semifirm Is slightly movable over the underlying structures	Presence of tenderness, thickening, or nodules Immobility
Scrotum		
10. Inspect the scrotum for appearance, general size, and symmetry. • To facilitate inspection of the scrotum during a physical examination, ask the client to hold the penis out of the way. • Inspect all skin surfaces by spreading the rugated surface skin and lifting the scrotum as needed to observe posterior surfaces.	Scrotal skin is darker in color than that of the rest of the body and is loose Size varies with temperature changes (the dartos muscles contract when the area is cold and relax when the area is warm) Scrotum appears asymmetric (left testis is usually lower than right testis)	Discolorations; any tightening of skin (may indicate edema or mass) Marked asymmetry in size
11. Palpate the scrotum to assess status of underlying testes, epididymis, and spermatic cord. Palpate both testes simultaneously for comparative purposes.	Testicles are rubbery, smooth, and free of nodules and masses Testis is about 2 × 4 cm (0.7 × 1.5 in.) Epididymis is resilient, normally tender, and softer than the spermatic cord Spermatic cord is firm	Testicles are enlarged, with uneven surface (possible tumor) Epididymis is nonresilient and painful
Inguinal Area		
12. Inspect both inguinal areas for bulges while the client is standing, if possible.	No swelling or bulges	Swelling or bulge (possible inguinal or femoral hernia)
13. Document findings in the client record using forms or checklists supplemented by narrative notes when appropriate.		

EVALUATION

- Perform a detailed follow-up examination based on findings that deviated from expected or normal for the client. Relate findings to previous assessment data if available.
- Report significant deviations to the primary care provider.

LIFESPAN CONSIDERATIONS   Assessing the Male Genitals and Inguinal Area

Infants

- The foreskin of the uncircumcised infant is normally tight at birth and should not be retracted. It will gradually loosen as the baby grows and is usually fully retractable by 2 to 3 years of age. Assess for cleanliness, redness, or irritation.
- Assess for placement of the urethral meatus.
- Palpate the scrotum to determine if the testes are descended; in the newborn and infant, the testes may retract into the inguinal canal, especially with stimulation of the cremasteric reflex.
- Assess the inguinal area for swelling or tenderness that may indicate presence of an inguinal hernia.

Children

- Ensure that you have the parent or guardian's approval to perform the examination and then tell the child what you are going to do. Preschool children are taught to not allow others to touch their "private parts."

- In young boys, the cremasteric reflex can cause the testes to ascend into the inguinal canal. If possible have the boy sit cross-legged, which stretches the muscle and decreases the reflex.

Older Adults

- The penis decreases in size with age; the size and firmness of the testes decrease.
- Testosterone is produced in smaller amounts.
- More time and direct physical stimulation are required for an older man to achieve an erection, but he can maintain the erection for a longer period before ejaculation than he could at a younger age.
- Seminal fluid is reduced in amount and viscosity.
- Urinary frequency, nocturia, dribbling, and problems with beginning and ending the stream are usually the result of prostatic enlargement.

THE RECTUM AND ANUS

Rectal examination, an essential part of every comprehensive physical examination, involves inspection and palpation (digital examination). The extent of the assessment of the rectum and anus depends on the rectal problems stated by the client in the nursing history. In many practice settings, the nurse performs only inspection of the anus.

Skill 17–18 describes how to assess the rectum and anus.

SKILL 17–18

ASSESSING THE RECTUM AND ANUS

PLANNING

Delegation
Assessment of the rectum and anus is not delegated to UAP. However, many aspects are observed during usual care and may be recorded by persons other than the nurse. Atypical findings must be validated and interpreted by the nurse.

EQUIPMENT
- Clean gloves
- Water-soluble lubricant

IMPLEMENTATION

Performance

1. Prior to performing the procedure, introduce self and verify the client's identity using agency protocol. Explain to the client what you are going to do, why it is necessary, and how he or she can cooperate. Discuss how the results will be used in planning further care or treatments. Because digital examination can cause apprehension and embarrassment in the client, it is important that the nurse help the client relax by encouraging the client to take slow, deep breaths and inform the client about potential sensations such as feelings of defecation or passing gas.
2. Perform hand hygiene, apply gloves, and observe appropriate infection control procedures for all rectal examinations.
3. Provide for client privacy. Drape the client appropriately to prevent undue exposure of body parts.

4. Inquire if the client has any history of the following: bright blood in stools, tarry black stools, diarrhea, constipation, abdominal pain, excessive gas, hemorrhoids, or rectal pain; family history of colorectal cancer; when last stool specimen for occult blood was performed and the results; and for males, if not obtained during the genitourinary examination, signs or symptoms of prostate enlargement.
5. Position the client. In adults, a left lateral or Sims' position with the upper leg acutely flexed is required for the examination. For females, a dorsal recumbent position with hips externally rotated and knees flexed or a lithotomy position may be used. ❶ For males, a standing position while the client bends over the examining table may also be used. This position is commonly used to examine the prostate gland.

Position		**Description**
Sims'	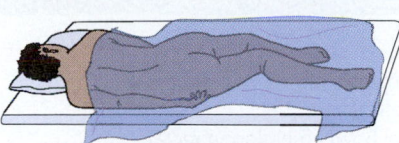	Side-lying position with lowermost arm behind the body, uppermost leg flexed at hip and knee, upper arm flexed at shoulder and elbow.
Lithotomy	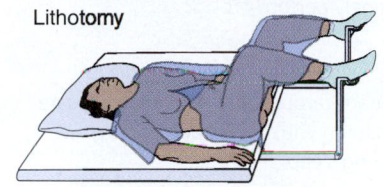	Back-lying position with feet supported in stirrups; the hips should be in line with the edge of the table.
Dorsal recumbent	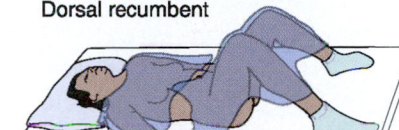	Back-lying position with knees flexed and hips externally rotated; small pillow under the head; soles of feet on the surface.

❶ Left Sims' lithotomy, and dorsal recumbent positions.

ASSESSMENT	**TYPICAL FINDINGS**	**ATYPICAL FINDINGS**
6. Inspect the anus and surrounding tissue for color, integrity, and skin lesions. Then, ask the client to bear down as though defecating. Bearing down creates slight pressure on the skin that may accentuate rectal abnormalities.	Intact perianal skin; usually slightly more pigmented than the skin of the buttocks Anal skin is typically more pigmented, coarser, and moister than perianal skin and is usually hairless	Presence of fissures (cracks), ulcers, excoriations, inflammations, abscesses, protruding hemorrhoids (dilated veins seen as reddened protrusions of the skin), lumps or tumors, fistula openings, or rectal prolapse (varying degrees of protrusion of the rectal mucous membrane through the anus)
7. Palpate the rectum for anal sphincter tonicity, nodules, masses, and tenderness.	Anal sphincter has good tone	Hypertonicity of the anal sphincter (may occur in the presence of an anal fissure or other lesion that causes contraction) Hypotonicity of anal sphincter (may occur after rectal surgery or result from a neurologic deficiency)
8. On withdrawing the finger from the rectum and anus, observe it for feces. If ordered, perform a test for occult blood on the stool (see Chapter 20 ∞). **9.** Document findings in the client record using forms or checklists supplemented by narrative notes when appropriate.	Brown color	Presence of mucus, blood, or black tarry stool

EVALUATION

• Perform a detailed follow-up examination based on findings that deviated from expected or normal for the client. Relate findings to previous assessment data if available.

• Report significant deviations to the primary care provider.

LIFESPAN CONSIDERATIONS   Assessing the Rectum and Anus

Infants

• Lightly touching the anus should result in a brief anal contraction ("wink" reflex).
• If the infant has normal bowel function, a rectal examination is not routinely performed.

Children

• Erythema and scratch marks around the anus may indicate a pinworm parasite. Children with this condition may be disturbed by itching during sleep.

• A rectal examination is not routinely performed on children.

Older Adults

• Chronic constipation and straining at stool cause an increase in the frequency of hemorrhoids and rectal prolapse.

CHAPTER HIGHLIGHTS

• The health examination is conducted to assess the function and integrity of the client's body parts.
• The health examination may entail a complete head-to-toe assessment or individual assessment of a body system or body part.
• The health assessment is conducted in a systematic manner that requires the fewest position changes for the client.
• Aspects of the physical assessment procedures should be incorporated in the assessment, intervention, and evaluation phases of the nursing process.
• Data obtained in the physical health examination supplement, confirm, or refute data obtained during the nursing history.
• Nursing history data help the nurse focus on specific aspects of the physical health examination.

• Data obtained in the physical health examination help the nurse establish nursing diagnoses, plan the client's care, and evaluate the outcomes of nursing care.
• Initial assessment findings provide baseline data about the client's functional abilities against which subsequent assessment findings are compared.
• Skills in inspection, palpation, percussion, and auscultation are required for the physical health examination; these skills are used in that order throughout the examination except during abdominal assessment, when auscultation follows inspection and precedes percussion and palpation.
• Knowledge of the anticipated structure and function of body parts and systems is an essential requisite to conducting physical assessment.

THINK ABOUT IT

Refer to the chapter-opening scenario and answer these questions.

1. When examining the client, how will the nurse document the location and types of bruises, lacerations, and abrasions?

2. Other than examining the client's skin for marks, what other aspects of the physical examination will

Mark perform to gather information regarding possible abuse?

3. How should Mark approach the nursing history to gather information about the client?

∞ *See suggested responses to Think About It on MyNursingKit.*

TEST YOUR KNOWLEDGE

1. Which of the following indicates a normal nursing assessment finding on auscultation of the lungs?
   1. Tympany over the right upper lobe
   2. Resonance over the left upper lobe
   3. Hyperresonance over the left lower lobe
   4. Dullness above the left 10th intercostal space

2. The nurse positions the client sitting upright during palpation of which of the following areas?
   1. Abdomen
   2. Genitals
   3. Breast
   4. Head and neck

3. After auscultating the abdomen, the nurse should report which of the following to the primary care provider?
1. Bruit over the aorta
2. Absence of bowel sounds for 60 seconds
3. Continuous bowel sounds over the ileocecal valve after a meal
4. A completely irregular pattern of bowel sounds

4. If unable to locate the client's popliteal pulse during a routine examination, the nurse should perform which of the following next?
1. Check for a pedal pulse.
2. Check for a femoral pulse.
3. Take the client's blood pressure on that thigh.
4. Ask another nurse to try to locate the pulse.

5. Which of the following is an expected finding during the nurse's assessment of the older adult?
1. Facial hair becomes finer and softer.
2. Decreased peripheral, color, and night vision
3. Increased sensitivity to odors
4. Respiratory rate and rhythm are irregular at rest.

6. List five aspects of the skin that the nurse assesses during a routine examination.
1.
2.
3.
4.
5.

7. If the client reports loss of short-term memory, the nurse would assess this using which one of the following?
1. Have the client repeat a series of three numbers, increasing to eight if possible.

2. Have the client describe his or her childhood illnesses.
3. Ask the client to describe how he or she arrived at this location.
4. Ask the client to count backward from 100 subtracting seven each time.

8. Refer back to Figure 17–7. If the client can accurately read only lines 1, 2, 3, and 4, an appropriate nursing diagnosis would be:
1. *Deficient Knowledge.*
2. *Impaired Memory.*
3. *Ineffective Tissue Perfusion.*
4. *Risk for Injury.*

9. In order to palpate lymph nodes, the nurse uses which of the following techniques?
1. Use the flat of all four fingers in a vertical and then side-to-side motion.
2. Use the back of the hand and feel for temperature variation between the right and left sides.
3. Use the pads of two fingers in a circular motion.
4. Compress the nodes between the index fingers of both hands.

10. For a client whose assessment of the musculoskeletal system is normal, the nurse checks which of the following on the medical record? Select all that apply.
1. Atrophied
2. Contractured
3. Crepitation
4. Equal
5. Firm

∞ *See answers to Test Your Knowledge in Appendix A.*

EXPLORE PEARSON **mynursingkit**™

MyNursingKit is your one stop for online chapter review materials and resources. Prepare for success with additional NCLEX®-style practice questions, interactive assignments and activities, web links, animations and videos, and more!

Register your access code from the front of your book at
www.mynursingkit.com.

REFERENCES AND SELECTED BIBLIOGRAPHY

Carter, K. F., Dufour, L. T., & Ballard, C. N. (2003). Wound & skin care. Identifying primary skin lesions. *Nursing, 33*(12), 68–69.

Carter, K. F., Dufour, L. T., & Ballard, C. N. (2004). Wound & skin care. Identifying secondary skin lesions. *Nursing, 34*(1), 68.

D'Amico, D., & Barbarito, C. (2007). *Health and physical assessment in nursing.* Upper Saddle River, NJ: Pearson Education.

Mehta, M. (2003). Assessing the abdomen. *Nursing, 33*(5), 54–55.

Mehta, M. (2003). Assessing respiratory status. *Nursing, 33*(2), 54–56.

Peacock, S. (2004). Systematic health assessment: A case study. *Practice Nursing, 15*(6), 270, 271–274.

Pullen, R. L. (2004). Clinical do's & don'ts. Neurologic assessment for pronator drift. *Nursing, 34*(3), 22.

Pullen, R. L. (2005). Clinical do's & don'ts. Testing the corneal reflex. *Nursing, 35*(11), 68.

Rushing, J. (2005). Clinical do's & don'ts. Assessing for ascites. *Nursing, 35*(2), 68.

Smith, R. A., Cokkinides, V., & Eyre, H. J. (2006). American Cancer Society recommendations for the early detection of cancer, 2006. *CA: A Cancer Journal for Clinicians, 56,* 11–25.

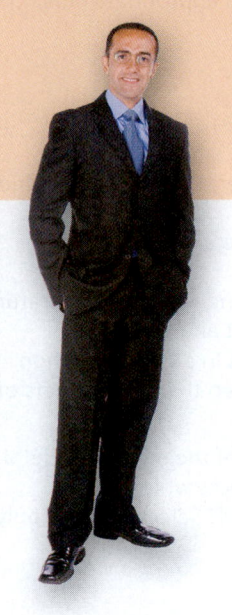

Frank is a 48-year-old Mexican American who is the senior partner in a large accounting practice. He spends a lot of his time sitting at his desk analyzing data and leads a fairly sedentary lifestyle, although he enjoys playing golf on the weekend and occasionally during the week with clients. While out on the course this past weekend he was enjoying a particularly competitive round of golf when he put his all into a swing on the 12th hole and felt a sudden sharp shooting pain in his back that traveled down his left leg. He tried to ignore it and continue the game, but the pain intensified until he could barely move. His friends took him to the local emergency room and called his wife to tell her what had happened. The doctor diagnosed him as having a herniated fourth lumbar vertebra and recommended he visit the pain clinic because his back pain was likely to be a lifelong issue.

LEARNING OUTCOMES

After completing this chapter, you will be able to:

1. Differentiate among pain threshold, pain tolerance, addiction, and dependence.

2. Discriminate between physiological and neuropathic pain categories.

3. List the four factors involved in nociception, and describe how nursing interventions can affect each factor.

4. Explain the gate control theory using the four physiologic processes involved in nociception.

5. List factors affecting the pain experience and nursing considerations for each.

6. Demonstrate a developmentally appropriate pain assessment.

7. Select appropriate nursing diagnoses for clients experiencing pain.

8. Develop a plan of care for clients in different stages of the lifespan who are experiencing pain.

9. Contrast the use of various pain management interventions for clients experiencing pain.

10. Demonstrate appropriate evaluation and documentation of pain management.

KEY TERMS

The widely agreed-upon definition of **pain** is "an unpleasant sensory and emotional experience associated with actual or potential tissue damage, or described in terms of such damage" (American Pain Society [APS], 2003; Gordon, 2009). Three parts of this definition have important implications for nurses. First, pain is a physical *and* emotional experience, not all in the body or all in the mind. Second, it is in response to actual *or* potential tissue damage, so there may not be abnormal lab or radiographic reports despite real pain. Finally, pain is described in terms of such damage. This final component is aligned with McCaffery's often-quoted definition of pain, "Pain is whatever the experiencing person says it is, existing whenever he says it does" (McCaffery & Pasero, 1999, p. 17). Given that some clients are reluctant to disclose the presence of pain unless prompted, nurses will not know of the client's pain until they assess for it. Additionally, it is clear that even nonverbal clients experience pain that demands nursing assessment and treatment even if clients are unable to "describe in terms" the nature of their discomfort.

Severe or persistent pain affects all body systems, causing potentially serious health problems while increasing the risk of complications, delays in healing, and an accelerated progression of fatal illnesses (Arnstein, 2003). Even if the original cause of the pain heals, the changes in the nervous system resulting from suboptimal pain management can result in the development of incurable chronic pain (Arnstein, 1997; Katz, Jackson, Kavanagh, & Sandler, 1996). Persistent pain also contributes to insomnia, weight gain, constipation, hypertension, deconditioning, chronic stress, and depression (Dodd et al., 2001; Monteiro-Cruz & Mattos-Pimenta, 2001; Wilson, Eriksson, D'Eon, Mikail, & Emery, 2002). These effects interfere with work, recreation, domestic activities, and personal care activities to the point that leads many sufferers to question if life is worth living (Hitchcock, Ferrell, & McCaffery, 1994). Effective pain management is an important aspect of nursing care to promote healing, prevent complications, reduce suffering, and prevent the development of incurable pain states.

Pain is more than a symptom of a problem; it is a high-priority problem in itself. Pain presents both physiologic and psychologic dangers to health and recovery. Severe pain is viewed as an emergency situation deserving attention and prompt professional treatment.

THE NATURE OF PAIN

Although pain is a universal experience, the nature of the experience is unique to the individual based, in part, on the type of pain experienced, the psychosocial context or meaning, and the response needed. Adding to the complexity, pain may be a physiological warning system alerting the nurse to a problem or unmet need demanding attention; or it may be a diseased, malfunctioning segment of the nervous system. Advances in the understanding of physiological mechanisms may someday replace the currently used categories of acute pain or chronic pain. In addition to the underlying mechanisms, nurses attuned to a holistic view of care need to consider how these physiological signals affect the mind, body, spirit, and social interactions. In this section, a review is included of the scientific, theoretical, and clinical concepts that form the foundation of knowledge needed by nurses to assess and treat clients with pain in a holistic, comprehensive fashion.

Types of Pain

Pain may be described in terms of location, duration, intensity, and etiology.

LOCATION   Classifications of pain based on where it is in the body may be useful in determining the client's underlying problems or needs; or it may be problematic given that most clients don't fit neatly into one of the categories. Location of pain is, however, a very important component to note. Complicating the categorization of pain by location is the fact that some pains radiate (spread or extend) to other areas. Pain may be **referred** (appear to arise in different areas) to other parts of the body. **Visceral pain** (pain arising from organs or hollow viscera) often presents this way, being perceived in an area remote from the organ causing the pain (Figure 18–1).

DURATION   When pain lasts only through the expected recovery period, it is described as **acute pain,** whether it has a sudden or slow onset and regardless of the intensity.

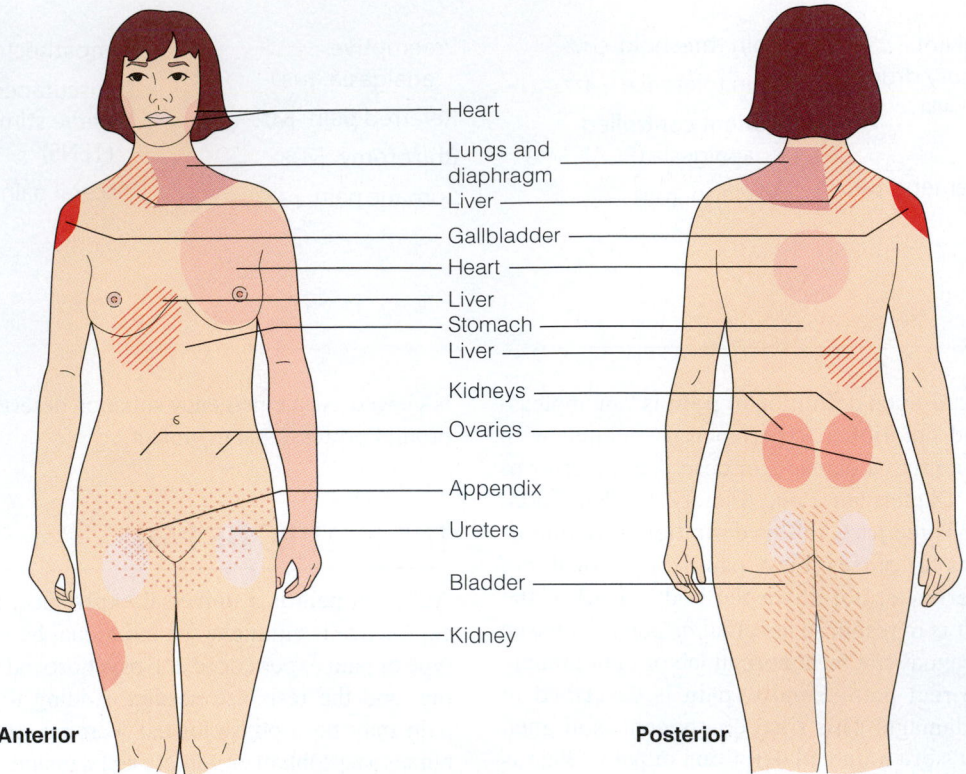

Anterior **Posterior**

Figure 18–1 ○ Common sites of referred pain from various body organs.

Chronic pain, on the other hand, is prolonged, usually recurring or persisting over 6 months or longer, and interferes with functioning. Acute and chronic pain results in different physiologic and behavioral responses, as shown in Table 18–1. Although experts may disagree on whether the cutoff point for chronic pain should be 1, 3, or 6 months

after onset, or expected healing time, NANDA specifies the accepted nursing diagnosis of *Chronic Pain* to be mild to severe, constant or recurring, without an anticipated or predictable end and a duration of greater than 6 months (Ackley & Ladwig, 2008).

The categories differentiating chronic cancer (malignant) pain from chronic nonmalignant pain have also been problematic. **Cancer pain** may result from the direct effects of the disease and its treatment, or it may be unrelated to the disease and its treatment in individuals with cancer. Over the years, other diagnoses have been included in the "malignant pain" category, such as HIV/AIDS or burn pain, which tend to be treated more aggressively than "nonmalignant pain."

INTENSITY To avoid ambiguity, categorizing pain according to intensity (mild, moderate, severe) or the underlying physiology (somatic, visceral, neuropathic) has emerged as a useful way to identify types of pain. Serlin, Mendoza, Nakamura, Edwards, and Cleeland (1995) conducted a large-scale international study that confirmed earlier classifications of pain by intensity using a standard 0 (no pain) to 10 (worst possible pain) scale. Linking the rating to health and functioning scores, pain in the 1–3 range is deemed mild pain, a rating of 4–6 is moderate pain, and pain reaching 7–10 is ranked severe pain and is associated with the worst outcomes.

ETIOLOGY Designating types of pain by etiology can be done under the broad categories of physiological pain and neuropathic pain. Physiological pain is experienced when an intact, properly functioning nervous system sends signals that tissues are damaged, requiring attention and proper care. Once stabi-

TABLE 18–1	Comparison of Acute and Chronic Pain
ACUTE PAIN	**CHRONIC PAIN**
Mild to severe	Mild to severe
Sympathetic nervous system responses:	Parasympathetic nervous system responses:
Increased pulse rate	Vital signs normal
Increased respiratory rate	
Elevated blood pressure	
Diaphoresis	Dry, warm skin
Dilated pupils	Pupils normal or dilated
Related to tissue injury; resolves with healing	Continues beyond healing
Client appears restless and anxious	Client appears depressed and withdrawn
Client reports pain	Client often does not mention pain unless asked
Client exhibits behavior indicative of pain: crying, rubbing area, holding area	Pain behavior often absent

| **BOX 18–1** | **Concepts Associated with Pain** |

Acute pain: Pain that is directly related to tissue injury and resolves when tissue heals.

Cancer pain: Pain associated with the disease, treatment, or some other factor in individuals with cancer.

Chronic pain: Pain that persists beyond 6 months secondary to chronic disorders or nerve malfunctions that produce ongoing pain after healing is complete.

Intractable pain: A pain state (generally severe) for which there is no cure possible after accepted medical evaluation and treatments have been implemented. The focus of treatment turns from cure to pain reduction, functional improvement, and the enhancement of quality of life.

Neuropathic pain: Pain that is related to damaged or malfunctioning nervous tissue in the peripheral and/or central nervous system.

Nociceptive pain: Pain that is directly related to tissue damage. May be somatic (e.g., damage to skin, muscle bone) or visceral (e.g., damage to organs).

Pain threshold: The process of recognizing, defining, and responding to pain.

Pain tolerance: The most pain an individual is willing or able to tolerate before taking evasive actions.

The following states indicate abnormal nerve functioning, and the associated cause needs to be identified/treated (as soon as possible) before irreversible damage occurs.

Allodynia: Sensation of pain from a stimulus that normally does not produce pain, e.g., light touch.

Dysesthesia: An unpleasant abnormal sensation that can be either spontaneous or evoked.

Hyperalgesia: Increased sensation of pain in response to a normally painful stimulus.

The following concepts are important reasons to prevent pain or treat it as soon as possible to prevent the amplification, spread, and persistence of pain.

Sensitization: An increased sensitivity of a receptor after repeated activation by noxious stimuli.

Windup: Progressive increase in excitability and sensitivity of spinal cord neurons, leading to persistent, increased pain.

---

lized or healed, the pain goes away; thus this pain is transient. There may also be persistent forms of physiological pain.

Subcategories of physiological pain include somatic or visceral. **Somatic pain** originates in the skin, muscles, bone, or connective tissue. Visceral pain results from activation of pain receptors in the organs and/or hollow viscera. Visceral pain tends to be poorly located, and may have a cramping, throbbing, pressing, or aching quality. Often visceral pain is associated with feeling sick (e.g., sweating, nausea, or vomiting).

Neuropathic pain is experienced by people who have damaged or malfunctioning nerves. The nerves may be abnormal due to illness, injury, or undetermined reasons. Subtypes of neuropathic pain are being developed based on the part of the nervous system believed to be damaged (Pasero, 2004).

Peripheral neuropathic pain follows damage and/or sensitization of peripheral nerves. Central neuropathic pain results from malfunctioning nerves in the central nervous system. Sympathetically maintained pain occurs occasionally when abnormal connections between pain fibers and the sympathetic nervous system perpetuate problems with both the pain and sympathetically controlled functions. Neuropathic pain is typically chronic; it is described as burning, "electric-shock," and/or tingling, dull, and aching. Episodes of sharp, shooting pain can also be experienced (Herr, 2004). Neuropathic pain tends to be difficult to treat. Unfortunately, evidence suggests that in some instances, neuropathic pain results from failure to treat pain effectively during the perioperative period (Manais, Bucknall, & Botti, 2005).

Concepts Associated with Pain

It is useful to differentiate pain threshold from pain tolerance. **Pain threshold** is the least amount of stimuli that is needed for a person to label a sensation as pain. Threshold studies are typically conducted in a laboratory with many controls and measured amounts of stimuli (typically electrically generated). Pain threshold may vary slightly from person to person, and may be related to age, gender, or race, but it changes little in the same individual over time. **Pain tolerance** is the maximum amount of painful stimuli that a person is willing to withstand without seeking avoidance of the pain or relief. Pain tolerance varies considerably from person to person, even within the same person at different times and in different circumstances.

Hyperalgesia, allodynia, hyperpathia, and dysesthesia are conditions of abnormal pain processing that may signal the development of neuropathic processes, which if caught early may be reversed, yet if ignored, may lead to the development of incurable pain syndromes. **Hyperalgesia** and **hyperpathia** are terms that may be used interchangeably to denote a heightened response to painful stimuli. This is differentiated from **allodynia**, in which nonpainful stimuli produce pain, and from **dysesthesia**, which is an unpleasant abnormal sensation. Dysesthesia mimics or imitates the pathology of a central neuropathic pain disorder. See Box 18–1 for a review of concepts associated with pain.

PHYSIOLOGY OF PAIN

How pain is transmitted and perceived is complex, in part because of the nature of the fully integrated, constantly changing structure of the central nervous system, and the symphony of chemical mediators, only a fraction of which are understood. The extent to which pain is perceived depends on the interaction between the body's analgesia system and the nervous system's transmission and the mind's interpretation of stimuli and its meaning.

Nociception

The peripheral nervous system includes primary sensory neurons specialized to detect mechanical, thermal, or chemical conditions associated with potential tissue damage. The signals, when these nociceptors are activated, must be transduced and transmitted to the spine and brain, where the signals are modified before they are ultimately understood and "felt." The physiologic processes related to pain perception are described as **nociception**. Four physiologic processes are involved in nociception: transduction, transmission, perception, and modulation (Paice, 2002).

TRANSDUCTION   Specialized pain receptors, or nociceptors, can be excited by mechanical, thermal, or chemical stimuli. During the transduction phase, noxious stimuli trigger the release of biochemical mediators that sensitize nociceptors. Noxious or painful stimulation also causes movement of ions across cell membranes, which excites nociceptors. Pain medications can work during this phase by blocking the production of prostaglandin or by decreasing the movement of ions across the cell membrane.

TRANSMISSION   The second process of nociception, transmission of pain, includes three segments (McCaffery & Pasero, 1999). During the first segment, the pain impulse travels from the peripheral nerve fibers to the spinal cord. Substance P serves as a neurotransmitter, enhancing the movement of impulses across the nerve synapse from the primary afferent neuron to the second-order neuron in the dorsal horn of the spinal cord. Two types of nociceptor fibers cause this transmission to the dorsal horn of the spinal cord: unmyelinated C fibers, which transmit dull, aching pain, and thin A-delta fibers, which transmit sharp, localized pain. In the dorsal horn, the pain signal is modified by modulating factors before the amplified or dampened signal travels via spinothalamic tracts. The second segment is transmission from the spinal cord, and ascension, via spinothalamic tracts, to the brain stem and thalamus. The third segment involves transmission of signals between the thalamus to the somatic sensory cortex where pain perception occurs.

Pain control can take place during this second process of transmission. For example, opioids block the release of neurotransmitters, particularly substance P, which stops the pain at the spinal level. Capsaicin may also deplete substance P and inhibit the transmission of pain signals.

PERCEPTION   The process of perception begins when the client becomes conscious of the pain. Pain perception is the sum of complex activities in the central nervous system that may shape the character and intensity of pain perceived and ascribes meaning to the pain. The psychosocial context of the situation, and the meaning of the pain based on past experiences and future hopes/dreams, help to shape the behavioral response that follows.

MODULATION   Often described as the "descending system," this process occurs when neurons in the thalamus and brain stem send signals back down to the dorsal horn of the spinal cord (Paice, 2002, p. 75). These descending fibers release substances such as endogenous opioids, serotonin, and norepinephrine, which can inhibit the ascending noxious impulses in the dorsal horn. In contrast, excitatory amino acids, and the upregulation of excitatory glial cells, can facilitate these pain signals. The effects of excitatory amino acids and glial cells tend to persist, while the effects of the inhibitory neurotransmitters tend to be short-lived as they are reabsorbed into the nerves. Tricyclic antidepressants block the reuptake of norepinephrine and serotonin; or NMDA antagonists may be used to help diminish the signals of pain.

Gate Control Theory

According to Melzack and Wall's gate control theory (1965), small-diameter, peripheral nerve fibers carry signals of noxious stimuli to the dorsal horn, where these signals are modified when they are exposed to the substantia gelatinosa (the milieu in the central nervous system) that may be imbalanced in an excitatory or inhibitory direction. Ion channels on the pre- and postsynaptic membranes serve as gates that, when open, permit positively charged ions to rush into the second order neuron, sparking an electrical impulse and sending signals of pain to the thalamus. Peripherally, large-diameter (A-delta) nerve fibers, which typically send messages of touch and temperature, have an inhibitory effect on the substantia gelatinosa and may activate descending mechanisms that can lessen the intensity of pain perceived or inhibit the transmission of those pain impulses—that is, close the (ion) gates.

Higher centers in the brain, especially those associated with affect and motivation, are capable of modifying the substantia gelatinosa and influence the opening or closing of the gates. Clinically, nurses can use this model to stop nociceptor firing (treat the underlying cause), apply topical therapies (e.g., heat, ice, electrical stimulation, or massage), and address the client's mood (e.g., reduce fear, anxiety, and anger) and goals (e.g., client education, anticipatory guidance).

Responses to Pain

The body's response to pain is a complex process rather than a specific action. It has both physiologic and psychosocial aspects. Initially the sympathetic nervous system responds, resulting in the fight-or-flight response, with a noticeable increase in pulse and blood pressure. The person may hold his or her breath, or have short, shallow breathing. There may also be some reflexive movements as the person withdraws from the painful stimuli. Over a matter of minutes, or hours, the pulse and blood pressure return to baseline despite the persistence of pain. Contrary to the adaptation noted in vital signs, the pain fibers themselves adapt very little and become sensitized in a way that intensifies, prolongs, and/or spreads the pain.

Unrelieved pain has been noted to have a potentially harmful effect on the person's well-being. Pain interferes with sleep, affects appetite, and lowers the quality of life for clients and their family members. A natural response to pain is to stop activity, tense muscles, and withdraw from the pain-provoking activities. This reduced mobility may produce muscle atrophy and painful spasm, putting the person at risk for complications related to immobility and/or cardiopulmonary deconditioning. Uncontrolled pain impairs immune function, which slows healing and increases susceptibility to infections and dermal ulcers. The short, shallow breathing that accompanies pain produces atelectasis, lowers circulating oxygen levels, and increases cardiac workload. Undertreated pain also increases morbidity and mortality for a wide variety of conditions, including metastasis of cancer and extending cardiac damage during a heart attack (Page, Ben-Eliyahu, Yirmiya, & Liebeskind, 1993; Puntillo & Weiss, 1994). The physical stress and emotional distress of severe or prolonged pain can contribute to the development of a wide variety of physical and emotional disorders.

Persistent, severe pain changes the nervous system in a way that intensifies, spreads, and prolongs the pain, risking the development of incurable chronic pain syndromes. Beginning at 24 hours, persistent unrelieved severe pain changes the structure and function of the nervous system in such a way that prolongs and intensifies the pain experience. A windup phenomenon occurs, tipping the balance in the substantia gelatinosa heavily in the direction of excitation, and establishing new nerve growth, including the development of reverberating loops, which further prolong, spread, and intensify the noxious stimuli (Arnstein, 1997). The pain threshold is lowered and the cells are said to be sensitized. Sensitization of the central nervous system is reflected by spontaneous neuron firing, reduced thresholds or increased responsiveness to afferent inputs, prolonged after-discharges to repeated stimulation, and the expan-

sion of the peripheral receptive field of dorsal horn neurons. A similar process can occur in the peripheral nerves, when sensitized, normally innocuous stimuli (e.g., light touch) may be perceived as painful. Thus to prevent the development of persistent pain and promote overall health and well-being, the nurse must act to promote optimal and expedient pain control.

Factors Affecting the Pain Experience

Numerous factors can affect a person's perception of, and reaction to, pain. These include the person's ethnic and cultural values, developmental stage, environment and support people, previous pain experiences, and the meaning of the current pain.

ETHNIC AND CULTURAL VALUES Ethnic background and cultural heritage have long been recognized as factors that influence both a person's reaction to pain and the expression of that pain. Behavior related to pain is a part of the socialization process.

Although there appears to be little variation in pain threshold, cultural background can affect the level of pain that an individual is willing to tolerate. In some Middle Eastern and African cultures, self-infliction of pain is a sign of mourning or grief. In other groups, pain may be anticipated as part of the ritualistic practices, and therefore tolerance of pain signifies strength and endurance. Additionally, there are significant variations in the expression of pain. Studies have shown that individuals of northern European descent tend to be more stoic and less expressive of their pain than individuals from southern European backgrounds.

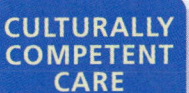

CULTURALLY COMPETENT CARE — Transcultural Differences in Responses to Pain

Expressions of pain vary from culture to culture and may vary from person to person *within* a culture.

African Americans

- Some believe pain and suffering is a part of life and is to be endured.
- Some may deny or avoid dealing with the pain till it becomes unbearable.
- Some believe that prayer and laying on of hands will free a person from suffering and pain.

Mexican Americans

- May tend to view pain as a part of life and as an indicator of the seriousness of an illness.
- Some believe that enduring pain is a sign of strength.

Puerto Ricans

- Many tend to be loud and outspoken in their expressions of pain. This is a socially learned way to cope and it is important for the nurse to not judge or disapprove.

Asian Americans

- Chinese culture values silence. As a result, some clients may be quiet when in pain because they do not want to cause dishonor to themselves and their family.
- Japanese may have a stoic (minimal verbal and nonverbal expressions) response to pain. They may even refuse pain medication.
- Filipino clients may believe that pain is "God's will." Some older adult Filipino clients may refuse pain medication.

Native Americans

- In general, Native Americans are quiet, less expressive verbally and nonverbally and may tolerate a high level of pain. They tend to not request pain medication and may tolerate pain until they are physically disabled.

Arab Americans

- Pain responses are considered private and reserved for immediate family, not with health professionals. As a result, this may lead to conflicting perceptions between the family members and the nurse regarding the effectiveness of the client's pain relief.

Note: From Transcultural Communication in Nursing, 2nd ed., by C. Munoz & J. Luckmann, 2005, Clifton Park: Delmar Learning, and Transcultural Concepts in Nursing Care, 4th ed., by M. M. Andrews & J. S. Boyle, 2003, Philadelphia: Lippincott Williams & Wilkins.

Nurses must realize they have their own attitudes and expectations about pain. Andrews and Boyle (2008) point out that health care has been dominated by white Anglo-Saxon Protestants and most nurses have been influenced by these values and beliefs. Nurses may place a higher value on silent suffering or self-control in response to pain. Nurses expect people to be objective about pain and to be able to provide a detailed description of the pain. Nurses who deny, refute, or downplay the pain they observe in others may be culturally incompetent. To become culturally competent, nurses must become knowledgeable about differences in the meaning of, and appropriate responses to, pain. They must be sympathetic to concerns and develop the skills needed to address pain in a culturally sensitive way.

DEVELOPMENTAL STAGE   The age and developmental stage of a client is an important variable that will influence both the reaction to and the expression of pain. Age variations and related nursing interventions are presented in Table 18–2.

The field of pain management for infants and children has grown significantly. It is now accepted that anatomic, physiologic, and biochemical elements necessary for pain

---

TABLE 18–2   **Lifespan Considerations Related to Pain**

AGE GROUP	EXAMPLES OF PAIN BEHAVIOR	SELECTED NURSING INTERVENTIONS
Infant	Responds to pain with increased sensitivity.	Give a glucose pacifier.
	Older infant tries to avoid pain.	Use tactile stimulation. Play music or tapes of a heartbeat.
Toddler and preschooler	Develops the ability to describe pain and its intensity and location.	Distract the child with toys, books, pictures. Involve the child in blowing bubbles as a way of "blowing away the pain."
	Responds with crying and anger because child perceives pain as a threat to security.	Appeal to the child's belief in magic by using a "magic" blanket or glove to take away pain.
	Reasoning with child at this stage is not always successful.	Hold the child to provide comfort.
	May consider pain a punishment.	Explore misconceptions about pain.
	Feels sad.	
	May learn there are gender differences in pain expression.	
	Tends to hold someone accountable for the pain.	
School-age child	Tries to be brave when facing pain.	Use imagery to turn off "pain switches."
	Rationalizes in an attempt to explain the pain.	Provide a behavioral rehearsal of what to expect and how it will look and feel.
	Responsive to explanations.	Provide support and nurturing.
	Can usually identify the location and describe the pain.	
	With persistent pain, may regress to an earlier stage of development.	
Adolescent	May be slow to acknowledge pain.	Provide opportunities to discuss pain.
	Recognizing pain or "giving in" may be considered weakness.	Provide privacy.
	Wants to appear brave in front of peers and not report pain.	Present choices for dealing with pain. Encourage music or TV for distraction.
Adult	Behaviors exhibited when experiencing pain may be gender-based behaviors learned as a child.	Deal with any misconceptions about pain.
	May ignore pain because to admit it is perceived as a sign of weakness or failure.	Focus on the client's control in dealing with the pain.
	Fear of what pain means may prevent some adults from taking action.	Allay fears and anxiety when possible.
Older adult	May have multiple conditions presenting with vague symptoms.	Thorough history and assessment is essential.
	May perceive pain as part of the aging process.	Spend time with the client and listen carefully.
	May have decreased sensations or perceptions of the pain.	
	Lethargy, anorexia, and fatigue may be indicators of pain.	
	May withhold complaints of pain because of fear of the treatment, of any lifestyle changes that may be involved, or of becoming dependent.	Clarify misconceptions.
	May describe pain differently, that is, as "ache," "hurt," or "discomfort."	Encourage independence whenever possible.
	May consider it unacceptable to admit or show pain.	

transmission are present in newborns, regardless of their gestational age. The American Academy of Pediatrics and the Canadian Paediatric Society (2000) recommend that environmental, nonpharmacologic, *and* pharmacologic interventions be used to prevent, reduce, or eliminate pain in neonates. Physiologic indicators may vary in infants, so behavioral observation is recommended for pain assessment (Ball & Bindler, 2007). Children may be less able than an adult to articulate their experience or needs related to pain, which may result in undertreatment of pain. However, children as young as 3 years can accurately report the location and intensity of their pain if it is evaluated properly.

With puberty comes the emergence of some pain syndromes, particularly for women. Men are more vulnerable to pain related to their occupational or risk-taking patterns. A needless disparity is that the very young, the very old, women, and ethnic minorities are undertreated for their pain more frequently than their adult male counterparts.

Studies have shown that chronic pain affects 25% to 50% of older clients living in the community and 45% to 80% of those in nursing homes (American Geriatrics Society [AGS], 1998). The prevalence of pain in the older population is generally higher due to both acute and chronic disease conditions. Pain threshold does not appear to change with aging, although the effect of analgesics may increase due to physiologic changes related to drug metabolism and excretion (Stanley, Blair, & Beare, 2005).

ENVIRONMENT AND SUPPORT PEOPLE   A strange environment can compound pain. The lonely person who is without a support network may perceive pain as severe, whereas the person who has supportive people around may perceive less pain. Some people prefer to withdraw when they are in pain, whereas others prefer the distraction of people and activity around them. Family caregivers can be a significant support for a person in pain. With the increase in outpatient and home care, families are assuming an increased responsibility for the management of pain. Education related to the assessment and management of pain can positively affect the perceived quality of life for both clients and their caregivers (McCaffery & Pasero, 1999).

Expectations of significant others can affect a person's perceptions of and responses to pain. Family role can also affect how a person perceives or responds to pain. The presence of support people often changes a client's reaction to pain.

PAST PAIN EXPERIENCES   Previous pain experiences alter a client's sensitivity to pain. People who have personally experienced pain or who have been exposed to the suffering of someone close are often more threatened by anticipated pain than people without a pain experience. In addition, the success or lack of success of pain relief measures influences a person's expectations for relief and future response to interventions.

MEANING OF PAIN   Some clients may accept pain more readily than others, depending on the circumstances and the client's interpretation of its significance. A client who asso-

ciates the pain with a positive outcome may withstand the pain amazingly well. These clients may view the pain as a temporary inconvenience rather than a potential threat or disruption to daily life.

Clients with unrelenting chronic pain may suffer more intensely. Chronic pain affects the body, mind, spirit, and social relationships in an undesirable way. Physically, the pain limits functioning and contributes to the disuse or deconditioning alluded to previously. For many, the change in activities of daily living also takes a toll. The side effects of the many medications used to try to control the pain also place a heavy burden on the body. Mentally, individuals with chronic pain change their outlook, becoming more pessimistic, often to the point of helplessness and hopelessness. Mood often becomes impaired when pain persists, because the sadness of being unable to do important or enjoyable activities combines with self-doubts and learned helplessness to produce depression. Anxiety, worry, and uncertainty about coping with the pain may escalate emotionally, to the point of panic. Spiritually, pain may be viewed in a variety of ways. It may be perceived as a punishment for wrongdoing, a betrayal by the higher power, a test of fortitude, or a threat to the essence of who the person is. Pain may be a source of spiritual distress, or it may be a source of strength and enlightenment. Socially, pain often strains valued relationships, in part because of the impaired ability to fulfill role expectations.

NURSING MANAGEMENT

ASSESSING

Accurate pain assessment is essential for effective pain management. Many health facilities are making pain assessment the fifth vital sign. The strategy of linking pain assessment to routine vital sign assessment and documentation represents a push to make pain assessment a routine aspect of care for all clients. Given the highly subjective and individually unique nature of pain, a comprehensive assessment of the pain provides the necessary foundation for optimal pain control.

The extent and frequency of the pain assessment varies according to the situation and the organizational policy. For clients experiencing acute, severe pain, the nurse may focus only on location, quality, and severity, and provide interventions to control the pain before conducting a more detailed evaluation. Clients with less severe or chronic pain can usually provide a more detailed description of the experience. As the fifth vital sign, pain should be screened for every time vital signs are evaluated.

Major barriers to better pain control for both nurses and clients relate to inadequate assessment of pain and fear of treatment-related problems (Horbury, Henderson, & Bromely, 2005). Given that many people will not voice their pain unless asked about it, pain assessments must be initiated by the nurse. Some of the many reasons clients may be reluctant to report pain are listed in Box 18–2. Because the words *pain* or *complain* may have emotional or sociocultural meaning

---

BOX 18–2   **Why Clients May Be Reluctant to Report Pain**

- Unwillingness to trouble staff who are perceived as busy
- Don't want to be labeled as a "complainer" or "bad"
- Fear of the injectable route of analgesic administration—especially children
- Belief that unrelieved pain is expected–normal part of recovery or aging
- Belief that others will think they are weak if they express pain
- Difficulty or inability to communicate their discomfort
- Concern about risks associated with opioid drugs (e.g., addiction)

- Concern about unwanted side effects, especially of opioid drugs
- Concern that use of drugs now will render the drug inefficient later in life
- Fear that reporting pain will lead to further tests and expenses
- Belief that nothing can be done to control pain
- Belief that enduring pain and suffering may lead to spiritual enlightenment

---

attached, it is better to ask, "Do you have any discomforts to report?" rather than "Do you have any complaints of pain?" It is also essential that nurses listen to and believe the client's perceptions of pain. Believing the person's perceptions is crucial in establishing the sense of trust needed to develop a therapeutic relationship.

Pain assessments consist of two major components: (a) a pain history to obtain facts from the client and (b) direct observation of behaviors, physical signs of tissue damage, and secondary physiologic responses of the client. The goal of assessment is to gain an objective understanding of a subjective experience. Box 18–3 provides one example of a helpful mnemonic to make a complete pain assessment.

Pain History

While taking pain histories, the nurse must provide an opportunity for clients to express how they view the pain and the situation. This will help the nurse understand what the pain means to the client and how the client is coping with it. Each person's pain experience is unique, and the client is the best interpreter. This history should be geared to the specific client. The initial pain assessment for someone in severe acute pain may consist of only a few questions before intervention occurs. In addition, the nurse may focus on previous pain treatment and its effectiveness, when and what analgesics were last taken, other medications being taken, and allergies. For a person with chronic pain, the nurse may focus on the client's coping mechanisms, effectiveness of current pain management, and ways in which the pain has affected the client's body, thoughts and feelings, activities, and relationships.

Data that should be obtained in a comprehensive pain history include pain location, intensity, quality, patterns, precipitating factors, alleviating factors, associated symptoms, effect on ADLs, past pain experiences, meaning of the pain to the person, coping resources, and affective responses.

LOCATION To ascertain the specific location of the pain, ask the individual to point to the site of the discomfort. A chart consisting of drawings of the body can assist in identifying pain locations. The client marks the location of pain on the chart. This tool can be especially effective with clients who have more than one source of pain. A client who has multiple pains of different character can use symbols to draw the distribution of different pain types.

When assessing the location of a child's pain, the nurse needs to understand the child's vocabulary. Asking the child to point to the pain helps clarify the child's word usage to identify location. The use of figure drawings can assist in identifying pain locations. Parents can also be helpful in interpreting the meaning of a child's words.

When documenting pain location, the nurse may use various body landmarks. Further clarification is possible with the use of terms such as *proximal*, *distal*, *medial*, *lateral*, and *diffuse*.

PAIN INTENSITY OR RATING SCALES The single most important indicator of the existence and intensity of pain is the client's report of pain. In practice, however, McCaffery, Ferrell, and Pasero (2000) found that nurses tend to use less reliable measures for assessing pain. The top factors identified by nurses were culturally influenced. In addition, studies have shown that health care providers may underrate or overrate the pain intensity (Bergh & Sjostrom, 1999). The use of pain intensity scales is an easy and reliable method of determining the client's pain intensity. Such scales provide consistency for nurses to communicate with the client and other health care providers. To avoid confusion, scales should use a 0 to 10 range with 0 indicating "no pain" and

---

BOX 18–3   **Mnemonic for Pain Assessment: COLDERR**

Character: describe the sensation (e.g., sharp, aching, burning),

Onset: when it started, how it has changed,

Location: where it hurts (all locations),

Duration: constant versus intermittent in nature,

Exacerbation: factors that make it worse,

Relief: factors that make it better (medications and other factors), and

Radiation: pattern of shooting/spreading/location of pain away from its origin.

Note: Reprinted from "Optimizing Perioperative Pain Management," 2002, by P. M. Arnstein. *AORN Journal, 76*(5), 812–818. Copyright © 2002 with permission of Elsevier.

Pain History

- Location: Where is your discomfort?
- Quality: Tell me what your discomfort feels like.
- Intensity: On a scale of 0 to 10, with 0 representing no pain and 10 representing the worst possible pain, how would you rate the degree of discomfort you are having right now?
- Pattern
  a. Time of onset: When did or does the pain start?
  b. Duration: How long have you had it, or how long does it usually last?
  c. Constancy: Do you have pain-free periods? When? And for how long?
- Precipitating factors: What triggers the pain or makes it worse?
- Alleviating factors: What measures or methods have you found helpful in lessening or relieving the pain? What pain medications do you use?
- Associated symptoms: Do you have any other symptoms before, during, or after your pain?
- Effects on ADLs: How does the pain affect your daily life?
- Past pain experiences: Tell me about past pain experiences you have had and what was done to relieve the pain.
- Meaning of pain: What does having this pain mean to you? Does it signal something about the future or past? What worries or scares you the most about your pain?
- Coping resources: What do you usually do to help you deal with pain?
- Affective response: How does the pain make you feel?

the highest number indicating the "worst pain possible" for that individual. The inclusion of word modifiers on the scale can assist some clients who find it difficult to apply a number level to their pain.

Another way to evaluate the intensity of pain for clients who are unable to use the numeric rating scales is to determine the extent of pain awareness and degree of interference with functioning. It is believed that the degree that pain interferes with functioning is a good marker for the severity of pain, especially for those with chronic pain.

CLINICAL ALERT

Perception is reality. The client's self-report of pain is what must be used to determine pain intensity. The nurse is obligated to record the pain intensity as reported by the client. By challenging the believability of the client's report, the nurse is undermining the therapeutic relationship and preventing the fulfillment of advocacy and helping people with pain, which is called for in the ANA 2005 Scope and Standards of Practice in Pain Management Nursing.

When noting pain intensity, it is important to determine any related factors that may be affecting the pain. The nurse needs to consider the possible cause when the intensity changes. Several factors affect the perception of intensity: (a) the amount of distraction, or the client's concentration on another event; (b) the client's state of consciousness; (c) the level of activity; and (d) the client's expectations.

Not all clients can understand or relate to numerical pain intensity scales. These include preverbal children, older adult clients with impairments in cognition or communication, and people who do not speak English. For these clients the Wong-Baker FACES Rating Scale (Figure 18–2) may be easier to use (Wong, Hockenberry-Eaton, Wilson, Winkelstein, & Schwartz, 2009). The face scale includes a number scale in relation to each expression so that the pain intensity can be documented. When clients are unable to verbalize their pain for reasons of age, mental capacity, medical interventions, or

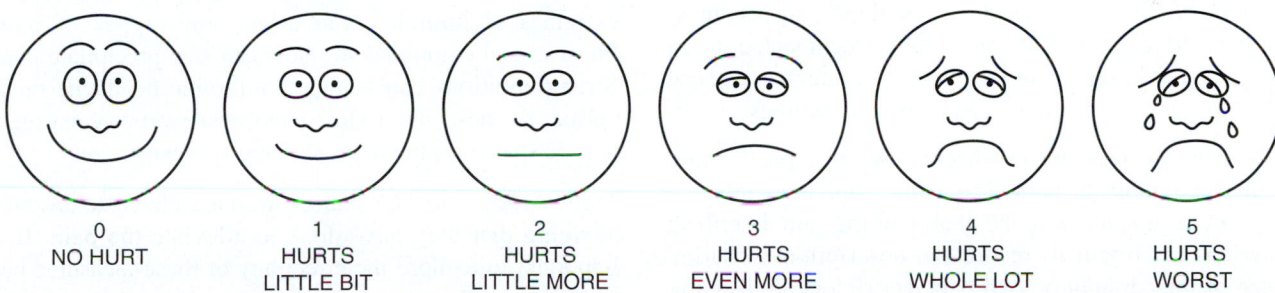

| 0 | 1 | 2 | 3 | 4 | 5 |
| NO HURT | HURTS LITTLE BIT | HURTS LITTLE MORE | HURTS EVEN MORE | HURTS WHOLE LOT | HURTS WORST |

Explain to the person that each face is for a person who feels happy because he has no pain (hurt) or sad because he has some or a lot of pain. Face 0 is very happy because he doesn't hurt at all. Face 1 hurts just a little bit. Face 2 hurts a little more. Face 3 hurts even more. Face 4 hurts a whole lot. Face 5 hurts as much as you can imagine, although you don't have to be crying to feel this bad. Ask the person to choose the face that best describes how he is feeling.

Rating scale is recommended for persons age 3 years and older.

Brief word instructions: Point to each face using the words to describe the pain intensity. Ask the child to choose the face that best describes own pain and record the appropriate number.

Figure 18–2 ● The Wong-Baker FACES Rating Scale.

Note: From *Wong's Essentials of Pediatric Nursing*, 6th ed. (p. 1301), by D. L. Wong, M. Hockenberry-Eaton, D. Wilson, M. L. Winkelstein, and P. Schwartz, 2001, St. Louis, MO: Mosby. Copyright by Mosby, Inc. Reprinted with permission.

other reasons, nurses need to accurately assess the intensity of each client's pain and the effectiveness of the pain management interventions. For these clients, the nurse must rely on observation of behavior.

Several validated behavioral pain rating scales can be used in specific populations. The FLACC scale has been validated in children 2 months to 7 years old and rates pain behaviors manifested in Facial expressions, Leg movement, Activity, Cry, and Consolability measures that yield a 0 to 10 score (Merkel, Voepel-Lewis, Shayevitz, & Malviya, 1997). Warden, Hurley, and Volicer (2003) tested a similar behavioral measure for older adults with dementia, which quantified respirations, vocalizations, facial expressions, body language, and consolability. Given the diversity of pain and behaviors among clients spanning a broad range of age and physical and mental capabilities, it is unrealistic to believe a single pain assessment tool can be applied across all populations. As an organization committed to improving the way pain is evaluated and treated, the American Society for Pain Management Nursing (ASPMN) has assembled a team of nurse experts to develop a position paper on assessing pain in the nonverbal patient.

For effective use of pain rating scales, clients need not only to understand the use of the scale but also to be educated about how the information will be used to determine changes in their condition and the effectiveness of pain management interventions. Clients should also be asked to indicate what level of comfort is acceptable so that they can perform specific activities (Acello, 2000). To align the client's goals and expectations with reality, it is important to note that acute pain can typically be cut by 50% and chronic pain can be cut by 25%. To ensure that optimal pain management is achieved, the client works together with professionals toward established goals of pain reduction and functional improvement.

The use of a pain rating scale together with a pain flow sheet has been shown to be effective in improving pain management (McCaffery & Pasero, 1999). Documentation can be completed by the nurse, the client, or a caregiver and can be used in acute, outpatient, and home care settings.

PAIN QUALITY   Descriptive adjectives help people communicate the quality of pain. The astute clinician can glean subtle clinical clues from the quality of the pain described; thus it is important to record the description verbatim. Some of the commonly used pain descriptors are listed in Table 18–3. Note that the term "unbearable" is listed as an affective term and "piercing" is a sensory term. Both pains are real physical conditions signaling an underlying condition, but the affective description "unbearable" suggests that there is a coexisting emotional distress that needs to be addressed as well. Pain described as burning or shock-like tends to be neuropathic in origin and may be responsive to anticonvulsants, with or without an opioid (e.g., morphine).

PATTERN   The pattern of pain includes time of onset, duration, and recurrence or intervals without pain. The nurse therefore determines when the pain began; how long the pain lasts; whether it recurs and, if so, the length of the

TABLE 18–3	Commonly Used Pain Descriptors	
TERM	SENSORY WORDS	AFFECTIVE WORDS
Pain	Searing	Unbearable
	Scalding	Killing
	Sharp	Intense
	Piercing	Torturing
	Drilling	Agonizing
	Wrenching	Terrifying
	Shooting	Exhausting
	Burning	Suffocating
	Crushing	Frightful
	Penetrating	Punishing
		Miserable
Hurt	Hurting	Heavy
	Pricking	
	Pressing	Throbbing
	Tender	
Ache	Numb	Annoying
	Cold	Nagging
	Flickering	Tiring
	Radiating	Troublesome
	Dull	Gnawing
	Sore	Uncomfortable
	Aching	Sickening
	Cramping	Tender

interval without pain; and when the pain last occurred. Attention to the pattern of pain helps the nurse anticipate and meet the needs of the client, as well as recognize patterns of grave concern.

PRECIPITATING FACTORS   Certain activities sometimes precede pain. For example, physical exertion may precede chest pain, or abdominal pain may occur after eating. These observations can help prevent pain and determine its cause. Environmental factors such as extreme cold or heat and extremes of humidity can affect some types of pain. Physical and emotional stressors can also precipitate pain. Strong emotions can trigger a migraine headache or an episode of chest pain. Extreme physical exertion can trigger muscle spasms in the neck, shoulders, or back.

ALLEVIATING FACTORS   Nurses must ask clients to describe anything that they have done to alleviate the pain. It is important to explore the effect any of these measures had on the pain, whether or not relief was obtained, or whether the pain became worse.

ASSOCIATED SYMPTOMS   Also included in the clinical appraisal of pain are associated symptoms such as nausea, vomiting, dizziness, and diarrhea. These symptoms may relate to the onset of the pain or they may result from the presence of the pain.

EFFECT ON ACTIVITIES OF DAILY LIVING (ADL)   Knowing how ADLs are affected by pain helps the nurse understand the client's perspective on the pain's severity. The nurse asks the client to describe how the pain has affected sleep, appetite, concentration, interpersonal relationships, marital relationships, driving, walking, home activities, leisure activities, and emotional status. A rating scale of none, a little, or a great deal, or another range can be used to determine the degree of alteration.

COPING RESOURCES Each individual will exhibit personal ways of coping with pain. Strategies may relate to earlier pain experiences or the specific meaning of the pain; some may reflect religious or cultural influences. Nurses can encourage and support the client's use of methods known to have helped in modifying pain, unless they are specifically contraindicated.

AFFECTIVE RESPONSES Affective responses vary according to the situation, the degree and duration of pain, the interpretation of it, and many other factors. The nurse needs to explore the client's feelings of anxiety, fear, exhaustion, depression, or sense of failure. Because many people with chronic pain become depressed and potentially suicidal, it may also be necessary to assess the client's suicide risk. In such situations, the nurse needs to ask the client, "Do you ever feel so bad that you want to die? Have you considered harming yourself or others recently?" Hitchcock, Ferrell, and McCaffery (1994) found that about half of the people with chronic pain surveyed have thought, at least at one time, they'd be better off dead. This fact may be reassuring to those who answer affirmatively to the first question. The vast majority of chronic pain sufferers, however, are not actively suicidal and do not have a specific, lethal plan. For those who express suicidal intent, nurses need to be familiar with state regulations, organizational policies, and resources available to guide practice in this area.

Observation of Behavioral and Physiologic Responses

There are wide variations in nonverbal responses to pain. For clients who are very young, aphasic, confused, or disoriented, nonverbal expressions may be the only means of communicating pain. Facial expression is often the first indication of pain, and it may be the only one. Vocalizations such as moaning and groaning or crying and screaming are sometimes associated with pain. Purposeless body movement or immobilization of the body or a part of the body may also indicate pain. Behavioral changes such as confusion and restlessness may be indicators of pain in both cognitively intact and cognitively impaired older adult clients (Ebersole, Hess, Touhy, & Jett, 2009). Older adults with chronic pain may become hostile or aggressive. Rhythmic body movements or rubbing may indicate pain.

It is important to note that behavioral responses can be controlled and so may not be very revealing. When pain is chronic there are rarely overt behavioral responses because the individual develops personal coping styles for dealing with pain, discomfort, or suffering.

Physiologic responses vary with the origin and duration of the pain. Early in the onset of acute pain the sympathetic nervous system is stimulated, resulting in increased blood pressure, pulse rate, respiratory rate, pallor, diaphoresis, and pupil dilation. The body does not sustain the increased sympathetic function over a prolonged period and, therefore, the sympathetic nervous system adapts, making the physiologic responses less evident or even absent. Physiologic responses are most likely to be absent in people with chronic pain because of autonomic nervous system adaptation. Thus, measures of physiologic responses are poor indicators of the presence, absence, or severity of pain and should not be used.

Daily Pain Diary

For clients who experience chronic pain, a daily diary may help the client and nurse identify pain patterns and factors that exacerbate or mediate the pain experience. Diary entries should be done three times a day at the same time each day to note time of day and day-to-day variability. The record can include time of onset of pain, activity or situation, physical pain characteristics and intensity, emotions experienced, and use of analgesics or other relief measures.

Recorded data can provide the basis for developing or modifying the plan for care. For this tool to be effective, it is important that the nurse educate the client and family about the value and use of the diary in achieving effective pain control. Review the diary each visit, asking questions, sharing observations, and providing hints. Determining the client's abilities to use the diary is essential.

| RESEARCH NOTES | **Is There a Relationship between Pain Control and Satisfaction with Care?** |

It has been suggested from prior research that there are health benefits for maintaining pain below the midpoint on pain scales (e.g., less than 5 on a 0–10 scale), but that client satisfaction does not always correlate to pain. This study was conducted to identify factors associated with the client's satisfaction with pain relief. A total of 207 subjects were enrolled in a clinical trial preoperatively to examine their patterns of pain control and related satisfaction with care. Clients who were "very satisfied" with pain control had pain intensity levels that averaged around 3, whereas those who were "somewhat satisfied" had pain of 4 on the 0–10 scale. Those having pain at or above the midpoint 5 were not satisfied.

Implications

This adds to the evidence that reducing pain below the midpoint of a pain scale is the target professionals should strive to achieve for overall health and well-being, as well as client satisfaction.

Note: Reprinted from *The Journal of Pain*, vol. 6, M. P. Jensen, S. A. Martin, and R. Cheung, pp. 400–406, Copyright 2005, with permission from Elsevier.

DIAGNOSING

NANDA includes the following diagnostic labels for clients experiencing pain or discomfort:

- *Acute Pain*
- *Chronic Pain*

When writing the diagnostic statement, the nurse should specify the location. Related factors should also be part of the diagnostic statement and can include both physiologic and psychologic factors. Examples of clinical application of these diagnoses using NANDA, NOC, and NIC designations are shown in Identifying Nursing Diagnoses, Outcomes, and Interventions. Because the presence of pain can affect so many facets of a person's functioning, pain may be the etiology of other nursing diagnoses.

PLANNING

The established goals for the client will vary according to the diagnosis and its defining characteristics. Specific nursing interventions can be selected to meet the individual needs of the client. Examples of clinical application of NOC

outcomes and NIC interventions are shown in the Identifying Nursing Diagnoses, Outcomes, and Interventions.

When planning, nurses need to choose pain relief measures appropriate for the client, based on the assessment data and input from the client or support persons. Nursing interventions may include a variety of pharmacologic and nonpharmacologic interventions. Developing a plan that incorporates a wide range of strategies is usually most effective. Whether in acute care or in home care, it is important for everyone involved in pain management to understand the plan of care. The plan should be documented in the client's record; in home care, a copy needs to be made available to the client, support persons, and caregivers. Involvement of the client and support persons is essential in pain management.

When the client's pattern and level of pain can be anticipated or is already known, regular or scheduled administration of analgesics can provide a steady serum level. With acute pain, this may be possible in the first 24 to 48 hours following surgery when the client is likely to have pain requiring opioid analgesics. Frequency of administration can be adjusted to prevent pain from recurring. When persistent, continuous pain exists, analgesics should be given around the clock (ATC), with additional as-needed (prn) doses

---

IDENTIFYING NURSING DIAGNOSES, OUTCOMES, AND INTERVENTIONS — **Clients Experiencing Pain**

DATA CLUSTER Mary Anderson, 75, fell and broke her right hip while shopping. She had surgery yesterday to repair the fracture. She rates her pain in the surgical site as 6 on a 0–10 scale and states the pain goes up to 9 when she is repositioned in bed. Morphine 10 mg q4h IV prn is ordered. She received a dose 5 hours ago. She states, "I try to hold out as long as I can before asking for a pain killer."

NURSING DIAGNOSIS/DEFINITION	SAMPLE DESIRED OUTCOMES*/*DEFINITION*	INDICATORS	SELECTED INTERVENTIONS*/*DEFINITION*	SAMPLE NIC ACTIVITIES
Acute Pain/Unpleasant sensory and emotional experience arising from actual or potential tissue damage or described in terms of such damage (International Association for the Study of Pain); sudden or slow onset of any intensity from mild to severe with an anticipated or predictable end and a duration of less than 6 months	Pain Control [1605]/*Personal actions to control pain*	Often demonstrated: • Describes causal factors • Uses analgesics appropriately • Reports uncontrolled symptoms to health care professional • Reports pain controlled	Analgesic Administration [2210]/*Use of pharmacologic agents to reduce or eliminate pain*	• Determine pain location, characteristics, quality, and severity before medicating client • Instruct to request prn pain medication before the pain is severe • Attend to comfort needs and other activities that assist relaxation to facilitate response to analgesia • Correct misconceptions/myths client or family members may hold regarding analgesics, particularly opioids (e.g., addiction and risk of overdose)

*The NOC # for desired outcomes and the NIC # for nursing interventions are listed in brackets following the appropriate outcome or intervention. Outcomes, indicators, interventions, and activities selected are only a sample of those suggested by NOC and NIC and should be further individualized for each client.

LONG-TERM CARE CONSIDERATION
Pain

While the prevalence of acute pain does not increase as a result of aging, chronic pain problems tend to increase in later life (Hadjistavropoulos & Fine, 2006). Furthermore, studies show that clients with dementia are less likely to receive analgesic medication than cognitively intact clients despite similar prevalence of pain-related conditions (Fuchs-Lacelle, 2007). This lack of pain control can lead to aggression and behavioral problems. A number of pain assessment scales exist including the Geriatric Pain Measure, the MPQ, and The Pain Assessment Checklist for Seniors with Dementia and Limited Ability to Communicate (PACSLAC). It is important that care planning for the long-term client include frequent pain assessment, especially when there are behavioral or cognitive changes. Asking the long-term care client about pain should be written into the plan of care and assessed at least daily.

available (Herr, 2002). Nonpharmacologic interventions should also be regularly scheduled. The additional advantage of scheduling measures is that the client spends less time in pain and does not experience as much anxiety or fear of the pain recurring, or the helplessness of not knowing what to do when pain flares.

IMPLEMENTING

Pain management is the alleviation of pain or a reduction in pain to a level of comfort that is acceptable to the client. It includes pharmacologic and nonpharmacologic interventions. Nursing management of pain consists of both independent and collaborative nursing actions. In general, noninvasive measures may be performed as an independent nursing function, whereas administration of analgesic medication generally requires a medical order from a primary care provider. However, because many analgesics are ordered to be administered on an "as needed" (prn) basis, the decision to administer the prescribed medication is frequently the nurse's, often requiring judgment as to the dose and the time of administration. Recent changes to the way range orders are written provide a little more structure than in the past; however, professional nursing judgment remains a key factor in relieving pain by determining which medication in what dosage would best meet the client's comfort needs (Gordon et al., 2005). See the Practice Guidelines for individualizing care for clients with pain.

Barriers to Pain Management

Misconceptions and biases can affect pain management. These may involve attitudes of the nurse or the client as well as knowledge deficits. Clients and families may lack knowledge of the adverse effects of pain and may have misinformation regarding the use of analgesics. Clients may not report pain because they expect nothing can be done, they think it is not severe enough, or they feel it would distract or prejudice the health care provider. Other common misconceptions are

shown in Table 18–4. Another barrier to effective pain management is the fear of becoming addicted, especially when long-term opioid use is prescribed. This fear is often held by both nurses and clients. It is important that all individuals know the difference between tolerance, dependence, and addiction (see Box 18–4). Pseudoaddiction is a condition that results from the undertreatment of pain where the client may become focused on obtaining medications, may "clock watch," and may otherwise seem inappropriately "drug seeking." Even behaviors such as illicit drug use and deception can occur in the client's efforts to obtain pain relief. Pseudoaddiction can be distinguished from true addiction in that the behaviors resolve when the pain is treated effectively.

Key Strategies in Pain Management

Key strategies to reduce pain include acknowledging and accepting the client's pain, assisting support persons, reducing misconceptions about pain, reducing fear and anxiety, and preventing pain.

ACKNOWLEDGING AND ACCEPTING CLIENT'S PAIN According to the professional standards of conduct, nurses have a duty to ask clients about their pain and to believe their reports of discomfort. Challenging the client's report of discomfort undermines the environment of trust that is an essential component in the therapeutic relationship. Consider these four ways of communicating this belief:

1. Acknowledge the possibility of the pain. "Many people with your condition are bothered by leg pain. Are you experiencing any leg discomfort? What does it feel like? How concerned/upset are you about it?"
2. Listen attentively to what the client says about the pain, restating your understanding of the reported discomfort. Adding an empathetic statement like, "I'm sorry you are hurting, it must be very upsetting. I want to help you feel better" lets the client know you believe the pain is real and intend to help.
3. Convey that you need to ask about the pain because, despite some similarities, everybody's experience is unique, for example, "Many people with your condition report having some discomforts. Do you have any pain or other discomforts now?"
4. Attend to the client's needs promptly. It is unconscionable to believe the client's report of pain and then do nothing. After determining the client has pain, discuss options and plan actions for providing relief.

CLINICAL ALERT

So what if you are fooled by a client's self-report of pain? Evidence suggests only 5% of people reporting pain are dishonest and seeking some secondary gain. By believing everyone, you will not shortchange the 95% of people who so desperately need to have help controlling their pain, providing them with competent, compassionate, and appropriate nursing care based on the best available information.

PRACTICE GUIDELINES

Individualizing Care for Clients with Pain

- Establish a trusting relationship. Convey your concern, and acknowledge that you believe that the client is experiencing pain. A trusting relationship promotes expression of the client's thoughts and feelings and enhances effectiveness of planned pain therapies.
- Consider the client's ability and willingness to participate actively in pain relief measures. Clients who are excessively fatigued or sedated or who have altered levels of consciousness are less able to participate actively. For example, a client with an altered level of consciousness or altered thought processes cannot safely or effectively use patient-controlled analgesia. In contrast, a fatigued client may express a willingness to use pain relief measures that require little effort, such as listening to music or performing relaxation techniques.
- Use a variety of pain relief measures. It is thought that using more than one measure has an additive, if not synergistic, effect in relieving pain. Two types of relief measures that should be part of any pain treatment plan are active (relief strategies that are self-initiated) and passive (relief strategies that require the assistance of others). Establishing rapport and client teaching are necessary components of all therapeutic encounters and may be implicit or explicit in the care plan. Because a client's pain may vary throughout a 24-hour period, different types of pain relief or preemptive interventions may need to be scheduled (e.g., administer medication 1 hour before dressing change, relaxation techniques with pleasant imagery after bedtime medication).
- Provide measures to relieve pain before it becomes severe. For example, providing an analgesic before the onset of pain is preferable to waiting for the client to complain of pain, when a larger dose may be required.
- Use pain-relieving measures that the client believes are effective. It has been recognized that clients are the authorities about their own pain. Thus, incorporating the client's preferred methods of relieving their pain into the treatment plan should be seriously considered.
- The selection of pain relief measures should be aligned with the client's report of the severity of the pain. If a client reports mild pain, an analgesic such as aspirin may be indicated, whereas a client who reports severe pain often requires a more potent relief measure. Telling a client to ignore the pain (e.g., through distraction techniques) when he or she is reporting severe pain is an example of a misalignment of the pain severity and intervention selected.
- If a pain relief measure is ineffective, encourage the client to try it again before abandoning it. Medications may need repeated doses to saturate plasma proteins before sufficient "free drug" is available to work on the intended target. Many nonpharmacologic measures require practice before they are effective.
- Maintain an unbiased attitude (open mind) about what may relieve the pain. New ways to relieve pain are continually being developed. It is not always possible to explain the effectiveness of particular pain relief measures; however, using approaches the client believes will work should be considered.
- Keep trying. Do not ignore a client because pain persists despite failed attempts to alleviate the discomfort. In these circumstances, reassess the pain and consider other relief measures.
- Prevent harm to the client. Pain therapy should not increase discomfort or harm the client. Some pain relief measures may have adverse untoward effects, such as fatigue, but they should not disable the client.
- Educate the client and caregivers about pain. Clients and support people need to be informed about possible causes of pain, precipitating and alleviating factors, and alternatives to drug therapy. Misconceptions also need to be corrected.

TABLE 18–4 Common Misconceptions about Pain

MISCONCEPTION	CORRECTION
Clients experience severe pain only when they have had major surgery.	Even after minor surgery, clients can experience intense pain.
The nurse or other health care professionals are the authorities about a client's pain.	The person who experiences the pain is the only authority about its existence and nature.
Administering analgesics regularly for pain will lead to addiction.	Clients are unlikely to become addicted to an analgesic provided to treat pain.
The amount of tissue damage is directly related to the amount of pain.	Pain is a subjective experience, and the intensity and duration of pain vary considerably among individuals.
Visible physiologic or behavioral signs accompany pain and can be used to verify its existence.	Even with severe pain, periods of physiologic and behavioral adaptation can occur.

ASSISTING SUPPORT PERSONS Support persons often need assistance to respond in a helpful manner to the person experiencing pain. Nurses can help by giving them accurate information about the pain and providing opportunities for them to discuss their emotional reactions, which may include anger, fear, frustration, and feelings of inadequacy. Teaching the support persons about the disease and medications (including warning signs to report) and nondrug pain-relieving techniques they can help with may diminish their feelings of helplessness and strengthen their relationship. Support persons also

BOX 18–4	Definitions

The American Academy of Pain Medicine, the American Pain Society, and the American Society of Addiction Medicine recognize the following definitions and recommend their use.

Addiction

Addiction is a primary, chronic, neurobiologic disease, with genetic, psychosocial, and environmental factors influencing its development and manifestations. It is characterized by one or more of the following behaviors: impaired control over drug use, compulsive use, craving, and continued use despite harm.

Physical Dependence

A state of adaptation manifested by withdrawal syndrome produced by abrupt cessation, rapid dose reduction, decreasing blood level of the drug, and/or administration of an antagonist.

Tolerance

Adaptation reducing drug's effects secondary to repeated exposure.

Note: From "Definitions Related to the Use of Opioids for the Treatment of Pain," *A Consensus Document from the American Academy of Pain Medicine, the American Pain Society, and the American Society of Addiction Medicine,* 2006, American Academy of Pain Medicine, American Pain Society, and the American Society of Addiction Medicine. Retrieved August 20, 2006, from http://www.ampainsoc.org/advocacy/opioids2.htm

---

may need the nurse's understanding, reassurance, and perhaps access to resources that will help them cope as they add the caregiver role to an already stressful life circumstance.

REDUCING MISCONCEPTIONS ABOUT PAIN Reducing a client's misconceptions about the pain and its treatment will remove one of the barriers to optimal pain relief. The nurse should explain to the client that pain is a highly individual experience and that it is only the client who really experiences the pain, although others can understand and empathize. Misconceptions are also dealt with when the nurse and client discuss the context of pain control as part of the healing process. For example, a client may refuse pain medicine out of concern for addiction, explaining that the pain is more tolerable as long as he or she remains totally still. This misconception overstates the risk of addiction (estimated at < 5% of clients without a history of substance abuse when treated for acute pain) while underestimating the risks associated with immobility (atelectasis, muscle atrophy, decubitus ulcers, infections, etc.).

CLINICAL ALERT

Emphasize to the client that at times, treatment may need to balance the demands of providing pain reduction with functional improvement. Too much pain medicine might impair alertness or gait; too much pain impairs alertness and ability to move. Thus a client may have to tolerate mild pain in order to do what is necessary to maximize functioning and recovery (e.g., cough, deep breathe, and walk).

REDUCING FEAR AND ANXIETY It is important to help relieve strong emotions capable of amplifying pain. When clients have no opportunity to talk about their pain and associated fears, their perceptions and reactions to the pain can be intensified. Often, these emotions are related to uncertainty about the future, feeling mistreated in the past, or having unmet expectations. By providing accurate information, the nurse can also reduce many of the client's fears or anxiety, while clarifying expectations can minimize frustration and anger. Specifically, client education about the range of pain that is considered normal for the condition as well as the types of discomforts that signal a potential for problems will help alleviate this fear and uncertainty.

PREVENTING PAIN A preventive approach to pain management involves the provision of measures to treat the pain before it occurs or before it becomes severe. **Preemptive analgesia** is the administration of analgesics prior to an invasive or operative procedure in order to treat pain before it occurs. Nurses can also use a preemptive approach by providing an analgesic around the clock (ATC), and supplementing with as needed prn doses prior to painful procedures. This strategy prevents the windup and sensitization described earlier that spreads, intensifies, and prolongs pain.

Pharmacologic Pain Management

Pharmacologic pain management involves the use of opioids (narcotics), nonopioids/nonsteroidal anti-inflammatory drugs (NSAIDs), and coanalgesic drugs (see Box 18–5). The principles of modern analgesic use are built on a foundation established by the World Health Organization (WHO) three-step approach to treating cancer pain. This approach focuses on aligning the proper analgesic with the intensity of pain. This approach has evolved into what is currently termed "rational polypharmacy," which demands that health professionals be aware of all ingredients of medications that alleviate pain and use combinations to reduce the need for high doses of any one medication, and to maximize pain control with a minimum of side effects or toxicity. These multidrug strategies, combined with multimodal therapy "may permit opioid dose reduction and improve patient outcomes" (APS, 2003, p. 34).

WORLD HEALTH ORGANIZATION (WHO) THREE-STEP APPROACH For clients with mild pain (1–3 on a 0–10 scale), step 1 of the analgesic ladder, nonopioid analgesics (with or without a coanalgesic), is the appropriate starting point. If the client has mild pain that persists or increases despite using full doses of step 1 medications, or if the pain is moderate (4–6 on a 0–10 scale), then a step 2 regimen is appropriate. At the second step, a weak opioid (e.g., codeine, tramadol, pentazocine) or a combination of opioid and nonopioid medicine (e.g., oxycodone with acetaminophen, hydrocodone with ibuprofen) is provided with or without coanalgesic medications. If the client has moderate pain that persists or increases despite using full doses of step 2 medications, or if the pain is severe (7–10 on a 0–10 scale), then a step 3 regimen is medically indicated. At the third step, strong opiates (e.g., morphine,

---

BOX 18–5 **Categories and Examples of Analgesics**

Nonopioid Analgesics/NSAIDs

- Acetaminophen (Tylenol, Datril)
- Acetylsalicylic acid (aspirin)
- Choline magnesium trisalicylate (Trilisate)
- Diclofenac sodium (Voltaren)
- Ibuprofen (Motrin, Advil)
- Indomethacin sodium trihydrate (Indocin)
- Naproxen (Naprosyn), naproxen sodium (Anaprox)
- Celecoxib (Celebrex)
- Piroxicam (Feldene)
- Meloxicam (Mobic)

Mixed or Weak Opioid Analgesics

- Butorphanol (Stadol)
- Hydrocodone (Lortab, Vicodin)
- Codeine (Tylenol No. 3, Empirin No. 3)

- Tramadol (Ultram, Ultracet)
- Propoxyphene napsylate (Darvon-N, Darvocet-N)

Strong Opioid Analgesics

- Fentanyl citrate (Sublimaze, transdermal patches)
- Hydromorphone hydrochloride (Dilaudid)
- Meperidine hydrochloride (Demerol)
- Morphine sulfate (morphine)
- Methadone (Dolophiné)

Coanalgesics

- Tricyclic antidepressants (nortriptyline)
- Anticonvulsants (gabapentin)
- Topical local anesthetic (Lidoderm)
- Hydroxyzine (Vistaril)

---

hydromorphone, fentanyl) are administered and titrated in around-the-clock scheduled doses until the pain is relieved or dose-limiting respiratory depression occurs.

CLINICAL ALERT

Combining opioid and nonopioid analgesics is frequently overlooked. Each has different side effects, mechanisms of action, and toxicity profile. Alternating the two or giving them at the same time creates no danger and often produces a synergistic rather than merely additive effect.

NONOPIOIDS/NSAIDS Nonopioids include acetaminophen and **nonsteroidal anti-inflammatory drugs (NSAIDs)** such as ibuprofen or aspirin. NSAIDs have anti-inflammatory, analgesic, and antipyretic effects, whereas acetaminophen has only analgesic and antipyretic effects. Individual NSAIDs vary little in their analgesic potency, but do vary in their anti-inflammatory properties, metabolism, excretion, and side effects. These drugs have a ceiling effect and a narrow therapeutic index. The *ceiling effect* means that once the maximum analgesic benefit is achieved, more drug will not produce more analgesia; however, more toxicity may occur. The *narrow therapeutic index* indicates that there's not much mar-

---

TABLE 18–5 **Misconceptions about Nonopioids**

MISCONCEPTION	CORRECTION
Regular daily use of NSAIDs is much safer than taking opioids.	Side effects from long-term use of NSAIDs are considerably more severe and life threatening than the side effects from daily doses of oral morphine or other opioids. The most common side effect from long-term use of opioids is constipation, whereas NSAIDs can cause gastric ulcers, increased bleeding time, and renal insufficiency. Acetaminophen can cause hepatotoxicity.
A nonopioid should not be given at the same time as an opioid.	It is safe to administer a nonopioid and opioid at the same time. Giving a dose of nonopioid at the same time as a dose of opioid poses no more danger than giving the doses at different times. In fact, many opioids are compounded with a nonopioid (e.g., Percocet [oxycodone and acetaminophen]).
Administering antacids with NSAIDs is an effective method of reducing gastric distress.	Administering antacids with NSAIDs can lessen distress but may be counterproductive. Antacids reduce the absorption and therefore the effectiveness of the NSAID by releasing the drug in the stomach rather than in the small intestine where absorption occurs.
Nonopioids are not useful analgesics for severe pain.	Nonopioids alone are rarely sufficient to relieve severe pain, but they are an important part in the total analgesic plan. One of the basic principles of analgesic therapy is: Whenever pain is severe enough to require an opioid, adding a nonopioid should be considered.
Gastric distress (e.g., abdominal pain) is indicative of NSAID-induced gastric ulceration.	Most clients with gastric lesions have no symptoms until bleeding or perforation occurs.

Note: Reprinted from *Pain: Clinical Manual,* 2nd ed., by M. McCaffery and C. Pasero, 1999, St. Louis, MO: Mosby. Copyright © 1999, Mosby, Inc. with permission from Elsevier.

gin for safety between the dose that produces a desired effect and the dose that may produce a toxic, even lethal effect. The most common side effect of nonopioid analgesics is gastrointestinal, such as heartburn or indigestion. These effects can become toxic or lethal when silent GI bleeding occurs.

Acetaminophen (Tylenol), on the other hand, has a different mechanism of action and side effect/toxicity profile. It does not affect platelet function and rarely causes GI distress, ulcers, or kidney, skin, or cardiovascular problems. Hepatotoxicity, and possible renal toxicity, does occur with high doses or with long-term use. Given that acetaminophen is so well tolerated, it is often a hidden ingredient in over-the-counter (OTC) remedies, so clients must be instructed to read the ingredient list of all OTC medicines they take. Table 18–5 lists common misconceptions about nonopioids.

OPIOIDS There are three primary types of opioids:

1. *Full agonists.* These pure opioid drugs produce maximum pain inhibition, an agonist effect. A full **agonist analgesic** includes morphine, oxycodone, and hydromorphone. There is no ceiling on the level of analgesia from these drugs; their dose can be steadily increased to relieve pain. There is also no maximum daily dose limit unless they are in a compound with a nonopioid analgesic drug.
2. *Mixed agonists-antagonists.* **Agonist-antagonist analgesic** drugs can act like opioids and relieve pain (agonist effect) when given to a client who has not taken any pure opioids. However, they can block or inactivate other opioid analgesics when given to a client who has been taking pure opioids (antagonist effect). These drugs include dezocine, pentazocine hydrochloride, butorphanol tartrate, and nalbuphine hydrochloride. These drugs also have a ceiling effect that limits the dose. They are not recommended for use with terminally ill clients. In the opioid naïve client with acute pain, these agents have a favorable effect and low side effect burden.
3. *Partial agonists.* Partial agonists have a ceiling effect in contrast to a full agonist. These drugs have good analgesic potency and are emerging as alternatives to methadone for opioid maintenance/narcotic treatment programs. The safety and favorable side effect profile make it an increasingly popular choice.

Box 18–6 presents a sedation scale for assessing clients receiving opioids. Box 18–7 lists common opioid side effects, preventive, and treatment measures.

BOX 18–6	**Sedation Scale**

S = Sleep, easy to arouse

1 = Awake and alert

2 = Slightly drowsy, easily aroused

3 = Frequently drowsy, arousable, drifts off to sleep during conversation

4 = Somnolent, minimal or no response to physical stimulation

Note: Reprinted from *Pain: Clinical Manual,* 2nd ed. (p. 267), by M. McCaffery and C. Pasero, 1999, St. Louis, MO. Mosby. Copyright © 1999, Mosby, Inc. with permission from Elsevier.

BOX 18–7	**Common Opioid Side Effects, Preventive, and Treatment Measures**

Constipation

- Increase fluid intake (e.g., 6 to 8 glasses daily).
- Increase fiber and bulk-forming agents to the diet (e.g., fresh fruits and vegetables). Increasing exercise is often ineffective in controlling this type of constipation.
- Administer daily stool softeners combined with a mild laxative (e.g., Senokot-S) as a first line of prevention against constipation for clients on opioid maintenance therapy.
- Stimulants (bisacodyl), osmotic laxatives (lactulose, sorbitol, and polyethylene glycol), enemas (tap water and sodium phosphate), and even prokinetic agents (metoclopramide) may be needed for refractory cases of constipation (Kurz & Sessler, 2003).

Nausea and Vomiting

- Inform client that tolerance to this emetic effect generally develops after several days of opiate therapy.
- Provide an antiemetic (antihistamines [e.g., Vistaril, Phenergan], antimuscarinics [e.g., cyclizine, hyoscine], and dopamine receptor antagonists [e.g., Haldol]) as indicated.
- Change the dose or analgesic agent as indicated.

Sedation

- Inform client that tolerance usually develops over 3 to 5 days.
- Consider the administration of a stimulant (e.g., Dexedrine or Ritalin) or an alternative route of administration (e.g., epidural) for clients with persistent pain and sedation.
- Observe client for evidence of respiratory depression that may occur with sedation.

Respiratory Depression

- Administer an opioid antagonist, such as naloxone hydrochloride (Narcan), cautiously by diluting 1 ampule in 10 mL of saline and then administering 1 cc per minute until the respirations are ≥ 10/min. Make provisions for repeat administration, continuous infusion, or a longer acting version of a reversal agent as the half-life of naloxone is considerably shorter than most opioids being reversed.
- Stop, change, or slow the administration of opioids until respirations are restored.

Pruritus

- Apply cool packs, lotion, and diversional activity.
- Administer an antihistamine (e.g., diphenhydramine hydrochloride [Benadryl]).
- Inform the client that tolerance also develops to pruritus.

Urinary Retention

- May need to catheterize client, or change or lower the analgesic dose.
- Administer narcotic antagonist (naloxone hydrochloride [Narcan]) or longer-acting reversal agent (methylnaltrexone is pending FDA approval). Extreme caution is urged with the use of Narcan.

CLINICAL ALERT

Constipation is an almost universal adverse effect of opioid use. All clients should receive prophylactic stimulant laxative therapy, unless contraindicated. Stool softeners are not useful alone, but are a good choice when combined with a stimulant laxative (e.g., Senokot-S). If those products are ineffective, a regimen of cathartic laxatives (e.g., bisacodyl), followed by more aggressive forms of treatment (e.g., osmotic laxatives, enema, manual disimpaction) may be necessary.

Older clients are particularly sensitive to the analgesic properties of opioids and may require less medication, or medication administered at less frequent intervals, than younger clients. This sensitivity may be related to reduced or delayed excretion of the drug in older adults. As such, the clinical pearl of "start low (25%–50% dose reduction) and go (titrate) slow" is often followed in the older population (AGS, 2002).

CLINICAL ALERT

Assessing for sedation and respiratory status is critical during the first 12 to 24 hours after starting opioid therapy. The most critical period is during the peak effect of the first dose (15 minutes if administered IV; first hour after IM, oral, or rectal route). An exception is with opioids administered via the spinal route. Respiratory depression may increase over time with epidural infusions and with intrathecal analgesia; respiratory depression may manifest 24 hours after the spinal injection even after the analgesic effect has worn off. In general, the longer the client receives opioids, the wider the safety margin as the client develops a tolerance to the sedative and respiratory depressive effects of the drug.

EQUIANALGESIC DOSING The term **equianalgesia** refers to the relative potency of various opioid analgesics compared to a standard dose of parenteral morphine. This tool helps professionals individualize the analgesic regimen by guiding the adjustment of medication, dose, time interval, and route of administration. An equianalgesic chart can be used to help provide doses of approximately equal ability to relieve pain. The two basic techniques for calculating doses based on equianalgesic equivalents are ratio and cross-multiplication methods. For example, with the ratio technique, it is known that the oral:IV morphine ratio is 3:1, meaning IV morphine is 3 times more potent than oral morphine. Thus, a client who has required 100 mg of IV morphine per day will require 300 mg of oral morphine per day to control the same level of pain.

CLINICAL ALERT

Many health care professionals underestimate the effectiveness of ordinary aspirin and acetaminophen. The ordinary dose of aspirin or acetaminophen relieves as much pain as 1.5 mg of parenteral morphine, whereas standard doses of mixed analgesics (e.g., Tylenol No. 3 or Percocet) are approximately equivalent to 2.5 to 5 mg of parenteral morphine.

COANALGESICS A **coanalgesic** agent (formerly known as an adjuvant) is a medication that is not classified as a pain medication. However, coanalgesics have properties that may reduce pain alone or in combination with other analgesics, relieve other discomforts, potentiate the effect of pain medications, or reduce the pain medication's side effects. Examples of coanalgesics that relieve pain are antidepressants (support the function of the pain-modulating system); anticonvulsants (stabilize nerve membranes, reducing excitability and spontaneous firing); and local anesthetics (block the transmission of pain signals). Anxiolytics, sedatives, and antispasmodics are examples of medicines that relieve other discomforts; however, they do not alleviate pain and thus should be used in addition to rather than instead of analgesics. Examples of medications used to reduce the side effects of analgesics include stimulants, laxatives, and antiemetics. Coanalgesics appear to be particularly beneficial for the management of neuropathic pain.

ADMINISTRATION OF PLACEBOS A **placebo** is "any medication or procedure, including surgery, which produces an effect in a client because of its implicit or explicit intent and not because of its specific physical or chemical properties" (McCaffery & Pasero, 1999). *Placebos* often take the form of sugar pills, saline injections, minuscule doses of drugs, or sham procedures designed to be void of any known therapeutic value. In contrast, the *placebo effect* is a perceptible, measurable, and desirable consequence that exceeds the anticipated biological changes and may occur as a result of interpersonal factors such as the presence of a caring person or a healing intent (Arnstein, 2003). Some professionals try to justify the use of placebos to elicit the desirable placebo effect or in a misguided attempt to determine if the client's pain is "real." The use of placebos, outside the context of an approved research study, is deceptive and represents fraudulent and unethical treatment. The American Society for Pain Management Nursing (2005) and other professional organizations have published position papers that adamantly oppose the use of placebos without consent.

ROUTES FOR OPIATE DELIVERY Opioids have traditionally been administered by oral, subcutaneous, intramuscular, and intravenous routes. In addition, newer methods of delivering opiates have been developed to circumvent potential obstacles that occur with these traditional routes. Examples are transnasal, transmucosal, and transdermal drug therapy, continuous subcutaneous infusions, and intraspinal infusion (Table 18–6).

CLINICAL ALERT

As a precaution, have naloxone (Narcan), sodium chloride 0.9% diluent, and injection equipment on hand for each client receiving an opioid-containing epidural infusion.

TABLE 18–6 Nursing Interventions for Clients Receiving Analgesics through an Epidural Catheter

NURSING GOALS	INTERVENTIONS
Maintain client safety	Label the tubing, the infusion bag, and the front of the pump with tape marked EPIDURAL to prevent confusion with similar-looking IV lines. Post sign above client's bed indicating epidural is in place. Secure all connections with tape. If there is no continuous infusion, apply tape over all injection ports on the epidural line to avoid the injection of substances intended for IV administration into the epidural catheter. Do not use alcohol in any care of catheter or insertion site as it can be neurotoxic. Ensure that any solution injected or infused intraspinally is sterile, preservative-free, and safe for intraspinal administration.
Maintain catheter placement	Secure temporary catheters with tape. When bolus doses are used, gently aspirate prior to medication administration to determine catheter has not migrated into the subarachnoid space. (Expect < 1 mL of fluid return in syringe.) Assist client in repositioning or moving out of bed. Teach client to avoid tugging on the catheter. Assess insertion site for leakage with each bolus dose or at least every 8–12 hours.
Prevent infection	Use strict aseptic techniques with all epidural-related procedures. Maintain sterile occlusive dressing over insertion site. Assess insertion site for signs of infection. Assess for increasing diffuse back pain or tenderness and/or paresthesia on intraspinal injection because these are cardinal signs of intraspinal infection (McCaffery & Pasero, 1999, p. 234).
Maintain urinary and bowel function	Monitor intake and output. Assess for bowel and bladder distention.
Prevent respiratory depression	Assess sedation level and respiratory status q1h for the first 24 hours and thereafter q4h. Do not administer other opioids or central nervous system depressants unless ordered. Keep an ampule of naloxone hydrochloride (0.4 mg) at the bedside. Notify the clinician in charge if the respiratory rate falls below 8 per minute or if the client is difficult to rouse.

Continuous Local Anesthetics   Continuous subcutaneous administration of long-acting local anesthetics into or near the surgical site is a technique being used to provide post-operative pain control. This technique has been used for a variety of surgical procedures, including knee arthroplasty, abdominal hysterectomy, hernia repair, and mastectomy. Nursing interventions for the client with infusion of a continuous local anesthetic include:

- Conduct pain assessment and documentation every 2 to 4 hours while the client is awake.
- Check the dressing every shift for intactness. The dressing is not usually changed in order to avoid dislodging the catheter. Contact the primary care provider if the dressing becomes loose.
- Check the site of the catheter. It should be clean and dry.
- Assess the client for signs of local anesthetic toxicity (e.g., cardiac arrhythmias, dizziness; ringing in the ears; a metallic taste; tingling or numbness of the lips, gums, or tongue) or neurological deficit distal to the catheter insertion site.
- Notify the primary care provider of signs of local anesthetic toxicity or neurological deficit. If detected early, prompt treatment can be initiated and serious complications avoided.

PATIENT-CONTROLLED ANALGESIA   **Patient-controlled analgesia (PCA)** is an interactive method of pain management that permits clients to treat their pain by self-administering doses of analgesics. The oral route for PCA is most common, but the subcutaneous, intravenous, and epidural routes are also used. The PCA mode of therapy minimizes the roller-coaster effect of peaks of sedation and valleys of pain that occur with the traditional method of prn dosing. With the parenteral routes, the client administers a predetermined dose of a narcotic by an electronic infusion pump. This allows the client to maintain a more constant level of comfort yet need less medication for pain relief. Patient-controlled analgesias can be effectively used for clients with acute pain related to a surgical incision, traumatic injury, or labor and delivery, and for chronic severe pain such as cancer. In some settings PCAs are used even if the client is unable to initiate a dose by pushing the button, as long as a caregiver is willing to accept the responsibility, but strict protocols and vigilant monitoring are required to prevent sentinel events.

The prescriber orders the analgesic dose, route, and frequency, with the client administering the medication. The nurse is responsible for the initial instruction regarding use of the PCA and for the ongoing monitoring of the therapy. The client's pain, ability to understand, and use of the device must be assessed at regular intervals, and analgesic use is documented in the client's record.

Patient-controlled analgesia pumps are designed with built-in safety mechanisms to prevent client overdosage, abusive use, and narcotic theft. The most significant adverse effects are respiratory depression and hypotension; however, they occur rarely. Although PCA pumps vary in design, they all have similar protective features. The line of the PCA pump, a syringe-type pump, is usually introduced into the injection port of a primary IV fluid line (Figure 18–3). When clients want a dose of analgesic, they can push a button attached to the infusion pump and the preset dose is delivered. A programmable lockout interval (usually 6 to 15 minutes) follows the dose, during which an additional dose cannot be given even if the client activates the button. It is also possible to program the maximum dose that can be delivered over a period of hours (usually 4). Many pumps

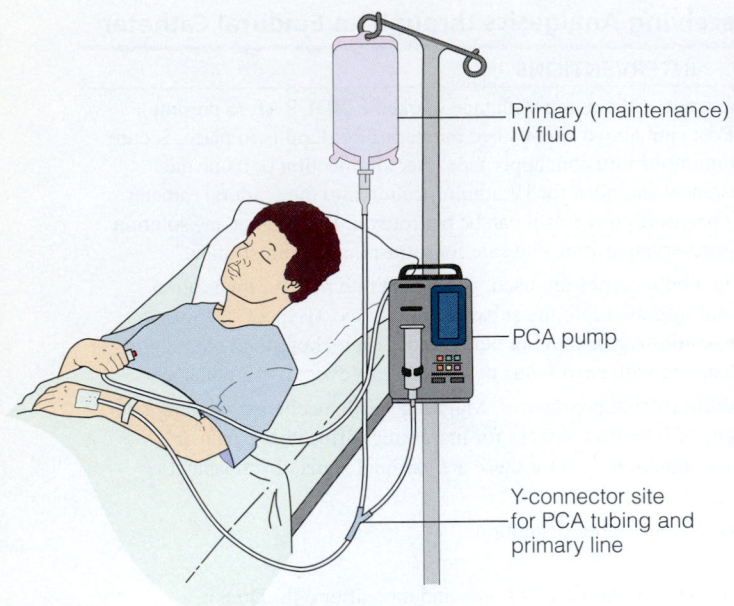

Primary (maintenance) IV fluid

PCA pump

Y-connector site for PCA tubing and primary line

Figure 18–3 ● PCA line introduced into the injection port of a primary line.

are capable of delivering a basal rate (continuous infusion), with or without additional PCA doses available.

Nonpharmacologic Pain Management

Nonpharmacologic pain management consists of a variety of physical, cognitive-behavioral, and lifestyle pain management strategies that target the body, mind, spirit, and social interactions. Physical modalities include cutaneous stimulation, ice or heat, immobilization or therapeutic exercises, transcutaneous electrical nerve stimulation (TENS), and acupuncture. Mind–body (cognitive-behavioral) interventions include distracting activities, relaxation techniques, imagery, meditation, biofeedback, hypnosis, cognitive-reframing, emotional counseling, and spiritually-directed approaches such as therapeutic touch or Reiki. Lifestyle management approaches include symptom monitoring, stress management, exercise, nutrition, pacing activities, disability management, and other approaches needed by many clients with persistent pain that has drastically changed their life. For further information on selected mind–body interventions and acupuncture, see Chapter 5 ∞.

PHYSICAL INTERVENTIONS The goals of physical intervention include providing comfort, altering physiologic responses to reduce pain perception, and optimizing functioning.

Cutaneous Stimulation Cutaneous stimulation can provide effective temporary pain relief. It distracts the client and focuses attention on the tactile stimuli, away from the painful sensations, thus reducing pain perception. Cutaneous stimulation is also believed to interfere with the transmission and perception of pain by stimulating the large-diameter A-beta sensory nerve fibers that activate the descending mechanisms that can reduce the intensity of pain, activate the endorphin system of pain control, and thus diminish conscious awareness of pain. Selected cutaneous stimulation techniques include massage, application of heat or cold, acupressure, and contralateral stimulation.

Cutaneous stimulation can be applied directly to the painful area, proximal to the pain or distal to the pain (along the nerve path or dermatome), and contralateral (exact location, opposite side of the body) to the pain. Cutaneous stimulation is contraindicated in areas of skin breakdown or impaired neurological functioning.

Massage Massage is a comfort measure that can aid relaxation, decrease muscle tension, and may ease anxiety because the physical contact communicates caring. It can also decrease pain intensity by increasing superficial circulation to the area. Massage can involve the back and neck, hands and arms, or feet. The use of ointments or liniments may provide localized pain relief with joint or muscle pain. Massage is contraindicated in areas of skin breakdown, suspected clots, or infections. See Skill 18–1.

SKILL 18–1

PROVIDING A BACK MASSAGE

Effleurage is a type of massage consisting of long, slow, gliding strokes. Research demonstrates that back massage can enhance client comfort and relaxation and have a positive effect on cardiovascular parameters such as blood pressure, heart rate, and respiratory rate (McNamara, Burnham, Smith, & Carroll, 2003).

PURPOSES
- To relieve muscle tension
- To decrease pain intensity
- To promote physical and mental relaxation

ASSESSMENT
Assess the following:
- Behaviors indicating potential need for a back massage, such as a complaint of stiffness, muscle tension in the back or shoulders, or difficulty sleeping related to tenseness or anxiety
- Whether the client is willing to have a massage (cultural considerations and personal preference may make massage uncomfortable or undesirable for some clients)
- Contraindications for back massage (e.g., coagulation issues, clots, impaired skin integrity, back surgery, vertebral issues, or risk of fracture)

PLANNING
Ensure that you have the full amount of time available for the massage. Although the actual technique may require only about 5 minutes, the entire process should be conducted in a calm and unhurried manner.

Delegation
The nurse can delegate this skill to UAP; however, the nurse should first assess for any contraindications and client willingness.

EQUIPMENT
- Lotion (assess client allergies prior to choosing lotion)
- Towel for excess lotion

IMPLEMENTATION

Preparation
Determine (a) previous assessments of the skin, (b) special lotions to be used, and (c) positions contraindicated for the client. Arrange for a quiet environment with no interruptions to promote maximum effect of the back massage.

Performance
1. Prior to performing the procedure, introduce self and verify the client's identity using agency protocol. Explain to the client what you are going to do, why it is necessary, and how he or she can cooperate. Encourage the client to give you feedback as to the amount of pressure you are using during the back rub. **Rationale:** *Client anxiety is reduced by knowing who you are, what you are planning to do, and involving the client in the process.*
2. Perform hand hygiene. **Rationale:** *Reduce the risk of pathogen exposure.*
3. Provide for client privacy. **Rationale:** *Reduce anxiety, allowing the client to relax without modesty concerns.*
4. Prepare the client.
   - Assist the client to move to the near side of the bed within your reach and adjust the bed to a comfortable working height. **Rationale:** *Placing the client close to you and at an appropriate height will prevent back strain.*
   - Establish which position the client prefers. The prone position is recommended for a back rub. The side-lying position can be used if a client cannot assume the prone position. **Rationale:** *Positioning the client for comfort based on physiological needs will improve the effectiveness of the massage.*
   - Expose the back from the shoulders to the inferior sacral area. Cover the remainder of the body. **Rationale:** *Prevent chilling and minimize exposure.*

5. Massage the back.
   - Pour a small amount of lotion onto the palms of your hands and hold it for a minute. The lotion bottle can also be placed in a bath basin filled with warm water. **Rationale:** *Lotions are often uncomfortably cold. Warming the solution facilitates client comfort and prevents chilling.*
   - Using your palm, begin in the sacral area using smooth, circular strokes.
   - Move your hands up the center of the back and then over both scapulae. **Rationale:** *Moving from distal to proximal improves venous blood return.*
   - Massage in a circular motion over the scapulae. **Rationale:** *Tension is often greatest in the upper back and shoulder areas.*
   - Move your hands down the sides of the back.
   - Massage the areas over the right and left iliac crests.
   - Apply firm, continuous pressure without breaking contact with the client's skin.
   - Repeat above for 3 to 5 minutes, obtaining more lotion as necessary. **Rationale:** *As lotion is absorbed into the skin apply more lotion to prevent friction injuries from hands moving over dry skin.*
   - While massaging the back, assess for skin redness and areas of decreased circulation. **Rationale:** *Learning to combine assessment skills with performance of procedures is effective and efficient. While the skin is exposed, assess for any abnormalities or unexpected findings.*
   - Pat dry any excess lotion with a towel. **Rationale:** *Allowing excess lotion to remain may be uncomfortable for the client and damp skin can be chilling.*
6. Document that a back rub was performed and the client's response. Record any unusual findings.

(continued)

PROVIDING A BACK MASSAGE *(continued)*

SAMPLE DOCUMENTATION

1/18/2010 1400 c/o aching, intermittent back pain. Wincing and grimacing when attempting to move in bed. Rates pain at 4–5 on 0–10 scale. States uses massage to help relieve pain when at home. Percocet given. Back massaged. Stated the massage helped him "to relax." Lights dimmed and door to room close.

——————————————— B. Burt, RN

1430 Rates pain at 1–2/10. States feels "much more comfortable." Moving in bed with ease. —————— D. Aubrey, RN

EVALUATION

Compare the client's current response to previous response. Is there a positive client outcome such as increased relaxation, decrease in pain, and/or decreased anxiety because of the back massage?

Heat and Cold Applications A warm bath, heating pads, ice bags, ice massage, hot or cold compresses, and warm or cold sitz baths in general relieve pain and promote healing of injured tissues (see Chapter 24 ∞).

Acupressure Acupressure developed from the ancient Chinese healing system of acupuncture. The therapist applies finger pressure to points that correspond to many of the points used in acupuncture (see Chapter 5 ∞).

Contralateral Stimulation Contralateral stimulation can be accomplished by stimulating the skin in an area opposite to the painful area. The contralateral area may be scratched for itching, massaged for cramps, or treated with cold packs or analgesic ointments. This method is particularly useful when the painful area cannot be touched because it is hypersensitive, when it is inaccessible by a cast or bandages, or when the pain is felt in a missing part (phantom pain).

Immobilization/Bracing Immobilizing or restricting the movement of a painful body part may help to manage episodes of acute pain. Splints or supportive devices should hold joints in the position of optimal function and should be removed regularly in accordance with agency protocol to provide range-of-motion (ROM) exercises. Prolonged immobilization can result in joint contracture, muscle atrophy, and cardiovascular problems. Therefore, clients should be encouraged to participate in self-care activities and remain as active as possible, with frequent ROM exercises.

Transcutaneous Electrical Nerve Stimulation Transcutaneous electrical nerve stimulation (TENS) is a method of applying low-voltage electrical stimulation directly over identified pain areas, at an acupressure point, along peripheral nerve areas that innervate the pain area, or along the spinal column. The TENS unit consists of a portable, battery-operated device with lead wire and electrode pads that are applied to the chosen area of skin (Figure 18–4). Cutaneous stimulation from the TENS unit is thought to activate large-diameter fibers that modulate the transmission of the nociceptive impulse in the peripheral and central nervous system (closing the pain "gate"), resulting in pain relief. This stimulation may also cause a release of endorphins from the CNS centers. The use of

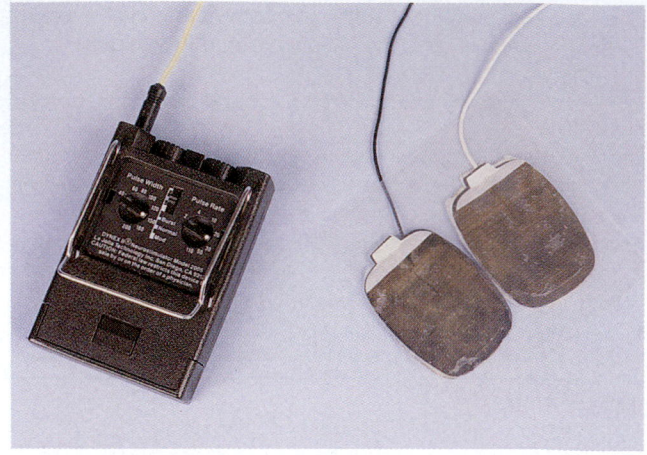

Figure 18–4 ⬤ A transcutaneous electric nerve stimulator.

TENS is contraindicated for clients with pacemakers or arrhythmias, or in areas of skin breakdown. It is generally not used on the head or over the chest.

COGNITIVE-BEHAVIORAL INTERVENTIONS The goals of cognitive-behavioral interventions include providing comfort, altering psychologic responses to reduce pain perception, and optimizing functioning. Selected cognitive-behavioral interventions include distraction, eliciting the relaxation response, repatterning thinking, and facilitating coping with emotions.

Distraction Distraction draws the person's attention away from the pain and lessens the perception of pain. In some instances, distraction can make a client completely unaware of pain. Distraction makes the person unaware of the pain only for the amount of time and to the extent that the distracting activity holds his or her "undivided" attention. For example, a client recovering from surgery may feel no pain while watching a football game on television, yet feel pain again during commercials or when the game is over. Different types of distractions are shown in Box 18–8. Using multiple forms of distraction simultaneously adds value to the activity. For example, listening to music can be distracting; however, the value can be added by tapping to the music, singing along, or playing along on a musical instrument.

BOX 18–8	**Types of Distraction**

Visual Distraction

- Reading or watching TV
- Watching a baseball game
- Guided imagery

Auditory Distraction

- Humor
- Listening to music

Tactile Distraction

- Slow, rhythmic breathing
- Massage
- Holding or stroking a pet or toy

Intellectual Distraction

- Crossword puzzles
- Card games (e.g., bridge)
- Hobbies (e.g., stamp collecting, writing a story)

Eliciting the Relaxation Response Stress increases pain, in part by increasing muscle tension, activating the sympathetic nervous system, and putting the client at risk for stress-related types of pain. The relaxation response decreases and counteracts the harmful effects of stress, including the effect it has on physical, cognitive, and emotional functioning. Eliciting this response requires more than simply helping a person relax; rather it involves a structured technique designed to focus the mind and relax muscle groups. Basic techniques with helpful scripts are detailed by McCaffery and Pasero (1999), with common techniques including progressive relaxation, breath-focus relaxation, and meditation. The nurse can coach the client, urge self-directed meditation, or provide an audiotaped guide to help elicit the relaxation response. Many clients can achieve the desired state after a few attempts, but mastery of this skill requires daily practice over a few weeks. In general, relaxation techniques by themselves do not have remarkable pain-relieving properties; however, they can reduce pain that may have been exacerbated by stress. Some clients may become more consciously aware of their pain while practicing relaxation techniques before they have learned mastery of controlling "mind chatter" and remaining mentally focused.

Once the client has mastered the basic skills for eliciting the relaxation response, techniques of imagery or self-hypnosis can be used. Both imagery and hypnosis begin with attaining a deep state of relaxation and are capable of altering the experience of pain; for example, having the client replace the pain with a feeling of pleasant numbness (Arnstein, 2004). Additional posthypnotic suggestions can then be made, linking these pleasant numb sensations to coping efforts used during the day.

Repatterning Unhelpful Thinking Some people harbor strong self-doubts, unrealistic expectations, rumination, helplessness, and magnification. These cognitive patterns have been identified as important contributors to treatment failures, the intensification of pain, disability, and depression (Arnstein, Caudill, Mandle, Norris, & Beasley, 1999; DeGood & Kiernan, 1997). Nurses can help by challenging the truthfulness and helpfulness of these thoughts, and replacing them with realistic and confidence-building ones that are particularly powerful predictors of more effective coping, better clinical outcomes, and improved quality of life (Caudill, 2002).

Facilitating Coping Nurses can help by intervening with clients who are anxious, are sad, or express overly pessimistic or helpless points of view. Awareness of the client's misperceptions or unrealistic expectations also helps the professional avoid a common cause of therapeutic failure. Therapeutic communication with an emphasis on listening, providing encouragement, teaching self-management skills, sharing vicarious experiences, and persuading them to act on their own behalf are strategies that enhance coping. Helping clients to better communicate with the professional staff, family members, and friends can also promote coping. Counseling from trained professionals may be indicated for those clients with severe emotional distress, but must be offered to them in a sensitive way that does not convey the notion that pain is "in their head."

Selected Spiritual Interventions The spiritual dimension encompasses a person's innermost concerns and values, including the ascribed purpose, meaning, and driving force in his or her life. It may include rituals that help the individual become part of a community, or feel a bond with the universe that is not necessarily religious in nature. For those who express their spirituality in a religious context, it is appropriate to offer prayer, intercessory prayer (being prayed for by others), or access to meaningful rituals. For some clients, a caring presence, attentive listening, and facilitating the process of acceptance can help reduce spiritual distress, whereas other clients benefit from manipulation of energy patterns.

Through improved spiritual insights, individuals with pain can find meaning in what seems incomprehensible and learn to cope with the intolerable. This process often begins by making peace with their past, being spiritually aware in the present, and making a commitment to go forward with life despite the pain (St. Marie & Arnold, 2002). By shifting awareness from within to external sources of power, pain sufferers can transcend the limits of their pain to find new energy and a renewed sense of purpose.

NONPHARMACOLOGIC INVASIVE THERAPIES A **nerve block** is a chemical interruption of a nerve pathway, effected by injecting a local anesthetic into the nerve. Nerve blocks are widely used during dental work. The injected drug blocks nerve pathways from the painful tooth, thus stopping the transmission of pain impulses to the brain. Nerve blocks are often used to relieve the pain of whiplash injury, lower back disorders, bursitis, and cancer. With the intention of quieting "pain generators" (irritable nerves that cause the pain), a combination of a long-acting local anesthetic and a steroid is injected adjacent to the problem nerve. The local anesthetic should provide relief for several hours, before the effect of the steroid begins a day or two later. Often a series of three injections are scheduled weeks or months apart. Each subsequent injection should result in a longer duration of pain relief. No more than three injections per year are recommended because of the mineral-robbing effect steroids have on bones in the area. For longer lasting results after a nerve block has worked, more permanent blocks may be attempted. The "permanent" blocks involve damaging nerves with alcohol, phenol, or radio frequency (heat). These nerve-killing procedures are controversial, as nerve fibers often regenerate and the pain returns in a significant proportion of clients.

Pain conduction pathways can be interrupted surgically. Because this disruption is permanent, surgery is performed only as a last resort, generally for intractable pain. A cordotomy obliterates pain. Temperature sensation below the level of the spinothalamic portion of the anterolateral tract is severed. This procedure is usually done for pain in the legs and trunk. **Rhizotomy** interrupts the anterior or posterior nerve root between the ganglion and the cord. Interruption of anterior motor nerve roots stops spasmodic movements that accompany paraplegia. Interruption of posterior sensory nerve roots eliminates pain in areas innervated by that specific nerve root. Rhizotomies are generally performed on cervical nerve roots to alleviate pain of the head and neck from cancer or neuralgia, and increasingly they use radio frequency technologies.

In **neurectomy**, peripheral or cranial nerves are interrupted to alleviate localized pain, such as pain in the lower leg or foot arising from a vascular occlusion. In a **sympathectomy**, pathways of the sympathetic division of the autonomic nervous system are severed. This procedure eliminates vasospasm, improves peripheral blood supply, and thus is effective in treating painful vascular disorders such as Raynaud's disease.

Spinal cord stimulation (SCS) is used with persistent pain that has not been controlled with less invasive therapies. SCS involves the insertion of an electrode (may be a single channel or multichannel device) adjacent to the spinal cord in the epidural space. The electrode(s) is attached to an impulse-generator (external or implanted) that sends electric impulses to the spinal cord to control pain. The client is awake during the insertion procedure to aid in the optimal placement of the electrodes.

EVALUATING

The goals established in the planning phase are evaluated according to specific desired outcomes, also established in that phase (see the Identifying Nursing Diagnoses, Outcomes, and Interventions box earlier in this chapter). To assist in the evaluation process, flow sheet records or a client diary may be helpful. A weekly log or diary can be structured in a similar fashion for the individual client.

LIFESPAN CONSIDERATIONS
Pain Management

Infants

- Giving an infant, particularly a very-low-birth-weight infant, a water and sucrose solution administered through a pacifier provides some evidence of pain reduction during procedures that may be painful, but should not be a substitute for anesthetic or analgesic medications.

Children

- Distract the child with toys, books, or pictures.
- Hold the child to console and promote comfort.
- Explore misconceptions about pain and correct in understandable "concrete" terms. Be aware of how your explanations may be misunderstood. For example, telling a child they won't hurt during surgery because they will be "put to sleep" will be very upsetting to a child who knows of an animal that was "put to sleep."
- Children can use their imagination during guided imagery. Ask the child to imagine a "pain switch" (even give it a color) and to visualize turning the switch off in the area where there is pain. A "magic glove" or "magic blanket" is an imaginary object that the child applies on areas of the body (e.g., hand, thigh, back, hip) to lessen discomfort.

Older Adults

- Promote the client's use of pain control measures that have worked in the past for them.
- Spend time with the client and listen carefully.
- Clarify misconceptions. Encourage independence whenever possible.
- Carefully review the treatment plan to avoid drug–drug, food–drug, or disease–drug interactions.

CLINICAL ALERT

The statement "Please tell me how I can best help you control your pain" sends a couple of subtle messages that are an important part of treatment planning and evaluation of care. First, it places the ownership and responsibility for controlling pain on the client. Second, it acknowledges that the client may be the best judge of what is needed, respecting the cultural meaning of pain and acceptable ways of expressing/controlling pain. Third, it establishes the nurse's role in helping the client be more comfortable and in control of his or her condition.

If outcomes are not achieved, the nurse and client need to explore the reasons before modifying the care plan. The nurse might consider the following questions:

- Is adequate analgesic being given? Would the client benefit from a change in dose or in the time interval between doses?
- Were the client's beliefs, expectations, and values about pain therapy considered?

- Did the client understate the pain experience for some reason?
- Were appropriate instructions provided to allay misconceptions about pain management?
- Did the client and support people understand the instructions about pain management techniques?

- Is the client receiving adequate support for both physical pain and emotional distress?
- Has the client's physical condition changed, necessitating modifications in interventions?
- Should selected intervention strategies be reevaluated?

See the Nursing Care Plan and the Concept Map.

Nursing Care Plan   Acute Pain

ASSESSMENT DATA	NURSING DIAGNOSIS	DESIRED OUTCOMES*
Nursing Assessment Mr. C. is a 57-year-old businessman who was admitted to the surgical unit for treatment of a possible strangulated inguinal hernia. Two days ago he had a partial bowel resection. Postoperative orders include NPO, intravenous infusion of D51/2 NS at 125 cc/hr left arm, nasogastric tube to low intermittent suction. Mr. C. is in a dorsal recumbent (supine) position and is attempting to draw up his legs. He appears restless and is complaining of abdominal pain (7 on a scale of 0–10).	*Acute Pain* related to tissue injury secondary to surgical intervention (as evidenced by restlessness; pallor; elevated pulse, respirations, and systolic blood pressure; dilated pupils; and report of 7/10 abdominal pain)	**Pain Control** [1605] as evidenced by often demonstrating ability to • Use analgesics appropriately • Use nonanalgesic relief measures • Report uncontrolled symptoms to health care professional **Pain Level** [2102] As evidenced by mild to no • Reported pain • Protective body positioning • Restlessness • Pupil dilation • Perspiration • Change in BP, HR, R from normal baseline data
Physical Examination Height: 188 cm (6' 3") Weight: 90.0 kg (200 lb) Temperature: 37°C (98.6°F) Pulse: 90 BPM Respirations: 24/minute Blood pressure: 158/82 mm Hg Skin pale and moist, pupils dilated. Midline abdominal incision, sutures dry and intact. **Diagnostic Data** Chest x-ray and urinalysis negative, WBC 12,000		

NURSING INTERVENTIONS*/SELECTED ACTIVITIES	RATIONALE
Pain Management [1400]	
Perform a comprehensive assessment of pain to include location, characteristics, onset, duration, frequency, quality, intensity or severity, and precipitating factors of pain.	*Pain is a subjective experience and must be described by the client in order to plan effective treatment.*
Consider cultural influences on pain response (e.g., cultural beliefs about pain may result in a stoic attitude).	*Each person experiences and expresses pain in an individual manner using a variety of sociocultural adaptation techniques.*
Reduce or eliminate factors that precipitate or increase Mr. C.'s pain experience (e.g., fear, fatigue, monotony, and lack of knowledge).	*Personal factors can influence pain and pain tolerance. Factors that may be precipitating or augmenting pain should be reduced or eliminated to enhance the overall pain management program.*
Teach the use of nonpharmacologic techniques (e.g., relaxation, guided imagery, music therapy, distraction, and massage) before, after, and if possible during painful activities; before pain occurs or increases; and along with other pain relief measures.	*The use of noninvasive pain relief measures can increase the release of endorphins and enhance the therapeutic effects of pain relief medications.*
Provide Mr. C. optimal pain relief with prescribed analgesics.	*Each client has a right to expect maximum pain relief. Optimal pain relief using analgesics includes determining the preferred route, drug, dosage, and frequency for each individual. Medications ordered on a prn basis should be offered to the client at the interval when the next dose is available.*
Medicate before an activity to increase participation, but evaluate the hazard of sedation.	*Turning and ambulation activities will be enhanced if pain is controlled or tolerable. Assessing level of sedation should precede the activity to ensure necessary safety precautions are put in place.*

(continued)

Nursing Care Plan   Acute Pain (continued)

NURSING INTERVENTIONS*/SELECTED ACTIVITIES	RATIONALE
Evaluate the effectiveness of the pain control measures used through ongoing assessment of Mr. C.'s pain experience.	Research shows that the most common reason for unrelieved pain is failure to routinely assess pain and pain relief. Many clients silently tolerate pain if not specifically asked about it.

Analgesic Administration [2210]

Check the medical order for drug, dose, and frequency of analgesic prescribed.	Ensures that the nurse has the right drug, right route, right dosage, right client, right frequency.
Determine analgesic selections (narcotic, nonnarcotic, or NSAID) based on type and severity of pain.	Various types of pain (e.g., acute, chronic, neuropathic, nociceptive) require different analgesic approaches. Some types of pain respond to nonopioid drugs alone, while others can be relieved by combining a low-dose opioid with a nonopioid.
Institute safety precautions as appropriate if Mr. C. receives narcotic analgesics.	Side effects of opioid narcotics include drowsiness and sedation.
Instruct Mr. C. to request prn pain medication before the pain is severe.	Severe pain is more difficult to control and increases the client's anxiety and fatigue. The preventive approach to pain management can reduce the total 24-hour analgesic dose.
Evaluate the effectiveness of analgesic at regular, frequent intervals after each administration and especially after the initial doses, also observing for any signs and symptoms of untoward effects (e.g., respiratory depression, nausea and vomiting, dry mouth, and constipation).	The analgesic dose may not be adequate to raise the client's pain threshold or may be causing intolerable or dangerous side effects or both. Ongoing evaluation will assist in making necessary adjustments for effective pain management.
Document Mr. C.'s response to analgesics and any untoward effects.	Documentation facilitates pain management by communicating effective and noneffective pain management strategies to the entire health care team.
Implement actions to decrease untoward effects of analgesics (e.g., constipation and gastric irritation).	Constipation is a common side effect of opioid narcotics, and a treatment plan to prevent occurrence should be instituted at the beginning of analgesic therapy. For Mr. C., constipation could result from his primary condition or his analgesia. Assess for overall GI functioning, possible complications of surgery (e.g., ileus), as well as opioid-induced constipation or NSAID-induced gastritis.

Simple Relaxation Therapy [6040]

Consider Mr. C.'s willingness and ability to participate, preference, past experiences, and contraindications before selecting a specific relaxation strategy.	The client must feel comfortable trying a different approach to pain management. To avoid ineffective strategies, the client should be involved in the planning process.
Elicit behaviors that are conditioned to produce relaxation, such as deep breathing, yawning, abdominal breathing, or peaceful imaging.	Relaxation techniques help reduce skeletal muscle tension, which will reduce the intensity of the pain.
Create a quiet, nondisruptive environment with dim lights and comfortable temperature when possible.	Comfort and a quiet atmosphere promote a relaxed feeling and permit the client to focus on the relaxation technique rather than external distraction.
Individualize the content of the relaxation intervention (e.g., by asking for suggestions about what Mr. C. enjoys or finds relaxing).	Each person may find different images or approaches to relaxation more helpful than others. The nurse should have a variety of relaxation scripts or audiovisual aids to help clients find the best one for them.
Demonstrate and practice the relaxation technique with Mr. C.	Return demonstrations by the participant provide an opportunity for the nurse to evaluate the effectiveness of teaching sessions.
Evaluate and document his response to relaxation therapy.	Conveys to the health care team effective strategies in reducing or eliminating pain.

EVALUATION

Outcomes partially met. The client verbalizes pain and discomfort, requesting analgesics at onset of pain. States "the pain is a 2" (on a scale of 0–10) 30 minutes after a parenteral analgesic administration. Requests analgesic 30 minutes before ambulation. States willingness to try relaxation techniques; however, has not attempted to do so.

The NOC # for desired outcomes and the NIC # for nursing interventions are listed in brackets following the appropriate outcome or intervention. Outcomes, indicators, interventions, and activities selected are only a sample of those suggested by NOC and NIC and should be further individualized for each client.

CRITICAL THINKING QUESTIONS

1. Is there any other assessment data you would want to gather to help plan Mr. C.'s pain management?

2. Mr. C. does not have a PCA. What nursing interventions are important?

3. What kind of data would you gather prior to having a discussion with the primary care provider about options for improving pain control in this client?

∞ *See Answers in MyNursingKit.*

CONCEPT MAP Acute Pain

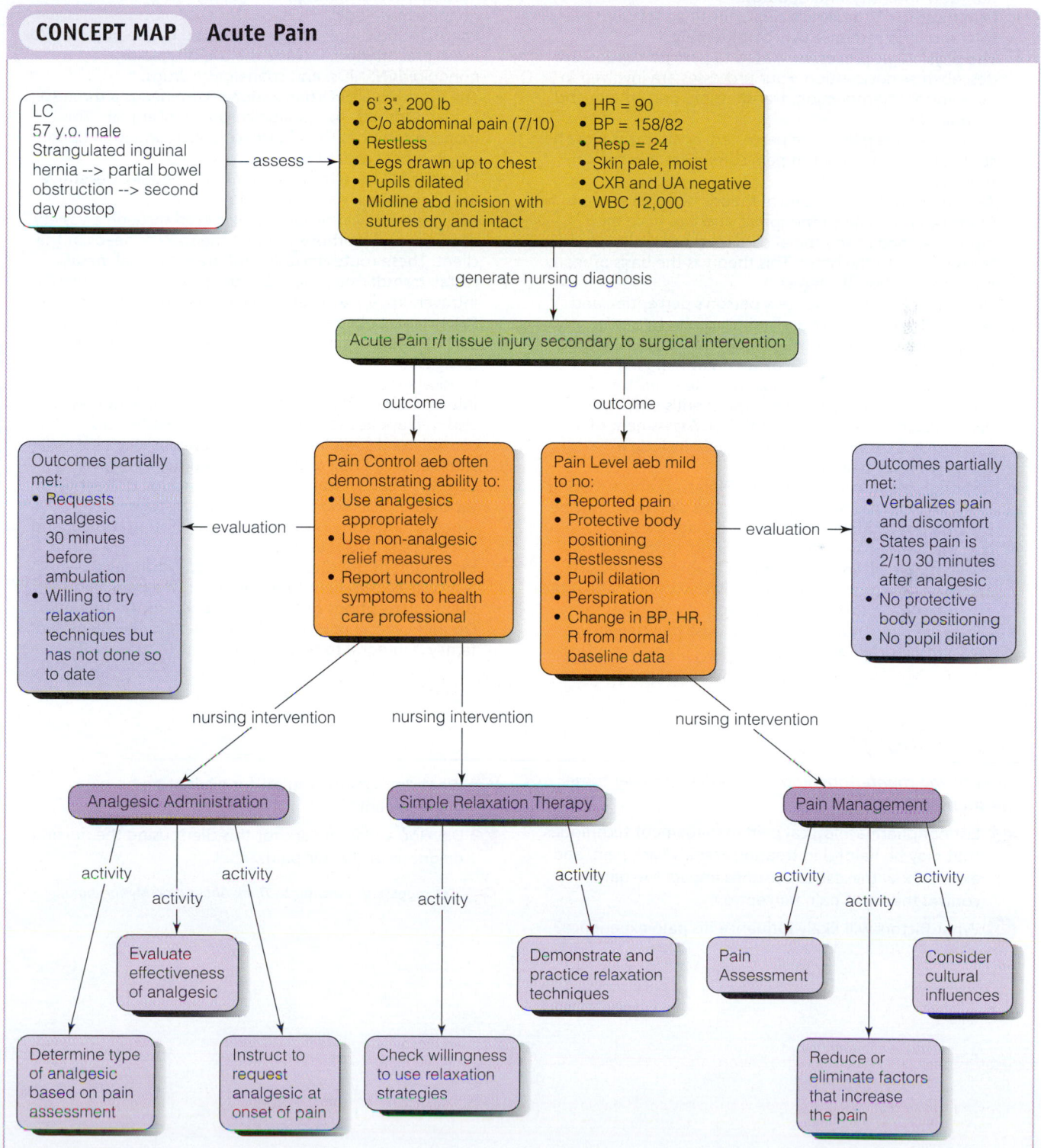

LC
57 y.o. male
Strangulated inguinal hernia --> partial bowel obstruction --> second day postop

assess

- 6' 3", 200 lb
- C/o abdominal pain (7/10)
- Restless
- Legs drawn up to chest
- Pupils dilated
- Midline abd incision with sutures dry and intact
- HR = 90
- BP = 158/82
- Resp = 24
- Skin pale, moist
- CXR and UA negative
- WBC 12,000

generate nursing diagnosis

Acute Pain r/t tissue injury secondary to surgical intervention

outcome   outcome

Outcomes partially met:
- Requests analgesic 30 minutes before ambulation
- Willing to try relaxation techniques but has not done so to date

Pain Control aeb often demonstrating ability to:
- Use analgesics appropriately
- Use non-analgesic relief measures
- Report uncontrolled symptoms to health care professional

Pain Level aeb mild to no:
- Reported pain
- Protective body positioning
- Restlessness
- Pupil dilation
- Perspiration
- Change in BP, HR, R from normal baseline data

Outcomes partially met:
- Verbalizes pain and discomfort
- States pain is 2/10 30 minutes after analgesic
- No protective body positioning
- No pupil dilation

evaluation   evaluation

nursing intervention   nursing intervention   nursing intervention

Analgesic Administration   Simple Relaxation Therapy   Pain Management

activity   activity   activity   activity   activity   activity   activity
    activity

Evaluate effectiveness of analgesic

Demonstrate and practice relaxation techniques

Pain Assessment

Consider cultural influences

Determine type of analgesic based on pain assessment

Instruct to request analgesic at onset of pain

Check willingness to use relaxation strategies

Reduce or eliminate factors that increase the pain

CHAPTER HIGHLIGHTS

- Pain is a subjective sensation to which no two people respond in the same way. It can directly impair health and prolong recovery from surgery, disease, and trauma.
- Types of pain may be described in terms of location, duration, intensity, and etiology.
- Pain threshold is generally similar in all people, but pain tolerance and response vary considerably.
- The physiologic processes related to pain perception are described as nociception. Four processes are involved in nociception: transduction, transmission, perception, and modulation.
- For nociceptive pain to be perceived, nociceptors must be stimulated. Three types of pain stimuli are mechanical, thermal, and chemical.
- According to the gate control theory, peripheral nerve fibers carrying pain to the spinal cord can have their input modified at the spinal cord level before transmission to the brain. This theory is the basis of many pain intervention strategies.
- Numerous factors influence a person's perception and reaction to pain: ethnic and cultural values, developmental stage, environment and support people, past pain experiences, and meaning of pain.
- Pain is subjective, and the most reliable indicator of the presence or intensity of pain is the client's self-report. Pain assessment is the fifth vital sign. Assessment of a client who is experiencing pain should include a comprehensive pain history.
- Although the nursing diagnosis given to clients suffering pain is *Acute Pain* or *Chronic Pain,* the pain itself may be the etiology of many other nursing diagnoses.
- Overall client goals include preventing, modifying, or eliminating pain so that the client is able to partly or completely resume usual daily activities and to cope more effectively with the pain experience.
- When planning, nurses need to choose pain relief measures appropriate for the client.

- Key strategies to reduce pain include acknowledging and accepting the client's pain, assisting support persons, reducing misconceptions about pain, reducing fear and anxiety, and preventing pain.
- Pain management includes two basic categories of nursing interventions: pharmacologic and nonpharmacologic.
- Pharmacologic interventions, ordered by the physician (or nurse practitioner), include the use of opioids, nonopioids/NSAIDs, and coanalgesic drugs.
- The World Health Organization recommends a three-step ladder approach to manage chronic cancer pain. This model establishes the pharmacologic foundation upon which other types of pain are managed.
- Placebos fail to relieve pain for many people. Deceptive use of placebos is an unethical practice.
- Analgesic medication can be delivered through a variety of routes and methods to meet the specific needs of the client. These routes include oral, transmucosal, nasal, rectal, transdermal, topical, subcutaneous, intramuscular, intravenous, intraspinal, and continuous local anesthetics.
- Patient-controlled analgesia enables the client to exercise control and treat the pain by self-administering doses of analgesics.
- Physical modalities of nonpharmacologic pain interventions include such cutaneous stimulation as hot and cold applications, massage, acupressure, and contralateral stimulation; transcutaneous electrical nerve stimulation (TENS); and immobilization/bracing.
- Cognitive-behavioral interventions include distraction techniques, eliciting the relaxation response, repatterning unhelpful thinking, facilitating coping, and selected spiritual interventions.
- Evaluation of the client's pain therapy includes the response of the client, the changes in the pain, and the client's perceptions of the effectiveness of the therapy. Ongoing verbal or written feedback from the client and family is integral to this process.

THINK ABOUT IT

Refer to the chapter-opening scenario and answer these questions.

1. List nonpharmacological pain management techniques that may be helpful in treating Frank's back pain, and explain how these interventions impact the gate control theory of pain perception.

2. What factors will likely influence his pain experience?

3. What goals might you set for evaluating his pain management?

4. Develop a plan of care for this client using the nursing diagnosis of chronic pain.

∞ *See suggested responses to Think About It on MyNursingKit.*

TEST YOUR KNOWLEDGE

1. The nurse would be most effective using what method of pain control during the transduction phase of nociception?
   1. Tricyclic antidepressants
   2. Opioids
   3. Ibuprofen
   4. Distraction

2. While collecting an admission pain assessment, the client tells the nurse that he begins to feel his back pain when it reaches a level of 3. He says he can handle that without intervention, but within 5 minutes the pain level increases to a 5. While he doesn't treat pain at this level, it interferes with his ability to function. When the pain level reaches an 8 he reports that he must use some method of pain control. The nurse assesses this client's pain threshold at which of the following?
   1. 3
   2. 5
   3. 8
   4. 5–8

3. The nurse classifies pain, reported by the client as 6 on a scale of 1 to 10, as which of the following?
   1. Mild pain
   2. Mild to moderate pain
   3. Moderate to severe pain
   4. Severe pain

4. A client who had abdominal surgery 4 hours ago is receiving a continuous epidural infusion of an analgesic. Which of the following observations indicates the nurse should monitor the client closely?
   1. Drowsy; drifts off to sleep before completing a sentence
   2. Respirations of 22/minute
   3. Drowsy; arouses with stimulation
   4. Pain rating 4 on 1–10 scale

5. The client has an order for morphine 2.5 to 5.0 mg IV every 4 hours. He received 2.5 mg IV 4 hours ago for pain rated at 3 on a scale of 0 to 10. He is now watching TV and visiting with family members. When you ask about his pain, he rates it as a 5. His VS are stable. What nursing intervention is the most appropriate?
   1. Give morphine 3.5 mg IV and inform him to continue watching TV because it is a distraction from the pain.
   2. Give 2.5 mg of morphine IV to avoid the client becoming addicted.
   3. Give nothing at this time because he is not exhibiting any signs of pain.
   4. Give morphine 5.0 mg IV and reassess in 20 minutes.

6. During an admission nursing assessment, a client with diabetes describes his leg pain as a "dull, burning sensation." The nurse recognizes this description to be characteristic of which type of pain?
   1. Physiological
   2. Somatic
   3. Visceral
   4. Neuropathic

7. Which of the following interventions, when implemented by the nurse, would apply the gate control theory of pain? Select all that apply.
   1. Oral analgesics around the clock (ATC)
   2. Massage
   3. Patient-controlled analgesia (PCA)
   4. Heat or cold application
   5. Teaching

8. Which statement best reflects the nurse's assessment of the fifth vital sign?
   1. "Do you have any complaints?"
   2. "Are you experiencing any discomfort right now?"
   3. "Is there anything I can do for you now?"
   4. "Do you have any complaints of pain?"

9. When planning care for pain control of older clients, the nurse should apply which of the following principles? Select all that apply.
   1. Pain is a natural outcome of the aging process.
   2. Pain perception increases with age.
   3. The client may deny pain.
   4. The nurse should avoid use of narcotics.
   5. The client may describe pain as an "ache" or "discomfort."

10. A client recovering from abdominal surgery refuses analgesia, saying that he is "fine, as long as he doesn't move." Which of the following nursing diagnoses should be a priority?
   1. *Deficient Knowledge* (pain control measures)
   2. *Ineffective Health Maintenance*
   3. *Risk for Ineffective Airway Clearance*
   4. *Impaired Physical Mobility*

∞ *See answers to Test Your Knowledge in Appendix A.*

REFERENCES AND SELECTED BIBLIOGRAPHY

Acello, B. (2000). Meeting JCAHO standards for pain control. *Nursing, 30*(3), 52–54.

Ackley, B. J., & Ladwig, G. B. (2008). *Nursing diagnosis handbook* (8th ed.). St. Louis: Mosby Elsevier.

Agency for Health Care Policy and Research (AHCPR). (1994). *Acute low back problems in adults. Clinical Practice Guideline No.14.* AHCPR Publication No. 94-0592. Rockville, MD: U.S. Department of Health and Human Services.

American Academy of Pain Medicine, American Pain Society, and the American Society of Addiction Medicine. (2006). *Definitions related to the use of opioids for the treatment of pain: A consensus document from the American Academy of Pain Medicine, the American Pain Society, and the American Society of Addiction Medicine.* Author Retrieved December 5, 2009, from http://www .ampaoinsoc.org

American Academy of Pediatrics & Canadian Paediatric Society. (2000). Prevention and management of pain and stress in the neonate. *Pediatrics, 105*(2), 454–461.

American Geriatrics Society (AGS) Clinical Practice Guidelines. (1998). The management of chronic pain in older persons. *Journal of the American Geriatrics Society, 46*, 635–651.

American Geriatrics Society (AGS). (2002). The management of persistent pain in older persons. *Journal of the American Geriatrics Society, 50* (6 Suppl.), S205–24.

American Nurses Association. (2005). *Scope and standards of practice: Pain management nursing.* Silver Spring, MD: NursingBooks.org.

American Pain Society (APS). (1999). *Chronic pain in America: Roadblocks to relief.* Retrieved December 5, 2009, from http:// www.ampainsoc.org

American Pain Society (APS). (2003). *Principles of analgesic use in the treatment of acute pain and cancer pain* (5th ed.). Glenview, IL: Author.

American Society for Pain Management Nursing. (2005). *Position paper: Use of placebos in pain management.* Retrieved June 22, 2006, from http://aspmn.org/ pdfs/Use%20of%20Placebos.pdf

American Society for Pain Management Nursing. (n.d.). *A position statement on the use of "as-needed" range orders for opioid analgesics in the management of acute pain.* Retrieved on June 22, 2006, from http://www.aspmn.org/pdfs/ As%20Needed%20Range%20Orders.pdf

Andrews, M. M., & Boyle, J. S. (2008). *Transcultural concepts in nursing care* (5th ed.). Philadelphia: Lippincott Williams & Wilkins.

Arnstein, P. (2006). Placebo: No relief for Ms. Mahoney's pain. *American Journal of Nursing, 106*(2), 54–57.

Arnstein, P. M. (1997). The neuroplastic phenomenon: A physiologic link between chronic pain and learning. *Journal of Neuroscience Nursing, 29*(3), 179–186.

Arnstein, P. M. (2002). Optimizing perioperative pain management. *AORN Journal, 76*(5), 812–818.

Arnstein, P. M. (2003). Comprehensive assessment and management of chronic pain. *Nursing Clinics of North America, 38*, 403–417.

Arnstein, P. M. (2004). Chronic neuropathic pain: Issues in patient education. *Pain Management Nursing, 5*(4), Suppl., 34–41.

Arnstein, P., Caudill, M., Mandle, C. L., Norris, A., & Beasley, R. (1999). Self efficacy as a mediator of the relationship between pain intensity, disability and depression in chronic pain patients. *Pain, 80*(3), 483–491.

Ball, J. W., & Bindler, R. C. (2007). *Pediatric nursing: Caring for children* (4th ed.). Upper Saddle River, NJ: Prentice Hall.

Bergh, I., & Sjostrom, B. (1999). A comparative study of nurses' and elderly patients' ratings of pain and pain tolerance. *Journal of Gerontological Nursing, 25*(5), 30–36.

Bines, A., & Paice, J. A. (2005). Are your pain management skills up-to-date? *Nursing, 35*(1), 36–37.

Bulechek, G. M., Butcher, H. K., & Dochterman, J. M. (Eds.). (2008) Nursing Interventions: Classification (NIC) (5th ed.) St. Louis, MO: Mosby.

Caudill, M. A. (2002). *Managing pain before it manages you* (Rev. ed.). New York: Guilford Press.

D'Arcy, Y. (2004). Assessing pain in patients who can't communicate. *Nursing, 34*(10), 27.

D'Arcy, Y. (2004). Using regional blockade for adjunct pain relief. *Nursing, 34*(11), 74–75.

D'Arcy, Y. (2005). Pain management standards, the law, and you. *Nursing, 35*(4), 17.

D'Arcy, Y. (2005). Liposomes: A new way to deliver pain medications. *Nursing, 35*(7), 17.

D'Arcy, Y. (2006). Hot topics in pain management: Using NSAIDs safely. *Nursing, 36*(2), 22–23.

DeGood, D. E., & Kiernan, B. D. (1997). Pain related cognitions as predictors of pain treatment outcomes. *Advances in Medical Psychotherapy, 9*, 73–90.

Dodd, M., Janson, S., Facione, N., Faucett, J., Froelicher, E. S., Humphreys, J., et al. (2001). Advancing the science of symptom management. *Journal of Advanced Nursing, 33*(5), 668–676.

Ebersole, P., Hess, P., Touhy, T., & Jett, K. (2009). *Gerontological nursing & healthy aging* (3rd ed.). St. Louis: Elsevier Mosby.

Elliott, A. M., Smith, B. H., Penny, K. I., Smith, W. C., & Chambers, W. A. (1999). The epidemiology of chronic pain in the community. *Lancet, 354,* 1248–1252.

Ernst, E. (2003). Massage treatment for back pain. *British Medical Journal, 326*(7389), 562–564.

FDA: U.S. Food and Drug Administration. (2005). *FDA Public Health Advisory: FDA announces important changes and additional warnings for COX-2 selective and non-selective non-steroidal anti-inflammatory drugs (NSAIDs).* Retrieved June 22, 2006, from http://www.fda.gov/cder/drug/advisory/COX2.htm

Fuchs-Lacelle, S.K. (2007). *Pain and dementia: The effects of systematic assessment on clinical practices and caregiver stress.* University of Regina: Canada.

Gordon, D. B., & Love, G. (2004). Pharmacologic management of neuropathic pain. *Pain Management Nursing, 5*(4, Suppl. 1), 19–33.

Gordon, D., Dahl, J., Phillips, P., Frandsen, J., Cowley, C., Foster, R., et al. (2005). The use of 'as-needed' range order for opioid analgesics in the management of acute pain: A consensus statement of the American Society for Pain Management Nursing and the American Pain Society. *Home Healthcare Nurse, 23*(6), 388–396.

Gordon, M. (2009). *The manual of nursing diagnosis* (12th ed.). St. Louis: Mosby.

Grace, P. J. (2006). The clinical use of placebos. *American Journal of Nursing, 106*(2), 58–61.

Guo, H. R., Tanaka, S., Halperin, W. E., & Cameron, L. L. (1999). Back pain prevalence in US industry and estimates of lost workdays. *American Journal of Public Health, 89*(7), 1029–1035.

Hadjistavropoulos, T., and Fine, P. G. (2006). Chronic pain in older persons: Prevalence, assessment, and management. *Reviews in Clinical Gerontology, 16*(3), 231–241.

Herr, K. (2002). Chronic pain in the older patient: Management strategies. *Journal of Gerontological Nursing, 28*(2), 28–34.

Herr, K. (2004). Neuropathic pain: A guide to comprehensive assessment. *Pain Management Nursing, 5*(4), Suppl., 1, 9–18.

Hitchcock, L. S., Ferrell, B. R., & McCaffery, M. (1994). The experience of chronic non-malignant pain. *Journal of Pain and Symptom Management, 9*(5), 312–318.

Horbury, C., Henderson, A., & Bromely, B. (2005). Influences of patient behavior on clinical nurses' pain assessment; Implications for continuing education. *Journal of Continuing Education in Nursing, 36*(1), 18–24.

Hutchison, R. (2004). COX-2-selective NSAIDs. A review and comparison with nonselective NSAIDs. *American Journal of Nursing, 104*(3), 52–54.

International Headache Society (IHS). (2004). The international classification of headache disorders (2nd ed.). *Cephalalgia: International Journal of Headache Disorders, 24* (Suppl. 1), 1–150.

Jensen, M. P., Martin, S. A., & Cheung, R. (2005). The meaning of pain relief in a clinical trial. *Journal of Pain, 6*(6), 400–406.

Joint Commission on Accreditation of Healthcare Organizations (JCAHO). (2004). *Patient controlled analgesia by proxy. Sentinel event alert.* Issue 33. Retrieved June 21, 2006, from http://www.jointcommission.org/SentinelEvents/SentinelEventAlert/sea_33.htm

Katz, J., Jackson, M., Kavanagh, B. P., & Sandler, A. N. (1996). Acute pain after thoracic surgery predicts long-term post-thoracotomy pain. *Clinical Journal of Pain, 12,* 50–55.

Keller, D. L. (2006). Pain relievers. *RN, 69*(4), 22–25.

Kurz, A., & Sessler, D. I. (2003). Opioid-induced bowel dysfunction: Pathophysiology and potential new therapies. *Drugs, 63*(7), 649–671.

Lafleur, K. J. (2004). Taking the fifth (vital sign). *RN, 67*(7), 30–36.

Lane, P. (2004). Assessing pain in patients with advanced dementia. *Nursing, 34*(8), 17.

Long, C. O. (2005). Seeking out pain-management resources. *Nursing, 35*(1), 74–75.

Manais, E., Bucknall, T., & Botti, M. (2005). Nursing strategies for managing pain in the postoperative setting. *Pain Management Nursing, 6*(1), 18–29.

Marders, J. (2004). PCA by proxy: Too much of a good thing. *Nursing, 34*(4), 24.

Mather, D. (2004). A low-tech approach to pain relief. *RN, 67*(3), 41–42.

McCaffery, M., & Arnstein, P. (2006). The debate over placebos in pain management. *American Journal of Nursing, 106*(2), 62–65.

McCaffery, M., Ferrell, B. R., & Pasero, C. (2000). Nurses' personal opinions about patients' pain and their effect on recorded assessments and titration of opioid doses. *Pain Management Nursing, 1*(3), 79–87.

McCaffery, M., & Pasero, C. (1999). *Pain: Clinical manual* (2nd ed.). St. Louis: Mosby.

McCaffery, M., & Pasero, C. (2003). Breakthrough pain: It's common in patients with chronic pain. *American Journal of Nursing, 103*(4), 83–85.

McNamara, M. E., Burnham, D. C., Smith, C., & Carroll, D. L. (2003). The effects of back massage before diagnostic cardiac catheterization. *Alternative Therapies in Health and Medicine, 9*(1), 50–57.

Melzack, R., & Wall, P. D. (1965). Pain mechanisms: A new theory. *Science, 150,* 971–979.

Merkel, S. I., Voepel-Lewis, T., Shayevitz, J. R., & Malviya, S. (1997). The FLACC: A behavioral scale for scoring postoperative pain in young children. *Pediatric Nursing, 23*(3), 293–297.

Monteiro-Cruz, D. A. L., & Mattos-Pimenta, C. A. (2001). Chronic pain: Nursing diagnosis or syndrome? *Nursing Diagnosis, 12*(4), 117–127.

Moorhead, S., Johnson, M., Maas, M. L., & Swanson, E. (Eds.). (2008). *Nursing outcomes classification (NOC)* (4th ed.). St. Louis: Mosby.

Munoz, C., & Luckmann, J. (2005). *Transcultural communication in nursing* (2nd ed.). Clifton Park, NY: Delmar Learning.

Murauski, J. D., & Gonzalez, K. R. (2002). Peripheral nerve blocks for postoperative analgesia. *AORN Journal, 75*(1), 136–147.

NANDA International. (2009). *NANDA nursing diagnoses: Definitions and classification 2009–2011.* West Sussex, U.K.: Wiley-Blackwell.

Nguyen, M., Ugarte, C., Fuller, I., Haas, G., & Portenoy, R. K. (2005). Access to care for chronic pain: Racial and ethnic differences. *Journal of Pain, 6*(5), 301–314.

Noah, V. (2003). PCA by proxy: Minimizing the risks. *Nursing, 103*(12), 17.

Page, G. G., Ben-Eliyahu, S., Yirmiya, R., & Liebeskind, J. C. (1993). Morphine attenuates surgery-induced enhancement of metastatic colonization in rats. *Pain, 54*(1), 21–28.

Paice, J. A. (2002). Controlling pain. Understanding nociceptive pain. *Nursing, 32*(3), 74–75.

Pasero, C. (2003). Lidocaine patch 5%: How to use a topical method of controlling localized pain. *American Journal of Nursing, 103*(9), 75–78.

Pasero, C. (2004). Pain relief for neonates. *American Journal of Nursing, 104,*(5), 44–47.

Pasero, C. (2004). Pathophysiology of neuropathic pain. *Pain Management Nursing, 5,* 4, (Suppl. 1), 3–8.

Pasero, C., & McCaffery, M. (2004). Controlled-release oxycodone: It's worth considering when treating around-the-clock pain. *American Journal of Nursing, 104*(1), 30–32.

Pasero, C., & McCaffery, M. (2005). Ketamine: Low doses may provide relief for some painful conditions. *American Journal of Nursing, 105*(4), 60–64.

Pasero, C., & McCaffery, M. (2005). Authorized and unauthorized use of PCA pumps. *American Journal of Nursing, 105*(7), 30–32.

Pasero, C., & McCaffery, M. (2005). No self-report means no pain-intensity rating. *American Journal of Nursing, 105*(10), 50–53.

Puntillo, K. A., & Weiss, S. J. (1994). Pain: Its mediators and associated morbidity in critically ill cardiovascular surgical patients. *Nursing Research, 43,* 31–36.

Purnell, L. D., & Paulanka, B. J. (2005). *Guide to culturally competent health care.* Philadelphia: Davis.

Reyes-Gibby, C. C., Aday, L., & Cleeland, C. (2002). Impact of pain on self-rated health in community-dwelling older adults. *Pain, 95,* 75–82.

Rhiner, M., & Kedziera, P. (1999). Managing breakthrough pain: A new approach. *American Journal of Nursing, 99*(3), Suppl. 3–12.

Schwartz, A. J. (2006). Learning the essentials of epidural anesthesia. *Nursing, 36*(1), 44–49.

Serlin, R. C., Mendoza, T. R., Nakamura, Y., Edwards, K. R., & Cleeland, C. S. (1995). When is cancer pain mild, moderate or severe? Grading pain severity by its interference with function. *Pain, 61,* 277–284.

Shapiro, R. S. (1996). Health care providers' liability exposure for inappropriate pain management. *Journal of Law and Medical Ethics, 24*(4), 360–364.

Siedlecki, S. (2004). Assessing chronic pain. *Nursing, 34*(5), 17.

Simons, J. M., & MacDonald, L. M. (2004). Pain assessment tools: Children's nurses' views. *Journal of Child Health Care, 8*(4), 264–278.

Spagrud, L. J., Piira, T., & von Baeyer, C. L. (2003). Children's self-report of pain intensity. *American Journal of Nursing, 103*(12), 62–64.

St. Marie, B., & Arnold, S. (2002). *When your pain flares up.* Minneapolis, MN: Fairview Press.

Stanley, M., Blair, K. A., & Beare, P. G. (2005). *Gerontological nursing: Promoting successful aging with older adults* (3rd ed.). Philadelphia: Davis.

vanDijk, M., Peters, W. B., vanDeventer, P., & Tibboel, D. (2005). The COMFORT behavior scale: A tool for assessing pain and sedation in infants. *American Journal of Nursing, 105*(1), 33–36.

Van Tudler, M., & Koes, B. (2004). Low back pain (acute). *Clinical Evidence, 12,* 1643–1658.

Warden, V., Hurley, A. C., & Volicer, L. (2003). Development and psychometric evaluation for the pain assessment in advanced dementia (PAINAD) scale. *Journal of the American Medical Directors Association, 4*(1), 9–15.

Wilson, K. G., Eriksson, M. Y., D'Eon, J. L., Mikail, S. F., & Emery, P. C. (2002). Major depression and insomnia in chronic pain. *Clinical Journal of Pain, 18*(2), 77–83.

Wong, D. L., Hockenberry-Eaton, M., Wilson, D., Winkelstein, M. L., & Schwartz, P. (2009). *Essentials of pediatric nursing* (8th ed.). St. Louis: Mosby.

World Health Organization. (1996). *Cancer pain relief* (2nd ed.). Geneva, Switzerland: Author.

Yezierski, R. P., Radson, E., & Vanderah, T. W. (2004). Understanding chronic pain. *Nursing, 34*(4), 22–23.

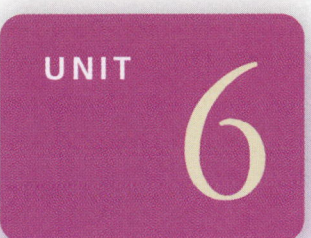

UNIT **6**

Integral Components of Client Care

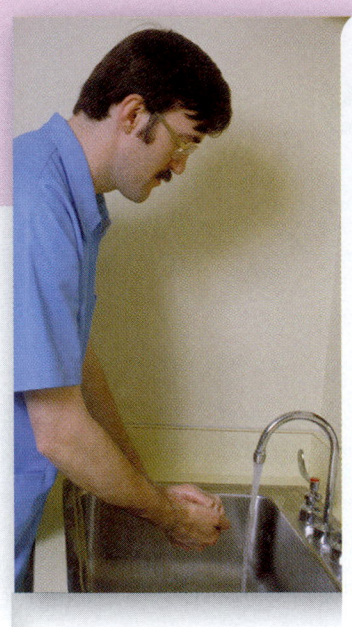

Frank, a senior nursing student, wants to work with neonates and is assigned to the Neonatal Intensive Care Unit to observe and assist with care. When entering the unit, he is stopped by a clerk who tells him he needs to change into hospital scrubs and perform thorough hand hygiene first. After changing and performing hand hygiene, he enters the unit and is surprised to see how small some of the babies are. He watches the nurses caring for them and how efficient and comfortable they are when handling these tiny things. The nurse caring for one of the tiniest infants calls Frank over and explains the baby was born 16 weeks early and is currently having respiratory problems exacerbated by septicemia. The nurse explains that premature infants are at high risk for infections because their immune systems are immature and their skin is fragile and easily torn. Altered skin integrity and invasive medical equipment combine to make the risk of infection very high. The nurse requires Frank to wash his hands before touching the baby, after touching the baby, and any time he touches anything not at that baby's bedside.

LEARNING OUTCOMES

After completing this chapter, you will be able to:

1. Contrast medical asepsis with surgical asepsis and describe situations when each would be used.

2. Categorize infections by microorganisms and types of infection.

3. Contrast risk factors and contributory factors for health care–associated infections.

4. Analyze commonly occurring factors in health care and diagram how they have the potential to maintain or break the chain of infection.

5. Contrast specific and nonspecific body defenses against infection and analyze how they interact together.

6. Identify factors that increase the client's susceptibility to infection.

7. Use the nursing process to develop an individualized plan of care to reduce the risk of infection for the client and others in contact with the client.

KEY TERMS

Acquired immunity p514	Cell-mediated defenses p514	Humoral immunity p514	Reservoirs p511
Active immunity p514	Cellular immunity p514	Hyperemia p513	Resident flora p509
Acute infections p510	Chronic infection p510	Iatrogenic infections p510	Sepsis p510
Airborne precautions p524	Circulating immunity p514	Immunoglobulins p514	Septicemia p510
Antibodies p514	Colonization p510	Infection p509	Specific defenses p513
Antigen p514	Contact precautions p524	Isolation p523	Sterilization p522
Antiseptic p522	Disease p509	Leukocytosis p514	Systemic infection p510
Asepsis p510	Disinfectants p522	Nonspecific defenses p513	Universal precautions p523
Autoantigen p514	Droplet nuclei p512	Opportunistic pathogen p510	Vector-borne transmission p512
Bacteria p510	Droplet precautions p524	Parasites p510	Vehicle-borne transmission p512
Bloodborne pathogen p523	Exudate p514	Passive immunity p514	Virulence p509
Body substance isolation p523	Fungi p510	Pathogenicity p509	Virus p510
	Health care–associated infection p510	Potency p509	

Nurses are directly involved in providing a safe environment, which includes an environment safe from pathogens. Microorganisms exist everywhere: in water, in soil, and on body surfaces such as the skin, intestinal tract, and other areas open to the outside. Most microorganisms are harmless, and some are even beneficial in that they perform essential functions in the body. Some microorganisms found in the intestines produce substances called *bacteriocins*, which are lethal to related strains of bacteria. Others produce substances that repress the growth of other microorganisms. Some microorganisms are normal **resident flora** (the collective vegetation in a given area) in one part of the body, yet produce infection in another. Table 19–1 provides a list of common resident microorganisms.

An **infection** is an invasion of body tissue by microorganisms. Such a microorganism is called an *infectious agent*. If the microorganism produces no clinical evidence of disease, the infection is called *asymptomatic* or *subclinical*. Some subclinical infections can cause considerable damage. A detectable alteration in normal tissue function, however, is called **disease**.

Microorganisms vary in their **virulence** (their ability to produce disease) and **potency** (their inherent capacity for growth and reproduction). Microorganisms also vary in the severity of the diseases they produce and their degree of communicability. If the infectious agent can be transmitted to an individual by direct or indirect contact or as an airborne infection, the resulting condition is called a communicable disease, such as swine flu or HIV.

Pathogenicity is the ability to produce disease; thus a pathogen is a microorganism that causes disease. Many microorganisms that are normally harmless can cause disease under certain circumstances. A "true" pathogen causes

TABLE 19–1 **Examples of Common Resident Microorganisms**

BODY AREA	MICROORGANISMS
Skin	*Staphylococcus epidermidis*
	Propionibacterium acnes
	Staphylococcus aureus
	Corynebacterium xerosis
	Pityrosporum oxale (yeast)
Nasal passages	*Staphylococcus aureus*
	Staphylococcus epidermidis
Oropharynx	*Streptococcus pneumoniae*
Mouth	*Streptococcus mutans*
	Lactobacillus
	Bacteroides
	Actinomyces
Intestine	*Bacteroides*
	Fusobacterium
	Eubacterium
	Lactobacillus
	Streptococcus
	Enterobacteriaceae
	Shigella
	Escherichia coli
Urethral orifice	*Staphylococcus epidermidis*
Urethra (lower)	*Proteus*
Vagina	*Lactobacillus*
	Bacteroides
	Clostridium
	Candida albicans

disease or infection in a healthy individual. An **opportunistic pathogen** causes disease only in a susceptible individual because the individual does not have adequate immune response to resist infection.

Infectious diseases are a major cause of death worldwide. The control of the spread of microorganisms and the protection of people from communicable diseases and infections are carried out on an international, national, state, community, and individual level. The World Health Organization is the major regulatory agency at the international level. In the United States, the Centers for Disease Control and Prevention (CDC) is the principal public health agency at the national level concerned with disease prevention and control. At the state level, health departments track epidemics and illnesses as reports are received from providers and organizations throughout that area.

Asepsis is the freedom from disease-causing microorganisms. To decrease the possibility of transferring microorganisms from one place to another, aseptic technique is used. There are two basic types of asepsis: medical and surgical. Medical asepsis includes all practices intended to confine a specific microorganism to a specific area, limiting the number, growth, and transmission of microorganisms. In medical asepsis, objects are referred to as clean, which means the absence of almost all microorganisms, or dirty (soiled, contaminated), which means likely to have microorganisms, some of which may be capable of causing infection.

Surgical asepsis, or sterile technique, refers to those practices that keep an area or object free of all microorganisms; it includes practices that destroy all microorganisms and spores (microscopic dormant structures formed by some pathogens that are very hardy and often survive common cleaning techniques). Surgical asepsis is used for all procedures involving the sterile areas of the body. **Sepsis** is the state of infection and can take many forms, including septic shock.

TYPES OF MICROORGANISMS CAUSING INFECTIONS

Four major categories of microorganisms cause infection in humans: bacteria, viruses, fungi, and parasites. **Bacteria** are by far the most common infection-causing microorganisms. Several hundred species can cause disease in humans and can live and be transported through air, water, food, soil, body tissues and fluids, and inanimate objects. Most of the microorganisms in Table 19–1 are bacteria. **Viruses** consist primarily of nucleic acid and therefore must enter living cells in order to reproduce. Common virus families include the rhinovirus, hepatitis, herpes, and human immunodeficiency virus. **Fungi** include yeasts and molds. *Candida albicans* is a yeast considered to be normal flora in the human vagina. **Parasites** live on other living organisms. They include protozoa such as the one that causes malaria, helminths (worms), and arthropods (mites, fleas, ticks).

TYPES OF INFECTIONS

Colonization is the process by which strains of microorganisms become resident flora. In this state, the microorganisms may grow and multiply but do not cause disease. Infection occurs when newly introduced or resident microorganisms succeed in invading a part of the body where the host's defense mechanisms are ineffective and the pathogen causes tissue damage. The infection becomes a disease when the signs and symptoms of the infection are unique and can be differentiated from other conditions.

Infections can be local or systemic. A local infection is limited to the specific part of the body where the microorganisms remain. If the microorganisms spread and damage different parts of the body, it is a **systemic infection**. When a culture of the person's blood reveals microorganisms, the condition is called bacteremia. When bacteremia results in systemic infection, it is referred to as **septicemia**. Unfortunately, these infections have become more common over time.

There are also **acute** or **chronic infections**. Acute infections generally have a sudden onset and short duration. A chronic infection may have a slower onset and longer duration lasting months or years in some cases.

Health care–associated infections (formerly called nosocomial infections) are classified as infections that are associated with the delivery of health care services in a health care facility. Health care–associated infections (HAI) can either develop during a client's stay in a facility or manifest after discharge. They may also be acquired by health personnel working in the facility and can cause significant illness and time lost from work. Health care workers may be carriers of certain pathogens and are capable of passing these infections to a susceptible host such as clients with weakened immune systems.

HAI have received increasing attention in recent years and are believed to involve about 2 million clients per year. The Joint Commission on Accreditation of Healthcare Organizations included reducing the risk of health care associated infections as one of the 2006 National Patient Safety Goals. The most common settings where HAI develop are hospital surgical or medical intensive care units. Reports from the National Nosocomial Infection Surveillance (NNIS) System have revealed that the urinary tract, the respiratory tract, bloodstream, and wounds are the most common health care–associated infection sites (see the NNIS website). The microorganisms that cause HAI can originate from the clients themselves (an endogenous source) or from the hospital environment and hospital personnel (exogenous sources). Most HAI appear to have endogenous sources. *Escherichia coli, Staphylococcus aureus,* and enterococci are the most common infecting microorganisms.

A number of factors contribute to HAI. **Iatrogenic infections** are the direct result of diagnostic or therapeutic procedures. Not all HAI are iatrogenic, nor are they all preventable. Another factor contributing to the development of HAI is the compromised host, that is, a client whose normal defenses have been lowered by surgery or illness.

TABLE 19–2 Health Care–Associated Infections

MOST COMMON MICROORGANISMS	CAUSES
Urinary Tract	
Escherichia coli	Improper catheterization technique
Enterococcus species	Contamination of closed drainage system
Pseudomonas aeruginosa	Inadequate hand cleansing
Surgical Sites	
Staphylococcus aureus (including methicillin-resistant strains—MRSA)	Inadequate hand cleansing
Enterococcus species (including vancomycin-resistant strains—VRE)	Improper dressing change technique
Pseudomonas aeruginosa	
Bloodstream	
Coagulase-negative staphylococci	Inadequate hand cleansing
Staphylococcus aureus *Enterococcus species*	Improper intravenous fluid, tubing, and site care technique
Pneumonia	
Staphylococcus aureus	Inadequate hand cleansing
Pseudomonas aeruginosa	Improper suctioning technique
Enterobacter species	

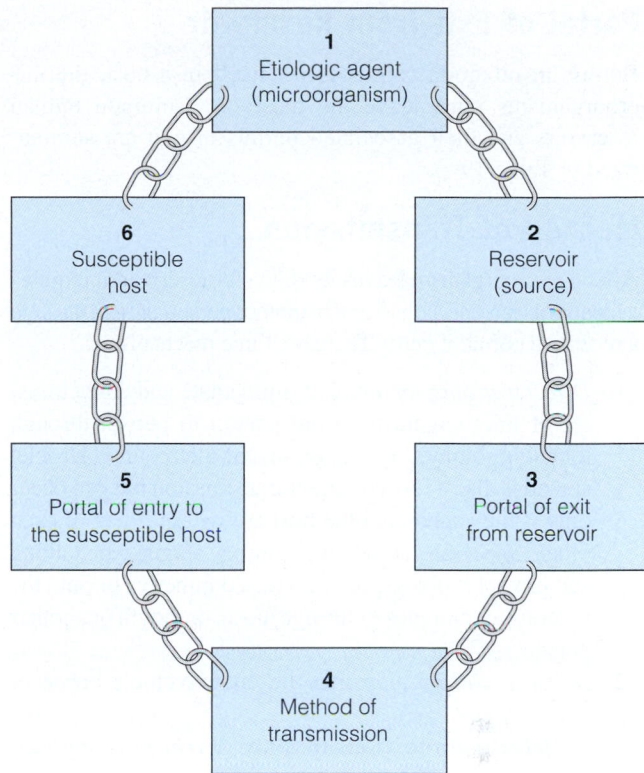

Figure 19–1 ● The chain of infection.

The hands of personnel are a common vehicle for the spread of microorganisms. Insufficient hand cleansing is thus an important factor contributing to the spread of health care–associated microorganisms.

CLINICAL ALERT

A person does not need to have an identified infection in order to pass potentially infective microorganisms to another person. Even normal microorganisms for one person can infect another person.

The cost of health care–associated infections to the client, the facility, and funding sources is large. HAI extend hospitalization time, increase clients' time away from work, cause disability and discomfort, and even result in loss of life (see Table 19–2).

CHAIN OF INFECTION

Six links make up the chain of infection (Figure 19–1): the etiologic agent, or microorganism; the place where the organism naturally resides (reservoir); a portal of exit from the reservoir; a method (mode) of transmission; a portal of entry into a host; and the susceptibility of the host.

Etiologic Agent

The extent to which any microorganism is capable of producing an infectious process depends on the number of microorganisms present, the virulence and potency of the microorganisms (pathogenicity), the ability of the microorganisms to enter the body, the susceptibility of the host, and the ability of the microorganisms to live in the host's body.

Some microorganisms, such as the smallpox virus, have the ability to infect almost all susceptible people after exposure. By contrast, microorganisms such as the tuberculosis bacillus infect a relatively small number of the population who are susceptible and exposed, usually people who are poorly nourished, who are living in crowded conditions, or whose immune systems are less competent (such as older adults or those with HIV or cancer).

Reservoir

There are many **reservoirs**, or sources, of microorganisms. Common sources are other humans, the client's own microorganisms, plants, animals, or the general environment. People are the most common source of infection for others and for themselves. A carrier is a person or animal reservoir of a specific infectious agent that usually does not manifest any clinical signs of disease. The *Anopheles* mosquito reservoir carries the malaria parasite but is unaffected by it. The carrier state may also exist in individuals with a clinically recognizable disease. Under either circumstance, the carrier state may be of short duration (temporary or transient carrier) or long duration (chronic carrier). Food, water, and feces also can be reservoirs.

Portal of Exit from Reservoir

Before an infection can establish itself in a host, the microorganisms must leave the reservoir. Common human reservoirs and their associated portals of exit are summarized in Table 19–3.

Method of Transmission

After a microorganism leaves its source or reservoir, it requires a means of transmission to reach another person or host through a receptive portal of entry. There are three mechanisms:

1. *Direct transmission* involves immediate and direct transfer of microorganisms from person to person through touching, biting, kissing, or sexual intercourse. Droplet spread is also a form of direct transmission but can occur only if the source and the host are within 3 feet of each other. Sneezing, coughing, spitting, singing, or talking can project droplet spray into the conjunctiva or onto the mucous membranes of the eye, nose, or mouth of another person.

2. *Indirect transmission* may be either vehicle borne or vector borne.
   a. **Vehicle-borne transmission.** A *vehicle* is any substance that serves as an intermediate means to transport and introduce an infectious agent into a susceptible host through a suitable portal of entry. Fomites (inanimate materials or objects), such as soiled clothes, cooking or eating utensils, and surgical instruments or dressings, can act as vehicles. Water, food, blood, serum, and plasma are other vehicles
   b. **Vector-borne transmission.** A *vector* is an animal or flying or crawling insect that serves as an intermediate means of transporting the infectious agent. Transmission may occur by injecting salivary fluid during biting or by depositing feces or other materials on the skin through the bite wound or a traumatized skin area, resulting in diseases such as Lyme's disease from ticks or malaria from mosquitoes.

3. *Airborne transmission.* Airborne transmission may involve droplets or dust. **Droplet nuclei**, the residue of evaporated droplets emitted by an infected host such as someone with tuberculosis, can remain in the air for long periods. Dust particles containing the infectious agent can also become airborne. The material is transmitted by air currents to a suitable portal of entry, usually the respiratory tract, of another person.

Portal of Entry to the Susceptible Host

Before a person can become infected, microorganisms must enter the body. The skin is a barrier to infectious agents and is the body's primary line of defense; however, any break in the skin can readily serve as a portal of entry.

TABLE 19–3   Human Body Area Reservoirs, Common Infectious Microorganisms, and Portals of Exit

BODY AREA RESERVOIR	COMMON INFECTIOUS ORGANISMS	PORTALS OF EXIT
Respiratory tract	Parainfluenza virus	Nose or mouth through sneezing, coughing, breathing, or talking
	Mycobacterium tuberculosis	
	Staphylococcus aureus	
Gastrointestinal tract	Hepatitis A virus	Mouth: saliva, vomitus; anus: feces; ostomies
	Salmonella species	
	Clostridium difficile	Anus: feces, colostomies
Urinary tract	*Escherichia coli* enterococci	Urethral meatus and urinary diversion
	Pseudomonas aeruginosa	
Reproductive tract	*Neisseria gonorrhoeae*	Vagina: vaginal discharge; urinary meatus: semen, urine
	Treponema pallidum	
	Herpes simplex virus type 2	
	Hepatitis B virus (HBV)	
Blood	Hepatitis B virus	Open wound, needle puncture site, any disruption of intact skin or mucous membrane surfaces
	Human immunodeficiency virus (HIV)	
	Staphylococcus aureus	
	Staphylococcus epidermidis	
Tissue	*Staphylococcus aureus*	Drainage from cut or wound
	Escherichia coli	
	Proteus species	
	Streptococcus beta-hemolytic A or B	

Often, microorganisms enter the body of the host by the same route they used to leave the source.

Susceptible Host

A susceptible host is any person who is at risk for infection. A compromised host is a person at increased risk, an individual who for one or more reasons is more likely than others to acquire an infection. Impairment of the body's natural defenses and a number of other factors can affect susceptibility to infection. Examples include age; clients receiving immune suppression treatment for cancer, for chronic illness, or following a successful organ transplant; and those with immune deficiency conditions.

BODY DEFENSES AGAINST INFECTION

Individuals normally have defenses that protect the body from infection. These defenses can be categorized as nonspecific and specific. **Nonspecific defenses** protect the person against all microorganisms, regardless of prior exposure. **Specific (immune) defenses**, by contrast, are directed against identifiable bacteria, viruses, fungi, or other infectious agents.

Nonspecific Defenses

Nonspecific body defenses include anatomic and physiologic barriers, and the inflammatory response.

ANATOMIC AND PHYSIOLOGIC BARRIERS Intact skin and mucous membranes are the body's first line of defense against microorganisms. Unless the skin and mucosa become cracked and broken, they are an effective barrier against bacteria. Fungi can live on the skin, but they cannot penetrate it. The dryness of the skin is also a deterrent to bacteria. Bacteria are most plentiful in moist areas of the body, such as the perineum and axillae. Resident bacteria of the skin also prevent other bacteria from multiplying. They use up the available nourishment, and the end products of their metabolism inhibit other bacterial growth. Normal secretions make the skin slightly acidic; acidity also inhibits bacterial growth.

The nasal passages have a defensive function. As entering air follows the tortuous route of the passage, it comes in contact with moist mucous membranes and cilia. These trap microorganisms, dust, and foreign materials. The lungs have alveolar macrophages (large phagocytes). Phagocytes are cells that ingest microorganisms, other cells, and foreign particles.

Each body orifice also has protective mechanisms. The oral cavity regularly sheds mucosal epithelium to rid the mouth of colonizers. The flow of saliva and its partially buffering action help prevent infections. Saliva contains microbial inhibitors, such as lactoferrin, lysozyme, and secretory IgA.

The eye is protected from infection by tears, which continually wash microorganisms away and contain inhibiting lysozyme. The gastrointestinal tract also has defenses against infection. The high acidity of the stomach normally prevents microbial growth. The resident flora of the large intestine help prevent the establishment of disease-producing microorganisms. Peristalsis also tends to move microbes out of the body.

The vagina also has natural defenses against infection. When a girl reaches puberty, lactobacilli ferment sugars in the vaginal secretions, creating a vaginal pH of 3.5 to 4.5. This low pH inhibits the growth of many disease-producing microorganisms. The entrance to the urethra normally harbors many microorganisms. It is believed that the urine flow has a flushing and bacteriostatic action that keeps the bacteria from ascending the urethra. An intact mucosal surface also acts as a barrier.

INFLAMMATORY RESPONSE Inflammation is a local and nonspecific defensive response of the tissues to an injurious or infectious agent. It is an adaptive mechanism that destroys or dilutes the injurious agent, prevents further spread of the injury, and promotes the repair of damaged tissue. It is characterized by five signs: (a) pain, (b) swelling, (c) redness, (d) heat, and (e) impaired function of the part, if the injury is severe. Commonly, words with the suffix *-itis* describe an inflammatory process.

Injurious agents can be categorized as physical agents, chemical agents, and microorganisms. *Physical agents* include mechanical objects causing trauma to tissues, excessive heat or cold, and radiation. *Chemical agents* include external irritants and internal irritants. *Microorganisms* include the broad groups of bacteria, viruses, fungi, and parasites. A series of dynamic events is commonly referred to as the three stages of the inflammatory response.

Vascular and Cellular Responses At the start of the first stage of inflammation, blood vessels at the site of injury constrict. This is rapidly followed by dilation of small blood vessels (occurring as a result of histamine released by the injured tissues). Thus, more blood flows to the injured area. This marked increase in blood supply is referred to as **hyperemia** and is responsible for the characteristic signs of redness and heat.

Vascular permeability increases at the site with dilation of the vessels in response to cell death, the release of chemical mediators (e.g., bradykinin, serotonin, and prostaglandin), and the release of histamine. Fluid, proteins, and leukocytes (white blood cells) leak into the interstitial spaces, and the signs of inflammation swelling (edema) and pain appear. Pain is caused by the pressure of accumulating fluid on nerve endings and the irritating chemical mediators. Fluid pouring into areas such as the pleural or pericardial cavity can seriously affect organ function. In other areas, such as joints, mobility is impaired.

Blood flow slows in the dilated vessels, allowing more leukocytes to arrive at the injured tissues. When the blood flow slows, leukocytes aggregate or line up along this inner surface of the blood vessels. This process is known as margination. Leukocytes then move through the blood vessel wall into the affected tissue spaces, a process called emigration.

In response to the exit of leukocytes from the blood, the bone marrow produces large numbers of leukocytes and releases them into the bloodstream. This is called **leukocytosis**. A normal leukocyte count of 4,500 to 11,000 per cubic millimeter of blood can rise to 20,000 or more when inflammation occurs.

Exudate Production In the second stage of inflammation, the inflammatory **exudate** is produced, consisting of fluid that escaped from the blood vessels, dead phagocytic cells, and dead tissue cells and products that they release. The plasma protein fibrinogen (which is converted to fibrin when it is released into the tissues), thromboplastin (released by injured tissue cells), and platelets together form an interlacing network to wall off the area, and prevent spread of the injurious agent. During this stage, the injurious agent is overcome, and the exudate is cleared away by lymphatic drainage. The nature and amount of exudate vary according to the tissue involved and the intensity and duration of the inflammation. The major types of exudate are serous, purulent, and hemorrhagic (sanguineous). Descriptions of these exudates are provided in Chapter 24 ∞.

REPARATIVE PHASE The third stage of the inflammatory response involves the repair of injured tissues by regeneration or replacement with fibrous tissue (scar) formation. Regeneration is the replacement of destroyed tissue cells by cells that are identical or similar in structure and function. Damaged cells are replaced one by one, but cells are organized so that the architectural pattern and function of the tissue are restored. The ability to regenerate cells varies considerably from one type of tissue to another. Tissues that have little regenerative capacity include nervous, muscular, and elastic tissues.

When regeneration is not possible, repair occurs by fibrous (scar) tissue formation. The inflammatory exudate with its interlacing network of fibrin provides the framework for this tissue to develop. Damaged tissues are replaced with the connective tissue elements of collagen, blood capillaries, lymphatics, and other tissue-bound substances. In the early stages of this process, the tissue is called granulation tissue. It is a fragile, gelatinous tissue, appearing pink or red because of the many newly formed capillaries. Later in the process, the tissue shrinks (the capillaries are constricted, even obliterated) and the collagen fibers contract, so that a firmer fibrous tissue remains. This is called cicatrix, or a scar.

Specific Defenses

Specific defenses of the body involve the immune system. An **antigen** is a substance that induces a state of sensitivity or immune responsiveness (immunity). If the proteins originate in a person's own body, the antigen is called an **autoantigen**.

The immune response has two components: antibody-mediated defenses and cell-mediated defenses. These two systems provide distinct but overlapping protection.

ANTIBODY-MEDIATED DEFENSES Another name for the *antibody-mediated defenses* is **humoral** (or **circulating**) **immunity** because these defenses reside ultimately in the B lymphocytes and are mediated by antibodies produced by B cells. **Antibodies,** also called **immunoglobulins,** are part of the body's plasma proteins. The antibody-mediated responses defend primarily against the extracellular phases of bacterial and viral infections.

There are two major types of immunity: active and passive (see Table 19–4). In **active immunity**, the host produces antibodies in response to natural antigens (e.g., infectious microorganisms) or artificial antigens (e.g., vaccines). B cells are activated when they recognize the antigen. They then differentiate into plasma cells, which secrete the antibodies and serum proteins that bind specifically to the foreign substance and initiate a variety of elimination responses. The B cell may produce antibody molecules of five classes of immunoglobulins designated by letters and usually written as IgM, IgG, IgA, IgD, and IgE. The presence of IgM in a laboratory analysis shows current infection. Before the antibody response can become effective, the phagocytic cells of the blood bind and ingest foreign substances. The rate of binding and phagocytosis increases if IgG antibodies (which indicate past infection and subsequent immunity) are present. With **passive** (or **acquired**) **immunity,** the host receives natural (e.g., from a nursing mother) or artificial (e.g., from an injection of immune serum) antibodies produced by another source.

CELL-MEDIATED DEFENSES The **cell-mediated defenses**, or **cellular immunity**, occur through the T-cell system. On exposure to an antigen, the lymphoid tissues release large numbers of activated T cells into the lymph system. These T cells pass into the general circulation. There are three main

TABLE 19–4	Types of Immunity	
TYPE	**ANTIGEN OR ANTIBODY SOURCE**	**DURATION**
1. Active	Antibodies are produced by the body in response to an antigen.	Long
a. Natural	Antibodies are formed in the presence of active infection in the body.	Lifelong
b. Artificial	Antigens (vaccines or toxoids) are administered to stimulate antibody production.	Many years; the immunity must be reinforced by booster
2. Passive	Antibodies are produced by another source, animal or human.	Short
a. Natural	Antibodies are transferred naturally from an immune mother to her baby through the placenta or in colostrum.	6 months to 1 year
b. Artificial	Immune serum (antibody) from an animal or another human is injected.	2 to 3 weeks

groups of T cells: (a) helper T cells, which help in the functions of the immune system; (b) cytotoxic T cells, which attack and kill microorganisms and sometimes the body's own cells; and (c) suppressor T cells, which can suppress the functions of the helper T cells and the cytotoxic T cells. When cell-mediated immunity is lost, as occurs with human immunodeficiency virus (HIV) infection, an individual is "defenseless" against most viral, bacterial, and fungal infections.

FACTORS INCREASING SUSCEPTIBILITY TO INFECTION

Whether a microorganism causes an infection depends on a number of factors already mentioned. One of the most important factors is host susceptibility, which is affected by age, heredity, level of stress, nutritional status, current medical therapy, and preexisting disease processes.

Age influences the risk of infection. Newborns and older adults have reduced defenses against infection. Infections are a major cause of death in newborns, who have immature immune systems and are protected only for the first 2 or 3 months by immunoglobulins passively received from the mother. Between 1 and 3 months of age, infants begin to synthesize their own immunoglobulins. Immunizations are usually started at 2 months, when the infant's immune system can respond.

With advancing age, the immune responses again become weak. Although there is still much to learn about aging, it is known that immunity to infection decreases with advancing age. Because of the prevalence of influenza and its potential for causing death, the CDC recommends annual immunization against influenza for older adults and for persons with chronic cardiac, respiratory, metabolic, and renal disease. Pneumococcal vaccine is recommended for older adults last vaccinated more than 5 years previously.

Heredity influences the development of infection in that some people have a genetic susceptibility to certain infections. People from specific areas may share similar genetic susceptibilities to certain infections.

The nature, number, and duration of physical and emotional stressors can influence susceptibility to infection. Stressors elevate blood cortisone. Prolonged elevation of blood cortisone decreases anti-inflammatory responses, depletes energy stores, leads to a state of exhaustion, and decreases resistance to infection.

Resistance to infection depends on adequate nutritional status. Because antibodies are proteins, the ability to synthesize antibodies may be impaired by inadequate nutrition, especially when protein reserves are depleted.

Some medical therapies predispose a person to infection. Some diagnostic procedures may also predispose the client to an infection, especially when the skin is broken or sterile body cavities are penetrated during the procedure.

Certain medications also increase susceptibility to infection. Antineoplastic (anticancer) medications may depress bone marrow function, resulting in inadequate production of white blood cells necessary to combat infections. Anti-inflammatory medications, such as adrenal corticosteroids, inhibit the inflammatory response, an essential defense against infection. Even some antibiotics used to treat infections can have adverse effects. Antibiotics may kill resident flora, allowing the proliferation of strains that would not grow and multiply in the body under normal conditions. Certain antibiotics can also induce resistance in some strains of organisms. This resistance has become so widespread that the CDC has created a 12-step Campaign to Prevent Antimicrobial Resistance in Healthcare Settings consisting of four strategies: preventing infection, diagnosing and treating infection effectively, using antimicrobials wisely, and preventing transmission.

Any disease that lessens the body's defenses against infection places the client at risk. Diabetes mellitus is a major underlying disease predisposing clients to infection because compromised peripheral vascular status and increased serum glucose levels increase susceptibility.

NURSING MANAGEMENT
ASSESSING

During the assessing phase of the nursing process, the nurse obtains the client's history, conducts the physical assessment, and gathers laboratory data.

Nursing History

During the nursing history, the nurse assesses (a) the degree to which a client is at risk of developing an infection and (b) any client complaints suggesting the presence of an infection. To identify clients at risk, the nurse reviews the client's chart and structures the nursing interview to collect data regarding the factors influencing the development of infection, especially existing disease process, history of recurrent infections, current medications and therapeutic measures, current emotional stressors, nutritional status, and history of immunizations. Collection of baseline data such as vital signs, height, and weight can help the nurse identify early signs and symptoms of a developing infection and the body's response to stressors.

Physical Assessment

Signs and symptoms of an infection vary according to the body area involved. Commonly the skin and mucous membranes are involved in a local infectious process, resulting in localized swelling, redness, pain or tenderness with palpation or movement, heat, or loss of function. In addition, open wounds may exude drainage of various colors. Signs of systemic infection may include fever, malaise, loss of energy, anorexia, nausea, vomiting, and enlargement and tenderness of lymph nodes draining the infected area. Older clients may present with confusion as an early manifestation of infection.

LIFESPAN CONSIDERATIONS   Infections

Children

Infections are an expected part of childhood, with most children experiencing some kind of infection from time to time. The majority of these infections are caused by viruses, and for the most part are transient, relatively benign, and able to be overcome by the body's natural defenses and supportive care. In some cases, severe, even life-threatening infections occur. Considerations related to children include the following:

- Newborns may not be able to respond to infections due to an underdeveloped immune system. As a result, in the first few months of life, infections may not be associated with typical signs and symptoms (e.g., an infant with an infection may not have a fever).
- Newborns are born with some naturally acquired immunity transferred from the mother across the placenta.
- Breast-fed infants enjoy higher levels of immunity against infections than formula-fed infants.
- Fevers less than 39°C (102.2°F) in children should not be treated, except for comfort of the child.
- Children between 6 months and 5 years are at higher risk for fever-induced (febrile) seizures. Febrile seizures are not associated with neurological seizure disorders (e.g., epilepsy).
- Children who are immune-compromised (e.g., leukemia, HIV) or have a chronic health condition (e.g., cystic fibrosis, sickle cell disease, congenital heart disease) need extra precautions to prevent exposure to infectious agents.
- Hand hygiene, comprehensive immunizations, good nutrition, adequate hydration, and appropriate rest are essential to preventing and/or treating infections in children.
- Hand washing and good hygiene in day care and schools are important to prevent the spread of infections.
- Adolescents are at high risk for sexually transmitted infections and should be well educated about how to prevent infections. Diseases such as mononucleosis and meningitis are also more commonly seen in adolescents, especially those in group living situations such as college dormitories.

Older Adults

Normal aging may predispose older adults to increased risk of infection and delayed healing. Anatomical and physiological agents that are protective when a person is younger often change in structure and function with increasing age and then provide a decrease in their protective ability. Changes take place in the skin, respiratory tract, gastrointestinal system, kidneys, and immune system. If unchallenged, these systems work well to maintain homeostasis for the individual, but if compromised by stress, illness, infections, treatments, or surgeries, they find it difficult to keep up and therefore are not able to provide adequate protection. Special considerations for older adults include the following:

- Nutrition is often poor in older adults. Certain components, especially adequate protein, are necessary to build up and maintain the immune system.
- Diabetes mellitus, which occurs more frequently in older adults, increases the risk of infection and delayed healing by causing an alteration in nutrition and impaired peripheral circulation, which decrease the oxygen transport to the tissues.
- The immune system reacts slowly to the introduction of antigens, allowing the antigen to reproduce itself several times before it is recognized by the immune system. T-cell effectiveness is often decreased due to immaturity.
- The normal inflammatory response is delayed. This often causes atypical responses to infections with unusual presentations. Instead of displaying redness, swelling, and fever usually associated with infections, atypical symptoms such as confusion and disorientation, agitation, incontinence, falls, lethargy, and general fatigue are often seen first.

Recognizing these changes in older adults is important in early detection and treatment of related potential for infections and delayed healing. Nursing interventions to promote prevention include the following:

- Provide and teach ways to improve nutritional status.
- Use strict aseptic technique to decrease chance of infections (especially health care–associated infections).
- Encourage older adults to have regular immunizations for flu and pneumonia.
- Be alert to subtle atypical signs of infection and act quickly to diagnose and treat.

Laboratory Data

Laboratory data that indicate the presence of an infection include the following:

- Elevated leukocyte count (4,500 to 11,000/mL is normal).
- Increases in specific types of leukocytes as revealed in the differential WBC count depending on the type of infection. See Chapter 20 ∞ for normal values for the adult.
- Elevated *erythrocyte sedimentation rate (ESR)*.

- Urine, blood, sputum, or other drainage cultures that indicate the presence of pathogenic microorganisms.
- Alterations in organ function studies may be altered if the organ system is impacted by an infection, such as altered liver function studies seen in infection of the liver.

DIAGNOSING

The NANDA nursing diagnostic label for problems associated with the transmission of microorganisms is *Risk for Infection:*

the state in which an individual is at increased risk for being invaded by pathogenic microorganisms.

When using this label, the nurse should identify risk factors:

1. Inadequate primary defenses
2. Inadequate secondary defenses

Clients who have or are at risk for an existing infection are prime candidates for other physical and psychologic problems. Examples of nursing diagnoses or collaborative problems that may arise from the actual presence of an infection include the following:

- *Potential Complication of Infection: Fever*
- *Imbalanced Nutrition: Less Than Body Requirements* if the client is too ill to eat adequately
- *Acute Pain* if the client is experiencing tissue damage and discomfort
- *Impaired Social Interaction or Social Isolation* if the client is required to be separated from others during a contagious episode
- *Anxiety* if the client is apprehensive regarding changes in life activities resulting from the infection or its treatment such as absence from work or inability to perform usual functions

Examples of nursing diagnoses and related outcomes and interventions are shown in Identifying Nursing Diagnoses, Outcomes, and Interventions.

PLANNING

The major goals for clients susceptible to infection are to

- Maintain or restore defenses.
- Avoid the spread of infectious organisms.
- Reduce or alleviate problems associated with the infection.

Desired outcomes depend on the individual client's condition. Examples of desired outcomes, established in the planning phase, are provided in Identifying Nursing Diagnoses, Outcomes, and Interventions. Nursing strategies to meet the three broad goals generally include using meticulous medical and surgical aseptic techniques to prevent the spread of potentially infectious microorganisms, implementing measures to support the defenses of a susceptible host, and teaching clients about protective measures to prevent infections and the spread of infectious agents when an infection is present.

IMPLEMENTING

Whenever possible, the nurse implements strategies to prevent infection. If infection cannot be prevented, the nurse's goal is to prevent the spread of the infection within and between persons, and to treat the existing infection. In the sections that follow, specific nursing activities are described that interfere in the chain of infection to prevent and control transmission of infectious organisms, and that promote care of the infected client. These activities are summarized in Table 19–5.

IDENTIFYING NURSING DIAGNOSES, OUTCOMES, AND INTERVENTIONS   **Client at Risk for Infection**

NURSING DIAGNOSIS/ DEFINITION	SAMPLE DESIRED OUTCOMES*/DEFINITION	INDICATORS†	SELECTED INTERVENTIONS*/ DEFINITION	SAMPLE ACTIVITIES
Risk for Infection/At increased risk for being invaded by pathogenic organisms	Knowledge: Infection Control [1807]/*Extent of understanding conveyed about prevention and control of infection*	• Description of factors contributing to transmission • Description of practices that reduce transmission • Description of activities to increase resistance to infection	Infection Control [6540]/*Minimizing the acquisition and transmission of infectious agents*	• Description of signs and symptoms • Description of treatment for diagnosed infection • Instruct patient on proper hand cleansing techniques • Institute standard precautions • Promote appropriate nutritional intake • Administer antibiotic therapy as indicated

*The NOC # for desired outcomes and the NIC # for nursing interventions are listed in brackets following the appropriate outcome or intervention. Outcomes, indicators, interventions, and activities are only a sample of those suggested by NOC and NIC and should be further individualized for each client.

†The measurement scale for these indicators ranges from None to Extensive. See MyNursingKit.

TABLE 19–5   **Nursing Interventions that Break the Chain of Infection**

LINK	INTERVENTIONS	RATIONALES
Etiologic agent (microorganism)	Ensure that articles are correctly cleaned and disinfected or sterilized before use.	Correct cleaning, disinfecting, and sterilizing reduce or eliminate microorganisms.
	Educate clients and support persons about appropriate methods to clean, disinfect, and sterilize articles.	Knowledge of ways to reduce or eliminate microorganisms reduces the numbers of microorganisms present and the likelihood of transmission.
Reservoir (source)	Change dressings and bandages when they are soiled or wet.	Moist dressings are ideal environments for microorganisms to grow and multiply.
	Assist clients to carry out appropriate skin and oral hygiene.	Hygienic measures reduce the numbers of resident and transient microorganisms and the likelihood of infection.
	Dispose of damp, soiled linens appropriately.	Damp, soiled linens harbor more microorganisms than dry linens.
	Dispose of feces and urine in appropriate receptacles.	Urine and feces in particular contain many microorganisms.
	Ensure that all fluid containers, such as bedside water jugs and suction and drainage bottles, are covered or capped.	Prolonged exposure increases the risk of contamination and promotes microbial growth.
	Empty suction and drainage bottles at the end of each shift or before they become full, or according to agency policy.	Drainage harbors microorganisms that, if left for long periods, proliferate and can be transmitted to others.
Portal of exit from the reservoir	Avoid talking, coughing, or sneezing over open wounds or sterile fields, and cover the mouth and nose when coughing and sneezing.	These measures limit the number of microorganisms that escape from the respiratory tract.
Method of transmission	Cleanse hands between client contacts, after touching body substances, and before performing invasive procedures or touching open wounds.	Hand cleansing is an important means of controlling and preventing the transmission of microorganisms.
	Instruct clients and support persons to cleanse hands before handling food or eating, after eliminating, and after touching infectious material.	Hand cleansing helps prevent transfer of microorganisms from one person to another.
	Wear gloves when handling secretions and excretions.	Gloves and gowns prevent soiling of the hands and clothing.
	Wear gowns if there is danger of soiling clothing with body substances.	
	Place discarded soiled materials in moisture-proof refuse bags.	Moisture-proof bags prevent the spread of microorganisms to others.
	Hold used bedpans steadily to prevent spillage, and dispose of urine and feces in appropriate receptacles.	Feces in particular contain many microorganisms.
	Initiate and implement aseptic precautions for all clients.	All clients may harbor potentially infectious microorganisms that can be transmitted to others.
	Wear masks and eye protection when in close contact with clients who have infections transmitted by droplets from the respiratory tract.	Masks and eyewear reduce the spread of droplet-transmitted microorganisms.
	Wear masks and eye protection when sprays of body fluid are possible (e.g., during irrigation procedures).	Masks and eye protection provide protection from microorganisms in clients' body substances.
Portal of entry to the susceptible host	Use sterile technique for invasive procedures (e.g., injections, catheterizations).	Invasive procedures penetrate the body's natural protective barriers to microorganisms.
	Use sterile technique when exposing open wounds or handling dressings.	Open wounds are vulnerable to microbial infection.
	Place used disposable needles and syringes in puncture-resistant containers for disposal.	Injuries from needles contaminated by blood or body fluids from an infected client or carrier are a primary cause of HBV and HIV transmission to health care workers.
	Provide all clients with their own personal care items.	People have less resistance to another person's microorganisms than to their own.
Susceptible host	Maintain the integrity of the client's skin and mucous membranes.	Intact skin and mucous membranes protect against invasion by microorganisms.
	Ensure that the client receives a balanced diet.	A balanced diet supplies proteins and vitamins necessary to build or maintain body tissues.
	Educate the public about the importance of immunizations.	Immunizations protect people against virulent infectious diseases.

Preventing Health Care–Associated Infections

Meticulous use of medical and surgical asepsis is necessary to prevent transport of potentially infectious microorganisms. Many HAI can be prevented using proper hand hygiene techniques, environmental controls, sterile technique when warranted, and identification and management of clients at risk for infections. A number of studies have shown a link between artificial fingernails and infection transmission, especially fungal. The nurse uses critical thinking and agency policy in implementing infection control procedures.

Hand Hygiene

Hand hygiene is important in every setting, including hospitals. It is considered one of the most effective infection control measures. Any client may harbor microorganisms that are currently harmless to the client yet potentially harmful to another person or to the same client if they find a portal of entry. It is important that both the nurses' and the clients' hands be cleansed at the following times to prevent the spread of microorganisms: before eating, after using the bedpan or toilet, and after the hands have come in contact with any body substances, such as sputum or drainage from a wound. In addition, health care workers should cleanse their hands before and after giving care of any kind.

For routine client care, the World Health Organization (2005) recommends hand washing under a stream of water for at least 20 seconds using plain granule soap, soap-filled sheets, or liquid soap when hands are visibly soiled, after using the restroom, after removing gloves, before handling invasive devices (such as intravenous tubing), and after contact with medical equipment or furniture. CDC guidelines also recommend hand hygiene when moving from dirty to clean areas.

However, soap and water are inadequate to sufficiently remove pathogens. The CDC recommends use of alcohol-based antiseptic hand rubs for use before and after direct client contact. Recently, placement of alcohol-based antiseptic hand rub dispensers has been approved for agency

---

| CLIENT TEACHING | **Infection Control** |

Environmental Management

- Discuss injury-proofing the home to prevent the possibility of further tissue injury (e.g., use of padding, handrails, removal of hazards).
- Explore ways to control the environmental temperature and airflow (especially if client has an airborne pathogen).
- Determine the advisability of visitors and family members in proximity to the client.
- Describe ways to manipulate the bed, the room, and other household facilities to prevent additional injury or to contain possible cross-contamination.
- Instruct to clean obviously soiled linen separately from other laundry. Rinse in cold water, wash in hot water if possible, and add a cup of bleach or phenol-based disinfectant such as Lysol concentrate to the wash.

Infection Control

- Based on assessment of client and family knowledge, teach proper hand hygiene (e.g., before handling foods, before eating, after toileting, before and after any required home care treatment, and after touching any body substances such as wound drainage) and related hygienic measures to all family members.
- Promote nail care: keep fingernails short, clean, and well manicured to eliminate rough edges or hangnails, which can harbor microorganisms.
- Instruct not to share personal care items such as toothbrushes, washcloths, and towels. Describe the rationale of how infections can be transmitted from shared personal items.

- Discuss antimicrobial soaps and effective disinfectants.
- Ensure access to and proper use of gloves and other barriers as indicated by the type of infection or risk.
- Discuss the relationship between hygiene, rest, activity, and nutrition in the chain of infection.
- Instruct about proper administration of medication.
- Instruct about cleaning reusable equipment and supplies. Use soap and water, and disinfect with a chlorine bleach solution.

Infection Protection

- Teach the client and family members the signs and symptoms of infection, and when to contact a health care provider. Determine by verbal questions the level of understanding on the topic after each teaching session.
- Teach the client and family members how to avoid infections.
- Suggest techniques for safe food preservation and preparation (e.g., wash raw fruits and vegetables before eating them, refrigerate all opened and unpackaged foods).
- Remind to avoid coughing, sneezing, or breathing directly on others. Cover the mouth and nose to prevent the transmission of airborne microorganisms.
- Inform of the importance of maintaining sufficient fluid intake to promote urine production and output. This helps flush the bladder and urethra of microorganisms.
- Emphasize the need for proper immunizations of all family members.

corridors (Centers for Medicare and Medicaid Services, 2005). Previous concerns that this represented a fire hazard have been addressed in the regulations. Proper application of alcohol-based products includes the following steps.

- Apply a palmful of the product to a cupped hand. An adequate amount to completely cover both hands, palms and backs, is essential.
- Rub palms against palms.
- Interlace fingers palm to palm.
- Rub palms to back of hands.
- Rub each finger individually on all sides with the other hand.
- Continue until product is dry—about 20 to 30 seconds.

Antimicrobial soaps are usually provided in high-risk areas, such as the newborn nursery, and are frequently supplied in dispensers at the sink. Studies have shown that the convenience of antimicrobial foams and gels, which do not require soap and water, may increase health care workers' adher-ence to hand cleansing. The CDC recommends antimicro-bial hand cleansing agents in the following situations:

- When there are known multiple resistant bacteria
- Before invasive procedures
- In special care units, such as nurseries and ICUs
- Before caring for severely immunocompromised clients

It is important to recognize that performing hand hygiene with either soap or alcohol-based cleansers can damage the skin through the drying effect of the detergents or chemicals. If the nurse develops dermatitis, the client may be at higher risk because hand washing does not decrease bacterial counts on skin with dermatitis. The nurse is also at higher risk be-cause the skin barrier has been broken. Although lotions, moisturizers, and emollients have been tried, no research has yet confirmed their effectiveness in decreasing the problem.

Skill 19–1 describes proper hand hygiene techniques using soap and water.

SKILL 19–1

HAND HYGIENE

PURPOSES
- To reduce the number of microorganisms on the hands
- To reduce the risk of transmission of microorganisms to clients
- To reduce the risk of cross-contamination among clients
- To reduce the risk of transmission of infectious organisms to oneself

ASSESSMENT
Determine the client's

- Risk for acquiring an infection.
- Use of immunosuppressive medications.
- Recent diagnostic procedures or treatments that penetrated the skin or a body cavity.
- Current nutritional status.

- Signs and symptoms indicating the presence of an infection:
  - Localized signs, such as swelling, redness, pain or tender-ness with palpation or movement, palpable heat at site, loss of function of affected body part, presence of exudate
  - Systemic indications, such as fever, increased pulse and respiratory rates, lack of energy, anorexia, enlarged lymph nodes

PLANNING
Determine the location of running water and soap or soap substitutes.

Delegation
The technique of hand hygiene is identical for all health care providers, including unlicensed assistive personnel (UAP). Health care team members are accountable for the implemen-tation of appropriate hand hygiene procedures.

EQUIPMENT
- Soap, foam, or alcohol gel sanitizer (for soap only)
- Warm running water
- Towels (for soap and water only)

IMPLEMENTATION
Preparation
Assess the hands.

- Nails should be kept short. **Rationale:** *Short, natural nails are less likely to harbor microorganisms, scratch a client, or puncture gloves. Most agencies do not permit health care workers in direct contact with clients to have any form of artificial nails.*
- Removal of jewelry is not thought to be necessary (Wongworawat & Jones, 2007), but is recommended. **Rationale:** *Microorganisms can lodge in the settings of jewelry and under rings. Removal facilitates proper cleaning of the hands and arms.*
- Check hands for breaks in the skin, such as hangnails or cuts. **Rationale:** *A nurse who has open sores may require a work assignment with decreased risk for transmission of infectious organisms due to the chance of acquiring or passing on an infection.*

Performance
1. If you are washing your hands where the client can observe you, introduce yourself and explain to the client what you are going to do and why it is necessary.
2. Turn on the water and adjust the flow.
   - There are five common types of faucet controls:
     a. Hand-operated handles.
     b. Knee levers. Move these with the knee to regulate flow and temperature.
     c. Foot pedals. Press these with the foot to regulate flow and temperature.

d. Elbow controls. Move these with the elbows instead of the hands.

e. Infrared control. Motion in front of the sensor causes water to start and stop flowing automatically.

- Adjust the flow so that the water is warm. **Rationale:** *Warm water removes less of the protective oil of the skin than hot water.*

3. Wet the hands thoroughly by holding them under the running water and apply soap to the hands.
   - Hold the hands lower than the elbows so that the water flows from the arms to the fingertips. **Rationale:** *The water should flow from the least contaminated to the most contaminated area; the hands are generally considered more contaminated than the lower arms.* Note that this is a different technique than is used when performing surgical hand washing. Nurses will learn to perform that level of hand washing if they are working in the operating room.
   - If the soap is liquid, apply 2 to 5 mL (1 tsp). If it is bar soap, granules, or sheets, rub them firmly between the hands.

4. Thoroughly wash and rinse the hands.
   - Use firm, rubbing, and circular movements to wash the palm, back, and wrist of each hand. Be sure to include the heel of the hand. Interlace the fingers and thumbs, and move the hands back and forth. ❶
     Continue this motion for at least 20 seconds (Houghton, 2006). **Rationale:** *The circular action creates friction that helps remove microorganisms mechanically. Interlacing the fingers and thumbs cleans the interdigital spaces.*
   - Rub the fingertips against the palm of the opposite hand. **Rationale:** *The nails and fingertips are commonly missed during hand hygiene.*
   - Rinse the hands.

5. Thoroughly pat dry the hands and arms.
   - Dry hands and arms thoroughly with a paper towel without scrubbing. **Rationale:** *Moist skin becomes chapped readily as does dry skin that is rubbed vigorously; chapping may produce lesions.*
   - Discard the paper towel in the appropriate container.

6. Turn off the water.
   - Use a new paper towel to grasp a hand-operated control. ❷ **Rationale:** *This prevents the nurse from picking up microorganisms from the faucet handles.*

VARIATION: HAND HYGIENE BEFORE STERILE SKILLS

- Apply the soap and wash as described in step 4, but hold the hands higher than the elbows during this hand wash. Wet the hands and forearms under the running water, letting it run from the fingertips to the elbows so that the hands

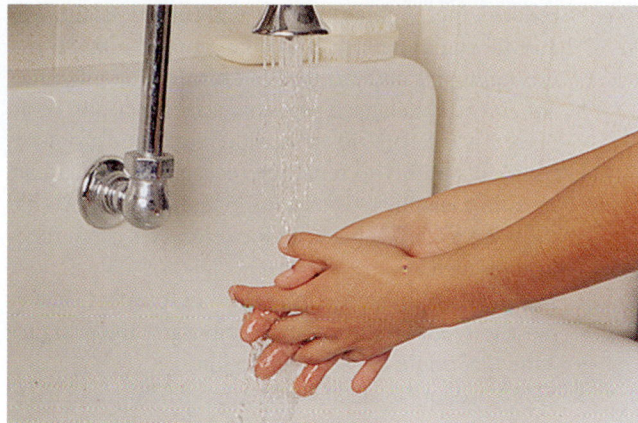

❶ Interlacing the fingers during hand washing.

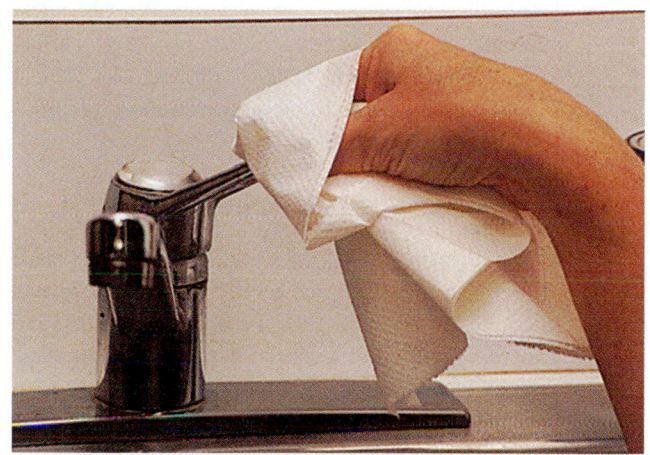

❷ Using a paper towel to grasp the handle of a hand-operated faucet.

become cleaner than the elbows. **Rationale:** *In this way, the water runs from the area that now has the fewest microorganisms to areas with a relatively greater number.*

- After washing and rinsing, use a towel to dry one hand thoroughly in a rotating motion from the fingers to the elbow. Use a new towel to dry the other hand and arm. **Rationale:** *A clean towel prevents the transfer of microorganisms from one elbow (least clean area) to the other hand (cleanest area).*

EVALUATION

There is no traditional evaluation of the effectiveness of the individual nurse's hand washing. Institutional quality control departments monitor the occurrence of client infections and investigate those situations in which health care providers are implicated in the transmission of infectious organisms. Research has repeatedly shown the positive impact of careful hand cleansing on client health associated with prevention of infection.

Supporting Defenses of a Susceptible Host

People are constantly in contact with microorganisms in the environment. Normally a person's natural defenses ward off the development of an infection. *Susceptibility* is the degree to which an individual can be affected. The following measures can reduce a person's susceptibility:

- *Hygiene.* Intact skin and mucous membranes are one barrier against microorganisms entering the body. In addition, good oral care, including flossing the teeth, reduces the likelihood of an oral infection. Regular and thorough bathing and shampooing remove microorganisms and dirt that can result in an infection.

- *Nutrition.* A balanced diet enhances the health of all body tissues, helps keep the skin intact, and promotes the skin's ability to repel microorganisms. Adequate nutrition enables tissues to maintain and rebuild themselves and helps keep the immune system functioning well.
- *Fluid.* Fluid intake permits fluid output that flushes out the bladder and urethra, removing microorganisms that could cause an infection.
- *Sleep.* Adequate sleep is essential to health and to renewing energy. See Chapter 31 ∞.
- *Stress.* Excessive stress predisposes people to infections. Nurses can assist clients to learn stress-reducing techniques. See Chapter 30 ∞.
- *Immunizations.* The use of immunizations has dramatically decreased the incidence of infectious diseases. It is recommended that immunizations begin shortly after birth and be completed in early childhood except for boosters.

Disinfecting and Sterilizing

The first links in the chain of infection, the etiologic agent and the reservoir, are interrupted by the use of **antiseptics** (agents that inhibit the growth of some microorganisms) and **disinfectants** (agents that destroy pathogens other than spores), and by sterilization.

DISINFECTING A disinfectant is a chemical preparation used on inanimate objects. Disinfectants are frequently caustic and toxic to tissues. An antiseptic is a chemical preparation used on skin or tissue. Disinfectants and antiseptics often have similar chemical components, but the disinfectant is a more concentrated solution.

Both antiseptics and disinfectants are said to have bactericidal or bacteriostatic properties. A *bactericidal* preparation destroys bacteria, whereas a *bacteriostatic* preparation prevents the growth and reproduction of some bacteria. An agent known to be effective against it should be selected. Spore-forming bacteria may be inhibited by only a few of the agents

normally effective against other forms of bacteria. Table 19–6 lists commonly used antiseptics and disinfectants.

When disinfecting articles, nurses need to follow agency protocol and consider the following:

1. The type and number of infectious organisms. Some microorganisms are readily destroyed, whereas others require longer contact with the disinfectant.
2. The recommended concentration of the disinfectant and the duration of contact.
3. The presence of soap. Some disinfectants are ineffective in the presence of soap or detergent.
4. The presence of organic materials. The presence of saliva, blood, pus, or excretions can readily inactivate many disinfectants.
5. The surface areas to be treated. The disinfecting agent must come into contact with all surfaces and areas.

STERILIZING **Sterilization** is a process that destroys all microorganisms, including spores and viruses. Four commonly used methods of sterilization are moist heat, gas, boiling water, and radiation.

Moist Heat To sterilize with moist heat, steam under pressure is used because it attains temperatures higher than the boiling point.

Gas Ethylene oxide gas destroys microorganisms by interfering with their metabolic processes. It is also effective against spores. Its advantages are good penetration and effectiveness for heat-sensitive items. Its major disadvantage is its toxicity to humans.

Boiling Water This is the most practical and inexpensive method for sterilizing in the home. The main disadvantage is that spores and some viruses are not killed by this method. Boiling a minimum of 15 minutes is advised for disinfection of articles in the home.

Radiation Both ionizing (such as alpha, beta, and x-rays) and nonionizing (ultraviolet light) radiation are used for disinfection and sterilization. The main drawback to ultraviolet light is that the rays do not penetrate deeply. Ionizing radiation is used effectively in industry to sterilize foods, drugs, and other items that are sensitive to heat. Its main advantage

TABLE 19–6 Commonly Used Antiseptics and Disinfectants, Effectiveness, and Use

AGENT	EFFECTIVE AGAINST					USE ON
	BACTERIA	TUBERCULOSIS	SPORES	FUNGI	VIRUSES	
Isopropyl and ethyl alcohol	X	X		X	X	Hands, vial stoppers
Chlorine (bleach)	X	X	X	X	X	Blood spills
Hydrogen peroxide	X	X	X	X	X	Surfaces
Iodophors	X	X	X	X	X	Equipment; intact skin and tissues if diluted
Phenol	X	X		X	X	Surfaces
Chlorhexidine gluconate (Hibiclens)	X				X	Hands
Triclosan (Bacti-Stat)	X					Hands, intact skin

is that it is effective for items difficult to sterilize; its chief disadvantage is that the equipment is very expensive.

Isolation Precautions

Isolation refers to measures designed to prevent the spread of infections or potentially infectious microorganisms to health personnel, clients, and visitors. Several sets of guidelines have been used in hospitals and other health care settings.

Category-specific isolation precautions use seven categories: strict isolation, contact isolation, respiratory isolation, tuberculosis isolation, enteric precautions, drainage/secretions precautions, and blood/body fluid precautions.

Disease-specific isolation precautions provide precautions for specific diseases. These precautions delineate use of private rooms with special ventilation, having the client share a room with other clients infected with the same organism, and gowning to prevent gross soilage of clothes for specific infectious diseases (Garner & Simmons, 1983).

Universal precautions (UP) are techniques to be used with all clients to decrease the risk of transmitting unidentified pathogens (CDC, 1987; U.S. Department of Health and Human Services [USDHHS], 1988). Universal precautions obstruct the spread of **bloodborne pathogens;** those microorganisms carried in blood and body fluids that are capable of infecting other persons with serious and difficult to treat viral infections, namely, hepatitis B virus, hepatitis C virus, and HIV. The CDC did not recommend that universal precautions replace disease-specific or category-specific precautions, but that they are used in conjunction with them.

The **body substance isolation (BSI)** system employs generic infection control precautions for all clients except those with the few diseases transmitted through the air. The BSI system (Jackson, 1993) is based on three premises:

1. All people have an increased risk for infection from microorganisms placed on their mucous membranes and nonintact skin.

2. All people are likely to have potentially infectious microorganisms in all of their moist body sites and substances.

3. An unknown portion of clients and health care workers will always be colonized or infected with potentially infectious microorganisms in their blood and other moist body sites and substances.

The term *body substance* includes blood, some body fluids, urine, feces, wound drainage, oral secretions, and any other body product or tissue.

In addition to other actions and precautions discussed in this chapter, significant emphasis is placed on avoiding injury due to sharp instruments (see Chapter 23 ∞), measures to be taken in case of exposure to bloodborne pathogens, and communication about biohazards to employees. Federal regulations require that in most cases warning labels be affixed to containers of regulated waste and to refrigerators and freezers containing blood or other potentially infectious materials. The labels required are fluorescent orange or orange-red and feature the biohazard legend.

CDC (HICPAC) ISOLATION PRECAUTIONS (1996) The Hospital Infection Control Practices Advisory Committee (HICPAC) of the CDC presented new guidelines for isolation precautions in hospitals in 1996 (Garner & HICPAC, 1996). These guidelines have since been updated in 2007 (HICPAC, 2007) (Boxes 19–1 and 19–2). These guidelines designate two tiers of precautions:

- Standard Precautions
- Transmission-Based Precautions

Standard Precautions These precautions are used in the care of all persons in any health care facility regardless of their diagnosis or possible infection status. They apply to blood, all body fluids, secretions, and excretions except sweat (whether or not blood is present or visible), nonintact skin, and mucous membranes. Thus they combine the

---

BOX 19–1 Types of Standard Precautions Depending on the Routes of Disease Transmission

Contact Precautions

- Methicillin-resistant *Staphylococcus aureus*
- Vancomycin-resistant *Enterococci*
- Clostridium difficile
- Norovirus (i.e., for institutional outbreaks)
- Respiratory syncytial virus

Airborne Precautions

- *Aspergillus* species
- *Mycobacterium* tuberculosis
- Rubeola virus (i.e., measles)
- Varicella virus (i.e., chickenpox)
- Variola (i.e., smallpox)
- Severe acute respiratory syndrome

Droplet Precautions

- *Bordetella pertussis* (i.e., whooping cough)
- Influenza virus (i.e., flu)
- *Mycoplasma pneumoniae*
- Severe acute respiratory syndrome*
- Group A *streptococcus***
- *Neisseria* meningitidis (i.e., bacterial meningitis)
- Rubella (i.e., German measles)

*If an airborne infection isolation room is not available
**For the first 24 hours after administration of antibiotics

From Tarrac, S. E. Application of the updated CDC isolation guidelines for health care facilities. *Association of periOperative Registered Nurses (AORN) Journal*, Mar; 87(3): 534–546. ISSN: 0001-2092 PMID: 18368742 CINAHL AN: 2009867648

BOX 19–2 **Summary of the Updated Centers for Disease Control and Prevention Isolation Guidelines**

Recommendation When to Use

Hand hygiene after touching

- blood,
- bloody fluids,
- secretions,
- excretions, or
- contaminated items

    Immediately after removing gloves

    Between patient contacts

    When moving from dirty to clean areas

Gloves when anticipating touching

- blood,
- body fluids,
- secretions,
- excretions,
- contaminated items,

- mucous membranes, or
- nonintact skin

Gown during procedures and patient-care activities when anticipating contact with

- clothing,
- blood,
- body fluids,
- secretions, or
- excretions

Mask/goggles/face shield during procedures and patient-care activities likely to generate splashes or sprays of

- blood,
- body fluid, or
- secretions (i.e., suctioning, endotracheal intubation)

From Tarrac, S. E. Application of the updated CDC isolation guidelines for health care facilities. *AORN Journal*, Mar; 87 (3): 534–546. ISSN: 0001-2092 PMID: 18368742 CINAHL AN: 2009867648

major features of UP and BSI. Recommended practices for standard precautions are shown in Box 19–3.

Transmission-Based Precautions These precautions are used in addition to standard precautions for clients with known or suspected infections that are spread in one of three ways: by airborne or droplet transmission, or by contact. The three types of transmission-based precautions may be used alone or in combination but always in addition to standard precautions. They encompass all of the conditions or diseases previously listed in the category-specific or disease-specific classifications developed by the CDC in 1983. Recommended practices for Transmission-Based Precautions are shown in Box 19–3.

Airborne precautions are used for clients known to have or suspected of having serious illnesses transmitted by airborne droplet nuclei smaller than 5 microns. Examples of such illnesses include measles (rubeola), varicella (including disseminated zoster), and tuberculosis. The CDC has prepared special guidelines for preventing the transmission of tuberculosis. The most current information may be found on the CDC Division of Tuberculosis Elimination website.

Droplet precautions are used for clients known or suspected to have serious illnesses transmitted by particle droplets larger than 5 microns. Examples of such illnesses are diphtheria (pharyngeal); mycoplasma pneumonia; pertussis; mumps; rubella; streptococcal pharyngitis, pneumonia, or scarlet fever in infants and young children; and pneumonic plague.

Contact precautions are used for clients known or suspected to have serious illnesses easily transmitted by direct client contact or by contact with items in the client's environment. According to the CDC (Garner & HICPAC, 1996), such illnesses include gastrointestinal, respiratory, skin, or wound infections or colonization with multidrug-resistant bacteria; specific enteric infections such as *C. difficile,* and enterohemorrhagic *Escherichia coli 0157:H7, Shigella,* and hepatitis A, for diapered or incontinent clients; respiratory syncytial virus,

parainfluenza virus, or enteroviral infections in infants and young children; and highly contagious skin infections such as herpes simplex virus, impetigo, pediculosis, and scabies.

In addition to the preceding conditions, special contact precautions are used for vancomycin-resistant enterococci (VRE) infections. The CDC recommends use of an antimicrobial soap for hand washing and no sharing of equipment among clients with and without VRE. The client should have a private room (or a room with other clients who have VRE), and such isolation should continue until at least three cultures taken 1 week apart are negative (HICPAC, 1995).

Some diseases require a combination of transmission-based precautions. For clients infected with the coronavirus that causes severe acute respiratory syndrome (SARS-CoV), standard (including eye protection), contact, and airborne precautions are indicated (CDC, 2005).

COMPROMISED CLIENTS Compromised clients (those highly susceptible to infection) are often infected by their own microorganisms, by microorganisms on the inadequately cleansed hands of health care personnel, and by nonsterile items. Clients who are severely compromised include those who:

- Have diseases that depress the client's resistance to infectious organisms.
- Have extensive skin impairments, such as severe dermatitis or major burns, which cannot be effectively covered with dressings.

The 2007 CDC guidelines for severely compromised (immunocompromised) clients include the use of standard precautions as described earlier.

Isolation Practices

Initiation of practices to prevent the transmission of microorganisms is generally a nursing responsibility and is based on a

| **BOX 19–3** | **Recommended Isolation Precautions in Hospitals** |

Standard Precautions

- Designed for use with all clients in any health care setting.
- These precautions apply to (a) blood; (b) all body fluids, excretions, and secretions except sweat; (c) nonintact (broken) skin; and (d) mucous membranes.
- Designed to reduce risk of transmission of microorganisms from recognized and unrecognized sources.
  1. Perform proper hand hygiene after contact with blood, body fluids, secretions, excretions, and contaminated objects whether or not gloves are worn.
     a. Perform proper hand hygiene immediately after removing gloves.
     b. Use a nonantimicrobial product for routine hand cleansing.
     c. Use an antimicrobial agent or an antiseptic agent for the control of specific outbreaks of infection.
  2. Wear clean gloves when touching blood, body fluids, secretions, excretions, contaminated items, or any item that came in contract with a client.
     a. Clean gloves can be unsterile unless their use is intended to prevent the entrance of microorganisms into the body. See the discussion of sterile gloves in this chapter.
     b. Remove gloves before touching noncontaminated items and surfaces.
     c. Perform proper hand hygiene immediately after removing gloves.
  3. Wear a mask, eye protection, or a face shield if splashes or sprays of blood, body fluids, secretions, or excretions can be expected. The new CDC guidelines recommend use of masks when performing any invasive procedure.
  4. Wear a clean, nonsterile gown if client care is likely to result in splashes or sprays of blood, body fluids, secretions, or excretions. The gown is intended to protect clothing.
     a. Remove a soiled gown carefully to avoid the transfer of microorganisms to others (i.e., clients or other health care workers).
     b. Cleanse hands after removing gown.
  5. Handle client care equipment that is soiled with blood, body fluids, secretions, or excretions carefully to prevent the transfer of microorganisms to others and to the environment.
     a. Make sure reusable equipment is cleaned and reprocessed correctly.
     b. Dispose of single-use equipment correctly.
  6. Handle, transport, and process linen that is soiled with blood, body fluids, secretions, or excretions in a manner to prevent contamination of clothing and the transfer of microorganisms to others and to the environment.
  7. Prevent injuries from used scalpels, needles, or other equipment, and place in puncture-resistant containers.
  8. Avoid using bags of IV solution as a common source of supply for multiple clients.

Respiratory Hygiene/Cough Etiquette

Use standard precautions as well as the following if the client has a cough or symptoms of a respiratory infection upon initial contact with the health care agency. Family or friends accompanying the client should also follow these recommendations:

1. Covering the mouth and nose with a tissue when coughing
2. Prompt and proper disposal of used tissues into no-touch receptacles
3. Observe hand hygiene after soiling of hands with respiratory secretions

4. Wear surgical mask if tolerated or maintain spatial separation of 3 feet if possible

Transmission-Based Precautions

Airborne Precautions

Use standard precautions as well as the following:

1. Place client in a private room that has negative air pressure, 6 to 12 air changes per hour, and either discharge of air to the outside or a filtration system for the room air.
2. If a private room is not available, place client with another client who is infected with the same microorganism.
3. Wear a respiratory device (N95 respirator) when entering the room of a client who is known or suspected of having primary tuberculosis.
4. Susceptible people should not enter the room of a client who has rubeola (measles) or varicella (chickenpox). If they must enter, they should wear a respirator.
5. Limit movement of client outside the room to essential purposes. Place a surgical mask on the client during transport.

Droplet Precautions

Use standard precautions as well as the following:

1. Place client in private room.
2. If a private room is not available, place client with another client who is infected with the same microorganism.
3. Wear a mask if working within 3 feet of the client.
4. Limit movement of client outside the room to essential purposes. Place a surgical mask on the client during transport.

Contact Precautions

Use standard precautions as well as the following:

1. Place client in private room.
2. If a private room is not available, place client with another client who is infected with the same microorganism.
3. Wear gloves as described in standard precautions.
   a. Change gloves after contact with infectious material.
   b. Remove gloves before leaving client's room.
   c. Cleanse hands immediately after removing gloves. Use an antimicrobial agent. Note: If the client is infected with *C. difficile*, do not use an alcohol-based hand rub as it may not be effective on these spores. Use soap and water.
   d. After hand cleansing, do not touch possibly contaminated surfaces or items in the room.
4. Wear a gown (see standard precautions) when entering a room if there is a possibility of contact with infected surfaces or items, or if the client is incontinent, or has diarrhea, a colostomy, or wound drainage not contained by a dressing.
   a. Remove gown in the client's room.
   b. Make sure uniform does not contact possible contaminated surfaces.
5. Limit movement of client outside the room.
6. Dedicate the use of noncritical client care equipment to a single client or to clients with the same infecting microorganisms.

Note: Adapted from "Guidelines for Isolation Precautions in Hospitals," by J. S. Garner and the Hospital Infection Control Practices Advisory Committee (HICPAC), 1996, *Infection Control Hospital Epidemiology, 17*, pp. 53–80, and 1996, *American Journal of Infection Control, 24*, pp. 24–52. And "Guidelines for Isolation Precautions: Preventing Transmission of Infectious Agents in Healthcare Settings 2007" by J. D. Siegel and the Healthcare Infection Control Practices Advisory Committee (HICPAC), 2007.

comprehensive assessment of the client. This assessment takes into account the status of the client's normal defense mechanisms, the client's ability to implement necessary precautions, and the source and mode of transmission of the infectious agent. The nurse then decides whether to wear gloves, gowns, masks, and protective eyewear. In all client situations, *nurses must cleanse their hands before and after giving care.*

In addition to the precautions cited within this chapter, the nurse implements aseptic precautions when performing many specific therapies discussed throughout this book. The following are some examples:

- Use strict aseptic technique when performing any invasive procedure and when changing surgical dressings. Use of a mask is recommended with any invasive procedure.
- Change intravenous tubing and solution containers according to hospital policy (e.g., every 48 to 72 hours).
- Check all sterile supplies for expiration date and intact packaging.
- Prevent urinary infections by maintaining a closed urinary drainage system with a downhill flow of urine. Keep the drainage bag and spout off the floor.
- Implement measures to prevent impaired skin integrity and to prevent accumulation of secretions in the lungs.

PERSONAL PROTECTIVE EQUIPMENT All health care providers must apply clean or sterile gloves, gowns, masks, and protective eyewear according to the risk of exposure to potentially infective materials.

Gloves Gloves are worn for three reasons: First, they protect the hands when the nurse is likely to handle any body substances, for example, blood, urine, feces, sputum, and nonintact skin. Second, gloves reduce the likelihood of nurses transmitting their own endogenous microorganisms to individuals receiving care. Nurses who have open sores or cuts on the hands must wear gloves for protection. Third, gloves reduce the chance that the nurse's hands will transmit microorganisms from one client or a fomite to another client. In all situations, gloves are changed between client contacts. The hands are cleansed each time gloves are removed for two primary reasons: (a) the gloves may have imperfections or be damaged during wearing so that they could allow microorganism entry and (b) the hands may become contaminated during glove removal.

Some of the gloves used in infection control may be made of latex rubber, as are various other items used in health care. Because of the frequent use of gloves, clients with chronic illnesses and health care workers have increasingly reported allergic reactions to latex. Latex gloves lubricated by powder or cornstarch are particularly allergenic because the latex allergen adheres to the powder, which is aerosolized during glove use and inhaled by the user. Latex gloves that are labeled "hypoallergenic" still contain measurable latex and should not be used by, or on, persons with known latex sensitivity. The people at greatest risk for developing latex allergies are those with other allergic conditions and those who have had frequent or long-term exposure to latex.

Latex allergies can be either local or systemic and may take the form of dermatitis, urticaria (hives), asthma, or anaphylaxis. Clients and health care workers should be assessed for possible allergies through a thorough history taking. People with significant allergies should have no contact with latex products. Most hospitals have eliminated latex products wherever possible and have established a "latex-free environment" goal.

Skill 19–2 describes application and removal of gloves.

SKILL 19–2

APPLYING AND REMOVING PERSONAL PROTECTIVE EQUIPMENT (GLOVES, GOWN, MASK, EYEWEAR)

PURPOSES
- To protect health care workers and clients from transmission of potentially infective materials

ASSESSMENT
Consider which activities will be required while the nurse is in the client's room at this time. **Rationale:** *This will determine which equipment is required.*

PLANNING
- Application and removal of personal protective equipment (PPE) can be time consuming. Prioritize care and arrange for personnel to care for your other clients if indicated.

- Determine which supplies are present within the client's room and which must be brought to the room.
- Consider whether special handling is indicated for removal of any specimens or other materials from the room.

Delegation
Use of PPE is identical for all health care providers. Clients whose care requires use of PPE may be delegated to UAP. Health care team members are accountable for proper implementation of these procedures by themselves and others.

EQUIPMENT
As indicated according to which activities will be performed. Ensure that extra supplies are easily available.

- Gown
- Mask
- Eyewear
- Clean gloves

IMPLEMENTATION

Preparation

Remove or secure all loose items such as name tags or jewelry.

Performance

1. Prior to performing the procedure, introduce self and verify the client's identity using agency protocol. Explain to the client what you are going to do, why it is necessary, and how he or she can participate.
2. Perform proper hand hygiene.
3. Apply a clean gown.
   - Pick up a clean gown, and allow it to unfold in front of you without allowing it to touch any area soiled with body substances.
   - Slide the arms and the hands through the sleeves.
   - Fasten the ties at the neck to keep the gown in place.
   - Overlap the gown at the back as much as possible, and fasten the waist ties or belt. ❶ **Rationale:** *Overlapping securely covers the uniform at the back. Waist ties keep the gown from falling away from the body, which can cause inadvertent soiling of the exposed uniform.*
4. Apply the face mask.
   - Locate the top edge of the mask. The mask usually has a narrow metal strip along the edge.
   - Hold the mask by the top two strings or loops.
   - Place the upper edge of the mask over the bridge of the nose, and tie the upper ties at the back of the head or secure the loops around the ears. If glasses are worn, fit the upper edge of the mask under the glasses. **Rationale:** *With the edge of the mask under the glasses, clouding of the glasses is less likely to occur.*
   - Secure the lower edge of the mask under the chin, and tie the lower ties at the nape of the neck. ❷ **Rationale:** *To be effective, a mask must cover both the nose and the mouth, because air moves in and out of both.*
   - If the mask has a metal strip, adjust this firmly over the bridge of the nose. **Rationale:** *A secure fit prevents both the escape and the inhalation of microorganisms around the edges of the mask and the fogging of eyeglasses.*
   - Wear the mask only once, and do not wear any mask longer than the manufacturer recommends or once it becomes wet. **Rationale:** *A mask should be used only once because it becomes ineffective when moist.*
   - Do not leave a used face mask hanging around the neck.
5. Apply protective eyewear if it is not combined with the face mask.
6. Apply clean gloves.
   - No special technique is required.
   - If wearing a gown, pull the gloves up to cover the cuffs of the gown. If not wearing a gown, pull the gloves up to cover the wrists.
7. To remove soiled PPE, remove the gloves first since they are the most soiled.
   - If wearing a gown that is tied at the waist in front, undo the ties before removing gloves.
   - Remove the first glove by grasping it on its palmar surface, taking care to touch only glove to glove. ❸ **Rationale:** *This keeps the soiled parts of the used gloves from touching the skin of the wrist or hand.*
   - Pull the first glove completely off by inverting or rolling the glove inside out.

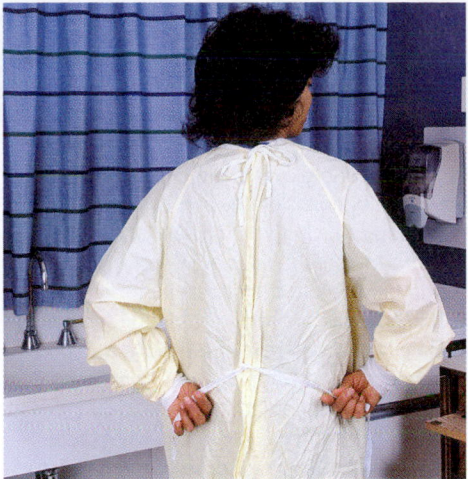

❶ Overlapping the gown at the back to cover the nurse's uniform.

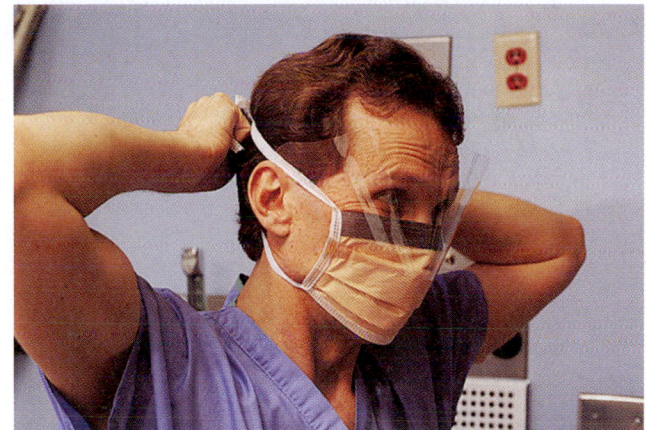

❷ A face mask and eye protection covering the nose, mouth, and eyes.

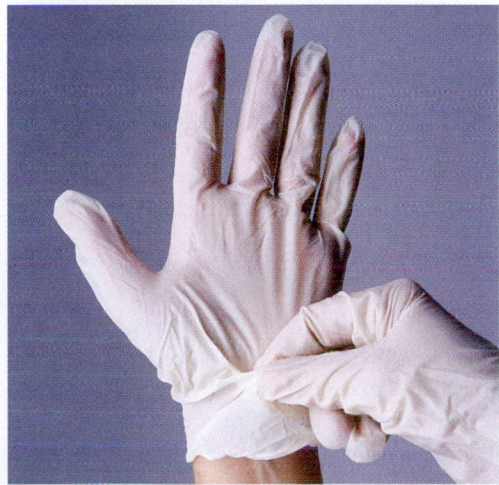

❸ Plucking the palmar surface below the cuff of a contaminated glove.

(continued)

SKILL 19–2

APPLYING AND REMOVING PERSONAL PROTECTIVE EQUIPMENT *(continued)*

- Continue to hold the inverted removed glove by the fingers of the remaining gloved hand. Place the first two fingers of the bare hand inside the cuff of the second glove. ❹ **Rationale:** *Touching the outside of the second soiled glove with the bare hand is avoided.*
- Pull the second glove off to the fingers by turning it inside out. This pulls the first glove inside the second glove. **Rationale:** *The soiled part of the glove is folded to the inside to reduce the chance of transferring any microorganisms by direct contact.*
- Using the bare hand, continue to remove the gloves, which are now inside out, and dispose of them in the refuse container. ❺

8. Perform hand hygiene.
9. Remove protective eyewear and dispose of properly or place in the appropriate receptacle for cleaning.
10. Remove the gown when preparing to leave the room. Unless a gown is grossly soiled with body substances, no special precautions are needed to remove it. If a gown is grossly soiled:
    - Avoid touching soiled parts on the outside of the gown, if possible. **Rationale:** *The top part of the gown may be soiled, for example, if you have been holding an infant with a respiratory infection.*
    - Grasp the gown along the inside of the neck and pull down over the shoulders. Do not shake the gown.
    - Roll up the gown with the soiled part inside, and discard it in the appropriate container.
11. Remove the mask.
    - Remove the mask at the doorway to the client's room. If using a respirator mask, remove it after leaving the room and closing the door.
    - If using a mask with strings, first untie the lower strings of the mask. **Rationale:** *This prevents the top part of the mask from falling onto the chest.*
    - Untie the top strings and, while holding the ties securely, remove the mask from the face. If side loops are present, lift the side loops up and away from the ears and face. Do not touch the front of the mask. **Rationale:** *The front*

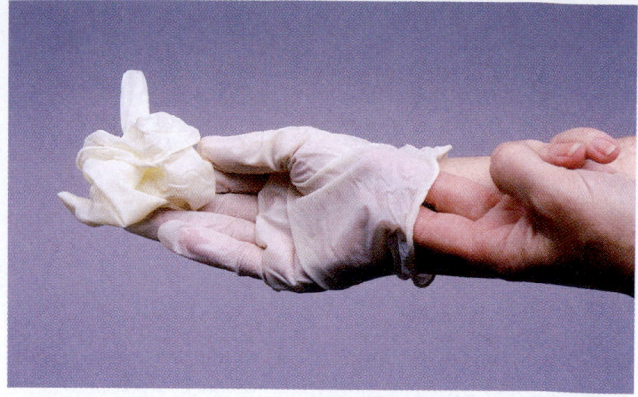

❹ Inserting fingers to remove the second contaminated glove.

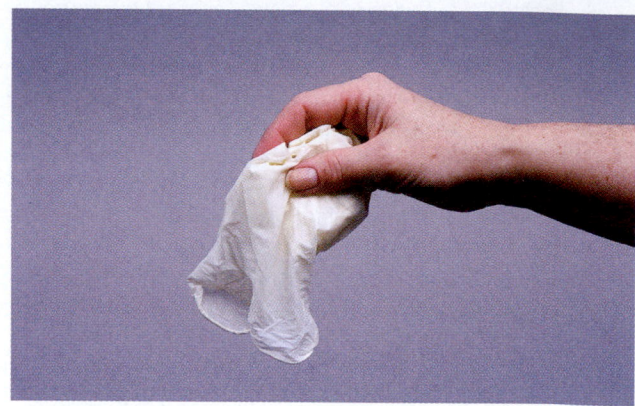

❺ Holding contaminated gloves, which are inside out.

of the mask through which the nurse has been breathing is contaminated.
- Discard a disposable mask in the waste container.
- Perform hand hygiene again.

EVALUATION

Conduct any follow-up indicated during your care of the client. If there has been any failure of the equipment and exposure to potentially infective materials is suspected, follow the procedure in the Practice Guidelines: "Steps to Follow after Exposure to Blood-borne Pathogens" later in this chapter.

Ensure that an adequate supply of equipment is available for the next health care provider.

Gowns Clean or disposable impervious (water-resistant) gowns or plastic aprons are worn during procedures when the nurse's uniform is likely to become soiled. Sterile gowns may be indicated when the nurse changes the dressings of a client with extensive wounds *Single-use gown technique* (using a gown only once before it is discarded or laundered) is the usual practice in hospitals. After the gown is worn, the nurse discards it or places it in a laundry hamper. See Skill 19–2. Before leaving the client's room, the nurse cleanses his or her hands.

CLINICAL ALERT

Wearing a client hospital gown over your uniform does not serve any infection control purpose.

Face Masks Masks are worn to reduce the risk for transmission of organisms by the droplet contact and airborne routes, and by splatters of body substances. The CDC recommends that masks be worn:

1. By those close to the client if the infection is transmitted by large-particle aerosols (droplets). Large-particle aerosols are transmitted by close contact and generally travel short distances (about 1 m, or 3 ft).
2. By all persons entering the room if the infection is transmitted by small-particle aerosols (droplet nuclei). Small-particle aerosols remain suspended in the air and thus travel greater distances by air. Special masks that provide a tighter face seal and better filtration may be used for these infections.
3. By anyone performing an invasive procedure such as inserting a urinary catheter, initiating an IV, or administering an injection (HICPAC, 2007)

Various types of masks differ in their filtration effectiveness and fit. Single-use disposable surgical masks are effective for use while the nurse provides care to most clients but should be changed if they become wet or soiled. These masks are discarded in the waste container after use. Disposable particulate respirators of different types may be effective for droplet transmission, splatters, and airborne microorganisms. Some respirators now available are effective in preventing inhalation of tuberculin organisms. The National Institute for Occupational Safety and Health (NIOSH) tests and certifies such respirators. Currently, the category "N" respirator at 95% efficiency (referred to as an N95 respirator) meets tuberculosis and SARS control criteria.

During certain techniques requiring surgical asepsis (sterile technique), masks are worn (a) to prevent droplet contact transmission of exhaled microorganisms to the sterile field or to a client's open wound and (b) to protect the nurse from splashes of body substances from the client. Guidelines for donning and removing face masks are shown in Skill 19–2.

Eyewear Protective eyewear (goggles, glasses, or face shields) and masks are indicated in situations where body substances may splatter the face (see Skill 19–2). If the nurse wears prescription eyeglasses, goggles must still be worn over the glasses because the protection must extend around the sides of the glasses.

DISPOSAL OF SOILED EQUIPMENT AND SUPPLIES Many pieces of equipment are supplied for single use only and are disposed of after use. Some items, however, are reusable. Agencies have specific policies and procedures for handling soiled equipment; the nurse needs to become familiar with these practices in the employing agency. Appropriate handling of soiled equipment and supplies is essential for these reasons:

- To prevent inadvertent exposure of health care workers to articles contaminated with body substances
- To prevent contamination of the environment

Bagging Articles contaminated, or likely to have been contaminated, with infective material such as pus, blood, body fluids, feces, or respiratory secretions need to be enclosed in a sturdy bag impervious to microorganisms before they are removed from the room of any client. Some agencies use labels or bags of a particular color that designates them as infective wastes.

CDC guidelines recommend the following methods:

- A single bag, if it is sturdy and impervious to microorganisms, and if the contaminated articles can be placed in the bag without soiling or contaminating its outside
- Double-bagging if the above conditions are not met

Follow agency protocol, or use the following CDC guidelines to handle and bag soiled items:

- Place garbage and soiled *disposable* equipment, including dressings and tissues, in the plastic bag that lines the waste container. Some agencies separate dry and wet waste material and incinerate dry items, such as paper towels and disposable items. No special precautions are required for disposable equipment that is not contaminated.
- Place *nondisposable* or *reusable* equipment that is visibly soiled in a labeled bag before removing it from the client's room or cubicle, and send it to a central processing area for decontamination. Some agencies may require that glass bottles or jars and metal items be placed in separate bags from rubber and plastic items. Glass and metal can be sterilized in an autoclave, but rubber and plastic are damaged by this process and must be cleaned by other methods, such as gas sterilization.
- Disassemble special procedure trays into component parts. Some components are disposable; others need to be sent to the laundry or central services for cleaning and decontaminating.
- Bag soiled clothing before sending it home or to the agency laundry.

Linens Handle soiled linen as little as possible and with the least agitation possible before placing it in the laundry hamper. This prevents gross microbial contamination of the air and persons handling the linen. Close the bag before sending it to the laundry in accordance with agency practice.

Laboratory Specimens Laboratory specimens, if placed in a leakproof container with a secure lid with a biohazard label, need no special precautions. Use care when collecting specimens to avoid contaminating the outside of the container. Containers that are visibly contaminated on the outside should be placed inside a sealable plastic bag before sending them to the laboratory. This prevents personnel from having hand contact with potentially infective material.

Dishes Dishes require no special precautions. Soiling of dishes can largely be prevented by encouraging clients to cleanse their hands before eating. Some agencies use paper dishes for convenience, which are disposed of in the refuse container.

Blood Pressure Equipment Blood pressure equipment needs no special precautions unless it becomes contaminated with infective material. If it does become contaminated, follow agency policy to decontaminate it. Cleaning procedures vary according to whether it is a wall or portable unit. In some agencies, a disposable cuff is used for clients placed on contact precautions.

Thermometers Nondisposable used thermometers are generally disinfected after use. Check agency practice.

Disposable Needles, Syringes, and Sharps Place needles, syringes, and "sharps" into a puncture-resistant container. To avoid puncture wounds, use approved safety or needleless systems and do not detach needles from the syringe or recap the needle before disposal. See Chapter 23 ∞ for how to prevent needlestick injuries.

CLINICAL ALERT

Federal rules protecting the privacy of personal health information may extend to the client labels placed on disposable supplies such as intravenous fluid containers. Agencies may require that these be returned to the pharmacy so that personal information may be removed before disposal. Check agency policy.

TRANSPORTING CLIENTS WITH INFECTIONS Transporting clients with infections outside their own rooms is avoided unless absolutely necessary. If a client must be moved, the nurse implements appropriate precautions and measures to prevent soilage of the environment. For example, the nurse ensures that any draining wound is securely covered or places a surgical mask on the client who has an airborne infection. In addition, the nurse notifies personnel at the receiving area of any infection risk so that they can maintain necessary precautions. Follow agency protocol.

PSYCHOSOCIAL NEEDS OF ISOLATION CLIENTS Clients requiring isolation precautions can develop several problems as a result of the separation from others and of the special precautions taken in their care. Two of the most common are sensory deprivation and decreased self-esteem related to feelings of inferiority. *Sensory deprivation* occurs when the environment lacks normal stimuli for the client, for example, communication with others. Nurses should therefore be alert to common clinical signs of sensory deprivation: boredom, inactivity, slowness of thought, daydreaming, increased sleeping, thought disorganization, anxiety, hallucinations, and panic.

Chapter 27 ∞ provides information on the development of self-esteem and self-esteem disturbances. A client's *feeling of inferiority* can be due to the perception of the infection itself or to the required precautions. In North America, many people place a high value on cleanliness, and the idea of being "soiled," "contaminated," or "dirty" can give clients the feeling that they are at fault and substandard. Al-

though this is obviously not true, the infected persons may feel "not as good" as others and blame themselves. An appropriate nursing diagnosis may be *Risk for Situational Low Self-Esteem.*

Nurses need to provide care that prevents these two problems or that deals with them positively. Nursing interventions include the following:

1. Assess the individual's need for stimulation.
2. Initiate measures to help meet the need, including regular communication with the client and diversionary activities, such as toys for a child, and books, television, or radio for an adult; provide a variety of foods to stimulate the client's sense of taste; stimulate the client's visual sense by providing a view or an activity to watch.
3. Explain the infection and the associated procedures to help clients and their support people understand and accept the situation.
4. Demonstrate warm, accepting behavior. Avoid conveying to the client any sense of annoyance about the precautions or any feelings of revulsion about the infection.
5. Do not use stricter precautions than are indicated by the diagnosis or the client's condition.

Sterile Technique

An object is sterile only when it is free of all microorganisms. It is well known that sterile technique is practiced in operating rooms and special diagnostic areas. Sterile technique is also employed for many procedures in general care areas. In these situations, all of the principles of surgical asepsis are applied as in the operating or delivery room; however, not all of the sterile techniques that follow are always required. The basic principles of surgical asepsis, and practices that relate to each principle, appear in Table 19–7.

STERILE FIELD A sterile field is a microorganism-free area. Nurses often establish a sterile field by using the innermost side of a sterile wrapper or by using a sterile drape. When the field is established, sterile supplies and sterile solutions can be placed on it. Sterile forceps are used in many instances to handle and transfer sterile supplies.

So that sterility can be maintained, supplies may be wrapped in a variety of materials. Commercially prepared items are frequently wrapped in plastic, paper, or glass. In the past, it was not unusual for sterile liquids to be supplied in large containers and used many times. This practice is considered undesirable today because once a container has been opened, there can be no assurance that it will remain sterile. Liquids are preferably packaged in amounts adequate for one use only. Any leftover liquid is discarded. The nurse should never use one container of fluid between multiple clients as this presents an increased risk of infection.

Skill 19–3 describes how to establish and maintain a sterile field.

TABLE 19–7	Principles and Practices of Surgical Asepsis
PRINCIPLES	**PRACTICES**
All objects used in a sterile field must be sterile.	All articles are sterilized appropriately by dry or moist heat, chemicals, or radiation before use.
	Always check a package containing a sterile object for intactness, dryness, and expiration date. Sterile articles can be stored for only a prescribed time; after that, they are considered unsterile. Any package that appears already open, torn, punctured, or wet is considered unsterile.
	Storage areas should be clean, dry, off the floor, and away from sinks.
	Always check chemical indicators of sterilization before using a package. The indicator is often a tape used to fasten the package or contained inside the package. The indicator changes color during sterilization, indicating that the contents have undergone a sterilization procedure. If the color change is not evident, the package is considered unsterile. Commercially prepared sterile packages may not have indicators but are marked with the word *sterile*.
Sterile objects become unsterile when touched by unsterile objects.	Handle sterile objects that will touch open wounds or enter body cavities only with sterile forceps or sterile gloved hands.
	Discard or resterilize objects that come into contact with unsterile objects.
	Whenever the sterility of an object is questionable, assume the article is unsterile.
Sterile items that are out of vision or below the waist or table level are considered unsterile.	Once left unattended, a sterile field is considered unsterile.
	Sterile objects are always kept in view. Nurses do not turn their backs on a sterile field.
	Only the front part of a sterile gown, from shoulder to waist (or table height, whichever is higher), and the cuff of the sleeves to 2 inches above the elbows are considered sterile.
	Always keep sterile gloved hands in sight and above waist/table level; touch only objects that are sterile.
	Sterile draped tables in the operating room or elsewhere are considered sterile only at surface level.
Sterile objects can become unsterile by prolonged exposure to airborne microorganisms.	Keep doors closed and traffic to a minimum in areas where a sterile procedure is being performed, because moving air can carry dust and microorganisms.
	Keep areas in which sterile procedures are carried out as clean as possible by frequent damp cleaning with detergent germicides to minimize contaminants in the area.
	Keep hair clean and short or enclose it in a net to prevent hair from falling on sterile objects. Microorganisms on the hair can make a sterile field unsterile.
	Wear surgical caps in operating rooms, delivery rooms, and burn units.
	Refrain from sneezing or coughing over a sterile field. This can make it unsterile because droplets containing microorganisms from the respiratory tract can travel 1 m (3 ft). Some agencies recommend that masks covering the mouth and the nose should be worn by anyone working over a sterile field or an open wound.
	Nurses with mild upper respiratory tract infections refrain from carrying out sterile procedures or wear masks.
	When working over a sterile field, keep talking to a minimum. Avert the head from the field if talking is necessary.
	To prevent microorganisms from falling over a sterile field, refrain from reaching over a sterile field unless sterile gloves are worn and refrain from moving unsterile objects over a sterile field.
Fluids flow in the direction of gravity.	Unless gloves are worn, always hold wet forceps with the tips below the handles. When the tips are held higher than the handles, fluid can flow onto the handle and become contaminated by the hands. When the forceps are again pointed downward, the contaminated fluid flows back down and contaminates the tips.
	During a surgical hand wash, hold the hands higher than the elbows to prevent contaminants from the forearms from reaching the hands.
Moisture that passes through a sterile object draws microorganisms from unsterile surfaces above or below to the sterile surface by capillary action.	Sterile moisture-proof barriers are used beneath sterile objects. Liquids (sterile saline or antiseptics) are frequently poured into containers on a sterile field. If they are spilled onto the sterile field, the barrier keeps the liquid from seeping beneath it.
	Keep the sterile covers on sterile equipment dry. Damp surfaces can attract microorganisms in the air.
	Replace sterile drapes that do not have a sterile barrier underneath when they become moist.
The edges of a sterile field are considered unsterile.	A 2.5-cm (1-in.) margin at each edge of an opened drape is considered unsterile because the edges are in contact with unsterile surfaces.
	Place all sterile objects more than 2.5 cm (1 in.) inside the edges of a sterile field.
	Any article that falls outside the edges of a sterile field is considered unsterile.
The skin cannot be sterilized and is unsterile.	Use sterile gloves or sterile forceps to handle sterile items.
	Prior to a surgical aseptic procedure, cleanse the hands to reduce the number of microorganisms on them.
Conscientiousness, alertness, and honesty are essential qualities in maintaining surgical asepsis.	When a sterile object becomes unsterile, it does not necessarily change in appearance.
	The person who sees a sterile object become contaminated must correct or report the situation.
	Do not set up a sterile field ahead of time for future use.

SKILL 19–3

ESTABLISHING AND MAINTAINING A STERILE FIELD

PURPOSES
* To ensure that sterile items remain sterile

ASSESSMENT
Review the client's record or discuss with the client or other health care team member exactly what procedure will be performed that requires a sterile field. Determine the client's presence or risk for infection and ability to participate with the procedure.

PLANNING
Determine, if possible, what supplies and techniques have been used in the past to perform the procedures for this client. Also, attempt to determine if the procedure will be performed again in the future, so appropriate client teaching can be done and adequate supplies will be available.

Schedule the procedure at a time consistent with the order, the need for the procedure, and the client's other activities.

> **Delegation**
> Sterile procedures are not delegated to UAP.

EQUIPMENT
* Package containing a sterile drape
* Sterile equipment as needed (e.g., wrapped sterile gauze, wrapped sterile bowl, antiseptic solution, sterile forceps)

IMPLEMENTATION
Preparation
* Ensure that the package is clean and dry; if moisture is noted on the inside of a plastic-wrapped package or the outside of a cloth-wrapped package, it is considered contaminated and must be discarded.
* Check the sterilization expiration dates on the package, and look for any indications that it has been previously opened. Spots or stains on cloth or paper-wrapped objects may indicate contamination, and the objects should not be used.
* Follow agency practice for disposal of possibly contaminated packages.

Performance
1. Prior to performing the procedure, introduce self and verify the client's identity using agency protocol. Explain to the client what you are going to do, why it is necessary, and how he or she can participate. Discuss how the results will be used in planning further care or treatments.
2. Observe other appropriate infection control procedures (see Skills 19–1 and 19–2).
3. Provide for client privacy if appropriate.
4. Open the package. If the package is inside a plastic cover, remove the cover.

   To Open a Wrapped Package on a Surface
   * Place the package in the work area so that the top flap of the wrapper opens away from you.
   * Reaching around the package (not over it), pinch the first flap on the outside of the wrapper between the thumb and index finger. ❶ **Rationale:** *Touching only the outside of the wrapper maintains the sterility of the inside of the wrapper.* Pull the flap open, laying it flat on the far surface.
   * Repeat for the side flaps, opening the outermost one first. Use the right hand for the right flap, and the left hand for the left flap. ❷ **Rationale:** *By using both hands, you avoid reaching over the sterile contents.*

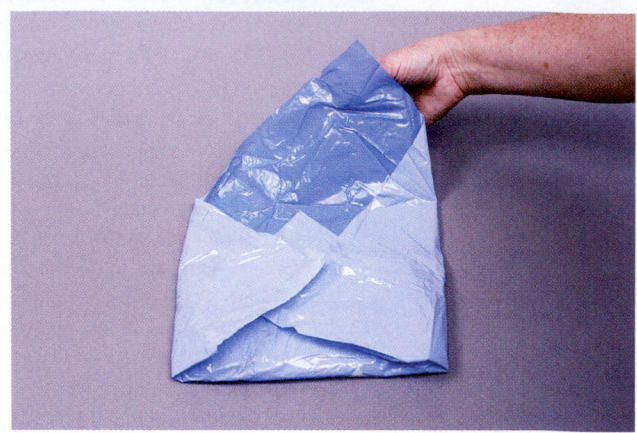

❶ Opening the first flap of a sterile wrapped package.

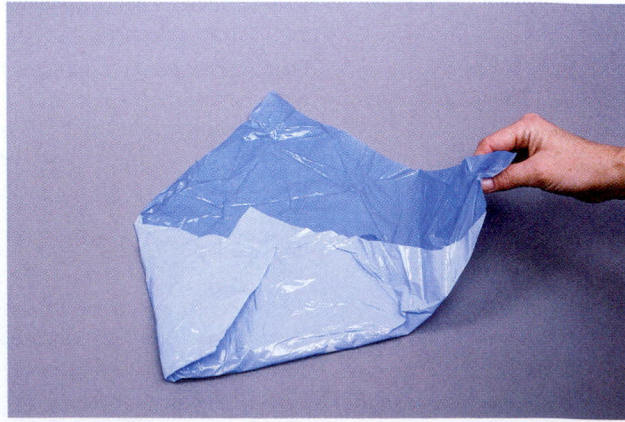

❷ Opening the second flap to the side.

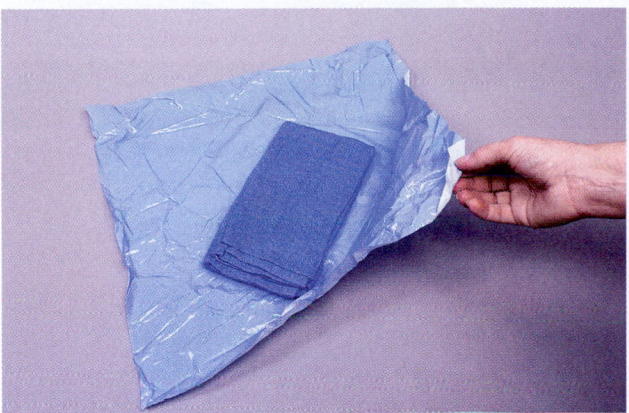

3 Pulling the last flap toward oneself by grasping the corner.

- Pull the fourth flap toward you by grasping the corner that is turned down. **3** Make sure that the flap does not touch any object. **Rationale:** *If the inner surface touches any unsterile article, it is contaminated.*

Variation: Opening a Wrapped Package While Holding It
- Hold the package in one hand with the top flap opening away from you.
- Using the other hand, open the package as described above, pulling the corners of the flaps well back. **4** Tuck each of the corners into the hand holding the package so that they do not flutter and contaminate sterile objects. **Rationale:** *The hands are considered contaminated, and at no time should they touch the contents of the package.*

Variation: Opening Commercially Prepared Packages
- If the flap of the package has an unsealed corner, hold the container in one hand, and pull back on the flap with the other hand. **5**
- If the package has a partially sealed edge, grasp both sides of the edge, one with each hand, and pull apart gently. **6**

5. Establish a sterile field by using a drape.
- Open the package containing the drape as described above.
- With one hand, pluck the corner of the drape that is folded back on the top touching only one side of the drape.

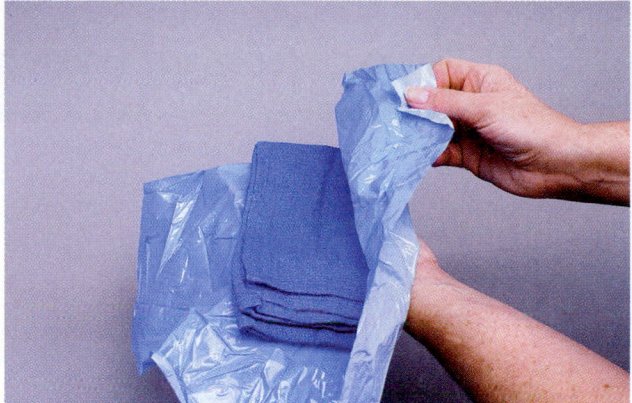

4 Opening a wrapped package while holding it.

- Lift the drape out of the cover, and allow it to open freely without touching any articles. **7** **Rationale:** *If the drape touches the outside of the package or any unsterile surface, it is considered contaminated.*
- With the other hand, carefully pick up another corner of the drape, holding it well away from you, and again, touching only the same side of the drape as the first hand.

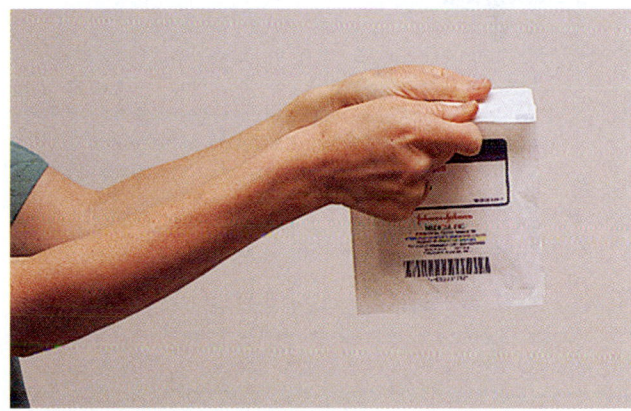

6 Opening a sterile package that has a partially sealed edge.

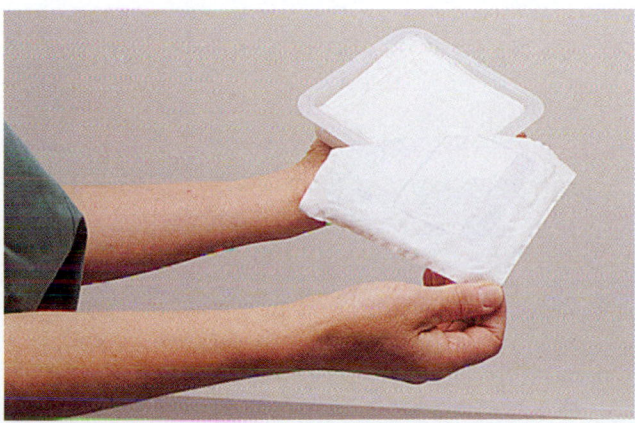

5 Opening a sterile package that has an unsealed corner.

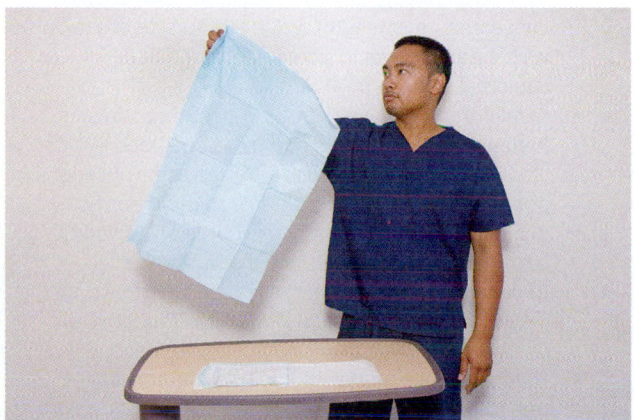

7 Allowing a drape to open freely without touching any objects.

(continued)

SKILL 19–3

ESTABLISHING AND MAINTAINING A STERILE FIELD *(continued)*

- Lay the drape on a clean and dry surface, placing the bottom (i.e., the freely hanging side) farthest from you. **Rationale:** *By placing the lowermost side farthest away, you avoid leaning over the sterile field and contaminating it.*

6. Add necessary sterile supplies, being careful not to touch the drape with the hands.

Adding Wrapped Supplies to a Sterile Field
- Open each wrapped package as described in the preceding steps.
- With the free hand, grasp the corners of the wrapper, and hold them against the wrist of the other hand. **8** **Rationale:** *The sterile wrapper now covers the unsterile hand.*
- Place the sterile bowl, drape, or other supply on the sterile field by approaching from an angle rather than holding the arm over the field.
- Discard the wrapper.

Variation: Adding Commercially Packaged Supplies to a Sterile Field
- Open each package as previously described.
- Hold the package 15 cm (6 in.) above the field, and allow the contents to drop on the field. **9** Keep in mind that 2.5 cm (1 in.) around the edge of the field is considered contaminated. **Rationale:** *At a height of 15 cm (6 in.), the outside of the package is not likely to touch and contaminate the sterile field.*

Adding Solution to a Sterile Bowl
Liquids (e.g., normal saline) may need to be poured into containers within a sterile field. Unwrapped bottles that contain sterile solution are considered sterile on the inside and contaminated on the outside because the bottle may have been handled. Bottles used in an operating room may be sterilized on the outside as well as the inside, however, and these are handled with sterile gloves.

- Before pouring any liquid, read the label three times to make sure you have the correct solution and concentration (strength). Wipe the outside of the bottle with a damp towel to remove any large particles that could fall into the bowl or field.
- Obtain the exact amount of solution, if possible. **Rationale:** *Once a sterile bottle has been opened, its sterility cannot be ensured for future use. Follow agency policy for reuse of opened sterile solution bottles.*
- Remove the lid or cap from the bottle and invert the lid before placing it on a surface that is not sterile. **Rationale:** *Inverting the lid maintains the sterility of the inside surface because it is not allowed to touch an unsterile surface.*
- Hold the bottle at a slight angle so that the label is uppermost. **10** **Rationale:** *Any solution that flows down the outside of the bottle during pouring will not damage or obliterate the label.*

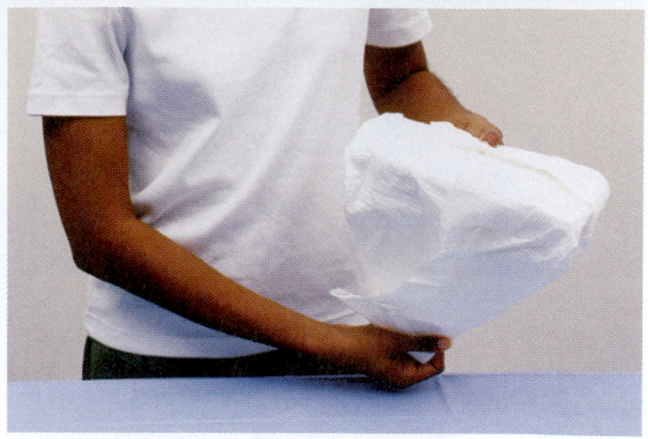

8 Adding wrapped sterile supplies to a sterile field.

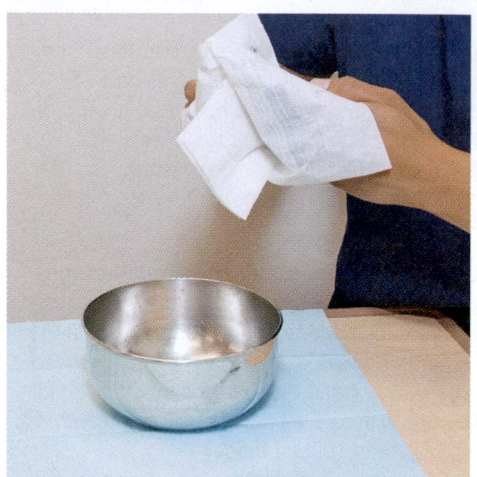

9 Adding commercially packaged gauze to a sterile field.

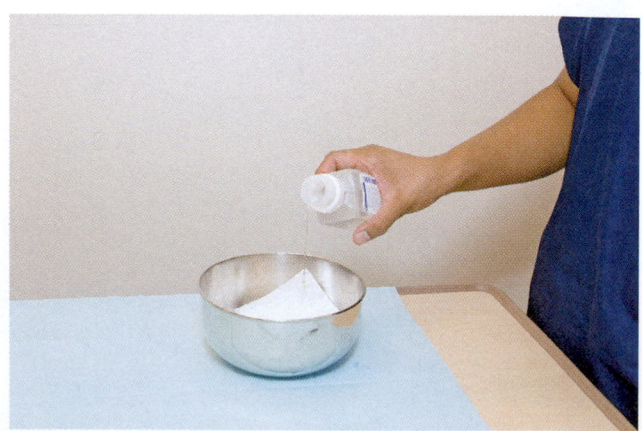

10 Adding a liquid to a sterile bowl.

- Hold the bottle of fluid at a height of 10 to 15 cm (4 to 6 in.) over the bowl and to the side of the sterile field so that as little of the bottle as possible is over the field. **Rationale:** *At this height, there is less likelihood of contaminating the sterile field by touching the field or by reaching an arm over it.*
- Pour the solution gently to avoid splashing the liquid. **Rationale:** *If a barrier drape (one that has a water-resistant layer) is not used and the drape is on an unsterile surface, moisture will contaminate the field by wicking microorganisms through the drape.*
- Tilt the neck of the bottle back to vertical quickly when done pouring so that none of the liquid flows down the outside of the bottle. **Rationale:** *Such drips would contaminate the sterile field if the outside of the bottle is not sterile.*
- If the bottle will be used again, replace the lid securely and write on the label the date and time of opening. **Rationale:** *Replacing the lid immediately maintains the sterility of the inner aspect of the lid and the solution.*
- Depending on agency policy, a sterile container of solution that is opened may be used only once and is then discarded (such as in the operating room). In other settings, policy may permit recapped bottles to be reused within 24 hours.

7. Use sterile forceps to handle sterile supplies. Forceps are usually used to move a sterile article from one place to another, for example, transferring sterile gauze from its package to a sterile dressing tray. Forceps may be disposable or resterilized after use. Commonly used forceps include hemostats and tissue forceps.
   - If forceps tips are wet, keep the tips lower than the wrist at all times, unless you are wearing sterile gloves. ⑪ **Rationale:** *Gravity prevents liquids on the tips of the forceps from flowing to the unsterile handles and later back to the tips.*
   - Hold sterile forceps above waist or table level, whichever is higher. **Rationale:** *Items held below waist or table level are considered contaminated.*

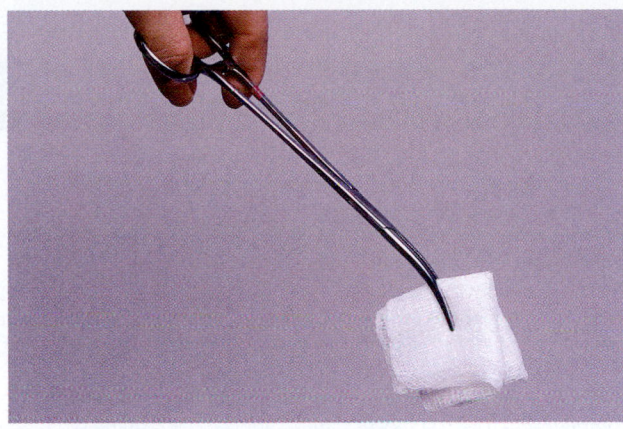

⑪ Holding forceps with an ungloved hand, keeping the tips lower than the wrist.

- Hold sterile forceps within sight. **Rationale:** *While out of sight, forceps may, unknown to the user, become unsterile. Any forceps that go out of sight should be considered unsterile.*
- When using forceps to lift sterile supplies, be sure that the forceps do not touch the edges or outside of the wrapper. **Rationale:** *The edges and outside of the sterile field are considered unsterile.*
- When placing forceps whose handles were in contact with the bare hand, position the handles outside the sterile area. **Rationale:** *The handles of these forceps harbor microorganisms from the bare hand.*
- Deposit a sterile item on a sterile field without permitting moist forceps to touch the sterile field when the surface under the absorbent sterile field is unsterile and a barrier drape is not used.

8. Document that sterile technique was used in the performance of the procedure.

EVALUATION

Conduct any follow-up indicated during your care of the client. Ensure that adequate numbers and types of sterile supplies are available for the next health care provider.

STERILE GLOVES Sterile gloves may be donned by the open method or the closed method. The open method is most frequently used outside the operating room because the closed method requires that the nurse wear a sterile gown. Gloves are worn during many procedures to maintain the sterility of equipment and to protect a client's wound.

Sterile gloves are packaged with a cuff of about 5 cm (2 in.) and with the palms facing upward when the package is opened. The package usually indicates the size of the glove.

Latex and latex-free sterile gloves are available to protect the nurse from contact with blood and body fluids. La-tex and nitrile are more flexible than vinyl, mold to the wearer's hands, allow freedom of movement, and have the added feature of resealing tiny punctures automatically. Therefore, wear latex or nitrile gloves when performing tasks (a) that demand flexibility, (b) that place stress on the material, and (c) that involve a high risk of exposure to pathogens. Vinyl gloves should be chosen for tasks unlikely to stress the glove material, requiring minimal precision, and with minimal risk of exposure to pathogens.

Skill 19–4 describes how to apply and remove sterile gloves by the open method.

APPLYING AND REMOVING STERILE GLOVES (OPEN METHOD)

PURPOSES
- To enable the nurse to handle or touch sterile objects freely without contaminating them
- To prevent transmission of potentially infective organisms from the nurse's hands to clients at high risk for infection

ASSESSMENT
Review the client's record and orders to determine exactly what procedure will be performed that requires sterile gloves. Check the client record and ask about latex allergies. Use nonlatex gloves whenever possible.

PLANNING
Think through the procedure, planning which steps need to be completed before the gloves can be applied. Determine what additional supplies are needed to perform the procedure for this client. Always have an extra pair of sterile gloves available.

EQUIPMENT
- Packages of sterile gloves

Delegation
Sterile procedures are not delegated to UAP in most states.

IMPLEMENTATION

Preparation
Ensure the sterility of the package of gloves.

Performance
1. Prior to performing the procedure, introduce self and verify the client's identity using agency protocol. Explain to the client what you are going to do, why it is necessary, and how he or she can participate. Discuss how the results will be used in planning further care or treatments.
2. Perform hard hygiene and observe other appropriate infection control procedures (see Skills 19–1, 19–2, and 19–3).
3. Provide for client privacy if appropriate.
4. Open the package of sterile gloves.
   - Place the package of gloves on a clean, dry surface. **Rationale:** *Any moisture on the surface could contaminate the gloves.*
   - Some gloves are packed in an inner as well as an outer package. Open the outer package without contaminating the gloves or the inner package. See Skill 19–3.
   - Remove the inner package from the outer package.
   - Open the inner package as in step 4 of Skill 19–3 or according to the manufacturer's directions. Some manufacturers provide a numbered sequence for opening the flaps and folded tabs to grasp for opening the flaps. If no tabs are provided, pluck the flap so that the fingers do not touch the inner surfaces. **Rationale:** *The inner surfaces, which are next to the sterile gloves, will remain sterile.*
5. Put the first glove on the dominant hand.
   - If the gloves are packaged so that they lie side by side, grasp the glove for the dominant hand by its folded cuff edge (on the palmar side) with the thumb and first finger of the nondominant hand. Touch only the inside of the cuff. ❶ **Rationale:** *The hands are not sterile. By touching only the inside of the glove, the nurse avoids contaminating the outside.*

     or
   - If the gloves are packaged one on top of the other, grasp the cuff of the top glove as above, using the opposite hand.

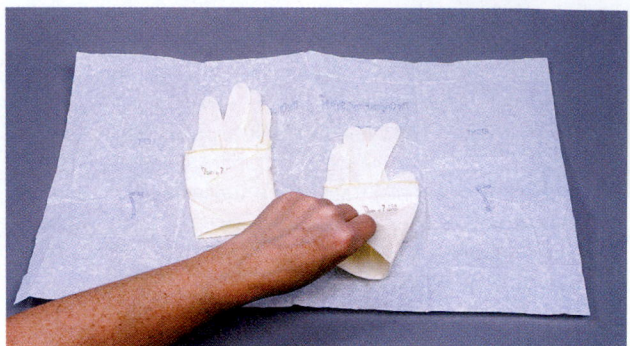
❶ Picking up the first sterile glove.

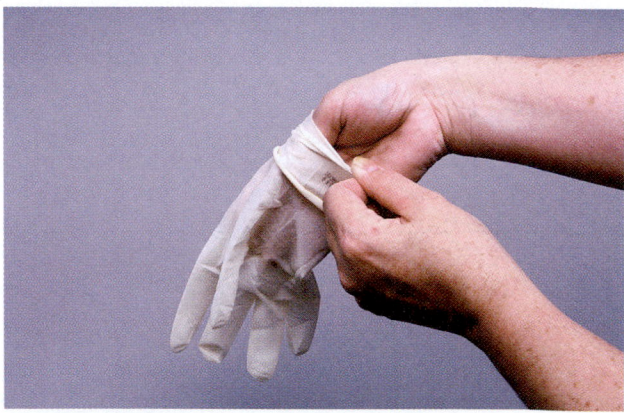
❷ Putting on the first sterile glove.

- Insert the dominant hand into the glove and pull the glove on. Keep the thumb of the inserted hand against the palm of the hand during insertion. ❷ **Rationale:** *If the thumb is kept against the palm, it is less likely to contaminate the outside of the glove.*
- Leave the cuff in place once the unsterile hand releases the glove. **Rationale:** *Attempting to further unfold the cuff is likely to contaminate the glove.*

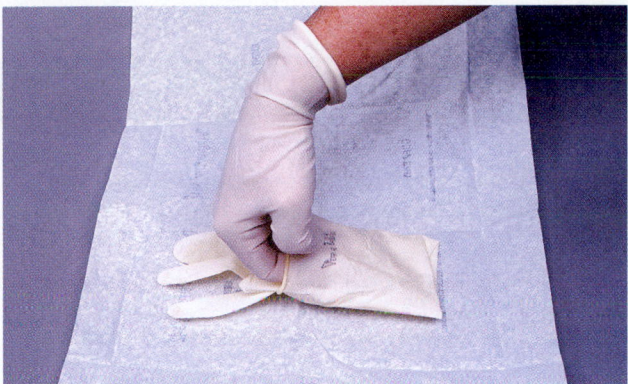

③ Picking up the second sterile glove.

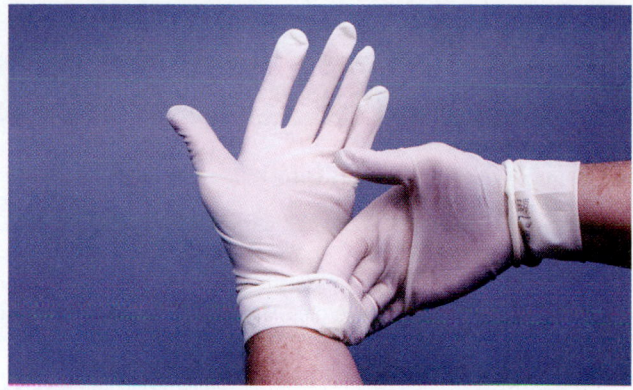

④ Putting on the second sterile glove.

6. Put the second glove on the nondominant hand.
   • Pick up the other glove with the sterile gloved hand, inserting the gloved fingers under the cuff and holding the gloved thumb close to the gloved palm. ③
     Rationale: *This helps prevent accidental contamination of the glove by the bare hand.*
   • Pull on the second glove carefully. Hold the thumb of the gloved first hand as far as possible from the palm. ④
     Rationale: *In this position, the thumb is less likely to touch the arm and become contaminated.*

   • Adjust each glove so that it fits smoothly, and carefully pull the cuffs up by sliding the fingers under the cuffs.
7. Remove and dispose of used gloves.
   • There is no technique for removing sterile gloves that is different from removing unsterile gloves. If they are soiled with secretions, remove them by turning them inside out. See removal of disposable gloves in Skill 19–2.
8. Document that sterile technique was used in the performance of the procedure.

EVALUATION

Conduct any follow-up indicated during your care of the client. Ensure that adequate numbers and types of sterile supplies are available for the next health care provider.

STERILE GOWNS Sterile gowning and closed gloving are chiefly carried out in operating or delivery rooms, where surgical asepsis is necessary. The closed method of gloving can be used only when a sterile gown is worn because the gloves are handled through the sleeves of the gown. Before these procedures, the nurse dons a hair cover and a mask, and performs a surgical hand wash.

Skill 19–5 describes the steps in applying a sterile gown and sterile gloves by the closed method.

Infection Control for Health Care Workers

NIOSH is part of the CDC and is a research agency of the U.S. Department of Health and Human Services. NIOSH investigates potentially hazardous working conditions and publishes recommendations for preventing workplace illnesses and injuries. For example, NIOSH published a study on preventing needlestick injuries in health care settings in 1999 that found that the majority of needlestick injuries were preventable. This, in part, led to the Needlestick Safety and Prevention Act that went into effect in April 2001.

The Occupational Safety and Health Administration (OSHA), an agency of the U.S. Department of Labor, publishes and enforces regulations to protect health care workers from occupational injuries, including exposure to bloodborne pathogens in the workplace. Occupational exposure is defined as skin, eye, mucous membrane, or parenteral contact with blood or other potentially infectious materials that may result from the performance of an employee's duties.

There are three major modes of transmission of infectious materials in the clinical setting:

• Puncture wounds from contaminated needles or other sharps
• Skin contact, which allows infectious fluids to enter through wounds and broken or damaged skin
• Mucous membrane contact, which allows infectious fluids to enter through mucous membranes of the eyes, mouth, or nose

Using proper precautions with general medical asepsis, appropriately using PPE (gloves, masks, gowns, goggles, special resuscitative equipment), and avoiding carelessness in the clinical area will place the caregiver at significantly

APPLYING A STERILE GOWN AND GLOVES (CLOSED METHOD)

PURPOSES
- To enable the nurse to work close to a sterile field and handle sterile objects freely
- To protect clients from becoming contaminated with microorganisms on the nurse's hands, arms, and clothing

ASSESSMENT
Review the client's record and orders to determine exactly what procedure will be performed that requires sterile gloves. Check the client record and ask about latex allergies. Use nonlatex gloves whenever possible.

PLANNING
Think through the procedure, planning which steps need to be completed before the gloves and gown can be applied. Determine what additional supplies are needed to perform the procedure for this client. Always have an extra pair of sterile gloves available.

EQUIPMENT
- Sterile pack containing a sterile gown
- Sterile gloves

> **Delegation**
> Sterile procedures are not delegated to UAP in most states.

IMPLEMENTATION

Preparation
Ensure the sterility of the package of gloves.

Performance
1. Perform surgical hand antisepsis/scrub.

Apply a Sterile Gown
1. Apply the sterile gown.
   - Grasp the sterile gown at the crease near the neck, hold it away from you, and permit it to unfold freely without touching anything, including the uniform. **Rationale:** *The gown will be unsterile if its outer surface touches any unsterile objects.*
   - Put the hands inside the shoulders of the gown without touching the outside of the gown. **❶**
   - Work the hands down the sleeves only to the beginning of the cuffs.
   - Have a co-worker grasp the neck ties without touching the outside of the gown and pull the gown upward to cover the neckline of your uniform in front and back. The co-worker ties the neck ties. Gowning continues on page 539.

Applying Sterile Gloves (Closed Method)
1. Open the sterile glove wrapper while the hands are still covered by the sleeves. **❷**
2. Put the glove on the nondominant hand. Figures **❸** through **❺** show a right-handed person.
   - With the dominant hand, pick up the opposite glove with the thumb and index finger, handling it through the sleeve.
   - Position the dominant hand palm upward inside the sleeve. Lay the glove on the opposite gown cuff, thumb side down, with the glove opening pointed toward the fingers. **❸**

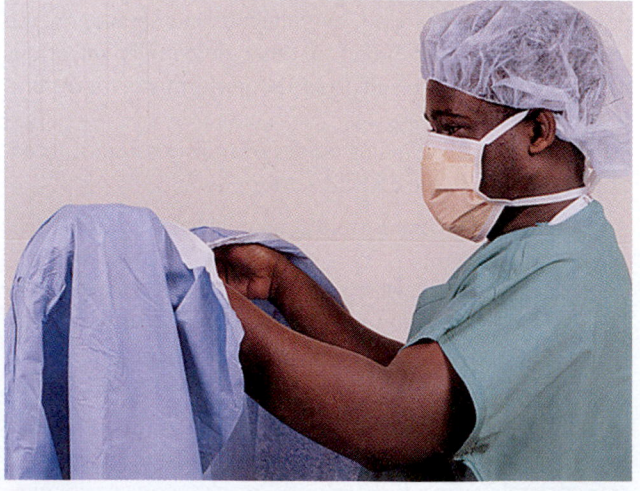

❶ Putting on a sterile gown.

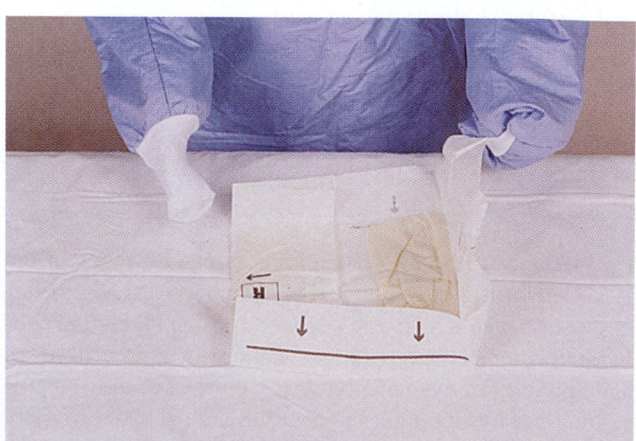

❷ Opening the sterile glove wrapper.

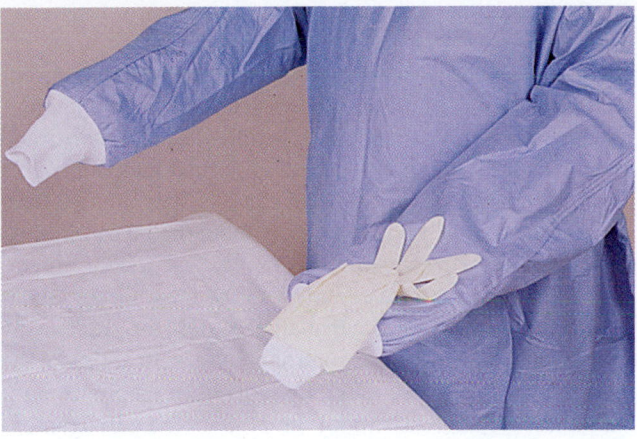

3 Positioning the first sterile glove for the nondominant hand.

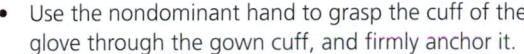

5 Extending the fingers into the second glove of the dominant hand.

- Use the nondominant hand to grasp the cuff of the glove through the gown cuff, and firmly anchor it.
- With the dominant hand working through its sleeve, grasp the upper side of the glove's cuff, and stretch it over the cuff of the gown.
- Pull the sleeve up to draw the cuff over the wrist as you extend the fingers of the nondominant hand into the glove's fingers. **4**

3. Put the glove on the dominant hand.
   - Place the fingers of the gloved hand under the cuff of the remaining glove.
   - Place the glove over the cuff of the second sleeve.
   - Extend the fingers into the glove as you pull the glove up over the cuff. **5**

Completion of Gowning

1. Complete gowning as follows.
   - Have a co-worker hold the waist tie of your gown, using sterile gloves or a sterile forceps or drape. **Rationale:** *This approach keeps the ties sterile.*
   - Make a three-quarter turn, then take the tie and secure it in front of the gown.

     or
   - Have a co-worker take the two ties at each side of the gown and tie them at the back of the gown, making sure that your uniform is completely covered.
   - When worn, sterile gowns should be considered sterile in front from the waist to the shoulder. Once the nurse approaches a table, the gown is considered contaminated from the waist or table down, whichever is higher. The sleeves should be considered sterile from the cuff to 5 cm (2 in.) above the elbow, since the arms of a scrubbed person must move across a sterile field. Moisture collection and friction areas such as the neckline, shoulders, underarms, back, and sleeve cuffs should be considered unsterile.

2. Remove and dispose of used gown and gloves.
   - If soiled, remove the attire by turning it inside out. See removal of disposable gowns and gloves in Skill 19–2 for the sequence of when to remove the gown.

3. If appropriate, document that sterile technique was used in the performance of the procedure.

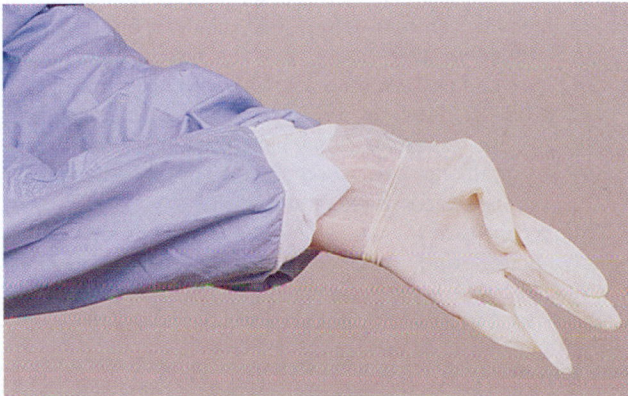

4 Pulling on the first sterile glove

EVALUATION

Conduct any follow-up indicated during your care of the client. Ensure that adequate numbers and types of sterile supplies are available for the next health care provider.

less risk for injury. The chance of a health care worker becoming infected following exposure to pathogens varies widely—estimates range from 30% for hepatitis B (nonimmune workers), to 1.8% for hepatitis C, to 0.3% for HIV (CDC, 2003). Measures to be taken in case of possible exposure to these viruses are delineated by the CDC and outlined in the accompanying Practice Guidelines feature. Hepatitis C, a worldwide epidemic greater than HIV, has become a significant concern to all health care workers since there is currently no vaccine against the virus or postexposure prophylaxis. Prevention remains the primary goal.

OSHA requires that health care employers make the hepatitis B vaccine and vaccination series available to all employees. Other vaccinations may also be made available.

CLINICAL ALERT

The nurse should consider in advance whether he or she would want prophylaxis for HIV exposure since this is optimally begun within 1 hour of exposure.

Role of the Infection Control Nurse

All health care organizations must have interdisciplinary infection control committees. Representatives from the clinical laboratory, housekeeping, maintenance, dietary, and client care areas are included. An important member of this committee is the infection control nurse. This nurse is specially trained to be knowledgeable about the latest research and practices in preventing, detecting, and treating infections. All infections are reported to the nurse in a manner that allows for recording and analyzing statistics that can assist in improving infection control practices. In addition, the infection control nurse may be involved in employee education and implementation of the bloodborne pathogen exposure control plan mandated by OSHA.

EVALUATING

Using data collected during care—vital signs, lung sounds, skin status, characteristics of urine or other drainage, laboratory blood values, and so on—the nurse judges whether

---

PRACTICE GUIDELINES — Steps to Follow after Exposure to Bloodborne Pathogens

- Report the incident immediately to appropriate personnel within the agency.
- Complete an injury report.
- Seek appropriate evaluation and follow-up. This includes:
  - Identification and documentation of the source individual when feasible and legal.
  - Testing of the source for hepatitis B, hepatitis C, and HIV when feasible and consent is given.
  - Making results of the test available to the source individual's health care provider.
  - Testing of blood of exposed nurse (with consent) for hepatitis B, hepatitis C, and HIV antibodies.
  - Postexposure prophylaxis if medically indicated.
  - Medical and psychologic counseling regarding personal risk of infection or risk of infecting others.
- For a puncture/laceration:
  - Encourage bleeding.
  - Wash/clean the area with soap and water.
  - Initiate first-aid and seek treatment if indicated.
  - For a mucous membrane exposure (eyes, nose, mouth), saline or water flush for 5 to 10 minutes.

Postexposure Protocol (PEP)

HIV

- Treatment should be started as soon as possible, preferably within hours after exposure. Treatment may be less effective

when started more than 24 hours after exposure. Starting treatment after a longer period (e.g., 1 week) should be considered for high-risk exposures previously untreated.
- For "high-risk" exposure (high blood volume *and* source with a high HIV titer): three-drug treatment is recommended.
- For "increased risk" exposure (high blood volume *or* source with a high HIV titer): three-drug treatment is recommended.
- For "low-risk" exposure (neither high blood volume nor source with a high HIV titer): two-drug treatment is considered.
- Drug prophylaxis continues for 4 weeks.
- Drug regimens vary and new drugs and regimens are continuously being developed.
- HIV antibody tests should be done shortly after exposure (baseline), and 6 weeks, 3 months, and 6 months afterward.

Hepatitis B

- Anti-HBs testing 1 to 2 months after last vaccine dose.
- HBIG and/or hepatitis B vaccine within 1 to 7 days following exposure for nonimmune workers.

Hepatitis C

- Anti-HCV and ALT at baseline and 4 to 6 months after exposure.

client outcomes have been achieved. Examples of client outcomes and indicators are shown in Identifying Nursing Diagnoses, Outcomes, and Interventions on page 517.

If outcomes are not achieved, the nurse may need to consider questions such as the following:

- Were appropriate measures implemented to prevent skin breakdown and lung infection?

- Was strict aseptic technique implemented for invasive procedures?
- Are prescribed medications affecting the immune system?
- Is client placement appropriate to reduce the risk of transmission of microorganisms?
- Did the client and family misunderstand or fail to comply with necessary instructions?

CHAPTER HIGHLIGHTS

- Microorganisms are everywhere. Most are harmless and some are beneficial; however, many can cause infection in susceptible persons.
- Effective control of infectious disease is an international, national, community, and individual responsibility.
- Asepsis is the freedom from infection or infectious material.
- Medical aseptic practices limit the number, growth, and transmission of microorganisms.
- Surgical aseptic practices keep an area or objects free of all microorganisms.
- The incidence of HAI is significant. Major sites for these infections are the respiratory and urinary tracts, the bloodstream, and wounds.
- Factors that contribute to health care–associated infection risks are invasive procedures, medical therapies, the existence of a large number of susceptible persons, inappropriate use of antibiotics, and insufficient hand cleansing after client contact and after contact with body substances.
- An infection can develop if the links in the chain of infection—infectious agent, reservoir, portal of exit, mode of transmission, portal of entry, and susceptible host—are not interrupted.
- Intact skin and mucous membranes are the body's first line of defense against microorganisms.
- Some normal body flora release bacteriocins and antibiotic-like substances that inhibit microbial growth and destroy foreign bacteria.

- Some body secretions (e.g., saliva and tears) contain enzymes that act as antibacterial agents.
- The inflammatory response limits physical, chemical, and microbial injury and promotes repair of injured tissue.
- Immunity is the specific resistance of the body to infectious agents.
- Acquired immunity is active or passive and in either case may be naturally or artificially induced.
- Especially at risk of acquiring an infection are the very young or old; those with poor nutritional status, a deficiency of serum immunoglobulins, multiple stressors, insufficient immunizations, or an existing disease process; and those receiving certain medical therapies.
- Preventing infections in healthy or ill persons and preventing the transmission of microorganisms from infected clients to others are major nursing functions.
- The nurse must be knowledgeable about sources and modes of transmission of microorganisms.
- Microorganisms are invisible, and nurses have an ethical obligation to ensure that appropriate aseptic measures are taken to protect clients, support people, and health personnel, including themselves.
- All health care providers must apply clean or sterile gloves, gowns, masks, and protective eyewear according to the risk of exposure to potentially infective materials.
- Should a health care worker be exposed to substances with high risk of transmitting bloodborne pathogens, postexposure practices and consideration of prophylactic treatment must be followed immediately.

THINK ABOUT IT

Refer to the chapter-opening scenario and answer these questions.

1. What procedures performed on the neonate would require Frank to wear clean gloves?

2. Frank learns that the infant's wound cultured positive for MRSA. What precautions would Frank anticipate to be initiated?

3. What interventions can Frank provide to reduce the risk of infection when caring for this infant, in addition to hand hygiene?

∞ *See suggested responses to Think About It on MyNursingKit.*

TEST YOUR KNOWLEDGE

1. The client is a chronic carrier of infection. To prevent the spread of the infection to other clients or health care providers, the nurse emphasizes interventions that do which of the following?
1. Eliminate the reservoir
2. Block the portal of exit from the reservoir
3. Block the portal of entry into the host
4. Decrease the susceptibility of the host

2. The most effective nursing action for controlling the spread of infection includes which of the following?
1. Thorough hand cleansing
2. Wearing gloves and masks when providing direct client care
3. Implementing appropriate isolation precautions
4. Administering broad-spectrum prophylactic antibiotics

3. In caring for a client requiring contact precautions for a draining infected foot ulcer, the nurse should perform which of the following?
1. Wear a mask during dressing changes
2. Provide disposable meal trays and silverware
3. Follow standard precautions in all interactions with the client
4. Use surgical aseptic technique for all direct contact with the client

4. When caring for a single client during one shift, it is appropriate for the nurse to reuse which of the following personal protective equipment?
1. Goggles
2. Gown
3. Surgical mask
4. Clean gloves

5. While donning sterile gloves (open method), the cuff of the first glove rolls under itself about 1/4 inch. The best action for the nurse is to:
1. Remove the glove and start over with a new pair.
2. Wait until the second glove is in place and then unroll the cuff with the other sterile hand.
3. Ask a colleague to assist by unrolling the cuff.
4. Leave the cuff rolled under.

6. After evaluating the client's chart, the nurse concludes that a 65-year-old client's immunizations are current. What evidence supports this conclusion? Select all that apply.
1. Last tetanus booster was at age 50
2. Receives a flu shot every year
3. Has not received the hepatitis B vaccine

4. Has not received the hepatitis A vaccine
5. Reports infection with rubella as a child

7. A client with poor nutrition enters the hospital for treatment of a puncture wound. An appropriate nursing diagnosis would be _____.

8. After teaching a client and family strategies to prevent infection, which statement by the client would indicate the nurse's teaching was effective?
1. "We will use antimicrobial soap and hot water to wash our hands at least three times per day."
2. "We must wash or peel all raw fruits and vegetables before eating."
3. "A wound or sore is not infected unless we see it draining pus."
4. "We should not share toothbrushes but it is OK to share towels and washcloths."

9. Which of the numbered areas is considered sterile on a person in the operating room? You may assume that all articles were sterile when applied. _____

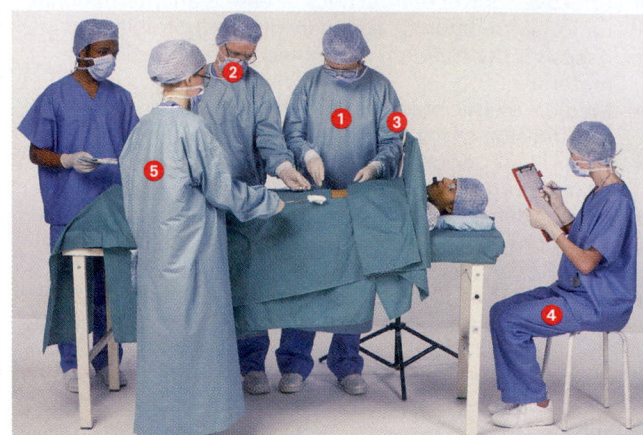

10. The nurse determines that a field remains sterile if which of the following conditions exist?
1. Tips of wet forceps are held upward when held in ungloved hands.
2. The field was set up 1 hour before the procedure.
3. Sterile items are 2 inches from the edge of the field.
4. The nurse reaches over the field rather than around the edges.

∞ *See answers to Test Your Knowledge in Appendix A.*

REFERENCES AND SELECTED BIBLIOGRAPHY

Arrowsmith, V. A., Maunder, J. A., Sargent, R. J., & Taylor, R. (2005). Removal of nail polish and finger rings to prevent surgical infection. *The Cochrane Library* (Oxford) (ID #CD003325).

Barbacane, J. L. (2004). Back to the basics: Handwashing. *Geriatric Nursing, 25*(2), 90–92.

Boyce, J. M., & Pittet, D. (2002). Guideline for hand hygiene in health-care settings: Recommendations of the Healthcare Infection Control Practices Advisory Committee and the HICPAC/SHEA/APIC/IDSA Hand Hygiene Task Force. *Morbidity and Mortality Weekly Report, 51*(RR-16), 1–44.

Carr, M. P. (2004). Waterless hand washing: A new era in hand hygiene. *Journal of Practical Hygiene, 13*(2), 33–36.

Centers for Disease Control. (1987). Recommendations for prevention of HIV transmission in health-care settings. *Morbidity and Mortality Weekly Report (suppl.), 36* (2s), 1S–18S.

Centers for Disease Control. (1997). 1997 USPHS/IDSA guidelines for the prevention of opportunistic infections in persons infected with human immunodeficiency virus. *Morbidity and Mortality Weekly Report, 46* (RR-12), 1–46.

Centers for Disease Control and Prevention. (2001). Updated U.S. Public Health Service guidelines for the management of occupational exposures to HBV, HCV, and HIV and recommendations for postexposure prophylaxis. *Morbidity and Mortality Weekly Report 50* (RR-11), 1–67.

Centers for Disease Control and Prevention. (2003). *Exposure to blood: What healthcare personnel need to know*. Atlanta, GA: Author.

Centers for Disease Control and Prevention. (2004). *Sequence for donning and removing personal protective equipment*. Retrieved July 16, 2006, from www.cdc.gov/ncidod/dhqp/ppe.html

Centers for Disease Control and Prevention. (2005). *Public health guidance for community-level preparedness and response to severe acute respiratory syndrome (SARS) version 2: Supplement I: Infection control in healthcare, home, and community settings*. Retrieved December 5, 2009, from http://www.cdc.gov/nip/recs/child-schedule.htm#printable

Centers for Disease Control and Prevention. (2006a). *Recommended childhood and adolescent immunization schedule, United States, 2005*. Retrieved December 5, 2009, from http://www.cdc.gov/nip/recs/child-schedule.htm#printable

Centers for Disease Control and Prevention. (2006b). *Recommended adult immunization schedule, United States, 2006*. Retrieved December 5, 2009, from http://www.cdc.gov/vaccines/recs/schedules/adult-schedule.htm

Centers for Medicare and Medicaid Services. (2005). Alcohol based hand rub solutions TIA 00-1 (101). *Federal Register, 70*(57), 15229–15239.

Garcia-Martin, M., Lardelli-Claret, P., Jimenez-Moleon, J. J., Bueno-Cavanillas, A., de Dios Luna del Castillo, J., & Galvez-Vargas, R. (2001). Proportion of hospital deaths potentially attributable to nosocomial infection. *Infection Control and Hospital Epidemiology, 22,* 708–714.

Garner, J. S., & Hospital Infection Control Practices Advisory Committee. (1996). Guidelines for isolation precautions in hospitals. *Infection Control Hospital Epidemiology, 17,* 53–80, and *American Journal of Infection Control, 24,* 24–52.

Garner, J. S., & Simmons, B. P. (1983). *CDC guideline for isolation precautions in hospitals* (HHS Publication No. CDC 83-8314). Atlanta, GA: U.S. Department of Health and Human Services, Public Health Service, Centers for Disease Control.

Goldrick, B. A. (2003). Adult respiratory infections. *American Journal of Nursing, 103*(10), 65–66.

Goldrick, B. A. (2004). 21st century emerging and reemerging infections. *American Journal of Nursing, 104*(1), 67–70.

Goldrick, B. A. (2004). MRSA, VRE, and VRSA: How do we control them in nursing homes? *American Journal of Nursing, 104* (8), 50–51.

Hospital Infection Control Practices Advisory Committee. (1995). Recommendations for preventing the spread of vancomycin resistance. *American Journal of Infection Control, 23,* 87–94; *Infection Control and Hospital Epidemiology, 16,* 105–113; and *Morbidity and Mortality Weekly Report, 44* (RR-12), 1–13.

Hospital Infection Control Practices Advisory Committee. (2007). Guidelines for Isolation Precautions: Preventing transmission of infectious agents in healthcare settings 2007. Retrieved December 18, 2008, from http://www.cdc.gov/ncidod/dhqp/pdf/guidelines/Isolation2007.pdf

Houghton, D. (2006). HAI prevention: The power is in your hands. *Nursing Management, 37*(Suppl.), 1–7.

Jackson, M. M. (1993). Infection precautions: What works and what does not. *CRNA: The Clinical Forum for Nurse Anesthetists, 4* (2), 77–82.

Jarvis, J. R. (2001). Infection control and changing health-care delivery systems. *Emerging Infectious Diseases, 7,* 170–173.

Joint Commission on Accreditation of Healthcare Organizations. (2006). *National patient safety goals*. Oakbrook Terrace, IL: Author. Retrieved December 5, 2009, from http://www.jointcommission.org/Standards/NationalPatientSafetyGoals

National Center for HIV, STD, and TB Prevention, Division of Tuberculosis Elimination. (2004). *Self-study modules on tuberculosis*. Retrieved July 16, 2006, from http://www.phppo.cdc.gov/phtn/tbmodules/Default.htm

National Institute for Occupational Safety and Health. (1999). *Preventing needlestick injuries in health care settings*. (DHHS Publication No. 2000-108) Cincinnati, OH: U.S. Department of Health and Human Services, Public Health Service, Centers for Disease Control and Prevention, National Institute for Occupational Safety and Health.

Occupational Safety & Health Administration. (2005). *Latex allergy*. Retrieved June 3, 2006, from http://www.osha.gov/SLTC/latexallergy/

Peate, I. (2004). Infection control. Occupational exposure of staff to HIV and prophylaxis therapy. *British Journal of Nursing, 13,* 1146–1150.

Raboud, J., Saskin, R., Wong, K., Moore, C., Parucha, G., Bennett, J., et al. (2004). Patterns of handwashing behavior and visits to patients on a general medical ward of healthcare workers. *Infection Control and Hospital Epidemiology, 25,* 198–202.

Sehulster, L. M., Chinn, R. Y. W., Arduino, M. J., Carpenter, J., Donlan, R., Ashford, D., et al. (2004). *Guidelines for environmental infection control in health-care facilities. Recommendations from CDC and the Healthcare Infection Control Practices Advisory Committee (HICPAC)*. Chicago: American Society for Healthcare Engineering/American Hospital Association.

Srinivasan, A., McDonald, L. C., Jernigan, D., Helfand, R., Ginsheimer, K., Jernigan, J., et al. (2004). Foundations of the severe acute respiratory syndrome preparedness and response plan for healthcare facilities. *Infection Control and Hospital Epidemiology, 25,* 1020–1025.

Stirling, B., Littlejohn, P., & Willbond, M. L. (2004). Nurses and the control of infectious disease: Understanding epidemiology and disease transmission is vital to nursing care. *Canadian Nurse, 100*(9), 16–20.

Sunenshine, R. H., & McDonald, L. C. (2006). *Clostridium difficile*-associated disease: New challenges from an established pathogen. *Cleveland Clinical Journal of Medicine, 73,* 187–197.

U.S. Department of Health and Human Services, Public Health Service. (1988). Update: Universal precautions for prevention of transmission of human immunodeficiency virus, hepatitis B virus, and other bloodborne pathogens in health care settings. *Morbidity and Mortality Weekly Report, 37* (24), 377–388.

Wongworawat, M. D., & Jones, S. G. (2007). Influence of rings on the efficacy of hand sanitization and residual bacterial contamination. *Infection Control and Hospital Epidemiology, 28*(3), 351–353.

World Health Organization. (2005). *WHO guidelines on hand hygiene in health care*. Geneva, Switzerland: Author.

Diagnostic Testing

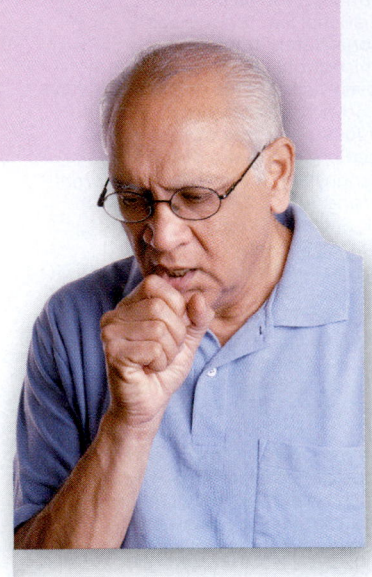

Martin Kohler, 63 years old, calls his provider to report he is coughing up blood. His provider wants to see him immediately and orders a chest x-ray be performed before the appointment. On examining the client and reviewing the radiological exam, the provider suspects Mr. Kohler may have lung cancer. He recommends admission to the local acute care facility for further testing, including an MRI of the lungs, the result of which reinforces the provider's suspicion. Mr. Kohler is scheduled for a bronchoscopy with biopsy of the mass, which then confirms oat cell carcinoma of the right lung. The physician orders further testing to determine possible metastasis, including MRI of the abdomen, liver enzymes, clotting studies, complete blood count, and serum electrolytes. A contrast MRI of the brain is also ordered. Mr. Kohler says he feels like a "pin cushion" and wonders if all these tests and procedures are really necessary. The provider assures him of their importance. When the provider leaves the room, Mr. Kohler turns to the nurse and asks for more information.

LEARNING OUTCOMES

After completing this chapter, you will be able to:

1. Describe the nurse's role in each phase of diagnostic testing.

2. Differentiate the purposes of commonly performed blood tests and the meaning of abnormal results.

3. Describe the nursing actions and rationales related to obtaining specimens using the nursing process.

4. Contrast various types of imaging procedures that may be used for clients with different medical diagnoses and issues.

5. Identify the nurse's role in assisting with and caring for the client undergoing biopsy and aspiration procedures.

KEY TERMS

Angiography p560
Anoscopy p559
Ascites p562
Aspiration p561
Blood chemistry p548
Clean-catch urine specimen p553

Colonoscopy p559
Computed tomography p560
Cystoscopy p560
Echocardiogram p560
Electrocardiogram p560
Guaiac test p552

Intravenous pyelography p559
Kidneys/ureters/bladder p559
Lumbar puncture p561
Magnetic resonance imaging p560

Manometer p562
Midstream urine specimen p553
Occult blood p552
Paracentesis p562
Phlebotomist p546

Diagnostic and laboratory tests (commonly called lab tests) are tools that provide assessment data about the client. Tests may be used as basic screening included in a wellness check or to help confirm a diagnosis, monitor an illness, and provide information about the client's response to treatment. Nurses require knowledge of the most common lab and diagnostic tests because one primary role of the nurse is to teach the client and family or significant other how to prepare for the test and provide care that may be required following the test. Nurses must also know the implications of the test results in order to provide the most appropriate nursing care for the client.

Diagnostic testing occurs in many environments. The traditional sites include hospitals, clinics, and the primary care provider's office. Many test sites, however, are moving to the community. More complex diagnostic tests are performed at diagnostic centers specifically built for those tests.

DIAGNOSTIC TESTING PHASES

Some diagnostic tests are simple, direct tests such as routine urinalysis, while others are invasive procedures that the client can find frightening. Understanding the three phases of diagnostic testing can help the nurse to anticipate the client's needs during each phase. Diagnostic testing involves pretest, intratest, and posttest phases.

Pretest

The major focus of the pretest phase is client preparation. A thorough assessment and data collection assist the nurse in determining communication and teaching strategies. Prior to radiologic studies it is important to ask female clients if pregnancy is possible because special precautions may be necessary or the test may need to be postponed.

The nurse also needs to know what equipment, supplies, and preparations are needed for the specific test. Nurses must also confirm a signed consent has been obtained if indicated. Assuring that all preparations have been anticipated can help avoid costly mistakes and reduce inconvenience to all involved. Most facilities have information about the tests available to the health care team. The laboratory at the facility can also act as a resource for information.

Intratest

This phase focuses on specimen collection and performing or assisting with certain diagnostic testing. Prior to beginning the test it is important for the nurse to determine that all

---

CULTURALLY COMPETENT CARE   **Drawing Blood Samples**

In Asian traditional medicine, blood is not drawn for medical purposes (Salimbene, 2000, p. 23). An Asian client practicing traditional medicine views blood as a source of life and believes that the body cannot replace lost blood (Spector, 2004). As a result, Asian clients may be upset by venipuncture or the drawing of blood for testing, especially if there are numerous tests. They may view this as upsetting the body's normal balance and weakening the body. Also, blood represents a person's essence and they may fear that their essence is being given away. Therefore, Asian clients may also need to be informed that their blood will not be given to anyone else.

Note: From *What Language Does Your Patient Hurt In? A Practical Guide to Culturally Competent Patient Care* by S. Salimbene, 2000, EMCParadigm; and *Cultural Diversity in Health & Illness* by R. E. Spector, 2004, Prentice Hall. Adapted with permission.

---

pretesting requirements were met. The nurse uses standard precautions and sterile technique as appropriate. During the procedure the nurse provides emotional and physical support while monitoring the client as needed. The nurse ensures correct labeling, storage, and transportation of the specimen to avoid invalid test results.

CLIENT TEACHING   **Preparing for Diagnostic Testing**

- Instruct the client and family about requirements or restrictions (e.g., when and what to eat or drink, how long to fast).
- Provide information about what the client may feel (e.g., a temporary flushing and feeling of warmth when the dye is injected).
- Ask the client if a description or pictures of the involved equipment would help prepare him or her for the test.
- Encourage questions and dialogue about fears and apprehensions. Find out what the client may have heard about the test from others.
- Inform the client of the time period before the results will be available.
- Document teaching. Include the client's response. Record names of audiovisual and reading materials, if used.

Note: From *A Manual of Laboratory & Diagnostic Tests*, 7th ed., by F. Fischbach, 2004, Philadelphia: Lippincott Williams & Wilkins. Reprinted with permission.

Posttest

The focus of this phase is on nursing care of the client and follow-up activities and observations. As appropriate, the nurse compares the previous and current test results and modifies nursing interventions as needed. The nurse also reports the results to appropriate health team members.

Nursing Diagnoses

Nursing diagnoses are based on client data and needs. Examples can include

- *Anxiety or Fear* related to the actual testing procedure or possible diagnosis of acute or chronic illness pending results of diagnostic testing.
- *Impaired Physical Mobility* related to prescribed bed rest and restricted movement that may be required by the diagnostic test.
- *Deficient Knowledge* (state diagnostic test) related to misperceptions or lack of information regarding process for test.

BLOOD TESTS

Blood tests are one of the most commonly used diagnostic tests and can provide valuable information about the hematologic system and many other body systems. A venipuncture (puncture of a vein for collection of a blood specimen) can be performed by various members of the health care team. Usually a **phlebotomist**, a person from a laboratory who performs venipuncture, collects the blood specimen for the tests ordered by the primary care provider. In some institutions, nurses may draw blood samples. The nurse needs to know the guidelines for drawing blood samples for the facility and also the state's nurse practice act.

Complete Blood Count

Specimens of venous blood are taken for a complete blood count (CBC), which includes hemoglobin and hematocrit measurements, erythrocyte (RBC) count, leukocyte (WBC) count, red blood cell (RBC) indices, and may also include a differential white cell count. The CBC is a basic screening test and one of the most frequently ordered blood tests (see Table 20–1).

Hemoglobin is the main intracellular protein of erythrocytes. It carries oxygen to and removes carbon dioxide from red blood cells (Van Leeuwen, Kranpitz, & Smith, 2006, p. 732). The hemoglobin test is a measure of the total amount of hemoglobin in the blood. The hematocrit measures the percentage of red blood cells in the total blood volume. Normal values for both hemoglobin and hematocrit vary, with males having higher levels than females. Hemoglobin and hematocrit increase with dehydration as the blood becomes more concentrated, and decrease with hypervolemia and resulting hemodilution. Hemoglobin and hematocrit are often ordered together and commonly referred to as "H & H" when ordering lab tests. Both the hemoglobin and hematocrit are related to the red blood cell (RBC) count, which is the number of RBCs per cubic millimeter of whole blood. It also varies by gender and age. Low RBC counts are indicative of anemia. Clients with chronic hypoxia may develop higher than normal counts, a condition known as polycythemia. Red blood cell (RBC) indices may be performed as part of the CBC to evaluate the size, weight, and hemoglobin concentration of RBCs.

The leukocyte or white blood cell (WBC) count determines the number of circulating WBCs per cubic millimeter of whole blood. High WBC counts are often seen in the presence of a bacterial infection; by contrast, WBC counts may be low if a viral infection is present. In the WBC differential, leukocytes are identified by type, and the percentage of each type is determined. This information is useful in diagnosing certain disorders that have characteristic patterns of distribution.

Serum Electrolytes

Serum electrolytes are often routinely ordered for any client admitted to a hospital as a screening test for electrolyte and acid–base imbalances or for clients seen in physician's offices that are receiving treatments or diagnosed with illnesses that can impact electrolyte levels. The most commonly ordered serum tests are for sodium, potassium, chloride, and bicarbonate ions. Serum electrolytes may be ordered as a Chem 7 or BMP (basic metabolic panel). The lab terminology varies depending on the lab. Normal values of commonly measured electrolytes are shown in Box 20–1.

Blood levels of two metabolically produced substances, urea and creatinine, are routinely used to evaluate renal function. The kidneys, through filtration and tubular secretion, normally eliminate both. Urea, the end product of protein metabolism, is measured as blood urea nitrogen (BUN). Creatinine is produced in relatively constant quantities by the muscles and is excreted by the kidneys. Thus, the amount of creatinine in the blood relates to renal excretory function.

Serum Osmolality

Serum osmolality is a measure of the solute concentration of the blood. The particles included are sodium ions, glucose, and BUN. Serum osmolality can be estimated by doubling the serum sodium, because sodium and its associated chloride ions are the major determinants of serum osmolality. Serum osmolality values are used primarily to evaluate fluid balance. Normal values are 280 to 300 mOsm/kg. An increase in serum

TABLE 20–1	Complete Blood Count with Clinical Implications	
COMPONENT	NORMAL FINDINGS (ADULT)	SIGNIFICANCE
Red blood cell count (RBC) The number of RBCs per cubic millimeter (mm^3).	M: 4.5–5.3 million/mm^3 F: 4.1–5.1 million/mm^3	RBCs are needed for the hemoglobin contained within them.
Hemoglobin (Hgb) Composed of a pigment (heme), which contains iron and a protein (globin).	M: 13.8–18 g/dL F: 12–16 g/DL	Hemoglobin is the molecule that oxygen binds to and is essential for oxygenation of cells.
Hematocrit (HCT) The hematocrit or packed cell volume (Hct, PCV, or crit) is a fast way to determine the percentage of RBCs in the plasma. The Hct is reported as a percentage because it is the proportion of RBCs to the plasma.	M: 37–49% F: 36–46%	Percentage of hematocrit is an indicator of hydration, percentage of RBCs circulating in bloodstream.
Red blood cell indices (RBC indices) *Mean corpuscular volume (MCV)* The mean or average size of the individual RBC.	M: 78–100 μm^3 F: 78–102 μm^3	Indicates the maturity and functional ability of the RBC
Mean corpuscular hemoglobin (MCH) Amount of Hgb present in one cell.	25–35 pg	Indicates oxygen carrying ability of the red blood cell
Mean corpuscular hemoglobin concentration (MCHC) The proportion of each cell occupied by Hgb.	31–37%	Indicates oxygen carrying ability of the red blood cell
White blood cell count (WBC) Count of the total number of WBCs in a cubic millimeter of blood.	4,500–11,000/mm^3	Indicator of the client's immune response
Differential count The proportion of each of the five types of WBCs in a sample of 100 WBCs.		
Neutrophils	55–70%	
Lymphocytes	20–40%	
Monocytes	2–8%	
Eosinophils	1–4%	
Basophils	0–2%	
Platelet count Platelets are fragments of cytoplasm that function in blood coagulation.	150,000–350,000/mm^3	Indicates ability of blood to clot

Source: Modified from *Laboratory Tests and Diagnostic Procedures with Nursing Diagnoses*, 6th ed., by J. V. Corbett, 2004, Upper Saddle River, NJ: Pearson Prentice Hall. Reproduced with permission of Pearson Education, Inc., Upper Saddle River, New Jersey.

BOX 20–1	Normal Electrolyte Ranges for Adults*

Venous Blood

Sodium	135–145 mEq/L
Potassium	3.5–5.0 mEq/L
Chloride	95–105 mEq/L
Calcium (total) (ionized)	4.5–5.5 mEq/L or 8.5–10.5 mg/dL 56% of total calcium (2.5 mEq/L or 4.0–5.0 mg/dL)
Magnesium	1.5–2.5 mEq/L or 1.6–2.5 mg/dL
Phosphate	1.8–2.6 mEq/L (phosphorus)
Serum osmolality	280–300 mOsm/kg water

*Normal laboratory values vary from agency to agency.

osmolality indicates a fluid volume deficit; a decrease reflects a fluid volume excess.

Drug Monitoring

Therapeutic drug monitoring is often conducted when a client is taking a medication with a narrow therapeutic range. This monitoring includes drawing blood samples for peak and trough levels to determine if the blood serum levels of a specific drug are at a therapeutic level and not a subtherapeutic or toxic level. The peak level indicates the highest concentration of the drug in the blood serum obtained shortly after administration of the drug, and the trough level represents the lowest concentration normally drawn within a specified period before the next dosage is administered. Specific therapeutic ranges exist for each medication.

Arterial Blood Gases

Measurement of arterial blood gases is another important diagnostic procedure (see Chapter 35 ∞). Specialty nurses, medical technicians, and respiratory therapists normally take specimens of arterial blood from the radial, brachial, or femoral arteries. Because of the relatively great pressure of the blood in these arteries, it is important to prevent hemorrhaging by applying pressure to the puncture side for about 5 to 10 minutes after removing the needle.

Blood Chemistry

A number of other tests may be performed on blood serum (the liquid portion of the blood). These are often referred to as **blood chemistry**. In addition to serum electrolytes, common chemistry examinations include determining certain enzymes that may be present, serum glucose, hormones, and other substances such as cholesterol and triglycerides. These tests provide valuable diagnostic cues.

A common lab test is the glycosylated hemoglobin or hemoglobin A1C (HbA_{1C}), which is a measurement of blood glucose that is bound to hemoglobin. Hemoglobin A_{1C} is a reflection of how well blood glucose levels have been controlled during the prior 3 to 4 months. The normal range is 4.0% to 5.5%. An elevated HbA_{1C} reflects hyperglycemia in diabetics.

The first specific blood test to detect and guide treatment for heart failure is the BNP (B-type natriuretic peptide) test. B-type natriuretic peptide is secreted primarily by the left ventricle in response to increased ventricular volume and pressure. BNP levels increase as the heart failure becomes more severe.

See Table 20–2 for normal values of common blood chemistry tests.

Metabolic Screening

Newborns are routinely screened for congenital metabolic conditions. Tests for phenylketonuria (PKU) and congenital hypothyroidism are required in all states in the United States. Other conditions that are frequently screened include sickle cell disease and galactosemia. Screening involves collecting peripheral venous blood (via a heel-stick) on a prepared blotting paper and sending the specimen to the state laboratory for analysis. Discovered abnormalities allow the provider and parents to plan early care (e.g., special diets for children with PKU) that can prevent long-term complications.

Capillary Blood Glucose

A capillary blood specimen is often taken to measure blood glucose when frequent tests are required or when a venipuncture cannot be performed. This technique is less painful than a venipuncture and easily performed. Hence, clients can perform this technique on themselves.

A number of manufacturers have developed blood glucose meters or monitors. Advances in technology have resulted in clients having greater choices for a glucose meter that meets their needs. There are software programs that analyze their trends in glucose control. Glucose meters can vary in amount of blood needed, testing speed, size, ability to store results, cost of the meter, and test strips (U.S. Food and Drug Administration, n.d.). Choosing the right glucose meter that matches the client's needs will help the client to be comfortable and confident in using the meter and thus promote control of his or her diabetes. Once the client chooses a blood glucose meter, it is imperative that the nurse or client review the manufacturer's operating guidelines. Being familiar with the proper use of the equipment helps ensure accurate readings.

Capillary blood specimens have commonly been obtained from the finger in adults but newer monitors allow for obtaining specimens from less sensitive areas on the arms, legs, or abdomen. If finger puncture is indicated, using the lateral aspect or side of the finger helps to avoid the nerve endings and calloused areas at the fingertip. The earlobe may be used if the client is in shock or the fingers are edematous.

Skill 20–1 describes how to obtain a capillary blood specimen and measure blood glucose using a portable meter.

TABLE 20–2 **Common Blood Chemistry Tests with Clinical Implications**

TEST	NORMAL FINDINGS (ADULT)*	SIGNIFICANCE
Liver Function Tests:		
ALT (alanine amino transferase), formerly known as serum pyretic transaminase (SGPT)	Men: 10–55 U/L Women: 7–30 U/L	Marker of hepatic injury; more specific of liver damage than AST.
AST (aspartate amino transferase), formerly known as serum glutamic oxaloacetic transaminase (SGOT)	Men: 10–40 U/L Women: 9–25 U/L	Found in heart, liver, and skeletal muscle. Can also be used to indicate liver injury.
Albumin	Adults: 3.5–4.8 g/dL or 35–48 g/L Panic value: <1.5 g/dL	Is a protein produced by the liver.
Alkaline phosphatase	Adults: 25–100 U/L	Found in the tissues of the liver, bone, intestine, kidney, and placenta. Used as an index of liver and bone disease when correlated with other clinical findings.
Ammonia	Adults: 35–65 µg/dL	The liver converts ammonia, a by-product of protein metabolism, into urea which is excreted by the kidneys.
Bilirubin	Adults: Total: 0.3–1.0 mg/dL Direct: 0.0–0.2 mg/dL Indirect: 0.1–1/0 mg/dL Panic value: >12 mg/dL	Results from the breakdown of hemoglobin in the red blood cells; removed from the body by the liver, which excretes it into the bile.
GGT (gamma-glutamyl transferase)	Men: 1–94 U/L Women: 1–70 U/L	Found primarily in the liver, kidney, prostate, and spleen. Is more specific for the hepatobiliary system.
Prothrombin	11–13 seconds Critical value: > 20 seconds for non-anticoagulated persons	A protein produced by the liver for clotting of blood.
Cardiac Markers:		
CK (creatine kinase)	Total: Men: 38–174 U/L Women: 26–140 U/L Isoenzymes: MM (CK$_3$): 96%–100% MB (CK$_2$): 0% –6% BB (CK$_1$): 0%	An enzyme found in the heart and skeletal muscles. Has three isoenzymes: BB or CK$_1$, MB or CK$_2$, and MM or CK$_3$.
Myoglobin	5–70 ng/mL	After an MI, serum levels of myoglobin rise in 2–4 hours, making it an early marker for muscle damage in MI.
Troponin I Troponin T	Troponin I: less than 1.0 ng/ml Critical value: >1.5 ng/mL Troponin T: less than 1.0 ng/mL	Cardiac troponin is highly concentrated in the heart muscle. This test is used in the early diagnosis of MI. After an MI, troponin I begins to increase in 4–6 hours and remains elevated for 5–7 days. Troponin T begins to increase in 3–4 hours and remains elevated for 10–14 days.
BNP (brain natriuretic peptide)	<100 pg/mL or <100 ng/L	A hormone produced by the ventricles of the heart and is a marker of ventricular systolic and diastolic dysfunction. This test is useful in diagnosing and guiding treatment of heart failure.
Lipoprotein Profile		
Cholesterol	Adults: Desirable: <. 200 mg/dL	This test is an important screening test for heart disease.
HDL-C (high-density lipoprotein cholesterol)	Men: 35–65 mg/dL Women: 35–80 mg/dL	A class of lipoproteins produced by the liver and intestines. The "good" cholesterol.
LDL (low-density lipoprotein)	Adults: Desirable: <130 mg/dL	Up to 70% of the total serum cholesterol is present in the LDL. The "bad" cholesterol.
Triglycerides	Desirable: <150 mg/dL	This test evaluates suspected atherosclerosis and measures the body's ability to metabolize fat.

*Normal values may vary based on laboratory process

OBTAINING A CAPILLARY BLOOD SPECIMEN TO MEASURE BLOOD GLUCOSE

PURPOSES

- To determine or monitor blood glucose levels of clients at risk for hyperglycemia or hypoglycemia
- To promote blood glucose regulation by the client
- To evaluate the effectiveness of insulin administration

ASSESSMENT

Before obtaining a capillary blood specimen, determine
- The policies and procedures for the facility.
- The frequency and type of testing.
- The client's understanding of the procedure.
- The client's response to previous testing.
- Assess the client's skin at the puncture site to determine if it is intact and the circulation is not compromised. Check color, warmth, and capillary refill.

- Review the client's record for medications that may prolong bleeding, such as anticoagulants, or medical problems that may increase the bleeding response.
- Assess the client's self-care abilities that may affect accuracy of test results, such as visual impairment and finger dexterity.

PLANNING

Delegation

Check the applicable nurse practice act and the facility policy and procedure manual to determine who can perform this skill. It is usually considered an invasive technique and one that requires problem solving and application of knowledge. It is the responsibility of the nurse to know the results of the test and supervise ancillary personnel responsible for assisting the nurse.

EQUIPMENT

- Blood glucose meter (glucometer)
- Blood glucose reagent strip compatible with the meter
- 2 × 2 inch gauze
- Antiseptic swab
- Clean gloves
- Sterile lancet
- Lancet injector

IMPLEMENTATION

Preparation

Review the type of meter and the manufacturer's instructions. Assemble the equipment at the bedside.

Performance

1. Prior to performing the procedure, introduce self and verify the client's identity using agency protocol. Explain to the client what you are going to do, why it is necessary, and how he or she can cooperate. Discuss how the results will be used in planning further care or treatments.
2. Perform hand hygiene and observe other appropriate infection control procedures (e.g., gloves).
3. Provide for client privacy.
4. Prepare the equipment.
   - Calibrate the meter and run a control sample according to the manufacturer's instructions.
5. Select and prepare the vascular puncture site.
   - Choose a vascular puncture site (e.g., the side of an adult's finger). Avoid sites beside bone. Hold a finger in a dependent position. If the earlobe is used, rub it gently with a small piece of gauze. **Rationale:** *These actions increase the blood flow to the area, ensure an adequate specimen, and reduce the need for a repeat puncture.*
   - Clean the site with the antiseptic swab or soap and water and allow it to dry completely. **Rationale:** *Alcohol can affect accuracy and the site burns when punctured when wet with alcohol.*
6. Obtain the blood specimen.
   - Apply clean gloves.
   - Place the injector, if used, against the site, and release the needle, thus permitting it to pierce the skin. Make sure the lancet is perpendicular to the site. **Rationale:** *The lancet is designed to pierce the skin at a specific depth when it is in a perpendicular position relative to the skin.*

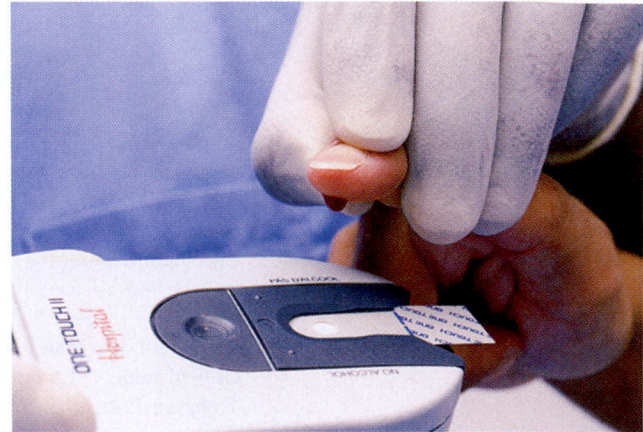

❶ Gently squeeze a drop of blood onto the reagent strip.

- Gently squeeze (but do not touch) the puncture site until a large drop of blood forms. ❶ The size of the drop of blood can vary depending on the meter. Some meters require as little as 0.3 mL (Passanza, 2001) or not much larger than the period at the end of this sentence (Mensing, 2004). **Rationale:** *An insufficient sample will result in an erroneous reading.*
- Hold the reagent strip under the puncture site until adequate blood covers the indicator square. The pad will absorb the blood and a chemical reaction will occur. Do not smear the blood. **Rationale:** *This will cause an inaccurate reading. Some meters wick the blood by just touching the puncture site with the strip.*
- Ask the client to apply pressure to the skin puncture site with a 2 × 2 or 4 × 4 inch gauze. **Rationale:** *Pressure will assist hemostasis.*

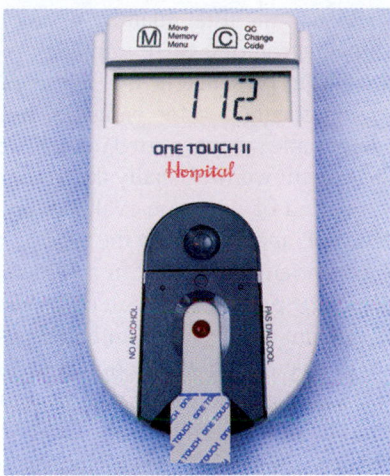

2 The glucose meter will display the glucose reading.

7. Expose the blood to the test strip for the period and the manner specified by the manufacturer. As soon as the blood is placed on the test strip:
   - Follow the manufacturer's recommendations on the glucose meter and monitor for the amount of time indicated by the manufacturer.

Some glucometers have the test strip placed in the machine before the specimen is obtained.

8. Measure the blood glucose.
   - Place the strip into the meter according to the manufacturer's instructions. Some devices require that the strip be wiped or blotted after a designated period of time before being inserted in the meter. Other strips do not require blotting or wiping. Refer to the specific manufacturer's recommendations for the specific procedure.
   - After the designated time, most glucose meters will display the glucose reading automatically. **2** Correct timing ensures accurate results.
   - Turn off the meter and discard the test strip and 2 × 2 inch gauze in a biohazard container. Discard the lancet into a sharps container.

9. Remove and discard gloves. Perform hand hygiene.

10. Document the method of testing and results on the client's record. If appropriate, record the client's understanding and ability to demonstrate the skill. The client's record may also include a flow sheet on which capillary blood glucose results and the amount, type, route, and time of insulin administration are recorded. Always check if a diabetic flow sheet is being used for the client.

11. Check for orders for sliding scale insulin based on capillary blood glucose results. Administer insulin as prescribed.

EVALUATION

- Compare glucose meter reading with normal blood glucose level, status of puncture site, and motivation of the client to perform the test independently.
- Relate blood glucose reading to previous readings and the client's current health status.
- Report abnormal results to the primary care provider.

- Conduct appropriate follow-up such as asking the client to explain the meaning of the results and/or demonstrating the procedure at the next scheduled test.
- Prepare the client for home glucose monitoring and review frequency, record keeping, and insulin administration if appropriate.

LIFESPAN CONSIDERATIONS   Capillary Blood Glucose

Infants
- The outer aspect of the heel is the most common site for neonates and infants. Placing a warm cloth on the infant's heel often increases the blood flow to the area.

Children
- Use the side of a fingertip for a young client older than age 2, unless contraindicated.
- Allow the child to choose the puncture site, when possible.
- Praise the young client for cooperating and assure the child that the procedure is not a punishment.

Older Adults
- Older adults may have arthritic joint changes, poor vision, or hand tremors and may need assistance using the glucose meter or obtaining a meter that accommodates their limitations.
- Older adults may have difficulty obtaining diabetic supplies due to financial concerns or homebound status.
- Older adults often have poor circulation. Warming the hands by wrapping with a warm washcloth for 3 to 5 minutes or placing the hand dependent for a few moments may help in obtaining a blood sample.

LONG-TERM CARE CONSIDERATION
Glucose Monitors

Clients in long-term care may use their own glucose monitors, requiring the nurse to be familiar with many different types of machines. The nurse should obtain a manual for the monitor that explains how to use it and how to test it for accuracy.

SPECIMEN COLLECTION

The nurse contributes to the assessment of a client's health status by collecting specimens of body fluids. Almost all hospitalized clients have at least one laboratory specimen collected during their stay at the health care facility. Laboratory examination of specimens such as urine, blood, stool, sputum, and wound drainage provides important adjunct information for diagnosing health care problems and also provides a measure of the responses to therapy.

Nurses often assume the responsibility for specimen collection. Depending on the type of specimen and skill required, the nurse may be able to delegate this task to unlicensed assistive personnel (UAP) under the supervision of the professional nurse.

Nursing responsibilities associated with specimen collection include the following:

- Explain the purpose of the specimen collection and the procedure for obtaining the specimen. Clients may experience anxiety about the procedure, especially if it is perceived as being intrusive or if they fear an unknown test result. A clear explanation will facilitate the client's cooperation in the collection of the specimen. With proper instruction, many clients are able to collect their own specimen, which promotes independence and reduces or avoids embarrassment.

- Provide client comfort, privacy, and safety. Clients may experience embarrassment or discomfort when providing a specimen. The nurse should provide the client with as much privacy as possible and handle the specimen discreetly. The nurse needs to be nonjudgmental and sensitive to possible sociocultural beliefs that may affect the client's willingness to participate in the specimen collection.

- Use the correct procedure for obtaining a specimen or ensure that the client or staff follows the correct procedure. Aseptic technique is used in specimen collection to prevent contamination that can cause inaccurate test results. A nursing procedure or laboratory manual is often available if the nurse is unfamiliar with the procedure. If there is any question about the procedure, the nurse calls the laboratory for directions before collecting the specimen.

- Note relevant information on the laboratory requisition slip, for example, medications the client is taking that may affect the results.

- Transport the specimen to the laboratory promptly. Fresh specimens provide more accurate results.

- Report abnormal laboratory findings to the health care provider in a timely manner consistent with the severity of the abnormal results.

Stool Specimens

Analysis of stool specimens can provide information about a client's health condition. Some of the reasons for testing feces include the following:

- To determine the presence of **occult** (hidden) **blood**, a test often referred to as the **guaiac test**, can be readily performed by the nurse in the clinical area or by the client at home. Guaiac paper used in the test is sensitive to fecal blood content.

- To analyze for dietary products and digestive secretions. For these kinds of tests, the nurse needs to col-

lect and send the total quantity of stool expelled at one time instead of a small sample.

- To detect the presence of ova and parasites. When collecting specimens for parasites, it is important that the sample be transported immediately to the lab while it is still warm. Usually three stool specimens, over a period of days, are evaluated to confirm the presence of, and to identify the type of, organism so that appropriate treatment can be ordered.

- To detect the presence of bacteria or viruses. Only a small amount of feces is required because the specimen will be cultured. Collection containers or tubes must be sterile and aseptic technique used during collection. Stools need to be sent immediately to the laboratory. The nurse needs to note on the lab requisition if the client is receiving any antibiotics.

The nurse is responsible for collecting stool specimens ordered for laboratory analysis. Before obtaining a specimen, the nurse needs to determine the reason for collecting the stool specimen and the correct method of obtaining and handling. It may be necessary to confirm this information by checking with the agency laboratory. In many situations only a single specimen is required; in others, timed specimens are necessary, and every stool passed is collected within a designated time period. UAP may obtain and collect stool specimen(s). The nurse, however, needs to consider the collection process before delegating this task. An incorrect collection technique can cause inaccurate test results. The task of obtaining and testing a stool specimen for occult blood may be performed by UAP. It is important that the nurse instruct the UAP to tell the nurse if blood is detected and/or whether the test is positive. In addition, the stool specimen should be saved to allow the nurse to repeat the test. See client teaching for instructions to the client.

When obtaining stool samples the nurse follows medical aseptic technique. Wear disposable gloves to prevent hand contamination and take care not to contaminate the outside of the specimen container. Use one or two clean tongue blades to transfer the specimen to the container and then wrap them in a paper towel before disposing of them in the waste container. This practice reduces the chance of contact with other articles and the spread of microorganisms. The amount of stool to be sent depends on the purpose for which the specimen is collected. Usually about 2.5 cm (1 in.) of formed stool or 15 to 30 mL of liquid stool is adequate. For some timed specimens, however, the entire stool passed may need to be sent. Visible pus, mucus, or blood should be included in sample specimens. For a stool culture, the nurse dips a sterile swab into the specimen, preferably where purulent fecal matter is present and, using sterile technique, places the swab in a sterile test tube.

Ensure that the specimen label and the laboratory requisition have the correct information on them and are securely attached to the specimen container. Inappropriate identification of the specimen risks errors of diagnosis or therapy for the client.

Because fresh specimens provide the most accurate results, the nurse sends the specimen to the laboratory immediately. If this is not possible, the nurse follows the directions on the specimen container. In some instances refrigeration is indicated, because bacteriologic changes take place in stool specimens left at room temperature. To prevent contamination, never place a stool specimen in a refrigerator that contains food or medication.

Document all relevant information. Record the collection of the specimen on the client's chart and on the nursing care plan. Include in the recording the date and time of the collection and all nursing assessments; presence of abnormal constituents, such as blood or mucus; results of test for occult blood if obtained; discomfort during or after defecation; status of perianal skin; and any bleeding from the anus after defecation.

TESTING FECES FOR OCCULT BLOOD A commonly used test product to measure occult blood is the Hemoccult test, which uses a chemical reagent (substance used in a chemical reaction to detect a specific substance). This reagent detects the presence of the enzyme peroxidase in the hemoglobin molecule. To perform the test, the nurse or client uses a tongue blade to place a small amount of stool on a slide or card and then closes the card. The card is turned over and a few drops of a reagent are placed onto the smear on the back of the card. The nurse then observes for a color change (Figure 20–1). A blue color indicates a guaiac positive result, that is, the presence of occult blood. No color change or any color other than blue is a negative finding, indicating the absence of blood in the stool.

Certain foods, medications, and vitamin C can produce inaccurate test results. False-positive results can occur if the client has recently ingested (a) red meat; (b) raw vegetables or fruits, particularly radishes, turnips, horseradish, and melons; or (c) certain medications that irritate the gastric mucosa and cause bleeding, such as aspirin or other nonsteroidal anti-inflammatory drugs, steroids, iron preparations, and anticoagulants. False-negative results can occur if the client has taken more than 250 mg per day of vitamin C from any sources up to 3 days before the test—even if bleeding is present. Guidelines for instructing clients to assess their stool for occult blood are listed in Client Teaching.

Urine Specimens

The nurse is responsible for collecting urine specimens for a number of tests: clean voided specimens for routine urinalysis, **clean-catch** or **midstream urine specimens** for urine culture, and timed urine specimens for a variety of tests that depend on the client's specific health problem. Urine specimen collection may require collection via straight catheter insertion. If this is necessary, refer to Chapter 33 ∞, Skill 33–2.

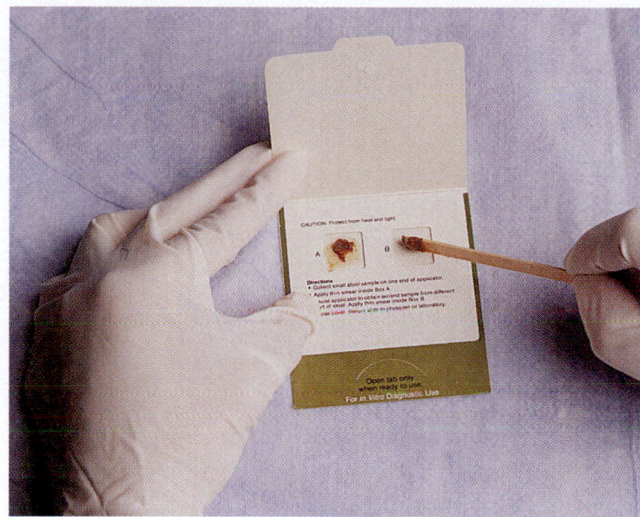

A

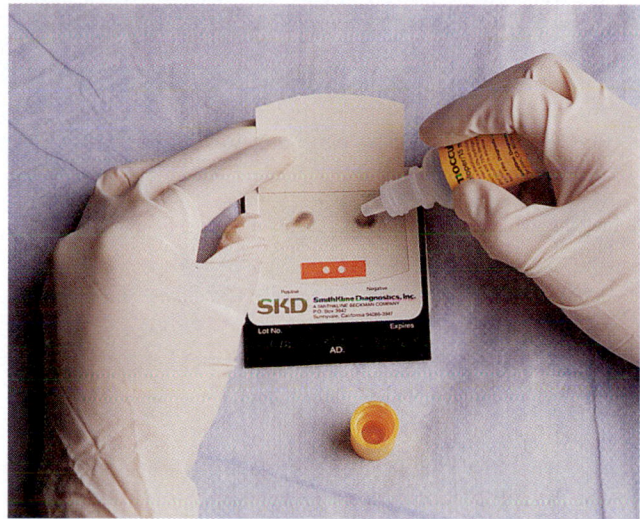

B

Figure 20–1 ◎ A, Opening the front cover of a Hemoccult slide and applying a thin smear of feces on the slide. **B**, Opening the flap on the back of the slide and applying two drops of developing fluid over each smear.

CLEAN VOIDED URINE SPECIMEN A clean voided specimen is usually adequate for routine examination. Many clients are able to collect a clean voided specimen and provide the specimen independently with minimal instructions. Male clients generally are able to void directly into the specimen container, and female clients usually sit or squat over the toilet, holding the container between their legs during voiding. Routine urine examination is usually done on the first voided specimen in the morning because it tends to have a higher, more uniform concentration and a more acidic pH than specimens later in the day.

At least 10 mL of urine is generally sufficient for a routine urinalysis. Clients who are seriously ill, physically

Assessing Stool for Occult Blood

- Avoid restricted foods and vitamin C for 3 days before the test and specified medications for 7 days before the test.
- Use a ballpoint pen to label the specimens with your name, address, age, and date of specimen. Each specimen must be dated accurately.
- Avoid collecting specimens during your menstrual period and for 3 days afterward, and while you have bleeding hemorrhoids or blood in your urine.
- Remove toilet bowl cleaners from the toilet bowl. Flush the toilet twice before proceeding with the test.
- Avoid contaminating the specimen with urine or toilet tissue. Empty your bladder before the test. To facilitate specimen collection, transfer the stool to a clean, dry container. Wear disposable gloves.
- Use the tongue blade provided to transfer the specimen to the test folder or tape. Only a small amount of stool is required. Take the sample from the center of a formed stool to ensure a uniform sample.
- Wrap the tongue blade in a paper towel and dispose of it in the waste receptacle.
- Follow the manufacturer's directions explicitly for the test product being used. Review procedure with client for the product being used.
- Consult your health care provider if there is any problem understanding the instructions.
- Return completed specimens to your primary care provider or laboratory as instructed.

LIFESPAN CONSIDERATIONS
Stool Specimen

Infants

- To collect a stool specimen for an infant, the stool is scraped from the diaper, being careful not to contaminate the stool with urine.

Children

- A child who is toilet trained should be able to provide a fecal specimen, but may prefer being assisted by a parent.
- When explaining the procedure to the child, use words appropriate for the child's age rather than medical terms. Ask the parent what words the family normally uses to describe a bowel movement.
- A specimen for pinworms is collected by the parent early in the morning, after sleep and before the child has a bowel movement. Scotch tape is attached to a tongue blade and the sticky side is laid flat against the perineum and anus to pick up any eggs or small worms. The tongue blade is then examined under a microscope.

Older Adults

- Older adults may need assistance if serial stool specimens are required.

---

incapacitated, or disoriented may need to use a bedpan or urinal in bed; others may require supervision or assistance in the bathroom. Whatever the situation, clear and specific directions are required:

- The specimen must be free of fecal contamination, so urine must be kept separate from feces.
- Female clients should discard the toilet tissue in the toilet or in a waste bag rather than in the bedpan because tissue in the specimen makes laboratory analysis more difficult.
- Put the lid tightly on the container to prevent spillage of the urine and contamination of other objects.
- If the outside of the container has been contaminated by urine, clean it with a disinfectant.

The nurse must (a) make sure that the specimen label and the laboratory requisition carry the correct information and (b) attach them securely to the specimen. Inappropriate identification of the specimen can lead to errors of diagnosis or therapy for the client.

UAP may be assigned to collect a routine urine specimen. Provide the UAP with clear directions on how to instruct the client to collect his or her own urine specimen or how to correctly collect the specimen for the client who may need to use a bedpan or urinal.

CLEAN-CATCH OR MIDSTREAM URINE SPECIMEN Clean-catch or midstream voided specimens are collected when a urine culture is ordered to identify microorganisms causing urinary tract infection. Although some contamination by skin bacteria may occur with a clean-catch specimen, the risk of introducing microorganisms into the urinary tract through catheterization is more significant. Care is taken to ensure that the specimen is as free as possible from contamination by microorganisms around the urinary meatus. Clean-catch specimens are collected into a sterile specimen container with a lid. Disposable clean-catch kits are available. Skill 20–2 explains how to collect a clean-catch urine specimen for culture.

SKILL 20–2

COLLECTING A URINE SPECIMEN FOR CULTURE AND SENSITIVITY BY CLEAN CATCH

PURPOSE
- To determine the presence of microorganisms, the type of organism(s), and the antibiotics to which the organisms are sensitive

ASSESSMENT
- Determine the ability of the client to provide the specimen.
- Assess the color, odor, and consistency of the urine and the presence of clinical signs of urinary tract infection

(e.g., frequency, urgency, dysuria, hematuria, flank pain, cloudy urine with foul odor).

PLANNING

> **Delegation**
> UAP may perform the collection of a clean-catch or midstream urine specimen. It is important, however, that the nurse inform the unlicensed person about how to instruct the client in the correct process for obtaining the specimen. Proper cleansing of the urethra should be emphasized to avoid contaminating the urine specimen.

EQUIPMENT
Equipment used varies from agency to agency. Some agencies use commercially prepared disposable clean-catch kits. Others are agency-prepared sterile trays. Both prepared trays and kits generally contain the following items:

- Clean gloves
- Antiseptic towelettes
- Sterile specimen container
- Specimen identification label

In addition the nurse needs to obtain the following:

- Completed laboratory requisition form
- Urine receptacle, if the client is not ambulatory
- Basin of warm water, soap, washcloth, and towel for the nonambulatory client

IMPLEMENTATION

Preparation
Gather the necessary equipment needed for the collection of the specimen. Use visual aids, if available, to assist the client to understand the midstream collection technique.

Performance
1. Prior to performing the procedure, introduce self and verify the client's identity using agency protocol. Explain to the client that a urine specimen is required, give the reason, and explain the method to be used to collect it. Discuss how the results will be used in planning further care or treatments.
2. Perform hand hygiene and observe other appropriate infection control procedures.
3. Provide for client privacy.
4. For an ambulatory client who is able to follow directions, instruct the client on how to collect the specimen.
   - Direct or assist the client to the bathroom.
   - Ask the client to wash and dry the genitals and perineal area with soap and water. **Rationale:** *Washing the perineal area reduces the number of skin and transient bacteria, decreasing the risk of contaminating the urine specimen.*
   - Instruct the client on how to clean the urinary meatus with antiseptic towelettes. **Rationale:** *The antiseptic further reduces bacterial contamination of the urinary meatus and the risk of contaminating the specimen.*

FOR FEMALE CLIENTS
- Use each towelette only once. Clean the perineal area from front to back and discard the towelette. Use all towelettes provided (usually two or three). **Rationale:** *Cleaning from front to back cleans the area of least contamination to the area of greatest contamination.*

FOR MALE CLIENTS
- If uncircumcised, retract the foreskin slightly to expose the urinary meatus.

- Using a circular motion, clean the urinary meatus and the distal portion of the penis. Use each towelette only once, then discard. Clean several inches down the shaft of the penis. **Rationale:** *This cleans from the area of least contamination to the area of greatest contamination.*
5. For a client who requires assistance, prepare the client and equipment. Apply clean gloves.
   - Wash the perineal area with soap and water, rinse, and dry.
   - Assist the client onto a clean commode or bedpan. If using a bedpan or urinal, position the client as upright as allowed or tolerated. **Rationale:** *Assuming a normal anatomic position for voiding facilitates urination.*
   - Remove and discard gloves. Perform hand hygiene.
   - Open the clean-catch kit, taking care not to contaminate the inside of the specimen container or lid. Place the lid in the upright position. **Rationale:** *It is important to maintain sterility of the specimen container to prevent contamination of the specimen.*
   - Put on clean gloves.
   - Clean the urinary meatus and perineal area as described in step 4.
6. Collect the specimen from a nonambulatory client or instruct an ambulatory client on how to collect it.
   - Instruct the client to start voiding. **Rationale:** *Bacteria in the distal urethra and at the urinary meatus are cleared by the first few milliliters of urine expelled.*
   - Place the specimen container into the midstream of urine and collect the specimen, taking care not to touch the container to the perineum or penis. **Rationale:** *It is important to avoid contaminating the interior of the specimen container and the specimen itself.*
   - Collect urine in the container.
   - Cap the container tightly, touching only the outside of the container and the cap. **Rationale:** *This prevents contamination or spilling of the specimen.*

(continued)

SKILL 20–2

COLLECTING A URINE SPECIMEN *(continued)*

- If necessary, clean the outside of the specimen container with disinfectant. **Rationale:** *This prevents transfer of microorganisms to others.*
- Remove and discard gloves. Perform hand hygiene.

7. Label the specimen and transport it to the laboratory.
- Ensure that the specimen label is attached to the specimen cup, not the lid, and the laboratory requisition provides the correct information. Place the specimen in a plastic bag that has a biohazard label on it. Attach the requisition securely to the bag. **Rationale:** *Inaccurate identification or information on the specimen container risks errors in diagnosis or therapy.*
- Arrange for the specimen to be sent to the laboratory immediately. **Rationale:** *Bacterial cultures must be started immediately before any contaminating organisms can grow, multiply, and produce false results.*

8. Document pertinent data.
- Record collection of the specimen, any pertinent observations of the urine such as color, odor, or consistency, and any difficulty in voiding that the client experienced.
- Indicate on the lab slip if the client is taking any current antibiotic therapy or if the client is menstruating.

SAMPLE DOCUMENTATION

1/15/2010 0800 Informed of MD order for clean catch urine for C&S. Instructed how to perform. Stated she understood. Urine specimen cloudy. States she continues to have burning on urination. Urine specimen sent to lab. Antibiotic started per MD orders. _____ T. Sanchez, RN

EVALUATION

- Report lab results to the primary care provider.
- Discuss findings of the laboratory test with primary care provider and client.
- Conduct appropriate follow-up nursing interventions as needed, such as administering *ordered* medications and client teaching.

LIFESPAN CONSIDERATIONS   Urine Specimen

Infants

- Clean the perineal area and the urethral opening as you would with an adult client. Apply a specimen bag that has an adhesive backing that attaches to the skin. After the infant has voided a desired amount, gently remove the bag from the skin.

Children

- When collecting a routine urine specimen, explain the procedure in simple nonmedical terms appropriate to the child and ask the child to void using a clean collecting receptacle (e.g., specimen cup, potty chair, bedpan, toilet collection device).

- Give the child a clean specimen container to play with.
- Allow a parent to assist the child, if possible. The child may feel more comfortable with a parent present.
- For sterile urine specimens, straight catheterization may be necessary, in which a urinary catheter is inserted using sterile technique, the specimen is obtained, and the catheter is removed.

Older Adults

- For a clean-catch urine specimen, older adults may have difficulty controlling the stream of urine.
- Older adult women with arthritis may have difficulty holding the labia apart during the collection of clean-catch urine.

TIMED URINE SPECIMEN   Some urine examinations require collection of all urine produced and voided over a specific period of time, ranging from 1 to 2 hours to 24 hours. Timed specimens generally either are refrigerated or contain a preservative to prevent bacterial growth or decomposition of urine components. Each voiding of urine is collected in a small, clean container and then emptied immediately into the large refrigerated bottle or carton.

CLINICAL ALERT

If the client or staff forgets and discards the client's urine during a timed collection, the procedure must be restarted from the beginning.

INDWELLING CATHETER SPECIMEN   Sterile urine specimens can be obtained from closed drainage systems by inserting a sterile needle attached to a syringe through a drainage port in the tubing. Aspiration of urine from catheters can be done only with self-sealing rubber catheters—not plastic, silicone, or Silastic catheters. When self-sealing rubber catheters are used, the needle is inserted just above the location where the catheter is attached to the drainage tubing. The area from which to obtain urine may be marked by a patch on the catheter (see Figure 20–2). Newer closed drainage urinary systems now have needleless ports, which avoids having to use a needle to obtain a sample. This protects the nurse from a needlestick injury and maintains the integrity and sterility of the catheter system by eliminating the need to puncture the tubing (Davis,

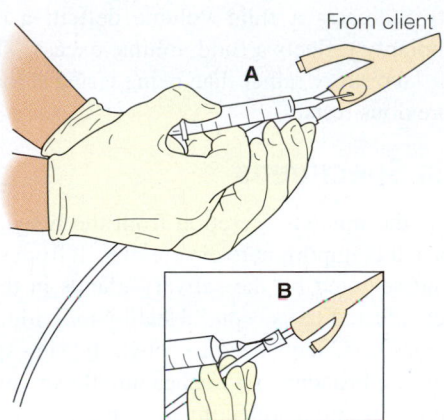

Figure 20–2 ○ Obtaining a urine specimen from a retention catheter. **A,** From a specific area near the end of the catheter; **B,** from an access port in the tubing.

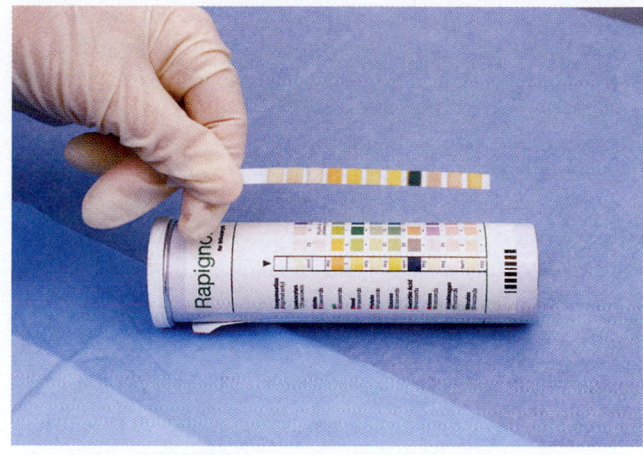

Figure 20–3 ○ After dipping the reagent strip (dipstick) into fresh urine, wait the stated time period and compare the results to the color chart.

2004). The needleless port accepts a Luer-Lok syringe. Position the syringe perpendicular to the center of the port and insert, twist, and lock into the port. When the specimen is obtained and the syringe removed, the port seals itself.

To collect a specimen from a Foley (retention) catheter or a drainage tube, follow these steps:

- Put on disposable gloves.
- If there is no urine in the catheter, clamp the drainage tubing at least 3 inches below the sampling port for about 30 minutes. This allows fresh urine to collect in the catheter.
- Wipe the area where the needle or Luer-Lok syringe will be inserted with a disinfectant swab. The site should be distal to the tube leading to the balloon to avoid puncturing this tube. Disinfecting the needle insertion site removes any microorganisms on the surface of the catheter, thereby avoiding contamination of the needle and the entrance of microorganisms into the catheter.
- Insert the needle at a 30- to 45-degree angle. This angle of entrance facilitates self-sealing of the rubber. Insert the Luer-Lok syringe at a 90-degree angle for the needleless port.
- Unclamp the catheter.
- Withdraw the required amount of urine, for example, 3 mL for a urine culture or 30 mL for a routine urinalysis.
- Transfer the urine to the specimen container. If a sterile culture tube is used, make sure the needle or syringe (depending on the system) does not touch the outside of the container.
- Discard the syringe and needle or syringe (depending on the system) in an appropriate sharps container.
- Cap the container.
- Remove gloves and discard appropriately.
- Label the container, and send the urine to the laboratory immediately for analysis or refrigeration.
- Record collection of the specimen and any pertinent observations of the urine on the appropriate records.

URINE TESTING Several simple urine tests are often done by nurses on the nursing units. These include tests for specific gravity, pH, and the presence of abnormal constituents such as glucose, ketones, protein, and occult blood.

Nurses in a health care facility or clients in the home setting can use commercially prepared kits to test abnormal constituents in the urine. These kits contain the required equipment and an appropriate reagent which may be in the form of a tablet, fluid, or paper test strip or dipstick. When the urine contacts the reagent a chemical reaction occurs, causing a color change that is then compared with a chart to interpret the significance of the color (Figure 20–3). Specific directions for the amount of urine needed, the time required for the chemical reaction, and the meaning of the colors produced vary among manufacturers. Thus it is essential that nurses and clients read and follow directions supplied by each manufacturer. In addition, testing materials need to be checked to ascertain that they are not outdated.

Urine testing may be performed by UAP. It is important that the UAP understands the specific specimen collection procedure and reports the results of the test to the nurse. Inform the UAP to save the urine sample to allow the nurse to repeat the test if necessary.

Specific gravity is an indicator of urine concentration, or the amount of solutes (metabolic wastes and electrolytes) present in the urine. The specific gravity of distilled water is 1.00; the specific gravity of urine normally ranges from 1.010 to 1.025. As urine becomes more concentrated, its specific gravity increases. Excess fluid intake or diseases affecting the ability of the kidneys to concentrate urine can result in low specific gravity readings. A high specific gravity may indicate fluid deficit or dehydration, or excess solutes such as glucose in the urine. Specific gravity can be measured with the use of a multiple-test dipstick that has a separate reagent area for specific gravity.

Urinary pH is measured to determine the relative acidity or alkalinity of urine and assess the client's acid–base status. Quantitative measurements of urine pH can be performed in the laboratory, but dipsticks or litmus paper often are used on nursing units or in clinics to obtain less precise pH measurements. Urine normally is slightly acidic, with an average pH of 6 (7 is neutral, less than 7 is acidic, greater than 7 is alkaline). Because the kidneys play a critical role in regulating acid–base balance, assessment of urine pH can be useful in determining whether the kidneys are responding appropriately to acid–base imbalances. In metabolic acidosis, urine pH should decrease as the kidneys excrete hydrogen ions; in metabolic alkalosis, the pH should increase (see Chapter 36 ∞).

Urine is tested for glucose to screen clients for diabetes mellitus and to assess clients during pregnancy for abnormal glucose tolerance. Normally, the amount of glucose in the urine is negligible, although individuals who have ingested large amounts of sugar may show small amounts of glucose in their urine.

Testing urine for glucose is not a measure of current blood glucose level and is considered an inadequate measurement. The American Diabetes Association (2000, p. 66) states that testing urine for glucose is *only* for people who *cannot or will not* test their blood glucose levels. It is important for clients to understand that urine testing is considered an inadequate measurement of blood glucose.

Ketone bodies, a product of the breakdown of fatty acids, normally are not present in the urine. They may, however, be found in the urine of clients with poorly controlled diabetes. Urine testing for ketone level is advised for type 1 diabetics who are at home and not feeling well, who are running a fever, or who have blood glucose consistently over 240 mg/dL (American Diabetes Association, 2000). Urine ketone testing with reagent tablets or a dipstick is also used to evaluate ketoacidosis in clients who are alcoholic, fasting, starving, or consuming high-protein diets.

Protein molecules normally are too large to escape from glomerular capillaries into the filtrate. If the glomerular membrane has been damaged, however (e.g., because of an inflammatory process such as glomerulonephritis), it can become "leaky," allowing proteins to escape. Urine testing for the presence of protein generally is done with a reagent strip (commonly referred to as a *dipstick*).

Normal urine is free from blood. When blood is present, it may be clearly visible or not visible (occult). Commercial reagent strips are used to test for occult blood in the urine.

CLINICAL ALERT

Blood in urine is always an indicator of damage to the kidney or urinary tract (Fischbach, 2004, p. 189).

Urine osmolality is a measure of the solute concentration of urine that is a more exact measurement of urine concentration than specific gravity. It is also used to monitor fluid and electrolyte balance. The particles included are nitrogenous wastes, such as creatinine, urea, and uric acid. Normal values are 500 to 800 mOsm/kg. An increased urine

osmolality indicates a fluid volume deficit; a decreased urine osmolality reflects a fluid volume excess. This test is sent to the laboratory rather than being tested at the bedside like the previous tests.

Sputum Specimens

Sputum is the mucous secretion from the lungs, bronchi, and trachea. It is important to differentiate it from saliva, the clear liquid secreted by the salivary glands in the mouth, sometimes referred to as "spit." Healthy individuals do not produce sputum. Clients need to cough to bring sputum up from the lungs, bronchi, and trachea into the mouth in order to expectorate it into a collecting container.

A UAP can obtain a sputum specimen that is expectorated by a client. It is important to instruct the UAP on when to collect the specimen, how to position the client, and how to correctly collect the specimen. Obtaining a sputum specimen by use of pharyngeal suctioning, however, should be performed by the nurse because it is an invasive, sterile process and requires knowledge application and problem solving. A "sputum trap" is used when the specimen is obtained by suctioning. (See Chapter 35 ∞ , Skill 35–2.)

Sputum specimens are usually collected for one or more of the following reasons:

- For culture and sensitivity to identify a specific microorganism and its drug sensitivities.
- For cytology to identify the origin, structure, function, and pathology of cells. Specimens for cytology often require serial collection of three early-morning specimens and are tested to identify cancer in the lung and its specific cell type.
- For acid-fast bacillus (AFB), which also requires serial collection, often for 3 consecutive days, to identify the presence of tuberculosis (TB). Some agencies use a special glass container when the presence of AFB is suspected.
- To assess the effectiveness of therapy.

Sputum specimens are often collected in the morning. Upon awakening, the client can cough up the secretions that have accumulated during the night. Sometimes specimens are collected during postural drainage, when the client can usually produce sputum. When a client cannot cough, the nurse must sometimes use pharyngeal suctioning to obtain a specimen.

To collect a sputum specimen, the nurse follows these steps:

- Offer mouth care so that the specimen will not be contaminated with microorganisms from the mouth.
- Ask the client to breathe deeply and then cough up 1 to 2 tablespoons, or 15 to 30 mL (4 to 8 fluid drams), of sputum.
- Wear gloves and personal protective equipment to avoid direct contact with the sputum. Follow special precautions if tuberculosis is suspected, obtaining the specimen in a room equipped with a special airflow system or ultraviolet light, or outdoors. If these

options are not available, wear a mask capable of filtering droplet nuclei.

- Ask the client to expectorate (spit out) the sputum into the specimen container. Make sure the sputum does not contact the outside of the container. If the outside of the container does become contaminated, wash it with a disinfectant.
- Following sputum collection, offer mouthwash to remove any unpleasant taste.
- Label and transport the specimen to the laboratory. Ensure that the specimen label and the laboratory requisition contain the correct information. Arrange for the specimen to be sent to the laboratory immediately or refrigerated. Bacterial cultures must be started immediately before any contaminating organisms can grow, multiply, and produce false results.
- Document the collection of the sputum specimen on the client's chart. Include the amount, color, consistency, presence of hemoptysis (blood in the sputum), odor of the sputum, any measures needed to obtain the specimen, and any discomfort experienced by the client.

Throat Culture

A throat culture sample is collected from the mucosa of the oropharynx and tonsillar regions using a culture swab. The sample is then cultured and examined for the presence of disease-producing microorganisms. Obtaining a throat culture is an invasive procedure that requires the application of scientific knowledge and potential problem solving to ensure client safety. Thus, it is best for the nurse to perform this procedure.

To obtain a throat culture specimen, the nurse puts on clean gloves, then inserts the swab into the oropharynx and runs the swab along the tonsils and areas on the pharynx that are reddened or contain exudate. The gag reflex, active in some clients, may be decreased by having the client sit upright if health permits, open the mouth, extend the tongue, and say "ah," and by taking the specimen quickly. The sitting position and extension of the tongue help expose the pharynx; saying "ah" relaxes the throat muscles and helps minimize contraction of the constrictor muscle of the pharynx (the gag reflex). If the posterior pharynx cannot be seen, use a light and depress the tongue with a tongue blade.

VISUALIZATION PROCEDURES

Visualization procedures include *indirect visualization* (noninvasive) and *direct visualization* (invasive) techniques for visualizing body organ and system functions.

Clients with Gastrointestinal Alterations

Direct visualization techniques include **anoscopy**, the viewing of the anal canal; **proctoscopy**, the viewing of the rec-

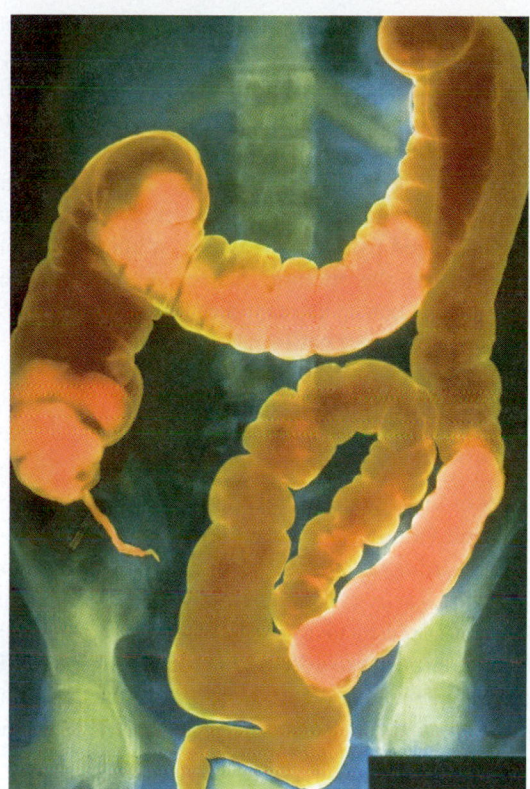

Figure 20–4 ● Enhanced-color x-ray of the colon during a barium enema exam.
(CNRI/Science Photo Library; Photo Researchers, Inc.)

tum; proctosigmoidoscopy, the viewing of the rectum and sigmoid colon; and **colonoscopy**, the viewing of the large intestine. Indirect visualization of the gastrointestinal tract is achieved by roentgenography. X-rays of the gastrointestinal tract can detect strictures, obstructions, tumors, ulcers, inflammatory disease, or other structural changes such as hiatal hernias. Visualization of the tract is enhanced by the introduction of a radiopaque substance such as barium. For examination of the upper gastrointestinal tract or small bowel, the client drinks the barium sulfate. This examination is often referred to as a *barium swallow.* For examination of the lower gastrointestinal tract, the client is given an enema containing the barium. This examination is commonly referred to as a *barium enema.* These x-rays usually include fluoroscopic examination; that is, projection of the x-ray films onto a screen, which permits continuous observation of the flow of barium (Figure 20–4). Nurses are responsible for preparing clients before these studies and for follow-up care, but the procedure is not performed by the nurse.

Clients with Urinary Alterations

Visualization procedures also may be used to evaluate urinary function. An x-ray of the **kidneys/ureters/bladder** is commonly referred to as a **KUB. Intravenous pyelography (IVP)** and **retrograde pyelography** also are radiographic studies used to evaluate the urinary tract. In an intravenous pyelogram, contrast medium is injected intravenously; during retrograde pyelography, the contrast medium is instilled directly into the kidney pelvis via the urethra, bladder, and ureters. Following injection or instillation of the contrast medium, x-rays are taken to evaluate urinary tract structures. Renal **ultrasonography** is a noninvasive test that uses reflected sound waves to visualize the kidneys. During a **cystoscopy**, the bladder, ureteral orifices, and urethra can be directly visualized using a cystoscope, a lighted instrument inserted through the urethra. Nurses are responsible for preparing clients before these studies and for follow-up care, but the procedure is not performed by the nurse.

Clients with Cardiopulmonary Alterations

A number of visualization procedures can be done to examine the cardiovascular system and respiratory tract.

Electrocardiography provides a graphic recording of the heart's electrical activity. Electrodes placed on the skin transmit the electrical impulses to an oscilloscope or graphic recorder. With the wave forms recorded, the **electrocardiogram (ECG)** can then be examined to detect dysrhythmias and alterations in conduction indicative of myocardial damage, enlargement of the heart, or drug effects.

Stress electrocardiography uses ECGs to assess the client's response to an increased cardiac workload during exercise. As the body's demand for oxygen increases with exercising, the cardiac workload increases, as does the oxygen demand of the heart muscle itself. Clients with coronary artery disease may develop chest pain and characteristic ECG changes during exercise.

Angiography is an invasive procedure requiring informed consent of the client. A radiopaque dye is injected into the vessels to be examined. Using fluoroscopy and x-rays, the flow through the vessels is assessed and areas of narrowing or blockage can be observed. Coronary angiography is performed to evaluate the extent of coronary artery disease; pulmonary angiography may be performed to assess the pulmonary vascular system, particularly if pulmonary emboli are suspected. Other vessels that may be studied include the carotid and cerebral arteries, the renal arteries, and the vessels of the lower extremities.

An **echocardiogram** is a noninvasive test that uses ultrasound to visualize structures of the heart and evaluate left ventricular function. Images are produced as ultrasound waves reflect back to a transducer after striking cardiac structures. The nurse should tell the client that this test causes no discomfort, although the conductive gel used may be cold.

X-ray examination of the chest is done both to diagnose disease and to assess the progress of a disease. For an x-ray examination, the nurse needs to inform the client that jewelry and clothing from the waist up must be removed.

A lung scan, also known as a V/Q (ventilation/perfusion) scan, records the emissions from radioisotopes that indicate how well gas and blood are traveling through the lungs. The *perfusion scan* (Q scan—P usually stands for "pulmonary," so apparently the next letter in the alphabet was used for "per-

fusion") is used to assess blood flow through the pulmonary vascular system. For this, the radioisotope is injected intravenously and measured as it circulates through the lung. The *ventilation scan* (V scan) detects ventilation abnormalities, particularly in clients with emphysema. For this scan, the client inhales a radioactive gas through a mask and then exhales it into room air. The client needs to be informed that no radiation precautions are necessary because the amount of radioactivity is very small. The scan may take 20 to 40 minutes.

Laryngoscopy and bronchoscopy are sterile procedures that are conducted with a laryngoscope and bronchoscope, respectively. Tissue samples may also be taken for biopsy. A local anesthetic is usually given before the examination. A local anesthetic is sprayed on the client's pharynx to prevent gagging; alternatively, the client gargles with an anesthetic to anesthetize the throat. The bronchoscope is then inserted to visualize the larynx or bronchi. Informed consent is required for these procedures.

While the nurse does not perform these studies, an important nursing role is preparation of the client. Fear of the unknown increases the client's anxiety level, and by adequately preparing the client the nurse can allay the client's fear as well as improve the outcome of the procedure by assuring pre-test preparation is accurately performed.

Computed Tomography

Computed tomography (CT), also called *CT scanning, computerized tomography,* or *computerized axial tomography (CAT),* is a painless, noninvasive x-ray procedure that has the unique capability of distinguishing minor differences in the density of tissues. The CT produces a three-dimensional image of the organ or structure, making it more sensitive than the x-ray machine.

Magnetic Resonance Imaging

Magnetic resonance imaging (MRI) is a noninvasive diagnostic scanning technique in which the client is placed in a magnetic field. Clients with implanted metal devices (e.g., pacemaker, metal hip prosthesis) cannot undergo an MRI because of the strong magnetic field. There is no exposure to radiation. If a contrast media is injected during the procedure, it is not an iodine contrast. Another advantage to the MRI is that it provides a better contrast between normal and abnormal tissue than the CT scan. It is, however, more costly.

Reports have shown that body art may cause problems to the client during an MRI (Armstrong & Elkins, 2005). Tattoo pigments may contain metal substances that create an electric current that can cause redness and swelling similar to a first-degree burn at the site of the tattoo. Permanent cosmetics (e.g., tattooed eyeliner, eyebrows, lip liner) may cause similar problems. The Society of Permanent Cosmetic Professionals (SPCP) (2005) states that the concentration of zinc oxide is low and the chances of diagnostic imaging problems are remote. Potential problems, however, can be avoided by wearing goggles to cover permanent cosmetics around the eyes. Metal body-piercing jewelry should be removed before an MRI. If the client is worried about the piercing tract closing, a sterile plastic IV catheter can be used to replace the jewelry and the pierced area can be covered by a sterile dressing during the MRI.

Many transdermal patches contain a foil backing that creates an electric current that can lead to intense heat and a burn (Karch, 2004). Again, it is important to ask clients if they are using a transdermal patch before undergoing an MRI. Because the patch may lose its adhesiveness, advise the client to apply a new patch after the MRI.

CLINICAL ALERT

Advise clients to inform the MRI operator if they have a tattoo or permanent makeup and to let the operator know of any unusual sensations felt at the site of the tattoo during the MRI.

The MRI is commonly used for visualization of the brain, spine, limbs and joints, heart, blood vessels, abdomen, and pelvis. The procedure involves the client lying on a platform that moves into either a narrow, closed, high-magnet scanner, or into an open, low-magnet scanner. The client must lie very still. A two-way communication system is used to monitor the client's response and to help relieve feelings of claustrophobia. Earplugs are offered to the client to reduce the discomfort from the loud noises that occur during the test. The procedure lasts between 60 and 90 minutes.

Nuclear Imaging Studies

Fischbach (2004, p. 655) states that nuclear scans study the "physiology or function" of an organ system in contrast to other studies (e.g., CT, MRI, x-ray) which visualize "anatomic" structures. A radiopharmaceutical, a pharmaceutical (targeted to a specific organ) labeled with a radioisotope, is administered through various routes for the test. Clients retain the radioisotope for a relatively short time with the most common radiopharmaceutical having a half-life of 6 hours. A gamma camera is placed over the part of the body under study. The camera, which is networked with a computer, converts the emission of the radioisotope and forms a detailed image. An equal distribution of color is normal; however, darker spots ("hot" spots) indicate hyperfunction and lighter areas ("cold" spots) indicate hypofunction (Fischbach, 2004). **Positron emission tomography (PET)** is a noninvasive radiologic study that involves the injection or inhalation of a radioisotope. Images are created as the radioisotope is distributed in the body. This allows study of various aspects of organ function and may include evaluation of blood flow and tumor growth, for example (Figure 20–5).

ASPIRATION/BIOPSY

Aspiration is the withdrawal of fluid that has abnormally collected (e.g., pleural cavity, abdominal cavity) or to obtain a specimen (e.g., cerebral spinal fluid). A biopsy is the removal and examination of tissue. Usually the biopsy is performed by the provider to determine a diagnosis or to detect malignancy. Both aspiration and biopsy are invasive procedures and require strict sterile technique.

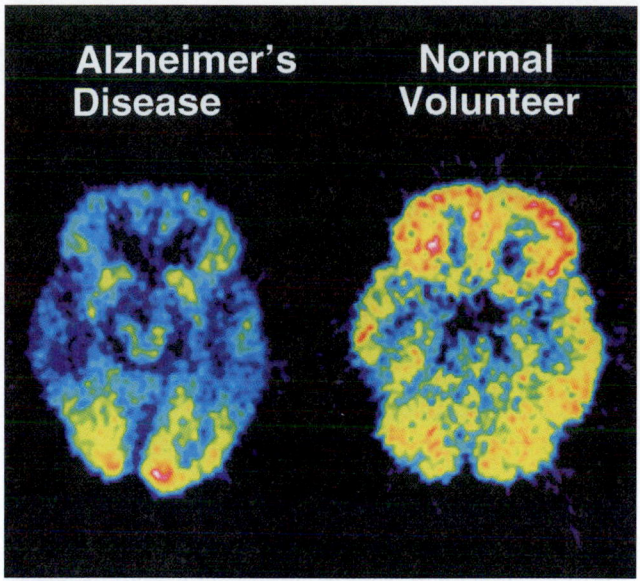

Figure 20–5 ⊙ PET scan comparing the metabolic activity levels of a normal brain and the brain of an individual with Alzheimer's disease. Red and yellow colors indicate high activity levels; blue colors represent low activity levels.
(Monte S. Buchsbaum, M.D.)

CLINICAL ALERT

Determine if the facility requires a signed informed-consent form for the aspiration/biopsy procedure.

Lumbar Puncture

In a **lumbar puncture** (LP, or spinal tap), cerebrospinal fluid (CSF) is withdrawn through a needle inserted into the subarachnoid space of the spinal canal between the third and fourth lumbar vertebrae or between the fourth and fifth lumbar vertebrae. At this level the needle avoids damaging the spinal cord and major nerve roots (Figure 20–6). The client

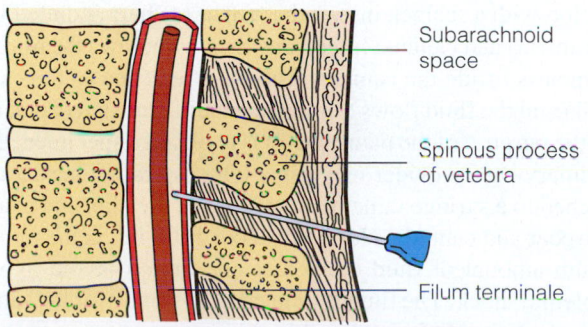

Figure 20–6 ⊙ A diagram of the vertebral column, indicating a site for insertion of the lumbar puncture needle into the subarachnoid space of the spinal canal.

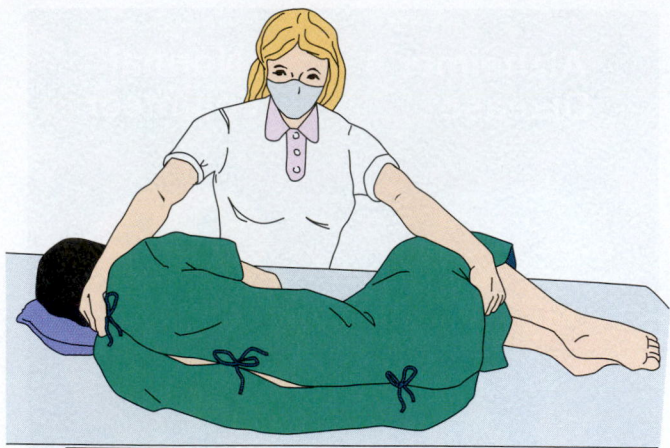

Figure 20–7 ◯ Supporting the client for a lumbar puncture.

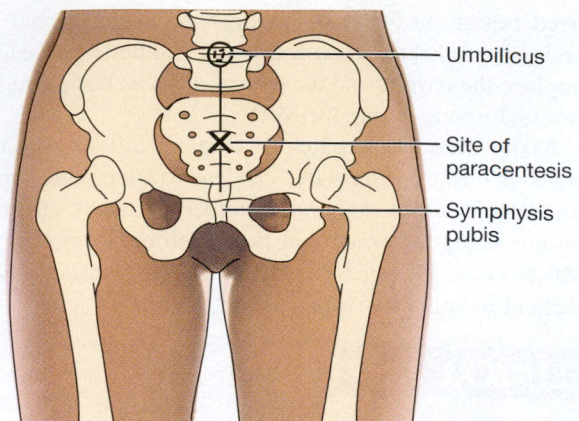

Umbilicus

Site of paracentesis

Symphysis pubis

Figure 20–8 ◯ A common site for an abdominal paracentesis.

is positioned laterally with the head bent toward the chest, the knees flexed onto the abdomen, and the back at the edge of the bed or examining table (Figure 20–7). In this position the back is arched, increasing the spaces between the vertebrae so that the spinal needle can be inserted readily. During a lumbar puncture, the primary care provider frequently takes CSF pressure readings using a **manometer**, a glass or plastic tube calibrated in millimeters. The nurse's role is to monitor the client and assist with the procedure.

Abdominal Paracentesis

Normally the body creates just enough peritoneal fluid for lubrication. The fluid is continuously formed and absorbed into the lymphatic system. However, in some disease processes, a large amount of fluid accumulates in the abdominal cavity; this condition is called **ascites**. Normal ascitic fluid is serous, clear, and light yellow in color. An abdominal **paracentesis** is carried out to obtain a fluid specimen for laboratory study and to relieve pressure on the abdominal organs due to the presence of excess fluid.

A primary care provider performs the procedure with the assistance of a nurse. Strict sterile technique is followed. A common site for abdominal paracentesis is midway between the umbilicus and the symphysis pubis on the midline (Figure 20–8). The primary care provider makes a small incision with a scalpel, inserts the **trocar** (a sharp, pointed instrument) and cannula (tube), and then withdraws the trocar, which is inside the cannula. Tubing is attached to the cannula and the fluid flows through the tubing into a receptacle. If the purpose of the paracentesis is to obtain a specimen, the primary care provider may use a long aspirating needle attached to a syringe rather than making an incision and using a trocar and cannula. Normally about 1500 mL is the maximum amount of fluid drained at one time to avoid hypovolemic shock. The fluid is drained very slowly for the same reason. Some fluid is placed in the specimen container before the cannula is withdrawn. The small incision may or may not be sutured; in either case, it is covered with a small sterile bandage.

Thoracentesis

Normally, only sufficient fluid to lubricate the pleura is present in the pleural cavity. However, excessive fluid can accumulate as a result of injury, infection, or other pathology. In such a case or in the case of pneumothorax, a primary care provider may perform a **thoracentesis** to remove the excess fluid or air to ease breathing. Thoracentesis is also performed to introduce chemotherapeutic drugs intrapleurally.

The nurse assists the client to assume a position that allows easy access to the intercostal spaces. This is usually a sitting position with the arms above the head, which spreads the ribs and enlarges the intercostal space. Two positions commonly used are one in which the arm is elevated and stretched forward and one in which the client leans forward over a pillow (Figure 20–9). To make sure that the needle is inserted below the fluid level when fluid is to be removed (or above any fluid if air is to be removed), the primary care provider will palpate and percuss the chest and select the exact site for insertion of the needle. A site on the lower posterior chest is often used to remove fluid, and a site on the upper anterior chest is used to remove air. A chest x-ray prior to the procedure will help pinpoint the best insertion site.

The primary care provider and the assisting nurse follow strict sterile technique. The primary care provider attaches a syringe and/or stopcock to the aspirating needle. The stopcock must be in the closed position so that no air

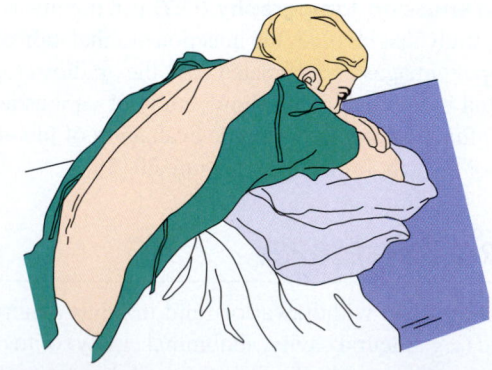

Figure 20–9 ◯ Preferred position for thoracentesis.

will enter the pleural space. The primary care provider inserts the needle through the intercostal space to the pleural cavity. In some instances, the primary care provider threads a small plastic tube through the needle and then withdraws the needle. (The tubing is less likely to puncture the pleura.)

If a syringe is used to collect the fluid, the plunger is pulled out to withdraw the pleural fluid as the stopcock is opened. If a large container is used to receive the fluid, the tubing is attached from the stopcock to the adapter on the receiving bottle. When the adapter and stopcock are opened, gravity allows fluid to drain from the pleural cavity into the container, which should be kept below the level of the client's lungs. After the fluid has been withdrawn, the primary care provider removes the needle or plastic tubing.

Bone Marrow Biopsy

Another type of diagnostic study is the *biopsy*. A biopsy is a procedure whereby tissue is obtained for examination. Biopsies are performed on many different types of tissues, for example, bone marrow, liver, breast, lymph nodes, and lung.

A bone marrow biopsy is the removal of a specimen of bone marrow for laboratory study. The biopsy is used to detect specific diseases of the blood, such as pernicious anemia and leukemia. The bones of the body commonly used for a bone marrow biopsy are the sternum, iliac crests, anterior or posterior iliac spines, and proximal tibia in children. The *posterior superior iliac crest* is the preferred site with the client placed prone or on the side.

After injecting a local anesthetic, a small incision may be made with a scalpel to avoid tearing the skin or pushing skin into the bone marrow with a needle. The primary care provider then introduces a bone marrow needle with stylet into the red marrow of the spongy bone (Figure 20–10).

<table>
<tr><td>

LIFESPAN CONSIDERATIONS
Bone Marrow Biopsy

Children
- Young clients need emotional support due to the pain and pressure associated with this procedure.
- Young clients may require gentle restraint to prevent movement during the procedure.

Older Adults
- Older adults with osteoporosis will experience less needle pressure.
- Ask the client to empty the bladder for comfort before the procedure.
- Provide pillows and blankets to help older adults remain comfortable during the procedure.

</td></tr>
</table>

Once the needle is in the marrow space, the stylet is removed and a 10-mL syringe is attached to the needle. The plunger is withdrawn until 1 to 2 mL of marrow has been obtained. The primary care provider replaces the stylet in the needle, withdraws the needle, and places the specimen in test tubes and/or on glass slides.

Liver Biopsy

A liver biopsy is a short procedure, generally performed at the client's bedside, in which a sample of liver tissue is aspirated. A primary care provider inserts a needle in the intercostal space between two of the right lower ribs and into the liver (Figure 20–11) or through the abdomen below the right rib cage (subcostally).

The client exhales and stops breathing while the primary care provider inserts the biopsy needle, injects a small

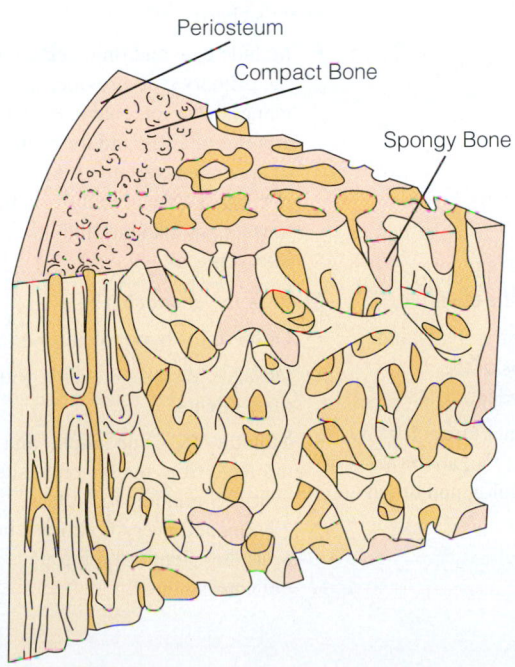

Figure 20–10 ⬤ A cross section of a bone.

Periosteum
Compact Bone
Spongy Bone

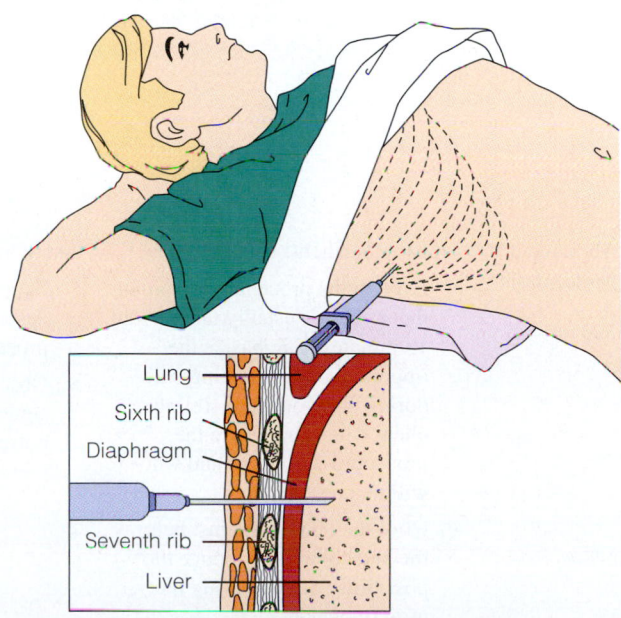

Figure 20–11 ⬤ A common site for a liver biopsy.

Lung
Sixth rib
Diaphragm
Seventh rib
Liver

amount of sterile normal saline to clear the needle of blood or particles of tissue picked up during insertion, and aspirates liver tissue by drawing back on the plunger of the syringe. After the needle is withdrawn, the nurse applies pressure to the site to prevent bleeding, often by positioning the client on the biopsy site.

Because many clients with liver disease have blood clotting defects and are prone to bleeding, prothrombin time and platelet count are normally taken well in advance of the test. If the test results are abnormal, the biopsy may be contraindicated.

Table 20–3 describes how the nurse assists with aspiration/biopsy procedures.

TABLE 20–3   Assisting with Aspiration and Biopsy

PROCEDURE	BEFORE THE PROCEDURE	DURING THE PROCEDURE	AFTER THE PROCEDURE
Lumbar puncture	Prepare the client: • Explain the procedure to the client and support persons. The primary care provider will be taking a small sample of spinal fluid from the lower spine. A local anesthetic will be given to minimize discomfort. Explain when and where the procedure will occur (e.g., the bedside or in a treatment room) and who will be present (e.g., the primary care provider and the nurse). Explain that it will be necessary to lie in a certain position without moving for about 15 minutes. A slight pinprick will be felt when the local anesthetic is injected and a sensation of pressure as the spinal needle is inserted. • Have the client empty the bladder and bowels prior to the procedure to prevent unnecessary discomfort. • Position and drape the client. • Open the lumbar puncture set.	Support and monitor the client throughout: • Stand in front of the client and support the back of the neck and knees if the client needs help remaining still. • Reassure the client throughout the procedure by explaining what is happening. Encourage normal breathing and relaxation. • Observe the client's color, respirations, and pulse during the procedure. Ask the client to report headache or persistent pain at the insertion site. Handle specimen tubes appropriately: • Wear gloves when handling test tubes. • Label the specimen tubes in sequence. • Send the CSF specimens to the lab immediately. Place a small sterile dressing over the puncture site.	Ensure the client's comfort and safety: • Assist the client to a dorsal recumbent position with only one head pillow. The client remains in this position for 1 to 12 hours, depending on the primary care provider orders. • Determine whether analgesics are ordered and can be given for headaches. • Offer oral fluids frequently, unless contraindicated, to help restore the volume of CSF. Monitor the client: • Observe for swelling or bleeding at the puncture site. • Monitor changes in neurologic status. • Determine whether the client is experiencing any numbness, tingling, or pain radiating down the legs. Document the procedure on the client's chart: • Include date and time performed; the primary care provider's name; the color, character, and amount of CSF; and the number of specimens obtained. Also document CSF pressure and the nurse's assessments and interventions.
Abdominal paracentesis	Prepare the client: • Explain the procedure: obtaining the specimen usually takes about 15 minutes. Emphasize the importance of remaining still during the procedure. Tell the client when and where the procedure will occur and who will be present. • Have the client void just before the paracentesis to reduce the possibility of puncturing the urinary bladder.	Assist and monitor the client: • Support the client verbally and describe the steps of the procedure as needed. • Observe the client closely for signs of distress (e.g., abnormal pulse rate, skin color, and blood pressure).	Monitor the client closely: • Observe for hypovolemic shock. • Observe for scrotal edema with male clients. • Monitor VS, urine output, and drainage from the puncture site every 15 minutes for at least 2 hours and every hour for 4 hours or as the client's condition indicates.

TABLE 20–3	Assisting with Aspiration and Biopsy *(continued)*		
PROCEDURE	**BEFORE THE PROCEDURE**	**DURING THE PROCEDURE**	**AFTER THE PROCEDURE**
Abdominal paracentesis *(continued)*	Prepare the client: • Help the client assume a sitting position in bed, in a chair, or on the edge of the bed supported by pillows. • Maintain the client's privacy and provide blankets for warmth.	Assist and monitor the client: • Observe for signs of hypovolemic shock induced by the loss of fluid: pallor, dyspnea, diaphoresis, drop in BP, and restlessness or increased anxiety. • Place a small sterile dressing over the site of the incision after the cannula or aspirating needle is withdrawn.	Monitor the client closely: • Measure the abdominal girth at the level of the umbilicus. Document all relevant information: • Include date and time performed; the primary care provider's name; abdominal girth before and after; the color, clarity, and amount of drained fluid; and the nurse's assessments and interventions. Transport the correctly labeled specimens to the laboratory.
Thoracentesis	Prepare the client: • Explain the procedure to the client. Normally, the client may experience some discomfort and a feeling of pressure when the needle is inserted. The procedure may bring considerable relief if breathing has been difficult. The procedure takes only a few minutes, depending primarily on the time it takes for the fluid to drain from the pleural cavity. To avoid puncturing the lungs, it is important for the client not to cough while the needle is inserted. Explain when and where the procedure will occur and who will be present. • Help position the client and cover the client as needed with a bath blanket.	Support and monitor the client throughout: • Support the client verbally and describe the steps of the procedure as needed. • Observe the client for signs of distress, such as dyspnea, pallor, and coughing. Collect drainage and laboratory specimens. Place a small sterile dressing over the site of the puncture.	Monitor the client: • Assess pulse rate and respiratory rate and skin color. • Don't remove more than 1,000 mL of fluid from the pleural cavity within the first 30 minutes. • Observe changes in the client's cough, sputum, respiratory depth, and breath sounds, and note complaints of chest pain. Position the client appropriately: • Some agency protocols recommend that the client lie on the unaffected side with the head of the bed elevated 30 degrees for at least 30 minutes because this position facilitates expansion of the affected lung and eases respirations. Document all relevant information: • Include date and time performed; the primary care provider's name; the amount, color, and clarity of fluid drained; and nursing assessments and interventions provided. Transport the specimens to the laboratory.
Bone marrow biopsy	Prepare the client: • Explain the procedure. The client may experience pain when the marrow is aspirated and hear a crunching sound as the needle is pushed through the cortex of the bone. The procedure usually takes 15 to 30 minutes. Explain when and where the procedure will occur, who will be present, and which site will be used.	Monitor and support the client throughout: • Describe the steps of the procedure as needed and provide verbal support. • Observe the client for pallor, diaphoresis, and faintness due to bleeding or pain.	Monitor the client: • Assess for discomfort and bleeding from the site. The client may experience some tenderness in the area. Bleeding and hematoma formation need to be assessed for several days. Report bleeding or pain to the nurse in charge.

(continued)

TABLE 20–3   **Assisting with Aspiration and Biopsy—continued**

PROCEDURE	BEFORE THE PROCEDURE	DURING THE PROCEDURE	AFTER THE PROCEDURE
Bone marrow biopsy *(continued)*	Prepare the client: • Help the client assume a supine position (with one pillow if desired) for a biopsy of the sternum (sternal puncture) or a prone position for a biopsy of either iliac crest. Fold the bedclothes back or drape the client to expose the area. • Administer a sedative as ordered.	Monitor and support the client throughout: Place a small dressing over the site of the puncture after the needle is withdrawn: • Some agency protocols recommend direct pressure over the site for 5 to 10 minutes to prevent bleeding. Assist with preparing specimens as needed.	Monitor the client: • Provide an analgesic as needed and ordered. Document all relevant information: • Include date and time of the procedure, the primary care provider's name; and any nursing assessments and interventions. Document any specimens obtained. Transport the specimens to the laboratory.
Liver biopsy	Prepare the client: • Give preprocedural medications as ordered. Vitamin K may be given for several days before the biopsy to reduce the risk of hemorrhage. • Explain the procedure and tell the client that the primary care provider will take a small sample of liver tissue by putting a needle into the client's side or abdomen. Explain that a sedative and local anesthetic will be given, so the client will feel no pain. Explain when and where the procedure will occur, who will be present, the time required, and what to expect as the procedure is being performed (e.g., the client may experience mild discomfort when the local anesthetic is injected and slight pressure when the biopsy needle is inserted). • Ensure that the client fasts for at least 2 hours before the procedure. • Administer the appropriate sedative about 30 minutes beforehand or at the specified time. • Help the client assume a supine position with the upper right quadrant of the abdomen exposed. Cover the client with the bedclothes so that only the abdominal area is exposed.	Monitor and support the client throughout: • Support the client in a supine position. • Instruct the client to take a few deep inhalations and exhalations and to hold the breath after the final exhalation for up to 10 seconds as the needle is inserted, the biopsy obtained, and the needle withdrawn. Holding the breath after exhalation immobilizes the chest wall and liver and keeps the diaphragm in its highest position, avoiding injury to the lung and laceration of the liver. • Instruct the client to resume breathing when the needle is withdrawn. • Apply pressure to the site of the puncture to help stop any bleeding. Apply a small dressing to the site of the puncture.	Position the client appropriately: • Assist the client to a right side-lying position with a small pillow or folded towel under the biopsy site. Instruct the client to remain in this position for several hours. Monitor the client: • Assess the client's VS every 15 minutes for the first hour following the test or until the signs are stable. Then monitor vital signs every hour for 24 hours or as needed. • Determine whether the client is experiencing abdominal pain. Severe abdominal pain may indicate bile peritonitis. • Check the biopsy site for localized bleeding. Pressure dressings may be required if bleeding does occur. Document all relevant information: • Include date and time performed; the primary care provider's name; and all nursing assessments and interventions. Transport the specimens to the laboratory.

LIFESPAN CONSIDERATIONS   General Considerations

Children

- Children may be frightened of even noninvasive procedures to collect specimens if they are not sure what is going to happen. Cooperation can be maximized by:
  - Demonstrating on dolls or teddy bears.
  - Allowing the child to examine and explore the collection materials being used.
  - Explaining in age-appropriate language what will be done.
  - Having parents actively involved in gently holding and comforting the child during and after the procedure.
  - Being well prepared to conduct the procedure.
  - Performing the procedure quickly, competently, and as gently as possible.

Older Adults

- In older adults, homeostatic mechanisms are not as efficient as in the younger person. When undergoing diagnostic tests that challenge these functions, care must be taken to accurately monitor functions and note any changes. Examples:
  - Dehydration and electrolyte imbalance can occur from laxative preps given before bowel diagnostic tests, such as a colonoscopy.
  - Fluid restrictions and NPO status for a length of time can lead to hypovolemia and electrolyte imbalances.
  - Many dye contrasts used for x-rays and scans can cause renal damage (especially in clients with diabetes).
  - Sedation used for certain procedures may require a longer recovery time for older clients.
  - Having several tests at a time or for several days compounds these potential problems and increases fatigue.

Interventions should focus on ensuring that the client is hydrated during and after these diagnostic tests, monitoring intake and output and vital signs frequently and accurately, and noting any mental status changes that might suggest electrolyte imbalance. Identification of clients at risk (persons with diabetes, kidney disease, or on certain medications) will help initiate measures to prevent injuries or complications from diagnostic tests.

CHAPTER HIGHLIGHTS

- Diagnostic testing involves three phases. Client preparation is the focus during the pretest phase. During the intratest phase, the nurse performs or assists with the diagnostic test and collects the specimen. Providing nursing care of the client and follow-up activities and observations are the role of the nurse during the posttest phase.
- Blood tests are one of the most commonly used diagnostic tests. Routinely ordered blood tests can include complete blood count (CBC) and serum electrolytes.
- A capillary blood glucose is a frequent test performed by nurses and clients. This test is used to monitor glucose levels of clients at risk for hyper- and hypoglycemia. It also evaluates the effectiveness of insulin administration.
- Nursing responsibilities associated with specimen collection include (a) providing client comfort, privacy, and safety; (b) explaining the purpose of and procedure for the specimen collection; (c) using correct procedure for obtaining the specimen; (d) noting relevant information on the laboratory requisition slip; (e) transporting the specimen promptly; and (f) reporting abnormal findings.
- Clients may need assistance to obtain stool specimens for laboratory analysis. In many agencies, nurses test the stool for occult blood.
- Nurses collect urine specimens for a number of tests. A clean voided specimen is used for routine examination. A clean-catch or midstream voided specimen is collected when a urine culture is ordered to identify microorganisms. Timed urine specimens are collected for a variety of tests, depending on the client's health problem. Nurses can complete some simple urine tests (e.g., specific gravity, pH, ketones, protein) at the bedside.
- Sputum and throat culture specimens help determine the presence of disease-producing organisms.
- Visualization procedures include indirect visualization (noninvasive) and direct visualization (invasive) techniques for visualizing body organs and system functions. Examples of invasive procedures include colonoscopy, barium enema, intravenous pyelography, and angiography. Noninvasive procedures include lung scan, echocardiogram, electrocardiography, x-ray, CT, and MRI.
- Examples of aspiration/biopsy tests include lumbar puncture, abdominal paracentesis, thoracentesis, bone marrow biopsy, and liver biopsy. These tests are invasive procedures and require strict sterile technique. After the procedure, the nurse assesses the client for possible complications and provides appropriate nursing interventions as needed.

THINK ABOUT IT

Refer to the chapter-opening scenario and answer these questions.

1. Mr. Kohler wants more information about the necessity for these tests to be performed. What would you tell him?

2. How would you prepare Mr. Kohler for the bronchoscopy and biopsy to be performed?

3. Prior to sending Mr. Kohler to the radiology department for his MRIs, what information would you assess?

∞ *See suggested responses to Think About It on MyNursingKit.*

TEST YOUR KNOWLEDGE

1. The nurse would call the primary care provider immediately for which of the following lab results?
1. Hgb = 16 g/dL for male client
2. Hct = 22% for female client
3. WBC = 9×10^3/mL^3
4. Platelets = 300×10^3/mL^3

2. Mr. Jones, 78, needs to complete a 24-hour urine specimen. In planning his care, which of the following is the highest priority nursing intervention?
1. At the beginning of the test, instruct him to empty his bladder and save this voiding to start the collection.
2. Use a sterile receptacle to collect the urine.
3. Place a sign stating "Save All Urine" in the bathroom.
4. Keep the urine specimen in the refrigerator.

3. The client has a urinary health problem of unknown origin. Which of the following indirect visualization tests would the nurse anticipate to be ordered?
1. IVP
2. KUB
3. Retrograde pyelography
4. Cystoscopy

4. When reviewing the client's radiographic results the nurse recognizes which of the following provides information regarding the physiology of an organ?
1. X-ray
2. Computerized tomography (CT)
3. Magnetic resonance imagery (MRI)
4. Nuclear scan

5. When assisting with a bone marrow biopsy, the nurse should take which of the following actions?
1. Assist the client to a right side-lying position after the procedure.
2. Observe for signs of dyspnea, pallor, and coughing.
3. Assess for bleeding and hematoma formation for several days after the procedure.
4. Stand in front of the client and support the back of the neck and knees.

6. During an assessment, the nurse learns that the client has a history of liver disease. Which of the following diagnostic tests might be indicated for this client? Select all that apply.
1. Alanine aminotransferase (ALT)
2. Myoglobin

3. Cholesterol
4. Ammonia
5. BNP

7. The nurse practitioner requests a laboratory blood test to determine how well a client has controlled her diabetes over the past three months. Which blood test will provide this information?
1. Fasting blood glucose
2. Capillary blood glucose
3. Glycosylated hemoglobin
4. Glucose tolerance test

8. A fecal occult blood test of a stool sample is ordered by the provider. The nurse is going to use the Hemoccult test. Which of the following indicates that the nurse is using the correct procedure? Select all that apply.
1. Mixes the reagent with the stool sample before applying to the card
2. Collects a sample from two different areas of the stool specimen
3. Assesses for a blue color change
4. Asks a colleague to verify the pink color results
5. Asks the client if he has taken vitamin C in the past few days

9. A primary care provider is preparing to perform a thoracentesis. The nurse's role will include which of the following?
1. Place the client supine in the Trendelenburg position.
2. Position the client in a seated position with elbows on the overbed table.
3. Instruct the unlicensed assistive personnel (UAP) to measure vital signs.
4. Administer narcotic analgesic.

10. The nurse needs to collect a sputum specimen to identify the presence of TB. Which of the following is indicated for this type of specimen? Select all that apply.
1. Collect the specimen in the evening.
2. Send the collected specimen to the lab immediately.
3. Ask the client to spit into the sputum container.
4. Offer mouth care before and after collection of the sputum specimen.
5. Collect a specimen for 3 consecutive days.

∞ *See answers to Test Your Knowledge in Appendix A.*

EXPLORE PEARSON **mynursingkit**™

MyNursingKit is your one stop for online chapter review materials and resources. Prepare for success with additional NCLEX®-style practice questions, interactive assignments and activities, web links, animations and videos, and more!

Register your access code from the front of your book at
www.mynursingkit.com.

REFERENCES AND SELECTED BIBLIOGRAPHY

Ahmed, D. S. (2000). Hidden factors in occult blood testing. *American Journal of Nursing, 100*(12), 25.

American Diabetes Association. (2000, January). Resource guide 2000: Urine testing. *Diabetes Forecast Supplement,* 66–67.

Anonymous. (2004). Blood glucose monitors and data management systems. *Diabetes Forecast, 57*(1), RG39–RG58.

Anonymous. (2004). Deciphering diagnostics: Every picture tells a story. *Nursing Made Incredibly Easy, 2*(6), 56–57.

Armstrong, M. L., & Elkins, L. (2005). Body art and MRI. *American Journal of Nursing, 105*(3), 65–66.

Ball, J. W., & Bindler, R. C. (2006). *Child health nursing.* Upper Saddle River, NJ: Prentice Hall Health.

Bindler, R. C., Ball, J. W., London, M. L., & Ladewig, P. W. (2007). *Clinical skills manual for maternal & child nursing care.* (2nd ed.). Upper Saddle River, NJ: Pearson Prentice Hall.

Corbett, J. V. (2008). *Laboratory tests and diagnostic procedures with nursing diagnoses* (7th ed.). Upper Saddle River, NJ: Pearson Prentice Hall.

Davis, K. (2004). Need urine from a catheter system? Forget the needle! *Nursing, 34*(12), 64.

DiNella, J. V. (2005). The ins and outs of pulmonary function testing. *Nursing, 35*(12), 70–71.

Fain, J. A. (2004). Blood glucose meters: Different strokes for different folks. *Nursing, 34*(11), 48–51.

Fischbach, F. T. (2004). *A manual of laboratory & diagnostic tests* (7th ed.). Philadelphia: Lippincott.

George, E. L., & Panos, A. (2005). Does a high WBC count signal infection? *Nursing, 35*(1), 20–21.

Karch, A. M. (2004). Don't get burnt by the MRI. *American Journal of Nursing, 104*(8), 31.

Kim, J. (2005). What does a B-type natriuretic peptide test show? *Nursing, 35*(1), 26.

Li, C. Z. (2004). Viewing the small intestine via capsule endoscopy. *Nursing, 34*(4), 70–71.

Mensing, C. (2004). Helping patients choose the right blood glucose meter. *Nurse Practitioner, 29*(5), 43–45.

NANDA International. (2009). *NANDA nursing diagnosis: Definitions and classification 2009–2010.* West Sussex, U. K.: Wiley-Blackwell.

Passanza, C. (2001). Diabetes update: Monitor options *RN, 64*(6), 36–42.

Penharlow, C., & Spader, C. (2005). Liver function tests: Pieces of a complex diagnostic puzzle. *NurseWeek-MountainWest, 6*(3), 13–15.

Pullen, R. L. (2005). Tips for safe, accurate occult blood testing. *Nursing, 35*(3), 28.

Rushing, J. (2006). Assisting with bone marrow aspiration and biopsy. *Nursing, 36*(3), 68.

Salimbene, S. (2000). *What language does your patient hurt in? A practical guide to culturally competent patient care.* Rockford, IL: EMC Paradigm.

Shatzer, M., & Saul, L. (2004). What does BNP tell you? *Nursing Made Incredibly Easy, 2*(3), 7.

Society of Permanent Cosmetic Professionals. (2005). *MRI facts.* Retrieved June 15, 2006, from http://www.spcp.org/MRIinfo.htm

Spector, R. E. (2008). *Cultural diversity in health and illness* (7th ed.). Upper Saddle River, NJ: Pearson Prentice Hall.

U.S. Food and Drug Administration. (n.d.). *Glucose meters & diabetes management.* Retrieved June 15, 2006, from http://www.fda.gov/diabetes/glucose.html

Van Leeuwen, A. M., Kranpitz, T. R., & Smith, L. (2006). *Laboratory and diagnostic tests with nursing implications* (2nd ed.). Philadelphia: Davis.

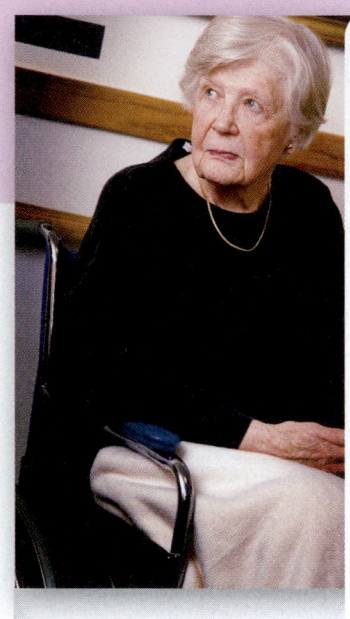

Bertha Pachekowski was a healthy, active 89-year-old widow. She played pinochle with a group every week, square-danced every Friday at the local senior citizen center, and enjoyed meeting her daughters for lunch on Saturday and walking through the mall afterward. Mrs. Pachekowski had lived alone since the death of her husband 11 years ago and was very independent, joking that she could even repair minor household problems.

She recently visited her provider's office because she was experiencing chest pain. She was taking medication for mild hypertension but was on no other medications and did not have a history of heart disease. After a thorough examination, her provider ordered some diagnostic tests and discovered she had valvular insufficiency. She was admitted to the hospital for valve replacement and was told she'd be home soon. From the operating room she was admitted to the coronary care unit for closer observation. She was receiving morphine sulfate for pain as needed.

At 3 AM she began displaying signs of confusion. At 5 AM the nurse responded to the cardiac monitor alarm and found Mrs. Pachekowski on the floor crying, with blood oozing from the incision site. Her leads had pulled out, and she said her buttocks hurt where she fell. After x-rays and a thorough assessment, she was diagnosed with a fractured right hip. Her incision required 4 sutures to close, and she developed a wound infection. When she recovered sufficiently from the hip repair, she was transferred to a rehabilitation facility, where she developed pneumonia and died a few months later.

LEARNING OUTCOMES

After completing this chapter, you will be able to:

1. Summarize factors that could impact a person's safety and place them at risk for injury.

2. Formulate a plan of care using the nursing process that promotes client safety.

3. Explain how the National Patient Safety Goals guide nursing practice.

4. Classify potential hazards within specific phases of the lifespan and indicate client teaching and nursing strategies to reduce the risk to the client.

5. Describe the legal implications of using restraints.

6. Differentiate when use of a restraint cannot be avoided because no alternative strategy would maintain client safety, and indicate what type of restraint you would employ.

A fundamental concern of nurses in any setting, whether on duty or off, is prevention of accidents and injury, as well as assisting the injured. Motor vehicle crashes, falls, drowning, fire and burns, poisoning, inhalation and ingestion of foreign objects, and use of firearms are major causes of injury and death. Nurses need to be aware of what constitutes a safe environment. Injuries are often caused by human conduct and can be prevented.

FACTORS AFFECTING SAFETY

The ability of people to protect themselves from injury is affected by many factors. Nurses need to assess each of these factors when they plan care or teach clients to protect themselves.

Age and Development

Through knowledge and accurate assessment of the environment, people learn to protect themselves from many injuries. For the very young, learning about the environment is essential. Only through knowledge and experience do children learn what is potentially harmful. Older adults can have difficulty with movement and diminished sensory acuity that contributes to the likelihood of injury. Specific age-related potential hazards and preventive measures are discussed later in this chapter. The Lifespan Considerations box summarizes selected hazards for each age group.

Lifestyle

Lifestyle factors that place people at risk include unsafe work environments; residence in neighborhoods with high crime rates; access to guns and ammunition; insufficient income to buy safety equipment or make necessary repairs; and access to illicit drugs, which may also be contaminated by harmful additives. Risk-taking behavior is a factor in some injuries.

Mobility and Health Status

People who have impaired mobility due to paralysis, muscle weakness, and poor balance or coordination are obviously prone to injury. Clients with spinal cord injury and

> **LIFESPAN CONSIDERATIONS**
> **Selected Hazards throughout the Lifespan**
>
> - *Developing fetus:* Exposure to maternal smoking, alcohol consumption, addictive drugs, x-rays (first trimester), certain pesticides
> - *Newborns and infants:* Falling, suffocation in crib, choking from aspirated milk or ingested objects, burns from hot water or other spilled hot liquids, automobile accidents, crib or playpen injuries, electric shock, poisoning
> - *Toddlers:* Physical trauma from falling, banging into objects, or getting cut by sharp objects; automobile crashes; burns; poisoning; drowning; and electric shock
> - *Preschoolers:* Injury from traffic, playground equipment, and other objects; choking, suffocation, and obstruction of airway or ear canal by foreign objects; poisoning; drowning; fire and burns; harm from other people or animals
> - *Adolescents:* Vehicular (automobile, bicycle) crashes, recreational accidents, firearms, substance abuse
> - *Older adults:* Falling, burns, and pedestrian and automobile crashes
>
> *Preventive measures are discussed later in this chapter.

paralysis of both legs may be unable to move even when they perceive discomfort. Hemiplegic clients or clients with leg casts often have poor balance and fall easily. Clients weakened by illness or surgery are not always fully aware of their condition.

Sensory-Perceptual Alterations

Accurate sensory perception of environmental stimuli is vital to safety. People with impaired touch perception, hearing, taste, smell, and vision are highly susceptible to injury.

Cognitive Awareness

Awareness is the ability to perceive environmental stimuli or body reactions and to respond appropriately through thought and action. Clients with impaired awareness include people lacking sleep; unconscious or semiconscious persons; disoriented people who may not understand where they are or what to do to help themselves; people who perceive stimuli that does not exist; and people whose judgment is altered by disease or medications, such as narcotics, tranquilizers, hypnotics, and sedatives. Mildly confused clients may momentarily forget where they are, wander from their rooms, misplace personal belongings, and risk potential injury.

Emotional State

Extreme emotional states can alter the ability to perceive environmental hazards. Stressful situations can reduce a person's level of concentration, cause errors of judgment, and decrease awareness of external stimuli. People with depression may think and react to environmental stimuli more slowly than usual. Those in a panic state may react without considering the consequences of their actions.

Ability to Communicate

Individuals with diminished ability to receive and convey information are at risk for injury because they cannot communicate their needs. This includes aphasic clients, people with language barriers, and those unable to read. For example, the person unable to interpret the sign "No smoking— oxygen in use" could cause a fire.

Safety Awareness

Information is crucial to safety. Clients in unfamiliar environments frequently need specific safety information. Lack of knowledge about unfamiliar equipment, such as medical equipment, pose a potential hazard. Healthy clients need information about water safety, car safety, fire prevention, ways to prevent the ingestion of harmful substances, and many preventive measures related to specific age-related hazards.

Environmental Factors

Depending on the client situation, the nurse may need to assess the environment of the home, workplace, or community. Client safety is affected by the health care setting. Bioterrorism has recently become a national safety concern.

HOME   A safe home requires well-maintained flooring and carpets, a nonskid bathtub or shower surface, functioning smoke alarms that are strategically placed, and knowledge of fire escape routes. Outdoor areas, such as swimming pools, need to be safely secured and maintained. Adequate lighting, both inside and out, will minimize the potential for injuries.

WORKPLACE   In the workplace, machinery, industrial belts and pulleys, and chemicals may create danger.

Worker fatigue, noise and air pollution, or working at great heights or in subterranean areas may also create occupational hazards. The work environment of the nurse may also be unsafe. Health care workers need to maintain an awareness of the potential risks of their work environment.

COMMUNITY   Adequate street lighting, safe water and sewage treatment, and regulation of sanitation in food buying and handling all contribute to a healthy, hazard-free community. A safe and secure community strives to be free of excess noise, crime, traffic congestion, dilapidated housing, or unprotected creeks and landfills.

HEALTH CARE SETTING   The 2000 Institute of Medicine (IOM) report *To Err Is Human: Building a Safer Health System* estimated that 44,000 to 98,000 people die in the United States each year due to medical errors in hospitals. This means that more people die in a given year as a result of medical errors than from motor vehicle crashes, breast cancer, or AIDS (Kohn, Corrigan, & Donaldson, 2000, p. 1). Client safety problems can include a variety of errors such as medication errors, wrong-site surgery, restraint-related injuries or death, falls, burns, pressure ulcers, or mistaken identity (p. 35). The IOM report defines *safety* as "freedom from accidental injury" (p. 58) and *error* as the "failure of a planned action to be completed as intended or the use of a wrong plan to achieve an aim" (p. 54).

The IOM reviewed many studies that investigated adverse events. An adverse event includes an injury caused by medical management rather than the underlying disease or condition of the client. It noted that over 50% of the adverse events were preventable. The committee who put together the report emphasized that while some of the errors were due to incompetent or impaired providers, the majority of the errors could have been avoided had better systems of care been in place (p. 30). Leonard, Frankel, Simmonds, and Vega (2004) echoed this belief by stating that an ever-increasing body of evidence indicates that at least 80% of medical error is system derived—meaning that system flaws set good people up to fail (p. 5). These same authors state that when people perform complex tasks, errors will occur.

The hospital environment is quite complex. Leonard et al. (2004) identified the following factors that increase the risk of human error:

- *Limited short-term memory.* Nurses have rapidly changing information coming at them continuously in busy hospital environments. Systems that rely on human memory are prone to failure.
- *Being late or in a hurry.* People start cutting corners when they are late or in a hurry. This may get the work done quicker; however, it also contributes to

the possibility of missing an important detail or piece of information that could cause client harm.

- *Limited ability to multitask.* People perform better at a single task.
- *Interruptions.* Many interruptions occur in complex environments such as a hospital. It is more difficult to get back on task or to remember what you were thinking with frequent interruptions.
- *Stress.* Stress causes anxiety, and anxiety affects performance. Also, stress affects a person's thinking by filtering information (e.g., only hearing the information you want to hear or missing all of the information), which subsequently affects problem-solving ability.
- *Fatigue and other physiological factors.* Studies show that fatigue affects a person's ability to process complex information.
- *Environmental factors.* Heat, noise, distractions, visual stimuli, and lighting can affect performance and lead to mistakes. Workplace design is a part of keeping clients and staff safe (pp. 18–22).

Another IOM report, *Keeping Patients Safe—Transforming the Work Environment of Nurses* (2004), established a link between nurses' work environment and client safety. The report found that the usual work environment of nurses is characterized by many serious threats to client safety (p. 3). Examples in this report include inconsistent staffing levels, long work hours, work processes, and physical design of the workplace.

Bioterrorism

In the past, being prepared for a disaster pertained to natural events such as hurricanes and earthquakes. However, the United States has significantly increased its preparedness for terrorism attacks since the events of September 11, 2001, and subsequent episodes where letters containing anthrax spores were sent through the U.S. postal system. Terrorism can include chemical, biological, or nuclear weapons. **Bioterrorism** is an intentional attack using weapons of viruses, bacteria, and other germs (Weber, 2004, p. 417). Nurses are important members of the community's disaster-preparedness team. As a result, nurses must be prepared and able to respond appropriately to all types of disasters.

NURSING MANAGEMENT

ASSESSING

Assessing clients at risk for injuries and injury involves (a) noting pertinent indicators in the nursing history and phys-

ical examination, (b) using specifically developed risk assessment tools, and (c) evaluating the client's environment.

Nursing History and Physical Examination

The nursing history and physical examination can reveal considerable data about the client's safety practices and risks for injury. Data including age and developmental level; general health status; mobility status; presence or absence of physiologic or perceptual deficits such as olfactory, visual, tactile, taste, or other sensory impairments; altered thought processes or other impaired cognitive or emotional capabilities; substance abuse; any indications of abuse or neglect; and an accident and injury history. A safety history also needs to include the client's awareness of hazards, knowledge of safety precautions both at home and at work, and any perceived threats to safety (Figure 21–1).

RISK ASSESSMENT TOOLS Risk assessment tools are available to determine clients at risk both for specific kinds of injury, such as falls, or for the general safety of the home and health care setting. In general, these tools direct the nurse to appraise the factors affecting safety as previously discussed. The tools summarize specific data contained in the client's nursing history and physical examination.

National Patient Safety Goals

As a result of IOM's report *To Err Is Human*, the health care industry and national organizations (e.g., National Patient Safety Foundation) increased their awareness of the need to improve client safety. For example, the Joint Commission requires its accredited agencies to meet specific National Patient Safety Goals (NPSG). See Box 21–1 for the 2008 National Patient Safety Goals. National Patient Safety Goals have been designed based on type of facility, such as critical access hospitals, long-term care facilities, or home care agencies. It is important to remember that the focus of the NPSG is on systemwide solutions. This is an important change from the traditional method of finding out who made the error to analyzing the system to find out why the error was made.

Bioterrorism Attacks

Nurses are considered frontline health care providers. As a result, they need education and training to be able to assess and detect potential bioterrorism attacks. The Centers for Disease Control and Prevention (CDC, 2001) defined three categories of biological pathogens that can be used for bioterrorism. The agents of highest concern are anthrax, botulism, plague, viral hemorrhagic fevers, smallpox, and

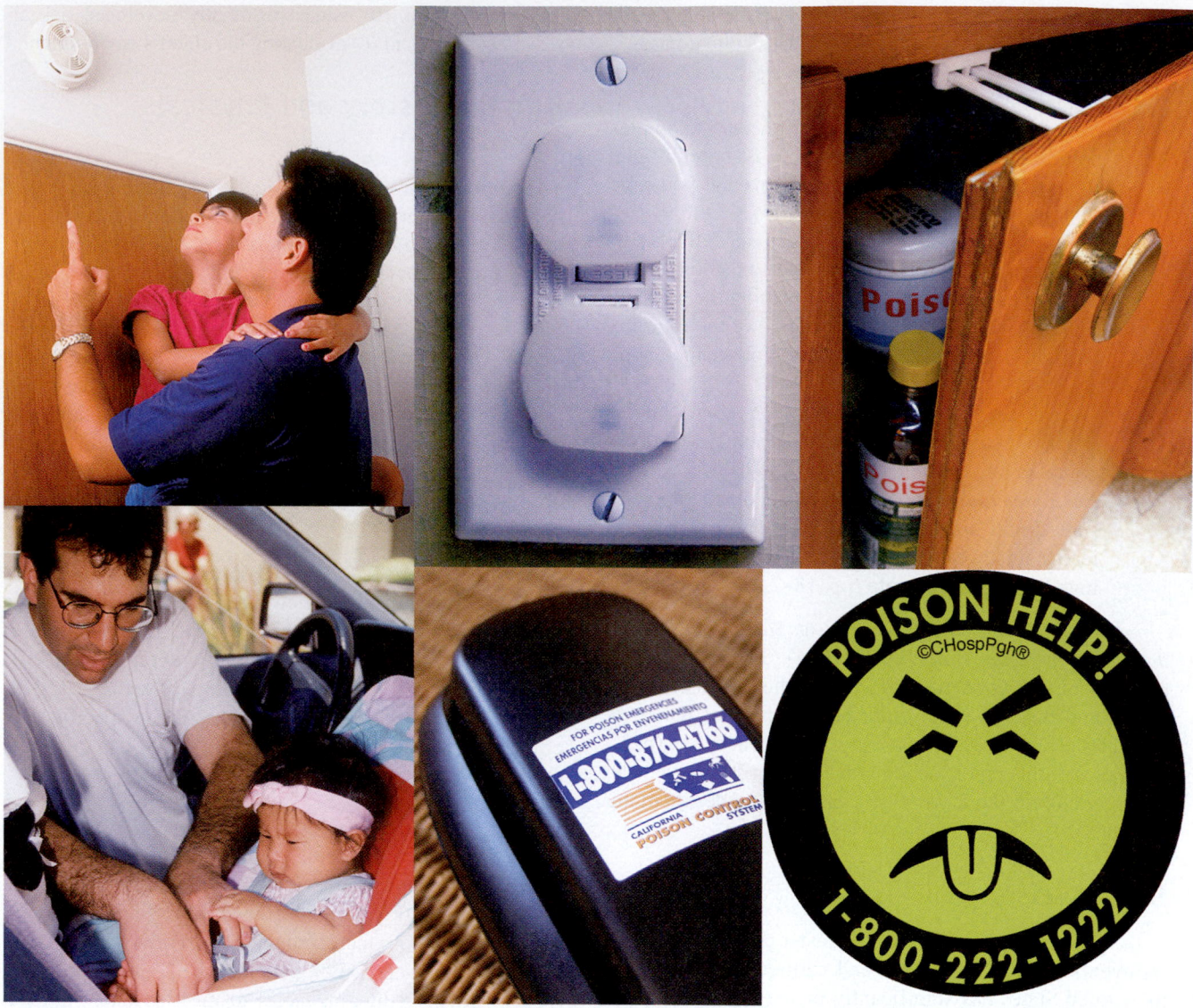

Figure 21–1 ○ Nurses need to teach clients about safety and how to prevent injuries such as using smoke detectors, safety covers for electrical outlets, childproof locks on drawers and cabinets, Mr. Yuk stickers on toxic substances, infant car seats, and by placing poison control information near or on the telephone.

(Top: Courtesy of Tony Freeman/PhotoEdit; Jerry Marshall; Michael Newman/PhotoEdit; Bottom: Grantpix/Photo Researchers Inc.; Geri Engberg; Children's Hospital Pittsburgh)

tularemia. See Table 21–1 for additional information on these agents.

Health care workers need to sustain a heightened awareness and alertness of circumstances or patterns that may indicate potential bioterrorism. The CDC (2001) and Massey (2004) have provided the following examples of when it is important to become suspicious:

- Is there an unusual geographic clustering of illness?
- Is the emergency department receiving an increase of clients with similar symptoms?

- Is the ICU caring for an unusual number of older adult clients with pneumonia?
- Is there an unusual age distribution for common diseases?

The health problems that nurses and other health care workers are seeing and caring for in one facility may only be one part of the big picture. Calling the local public health department and reporting observations and suspicions may reveal a larger pattern. Early detection and management is needed to help stop a bioterrorism attack.

BOX 21–1	Joint Commission 2008 National Patient Safety Goals

Improve the accuracy of patient identification.

- Use at least two patient identifiers (neither to be the patient's room number) whenever administering medications or blood products, taking blood samples and other specimens for clinical testing, or providing any other treatments or procedures.
- Eliminate transfusion errors related to patient misidentification.
- Prior to the start of any invasive procedure, conduct a final verification process to confirm the correct patient, procedure, site, and availability of appropriate documents. This verification process uses active—not passive—communication techniques.

Improve the effectiveness of communication among caregivers.

- For verbal or telephone orders or for telephone reporting of critical test results, the individual giving the order or test result verifies the complete order or test result by having the person receiving the information record and "read back" the complete order or test result.
- Standardize a list of abbreviations, acronyms, and symbols that are not to be used throughout the organization.
- Measure, assess, and, if appropriate, take action to improve the timeliness of reporting, and the timeliness of receipt by the responsible licensed caregiver of critical test results and values.
- All values defined as critical by the laboratory are reported to a responsible licensed caregiver within time frames established by the laboratory (defined in cooperation with nursing and medical staff). When the patient's responsible licensed caregiver is not available within the time frames, there is a mechanism to report the critical information to an alternative responsible caregiver.
- Implement a standardized approach to "hand off" communications, including an opportunity to ask and respond to questions.

Improve the safety of using medications.

- Standardize and limit the number of drug concentrations available in the organization.
- Identify and, at a minimum, annually review a list of look-alike/sound-alike drugs used in the organization, and take action to prevent errors involving the interchange of these drugs.
- Label all medications, medication containers (e.g., syringes, medicine cups, basins), or other solutions on and off the sterile field in perioperative and other procedural settings.
- Reduce the likelihood of patient harm associated with the use of anticoagulant therapy by implementing a defined anticoagulation management program to individualize the care provided to each patient receiving anticoagulant therapy; use only oral unit dose products, pre-filled syringes, or pre-mixed infusion bags when these products are available; use approved protocols to initiate and maintain anticoagulant therapy with a baseline INR for any client started on warfarin; notify dietary services of patients receiving warfarin to eliminate food interactions; use programmable pumps to deliver IV heparin, develop a written policy addressing baseline and ongoing lab tests required; and provide education to prescribers, staff, patients and families about the anticoagulation therapy.

Reduce the risk of health care–associated infections.

- Comply with current Centers for Disease Control and Prevention (CDC) hand hygiene guidelines.
- Manage as sentinel events all identified cases of unanticipated death or major permanent loss of function associated with a health care–associated infection.
- Implement evidence-based practices to prevent health care–associated infections due to multidrug-resistant organisms.
- Implement best practices or evidence-based guidelines to prevent central line-associated bloodstream infections and surgical site infections.

Accurately and completely reconcile medications across the continuum of care.

- Implement a process for obtaining and documenting a complete list of the patient's current medications upon the patient's admission to the organization and with the involvement of the patient. This process includes a comparison of the medications the organization provides to those on the list.
- A complete list of the patient's medications is communicated to the next provider of service when it refers or transfers a patient to another setting, service, practitioner, or level of care within or outside the organization.

Reduce the risk of patient harm resulting from falls.

- Implement a fall reduction program and evaluate the effectiveness of the program.

Improve recognition and response to change in a patient's condition

- Health care staff members will directly request additional assistance from a specially trained individual when the patient's condition appears to be worsening.

The organization meets the expectations of the Universal protocol

- Identify the proper client, correct site, and correct procedure is performed on patients at the time the procedure is scheduled, at preadmission testing and assessment, upon admission to the facility, before the patient leaves the preprocedure area or enters the procedure room, and anytime responsibility for the client's care is passed to another provider while the patient is awake and aware.
- Mark the procedure site.
- A time-out is performed immediately prior to starting procedures so all members of the health care team can address the following: correct patient and procedure site, signed consent form is accurate, agreement on the procedure to be performed, correct patient position, relevant images and results are properly labeled and appropriately displayed, need to administer antibiotics or fluids for irrigation, and safety precautions based on patient history or medication use.

© The Joint Commission, 2009: *Accreditation Program: Critical Access Hospital National Patient Safety Goals.* Accessed December 19, 2008, from http://www.jointcommission.org/NR/rdonlyres/4BAD7889-79DE-493F-A6FD-CEB9F003434D/0/CAH_NPSG.pdf Reprinted with permission.

TABLE 21-1 Biological Pathogens of Highest Concern for Bioterrorism Attacks

Anthrax	Cause	Spore-forming bacterium—*Bacillus anthracis*
	Transmission	• Not known to spread from one person to another • Cutaneous/skin: direct skin contact with spores (most common) • Respiratory: inhalation of aerosolized spores (rare) • GI: consumption of undercooked or raw meat products or dairy products from infected animals (rare)
	Symptoms of cutaneous anthrax	• Localized itching followed by a lesion that turns vesicular and subsequent development of black eschar (scab) within 7 to 10 days of initial lesion • Fever, flulike symptoms, nonproductive cough, sore throat
Botulism	Cause	By a toxin made by a bacterium called *Clostridium botulinum*
	Transmission	• Not spread from one person to another • Foodborne—person ingests preformed toxin • Infant—occurs in small number of infants who harbor *C. botulinum* in their intestinal tract • Wound—occurs when wounds are infected with *C. botulinum*
	Symptoms of foodborne botulism	Between 12 and 36 hours after eating toxin-containing food: double and blurred vision, slurred speech, difficulty swallowing, muscle weakness that always descends through the body
Viral Hemorrhagic Fevers (VHF)	Cause	• Virus. Ebola and yellow fever are two examples. • Viruses of most VHFs reside in an animal reservoir host or arthropod host (e.g., rodents are hosts and ticks and mosquitoes can be vectors). However, the hosts of some VHF (e.g., Ebola and Marburg) are unknown.
	Transmission	Humans are not natural reservoirs for VHFs. People are infected when they come in contact with infected hosts. However, with some VHFs, after the accidental transmission from the host, humans can transmit the virus to one another.
	Symptoms	After an incubation period of 5 to 10 days: abrupt onset of fever, myalgia, headache, nausea and vomiting, abdominal pain, diarrhea, chest pain. A rash on the trunk develops approximately 5 days after onset. Bleeding (e.g., petechiae, bruises, and hemorrhages) occur as disease progresses.
Smallpox	Cause	Variola virus
	Transmission	Droplet nuclei expelled from the mouth of an infected person or by aerosol. Contaminated clothing or bed linen could also spread the disease. Humans are the only natural host of variola.
	Symptoms	• Incubation period can range from 7 to 17 days where the person has no symptoms and is not contagious. • Initial symptoms include high fever, head and body aches, and possibly vomiting. These symptoms last 2 to 4 days and the person may be contagious. • A rash then appears—first on the tongue and in the mouth. These red spots develop into sores that break open and spread large amounts of the virus into the mouth and throat. The person is highly contagious at this point. • The rash then spreads to the entire body. By the third day of the rash, the rash becomes raised bumps which fill with thick, opaque fluid and have a depression in the center. The bumps become pustules which begin to form a crust and then scab. • The scabs fall off leaving pitted scars. The person is contagious until all the scabs have fallen off.

DIAGNOSING

NANDA offers a broad diagnostic label related to safety issues:

• *Risk for Injury:* A state in which the individual is at risk for injury as a result of environmental conditions interacting with the individual's adaptive and defense resources.

This broad label consists of seven subcategories that may be preferred when the nurse wants to describe injury more specifically or isolate suitable interventions (Wilkinson, 2009):

• *Risk for Poisoning:* Accentuated risk of accidental exposure to, or ingestion of, drugs or dangerous products in doses sufficient to cause poisoning
• *Risk for Suffocation:* Accentuated risk of accidental suffocation (inadequate air available for inhalation)
• *Risk for Trauma:* Accentuated risk of accidental tissue injury (e.g., wound, burn, or fracture)

- *Latex Allergy Response:* A hypersensitive reaction to natural latex rubber products
- *Risk for Latex Allergy Response:* Risk of hypersensitivity to natural latex rubber products
- *Contamination:* Exposure to environmental contaminants in doses sufficient to cause adverse health effects
- *Risk for Contamination:* Accentuated risk of exposure to environmental contaminants in doses sufficient to cause adverse health effects
- *Risk for Aspiration:* At risk for the entry of gastrointestinal secretions, oropharyngeal secretions, solids, or fluids into tracheobronchial passages

- *Risk for Disuse Syndrome:* At risk for deterioration of body systems as the result of prescribed or unavoidable musculoskeletal inactivity

Another diagnosis the nurse may choose to use is

- *Deficient Knowledge (Injury Prevention):* Inability to state or explain information or demonstrate a required skill related to safety of self and others

See Identifying Nursing Diagnoses, Outcomes, and Interventions for examples of applying the nursing process for clients at risk for injury.

IDENTIFYING NURSING DIAGNOSES, OUTCOMES, AND INTERVENTIONS   **Client Injury**

DATA CLUSTER Mrs. H. has adopted a toddler. Home assessment reveals many cleaning supplies at floor level, and paint peeling off the walls.

NURSING DIAGNOSIS/DEFINITION	SAMPLE DESIRED OUTCOMES*/DEFINITION	INDICATORS	SELECTED INTERVENTIONS*/DEFINITION	SAMPLE NIC ACTIVITIES
Risk for Poisoning related to dangerous products within reach of a child/ *Accentuated risk of accidental exposure to, or ingestion of, drugs or dangerous products in doses sufficient to cause poisoning*	Safe Home Physical Environment[1910]/ *Physical arrangements to minimize environmental factors that might cause physical harm or injury in the home*	Totally adequate • Placement of appropriate hazard warning labels • Storage of hazardous materials to prevent injury • Correction of lead hazard risks • Provision of safe play area	Environmental Management: Safety[6486]/ *Monitoring and manipulation of the physical environment to promote safety*	• Identify safety hazards • Remove hazards from the environment, when possible • Initiate and/or conduct screening programs for environmental hazards (e.g., lead) • Educate about environmental hazards • Provide emergency phone numbers (e.g., poison control center)

DATA CLUSTER Mr. P. suffered a stroke resulting in left-sided weakness. As a result, his gait is unsteady. The nurse noticed that his home has several throw rugs and much furniture impeding his mobility. The bathroom does not have grab bars by the toilet or shower.

NURSING DIAGNOSIS/DEFINITION	SAMPLE DESIRED OUTCOMES*/DEFINITION	INDICATORS	SELECTED INTERVENTIONS*/DEFINITION	SAMPLE NIC ACTIVITIES
Risk for Injury related to impaired mobility and potential home hazards/ *At risk of injury as a result of environmental conditions interacting with the individual's adaptive and defense resources*	Safe Home Environment[1910]/ *Physical arrangements to minimize environmental factors that might cause physical harm or injury in the home*	Totally adequate • Placement of handrails in bathroom • Arrangement of furniture to reduce risks	Environmental Management: Safety[6486]/*Monitoring and manipulation of the physical environment to promote safety*	• Identify safety needs of client • Identify safety hazards • Modify the environment to minimize hazards and risks • Provide adaptive devices (e.g., handrails) to increase safety of the environment • Monitor the environment for changes in safety status • Educate about environmental hazards

*The NOC # for desired outcomes and the NIC # for nursing interventions are listed in brackets following the appropriate outcome or intervention. Outcomes, indicators, interventions, and activities selected are only a sample of those suggested by NOC and NIC and should be further individualized for each client.

PLANNING

When planning care to prevent accidents and injury, the nurse considers all factors affecting the client's safety, specifies desired outcomes, and selects nursing activities to meet these outcomes. The major goal for clients with safety risks is to prevent accidents and injury. To meet this goal, clients often need to change their health behavior and may need to modify the environment.

Desired outcomes associated with preventing injury depend on the individual client. Examples of desired outcomes, although established in the planning phase, are provided in the "Evaluating" section on page 596.

Nursing interventions to meet desired outcomes are largely directed toward helping the client and family to accomplish the following:

- Identify environmental hazards in the home and community.

- Demonstrate safety practices appropriate to the home health care agency, community, and workplace.
- Experience a decrease in the frequency or severity of injury.
- Demonstrate safe child-rearing practices or lifestyle practices.

IMPLEMENTING

Hazards to safety occur at all ages and vary according to the age and development level of the individual.

Promoting Safety across the Life Span

Measures to ensure the safety of people of all ages focus on (a) observation or prediction of potentially harmful situations so that harm can be avoided and (b) client education that empowers clients to protect themselves and their families from injury. Safety measures covering the life span from infancy to older adults are listed in the accompanying Client Teaching.

CLIENT TEACHING   **Safety Measures throughout the Life Span**

Newborns and Infants

- Use a federally approved car seat at all times (including coming home from hospital). It should be in the back seat, facing backward.
- Never leave the infant unattended on a raised surface.
- Check the temperature of the infant's bath water and formula prior to using.
- Hold the infant upright during feeding. Do not prop the bottle. Cut food in small pieces, and do not feed the infant peanuts or popcorn.
- Investigate the infant's crib for compliance with federal safety regulations: slats no more than 2 3/8 inches apart, lead-free paint, height of crib sides, tight fit of mattress to crib.
- Use a playpen with sides made of small-size netting. Never leave playpen sides down.
- Provide large soft toys with no small detachable or sharp-edged parts.
- Use guard gates on stairs and screens on windows. Supervise the infant in swings and highchairs.
- Cover electric outlets. Coil cords out of reach.
- Place plants, household cleaners, and wastebaskets out of reach. Lock away potential poisons, such as medicines, paint, and gasoline.

Toddlers

- Continue to use federally approved car seats at all times. Place children in back seat when traveling in a car.
- Teach children not to put objects in the mouth, including pills (unless given by parent).
- Keep objects with sharp edges out of children's reach.
- Place hot pots on back burners with handles turned inward.
- Keep cleaning solutions, insecticides, and medicines in locked cupboards.
- Keep windows and balconies screened.

- Supervise toddlers in the tub.
- Fence in pools, and supervise toddlers at all times when in or near pools. Do not overfill bathtub. Do not let toddlers play near ditches or wells.
- Teach children not to run or ride a tricycle into the street.
- Obtain a low bed when the child begins to climb.
- Cover outlets with safety covers or plugs.

Preschoolers

- Do not allow children to run with candy or other objects in the mouth.
- Teach children not to put small objects in the mouth, nose, and ears.
- Remove doors from unused equipment such as refrigerators or safes.
- Always supervise preschoolers crossing streets and begin safety teaching about obeying traffic signals and looking both ways.
- Check Halloween treats before allowing children to eat them. Discard loose or open candy.
- Teach children to play in "safe" areas, not on streets and railroad tracks.
- Teach preschoolers the dangers of playing with matches and playing near charcoal, fire, and heating appliances.
- Teach children to avoid strangers and keep parents informed of their whereabouts.
- Teach preschoolers not to walk in front of swings and not to push others off playground equipment.

School-Age Children

- Teach children safety rules for recreational and sports activities: never swim alone, always wear a life jacket when in a boat, and wear a protective helmet and knee and elbow pads when needed.

- Supervise contact sports and activities in which children aim at a target.
- Teach children to obey all traffic and safety rules for bicycling, skateboarding, and roller skating.
- Teach children to use light or reflective clothing when walking or cycling at night.
- Teach children safe ways to use the stove, garden tools, and other equipment.
- Supervise children when they use saws, electric appliances, tools, and other potentially dangerous equipment.
- Teach children not to play with fireworks, gunpowder, or firearms. Keep firearms unloaded, locked up, and out of reach.
- Teach children to avoid excavations, quarries, vacant buildings, and playing around heavy machinery.
- Teach children the health hazards of smoking. If you smoke, stop.
- Teach children the effects of drugs and alcohol on judgment and coordination.

Adolescents

- Have adolescents complete a drivers' education course, and take practice drives with them in various kinds of weather.
- Set firm limits on automobile use, namely, never to drive after drinking or using drugs, and never to ride with a driver who has done so. Encourage adolescents to call home for a ride if they have been drinking, assuring them they can do so without a reprimand.
- Restrict number of passengers in car during the first year of driving.
- Teach adolescents to wear a safety helmet when riding motorcycles, scooters, and other sports vehicles. Teach safety rules for water sports.
- Encourage adolescents to use proper equipment when participating in sports. Schedule a physical examination before participation, and be certain there is medical supervision for all athletic activities.
- Encourage adolescents to swim, jog, and go boating in groups so they can obtain help in case of an accident.
- Teach safety measures for use of power tools.
- Teach rules for hunting and the proper care and use of firearms.
- Inform the adolescent of the dangers of drugs, alcohol, and unprotected sex. Include teaching about date rape prevention and defense.
- Teach dangers of sunbathing and tanning beds, as well as use of sun block and protective clothing when doing outdoor activities.
- Be alert to changes in the adolescent's mood and behavior. Listen to and maintain open communication with the adolescent. Open communication is a powerful preventive measure.
- Set a good example of behavior that the adolescent can follow.

Young Adults

- Reinforce motor vehicle safety: Drive defensively, use "designated drivers" if alcohol is consumed, routinely check brakes and tires, and use seat and shoulder belts or car seats for all passengers.
- Remind the young adult to repair potential fire hazards, such as electric wiring.
- Reinforce water safety: Know the depth of a pool or lake before diving; supervise backyard pools and other water activities.

- Discuss evaluating the potential for workplace injuries or death when making decisions about a career or occupation. Encourage the young adult to participate actively in programs that reduce occupational hazards.
- Discuss avoiding excessive sun radiation by limiting exposure, using sun-blocking agents, and wearing protective clothing. Explain the skin changes that may indicate a cancerous condition.
- Encourage young adults who are unable to cope with the pressures, responsibilities, and expectations of adulthood to seek counseling.

Middle-Aged Adults

- Reinforce motor vehicle safety: Use seat belts and drive within the speed limit, especially at night. Test visual acuity periodically.
- Make certain stairways are well lighted and uncluttered.
- Equip bathrooms with hand grasps and nonskid bath mats.
- Test smoke detectors and fire alarms regularly.
- Keep all machines and tools in good working condition at work and at home. Follow safety precautions when using machinery.
- Reinforce safety measures taught earlier in life, such as the hazards of excessive sun exposure.

Older Adults

- Encourage the client to have regular vision and hearing tests.
- Assist the client to have a home hazard appraisal.
- Encourage the client to keep as active as possible.

Preventive Measures

- Ensure eyeglasses are functional.
- Ensure appropriate lighting.
- Mark doorways and edges of steps as needed.
- Keep environment tidy and uncluttered.
- Set safe limits to activities.
- Remove unsafe objects.
- Wear shoes or well-fitted slippers with nonskid soles.
- Use ambulatory devices as necessary (cane, crutches, walker, braces, wheelchair).
- Provide assistance with ambulation as needed.
- Monitor gait and balance.
- Adapt living arrangements to one floor if necessary.
- Encourage exercise and activity as tolerated to maintain muscle strength, joint flexibility, and balance.
- Ensure uncluttered environment with securely fastened rugs.
- Encourage client to request assistance.
- Keep bed in the low position.
- Install grab bars in bathroom.
- Provide raised toilet seat.
- Instruct client to rise slowly from a lying to sitting to standing position, and to stand in place for several seconds before walking.
- Provide a bedside commode as needed.
- Assist with voiding on a frequent and scheduled basis.
- Encourage client to summon help.
- Monitor activity tolerance.
- Attach side rails to the bed.
- Keep rails in place when the bed is in the lowest position.
- Monitor orientation and alertness status.
- Encourage annual or more frequent review of all medications prescribed.

NEWBORNS AND INFANTS Injuries are a leading cause of death during infancy, especially during the first year of life. Infants are completely dependent on others for care; they are oblivious to such dangers as falling or ingesting harmful substances. Parents need to learn the amount of observation necessary to maintain infant safety. They also need help to identify and remove common hazards in and around the home, and first-aid information that includes cardiopulmonary resuscitation and interventions for airway obstruction. Common injuries during infancy include burns, suffocation or choking, motor vehicle crashes, falls, and poisoning. Education and support of parents can make them more knowledgeable and better prepared to protect their children from injuries.

TODDLERS Toddlers are curious and like to feel and taste everything. They are fascinated by potential dangers, such as pools and busy streets, so they need constant supervision and protection (Figure 21–2). Parents prevent many injuries by "toddler-proofing" the home or other setting where the child will be. This practice extends to the use of federally approved car restraints and removing or securing all items that can pose a safety hazard to the child in any setting. It may be necessary to inspect for and remove sources of lead from the environment. Lead poisoning (plumbism) is a risk for children exposed to lead paint chips, fumes from leaded gasoline, or any "leaded" substances. The ingestion of lead-based paint chips is the most common cause of lead poisoning in children.

CLINICAL ALERT

The remodeling and renovation of older homes (e.g., those built before 1978) accounts for most of the lead poisoning seen today. Nurses need to educate families living in older homes about their children's risk for lead poisoning and provide lead poisoning prevention advice.

PRESCHOOLERS Children of preschool age are active and often very clumsy, making them susceptible to injury. Control of the environment must continue, keeping hazards such as matches, medicines, and other potential poisons out of reach. Safety education for the child must begin now. Education of the preschooler involves learning how to cross streets, what traffic signals mean, and how to ride bicycles and other wheeled toys safely. Children must be cautioned to avoid hazards, such as busy streets, swimming pools, and other potentially dangerous areas. Parents must maintain careful surveillance; the developmental level of the preschooler does not allow for self-reliance in matters of safety. Parents must also keep in mind that their child's cognitive and motor skills increase quickly; hence, safety measures must keep up with the acquisition of new skills.

SCHOOL-AGE CHILDREN By the time children attend school, they are learning to think before they act. They often prefer adult equipment to toys. They want to play with other children in such activities as bicycling, hiking, swimming, and

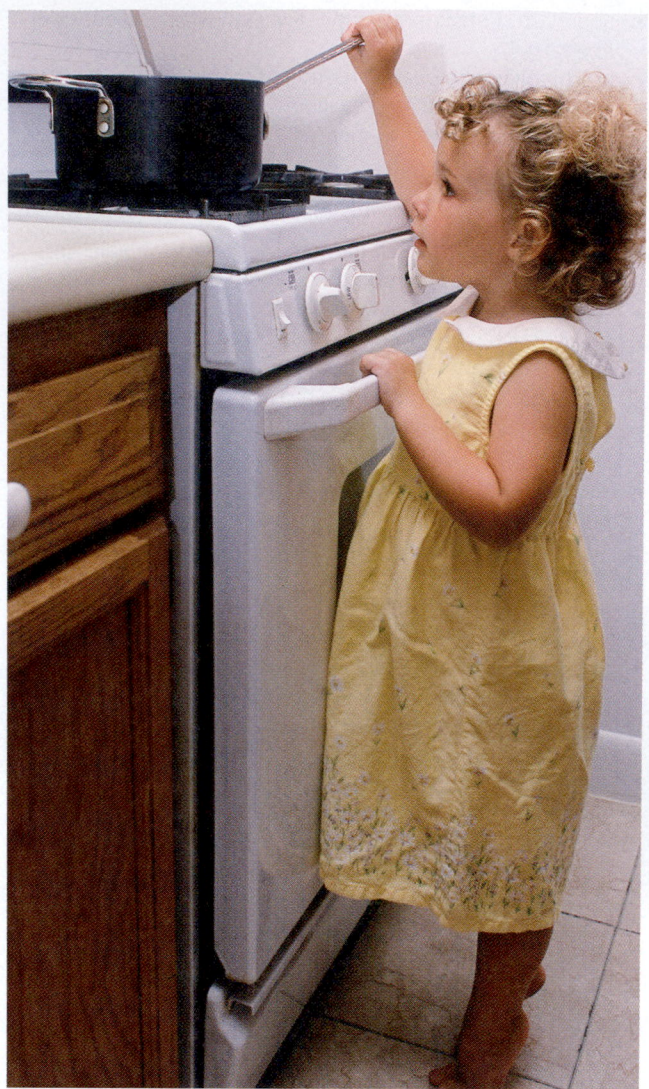

Figure 21–2 ● Promoting safety (e.g., by placing hot pots on back burners with handles turned inward) is required to keep children from injury.

boating. Although sensitive to peer pressure, the school-age child will respond to rules. Children of this age engage in fantasy and magical thinking. They often imitate actions of parents and superheroes with whom they identify.

Injuries are the leading cause of death in school-age children. The most frequent causes of fatalities, in descending order, are motor vehicle crashes, drownings, fires, and firearms. School-age children are also involved in many minor injuries, frequently resulting from outdoor activities and recreational equipment such as swings, bicycles, skateboards, and swimming pools.

ADOLESCENTS Obtaining a driver's license is an important event in the life of an adolescent in the United States, but the privilege is not always wisely handled. Teenagers may use driving as an outlet for stress, as a way to assert independence, or as a way to impress peers. When setting limits on automobile use, parents need to assess the teenager's level of responsibility, common sense, and ability to resist peer pressure. The age of the teenager alone does not determine readiness to handle this responsibility.

Adolescents are at risk for sports injuries because their coordination skills are not fully developed. However, sports activities are important to the adolescent's self-esteem and overall development. In addition to providing beneficial exercise, sports activities enhance social and personal development. They help the adolescent experience competition, teamwork, and conflict resolution.

Suicide and homicide are two leading causes of death among teenagers. Adolescent males commit suicide at a higher rate than adolescent females, and African Americans commit homicide at a higher rate than European Americans. Suicides by firearms, drugs, and automobile exhaust gases are the most common. Factors influencing the high suicide and homicide rates include economic deprivation, family breakup, and the availability of firearms, which are the most frequently used weapons. Cutting or stabbing tools are the next most frequently used weapons.

YOUNG ADULTS Motor vehicle crashes are by far the leading cause of mortality for this group; other causes of death for young adults include drowning, fires, burns, and firearms.

One safety hazard for many young adults is exposure to natural radiation from sunbathing or outdoor activities. Exposure to the sun is directly related to skin cancer. Suicide is another leading cause of death in young adults. Many suicides may actually be mistaken for unintentional death (automobile crashes, alcohol intoxication, and drug overdose). In general, suicide results from the young adult's inability to cope with the pressures, responsibilities, and expectations of adulthood.

The nurse's role in the prevention of suicide includes identifying behaviors that may indicate potential problems: depression; a variety of physical complaints including weight loss, sleep disturbances, and digestive disorders; and decreased interest in social and work roles along with an increase in isolation. A young adult identified as at risk for suicide should be referred to a mental health professional or a crisis center. Nurses can also reduce the incidence of suicide by participating in educational programs that provide information about the early signs of suicide.

MIDDLE-AGED ADULTS Changing physiologic factors, as well as concern over personal and work-related responsibilities, may contribute to the injury rate of middle-aged persons. Motor vehicle crashes are the most common cause of accidental death in this age group. Decreased reaction times and visual acuity may make the middle-aged adult prone to injuries. Other unintentional causes of death for middle-aged adults include falls, fires, burns, poisonings, and drownings. Occupational injuries continue to be a significant safety hazard during the middle years.

OLDER ADULTS Injury prevention is a major concern for older adults. Because vision is limited, reflexes are slowed, and bones are brittle, climbing stairs, driving a car, and even walking require caution. Driving, particularly night driving, requires caution because accommodation of the eye to light is impaired and peripheral vision is diminished. Older adults need to learn to turn their head before changing lanes and should not rely on side vision, for example, when crossing a street or changing lanes. Driving in fog or other hazardous conditions should be avoided.

Fires are a hazard for the older adult with a failing memory. The older person may forget that the iron or stove has been left on or may not extinguish a cigarette completely. Because of reduced sensitivity to pain and heat, care must be taken to prevent burns when the person bathes or uses heating devices.

Older adults at risk for wandering due to organic brain syndromes need to wear identification devices. They can also be registered with the local Alzheimer's Association's Wanderer's Alert Program.

Because older adults who take analgesics or sedatives may become lethargic or confused, they should be monitored regularly and closely. Other measures to induce sleep should be used whenever possible. Nurses can help older adult clients make the home environment safer by identifying and correcting specific hazards; for example, handrails can be installed on staircases. The nurse teaches the importance of taking prescribed medications as directed and contacting a health professional at the first indication of medication intolerance.

CLINICAL ALERT

Older adults have trouble seeing the edges of stairs. Painting white stripes on the edges of the steps will help increase contrast and may prevent falls.

The incidence of suicide in older adults is increasing and often goes unnoticed when the causes are due to hidden self-destructive behaviors, such as starvation, overdosing with medications, and noncompliance with medical care, treatments, and medications. In older individuals, the suicide attempt is usually more serious, because it is truly intended to end the life, not just to get attention as is often seen in other age groups. Also, the method of suicide is generally more violent in older adults, such as a gunshot wound to the head, or hanging.

Ebersole, Hess, Touhy, and Jett (2009) have listed important facts regarding suicide of the older adult: (a) White men are the most likely to commit suicide; (b) uncontrollable pain, loss of a loved one, and major life changes can be contributing factors; (c) major depression and social isolation increase the risk of suicide; and (d) older adults rarely threaten to commit suicide; they just do it.

Nurses need to be aware of the symptoms and risk factors of suicide. They should direct the client to the appropriate professional or agency for treatment and counseling.

VIOLENCE HAZARDS ACROSS THE LIFE SPAN Domestic violence is increasing at an alarming rate and involving individuals of all ages. It includes child abuse, intimate partner abuse, and elder abuse and affects the health and safety of families and the community. Statistics are inaccurate due to the underreporting of incidents. Nurses should be involved in working with all phases of domestic violence: prevention, screening, referrals for treatment, and follow-up care. This usually necessitates collaborative planning with primary care providers, law enforcement agencies, social services, and other community agencies. Nurses also have the opportunity to become advocates for community support programs for the prevention of domestic violence and can become involved in educating other professionals regarding prevention, screening, and treatment.

Domestic violence takes on extra importance because it is known that people who were abused as children often display abusive behavior as an adult. This points to the need for prevention and early intervention to prevent the cycle from continuing. Nurses can be of assistance in restoring dignity, health, and safety to vulnerable individuals.

Promoting Safety in the Health Care Setting

As stated previously, the IOM report *To Err Is Human* provided proof that errors in the health care industry are at an unacceptably high level (p. 69). Recent health care literature (Kohn et al., 2000; Leonard et al., 2004; Page, 2004) suggests that new systems to improve client safety are needed. Examples include:

- Establishing a National Center for Patient Safety to provide leadership for safety improvements and expand the knowledge base for improving safety and preventing errors in health care (Kohn et al., 2000).
- Establishing a reporting system. This information would be used to design systems that are safer for clients. Literature discussions (Berntsen, 2004; Kohn et al., 2000) suggest both a mandatory reporting system for errors causing serious injury or death and a voluntary reporting system for errors that result in no harm, sometimes called "near misses" or "close calls."
- Promoting effective teamwork and communication. Health care practitioners are part of a team and client safety may be at risk if critical, relevant information is not communicated appropriately. Successful nurse–primary care provider communication is critical. See Chapter 13 ∞.
- Creating a culture of trust. There is a need to change the culture in health care from placing blame to examining how to improve. Trust needs to be developed and sustained for people to feel open to discuss and share experiences about their safety near misses and/or errors.
- Involving health care workers in the design of work processes and work spaces to promote efficiency and safety of the staff who will work here.

Preventing Specific Hazards

Implementing measures to prevent specific hazards or injuries such as burns, fires, falls, poisoning, suffocation, electrocution, and so on are critical aspects of nursing care. Teaching clients about safety is another important aspect. Nurses usually have opportunities to teach while providing care.

SCALDS AND BURNS A scald is a burn from a hot liquid or vapor, such as steam. A burn results from excessive exposure to thermal, chemical, electric, or radioactive agents.

Common home hazards causing scalds include the following:

- Pot handles that protrude over the edge of a stove
- Electric appliances used to heat liquids or oils, especially those with dangling cords that are within reach of crawling infants and young children
- Excessively hot bath water

In health care agencies, the risk of scalds and burns is greater for clients whose skin sensitivity to temperature is impaired. Scalds can occur from overly hot bath water, and burns can occur from therapeutic applications of heat (see Chapter 24 ∞). It is important for the nurse to assess how well clients can protect themselves and what special precautions, if any, need to be taken.

FIRES Fires continue to be a constant risk in both health care settings and homes. Agency fires usually result from malfunctioning electric equipment or combustion of anesthetic gas. Home fires most frequently result from careless disposal of burning cigarettes or matches, from grease, or from faulty electric wiring.

Agency Fires In health care agencies, fire is particularly hazardous when people are incapacitated and unable to leave the building without assistance. This incapacity makes it extremely important for nurses to be aware of the fire safety regulations and fire prevention practices of the agency in which they work. When a fire occurs the nurse follows four sequential priorities:

1. Protect and evacuate clients who are in immediate danger.
2. Report the fire.
3. Contain the fire.
4. Extinguish the fire.

Extinguishing the fire requires knowledge of three categories of fire, classified according to the type of material that is burning:

Class A: Paper, wood, upholstery, rags, ordinary rubbish
Class B: Flammable liquids and gases
Class C: Electrical

The right type of extinguisher must be used to fight the fire. Extinguishers have picture symbols showing the type of fire for which they are to be used. Directions for use are also attached.

Home Fires Nursing interventions for home fires focus on teaching fire safety. Preventive measures include the following:

- Keep emergency numbers near the telephone, or stored for speed dialing.

- Be sure the smoke alarms are operable and appropriately located.
- Teach clients to change the batteries in their smoke alarms annually on a special day such as a birthday or January 1.
- Have a family "fire drill" plan. Every member needs to know the plan for the nearest exit from different locations of the home.
- Keep fire extinguishers available and in working order.
- Close windows and doors if possible; cover the mouth and nose with a damp cloth when exiting through a smoke-filled area; and avoid heavy smoke by assuming a bent position with the head as close to the floor as possible.

FALLS People of any age can fall, but infants and older adults are particularly prone to falling and causing serious injury. Falls are the leading cause of injuries among older adults. They are also a major cause of hospital and nursing home admissions. Most falls occur in the home and are a major threat to the independence of older adults. Fear of falling is common in older adults, even in those who have not experienced a fall. This fear is of particular concern for those who live alone and who anticipate being helpless and unable to summon help after a fall. For these individuals the nurse should encourage daily or more frequent contact with a friend or family member, installation of a personal emergency response system, and measures to maintain a physical environment that prevents falls. Risk factors and associated preventive measures are shown in Table 21–2.

CLINICAL ALERT

Falls can break bones and self-confidence, leading to fear of falling causing a decreased activity level and decreased muscle strength. All increase the risk of falling.

TABLE 21–2   **Risk Factors and Preventive Measures for Falls**

RISK FACTOR	PREVENTIVE MEASURES
Poor vision	Ensure eyeglasses are functional.
	Ensure appropriate lighting.
	Mark doorways and edges of steps as needed.
	Keep the environment tidy.
Cognitive dysfunction (confusion, disorientation, impaired memory, or judgment)	Set safe limits to activities.
	Remove unsafe objects.
Impaired gait or balance and difficulty walking because of lower extremity dysfunction (e.g., arthritis)	Wear shoes or well-fitted slippers with nonskid soles.
	Use ambulatory devices as necessary (cane, crutches, walker, braces, wheelchair).
	Provide assistance with ambulation as needed.
	Monitor gait and balance.
	Adapt living arrangements to one floor if necessary.
	Encourage exercise and activity as tolerated to maintain muscle strength, joint flexibility, and balance.
	Ensure uncluttered environment with securely fastened rugs.
Difficulty getting in and out of chair or in and out of bed	Encourage client to request assistance.
	Keep the bed in the low position.
	Install grab bars in bathroom.
	Provide raised toilet seat.
Orthostatic hypotension	Instruct client to rise slowly from a lying to sitting to standing position, and to stand in place for several seconds before walking.
Urinary frequency or receiving diuretics	Provide a bedside commode.
	Assist with voiding on a frequent and scheduled basis.
Weakness from disease process or therapy	Encourage client to summon help.
	Monitor activity tolerance.
Current medication regimen that includes sedatives, hypnotics, tranquilizers, narcotic analgesics, diuretics	Attach side rails to the bed if appropriate.
	Keep the rails in place when the bed is in the lowest position.
	Monitor orientation and alertness status.
	Discuss how alcohol contributes to fall-related injuries.
	Encourage client not to mix alcohol and medications and to avoid alcohol when necessary.
	Encourage annual or more frequent review of all medications prescribed.

Weak leg muscles, weak knees, poor balance, and loss of flexibility contribute to falls in older adults. The nurse can use an assessment tool, called the "Get Up and Go" test, in a hospital, subacute, or home setting. Kimbell (2001) describes the following steps of the test:

1. Observe the client's posture while he sits in a straight-backed chair.
2. Ask the client to stand. Observe if the client stands using only his leg muscles or if he needs to push himself up with his hands.
3. Once the client is comfortable standing, ask him to close his eyes. Does he sway?
4. Ask him to open his eyes, walk 10 feet, turn around, and return to the chair. Observe his gait, balance, speed, and stability. How smoothly does he turn?
5. When he gets to the chair, ask him to turn and sit down. Observe how smoothly the client performs this motion.

This quick assessment along with an assessment of the client's environment can help the nurse recommend safety measures to the client and family.

Prevention of falls in health care agencies is an ongoing concern. Health care environments are designed with many safety features to reduce the risk of falls, such as railings along corridors; call bells at each bedside; safety bars in toilet areas; locks on beds, wheelchairs, and stretchers; side rails on beds; night-lights; and so on. In addition, nurses can implement measures to decrease the incidence of falls (see the Long-Term Care Considerations box).

CLINICAL ALERT

When a client falls, the nurse's first duty is to the client. First, assess for injuries. Then, notify the primary care provider.

Although it may seem that raising the side rails on a bed is an effective method of preventing falls, rails should not be

LONG-TERM CARE CONSIDERATIONS
Preventing Falls in Health Care Agencies

- On admission, orient clients to their surroundings and explain the call system.
- Carefully assess the client's ability to ambulate and transfer. Provide walking aids and assistance as required.
- Closely supervise the clients at risk for falls, especially at night.
- Encourage the client to use the call bell to request assistance. Ensure that the bell is within easy reach.
- Place bedside tables and overbed tables near the bed or chair so that clients do not overreach and consequently lose their balance.
- Always keep hospital beds in the low position and wheels locked when not providing care so that clients can move in or out of bed easily.
- Encourage clients to use grab bars mounted in toilet and bathing areas and railings along corridors.
- Make sure nonskid bath mats are available in tubs and showers.
- Encourage the client to wear nonskid footwear.
- Keep the environment tidy; especially keep light cords from underfoot and furniture out of the way.
- Use individualized interventions (e.g., alarm sensitive to client position) rather than side rails for confused clients.

raised routinely for this purpose. Research has shown that persons with memory impairment, altered mobility, nocturia, and other sleep disorders are prone to becoming entrapped in side rails and may, in fact, be more likely to fall trying to get out of bed by going around or over the raised rails (Marcy-Edwards, 2005).

Electronic devices are available to detect that clients are attempting to move or get out of bed. A bed or chair **safety monitoring device** has a position-sensitive switch that triggers an audio alarm when the client attempts to get out of the bed or chair. Skill 21–1 describes how to use these devices.

SKILL 21–1

USING A BED OR CHAIR EXIT SAFETY MONITORING DEVICE

PURPOSES
- To alert the nurse that the client is attempting to get out of bed
- To help decrease the risk of client falls

ASSESSMENT
Assess
- Mobility status
- Judgment about ability to get out of bed safely
- Proximity of client's room to nurses' station
- Position of side rails
- Functioning status of call light

PLANNING

Determine the appropriate location for the device. If the device will be applied to a thigh, ensure that the location has intact skin.

> ### Delegation
> Risk factors for falls may be observed and recorded by persons other than the nurse. The nurse is responsible for assessing the client and confirming that there is a risk of the client falling when getting out of a chair or bed unassisted. The nurse develops a plan of care that includes a variety of interventions that will protect the client. If indicated, use of a safety monitoring device may be delegated to unlicensed assistive personnel (UAP) who have been trained in their application and monitoring.

EQUIPMENT

- Alarm and control device
- Sensor
- Connection to nurse call system

IMPLEMENTATION

Performance

1. Prior to performing the procedure, introduce self and verify the client's identity using agency protocol. Explain to client and family the purpose and procedure of using a safety monitoring device. Explain that the device does not limit mobility in any manner; rather, it alerts the staff when the client is about to get out of bed. Explain that the nurse must be called when the client needs to get out of bed.
2. Perform hand hygiene and observe appropriate infection control procedures.
3. Provide for client privacy.
4. Test the battery device and alarm sound. **Rationale:** *Testing ensures that the device is functioning properly prior to use.*
5. Apply the sensor pad or leg band.
   - Place the leg band according to the manufacturer's recommendation. ❶ Place the client's leg in a straight horizontal position. **Rationale:** *The alarm device is position sensitive; that is, when it approaches a near-vertical position (such as in walking, crawling, or kneeling as the client attempts to get out of bed), the audio alarm will be triggered.*
   - For the bed or chair device, the sensor is usually placed under the buttocks area. ❷
   - For a bed or chair device, set the time delay for determining the client's movement patterns from 1 to 12 seconds.
   - Connect the sensor pad to the control unit and the nurse call system.
6. Instruct the client to call the nurse when the client wants or needs to get up, and assist as required.
   - When assisting the client up, deactivate the alarm.
   - Assist the client back to bed, and reattach the alarm device.
7. Ensure client safety with additional safety precautions.
   - Place call light within client reach, lift side rails per agency policy, and lower the bed to its lowest position. **Rationale:** *The alarm device is not a substitute for other precautionary measures.*
   - Place ambulation monitoring stickers on the client's door, chart, and other relevant locations.
8. Document the type of alarm used, where it was placed, and its effectiveness in the client record using forms or checklists

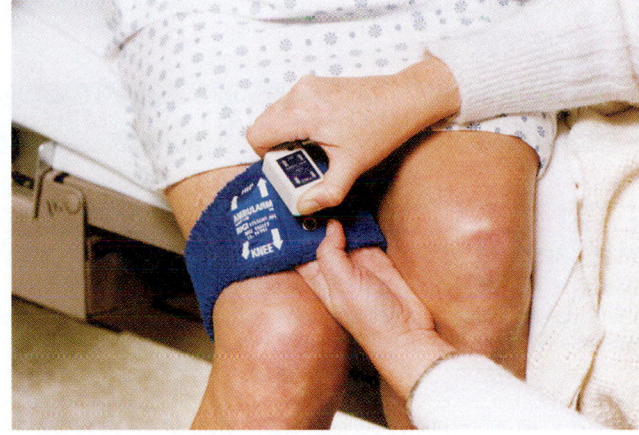

❶ Placing the leg band alarm.
(Courtesy of Alert Care, Mill Valley, CA.)

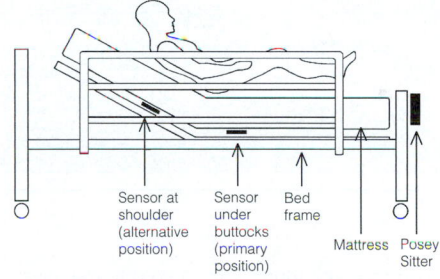

❷ Placement of a bed exit monitoring device.

supplemented by narrative notes when appropriate. Record all additional safety precautions and interventions discussed and employed.

SAMPLE DOCUMENTATION

1/12/2010 Found out of bed again despite frequent reminders given to use call light for assistance. Explained about using a leg band alarm to ensure own safety from possible fall. Verbalized agreement. Alarm device applied. Reminded again of importance to call the nurse for assistance. —————— T. Kyle, RN

EVALUATION

- If the alarm is too sensitive to client movement that is not an attempt to move from bed or chair, reassess and modify alarm controls accordingly.
- Conduct appropriate follow-up relating to effectiveness of safety precautions.
- Report any difficulties using the device or any falls to the primary care provider.

SEIZURES A seizure is a sudden onset of excessive electrical discharges in one or more areas of the brain. Seizures can develop at any time during a person's life and can occur at any time (Gambrell & Flynn, 2004). Clients may be prone to seizures due to permanent or temporary medical conditions such as drug reactions, epilepsy, or extreme fever. However, about 50% of seizures have no known cause (Cross, 2004).

Seizures are classified into two categories: partial and generalized. Partial seizures (also called focal) involve electrical discharges from one area of the brain. In contrast, generalized seizures affect the whole brain. Each of these seizure categories includes different types of seizure, depending on the characteristics of the seizure activity (e.g., loss of consciousness versus no impairment to consciousness). Thus, it is important for nurses to thoroughly describe their observations before, during, and after a client's seizure episode. Clients are at risk for injury if they experience seizures that involve the entire body such as *grand mal* (tonic-clonic) seizures or any seizure that includes loss of consciousness. **Seizure precautions** are safety measures taken by the nurse to protect clients from injury should they have a seizure. Skill 21–2 describes how to implement seizure precautions.

SKILL 21–2

IMPLEMENTING SEIZURE PRECAUTIONS

PURPOSE
• Protect the client from injury

ASSESSMENT
Assess history of seizures during the admission assessment. If the client has experienced a seizure previously, ask for detailed information, including characteristics of an aura or warning symptoms that indicate the seizure is beginning, duration and frequency of the seizures, consequences of the seizures (e.g., incontinence or difficulty breathing), and actions that should be taken to prevent or reduce seizure activity.

PLANNING
Review emergency procedures as a respiratory arrest or other injury can result from a seizure.

Delegation
UAP should be familiar with establishing and implementing seizure precautions and methods of obtaining assistance during a client's seizure. Care of the client during a seizure, however, is the responsibility of the nurse due to the importance of careful assessment of respiratory status and potential need for intervention.

EQUIPMENT
• Blankets or other linens to pad side rails
• Oral suction equipment and clean gloves
• Oxygen equipment

IMPLEMENTATION
Performance
1. Prior to performing the procedure, introduce self and verify the client's identity using agency protocol. Explain to the client what you are going to do, why it is necessary, and how he or she can participate.
2. Perform hand hygiene and observe appropriate infection control procedures. If the client is actively seizing, apply clean gloves in preparation for performing respiratory care measures.
3. Provide for client privacy.
4. Pad the bed of any client who might have a seizure. Secure blankets or other linens around the head, foot, and side rails of the bed. ❶
5. Put oral suction equipment in place and test to ensure that it is functional. **Rationale:** *Suctioning may be needed to prevent aspiration of oral secretions.*
6. If a seizure occurs:
   • Remain with the client and call for assistance. Do not restrain the client.
   • If the client is not in bed, assist client to the floor and protect the client's head by holding it in your lap or on a pillow. Loosen any clothing around the neck and chest.

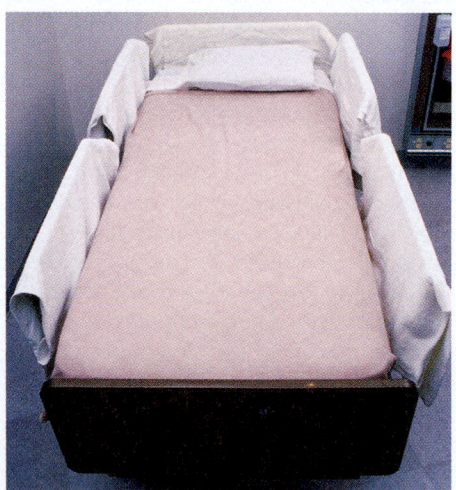

❶ Padding a bed for seizure precautions.

• Turn the client to a lateral position if possible. **Rationale:** *Turning to the side allows secretions to drain out of the mouth, decreasing the risk of aspiration, and helps keep the tongue from occluding the airway.*

- Move items in the environment to ensure the client does not experience an injury.
- Do not insert anything into the client's mouth.
- Time the seizure duration.
- Observe the progression of the seizure, noting the sequence and type of limb involvement. Observe skin color. When the seizure allows, check pulse and respirations.
- Apply oxygen via mask or nasal cannula.
- Use equipment to suction the oral airway if the client vomits or has excessive oral secretions.
- Administer anticonvulsant medications, as ordered.
- When the seizure has subsided, assist client to a comfortable position. Reorient. Explain what happened. Reassure the client. Provide hygiene as necessary. Allow the client to verbalize feelings about the seizure.

- If applied, remove and discard gloves. Perform hand hygiene.
7. Document the event in the client record using forms or checklists supplemented by narrative notes when appropriate.

SAMPLE DOCUMENTATION

1/8/2010 1815 Upon entering room, observed generalized muscle spasms/contractions of arms and legs lasting 25 seconds. Seizure padding previously placed on bed. Incontinent of urine. Cyanotic. Placed on left side. Suctioned. Airway clear. Respirations slightly irregular at 14/min. Oxygen applied at 4L/min via mask. Oxygen sat 90% on O2. Not currently responding to verbal stimuli. Dr. Smith notified. Diazepam 10 mg given IV per order. VS taken every 15 min. See neuro flow sheet. —————————————— B. Gill, RN

EVALUATION

- Perform a detailed follow-up examination of the client. Administer medications if indicated and ordered.

- Report significant deviations from normal to the primary care practitioner.

LIFESPAN CONSIDERATION
Implementing Seizure Precautions

Infants

- About 24% of children experience seizures, most during infancy (Ball & Bindler, 2008).

Children

- Febrile seizures occur more commonly than in adults and are usually preventable through antipyretics and tepid baths.
- Determine oxygenation. Apply oxygen if pulse oximetry reading is less than 95% (see Chapter 35 ∞).
- Children who have frequent seizures may need to wear helmets for protection.
- Children on anticonvulsant medications should wear a medical identification tag (bracelet or necklace).

POISONING Inadequate supervision and improper storage of many household toxic substances are the major reasons for poisoning in children. Implementing poison prevention for children is focused on teaching parents to "childproof" the environment, including disposing of unused medications safely. Flushing medications down a drain has led to increased levels of drugs in municipal water supplies so they are most safely disposed of in the trash, with care taken to prevent children from retrieving them once discarded. Adolescent and adult poisonings are usually caused by insect or snake bites and drugs used for recreation or in suicide attempts. Implementing poison prevention in these age groups focuses on providing information and counseling. Poisoning in older adults usually results from accidental ingestion of a toxic substance (e.g., due to failing eyesight) or an overdose of a prescribed medication (e.g., due to impaired memory). Implementing poison prevention with older adults focuses on safeguarding the environment and monitoring the underlying problems.

In older adults who have dementia, poisoning is often a safety problem. As cognitive abilities deteriorate, the same precautions need to be taken as with children. Older adults who have dementia have the need to feel everything and will put anything in their mouths, including plants, flowers, candles, small objects, and medications. These and other potentially dangerous items need to be locked up or kept out of reach. A telephone number for the nearest poison control center should be readily available. These precautions are important whether the individual with dementia is being cared for at home or in an institution.

In response to the ever-increasing number of poison hazards, many countries have established poison control centers that provide accurate, up-to-date information about potential hazards and recommend treatment as needed. For certain poisons, specific antidotes or treatments are available; for many, there is no specific therapy.

Nurses intervene in community settings by educating the public about what to do in the event of poisoning: Identify the specific poison by searching for an opened container, empty bottle, or other evidence. Contact the poison control center, indicate the exact quantity of poison the person ingested, and state the person's age and apparent symptoms. Keep the person as quiet as possible and lying on the side or sitting with head placed between the legs to prevent aspiration of vomitus. The Client Teaching feature provides additional guidelines for teaching clients to prevent poisoning.

Carbon Monoxide Poisoning Carbon monoxide (CO) is an odorless, colorless, tasteless gas that is very toxic. Exposure to CO can cause symptoms including headaches, dizziness, weakness, nausea, vomiting, or loss of muscle control. Prolonged exposure to CO can lead to unconsciousness, brain damage, or death. Learning the steps to prevent CO exposure is particularly important because all gasoline-powered vehicles, lawn mowers, kerosene stoves, barbecues, and burning wood emit CO. Incomplete or faulty combustion of any fuel, including natural gas used in

---

CLIENT TEACHING

Preventing Poisoning

- Lock potentially toxic agents, including drugs and cleaning agents, in a cupboard, or attach special plastic hooks to the insides of cabinet doors to keep them securely closed. Unlatching these hooks requires firmer thumb pressure than small children can usually exert. Don't let children watch you open the latches. Kids learn fast!
- Avoid storing toxic liquids or solids in food containers, such as soft drink bottles, peanut butter jars, or milk cartons.
- Do not remove container labels or reuse empty containers to store different substances. Laws mandate that the labels of all poisons specify antidotes.
- Do not rely on cooking to destroy toxic chemicals in plants. Never use anything prepared from nature as a medicine or "tea."
- Teach children never to eat any part of an unknown plant or mushroom and not to put leaves, stems, bark, seeds, nuts, or berries from any plant into their mouths.

- Place poison warning stickers designed for children on containers of bleach, lye, kerosene, solvent, and other toxic substances.
- Do not refer to medicine as candy or pretend false enjoyment when taking medications in front of children; allow them to see the necessity of the medicine without glamorizing it.
- Read and follow label directions on all products before using them.
- Do not keep poisonous plants in the home, and avoid planting poisonous plants in the yard. The cooperative extension agency in your county can provide a list of poisonous plants.
- Display the phone number of the poison control center near or on all telephones in the home so that it is available to babysitters, family, and friends.

---

furnaces, also produces CO. Carbon monoxide detectors are available for the home.

SUFFOCATION OR CHOKING Suffocation, or **asphyxiation,** is lack of oxygen due to interrupted breathing. Suffocation occurs when the air source is cut off for any reason. One common reason for choking is that food or a foreign object has become lodged in the throat. The universal sign of distress is the victim's grasping the anterior neck and being unable to speak or cough. The emergency response is the Heimlich maneuver or abdominal thrust, which can dislodge the foreign object and reestablish an airway.

Other causes of suffocation are drowning, gas or smoke inhalation, accidental coverage of the nose and mouth by a piece of plastic, accidental strangulation by the shoulder harness of a seat belt, and being trapped in a confined space (e.g., a discarded refrigerator). If a person does not receive immediate relief from suffocation, the interrupted breathing leads to respiratory and cardiac arrest and death. Any obstruction to the air passages must be immediately removed and life-support measures instituted when an arrest occurs.

EXCESSIVE NOISE Excessive noise is a health hazard that can cause hearing loss, depending on (a) the overall level of noise, (b) the frequency range of the noise, and (c) the duration of exposure and individual susceptibility. Tolerance of noise is largely individual. When ill or injured, people are frequently sensitive to noises that normally would not disturb them. It is important for nurses to minimize noise in the hospital setting and to encourage clients to protect their hearing as much as possible.

ELECTRICAL HAZARDS All electric equipment must be properly grounded. The electric plug of grounded equipment has three prongs. The two short prongs transmit the power to the equipment. The third, longer prong is the grounding device, which carries short circuits or stray elec-

tric current to the ground. Grounding prongs offer a path of least resistance to stray electric currents.

Faulty equipment such as equipment with a frayed cord presents a danger of electric shock or may start a fire. For example, an electric spark near certain anesthetic gases or a high concentration of oxygen can cause a serious fire. Actions to reduce electrical hazards are described in Client Teaching.

CLIENT TEACHING

Reducing Electrical Hazards

- Check cords for fraying or other signs of damage before using an appliance. Do not use if damage is apparent.
- Avoid overloading outlets and fuse boxes with too many appliances.
- Use only grounded outlets and plugs.
- Always pull a plug from the wall outlet by firmly grasping the plug and pulling it straight out. Pulling a plug by its cord can damage the cord and plug unit.
- Never use electric appliances near sinks, bathtubs, showers, or other wet areas, because water readily conducts electricity.
- Keep electric cords and appliances out of the reach of young children.
- Place protective covers over wall outlets to protect young children.
- Have all noninsulated wiring in the home altered to meet safety standards.
- Carefully read instructions before operating electric equipment. Clients who do not understand how to operate the equipment should seek advice.
- Always disconnect appliances before cleaning or repairing them.
- Unplug any appliance that has given a tingling sensation or shock and have an electrician evaluate it for stray current.
- Keep electric cords coiled or taped to the ground away from areas of traffic to prevent others from damaging the cords or tripping over them.

When major electrical injury (macroshock) does occur, the victim may sustain both superficial and deep burns, muscle contractions, and cardiac and respiratory arrest, necessitating cardiopulmonary resuscitation and life support. Electric shock occurs when a current travels through the body to the ground rather than through electric wiring, or from static electricity that builds up on the body. Using machines in good repair, wearing shoes with rubber soles, standing on a nonconductive floor, and using nonconductive gloves can prevent macroshock. However, even with such precautions the rescuer must know that the victim is not to be touched until the electricity is shut off or the victim has been removed from contact with the electric current; otherwise the rescuer may also receive electrical injury.

FIREARMS Parents who bring a handgun into the home must accept full responsibility for teaching safety rules to any children who have knowledge of the presence of firearms. The following basic firearm safety rules must be implemented for any gun:

- Store all guns in sturdy locked cabinets without glass and make sure the keys are inaccessible to children.
- Store the bullets in a different location from the guns.
- Tell children never to touch a gun or stay in a friend's house where a gun is accessible.
- Teach children never to point the barrel of a gun at anyone.
- Ensure the firearm is unloaded and the action is open when handing it to someone else.
- Don't handle firearms while affected by alcohol or drugs of any kind, including pharmaceuticals.
- When cleaning or dry firing a firearm, remove all ammunition to another room, and double-check the firearm when you enter the room in which you will be cleaning the firearm.
- Have firearms that are regularly used inspected by a qualified gunsmith at least every 2 years.

RADIATION Radiation injury can occur from overexposure to radioactive materials used in diagnostic and therapeutic procedures. Clients being examined using radiography or fluoroscopy generally receive minimal exposure and few precautions are necessary. Nurses need to protect themselves, however, from radiation when some clients are receiving radiation therapy. Exposure to radiation can be minimized by (a) limiting the time near the source, (b) providing as much distance as possible from the source, and (c) using shielding devices such as lead aprons when near the source. Nurses need to become familiar with agency protocols related to radiation therapy.

Bioterrorism Attack

No one knows when a bioterrorism attack will occur. Thus, it is important that health care personnel and facilities plan and prepare for the unknown. The Joint Commission requires its accredited health care organizations to meet established disas-

BOX 21–2 **Key Knowledge Content about Bioterrorism**

- Detection and reporting of an unusual outbreak or syndrome (e.g., CDC's categorization of biological agents and the process for reporting to public health authorities)
- Treatment of casualties (e.g., basic prophylactic guidelines, nursing care needs for each biological agent)
- Implementation of control measures (e.g., using standard precautions for every patient, isolation procedures, cleaning, disinfection and sterilization of equipment, linen, and the environment)
- Resource acquisition and preparedness planning (e.g., how to obtain resources such as medical equipment, medications, personnel during a crisis)
- Management of public reactions to bioterrorism (e.g., clear communication to victims, mental health professional support, treatment of anxiety in people not exposed but concerned)

Note: From "Integrating Bioterrorism Education into Nursing School Curricula," by C. Steed, L. Howe, R. Pruitt, and W. Sherrill, 2004, *Journal of Nursing Education.* Copyright © 2004 SLACK, Inc. Reprinted with permission.

ter preparedness standards. In 2001, these standards were expanded to introduce the concepts of emergency management and community involvement in the preparedness process. Health care organizations are now expected to address four specific phases of disaster planning—mitigation, preparedness, response, and recovery—as well as to participate annually in at least one community-wide practice drill (The Joint Commission, 2005a, p. 4). A major part of being prepared is knowledge. See Box 21–2 for a list of content that nurses should know about terrorism. These elements are imperative for an appropriate response to a potential bioterrorism attack.

Procedure- and Equipment-Related Injuries

Risk assessment in the health care setting must include risks related to procedures and equipment. Whether giving a medication or assisting a client out of bed, nurses need to follow safeguards to prevent errors or injuries. Most health care agencies establish protocols that are designed to prevent injuries. When in doubt about a course of action, the nurse should consult the appropriate written guidelines before proceeding.

When an injury or error does occur, most agencies require that the incident be reported. The nurse completes the report immediately after taking whatever action is required to safeguard the client and notifying the charge nurse. For additional information about incident reports, see Chapter 2 ∞.

Restraining Clients

Restraints are protective devices used to limit the physical activity of the client or a part of the body. They can be classified as physical or chemical. **Physical restraints** are any manual method or physical or mechanical device, material, or equipment attached to the client's body; they cannot be removed easily and they restrict the client's movement. **Chemical restraints** are medications such as neuroleptics, anxiolytics, sedatives, and psychotropic agents used to control socially disruptive behavior. The purpose of restraints is to prevent the client from injuring self or others.

Restraints, however, can injure. In 1998, the Joint Commission sent out a sentinel event alert warning of the need to prevent restraint deaths. This alert resulted after a tracking study of sentinel events, which are unexpected occurrences that resulted in death or serious injury. The results indicated that 20 clients who were being physically restrained had died, with the majority of deaths caused by asphyxiation and strangulation. In addition to the physical safety concerns, many consider restraints to be demeaning and psychologically harmful. Some believe they limit a client's autonomy. The current focus in health care is to explore ways to prevent, reduce, and hopefully eliminate the use of restraints while protecting a client's safety, rights, and dignity.

LEGAL IMPLICATIONS OF RESTRAINTS Increasingly, determining the need for safety measures is viewed as an independent nursing function. However, because restraints restrict the individual's freedom, their use has legal implications. Nurses need to know their agency's policies and state laws about restraining clients. The U.S. Centers for Medicare and Medicaid Services (CMS) published revised standards for use of restraints in the United States in 2001. CMS updated the rules applying to the use of restraints in 2007 to include vigorous training of health care workers to ensure the appropriate use of restraints as well as to protect patient rights. The updated rule also requires mandatory reporting of all deaths occurring while a client is subjected to the use of a restraint. On the client's admission to the facility, the family or client must be provided with their rights including freedom from restraints and seclusion in any form when used as a means of coercion, discipline, convenience for the staff, or retaliation (Centers for Medicare and Medicaid Services, 2006). These standards apply to all health care organizations and specify two standards for applying restraints: the behavior management standard when the client is a danger to self or others, and the acute medical and surgical care standard when temporary immobilization of a client is required to perform a procedure.

In the case of the behavior management standard, the nurse may apply restraints but the primary care provider or other licensed independent practitioner must see the client within 1 hour for evaluation. A written restraint order for an adult, following evaluation, is valid for only 4 hours. If the client must be restrained and secluded, there must be continual visual and audio monitoring of the client's status. The medical surgical care standard permits up to 12 hours for obtaining the primary care provider written order for the restraints. All orders must be renewed daily.

Standards require that a primary care provider's order for restraints state the reason and time period. The use of a prn order for restraints is prohibited. In all cases, restraints should be used *only* after every other possible means of ensuring safety have been unsuccessful and documented. See alternatives to the use of restraints in Box 21–3. Restrained clients often become more restless and anxious as a result of the loss of self-control. Nurses must document that the need for the restraint was made clear both to the client and family.

Clients have the right to be free from restraints that are not medically necessary. As a result, there must be justification that the use of restraints will protect the client and that less restrictive measures were attempted and found not effective. Restraints *cannot* be used for staff convenience or client punishment. Given that the above conditions are met and restraints are needed, it is important for

---

BOX 21–3   Alternatives to Restraints

- Assign nurses in pairs to act as "buddies" so that one nurse can observe the client when the other leaves the unit.
- Place unstable clients in an area that is constantly or closely supervised.
- Prepare clients before a move to limit relocation shock and resultant confusion.
- Stay with a client using a bedside commode or bathroom if the client is confused or sedated or has a gait disturbance or a high risk score for falling.
- Monitor all the client's medications and, if possible, attempt to lower or eliminate dosages of sedatives or psychotropics.
- Position beds at their lowest level to facilitate getting in and out of bed.
- Replace full-length side rails with half- or three-quarter-length rails to prevent confused clients from climbing over rails or falling from the end of the bed.
- Use rocking chairs to help confused clients expend some of their energy so that they will be less inclined to wander.

- Wedge pillows or pads against the sides of wheelchairs to keep clients well positioned.
- Place a removable lap tray on a wheelchair to provide support and help keep the client in place.
- To quiet agitated clients, try a warm beverage, soft lights, a back rub, or a walk.
- Use "environmental restraints," such as pieces of furniture or large plants as barriers, to keep clients from wandering beyond appropriate areas.
- Place a picture or other personal item on the door to clients' rooms to help them identify their room.
- Try to determine the causes of the client's sundowner syndrome (nocturnal wandering and disorientation as darkness falls, associated with dementia). Possible causes include poor hearing, poor eyesight, or pain.
- Establish ongoing assessment to monitor changes in physical and cognitive functional abilities and risk factors.

RESEARCH NOTES

Does the Use of Restraints Vary between Hospitals in the United States and Other Countries?

This observational research study used a descriptive, correlational design to compare the relationship between clients' characteristics, environment, and actual use of restraints in critical care units in Norway and the United States. Fifty ICU clients in each country were observed for 10 weeks. During this time the researchers collected data on the level of activity and use of physical restraints. Other collected data included a description of the ICU environment, the nurse-to-client ratio, and nursing workload.

The results indicated that the use of restraints was associated with client activity. Restraints were used 40% of the time in U.S. subjects and not at all in the Norwegian sample. The Norwegian subjects were more sedated. The client characteristics between the two countries did not significantly differ. The activity level, however, differed significantly. The clients in the United States were more active, and the most common restraint used was soft wrist restraints. The activity that led to restraints being applied was interference with an invasive device. Seven incidents of unplanned removal of an invasive device occurred in the United States sample—all in restrained clients. The activity level was less in the Norwegian sample as morphine sulfate was administered at a substantially higher dose.

The nursing workload per client and nurse-to-client ratio differed significantly between the two samples. The nursing workload was higher in the Norwegian sample, and the Norwegian nurse-to-client ratio remained higher than the ratio in the U.S. critical care units.

In the discussion of the study, the researchers pointed out that there was a cultural norm in Norway for nurses to remain within a distance that allows direct visual observation of clients, respiratory therapists are not used at all, and unlicensed personnel are used infrequently.

Implications

Additional research and larger scale studies are needed to determine the effectiveness of restraint-free care. Comparing health care practices in different cultural settings helps nurses become more aware of their own environment.

Note: American Journal of Critical Care by B. Martin and L. Mathisen. Copyright 2005 by American Association of Critical-Care Nurses. Reproduced with permission of American Association of Critical Care Nurses in the Format Textbook via Copyright Clearance Center.

---

the nurse to be able to correctly apply restraints without endangering client safety.

SELECTING A RESTRAINT Before selecting a restraint, nurses need to understand its purpose clearly and measure it against the following five criteria:

1. It restricts the client's movement as little as possible. If a client needs to have one arm restrained, do not restrain the entire body.
2. It does not interfere with the client's treatment or health problem. If a client has poor blood circulation to the hands, apply a restraint that will not aggravate that circulatory problem.
3. It is readily changeable. Restraints need to be changed frequently, especially if they become soiled. Keeping other guidelines in mind, choose a restraint that can be changed with minimal disturbance to the client.
4. It is safe for the particular client. Choose a restraint with which the client cannot self-inflict injury. For example, a physically restrained person could be injured trying to climb out of bed if one wrist is tied to the bed frame. A jacket restraint would restrain the person more safely.
5. It is the least obvious to others. Both clients and visitors are often embarrassed by a restraint, even though they understand why it is being used. The less obvious the restraint, the more comfortable people feel.

KINDS OF RESTRAINTS There are several kinds of restraints. Among the most common for adults are jacket restraints, belt

restraints, mitt or hand restraints, and limb restraints. Geri chairs, wheelchairs with lap trays, and bed rails can also be considered restraints. Restraints for infants and children include mummy restraints, elbow restraints, and crib nets (see Lifespan Considerations later in the chapter). When using restraints, the nurse may find the Practice Guidelines box helpful.

When evaluating if a device is a restraint or not, determine the intended use (e.g., physical restriction), its involuntary application, and/or the client need for the restraint (The Joint Commission, 2005b). For example, if all of the bed's side rails are up and restrict the client's freedom to leave the bed, and the client did not voluntarily request all rails to be up, they are a restraint. If, however, one side rail is up to assist the client to get in and out of the bed, it is not a restraint. Also, if the client can release or remove a device, it would not be considered a restraint.

There are several types of vest restraints, but all are essentially sleeveless jackets or vests with straps (tails) that can be tied to the bed frame under the mattress. These body restraints are used to ensure the safety of confused or sedated clients in beds or wheelchairs. The U.S. Food and Drug Administration (FDA) advises that manufacturers place "front" and "back" labels on vest restraints.

Belt or safety strap body restraints (Figure 21–3) are used to ensure the safety of all clients who are being moved on stretchers or in wheelchairs. Some wheelchairs have a soft, padded safety bar that attaches to side brackets that are installed under the arm rests. To prevent the person from slumping forward, the nurse then attaches a shoulder "Y"

PRACTICE GUIDELINES | Applying Restraints

- Obtain consent from the client or guardian.
- Ensure that a primary care provider's order has been provided or, in an emergency, obtain one within 24 hours after applying the restraint.
- Assure the client and the client's support people that the restraint is temporary and protective. A restraint must never be applied as punishment for any behavior or merely for the nurse's convenience.
- Apply the restraint in such a way that the client can move as freely as possible without defeating the purpose of the restraint.
- Ensure that limb restraints are applied securely but not so tightly that they impede blood circulation to any body area or extremity.
- Pad bony prominences (e.g., wrists and ankles) before applying a restraint over them. The movement of a restraint without padding over such prominences can quickly abrade the skin.
- Always tie a limb restraint with a knot (e.g., a clove hitch) that will not tighten when pulled.
- Tie the ends of a body restraint to the part of the bed that moves to elevate the head. Never tie the ends to a side rail or to the fixed frame of the bed if the bed position is to be changed.
- Assess the restraint per agency protocol time frame. Some facilities have specific forms to be used to record ongoing assessment. This may be a visual check to ensure client safety and no signs of injury.
- Assess skin integrity per agency protocol (e.g., every 2 hours), and provide range-of-motion (ROM) exercises (see Chapter 31 ∞) and skin care when restraints are removed (see Chapter 24 ∞).
- Assess and assist with basic needs: nutrition, hydration, hygiene, elimination.
- Reassess the continued need for the restraint. Include an assessment of the underlying cause of the behavior necessitating use of the restraints.
- When a restraint is temporarily removed, do not leave the client unattended.
- Immediately report to the nurse in charge and record on the client's chart any persistent reddened or broken skin areas under the restraint.
- At the first indication of cyanosis or pallor, coldness of a skin area, or a client's complaint of a tingling sensation, pain, or numbness, loosen the restraint and exercise the limb.
- Apply a restraint so that it can be released quickly in case of an emergency and with the body part in a normal anatomic position.
- Provide emotional support verbally and through touch.

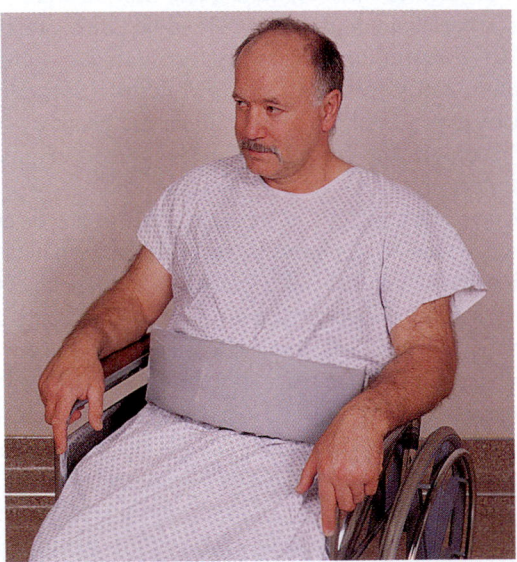

Figure 21–3 ○ A belt restraint.

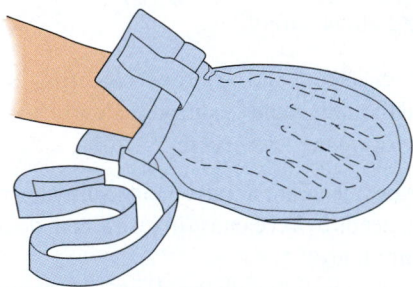

Figure 21–4 ○ A mitt restraint.

A mitt or hand restraint (Figure 21–4) is used to prevent confused clients from using their hands or fingers to scratch and injure themselves. For example, a confused client may need to be prevented from pulling at intravenous tubing or a head bandage following brain surgery. Hand or mitt restraints allow the client to be ambulatory and/or to move the arm freely rather than be confined to a bed or a chair. Mittens need to be removed on a regular basis to permit the client to wash and exercise the hands. The nurse also needs to take off the mitten to check the circulation to the hand.

Limb restraints, which are generally made of cloth, may be used to immobilize a limb, primarily for therapeutic reasons (e.g., to maintain an intravenous infusion). See Skill 21–3 for applying restraints.

strap to the bar and over the client's shoulders to the rear handles. Other safety belt models have a three-loop design. One loop surrounds the person's waist and attaches to the rear handles. If such restraints are unavailable, the nurse can place a folded towel or small sheet around the client's waist and fasten it at the back of the wheelchair. Belt restraints may also be used for certain clients confined to bed or to chairs.

APPLYING RESTRAINTS

PURPOSES
- To promote safety and prevent injury
- To allow a medical or surgical treatment to proceed without client interference (e.g., to prevent movements that would disrupt therapy to a limb connected to tubes or appliance)

ASSESSMENT
Assess
- The behavior indicating the possible need for a restraint
- Underlying cause for assessed behavior

- What other protective measures may be implemented before applying a restraint
- Status of skin to which restraint is to be applied
- Circulatory status distal to restraints and of extremities
- Effectiveness of other available safety precautions

PLANNING
Review institutional policy for restraints and seek consultation as appropriate before independently deciding to apply a restraint. All other possible interventions that are less restrictive *must* have been tried and their failure documented. The primary care provider must be notified prior to using a restraint, unless there is a danger to self or others. In that case the primary care provider must be notified within the prescribed time frame per the agency protocol.

Delegation
The nurse must make the determination that restraints are appropriate in specific situations, select the proper type of restraints, evaluate the effectiveness of the restraints, and assess for potential complications from their use. Application of ordered restraints and their temporary removal for skin assessment and care may be delegated to UAP who have been trained in their use.

EQUIPMENT
- Appropriate type and size of restraint

IMPLEMENTATION
Performance
1. Prior to performing the procedure, introduce self and verify the client's identity using agency protocol. Explain to the client and family what you are going to do, why it is necessary, and how they can participate. Discuss how the results will be used in planning further care or treatments. Allow time for the client to express feelings about being restrained. Provide needed emotional reassurance that the restraints will be used only when absolutely necessary and that there will be close contact with the client in case assistance is required.
2. Perform hand hygiene and observe appropriate infection control procedures.
3. Provide for client privacy if indicated.
4. Apply the selected restraint.

   Belt Restraint (Safety Belt)
   - Determine that the safety belt is in good order. If a Velcro safety belt is to be used, make sure that both pieces of Velcro are intact.
   - If the belt has a long portion and a shorter portion, place the long portion of the belt behind (under) the bedridden client and secure it to the movable part of the bed frame. **Rationale:** *The long attached portion will then move up when the head of the bed is elevated and will not tighten around the client.* Place the shorter portion of the belt around the client's waist, over the gown. There should be a finger's width between the belt and the client.

     or
   - Attach the belt around the client's waist, and fasten it at the back of the chair.

     or
   - If the belt is attached to a stretcher, secure the belt firmly over the client's hips or abdomen. **Rationale:** *Belt*

restraints must be applied to all clients on stretchers even when the side rails are up.

Jacket Restraint
- Place vest on client, with opening at the front or the back, depending on the type.
- Pull the tie on the end of the vest flap across the chest, and place it through the slit in the opposite side of the chest.
- Repeat for the other tie.

Use a half-bow knot to secure each tie around the movable bed frame or behind the chair to a chair leg. ❶ ❷

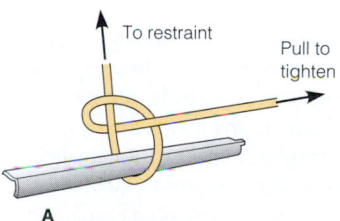

A

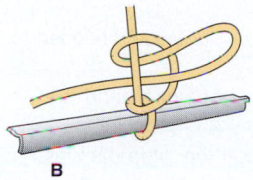

B

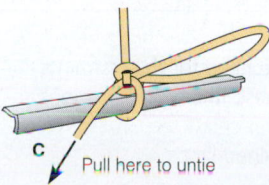

C ↓ Pull here to untie

❶ To make a half-bow knot (quick-release knot), first place the restraint tie under the side frame of the bed (or around a chair leg). **A**, Bring the free end up, around, under, and over the attached end of the tie and pull it tight. **B**, Again take the free end over and under the attached end of the tie, but this time make a half-bow loop. **C**, Tighten the free end of the tie and the bow until the knot is secure. To untie the knot, pull the end of the tie and then loosen the first cross over the tie.

(continued)

SKILL 21–3

APPLYING RESTRAINTS *(continued)*

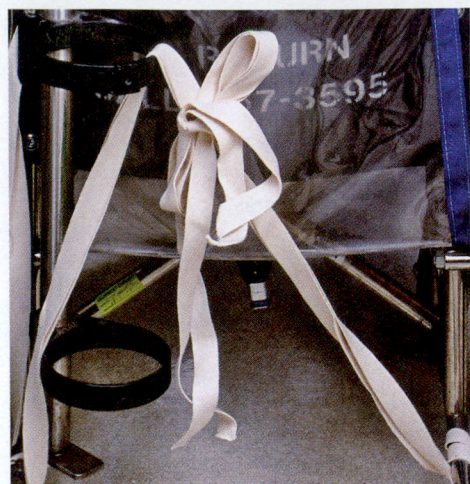

2 Quick-release knot.

Rationale: *A half-bow knot does not tighten or slip when the attached end is pulled but unties easily when the loose end is pulled.*

or

- Fasten the ties together behind the chair using a slip or quick-release knot.
- Ensure that the client is positioned appropriately to enable maximum chest expansion for breathing.

Mitt Restraint

- Apply the commercial thumbless mitt (Figure 21–4) to the hand to be restrained. Make sure the fingers can be slightly flexed and are not caught under the hand.
- Follow the manufacturer's directions for securing the mitt.
- If a mitt is to be worn for several days, remove it at regular intervals per agency protocol. Wash and exercise the client's hand, then reapply the mitt. Check agency practices about recommended intervals for removal.
- Assess the client's circulation to the hands shortly after the mitt is applied and at regular intervals. **Rationale:** *Client complaints of numbness, discomfort, or inability to move the fingers could indicate impaired circulation to the hand.*

Wrist or Ankle Restraint

- Pad bony prominences on the wrist or ankle if needed to prevent skin breakdown.
- Apply the padded portion of the restraint around the ankle or wrist.
- Pull the tie of the restraint through the slit in the wrist portion or through the buckle and ensure the restraint is not too tight. **3**

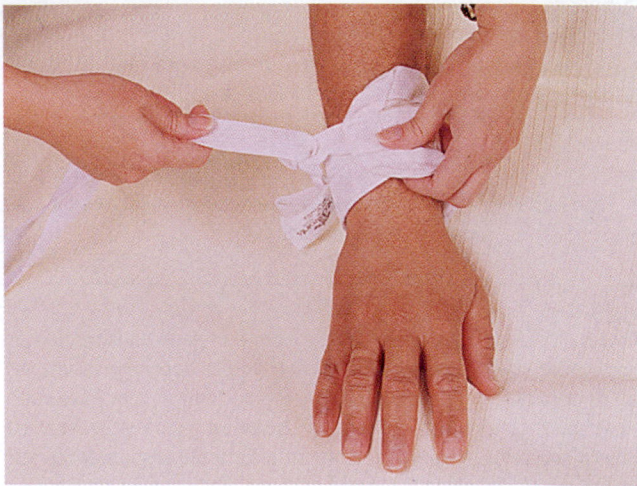

3 Ensure that a finger can be inserted between the restraint and the wrist or ankle.

- Using a half-bow knot (quick-release knot), attach the other end of the restraint to the movable portion of the bed frame. **Rationale:** *If the ties are attached to the movable portion, the wrist or ankle will not be pulled when the bed position is changed.*

5. Adjust the plan of care as required, for example, to include releasing the restraint, providing skin care, range-of-motion exercises, and attending to the client's physical needs by providing fluids, nutrition, and toileting.

6. Record on the client's chart the behavior(s) indicating the need for the restraint, all other interventions implemented in an attempt to avoid the use of restraints and their outcomes, and the time the primary care provider was notified of the need for restraint. Also record:

- The type of restraint applied, the time it was applied, and the goal for its application.
- The client's response to the restraint including a rationale for its continued use. (Anistine, 2007).
- The times that the restraints were removed and skin care given.
- Any other assessments and interventions.
- Explanations given to the client and significant others.

SAMPLE DOCUMENTATION

1/11/2010 Confused. Disoriented to time and place. Reoriented frequently. Pulling at central IV line, NG tube and chest tube. Medicated for pain relief. Lights dimmed. Continues to pull at IV and tubes. Dr. Jones called. Received an order to apply mitt restraints. Family called and explained the situation. Stated someone will come in and sit with the client. Mitt restraints applied till family member arrives. ———————— C. Murphy, RN

EVALUATION

- Perform a detailed follow-up of the need for the restraints and the client's response. Relate these findings to previous data if available.
- Evaluate circulatory status of restrained limbs.

- Evaluate skin status beneath restraints.
- Remove the restraints as soon as they are no longer needed and document.
- Report significant deviations from normal to the primary care provider.

LIFESPAN CONSIDERATIONS   Restraints

Infants

Elbow restraints (Figure 21–5) are used to prevent infants or small children from flexing their elbows to touch or reach their face or head, especially after surgery. Ready-made elbow restraints are available commercially.

A mummy restraint (Figure 21–6) is a special folding of a blanket or sheet around the infant to prevent movement during a procedure such as gastric washing, eye irrigation, or collection of a blood specimen.

- Obtain a blanket or sheet large enough so that the distance between opposite corners is about twice the length of the infant's body. Lay the blanket or sheet on a flat, dry surface.
- Fold down one corner, and place the baby on it in the supine position.
- Fold the right side of the blanket over the infant's body, leaving the left arm free (Figure 21–6, *A*). The right arm is in a natural position at the side.

- Fold the excess blanket at the bottom up under the infant (Figure 21–6, *B,2*).
- With the left arm in a natural position at the baby's side, fold the left side of the blanket over the infant, including the arm, and tuck the blanket under the body (Figure 21–6, *B,3*).
- Remain with the infant who is in a mummy restraint until the specific procedure is completed.

Children

A crib net is simply a device placed over the top of a crib to prevent active young children from climbing out of the crib. At the same time, it allows them freedom to move about in the crib. The crib net or dome is not attached to the movable parts of the crib so that the caregiver can have access to the child without removing the dome or net.

- Place the net over the sides and ends of the crib.
- Secure the ties to the springs or frame of the crib. The crib sides can then be freely lowered without removing the net.
- Test with your hand that the net will stretch if the child stands against it in the crib.

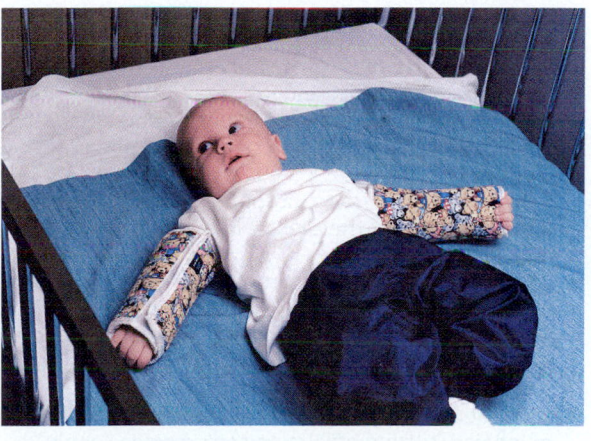

Figure 21–5 ○ Infant with elbow restraints.

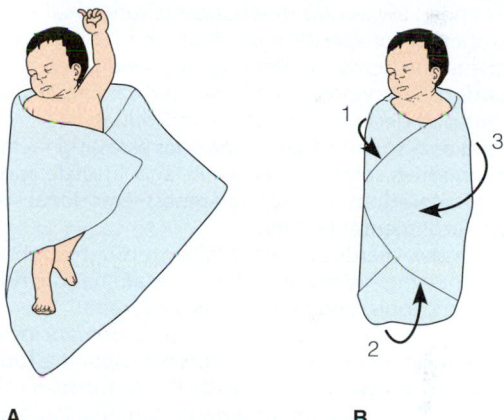

A   B

Figure 21–6 ○ Making a mummy restraint.

LIFESPAN CONSIDERATIONS   Safety

Older Adults

Some of the changes due to aging that place the older adult at higher risk for safety concerns are:

- Decrease in hearing and sight.
- Decrease in response of reflexes.
- Fragility of bones and decrease in flexibility of joints and muscles.
- Decrease in temperature regulation, increasing the risk of hypothermia and hyperthermia.

- Decrease in kidney function, which increases risk of toxicity from medications.

A home environment that was safe when they were younger may need modifications for older adults to decrease the risk of injury. A plan and telephone numbers of those to call should be available for emergency situations.

EVALUATING

To prevent client injury, the nurse's role is largely educative and desired outcomes reflect the client's acquisition of knowledge of hazards, behaviors that incorporate safety practices, and skills to perform in the event of certain emergencies. The nurse needs to individualize these for clients. Examples of desired outcomes include the client being able to do the following:

- Describe methods to prevent specific hazards (e.g., falls, suffocation, choking, fires, drowning, electric shock).
- Report use of home safety measures (e.g., fire safety measures, smoke detector maintenance, fall prevention strategies, burn prevention measures, poison prevention measures, safe storage of hazardous materials, firearm safety precautions, electrocution prevention, water safety precautions, bicycle safety, motor vehicle safety).
- Alter home physical environment to reduce the risk of injury.
- Describe emergency procedures for poisoning and fire.
- Describe age-specific risks, work safety risks, or community safety risks.
- Demonstrate correct use of child safety seats.
- Demonstrate correct administration of cardiopulmonary resuscitation.

CHAPTER HIGHLIGHTS

- Injuries are a major cause of death among individuals of all ages in the United States.
- Nurses need awareness of what constitutes a safe environment for specific individuals and for groups of people in the home, community, and workplace.
- Hazards to safety occur at all ages and vary according to the age and development of the individual.
- Nursing assessment of safety includes assessing factors that can affect safety, for example, age, lifestyle, mobility, sensory alterations, level of awareness, emotional state, and environmental factors.
- Nurses assess clients at risk for injury through methods such as nursing history and physical examination, risk assessment tools, and home hazard appraisal.
- Recent studies and reports (e.g., *To Err Is Human*) indicate that the incidence of medical errors in hospitals is too high and half are preventable. At least 80% of the medical errors are system related. As a result, National Patient Safety Goals (NPSG) were initiated and are required to be implemented by Joint Commission–accredited agencies. The focus of the NPSG is on systemwide solutions.
- Nurses need to sustain a heightened awareness and alertness of circumstances or patterns that may indicate potential bioterrorism. Early detection and management is needed to help stop a bioterrorism attack.
- Major nursing diagnoses for clients at risk for injury can be categorized as *Risk for Injury*, with seven subcategories: *Risk for Poisoning, Risk for Suffocation, Risk for Trauma, Latex Allergy Response, Risk for Latex Allergy Response, Contamination, Risk for Contamination, Risk for Aspiration,* and *Risk for Disuse Syndrome.*
- When planning to meet safety needs of clients, nurses need to consider physical factors in the environment and the psychologic and physiologic state of the individual. Clients often need to change their health behavior and may need to modify the environment.
- Measures to ensure the safety of people of all ages focus on (a) observation or prediction of situations that are potentially harmful and (b) client education that empowers clients to safeguard themselves and their families from injury. Education is a major health protection strategy in preventing injuries.
- Nurses must be familiar with the fire procedures in the health care agency where they practice. In the event of a fire, the nurse must (a) protect clients from injury, (b) report, (c) contain, and (d) put out the fire.
- Falls are a common cause of injury among older adults.
- Prevention of falls in health care agencies is a continuous concern.
- Side rails do not protect hospitalized clients from falls. It is more likely that the client will fall trying to get around or over the side rail.
- Seizure precautions are safety measures taken by the nurse to protect clients from injury should they have a seizure.
- Major reasons for poisoning in children are inadequate supervision and improper storage of household toxic substances.
- Suffocation can occur when foreign objects are swallowed or inhaled, cutting off the person's oxygen supply.
- Prolonged exposure to excessive noise can produce hearing loss.
- Faulty electric equipment and improper grounding pose health hazards in the hospital and the home. Injuries can be prevented by using grounded outlets and plugs, putting protective covers over outlets, keeping appliances in good repair, and making sure that electric wiring and circuits meet safety standards.
- Firearms pose a risk to individuals of all ages. Adults must take full responsibility for following safety procedures when keeping firearms in the home, including storage of ammunition in a separate location.
- In hospitals, radioactive substances are used for both diagnostic and treatment purposes; agency policy should be followed to safeguard clients and staff from unsafe exposure.
- Various alternatives to restraints must be considered before a restraint is applied.
- Because restraints restrict a client's basic freedom to move, careful assessment and accurate, complete documentation are important when restraints are used.

THINK ABOUT IT

Refer to the chapter-opening scenario and answer these questions.

1. What factors increased Mrs. Pachekowski's risk for injury?

2. What could the nurse have done to reduce these risk factors?

3. Should the nurse have applied a jacket restraint to Mrs. Pachekowski? Why or why not?

∞ *See suggested responses to Think About It on MyNursingKit.*

TEST YOUR KNOWLEDGE

1. The nurse enters the client's room and finds a fire in the trash can. Place the following nursing priorities in correct sequence if a fire occurs in a health setting.
1. Report the fire.
2. Extinguish the fire.
3. Protect the clients.
4. Contain the fire.

2. The nurse is teaching a course on safety and explains that which of the following is the leading cause of accidents in young and middle-aged adults?
1. Automobile crashes
2. Drowning and firearms
3. Falls
4. Suicide and homicide

3. Because a hospitalized older female client, who ambulates with a walker, is receiving diuretics, the nurse should perform which of the following?
1. Leave the bathroom light on.
2. Withhold the client's diuretic medication.
3. Provide a bedside commode.
4. Keep the side rails up.

4. Which NANDA nursing diagnosis is most specifically applicable for toddlers?
1. *Risk for Suffocation*
2. *Risk for Injury*
3. *Risk for Poisoning*
4. *Risk for Disuse Syndrome*

5. A 75-year-old client, hospitalized following a cerebral vascular accident (stroke), becomes disoriented at times and tries to get out of bed, but is unable to ambulate without help. What is the most appropriate safety measure?
1. Restrain the client in bed.
2. Ask a family member to stay with the client.
3. Check the client every 15 minutes.
4. Use a bed exit safety monitoring device.

6. A client is being admitted to the hospital following a seizure that occurred at his home. The client has no previous history of seizures. In planning the client's nursing care, which of the following measures is most essential at the time of admission? Select all that apply.
1. Place a padded tongue depressor at the head of the bed.
2. Pad the side rails.
3. Inform the client about the importance of wearing a medical identification tag.
4. Teach the client about epilepsy.
5. Test oral suction equipment.

7. Which of the following nursing interventions is the highest priority for a client at risk for falls in a hospital setting?
1. Keep all of the side rails up.
2. Review prescribed medications.
3. Complete the "get up and go" test.
4. Place the bed in the lowest position.

8. Which of the following nursing practices will help decrease the risk of medication errors? Select all that apply.
1. Hire only competent nurses.
2. Improve the nurse's ability to multitask.
3. Establish a reporting system for "near misses."
4. Communicate effectively.
5. Create a culture of trust.

9. When planning to teach health care topics to a group of male adolescents, the nurse should consider which of the following topics a priority?
1. Sports contribute to an adolescent's self-esteem.
2. Sunbathing and tanning beds can be dangerous.
3. Guns are the most frequently used weapon for adolescent suicide.
4. A driver's education course is mandatory for safety.

10. The nurse, at change-of-shift report, learns that one of the assigned clients has bilateral soft wrist restraints currently in place. The client is confused, is trying to get out of bed, and had pulled out the IV line, which was subsequently reinserted. Which of the following actions by the nurse is appropriate? Select all that apply.
1. Document the behavior(s) that require continued use of the restraints.
2. Ensure that the restraints are tied to the side rails.
3. Provide range-of-motion exercises when the restraints are removed.
4. Orient the client.
5. Assess the tightness of the restraints.

∞ *See answers to Test Your Knowledge in Appendix A.*

EXPLORE PEARSON **mynursingkit**™

MyNursingKit is your one stop for online chapter review materials and resources. Prepare for success with additional NCLEX®-style practice questions, interactive assignments and activities, web links, animations and videos, and more!

Register your access code from the front of your book at
www.mynursingkit.com.

REFERENCES AND SELECTED BIBLIOGRAPHY

American Geriatrics Society. (2006). *Falls in older adults. Management in primary practice.* Retrieved June 18, 2006, from http://www.americangeriatrics.org/education/falls.shtml

Anistine, J.P. (2007). Understanding the new standards for patient restraint and seclusion. *American Nurse Today, 2*(6), 15–17.

Ball, J., & Bindler, R. (2008). *Pediatric nursing: Caring for children* (4th ed.). Upper Saddle River, NJ: Pearson Education.

Berntsen, K. J. (2004). Valuable lessons in patient safety. Reporting near misses in healthcare. *Journal of Nursing Care Quality, 19*(3), 177–179.

Beyea, S. C. (2004). A critical partnership–Safety for nurses and patients. *AORN Journal, 79*(6), 1299–1302.

Beyea, S. C. (2005). Patient advocacy—Nurses keeping patients safe. *AORN Journal, 81*(5), 1046–1047.

Bulechek, G. M., Butcher, H. K., & Dochterman, J. M. (Eds.). (2008). Nursing interventions: Classification (NIC) (5th ed.). St. Louis, MO: Mosby.

Centers for Disease Control and Prevention. (2001). Recognition of illness associated with the intentional release of a biologic agent. *Morbidity and Mortality Weekly Report, 50*(41), 893–897.

Centers for Disease Control and Prevention. (2001). *Facts about botulism.* Retrieved June 18, 2006, from http://www.bt.cdc.gov/agent/botulism/factsheet.asp

Centers for Disease Control and Prevention. (2002). *Fact sheet: Anthrax information for health care providers.* Retrieved June 18, 2006, from http://www.bt.cdc.gov/agent/anthrax/anthrax-hcp-factsheet.asp

Centers for Disease Control and Prevention. (2003). *Key facts about tularemia.* Retrieved June 18, 2006, from http://www.bt.cdc.gov/agent/tularemia/facts.asp

Centers for Disease Control and Prevention. (2003). *Frequently asked questions (FAQ) about tularemia.* Retrieved June 18, 2006, from http://www.bt.cdc.gov/agent/tularemia/faq.asp

Centers for Disease Control and Prevention. (2004). *Viral hemorrhagic fevers.* Retrieved June 19, 2006, from http://www.cdc.gov/ncidod/dvrd/spb/mnpages/dispages/Fact_Sheets/Viral_Hemorrhagic_Fevers_Fact_ Sheet.pdf

Centers for Disease Control and Prevention. (2004). *Frequently asked questions about smallpox.* Retrieved June 19, 2006, from http://www.bt.cdc.gov/agent/smallpox/disease/faq.asp

Centers for Disease Control and Prevention. (2004). *Smallpox disease overview.* Retrieved June 18, 2006, from http://www.bt.cdc.gov/agent/smallpox/overview/disease-facts.asp

Centers for Disease Control and Prevention. (2005). *Frequently asked questions (FAQ) about plague.* Retrieved June 19, 2006, from http://www.bt.cdc.gov/agent/plague/faq.asp

Centers for Disease Control and Prevention. (2005). *Questions and answers about anthrax.* Retrieved June 18, 2006, from http://www.bt.cdc.gov/agent/anthrax/faq/index.asp

Centers for Medicare and Medicaid Services. (2006, December 8). *CMS Publishes final patient rights rule on use of restraints and seclusion.* Retrieved June 15, 2009, from http://www.cms.hhs.gov/apps/media/press/release.asp?Counter=2057

Cross, C. (2004). Seizures. Regaining control. *RN, 67*(12), 44–50.

Ebersole, P., Hess, P., Touhy, T., & Jett, K. (2009). *Gerontological nursing & healthy aging* (3rd ed.). St. Louis: Mosby.

Gambrell, M., & Flynn, N. (2004). Seizures 101: Brush up on the essentials about seizures, so you can remain calm and provide effective care. *Nursing, 34*(8), 36–41.

Institute of Medicine. (2000). *To err is human. Building a safer health system.* Washington, DC: National Academy of Sciences.

Institute of Medicine. (2004). *Keeping patients safe. Transforming the work environment of nurses.* Washington, DC: National Academies Press.

Jasniewski, J. (2006). Take steps to protect your patient from falls. *Nursing, 36*(4), 24–25.

The Joint Commission, 2009: *Accreditation Program: Critical Access Hospital National Patient Safety Goals.* Retrieved December 19, 2008, from http://www.jointcommission.org/NR/rdonlyres/4BAD7889-79DE-493F-A6FD-CEB9F003434D/0/CAH_NPSG.pdf

Joint Commission on Accreditation of Healthcare Organizations. (2003). *Health care at the crossroads. Strategies for creating and sustaining community-wide emergency preparedness systems.* Oakbrook Terrace, IL: Author.

Joint Commission on Accreditation of Healthcare Organizations. (2005a).

Setting the standard. Oakbrook Terrace, IL: Author.

Joint Commission on Accreditation of Healthcare Oganizations. (2005b). *Restraint and seclusion.* Retrieved June 11, 2006, from http://www.jointcommission.org/AccreditationPrograms/BehavioralHealthCare/Standards/FAQs/Provision+of+Care+Treatment+and+Services/Restraint+and+Seclusion/Restraint_Seclusion.htm

Joint Commission on Accreditation of Healthcare Organizations. (2006). *2007 critical access hospital and hospital national patient safety goals.* Retrieved June 19, 2006, from http://www.jointcommission.org/PatientSafety/NationalPatientSafetyGoals/07_hap_cah_npsgs.htm

Joint Commission on Accreditation of Healthcare Organizations. (2006). *2007 Long term care national patient safety goals.* Retrieved June 19, 2006, from http://www.jointcommission.org/PatientSafety/NationalPatientSafetyGoals/07_ltc_npsgs.htm

Joint Commission on Accreditation of Healthcare Organizations. (2006). *Facts about 2006 National Patient Safety Goals.* Retrieved June 19, 2006, from http://www.jointcommission.org/PatientSafety/NationalPatientSafetyGoals/06_npsg_facts.htm

Karber, S., & Fasano, N. (2003). What you need to know about the smallpox vaccine. *Nursing, 33*(6), 36–42.

Kimbell, S. (2001). Before the fall. Keeping your patient on his feet. *Nursing, 3*(8), 44–45.

Kleen, K. (2004). Restraint regulation: The tie that binds. *Nursing Management, 35*(11), 36–38.

Kohn, L. T., Corrigan, J. M., & Donaldson, M. S. (Eds.). (2000). *To err is human. Building a safer health system.* Washington, DC: National Academy Press.

Leonard, M., Frankel, A., Simmonds, T., & Vega, K. B. (2004). *Achieving safe and reliable healthcare.* Chicago: Health Administration Press.

Lyons, S. S. (2005). Evidence-based protocol: Fall prevention for older adults. *Journal of Gerontological Nursing, 31*(11), 9–14.

Manno, M., Hogan, P., Heberlein, V., Nyakiti, J., & Mee, C. L. (2006). Patient-safety survey report. *Nursing, 36*(3), 54–63.

Marcy-Edwards, D. (2005). Bed rails: Is there an up side? *Canadian Nurse, 101*(1), 30–34.

Marthaler, M. T. (2004). Seizures revisited. *Nursing Management, 35*(4), 71–74.

Martin, B., & Mathisen, L. (2005). Use of physical restraints in adult critical care: A bicultural study. *American Journal of Critical Care, 14*(2), 133–142.

Massey, M. (2004, October 11). Battling bioterrorism. *Advance for Nurses– Northern California and Reno, NV,* 30–31.

McBeth, S. (2004). Get a firmer grasp on restraints. *Nursing Management, 35*(10), 20–22.

Moorhead, S., Johnson, M., & Maas, M. L., & Swanson, E. (Eds.). (2008). *Nursing outcomes classification (NOC)* (4th ed.). St. Louis: Mosby.

Morath, J., & Leary, M. (2004). Creating safe spaces in organizations to talk about safety. *Nursing Economics, 22*(6), 344–354.

Murphy, J. K. (2004). After 9/11: Priority focus areas for bioterrorism preparedness in hospitals. *Journal of Healthcare Management, 49*(4), 227–235.

NANDA International. (2009). *NANDA nursing diagnoses: Definitions and classification* 2009–2011. West Sussex, U.K.: Wiley-Blackwell.

Napierkowski, D. (2002). Using restraints with restraint. *Nursing, 32*(11), 58–62.

National Safety Council. (2004). How to prevent poisonings in your home. Retrieved December 5, 2009, from http://www.nsc. org/news_resources/Resources/ Documents/How_to_Prevent_Poisonings_ in_Your_Home.pdf

National Safety Council. (2004). *Carbon monoxide.* Retrieved December 5, 2009, from http://www.nsc.org/news_ resources/Resources_Documents/ Carbon_monoxide.pdf

National Safety Council. (2004). *Lead poisoning.* Retrieved December 5, 2009, from http://nursingworld.org/ MainMenuCategories/ANAMarketplace/ ANAPeriodicals/OJIN/TableofContents/ Volume82003/No3Sept2003/ AssociationsRole.aspx

Page, A. (Ed.). (2004). *Keeping patients safe. Transforming the work environment of nurses.* Washington, DC: National Academies Press.

Pena, C. G. (2003). Seizure. A calm response and careful observation are crucial. *American Journal of Nursing, 103*(11), 73–81.

Rowell, P. (2003, September 30). The professional nursing association's role in patient safety. *Online Journal of Issues in Nursing, 8*(3), manuscript 3. Retrieved June 18, 2006, from http://nursingworld .org/ojin/topic22/tpc22_3.htm

Steed, C. J., Howe, L. A., Pruitt, R. H., & Sherrill, W. W. (2004). Integrating bioterrorism education into nursing school curricula. *Journal of Nursing Education, 43*(8), 362–367.

Todd, J. F. (2004). Burning beds. *Nursing, 34*(9), 23.

Weber, C. J. (2004). Update on bioterrorism preparedness. *Urologic Nursing, 24*(5), 417–419.

Wilkinson, J. M. (2009). *Prentice Hall Nursing Diagnosis Handbook* (9th ed.). Upper Saddle River, NJ: Pearson Education.

Hygiene

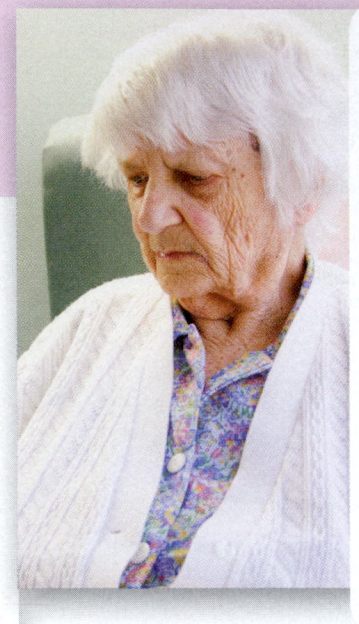

Cece Roker, 88 years old, lives with her 21-year-old granddaughter. She is admitted to the hospital after police find her in her bed showing signs of neglect. Ms. Roker experienced a cerebrovascular accident 3 years ago that left her bedridden, occasionally confused, and experiencing intermittent aphasia. Due to lack of medical insurance and the inability to pay for services, Ms. Roker was not sent to a rehabilitation facility but was discharged to her home and the care of her then-18-year-old granddaughter, Brenda. When her granddaughter started a new job, Ms. Roker was left at home alone for 10 to 12 hours a day. She is admitted to the medical unit for treatment of dehydration and hypertension and care of the pressure ulcers she developed as a result of malnutrition and inadequate care.

LEARNING OUTCOMES

After completing this chapter, you will be able to:

1. Describe hygienic care that nurses provide to clients and the factors influencing clients' needs.

2. Describe the use of the nursing process to meeting hygienic needs of the client.

3. Demonstrate the proper delivery of hygienic-care procedures.

4. Identify steps in removing contact lenses and inserting and removing artificial eyes.

5. Describe steps for removing, cleaning, and inserting hearing aids.

6. Identify safety and comfort measures underlying bed-making procedures.

KEY TERMS

Alopecia p628
Callus p614
Cerumen p634
Cleaning bath p605
Dandruff p628

Dental caries p618
Gingivitis p619
Hygiene p601
Ingrown toenail p614
Pediculosis p628

Periodontal disease p618
Plaque p619
Pyorrhea p619
Scabies p628
Sebum p601

Tartar p619
Therapeutic bath p605
Ticks p628
Xerostomia p625

Hygiene is the science of health and its maintenance. Personal **hygiene** is the self-care by which people attend to such functions as bathing, toileting, general body hygiene, and grooming. Hygiene is a highly personal matter determined by individual values and practices. It involves care of the skin, hair, nails, teeth, oral and nasal cavities, eyes, ears, and perineal-genital areas.

It is important for nurses to know exactly how much assistance a client needs for hygienic care. Clients may require help after urinating or defecating, after vomiting, and whenever they become soiled, for example, from wound drainage or from profuse perspiration. Table 22–1 lists factors that influence hygiene practices.

HYGIENIC CARE

Nurses commonly use the following terms to describe types of hygienic care. *Early morning care* is provided to clients as they awaken in the morning. This care consists of providing a urinal or bedpan to the client confined to bed, washing the face and hands, and giving oral care. *Morning care* is often provided after clients have breakfast, although it may be provided before breakfast. It usually includes providing for elimination needs, a bath or shower, perineal care, back massages, and oral, nail, and hair care. Making the client's bed is part of morning care. *Hour of sleep (HS)* or *PM care* is provided to clients before they retire for the night. It usually involves providing for elimination needs, washing face and hands, giving oral care, and giving a back massage. *As-needed (prn) care* is provided as required by the client. For example, a client who is diaphoretic (sweating profusely) may need more frequent bathing and a change of clothes and linen.

SKIN

The skin is the largest organ of the body. It serves five major functions:

1. It protects underlying tissues from injury by preventing the passage of microorganisms. The skin and mucous membranes are considered the body's first line of defense.
2. It regulates the body temperature. Cooling of the body occurs through the heat loss processes of evaporation of perspiration, and by radiation and conduction of heat from the body when the blood vessels of the skin are vasodilated. Body heat is conserved through lack of perspiration and vasoconstriction of the blood vessels. See Chapter 17 ∞.
3. It secretes **sebum**, an oily substance that (a) softens and lubricates the hair and skin, (b) prevents the hair from becoming brittle, and (c) decreases water loss from the skin when the external humidity is low. Because fat is a poor conductor of heat, sebum (d) lessens the amount of heat lost from the skin. Sebum also (e) has a bactericidal (bacteria-killing) action.
4. It transmits sensations through nerve receptors, which are sensitive to pain, temperature, touch, and pressure.
5. It produces and absorbs vitamin D in conjunction with ultraviolet rays from the sun, which activate a vitamin D precursor present in the skin.

The normal skin of a healthy person has transient and resident microorganisms that are not usually harmful. See Chapter 24 ∞.

Sudoriferous (sweat) glands are on all body surfaces except the lips and parts of the genitals. The body has from 2 to 5 million, which are all present at birth. They are most

TABLE 22–1	Factors Influencing Individual Hygienic Practices
FACTOR	**VARIABLES**
Culture	North American culture places a high value on cleanliness. Many North Americans bathe or shower once or twice a day, whereas people from some other cultures bathe once a week. Some cultures consider privacy essential for bathing, whereas others practice communal bathing. Body odor is offensive in some cultures and accepted as normal in others.
Religion	Ceremonial washings are practiced by some religions.
Environment	Finances may affect the availability of facilities for bathing. For example, homeless people may not have warm water available; soap, shampoo, shaving lotion, and deodorants may be too expensive for people who have limited resources.
Developmental level	Children learn hygiene in the home. Practices vary according to the individual's age; for example, preschoolers can carry out most tasks independently with encouragement.
Health and energy	Ill people may not have the motivation or energy to attend to hygiene. Some clients who have neuromuscular impairments may be unable to perform hygienic care.
Personal preferences	Some people prefer a shower to a tub bath. People have different preferences regarding the time of bathing (e.g., morning versus evening).

numerous on the palms of the hands and the soles of the feet. Sweat glands are classified as apocrine and eccrine. The apocrine glands, located largely in the axillae and anogenital areas, begin to function at puberty under the influence of androgens. Although they produce sweat almost constantly, apocrine glands are of little use in thermoregulation. The secretion of these glands is odorless, but when decomposed or acted on by bacteria on the skin, it takes on a musky, unpleasant odor. The eccrine glands are important physiologically. They are more numerous than the apocrine glands and are found chiefly on the palms of the hands, the soles of the feet, and the forehead. The sweat they produce cools the body through evaporation. Sweat is made up of water, sodium, potassium, chloride, glucose, urea, and lactate.

> **CULTURALLY COMPETENT CARE**
>
> ## Biocultural Variations in Body Secretions
>
> - Most Asians and Native North Americans have a mild to absent body odor, whereas Whites and African Americans tend to have strong body odor.
> - Eskimos have made an environmental adaptation where they sweat less than Whites on their trunks and extremities but more on their faces. This adaptation allows for temperature regulation without the need to change clothes because of perspiration.
> - The amount of chloride excreted by sweat glands varies widely. African Americans have lower salt concentrations in their sweat than Whites.
>
> *Note:* From M. M. Andrews and J. S. Boyle, *Transcultural Concepts in Nursing Care,* 4th ed. Lippincott, Williams & Wilkins, 2003. Reprinted with permission.

NURSING MANAGEMENT

ASSESSING

Assessment of the client's skin and hygienic practices includes (a) a nursing health history to determine the client's skin care practices, self-care abilities, and past or current skin problems; (b) physical assessment of the skin; and (c) identification of clients at risk for developing skin impairments.

Nursing History

Data about the client's skin care practices enable the nurse to incorporate the client's needs and preferences as much as possible in the plan of care. According to Andrews and Boyle (2008), people in most cultures in the United States try to disguise natural body odors by bathing frequently and using deodorant, cologne, or perfumes. Immigrants from other countries where water is scarce may bathe less often than people from countries where water is more accessible.

Assessment of the client's self-care abilities determines the amount of nursing assistance and the type of bath best suited for the client. Important considerations include the client's balance, ability to sit unsupported, activity tolerance, coordination, adequate muscle strength, appropriate joint range of motion, vision, and the client's preferences. Cognition and motivation are also essential. Clients whose cognitive function is impaired or whose illness alters energy levels and motivation will usually need more assistance. It is important for the nurse to determine the client's functional level and to maintain and promote as much client independence as possible. This also enables the nurse to identify the client's potential for growth and rehabilitation. There are several models of functional levels of self-care.

The presence of past or current skin problems alerts the nurse to specific nursing interventions or referrals the client may require. Many skin care conditions have implications for hygienic care. The client may provide descriptions of these problems during the nursing health history, or the nurse may observe some during the physical examination that follows. Common skin problems and implications for nursing interventions are shown in Table 22–2.

Physical Assessment

Physical assessment of the skin, which involves inspection and palpation, is described in Chapter 17 ∞. When assisting with bathing and other hygienic care, the nurse often has the opportunity to collect data about skin color, uniformity of color, texture, turgor, temperature, intactness, and lesions.

DIAGNOSING

Self-Care Deficit diagnoses are used for clients who have problems performing hygiene care. Three of NANDA's four self-care deficit diagnoses, specified as *Self-Care Deficit: Bathing/Hygiene, Self-Care Deficit: Dressing/Grooming,* and *Self-Care Deficit: Toileting* are discussed in this chapter. The fourth diagnosis, *Self-Care Deficit: Feeding,* is discussed in Chapter 32 ∞.

Difficulties encountered by the client in performing bathing activities include the inability to wash the body or body parts, to obtain or get to a water source, and to regulate water temperature or flow. Difficulties in dressing and grooming include inability to obtain, put on, take off, fasten, or replace articles of clothing; and to maintain appearance at a satisfactory level. Toileting problems may involve difficulties getting to the toilet or commode or sitting on and rising from it. In addition, the client may experience problems manipulating clothing for toileting, carrying out proper toilet hygiene, or flushing the toilet or emptying the commode. The reasons (etiologies or related factors) for these problems are varied.

TABLE 22–2 Common Skin Problems

PROBLEM AND APPEARANCE	NURSING IMPLICATIONS
Abrasion Superficial layers of the skin are scraped or rubbed away. Area is reddened and may have localized bleeding or serous weeping.	1. Prone to infection; therefore, wound should be kept clean and dry. 2. Do not wear rings or jewelry when providing care to avoid causing abrasions to clients. 3. Lift, do not pull, a client across a bed. 4. Use two or more people for assistance.
Excessive Dryness Skin can appear flaky and rough.	1. Prone to infection if the skin cracks; therefore, provide alcohol-free lotions to moisturize the skin and prevent cracking. 2. Bathe client less frequently; use no soap, or use nonirritating soap and limit its use. Rinse skin thoroughly because soap can be irritating and drying. 3. Encourage increased fluid intake if health permits to prevent dehydration.
Ammonia Dermatitis (Diaper Rash) Caused by skin bacteria reacting with urea in the urine. The skin becomes reddened and is sore.	1. Keep skin dry and clean by applying protective ointments containing zinc oxide to areas at risk (e.g., buttocks and perineum). 2. Boil an infant's diapers or wash them with an antibacterial detergent to prevent infection. Rinse diapers well because detergent is irritating to an infant's skin.
Acne Inflammatory condition with papules and pustules.	1. Keep the skin clean to prevent secondary infection. 2. Treatment varies widely.
Erythema Redness associated with a variety of conditions, such as rashes, exposure to sun, elevated body temperature.	1. Wash area carefully to remove excess microorganisms. 2. Apply antiseptic spray or lotion to prevent itching, promote healing, and prevent skin breakdown.
Hirsutism Excessive hair on a person's body and face, particularly in women.	1. Remove unwanted hair by using depilatories, shaving, electrolysis, or tweezing. 2. Enhance client's self-concept.

Examples of associated diagnoses include the following:

- *Deficient Knowledge* related to
  a. Lack of experience with skin condition (acne) and need to prevent secondary infection
  b. New therapeutic regimen to manage skin problems
  c. Lack of experience in providing hygiene care to dependent person
  d. Unfamiliarity with devices available to facilitate sitting on or rising from toilet
- *Situational Low Self-Esteem* related to
  a. Visible skin problem (e.g., acne or alopecia)
  b. Body odor

The diagnoses *Risk for Impaired Skin Integrity* and *Impaired Skin Integrity* are discussed in Chapter 24 ∞.

PLANNING

In planning care, the nurse and, if appropriate, the client and/or family set outcomes for each nursing diagnosis. The nurse then performs nursing interventions and activities to achieve the client outcomes.

The specific, detailed nursing activities taken by the nurse may include assisting dependent clients with bathing, skin care, and perineal care; providing back massages to promote circulation; instructing clients/families about appropriate hygienic practices and alternative methods for dressing; and demonstrating use of assistive equipment and adaptive activities. Although the nursing interventions discussed in this chapter focus on hygienic measures, the etiology of the nursing diagnoses established may point to other interventions that promote circulation, promote self-esteem, restore nutritional status, correct fluid deficits or excesses, or prevent problems associated with immobility. Nursing strategies to deal with these etiologies are provided in other chapters.

Planning to assist a client with personal hygiene includes consideration of the client's personal preferences, health, and limitations; the best time to give the care; and the equipment, facilities, and personnel available. A client's personal preferences—about when and how to bathe, for example—should be followed as long as they are compatible with the client's health and the equipment available. Another consideration for the nurse is to assess the client's comfort level with the gender of the caregiver.

Hygienic care, particularly bathing, can be embarrassing and stressful to modest individuals. Women in some cultures are generally modest. Nurses must respect a person's modesty, whether male or female, and provide adequate privacy and sensitivity. If possible, try to provide a caregiver of the same gender (Purnell & Paulanka, 2005). Nurses need to provide whatever assistance the client requires, either directly or by delegating this task to other nursing personnel.

IMPLEMENTING

The nurse applies the general guidelines for skin care while providing one of the various types of baths available to clients. Skill 22–1 describes how to bathe an adult or pediatric client.

General Guidelines for Skin Care

1. *An intact, healthy skin is the body's first line of defense.* Nurses need to ensure that all skin care measures prevent injury and irritation. Scratching the skin with jewelry or long, sharp fingernails must be avoided. Harsh rubbing or use of rough towels and washcloths can cause tissue damage, particularly when the skin is irritated or when circulation or sensation is diminished. Bottom bedsheets are kept taut and free from wrinkles to reduce friction and abrasion to the skin. Top bed linens are arranged to prevent undue pressure on the toes. When necessary, bed cradles on footboards are used to keep bedclothes off the feet.

2. *The degree to which the skin protects the underlying tissues from injury depends on the general health of the cells, the amount of subcutaneous tissue, and the dryness of the skin.* Skin that is poorly nourished and dry is less easily protected and more vulnerable to injury. When the skin is dry, lotions or creams with lanolin can be applied, and bathing is limited to once or twice a

week because frequent bathing removes the natural oils of the skin and causes dryness.

3. *Moisture in contact with the skin for more than a short time can result in increased bacterial growth and irritation.* After a bath, the client's skin is dried carefully. Particular attention is paid to areas such as the axillae, the groin, beneath the breasts, and between the toes, where the potential for irritation is greatest. A nonirritating dusting powder tends to reduce moisture and can be applied to these areas after they are dried. Clients who are incontinent of urine or feces or who perspire excessively are provided with immediate skin care to prevent skin irritation.

4. *Body odors are caused by resident skin bacteria acting on body secretions.* Cleanliness is the best deodorant. Commercial deodorants and antiperspirants can be applied only after the skin is cleaned. Deodorants diminish odors, whereas antiperspirants reduce the amount of perspiration. Neither is applied immediately after shaving, because of the possibility of skin irritation, nor are they used on skin that is already irritated.

5. *Skin sensitivity to irritation and injury varies among individuals and in accordance with their health.* Generally speaking, skin sensitivity is greater in infants, very young children, and older people. A person's nutritional status also affects sensitivity. Emaciated and obese persons tend to experience more skin irritation and injury. The same tendency is seen in individuals with poor dietary habits and insufficient fluid intake. Even in healthy persons, skin sensitivity is highly variable. Some people's skin is sensitive to chemicals in skin care agents and cosmetics. Hypoallergenic cosmetics and soaps or soap substitutes are now available for these people. The nurse needs to ascertain whether the client has any sensitivities and what agents are appropriate to use.

6. *Agents used for skin care have selective actions and purposes.* Commonly used agents are described in Table 22–3.

TABLE 22–3	Agents Commonly Used on the Skin	
Soap	Lowers surface tension and thus helps in cleaning. Some soaps contain antibacterial agents, which can change the natural flora of the skin.
Detergent	Used instead of soap for cleaning. Some people who are allergic to soaps may not be allergic to detergents, and vice versa. Do not use on older clients.
Bath oil	Used in bathwater; provides an oily film on the skin that softens and prevents chapping. Oils can make the tub surface slippery, and clients should be instructed about safety measures (e.g., using nonskid tub surface or mat).
Skin cream, lotion	Provides a film on the skin that prevents evaporation and therefore chapping.
Powder	Can be used to absorb water and prevent friction. For example, powder under the breasts can prevent skin irritation. Some powders are antibacterial.
Deodorant	Masks or diminishes body odors.
Antiperspirant	Reduces the amount of perspiration.

Bathing

Bathing removes accumulated oil, perspiration, dead skin cells, and some bacteria. The nurse can appreciate the quantity of oil and dead skin cells produced when observing a person after the removal of a cast in place for 6 weeks. The skin is crusty, flaky, and dry underneath the cast. An application of oil over several days is usually necessary to remove the debris.

Excessive bathing, however, can interfere with the intended lubricating effect of the sebum, causing dryness of the skin. This is an important consideration, especially for older adults, who produce less sebum.

In addition to cleaning the skin, bathing also stimulates circulation. A warm or hot bath dilates superficial arterioles, bringing more blood and nourishment to the skin. Vigorous rubbing has the same effect. Rubbing with long smooth strokes from the distal to proximal parts of extremities (from the point farthest from the body to the point closest) is particularly effective in facilitating venous blood flow unless there is some underlying condition that would preclude this.

Bathing also produces a sense of well-being. It is refreshing and relaxing and frequently improves morale, appearance, and self-respect. Some people take a morning shower for its refreshing, stimulating effect. Others prefer an evening bath because it is relaxing. These effects are more evident when a person is ill.

Bathing offers an excellent opportunity for the nurse to assess all clients. The nurse can observe the condition of the client's skin and physical conditions such as sacral edema or rashes. While assisting a client with a bath, the nurse can also assess the client's psychosocial needs, such as orientation to time and ability to cope with the illness. Learning needs, such as a diabetic client's need to learn foot care, can also be assessed.

CATEGORIES Two categories of baths are given to clients: cleaning and therapeutic. **Cleaning baths** are given chiefly for hygiene purposes and include these types:

- *Complete bed bath:* The nurse washes the entire body of a dependent client in bed.
- *Self-help bed bath:* Clients confined to bed are able to bathe themselves with help from the nurse for washing the back and perhaps the feet.
- *Partial bath (abbreviated bath):* Only the parts of the client's body that might cause discomfort or odor, if neglected, are washed: the face, hands, axillae, perineal area, and back. Omitted are the arms, chest, abdomen, legs, and feet. The nurse provides this care for dependent clients and assists self-sufficient clients confined to bed by washing their backs. Some ambulatory clients prefer to take a partial bath at the sink. The nurse can assist them by washing their backs.
- *Bag bath:* This bath is a commercially prepared product that contains 10 to 12 presoaked disposable washcloths that contain no-rinse cleanser solution.

The package is warmed in a microwave. The warming time is about 1 minute, but the nurse needs to determine how long it takes to attain a desirable temperature. Each area of the body is cleaned with a different cloth and then air dried. Because the body is not rubbed dry, the emollient in the solution remains on the skin.
- *Tub bath:* Tub baths are often preferred to bed baths because it is easier to wash and rinse in a tub. Tubs are also used for therapeutic baths. The amount of assistance the nurse offers depends on the abilities of the client. There are specially designed tubs for dependent clients. These tubs greatly reduce the work of the nurse in lifting clients in and out of the tub and offer greater benefits than a sponge bath in bed.

Sponge baths are suggested for the newborn because daily tub baths are not considered necessary. After the bath, the infant should be immediately dried and wrapped to prevent heat loss. Parents need to be advised that the infant's ability to regulate body temperature has not yet fully developed. Infants perspire minimally, and shivering starts at a lower temperature than it does in adults; therefore, infants lose more heat before shivering begins. In addition, because the infant's body surface area is very large in relation to body mass, the body loses heat readily.

- *Shower:* Many ambulatory clients are able to use shower facilities and require only minimal assistance from the nurse. Clients in long-term care settings are often given showers with the aid of a shower chair. The wheels on the shower chair allow clients to be transported from their room to the shower. The shower chair also has a commode seat to facilitate cleansing of the client's perineal area during the shower process.

The water for a bath should feel comfortably warm to the client. People vary in their sensitivity to heat; generally, the temperature should be 43°C to 46°C (110°F to 115°F). Most clients will verify a suitable temperature. Clients with decreased circulation or cognitive problems will not be able to verify the temperature. Therefore, the nurse must check the water temperature to avoid burning the client with water that is too hot. The water for a bed bath should be changed when it becomes dirty or cold.

Therapeutic baths are given for physical effects, such as to soothe irritated skin or to treat an area. Medications may be placed in the water. A therapeutic bath is generally taken in a tub one-third or one-half full. The client remains in the bath for a designated time, often 20 to 30 minutes. If the client's back, chest, and arms are to be treated, these areas need to be immersed in the solution. The bath temperature is generally included in the order; 37.7°C to 46°C (100°F to 115°F) may be ordered for adults, and 40.5°C (105°F) is usually ordered for infants. Skill 22–1 provides guidelines for bathing clients.

SKILL 22–1

BATHING AN ADULT OR PEDIATRIC CLIENT

PURPOSES
- To remove transient microorganisms, body secretions and excretions, and dead skin cells
- To stimulate circulation to the skin
- To promote a sense of well-being
- To produce relaxation and comfort
- To prevent and eliminate unpleasant body odors

ASSESSMENT
- Condition of the skin (color, texture and turgor, presence of pigmented spots, temperature, lesions, excoriations, abrasions, and bruises)
- Physical or emotional factors (e.g., fatigue, sensitivity to cold, need for control, anxiety or fear)
- Presence of pain and need for adjunctive measures (e.g., an analgesic) before the bath
- Range of motion of the joints
- Any other aspect of health that may affect the client's bathing process (e.g., mobility, strength, cognition)

PLANNING

Delegation

The nurse often delegates the skill of bathing to UAP. However, the nurse remains responsible *for assessment and client care.* The nurse needs to do the following:

- Inform the UAP of the type of bath appropriate for the client and precautions, if any, specific to the needs of the client.
- Remind the UAP to notify the nurse of any concerns or changes (e.g., redness, skin breakdown, rash) so the nurse can assess, intervene if needed, and document.
- Instruct the UAP to encourage the client to perform as much self-care as appropriate in order to promote independence and self-esteem.
- Obtain a complete report about the bathing experience from the UAP.

EQUIPMENT
- Basin or sink with warm water (between 43°C and 46°C or 110°F and 115°F)
- Soap and soap dish
- Linens: bath blanket, two bath towels, washcloth, clean gown or pajamas or clothes as needed, additional bed linen and towels, if required
- Gloves, if appropriate (e.g., presence of body fluids or open lesions)
- Personal hygiene articles (e.g., deodorant, powder, lotions)
- Shaving equipment
- Table for bathing equipment
- Laundry bag

IMPLEMENTATION

Preparation

Before bathing a client, determine (a) the purpose and type of bath the client needs; (b) self-care ability of the client; (c) any movement or positioning precautions specific to the client; (d) other care the client may be receiving, such as physical therapy or x-rays, in order to coordinate all aspects of health care and prevent unnecessary fatigue; (e) the client's comfort level with being bathed by someone else; and (f) necessary bath equipment and linens.

Caution is needed when bathing clients who are receiving intravenous therapy. Easy-to-remove gowns that have Velcro or snap fasteners along the sleeves may be used. If a special gown is not available, the nurse needs to pay special attention when changing the client's gown after the bath (or whenever the gown becomes soiled).

Performance

1. Prior to performing the procedure, introduce self and verify the client's identity using agency protocol. Explain to the client what you are going to do, why it is necessary, and how he or she can participate. Discuss with the client the plan for bathing and explain any unfamiliar procedures to the client.
2. Perform hand hygiene and observe other appropriate infection control procedures.
3. Provide for client privacy by drawing the curtains around the bed or closing the door to the room. Some agencies provide signs indicating the need for privacy. **Rationale:** *Hygiene is a personal matter.*

4. Prepare the client and the environment.
   - Invite a family member or significant other to participate if desired.
   - Close windows and doors to ensure the room is a comfortable temperature. **Rationale:** *Air currents increase loss of heat from the body by convection.*
   - Offer the client a bedpan or urinal or ask whether the client wishes to use the toilet or commode. **Rationale:** *Warm water and activity can stimulate the need to void. The client will be more comfortable after voiding, and voiding before cleaning the perineum is advisable.*
   - Encourage the client to perform as much personal self-care as possible. **Rationale:** *This promotes independence, exercise, and self-esteem.*
   - During the bath, assess each area of the skin carefully.

FOR A BED BATH

5. Prepare the bed and position the client appropriately.
   - Position the bed at a comfortable working height. Lower the side rail on the side close to you. Keep the other side rail *up.* Assist the client to move near you. **Rationale:** *This avoids undue reaching and straining and promotes good body mechanics.*
   - Place a bath blanket over the top sheet. Remove the top sheet from under the bath blanket by starting at the client's shoulders and moving linen down toward the client's feet. Ask the client to grasp and hold the top of the bath blanket while pulling linen to the foot of the bed. **Rationale:** *The bath blanket provides comfort,*

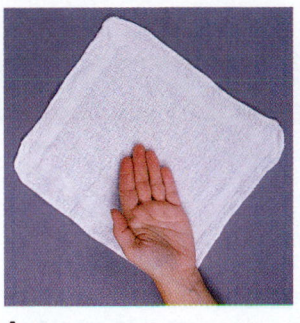 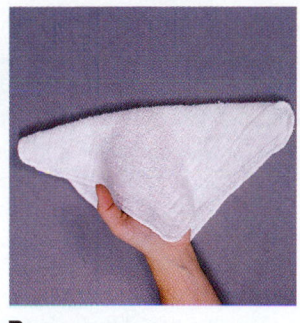 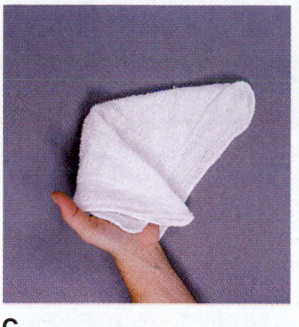 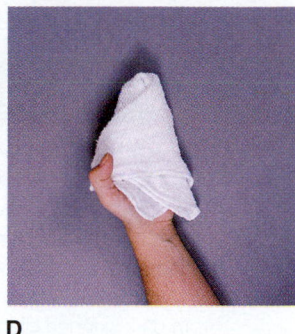

A **B** **C** **D**

❶ Making a bath mitt, triangular method. **A,** Lay your hand on the washcloth; **B,** fold the top corner over your hand; **C,** fold the side corners over your hand; **D,** tuck the second corner under the cloth on the palm side to secure the mitt.

warmth, and privacy. Note: If the bed linen is to be reused, place it over the bedside chair. If it is to be changed, place it in the linen hamper, not on the floor.
- Remove client's gown while keeping the client covered with the bath blanket. Place gown in linen hamper.

6. Make a bath mitt with the washcloth. **Rationale:** *A bath mitt retains water and heat better than a cloth loosely held and prevents ends of washcloth from dragging across the skin.* See ❶ for the triangular method.

7. Wash the face. **Rationale:** *Begin the bath at the cleanest area and work downward toward the feet.*
- Place towel under client's head.
- Wash the client's eyes with water only and dry them well. Use a separate corner of the washcloth for each eye. **Rationale:** *Using separate corners prevents transmitting microorganisms from one eye to the other.* Wipe from the inner to the outer canthus. **Rationale:** *This prevents secretions from entering the nasolacrimal ducts.*
- Ask whether the client wants soap used on the face. **Rationale:** *Soap has a drying effect, and the face, which is exposed to the air more than other body parts, tends to be drier.*
- Wash, rinse, and dry the client's face, ears, and neck.
- Remove the towel from under the client's head.

8. Wash the arms and hands. (Omit the arms for a partial bath.)
- Place a towel lengthwise under the arm away from you. **Rationale:** *It protects the bed from becoming wet.*
- Wash, rinse, and dry the arm by elevating the client's arm and supporting the client's wrist and elbow. Use long, firm strokes from wrist to shoulder, including the axillary area. **Rationale:** *Firm strokes from distal to proximal areas promote circulation by increasing venous blood return.*
- Apply deodorant or powder if desired.
- (Optional) Place a towel on the bed and put a washbasin on it. Place the client's hands in the basin. **Rationale:** *Many clients enjoy immersing their hands in the basin and washing themselves. Soaking loosens dirt under the nails.* Assist the client as needed to wash, rinse, and dry the hands, paying particular attention to the spaces between the fingers.
- Repeat for hand and arm nearest you. Exercise caution if an intravenous infusion is present, and check its flow after moving the arm.

9. Wash the chest and abdomen. (Omit the chest and abdomen for a partial bath. However, the areas under a woman's breast may require bathing if this area is irritated or if the client has significant perspiration under the breast.)
- Place the bath towel lengthwise over the chest. Fold the bath blanket down to the client's pubic area. **Rationale:** *This keeps the client warm while preventing unnecessary exposure of the chest.*
- Lift the bath towel off the chest, and bathe the chest and abdomen with your mitted hand using long, firm strokes. Give special attention to the skin under the breasts and any other skin folds particularly if the client is overweight. Rinse and dry well.
- Replace the bath blanket when the areas have been dried.

10. Wash the legs and feet. (Omit legs and feet for a partial bath.)
- Expose the leg farthest from you by folding the bath blanket toward the other leg being careful to keep the perineum covered. **Rationale:** *Covering the perineum promotes privacy and maintains the client's dignity.*
- Lift leg and place the bath towel lengthwise under the leg. Wash, rinse, and dry the leg using long, smooth, firm strokes from the ankle to the knee to the thigh. **Rationale:** *Washing from the distal to proximal areas promotes circulation by stimulating venous blood flow.*
- Reverse the coverings and repeat for the other leg.
- Wash the feet by placing them in the basin of water. ❷

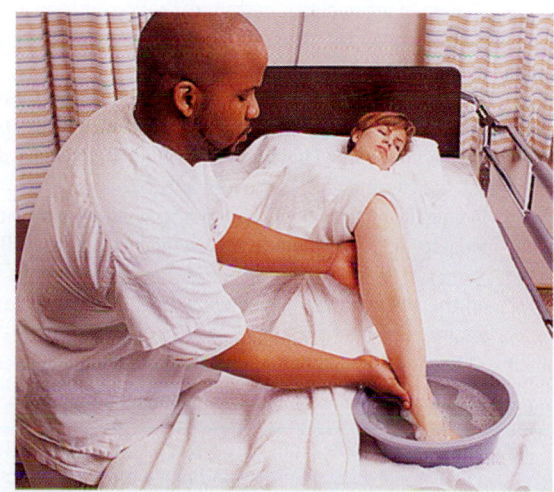

❷ Soaking a foot in a basin.

(continued)

BATHING AN ADULT OR PEDIATRIC CLIENT *(continued)*

- Dry each foot. Pay particular attention to the spaces between the toes. If preferred, wash one foot after that leg before washing the other leg.
- Obtain fresh, warm bath water now or when necessary. **Rationale:** *Water may become dirty or cold.* Because surface skin cells are removed with washing, the bathwater from dark-skinned clients may be dark, however, this does not mean the client is dirty. Lower the bed when refilling basin. **Rationale:** *This ensures the safety of the client.*

11. Wash the back and then the perineum.
    - Assist the client into a prone or side-lying position facing away from you. Place the bath towel lengthwise alongside the back and buttocks while keeping the client covered with the bath blanket as much as possible. **Rationale:** *This provides warmth and prevents undue exposure.*
    - Wash and dry the client's back, moving from the shoulders to the buttocks, and upper thighs, paying attention to the gluteal folds.
    - Perform a back massage now or after completion of bath. (See Skill 18–1 in Chapter 18 ∞.)
    - Assist the client to the supine position and determine whether the client can wash the perineal area independently. If the client cannot do so, drape the client as shown in Skill 22–2 and wash the area.

12. Assist the client with grooming aids such as powder, lotion, or deodorant.
    - Use powder sparingly. Release as little as possible into the atmosphere. **Rationale:** *This will avoid irritation of the respiratory tract by powder inhalation. Excessive powder can cause caking, which leads to skin irritation.*
    - Help the client put on a clean gown or pajamas.
    - Assist the client to care for hair, mouth, and nails. Some people prefer or need mouth care prior to their bath.

FOR A TUB BATH OR SHOWER

13. Prepare the client and the tub.
    - Fill the tub about one-third to one-half full of water at 43°C to 46°C (110°F to 115°F). **Rationale:** *Sufficient water is needed to cover the perineal area.*
    - Cover all intravenous catheters or wound dressings with plastic coverings, and instruct the client to prevent wetting these areas if possible.
    - Put a rubber bath mat or towel on the floor of the tub if safety strips are not on the tub floor. **Rationale:** *These prevent slippage of the client during the bath or shower.*

14. Assist the client into the shower or tub.
    - Assist the client taking a standing shower with the initial adjustment of the water temperature and water flow pressure, as needed. Some clients need a chair to sit on in the shower because of weakness. Hot water can cause older people to feel faint.
    - If the client requires considerable assistance with a tub bath, a hydraulic bathtub chair may be required (see "Variation").
    - Explain how the client can signal for help, leave the client for 2 to 5 minutes, and place an "occupied" sign on the door. For safety reasons, do not leave a client

with decreased cognition or clients who may be at risk (e.g., history of seizures, syncope).

15. Assist the client with washing and getting out of the tub.
    - Wash the client's back, lower legs, and feet, if necessary.
    - Assist the client out of the tub. If the client is unsteady, place a bath towel over the client's shoulders and drain the tub of water before the client attempts to get out of it. **Rationale:** *Draining the water first lessens the likelihood of a fall. The towel prevents chilling.*

16. Dry the client, and assist with follow-up care.
    - Follow step 12.
    - Assist the client back to his or her bed.
    - Clean the tub or shower in accordance with agency practice, discard the used linen in the laundry hamper, and place the "unoccupied" sign on the door.

17. Document
    - Type of bath given (i.e., complete, partial, or self-help). This is usually recorded on a flow sheet.
    - Skin assessment, such as excoriation, erythema, exudates, rashes, drainage, or skin breakdown.
    - Nursing interventions related to skin integrity.
    - Ability of the client to assist or cooperate with bathing.
    - Client response to bathing.
    - Educational needs regarding hygiene.
    - Information or teaching shared with the client or the family.

VARIATION: BATHING USING A HYDRAULIC BATHTUB CHAIR

A hydraulic lift, often used in long-term care or rehabilitation settings, can facilitate the transfer of a client who is unable to ambulate to a tub. The lift also helps eliminate strain on the nurse's back.

- Bring the client to the tub room in a wheelchair or shower chair.
- Fill the tub and check the water temperature with a bath thermometer *to avoid thermal injury to the client.*
- Lower the hydraulic chair lift to its lowest point, outside the tub.
- Transfer the client to the chair lift and secure the seat belt. ❸
- Raise the chair lift above the tub.

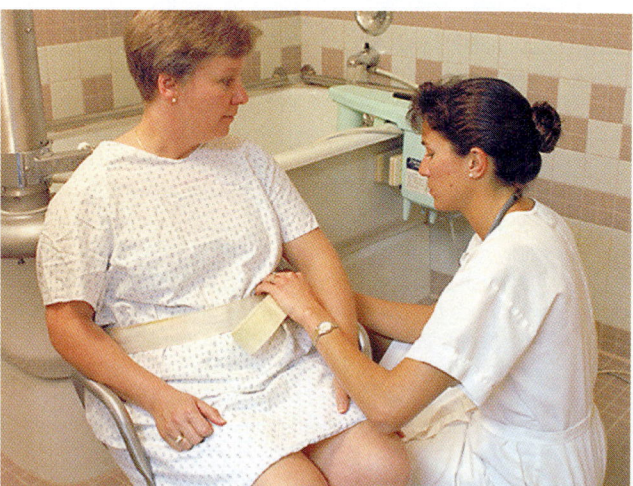

❸ Secure the seat belt before moving the client in a hydraulic bathtub chair.

- Support the client's legs as the chair is moved over the tub *to avoid injury to the legs.*
- Position the client's legs down into the water and slowly lower the chair lift into the tub.

- Assist in bathing the client, if appropriate.
- Reverse the procedure when taking the client out of the tub.
- Dry the client and transport him or her to the room.

EVALUATION

- Note the client's tolerance of the procedure (e.g., respiratory rate and effort, pulse rate, behaviors of acceptance or resistance, statements regarding comfort).
- Conduct appropriate follow-up, such as:
  - Condition and integrity of skin (dryness, turgor, redness, lesions, and so on).

- Client strength.
- Percentage of bath done without assistance.
- Relate to prior assessment data, if available.

LIFESPAN CONSIDERATIONS   Bathing

Infants

- Sponge baths are suggested for the newborn because daily tub baths are not considered necessary. After the bath, the infant should be immediately dried and wrapped. Parents need to be advised that the infant's ability to regulate body temperature has not yet fully developed and newborns' bodies lose heat readily.

Children

- Encourage a child's participation appropriate for developmental level.
- Closely supervise children in the bathtub. Do not leave them unattended.

Adolescents

- Assist adolescents as needed to choose deodorants and antiperspirants. Secretions from newly active sweat glands react with bacteria on the skin, causing a pungent odor.

Older Adults

- Changes of aging can decrease the protective function of the skin in older adults. These changes include fragile skin, less oil and moisture, and a decrease in elasticity.
- To minimize skin dryness in older adults, avoid excessive use of soap. The ideal time to moisturize the skin is immediately after bathing.
- Avoid powder because it causes moisture loss and is a hazardous inhalant. Cornstarch should also be avoided because in the presence of moisture it breaks down into glucose and can facilitate the growth of organisms.
- Protect older adults and children from injury related to hot water burns.

LONG-TERM CARE CONSIDERATIONS
Hygiene

Assess:

- Cultural considerations and preferences of the client in regard to bathing and hygiene needs.
- Client's self-care ability.
- Client's skin for any altered integrity, condition, and hydration status to determine frequency of bathing.

When bathing the resident:

- Avoid making bath-time a routine depersonalized time. During the bath, talk with client and learn about any concerns or issues. This can be an excellent time to learn more about the client.
- Clients who become aggressive or combative during a bath may be reacting to feeling depersonalized. Involve the client in the process, even if total care is required.
- Carefully monitor the temperature of the bathwater and refresh the water when it gets cold. Older residents are more temperature insensitive.

LONG-TERM CARE SETTING From a historical perspective, the bath has always been a part of nursing care and considered a component of the "art" of nursing. In today's nursing world, however, the bath is seen as a necessary, routine task and is often delegated to nonprofessionals.

In spite of the previously listed beneficial values associated with bathing, the choice of bathing procedure often depends on the amount of time available to the nurse or unlicensed assistive personnel (UAP) and the client's self-care ability. Nursing authors (Barrick & Rader, 2000; Dunn, Thiru-Chelvam, & Beck, 2002; Rader et al., 2006; Rasin & Barrick, 2004) have challenged nurses to switch from a task-centered approach to a person-centered approach to bathing, especially for the older person in a long-term care setting. The bath routine (e.g., day, time, and number/week) for clients in health care settings is often determined by agency policy, which often results in the bath becoming routine and depersonalized versus therapeutic, satisfying, and person focused.

Rader et al. (2006) encourage nurses in the long-term care setting to view the bath from the individual's perspective. Rader, who was showered during a preliminary study, realized that behaviors previously labeled "aggressive" or "resistive" were actually defensive actions from feeling threatened and anxious during a cold and distressing shower experience (p. 44). A nurse who provides person-centered care asks such questions as: What is the client's usual method of maintaining cleanliness? Are there any past negative experiences related to bathing? Are factors such as pain or fatigue increasing the client's difficulty with the demands and stimuli associated with bathing or showering? A client's resistance to the bathing experience can be a cue to the nurse to consider other methods of maintaining cleanliness. For example, if the shower causes distress, is there another form of bathing (such as the bag bath) that may be more therapeutic and comforting?

An individualized approach focusing on therapeutic and comforting outcomes of bathing is especially important for clients with dementia. Alzheimer's disease is the most common cause of dementia among people age 65 and older. Given the current population trends, it is estimated that 14 million Americans will have Alzheimer's disease by 2050 (Alzheimer's Disease Education & Referral Center, n.d.). This statistic has implications for nursing care. For example, Rasin and Barrick (2004) reported that in an observational study of people with dementia, more than 90% became agitated as soon as they were told it was time to bathe (p. 30). See Box 22–1 for possible strategies that can reduce the stress of the bathing experience for both the person with dementia and the caregiver.

Providing personal hygiene to clients with dementia is often an ongoing challenge. Being sensitive to the rhythm of their behavior and looking for cues can often offset problems related to this. Clients with dementia, whether they are at home or in a health care facility, often have certain times of the day when they are more agitated—these are times to avoid doing things that will increase their fear and agitation. It is sometimes helpful to wait (e.g., half an hour or so) and then try giving the bath because they may forget that they were protesting and be willing to participate.

In addition, collaboration between the nurse and UAP is a critical element to implementing the individualized person-focused approach for cognitively impaired clients who exhibit aggressive behavior during bathing. The nurse, after observing a difficult bathing situation, should discuss with the UAP possible alternative strategies or methods they might implement for the client. More than one intervention may be required. It is important for the nurse to subsequently evaluate the person's response to the new intervention(s).

PERINEAL-GENITAL CARE Perineal-genital care is also referred to as *perineal care* or *pericare*. Perineal care as part of the bed bath is embarrassing for many clients. Nurses may also find it embarrassing initially, particularly with clients of the opposite sex. Most clients who require a bed bath from the nurse are able to clean their own genital areas with minimal assistance. The nurse may need to hand a moistened washcloth and soap to the client, rinse the washcloth, and provide a towel.

Because some clients are unfamiliar with terminology for the genitals and perineum, it may be difficult for nurses to explain what is expected. Most clients, however, understand what is meant if the nurse simply says, "I'll give you a washcloth to finish your bath." The nurse needs to provide perineal care efficiently and matter-of-factly. Nurses should wear gloves while providing this care for the comfort of the client and to protect themselves from infection. Skill 22–2 explains how to provide perineal-genital care.

BOX 22–1   **General Guidelines for Bathing Persons with Dementia**

- Focus on the person rather than the task.
  - Cover! Keep the person covered as much as possible to keep him or her warm.
  - Time the bath to fit the person's history, preferences, and mood.
  - Move slowly and let the person know when you are going to move him or her.
  - Evaluate to determine if the person needs pain control before the bath.
  - Use a gentle touch. Use soft cloths. Pat dry rather than rubbing.
- Be flexible. Adapt your approach to meet the needs of the person.
  - Consider adapting your methods (e.g., distracting the person with singing while bathing), the environment (e.g., correct size of shower chair, reducing noise, playing music), and the procedure (e.g., consistently assigning same caregiver, inviting family to help).
  - Encourage flexibility in scheduling of bath based on person's preference.
- Use persuasion, not coercion.
  - Give choices and respond to individual requests.

- Help the person feel in control.
  - Use a supportive, calm approach and praise the person often.
- Be prepared.
  - Gather everything that you will need for the bath (e.g., towels, washcloths, clothes) before approaching the person.
- Stop when a person becomes distressed. It is *not* normal to have cries, screams, or protests from the person.
  - Stop what you are doing and assess for causes of the distress.
  - Adjust your approach.
  - Shorten or stop the bath.
  - Try to end on a positive note.
  - Reapproach later to wash critical areas if necessary.
- Ask for help.
  - Talk with others, including the family, about different ways to help make the bath more comfortable for the person.

Note: Adapted From *Bathing Without a Battle: Personal Care of Individuals with Dementia*, by A. L. Barrick, J. Rader, B. Hoeffer, & P. D. Sloane, 2002. Copyright © 2002 Springer Publishing Company, Inc., New York, New York, 10036. Used by permission.

SKILL 22–2

PROVIDING PERINEAL-GENITAL CARE

PURPOSES

- To remove normal perineal secretions and odors
- To promote client comfort

ASSESSMENT

Assess for the presence of:

- Irritation, excoriation, inflammation, swelling
- Excessive discharge
- Odor; pain or discomfort
- Urinary or fecal incontinence
- Recent rectal or perineal surgery
- Indwelling catheter

Determine:

- Perineal-genital hygiene practices
- Self-care abilities

PLANNING

> **Delegation**
>
> Perineal-genital care can be delegated to UAP. If the client has recently had perineal, rectal, or genital surgery, the nurse needs to assess if it is appropriate for the UAP to perform perineal-genital care.

EQUIPMENT

Perineal-genital care provided in conjunction with the bed bath:

- Bath towel
- Bath blanket
- Clean gloves

- Bath basin with water at 43°C to 46°C (110°F to 115°F)
- Soap
- Washcloth

Special perineal-genital care:

- Bath towel
- Bath blanket
- Clean gloves
- Cotton balls or swabs
- Solution bottle, pitcher, or container filled with warm water or a prescribed solution
- Bedpan to receive rinse water
- Moisture-resistant bag or receptacle for used cotton swabs
- Perineal pad

IMPLEMENTATION

Preparation

- Determine whether the client is experiencing any discomfort in the perineal-genital area.
- Obtain and prepare the necessary equipment and supplies.

Performance

1. Prior to performing the procedure, introduce self and verify the client's identity using agency protocol. Explain to the client what you are going to do, why it is necessary, and how he or she can participate, being particularly sensitive to any embarrassment felt by the client.
2. Perform hand hygiene and observe other appropriate infection control procedures (e.g., clean gloves).
3. Provide for client privacy by drawing the curtains around the bed or closing the door to the room. Some agencies provide signs indicating the need for privacy. **Rationale:** *Hygiene is a personal matter.*
4. Prepare the client:
   - Fold the top bed linen to the foot of the bed and fold the gown up to expose the genital area.
   - Place a bath towel under the client's hips. **Rationale:** *The bath towel prevents the bed from becoming soiled.*
5. Position and drape the client and clean the upper inner thighs.

For Females

- Position the female in a back-lying position with the knees flexed and spread well apart.
- Cover her body and legs with the bath blanket positioned so a corner is at her head, the opposite corner at her feet, and the other two on the sides. Drape the legs by tucking the bottom corners of the bath blanket under the inner sides of

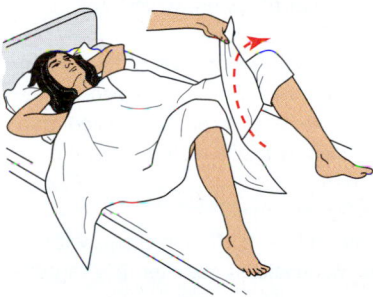

❶ Draping the client for perineal-genital care.

the legs. ❶ **Rationale:** *Minimum exposure lessens embarrassment and helps to provide warmth.* Bring the middle portion of the base of the blanket up over the pubic area.

- Put on gloves, wash and dry the upper inner thighs.

For Males

- Position the male client in a supine position with knees slightly flexed and hips slightly externally rotated.
- Put on gloves; wash and dry the upper inner thighs.
6. Inspect the perineal area.
   - Note particular areas of inflammation, excoriation, or swelling, especially between the labia in females and the scrotal folds in males.
   - Also note excessive discharge or secretions from the orifices and the presence of odors.
7. Wash and dry the perineal-genital area.

(continued)

SKILL 22–2

PROVIDING PERINEAL-GENITAL CARE *(continued)*

For Females

- Clean the labia majora. Then spread the labia to wash the folds between the labia majora and the labia minora. ❷ **Rationale:** *Secretions that tend to collect around the labia minora facilitate bacterial growth.*
- Use separate quarters of the washcloth for each stroke, and wipe from the pubis to the rectum. For menstruating women and clients with indwelling catheters, use clean wipes. Take a clean wipe for each stroke. **Rationale:** *Using separate quarters of the washcloth or new wipes prevents the transmission of microorganisms from one area to the other. Wipe from the area of least contamination (the pubis) to that of greatest (the rectum).*
- Rinse the area well. You may place the client on a bedpan and use a periwash or solution bottle to pour warm water over the area. Dry the perineum thoroughly, paying particular attention to the folds between the labia. **Rationale:** *Moisture supports the growth of many microorganisms.*

For Males

- Wash and dry the penis, using firm strokes.
- If the client is uncircumcised, retract the prepuce (foreskin) to expose the glans penis (the tip of the penis) for cleaning. Replace the foreskin after cleaning the glans penis. ❸ **Rationale:** *Retracting the foreskin is necessary to remove the smegma (thick, cheesy secretion) that collects under the foreskin and facilitates bacterial growth. Replacing the foreskin prevents constriction of the penis, which may cause edema.*
- Wash and dry the scrotum. The posterior folds of the scrotum may need to be cleaned when the buttocks are cleaned (see step 9). **Rationale:** *The scrotum tends to be more soiled than the penis because of its proximity to the rectum; thus it is usually cleaned after the penis.*
8. Inspect perineal orifices for intactness.
   - Inspect particularly around the urethra in clients with indwelling catheters. **Rationale:** *A catheter may cause excoriation around the urethra.*

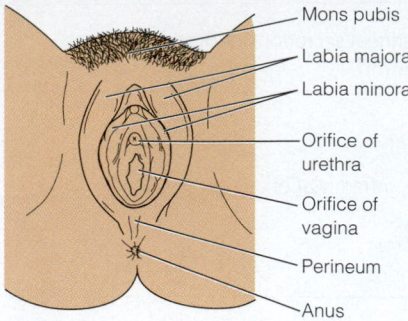

❷ Female genitals.

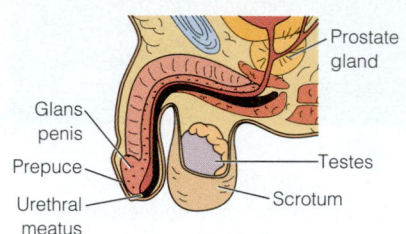

❸ Male genitals.

9. Clean between the buttocks.
   - Assist the client to turn onto the side facing away from you.
   - Pay particular attention to the anal area and posterior folds of the scrotum in males. Clean the anus with toilet tissue before washing it, if necessary.
   - Dry the area well.
   - For postdelivery or menstruating females, apply a perineal pad as needed from front to back. **Rationale:** *This prevents contamination of the vagina and urethra from the anal area.*
10. Document any unusual findings such as redness, excoriation, skin breakdown, discharge or drainage, and any localized areas of tenderness.

EVALUATION

- Relate current assessments to previous assessments.
- Conduct appropriate follow-up such as prescribed ointment for excoriation.
- Report any deviation from normal to the primary care provider.

CLINICAL ALERT

Always wash or wipe from "clean to dirty." For a female, cleanse the perineal area from front to back. For a male, cleanse the urinary meatus by moving in a circular motion from center of urethral opening around the glans.

CLIENT TEACHING Clients often need information about dry skin, skin rashes, and acne.

EVALUATING

Using data collected during care, the nurse judges whether desired outcomes have been achieved. If the outcomes are not achieved, the nurse explores reasons why. For example:

- Did the nurse overestimate the client's functional abilities (physical, mental, emotional) for self-care?
- Were provided instructions not clear?
- Were appropriate assistive devices or supplies not available to the client?

Skin Problems and Care

Dry Skin

- Use cleansing creams to clean the skin rather than soap or detergent, which cause drying and, in some cases, allergic reactions.
- Use bath oils, but take precautions to prevent falls caused by slippery tub surfaces.
- Thoroughly rinse soap or detergent, if used, from the skin.
- Bathe less frequently when environmental temperature and humidity are low.
- Increase fluid intake.
- Humidify the air with a humidifier or by keeping a tub or sink full of water.
- Use moisturizing or emollient creams that contain lanolin, petroleum jelly, or cocoa butter to retain skin moisture.

Skin Rashes

- Keep the area clean by washing it with a mild soap. Rinse the skin well, and pat it dry.

- To relieve itching, try a tepid bath or soak. Some over-the-counter preparations, such as Caladryl lotion, may help but should be used with full knowledge of the product.
- Avoid scratching the rash to prevent inflammation, infection, and further skin lesions.
- Choose clothing carefully. Too much can cause perspiration and aggravate a rash.

Acne

- Wash the face frequently with soap or detergent and hot water to remove oil and dirt.
- Avoid using oily creams, which aggravate the condition.
- Avoid using cosmetics that block the ducts of the sebaceous glands and the hair follicles.
- Never squeeze or pick at the lesions. This increases the potential for infection and scarring.

- Did the client's condition change?
- Were required analgesics provided before hygienic care?
- What currently prescribed medications and therapies could affect the client's abilities or tissue integrity?
- Is the client's fluid and food intake adequate or appropriate to maintain skin and mucous membrane moisture and integrity?

FEET

The feet are essential for ambulation and merit attention even when people are confined to bed. Each foot contains 26 bones, 107 ligaments, and 19 muscles. These structures function together for both standing and walking.

Developmental Variations

At birth, a baby's foot is relatively unformed. The arches are supported by fatty pads and do not take their full shape until 5 to 6 years of age. During childhood, the bones and small muscles of the feet are easily damaged by tight, binding stockings and ill-fitting shoes. For normal development, it is important that the arches be supported and that the bony structure and the feet grow with no external restrictions. Feet are not fully grown until about age 20. The average person takes 10,000 steps per day. Each step places 2 to 3 times the force of the body weight on the feet. This repetitive use leads to normal changes associated with aging. These include wider and longer feet, mild settling of the arches, and loss of natural padding on the bottom of the heels. The cartilage around the joints also deteriorates, producing loss of normal range of motion of the foot and ankle

(Pattillo, 2004, p. 27). All older persons should know about foot care. However, some older individuals require special attention for their feet. For example, reduced blood supply and accompanying arteriosclerosis can make a foot prone to ulcers and infection following trauma.

> **CLINICAL ALERT**
>
> Clients with diabetes are at high risk for lower extremity amputations (LEA). Routine foot assessment and client education in proper foot care can significantly reduce the risk for LEA.

NURSING MANAGEMENT

ASSESSING

Assessment of the client's feet includes a nursing health history, physical assessment of the feet, and identifying clients at risk for foot problems.

Nursing Health History

The nurse determines the client's history of (a) normal nail and foot care practices, (b) type of footwear worn, (c) self-care abilities, (d) presence of risk factors for foot problems, (e) any foot discomfort, and (f) any perceived problems with foot mobility.

Physical Assessment

Each foot and toe is inspected for shape, size, and presence of lesions and is palpated to assess areas of tenderness, edema, and circulatory status. Normally, the toes are straight

TABLE 22-4 Assessment of the Feet

METHOD	NORMAL FINDINGS	DEVIATIONS FROM NORMAL
Inspect all skin surfaces, particularly between the toes, for cleanliness, odor, dryness, inflammation, swelling, abrasions, or other lesions.	Intact skin	Excessive dryness
	Absence of swelling or inflammation	Areas of inflammation or swelling (e.g., corns, calluses)
		Fissures
		Scaling and cracking of skin (e.g., athlete's foot) Plantar warts
Palpate anterior and posterior surfaces of ankles and feet for edema.	No swelling	Swelling or pitting edema
Palpate the dorsalis pedis pulse on the dorsal surface of the foot.	Strong, regular pulses in both feet	Weak or absent pulses
Compare skin temperature of both feet.	Warm skin temperature	Cool skin temperature in one or both feet

and flat. Table 22–4 lists physical assessment methods for the feet. Common foot problems include calluses, corns, unpleasant odors, plantar warts, fissures between the toes, and fungal infections such as athlete's foot.

A **callus** is a thickened portion of epidermis, a mass of keratotic material. Most calluses are painless and flat and are found on the bottom or side of the foot over a bony prominence. Calluses are usually caused by pressure from shoes. They can be softened by soaking the foot in warm water with Epsom salts, and abraded with pumice stones or similar abrasives. Creams with lanolin help to keep the skin soft and prevent the formation of calluses.

A corn is a keratosis caused by friction and pressure from a shoe. It commonly occurs on the fourth or fifth toe, usually on a bony prominence such as a joint. Corns are usually conical (circular and raised). The base is the surface of the corn. The apex is in deeper tissues, sometimes even attached to bone. Corns are generally removed surgically. They are prevented from re-forming by relieving the pressure on the area (i.e., wearing comfortable shoes) and massaging the tissue to promote circulation. The use of oval corn pads should be avoided because they increase pressure and decrease circulation.

Unpleasant odors occur as a result of perspiration and its interaction with microorganisms. Regular and frequent washing of the feet and wearing clean hosiery help to minimize odor. Foot powders and deodorants also help to prevent this problem.

Fissures, or deep grooves, frequently occur between the toes as a result of dryness and cracking of the skin. The treatment of choice is good foot hygiene and application of an antiseptic to prevent infection. Often a small piece of gauze is inserted between the toes in applying the antiseptic and left in place to assist healing by allowing air to reach the area.

CLINICAL ALERT

Clients with diabetes often have extremely dry skin. Tell them to use a nonperfumed lotion and to avoid putting lotion between the toes. Advise to not soak their feet in water because it is drying to the skin.

An **ingrown toenail**, the growing inward of the nail into the soft tissues around it, most often results from improper nail trimming. Pressure applied to the area causes localized pain. Treatment involves frequent, hot antiseptic soaks and surgical removal of the portion of nail embedded in the skin. Preventing recurrence involves appropriate instruction and adherence to proper nail-trimming techniques.

Identifying Clients at Risk

Because of reduced peripheral circulation to the feet, clients with diabetes or peripheral vascular disease are particularly prone to infection if skin breakage occurs. Many foot problems can be prevented by teaching the client simple foot care guidelines (see Client Teaching).

DIAGNOSING

A number of nursing diagnoses may apply to clients with foot or foot care problems. The most common diagnostic labels, along with possible related or contributing factors, are as follows:

- *Self-Care Deficit: Hygiene* (foot care) related to
  a. Visual impairment
  b. Impaired hand coordination
  c. Other related or contributing factors
- *Risk for Impaired Skin Integrity* related to
  a. Altered tissue perfusion: peripheral (associated with edema, inadequate arterial circulation)
  b. Poorly fitting shoes
- *Risk for Infection* related to
  a. Impaired skin integrity (ingrown toenail, corn, trauma)
  b. Deficient nail or foot care
- *Deficient Knowledge* (diabetic foot care) related to
  a. Lack of teaching/learning activities about diabetic foot care
  b. Newly established medical diagnosis (diabetes) and necessary foot hygiene practices.

Examples of assessment data clusters, related nursing diagnoses, outcomes, and interventions are shown in Identifying Nursing Diagnoses, Outcomes, and Interventions.

CLIENT TEACHING   Foot Care

- Wash the feet daily, and dry them well, especially between the toes.
- When washing, inspect the skin of the feet for breaks or red or swollen areas. Use a mirror if needed to visualize all areas.
- To prevent burns, check the water temperature before immersing the feet.
- Cover the feet, except between the toes, with creams or lotions to moisten the skin. Lotion will also soften calluses. A lotion that reduces dryness effectively is a mixture of lanolin and mineral oil.
- To prevent or control an unpleasant odor due to excessive foot perspiration, wash the feet frequently and change socks and shoes at least daily. Special deodorant sprays or absorbent foot powders are also helpful.
- File the toenails rather than cutting them to avoid skin injury. File the nails straight across the ends of the toes. If the nails are too thick or misshapen to file, consult a podiatrist.
- Wear clean stockings or socks daily. Avoid socks with holes or darns that can cause pressure areas.
- Wear comfortable, well-fitting shoes that neither restrict the foot nor rub on any area; rubbing can cause corns and calluses. Check worn shoes for rough spots in the lining.

Break in new shoes gradually by increasing the wearing time 30 to 60 minutes each day.
- Avoid walking barefoot, because injury and infection may result. Wear slippers in public showers and in change areas to avoid contracting athlete's foot or other infections.
- Several times each day exercise the feet to promote circulation. Point the feet upward, point them downward, and move them in circles.
- Avoid wearing constricting garments such as knee-high elastic stockings and avoid sitting with the legs crossed at the knees, which may decrease circulation.
- When the feet are cold, use extra blankets and wear warm socks rather than using heating pads or hot water bottles, which may cause burns. Test bathwater before stepping into it.
- Wash any cut on the foot thoroughly, apply a mild antiseptic, and notify the primary care provider.
- Avoid self-treatment for corns or calluses. Pumice stones and some callus and corn applications are injurious to the skin. Do not cut calluses or corns. Consult a podiatrist or primary care provider first.
- Notify the primary care provider if you notice abnormal sores or drainage, pain, or changes in temperature, color, and sensation of the foot.

IDENTIFYING NURSING DIAGNOSES, OUTCOMES, AND INTERVENTIONS   Clients with Foot Problems

DATA CLUSTER Sally Brown, an 83-year-old widow, lives alone. Has home-maker services twice a week and Meals on Wheels service daily. Manages to shower once a week with daughter's help. Has pronounced hand tremors and obvious cataracts. States, "I can't see well enough to cut my nails and even if I could see, my hands shake so badly."

NURSING DIAGNOSIS/DEFINITION	SAMPLE DESIRED OUTCOME*/*DEFINITION*	INDICATORS	SELECTED INTERVENTIONS*/ *DEFINITION*	SAMPLE NIC ACTIVITIES
Self-Care Deficit: Hygiene (Foot Care) related to impaired hand coordination and visual impairment/*Impaired ability to perform or complete bathing/hygiene activities for oneself*	Self-Care: Hygiene [0305]/*Ability to maintain own personal cleanliness and kempt appearance independently with or without assistive device*	Severely compromised: • Cares for nails	Foot Care [1660]/ *Cleansing and inspecting the feet for the purposes of relaxation, cleanliness, and healthy skin*	• Inspect skin for irritation, cracking, lesions, corns, calluses, or edema • Instruct family on the importance of foot care • Cut normal-thickness toenails when soft, using a toenail clipper and using the curve of the toe as a guide • Refer to podiatrist for trimming of thickened nails, as appropriate

*The NOC # for desired outcomes and the NIC# for nursing interventions are listed in brackets following the appropriate outcome or intervention. Outcomes, indicators, interventions, and activities selected are only a sample of those suggested by NOC and NIC and should be further individualized for each client.

PLANNING

Planning involves (a) identifying nursing interventions that will help the client maintain or restore healthy foot care practices and (b) establishing desired outcomes for each client. Interventions may include teaching the client about correct nail and foot care, proper footwear, wearing the correct size, and ways to prevent potential foot problems (e.g., infection, injury, and decreased circulation). For clients with self-care difficulties, the nurse plans a schedule for soaking the client's feet and assisting with regular cleaning and trimming of nails (if not contraindicated). Foot and nail care is often provided during the client's bath but may be provided at any time in the day to accommodate the client's preference or schedule. The frequency of foot care is determined by the nurse and client and is based on objective assessment data and the client's specific problems. For some clients, the feet need to be bathed daily; for those whose feet perspire excessively, bathing more than once a day may be necessary.

IMPLEMENTING

Skill 22–3 describes how to provide foot care. See also the discussion of nails. During these procedures, the nurse has the opportunity to teach the client appropriate methods for foot care, that is, methods designed to prevent tissue injury and infection (see earlier Client Teaching feature).

SKILL 22–3

PROVIDING FOOT CARE

PURPOSES
- To maintain the skin integrity of the feet
- To prevent foot infections
- To prevent foot odors
- To assess or monitor foot problems

ASSESSMENT
Determine
- History of any problems with foot discomfort, foot odor, foot mobility, circulatory problems (e.g., swelling, changes in skin color and/or temperature, and pain), structural problems (e.g., bunion, hammer toe, or overlapping digits)
- Usual foot care practices (e.g., frequency of washing feet and cutting nails, foot hygiene products used, how often socks are changed, whether the client ever goes barefoot, whether the client sees a podiatrist)

Assess
- Skin surfaces for cleanliness, odor, dryness, and intactness
- Each foot and toe for shape, size, presence of lesions (e.g., corn, callus, wart, or rash), and areas of tenderness, ankle edema
- Skin temperatures of both feet to assess circulatory status
- Pedal pulses: dorsalis pedis and posterior tibialis
- Self-care abilities (e.g., any problems managing foot care)

PLANNING

Delegation
Foot care for the *nondiabetic* client can be delegated to UAP. Remind the UAP to notify the nurse of anything that looks out of the ordinary. Review with the UAP the agency policy about cutting or trimming nails.

EQUIPMENT
- Washbasin containing warm water
- Pillow
- Moisture-resistant disposable pad
- Towels
- Soap
- Washcloth
- Toenail cleaning and trimming equipment, if agency policy permits
- Lotion or foot powder

IMPLEMENTATION
Performance
1. Prior to performing the procedure, introduce self and verify the client's identity using agency protocol. Explain to the client what you are going to do, why it is necessary, and how he or she can participate.
2. Perform hand hygiene and observe other appropriate infection control procedures.
3. Provide for client privacy by drawing the curtains around the bed or closing the door to the room. Some agencies provide signs indicating the need for privacy. **Rationale:** *Hygiene is a personal matter.*
4. Prepare the equipment and the client.
   - Fill the washbasin with warm water at about 40°C to 43°C (105°F to 110°F). **Rationale:** *Warm water promotes circulation, comforts, and refreshes.*
   - Assist the ambulatory client to a sitting position in a chair, or the bed client to a supine or semi-Fowler's position.
   - Place a pillow under the bed client's knees. **Rationale:** *This provides support and prevents muscle fatigue.*
   - Place the washbasin on the moisture-resistant pad at the foot of the bed for a bed client or on the floor in front of the chair for an ambulatory client.
   - For a bed client, pad the rim of the washbasin with a towel. **Rationale:** *The towel prevents undue pressure on the skin.*
5. Wash the foot and soak it.
   - Place one of the client's feet in the basin and wash it with soap, paying particular attention to the interdigital areas. Prolonged soaking is generally not recommended

for diabetic clients or individuals with peripheral vascular disease. **Rationale:** *Prolonged soaking may remove natural skin oils, thus drying the skin and making it more susceptible to cracking and injury.*

- Rinse the foot well to remove soap. **Rationale:** *Soap irritates the skin if not completely removed.*
- Rub callused areas of the foot with the washcloth. **Rationale:** *This helps remove dead skin layers.*
- If the nails are brittle or thick and require trimming, replace the water and allow the foot to soak for 10 to 20 minutes. **Rationale:** *Soaking softens the nails and loosens debris under them.*
- Clean the nails as required with an orange stick. **Rationale:** *This removes excess debris that harbors microorganisms.*
- Remove the foot from the basin and place it on the towel.

6. Dry the foot thoroughly and apply lotion or foot powder.
   - Blot the foot gently with the towel to dry it thoroughly, particularly between the toes. **Rationale:** *Harsh rubbing can damage the skin. Thorough drying reduces the risk of infection.*

- Apply lotion or lanolin cream to the foot but not between the toes. **Rationale:** *This lubricates dry skin and keeps the area between the toes dry.*
      or
- Apply a foot powder containing a nonirritating deodorant if the feet tend to perspire excessively. **Rationale:** *Foot powders have greater absorbent properties than regular bath powders; some also contain menthol, which makes the feet feel cool.*

7. If agency policy permits, trim the nails of the first foot while the second foot is soaking.
   - See the discussion on nails for the appropriate method to trim nails. Note that in many agencies, toenail trimming requires a primary care provider's order or is contraindicated for clients with diabetes mellitus, toe infections, and peripheral vascular disease, unless performed by a podiatrist, general practice physician, or advanced practice provider such as a nurse practitioner.

8. Document any foot problems observed.
   - Foot care is not generally recorded unless problems are noted.
   - Record any signs of inflammation, infection, breaks in the skin, corns, troublesome calluses, bunions, and pressure areas. This is of particular importance for clients with peripheral vascular disease and diabetes.

EVALUATION
- Inspect nails and skin after the soak.
- Compare to prior assessment data.
- Report any abnormalities to the primary care provider.

EVALUATING

Examples of desired outcomes for foot hygiene include the client being able to:

- Participate in self-care (foot hygiene) to optimal level of capacity (specify).
- Describe hygienic and other interventions (e.g., proper footwear) to maintain skin integrity, prevent infection, and maintain peripheral tissue perfusion.
- Demonstrate optimal foot hygiene, as evidenced by:
  a. Intact, pink, smooth, soft, hydrated, and warm skin.
  b. Intact cuticles and skin surrounding nails.
  c. Correct foot care and nail care practices.

NAILS

Nails are normally present at birth. They continue to grow throughout life and change very little until people are older. At that time, the nails tend to be tougher, more brittle, and in some cases thicker. The nails of an older person normally grow less quickly than those of a younger person and may be ridged and grooved.

NURSING MANAGEMENT

ASSESSING

During the nursing health history, the nurse explores the client's usual nail care practices, self-care abilities, and any problems associated with them. Physical assessment involves inspection of the nails. See Chapter 17 ∞.

DIAGNOSING

Nursing diagnoses related to nail care and nail problems include *Self-Care Deficit* and *Risk for Infection.* Examples of these nursing diagnoses and contributing factors follow:

- *Self-Care Deficit: Grooming* related to
  a. Impaired vision
- *Risk for Infection* around the nail bed related to
  a. Impaired skin integrity of cuticles
  b. Altered peripheral circulation

PLANNING

The nurse identifies measures that will assist the client to develop or maintain healthy nail care practices. A schedule of nail care needs to be established.

IMPLEMENTING

To provide nail care, the nurse needs a nail cutter or sharp scissors, a nail file, an orange stick to push back the cuticle, hand lotion or mineral oil to lubricate any dry tissue around the nails, and a basin of water to soak the nails if they are particularly thick or hard. Check the agency's policy regarding nail care. Often, podiatrists must be consulted for clients with diabetes or peripheral vascular disease.

One hand or foot is soaked, if needed, and dried; then the nail is cut or filed straight across beyond the end of the finger or toe (see Figure 22–1). Avoid trimming or digging into nails at the lateral corners. This predisposes the client to ingrown toenails. Clients who have diabetes or circulatory problems should have their nails filed rather than cut; inadvertent injury to tissues can occur if scissors are used. After the initial cut or filing, the nail is filed to round the corners, and the nurse cleans under the nail. The nurse then gently pushes back the cuticle, taking care not to injure it. The next finger or toe is cared for in the same manner. Any abnormalities, such as an infected cuticle or inflammation of the tissue around the nail, are recorded and reported.

EVALUATING

Examples of desired outcomes for nail hygiene include the client being able to:

- Demonstrate healthy nail care practices, as shown by:
  a. Clean, short nails with smooth edges.
  b. Intact cuticles and hydrated surrounding skin.
- Describe factors contributing to the nail problem.
- Describe preventive interventions for the specific nail problem.
- Demonstrate nail care as instructed.

MOUTH

Each tooth has three parts: the crown, the root, and the pulp cavity (Figure 22–2). The crown is the exposed part of the tooth, which is outside the gum. It is covered with a hard substance called enamel. The ivory-colored internal part of the crown below the enamel is the dentin. The root of a tooth is embedded in the jaw and covered by a bony tissue called cementum. The pulp cavity in the center of the tooth contains the blood vessels and nerves.

Developmental Variations

Teeth usually appear 5 to 8 months after birth. Baby-bottle syndrome may result in decay of all of the upper teeth and the lower posterior teeth (Pillitteri, 2010). This syndrome occurs when an infant is put to bed with a bottle of sugar water, formula, milk, or fruit juice. The carbohydrates in the solutions cause demineralization of the tooth enamel, which leads to tooth decay.

The incidence of periodontal disease increases during pregnancy because the rise in female hormones affects gingival tissue and increases its reaction to bacterial plaque. Many pregnant women experience more bleeding from the gingival sulcus during brushing and increased redness and swelling of the gingiva (the gum).

Teeth turn yellowish in color as a part of the aging process. Teeth are normally off-white. With age, the enamel thins and the yellow-gray color of the inner portion of the teeth begins to show. In addition, coffee drinking and cigarette smoking can stain the teeth. Commercial teeth whitening products and whitening treatments offered at dental offices are available to consumers who desire whiter teeth for cosmetic reasons.

Lack of fluoridated water and preventive dentistry during their developmental years caused tooth and gum problems in older adults (Edelman & Mandle, 2010). As a result, some older adults may have few permanent teeth left, and some have dentures. Loss of teeth occurs mainly because of **periodontal disease** (gum disease) rather than **dental caries** (cavities); however, caries are also common in middle-aged adults.

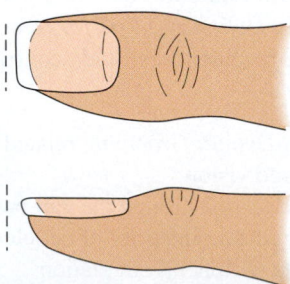

Figure 22–1 ● Fingernails are trimmed straight across.

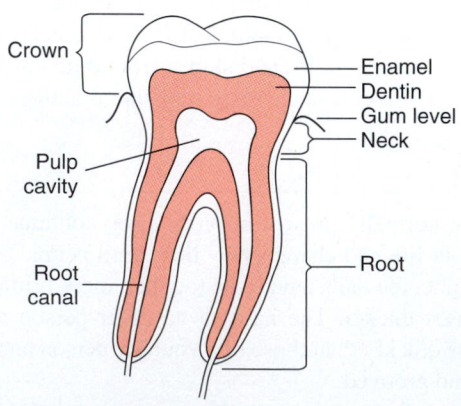

Figure 22–2 ● The anatomic parts of a tooth.

Some receding of the gums and a brownish pigmentation of the gums occur with age. Because saliva production decreases with age, dryness of the oral mucosa is a common finding in older people.

NURSING MANAGEMENT

ASSESSING

Assessment of the client's mouth and hygiene practices includes (a) a nursing health history, (b) physical assessment of the mouth, and (c) identification of clients at risk for developing oral problems.

Nursing History

During the nursing health history, the nurse obtains data about the client's oral hygiene practices, including dental visits, self-care abilities, and past or current mouth problems. Data about the client's oral hygiene help the nurse determine learning needs and incorporate the client's needs and preferences in the plan of care. Assessment of the client's self-care abilities determines the amount and type of nursing assistance to provide. Clients whose hand coordination is impaired, whose cognitive function is impaired, whose illness alters energy levels and motivation, or whose therapy imposes restrictions on activities will need assistance from the nurse. Information about past or current problems alerts the nurse to specific interventions required or referrals that may be necessary.

Physical Assessment

For information about mouth assessment, see Chapter 17 ∞. Dental caries (cavities) and periodontal disease are the two problems that most frequently affect the teeth. Both problems are commonly associated with plaque and tartar deposits. **Plaque** is an *invisible* soft film that adheres to the enamel surface of teeth; it consists of bacteria, molecules of saliva, and remnants of epithelial cells and leukocytes. When plaque is unchecked, tartar (dental calculus) is formed. **Tartar** is a visible, hard deposit of plaque and dead bacteria that forms at the gum lines. Tartar buildup can alter the fibers that attach the teeth to the gum and eventually disrupt bone tissue. Periodontal disease is characterized by **gingivitis** (red, swollen gingiva), bleeding, receding gum lines, and the formation of pockets between the teeth and gums. In advanced periodontal disease (**pyorrhea**), the teeth are loose and pus is evident when the gums are pressed.

Identifying Clients at Risk

Certain clients are prone to oral problems because of lack of knowledge or the inability to maintain oral hygiene. Among these are seriously ill, confused, comatose, depressed, and dehydrated clients. In addition, people with nasogastric tubes or receiving oxygen are likely to develop dry oral mucous membranes, especially if they breathe through their mouths. Clients who have had oral or jaw surgery must have meticulous oral hygiene care to prevent the development of infections.

CLINICAL ALERT

Clients in long-term care settings are at high risk for oral health problems. The nurse must assess the client's oral health and teach the UAP about the importance of and methods to promote oral hygiene.

Healthy-appearing individuals, too, may be at risk. High-risk variables such as inadequate nutrition, lack of money and/or insurance for dental care, excessive intake of refined sugars, and family history of periodontal disease also need to be identified. Some older people may also be at risk, for example, those who choose salty and enamel-eroding sugary foods because of a decline in their number of taste buds. The decreased saliva production in older adults, which produces a dry mouth and thinning of the oral mucosa, is another factor.

A dry mouth can be aggravated by poor fluid intake, heavy smoking, alcohol use, high salt intake, anxiety, and many medications. Medications that can cause dryness of the mouth include diuretics; laxatives, if used excessively; and tranquilizers. Some chemotherapeutic agents used to treat cancer also cause oral dryness and lesions. A common side effect of the anticonvulsant drug phenytoin (Dilantin) is gingival hyperplasia. Optimal oral hygiene is needed.

Clients who are receiving or have received radiation treatments to the head and neck may have permanent damage to salivary glands. This results in a very dry mouth and can often be treated by providing a thick liquid called *artificial saliva.* Some clients prefer to just sip on liquids to moisten their mouth. Radiation can also cause damage to teeth and jaw structure, with actual damage occurring years after the radiation.

DIAGNOSING

Three nursing diagnoses related to problems with oral hygiene and the oral cavity are *Self-Care Deficit, Impaired Oral Mucous Membrane,* and *Deficient Knowledge.* Note that the North American Nursing Diagnosis Association (NANDA, 2009) includes oral hygiene in the diagnostic label *Self-Care Deficit: Bathing/Hygiene.* In this book the diagnosis *Self-Care Deficit: Oral Hygiene* will be used for clients unable to perform oral care independently. This includes the inability to brush or floss teeth or clean dentures.

The nursing diagnosis *Impaired Oral Mucous Membrane* refers to the state in which an individual experiences disruptions in the tissue layers of the oral cavity. Manifestations include a coated tongue; dry mouth; halitosis; gingivitis; oral pain, discomfort, erythema, oral lesions, or ulcers; and dry mouth. These may be the result of ineffective oral hygiene, physical injury or drying effect, mechanical trauma, chemical trauma, or radiation therapy. The diagnosis *Deficient Knowledge* is discussed in Chapter 14 ∞.

Clinical examples of assessment data, related nursing diagnosis, outcome, and interventions are shown in the Identifying Nursing Diagnoses, Outcomes, and Interventions box.

PLANNING

In planning care, the nurse and, if appropriate, the client and/or family set outcomes for each nursing diagnosis. The nurse then performs nursing interventions and activities to achieve the client outcomes.

During the planning phase, the nurse also identifies interventions that will help the client achieve these goals. Specific, detailed nursing activities taken by the nurse may include the following:

- Monitor every shift for dryness of the oral mucosa.
- Monitor for signs and symptoms of glossitis (inflammation of the tongue) and stomatitis (inflammation of the mouth).
- Assist dependent clients with oral care.
- Provide special oral hygiene for clients who are debilitated, are unconscious, or have lesions of the mucous membranes or other oral tissues.
- Teach clients about good oral hygiene practices and other measures to prevent tooth decay.
- Reinforce the oral hygiene regimen as part of discharge teaching.

IMPLEMENTING

Good oral hygiene includes daily stimulation of the gums, mechanical brushing and flossing of the teeth, and flushing of the mouth. The nurse is often in a position to help people maintain oral hygiene by helping or teaching them to clean the teeth and oral cavity, by inspecting whether clients (especially children) have done so, or by actually providing mouth care to clients who are ill or incapacitated. The nurse can also be instrumental in identifying problems that require the intervention of a dentist or oral surgeon and arranging a referral.

Promoting Oral Health through the Life Span

A major role of the nurse in promoting oral health is to teach clients about specific oral hygienic measures.

IDENTIFYING NURSING DIAGNOSES, OUTCOMES, AND INTERVENTIONS — **Clients with Oral Cavity Problems**

DATA CLUSTER Mary Brown, 77 years old, suffered a cerebrovascular accident. Is unconscious and breathing through the mouth via O_2 face mask. 2500 mL intravenous fluid ordered daily.

NURSING DIAGNOSIS/DEFINITION	SAMPLE DESIRED OUTCOME*/*DEFINITION*	INDICATORS	SELECTED INTERVENTIONS*/ *DEFINITION*	SAMPLE NIC ACTIVITIES
Self-Care Deficit: Oral Hygiene related to cognitive inability (unconsciousness)/*Impaired ability to perform or complete bathing/hygiene activities for oneself*	Self-Care: Oral Hygiene [0308]/*Ability to care for own mouth and teeth independently with or without assistive device*	Severely compromised: • Cleans mouth, gums, and tongue	Oral Health Maintenance [1710]/*Maintenance and promotion of oral hygiene and dental health for the client at risk for developing oral or dental lesions*	• Establish a mouth care routine • Apply lubricant to moisten lips and oral mucosa, as needed • Monitor for signs and symptoms of glossitis and stomatitis

*The NOC # for desired outcomes and the NIC # for nursing interventions are listed in brackets following the appropriate outcome or intervention. Outcomes, indicators, interventions, and activities selected are only a sample of those suggested by NOC and NIC and should be further individualized for each client.

INFANTS AND TODDLERS Most dentists recommend that dental hygiene should begin when the first tooth erupts and be practiced after each feeding. Cleaning can be accomplished by using a wet washcloth or small gauze moistened with water.

Dental caries occur frequently during the toddler period, often as a result of the excessive intake of sweets or a prolonged use of the bottle during naps and at bedtime. The nurse should give parents the following instructions to promote and maintain dental health:

- Beginning at about 18 months of age, brush the child's teeth with a soft toothbrush. Use only a toothbrush moistened with water at first and introduce toothpaste later. Use one that contains fluoride.
- Give a fluoride supplement daily or as recommended by the primary care provider or dentist, unless the drinking water is fluoridated.
- Schedule an initial dental visit for the child at about 2 or 3 years of age, as soon as all 20 primary teeth have erupted.
- Some dentists recommend an inspection type of visit when the child is about 18 months old to provide an early pleasant introduction to the dental examination.
- Seek professional dental attention for any problems such as discoloring of the teeth, chipping, or signs of infection such as redness and swelling.

PRESCHOOLERS AND SCHOOL-AGE CHILDREN Because deciduous teeth guide the entrance of permanent teeth, dental care is essential to keep these teeth in good repair. Abnormally placed or lost deciduous teeth can cause misalignment of permanent teeth. Fluoride remains important at this stage to prevent dental caries. Preschoolers need to be taught to brush their teeth after eating and to limit their intake of refined sugars. Parental supervision may be needed to ensure the completion of these self-care activities. Regular dental checkups are required during these years when permanent teeth appear.

ADOLESCENTS AND ADULTS Proper diet and tooth and mouth care should be evaluated and reinforced to adolescents and adults. Specific measures to prevent tooth decay and periodontal disease are listed in Client Teaching.

OLDER ADULTS Over 50% of older adults have their own teeth (Gooch, Eke, & Malvitz, 2004). As a result, older adults are at risk for dental cavities and periodontal disease. Older adults who have self-care deficits are at an increased risk because they cannot maintain their oral hygiene practices and/or may not be able to visit the dentist on a routine basis. Furthermore, those who suffer the worst oral health and hygiene include older adults residing in nursing homes (Coleman, 2002, 2004). Coleman (2004) reported that poor oral hygiene among the frail and dependent nursing home residents can place them at risk for serious illness such as pneumonia (p. 3). Nurses have an important role in promoting optimal geriatric oral health care.

CLIENT TEACHING — **Measures to Prevent Tooth Decay**

- Brush the teeth thoroughly after meals and at bedtime. Assist children or inspect their mouths to be sure the teeth are clean. If the teeth cannot be brushed after meals, vigorous rinsing of the mouth with water is recommended.
- Floss the teeth daily.
- Ensure an adequate intake of nutrients, particularly calcium, phosphorus, vitamins A, C, and D, and fluoride.
- Avoid sweet foods and drinks between meals. Take them in moderation at meals.
- Eat coarse, fibrous foods (cleansing foods), such as fresh fruits and raw vegetables.
- Have topical fluoride applications as prescribed by the dentist.
- Have a checkup by a dentist every 6 months.

Brushing and Flossing the Teeth

Thorough brushing of the teeth is important in preventing tooth decay. The mechanical action of brushing removes food particles that can harbor and incubate bacteria. It also stimulates circulation in the gums, thus maintaining their healthy firmness. One of the techniques recommended for brushing teeth is called the sulcular technique, which removes plaque and cleans under the gingival margins. Many toothpastes are marketed. Fluoride toothpaste is often recommended because of its antibacterial protection.

Caring for Artificial Dentures

Some people have artificial teeth in the form of a plate—a complete set of teeth for one jaw. A person may have a lower plate or an upper plate or both. When only a few artificial teeth are needed, the individual may have a bridge rather than a plate. A bridge may be fixed or removable. Artificial teeth are fitted to the individual and usually will not fit another person. People who wear dentures or other types of oral prostheses should be encouraged to use them. Ill-fitting dentures or other oral prostheses can cause discomfort and chewing difficulties. They may also contribute to oral problems as well as poor nutrition and enjoyment of food. Those who do not wear their prostheses are prone to shrinkage of the gums, which results in further tooth loss.

Like natural teeth, artificial dentures collect microorganisms and food. They need to be cleaned regularly, at least once a day. They can be removed from the mouth, scrubbed with a toothbrush, rinsed, and reinserted. Some people use a dentifrice for cleaning teeth, and others use commercial cleaning compounds for plates.

Assisting Clients with Oral Care

When providing mouth care for partially or totally dependent clients, the nurse should wear gloves to guard against infections. Other required equipment includes a curved basin that fits snugly under the client's chin to receive the rinse water, and a towel to protect the client and the bed-clothes. See Skill 22–4.

Foam swabs are often used in health care agencies to clean the mouths of dependent clients (Figure 22–3). These swabs are convenient and effective in removing excess debris from the teeth and mouth but should be used infrequently and for short periods because they do not remove plaque that is at the base of the teeth.

Most people prefer privacy when they take their artificial teeth out to clean them. Many do not like to be seen without their teeth; one of the first requests of many post-operative clients is "May I have my teeth in, please?" The "Variation" section in Skill 22–4 describes how to clean artificial dentures.

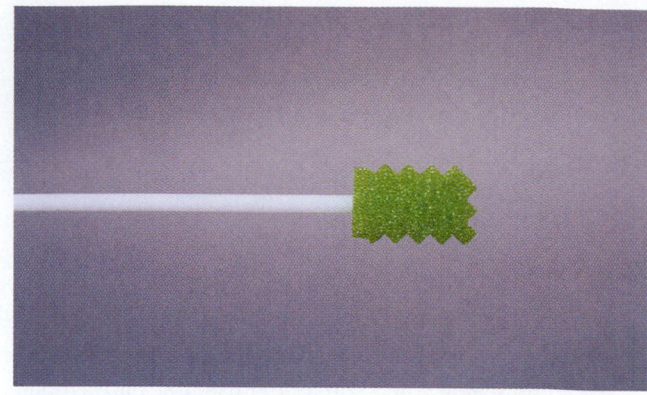

Figure 22–3 ◯ Example of a foam swab used to clean the mouth of a dependent client.

SKILL 22–4

BRUSHING AND FLOSSING THE TEETH

PURPOSES
- To remove food particles from around and between the teeth
- To remove dental plaque
- To promote the client's feelings of well-being
- To prevent sores and infection of the oral tissues

ASSESSMENT
- Determine the extent of the client's self-care abilities.
- Assess the client's usual mouth care practices.
- Inspect lips, gums, oral mucosa, and tongue for deviations from normal.
- Identify presence of oral problems such as tooth caries, halitosis, gingivitis, and loose or broken teeth.
- Check if the client has bridgework or wears dentures. If the client has dentures, ask if any tenderness or soreness is present and, if so, the location of the area(s) for ongoing assessment.

PLANNING

> **Delegation**
> Oral care, brushing and flossing of teeth, and denture care can be delegated to the UAP. After performing the above assessment, the nurse should instruct the UAP as to the type of oral care and amount of assistance needed by the client. Remind the UAP to report changes in the client's oral mucosa.

EQUIPMENT
Brushing and Flossing
- Towel
- Disposable gloves
- Curved basin (emesis basin)
- Toothbrush (soft bristle)
- Cup of tepid water

- Dentifrice (toothpaste)
- Mouthwash
- Dental floss, at least two pieces 20 cm (8 in.) in length
- Floss holder (optional)

For Cleaning Artificial Dentures
- Disposable gloves
- Tissue or piece of gauze
- Denture container
- Clean washcloth
- Toothbrush or stiff-bristled brush
- Dentifrice or denture cleaner
- Tepid water
- Container of mouthwash
- Curved basin (emesis basin)
- Towel

IMPLEMENTATION

Preparation
Assemble all the necessary equipment.

Performance
1. Prior to performing the procedure, introduce self and verify the client's identity using agency protocol. Explain to the client what you are going to do, why it is necessary, and how he or she can participate.
2. Perform hand hygiene and observe other appropriate infection control procedures (e.g., disposable gloves). **Rationale:** *Wearing gloves while providing mouth care prevents the nurse from acquiring infections. Gloves also prevent transmission of microorganisms to the client.*
3. Provide for client privacy by drawing the curtains around the bed or closing the door to the room. Some agencies provide signs indicating the need for privacy. **Rationale:** *Hygiene is a personal matter.*
4. Prepare the client.
   - Assist the client to a sitting position in bed, if health permits. If not, assist the client to a side-lying position with the head turned *so liquid may be prevented from draining down the client's throat.*
5. Prepare the equipment.
   - Place the towel under the client's chin.
   - Put on disposable gloves.
   - Moisten the bristles of the toothbrush with tepid water and apply the dentifrice to the toothbrush.

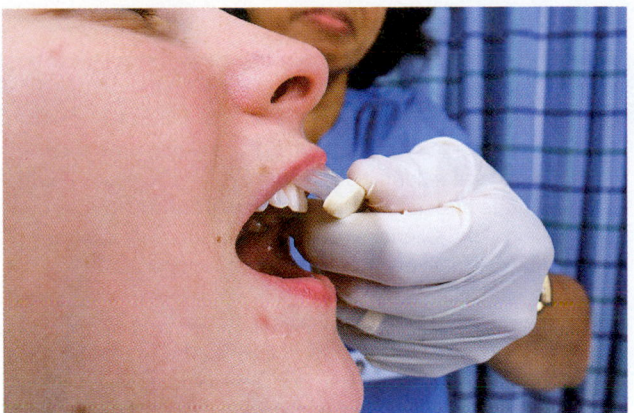

❶ The sulcular technique: Place the bristles at a 45-degree angle with the tips of the outer bristles under the gingival margins.

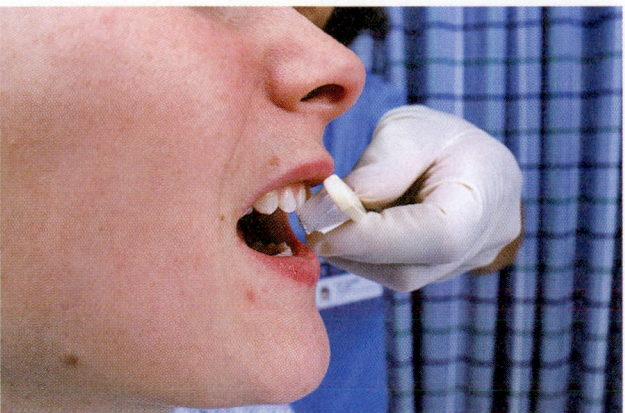

❷ Brushing from the sulcus to the crown of the teeth.

- Use a soft toothbrush (a small one for a child) and the client's choice of dentifrice.
- For the client who must remain in bed, place or hold the curved basin under the client's chin, fitting the small curve around the chin or neck.
- Inspect the mouth and teeth.

6. Brush the teeth.
   - Hand the toothbrush to the client, or brush the client's teeth as follows:
     a. Hold the brush against the teeth with the bristles at a 45-degree angle. The tips of the outer bristles should rest against and penetrate under the gingival sulcus. ❶ The brush will clean under the sulcus of two or three teeth at one time. **Rationale:** *This sulcular technique removes plaque and cleans under the gingival margins.*
     b. Move the bristles up and down gently in short strokes from the sulcus to the crowns of the teeth. ❷
     c. Repeat until all outer and inner surfaces of the teeth and sulci of the gums are cleaned.
     d. Clean the biting surfaces by moving the brush back and forth over them in short strokes. ❸
     e. Brush the tongue gently with the toothbrush. **Rationale:** *Brushing removes bacteria and freshens breath. A coated tongue may be caused by poor oral hygiene and low fluid intake. Brushing gently and carefully helps prevent gagging or vomiting.*
   - Hand the client the water cup or mouthwash to rinse the mouth vigorously. Then ask the client to spit the water and excess dentifrice into the basin. Some agencies supply a standard mouthwash. Alternatively, a mouth rinse of normal saline can be an effective cleaner and moisturizer. **Rationale:** *Vigorous rinsing loosens food particles and washes out already loosened particles.*
   - Repeat the preceding steps until the mouth is free of dentifrice and food particles.
   - Remove the curved basin and help the client wipe the mouth.

7. Floss the teeth.
   - Assist the client to floss independently, or floss the teeth of an alert and cooperative client as follows. Waxed floss is less likely to fray than unwaxed floss; particles between the teeth attach more readily to unwaxed floss than to waxed floss.

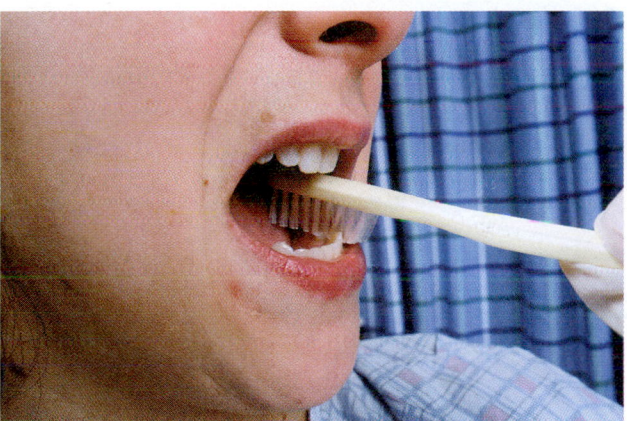

❸ Brushing the biting surfaces.

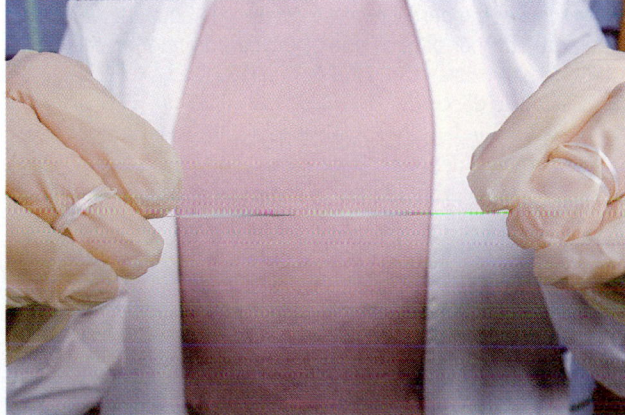

❹ Stretching the floss between the third finger of each hand.

   a. Wrap one end of the floss around the third finger of each hand. ❹
   b. To floss the upper teeth, use your thumb and index finger to stretch the floss. Move the floss up and down between the teeth. When the floss reaches the gum line, gently slide the floss into the space

(continued)

SKILL 22–4

BRUSHING AND FLOSSING THE TEETH *(continued)*

between the gum and the tooth. Gently move the floss away from the gum with up and down motions (American Dental Association, n.d.). Start at the back on the right side and work around to the back of the left side, or work from the center teeth to the back of the jaw on either side.

  c. To floss the lower teeth, use your index fingers to stretch the floss.

- Give the client tepid water or mouthwash to rinse the mouth and a curved basin in which to spit the water.
- Assist the client in wiping the mouth.

8. Remove and dispose of equipment appropriately.
   - Remove and clean the curved basin.
   - Remove and discard the gloves.

9. Document assessment of the teeth, tongue, gums, and oral mucosa. Include any problems such as sores or inflammation, bleeding, and swelling of the gums. Brushing and flossing teeth are not usually recorded.

VARIATION: ARTIFICIAL DENTURES

1. Remove the dentures.
   - Put on gloves. **Rationale:** *Wearing gloves decreases the likelihood of spreading infection.*
   - If the client cannot remove the dentures, take the tissue or gauze, grasp the upper plate at the front teeth with your thumb and second finger, and move the denture up and down slightly. ❺ **Rationale:** *The slight movement breaks the suction that holds the plate on the roof of the mouth.*
   - Lower the upper plate, move it out of the mouth, and place it in the denture container.
   - Lift the lower plate, turning it so that the left side, for example, is slightly lower than the right, to remove the plate from the mouth without stretching the lips. Place the lower plate in the denture container.
   - Remove a partial denture by exerting equal pressure on the border of each side of the denture, not on the clasps, which can bend or break.

2. Clean the dentures.
   - Take the denture container to a sink. Take care not to drop the dentures. Place a washcloth in the bowl of the sink *to prevent damage if the dentures are dropped.*
   - Using a toothbrush or special stiff-bristled brush, scrub the dentures with the cleaning agent and tepid water.
   - Rinse the dentures with tepid running water. **Rationale:** *Rinsing removes the cleaning agent and food particles.*
     a. If the dentures are stained, soak them in a commercial cleaner. Be sure to follow the manufacturer's directions. To prevent corrosion, dentures with metal parts should not be soaked overnight.

3. Inspect the dentures and the mouth.
   - Observe the dentures for any rough, sharp, or worn areas that could irritate the tongue or mucous membranes of the mouth, lips, and gums.
   - Inspect the mouth for any redness, irritated areas, or indications of infection.

- Assess the fit of the dentures. People who have them should see a dentist at least once a year to check the fit and the presence of any irritation to the soft tissues of the mouth. Clients who need repairs to their dentures or new dentures may need a referral for financial assistance.

4. Return the dentures to the mouth.
   - Offer some mouthwash and a curved basin to rinse the mouth. If the client cannot insert the dentures independently, insert the plates one at a time. Hold each plate at a slight angle while inserting it, to avoid injuring the lips. ❻

5. Assist the client as needed.
   - Wipe the client's hands and mouth with the towel.
   - If the client does not want to or cannot wear the dentures, store them in a denture container with water. Label the container with the client's name and identification number.

6. Remove and discard gloves.

7. Document all assessments and include any problems such as an irritated area on the mucous membrane.

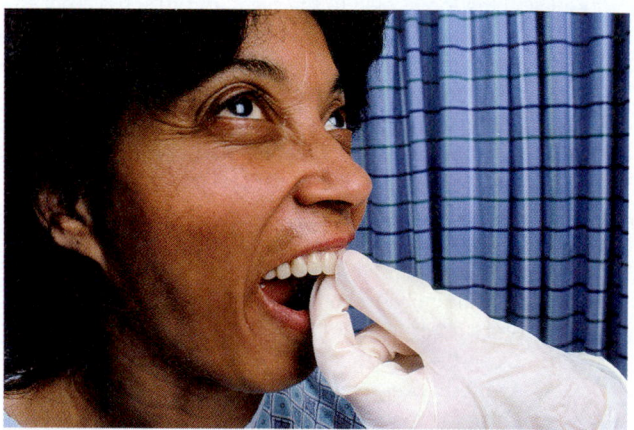

❺ Removing the top dentures by first breaking the suction.

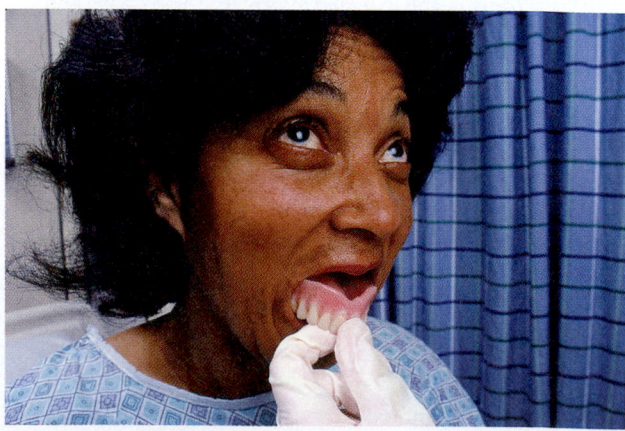

❻ Inserting the dentures at a slight angle.

Clients with Special Oral Hygiene Needs

For the client who is debilitated or unconscious or who has excessive dryness, sores, or irritations of the mouth, it may be necessary to clean the oral mucosa and tongue in addition to the teeth. Agency practices differ in regard to special mouth care and the frequency with which it is provided. Depending on the health of the client's mouth, special care may be needed every 2 to 8 hours.

Mouth care for unconscious or debilitated people is important because their mouths tend to become dry and consequently predisposed to tooth decay and infections. Saliva has antiviral, antibacterial, and antifungal effects (Walton, Miller, & Tordecilla, 2001, p. 40). Dry mouth—called **xerostomia**—occurs when the supply of saliva is reduced (American Dental Association, n.d.). This condition can be caused by side effects of certain medications, oxygen therapy, tachypnea, and NPO status when the client cannot take fluids by mouth (Anonymous, 2003).

For clients with special oral hygiene needs, the nurse needs to focus on removal of plaque and microorganisms as well as client comfort. If possible, a soft-bristled toothbrush should be used as it provides the best means of plaque removal. A sodium bicarbonate toothpaste will help dissolve mucus and reduce the saliva's acidity, which helps decrease bacteria (Nainar & Mohummed, 2004). If the client cannot tolerate the use of a toothbrush, the nurse can use an oral swab or a gauze soaked with saline to swab the teeth and tongue. A foam swab (Figure 22–3) can be used to provide oral hygiene to dependent clients. The swab, however, is not effective for plaque removal (Munro, Grap, & Kleinpell, 2004). Lemon-glycerin swabs are not recommended as they irritate and dry the oral mucosa and can decalcify teeth. Mouthwashes containing alcohol can irritate the oral mucosa as well as cause dryness. Hydrogen peroxide is approved as a mouth rinse by the Food and Drug Administration (Anonymous, 2003, p. 12). It provides a cleaning action as well as an antimicrobial effect. Diluting the hydrogen peroxide with saline or a non-alcohol–based mouthwash will help decrease a possible burning sensation experienced by the client. Mineral oil is contraindicated as a moisturizer for the lips or inside the mouth because aspiration of it can initiate an infection. A water-soluble moisturizer, absorbed by the skin and tissue, provides important hydration. Saliva substitutes can also help moisturize the oral cavity.

Skill 22–5 focuses on oral care for the unconscious person but may be adapted for conscious persons who are seriously ill or have mouth problems.

SKILL 22–5

PROVIDING SPECIAL ORAL CARE FOR THE UNCONSCIOUS CLIENT

PURPOSES
- To maintain the intactness and health of the lips, tongue, and mucous membranes of the mouth
- To prevent oral infections
- To clean and moisten the membranes of the mouth and lips

ASSESSMENT
- Inspect lips, gums, oral mucosa, and tongue for deviations from normal.
- Identify presence of oral problems such as tooth caries, halitosis, gingivitis, and loose or broken teeth.
- Assess for gag reflex, when appropriate.

PLANNING

> **Delegation**
> Special oral care may be delegated to UAP; however, the nurse needs to assess for the gag reflex. Dependent on this assessment, the nurse needs to inform the UAP of the correct positioning of the client and how to use the oral suction catheter, if needed. Remind the UAP to report changes in the client's oral mucosa.

EQUIPMENT
- Towel
- Curved basin (emesis basin)
- Disposable clean gloves
- Bite-block to hold the mouth open and teeth apart (optional)
- Toothbrush
- Cup of tepid water
- Dentifrice or denture cleaner
- Tissue or piece of gauze to remove dentures (optional)
- Denture container as needed
- Mouthwash
- Rubber-tipped bulb syringe
- Suction catheter with suction apparatus when aspiration is a concern
- Foam swabs and cleaning solution for cleaning the mucous membranes
- Water-soluble lip moisturizer

Performance

1. Prior to performing the procedure, introduce self and verify the client's identity using agency protocol. Explain to the client and the family what you are going to do and why it is necessary.

2. Perform hand hygiene and observe other appropriate infection control procedures (e.g., disposable gloves).

3. Provide for client privacy by drawing the curtains around the bed or closing the door to the room. Some agencies provide

(continued)

SKILL 22–5

PROVIDING SPECIAL ORAL CARE FOR THE UNCONSCIOUS CLIENT *(continued)*

signs indicating the need for privacy. **Rationale:** *Hygiene is a personal matter.*

4. Prepare the client.
   • Position the unconscious client in a side-lying position, with the head of the bed lowered. **Rationale:** *In this position, the saliva automatically runs out by gravity rather than being aspirated into the lungs.* This position is chosen for the unconscious client receiving mouth care. If the client's head cannot be lowered, turn it to one side. **Rationale:** *The fluid will readily run out of the mouth or pool in the side of the mouth, where it can be suctioned.*
   • Place the towel under the client's chin.
   • Place the curved basin against the client's chin and lower cheek to receive the fluid from the mouth. ❶
   • Put on gloves.
5. Clean the teeth and rinse the mouth.
   • If the person has natural teeth, brush the teeth as described in Skill 22–4. Brush gently and carefully to avoid injuring the gums. If the client has artificial teeth, clean them as described in the "Variation" component of Skill 22–4.
   • Rinse the client's mouth by drawing about 10 mL of water or alcohol-free mouthwash into the syringe and injecting it gently into each side of the mouth. **Rationale:** *If the solution is injected with force, some of it may flow down the client's throat and be aspirated into the lungs.*
   • Watch carefully to make sure that all the rinsing solution has run out of the mouth into the basin. If not, suction the fluid from the mouth. **Rationale:** *Fluid remaining in the mouth may be aspirated into the lungs.*
   • Repeat rinsing until the mouth is free of dentifrice, if used.
6. Inspect and clean the oral tissues.
   • If the tissues appear dry or unclean, clean them with the foam swabs or gauze and cleaning solution following agency policy.
   • Picking up a moistened foam swab, wipe the mucous membrane of one cheek. Discard the swab in a waste container; use a fresh one to clean the next area.

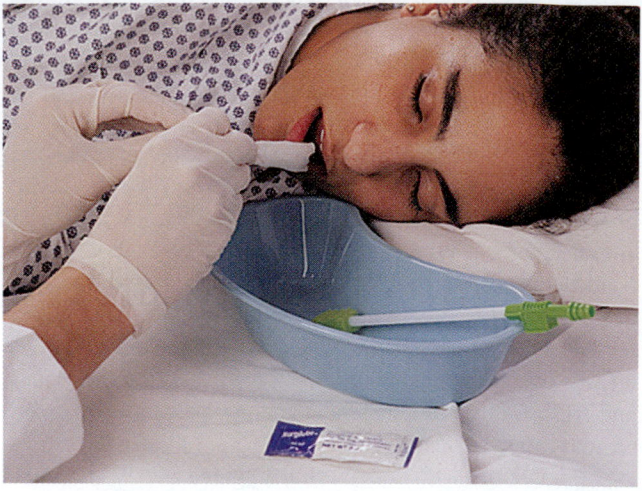

❶ Position of client and placement of curved basin when providing special mouth care.

Rationale: *Using separate applicators for each area of the mouth prevents the transfer of microorganisms from one area to another.*
   • Clean all mouth tissues in an orderly progression, using separate applicators: the cheeks, roof of the mouth, base of the mouth, and tongue.
   • Observe the tissues closely for inflammation and dryness.
   • Rinse the client's mouth as described in step 5.
   • Remove and discard gloves.
7. Ensure client comfort.
   • Remove the basin, and dry around the client's mouth with the towel. Replace artificial dentures, if indicated.
   • Lubricate the client's lips with water-soluble moisturizer. **Rationale:** *Lubrication prevents cracking and subsequent infection.*
8. Document assessment of the teeth, tongue, gums, and oral mucosa. Include any problems such as sores or inflammation and swelling of the gums.

EVALUATION

• Consider the client's medical diagnosis and treatment (e.g., chemotherapy, oxygen) and the necessary nursing interventions related to oral hygiene.

• Conduct an ongoing assessment, if appropriate, of the oral mucosa, gums, tongue, and lips.
• Report deviations from normal to the primary care provider.
• Conduct appropriate follow-up such as a referral to a dentist for dental caries.

LIFESPAN CONSIDERATIONS   Oral Hygiene

Infants

- Most dentists recommend that dental hygiene should begin when the first tooth erupts and be practiced after each feeding. Cleaning can be accomplished by using a wet washcloth or small gauze moistened with water.

Children

- Beginning at about 18 months of age, brush the child's teeth with a soft toothbrush. Use only a toothbrush moistened with water. Introduce toothpaste later and use one that contains fluoride.
- Frequent snacking of products containing sugar increases the child's risk for developing cavities.

Older Adults

- Oral care is often difficult for certain older adults to perform due to problems with dexterity or cognitive problems with dementia.
- Most long-term health care facilities have dentists that come on a regular basis to see clients with special needs.
- Dryness of the oral mucosa is a common finding in older adults. Because this can lead to tooth decay, advise clients to discuss it with their dentist or primary care provider.
- Decay of the tooth root is common among older adults. When the gums recede, the tooth root is more vulnerable to decay.
- Promoting good oral hygiene can have a positive effect on the older adults' ability to eat.

EVALUATING

Using data collected during care—status of oral mucosa, lips, tongue, teeth, and so on—the nurse judges whether desired outcomes have been achieved.

If outcomes are not achieved, the nurse and client need to explore the reasons before modifying the care plan. Examples of questions to consider are as follows:

- Did the nurse overestimate the client's functional abilities?
- Is the client's hand coordination or cognitive function impaired?
- Did the client's condition change?
- Has there been a change in the client's energy level and/or motivation?

HAIR

The appearance of the hair often reflects a person's feelings of self-concept and sociocultural well-being. Becoming familiar with hair care needs and practices that may be different from our own is an important aspect of providing competent nursing care to all clients. People who feel ill may not groom their hair as before. A dirty scalp and hair are itchy and uncomfortable, and can have an odor. The hair may also reflect state of health (e.g., excessive coarseness and dryness may be associated with endocrine disorders such as hypothyroidism).

Each person has particular ways of caring for hair. Many dark-skinned people need to oil their hair daily because it tends to be dry. Oil prevents the hair from breaking and the scalp from drying. A wide-toothed comb is usually used because finer combs pull and break the hair. Some people brush their hair vigorously before retiring; others comb their hair frequently.

Developmental Variations

Newborns may have lanugo (the fine hair on the body of the fetus, also referred to as *down* or *woolly hair*) over their shoulders, back, and sacrum. This generally disappears, and the hair distribution on the eyebrows, head, and eyelashes of young children subsequently becomes noticeable. Some newborns have hair on their scalps; others are free of hair at birth but grow hair over the scalp during the first year of life.

Pubic hair usually appears in early puberty, followed in about 6 months by the growth of axillary hair. Boys develop facial hair in later puberty.

In adolescence, the sebaceous glands increase in activity as a result of increased hormone levels. As a result, hair follicle openings enlarge to accommodate the increased amount of sebum, which can make the adolescent's hair more oily.

In older adults, the hair is generally thinner, grows more slowly, and loses its color as a result of aging tissues and diminishing circulation. Men often lose their scalp hair and may become completely bald. This phenomenon may occur even when a man is relatively young. The older person's hair also tends to be drier than normal. With age, axillary and pubic hair becomes finer and scanter, in contrast to the eyebrows, which become bristly and coarse. Many women develop hair on their faces, which may be a concern to them.

NURSING MANAGEMENT

ASSESSING

Assessment of the client's hair, hair care practices, and potential problems includes a nursing health history and physical assessment.

Nursing History

During the nursing history the nurse elicits data about usual hair care, self-care abilities, history of hair or scalp problems, and conditions known to affect the hair. Chemotherapeutic agents and radiation of the head may cause **alopecia** (hair loss). Hypothyroidism may cause the hair to be thin, dry, and/or brittle. Use of some hair dyes and curling or straightening preparations can cause the hair to become dry and brittle.

Physical Assessment

Physical assessment of the hair is discussed in Chapter 17 ∞. Problems include dandruff, hair loss, ticks, pediculosis, scabies, and hirsutism.

DANDRUFF Often accompanied by itching, **dandruff** appears as a diffuse scaling of the scalp. In severe cases it involves the auditory canals and the eyebrows. Dandruff can usually be treated effectively with a commercial shampoo. In severe or persistent cases, the client may need the advice of a primary care provider.

HAIR LOSS Hair loss and growth are continual processes. Some permanent thinning of hair normally occurs with aging. Baldness, common in men, is thought to be a hereditary problem for which there is no known remedy other than the wearing of a hairpiece or a costly surgical hair transplant, in which hair is taken from the back or the sides of the scalp and surgically moved to the hairless area. Although some medications are being developed, their long-term outcomes are unknown.

TICKS Small gray-brown parasites that bite into tissue and suck blood, **ticks** transmit several diseases to people, in particular Rocky Mountain spotted fever, Lyme disease, and tularemia. To remove a tick, use a blunt tweezers or gloved fingers and grasp the tick as close to the skin as possible. Gently pull the tick away using perpendicular traction to remove the tick. Be careful to not twist or squeeze the tick's body. If the head breaks off and remains in the skin, use tweezers to remove in a manner similar to that used for removing a splinter. Wash the area with antibacterial soap. Save the tick in a bottle of rubbing alcohol in case the primary care provider wants to identify the type of tick.

PEDICULOSIS (LICE) Lice are parasitic insects that infest mammals. Infestation with lice is called **pediculosis**. Hundreds of varieties of lice infest humans. Three common kinds are *Pediculus capitis* (the head louse), *Pediculus corporis* (the body louse), and *Pediculus pubis* (the crab louse).

Pediculus capitis is found on the scalp and tends to stay hidden in the hairs; similarly, *Pediculus pubis* stays in pubic hair. *Pediculus corporis* tends to cling to clothing, so that when a client undresses, the lice may not be evident on the body; these lice suck blood from the person and lay their eggs on the clothing. The nurse can suspect their presence in the clothing if (a) the person habitually scratches, (b) there are scratches on the skin, and (c) there are hemorrhagic spots on the skin where the lice have sucked blood.

Head and pubic lice lay their eggs on the hairs; the eggs look like oval particles, similar to dandruff, clinging to the hair. Bites and pustular eruptions may also be noticed at the hair lines and behind the ears. Lice are very small, grayish white, and difficult to see. The crab louse in the pubic area has red legs. Lice may be contracted from infested clothes and direct contact with an infested person.

The treatment often includes topical pediculicides such as pyrethrins, permethrin, and lindane. The current recommended treatment of choice for head lice is Nix because it is the least toxic (Frankowski & Weiner, 2002; Goldsmith, 2003). Natural products offered by health food stores are also available. Moses (2003) advocates using these natural vegetable extracts first because they are nontoxic, safe for children and pregnant or nursing women, inexpensive, and effective (p. 11). Clients, however, need to be reminded that natural products are not required to meet the Food and Drug Administration standards. Some home remedies suggest applying an oily substance such as olive oil or petroleum jelly to smother the lice. This practice, according to the Centers for Disease Control and Prevention, can be dangerous or cause infections (Goldsmith, 2003, p. 23).

Removal of nits (eggs) after applying the treatment is not necessary to prevent spread but most people remove them for aesthetic reasons (Frankowski & Weiner, 2002). Fine-toothed "nit" combs are available. Transmission is from head-to-head contact, and it is suggested that the hair care items and bedding of the person who has the lice infestation be washed with hot water or tightly bagged in plastic for 2 weeks if they cannot be washed.

SCABIES **Scabies** is a contagious skin infestation by the itch mite. The characteristic lesion is the burrow produced by the female mite as it penetrates into the upper layers of the skin. Burrows are short, wavy, brown or black, threadlike lesions most commonly observed between the fingers, in the creases of the wrists and elbows, beneath breast tissue, and in the groin area (Stewart, 2000). The mites cause intense itching that is more pronounced at night because the increased warmth of the skin has a stimulating effect on the parasites. Secondary lesions caused by scratching include vesicles, papules, pustules, excoriations, and crusts. Treatment involves thorough cleansing of the body with soap and water to remove scales and debris from crusts, and then an application of a scabicide lotion. All bed linens and clothing should be washed in very hot or boiling water.

HIRSUTISM The growth of excessive body hair is called hirsutism. The acceptance of body hair in the axillae and on the legs is largely dictated by culture. In North America, the well-groomed woman, as depicted in magazines, has no hair on her legs or under her axillae. In many European cultures, it is not customary for well-groomed women to remove this hair. Excessive facial hair on a woman is thought unattractive in most Western and Asian cultures.

DIAGNOSING

Nursing diagnoses related to hair hygiene and hair and scalp problems include *Self-Care Deficit: Grooming, Impaired Skin Integrity, Risk for Infection,* and *Disturbed Body Image.* Examples of these nursing diagnoses with contributing factors follow:

- *Self-Care Deficit: Grooming* related to
  a. Activity intolerance
  b. Imposed immobility (bed rest)
  c. Pain in upper extremities
  d. Altered level of consciousness
  e. Lack of motivation associated with depression
- *Impaired Skin Integrity* related to
  a. Scalp laceration
  b. Insect bite
- *Risk for Infection* related to
  a. Scalp laceration
  b. Insect bite
- *Disturbed Body Image* related to alopecia

PLANNING

In planning care, the nurse and, if appropriate, the client and/or family set outcomes for each nursing diagnosis. The nurse then performs nursing interventions and activities to achieve the client outcomes.

The specific, detailed nursing activities taken by the nurse to assist the client should take into account the client's personal preferences, health, and energy resources as well as the time, equipment, and personnel available. Often, clients like to receive hair care after a bath, before receiving visitors, and before retiring. Nursing interventions may include instructing the client/family in alternative methods for hair care including facilitating the assistance of a barber or beautician, as necessary. At some agencies, shampoos can be given to clients only after a primary care provider's order.

IMPLEMENTING

Hair needs to be brushed or combed daily and washed, as needed, to keep it clean. Nurses may need to provide hair care for clients who cannot meet their own self-care needs.

Brushing and Combing Hair

To be healthy, hair needs to be brushed daily. Brushing has three major functions: It stimulates the circulation of blood in the scalp, it distributes the oil along the hair shaft, and it helps to arrange the hair.

Long hair may present a problem for clients confined to bed because it may become matted. It should be combed and brushed at least once a day to prevent this. A brush with stiff bristles provides the best stimulation to blood circulation in the scalp. The bristles should not be so sharp that they injure the client's scalp, however. A comb with dull, even teeth is advisable. A comb with sharp teeth might injure the scalp; combs that are too fine can pull and break the hair. Some clients are pleased to have their hair tied neatly in the back or braided until other assistance is available or until they feel better and can look after it themselves. Braiding also prevents tangling and matting for clients confined to bed.

Dark-skinned people often have thicker, drier, curlier hair than light-skinned people. Very curly hair may stand out from the scalp. Although the shafts of curly or kinky hair look strong and wiry, they have less strength than straight hair shafts and can break easily. Many African American people have hair that is naturally curly, and it can easily become matted and tangled in a short period of time (Jackson, 1998). African Americans generally wash their hair less often than other ethnic groups because the hair is drier. Shampooing often could damage their hair.

Some African Americans have their hair straightened. Even if straightened, the hair tends to tangle and mat easily, especially at the back and the sides if the client is confined to bed. Other African Americans style their hair in small braids. These braids do not have to be unbraided for shampooing and washing. If, however, unbraiding becomes necessary, the nurse should obtain the client's permission to do so. Some African American clients may use oil by applying it between the braids and massaging it into the scalp. The oil prevents the hair strands from breaking and the scalp from becoming too dry. Not all African American individuals have curly or kinky hair. Some have naturally straight hair. Keeping the scalp and hair clean and oiled remains important and necessary.

Shampooing the Hair

Hair should be washed as often as needed to keep it clean. There are several ways to shampoo clients' hair, depending on their health, strength, and age. The client who is well enough to take a shower can shampoo while in the shower. The client who is unable to shower may be given a shampoo while sitting on a chair in front of a sink. The back-lying client who can move to a stretcher can be given a shampoo on a stretcher wheeled to a sink. The client who must remain in bed can be given a shampoo with water brought to the bedside. A commercial product, similar to the bag bath, called a "head bath" is another approach. It consists of a specially designed cap (looks like a shower cap) placed over the hair. The cap contains shampoo and conditioner, and gently massaging the cap cleans the hair and scalp. In some agencies, volunteer beauticians with portable shampoo chairs may be available to assist with hair care. Skill 22–6 describes how to shampoo the hair of a client confined to bed.

SKILL 22–6

SHAMPOOING THE HAIR OF A CLIENT CONFINED TO BED

PURPOSES
- To stimulate the blood circulation to the scalp through massage
- To clean the hair and increase the client's sense of well-being

ASSESSMENT
- Determine routinely used shampoo products
- Assess:
- Any scalp problems
- Activity tolerance of the client

PLANNING

Delegation (see Skill 22–5)

EQUIPMENT
- Comb and brush
- Plastic sheet or pad
- Two bath towels
- Shampoo basin
- Washcloth or pad
- Bath blanket
- Receptacle for the shampoo water
- Pitcher of water
- Bath thermometer
- Liquid or cream shampoo
- Hair dryer

IMPLEMENTATION

Preparation
- Determine whether a primary care provider's order is needed before a shampoo can be given. **Rationale:** *Some agencies require an order.*
- Determine the type of shampoo to be used (e.g., medicated shampoo).
- Determine the best time of day for the shampoo. Discuss this with the client. A person who must remain in bed may find the shampoo tiring. Choose a time when the client is rested and can rest after the procedure.

Performance
1. Prior to performing the procedure, introduce self and verify the client's identity using agency protocol. Explain to the client what you are going to do, why it is necessary if appropriate, and how he or she can participate.
2. Perform hand hygiene and observe other appropriate infection control procedures as needed.
3. Provide for client privacy by drawing the curtains around the bed or closing the door to the room. Some agencies provide signs indicating the need for privacy. **Rationale:** *Hygiene is a personal matter.*
4. Position and prepare the client appropriately.
   - Assist the client to the side of the bed from which you will work.
   - Remove pins and ribbons from the hair, and brush and comb it to remove any tangles.
5. Arrange the equipment.
   - Put the plastic sheet or pad on the bed under the head. **Rationale:** *The plastic keeps the bedding dry.*
   - Remove the pillow from under the client's head, and place it under the shoulders unless there is some underlying condition (e.g., neck surgery, arthritis of the neck). **Rationale:** *This hyperextends the neck.*
   - Tuck a bath towel around the client's shoulders. **Rationale:** *This keeps the shoulders dry.*
   - Place the shampoo basin under the head, ❶ putting a folded washcloth or pad where the client's neck rests on the edge of the basin. If the client is on a stretcher, the neck can rest on the edge of the sink with the washcloth

as padding. **Rationale:** *Padding supports the muscles of the neck and prevents undue strain and discomfort.*
   - Fanfold the top bedding down to the waist, and cover the upper part of the client with the bath blanket. **Rationale:** *The folded bedding will stay dry, and the bath blanket, which can be discarded after the shampoo, will keep the client warm.*
   - Place the receiving receptacle on a table or chair at the bedside. Put the spout of the shampoo basin over the receptacle.
6. Protect the client's eyes.
   - Place a damp washcloth over the client's eyes. **Rationale:** *The washcloth protects the eyes from soapy water. A damp washcloth will not slip.*
7. Shampoo the hair.
   - Wet the hair thoroughly with the water.
   - Apply shampoo to the scalp. Make a good lather with the shampoo while massaging the scalp with the pads of your fingertips. Massage all areas of the scalp systematically, for

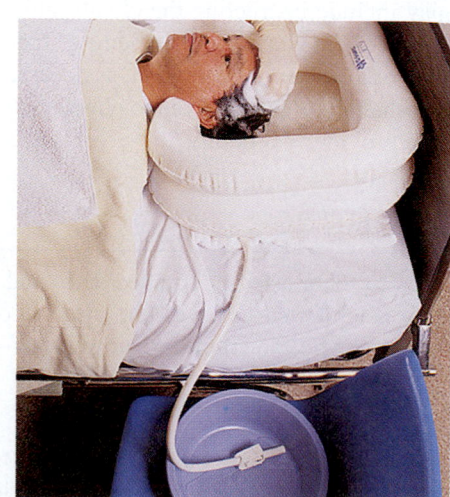

❶ Shampooing the hair of a client confined to bed.
Note the shampoo basin and the receptacle below.

example, starting at the front and working toward the back of the head. **Rationale:** *Massaging stimulates the blood circulation in the scalp. The pads of the fingers are used so that the fingernails will not scratch the scalp.*

- Rinse the hair briefly, and apply shampoo again.
- Make a good lather and massage the scalp as before.
- Rinse the hair thoroughly this time to remove all shampoo. **Rationale:** *Shampoo remaining in the hair may dry and irritate the hair and scalp.*
- Squeeze as much water as possible out of the hair with your hands.

8. Dry the hair thoroughly.
   - Rub the client's hair with a heavy towel.
   - Dry the hair with the dryer. Set the temperature at "warm."
   - Continually move the dryer to prevent burning the client's scalp.
9. Ensure client comfort.
   - Assist the person confined to bed to a comfortable position.
   - Arrange the hair using a clean brush and comb.
10. Document the shampoo and any assessments.

EVALUATION

- Conduct ongoing assessments such as any scalp problems or intolerance to the procedure. Report any problems noted to the nurse in charge.

LIFESPAN CONSIDERATIONS
Hair Care

Infants

- Shampoo an infant's hair daily to prevent seborrhea.

Children

- Monitor school-age children for nits (pediculosis).

Older Adults

- Ensure adequate warmth for older adults when shampooing their hair, because they are susceptible to chilling.

Beard and Mustache Care

Beards and mustaches also require daily care. The most important aspect of the care is to keep them clean. Food particles tend to collect in beards and mustaches, and they need washing and combing periodically. Clients may also wish for a beard or mustache trim to maintain a well-groomed appearance.

CLINICAL ALERT

A beard or mustache should not be shaved off without the client's consent.

Male clients often shave or are shaved after a bath (Figure 22–4). Frequently clients supply their own electric or safety razors. See Box 22–2 for the steps involved in shaving facial hair with a safety razor. If a client is taking an anticoagulant (e.g., Warfarin [Coumadin], heparin), an electric shaver should be used.

EVALUATING

Using data collected during care, the nurse judges whether desired outcomes have been achieved. Examples of client

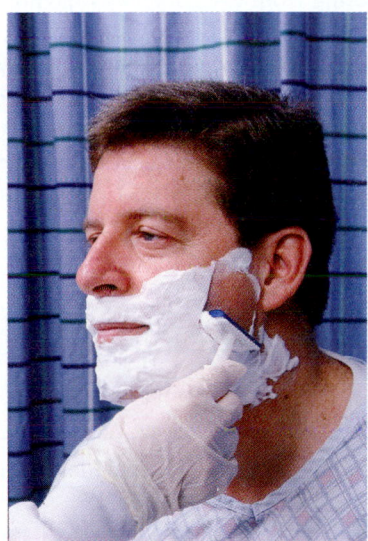

Figure 22–4 ◯ Shaving in the direction of hair growth.

BOX 22–2	Using a Safety Razor to Shave Facial Hair

- Wear gloves in case facial nicks occur and you come in contact with blood.
- Apply shaving cream or soap and water to soften the bristles and make the skin more pliable.
- Hold the skin taut, particularly around creases, to prevent cutting the skin.
- Hold the razor so that the blade is at a 45-degree angle to the skin, and shave in short, firm strokes in the direction of hair growth (Figure 22–4).
- After shaving the entire area, wipe the client's face with a wet washcloth to remove any remaining shaving cream and hair.
- Dry the face well, then apply aftershave lotion or powder as the client prefers.
- To prevent irritating the skin, pat on the lotion with the fingers and avoid rubbing the face.

outcomes that are measurable or observable include the client being able to:

- Perform hair grooming with assistance (specify).
- Exhibit clean, well-groomed, resilient hair with a healthy sheen.
- Reduce or get rid of scalp lesions or infestations.
- Describe factors, interventions, and preventive measures for a specific hair problem (e.g., dandruff).

EYES

Normally eyes require no special hygiene, because lacrimal fluid continually washes the eyes, and the eyelids and lashes prevent the entrance of foreign particles. Special interventions are needed, however, for unconscious clients and for clients recovering from eye surgery or having eye injuries, irritations, or infections. In unconscious clients, the blink reflex may be absent, and excessive drainage may accumulate along eyelid margins. In clients with eye trauma or eye infections, excessive discharge or drainage is common. Excessive secretions on the lashes need to be removed before they dry on the lashes as crusts. Clients who wear eyeglasses, contact lenses, or an artificial eye also may require instruction from and care by the nurse.

NURSING MANAGEMENT

ASSESSING

Assessment of the client's eyes includes a nursing health history and physical assessment.

Nursing Health History

During the nursing history, the nurse obtains data about the client's eyeglasses or contact lenses, recent examination by an ophthalmologist, and any history of eye problems and related treatments.

Physical Assessment

In physical assessment, all external eye structures are inspected for signs of inflammation, excessive drainage, encrustations, or other obvious abnormalities. Inspection of the external eye structures is discussed in Chapter 17 ∞.

DIAGNOSING

Nursing diagnoses related to eye problems may include *Self-Care Deficit*, *Risk for Infection*, and *Risk for Injury*. Examples of these diagnoses and possible contributing factors follow:

- *Self-Care Deficit* (contact lens insertion, removal, and cleaning) related to
  a. Deficient knowledge
  b. Impaired vision associated with cataracts

- *Risk for Infection* related to
  a. Improper contact lens hygiene
  b. Accumulation of secretions on eyelids
- *Risk for Injury* related to
  a. Prolonged wearing of contact lenses
  b. Absence of blink reflex associated with unconsciousness

PLANNING

In planning care, the nurse identifies nursing activities that will assist the client to maintain the integrity of the eye structures or prosthesis and to prevent eye injury and infection.

IMPLEMENTING

Nursing activities may include teaching clients about how to insert, clean, and remove contact lenses or a prosthesis and ways to protect the eyes from injury and strain.

Eye Care

Dried secretions that have accumulated on the lashes need to be softened and wiped away. Soften dried secretions by placing a sterile cotton ball moistened with sterile water or normal saline over the lid margins. Wipe the loosened secretions from the inner canthus of the eye to the outer canthus to prevent the particles and fluid from draining into the lacrimal sac and nasolacrimal duct.

If the client is unconscious and lacks a blink reflex or cannot close the eyelids completely, drying and irritation of the cornea must be prevented. Lubricating eye drops may be ordered. Box 22–3 gives suggestions for providing eye care for the comatose client.

Eyeglass Care

It is essential that the nurse exercise caution when cleaning eyeglasses to prevent breaking or scratching the lenses.

BOX 22–3 **Eye Care for the Comatose Client**

When a comatose client's corneal reflex is impaired, eye care is essential to keep moist the areas of the cornea that are exposed to air.

- Administer moist compresses to cover the eyes every 2 to 4 hours.
- Clean the eyes with saline solution and cotton balls. Wipe from the inner to outer canthus. This prevents debris from being washed into the nasolacrimal duct.
- Use a new cotton ball for each wipe. This prevents extending infection in one eye to the other eye.
- Instill ophthalmic ointment or artificial tears into the lower lids as ordered. This keeps the eyes moist.
- If the client's corneal reflex is absent, keep the eyes moist with artificial tears and protect the eye with a protective shield. These should be ordered by a primary care provider.
- Monitor the eyes for redness, exudate, or ulceration.

Glass lenses can be cleaned with warm water and dried with a soft tissue that will not scratch the lenses. Plastic lenses are easily scratched and may require special cleaning solutions and drying tissues. When not being worn, all glasses should be placed in an appropriately labeled case and stored in the client's bedside table drawer.

Contact Lens Care

Contact lenses, thin curved discs of hard or soft plastic, fit on the cornea of the eye directly over the pupil. They float on the tear layer of the eye. For some people, contact lenses offer several advantages over eyeglasses: (a) They cannot be seen and thus have cosmetic value; (b) they are highly effective in correcting some astigmatisms; (c) they are safer than glasses for some physical activities; (d) they do not fog, as eyeglasses do; and (e) they provide better vision in many cases.

Contact lenses may be either hard or soft or a compromise between the two types—gas-permeable lenses. *Hard contact lenses* are made of a rigid, unwettable, airtight plastic that does not absorb water or saline solutions. They usually cannot be worn for more than 12 to 14 hours and are rarely recommended for first-time wearers.

Soft contact lenses cover the entire cornea. Being more pliable and soft, they mold to the eye for a firmer fit. The duration of extended wear varies by brand from 1 to 30 days or more. Eye specialists recommend that long-wear brands be removed and cleaned at least once a week. These lenses require scrupulous care and handling.

Gas-permeable lenses are rigid enough to provide clear vision but are more flexible than the traditional hard lens. They permit oxygen to reach the cornea, thus providing greater comfort, and will not cause serious damage to the eye if left in place for several days.

Most clients normally care for their own contact lenses. In general, each lens manufacturer provides detailed cleaning instructions. Depending on the type of lens and cleaning method used, warm tap water, normal saline, or special rinsing or soaking solutions may be used.

All users should have a special container for their lenses. Some contain a solution so that the lenses are stored wet; in others, the lenses are dry. Each lens container has a slot or cup with a label indicating whether it is for the right or left lens. It is essential that the correct lens be stored in the appropriate slot so that it will be placed in the correct eye.

REMOVING CONTACT LENSES Hard contact lenses must be positioned directly over the cornea for proper removal. If the lens is displaced, the nurse asks the client to look straight ahead, and gently exerts pressure on the upper and lower lids to move the lens back onto the cornea. Figure 22–5 shows the steps needed to remove a hard lens. To avoid lens mixups, the nurse places the first lens in its designated cup in the storage base before removing the second lens.

Removal of soft lenses differs in two ways. First, have the client look forward. Retract the lower lid with one hand. Using the pad of the index finger of the other hand, move the lens down to the inferior part of the sclera. This reduces the risk of damage to the cornea. Second, remove the lens by gently pinching the lens between the pads of the thumb and index finger. Pinching causes the lens to double up, so that air enters underneath the lens, overcoming the suction and allowing removal. Use the pads of the fingers to prevent scratching the eye or the lens with the fingernails. Figure 22–6 shows a client removing her own contact lens using the method described. Please note that a nurse would need to wear gloves.

INSERTING CONTACT LENSES Seriously ill clients whose contact lenses have been removed will not need them reinserted until the client becomes more active and require the lenses to see properly. Contact lenses need to be lubricated in a sterile, nonirritating wetting solution (usually a saline solution) before they are inserted. The wetting solution helps the lens glide over the cornea, thus reducing the risk of injury. Most clients, when well, will reinsert the lenses independently.

Artificial Eyes

Artificial eyes are usually made of glass or plastic. Some are permanently implanted; others are removed regularly for

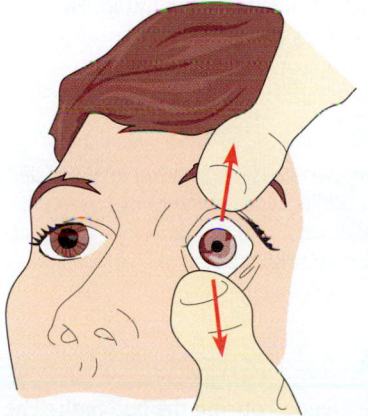
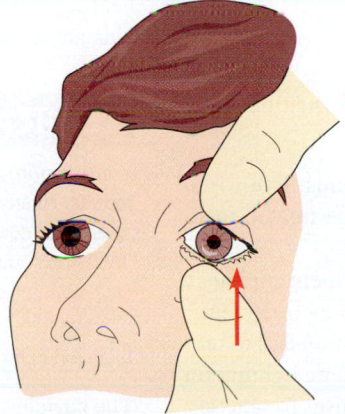
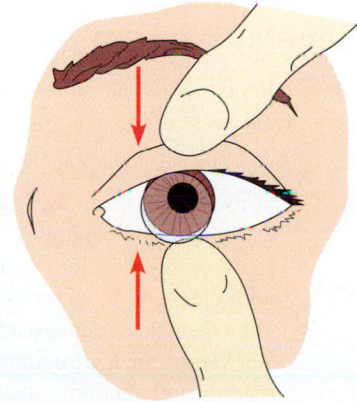

A   B   C

Figure 22–5 ○ Removing hard contact lenses.

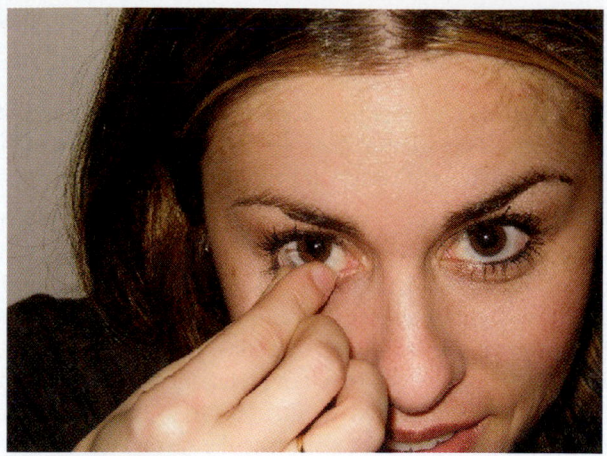

Figure 22–6 ◯ Removing a soft lens by pinching it between the pads of the thumb and index finger.
(Lester Lefkowitz/Corbis.)

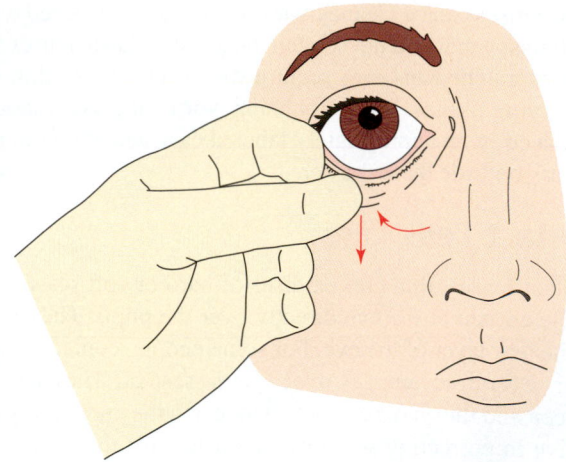

Figure 22–7 ◯ Removing an artificial eye by retracting the lower eyelid and exerting slight pressure below the eyelid.

cleaning. Most clients who wear a removable artificial eye follow their own care regimen. Even for an unconscious client, daily removal and cleaning are not necessary.

To remove an artificial eye, the nurse puts on clean gloves and retracts the client's lower eyelid down over the infraorbital bone while exerting slight pressure below the eyelid to overcome the suction (Figure 22–7). An alternative method is to compress a small rubber bulb and apply the tip directly to the eye. As the nurse gradually releases the finger pressure on the bulb, the suction of the bulb counteracts the suction holding the eye in the socket and draws the eye out of the socket.

The eye is cleaned with warm normal saline and placed in a container filled with water or saline solution. The socket and tissues around the eye are usually cleaned with cotton wipes and normal saline. To reinsert the eye, the nurse uses the thumb and index finger of one hand to retract the eyelids, exerting pressure on the supraorbital and infraorbital bones. Holding the eye between the thumb and index finger of the other hand, the nurse slips the eye gently into the socket.

General Eye Care

Many clients may need to learn specific information about care of the eyes. Some examples follow:

- Avoid home remedies for eye problems. Eye irritations or injuries at any age should be treated medically and immediately.
- If dirt or dust gets into the eyes, clean them copiously with clean, tepid water as an emergency treatment.
- Take measures to guard against eyestrain and to protect vision, such as maintaining adequate lighting for reading and obtaining shatterproof lenses for glasses.
- Schedule regular eye examinations, particularly after age 40, to detect problems such as cataracts and glaucoma.

EVALUATING

Using data collected during care, the nurse judges whether desired outcomes have been achieved. Examples of desired outcomes to evaluate the effectiveness of nursing interventions follow:

- Conjunctiva and sclera free of inflammation
- Eyelids free of secretions
- No tearing
- No eye discomfort
- Demonstrates appropriate methods of caring for contact lenses
- Describes interventions to prevent eye injury and infection

EARS

Normal ears require minimal hygiene. Clients who have excessive **cerumen** (earwax) and dependent clients who have hearing aids may require assistance from the nurse. Hearing aids are usually removed before surgery.

CLINICAL ALERT

Cerumen impaction is a common cause of hearing loss in older adults. Nearly 35% of older adults in the community have cerumen impaction in one or both ears, and the incidence is higher in institutionalized older adults (Stone, 1999).

Cleaning the Ears

The auricles of the ear are cleaned during the bed bath. The nurse or client must remove excessive cerumen that is visible or that causes discomfort or hearing difficulty. Visible cerumen may be loosened and removed by retracting the auricle up and back. If this measure is ineffective, irrigation is necessary. Clients need to be advised never to use bobby pins, toothpicks, or cotton-tipped applicators to remove cerumen. Bobby pins and toothpicks can injure the ear canal and rupture the tympanic membrane; cotton-tipped applicators can cause wax to become impacted within the canal.

Care of Hearing Aids

A hearing aid is a battery-powered, sound-amplifying device used by persons with hearing impairments. It consists of a microphone that picks up sound and converts it to electric energy, an amplifier that magnifies the electric energy electronically, a receiver that converts the amplified energy back to sound energy, and an earmold that directs the sound into the ear. There are several types of hearing aids:

- *Behind-the-ear (BTE, or postaural) aid.* This is the most widely used type because it fits snugly behind the ear. The hearing aid case, which holds the microphone, amplifier, and receiver, is attached to the earmold by a plastic tube (Figure 22–8).
- *In-the-ear aid (ITE, or intra-aural).* This one-piece aid has all its components housed in the earmold.
- *In-the-canal (ITC) aid.* This is the most compact and least visible aid, fitting completely inside the ear canal. In addition to having cosmetic appeal, the ITC does not interfere with telephone use or the wearing of eyeglasses. However, it is not suitable for clients with progressive hearing loss; it requires adequate ear canal diameter and length for a good fit; and it tends to plug with cerumen more than other aids.
- *Eyeglasses aid.* This is similar to the behind-the-ear aid, but the components are housed in the temple of the eyeglasses. A hearing aid can be in one or both temples of the glasses.
- *Body hearing aid.* This pocket-sized aid, used for more severe hearing losses, clips onto an undergarment, shirt pocket, or harness carrier supplied by the manufacturer. The case, containing the microphone

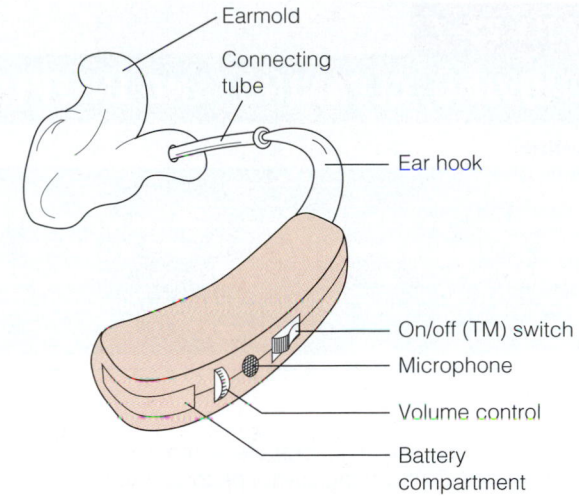

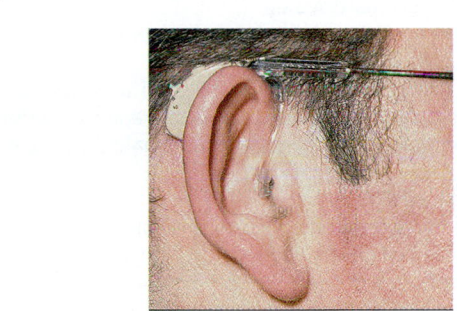

Figure 22–8 ⭘ **A,** A behind-the-ear hearing aid. **B,** A behind-the-ear hearing aid attached to glasses.
(Jane Schemilt/Science Photo Library, Photo Researchers, Inc.)

and amplifier, is connected by a cord to the receiver, which snaps into the earpiece.

For correct functioning, hearing aids require appropriate handling during insertion and removal, regular cleaning of the earmold, and replacement of dead batteries. With proper care, hearing aids generally last 5 to 10 years. Earmolds generally need readjustment every 2 to 3 years. Skill 22–7 describes how to remove, clean, and insert a hearing aid.

SKILL 22-7

REMOVING, CLEANING, AND INSERTING A HEARING AID

PURPOSE
- To maintain proper hearing aid function

ASSESSMENT
Determine if the client has experienced any problems with the hearing aid and hearing aid practices. Assess for the presence of inflammation, excessive wax, drainage, or discomfort in the external ear.

(continued)

REMOVING, CLEANING, AND INSERTING A HEARING AID (continued)

PLANNING

Delegation
A nurse can delegate the task of caring for a hearing aid to the UAP. It is important, however, for the nurse to first determine that the UAP knows the correct way to care for a hearing aid. Inform the UAP to report the presence of ear inflammation, discomfort, excess wax, or drainage to the RN.

EQUIPMENT
- Client's hearing aid
- Soap, water, and towels or a damp cloth
- Pipe cleaner or toothpick (optional)
- New battery (if needed)

IMPLEMENTATION

Performance

1. Prior to performing the procedure, introduce self and verify the client's identity using agency protocol. Explain to the client what you are going to do, why it is necessary, and how he or she can participate.
2. Perform hand hygiene and observe other appropriate infection control procedures.
3. Provide for client privacy by drawing the curtains around the bed or closing the door to the room. Some agencies provide signs indicating the need for privacy. **Rationale:** *Hygiene is a personal matter.*
4. Remove the hearing aid.
   - Turn the hearing aid off and lower the volume. The on/off switch may be labeled "O" (off), "M" (microphone), "T" (telephone), or "TM" (telephone/microphone). **Rationale:** *The batteries continue to run if the hearing aid is not turned off.*
   - Remove the earmold by rotating it slightly forward and pulling it outward.
   - If the hearing aid is not to be used for several days, remove the battery. **Rationale:** *Removal prevents corrosion of the hearing aid from battery leakage.*
   - Store the hearing aid in a safe place and label with client's name. Avoid exposure to heat and moisture. **Rationale:** *Proper storage prevents loss or damage.*
5. Clean the earmold.
   - Detach the earmold if possible. Disconnect the earmold from the receiver of a body hearing aid or from the hearing aid case of behind-the-ear and eyeglass hearing aids where the tubing meets the hook of the case. Do not remove the earmold if it is glued or secured by a small metal ring. **Rationale:** *Removal facilitates cleaning and prevents inadvertent damage to the other parts.*
   - If the earmold is detachable, soak it in a mild soapy solution. Rinse and dry it well. Do not use isopropyl alcohol. **Rationale:** *Alcohol can damage the hearing aid.*
   - If the earmold is not detachable or is for an in-the-ear aid, wipe the earmold with a damp cloth.
   - Check that the earmold opening is patent. Blow any excess moisture through the opening or remove debris (e.g., earwax) with a pipe cleaner or toothpick.
   - Reattach the earmold if it was detached from the rest of the hearing aid.
6. Insert the hearing aid.
   - Determine from the client if the earmold is for the left or the right ear.

- Check that the battery is inserted in the hearing aid. Turn off the hearing aid, and make sure the volume is turned all the way down. **Rationale:** *A volume that is too loud is distressing.*
- Inspect the earmold to identify the ear canal portion. Some earmolds are fitted for only the ear canal and concha; others are fitted for all the contours of the ear. The canal portion, common to all, can be used as a guide for correct insertion.
- Line up the parts of the earmold with the corresponding parts of the client's ear.
- Rotate the earmold slightly forward, and insert the ear canal portion.
- Gently press the earmold into the ear while rotating it backward.
- Check that the earmold fits snugly by asking the client if it feels secure and comfortable.
- Adjust the other components of a behind-the-ear or body hearing aid.
- Turn the hearing aid on, and adjust the volume according to the client's needs.
7. Correct problems associated with improper functioning.
   - If the sound is weak or there is no sound:
     a. Ensure that the volume is turned high enough.
     b. Ensure that the earmold opening is not clogged.
     c. Check the battery by turning the hearing aid on, turning up the volume, cupping your hand over the earmold, and listening. A constant whistling sound indicates the battery is functioning. If necessary, replace the battery. Be sure that the negative (–) and positive (+) signs on the battery match those where indicated on the hearing aid.
     d. Ensure that the ear canal is not blocked with wax, which can obstruct sound waves.
   - If the client reports a whistling sound or squeal after insertion:
     a. Turn the volume down.
     b. Ensure that the earmold is properly attached to the receiver.
     c. Reinsert the earmold.
8. Document pertinent data.
   - The removal and the insertion of a hearing aid are not normally recorded.
   - Report and record any problems the client has with the hearing aid.

EVALUATION
- Speak to the client in a normal conversational tone and observe client behaviors.
- Compare the client's hearing ability to previous assessments.
- Report to the primary care provider any deviations from normal for the client.

NOSE

Nurses usually need not provide special care for the nose, because clients can ordinarily clear nasal secretions by blowing gently into a soft tissue. When the external nares are encrusted with dried secretions, they should be cleaned with a cotton-tipped applicator or moistened with saline or water. The applicator should not be inserted beyond the length of the cotton tip; inserting it further may cause injury to the mucosa.

SUPPORTING A HYGIENIC ENVIRONMENT

Because people are usually confined to bed when ill, often for long periods, the bed becomes an important element in the client's life. A place that is clean, safe, and comfortable contributes to the client's ability to rest and sleep and to a sense of well-being. Basic furniture in a health care facility includes the bed, bedside table, overbed table, one or more chairs, and a storage space for clothing. Most bed units also have a call light, light fixtures, electric outlets, and hygienic equipment in the bedside table. Three types of equipment often installed in an acute care facility are a suction outlet for several kinds of suction, an oxygen outlet for most oxygen equipment, and a sphygmomanometer to measure the client's blood pressure. Some long-term care agencies also permit clients to have personal furniture, such as a television, a chair, and lamps, at the bedside. In the home a client often has personal and medical equipment.

Environment

When providing a comfortable environment it is important to consider the client's age, severity of illness, and level of activity. The very young, the very old, and the acutely ill frequently need a room temperature higher than normal. A room temperature between 20°C and 23°C (68°F and 74°F) is comfortable for most clients. Good ventilation is important to remove unpleasant odors and stale air. Room deodorizers can help eliminate odors. Ill persons are sensitive to noise such as clanging of metal equipment, loud talking, and laughter. Nurses should try to control noise in health care settings.

Hospital Beds

The frame of a hospital bed is divided into three sections. This permits the head and the foot to be elevated separately. Most hospital beds have electric motors to operate the movable joints. The motor is activated by pressing a button or moving a small lever, located either at the side of the bed or on a small panel separate from the bed but attached to it by a cable, which the client can readily use.

Hospital beds are usually 66 cm (26 in.) high and 0.9 m (3 ft) wide, narrower than the usual bed, so that the nurse can reach the client from either side of the bed without undue stretching. The length is usually 1.9 m (6.5 ft). Some beds can be extended in length to accommodate very tall clients.

Long-term care facilities for ambulatory clients usually have low beds to facilitate movement in and out of bed. Most hospital beds have "high" and "low" positions that can be adjusted either mechanically or electrically by a button or lever. The high position permits the nurse to reach the client without undue stretching or stooping. The low position allows the client to step easily to the floor.

Mattresses

Mattresses are usually covered with a water-repellent material that resists soiling and can be cleaned easily. Most mattresses have handles on the sides called lugs by which the mattress can be moved. Many special mattresses are also used in hospitals to relieve pressure on the body's bony prominences, such as the heels. They are particularly helpful for clients confined to bed for a long time. For additional information about mattresses, see Chapter 24 ∞.

Side Rails

Side rails, or safety sides, are used on both hospital beds and stretchers. They are of various shapes and sizes and are usually made of metal. A bed can have two full-length side rails or four half- or quarter-length side rails (also called split rails). Devices to raise and lower side rails differ. When side rails are being used, it is important that the nurse never leave the bedside while the rail is lowered.

For decades, the use of side rails has been routine practice with the rationale that the side rails serve as a safe and effective means of preventing clients from falling out of bed. Research, however, has not validated this assumption. In fact, several studies have shown that raised side rails do not deter older clients from getting out of bed unassisted and have led to more serious falls, injuries, and even death (Capezuti, 2004; Talerico & Capezuti, 2001). The Health Care Financing Administration now mandates that nurses in both acute care and long-term care decrease the routine use of side rails. Alternatives to side rails do exist and can include low-height bed, mats placed at the side of the beds, motion sensors, and bed alarms (see Chapter 21 ∞).

> **CLINICAL ALERT**
>
> Side rail entrapment, injuries, and deaths do occur. When side rails are used, the nurse must assess the client's physical and mental status and closely monitor high-risk (frail, older, or confused) clients.

Footboard or Footboot

These are used to support the immobilized client's foot in a normal right angle to the legs to prevent plantar flexion contractures (see Chapter 31 ∞).

Bed Cradles

A bed cradle is a device designed to keep the top bedclothes off the feet, legs, and even abdomen of a client. The bedclothes are arranged over the device and may be pinned in place. There are several types of bed cradles. One of the most common is a curved metal rod that fits over the bed. Part of the cradle fits under the mattress, and small metal brackets press down on each side of the mattress to keep the cradle in place. The frame of some cradles extends over half of the width of the bed, above one leg.

MAKING BEDS

Nurses need to be able to prepare hospital beds in different ways for specific purposes. In most instances, beds are made after the client receives certain care and when beds are unoccupied. At times, however, nurses need to make an occupied bed or prepare a bed for a client who is having surgery.

Unoccupied Bed

An unoccupied bed can be either closed or open. Generally the top covers of an open bed are folded back (thus the term *open bed*) to make it easier for a client to get in. Open and closed beds are made the same way, except that the top sheet, blanket, and bedspread of a *closed bed* are drawn up to the top of the bed and under the pillows.

Beds are often changed after bed baths. The linen can be collected before the bath. The linen is not usually changed unless it is soiled. Check the policy at each clinical agency.

Unfitted sheets, blankets, and bedspreads are mitered at the corners of the bed. The purpose of mitering is to secure the bedclothes while the bed is occupied. Figure 22–9 shows how to miter the corner of a bed. Skill 22–8 explains how to change an unoccupied bed.

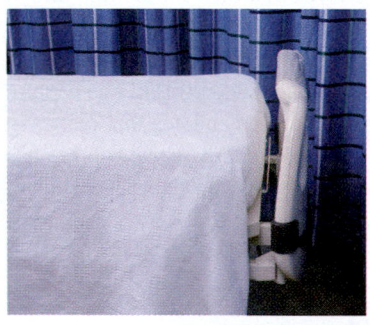
A

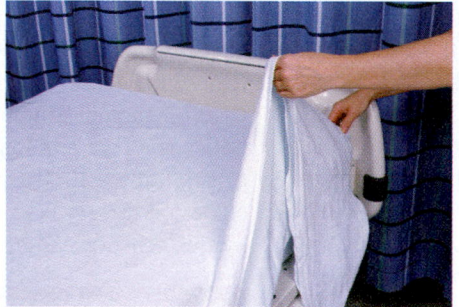
B

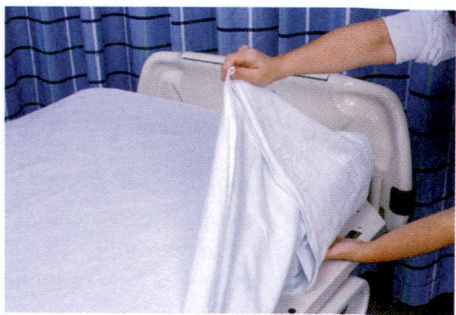
C

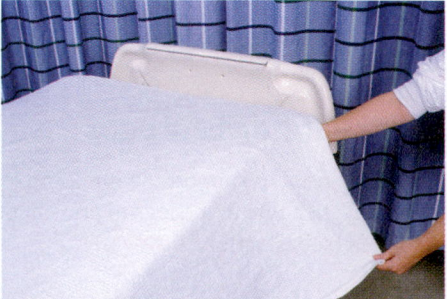
D

E

Figure 22–9 ⭕ Mitering the corner of a bed. **A,** Tuck the ends of the sheet first. **B,** Make a triangular fold. **C,** Tuck the corner of the sheet under the mattress. **D,** Bring down the top of the triangle. **E,** Tuck the sides in tightly.

SKILL 22–8

CHANGING AN UNOCCUPIED BED

PURPOSES
- To provide a clean neat environment for the client
- To provide a smooth, wrinkle-free bed foundation, thus minimizing sources of skin irritation

ASSESSMENT
- Assess the client's health status to determine that the person can safely get out of bed. In some hospitals it is necessary to have a written order if the client has been in bed continuously.
- Assess the client's pulse and respirations if indicated.

- Note all the tubes and equipment connected to the client. **Rationale:** *This may influence the need for additional linens or waterproof pads.*

PLANNING

> ### Delegation
> Bed-making is usually delegated to UAP. If appropriate, inform the UAP of the proper disposal method of linens that contain drainage. Ask the UAP to inform you immediately if any tubes or dressings become dislodged or removed. Stress the importance of the call light being readily available while the client is out of bed.

EQUIPMENT
- Two flat sheets or one fitted and one flat sheet
- Cloth drawsheet (optional)
- One blanket
- One bedspread
- Waterproof pads (optional)
- Pillowcase(s) for the head pillow(s)
- Plastic laundry bag or portable linen hamper, if available

IMPLEMENTATION

Preparation
Determine what linens the client may already have in the room *to avoid stockpiling of unnecessary extra linens.*

Performance
1. If the client is in the bed prior to performing the procedure, introduce self and verify the client's identity using agency protocol. Explain to the client what you are going to do, why it is necessary, and how he or she can participate.
2. Perform hand hygiene and observe other appropriate infection control procedures.
3. Provide for client privacy.
4. Place the fresh linen on the client's chair or overbed table; do not use another client's bed. **Rationale:** *This prevents cross-contamination (the movement of microorganisms from one client to another) via soiled linen.*
5. Assess and assist the client out of bed.
   - Make sure that this is an appropriate and convenient time for the client to be out of bed.
   - Assist the client to a comfortable chair.
6. Raise the bed to a comfortable working height.
7. Strip the bed.
   - Check bed linens for any items belonging to the client, and detach the call bell or any drainage tubes from the bed linen.
   - Loosen all bedding systematically, starting at the head of the bed on the far side and moving around the bed up to the head of the bed on the near side. **Rationale:** *Moving around the bed systematically prevents stretching and reaching and possible muscle strain.*
   - Remove the pillowcases, if soiled, and place the pillows on the bedside chair near the foot of the bed.
   - Fold reusable linens, such as the bedspread and top sheet on the bed, into fourths. First, fold the linen in half by bringing the top edge even with the bottom edge, and then grasp it at the center of the middle fold and bottom edges. **Rationale:** *Folding linens saves time and*

energy when reapplying the linens on the bed and keeps them clean.
   - Remove the waterproof pad and discard it if soiled.
   - Roll all soiled linen inside the bottom sheet, hold it away from your uniform, and place it directly in the linen hamper, not on the floor. **Rationale:** *These actions are essential to prevent the transmission of microorganisms to the nurse and others.*
   - Grasp the mattress securely, using the lugs if present, and move the mattress up to the head of the bed.
8. Apply the bottom sheet and drawsheet.
   - Place the folded bottom sheet with its center fold on the center of the bed. Make sure the sheet is hem side down for a smooth foundation. Spread the sheet out over the mattress, and allow a sufficient amount of sheet at the top to tuck under the mattress. ❶ **Rationale:** *The top of the sheet needs to be well tucked under to remain securely in place, especially when the head of the bed is elevated.* Place the sheet along the edge of the mattress

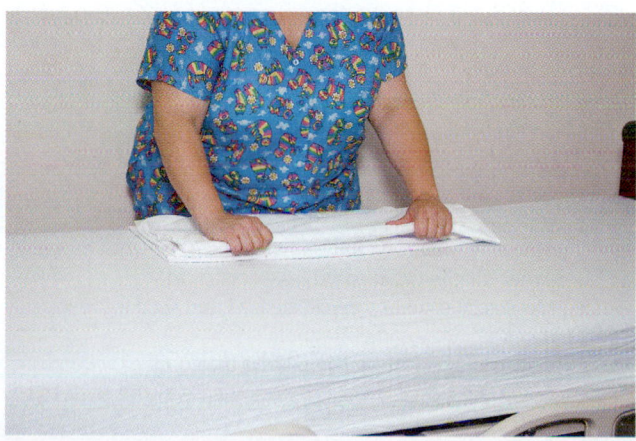

❶ Placing bottom sheet on bed.

(continued)

CHANGING AN UNOCCUPIED BED *(continued)*

at the foot of the bed and do not tuck it in (unless it is a contour or fitted sheet).

- Miter the sheet at the top corner on the near side (Figure 22–9, earlier) and tuck the sheet under the mattress, working from the head of the bed to the foot.

- If a waterproof drawsheet is used, place it over the bottom sheet so that the centerfold is at the centerline of the bed and the top and bottom edges extend from the middle of the client's back to the area of the midthigh or knee. Fanfold the uppermost half of the folded drawsheet at the center or far edge of the bed and tuck in the near edge.

- Lay the cloth drawsheet over the waterproof sheet in the same manner.

- *Optional:* Before moving to the other side of the bed, place the top linens on the bed hemside up, unfold them, tuck them in, and miter the bottom corners. **Rationale:** *Completing one entire side of the bed at a time saves time and energy.*

9. Move to the other side and secure the bottom linens.
   - Tuck in the bottom sheet under the head of the mattress, pull the sheet firmly, and miter the corner of the sheet.
   - Pull the remainder of the sheet firmly so that there are no wrinkles. **Rationale:** *Wrinkles can cause discomfort for the client and breakdown of skin. Tuck the sheet in at the side.*
   - Complete this same process for the drawsheet(s).

10. Apply or complete the top sheet, blanket, and spread.
    - Place the top sheet, hemside up, on the bed so that its centerfold is at the center of the bed and the top edge is even with the top edge of the mattress.
    - Unfold the sheet over the bed.
    - *Optional:* Make a vertical or a horizontal toe pleat in the sheet to provide additional room for the client's feet.
      a. *Vertical toe pleat:* Make a fold in the sheet 5 to 10 cm (2 to 4 in.) perpendicular to the foot of the bed. ②
      b. *Horizontal toe pleat:* Make a fold in the sheet 5 to 10 cm (2 to 4 in.) across the bed near the foot. ③
         Loosening the top covers around the feet after the client is in bed is another way to provide additional space.
    - Follow the same procedure for the blanket and the spread, but place the top edges about 15 cm (6 in.) from the head of the bed to allow a cuff of sheet to be folded over them.
    - Tuck in the sheet, blanket, and spread at the foot of the bed, and miter the corner, using all three layers of linen. Leave the sides of the top sheet, blanket, and spread hanging freely unless toe pleats were provided.
    - Fold the top of the top sheet down over the spread, providing a cuff. ④ **Rationale:** *The cuff of sheet makes it easier for the client to pull the covers up.*
    - Move to the other side of the bed and secure the top bedding in the same manner.

11. Put clean pillowcases on the pillows as required.
    - Grasp the closed end of the pillowcase at the center with one hand.

- Gather up the sides of the pillowcase and place them over the hand grasping the case. Then grasp the center of one short side of the pillow through the pillowcase. ⑤

- With the free hand, pull the pillowcase over the pillow.

- Adjust the pillowcase so that the pillow fits into the corners of the case and the seams are straight. **Rationale:** *A smoothly fitting pillowcase is more comfortable than a wrinkled one.*

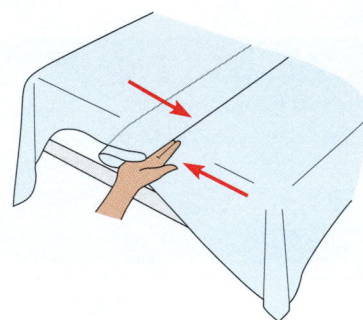

② A vertical toe pleat.

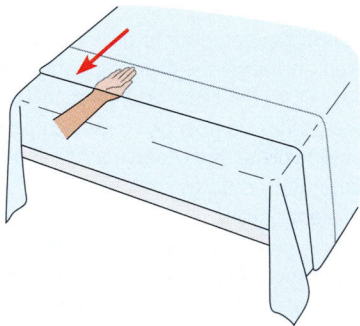

③ A horizontal toe pleat.

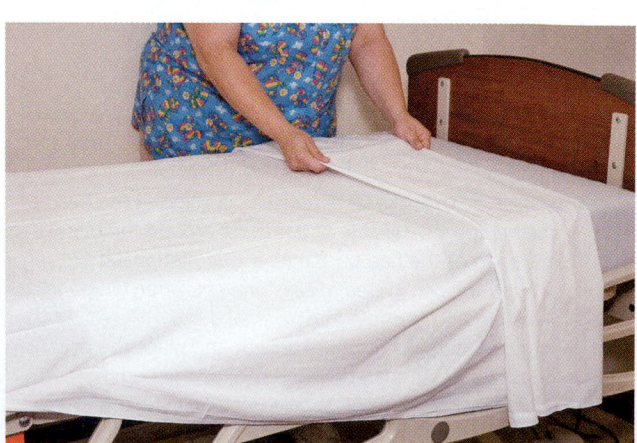

④ Making a cuff of the top linens.

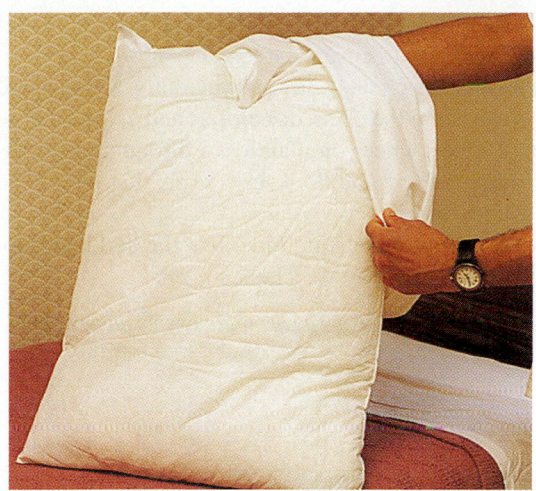

5 Method for putting a clean pillowcase on a pillow.

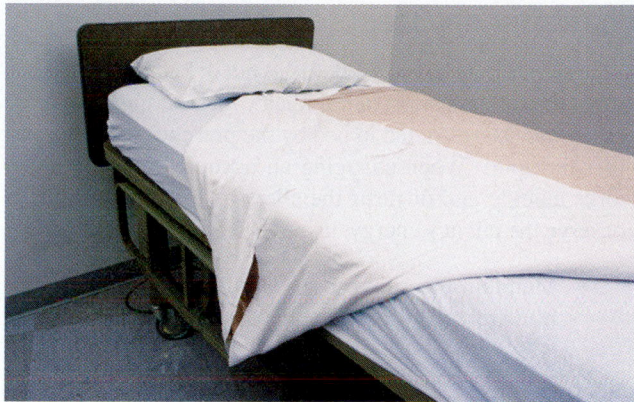

6 Fold up the two outer corners of the top linens, forming a triangle.

- Place the pillows appropriately at the head of the bed.
12. Provide for client comfort and safety.
   - Attach the signal cord so that the client can conveniently reach it. Some cords have clamps that attach to the sheet or pillowcase. Others are attached by a safety pin.
   - If the bed is currently being used by a client, either fold back the top covers at one side or fanfold them down to the center of the bed. **Rationale:** *This makes it easier for the client to get into the bed.*
   - Place the bedside table and the overbed table so that they are available to the client.
   - Leave the bed in the high position if the client is returning by stretcher, or place in the low position if the client is returning to bed after being up.
13. Document and report pertinent data.
   - Bed-making is not normally recorded.
   - Record any nursing assessments, such as the client's physical status and pulse and respiratory rates before and after being out of bed, as indicated.

VARIATION: SURGICAL BED
While the client is in the operating room, the client's bed is prepared for the postoperative phase. In some agencies, the client is brought back to the unit on a stretcher and transferred to the bed in the room. In other agencies, the client's bed is brought to the surgery suite and the client is transferred there. In the latter situation, the bed needs to be made with clean linens as soon as the client goes to surgery so that it can be taken to the operating room when needed.

- Strip the bed.
- Place and leave the pillows on the bedside chair. **Rationale:** *Pillows are left on a chair to facilitate transferring the client into the bed.*

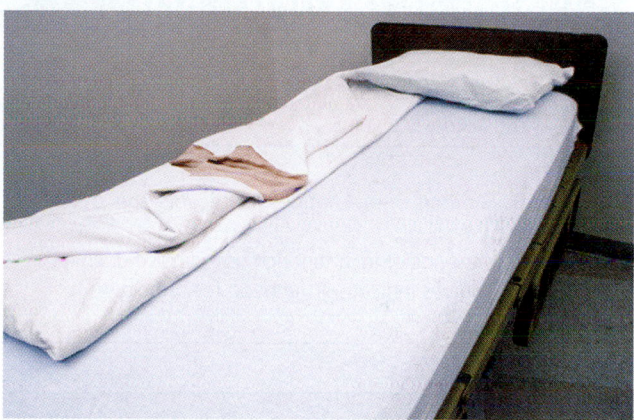

7 Surgical bed. The linens are horizontally fanfolded to the other side of the bed to facilitate transfer of the client into the bed.

- Apply the bottom linens as for an unoccupied bed. Place a bath blanket on the foundation of the bed if this is agency practice. **Rationale:** *A flannel bath blanket provides additional warmth.*
- Place the top covers (sheet, blanket, and bedspread) on the bed as you would for an unoccupied bed. Do not tuck them in, miter the corners, or make a toe pleat.
- Make a cuff at the top of the bed as you would for an unoccupied bed. Fold the top linens up from the bottom.
- On the side of the bed where the client will be transferred, fold up the two outer corners of the top linens so they meet in the middle of the bed forming a triangle. **6**
- Pick up the apex of the triangle and fanfold the top linens lengthwise to the other side of the bed *to facilitate the client's transfer into the bed.* **7**
- Leave the bed in high position with the side rails down. **Rationale:** *The high position facilitates the transfer of the client.*
- Lock the wheels of the bed if the bed is not to be moved. **Rationale:** *Locking the wheels keeps the bed from rolling when the client is transferred from the stretcher to the bed.*

EVALUATION
- Make sure the call light is accessible to the client.
- Relate client parameters of activity (e.g., pulse and respirations) to previous assessment data, particularly if the client has been on bed rest for an extended period of time or if it is the first time that the client is getting out of bed after surgery.

Changing an Occupied Bed

Some clients may be too weak to get out of bed. Either the nature of their illness may contraindicate their sitting out of bed, or they may be restricted in bed by the presence of traction or other therapies. When changing an occupied bed, the nurse works quickly and disturbs the client as little as possible to conserve the client's energy, using the following guidelines:

- Maintain the client in good body alignment. Never move or position a client in a manner that is con-

traindicated by the client's health. Obtain help if necessary to ensure safety.
- Move the client gently and smoothly. Rough handling can cause the client discomfort and abrade the skin.
- Explain what you plan to do throughout the procedure before you do it. Use terms that the client can understand.
- Use the bed-making time, like the bed bath time, to assess and meet the client's needs.

See Skill 22–9 for instructions on changing an occupied bed.

SKILL 22–9

CHANGING AN OCCUPIED BED

PURPOSES
- To conserve the client's energy
- To promote client comfort
- To provide a clean, neat environment for the client
- To provide a smooth, wrinkle-free bed foundation, thus minimizing sources of skin irritation

ASSESSMENT
- Note specific orders or precautions for moving and positioning the client.
- Determine presence of incontinence or excessive drainage from other sources indicating the need for protective waterproof pads.
- Assess skin condition and need for special mattress (e.g., egg crate), footboard, or heel protectors.

PLANNING

> **Delegation**
> Bed-making is usually delegated to UAP. Inform the UAP to what extent the client can assist or if another person will be needed to assist the UAP. Instruct the UAP about the handling of any dressings and/or tubes of the client and also the need for special equipment (e.g., footboard, heel protectors), if appropriate.

EQUIPMENT
- Two flat sheets or one fitted and one flat sheet
- Cloth drawsheet (optional)
- One blanket
- One bedspread
- Waterproof drawsheet or waterproof pads (optional)
- Pillowcase(s) for the head pillow(s)
- Plastic laundry bag or portable linen hamper, if available

IMPLEMENTATION

Performance

1. Explain to the client what you are going to do, why it is necessary, and how he or she can participate.
2. Perform hand hygiene and observe other appropriate infection control procedures. Put on disposable gloves if linen is soiled with body fluids.
3. Provide for client privacy.
4. Remove the top bedding.
   - Remove any equipment attached to the bed linen, such as a signal light.
   - Loosen all the top linen at the foot of the bed, and remove the spread and the blanket.
   - Leave the top sheet over the client (the top sheet can remain over the client if it is being changed and if it will provide sufficient warmth), or replace it with a bath blanket as follows:
     Spread the bath blanket over the top sheet.
     a. Ask the client to hold the top edge of the blanket.
     b. Reaching under the blanket from the side, grasp the top edge of the sheet and draw it down to the foot of the bed, leaving the blanket in place.
     c. Remove the sheet from the bed and place it in the soiled linen hamper.

5. Change the bottom sheet and drawsheet.
   - Assist the client to turn on the side facing away from the side where the clean linen is.
   - Raise the side rail nearest the client. **Rationale:** *This protects the client from falling.* If there is no side rail, have another nurse support the client at the edge of the bed.
   - Loosen the foundation of the linen on the side of the bed near the linen supply.
   - Fanfold the drawsheet and the bottom sheet at the center of the bed ❶, as close to and under the client as possible. **Rationale:** *Doing this leaves the near half of the bed free to be changed.*
   - Place the new bottom sheet on the bed, and vertically fanfold the half to be used on the far side of the bed as close to the client as possible. ❷ Tuck the sheet under the near half of the bed and miter the corner if a contour sheet is not being used.
   - Place the clean drawsheet on the bed with the center fold at the center of the bed. Fanfold the uppermost half vertically at the center of the bed and tuck the near side edge under the side of the mattress. ❸
   - Assist the client to roll over toward you onto the clean side of the bed. The client rolls over the fanfolded linen at the center of the bed.

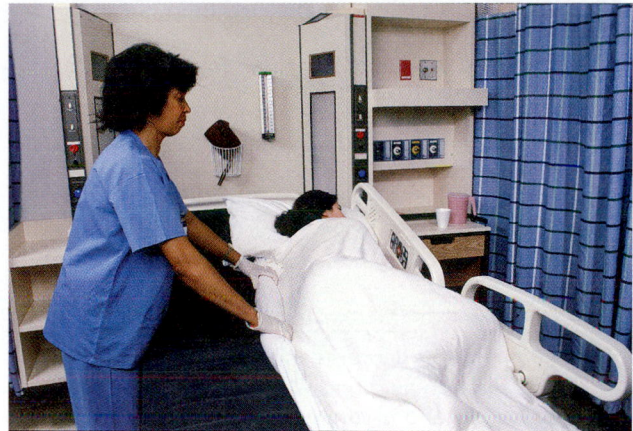

1 Moving soiled linen as close to the client as possible.

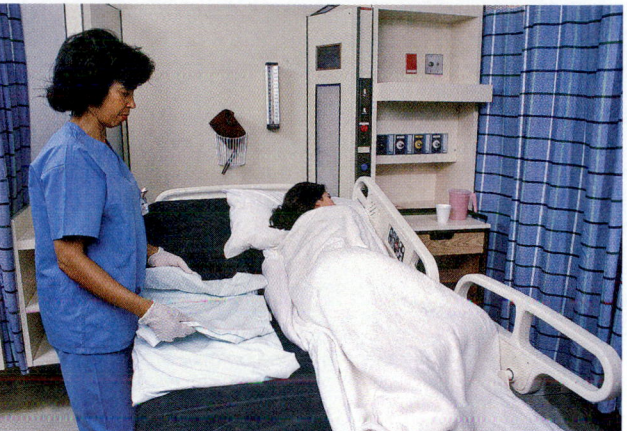

2 Placing a new bottom sheet on half of the bed.

- Move the pillows to the clean side for the client's use. Raise the side rail before leaving the side of the bed.
- Move to the other side of the bed and lower the side rail.
- Remove the used linen and place it in the portable hamper.
- Unfold the fanfolded bottom sheet from the center of the bed.
- Facing the side of the bed, use both hands to pull the bottom sheet so that it is smooth and tuck the excess under the side of the mattress.
- Unfold the drawsheet fanfolded at the center of the bed and pull it tightly with both hands. Pull the sheet in three sections: (a) Face the side of the bed to pull the middle section, (b) face the far top corner to pull the bottom section, and (c) face the far bottom corner to pull the top section.
- Tuck the excess drawsheet under the side of the mattress.

6. Reposition the client in the center of the bed.
   - Reposition the pillows at the center of the bed.
   - Assist the client to the center of the bed. Determine what position the client requires or prefers and assist the client to that position.

7. Apply or complete the top bedding.
   - Spread the top sheet over the client and either ask the client to hold the top edge of the sheet or tuck it under the shoulders. The sheet should remain over the client when the bath blanket or used sheet is removed.

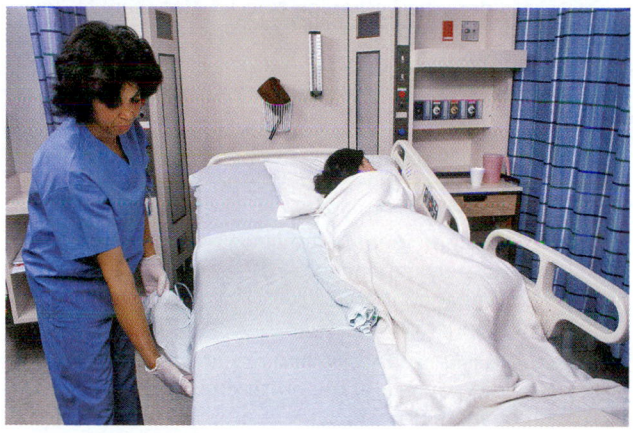

3 Placing a clean drawsheet on the bed.

   - Complete the top of the bed.
8. Ensure continued safety of the client.
   - Raise the side rails. Place the bed in the low position before leaving the bedside.
   - Attach the signal cord to the bed linen within the client's reach.
   - Put items used by the client within easy reach.
9. Bed-making is not normally recorded.

EVALUATION
- Conduct appropriate follow-up, such as determining client's comfort and safety, patency of all drainage tubes, and client's access to call light to summon help when needed.

CHAPTER HIGHLIGHTS

- Clients' hygienic practices are influenced by numerous factors, including culture, religion, environment, developmental level, health and energy, and personal preferences.
- The major functions of the skin are to protect underlying tissues, to help regulate body temperature,

to secrete sebum, to transmit sensations through nerve receptors for sensory perception, and to produce and absorb vitamin D in conjunction with ultraviolet rays from the sun.
- When planning hygiene care, the nurse must take the client's preferences into consideration.

- Nurses provide perineal-genital care for clients who are unable to do so for themselves.
- Nurses can often teach clients how to prevent foot problems.
- Oral hygiene should include daily dental flossing and mechanical brushing of the teeth.
- Regular dental checkups and fluoride supplements are recommended to maintain healthy teeth.
- Nurses provide special oral care to clients who are unconscious or debilitated.

- Hair care includes daily combing and brushing and regular shampooing.
- African American clients' hair may require special care.
- Nurses may need to assist dependent clients with their artificial eyes, eyeglasses, and contact lenses.
- Clients with a hearing aid may require nursing assistance with the device.
- Changing bed linens is a part of maintaining hygiene.
- It is important to keep beds clean and comfortable for clients.

THINK ABOUT IT

Refer to the chapter-opening scenario and answer these questions.

1. After admitting Ms. Roker to the unit, what hygiene care would you perform first?

2. What special developmental and physical factors would you consider when planning care for this client?

3. Ms. Roker wears dentures and has acute halitosis as well as sores on her gums when the dentures are removed. What oral care would you provide her?

∞ *See suggested responses to Think About It on MyNursingKit.*

TEST YOUR KNOWLEDGE

1. A client can bathe independently except for the back and feet, walk to and from the bathroom, and dress if the clothing is provided. What is the most appropriate functional level for this client?
   1. Totally dependent (+4)
   2. Moderately dependent (+3)
   3. Semidependent (+2)
   4. Independent (0)

2. The client is unresponsive and requires total care. Prior to providing oral care, the nurse should assess for which of the following?
   1. Presence of pain
   2. Condition of the skin
   3. Gag reflex
   4. Range of motion

3. A client with diabetes has very dry skin on her feet and lower extremities. To maintain intact skin the nurse teaches which of the following?
   1. Soak her feet frequently.
   2. Use a nonperfumed lotion.
   3. Apply foot powder.
   4. Avoid knee-high elastic stockings.

4. The client wears an in-the-ear hearing aid and because of arthritis needs someone to insert the hearing aid. The nurse teaches the unlicensed assistive personnel (UAP) to do which of the following actions before inserting the client's hearing aid?
   1. Turn the hearing aid off.
   2. Soak the hearing aid in soapy solution to clean it.
   3. Turn the volume all the way up.
   4. Remove the batteries.

5. The client is in surgery and will be returning to his bed via a stretcher. The nurse plans ahead by making which type of bed and placing the bed in which position?
   1. An open bed in low position
   2. An occupied bed in low position
   3. A closed bed in high position
   4. A surgical bed in high position

6. Which of the following strategies are most appropriate for client with dementia? Select all that apply.
   1. Cover the client as much as possible.
   2. Sing or talk to the client.
   3. Complete the bath as quickly as possible.
   4. Be organized.
   5. Expect the client to protest—finish quickly.

7. The nurse observed the UAP performing perineal care for a client. Which of the following actions indicates that further teaching is required?
   1. Used a clean portion of the washcloth for each stroke.
   2. Wiped from the pubis to the rectum.
   3. Used clean gloves.
   4. Did not retract the foreskin.

8. Which of the following statements will be important to include during a presentation on oral health at an intergenerational community center? Select all that apply.
   1. Using a bottle during naps and at bedtime can cause dental caries in a toddler.
   2. Schedule a visit to the dentist when your child is ready to go to school.
   3. It is important for parents to supervise a child's tooth-brushing.
   4. Most older adults have dentures and don't need to worry about oral care.
   5. Older adults are at risk for periodontal disease.

9. The nurse is discussing foot care with a client who was recently diagnosed with diabetes. Which of the following statements indicates a need for further teaching?
   1. "I am going to use a mirror to check my feet."
   2. "I enjoy walking barefoot around the house."
   3. "I will file my nails."
   4. "I will increase the time that I wear new shoes each day."

10. The client experiencing labored, shortness of breath has a respiratory rate of 28. The bed is currently in the flat position. The best nursing intervention includes putting the bed in which of the following positions?
    1. Fowler's
    2. Semi-Fowler's
    3. Trendelenburg
    4. Reverse Trendelenburg

∞ *See answers to Test your knowledge in Appendix A.*

REFERENCES AND SELECTED BIBLIOGRAPHY

Alzheimer's Disease Education & Referral Center. (n.d.). *2001–2002 Alzheimer's disease progress report.* Retrieved June 13, 2006, from http://www.nia.nih.gov/NR/rdonlyres?7049AF18-6827-4DCE-95FA-B853D171C974/0/2002_ALZ_PR.pdf

American Dental Association. (n.d.). *Cleaning your teeth and gums (oral hygiene).* Retrieved June 13, 2006, from http://www.ada.org/public/topics/cleaning_faq.asp

American Dental Association. (n.d.). *Oral changes with age.* Retrieved June 13, 2006, from http://www.ada.org/public/topics/oral_changes_faq.asp

Anderson, E. G. (1998). Deafness is a scourge and you can say that again. *Geriatrics, 53*(8), 65–69.

Andrews, M. M., & Boyle, J. S. (2008). *Transcultural concepts in nursing care* (5th ed.). Philadelphia: Lippincott Williams & Wilkins.

Anonymous. (2003). Oral care update. *Nursing Management, 34*(5), S1–S16.

Barrick, A. L., & Rader, J. (2000). Bathing without a battle [Electronic Version]. *Alzheimer's Care Quarterly, 1*(4), 35–49.

Barrick, A. L., Rader, J., Hoeffer, B., & Sloane, P. (Eds.). (2002). *Bathing without a battle: Personal care of individuals with dementia.* New York: Springer.

Bulechek, G. M., Butcher, H. K., & Dochterman, J. M. (Eds.). (2008). *Nursing interventions: Classification (NIC)* (5th ed.). St. Louis, MO: Mosby.

Capezuti, E. (2004). Guidelines address side rail entrapment. *American Journal of Nursing, 104*(5), 74.

Chalmer, J., Johnson, V., Hsiao-Chen, J., & Titler, M. G. (2004). Evidence-based protocol: Oral hygiene care for functionally dependent and cognitively impaired older adults. *Journal of Gerontological Nursing, 30*(11), 5–12.

Coleman, P. R. (2002). Improving oral health care for the frail elderly: A review of widespread problems and best practices. *Geriatric Nursing, 23,* 189–199.

Coleman, P. R. (2004). Promoting oral health in elder care: Challenges and opportunities. *Journal of Gerontological Nursing, 30*(4), 3.

Dougherty, J., & Long, C. O. (2003). Techniques for bathing without a battle. *Home Healthcare Nurse, 21*(1), 38–39.

Dunn, J. C., Thiru-Chelvam, B., & Beck, C. H. M. (2002). Bathing: Pleasure or pain? *Journal of Gerontological Nursing, 28*(11), 6–13.

Edelman, C. L., & Mandle, C. L. (2010). *Health promotion throughout the life span* (7th ed.). St. Louis: Mosby Elsevier.

Ficorelli, C. T., & Edelman, M. (2005). Foot care for patients with diabetes. *Nursing, 35*(10), 43.

Forrester, D. A., Nash-Luchenback, D., & Tistler, M. (2004). Help your patient manage dry mouth. *Nursing, 34*(4), 32hn10-11.

Frankowski, B. L., & Weiner, L. B. (2002). Head lice. *Pediatrics, 110*(3), 638–643.

Gammons, M., & Salam, G. (2002). Tick removal. *American Family Physician, 66*(4), 643–645.

Goldsmith, J. (2003). Nit-picking. *American Journal of Nursing, 103*(9), 22–23.

Gooch, B. F., Eke, P. I., & Malvitz, D. M. (2004). Public health and aging: Retention of natural teeth among older adults—United States, 2002. *Journal of the American Medical Association, 291*(3), 292.

Hilgers, J. (2003). Comforting a confused patient. *Nursing, 33*(1), 48–50.

Hoffman, S. B., Powell-Cope, G., MacClellan, L., & Bero, K. (2003). BedSAFE: A bed safety project for frail older adults. *Journal of Gerontological Nursing, 29*(11), 34–42.

Jackson, F. (1998). The ABC's of black hair and skin care. *ABNF Journal, 9*(5), 100–104.

Kelly, S. E., Binkley, C. J., Neace, W. P., & Gale, B. S. (2005). Barriers to care-seeking for children's oral health among low-income caregivers. *American Journal of Public Health, 95*(8), 1345–1351.

Lamster, I. B. (2004). Oral health care services for older adults: A looming crisis. *American Journal of Public Health, 94*(5), 699–703.

Lucas, L. J., & Mathews-Flint, L. J. (2003). Heed the word about hearing impairment. *Nursing, 33*(10), 32hn1–32hn1-4.

Moorhead, S., Johnson, M., Maas, M. L., & Swanson, E. (Eds.). (2008). *Nursing outcomes classification (NOC)* (4th ed.). St. Louis, MO: Mosby.

Moses, M. (2003). A simple matter of grooming. Stop using toxic pesticides to treat head lice. *American Journal of Nursing, 103*(9), 11.

Munro, C. L., Grap, M. J., & Kleinpell, R. (2004). Oral health and care in the intensive care unit: State of the science. *American Journal of Critical Care, 13*(1), 25–34.

Nainar, S. M., & Mohummed, S. (2004). Role of infant feeding practices on the dental health of children. *Clinical Pediatrics, 43*(2), 129–133.

NANDA International (2009). *NANDA nursing diagnoses: Definitions & Classification 2009–2010.* West Sussex, U. K.: Wiley-Blackwell.

Parker, L. (2004). Infection control: Maintaining the personal hygiene of patients and staff. *British Journal of Nursing, 13*(8), 474–478.

Pattillo, M. M. (2004). Therapeutic and healing foot care: A healthy feet clinic for older adults. *Journal of Gerontological Nursing, 30*(12), 25–32.

Perlmutter, J. S., & Camberg, L. (2004). Better bathing for residents with Alzheimer's. *Nursing Homes, 53*(4), 40–43.

Pillitteri, A. (2010). *Maternal and child health nursing: Care of the childbearing and childrearing family* (5th ed.). Philadelphia: Lippincott Williams & Wilkins.

Purnell, L. D., & Paulanka, B. J. (2005). *Guide to culturally competent health care.* Philadelphia: Davis.

Rader, J., Barrick, A. L., Hoeffer, B., Sloane, P. D., McKenzie, D., Talerico, K. A., et al. (2006). The bathing of older adults with dementia. Easing the unnecessarily unpleasant aspects of assisted bathing. *American Journal of Nursing, 106*(4), 40–48.

Rasin, J., & Barrick, A. L. (2004). Bathing patients with dementia: Concentrating on the patient's needs rather than merely the task. *American Journal of Nursing, 104*(3), 30–33.

Sieggreen, M. Y. (2005). Stepping up care for diabetic foot ulcers. *Nursing, 35*(10), 36–41.

Stewart, K. B. (2000). Stopping the itch of scabies and lice. *Nursing, 30*(7), 30–31.

Stone, C. M. (1999). Preventing cerumen impaction in nursing facility residents. *Journal of Gerontological Nursing, 25*(5), 43–45.

Talerico, K. A., & Capezuti, E. (2001). Myths and facts about side rails. *American Journal of Nursing, 101*(7), 43–48.

Walton, J. C., Miller, J., & Tordecilla, L. (2001). Elder oral assessment and care. *Medsurg Nursing, 10*(1), 37–44.

Wilkinson, J. M. (2009). *Nursing diagnosis handbook with NIC interventions and NOC outcomes* (9th ed.). Upper Saddle River, NJ: Prentice Hall Health.

Yetzer, E. A. (2004). Incorporating foot care education into diabetic foot screening. *Rehabilitation Nursing, 29*(3), 80–84.

Zulkowski, K., & Albrecht, D. (2003). How dental status affects healing in older adults. *Nursing, 33*(10), 22.

Medications

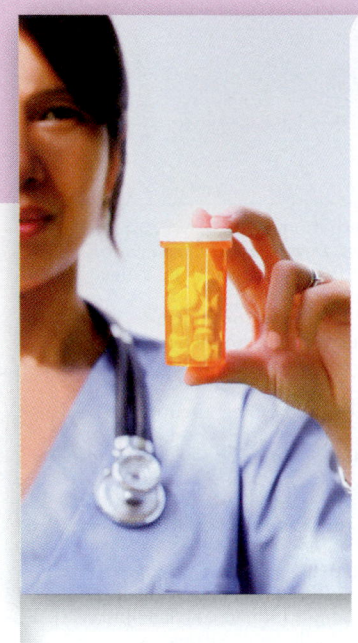

Brittany is the medication nurse today on a busy skilled care unit in the long-term care facility. After receiving report she is checking the medication administration records (MAR) against the clients' medical records when an unlicensed assistive personnel reports that a client's blood glucose is elevated. Brittany stops to administer insulin on an ordered sliding scale and then returns to checking the MARs. She is almost finished when a client on the unit stops breathing and she is called to administer medications during the client's resuscitation efforts. Afterwards, she sees it is almost 9:00 and she has yet to begin preparing the 9:00 medications. She rushes to the medication cart and begins passing medications. She enters each client's room and asks if their name is . . . and when they say yes she administers the medication. A staff member interrupts her when she has given only half of her 9:00 medications and reports that a client is in pain and requires PRN analgesia. Then when she returns to giving 9:00 medications, a family member stops to discuss a loved one's condition and response to therapy. It is almost 10:00 before she finishes the medication administration due an hour ago. She has documented medications as she administered them, but now she needs to assess and document the client's responses to the PRN medication she administered. At 11:00 she prepares to administer an IM injection. The order reads, "Administer ampicillin 725 mg. IM every 6 hours." She looks in the drawer and finds ampicillin 500 mg per 2 mL, ampicillin 1 Gram per 2 ml, and ampicillin 250 mg per 1 mL. She pauses to consider how to prepare this medication.

LEARNING OUTCOMES

After completing this chapter, you will be able to:

1. Describe legal considerations for nurses when administering medications.

2. Identify factors that could impact medication actions in different clients.

3. Contrast various routes used for medication administration.

4. Identify the different parts and types of medication orders.

5. Calculate proper medication dosages using different systems of measurement.

6. Identify the contribution to safe medication administration of each of the six steps to follow when administering medications.

7. Describe how each of the "rights" to medication administration is performed and how each improves client safety.

8. Diagram the steps required to administer medications via oral, nasogastric, or gastrostomy tube.

9. Describe the safe use of equipment required to administer medications via parenteral routes and how the choice of equipment depends on the route and circumstances.

10. State the essential steps for administering parenteral medications safely, including selection of the best site, via intradermal, subcutaneous, intramuscular, or intravenous routes.

11. State the essential steps for administering medications via the topical, ophthalmic, otic, nasal, vaginal, rectal, and respiratory inhalation routes.

KEY TERMS

Absorption p651

Adverse effects p650

Agonist p651

Ampule p675

Antagonist p651

Bevel p674

Biotransformation p652

Brand name p647

Buccal p654

Chemical name p647

Cumulative effect p650

Desired effect p649

Distribution p652

Dependence p650

Drug abuse p650

Drug allergy p650

Drug interaction p650

Drug toxicity p650

Excretion p652

Gauge p674

Generic name p647

Habituation p650

Half-life p651

Hub p674

Iatrogenic disease p650

Idiosyncratic effect p650

Inhibiting effect p650

Intradermal p655

Intramuscular p655

Intrathecal p655

Intravenous p655

Medication p647

Meniscus p669

Metabolism p652

Metered-dose inhaler p706

Official name p647

Onset of action p651

Parenteral p655

Peak plasma level p651

Pharmacodynamics p651

Pharmacogenetics p652

Pharmacokinetics p651

Pharmacology p647

Piggyback p693

Plateau p651

Potentiating effect p650

Prescription p647

PRN order p657

Reconstitution p676

Shaft p674

Side effect p650

Single order p657

Standing order p657

Stat order p657

Subcutaneous p655

Sublingual p654

Synergistic p650

Therapeutic effect p649

Tolerance p650

Topical p656

Trade name p647

Transdermal p697

Vial p675

Volume-control infusion set p688

A **medication** is a substance administered for the diagnosis, cure, treatment, or relief of a symptom or for prevention of disease. In the health care context, the words *medication* and *drug* are generally used interchangeably. The term drug also has the connotation of an illicitly obtained substance such as heroin, cocaine, or amphetamines. Medications have been known and used since antiquity. Over the centuries the number of drugs available has increased greatly, and knowledge about these drugs has become correspondingly more accurate and detailed.

In the United States and Canada, medications are usually dispensed on the order of physicians and dentists. In some U.S. states, specially qualified nurse practitioners or other advanced practice nurses and physician's assistants may prescribe drugs. The written direction for the preparation and administration of a drug is called a **prescription**. One drug can have as many as four kinds of names: its generic name, official name, chemical name, and trademark or brand name. The **generic name** is given before a drug be-

comes officially an approved medication. The generic name is generally used throughout the drug's use. The **official name** is the name under which it is listed in one of the official publications (e.g., the *United States Pharmacopeia*). The **chemical name** is the name by which a chemist knows it; this name describes the constituents of the drug precisely. A drug's **trade name** is the name given by the drug manufacturer. The name is usually selected to be short and easy to remember. The trade name is sometimes called the **brand name**. Because one drug may be manufactured by several companies, it can have several trade names; for example, the drug hydrochlorothiazide (official name) is known by the trade names Esidrix and HydroDIURIL. Medications are often available in a variety of forms (see Table 23–1).

Pharmacology is the study of the effect of drugs on living organisms. Pharmacy is the art of preparing, compounding, and dispensing drugs. The word also refers to the place where drugs are prepared and dispensed. Drugs are prepared by a pharmacist, a person licensed to prepare

TABLE 23–1	Types of Drug Preparation
TYPE	**DESCRIPTION**
Aerosol spray or foam	A liquid, powder, or foam deposited in a thin layer on the skin by air pressure
Aqueous solution	One or more drugs dissolved in water
Aqueous suspension	One or more drugs finely divided in a liquid such as water
Caplet	A solid form, shaped like a capsule, coated and easily swallowed
Capsule	A gelatinous container to hold a drug in powder, liquid, or oil form
Cream	A nongreasy, semisolid preparation used on the skin
Elixir	A sweetened and aromatic solution of alcohol used as a vehicle for medicinal agents
Extract	A concentrated form of a drug made from vegetables or animals
Gel or jelly	A clear or translucent semisolid that liquefies when applied to the skin
Liniment	A medication mixed with alcohol, oil, or soapy emollient and applied to the skin
Lotion	A medication in a liquid suspension applied to the skin
Lozenge (troche)	A flat, round, or oval preparation that dissolves and releases a drug when held in the mouth
Ointment (salve, unction)	A semisolid preparation of one or more drugs used for application to the skin and mucous membrane
Paste	A preparation like an ointment, but thicker and stiff, that penetrates the skin less than an ointment
Pill	One or more drugs mixed with a cohesive material, in oval, round, or flattened shapes
Powder	A finely ground drug or drugs; some are used internally, others externally
Suppository	One or more drugs mixed with a firm base such as gelatin and shaped for insertion into the body (e.g., the rectum); the base dissolves gradually at body temperature, releasing the drug
Syrup	An aqueous solution of sugar often used to disguise unpleasant-tasting drugs
Tablet	A powdered drug compressed into a hard small disc; some are readily broken along a scored line; others are enteric coated to prevent them from dissolving in the stomach
Tincture	An alcoholic or water-and-alcohol solution prepared from drugs derived from plants
Transdermal patch	A semipermeable membrane shaped in the form of a disc or patch that contains a drug to be absorbed through the skin over a long period of time

and dispense drugs and to make up prescriptions. A clinical pharmacist is a specialist who often guides the physician in prescribing drugs. A pharmacy technician is a member of the health team who in some states administers drugs to clients or assists the pharmacist in preparing medications.

DRUG STANDARDS

Drugs may have natural sources, or they may be synthesized in the laboratory. Early drugs were derived from natural sources only. More and more drugs are being produced synthetically.

Drugs vary in strength and activity. Drugs derived from plants, for example, vary in strength according to the age of the plant, the variety, the place in which it is grown, and the method by which it is preserved. Drugs must be pure and of uniform strength if drug dosages are to be predictable in their effect. Drug standards have therefore been developed to ensure uniform quality. In the United States, official drugs are those so designated by the federal Food, Drug, and Cosmetic Act. These drugs are officially listed in the *United States Pharmacopeia (USP)* and described according to their source, physical and chemical properties, tests for purity and identity, method of storage, assay, category, and

normal dosages. In Canada, the *British Pharmacopoeia* is used for the same purpose, although some drugs used in Canada conform to the *USP* because they are obtained from the United States. There is a trend for people to purchase "natural" vitamins and supplements from health food stores or over the counter at pharmacies.

A pharmacopoeia (also spelled *pharmacopeia*) is a book containing a list of products used in medicine, with descriptions of the product, chemical tests for determining identity and purity, and formulas and prescriptions. The United States' *National Formulary* lists drugs and their therapeutic value and can include drugs that may still be used but not listed in the *USP*. The *Canadian Formulary* lists drugs used extensively in Canada but not necessarily listed in the *British Pharmacopoeia.*

Pharmacopoeias and formularies are invaluable reference sources for nurses and nursing students. Nurses not only administer thousands of medications but also are responsible for assessing their effectiveness and recognizing unfavorable reactions to drugs. Medication or drug handbooks and agency formularies are valuable resources for nurses. Because it is impossible to commit to memory all pertinent information about a very large number of drugs, nurses must have a reliable reference readily available.

LEGAL ASPECTS OF DRUG ADMINISTRATION

The administration of drugs in both the United States and Canada is controlled by law. Nurses need to (a) know how nursing practice acts in their areas define and limit their functions and (b) be able to recognize the limits of their own knowledge and skill. To function beyond the limits of nursing practice acts or one's ability is to endanger clients' lives and leave oneself open to malpractice suits. Under the law, nurses are responsible for their own actions regardless of whether there is a written order. If a physician writes an incorrect order, *a nurse who administers the written incorrect dosage is responsible for the error as well as the physician.* Therefore, nurses should question any order that appears unreasonable and refuse to give the medication until the order is clarified.

Another aspect of nursing practice governed by law is the use of controlled substances. In hospitals, controlled substances are kept in a double locked drawer, cupboard, medication cart, or computer-controlled dispensing system. Agencies may have special inventory forms for recording the use of controlled substances. The information required usually includes the name of the client, the date and time of administration, the name of the drug, the dosage, and the signature of the person who prepared and gave the drug. The name of the physician who ordered the drug may also be part of the record. Some agencies may require a verifying signature of another registered nurse for administration of a controlled substance. Most health care agencies maintain a list of high-alert medications, including controlled substances, which require the verification of two registered nurses. Before removing a controlled substance, the nurse verifies the number actually available with the number indicated on the narcotic or controlled substance inventory record (Figure 23–1). If the number is not the same, the nurse must investigate and correct the discrepancy before proceeding.

Included on the record are the controlled substances wasted during preparation. When a portion or all of a controlled substance dose is discarded, the nurse must ask a second nurse to witness the discarding. Both nurses must sign the control inventory form.

In most agencies, counts of controlled substances are taken at the end of each shift. The count total should tally with the total at the end of the last shift minus the number used. If the totals do not tally and the discrepancy cannot be resolved, it must be reported immediately to the nurse manager, nursing supervisor, and pharmacy according to agency policy. In facilities that use a computerized dispensing system, manual counts may not be required, because the dispensing system runs a continuous count; however, discrepancies must be accounted for.

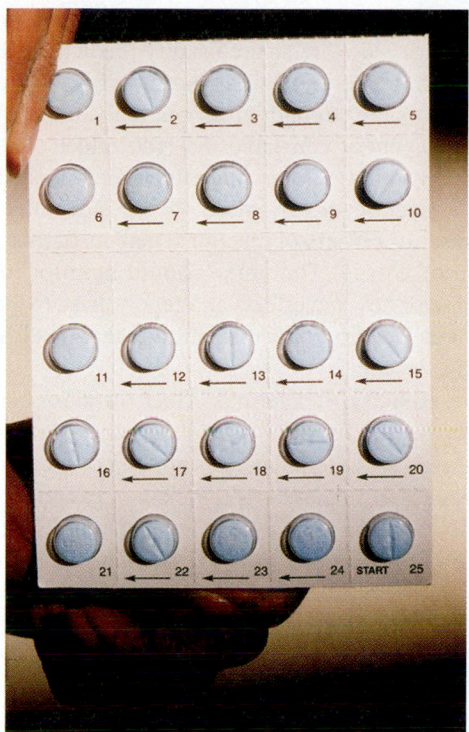

Figure 23–1 ● Some narcotics are kept in specially designed packages or plastic containers that are sectioned and numbered.

EFFECTS OF DRUGS

The **therapeutic effect** of a drug, also referred to as the **desired effect**, is the primary effect intended, that is, the reason the drug is prescribed. See Table 23–2 for kinds of therapeutic actions.

TABLE 23–2   Therapeutic Actions of Drugs

DRUG TYPE	DESCRIPTION	EXAMPLES
Palliative	Relieves the symptoms of a disease but does not affect the disease itself.	Morphine sulfate, aspirin for pain
Curative	Cures a disease or condition.	Penicillin for infection
Supportive	Supports body function until other treatments or the body's response can take over.	Norepinephrine bitartrate for low blood pressure; aspirin for high body temperature
Substitutive	Replaces body fluids or substances.	Thyroxine for hypothyroidism, insulin for diabetes mellitus
Chemotherapeutic	Destroys malignant cells.	Busulfan for leukemia
Restorative	Returns the body to health.	Vitamin, mineral supplements

A **side effect**, or secondary effect, of a drug is one that is unintended. Side effects are usually predictable and may be either harmless or potentially harmful. For example, digitalis increases the strength of myocardial contractions (desired effect), but it can have the side effect of inducing nausea and vomiting. Some side effects are tolerated for the drug's therapeutic effect; more severe side effects, also called **adverse effects** or reactions, may justify the discontinuation of a drug. The nurse should monitor for dose-related side or adverse effects and report these to the health care provider, who may discontinue the medication or change the dosage.

Drug toxicity (deleterious effects of a drug on an organism or tissue) results from overdosage, ingestion of a drug intended for external use, or buildup of the drug in the blood because of impaired metabolism or excretion (cumulative effect). Some toxic effects are apparent immediately; some are not apparent for weeks or months. Fortunately, most drug toxicity is avoidable if careful attention is paid to dosage and monitoring for toxicity. An example of a toxic effect is respiratory depression due to the cumulative effect of morphine sulfate in the body.

A **drug allergy** is an immunologic reaction to a drug. When a client is first exposed to a foreign substance (antigen), the body may react by producing antibodies. A client can react to a drug as to an antigen and thus develop symptoms of an allergic reaction.

Allergic reactions can be either mild or severe. A mild reaction has a variety of symptoms, from skin rashes to diarrhea. An allergic reaction can occur anytime from a few minutes to 2 weeks after the administration of the drug. A severe allergic reaction usually occurs immediately after the administration of the drug and is called an anaphylactic reaction. This response can be fatal if the symptoms are not noticed immediately and treatment is not initiated promptly. The earliest symptoms are a subjective feeling of swelling in the mouth and tongue, acute shortness of breath, acute hypotension, and tachycardia.

Drug **tolerance** exists in a person who has unusually low physiologic response to a drug and who requires increases in the dosage to maintain a given therapeutic effect. Drugs that commonly produce tolerance are opiates, barbiturates, ethyl alcohol, and tobacco. A **cumulative effect** is the increasing response to repeated doses of a drug that occurs when the rate of administration exceeds the rate of metabolism or excretion. As a result, the amount of the drug builds up in the client's body unless the dosage is adjusted. Toxic symptoms may occur. An **idiosyncratic effect** is one that is unexpected and may be individual to a client. Underresponse and overresponse to a drug may be idiosyncratic. Also, the drug may have a completely different effect from the normal one or cause unpredictable and unexplainable symptoms in a particular client.

A **drug interaction** occurs when the administration of one drug before, at the same time as, or after another drug alters the effect of one or both drugs. Drug interactions may be beneficial or harmful. The effect of one or both drugs may be either increased (**potentiating effect**) or decreased (**inhibiting effect**). Potentiating effects may be additive or synergistic. When two of the same types of drug increase the action of each other it is known as additive. **Synergistic** is when two different drugs increase the action of one or another drug. For example, probenecid, which blocks the excretion of penicillin, can be given with penicillin to increase blood levels of the penicillin for longer periods (synergistic effect). Two analgesics, such as aspirin and codeine, are often given together because together they provide greater pain relief (additive effect). In this example of aspirin and codeine, using a combination of drugs often decreases the total dose of narcotics needed. In addition, certain foods may interact adversely with a medication.

Iatrogenic disease (disease caused unintentionally by medical therapy) can be due to drug therapy. Hepatic toxicity resulting in biliary obstruction, renal damage, and malformations of the fetus as a result of specific drugs taken during pregnancy are examples.

DRUG MISUSE

Drug misuse is the improper use of common medications in ways that lead to acute and chronic toxicity. Both over-the-counter drugs and prescription drugs may be misused. Laxatives, antacids, vitamins, headache remedies, and cough and cold medications are often self-prescribed and overused. Most people suffer no harmful effects from these drugs, but some people do. A persistent cough may go undiagnosed until the underlying problem becomes serious and advanced.

Drug abuse is inappropriate intake of a substance, either continually or periodically. By definition, drug use is abusive when society considers it abusive. For example, the intake of alcohol at work may be considered alcohol abuse, but intake at a social gathering may not. Drug abuse has two main facets, drug dependence and habituation. Drug **dependence** is a person's reliance on or need to take a drug or substance. The two types of dependence, physiologic and psychologic, may occur separately or together. Physiologic dependence is due to biochemical changes in body tissues, especially the nervous system. These tissues come to require the substance for normal functioning. A dependent person who stops using the drug experiences withdrawal symptoms. Psychologic dependence is emotional reliance on a drug to maintain a sense of well-being, accompanied by feelings of need or cravings for that drug. There are varying degrees of psychologic dependence, ranging from mild desire to craving and compulsive use of the drug.

Drug **habituation** denotes a mild form of psychologic dependence. The individual develops the habit of taking the substance and feels better after taking it. The habituated individual tends to continue the habit even though it may be injurious to health.

Illicit drugs, also called *street drugs,* are those sold illegally. Illicit drugs are of two types: (a) drugs unavailable for purchase under any circumstances, such as heroin (in the

United States), and (b) drugs normally available with a prescription that are being obtained through illegal channels. Illicit drugs are often taken because of their mood-altering effect.

ACTIONS OF DRUGS ON THE BODY

The action of a drug in the body can be described in terms of its half-life, the time interval required for the body's elimination processes to reduce the concentration of the drug in the body by one-half. For example, if a drug's half-life is 8 hours, then the amount of drug in the body is as follows:

Initially: 100%
After 8 hours: 50%
After 16 hours: 25%
After 24 hours: 12.5%
After 32 hours: 6.25%

Because the purpose of most drug therapy is to maintain a constant drug level in the body, repeated doses are required to maintain that level. When an orally administered drug is absorbed from the gastrointestinal tract into the blood plasma, its concentration in the plasma increases until the elimination rate equals the rate of absorption. This point is known as the *peak plasma level* (Figure 23–2). When a drug is given intravenously (IV), its level is high immediately after administration and decreases through time. Another dose is given in order to maintain therapeutic levels. If the client does not receive another dose of the drug (either orally or IV), the concentration steadily decreases. Key terms related to drug actions are as follows:

- **Onset of action**: The time after administration when the body initially responds to the drug
- **Peak plasma level**: The highest plasma level achieved by a single dose when the elimination rate of a drug equals the absorption rate
- Drug **half-life** (elimination half-life): The time required for the elimination process to reduce the concentration of the drug to one-half what it was at initial administration
- **Plateau**: A maintained concentration of a drug in the plasma during a series of scheduled doses

Pharmacodynamics

Pharmacodynamics is the process by which a drug changes the body (e.g., alters cell physiology). Such changes require that the drug interact with specific molecules and chemicals normally found in the body (Adams, Josephson, & Holland, 2005). A receptor, usually a protein, is located on the surface of a cell membrane or within the cell. A cell membrane contains receptors for physiologic or endogenous substances such as hormones and neurotransmitters (Abrams, 2009).

Most drugs exert their effects by chemically binding with receptors at the cellular level. When a drug binds to its receptor, the pharmacologic effects are either agonism or antagonism. A drug that produces the same type of response as the physiologic or endogenous substance is called an **agonist**. Conversely, a drug that inhibits cell function by occupying receptor sites is called an **antagonist**. The antagonist prevents natural body substances or other drugs from activating the functions of the cell by occupying the receptor sites.

Pharmacokinetics

Pharmacokinetics is the study of the absorption, distribution, biotransformation, and excretion of drugs.

Absorption is the process by which a drug passes into the bloodstream. Unless the drug is administered directly into the bloodstream, absorption is the first step in the movement of the drug through the body. For absorption to occur, the correct form of the drug must be given by the route intended.

The rate of absorption of a drug in the stomach is variable. Food, for example, can delay the dissolution and absorption of some drugs as well as their passage into the small intestine, where most drug absorption occurs. Food can also combine with molecules of certain drugs, thereby changing their molecular structure and subsequently inhibiting or preventing their absorption. Another factor that affects the absorption of some drugs is the acid medium in the stomach. Acidity can vary according to the time of day, foods ingested, use of antacid medications, and the age of the client. Some drugs do not dissolve or have limited ability to dissolve in the gastrointestinal fluids, decreasing their absorption into the bloodstream. Some drugs are absorbed by tissues before they reach the stomach. The first-pass effect occurs when oral drugs first pass through the liver and are partially metabolized prior to reaching the target organ requiring higher oral doses in order to achieve the appropriate effect.

A drug administered directly into the bloodstream, that is, intravenously, is immediately placed into the vascular system without having to be absorbed. This, then, is the route of choice for rapid action. The intramuscular route is the next most rapid route due to the highly vascular nature of muscle tissue. Because subcutaneous tissue has a poorer blood supply than muscle tissue, absorption

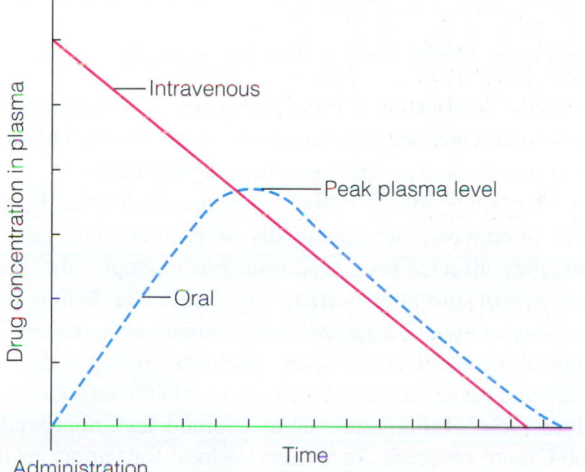

Figure 23–2 ○ A graphic plot of drug concentration in the blood plasma following a single dose.

MyNursingKit | Agonist and Antagonist

from subcutaneous tissue is slower. The rate of absorption of a drug can be accelerated by the application of heat, which increases blood flow to the area; conversely, absorption can be slowed by the application of cold. In addition, the injection of a vasoconstrictor drug such as epinephrine into the tissue can slow absorption of other drugs. Some drugs intended to be absorbed slowly are suspended in a low-solubility medium, such as oil. The absorption of drugs from the rectum into the bloodstream tends to be unpredictable. Therefore, this route is normally used when other routes are unavailable or when the intended action is localized to the rectum or sigmoid colon.

Distribution is the transportation of a drug from its site of absorption to its site of action. When a drug enters the bloodstream, it is carried to the most vascular organs— that is, liver, kidneys, and brain. Body areas with lower blood supply—that is, skin and muscles—receive the drug later. The chemical and physical properties of a drug largely determine the area of the body to which the drug will be attracted. For example, fat-soluble drugs will accumulate in fatty tissue, whereas other drugs may bind with plasma proteins.

Biotransformation, also called detoxification, or **metabolism**, is a process by which a drug is converted to a less active form. Most biotransformation takes place in the liver, where many drug-metabolizing enzymes in the cells detoxify the drugs. The products of this process are called metabolites. There are two types of metabolites: active and inactive. An *active metabolite* has a pharmacologic action itself, whereas an *inactive metabolite* does not.

Biotransformation may be altered if a person is very young, is older, or has an unhealthy liver. Nurses must be alert to the accumulation of the active drug in these clients and to subsequent toxicity.

Excretion is the process by which metabolites and drugs are eliminated from the body. Most metabolites are eliminated by the kidneys in the urine; however, some are excreted in the feces, the breath, perspiration, saliva, and breast milk. Certain drugs, such as general anesthetic agents, are excreted in an unchanged form via the respiratory tract. The efficiency with which the kidneys excrete drugs and metabolites diminishes with age. Older people may require smaller doses of a drug because the drug and its metabolites may accumulate in the body.

FACTORS AFFECTING MEDICATION ACTION

A number of factors other than the drug itself can affect its action. A person may not respond in the same manner to successive doses of a drug. In addition, the identical drug and dosage may affect different clients differently.

Development

During pregnancy women must be very careful about taking medications. Drugs taken during pregnancy pose a risk throughout the pregnancy, but pose the highest risk during the first trimester, due to the formation of vital organs and func-

---

tions of the fetus during this time. Most drugs are contraindicated because of the possible adverse effects on the fetus.

Infants usually require small dosages because of their body size and the immaturity of their organs, especially the liver and kidneys. Differences in gastric acidity and liver enzymes required for drug metabolism may require different medication choices and dosages than adults. In adolescence or adulthood, allergic reactions may occur to drugs formerly tolerated. Children may have an idiosyncratic effect from medications as compared with adults.

Older adults have different responses to medications due to physiologic changes that accompany aging. These changes include decreased liver and kidney function, which can result in the accumulation of the drug in the body. In addition, the older person may be on multiple drugs (polypharmacy) and incompatibilities may occur.

Gender

Differences in the way men and women respond to drugs are chiefly related to the distribution of body fat and fluid and hormonal differences. Because most drug research is done on men, more research on women is required to reflect the effects of hormonal changes on drug actions in women.

Culture, Ethnicity, and Genetics

A client's response to a drug is influenced by genetic variations such as gender, size, and body composition. This variation in response is called **pharmacogenetics**.

According to Lea (2005), drug metabolism and variations in enzymes are genetically determined and, as a result, may affect a drug response. For example, the genes that control liver metabolism vary. Some clients may have slow liver metabolism and not achieve an adequate response to a medication, whereas others are rapid metabolizers and may require lower doses of a medication to avoid adverse reactions. A new genetic blood test, approved in 2004, analyzes genes in a client's blood for variations that could cause the variations in metabolism of certain drugs. This information can help health care providers to individualize medication treatment and avoid adverse reactions.

A new field of study, ethnopharmacology, is the study of the effect of ethnicity on responses to prescribed medication (Munoz & Hilgenberg, 2005). Research has shown that certain medications may work well at usual therapeutic dosages for certain ethnic groups but be toxic for others. Ethnopharmacology also incorporates pharmacogenetics, which is the study of the genetic ability to produce enzymes that affect drug metabolism. Pharmacogenetics can also vary by race or ethnic group.

Cultural factors and practices can also affect a drug's action. The Culturally Competent Care feature provides guidelines for nurses who care for clients from other cultures.

Diet

Nutrients can affect the action of a medication. For example, vitamin K found in green leafy vegetables can counteract the effect of an anticoagulant such as warfarin (Coumadin).

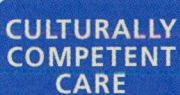

CULTURALLY COMPETENT CARE — Ethnopharmacology

Knowing that ethnicity can affect drug response helps the nurse provide culturally competent care. In the past, clinical drug research was conducted on Caucasian males even when the health disorder being studied was prevalent in other ethnic groups. Ethnopharmacologic research has focused on two major classifications: psychotropic and antihypertensive medications.

Psychotropic Medications

Research has found that African American clients experienced faster therapeutic responses, to tricyclic antidepressants, higher serum concentrations, and more adverse reactions than Caucasian clients.

African American clients may require lower doses of lithium than white clients.

Antihypertensive Medications

Studies have shown that certain angiotensin-converting enzyme (ACE) inhibitors (i.e., captopril and enalapril) and the angiotensin II receptor antagonist (i.e., losartan) were found to be less effective in African Americans than in Whites.

Thiazide diuretics appear to be more effective antihypertensives in African Americans than in Whites.

Beta blockers can vary among ethnic groups. African Americans may require higher dosages than Whites, and Asians usually require lower doses than Whites.

Implications for Nursing Interventions

Remember that there may be differences in medication responses among different ethnic groups and differences *within* ethnic groups.

Ask about health beliefs, values, and customs/practices.

Conduct a cultural assessment with each client.

Learn about drugs that are likely to elicit varied responses in people from different ethnic groups, as well as the potential for adverse effects.

Ask the client direct, specific questions to reveal the presence or absence of potential adverse effects of medications.

Monitor the client and document findings carefully as it may be possible to maintain therapeutic benefit at a lower dosage of a given drug.

Keep cultural context in mind when planning education for clients and families.

Note: From "Ethnopharmacology" by C. Munoz and C. Hilgenberg, 2005, *American Journal of Nursing, 105*(8), pp. 40–48. Adapted with permission.

RESEARCH NOTES — Is There an Intervention to Improve Medication Adherence in Minority Women?

The purpose of this 12-month study was to determine the effectiveness of several strategies to promote medication adherence in older women from a variety of minority groups. The total sample of 109 women older than 65 years from Caucasian, African American, and Hispanic origins received standardized teaching about osteoporosis and their medication (estrogen and calcium) and provided opportunities for questions and clarification.

The Caucasian women used pillboxes marked with the days of the week and times of the day for 12 months. The African American and Hispanic women used the pillboxes for 6 months and then switched to using electronic monitoring medication bottles that recorded each bottle opening and closing as the administration of a dose for the remaining 6 months. A nurse contacted each participant on a monthly basis.

Results: Caucasian women were found to be the most adherent to their medication regimen. Hispanic women demonstrated significantly higher levels of adherence using the electronic bottles than using pillboxes, while the African American women had higher levels of adherence using both the pillboxes and electronic monitoring devices.

Implications

Older clients, especially those from minority groups, may benefit from innovative medication adherence programs.

Note: From "Multicultural Medication Adherence: A Comparative Study," by B. Robbins, K. J. Rausch, R. I. Garcia, & K. W. Prestwood, 2004, *Journal of Gerontological Nursing, 30*(7), 25–32. Copyright © 2004 SLACK, Inc. Reprinted with permission.

Environment

The client's environment can affect the action of drugs, particularly those used to alter behavior and mood. Therefore, nurses assessing the effects of a drug need to consider the drug in the context of the client's personality and milieu.

Environmental temperature may also affect drug activity. When environmental temperature is high, the peripheral blood vessels dilate, thus intensifying the action of vasodilators. In contrast, a cold environment and the consequent vasoconstriction inhibit the action of vasodilators but enhance the action of vasoconstrictors. A client who takes a sedative or analgesic in a busy, noisy environment may not benefit as fully as if the environment were quiet and peaceful.

Psychology

A client's expectations about what a drug can do can affect the response to the medication. Research studies have been performed that show the "placebo effect" of medications. For example, a client who believes that codeine is a very strong and potent pain reliever may experience greater relief from pain after it is given.

Illness and Disease

Illness and disease can also affect the action of drugs. For example, aspirin can reduce the body temperature of a feverish client but has no effect on the body temperature of a client without fever. Drug action is altered in clients with circulatory, liver, or kidney dysfunction.

Time of Administration

The time of administration of oral medications affects the relative speed with which they act. Orally administered medications are absorbed more quickly if the stomach is empty. Thus, oral medications taken 2 hours before meals act faster than those taken after meals. However, some medications irritate the gastrointestinal tract and are given after a meal, when they will be better tolerated.

ROUTES OF ADMINISTRATION

Pharmaceutical preparations are generally designed for one or two specific routes of administration (see Table 23–3). The route of administration should be indicated when the drug is ordered. When administering a drug, the nurse should ensure that the pharmaceutical preparation is appropriate for the route specified.

Oral

Oral administration is the most common, least expensive, and most convenient route for most clients. In oral administration, the drug is swallowed. Because the skin is not broken as it is for an injection, oral administration is also a safe method.

The major disadvantages may include unpleasant taste of the drugs, irritation of the gastric mucosa, irregular absorption from the gastrointestinal tract, slow absorption, and, in some cases, harm to the client's teeth.

Sublingual

In **sublingual** administration a drug is placed under the tongue, where it dissolves (Figure 23–3, *A*). In a relatively short time, the drug is largely absorbed into the blood vessels on the underside of the tongue. The medication should not be swallowed. Nitroglycerin is one example of a drug commonly given in this manner.

Buccal

Buccal means "pertaining to the cheek." In buccal administration, a medication is held in the mouth against the mucous membranes of the cheek until the drug dissolves (Figure 23–3, *B*). The drug may act locally on the mucous membranes of the mouth or systemically when it is swallowed in the saliva.

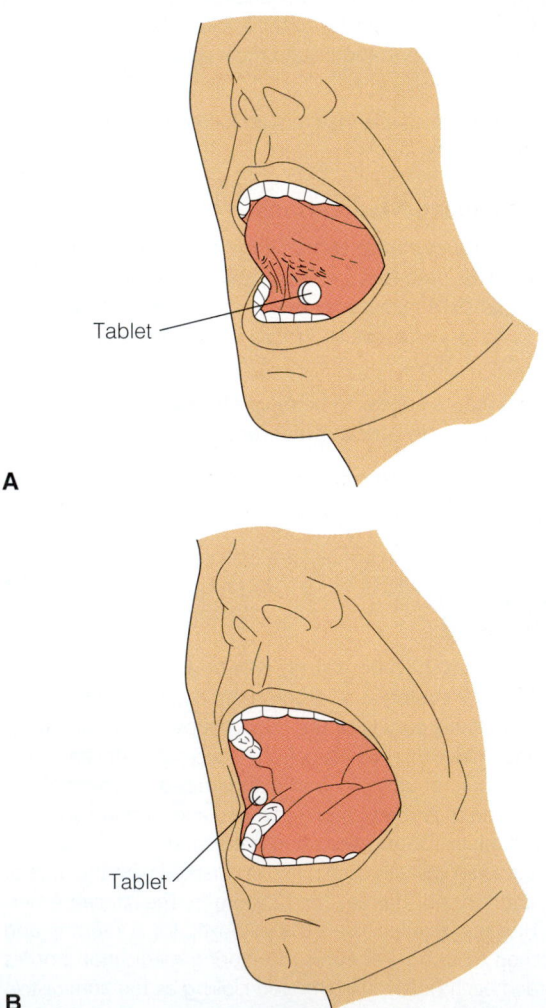

Tablet

A

Tablet

B

Figure 23–3 ⬤ *A*, Sublingual administration of a tablet.
B, Buccal administration of a tablet.

TABLE 23–3	Routes of Administration	
ROUTE	**ADVANTAGES**	**DISADVANTAGES**
Oral	Most convenient	Inappropriate for clients with nausea or vomiting
	Usually least expensive	Drug may have unpleasant taste or odor
	Safe, does not break skin barrier	Inappropriate when gastrointestinal tract has reduced motility
	Administration usually does not cause stress	Inappropriate if client cannot swallow or is unconscious
	Some new oral medications are designed to rapidly dissolve on the tongue, allowing for faster absorption and action	Cannot be used before certain diagnostic tests or surgical procedures
		Drug may discolor teeth, harm tooth enamel
		Drug may irritate gastric mucosa
		Drug can be aspirated by seriously ill clients
Sublingual	Same as for oral, *plus:*	If swallowed, drug may be inactivated by gastric juice
	Drug can be administered for local effect	Drug must remain under tongue until dissolved and absorbed. May cause stinging or irritation of the mucous membranes
	More potent than oral route because drug directly enters the blood and bypasses the liver	Drug is rapidly absorbed into the bloodstream
Buccal	Same as for sublingual	Same as for sublingual
Rectal	Can be used when drug has objectionable taste or odor	Dose absorbed is unpredictable
	Drug released at slow, steady rate	May be perceived as unpleasant by the client
	Provides a local therapeutic effect	Limited use
Vaginal	Provides a local effect	May be messy and may soil clothes
Topical	Few side effects	Drug can enter body through abrasions and cause systemic effects
	Prolonged systemic effect	Leaves residue on the skin that may soil clothes
Transdermal	Few side effects	Can cause skin irritation
	Avoids gastrointestinal absorption problems	
	Onset of drug action faster than oral	
Subcutaneous		More expensive than oral
		Can administer only small volume
		Slower absorption rate as compared to intramuscular administration
		Some drugs can irritate tissues and cause pain
		Can produce anxiety
		Breaks skin barrier
Intramuscular	Can administer larger volume than subcutaneous	Can produce anxiety
	Drug is rapidly absorbed	
Intradermal	Absorption is slow (this is an advantage in testing for allergies)	Amount of drug administered must be small
		Breaks skin barrier
Intravenous	Rapid effect	Limited to highly soluble drugs
		Drug distribution inhibited by poor circulation
Inhalation	Introduces drug throughout respiratory tract	Drug intended for localized effect can have systemic effect
	Rapid localized relief	Of use only for the respiratory system
	Drug can be administered to unconscious client	

Parenteral

The **parenteral** route is defined as other than through the alimentary or respiratory tract; that is, by needle. The following are some of the more common routes for parenteral administration:

- **Subcutaneous (hypodermic)**—into the subcutaneous tissue, just below the skin
- **Intramuscular**—into a muscle

- **Intradermal**—under the epidermis (into the dermis)
- **Intravenous**—into a vein

Some of the less commonly used routes for parenteral administration are intra-arterial (into an artery), intracardiac (into the heart muscle), intraosseous (into a bone), **intrathecal** or intraspinal (into the spinal canal), intrapleural (into the pleural space), epidural (into the epidural space), and intra-articular (into a joint). Sterile equipment and sterile drug solution are essential for all parenteral therapy. The main advantage is fast absorption.

Topical

Topical applications are those applied to a circumscribed surface area of the body. They affect only the area to which they are applied. Topical applications include the following:

- Dermatologic preparations—applied to the skin
- Instillations and irrigations—applied into body cavities or orifices, such as the urinary bladder, eyes, ears, nose, rectum, or vagina
- Inhalations—administered into the respiratory tract by a nebulizer or positive pressure breathing apparatus. Air, oxygen, and vapor are generally used to carry the drug into the lungs.

MEDICATION ORDERS

A physician usually determines the client's medication needs and orders medications, although in some settings nurse practitioners and physician's assistants now order some drugs. Each health agency will have its own policies. Usually the order is written, although telephone and verbal orders are acceptable in a number of agencies. Nursing students need to know the school and agency policies about medication orders. In some hospitals, for example, only licensed nurses are permitted to accept telephone and verbal orders.

Policies about primary care providers' orders vary considerably from agency to agency. For example, a client's orders may be automatically canceled after surgery or an examination involving an anesthetic agent. The primary care provider must then write new orders. Most agencies also have lists of abbreviations officially accepted for use in the agency. Recently, in order to prevent medication errors, the Joint Commission mandated that agencies must standardize abbreviations, acronyms, and symbols used throughout the organization and *must* list abbreviations that are never to be used (Karch, 2004; The Joint Commission, 2009). See Table 23–4 for the list of unacceptable abbreviations.

TABLE 23–4 Unacceptable Abbreviations—"Do Not Use" List

ABBREVIATION	POTENTIAL PROBLEM	USE INSTEAD
U (unit)	Mistaken for "0" (zero), the number "4" (four), or "cc"	Write "unit"
IU (international unit)	Mistaken for IV (intravenous) or the number 10 (ten)	Write "International Unit"
Q.D., QD, q.d., qd (daily)	Mistaken for each other	Write "daily"
Q.O.D., QOD, q.o.d., qod (every other day)	Period after the Q mistaken for "I" and the "O" mistaken for "I"	Write "every other day"
Trailing zero (X.0 mg)	Decimal point is missed	Write X mg
Lack of leading zero (.X mg)		Write 0.X mg
MS	Can mean morphine sulfate or magnesium sulfate	Write "morphine sulfate"
MSO_4 and $MgSO_4$		Write "magnesium sulfate"
For Possible Future Inclusion in the Official "Do Not Use" List		
> (greater than)	Misinterpreted as the number "7" (seven) or the letter "L"	Write "greater than"
< (less than)	Confused for one another	Write "less than"
Abbreviations for drug names	Misinterpreted due to similar abbreviations for multiple drugs	Write drug names in full
Apothecary units	Unfamiliar to many practitioners Confused with metric units	Use metric units
@	Mistaken for the number "2" (two)	Write "at"
cc	Mistaken for U (units) when poorly written	Write "mL" or "milliliters"
µg	Mistaken for mg (milligrams) resulting in one thousand-fold overdose	Write "mcg" or "micrograms"
Others to Consider		
TIW (three times a week)	Has been misinterpreted as "two times a week" or "three times a day" resulting in misdosing	Write "three times weekly"
AS (left ear) AD (right ear) AU (both ears)	Mistaken for OS (left eye), OD (either "overdose" or "optic density"), and OU ("each eye" or "both eyes")	Write "left ear," "right ear," or "both ears," as appropriate
HS	Has been used to indicate "half strength" and "bedtime" or "hour of sleep"	Write out "half strength" or "at bedtime," as appropriate
SC and SQ (subcutaneous)	Have been read as "SL" (sublingual) and as "5 every hour"	Write "subq" or "subcutaneous"
D/C	Can mean either "discharge" or "discontinue"	Write "discharge" or "discontinue" as appropriate

Types of Medication Orders

Four common medication orders are the stat order, the single order, the standing order, and the prn order.

1. A **stat order** indicates that the medication is to be given immediately and only once.
2. The **single order** or *one-time order* is for medication to be given once at a specified time.
3. The **standing order** may or may not have a termination date. A standing order may be carried out indefinitely until an order is written to cancel it, or it may be carried out for a specified number of days. In some agencies, standing orders are automatically canceled after a specified number of days and must be reordered.
4. A **prn order**, or *as-needed order,* permits the nurse to give a medication when, in the nurse's judgment, the client requires it. The nurse must use good judgment about when the medication is needed and when it can be safely administered.

Essential Parts of a Drug Order

The drug order has seven essential parts, as listed in Box 23–1. In addition, unless it is a standing order it should state the number of doses or the number of days the drug is to be administered.

The signature of the ordering primary care provider or nurse makes the drug order a legal request. *An unsigned order has no validity,* and the ordering physician or nurse practitioner needs to be notified if the order is unsigned.

When a primary care provider writes a prescription for a client, the prescription also includes information for the pharmacist. Therefore, a prescription's content differs from that of a medication order in a hospital (Box 23–2).

Communicating a Medication Order

A drug order is written on the client's chart by a primary care provider or by a nurse receiving a telephone or verbal order from a primary care provider. Most acute care agencies have a specified time frame in which the primary care provider issuing the telephone or verbal order must cosign the order written by the nurse. The medication order is then copied by a nurse or clerk to a Kardex or medication administration

BOX 23–1 Essential Parts of a Drug Order

- Full name of the client
- Date and time the order is written
- Name of the drug to be administered
- Dosage of the drug
- Frequency of administration
- Route of administration
- Signature of the person writing the order

BOX 23–2 Parts of a Prescription

- Descriptive information about the client: name, address, and sometimes age
- Date on which the prescription was written
- The Rx symbol, meaning "take thou"
- Medication name, dosage, and strength
- Route of administration
- Dispensing instructions for the pharmacist, for example, "Dispense 30 capsules"
- Directions for administration to be given to the client, for example, "one tablet with meals"
- Refill and/or special labeling, for example, "Refill × 1"
- Prescriber's signature

record (MAR). Increasingly, nurses receive computer printouts of a client's medications instead of a copy of the primary care provider's order. This method avoids errors and saves nursing time.

CLINICAL ALERT

If your assigned client receives new medication orders, double-check the transcribed information with the primary care provider's order. This ensures client safety.

Medication administration records (MARs) vary in form, but all include the client's name, room, and bed number; drug name and dose; and times and method of administration (Figure 23–4). In some agencies, the date the order was prescribed and the date the order expires are also included.

The nurse should always question the primary care provider about any order that is ambiguous, unusual, or contraindicated by the client's condition. When the nurse judges a primary care provider–ordered medication inappropriate, the following actions are required:

- Contact the primary care provider and discuss the rationale for believing the medication or dosage to be inappropriate.
- Document the following: when the primary care provider was notified, what was conveyed to the primary care provider, and the primary care provider's response.
- If the primary care provider cannot be reached, document all attempts to contact the primary care provider and the reason for withholding the medication. Facility policy dictates whether a different physician is contacted to avoid having the client miss a dose.
- If someone else gives the medication, document data about the client's condition before and after the medication.
- If an incident report (see Chapter 2 ∞) is indicated, clearly document factual information.

MEDICATION ADMINISTRATION RECORD

PAGE 1 OF 1

PRN#:
MRN#:   AGE:
ADM: 08-04-07   SEX:
DOB: HT:
DR.   HT:

VERIFIED BY: _____ DATE: _____

DIAGNOSIS: ALOC
          PNEUMONIA

ALLERGIES: NO KNOWN DRUG ALLERGIES

GENERATED: 08-07-07   07:32
FOR PERIOD: 08-07-07   08:00
THROUGH: 08-08-07   07:59

START	STOP	MEDICATION/I.V./IVPB/IRRIGATION		0800-1559	1600-2359	0000-0759
08-06	09-05	FERROUS SULFATE 300MG=5ML TWICE A DAY PO (FESO4)	(973539)	09	17	
08-06	09-05	DOCUSATE SODIUM 100MG=1UDCUP TWICE A DAY PO (COLACE) 100MG/30ML UD HOLD FOR LOOSE STOOL	(973532)	09	17	
08-05	09-04	ASCORBIC ACID 500MG=1TAB TWICE A DAY PO (VITAMIN C) 500MG TAB	(972096)	09	17	
08-05	09-04	LEVOTHYROXINE 0.05MG=1TAB DAILY PO (SYNTHROID) 0.05MG TAB	(972095)	09		
08-05	09-04	ASPIRIN 325MG=1 TAB DAILY PO (ASPIRIN) 325MG TAB *W/FOOD TO AVOID GI UPSET	(972094)	09		
08-04	08-14	CEFUROXIME ADDV. 1.500GM=1VIAL EVERY 8 HOURS IV (KEFUROX) 1.5GM ADDV *ATTACH TO D5W 50ML ADDV BAG *ACTIVATE BEFORE INFUSION* * INFUSE OVER 30 MINS*	(971776)	14	22	06

———— PRN ORDERS ————

START	STOP	MEDICATION/I.V./IVPB/IRRIGATION		0800-1559	1600-2359	0000-0759
08-04	09-03	ACETAMINOPHEN 650MG=1SUPP EVERY 4 HOURS AS NEEDED PR (TYLENOL) 650MG SUPP	(971779)			

INITIALS	SIGNATURE	SHIFT	INITIALS	SIGNATURE	SHIFT	INITIALS	SIGNATURE	SHIFT

SITE CODES: A. Right Upper Outer Quadrant Gluteus   C. Right Outer Aspect Arm   E. Right Ventrogluteal   G. Abdomen   I. Left Thigh
B. Left Upper Outer Quadrant Gluteus   D. Left Outer Aspect Arm   F. Left Ventrogluteal   H. Right Thigh

Figure 23–4 ● Sample medication administration record (MAR).

SYSTEMS OF MEASUREMENT

Three systems of measurement are used in North America: the metric system, the apothecaries' system, and the household system, which is similar to the apothecaries' system.

Metric System

The metric system, devised by the French in the latter part of the 18th century, is the system prescribed by law in most European countries and in Canada. The metric system is logically organized into units of 10; it is a decimal system. Basic units can be multiplied or divided by 10 to form secondary units. Multiples are calculated by moving the decimal point to the right, and division is accomplished by moving the decimal point to the left.

Basic units of measurement are the *meter,* the *liter,* and the *gram.* Prefixes derived from Latin designate subdivisions of the basic unit: *deci* (1/10 or 0.1), *centi* (1/100 or 0.01), and *milli* (1/1,000 or 0.001). Multiples of the basic unit are designated by prefixes derived from Greek: *deka* (10), *hecto* (100), and *kilo* (1,000). Only the measurements of volume (the liter) and of weight (the gram) are discussed in this chapter. These are the measures used in medication administration (see Figure 23–5). The *kilogram* (kg) is the only multiple of the gram used, and the *milligram* (mg) and *microgram* (mcg) are subdivisions. Fractional parts of the liter are usually expressed in *milliliters* (mL), for example, 600 mL; multiples of the liter are usually expressed as *liters* or milliliters, for example, 2.5 liters or 2,500 mL. In nursing practice it is important to understand the difference between weight and volume. A drug dosage may be ordered by weight (i.e., grams, mg, mcg) and administered by volume (mL). For example, a health care provider prescribes 20 mg (weight) of codeine elixir. The codeine elixir bottle is labeled 10 mg per 5 mL. The nurse administers 10 mL (volume) of codeine elixir.

Apothecaries' System

The apothecaries' system, older than the metric system, was brought to the United States from England during the colo-nial period. The basic unit of weight in the apothecaries' system is the *grain* (gr), likened to a grain of wheat, and the basic unit of volume is the *minim,* a volume of water equal in weight to a grain of wheat. The word *minim* means "the least." In ascending order, the other units of weight are the *scruple,* the *dram,* the *ounce,* and the *pound.* Today, the scruple is seldom used. The units of volume are, in ascending order, the fluid dram, the fluid ounce, the pint, the quart, and the gallon.

Quantities in the apothecaries' system are often expressed by lowercase Roman numerals, particularly when the unit of measure is abbreviated. The Roman numeral follows rather than precedes the unit of measure. For example, two grains are written as gr ii. Quantities less than 1 are expressed as a fraction, for example, gr 1/6. As stated earlier, apothecary units are unfamiliar to many practitioners and they may be confused with metric units. It is advisable to *not* use apothecary units. Use metric units instead to avoid medication errors.

Household System

Household measures may be used when more accurate systems of measure are not required. Included in household measures are drops, teaspoons, tablespoons, cups, and glasses. Although pints and quarts are often found in the home, they are defined as apothecaries' measures.

Converting Units of Weight and Measure

Sometimes drugs are dispensed from the pharmacy in grams when the order specifies milligrams, or they are dispensed in milligrams though ordered in grains. For example, a physician orders morphine gr 1/4. The medication is available labeled only in milligrams. The nurse knows that 1 mg = 1/60 gr or 60 mg = 1 grain. To convert the ordered dose to milligrams, the nurse calculates as follows:

$$\text{If } 60 \text{ mg} = 1 \text{ gr}$$
$$\text{Then } x \text{ mg} = 1/4 \text{ gr } (0.25 \text{ gr})$$
$$x = \frac{(60 \times 0.25)}{1}$$
$$x = 15 \text{ mg}$$

CONVERTING WEIGHTS WITHIN THE METRIC SYSTEM   It is relatively simple to arrive at equivalent units of weight within the metric system because the system is based on units of 10. Only three metric units of weight are used for drug dosages, the gram (g), milligram (mg), and microgram (mcg): 1,000 mg or 1,000,000 mcg equals 1 gram (g). Equivalents are computed by dividing or multiplying; for example, to change milligrams to grams, the nurse divides the number of milligrams by 1,000. The simplest way to divide by 1,000 is to move the decimal point three places to the left:

$$500 \text{ mg} = ? \text{ g}$$

Move the decimal point three places to the *left:*

$$\text{Answer} = 0.5 \text{ g}$$

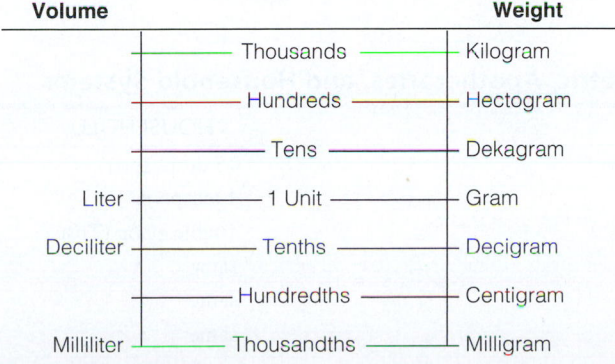

Volume		Weight
	Thousands	Kilogram
	Hundreds	Hectogram
	Tens	Dekagram
Liter	1 Unit	Gram
Deciliter	Tenths	Decigram
	Hundredths	Centigram
Milliliter	Thousandths	Milligram

Figure 23–5 Basic metric measurements of volume and weight.

Conversely, to convert grams to milligrams, multiply the number of grams by 1,000, or move the decimal point three places to the right:

$$0.006 \text{ g} = ? \text{ mg}$$

Move the decimal point three places to the *right*:

$$\text{Answer} = 6 \text{ mg}$$

CONVERTING WEIGHTS AND MEASURES BETWEEN SYSTEMS When preparing client medications, a nurse may need to convert weights or volumes from one system to another. As an example, the pharmacy may dispense milligrams or grams of chloral hydrate, yet the nurse must administer an order that reads "chloral hydrate gr viiss." To prepare the correct dose, the nurse must convert from the apothecaries' to the metric system. To give clients a useful, realistic measure for home use, the nurse may have to convert from the apothecaries' or metric system to the household system. All conversions are approximate, that is, not totally precise.

CONVERTING UNITS OF VOLUME Commonly used approximate equivalents are shown in Table 23–5. By learning these equivalents, the nurse can make many conversions readily. For example, 15 minims = approximately 15 drops (gtt); therefore, 1 minim is approximately 1 drop. Similarly, 1 quart approximates 1,000 mL, and 1 gallon approximates 4,000 mL.

The following are some situations in which nurses need to apply knowledge of volume conversion:

- Fluid drams and ounces are commonly used in prescribing liquid medications, such as cough syrups, laxatives, antacids, and antibiotics for children. The fluid ounce is frequently converted to milliliters when measuring a client's fluid intake or output.
- Liters and milliliters are the volumes commonly used in preparing solutions for enemas, irrigating solutions for bladder irrigations, and solutions for cleaning open wounds. In some situations, the nurse needs to convert the volumes of such solutions.

CONVERTING UNITS OF WEIGHT The units of weight most commonly used in nursing practice are the gram, milligram,

TABLE 23–6 Approximate Weight Equivalents: Metric and Apothecaries' Systems

METRIC		APOTHECARIES
1 mg	=	1/60 grain
60 mg	=	1 grain
1 g	=	15 grains
4 g	=	1 dram
30 g	=	1 ounce
500 g	=	1.1 pound (lb)
1,000 g (1 kg)	=	2.2 lb

and kilogram and the grain and the pound. Household units of weight are generally not applicable.

Table 23–6 shows metric and apothecaries' approximate equivalents. Learning these equivalents helps the nurse make weight conversions readily, as for example in the following situations:

- Converting milligrams to grains and vice versa, for example, when preparing medications
- Converting pounds to kilograms and vice versa, for example, a person's weight

When converting units of weight from the metric system to the apothecaries' system, the nurse should keep in mind that a milligram is smaller than a grain (1 mg = 1/60 grain and 1 grain = 60 mg). The result of converting a smaller unit (milligram) to a larger unit (grain) is a smaller number. Thus, the nurse must divide (by 60 if converting from milligrams to grains). Conversely, when converting from a larger unit to a smaller unit, the nurse multiplies (by 60 if converting from grains to milligrams), and the product is a larger number. In other words:

Small units (mg) to large units (grains) = a smaller number

Large units (grains) to small units (mg) = larger number

$$\frac{3,000 \text{ mg}}{60} = 50 \text{ grains}$$

$$50 \text{ grains} \times 60 = 3,000 \text{ mg}$$

TABLE 23–5 Approximate Volume Equivalents: Metric, Apothecaries, and Household Systems

METRIC		APOTHECARIES		HOUSEHOLD
1 mL	=	15 minims (min or m)	=	15 drops (gtt)
4–5 mL	=	1 fluid dram	=	1 teaspoon
15 mL	=	4 fluid drams	=	1 tablespoon (Tbsp)
30 mL	=	1 fluid ounce	=	same
500 mL	=	1 pint (pt)	=	same
1,000 mL	=	1 quart (qt)	=	same
4,000 mL	=	1 gallon (gal)	=	same

When converting pounds to kilograms, the nurse applies the same rule. The pound is a smaller unit than the kilogram, and the nurse converts by dividing or multiplying by 2.2:

$$2.2 \text{ lb} = 1 \text{ kg}$$
$$110 \text{ lb} = x \text{ kg}$$
$$x = \frac{110 \times 1}{2.2}$$
$$= 50 \text{ kg}$$

or

$$50 \text{ kg} = x \text{ lb}$$
$$1 \text{ kg} = 2.2 \text{ lb}$$
$$x = \frac{2.2 \times 50}{1}$$
$$= 110 \text{ lb}$$

The conversion of milligrams to grams was previously discussed. The decimal point is moved three spaces to the left:

$$3,000 \text{ mg} = 3 \text{ g}$$

Calculating Dosages

Several formulas can be used to calculate drug dosages. One formula uses ratios:

$$\frac{\text{Dose on hand}}{\text{Quantity on hand}} = \frac{\text{desired dose}}{\text{quantity desired } (x)}$$

For example, erythromycin 500 mg is ordered. It is supplied in a liquid form containing 250 mg in 5 mL. To calculate the dosage, the nurse uses the formula

$$\frac{\text{Dose on hand } (250 \text{ mg})}{\text{Quantity on hand } (5 \text{ mL})} = \frac{\text{desired dose } (500 \text{ mg})}{\text{quantity desired } (x)}$$

Then the nurse cross multiplies:

$$250\, x = 5 \text{ mL} \times 500 \text{ mg}$$
$$x = \frac{5 \text{ mL} \times 500 \text{ mg}}{250 \text{ mg}}$$
$$x = 10 \text{ mL}$$

Therefore, the dose ordered is 10 mL. The nurse can also use this formula to calculate dosages:

$$\text{Amount to administer } (x) =$$
$$\frac{\text{desired dose}}{\text{dose on hand}} \times \text{quantity on hand}$$

For example, heparin is often distributed in vials in prepared dilutions of 10,000 units per milliliter. If the order calls for 5,000 units, the nurse can use the preceding formula to calculate

$$x = \frac{5,000}{10,000} \times 1$$
$$x = 1/2 \text{ mL}$$

Therefore, the nurse injects 0.5 mL for a 5,000-unit dose.

DOSAGES FOR CHILDREN   Although dosage is stated in the medication order, nurses must understand something about the safe dosage for children and verify dosages as within a safe range. Unlike adult dosages, children's dosages are not always standard. Body size significantly affects dosage; therefore, dosages are calculated. Dosages based on weight use kilograms of body weight and per kilogram medication recommendations to arrive at appropriate and safe doses. Recommendations for surface area dosing are also standardized.

BODY SURFACE AREA   Body surface area is determined by using a nomogram and the child's height and weight. This is considered to be the most accurate method of calculating a child's dose. Standard nomograms give a child's body surface area according to weight and height (Figure 23–6). The formula is the ratio of the child's body surface area to the surface area of an average adult

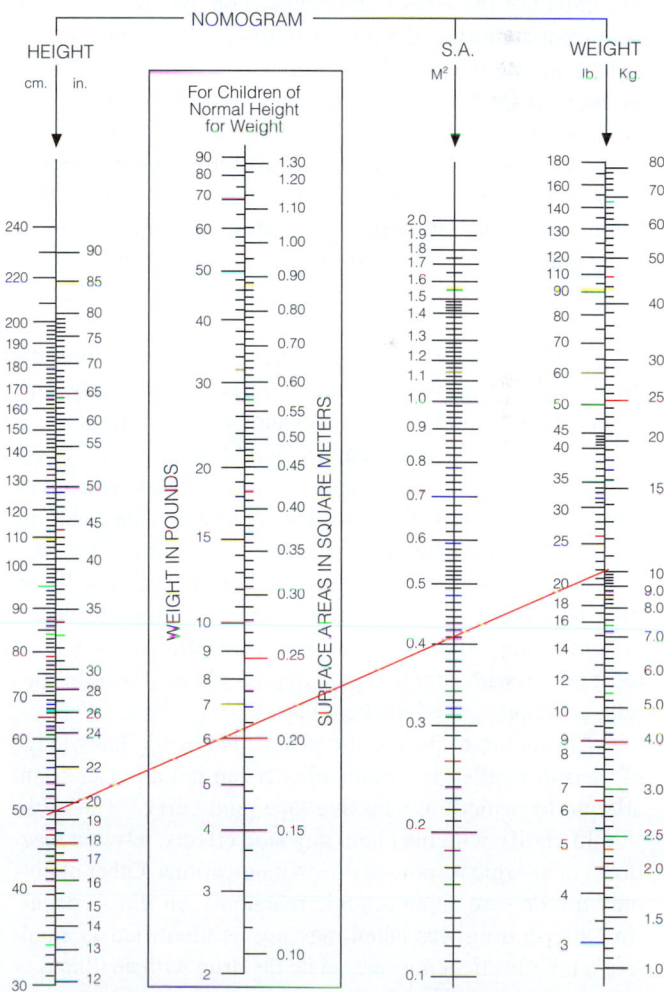

Figure 23–6 ◉ Nomogram with estimated body surface area. A straight line is drawn between the child's height (on the left) and the child's weight (on the right). The point at which the line intersects the surface area column is the estimated body surface area.

(1.7 square meters, or 1.7 m²), multiplied by the normal adult dose of the drug:

$$\text{Child's dose} = \frac{\text{surface area of child } (m^2)}{1.7 \text{ m}^2} \times \text{normal adult dose}$$

For example, a child who weighs 10 kg and is 50 cm tall has a body surface area of 0.4 m². Therefore, the child's dose of tetracycline corresponding to an adult dose of 250 mg would be as follows:

$$\text{Child's dose} = \frac{0.4 \text{ m}^2}{1.7 \text{ m}^2} \times 250 \text{ mg}$$
$$= 0.23 \times 250 = 58.82 \text{ mg}$$

ADMINISTERING MEDICATIONS SAFELY

The nurse should always assess a client's health status and obtain a medication history prior to giving any medication. The extent of the assessment depends on the client's illness or current condition, the intended drug, and the route of administration. For example, if a client has dyspnea, the nurse assesses respirations carefully before administering any medication that might affect breathing. It is important to determine whether the route of administration is suitable. For example, a client who is nauseated may not be able to take a drug administered orally. In general, the nurse assesses the client *prior* to administering any medication to obtain baseline data by which to evaluate the effectiveness of the medication.

The medication history includes information about the drugs the client is taking currently or has taken recently. This includes prescription drugs; over-the-counter drugs such as antacids, alcohol, and tobacco; and nonsanctioned drugs such as marijuana. Sometimes an incompatibility with one or more of these drugs affects the choice of a new medication.

Older adults often take vitamins, herbs, and food supplements, and/or use folk remedies that they do not list in their medication history. Because many of these have unknown or unpredictable actions and side effects, they need to be noted, with attention paid to possible incompatibilities with other prescribed medications.

An important part of the history is clients' knowledge of their drug allergies. Some clients can tell a nurse, "I am allergic to penicillin, adhesive tape, and curry." The nurse should clarify with the client any side effects, adverse reactions, or allergic responses due to medications. Other clients may not be sure about allergic reactions. An illness occurring after a drug was taken may not be identified as an allergy, but the client may associate the drug with an illness or unusual reaction. The client's primary care provider can often give information about allergies. During the history, the nurse tries to elicit information about drug dependencies. How often drugs are taken and the client's perceived need for them are measures of dependence.

PRACTICE GUIDELINES — Administering Medications

- Nurses who administer medications are responsible for their own actions. Question any order that is illegible or that you consider incorrect. Call the person who prescribed the medication for clarification.
- Be knowledgeable about the medications you administer. You need to know why the client is receiving the medication. Look up the necessary information if you are not familiar with the medication. Under no circumstances should a nurse give a medication they are not familiar with.
- Federal laws govern the use of narcotics and barbiturates. Keep these medications in a locked place.
- Use only medications that are in a clearly labeled container.
- Do not use liquid medications that are cloudy or have changed color.
- Calculate drug doses accurately. If you are uncertain, ask another nurse to double-check your calculations.
- Administer only medications personally prepared.
- Before administering a medication, identify the client correctly using the appropriate means of identification, such as checking the identification bracelet.
- Do not leave medications at the bedside, with certain exceptions that generally require a physician's order giving permission for the client to self-administer. Check agency policy.
- If a client vomits after taking an oral medication, report this to the nurse in charge, or the primary care provider, or both.
- Take special precautions when administering certain medications; for example, have another nurse check the dosages of anticoagulants, insulin, and certain IV preparations.
- Most hospital policies require new orders from the primary care provider for a client's postsurgery care.
- When a medication is omitted for any reason, record the fact together with the reason.
- When a medication error is made, report it immediately to the nurse in charge, the primary care provider, or both.

Also included in the history are the client's normal eating habits. Sometimes the medication schedule needs to be coordinated with mealtimes or the ingestion of foods. Where a medication must be taken with food on a specified schedule, clients can often adjust their mealtime or have a snack (e.g., with a bedtime medication). In addition, certain foods are incompatible with certain medications.

It is also important for the nurse to identify any problems the client may have in self-administering a medication. A client with poor eyesight, for example, may require special labels for the medication container; older adults with unsteady hands may not be able to hold a syringe or to inject themselves or another person. Obtaining information as to how and where clients store their medications is also important. If clients have difficulty opening certain containers, they may change containers, but leave old labels on, which increases the risk of medication errors.

The nurse needs to consider socioeconomic factors for all clients, but especially for older adults. Two common problems are lack of transportation to obtain medications and inadequate finances to purchase medications. The nurse can provide referrals to available resources when these concerns arise.

Medication Reconciliation

Another safety issue that affects the nurse is to ensure that clients receive the appropriate medications and dosages on admission, during transfer, and at discharge. According to the Institute for Healthcare Improvement (IHI), poorly communicated medical information at admission and other health care transition points is responsible for as many as 50% of all medication errors in hospitals (Manno & Hayes, 2006, p. 63). Furthermore, one out of five drugs administered in hospitals and skilled nursing facilities is in error and nearly 34% of preventable adverse drug events (ADEs) can be traced back to the administration process (Ketchum, Grass, & Padwojski, 2005, p. 78).

As a result, the IHI campaigned for medication reconciliation, and the Joint Commission incorporated medication reconciliation into their National Patient Safety Goals. The IHI defines medication reconciliation as "the process of creating the most accurate list possible of all medications a patient is taking—including drug name, dosage, frequency, and route—and comparing that list against the physician's admission, transfer, and/or discharge orders, with the goal of providing correct medications to the patient at all transition points within the hospital" (IHI, n.d.).

As of January 2006, all Joint Commission accredited facilities must have protocols and processes in place for medication reconciliation, particularly in three transition areas: on admission; during transfer between units, in shift reports, and in new MARs; and at discharge. The nurse needs to make a complete list of the client's medications (including prescriptions, vitamins, supplements, and over-the-counter) on admission. This current list needs to be compared to any new medications ordered by the physician on admission and during the client's hospital stay. Medications that are to be administered around the time of shift report need to be discussed at the report. It is important that the oncoming nurse know if the medication was given or not. If a client is transferred to another setting, within or outside of the facility, a complete list of the client's medications must be communicated to the next provider of care. This list is also provided to clients on discharge from the facility. In addition, the client should receive, at discharge, written and oral information on each medication to be taken at home. It is important for the nurse to emphasize to the client the importance of keeping the list of their medications and taking it with them to their follow-up visits and to future hospitalizations, if any. Maintaining their list of current medications helps improve communication and avoid potential errors in medication administration.

Medication Dispensing Systems

Medical facilities vary in their medication dispensing systems. The systems can include the following:

- *Medication cart:* The medication cart is on wheels allowing the nurse to move the cart to outside the

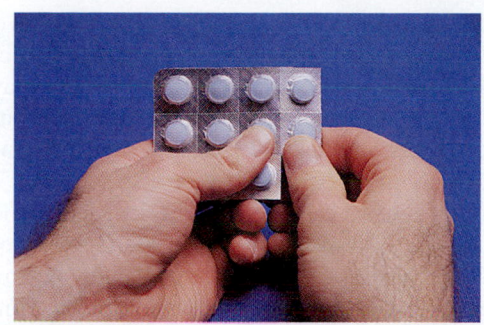

A

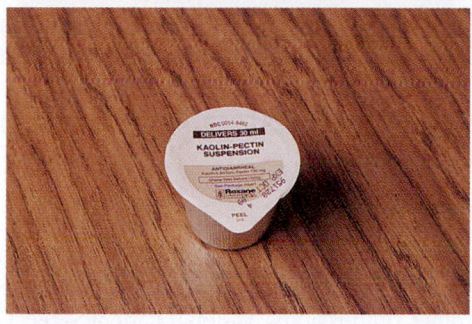

B

Figure 23–7 ● Unit-dose packages: **A,** tablets; **B,** liquid medications.

client's room. The cart contains small numbered drawers that correlate to the room numbers on the nursing unit. The small drawer is labeled with the name of the client currently in that room and holds the client's medications for the shift or 24 hours. The medication is usually in unit-dose packaging; that is, the individual drug package states the drug name, dose, and expiration date (Figure 23–7). A larger locked drawer in the cart contains the controlled substances rather than keeping them in the client's individual drawer. The cart may also include a supply drawer that contains client-labeled bulk containers, such as Metamucil, that are too large for the small individual drawer. The MAR is usually located in a binder or a computer located on top of the medication cart. The nurse either carries a key for the medication cart or enters a special code to open the cart, because it must be kept locked when not in use.

- *Medication cabinet:* Some facilities have a locked cabinet in the client's room. This cabinet holds the client's unit-dose medications and MAR. Controlled substances are not kept in this cabinet but at another location on the nursing unit. The nurse uses either a key or a special code for opening the client's medication cabinet, because it must be locked when not in use.

- *Medication room:* Depending on the facility, a medication room may be used for a variety of purposes. For example, the medication carts, when not in use, may be placed in this room. The medication room may also be the central location for stock medications, controlled medications, and/or drugs used for emergencies. The medication room may have a refrigerator for intravenous and other medications needing a cold environment. The room may also contain other medication administration supplies (syringes, needles, etc.). Nurses access the medication room by either a key or a special code as the room is often kept locked. Check agency policy.

- *Automated dispensing cabinet (ADC).* This computerized access system automates the distribution, management, and control of medications. Similar to automated teller machines, the nurse uses a password to access the system, selects the client's name from an on-screen list, and selects the medication(s).

Process of Administering Medications

When administering any drug, regardless of the route of administration, the nurse must do the following:

1. *Identify the client.* Errors can and do occur, usually because one client gets a drug intended for another. One of the Joint Commission's National Patient Safety Goals is to improve the accuracy of client identification. This goal requires a nurse to use at least two client identifiers whenever administering medications. Neither identifier can be the client's room number. Acceptable identifiers may be the person's name, assigned identification number, telephone number, photograph, or other person-specific identifier (The Joint Commission, 2006). In hospitals, most clients wear some sort of identification, such as a wristband with name and hospital identification number. Before giving the client any drug, always check the client's identification band. Some hospitals use bar-code technology for medication administration. A nurse preparing to administer a medication using bar-code technology scans or enters the nurse's own ID, the client's wristband, and each package of medication to be administered (Grissinger & Globus, 2004, p. 39). Bar coding often includes two or more person-specific identifiers, which meets the identifier requirement (Figure 23–8).

CLINICAL ALERT

Do not ask "Are you John Jones?" because the client may answer "yes" to the wrong name.

2. *Inform the client.* If the client is unfamiliar with the medication, the nurse should explain the intended action as well as any side effects or adverse effects that might occur. Listen to the client. It is easy to get so focused on the task of timely medication administration that the nurse may miss relevant information provided by the client. For example, if the client says that he doesn't take a pill for high blood pressure, this should be an "alert" for the nurse to stop and check if this is the correct medication for that client.

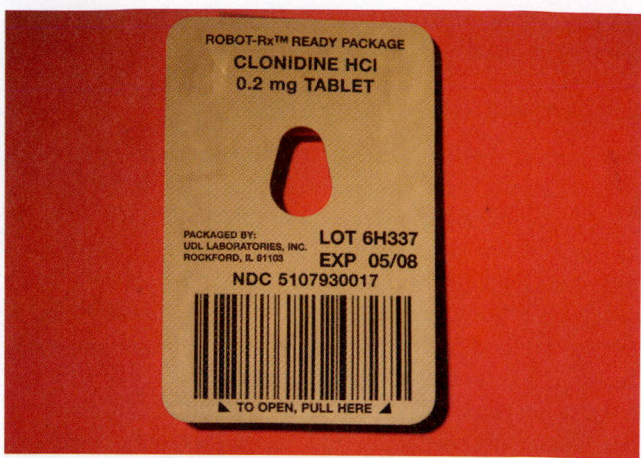

A

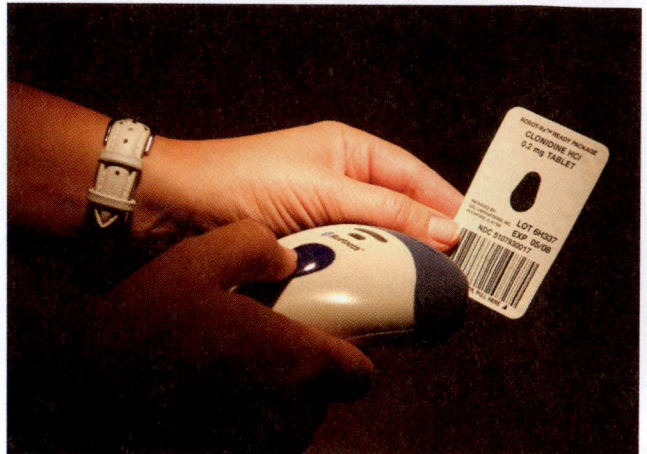

B

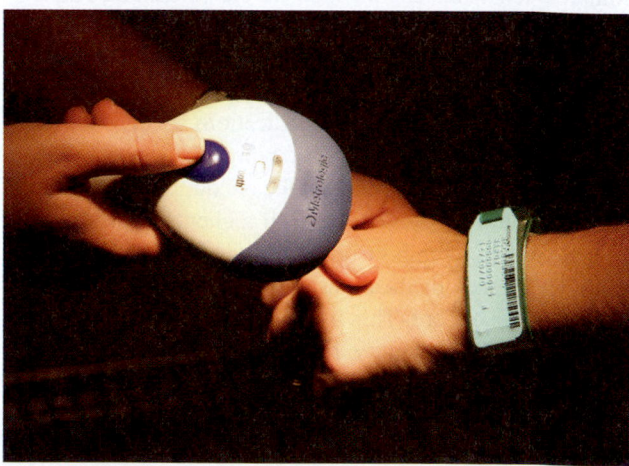

C

Figure 23–8 ● *A,* A sample bar code. *B,* The nurse scans the bar code on the medication package and *C,* the bar code on the client's wristband before administering the medication.

3. *Administer the drug.* Read the MAR carefully and perform three checks with the labeled medications (see Box 23–3). Then administer the medication in the prescribed dosage, by the route ordered, at the correct time. There are aspects of medication administration that are

Check Three Times for Safe Medication Administration

First Check

- Read the medication administration record (MAR) and remove the medication(s) from the client's drawer. Verify that the client's name and room number match the MAR.
- Compare the label of the medication against the MAR.
- If the dosage does not match the MAR, determine if you need to do a math calculation.
- Check the expiration date of the medication.

Second Check

- While preparing the medication (e.g., pouring, drawing up, or placing unopened package in a medication cup), look at the medication label and check against the MAR.

Third Check

- Recheck the label on the container (e.g., vial, bottle, or unused unit-dose medications) before returning to its storage place.

or

- Check the label on the medication against the MAR before opening the package at the bedside.

Note: Reprinted from *"Safe Meds: An Interactive Guide to Safe Medication Practices,"* by P. Przybycien. Copyright © 2005, with permission of Elsevier.

important for the nurse to check each time a medication is administered. These are referred to as the "rights." Traditionally, there were five rights to medication administration. More rights have been added over the last few years with the latest being the ten rights (Przybycien, 2005). See Box 23–4.

4. *Provide adjunctive interventions as indicated.* Clients may need help when receiving medications. They may require physical assistance, for instance, in assuming positions for intramuscular injections, or they may need guidance about measures to enhance drug effectiveness and prevent complications, such as drinking fluids. Some clients convey fear about their medications. The nurse can allay fears by listening carefully to clients' concerns and giving correct information.

5. *Record the drug administered.* The facts recorded in the chart, in ink or by computer printout, are name of the drug, dosage, method of administration, specific relevant data such as pulse rate (taken in most settings prior to the administration of digitalis), and any other pertinent information. The record should also include the exact time of administration and the signature of the nurse providing the medication. Many medication records are designed so that the nurse signs once on the page and initials each medication administered. Often,

Ten "Rights" of Medication Administration

Right Medication

- The medication given was the medication ordered.

Right Dose

- The dose ordered is appropriate for the client.
- Give special attention if the calculation indicates multiple pills/tablets or a large quantity of a liquid medication. This can be a "cue" that the math calculation may be incorrect.
- Double-check calculations that appear questionable.
- Know the usual dosage range of the medication.
- Question a dose outside of the usual dosage range.

Right Time

- Give the medication at the right frequency and at the time ordered according to agency policy.
- Medications given within 30 minutes before or after the scheduled time are considered to meet the right time standard.

Right Route

- Give the medication by the ordered route.
- Make certain that the route is safe and appropriate for the client.

Right Client

- Medication is given to the intended client.
- Check the client's identification band with each administration of a medication.
- Know the agency's name alert procedure when clients with the same or similar last names are on the nursing unit.

Right Client Education

- Explain information about the medication to the client (e.g., why receiving, what to expect, any precautions).

Right Documentation

- Document medication administration after giving it, not before.
- If time of administration differs from prescribed time, note the time on the MAR and explain reason and follow-through activities (e.g., pharmacy states medication will be available in 2 hours) in nursing notes.
- If a medication is not given, follow the agency's policy for documenting the reason why.

Right to Refuse

- Adult clients have the right to refuse any medication.
- The nurse's role is to ensure that the client is fully informed of the potential consequences of refusal and to communicate the client's refusal to the health care provider.

Right Assessment

- Some medications require specific assessments prior to administration (e.g., apical pulse, blood pressure, lab results).
- Medication orders may include specific parameters for administration (e.g., do not give if pulse less than 60 or systolic blood pressure less than 100).

Right Evaluation

- Conduct appropriate follow-up (e.g., was the desired effect achieved or not? Did the client experience any side effects or adverse reactions?).

medications that are given regularly are recorded on a special flow record. PRN (as needed) or stat (at once) medications are recorded separately.

6. *Evaluate the client's response to the drug.* The kinds of behavior that reflect the action or lack of action of a drug and its untoward effects (both minor and major) are as variable as the purposes of the drugs themselves. The anxious client may show the desired effects of a tranquilizer by behavior that reflects a lowered stress level (e.g., slower speech or fewer random movements). The effectiveness of a sedative can often be measured by how well a client slept, and the effectiveness of an antispasmodic by how much pain the client feels. In all nursing activities, nurses need to be aware of the medications that a client is taking and record their effectiveness as assessed by the client and the nurse on the client's chart. The nurse may also report the client's response directly to the nurse manager and primary care provider.

Developmental Considerations

It is important for the nurse to be aware of how growth and development affects administration of medications for all age groups, particularly the very young and the very old.

INFANTS AND CHILDREN Knowledge of growth and development is essential for the nurse administering medications to children. Oral medications for children are usually prepared in sweetened liquid form to make them more palatable. The parents may provide suggestions about what method is best for their child. Do not use necessary foods such as milk or orange juice to mask the taste of medications, because the child may develop unpleasant associations and refuse that food in the future.

Children tend to fear any procedure in which a needle is used because they anticipate pain or because the procedure is unfamiliar and threatening. The nurse needs to acknowledge that the child will feel some pain; denying this fact only deepens the child's distrust. After the injection, the nurse (or the parent) can cuddle and speak softly to the infant and give the child a toy to dispel the child's association of the nurse only with pain.

OLDER ADULTS Older adults can have special problems, most of which are related to physiologic changes, to past experiences, and to established attitudes toward medications. See Box 23–5 for a list of the physiologic changes in older adults that may affect the administration and effectiveness of medications.

Many of these changes enhance the possibility of cumulative effects and toxicity. For example, impaired circulation delays the action of medications given intramuscularly or subcutaneously. Digitalis, which is frequently taken by older adults, can accumulate to toxic levels and be lethal. It is not uncommon for older adults to take several different medications daily. The possibility of error increases with the number of medications taken, whether self-administered at home or administered in a hospital. The greater number of medica-

BOX 23–5	**Physiologic Changes Associated with Aging That Influence Medication Administration and Effectiveness**

- Altered memory
- Decreased visual acuity
- Decrease in renal function, resulting in slower elimination of drugs and higher drug concentrations in the bloodstream for longer periods
- Less complete and slower absorption from the gastrointestinal tract
- Increased proportion of fat to lean body mass, which facilitates retention of fat-soluble drugs and increases potential for toxicity
- Decreased liver function, which hinders biotransformation of drugs
- Decreased organ sensitivity, which means that the response to the same drug concentration in the vicinity of the target organ is less in older people than in the young
- Altered quality of organ responsiveness, resulting in adverse effects becoming pronounced before therapeutic effects are achieved
- Decrease in manual dexterity due to arthritis and/or decrease in flexibility

tions also compounds the problem of drug interactions. A general rule to follow is that older adults should take as few medications as possible.

Older adults usually require smaller dosages of drugs, especially sedatives and other central nervous system depressants. Reactions of older adults to medications, particularly sedatives, are unpredictable and often bizarre. It is not uncommon to see irritability, confusion, disorientation, restlessness, and incontinence as a result of sedatives. Nurses therefore need to observe clients carefully for untoward reactions. Prescribers often follow the unwritten rule to "start low and go slow" when prescribing medications for older adults. The initial prescribed dosage will often be low and then gradually increased with careful monitoring of actions and side effects of the drug.

Attitudes of older adults toward medical care and medications vary. Older adults tend to believe in the wisdom of the health care provider more readily than younger people. Some older people are bewildered by the prescription of several medications and may passively accept their medications from nurses but not swallow them, spitting out tablets or capsules after the nurse leaves the room. For this reason, the nurse is advised to stay with clients until they have swallowed the medications. Others may be suspicious of medications and actively refuse them.

Older adults are mature adults capable of reasoning. Therefore, the nurse needs to explain the reasons for and the effects of medications. This education can prevent clients from continuing to take a medication long after there is a need for it or discontinuing a drug too quickly. For example, clients should know that diuretics will cause them to urinate

RESEARCH NOTES

Can Changing the Health Care Workplace to Avoid Interruptions Prevent Medication Errors?

Nursing units are complex units in which nurses are often hurried, distracted, and interrupted during medication administration. This process improvement project implemented a program to decrease distractions on the nursing unit through "Do Not Disturb" reminder signs at medication carts and medication dispensing machines. They also designed a medication administration protocol checklist that was given to the nurses and also placed on medication carts. Nurses were asked to avoid conversation and prevent distractions during medication administration.

Researchers conducted medication administration observations during 7 AM to 7 PM shifts during the week. The observations revealed decreased episodes of distraction, more focus on the administration process, and decreased reported medication errors.

The researchers found that interruptions by other nurses and personnel, conversation, and loud noises caused the highest number of distractions when nurses administered medications.

Implications

"Do Not Disturb" signs and protocol checklists represent easy and inexpensive strategies to reduce distractions and keep nurses focused during the process of medication administration with the outcome of enhancing client safety.

Note: From: "Innovative Approaches to Reducing Nurses' Distractions during Medication Administration," by T. M. Pape et al., 2005, *Journal of Continuing Education in Nursing, 36*(3), 108–116. Copyright © 2005 SLACK, Inc. Reprinted with permission.

more frequently and may reduce ankle edema. All clients need instructions about medications. These instructions should include when to take the drugs, what effects to expect, and when to consult a primary care provider.

Because some clients are required to take several medications daily and because visual acuity and memory may be impaired, the nurse needs to develop simple, realistic plans for clients to follow at home. For example, remembering to take drugs can be difficult for most people, including older adults. Scheduling medications at mealtime or at bedtime helps clients to remember to take their medications. Some clients may take their medications and then an hour later not remember whether they took them. One solution to forgetfulness is to use a special container or glass strictly for medications. An empty glass or container indicates that the person took the pills. Special containers with individual slots and markings for each day can reduce confusion. Loss of visual acuity presents problems that can be overcome by writing out the plan in block letters large enough to be read.

In some situations, enlisting the help of a spouse, son, or daughter can be helpful.

Older adults often have a decrease in dexterity due to arthritis or stiffness of their hands and fingers due to aging. This causes difficulty in opening medication containers or in self-administration of other medications such as eyedrops, eardrops, insulin injections, and inhalers. Nurses can help clients make the necessary changes or enlist the assistance of another person to help them administer their medications.

ORAL MEDICATIONS

The oral route is the most common route by which medications are given. As long as a client can swallow and retain the drug in the stomach, this is the route of choice (see Skill 23–1). Oral medications are contraindicated when a client is vomiting, has gastric or intestinal suction, or is unconscious and unable to swallow. Such clients in a hospital are usually on orders for "nothing by mouth" (Latin is *nil per os:* NPO).

SKILL 23–1

ADMINISTERING ORAL MEDICATIONS

PURPOSE
- To provide a medication that has systemic effects or local effects on the gastrointestinal tract or both (see specific drug action).

ASSESSMENT
Assess
- Allergies to medication(s)
- Client's ability to swallow the medication
- Presence of vomiting or diarrhea that would interfere with the ability to absorb the medication
- Specific drug action, side effects, interactions, and adverse reactions

- Client's knowledge of and learning needs about the medication

Perform appropriate assessments (e.g., vital signs, laboratory results) specific to the medication.

Determine if the assessment data influence administration of the medication (i.e., is it appropriate to administer the medication or does the medication need to be held and the prescriber notified?).

(continued)

ADMINISTERING ORAL MEDICATIONS *(continued)*

PLANNING

Delegation
In acute care settings, administration of oral/enteral medications is performed by the nurse and is not delegated to unlicensed assistive personnel (UAP). The nurse can inform the UAP of the intended therapeutic effects and/or specific side effects of the medication and request the UAP to report specific client observations to the nurse for follow-up. In some long-term care settings, trained UAP may administer certain medications to stable clients. It is important, however, for the nurse to remember that the medication knowledge of the UAP is limited and *assessment and evaluation of the effectiveness of the medication remains the responsibility of the nurse.*

EQUIPMENT
- Dispensing system
- Disposable medication cups: small paper or plastic cups for tablets and capsules, waxed or plastic calibrated medication cups for liquids
- MAR or computer printout
- Pill crusher/cutter
- Straws to administer medications that may discolor the teeth or to facilitate the ingestion of liquid medication for certain clients
- Drinking glass and water or juice
- Applesauce or pudding to use for crushed medications for clients who may choke on liquids

IMPLEMENTATION

Preparation
1. Know the reason why the client is receiving the medication, the drug classification, contraindications, usual dosage range, side effects, and nursing considerations for administering and evaluating the intended outcomes for the medication.
2. Check the medication administration record (MAR).
   - Check the MAR for the drug name, dosage, frequency, route of administration, and expiration date for administering the medication, if appropriate. **Rationale:** *Certain medications (e.g., narcotics, antibiotics) have a specified time frame at which they expire and need to be reordered by the primary care provider.*
   - If the MAR is unclear or pertinent information is missing, compare the MAR with the most recent prescriber's written order.
   - Report any discrepancies to the charge nurse or the prescriber, as agency policy dictates.
3. Verify the client's ability to take medication orally.
   - Determine whether the client can swallow, is NPO, is nauseated or vomiting, has gastric suction, or has diminished or absent bowel sounds.
4. Organize the supplies.
   - Assemble the MAR(s) for each client together so that medications can be prepared for one client at a time. **Rationale:** *Organization of supplies saves time and reduces the chance of error.*

Performance
1. Perform hand hygiene and observe other appropriate infection control procedures.
2. Unlock the dispensing system.
3. Obtain appropriate medication.
   - Read the MAR and take the appropriate medication from the shelf, drawer, or refrigerator. The medication may be dispensed in a bottle, box, or unit-dose package.
   - Compare the label of the medication container or unit-dose package against the order on the MAR or computer printout. **Rationale:** *This is a safety check to ensure that the right medication is given.* If these are not identical, recheck the prescriber's written order in the client's chart. If

there is still a discrepancy, check with the nurse in charge or the pharmacist.
   - Check the expiration date of the medication. Return expired medications to the pharmacy. **Rationale:** *Outdated medications are not safe to administer.*
   - Use only medications that have clear, legible labels *to ensure accuracy.*
4. Prepare the medication.
   - Calculate the medication dosage accurately.
   - Prepare the correct amount of medication for the required dose, without contaminating the medication. **Rationale:** *Aseptic technique maintains drug cleanliness.*
   - While preparing the medication, recheck each prepared drug and container with the MAR again. **Rationale:** *This second safety check reduces the chance of error.*

TABLETS OR CAPSULES
- Place packaged unit-dose capsules or tablets directly into the medicine cup. Do not remove the medication from the package until at the bedside. **Rationale:** *The wrapper keeps the medication clean. Not removing the medication facilitates identification of the medication in the event the client refuses the drug or assessment data indicate to hold the medication. Unopened unit-dose packages can usually be returned to the medication cart.*
- If using a stock container, pour the required number into the bottle cap, and then transfer the medication to the disposable cup without touching the tablets.
- Keep narcotics and medications that require specific assessments, such as pulse measurements, respiratory rate or depth, or blood pressure, separate from the others. **Rationale:** *This reminds the nurse to complete the needed assessment(s) in order to decide whether to give the medication or to withhold the medication if indicated.*
- Break only scored tablets if necessary to obtain the correct dosage. Use a cutting or splitting device if needed. Check the agency policy as to whether unused portions of a medication can be discarded and, if so, how they are to be discarded. **1**
- If the client has difficulty swallowing, check if the medication can be crushed. If this is acceptable, crush the tablets to a fine powder with a pill crusher or between two medication cups.

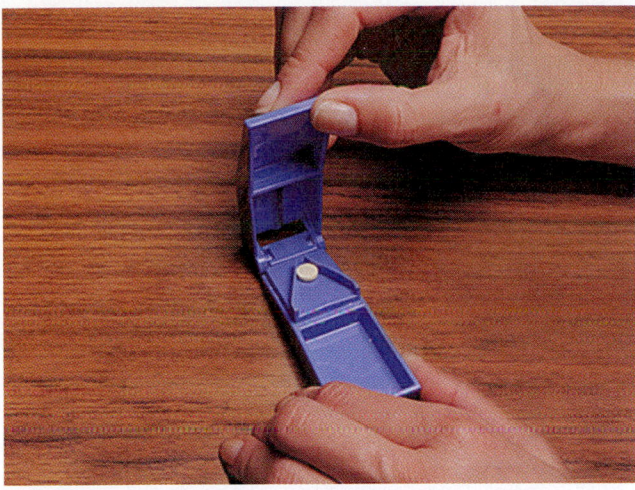

❶ A cutting device can be used to divide tablets.

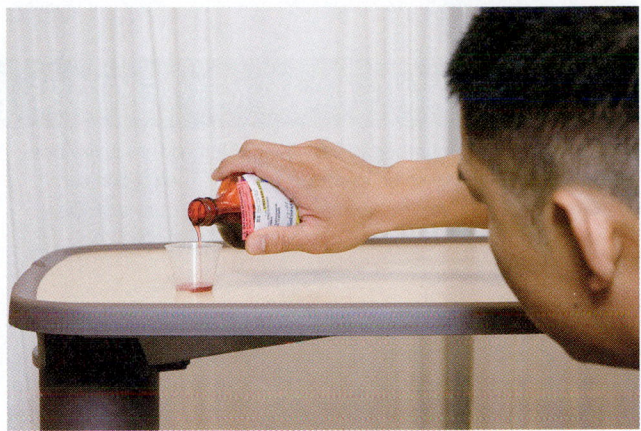

❷ Pouring a liquid medication from a bottle.

Then, mix the powder with a small amount of soft food (e.g., custard, applesauce). Some medications should not be crushed (e.g., time-released and enteric coated). An example of tablets that should not be crushed is oxycodone (OxyContin), a long-acting narcotic that normally lasts 12 hours after administration. If the tablet is crushed, the client gets a surge of action in the first 2 hours, then may start having severe pain again in 4 to 6 hours, as the effects wear off too soon. The crushing of these tablets causes an uneven effect, and the long action of the medication is lost.

CLINICAL ALERT

Check with the pharmacy before crushing tablets. Sustained-action, enteric-coated, buccal, or sublingual tablets should not be crushed.

LIQUID MEDICATION
- Thoroughly mix the medication before pouring. Discard any medication that has changed color or turned cloudy.
- Remove the cap and place it upside down on the countertop **Rationale:** *This avoids contaminating the inside of the cap.*
- Hold the bottle so the label is next to your palm and pour the medication away from the label. **Rationale:** *This prevents the label from becoming soiled and illegible as a result of spilled liquids.* ❷
- Place the medication cup on a flat surface at eye level and fill it to the desired level, using the *bottom* of the **meniscus** (crescent-shaped upper surface of a column of liquid) to align with the container scale. ❸ **Rationale:** *This method ensures accuracy of measurement.*
- Before capping the bottle, wipe the lip with a paper towel. **Rationale:** *This prevents the cap from sticking.*
- When giving small amounts of liquids (e.g., < 5 mL), prepare the medication in a sterile syringe without the needle or in a specially designed oral syringe. Label the syringe with the name of the medication and the route (PO). **Rationale:** *Any oral solution removed from the original container and placed into a syringe should be labeled to avoid medications being given by the wrong route (e.g., IV). This practice facilitates client safety and avoids tragic errors.*

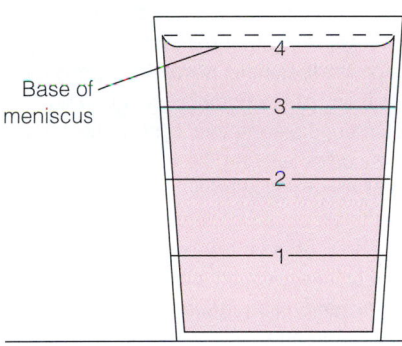

Base of meniscus

❸ The bottom of the meniscus is the measuring guide.

- Keep unit-dose liquids in their package and open them at the bedside.

ORAL NARCOTICS
- If an agency uses a manual recording system for controlled substances, check the narcotic record for the previous drug count and compare it with the supply available. Some medications, including narcotics, are kept in plastic containers that are sectioned and numbered.
- Remove the next available tablet and drop it in the medicine cup.
- After removing a tablet, record the necessary information on the appropriate narcotic control record and sign it.
- **Note:** Computer-controlled dispensing systems allow access only to the selected drug and automatically record its use.

ALL MEDICATIONS
- Place the prepared medication and MAR together on the medication cart.
- Recheck the label on the container before returning the bottle, box, or envelope to its storage place. **Rationale:** *This third check further reduces the risk of error.*
- Avoid leaving prepared medications unattended. **Rationale:** *This precaution prevents potential mishandling errors.*
- Lock the medication cart before entering the client's room. **Rationale:** *This is a safety measure because medication carts are not to be left open when unattended.*

(continued)

SKILL 23–1

ADMINISTERING ORAL MEDICATIONS *(continued)*

- Check the room number against the MAR if agency policy does not allow the MAR to be removed from the medication cart. **Rationale:** *This is another safety measure to ensure that the nurse is entering the correct client room.*

5. Provide for client privacy.
6. Prepare the client.
   - Check the client's identification band. **Rationale:** *This ensures that the right client receives the medication.*
   - Assist the client to a sitting position or, if not possible, to a side-lying position. **Rationale:** *These positions facilitate swallowing and prevent aspiration.*
   - If not previously assessed, take the required assessment measures, such as pulse and respiratory rates or blood pressure. Take the apical pulse rate before administering digitalis preparations. Take blood pressure before giving antihypertensive drugs. Take the respiratory rate prior to administering narcotics. **Rationale:** *Narcotics depress the respiratory center.* If any of the findings are above or below the predetermined parameters, consult the primary care provider before administering the medication.
7. Explain the purpose of the medication and how it will help, using language that the client can understand. Include relevant information about effects; for example, tell the client receiving a diuretic to expect an increase in urine output. **Rationale:** *Information can facilitate acceptance of and compliance with the therapy.*
8. Administer the medication at the correct time.
   - Take the medication to the client within the period of 30 minutes before or after the scheduled time.
   - Give the client sufficient water or preferred juice to swallow the medication. Before using juice, check for any food and medication incompatibilities. **Rationale:** *Fluids ease swallowing and facilitate absorption from the gastrointestinal tract.* Liquid medications other than antacids or cough preparations may be diluted with 15 mL (1/2 oz) of water to facilitate absorption.
   - If the client is unable to hold the pill cup or use the pill cup to introduce the medication into the mouth, then give only one tablet or capsule at a time. **Rationale:** *Putting the cup to the client's mouth maintains the cleanliness of the nurse's hands. Giving one medication at a time eases swallowing.*
   - If an older child or adult has difficulty swallowing, ask the client to place the medication on the back of the tongue before taking the water. **Rationale:** *Stimulation of the back of the tongue produces the swallowing reflex.*
   - If the medication has an objectionable taste, ask the client to suck a few ice chips beforehand, or give the medication with juice, applesauce, or bread if there are no contraindications. **Rationale:** *The cold of the ice chips will desensitize the taste buds, and juices or bread can mask the taste of the medication.*
   - If the client says that the medication you are about to give is different from what the client has been receiving, do not give the medication without first checking the original order. **Rationale:** *Most clients are familiar with the appearance of medications taken previously. Unfamiliar medications may signal a possible error.*
   - Stay with the client until all medications have been swallowed. **Rationale:** *The nurse must see the client swallow the medication before the drug administration can be recorded.* The nurse may need to check the client's mouth to ensure that the medication was swallowed and not hidden inside the cheek. A primary care provider's order or agency policy is required for medications left at the bedside.
9. Document each medication given.
   - Record the medication given, dosage, time, any complaints or assessments of the client, and your signature.
   - If medication was refused or omitted, record this fact on the appropriate record; document the reason, when possible, and the nurse's actions according to agency policy.
10. Dispose of all supplies appropriately.
    - Replenish stock (e.g., medication cups) and return the cart to the appropriate place.
    - Discard used disposable supplies.

EVALUATION
- Conduct appropriate follow-up.
- Observe for desired effect (e.g., relief of pain or decrease in body temperature).
- Note any adverse effects or side effects (e.g., nausea, vomiting, skin rash, change in vital signs).
- Relate to previous findings, if available.
- Report significant deviations from normal to the primary care provider.

LIFESPAN CONSIDERATIONS   Administering Oral Medications

- Knowledge of growth and development is essential for the nurse administering medications to infants and children.
- Nurses must know the range of safe medication dosages for infants and children.

Infants

- Oral medications can be effectively administered in several ways:
  - A syringe or dropper
  - A medication nipple, which allows the infant to suck the medication
  - Mixed in small amounts of food
  - A spoon or medication cup, for older children
- Never mix medications into foods that are essential, since the infant may associate the food with an unpleasant taste and refuse that food in the future. Never mix medications with formula.
- Place a small amount of liquid medication along the inside of the baby's cheek and wait for the infant to swallow before giving more to prevent aspiration or spitting out.
- When using a spoon, retrieve and refeed medication that is thrust outward by the infant's tongue.

Children

- Whenever possible, give children a choice between the use of a spoon, dropper, or syringe.
- Dilute the oral medication, if indicated, with a small amount of water. Many oral medications are readily swallowed if they are diluted with a small amount of water. If large quantities of water are used, the child may refuse to drink the entire amount and receive only a portion of the medication.
- Oral medications for children are usually prepared in sweetened liquid form to make them more palatable. Crush medications that are not supplied in liquid form and mix them with substances available on most pediatric units, such as honey, flavored syrup, jam, or a fruit puree.
- Necessary foods such as milk or orange juice should not be used to mask the taste of medications because the

child may develop unpleasant associations and refuse that food in the future.
- Disguise disagreeable-tasting medications with sweet-tasting substances mentioned previously. However, present any altered medication to the child honestly and not as a food or treat.
- Place the young child or toddler on your lap or a parent's lap in a sitting position.
- Administer the medication slowly with a measuring spoon, plastic syringe, or medicine cup.
- To prevent nausea, pour a carbonated beverage over finely crushed ice and give it before or immediately after the medication is administered.
- Follow medication with a drink of water, juice, a soft drink, or a Popsicle or frozen juice bar. This removes any unpleasant aftertaste.
- For children who take sweetened medications on a long-term basis, follow the medication administration with oral hygiene. These children are at high risk for dental caries.

Older Adults

- The physiologic changes associated with aging influence medication administration and effectiveness. Examples include altered memory, less acute vision, decrease in renal function, less complete and slower absorption from the gastrointestinal tract, and decreased liver function. Many of these changes enhance the possibility of cumulative effects and toxicity.
- Older adults usually require smaller dosages of drugs, especially sedatives and other central nervous system depressants.
- Older adults are mature adults capable of reasoning. The nurse, therefore, needs to explain the reasons for and the effects of the client's medications.
- Socioeconomic factors such as lack of transportation and decreased finances may influence obtaining medications when needed.
- An increase in marketing and availability of vitamins, herbs, and supplements alerts the nurse to include this information in a medication history.

NASOGASTRIC AND GASTROSTOMY MEDICATIONS

For clients who cannot take anything by mouth (NPO) and have a nasogastric tube or a gastrostomy tube in place, an alternative route for administering medications is through the nasogastric or gastrostomy tube. A nasogastric (NG) tube is inserted by way of the nasopharynx and is placed into the client's stomach for the purpose of feeding the client or to remove gastric secretions. A gastrostomy tube is surgically placed directly into the client's stomach and provides an-

other route for administering medications and nutrition (see Chapter 32 ∞). Guidelines for administering medications by nasogastric tubes and gastrostomy tubes are shown in the Practice Guidelines box.

PARENTERAL MEDICATIONS

Parenteral administration of medications is a common nursing procedure. Nurses give parenteral medications intradermally (ID), subcutaneously, intramuscularly (IM), or intravenously

- Always check with the pharmacist to see if the client's medications come in a liquid form because these are less likely to cause tube obstruction.
- If medications do not come in liquid form, check to see if they may be crushed. (Note that enteric-coated, sustained action, buccal, and sublingual medications should never be crushed.)
- Crush a tablet into a fine powder and dissolve in at least 30 mL of warm water. Cold liquids may cause client discomfort. Use only water for mixing and flushing. Some medications are mixed with other fluids, such as normal saline, in order to maximize dissolution. Nurses are encouraged to consult with a pharmacist.
- Read medication labels carefully before opening a capsule. Open capsules and mix the contents with water only with the pharmacist's advice.
- Do not administer whole or undissolved medications because they will clog the tube.
- Assess tube placement (see Chapter 32 ∞ for methods to verify tube placement).
- Before giving the medication, aspirate all the stomach contents and measure the residual volume. Check agency policy if residual volume is greater than 100 mL.

- When administering the medication(s):
  - Remove the plunger from the syringe and connect the syringe to a pinched or kinked tube. *Pinching or kinking the tube prevents excess air from entering the stomach and causing distention.*
  - Put 15 to 30 mL (5 to 10 mL for children) of water into the syringe barrel to flush the tube before administering the first medication. Raise or lower the barrel of the syringe to adjust the flow as needed. Pinch or clamp the tubing before all the water is instilled to avoid excess air entering the stomach.
  - Pour liquid or dissolved medication into the syringe barrel and allow to flow by gravity into the enteral tube.
  - If you are giving several medications, administer each one separately and flush with at least 15 to 30 mL (5 mL for children) of tap water between each medication.
  - When you have finished administering all medications, flush with another 15 to 30 mL (5 to 10 mL for children) of warm water to clear the tube and prevent blockage.
- If the tube is connected to suction, disconnect the suction and keep the tube clamped for 20 to 30 minutes after giving the medication to allow for absorption.

(IV). Because these medications are absorbed more quickly than oral medications and are irretrievable once injected, the nurse must prepare and administer them carefully and accurately. Administering parenteral drugs requires the same nursing knowledge as for oral and topical drugs; however, because injections are invasive procedures, aseptic technique must be used to minimize the risk of infection.

Equipment

To administer parenteral medications, nurses use syringes and needles to withdraw medication from ampules and vials.

SYRINGES   Syringes have three parts: the tip, which connects with the needle; the barrel, or outside part, on which the scales are printed; and the plunger, which fits inside the barrel (Figure 23–9). When handling a syringe, the nurse may touch the outside of the barrel and the handle of the plunger; however, the nurse must *avoid letting any unsterile object touch the tip or inside of the barrel, the shaft of the plunger, or the shaft or tip of the needle.*

There are several kinds of syringes, differing in size, shape, and material. The three most commonly used types are the standard hypodermic syringe, the insulin syringe, and the tuberculin syringe (Figure 23–10). A hypodermic syringe comes in 2-, 2.5-, 3-, and 5-mL sizes. The syringe may have two scales marked on it: the minim and the milliliter. The milliliter scale is the one normally used; the minim scale is used for very small dosages.

An insulin syringe is similar to a hypodermic syringe, but the scale is specially designed for insulin: a 100-unit cal-

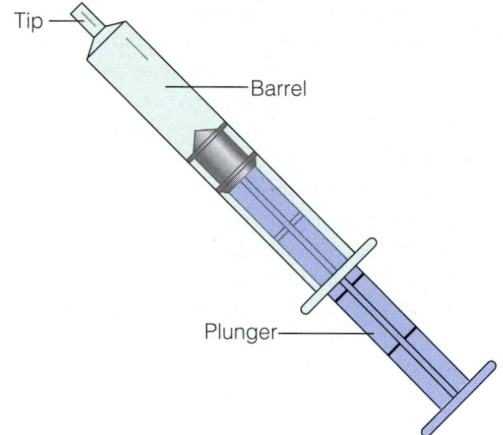

Figure 23–9 ◯ The three parts of a syringe.

ibrated scale intended for use with U-100 insulin. This is the only syringe that should be used to administer insulin. Several low-dose insulin syringes are also available. These syringes frequently have a nonremovable needle. All insulin syringes are calibrated on the 100-unit scale in North America. The correct choice of syringe is based on the amount of insulin required.

The tuberculin syringe was originally designed to administer tuberculin solution. It is a narrow syringe, calibrated in tenths and hundredths of a milliliter (up to 1 mL) on one scale and in sixteenths of a minim (up to 1 minim) on the other scale. This type of syringe can also be useful in

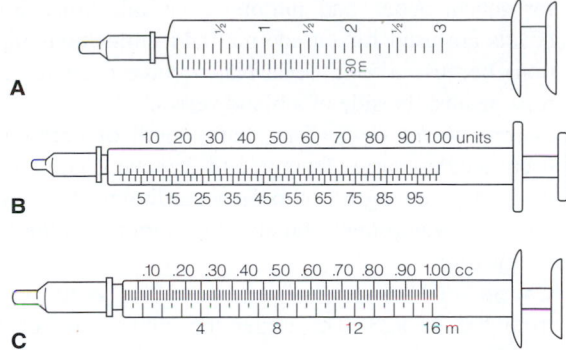

Figure 23–10 ● Three kinds of syringes: **A,** hypodermic syringe marked in tenths (0.1) of milliliters and in minims; **B,** insulin syringe marked in 100 units; **C,** tuberculin syringe marked in tenths and hundredths (0.01) of cubic millimeters and in minims.

administering other drugs, particularly when small or precise measurement is indicated.

Syringes are made in other sizes as well (e.g., 10, 20, and 50 mL). These are not generally used to administer drugs directly but can be useful for adding medications to intravenous solutions or for irrigating wounds. The tip of a syringe varies and is classified as either a Luer-Lok or non-Luer-Lok. A Luer-Lok syringe has a tip that requires the needle to be twisted onto it to avoid accidental removal of the needle (see Figure 23–11). The non-Luer-Lok syringe has a smooth graduated tip, and needles are slipped onto it. The larger 50-mL non-Luer-Lok syringe is often used for irrigation purposes (e.g., wounds, tubes).

Most syringes used today are made of plastic, are individually packaged for sterility in a paper wrapper or a rigid plastic

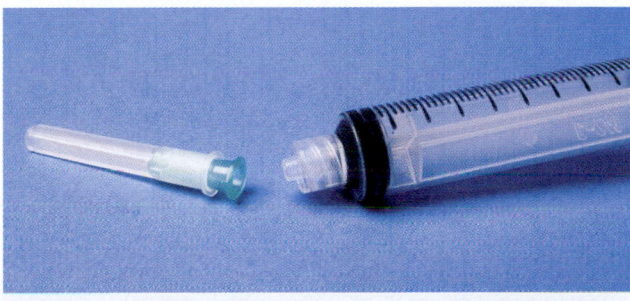

A

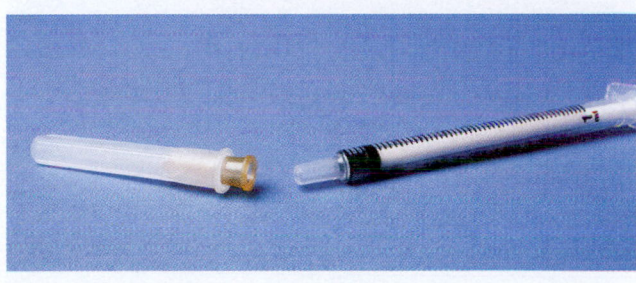

B

Figure 23–11 ● Tips of syringes: **A,** Luer-Lok syringe (note threaded tip); **B,** non-Luer-Lok syringe (note the smooth graduated tip).

container, and are disposable. The syringe and needle may be packaged together or separately. Needleless systems are also available in which the needle is replaced by a plastic cannula.

Injectable medications are frequently supplied in disposable prefilled unit-dose systems. These are available as (a) prefilled syringes ready for use or (b) prefilled sterile cartridges and needles that require the attachment of a reusable holder (injection system) before use (Figure 23–12). Examples of the latter system are the Tubex and Carpuject injection systems. The manufacturers provide specific directions for use. Because most prefilled

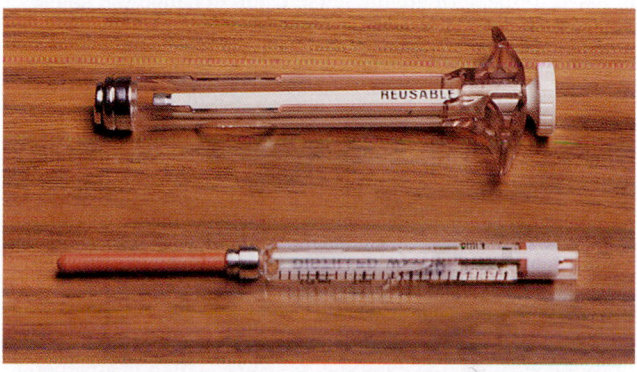

A

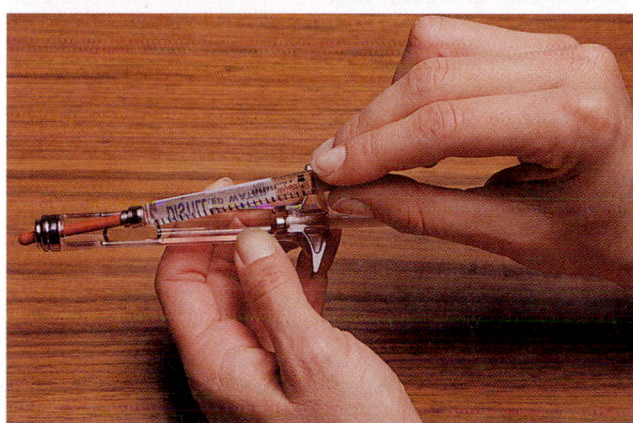

B

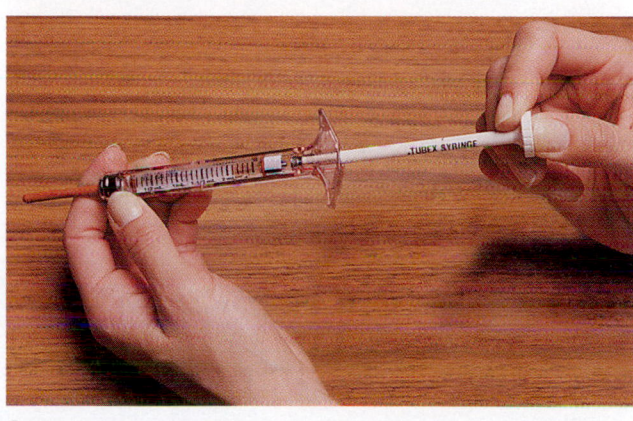

C

Figure 23–12 ● **A,** Syringe and prefilled sterile cartridge with needle; **B,** assembling the device; **C,** the cartridge slides into the syringe barrel, turns, and locks at the needle end. The plunger then screws into the cartridge end.

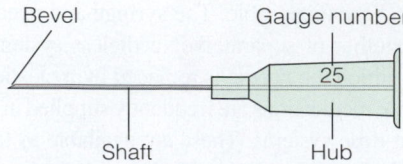

Figure 23–13 ● The parts of a needle.

cartridges are overfilled, excess medication must be ejected before the injection to ensure the right dosage. Because the needle is fused to the syringe, the nurse cannot change the gauge or length of the needle. The nurse, however, can transfer the medication into a regular syringe if the assessment of the client necessitates a different needle gauge or length.

NEEDLES   Needles are made of stainless steel, and most are disposable. Reusable needles (e.g., for special procedures) need to be sharpened periodically before resterilization because the points become dull with use and are occasionally damaged or acquire burrs on the tips. A dull or damaged needle should *never* be used.

A needle has three discernible parts: the **hub**, which fits onto the syringe; the cannula, or **shaft**, which is attached to the hub; and the **bevel**, which is the slanted part at the tip of the needle (Figure 23–13). A disposable needle has a plastic hub. Needles used for injections have three variable characteristics:

1. *Slant or length of the bevel:* The bevel of the needle may be short or long. Longer bevels provide the sharpest needles and cause less discomfort. They are commonly used

for subcutaneous and intramuscular injections. Short bevels are used for intradermal and intravenous injections because a long bevel can become occluded if it rests against the side of a blood vessel.

2. *Length of the shaft:* The shaft length of commonly used needles varies from 1/2 to 2 inches. The appropriate needle length is chosen according to the client's muscle development, the client's weight, and the type of injection.

3. **Gauge** *(or diameter) of the shaft:* The gauge varies from #18 to #28. The larger the gauge number, the smaller the diameter of the shaft. Smaller gauges produce less tissue trauma, but larger gauges are necessary for viscous medications, such as penicillin.

For an adult requiring a subcutaneous injection, it is appropriate to use a needle of #24 to #26 gauge and 3/8 to 5/8 inch long. Obese clients may require a 1-inch needle. For intramuscular injections, a longer needle (e.g., 1 to 1 1/2 inches) with a larger gauge (e.g., #20 to #22 gauge) is used. Slender adults and children usually require a shorter needle. The nurse must assess the client to determine the appropriate needle length.

PREVENTING NEEDLESTICK INJURIES   One of the most potentially hazardous procedures that health care personnel face is using and disposing of needles and sharps. Needlestick injuries present a major risk for infection with hepatitis B virus, human immunodeficiency virus (HIV), and many other pathogens. Standards have been set by OSHA to prevent such injuries. Some of these are summarized in Box 23–6. If an accidental needlestick injury

---

BOX 23–6   Avoiding Puncture Injuries

- Use appropriate puncture-proof disposal containers to dispose of uncapped needles and sharps. These are provided in all client areas. Never throw sharps in wastebaskets. Sharps include any items that can cut or puncture skin such as:
  Needles
  Surgical blades
  Lancets
  Razors
  Broken glass
  Broken capillary pipettes
  Exposed dental wires
  Reusable items (e.g., large-bore needles, hooks, rasps, drill points)
  ANY SHARP INSTRUMENT!
- Never bend or break needles before disposal.
- Never recap *used* needles (i.e., has been inserted into a client) except under specified circumstances (e.g., when transporting a syringe to the laboratory for an arterial blood gas or blood culture).
- When recapping a needle (i.e., drawing up a medication into a syringe *prior* to administration):
  - Use a safety mechanical device that firmly grips the needle cap and holds it in place until it is ready to recap.

- Use a one-handed "scoop" method. This is performed by (a) placing the needle cap and syringe with needle horizontally on a flat surface, (b) inserting the needle into the cap, using one hand (Figure 23–14), and then (c) using your other hand to pick up the cap and tighten it to the needle hub. Be careful not to contaminate the needle. If the needle becomes contaminated, replace the needle with a new one.

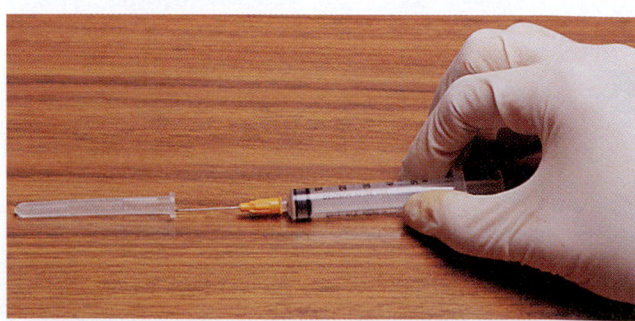

Figure 23–14 ● Recapping a used needle using the one-handed scoop method.

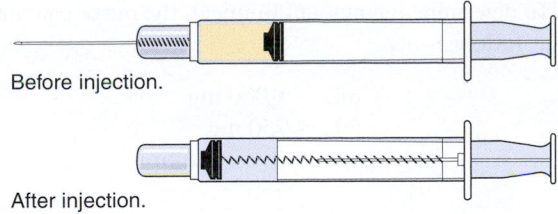

Figure 23–15 ◯ Passive safety device. The needle retracts immediately into the barrel after injection.

occurs, the nurse needs to follow specific steps outlined by the agency.

Safety syringes have been designed in recent years to protect health care workers. Safety devices are categorized as either *passive* or *active*. The nurse does not need to activate the passive safety device. For example, for some syringes, after injection, the needle retracts immediately into the barrel (Figure 23–15). In contrast, the active safety device requires the nurse to manually activate the safety feature. For example, the nurse activates a mechanism to retract the needle into the syringe barrel, or the nurse, after injection, manually pulls a plastic sheath or guard over the needle (Figure 23–16).

Preparing Injectable Medications

Injectable medications can be prepared by withdrawing the medication from an ampule or vial into a sterile syringe, using prefilled syringes, or using needleless injection systems.

AMPULES AND VIALS Ampules and vials (Figure 23–17) are frequently used to package sterile parenteral medications. An **ampule** is a glass container usually designed to hold a single dose of a drug. It is made of clear glass and has a distinctive shape with a constricted neck. Ampules vary in size from 1 to 10 mL or more. Most ampule necks have colored marks around them, indicating where they are prescored for easy opening.

To access the medication in an ampule, the ampule must be broken at its constricted neck. Traditionally, files have been used to score the ampule. Today plastic ampule openers are available that prevent injury from broken

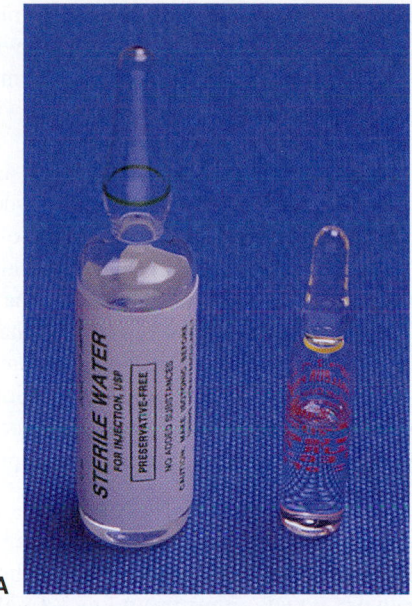

A

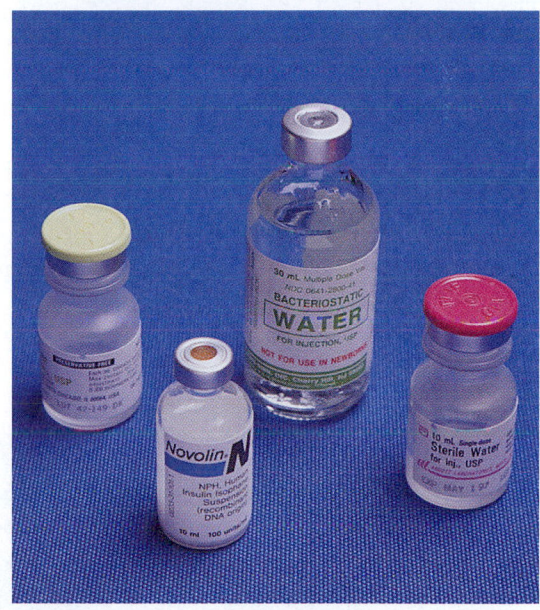

B

Figure 23–17 ◯ *A,* Ampules; *B,* vials.

glass. The device consists of a plastic cap that fits over the top of an ampule. The head of the ampule, when broken, remains inside the cap and is placed into a sharps container. If an ampule opener is not available, the neck should be filed with a small file, then broken off at that point. Once the ampule is broken, the fluid is aspirated into a syringe using a filter needle. This prevents aspiration of any glass particles.

A **vial** is a small glass bottle with a sealed rubber cap. Vials come in different sizes, from single to multidose vials. They usually have a metal or plastic cap that protects the rubber seal and must be removed to access the medication. To access the medication in a vial, the vial

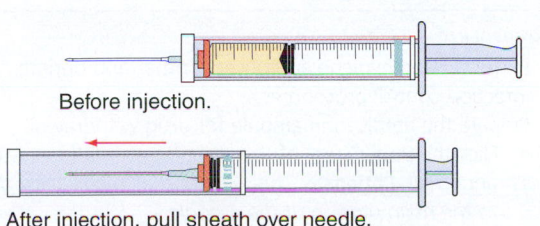

Figure 23–16 ◯ Active safety device. The nurse manually pulls the sheath or guard over the needle after injection.

must be pierced with a needle. In addition, air must be injected into a vial before the medication can be withdrawn. Failure to inject air before withdrawing the medication leaves a vacuum within the vial that makes withdrawal difficult.

Several drugs (e.g., penicillin) are dispensed as powders in vials. A liquid (diluent) must be added to a powdered medication before it can be injected. The technique of adding a diluent to a powdered drug to prepare it for administration is called **reconstitution**. Powdered drugs usually have printed instructions (enclosed with each packaged vial) that describe the amount and kind of solvent to be added. Commonly used diluents are sterile water or sterile normal saline. Some preparations are supplied in individual-dose vials; others come in multidose vials. The following are two examples of the preparation of powdered drugs:

1. *Single-dose vial:* Instructions for preparing a single-dose vial state that 1.5 mL of sterile water be added to the sterile dry powder, thus providing a single dose of 2 mL. The volume of the drug powder was 0.5 mL. Therefore, the 1.5 mL of water plus the 0.5 mL of powder results in 2 mL of solution. In other instances, the addition of a solution does not increase the volume. Therefore, it is important to follow the manufacturer's directions.

2. *Multidose vial:* A dose of 750 mg of a certain drug is ordered for a client. On hand is a 10-g multidose vial. The directions for preparation read: "Add 8.5 mL of sterile water, and each milliliter will contain 1.0 g or 1,000 mg."

To determine the amount to inject, the nurse calculates as follows:

$$1 \text{ mL} = 1,000 \text{ mg}$$
$$x \text{ mL} = 750 \text{ mg}$$
$$\text{(cross multiply)}$$
$$x = \frac{750 \times 1}{1,000}$$
$$x = 0.75$$

The nurse will give 0.75 mL of the medication.

Glass and rubber particulate have been found in medications withdrawn from ampules and vials using a regular needle. As a result, it is strongly recommended that the nurse use a filter needle when withdrawing medications from ampules and vials to prevent withdrawing glass and rubber particles. After drawing the medication into the syringe, the filter needle is replaced with the regular needle for injection. This prevents tracking of the medication through the client's tissues during the insertion of the needle, which minimizes discomfort. Research validates this practice, especially in clients receiving intramuscular injections on a repeated basis or with injections that use larger bore needles (Preston & Hegadoren, 2004).

Skills 23–2 and 23–3 describe how to prepare medications from ampules and vials. Additionally, it is important to remember that when powdered drugs have been reconstituted, the date and time should be written on the label of the vial. Many of these drugs have to be used within a certain time period following reconstitution, so nurses need to know the expiration time after it has been reconstituted.

SKILL 23–2

PREPARING MEDICATIONS FROM AMPULES

PLANNING

Delegation
Preparing medications from ampules and vials involves knowledge and use of sterile technique. Therefore, these techniques are not delegated to UAP.

EQUIPMENT
- MAR or computer printout
- Ampule of sterile medication
- File (if ampule is not scored) and small gauze square or plastic ampule opener
- Antiseptic swabs
- Syringe
- Needle for administering the medication
- Filter needle for withdrawing medication from the ampule

IMPLEMENTATION
Preparation
1. Check the medication administration record (MAR).
   - Check the label on the ampule carefully against the MAR to make sure that the correct medication is being prepared.
   - Follow the three checks for administering medications. Read the label on the medication (1) when it is taken from the medication cart, (2) before withdrawing the medication, and (3) after withdrawing the medication.
2. Organize the equipment.

Performance
1. Perform hand hygiene and observe other appropriate infection control procedures.
2. Prepare the medication ampule for drug withdrawal.
   - Flick the upper stem of the ampule several times with a fingernail. **Rationale:** *This will bring all medication down to the main portion of the ampule.*
   - Use an ampule opener or place a piece of sterile gauze or alcohol wipe between your thumb and the ampule neck or around the ampule neck, and break off the top by *bending*

it toward you to ensure the ampule is broken away from yourself and away from others. **Rationale:** *The sterile gauze protects the fingers from the broken glass, and any glass fragments will spray away from the nurse.* ❶

or

- Place the antiseptic wipe packet over the top of the ampule before breaking off the top. **Rationale:** *This method ensures that all glass fragments fall into the packet and reduces the risk of cuts.*
- Dispose of the top of the ampule in the sharps container.

3. Withdraw the medication.
   - Place the ampule on a flat surface.
   - Attach the filter needle to the syringe. **Rationale:** *The filter needle prevents glass particles from being withdrawn with the medication.*
   - Remove the cap from the filter needle and insert the needle into the center of the ampule. Do not touch the rim of the ampule with the needle tip or shaft. **Rationale:** *This will keep the needle sterile.* Withdraw the amount of drug required for the dosage.
   - With a single-dose ampule, hold the ampule slightly on its side, if necessary, to obtain more than the ordered amount of medication.

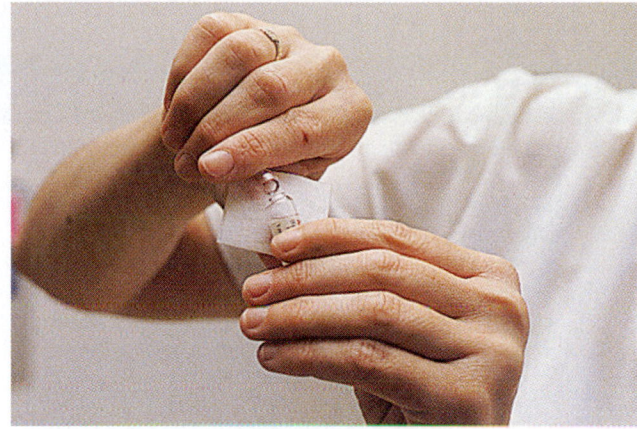

❶ Breaking the neck of an ampule.

- Dispose of the filter needle by placing in a sharps container.
- If giving an injection replace the filter needle with a regular needle, tighten the cap at the hub of the needle, and push solution into the needle, to the prescribed amount.

SKILL 23–3

PREPARING MEDICATIONS FROM VIALS

PLANNING
Medication preparation should not be delegated because it requires knowledge and use of sterile technique.

EQUIPMENT
- MAR or computer printout

- Vial of sterile medication
- Antiseptic swabs
- Safety needle and syringe
- Filter needle (check agency policy)
- Sterile water or normal saline, if drug is in powdered form

---

IMPLEMENTATION

Preparation
- Follow the same preparation as described in Skill 23–2.

Performance
1. Perform hand hygiene and observe other appropriate infection control procedures.
2. Prepare the medication vial for drug withdrawal.
   - Mix the solution, if necessary, by rotating the vial between the palms of the hands, not by shaking. **Rationale:** *Some vials contain aqueous suspensions, which settle when they stand. In some instances, shaking is contraindicated because it may cause the mixture to foam.*
   - Remove the protective cap, or clean the rubber cap of a previously opened vial with an antiseptic wipe by rubbing in a circular motion. **Rationale:** *The antiseptic cleans the cap and reduces the number of microorganisms.*
3. Withdraw the medication.
   - Attach a filter needle, as agency practice dictates, to draw up premixed liquid medications from multidose vials. **Rationale:** *Using the filter needle prevents any solid particles from being drawn up through the needle.*
   - Ensure that the needle is firmly attached to the syringe.
   - Remove the cap from the needle, then draw up into the syringe the amount of air equal to the volume of the medication to be withdrawn.

- Carefully insert the needle into the upright vial through the center of the rubber cap, maintaining the sterility of the needle.
- Inject the air into the vial, keeping the bevel of the needle above the surface of the medication. ❶ **Rationale:** *The air will allow the medication to be drawn out easily because negative pressure will not be created*

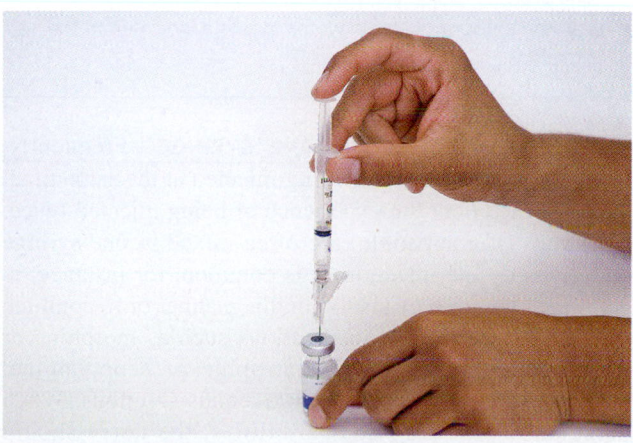

❶ Injecting air into a vial.

(continued)

SKILL 23–3

PREPARING MEDICATIONS FROM VIALS *(continued)*

inside the vial. The bevel is kept above the medication to avoid creating bubbles in the medication.

- Withdraw the prescribed amount of medication using either of the following methods:

  a. Hold the vial down (i.e., with the base lower than the top), move the needle tip so that it is below the fluid level, and withdraw the medication. Avoid drawing up the last drops of the vial. **Rationale:** *Proponents of this method say that keeping the vial in the upright position while withdrawing the medication allows particulate matter to precipitate out of the solution. Leaving the last few drops reduces the chance of withdrawing foreign particles.* ❷

    or

  b. Invert the vial, ensure the needle tip is *below* the fluid level; and gradually withdraw the medication. **Rationale:** *Keeping the tip of the needle below the fluid level prevents air from being drawn into the syringe.* ❸

- Hold the syringe and vial at eye level to determine that the correct dosage of drug is drawn into the syringe. Eject air remaining at the top of the syringe into the vial.

- When the correct volume of medication plus a little more (e.g., 0.25 mL) is obtained, withdraw the needle from the vial, and replace the cap over the needle using the scoop method, thus maintaining its sterility.

- If necessary, tap the syringe barrel to dislodge any air bubbles present in the syringe. **Rationale:** *The tapping motion will cause the air bubbles to rise to the top of the syringe where they can be ejected out of the syringe.*

- If giving an injection, replace the filter needle, if used, with a regular or safety needle of the correct gauge and length. Eject air from the new needle and verify correct medication volume before injecting the client.

VARIATION: PREPARING AND USING MULTIDOSE VIALS

- Read the manufacturer's directions.
- Withdraw an equivalent amount of air from the vial before adding the diluent, unless otherwise indicated by the directions.
- Add the amount of sterile water or saline indicated in the directions.

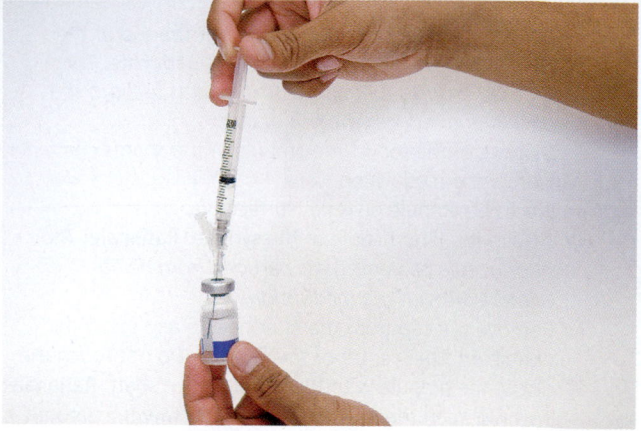

❷ Withdrawing a medication from a vial that is held with the base down.

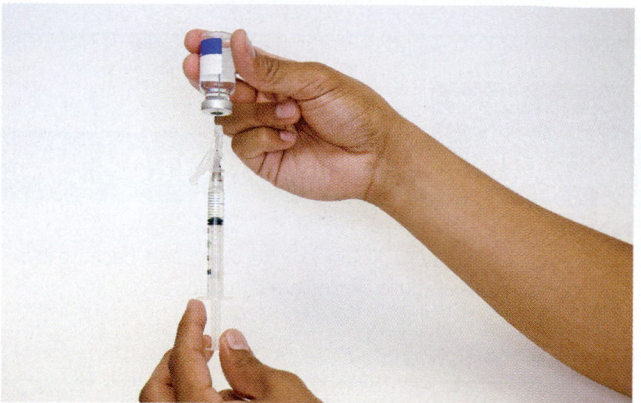

❸ Withdrawing a medication from an inverted vial.

- If a multidose vial is reconstituted, label the vial with the date and time it was prepared, the amount of drug contained in each milliliter of solution, and your initials. **Rationale:** *Time is an important factor to consider in the expiration of these medications.*
- Once the medication is reconstituted, store it in a refrigerator or as recommended by the manufacturer.

MIXING MEDICATIONS IN ONE SYRINGE Frequently, clients need more than one drug injected at the same time. To spare the client the experience of being injected twice, two drugs (if compatible) are often mixed in one syringe and given as one injection. It is common, for instance, to combine two types of insulin in this manner or to combine injectable preoperative medications such as morphine or meperidine (Demerol) with atropine or scopolamine. Drugs can also be mixed in intravenous solutions. When uncertain about drug compatibilities, the nurse should consult a pharmacist or check a compatibility chart before mixing the drugs.

The nurse must also exercise caution when mixing short- and long-acting insulins, because they vary in content. Chemically, insulin is a protein that, when hydrolyzed in the body, yields a number of amino acids. Some insulin preparations contain an additional modifying protein, such as globulin or protamine, that slows absorption. This fact is particularly relevant to mixing two insulin preparations for injection because many insulin syringes have needles that cannot be changed. A vial of insulin that does not have the added protein (i.e., regular insulin) should *never* be contaminated with insulin that does have the added protein (i.e., Lente or NPH insulin). Skill 23–4 describes how to mix medications in one syringe.

MIXING MEDICATIONS USING ONE SYRINGE

PLANNING

Delegation
Mixing medications in one syringe involves knowledge and use of aseptic technique. Therefore, this procedure is not delegated to UAP.

EQUIPMENT
- MAR or computer printout
- Two vials of medication; one vial and one ampule; two ampules; or one vial or ampule and one cartridge
- Antiseptic swabs
- Sterile syringe and safety needle or insulin syringe and needle (If insulin is being given, use a small-gauge hypodermic needle, e.g., #26 gauge.)
- Additional sterile subcutaneous or intramuscular safety needle (optional)

IMPLEMENTATION

Preparation
1. Check the medication administration record (MAR).
   - Check the label on the medications carefully against the MAR to make sure that the correct medication is being prepared.
   - Follow the three checks for administering medications. Read the label on the medication (1) when it is taken from the medication cart, (2) before withdrawing the medication, and (3) after withdrawing the medication.
   - Before preparing and combining the medications, ensure that the total volume of the injection is appropriate for the injection site.
2. Organize the equipment.

Performance
1. Perform hand hygiene and observe other appropriate infection control procedures.
2. Prepare the medication ampule or vial for drug withdrawal.
   - See Skill 23–2, step 2, for an ampule.
   - Inspect the appearance of the medication for clarity. Some medications are always cloudy. **Rationale:** *Preparations that have changed in appearance should be discarded.*
   - If using insulin, thoroughly mix the solution in each vial prior to administration. Rotate the vials between the palms of the hands and invert the vials. **Rationale:** *Mixing ensures an adequate concentration and thus an accurate dose. Shaking insulin vials can make the medication frothy, making precise measurement difficult.*
   - Clean the tops of the vials with antiseptic swabs.
3. Withdraw the medications.

MIXING MEDICATIONS FROM TWO VIALS
- Take the syringe and draw up a volume of air equal to the volume of medications to be withdrawn from both vials A *and* B.
- Inject a volume of air equal to the volume of medication to be withdrawn into vial A. Make sure the needle does not touch the solution. **Rationale:** *This prevents cross-contamination of the medications.*
- Withdraw the needle from vial A and inject the remaining air into vial B.
- Withdraw the required amount of medication from vial B. **Rationale:** *The same needle is used to inject air into and withdraw medication from the second vial. It must not be contaminated with the medication in vial A.*

- Using a newly attached sterile needle, withdraw the required amount of medication from vial A. Avoid pushing the plunger as that will introduce medication B into vial A. If using a syringe with a fused needle, withdraw the medication from vial A. The syringe now contains a mixture of medications from vials A and B. **Rationale:** *With this method, neither vial is contaminated by microorganisms or by medication from the other vial.* Be careful to withdraw only the ordered amount and to not create air bubbles. **Rationale:** *The syringe now contains two medications and an excess amount cannot be returned to the vial.*

See also "Variation" later in this Skill.

MIXING MEDICATIONS FROM ONE VIAL AND ONE AMPULE
- First prepare and withdraw the medication from the vial. **Rationale:** *Ampules do not require the addition of air prior to withdrawal of the drug.*
- Then withdraw the required amount of medication from the ampule.

MIXING MEDICATIONS FROM ONE CARTRIDGE AND ONE VIAL OR AMPULE
- First ensure that the correct dose of the medication is in the cartridge. Discard any excess medication and air.
- Draw up the required medication from a vial or ampule into the cartridge. Note that when withdrawing medication from a vial, an equal amount of air must first be injected into the vial.
- If the total volume to be injected exceeds the capacity of the cartridge, use a syringe with sufficient capacity to withdraw the desired amount of medication from the vial or ampule, and transfer the required amount from the cartridge to the syringe.

VARIATION: MIXING INSULINS
The following is an example of mixing 10 units of regular insulin and 30 units of neutral protamine Hagedorn (NPH) insulin, which contains protamine.

- Inject 30 units of air into the NPH vial and withdraw the needle. (There should be no insulin in the needle.) The needle should not touch the insulin.
- Inject 10 units of air into the regular insulin vial and immediately withdraw 10 units of regular insulin. Always withdraw the regular insulin first *to minimize the possibility of the regular insulin becoming contaminated with the additional protein in the NPH.*
- Reinsert the needle into the NPH insulin vial and withdraw 30 units of NPH insulin. (The air was previously injected into

(continued)

SKILL 23–4

MIXING MEDICATIONS USING ONE SYRINGE *(continued)*

the vial.) Be careful to withdraw only the ordered amount and to not create air bubbles. If excess medication has been drawn up, discard the syringe and begin the procedure over again. **Rationale:** *The syringe now contains two medications, and an excess amount cannot be returned to the vial because the syringe contains regular insulin, which, if returned to the NPH vial, would dilute the NPH with regular insulin. The NPH vial would not provide accurate future dosages of NPH insulin.*

By using this method, you avoid adding NPH insulin to the regular insulin.

CLINICAL ALERT

One way to determine which insulin to *withdraw* first is to remember the saying "Clear before cloudy." (Regular insulin is clear and NPH is cloudy due to the proteins in the insulin.)

Intradermal Injections

An intradermal (ID) injection is the administration of a drug into the dermal layer of the skin just beneath the epidermis. Usually only a small amount of liquid is used, for example, 0.1 mL. This method of administration is frequently used for allergy testing and tuberculosis (TB) screening. Common sites for intradermal injections are the inner lower arm, the upper chest, and the back beneath the scapulae (Figure 23–18). The left arm is commonly used for TB screening and the right arm is used for all other tests. The steps for administering an intradermal are described in Skill 23–5.

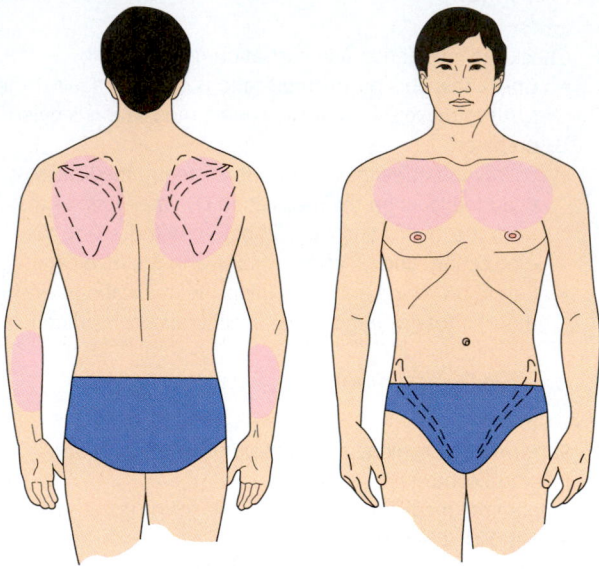

Figure 23–18 ◉ Body sites commonly used for intradermal injections.

SKILL 23–5

ADMINISTERING AN INTRADERMAL INJECTION FOR SKIN TESTS

PURPOSE
- To provide a medication that the client requires for allergy testing and TB screening

ASSESSMENT
Assess
- Appearance of injection site
- Specific drug action and expected response
- Client's knowledge of drug action and response

  Check agency protocol about sites to use for skin tests.

PLANNING

Delegation
The administration of intradermal injections is an invasive technique that involves the application of nursing knowledge, problem solving, and sterile technique. This technique is not delegated to UAP. The nurse, however, can inform the UAP about symptoms of allergic reactions and the necessity to report those observations immediately to the nurse.

EQUIPMENT
- Vial or ampule of the correct medication
- Sterile 1-mL syringe calibrated into hundredths of a milliliter (i.e., tuberculin syringe) and a #25- to #27-gauge safety needle that is 1/4 to 5/8 inch long
- Alcohol swabs
- 2-in. × 2-in. sterile gauze square (optional)
- Clean gloves (according to agency protocol)
- Bandage (optional)
- Epinephrine on hand in case of allergic anaphylactic reaction

IMPLEMENTATION

Preparation

1. Check the medication administration record (MAR).
   - Check the label on the medication carefully against the MAR to make sure that the correct medication is being prepared.
   - Follow the three checks for administering medications. Read the label on the medication (1) when it is taken from the medication cart, (2) before withdrawing the medication, and (3) after withdrawing the medication.
2. Organize the equipment.

Performance

1. Perform hand hygiene and observe other appropriate infection control procedures (e.g., clean gloves).
2. Prepare the medication from the vial or ampule for drug withdrawal.
   - See Skills 23–2 and 23–3.
3. Prepare the client
   - Prior to performing the procedure, introduce self and verify the client's identity using agency protocol. **Rationale:** *This ensures that the right client receives the medication.*
4. Explain to the client that the medication will produce a small wheal, sometimes called a *bleb*. A *wheal* is a small raised area, like a blister. The client will feel a slight prick as the needle enters the skin. Some medications are absorbed slowly through the capillaries into the general circulation, and the bleb gradually disappears. Other drugs remain in the area and interact with the body tissues to produce redness and induration (hardening), which will need to be interpreted at a particular time (e.g., in 24 or 48 hours). This reaction will also gradually disappear. **Rationale:** *Information can facilitate acceptance of and compliance with the therapy.*
5. Provide for client privacy.
6. Select and clean the site.
   - Select a site (e.g., the forearm about a hand's width above the wrist and three or four fingerwidths below the antecubital space).
   - Avoid using sites that are tender, inflamed, or swollen and those that have lesions.
   - Put on gloves as indicated by agency policy.
   - Cleanse the skin at the site using a firm circular motion starting at the center and widening the circle outward. Allow the area to dry thoroughly.
7. Prepare the syringe for the injection.
   - Remove the needle cap while waiting for the antiseptic to dry.
   - Expel any air bubbles from the syringe. Small bubbles that adhere to the plunger are of no consequence. **Rationale:** *A small amount of air will not harm the tissues.*
   - Grasp the syringe in your dominant hand, close to the hub, holding it between thumb and forefinger. Hold the needle almost parallel to the skin surface, with the bevel of the needle up. **Rationale:** *The possibility of the medication entering the subcutaneous tissue increases when using an angle greater than 15 degrees. The bevel up position provides more comfort for the nurse and is faster to administer* (Tarnow & King, 2004).
8. Inject the fluid.
   - With the nondominant hand, pull the skin at the site until it is taut. For example, if using the ventral forearm, grasp the client's dorsal forearm and gently pull it to tighten the ventral skin. **Rationale:** *Taut skin allows for easier entry of the needle and less discomfort for the client.*
   - Insert the tip of the needle far enough to place the bevel through the epidermis into the dermis. The outline of the bevel should be visible under the skin surface.
   - Stabilize the syringe and needle. Inject the medication carefully and slowly so that it produces a small wheal on the skin. **Rationale:** *This verifies that the medication entered the dermis.* ❶
   - Withdraw the needle quickly at the same angle at which it was inserted. Activate the needle safety device. Apply a bandage if indicated.
   - Do not massage the area. **Rationale:** *Massage can disperse the medication into the tissue or out through the needle insertion site.*
   - Dispose of the syringe and needle into the sharps container. **Rationale:** *Do not recap the needle in order to prevent needlestick injuries.*
   - Remove gloves.
   - Circle the injection site with ink to observe for redness or induration (hardening), per agency policy.
9. Document all relevant information.
   - Record the testing material given, the time, dosage, route, site, and nursing assessments.

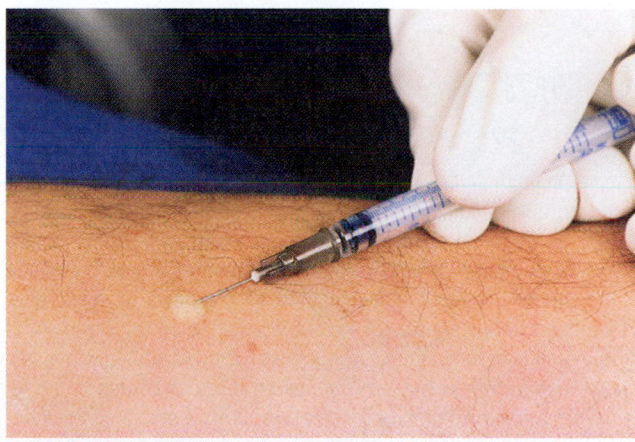

❶ The medication forms a bleb or wheal under the epidermis.

EVALUATION

- Evaluate the client's response to the testing substance. **Rationale:** *Some medications used in testing may cause allergic reactions.* Epinephrine may need to be used.

- Evaluate the condition of the site in 24 or 48 hours, depending on the test. Measure the area of redness and induration in millimeters at the largest diameter and document findings.

Subcutaneous Injections

Among the many kinds of drugs administered subcutaneously (just beneath the skin) are vaccines, insulin, and heparin. Common sites for subcutaneous injections are the outer aspect of the upper arms and the anterior aspect of the thighs. These areas are convenient and normally have good blood circulation. Other areas that can be used are the abdomen, the scapular areas of the upper back, and the upper ventrogluteal and dorsogluteal areas (Figure 23–19). Only small doses (0.5 to 1 mL) of medication are usually injected via the subcutaneous route. Check agency policy.

Use of an air bubble when injecting heparin subcutaneously has been found to be contraindicated and can lead to an increased incidence of bruising and hematoma formation. Bruising and hematoma formation can best be minimized by injecting the heparin over 30 seconds, changing the needle after drawing up the medication, and inserting into the abdomen at a 90-degree angle (Zaybak & Khorshid, 2007).

The type of syringe used for subcutaneous injections depends on the medication to be given. Generally a 2-mL

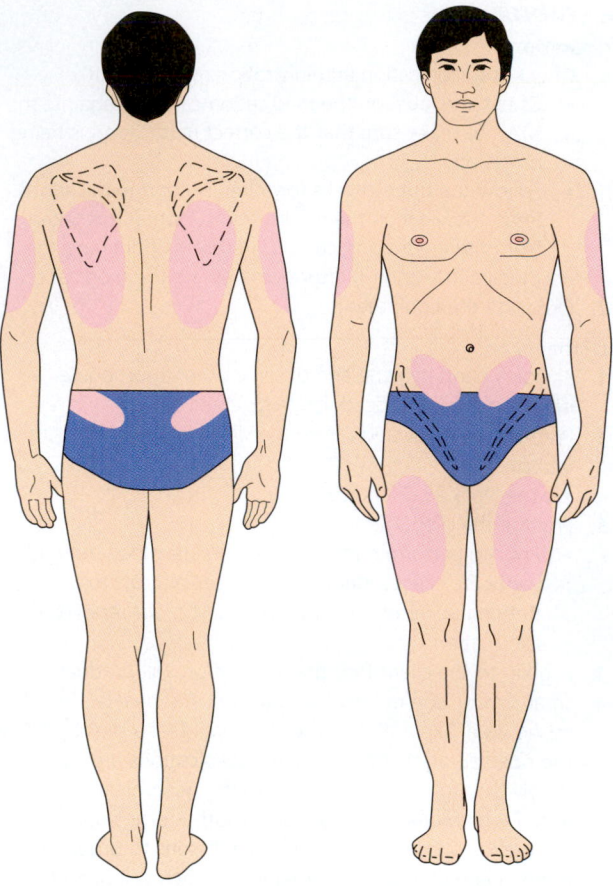

Figure 23–19 ● Body sites commonly used for subcutaneous injections.

syringe is used for most subcutaneous injections. However, if insulin is being administered, an insulin syringe is used; and if heparin is being administered, a tuberculin syringe or prefilled cartridge may be used.

RESEARCH NOTES   **Should the Bevel Be Up or Down?**

The tradition in nursing practice is to administer an intradermal injection with the bevel up. The authors point out that only one 1997 study investigated intradermal technique and it found the bevel-down technique to be superior to the bevel-up technique. However, the sample size of that study was small (e.g., three volunteers). Therefore, these researchers decided to replicate the study with tighter control and improved research methods.

This study used qualitative and quantitative methods to examine differences regarding correct placement of injectate, leaking or bleeding, time to administer injection, and comfort of persons administering and receiving an intradermal injection. Each of the 98 subjects administered and received two injections. The subjects evaluated their comfort in administering and in receiving a bevel-up injection and a bevel-down injection using a Likert scale.

The results indicated that there was no significant difference related to comfort for client preference for bevel up or bevel down.

There was, however, a statistically significant difference for the subjects in the nurse role citing that there was more comfort with the bevel being up. The subjects administered the bevel-up injections faster than the bevel-down injections. Client outcomes (e.g., wheal, leakage, and bleeding) with regard to bevel-up or bevel-down technique were equivalent. There was no statistical difference.

Implications

The researchers suggest that nurses continue to use bevel-up technique as the preferred way to administer intradermal injections because of the increased comfort for the person in the nurse role and because it was faster to administer. They also suggest that more research be done as there are only two studies and they differ in results.

Note: Reprinted from *Applied Nursing Research, 17*(4) K. Tarnow and N. King, "Intradermal Injections: Traditional Bevel Up Versus Bevel Down," pp. 275–282. Copyright 2004, with permission from Elsevier.

Needle sizes and lengths are selected based on the client's body mass, the intended angle of insertion, and the planned site. Generally a #25-gauge, 5/8-inch needle is used for adults of normal weight and the needle is inserted at a 45-degree angle; a 3/8-inch needle is used at a 90-degree angle. A child may need a 1/2-inch needle inserted at a 45-degree angle.

One method nurses use to determine length of needle is to pinch the tissue at the site and select a needle length that is half the width of the skinfold. To determine the angle of insertion, a general rule to follow relates to the amount of tissue that can be pinched or grasped at the site. A 45-degree angle is used when 1 inch of tissue can be grasped at the site; a 90-degree angle is used when 2 inches of tissue can be grasped.

When administering insulin to adults, the current standard needle gauge is #30 gauge. Short needles (5/16 inch) are available with 0.3-, 0.5-, 1.0-, and 2.0-mL capacities (American Diabetes Association, 2004). Most clients prefer the shorter and thinner needles because they are less painful. The risk of injecting into the muscle is lessened with the shorter needle.

Subcutaneous injection sites need to be rotated in an orderly fashion to minimize tissue damage, aid absorption, and avoid discomfort. This is especially important for clients who must receive repeated injections, such as diabetics. Because insulin is absorbed at different rates at different parts of the body, the diabetic client's blood glucose levels can vary when various sites are used. Insulin is absorbed most quickly when injected into the abdomen and then into the arms, and most slowly when injected into the thighs and buttocks. Current recommendations include rotating injections within one area to prevent lipoatrophy and lipohypertrophy (American Diabetes Association, 2004).

Nurses have traditionally been taught to aspirate by pulling back on the plunger after inserting the needle and before injecting the medication. The nurse could then determine whether the needle had entered a blood vessel. Absence of blood was believed to indicate that the needle was in subcutaneous tissue and not in the more vascular muscular tissue. According to the American Diabetes Association (2004), routine aspiration is no longer recommended with insulin administration. It is likely that students will observe that the practice of aspirating subcutaneous injections will vary among nurses.

The steps for administering a subcutaneous injection are described in Skill 23–6.

ADMINISTERING A SUBCUTANEOUS INJECTION

PURPOSES
- To provide a medication the client requires (see specific drug action)
- To allow slower absorption of a medication compared with either the intramuscular or intravenous route

ASSESSMENT
Assess
- Allergies to medication
- Specific drug action, side effects, and adverse reactions
- Client's knowledge and learning needs about the medication
- Status and appearance of subcutaneous site for lesions, erythema, swelling, ecchymosis, inflammation, and tissue damage from previous injections
- Ability of client to cooperate during the injection
- Previous injection sites used

PLANNING

Delegation
The administration of subcutaneous injections is an invasive technique that involves the application of nursing knowledge, problem solving, and sterile technique. Therefore, this skill is not delegated to UAP. The nurse, however, can inform the UAP of the intended therapeutic effects and/or specific side effects of the medication and direct the UAP to report specific client observations to the nurse for follow-up.

EQUIPMENT
- Client's MAR or computer printout
- Vial or ampule of the correct sterile medication
- Syringe and needle (e.g., 3-mL syringe, #25-gauge needle or smaller, 3/8 or 5/8 inch long)
- Antiseptic swabs
- Dry sterile gauze for opening an ampule (optional)
- Clean gloves

IMPLEMENTATION
Preparation
1. Check the medication administration record (MAR).
   - Check the label on the medication carefully against the MAR to make sure that the correct medication is being prepared.
   - Follow the three checks for administering medications. Read the label on the medication (1) when it is taken from the medication cart, (2) before withdrawing the medication, and (3) after withdrawing the medication.
2. Organize the equipment.

Performance
1. Perform hand hygiene and observe other appropriate infection control procedures (e.g., clean gloves).
2. Prepare the medication from the ampule or vial for drug withdrawal.
   - See Skill 23–2 (ampule) or 23–3 (vial).
3. Provide for client privacy.
4. Prepare the client.
   - Prior to performing the procedure, introduce self and verify the client's identity using agency protocol. **Rationale:** *This ensures that the right client receives the medication.*

(continued)

SKILL 23-6

ADMINISTERING A SUBCUTANEOUS INJECTION *(continued)*

- Assist the client to a position in which the arm, leg, or abdomen can be relaxed, depending on the site to be used. **Rationale:** *A relaxed position of the site minimizes discomfort.*
- Obtain assistance in holding an uncooperative client. **Rationale:** *This prevents injury due to sudden movement after needle insertion.*

5. Explain the purpose of the medication and how it will help, using language that the client can understand. Include relevant information about effects of the medication. **Rationale:** *Information can facilitate acceptance of and compliance with the therapy.*

6. Select and clean the site.
   - Select a site free of tenderness, hardness, swelling, scarring, itching, burning, or localized inflammation. Select a site that has not been used frequently. **Rationale:** *These conditions could hinder the absorption of the medication and may also increase the likelihood of injury and discomfort at the injection site.*
   - Put on clean gloves.
   - As agency protocol indicates, clean the site with an antiseptic swab. Start at the center of the site and clean in a widening circle to about 5 cm (2 in.). Allow the area to dry thoroughly. **Rationale:** *The mechanical action of swabbing removes skin secretions, which contain microorganisms.*
   - Place and hold the swab between the third and fourth fingers of the nondominant hand, or position the swab on the client's skin above the intended site. **Rationale:** *Using this technique keeps the swab readily accessible when the needle is withdrawn.*

7. Prepare the syringe for injection.
   - Remove the needle cap while waiting for the antiseptic to dry. Pull the cap straight off to avoid contaminating the needle by the outside edge of the cap. **Rationale:** *The needle will become contaminated if it touches anything but the inside of the cap, which is sterile.*
   - Dispose of the needle cap.

8. Inject the medication.
   - Grasp the syringe in your dominant hand by holding it between your thumb and fingers. With palm facing to the side or upward for a 45-degree angle insertion, or with the palm downward for a 90-degree angle insertion, prepare to inject. ❶

- Using the nondominant hand, pinch or spread the skin at the site, and insert the needle using the dominant hand and a firm steady push. Recommendations vary about whether to pinch or spread the skin and at what angle to administer subcutaneous injections. The most important consideration is the depth of the subcutaneous tissue in the area to be injected. If the client has more than 1/2 inch of adipose tissue in the injection site, it would be safe to administer the injection at a 90-degree angle with the skin spread. If the client is thin or lean and lacks adipose tissue, the subcutaneous injection should be given with the skin pinched and at a 45- to 60-degree angle. One way to check that the pinch of skin is subcutaneous tissue is to ask the client to flex and extend the elbow. If any muscle is being held in the pinch, you will feel it contract and relax. If so, release the pinch and try again. ❷
- When the needle is inserted, move your nondominant hand to the end of the plunger. Some nurses find it easier to move the nondominant hand to the barrel of the syringe and the dominant hand to the end of the plunger.
- Inject the medication by holding the syringe steady and depressing the plunger with a slow, even pressure. **Rationale:** *Holding the syringe steady and injecting the medication at an even pressure minimizes discomfort for the client.*
- It is recommended that with many subcutaneous injections, especially insulin, the needle "should be embedded within the skin for five seconds after complete depression of the plunger to ensure complete delivery of the dose" (American Diabetes Association, 2004, p. S108).

9. Remove the needle.
   - Remove the needle smoothly, pulling along the line of insertion while depressing the skin with your nondominant hand. **Rationale:** *Depressing the skin places countertraction on it and minimizes the client's discomfort when the needle is withdrawn.*

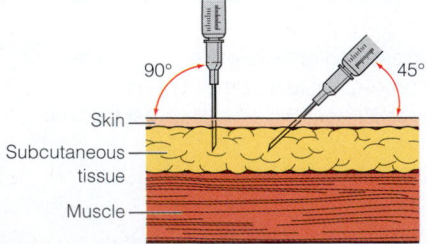

❶ Inserting a needle into the subcutaneous tissue using 90- and 45-degree angles.

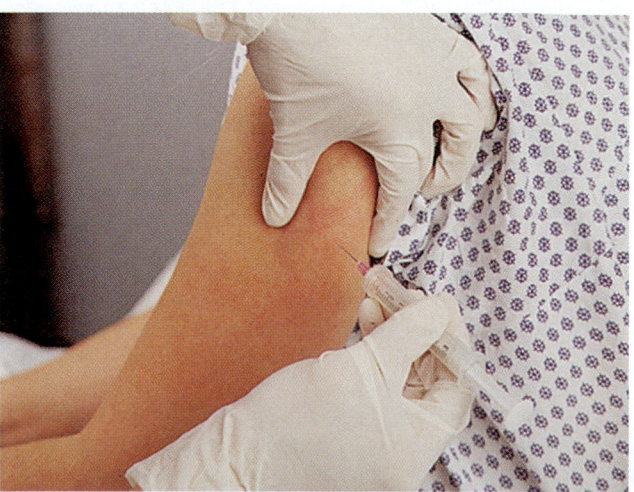

❷ Administering a subcutaneous injection into pinched tissue.

- If bleeding occurs, apply pressure to the site with dry sterile gauze until it stops. *Bleeding rarely occurs after subcutaneous injection.*
10. Dispose of supplies appropriately.
    - Activate the needle safety device or discard the uncapped needle and attached syringe into designated receptacles. **Rationale:** *Proper disposal protects the nurse and others from injury and contamination. The Centers for Disease Control and Prevention (CDC) recommends not capping the needle before disposal to reduce the risk of needlestick injuries.*
    - Remove gloves and perform hand hygiene.
11. Document all relevant information.
    - Document the medication given, dosage, time, route, and any assessments.
    - Many agencies prefer that medication administration be recorded on the medication record. The nurse's notes are used when prn medications are given or when there is a special problem.
12. Assess the effectiveness of the medication at the time it is expected to act and document it.

EVALUATION

- Conduct appropriate follow-up such as desired effect (e.g., relief of pain, sedation, lowered blood sugar, a prothrombin

VARIATION: ADMINISTERING A HEPARIN INJECTION

The subcutaneous administration of heparin and low molecular weight heparin (i.e., enoxaparin [Lovenox]) requires special precautions because of the drug's anticoagulant properties.

- Select a site on the abdomen at least 2 inches *away* from the umbilicus and above the level of the iliac crests. Some agencies support the practice of subcutaneous injection of heparin in the thighs or arms as alternate sites to the abdomen.
- Use a 3/8-inch, #25- or #26-gauge needle or smaller, and insert it at a 90-degree angle. If a client is very lean or wasted, use a needle longer than 3/8 inch and insert it at a 45-degree angle. The arms or thighs may be used as alternate sites.
- Do *not* aspirate when giving heparin by subcutaneous injection. **Rationale:** *Aspiration can possibly damage the surrounding tissue and cause bleeding as well as bruising.*
- Do not massage the site after the injection. **Rationale:** *Massaging could cause bleeding and ecchymoses (bruises) and hasten drug absorption.*
- Alternate the sites of subsequent injections.

time within preestablished limits), any adverse effects (e.g., nausea, vomiting, skin rash), and clinical signs of side effects.
- Relate to previous findings if available.
- Report deviations from normal to the primary care provider.

Intramuscular Injections

Injections into muscle tissue, or intramuscular (IM) injections, are absorbed more quickly than subcutaneous injections because of the greater blood supply to the body muscles. Muscles can also take a larger volume of fluid without discomfort than subcutaneous tissues can, although the amount varies among individuals, chiefly based on muscle size and condition and the site used. An adult with well-developed muscles can usually safely tolerate up to 3 mL of medication in the gluteus medius and gluteus maximus muscles (Figure 23–20). A volume of 1 to 2 mL is usually recommended for adults with less developed muscles. In the deltoid muscle, volumes of 0.5 to 1 mL are recommended.

Usually a 3- to 5-mL syringe is needed. The size of syringe used depends on the amount of medication being administered. The standard prepackaged intramuscular needle is 1 1/2 inches and #21 or #22 gauge. Several factors indicate the size and length of the needle to be used:

- The muscle
- The type of solution
- The amount of adipose tissue covering the muscle
- The age of the client

For example, a smaller needle such as a #23– to #25-gauge needle 1 inch long is commonly used for the deltoid muscle. More viscous solutions require a larger gauge (e.g., #20 gauge). Very obese clients may require a needle longer than 1 1/2 inches (e.g., 2 inches), and emaciated clients may require a shorter needle (e.g., 1 inch).

Introduction of an air bubble to reduce pain at the injection site has been shown to be a dangerous practice and should

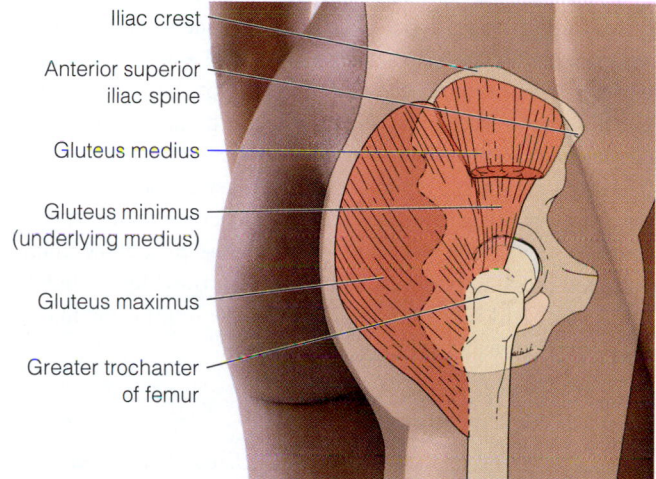

Iliac crest
Anterior superior iliac spine
Gluteus medius
Gluteus minimus (underlying medius)
Gluteus maximus
Greater trochanter of femur

Figure 23–20 ⬤ Lateral view of the right buttock showing the three gluteal muscles used for intramuscular injections.
(Custom Medical Stock Photo, Inc.)

be discouraged unless the medication specifically indicates the need for this technique. Medications such as Inferon or immunizations containing aluminum adjuvant recommend use of an air bubble to prevent skin staining or abscess formation. However, use with other medications can result in an increased dosage of medication administered, because the measurements on the syringe anticipate some fluid will remain in the dead space of the hub and needle after injection, but this extra amount is administered when an air bubble is used (Chapin & Welk, 1985; Rodger & King, 2000).

A major consideration in the administration of intramuscular injections is the selection of a safe site located away from large blood vessels, nerves, and bone. Several body sites can be used for intramuscular injections. These sites are discussed in detail next. Contraindications for using a specific site include tissue injury and the presence of nodules, lumps, abscesses, tenderness, or other pathology.

VENTROGLUTEAL SITE   The ventrogluteal site is in the gluteus medius muscle, which lies over the gluteus minimus (Figure 23–20). The ventrogluteal site is the *preferred* site for intramuscular injections because the area:

- Contains no large nerves or blood vessels.
- Provides the greatest thickness of gluteal muscle consisting of both the gluteus medius and gluteus minimus.
- Is sealed off by bone.
- Contains consistently less fat than the buttock area, thus eliminating the need to determine the depth of subcutaneous fat.

This site is suitable for children over 1 year and adults (Nicoll & Hesby, 2002). The client position for the injection can be a back, prone, or side-lying position. The side-lying position, however, helps locate the ventrogluteal site more easily. Position the client on his or her side with the knee bent and raised slightly toward the chest. The trochanter will protrude, which facilitates locating the ventrogluteal site. To establish the exact site, the nurse places the heel of the hand on the client's greater trochanter, with the fingers pointing toward the client's head. The right hand is used for the left hip, and the left hand for the right hip. With the index finger on the client's anterior superior iliac spine, the nurse stretches the middle finger dorsally (toward the buttocks), palpating the crest of the ilium and then pressing below it. The triangle formed by the index finger, the third finger, and the crest of the ilium is the injection site (Figures 23–21 and 23–22).

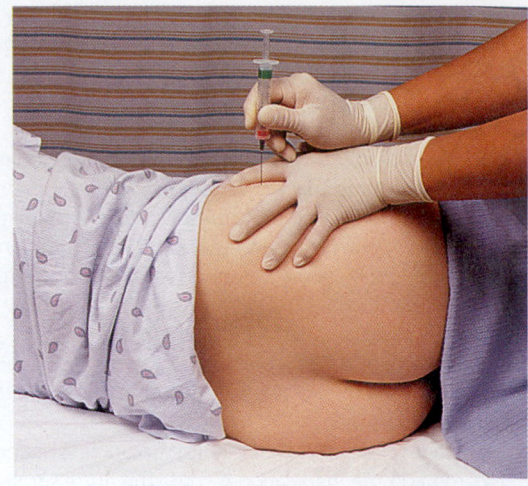

Figure 23–22 ○ Administering an intramuscular injection into the ventrogluteal site.

VASTUS LATERALIS SITE   The vastus lateralis muscle is usually thick and well developed in both adults and children. It is recommended as the site of choice for intramuscular injections for infants 1 year and younger (Nicoll & Hesby, 2002). Because there are no major blood vessels or nerves in the area, it is desirable for infants whose gluteal muscles are poorly developed. It is situated on the anterior lateral aspect of the infant's thigh (Figure 23–23). The middle third of the muscle is suggested as the site. In the adult, the landmark is established by dividing the area between the greater trochanter of the femur and the lateral femoral condyle into thirds and selecting the middle third (Figures 23–24 and 23–25). The client can assume a back-lying or a sitting position for an injection into this site.

DORSOGLUTEAL SITE   The dorsogluteal site is composed of the thick gluteal muscles of the buttocks (Figure 23–20).

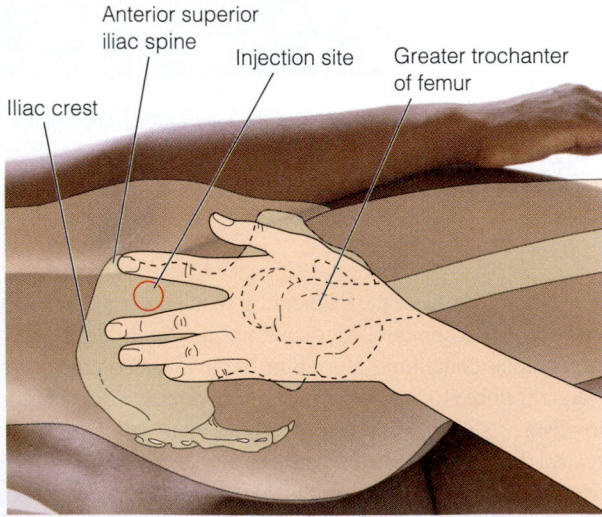

Figure 23–21 ○ Landmarks for the ventrogluteal site for an intramuscular injection.

Labels in figure: Anterior superior iliac spine; Injection site; Greater trochanter of femur; Iliac crest

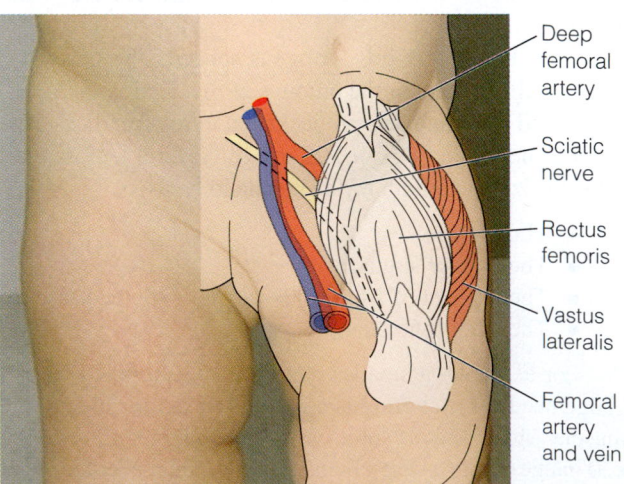

Figure 23–23 ○ The vastus lateralis muscle of an infant's upper thigh, used for intramuscular injections.
(Custom Medical Stock Photo, Inc.)

Labels in figure: Deep femoral artery; Sciatic nerve; Rectus femoris; Vastus lateralis; Femoral artery and vein

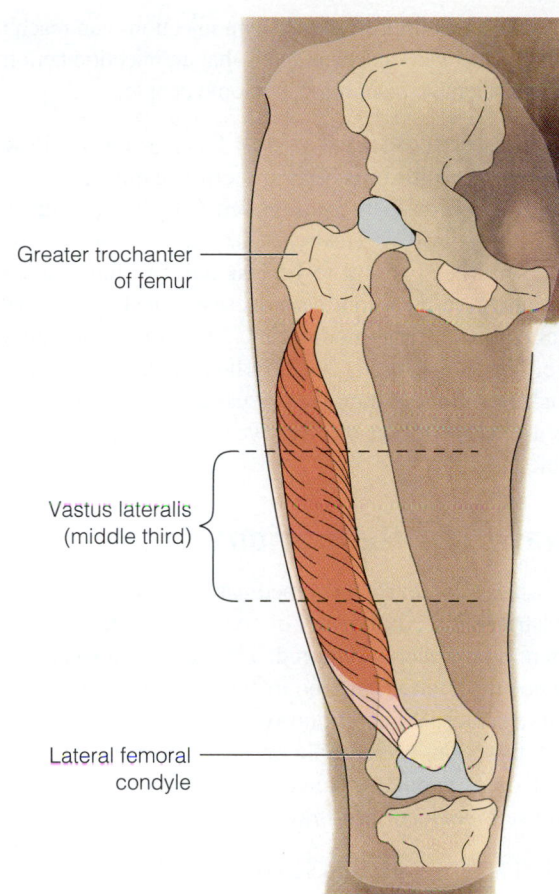

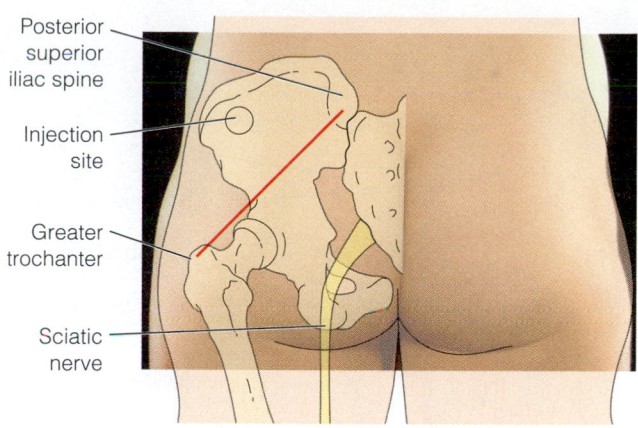

Figure 23–26 ◉ Landmarks for the dorsogluteal site for an intramuscular injection.

(Custom Medical Stock Photo, Inc.)

of medication compared to other sites because of the thick layer of adipose tissue making it problematic, and is not recommended for use (Bolander, 1994; Rosdahl, 1995). This site should never be used when the client is standing (Bolander, 1994). The nurse must choose the injection site carefully to avoid striking the sciatic nerve, major blood vessels, or bone.

The nurse palpates the posterior superior iliac spine, and then draws an imaginary line to the greater trochanter of the femur. This line is lateral to and parallel to the sciatic nerve. The injection site is lateral and superior to this line (Figure 23–26). Palpating the ilium and the trochanter is important; visual calculations alone can result in an injection that is placed too low and injures other structures.

The client needs to assume a prone position with the toes pointed inward or a side-lying position with the upper knee flexed and in front of the lower leg. These positions promote muscle relaxation and therefore minimize discomfort from the injection.

Greater trochanter of femur

Vastus lateralis (middle third)

Lateral femoral condyle

Figure 23–24 ◉ Landmarks for the vastus lateralis site of an adult's right thigh, used for an intramuscular injection.

(Custom Medical Stock Photo, Inc.)

DELTOID SITE The deltoid muscle is found on the lateral aspect of the upper arm. It is not used often for intramuscular injections because it is a relatively small muscle and is very close to the radial nerve and radial artery. It is sometimes considered for use in adults because of rapid absorption from the deltoid area, but no more than 1 mL of solution can be administered. This site is recommended for the administration of hepatitis B vaccine in adults.

The upper landmark for the deltoid site is located by the nurse placing four fingers across the deltoid muscle with the first finger on the acromion process. The top of the axilla is the line that marks the lower border landmark (Figure 23–27). A triangle within these boundaries indicates the deltoid muscle about 5 cm (2 in.) below the acromion process.

Nicoll and Hesby (2002) reported that researchers found that "applying pressure to the site for ten seconds prior to injection reduced injection pain" (p. 158). Further research is needed to determine additional techniques that will minimize the degree of pain at the time of injection.

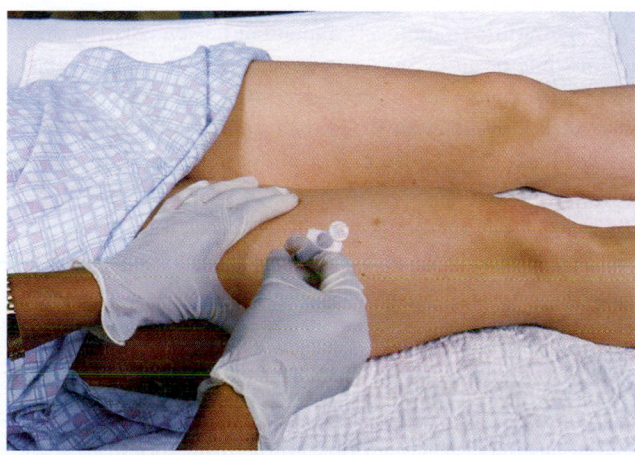

Figure 23–25 ◉ Administering an intramuscular injection into the vastus lateralis site.

The dorsogluteal site can be used for adults and for children with well-developed gluteal muscles. Because these muscles are developed by walking, this site should not be used for children under 3 years unless the child has been walking for at least 1 year. However, this site is in the presence of major nerves and blood vessels, has relatively slow uptake

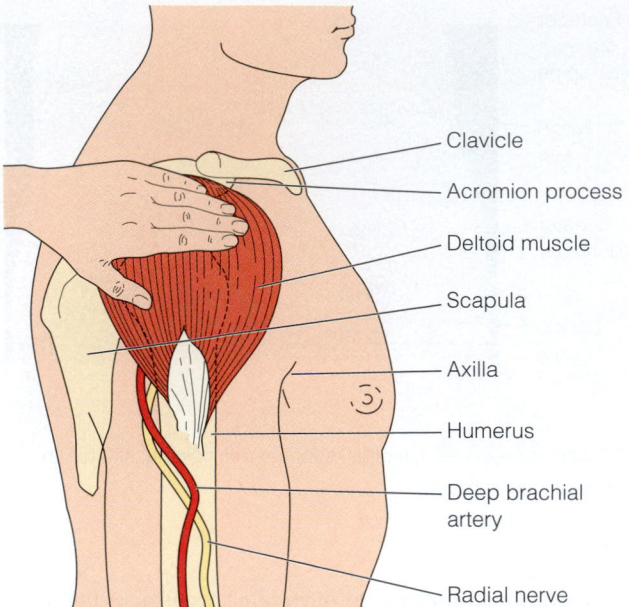

Figure 23–27 ⬤ A method of establishing the deltoid muscle site for an intramuscular injection.

RECTUS FEMORIS SITE The rectus femoris muscle, which belongs to the quadriceps muscle group, is used only occasionally for intramuscular injections. It is situated on the anterior aspect of the thigh (Figure 23–28). Its chief advantage is

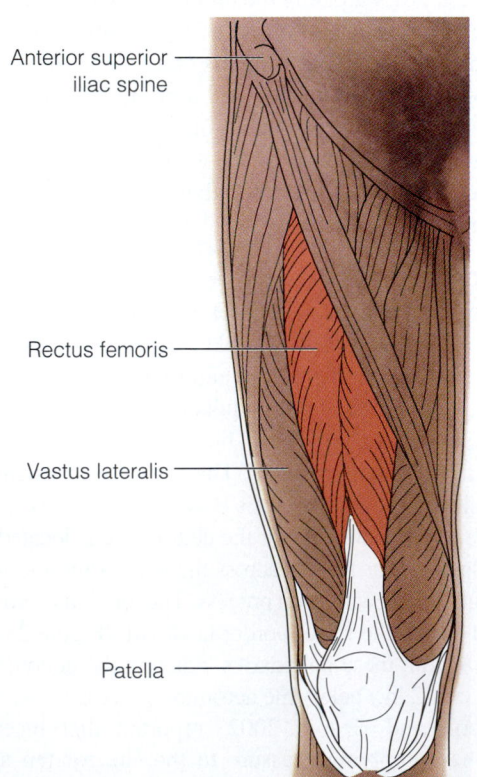

Figure 23–28 ⬤ Landmarks for the rectus femoris muscle of the upper right thigh, used for intramuscular injections.

that clients who administer their own injections can reach this site easily. Its main disadvantage is that an injection here may cause considerable discomfort for some people.

IM INJECTION TECHNIQUE Skill 23–7 describes how to administer an intramuscular injection using the Z-track technique, which is recommended for all intramuscular injections (Nicoll & Hesby, 2002, p. 157). The Z-track method has been found to be less painful than the traditional injection technique and decreases leakage of irritating and discoloring medications into the subcutaneous tissue (Nicoll & Hesby, 2002; Pullen, 2005). Although the Z-track technique is not always used in practice, research evidence does support its effectiveness and recommends its routine use.

Intravenous Medications

Because intravenous (IV) medications enter the client's bloodstream directly by way of a vein, they are appropriate when a rapid effect is required. This route is also appropriate when medications are too irritating to tissues to be given by other routes. When an intravenous line is already established, this route is desirable because it avoids the discomfort of other parenteral routes. Following are methods to administer medications intravenously:

- Large-volume infusion of intravenous fluid
- Intermittent intravenous infusion (piggyback or tandem setups)
- **Volume-controlled infusion** (often used for children)
- Intravenous push or bolus
- Intermittent injection ports (device)

In all of these methods, the client has an existing intravenous line or an IV access site such as a saline or heparin lock. Most agencies have procedures and policies about who may administer an IV medication. Chapter 36 ∞ describes the technique for performing a venipuncture and establishing an IV line.

With all IV medication administration, it is very important to observe clients closely for signs of adverse reactions. Because the drug enters the bloodstream directly and acts immediately, there is no way it can be withdrawn or its action terminated. Therefore, the nurse must take special care to avoid any errors about the preparation of the drug and the calculation of the dosage. When the administered drug is particularly potent, an antidote to the drug should be available. In addition, assess the vital signs before, during, and after infusion of the drug.

Before adding any medications to an existing intravenous infusion, the nurse must check for the "rights" and check compatibility of the drug and the existing intravenous fluid. Be aware of any incompatibilities of the drug and the fluid that is infusing. For example, the drug phenytoin (Dilantin) is incompatible with glucose and will form a precipitate if injected through a port in an intravenous line with glucose/dextrose infusing.

ADMINISTERING AN INTRAMUSCULAR INJECTION

PURPOSE
- To provide a medication the client requires (see specific drug action)

ASSESSMENT
Assess
- Client allergies to medication(s)
- Specific drug action, side effects, and adverse reactions
- Client's knowledge of and learning needs about the medication
- Tissue integrity of the selected site
- Client's age and weight to determine site and needle size
- Client's ability or willingness to cooperate

Determine whether the size of the muscle is appropriate to the amount of medication to be injected. An average adult's deltoid muscle can usually absorb 0.5 mL of medication, although some authorities believe 1 mL can be absorbed by a well-developed deltoid muscle. The gluteus medius muscle can often absorb 1 to 4 mL, although 4 mL may be very painful and may be contraindicated by agency protocol.

PLANNING

Delegation
The administration of IM injections is an invasive technique that involves the application of nursing knowledge, problem solving, and sterile technique. Delegation to UAP would be inappropriate. The nurse, however, can inform the UAP of the intended therapeutic effects and/or specific side effects of the medication and direct the UAP to report specific client observations to the nurse for follow-up.

EQUIPMENT
- MAR or computer printout
- Sterile medication (usually provided in an ampule or vial or prefilled syringe)
- Syringe and needle of a size appropriate for the amount and type of solution to be administered
- Antiseptic swabs
- Clean gloves

IMPLEMENTATION

Preparation
1. Check the medication administration record (MAR).
   - Check the label on the medication carefully against the MAR to make sure that the correct medication is being prepared.
   - Follow the three checks for administering the medication and dose. Read the label on the medication (1) when it is taken from the medication cart, (2) before withdrawing the medication, and (3) after withdrawing the medication.
   - Confirm that the dose is correct.
2. Organize the equipment.

Performance
1. Perform hand hygiene and observe other appropriate infection control procedures (e.g., clean gloves).
2. Prepare the medication from the ampule or vial for drug withdrawal.
   - See Skill 23–2 (ampule) or 23–3 (vial).
   - Whenever feasible, change the needle on the syringe before the injection. **Rationale:** *Because the outside of a new needle is free of medication, it does not irritate subcutaneous tissues as it passes into the muscle.*
   - Invert the syringe needle uppermost and expel all excess air.
3. Provide for client privacy.
4. Prepare the client.
   - Prior to performing the procedure, introduce self and verify the client's identity using agency protocol. **Rationale:** *This ensures that the right client receives the medication.*
   - Assist the client to a supine, lateral, prone, or sitting position, depending on the chosen site. If the target

muscle is the gluteus medius (ventrogluteal site), have the client in the supine position flex the knee(s); in the lateral position, flex the upper leg; and in the prone position, toe in. **Rationale:** *Appropriate positioning promotes relaxation of the target muscle.*
   - Obtain assistance in holding an uncooperative client. **Rationale:** *This prevents injury due to sudden movement after needle insertion.*
5. Explain the purpose of the medication and how it will help, using language that the client can understand. Include relevant information about effects of the medication. **Rationale:** *Information can facilitate acceptance of and compliance with the therapy.*
6. Select, locate, and clean the site.
   - Select a site free of skin lesions, tenderness, swelling, hardness, or localized inflammation and one that has not been used frequently.
   - If injections are to be frequent, alternate sites. Avoid using the same site twice in a row. **Rationale:** *This is to reduce the discomfort of intramuscular injections.* If necessary, discuss with the prescribing primary care provider an alternative method of providing the medication.
   - Locate the exact site for the injection. See the discussion of sites earlier in this chapter.
   - Apply clean gloves.
   - Clean the site with an antiseptic swab. Using a circular motion, start at the center and move outward about 5 cm (2 in.).
   - Transfer and hold the swab between the third and fourth fingers of your nondominant hand in readiness for needle withdrawal, or position the swab on the client's skin above the intended site. Allow skin to dry prior to injecting medication. **Rationale:** *This will help reduce the discomfort of the injection.*

(continued)

SKILL 23–7

ADMINISTERING AN INTRAMUSCULAR INJECTION *(continued)*

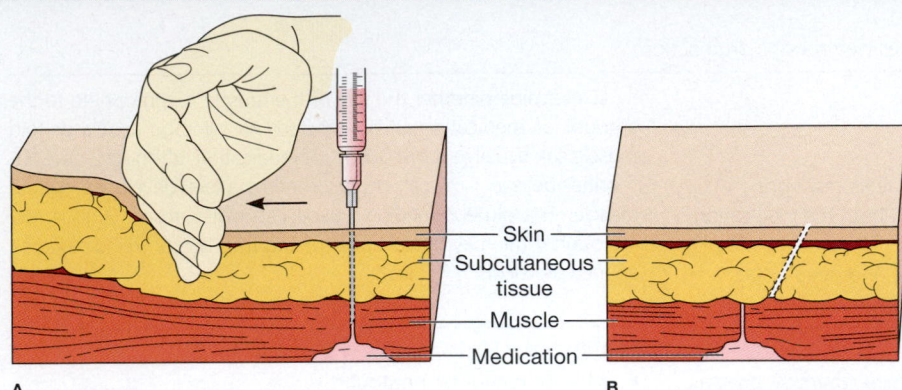

Skin
Subcutaneous tissue
Muscle
Medication

A   **B**

❶ Inserting an intramuscular needle at a 90-degree angle using the Z-track method: *A,* skin pulled to the side; *B,* skin released. Note: When the skin returns to its normal position after the needle is withdrawn, a seal is formed over the intramuscular site. This prevents seepage of the medication into the subcutaneous tissues and subsequent discomfort.

7. Prepare the syringe for injection.
- Remove the needle cover and discard without contaminating the needle.
- If using a prefilled unit-dose medication, take caution to avoid dripping medication on the needle prior to injection. If this does occur, wipe the medication off the needle with a sterile gauze. Some sources recommend changing the needle if possible. **Rationale:** *Medication left on the needle can cause pain when it is tracked through the subcutaneous tissue* (Nicoll & Hesby, 2002, p. 156).

8. Inject the medication using a Z-track technique.
- Use the ulnar side of the nondominant hand to pull the skin approximately 2.5 cm (1 inch) to the side. Under some circumstances, such as for an emaciated client or an infant, the muscle may be pinched. **Rationale:** *Pulling the skin and subcutaneous tissue or pinching the muscle makes it firmer and facilitates needle insertion.* **❶**
- Holding the syringe between the thumb and forefinger (as if holding a pencil), pierce the skin quickly and smoothly at a 90-degree angle, and insert the needle into the muscle. **Rationale:** *Using a quick motion lessens the client's discomfort.*
- Hold the barrel of the syringe steady with your nondominant hand and aspirate by pulling back on the plunger with your dominant hand. Aspirate for 5 to 10 seconds. **Rationale:** *If the needle is in a small blood vessel, it takes time for the blood to appear.* If blood appears in the syringe, withdraw the needle, discard the syringe, and prepare a new injection. **Rationale:** *This step determines whether the needle has been inserted into a blood vessel.* Although some controversy exists with

subcutaneous aspiration practices, aspiration continues to be recommended with IM injection to avoid medication injection into the bloodstream (Barr & Thomas, 2005).
- If blood does not appear, inject the medication steadily and slowly (approximately 10 seconds per milliliter) while holding the syringe steady. **Rationale:** *Injecting medication slowly promotes comfort and allows time for tissue to expand and begin absorption of the medication (Nicoll & Hesby, 2002). Holding the syringe steady minimizes discomfort.*
- After injection, wait 10 seconds *to permit the medication to disperse into the muscle tissue, thus decreasing the client's discomfort.*

9. Withdraw the needle.
- Withdraw the needle smoothly at the same angle of insertion. **Rationale:** *This minimizes tissue injury. Release the skin.*
- Apply gentle pressure at the site with a dry sponge. **Rationale:** *Use of an alcohol swab may cause pain or a burning sensation.*
- If bleeding occurs, apply pressure with a dry sterile gauze until it stops.

10. Activate the needle safety device or discard the uncapped needle and attached syringe into the proper receptacle.
- Remove gloves. Perform hand hygiene.

11. Document all relevant information.
- Include the time of administration, drug name, dose, route, and the client's reactions.

12. Assess effectiveness of the medication at the time it is expected to act.

EVALUATION
- Conduct appropriate follow-up, such as:
  - Desired effect (e.g., relief of pain or vomiting).
  - Any adverse reactions or side effects.
  - Local skin or tissue reactions at injection site (e.g., redness, swelling, pain, or other evidence of tissue damage).
- Relate to previous findings, if available.
- Report significant deviation from normal to the primary care provider.

| LIFESPAN CONSIDERATIONS | Intramuscular Injections |

Infants

- The vastus lateralis site is recommended as the site of choice for intramuscular injections for infants. There are no major blood vessels or nerves in this area, and it is the infant's largest muscle mass. It is situated on the anterior lateral aspect of the thigh.
- Obtain assistance to immobilize an infant or young child. The parent may hold the child. This prevents accidental injury during the procedure.

Children

- Use needles that will place medication in the main muscle mass; infants and children usually require smaller, shorter

needles (#22 to #25 gauge, 5/8 to 1 inch long) for intramuscular injections.
- The vastus lateralis is recommended as the site of choice for toddlers and children.
- For the older child and adolescent, the recommended sites are the same as for the adult: ventrogluteal or deltoid. Ask which arm they would like the injection in.

Older Adults

- Older clients may have a decreased muscle mass or muscle atrophy. A shorter needle may be needed. Assessment of appropriate injection site is critical. Absorption of medication may occur more quickly than expected.

LARGE-VOLUME INFUSIONS Mixing a medication into a large-volume IV container is the safest and easiest way to administer a drug intravenously. The drugs are diluted in volumes of 1,000 mL or 500 mL of compatible fluids. It may be necessary to consult a pharmacist to confirm compatibility. Fluids such as IV normal saline or Ringer's lactate are frequently used. Commonly added drugs are potassium chloride and vitamins. It may also be necessary to ensure the compatibility of some drugs with the plastic IV bag and tubing. A glass IV bottle and special tubing may be used in special situations. See Skill 23–8.

The main danger of infusing a large volume of fluid is circulatory overload (hypervolemia) (see Chapter 36 ∞).

The nurse adds the medication to the infusing fluid container or before it is hung for infusion. In some hospitals, the pharmacist adds the medication to the IV container.

SKILL 23–8

ADDING MEDICATIONS TO INTRAVENOUS FLUID CONTAINERS

PURPOSES
- To provide and maintain a constant level of a medication in the blood
- To administer well-diluted medications at a continuous and slow rate

ASSESSMENT
- Inspect and palpate the intravenous insertion site for signs of infection, infiltration, or a dislocated catheter.
- Inspect the surrounding skin for redness, pallor, or swelling.
- Palpate the surrounding tissues for coldness and the presence of edema, which could indicate leakage of the IV fluid into the tissues.

- Take vital signs for baseline data for medication that is particularly potent.
- Determine if the client has allergies to the medication(s).
- Check the compatibility of the medication(s) and IV fluid.

PLANNING

Delegation
Adding medications to IV fluid containers involves the application of nursing knowledge and critical thinking. The nurse does not delegate this procedure to UAP. However, the nurse can inform the UAP of the intended therapeutic effects and/or specific side effects of the medication(s) in the IV and direct the UAP to report specific client observations to the nurse for follow-up.

EQUIPMENT
- MAR or computer printout
- Correct sterile medication
- Diluent for medication in powdered form (see manufacturer's instructions)
- Correct solution container, if a new one is to be attached
- Antiseptic swabs
- Sterile syringe of appropriate size (e.g., 5 or 10 mL) and a 1- to 1 1/2-inch, #20- or #21-gauge sterile safety needle if not using a needleless system
- IV additive label

(continued)

SKILL 23–8

ADDING MEDICATIONS TO INTRAVENOUS FLUID CONTAINERS *(continued)*

IMPLEMENTATION

Preparation

1. Check the medication administration record (MAR).
   - Check the label on the medication carefully against the MAR to make sure that the correct medication is being prepared.
   - Follow the three checks for administering medications. Read the label on the medication (1) when it is taken from the medication cart, (2) before withdrawing the medication, and (3) after withdrawing the medication.
   - Confirm that the dosage and route is correct.
   - Verify which infusion solution is to be used with the medication.
   - Consult a pharmacist, if required, to confirm compatibility of the drugs and solutions being mixed.
2. Organize the equipment.

Performance

1. Perform hand hygiene and observe other appropriate infection control procedures.
2. Prepare the medication ampule or vial for drug withdrawal.
   - See Skill 23–2 (ampule) or 23–3 (vial).
   - Check the agency's practice for using a filter needle to withdraw premixed liquid medications from multidose vials or ampules.
3. Add the medication.

   To New IV Container
   - Locate the injection port. Clean the port with the antiseptic or alcohol swab. **Rationale:** *This reduces the risk of introducing microorganisms into the container when the needle is inserted.*
   - Remove the needle cap from the syringe, insert the needle through the center of the injection port, and inject the medication into the bag. Activate the needle safety device. ❶
   - Mix the medication and solution by gently rotating the bag or bottle. **Rationale:** *This should disperse the medication throughout the solution.*
   - Complete the IV additive label with name and dose of medication, date, time, and nurse's initials. Attach it upside down on the bag or bottle. **Rationale:** *This documents that medication has been added to the solution. When the label is attached upside down, it is easily read when the bag is hanging up.*
   - Clamp the IV tubing. Spike the bag or bottle with IV tubing and hang the IV. **Rationale:** *Clamping prevents rapid infusion of the solution.*
   - Regulate infusion rate as ordered.

   To an Existing Infusion
   - Determine that the IV solution in the container is sufficient for adding the medication. **Rationale:**

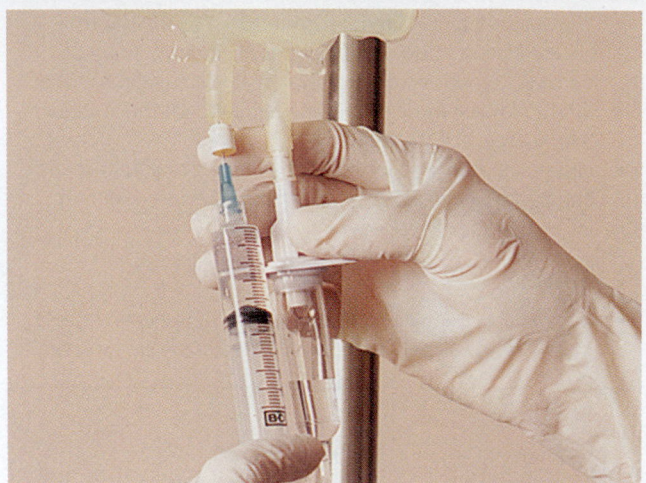

❶ Inserting a medication through the injection port of an infusing container.

Sufficient volume is necessary to dilute the medication adequately.
   - Confirm the desired dilution of the medication, that is, the amount of medication per milliliter of solution.
   - Close the infusion clamp. **Rationale:** *This prevents the medication from infusing directly into the client as it is injected into the bag or bottle.*
   - Wipe the medication port with the alcohol or disinfectant swab. **Rationale:** *This reduces the risk of introducing microorganisms into the container when the needle is inserted.*
   - Remove the needle cover from the medication syringe.
   - While supporting and stabilizing the bag with your thumb and forefinger, carefully insert the syringe needle through the port and inject the medication. **Rationale:** *The bag is supported during the injection of the medication to avoid punctures.* If the bag is too high to reach easily, lower it from the IV pole. Activate the needle safety device.
   - Remove the bag from the pole and gently rotate the bag. **Rationale:** *This will mix the medication and solution.*
   - Rehang the container and regulate the flow rate. **Rationale:** *This establishes the correct flow rate.*
   - Complete the medication label and apply to the IV container.
4. Dispose of the equipment and supplies according to agency practice. **Rationale:** *This prevents inadvertent injury to others and the spread of microorganisms.*
5. Document the medication(s) on the appropriate form in the client's record.

INTERMITTENT INTRAVENOUS INFUSIONS   An intermittent infusion is a method of administering a medication mixed in a small amount of IV solution, such as 50 or 100 mL. The drug is administered at regular intervals, such as every 4 hours, with the drug being infused for a short period of time such as 30 to 60 minutes. Two commonly used additive or secondary IV setups are the tandem and the **piggyback**.

In a tandem setup, a second container is attached to the line of the first container at the lower, secondary port. It permits medications to be administered intermittently or simultaneously with the primary solution.

In the piggyback alignment, a second set connects the second container to the tubing of the primary container at the upper port. This setup is used solely for intermittent drug administration. Various manufacturers describe these sets differently, so the nurse must check the manufacturer's labeling and directions carefully. Traditionally the tubing of the secondary set has been attached to ports of the primary infusion by inserting a needle through the port and taping it in place. Needleless systems are now available. These needleless systems can use threaded-lock or lever-lock cannulae to connect the secondary set to the ports of the primary infusion (Figure 23–29). This design prevents

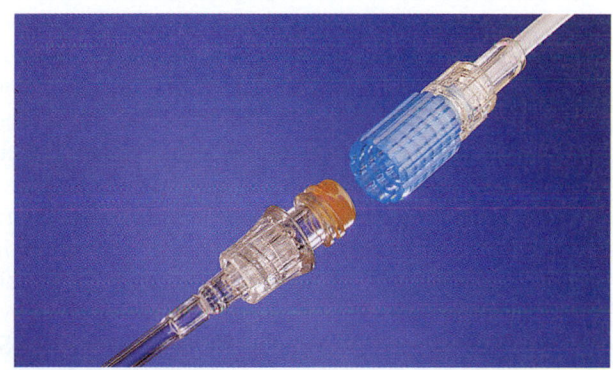

A

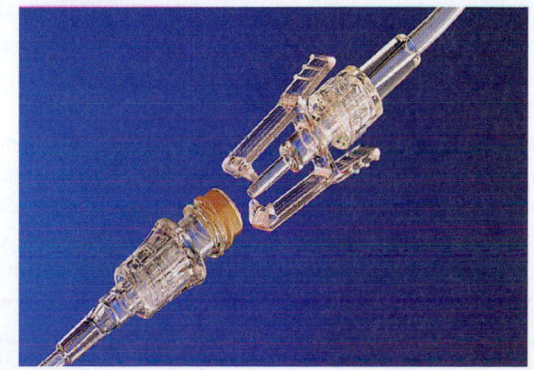

B

Figure 23–29 ⬤ Needleless cannulae used to connect the tubing of secondary sets to primary infusions: *A,* threaded-lock cannula; *B,* lever-lock cannula.

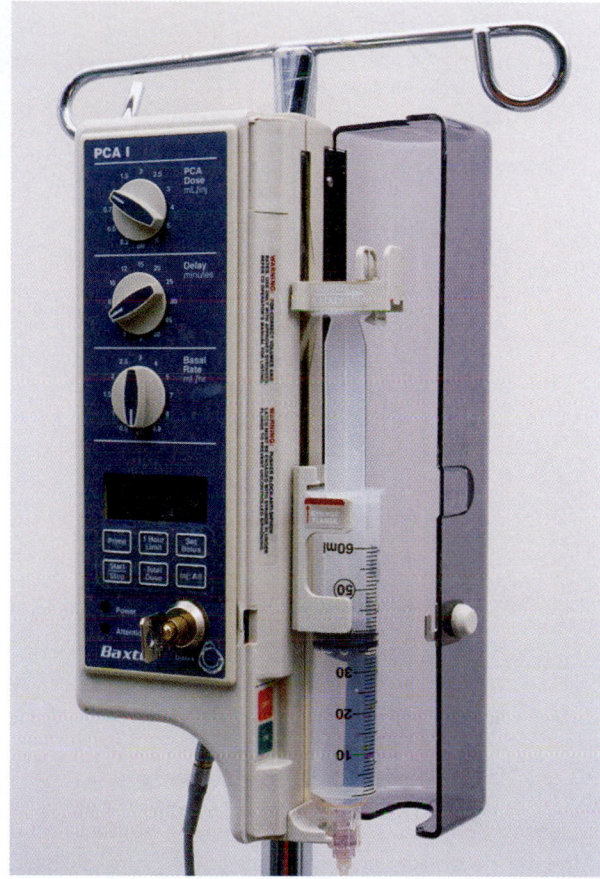

Figure 23–30 ⬤ Syringe pump or mini-infuser for administration of IV medications.

needlestick injuries and also prevents touch contamination at the IV connection site.

Another method of intermittently administering an IV medication is by a syringe pump or mini-infuser. The medication is mixed in a syringe that is connected to the primary IV line via a mini-infuser (see Figure 23–30).

VOLUME-CONTROL INFUSIONS   Intermittent medications may also be administered by a volume-control infusion set such as Buretrol, Soluset, Volutrol, and Pediatrol (Figure 23–31). They are small fluid containers (100 to 150 mL in size) attached below the primary infusion container so that the medication is administered through the client's IV line. Volume-control sets are frequently used to infuse solutions into children and older clients when the volume administered is critical and must be carefully monitored. Box 23–7 provides additional information.

INTRAVENOUS PUSH   Intravenous push (IVP) (bolus) is the intravenous administration of an undiluted drug directly into the systemic circulation. It is used when a medication cannot be diluted or in an emergency. An IV bolus can be introduced directly into a vein by venipuncture or into

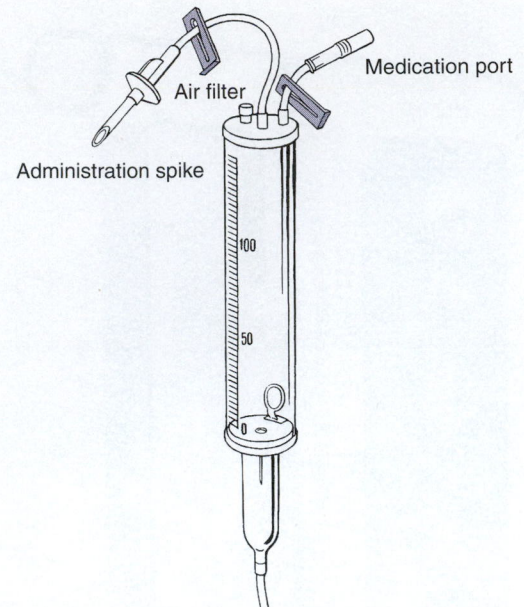

Figure 23–31 ⬤ A volume-control infusion set.

BOX 23–7 | **Adding a Medication to a Volume-Control Infusion Set**

- Withdraw the required dose of the medication into a syringe.
- Ensure that there is sufficient fluid in the volume-control fluid chamber to dilute the medication. Generally, at least 50 mL of fluid is used. Check the directions from the drug manufacturer or consult the pharmacist.
- Close the inflow to the fluid chamber by adjusting the upper roller or slide clamp above the fluid chamber; also ensure that the clamp on the air vent of the chamber is open.
- Clean the medication port on the volume-control fluid chamber with an antiseptic swab.
- Inject the medication into the port of the partially filled volume-control set.
- Gently rotate the fluid chamber until the fluid is well mixed.
- Open the line's upper clamp, and regulate the flow by adjusting the lower roller or slide clamp below the fluid chamber.
- Attach a medication label to the volume-control fluid chamber.
- Document relevant data, and monitor the client and the infusion.

---

an existing IV line through an injection port or through an IV lock.

There are two major disadvantages to this method of drug administration: Any error in administration cannot be corrected after the drug has entered the client, and the drug may be irritating to the lining of the blood vessels. Before administering a bolus, the nurse should look up the maxi-

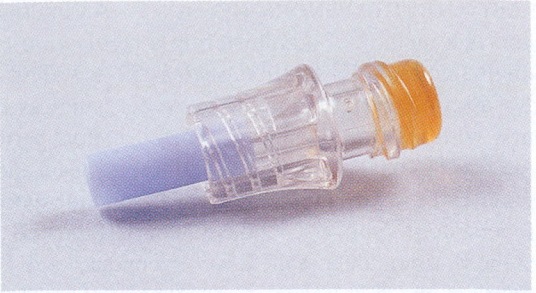

Figure 23–32 ⬤ Intermittent infusion device with injection port. (Courtesy of Baxter Healthcare Corporation. All rights reserved.)

mum concentration recommended for the particular drug and the rate of administration. The administered medication takes effect immediately (see Skill 23–9).

INTERMITTENT INFUSION DEVICES Intermittent infusion devices (Figure 23–32) may be affixed to an intravenous catheter or needle to allow medications to be administered intravenously without requiring repeated needlesticks or a continuous intravenous infusion.

Intermittent injection ports have either a resealable latex injection site for needle access or a port that allows a syringe or a needleless adapter to be connected for administering medications. Needleless systems are preferred, because they significantly reduce the risk of needlestick injuries among health care workers. With the needleless system, the injection adapter may be attached at the time of intravenous catheter placement, allowing a closed system to be maintained.

Intermittent injection ports may be flushed with sterile saline prior to and after medication. Most agencies use saline flushes with medication administration through peripheral IV lines. When administering a medication through a central venous access device (CVAD), some agencies use the SASH (flush with Saline–Adminster drug–flush with Saline–then flush with Heparin) flushing procedure (Bunce, 2003). Flushing the port maintains patency of the intravenous catheter and port, and reduces the risks of mixing incompatible medications within the system (see Skill 23–9).

Clients who require long-term venous access for administering medications (e.g., people receiving chemotherapy for cancer treatment) may have a specialized catheter or port to allow central venous access. The catheter may be tunneled subcutaneously and accessed through an intermittent injection port attached to the distal end of the venous catheter. Other devices have an implantable port or vascular access port surgically inserted under the skin so that no portion of the device exits the body. To administer medications, the port is accessed using a specialized needle through the skin. See Chapter 36 ∞ for more information about central venous lines.

ADMINISTERING INTRAVENOUS MEDICATIONS USING IV PUSH

PURPOSE

- To achieve immediate and maximum effects of a medication

ASSESSMENT

- Inspect and palpate the IV insertion site for signs of infection, infiltration, or a dislocated catheter.
- Inspect the surrounding skin for redness, pallor, or swelling.
- Palpate the surrounding tissues for coldness and the presence of edema, which could indicate leakage of the IV fluid into the tissues.

- Take vital signs for baseline data if the medication being administered is particularly potent.
- Determine if the client has allergies to the medication(s).
- Check the compatibility of the medication(s) and IV fluid.
- Determine specific drug action, side effects, normal dosage, recommended administration time, and peak action time.
- Check patency of IV.

PLANNING

Delegation

The administration of intravenous medication via IV push involves the application of nursing knowledge and critical thinking. This procedure is not delegated to UAP. The nurse, however, can inform the UAP of the intended therapeutic effects and/or specific side effects of the medication and direct the UAP to report specific client observations to the nurse for follow-up. *Note:* Administration of IV push medications varies by state nurse practice acts. For example, some states may allow the RN to delegate certain medications to be given by an LPN/LVN while other states may allow only the RN to administer IV push medications. The nurse needs to know his or her scope of practice according to the state's nurse practice act and agency policies.

- Sterile needles #21 to #25 gauge, 2.5 cm (1 in.) (needle not needed if using a needleless system)
- Antiseptic swabs
- Watch with a digital readout or second hand
- Clean gloves

IV Push for an IV Lock

- Medication in a vial or ampule
- Sterile syringe (3 to 5 mL) (to prepare the medication)
- Sterile syringe (3 mL) (for the saline or heparin flush)
- Vial of normal saline to flush the IV catheter or vial of heparin flush solution or both depending on agency practice. **Rationale:** *These maintain the patency of the IV lock. Saline is frequently used for peripheral locks.*
- Sterile needles (#21 gauge) (needle not needed if using a needleless system)
- Antiseptic swabs
- Watch with a digital readout or second hand
- Disposable gloves

EQUIPMENT

IV Push for an Existing Line

- Medication in a vial or ampule
- Sterile syringe (3 to 5 mL) (to prepare the medication)

IMPLEMENTATION

Preparation

1. Check the medication administration record (MAR).
   - Check the label on the medication carefully against the MAR to make sure that the correct medication is being prepared.
   - Follow the three checks for correct medication and dose. Read the label on the medication (1) when it is taken from the medication cart, (2) before withdrawing the medication, and (3) after withdrawing the medication.
   - Calculate medication dosage accurately.
   - Confirm that the route is correct.
2. Organize the equipment.

Performance

1. Perform hand hygiene and observe other appropriate infection control procedures.
2. Prepare the medication.

   Existing Line
   - Prepare the medication according to the manufacturer's direction. **Rationale:** *It is important to have the correct dose and the correct dilution.*

   IV Lock
   a. Flushing with saline
      - Prepare two syringes, each with 1 mL of sterile normal saline (or as facility policy dictates).

   b. Flushing with heparin (if indicated by agency policy) and saline
      - Prepare one syringe with 1 mL of heparin flush solution (if indicated by agency policy).
      - Prepare two syringes with 1 mL each of sterile, normal saline.
      - Draw up the medication into a syringe.
3. Put a small-gauge needle on the syringe if using a needle system.
4. Perform hand hygiene and put on clean gloves. **Rationale:** *This reduces the transmission of microorganisms and reduces the likelihood of the nurse's hands contacting the client's blood.*
5. Provide for client privacy.
6. Prepare the client.
   - Prior to performing the procedure, introduce self and verify the client's identity using agency protocol. **Rationale:** *This ensures that the right client receives the medication.*
   - If not previously assessed, take the appropriate assessment measures necessary for the medication. If any of the findings are above or below the predetermined parameters, consult the primary care provider before administering the medication.
7. Explain the purpose of the medication and how it will help, using language that the client can understand. Include relevant information about the effects of the medication.

(continued)

ADMINISTERING INTRAVENOUS MEDICATIONS USING IV PUSH *(continued)*

8. Administer the medication by IV push. Bunce (2003) reported that the use of the "push-stop-push-stop" technique is helpful, especially for central venous catheters. **Rationale:** *This creates a turbulence in the flow through the catheter which reduces the residue buildup in the line and the potential for occlusion.*

IV Lock with Needle
- Clean the diaphragm with the antiseptic swab. **Rationale:** *This prevents microorganisms from entering the circulatory system during the needle insertion.*
- Insert the needle of the syringe containing normal saline through the center of the diaphragm and aspirate for blood. **Rationale:** *The presence of blood confirms that the catheter or needle is in the vein. In some situations, blood will not return even though the lock is patent.*
- Flush the lock by injecting 1 mL of saline slowly. **Rationale:** *This removes blood and heparin (if present) from the needle and the lock.*
- Remove the needle and syringe. Activate the needle safety device.
- Clean the lock's diaphragm with an antiseptic swab. **Rationale:** *This prevents the transfer of microorganisms.*
- Insert the needle of the syringe containing the prepared medication through the center of the diaphragm.
- Inject the medication slowly at the recommended rate of infusion. Use a watch or digital readout to time the injection. Observe the client closely for adverse reactions. Remove the needle and syringe when all medication is administered. **Rationale:** *Injecting the drug too rapidly can have a serious untoward reaction.*
- Activate the needle safety device.
- Clean the diaphragm of the lock.
- Attach the second saline syringe, and inject 1 mL of saline. **Rationale:** *The saline injection flushes the medication through the catheter and prepares the lock for heparin if this medication is used. Heparin is incompatible with many medications.*
- If heparin is to be used, insert the heparin syringe and inject the heparin slowly into the lock.

IV Lock with Needleless System
- Remove the protective cap from the needleless port.
- Insert syringe containing normal saline into the lock.
- Flush the lock with 1 mL of sterile saline. **Rationale:** *This clears the lock of blood.*
- Remove the syringe.
- Insert the syringe containing the medication into the valve.
- Inject the medication following the precautions described previously.
- Withdraw the syringe.
- Repeat injection of 1 mL of saline.
- Place a new sterile cap over the lock.

Existing Line
- Identify the injection port closest to the client. Some ports have a circle indicating the site for the needle insertion. **Rationale:** *An injection port must be used because it is self-sealing. Any puncture to the plastic tubing will leak.*

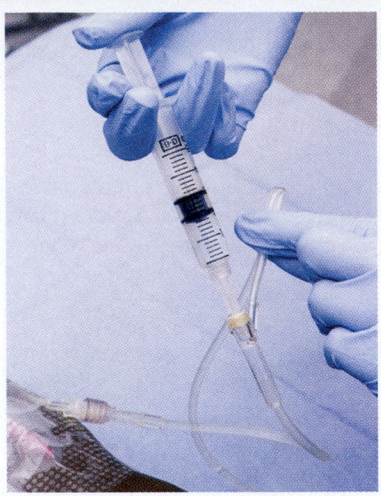

1 Injecting a medication by IV push to an existing IV using a needleless system.

- Clean the port with an antiseptic swab.
- Stop the IV flow by closing the clamp or pinching the tubing above the injection port.
- Connect the syringe to the IV system.
  a. Needle system
     - Hold the port steady.
     - Insert the needle of the syringe that contains the medication through the center of the port. **Rationale:** *This prevents damage to the IV line and to the diaphragm of the port.*
  b. Needleless system
     - Remove the cap from the needleless injection port. Connect the tip of the syringe directly to the port. **1**
     - Inject the medication at the ordered rate. Use the watch or digital readout to time the medication administration. **Rationale:** *This ensures safe drug administration because a too rapid injection could be dangerous.*
     - Release the clamp or tubing.
     - After injecting the medication, withdraw the needle and activate the needle safety device. For a needleless system, detach the syringe and attach a new sterile cap to the port.

9. Dispose of equipment according to agency practice. **Rationale:** *This reduces needlestick injuries and spread of microorganisms.*
10. Remove and dispose of gloves. Perform hand hygiene.
11. Observe the client closely for adverse reactions.
12. Determine agency practice about recommended times for changing the IV lock. Some agencies advocate a change every 48 to 72 hours for peripheral IV devices.
13. Document all relevant information.
    - Record the date, time, drug, dose, and route; client response; and assessments of infusion or heparin lock site if appropriate.

EVALUATION
- Conduct appropriate follow-up such as desired effect of medication, any adverse reactions or side effects, or change in vital signs.
- Reassess status of IV lock site and patency of IV infusion, if running.

- Relate to previous findings, if available.
- Report significant deviations from normal to the primary care provider.

Topical Medications

A topical medication is applied locally to the skin or to mucous membranes in areas such as the eye, external ear canal, nose, vagina, and rectum. Most topical applications used therapeutically are not absorbed well, completely, or predictably when applied to intact skin because the skin's thick outer layer serves as a natural barrier to drug diffusion. This route of absorption through the skin, called percutaneous, can be increased if the skin is altered by a laceration, burn, or some other problem. However, if high concentrations or large amounts of a topical medication are applied to the skin, especially if it is done repeatedly, sufficient amounts of the drug can enter the bloodstream to cause systemic effects, usually undesirable ones.

A particular type of topical or dermatologic medication delivery system is the **transdermal** patch. This system administers sustained-action medications (e.g., nitroglycerin, estrogen, and nicotine) via multilayered films containing the drug and an adhesive layer. The rate of delivery of the drug is controlled and varies with each product (e.g., from 12 hours to 1 week). Generally, the patch is applied to a hairless, clean area of skin that is not subject to excessive movement or wrinkling (i.e., the trunk or lower abdomen). It may also be applied on the side, lower back, or buttocks. Patches should not be applied to areas with cuts, burns, or abrasions, or on distal parts of extremities (e.g., the forearms). If hair is likely to interfere with patch adhesion or removal, clipping (not shaving) may be necessary before application.

CLINICAL ALERT

It is important to keep track of the transdermal patches. Some patches are clear and may be difficult to see and, as a result, be overlooked. If the client is obese, patches may be difficult to find in the skin folds. Duplication of patches may cause adverse reactions. Remove the old patch before applying a new one.

Reddening of the skin with or without mild local itching or burning, as well as allergic contact dermatitis, may occasionally occur. Upon removal of the patch, any slight reddening of the skin usually disappears within a few hours. All applications should be changed regularly to prevent local irritation, and each successive application should be placed on a different site. All clients need to be assessed for allergies to the drug and to materials in the patch before the patch is applied. If a client has a transdermal patch on and develops a fever, the medication may be absorbed and metabolized at a faster rate than normal. The client will need to be monitored for changes in effects of the medication.

When transdermal patches are removed, care needs to be taken as to how and where they are discarded. In the home environment, if they are simply discarded into a trash can, pets or children can be exposed to them, causing effects from any drug remaining on the patch. When removed, they should be folded with the medication side to the inside, put into a closed container, and kept out of reach of children and pets.

CLINICAL ALERT

The nurse should wear gloves when applying a transdermal patch to avoid getting any of the medication on his or her skin, which can result in the nurse receiving the effect of the medication.

SKIN APPLICATIONS   Topical skin or dermatologic preparations include ointments, pastes, creams, lotions, powders, sprays, and patches. See Table 23–1 earlier in this chapter. See Practice Guidelines for applying topical medications. Before applying a dermatologic preparation, thoroughly clean the area with soap and water and dry it with a patting motion. Skin encrustations harbor microorganisms and these as well as previously applied applications can prevent the medication from coming in contact with the area to be treated. Nurses should wear gloves when administering skin applications and always use surgical asepsis when an open wound is present.

OPHTHALMIC MEDICATIONS   Medications may be administered to the eye using irrigations or instillations. An eye irrigation is administered to wash out the conjunctival sac to remove secretions or foreign bodies or to remove chemicals that may injure the eye. Medications for the eyes, called ophthalmic medications, are instilled in the form of liquids or ointments. Eyedrops are packaged in monodrip plastic containers that are used to administer the preparation. Ointments are usually supplied in small tubes. All containers must state that the medication is for ophthalmic use. Sterile preparations and sterile technique are indicated. Prescribed liquids are usually dilute, for example, less than 1% strength.

Skill 23–10 illustrates how to administer ophthalmic instillations.

Applying Skin Preparations

Powder

Make sure the skin surface is dry. Spread apart any skin folds, and sprinkle the site until the area is covered with a fine *thin* layer. Cover the site with a dressing if ordered.

Suspension-Based Lotion

Shake the container before use to distribute suspended particles. Put a little lotion on a small gauze dressing or pad, and apply the lotion to the skin by stroking it evenly in the direction of the hair growth.

Creams, Ointments, Pastes, and Oil-Based Lotions

Warm and soften the preparation in gloved hands to make it easier to apply and to prevent chilling (if a large area is to be treated). Smear it evenly over the skin using long strokes that follow the direction of the hair growth. Explain that the skin may feel somewhat greasy after application. Apply a sterile dressing if ordered by the primary care provider.

Aerosol Spray

Shake the container well to mix the contents. Hold the spray container at the recommended distance from the area (usually about 15 to 30 cm [6 to 12 inches] but check the label). Cover the client's face with a towel if the upper chest or neck is to be sprayed. Spray the medication over the specified area.

Transdermal Patches

Select a clean, dry area that is free of hair and matches the manufacturer's recommendations. Remove the patch from its protective covering, holding it without touching the adhesive edges, and apply it by pressing firmly with the palm of the hand for about 10 seconds. Advise the client to avoid using a heating pad over the area to prevent an increase in circulation and the rate of absorption. Remove the patch at the appropriate time, folding the medicated side to the inside so it is covered.

SKILL 23–10

ADMINISTERING OPHTHALMIC INSTILLATIONS

PURPOSE
- To provide an eye medication the client requires (e.g., an antibiotic) to treat an infection or for other reasons (see specific drug action)

ASSESSMENT
In addition to the assessment performed by the nurse related to the administration of any medication, prior to applying ophthalmic medications, assess:

- Appearance of eye and surrounding structures for lesions, exudate, erythema, or swelling
- The location and nature of any discharge, lacrimation, and swelling of the eyelids or of the lacrimal gland

- Client complaints (e.g., itching, burning pain, blurred vision, and photophobia)
- Client behavior (e.g., squinting, blinking excessively, frowning, or rubbing the eyes)

  Determine if assessment data influence administration of the medication (i.e., is it appropriate to administer the medication or does the medication need to be held and the primary care provider notified?).

PLANNING

Delegation
Due to the need for assessment, interpretation of client status, and use of sterile technique, ophthalmic medication administration is not delegated to UAP.

EQUIPMENT
- Clean gloves
- Sterile absorbent sponges soaked in sterile normal saline

- Medication
- Sterile eye dressing (pad) as needed and paper tape to secure it

  For irrigation, add:

- Irrigating solution (e.g., normal saline) and irrigating syringe or tubing
- Dry sterile absorbent sponges
- Moisture-resistant towel
- Basin (e.g., emesis basin)

IMPLEMENTATION

Preparation
1. Check the medication administration record (MAR).
   - Check the MAR for the drug name, dose, and strength. Also confirm the prescribed frequency of the instillation and which eye is to be treated.
   - If the MAR is unclear or pertinent information is missing, compare it with the most recent primary care provider's written order.
   - Report any discrepancies to the charge nurse or physician, as agency policy dictates.

2. Know the reason why the client is receiving the medication, the drug classification, contraindications, usual dose range, side effects, and nursing considerations for administering and evaluating the intended outcomes of the medication.

Performance
1. Compare the label on the medication tube or bottle with the medication record and check the expiration date.
2. If necessary, calculate the medication dosage.
3. Introduce self and explain to the client what you are going to do, why it is necessary, and how he or she can cooperate. The administration of an ophthalmic medication is not

usually painful. Ointments are often soothing to the eye, but some liquid preparations may sting initially. Discuss how the results will be used in planning further care or treatments.

4. Perform hand hygiene and observe appropriate infection control procedures.

5. Provide for client privacy.

6. Prepare the client.
   - Prior to performing the procedure, verify the client's identity using agency protocol. **Rationale:** *This ensures that the right client receives the medication.*
   - Assist the client to a comfortable position, either sitting or lying.

7. Clean the eyelid and the eyelashes.
   - Put on clean gloves.
   - Use sterile cotton balls moistened with sterile irrigating solution or sterile normal saline, and wipe from the inner canthus to the outer canthus. **Rationale:** *If not removed, material on the eyelid and lashes can be washed into the eye. Cleaning toward the outer canthus prevents contamination of the other eye and the lacrimal duct.*

8. Administer the eye medication.
   - Check the ophthalmic preparation for the name, strength, and number of drops if a liquid is used. **Rationale:** *Checking medication data is essential to prevent a medication error.* Draw the correct number of drops into the shaft of the dropper if a dropper is used. If ointment is used, discard the first bead. **Rationale:** *The first bead of ointment from a tube is considered to be contaminated.*
   - Instruct the client to look up to the ceiling. Give the client a dry sterile absorbent sponge. **Rationale:** *The person is less likely to blink if looking up. While the client looks up, the cornea is partially protected by the upper eyelid. A sponge is needed to press on the nasolacrimal duct after a liquid instillation to prevent systemic absorption or to wipe excess ointment from the eyelashes after an ointment is instilled.*
   - Expose the lower conjunctival sac by placing the thumb or fingers of your nondominant hand on the client's cheekbone just below the eye and gently drawing down the skin on the cheek. If the tissues are edematous, handle the tissues carefully to avoid damaging them. **Rationale:** *Placing the fingers on the cheekbone minimizes the possibility of touching the cornea, avoids putting any pressure on the eyeball, and prevents the person from blinking or squinting.*
   - Holding the medication in the dominant hand, place hand on client's forehead to stabilize hand. Approach the eye from the side and instill the correct number of drops onto the outer third of the lower conjunctival sac. Hold the dropper 1 to 2 cm (0.4 to 0.8 in.) above the sac. ❶ **Rationale:** *The client is less likely to blink if a side approach is used. When instilled into the conjunctival sac, drops will not harm the cornea as they might if dropped directly on it. The dropper must not touch the sac or the cornea.*

   or
   - Holding the tube above the lower conjunctival sac, squeeze 2 cm (0.8 in.) of ointment from the tube into the lower conjunctival sac from the inner canthus outward. ❷
   - Instruct the client to close the eyelids but not to squeeze them shut. **Rationale:** *Closing the eye spreads the*

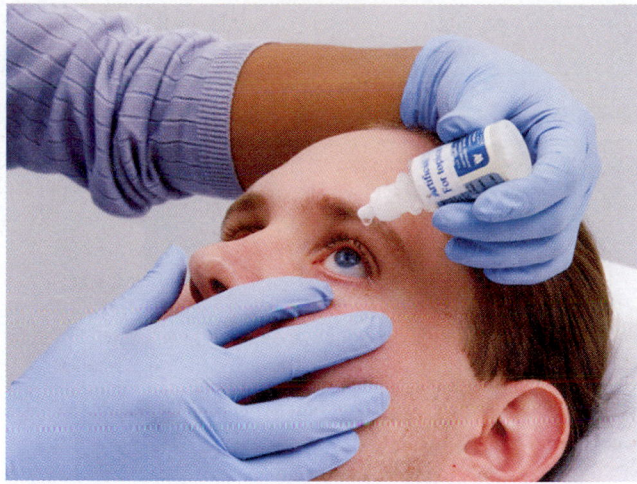

❶ Instilling an eyedrop into the lower conjunctival sac.

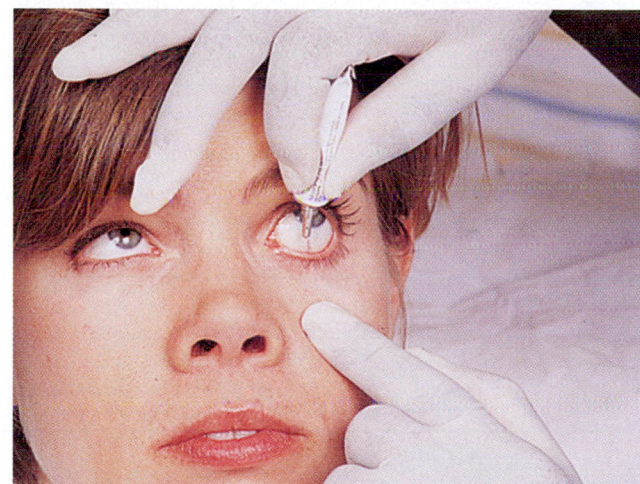

❷ Instilling an eye ointment into the lower conjunctival sac.

medication over the eyeball. Squeezing can injure the eye and push out the medication.
   - For liquid medications, press firmly or have the client press firmly on the nasolacrimal duct for at least 30 seconds. **Rationale:** *Pressing on the nasolacrimal duct prevents the medication from running out of the eye and down the duct, preventing systemic absorption.* ❸

Variation: Irrigation
   - Place absorbent pads under the head, neck, and shoulders. Place an emesis basin next to the eye to catch drainage. Some eye medications cause systemic reactions such as confusion or a decrease in heart rate and blood pressure if the eyedrops go down the nasolacrimal duct and get into the systemic circulation.
   - Expose the lower conjunctival sac. Or, to irrigate in stages, first hold the lower lid down, then hold the upper lid up. Exert pressure on the bony prominences of the cheekbone and beneath the eyebrow when holding the eyelids. **Rationale:** *Separating the lids prevents reflex blinking. Exerting pressure on the bony prominences minimizes the possibility of pressing the eyeball and causing discomfort.*

(continued)

SKILL 23–10

ADMINISTERING OPHTHALMIC INSTILLATIONS *(continued)*

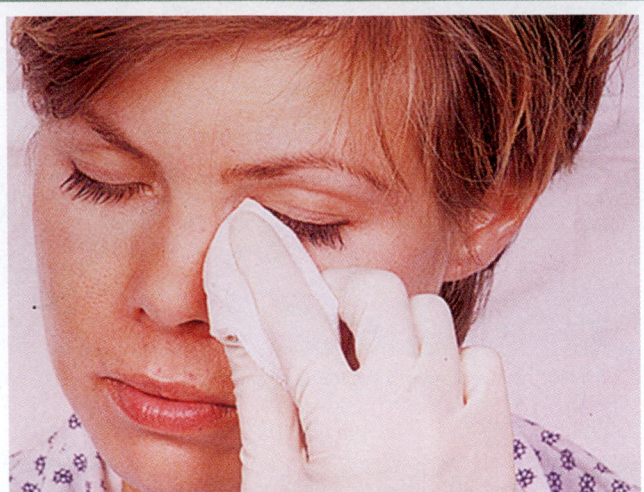

❸ Pressing on the nasolacrimal duct.

- Fill and hold the eye irrigator about 2.5 cm (1 in.) above the eye. **Rationale:** *At this height the pressure of the solution will not damage the eye tissue, and the irrigator will not touch the eye.*

- Irrigate the eye, directing the solution onto the lower conjunctival sac and from the inner canthus to the outer canthus. **Rationale:** *Directing the solution in this way prevents possible injury to the cornea and prevents fluid and contaminants from flowing down the nasolacrimal duct.*
- Irrigate until the solution leaving the eye is clear (no discharge is present) or until all the solution has been used.
- Instruct the client to close and move the eye periodically. **Rationale:** *Eye closure and movement help to move secretions from the upper to the lower conjunctival sac.*

9. Clean and dry the eyelids as needed. Wipe the eyelids gently from the inner to the outer canthus to collect excess medication.
10. Apply an eye pad if needed, and secure it with paper eye tape.
11. Assess the client's response immediately after the instillation or irrigation and again after the medication should have acted.
12. Document all relevant assessments and interventions. Include the name of the drug or irrigating solution, the strength, the number of drops if a liquid medication, the time, and the response of the client.

EVALUATION
- Perform follow-up based on findings of the effectiveness of the administration or outcomes that deviated from expected or normal for the client. Relate findings to previous data if available.
- Report significant deviations from normal to the primary care provider.

LIFESPAN CONSIDERATIONS   Administering Ophthalmic Medications

Infants/Children
- Explain the technique to the parents of an infant or child.
- For a young child or infant, obtain assistance to immobilize the arms and head. The parent may hold the infant or young child. *This prevents accidental injury during medication administration.*
- For a young child, use a doll to demonstrate the procedure. *This facilitates cooperation and decreases anxiety.*
- Drops may be tolerated better by children than ointment since they are less likely to cause blurred vision.
- An intravenous (IV) bag and tubing may be used to deliver irrigating fluid to the eye (Figure 23–33).

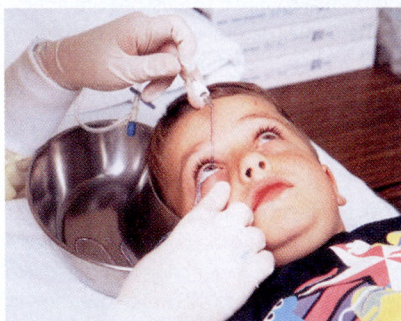

Figure 23–33 ⬤ Eye irrigation using IV tubing.

OTIC MEDICATIONS Instillations or irrigations of the external auditory canal are referred to as otic and are generally carried out for cleaning purposes. Sometimes applications of heat and antiseptic solutions are prescribed. Irrigations performed in a hospital require aseptic technique so that microorganisms will not be introduced into the ear.

Sterile technique is used if the eardrum is perforated. The position of the external auditory canal varies with age. In the child under 3 years of age, it is directed upward. In the adult, the external auditory canal is an S-shaped structure about 2.5 cm (1 inch) long.

Skill 23–11 explains how to administer otic instillations.

SKILL 23-11

ADMINISTERING OTIC INSTILLATIONS

PURPOSE
- To soften earwax so that it can be readily removed at a later time
- To provide local therapy to reduce inflammation, destroy infective organisms in the external ear canal, or both
- To relieve pain

ASSESSMENT
In addition to the assessment performed by the nurse related to the administration of any medications, prior to applying otic medications, assess:

- Appearance of the pinna of the ear and meatus for signs of redness and abrasions
- Type and amount of any discharge

Determine if assessment data influence administration of the medication (i.e., is it appropriate to administer the medication or does the medication need to be held and the primary care provider notified?).

PLANNING

> **Delegation**
> Due to the need for assessment, interpretation of client status, and use of sterile technique, otic medication administration is not delegated to UAP.

EQUIPMENT
- Clean gloves
- Cotton-tipped applicator
- Correct medication bottle with a dropper

- Flexible rubber tip (optional) for the end of the dropper, which prevents injury from sudden motion, for example, by a disoriented client
- Cotton fluff

  For irrigation, add:

- Moisture-resistant towel
- Basin (e.g., emesis basin)
- Irrigating solution at the appropriate temperature, about 500 mL (16 oz) or as ordered
- Container for the irrigating solution
- Syringe (rubber bulb or Asepto syringe is frequently used)

IMPLEMENTATION

Preparation

1. Check the medication administration record (MAR).
   - Check the MAR for the drug name, strength, number of drops, and prescribed frequency.
   - If the MAR is unclear or pertinent information is missing, compare it with the most recent primary care provider's written order.
   - Report any discrepancies to the charge nurse or physician, as agency policy dictates.
2. Know the reason why the client is receiving the medication, the drug classification, contraindications, usual dose range, side effects, and nursing considerations for administering and evaluating the intended outcomes of the medication.

Performance

1. Compare the label on the medication container with the medication record and check the expiration date.
2. If necessary, calculate the medication dosage.
3. Explain to the client what you are going to do, why it is necessary, and how he or she can cooperate. The administration of an otic medication is not usually painful. Discuss how the results will be used in planning further care or treatments.
4. Perform hand hygiene and observe appropriate infection control procedures.
5. Provide for client privacy.
6. Prepare the client.
   - Prior to performing the procedure, introduce self and verify the client's identity using agency protocol. **Rationale:** *This ensures that the right client receives the medication.*

   - Assist the client to a comfortable position for eardrops, lying with the ear being treated uppermost.
7. Clean the pinna of the ear and the meatus of the ear canal.
   - Put on gloves if infection is suspected.
   - Use cotton-tipped applicators and solution to wipe the pinna and auditory meatus. **Rationale:** *This removes any discharge present before the instillation so that it won't be washed into the ear canal.*
8. Administer the ear medication.
   - Warm the medication container in your hand, or place it in warm water for a short time. **Rationale:** *This promotes client comfort.*
   - Partially fill the ear dropper with medication.
   - Straighten the auditory canal. Pull the pinna upward and backward for clients over 3 years of age. **Rationale:** *The auditory canal is straightened so that the solution can flow the entire length of the canal.* ❶

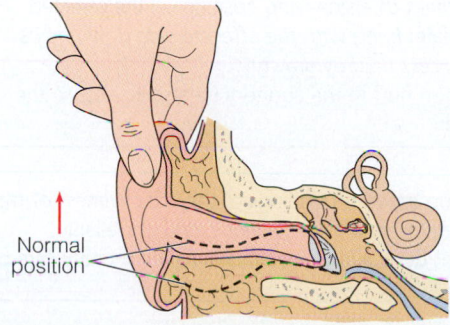

Normal position

❶ Straightening the adult ear canal by pulling pinna upward and backward.

(continued)

SKILL 23–11

ADMINISTERING OTIC INSTILLATIONS *(continued)*

- Instill the correct number of drops along the side of the ear canal. ❷
- Press gently but firmly a few times on the tragus of the ear (the cartilaginous projection in front of the exterior meatus of the ear). **Rationale:** *Pressing on the tragus assists the flow of medication into the ear canal.*
- Ask the client to remain in the side-lying position for about 5 minutes. **Rationale:** *This prevents the drops from escaping and allows the medication to reach all sides of the canal cavity.*
- Insert a small piece of cotton fluff loosely at the meatus of the auditory canal for 15 to 20 minutes. Do not press it into the canal. **Rationale:** *The cotton helps retain the medication when the client is up. If pressed tightly into the canal, the cotton would interfere with the action of the drug and the outward movement of normal secretions.*

Variation: Ear Irrigation
- Explain that the client may experience a feeling of fullness, warmth, and, occasionally, discomfort when the fluid comes in contact with the tympanic membrane.
- Assist the client to a sitting or lying position with head tilted toward the affected ear. **Rationale:** *The solution can then flow from the ear canal to a basin.* ❸
- Place the moisture-resistant towel around the client's shoulder under the ear to be irrigated, and place the basin under the ear to be irrigated.
- Fill the syringe with solution.

  or

- Hang up the irrigating container, and run solution through the tubing and the nozzle. **Rationale:** *Solution is run through to remove air from the tubing and nozzle.*
- Straighten the ear canal.
- Insert the tip of the syringe into the auditory meatus, and direct the solution gently upward against the top of the canal. **Rationale:** *The solution will flow around the entire canal and out at the bottom. The solution is instilled gently because strong pressure from the fluid can cause discomfort and damage the tympanic membrane.*
- Continue instilling the fluid until all the solution is used or until the canal is cleaned, depending on the purpose of the irrigation. Take care not to block the outward flow of the solution with the syringe.
- Assist the client to a side-lying position on the affected side. **Rationale:** *Lying with the affected side down helps drain the excess fluid by gravity.*
- Place a cotton fluff in the auditory meatus to absorb the excess fluid.

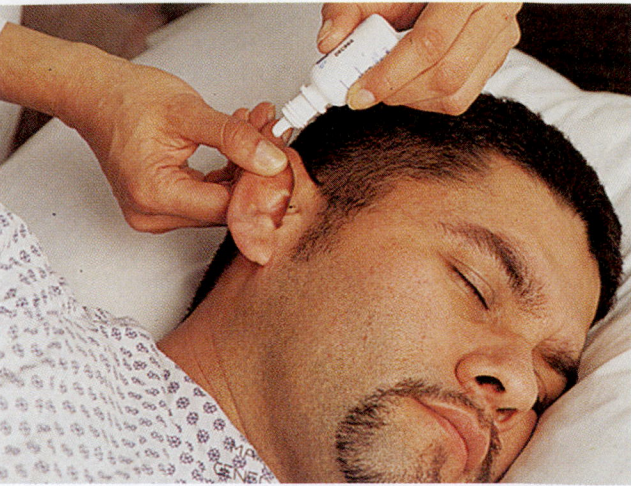

❷ Instilling eardrops.

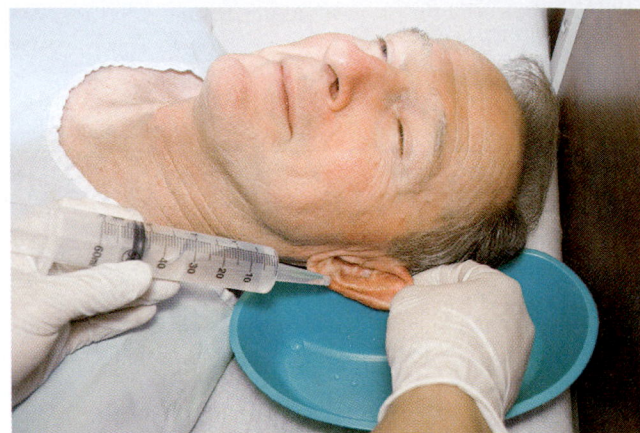

❸ Ear irrigation.

9. Assess the client's response and the character and amount of discharge, appearance of the canal, discomfort, and so on, immediately after the instillation and again when the medication is expected to act. Inspect the cotton ball for any drainage.
10. Document all nursing assessments and interventions relative to the procedure. Include the name of the drug or irrigating solution, the strength, the number of drops if a liquid medication, the time, and the response of the client.

EVALUATION
- Perform follow-up based on findings of the effectiveness of the administration or outcomes that deviated from expected or normal for the client. Relate findings to previous data if available.
- Report significant deviations from normal to the primary care provider.

LIFESPAN CONSIDERATIONS   Administering Otic Medications

Infants/Children

- Obtain assistance to immobilize an infant or young child. This prevents accidental injury due to sudden movement during the procedure.
- Because in infants and children under 3 years of age, the ear canal is directed upward, to administer medication, gently pull the pinna down and back (Figure 23–34). For a child *older* than 3 years of age, pull the pinna upward and backward.

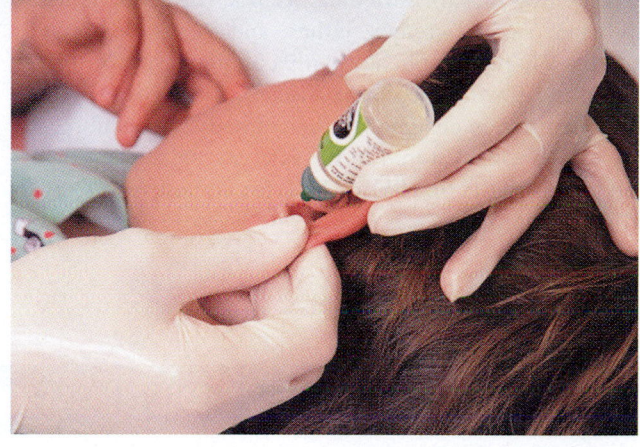

Figure 23–34 ○ Straightening the ear canal of a child by pulling the pinna down and back.

NASAL MEDICATIONS   Nasal instillations (nose drops and sprays) usually are instilled for their astringent effect (to shrink swollen mucous membranes), to loosen secretions and facilitate drainage, or to treat infections of the nasal cavity or sinuses. Nasal decongestants are the most common nasal instillations. Many of these products are available without a prescription. Clients need to be taught to use these agents with caution. Chronic use of nasal decongestants may lead to a rebound effect, that is, an increase in nasal congestion. If excess decongestant solution is swallowed, serious systemic effects may also develop, especially in children. Saline drops are safer as a decongestant for children.

Usually clients self-administer sprays. In the supine position with the head tilted back, the client holds the tip of the container just inside the nares and inhales as the spray enters the nasal passages. For clients who use nasal sprays repeatedly, the nares need to be assessed for irritation. In children, nasal sprays are given with the head in an upright position to prevent excess spray from being swallowed.

Nasal drops may be used to treat sinus infections. Clients need to learn ways to position themselves to effectively treat the affected sinus:

- To treat the ethmoid and sphenoid sinuses, instruct the client to lie back with the head over the edge of the bed or a pillow under the shoulders so that the head is tipped backward (Figure 23–35).
- To treat the maxillary and frontal sinuses, instruct the client to assume the same back-lying position, with the head turned toward the side to be treated (Figure 23–36). The client should also be instructed to (a) breathe through the mouth to prevent aspiration of medication into the trachea and bronchi, (b) remain in a back-lying position for at least 1 minute so that the solution will come into contact with all of the nasal surface, and (c) avoid blowing the nose for several minutes.

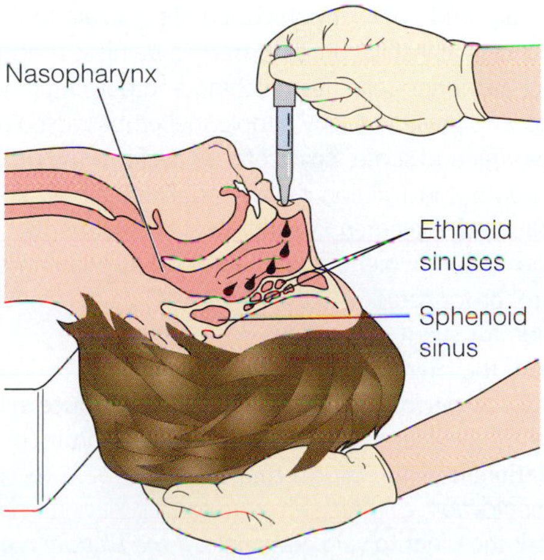

Nasopharynx

Ethmoid sinuses

Sphenoid sinus

Figure 23–35 ○ Position of the head to instill drops into the ethmoid and sphenoid sinuses.

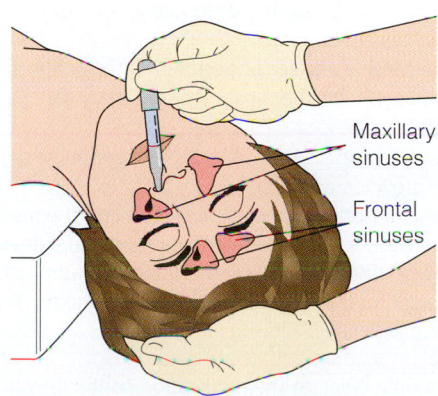

Maxillary sinuses

Frontal sinuses

Figure 23–36 ○ Position of the head to instill drops into the maxillary and frontal sinuses.

VAGINAL MEDICATIONS   Vaginal medications, or installations, are inserted as creams, jellies, foams, or suppositories to treat infection or to relieve vaginal discomfort (e.g., itching or pain). Medical aseptic technique is usually used. Vaginal creams, jellies, and foams are applied by using a tubular applicator with a plunger. Suppositories are inserted with the index finger of a gloved hand. Suppositories are designed to melt at body temperature, so they are generally stored in the refrigerator to keep them firm for insertion. See Skill 23–12 for administering vaginal installations.

A vaginal irrigation (douche) is the washing of the vagina by a liquid at a low pressure. Vaginal irrigations are not necessary for ordinary female hygiene but are used to prevent infection by applying an antimicrobial solution that discourages the growth of microorganisms, to remove an offensive or irritating discharge, and to reduce inflammation or prevent hemorrhage by the application of heat or cold. In hospitals, sterile supplies and equipment are used; in a home, sterility is not usually necessary because people are accustomed to the microorganisms in their environments. Sterile technique, however, is indicated if there is an open wound.

SKILL 23–12

ADMINISTERING VAGINAL INSTILLATIONS

PURPOSE
- To treat or prevent infection
- To reduce inflammation
- To relieve vaginal discomfort

ASSESSMENT
In addition to the assessment performed by the nurse related to the administration of any medications, prior to applying vaginal medications, assess:

- The vaginal orifice for inflammation; amount, character, and odor of vaginal discharge
- For complaints of vaginal discomfort (e.g., burning or itching)

Determine if assessment data influence administration of the medication (i.e., is it appropriate to administer the medication or does the medication need to be held and the primary care provider notified?).

PLANNING

> **Delegation**
> Due to the need for assessments and interpretation of client status, vaginal medication administration is not delegated to UAP.

EQUIPMENT
- Drape
- Correct vaginal suppository or cream
- Applicator for vaginal cream

- Clean gloves
- Lubricant for a suppository
- Disposable towel
- Clean perineal pad

  For an irrigation, add:

- Moisture-proof pad
- Vaginal irrigation set (these are often disposable) containing a nozzle, tubing and a clamp, and a container for the solution
- Irrigating solution

IMPLEMENTATION

Preparation

1. Check the medication administration record (MAR).
   - Check the MAR for the drug name, strength, and prescribed frequency.
   - If the MAR is unclear or pertinent information is missing, compare it with the most recent primary care provider's written order.
   - Report any discrepancies to the charge nurse or primary care provider, as agency policy dictates.
2. Know the reason why the client is receiving the medication, the drug classification, contraindications, usual dose range, side effects, and nursing considerations for administering and evaluating the intended outcomes of the medication.

Performance

1. Compare the label on the medication container with the medication record and check the expiration date.
2. If necessary, calculate the medication dosage.

3. Explain to the client what you are going to do, why it is necessary, and how she can cooperate. Explain to the client that a vaginal instillation is normally a painless procedure, and in fact may bring relief from itching and burning if an infection is present. Many people feel embarrassed about this procedure, and some may prefer to perform the procedure themselves if instruction is provided. Discuss how the results will be used in planning further care or treatments.
4. Perform hand hygiene and observe appropriate infection control procedures.
5. Provide for client privacy.
6. Prepare the client.
   - Prior to performing the procedure, introduce self and verify the client's identity using agency protocol. **Rationale:** *This ensures that the right client receives the medication.*
   - Ask the client to void. **Rationale:** *If the bladder is empty, the client will have less discomfort during the treatment, and the possibility of injuring the vaginal lining is decreased.*

- Assist the client to a back-lying position with the knees flexed and the hips rotated laterally.
- Drape the client appropriately so that only the perineal area is exposed.

7. Prepare the equipment.
   - Unwrap the suppository, and put it on the opened wrapper.

   or

   - Fill the applicator with the prescribed cream, jelly, or foam. Directions are provided with the manufacturer's applicator.

8. Assess and clean the perineal area.
   - Put on gloves. **Rationale:** *Gloves prevent contamination of the nurse's hands from vaginal and perineal microorganisms.*
   - Inspect the vaginal orifice, note any odor of discharge from the vagina, and ask about any vaginal discomfort.
   - Provide perineal care to remove microorganisms. **Rationale:** *This decreases the chance of moving microorganisms into the vagina.*

9. Administer the vaginal suppository, cream, foam, jelly, or irrigation.

   Suppository
   - Lubricate the rounded (smooth) end of the suppository, which is inserted first. **Rationale:** *Lubrication facilitates insertion.*
   - Lubricate your gloved index finger.
   - Expose the vaginal orifice by separating the labia with your nondominant hand.
   - Insert the suppository about 8 to 10 cm (3 to 4 in.) along the posterior wall of the vagina, or as far as it will go. **Rationale:** *The posterior wall of the vagina is about 2.5 cm (1 in.) longer than the anterior wall because the cervix protrudes into the uppermost portion of the anterior wall.* ❶
   - Ask the client to remain lying in the supine position for 5 to 10 minutes following insertion. The hips may also be elevated on a pillow. **Rationale:** *This position allows the medication to flow into the posterior fornix after it has melted.*

   Vaginal Cream, Jelly, or Foam
   - Gently insert the applicator about 5 cm (2 in.).
   - Slowly push the plunger until the applicator is empty. ❷
   - Remove the applicator and place it on the towel. **Rationale:** *The applicator is put on the towel to prevent the spread of microorganisms.*
   - Discard the applicator if disposable or clean it according to the manufacturer's directions.
   - Ask the client to remain lying in the supine position for 5 to 10 minutes following the insertion.

   Irrigation
   - Place the client on a bedpan.
   - Clamp the tubing. Hold the irrigating container about 30 cm (12 in.) above the vagina. **Rationale:** *At this height, the pressure of the solution should not be great enough to injure the vaginal lining.*

- Run fluid through the tubing and nozzle into the bedpan. **Rationale:** *Fluid is run through the tubing to remove air and to moisten the nozzle.*
- Insert the nozzle carefully into the vagina. Direct the nozzle toward the sacrum, following the direction of the vagina.
- Insert the nozzle about 7 to 10 cm (3 to 4 in.), start the flow, and rotate the nozzle several times. **Rationale:** *Rotating the nozzle irrigates all parts of the vagina.*
- Use all of the irrigating solution, permitting it to flow out freely into the bedpan.
- Remove the nozzle from the vagina.
- Assist the client to a sitting position on the bedpan. **Rationale:** *Sitting on the bedpan will help drain the remaining fluid by gravity.*

10. Ensure client comfort.
    - Dry the perineum with tissues as required.
    - Apply a clean perineal pad if there is excessive drainage.

11. Document all nursing assessments and interventions relative to the Skill. Include the name of the drug or irrigating solution, the strength, the time, and the response of the client.

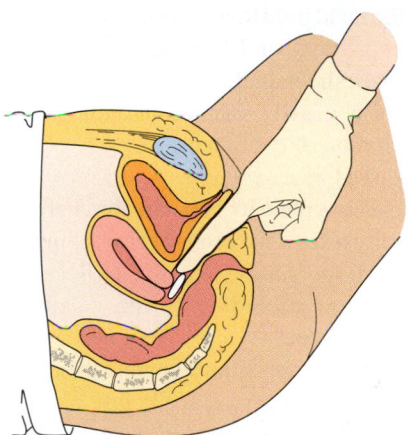

❶ Instilling a vaginal suppository.

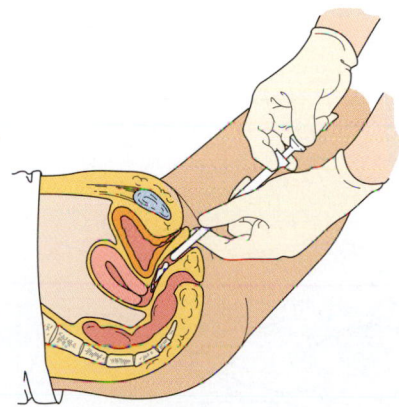

❷ Using an applicator to instill a vaginal cream.

EVALUATION

- Perform follow-up based on findings of the effectiveness of the administration or outcomes that deviated from expected or normal for the client. Relate findings to previous data if available.
- Report significant deviations from normal to the primary care provider.

RECTAL MEDICATIONS   Insertion of medications into the rectum in the form of suppositories is a frequent practice. Rectal administration is a convenient and safe method of giving certain medications. Advantages include the following:

- It avoids irritation of the upper gastrointestinal tract in clients who encounter this problem (e.g., in clients who are nauseated or vomiting).
- It is advantageous when the medication has an objectionable taste or odor.
- The drug is released at a slow but steady rate.
- Rectal suppositories are thought to provide higher bloodstream levels (titers) of medication because the venous blood from the lower rectum is not transported through the liver.

To insert a rectal suppository:

- Assist the client to a left lateral or left Sims' position, with the upper leg flexed.
- Fold back the top bedclothes to expose the buttocks.
- Put a glove on the hand used to insert the suppository.
- Unwrap the suppository and lubricate the smooth rounded end, or see the manufacturer's instructions. The rounded end is usually inserted first and lubricant reduces irritation of the mucosa.
- Lubricate the gloved index finger.
- Encourage the client to relax by breathing through the mouth. This usually relaxes the external anal sphincter.
- Insert the suppository gently into the anal canal, rounded end first (or according to the manufacturer's instructions), using your gloved index finger. For an adult, insert the suppository beyond the internal sphincter (i.e., 10 cm [4 in.]) (see Figure 23–37).
- Avoid embedding the suppository in feces in order for the suppository to be absorbed effectively.
- Press the client's buttocks together for a few minutes.

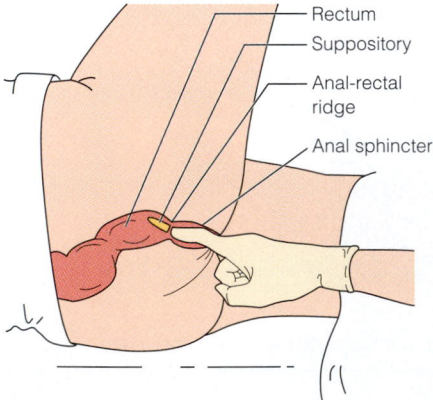

Figure 23–37 Inserting a rectal suppository beyond the internal sphincter and along the rectal wall.

> ### LIFESPAN CONSIDERATIONS
> **Administering Rectal Medications**
>
> **Infants/Children**
> - Obtain assistance to immobilize an infant or young child. This prevents accidental injury due to sudden movement during the procedure.
> - For a child under 3 years, the nurse should use the gloved fifth finger for insertion. After this age, the index finger can usually be used.
> - For a child or infant, insert a suppository 5 cm (2 in.) or less.

- Ask the client to remain in the left lateral or supine position for at least 5 minutes (or longer as directed by manufacturer's instructions) to allow the medication to be absorbed.

RESPIRATORY INHALATION

Nebulizers deliver most medications administered through the inhaled route. A nebulizer is used to deliver a fine spray (fog or mist) of medication or moisture to a client. There are two kinds of nebulization: *atomization* and *aerosolization*. In atomization, a device called an *atomizer* produces rather large droplets for inhalation. In aerosolization, the droplets are suspended in a gas, such as oxygen. The smaller the droplets, the further they can be inhaled into the respiratory tract. When a medication is intended for the nasal mucosa, it is inhaled through the nose; when it is intended for the trachea, bronchi, and/or lungs, it is inhaled through the mouth.

A large-volume nebulizer can provide a heated or cool mist. It is used for long-term therapy, such as that following a tracheostomy. The ultrasonic nebulizer provides 100% humidity and can provide particles small enough to be inhaled deeply into the respiratory tract.

The **metered-dose inhaler (MDI)**, a handheld nebulizer (Figure 23–38), is a pressurized container of medica-

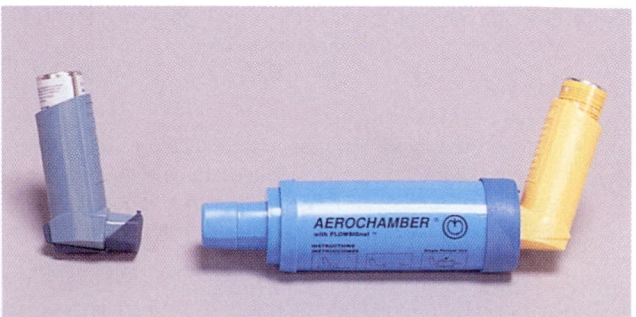

Figure 23–38 Metered-dose inhaler.

Children

- Spacers hold a medication in suspension and provide the child an opportunity to take several deep breaths in order to inhale all the medication.
- A mask is used for nebulizer treatments, allowing the child to breathe naturally. Some infants and children may be

frightened or uncomfortable with the mask and become resistant. Use a doll or stuffed animal to demonstrate its use, and allow them to play with the equipment before putting it in place. Having the child sit in the parent's lap during the procedure can help the child relax and be more cooperative.

---

tion that can be used by the client to release the medication through a nosepiece or mouthpiece. The force with which the air moves through the nebulizer causes the large particles of medicated solution to break up into finer particles, forming a mist or fine spray. According to Bower (2005), metered-dose inhalers can deliver accurate doses, provide for target action at the needed sites, and sustain less systemic effects than medication delivered by other routes. Some inhalers deliver medication in powdered form and are referred to as metered powder inhalers (MPI).

To ensure correct delivery of the prescribed medication by MDIs, nurses need to instruct clients to use aerosol inhalers correctly. The client compresses the medication canister by hand to release medication through a mouthpiece. An extender or spacer may be attached to the mouthpiece to facilitate medication absorption for better results. Spacers are holding chambers into which the medication is fired and from which the client inhales, so that the dose is not lost by exhalation. The Client Teaching feature provides instructions for clients about using an MDI. Newer breath-activated MDIs are being produced in which inhalation triggers the release of a premeasured dose of medication.

CLINICAL ALERT

It is important for the nurse to assess if the client is using the MDI correctly. A client's ability to use an MDI correctly can decrease over time.

IRRIGATIONS

An irrigation (lavage) is the washing out of a body cavity by a stream of water or other fluid that may or may not be medicated. Irrigation is performed for one or more of the following reasons:

- To clean the area, that is, to remove a foreign object or excessive secretions or discharge

- To apply heat or cold
- To apply a medication, such as an antiseptic
- To reduce inflammation
- To relieve discomfort

Surgical asepsis is required when there is a break in the skin (e.g., in a wound irrigation) or whenever a sterile body cavity (e.g., the bladder) is entered. Some irrigations (e.g., a vaginal, rectal, or gastric irrigation) are often safely conducted using medical asepsis.

Different kinds of syringes are used for irrigations. The most common are the Asepto and the rubber bulb (Figure 23–41). The syringes are often calibrated, permitting the nurse to determine the amount of irrigant being delivered at any given time.

The Asepto syringe is a plastic (or glass) syringe with a rubber bulb. Squeezing the air out of the bulb produces negative pressure, and fluid can be sucked into the syringe. When the bulb is squeezed again, the fluid is ejected from the syringe. Asepto syringes come in several sizes ranging from 30 mL (1 oz) to 120 mL (4 oz).

The rubber bulb syringe is often used for irrigating the ears. Like the Asepto syringe, the rubber bulb syringe comes in a range of sizes.

Other syringes that can be used are the piston syringe, which has a tip to which a catheter can be attached, and the Pomeroy syringe. Catheters may be used for deep-wound irrigations and for some types of bladder irrigations. The Pomeroy syringe is a metal syringe commonly used for ear irrigations. A shield near the tip prevents the solution from spraying outward. Plastic squeezable bottles are also available for irrigations. These are commonly used for perineal irrigations and some wound irrigations.

The type, amount, temperature, and strength of the solution and the frequency of the irrigation are ordered by the primary care provider. Generally, normal saline at body temperature (37°C [98.6°F]) is used unless specified otherwise. The amount of solution used varies with the site and purpose of the irrigation. Guidelines for administering eye and ear irrigations are given in Skills 23–10 (eye) and 23–11 (ear).

- Ensure that the canister is firmly and fully inserted into the inhaler.
- Remove the mouthpiece cap. Holding the inhaler upright, shake the inhaler vigorously for 3 to 5 seconds to mix the medication evenly.
- Exhale comfortably (as in a normal full breath).
- Hold the canister upside down.
  a. Hold the MDI 2 to 4 cm (1 to 2 in.) from the open mouth (Figure 23–39).

    or

  b. Put the mouthpiece far enough into the mouth with its opening toward the throat such that the lips can tightly close around the mouthpiece. An MDI with a spacer or extender is always placed in the mouth (Figure 23–40). This method should not be used for steroid medications via an MDI because it is not considered as efficient in delivery of the medication (Bower, 2005).

Administering the Medication

- Press down *once* on the MDI canister (which releases the dose) and inhale slowly (for 3 to 5 seconds) and deeply through the mouth.
- Hold your breath for 10 seconds or as long as possible. *This allows the aerosol to reach deeper airways.*
- Remove the inhaler from or away from the mouth.
- Exhale slowly through *pursed* lips. *Controlled exhalation keeps the small airways open during exhalation.*

- Repeat the inhalation if ordered. Wait 20 to 30 seconds between inhalations of bronchodilator medications *so the first inhalation has a chance to work and the subsequent dose reaches deeper into the lungs.*
- Following use of the inhaler, rinse mouth with tap water to remove any remaining medication and reduce irritation and risk of infection.
- Clean the MDI mouthpiece after each use. Use mild soap and water, rinse it, and let it air dry before replacing it on the device.
- Store the canister at room temperature. Avoid extremes of temperature.
- Report adverse reactions such as restlessness, palpitations, nervousness, or rash to the physician.
- Many MDIs contain steroids for an anti-inflammatory effect. Prolonged use increases the risk of fungal infections in the mouth, indicating a need for attentive mouth care.

If two inhalers are to be used, the bronchodilator medication (which opens the airways) should be given prior to other medications. Bower (2005) recommends the use of the mnemonic *B before C* to remember bronchodilator before corticosteroid.

Inhaled steroids may not be correctly used by clients because they do not associate these medications with immediate symptom relief. The bronchodilators act to open the airways in the short term. However, it is the inhaled steroids that act as "chemical Band-Aids" to keep airway inflammation under control.

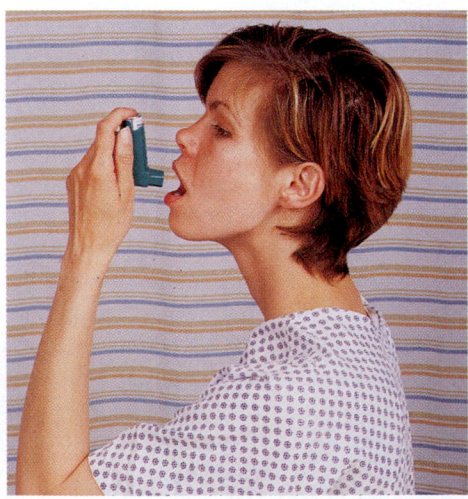

Figure 23–39 ◉ Inhaler positioned away from the open mouth.

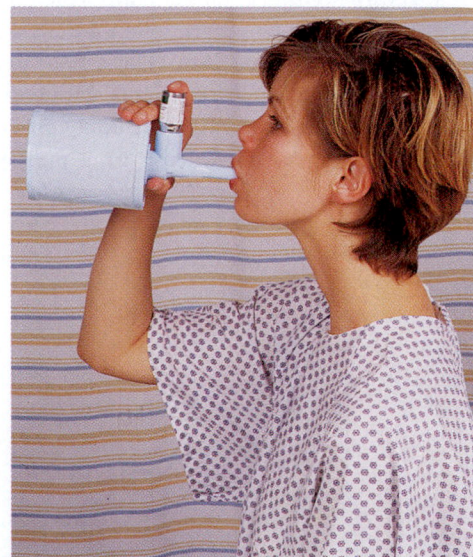

Figure 23–40 ◉ An extender spacer attached to a mouthpiece placed in the mouth.

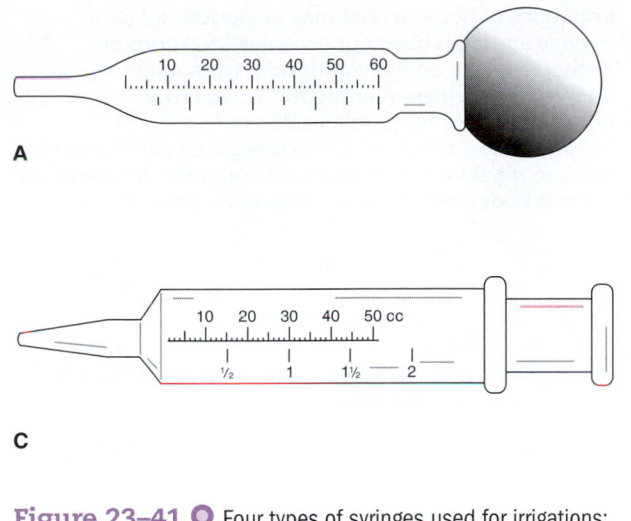

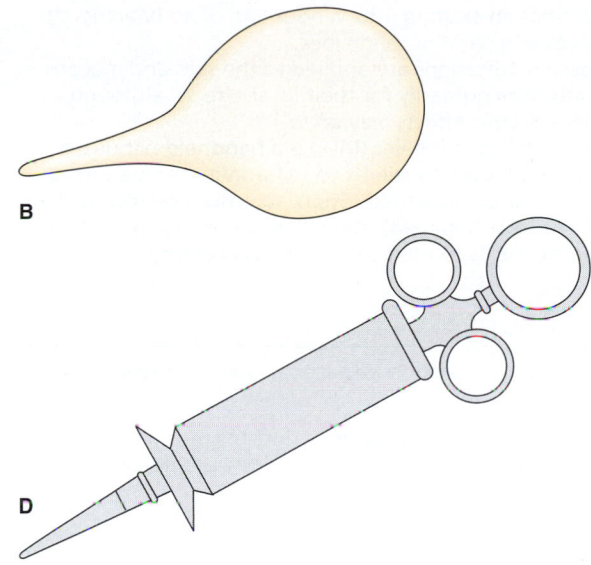

Figure 23–41 ⬤ Four types of syringes used for irrigations: *A*, Asepto; *B*, rubber bulb; *C*, piston syringe; *D*, Pomeroy.

CHAPTER HIGHLIGHTS

- Federal drug legislation regulates the production, prescription, distribution, and administration of drugs.
- Nursing practice acts define limits on the nurse's responsibilities regarding medications.
- Medications have several names. Nurses need to know the generic and trade names of a medication and be aware of both its therapeutic and side effects.
- Adverse effects of medications include drug toxicity, drug allergy, drug tolerance, idiosyncratic effect, and drug interactions.
- Several factors other than the drug itself can affect its action. These include pregnancy; age; gender; cultural, ethnic, and genetic factors; diet; client environment; psychologic factors; illness and disease; and time of administration.
- Various routes are used to administer medications: oral, sublingual, buccal, parenteral, topical, or via a nasogastric or gastrostomy tube. When administering a medication, the nurse must ensure that it is appropriate for the route specified.
- Medication orders must include the client name, date and time the order is written, name of the medication, dosage, route, frequency of administration, and signature of the person writing the order. Nurses must question any unclear orders before implementing the order.
- Telephone or verbal orders must be cosigned by the primary care provider within a time specified by agency policy (usually 24 to 48 hours).
- Three systems of measurement are used in North America: the metric system, the apothecaries' system, and the household system. Weights and measures may need to be converted by the nurse within these three systems.
- Several formulas can be used to calculate dosages. Pediatric dosages are calculated by the child's weight or body surface area.
- Nurses must always assess a client's physical status before giving any medication and obtain a medication history.
- Medication reconciliation is another method that the nurse uses to ensure that clients receive the appropriate

medications and dosages. Three important areas for medication reconciliation to occur are (a) on admission, (b) during shift reports, transfers, and with new medication orders, and (c) upon discharge.
- When administering medications the nurse observes specified "rights" to ensure accurate administration. When preparing medications, the nurse checks the medication container label against the medication administration record (MAR) three times.
- The nurse who prepares the medication administers it and must never leave a prepared medication unattended.
- The nurse always identifies the client appropriately before administering a medication and stays with the client until the medication is taken.
- Medications, once given, are documented as soon as possible after administration.
- Medications given parenterally act more quickly than those given orally or topically and must be prepared using sterile technique.
- When preparing two insulins to be mixed in the same syringe, a vial of unmodified insulin should never be contaminated with modified insulin.
- Proper site selection is essential for an intramuscular injection to prevent tissue, bone, and nerve damage. The nurse should always palpate anatomic landmarks when selecting a site.
- The Z-track method for intramuscular injection is recommended to prevent discomfort caused by leakage of irritating or staining medication into subcutaneous tissues.
- Clients receiving a series of injections should have the injection sites rotated.
- After use, needles should *not* be recapped but must be placed in puncture-resistant containers.
- Intravenous medications can be administered by various methods: in a large-volume infusion of intravenous fluid, by intermittent intravenous infusion, by volume-controlled infusion, by intravenous push (IVP) or bolus, or by intermittent venous access. In all of these methods the

client has an existing intravenous line or an IV access site such as a heparin or saline lock.
- Topical medications are applied to the skin and mucous membranes primarily for their local effects, although some systemic effects may occur.
- A metered-dose inhaler (MDI) is a handheld nebulizer that can be used by clients to self-administer measured doses of an aerosol medication. To ensure correct delivery of the prescribed medication by MDIs, nurses need to instruct clients to use aerosol inhalers correctly.

- Irrigations of body cavities may be performed (a) to remove a foreign object or excessive secretions or discharge, (b) to apply heat or cold, (c) to apply a medication, such as an antiseptic, (d) to reduce inflammation, or (e) to relieve discomfort.
- Surgical asepsis for an irrigation is required when there is a break in the skin (e.g., in a wound irrigation), or whenever a sterile body cavity (e.g., the bladder) is entered.

THINK ABOUT IT

Refer to the chapter-opening scenario and answer these questions.

1. When preparing the IM injection of ampicillin, which vial of medication will she choose, and how many mL will she prepare?

2. Evaluate Brittany's medication administration practice. What practices performed by Brittany are safe medication practices?

3. What practices performed by Brittany could potentially result in medication errors?

∞ *See suggested responses to Think About It on MyNursingKit.*

TEST YOUR KNOWLEDGE

1. A client tells the nurse, "This pill is a different color than the one that I usually take at home." Which is the best response by the nurse?
   1. "You can take this. Manufacturers of generic drugs sometimes make medications in different colors."
   2. "I will recheck your medication orders."
   3. "Maybe the doctor ordered a different medication."
   4. "I'll leave the pill here while I check with the doctor."

2. If the following medications are listed on a client's medication administration record (MAR), which one should the nurse question?
   1. Lasix 40 mg, po, STAT
   2. Ampicillin 500 mg, q 6 hr, IVPB
   3. Humulin L (Lente) insulin 36 units, subcutaneous, q am, ac.
   4. Codeine q 4–6 hr, po, prn for pain.

3. The primary care provider prescribed 5 mL of a medication to be given deep IM for a 40-year-old female who is 5'7" tall and weighs 135 pounds. Which of the following is the most appropriate method of administration?
   1. A tuberculin syringe, #25–#27 gauge, 1/4- to 5/8-inch needle
   2. Two 3-mL syringes, #20–#23 gauge, 1 1/2-inch needle
   3. Two 2-mL syringes, #25 gauge, 5/8-inch needle
   4. Two 2-mL syringes, #20–#23 gauge, 1-inch needle

4. The nurse is to administer 0.75 mL of medication sub-cutaneously in the upper arm to a 50-year-old 300-pound client. The nurse can grasp approximately 2 inches of the client's tissue at the upper arm. Which of the following is the most appropriate for the nurse to use?
   1. A tuberculin syringe, #25–#27 gauge, 1/4- to 5/8-inch needle
   2. Two 3-mL syringes, #20–#23 gauge, 1 1/2-inch needle
   3. 1-mL syringe, #25 gauge, 5/8-inch needle
   4. 1-mL syringe, #20--#23 gauge, 1-inch needle

5. The nurse is to administer a tuberculin test to a 22-year-old male who is 6 feet tall and weighs 180 pounds. Which of the following is the most appropriate for the nurse to use?
   1. A tuberculin syringe, #25–#27 gauge, 1/4- to 5/8-inch needle
   2. Two 3-mL syringes, #20–#23 gauge, 1 1/2-inch needle
   3. 2-mL syringe, #25 gauge, 5/8-inch needle
   4. 2-mL syringe, #20–#23 gauge, 1-inch needle

6. The nurse is to administer 0.5 mL of a medication by IM injection to an older emaciated client. Which of the following is the most appropriate site for the nurse to use?
   1. Ventrogluteal
   2. Deltoid
   3. Abdomen
   4. Outer aspect of the upper arm

7. An older adult client with renal insufficiency is to receive a cardiac medication. The nurse is most likely to receive an order to administer which of the following?
   1. A decreased dosage
   2. The standard dosage
   3. An increased dosage
   4. Divided dosages

8. Proper administration of an otic medication to a 2-year-old client includes which of the following nursing action?
   1. Pull the ear straight back
   2. Pull the ear down and back
   3. Pull the ear up and back
   4. Pull the ear straight upward

9. A primary care provider writes a prescription for 0.15 milligrams of digoxin intravenously every day. The medication is available in a concentration of 400 micrograms per mL. How many mL will the nurse administer? _____

10. A student nurse is preparing to administer insulin to a client with diabetes. Indicate the correct order for the administration of this medication:

1. Cleanse the site with alcohol.
2. Insert the needle quickly into the subcutaneous tissue.
3. Prepare the insulin in the correct syringe.
4. Assess the site chosen for the injection.
5. Pinch the skin lightly.
6. Inject the medication.
7. Count to five.
8. Remove the syringe.
   Correct sequence: _____

∞ *See Answers to Test Your Knowledge in Appendix A.*

EXPLORE PEARSON **mynursingkit™**

MyNursingKit is your one stop for online chapter review materials and resources. Prepare for success with additional NCLEX®-style practice questions, interactive assignments and activities, web links, animations and videos, and more!

Register your access code from the front of your book at
www.mynursingkit.com.

REFERENCES AND SELECTED BIBLIOGRAPHY

Abrams, A. C. (2009). *Clinical drug therapy: Rationales for nursing practice* (8th ed.). Philadelphia: Lippincott Williams & Wilkins.

Adams, M. P., Josephson, D. L., & Holland, L. N. (2005). *Pharmacology for nurses: A pathophysiologic approach*. Upper Saddle River, NJ: Pearson Prentice Hall.

American Diabetes Association. (2004). Insulin administration. *Diabetes Care, 27*(1), S106–S109.

Barr, D. H., & Thomas, C. H. (2005). Is aspiration necessary during intramuscular injection? *Advance Online Editions for Nurses 7*(18), 27.

Bastable, S. B. (2008). *Nurse as educator* (3rd ed.). Boston: Jones & Bartlett.

Bindler, R. C., & Ball, J. W. (2007). *Clinical skills manual for pediatric nursing: Caring for children* (4th ed.). Upper Saddle River, NJ: Prentice Hall.

Bolander V. R. (1994). *Sorenson and Luckmann's Basic Nursing, a Psycho Physiological Approach*, 3rd ed. Saunders, Philadelphia, PA.

Bower, L. M. (2005). Is your patient's metered-dose inhaler technique up to snuff? *Nursing, 35*(8), 50–51.

Bunce, M. (2003). Troubleshooting central lines. *RN, 66*(12), 28–34.

Burke, K. G. (2005). The state of the science on safe medication administration symposium. *American Journal of Nursing, 105*(3), 73–78.

Chapin, G., & Welk, P. C. (1985). How safe is the air bubble technique for IM injections. *Nursing, 15*(9), 59.

Cohen, H., Robinson, E. S., & Mandrack, M. (2003). Getting to the root of medication errors: Survey results. *Nursing, 33*(9), 36–45.

Cohen, M. R. (2005). Reconciling medications: Safeguarding transitions. *Nursing, 35*(7), 14.

Douglas, J., & Larrabee, S. (2003). Bring barcoding to the bedside. *Nursing Management, 34*(5), 36–40.

Greenway, K. (2004). Using the ventrogluteal site for intramuscular injection. *Nursing Standard, 18*(25), 39–42.

Grissinger, M., & Globus, N. J. (2004). Technology affects your risk of medication errors. *Nursing, 34*(1), 36–42.

Hughes, R. G., & Edgerton, E. A. (2005). Reducing pediatric medication errors. *American Journal of Nursing, 105*(5), 79–91.

Institute for Healthcare Improvement (IHI). (n.d.). *Reconcile medications at all transition points*. Retrieved June 18, 2006, from

http://www.ihi.org/IHI/Topics/PatientSafety/MedicationSystems/Changes/Reconcile+Medications+at+All+Transition+Points.htm

Joint Commission on Accreditation of Healthcare Organizations. (2009). *Official do not use abbreviations list*. Retrieved December 6, 2009, from http://www.jointcommission.org/NR/rdonlyres/2329F8F5-6EC5-4E21-B932-54B2B7D53F00/0/06_dnu_list.pdf

Joint Commission on Accreditation of Healthcare Organizations. (2006). *2007 hospital/critical access hospital national patient safety goals*. Retrieved June 18, 2006, from http://www.jointcommission.org/PatientSafety/NationalPatientSafetyGoals/07_hap_cah_npsgs.htm

Karch, A. (2004). What's wrong with U? *American Journal of Nursing, 104*(6), 65–66.

Kennedy, S. (2005). To err is not surprising. *American Journal of Nursing, 105*(6), 19.

Ketchum, K., Grass, C. A., & Padwojski, A. (2005). Medication reconciliation. *American Journal of Nursing, 105*(11), 78–85.

Lafleur, K. J. (2004). Tackling med errors with technology. *RN, 67*(5), 29–35.

Lea, D. H. (2005). Tailoring drug therapy with pharmacogenetics. *Nursing, 35*(4), 22–23.

Macdonald, F. (2004). Iatrogenic prescribing in acute care: Learning from our mistakes. *Journal of Gerontological Nursing, 34,* 20–25.

Manno, M. S., & Hayes, D. D. (2006). Best-practice interventions: How medication reconciliation saves lives. *Nursing, 36*(3), 63.

McErlane, K. (2005). Keeping track of the patch. *American Journal of Nursing, 105*(6), 36–37.

Molony, S. L. (2003). Beers' criteria for potentially inappropriate medication use in the elderly. *Journal of Gerontological Nursing, 29*(11), 6–7.

Munoz, C., & Hilgenberg, C. (2005). Ethnopharmacology. *American Journal of Nursing, 105*(8), 40–48.

Nelson, R. (2004). Needlestick injuries: Going but not gone? *American Journal of Nursing, 104*(11), 25–26.

Nicoll, L. H., & Hesby, A. (2002). Intramuscular injection: An integrative research review and guideline for evidence-based practice. *Applied Nursing Research, 16*(2), 149–162.

Pape, T. M., Guerra, D. M., Muzquiz, M., Bryant, J. B., Ingram, M., Schranner, B., et al. (2005). Innovative approaches to reducing nurses' distraction during medication administra-

tion. *Journal of Continuing Education in Nursing, 36*(3), 108–116.

Perry, J., & Jagger, J. (2005). Sharps safety update: "Are we there yet?" *Nursing, 35*(6), 17.

Perry, J., Robinson, E. S., & Jagger, J. (2004). Needle-stick and sharps-safety survey. *Nursing, 34*(4), 43–47.

Preston, S. T., & Hegadoren, K. (2004). Glass contamination in parenterally administered medication. *Journal of Advanced Nursing, 48*(3), 266–270.

Prettyman, J. (2005). Subcutaneous or intramuscular? Confronting a parenteral administration dilemma. *Medsurg Nursing, 14*(2), 93–99.

Przybycien, P. (2005). *Safe meds*. St. Louis: Elsevier Mosby.

Pullen, R. L. (2005). Administering medication by the z-track method. *Nursing, 35*(7), 24.

Roark, D. C. (2004). Bar codes and drug administration. *American Journal of Nursing, 104*(1), 63–66.

Robbins, B., Rausch, K. J., Garcia, R. I., & Prestwood, K. W. (2004). Multicultural medication adherence: A comparative study. *Journal of Gerontological Nursing, 30*(7), 25–32.

Rodger, M., & King, L. (2000). Drawing up and administering intramuscular injections: a review of the literature. *Journal of Advanced Nursing, 31*(3), 574–582.

Rosdahl C.B. (1995) *Textbook of Basic Nursing*, 6th edn. Lippincott, Philadelphia, PA.

Rushing, J. (2004). How to administer a subcutaneous injection. *Nursing, 34*(6), 32.

Schlenk, E. A., Dunbar-Jacob, J., & Engberg, S. (2004). Medication non-adherence among older adults. *Journal of Gerontological Nursing, 35,* 33–43.

Small, S. P. (2004). Preventing sciatic nerve injury from intramuscular injections: Literature review. *Journal of Advanced Nursing, 47*(3), 287–296.

Tarnow, K., & King, N. (2004). Intradermal injections: Traditional bevel up versus bevel down. *Applied Nursing Research, 17*(4), 275–282.

Woods, A. (2003). How to use your medicine safely. *Nursing, 33*(12), 50–51.

Wooten, J., & Galavis, J. (2005). Polypharmacy: Keeping the elderly safe. *RN, 68*(8), 45–50.

Zaybak, A., & Khorshid, L. (2007). A study on the effect of the duration of subcutaneous heparin injection on bruising and pain. *Journal of Clinical Nursing, 17*(3), 378–386.

Skin Integrity and Wound Care

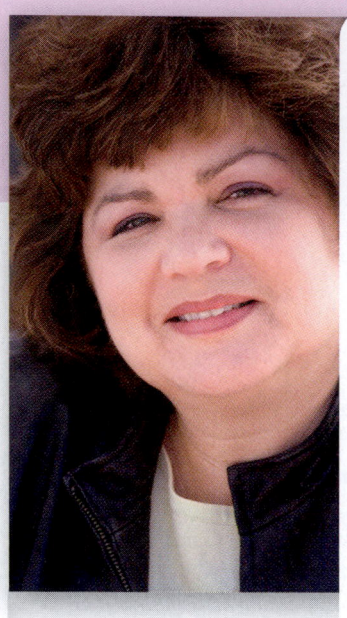

Kate Cassidy, 42 years old, is an obese woman admitted to the acute care facility for surgery to remove her gallbladder. She is not a candidate for laparoscopic surgery because of past surgeries that resulted in adhesions. Postoperatively she returns to the surgical floor with a Jackson Pratt wound vac and a medial abdominal wound with both staples and sutures. The surgeon orders her to be NPO until bowel sounds resume. Morphine sulfate is administered via patient-controlled anesthesia. Three days after surgery the nurse notes purulent drainage from the abdominal wound. Upon changing the dressing, the nurse notes that a 2 cm area on the inferior aspect of the incision is red, warm to touch, and edematous, and the client is reporting increased pain.

LEARNING OUTCOMES

After completing this chapter, you will be able to:

1. Identify factors that place specific clients at increased risk for alterations in skin integrity.

2. Differentiate the four stages of pressure ulcer development.

3. Contrast primary and secondary wound healing and describe situations in which each may be anticipated.

4. Describe the four phases of wound healing with appropriate assessment findings.

5. Identify the three major types of wound exudate.

6. Categorize the main complications of wound healing and the factors that may contribute.

7. Create a plan of care for clients with various types of wounds using each step of the nursing process.

8. Propose both independent and collaborative nursing interventions that could be employed to prevent or resolve a client's wounds and support wound healing.

9. Compare and contrast types of commonly used wound dressings, bandages, and binders according to purpose, situations in which they may be useful, and the nursing care required.

10. Explain the physiologic responses to, the purposes of, and the techniques for applying heat and cold applications.

KEY TERMS

Approximated p715
Bandage p731
Binder p733
Collagen p718

Compress p737
Debridement p726
Decubitus ulcer p714
Dehiscence p719

Eschar p718
Evisceration p719
Excoriation p714
Exudate p719

Fibrin p718
Granulation tissue p718
Hematoma p719
Hemorrhagic exudate p719

The skin is the largest organ in the body and serves a variety of important functions in maintaining health and protecting the individual from injury. Important nursing functions are maintaining skin integrity and promoting wound healing. Impaired skin integrity is not a frequent problem for most healthy people but is a threat to older adults; to clients with restricted mobility, chronic illnesses, malnutrition, or trauma; and to those undergoing invasive health care procedures. To protect the skin and manage wounds effectively, the nurse must understand the factors affecting skin integrity, the physiology of wound healing, and specific measures that promote optimal skin conditions.

SKIN INTEGRITY

Intact skin refers to the presence of normal skin and skin layers uninterrupted by wounds. Chapter 17 ∞ provides details regarding physical examination of the integumentary system. The appearance of the skin and skin integrity are influenced by internal factors such as genetics, age, and the underlying health of the individual as well as external factors such as activity.

Genetics and heredity determine many aspects of a person's skin. Age influences skin integrity in that the skin of both the very young and the very old is more fragile and susceptible to injury. Wounds tend to heal more rapidly in infants and children.

Many chronic illnesses and their treatments affect skin integrity. Some medications cause thinning of the skin and allow it to be much more readily harmed. Many medications increase sensitivity to sunlight and can predispose one to severe sunburns. Poor nutrition can interfere with the appearance and function of normal skin.

TYPES OF WOUNDS

Body wounds are either intentional or unintentional. Intentional trauma occurs during therapy. Unintentional wounds are accidental. If the tissues are traumatized without a break in the skin, the wound is closed. The wound is open when the skin or mucous membrane surface is broken.

Wounds may be described according to how they are acquired (see Table 24–1). They also can be described according to the likelihood and degree of wound contamination.

- *Clean wounds* are uninfected wounds in which minimal inflammation is encountered and the respiratory, alimentary, genital, and urinary tracts are not entered. Clean wounds are primarily closed wounds.
- *Clean-contaminated wounds* are surgical wounds in which the respiratory, alimentary, genital, or urinary tract has been entered. Such wounds show no evidence of infection.
- *Contaminated wounds* include open, fresh, accidental wounds and surgical wounds involving a major break in sterile technique or a large amount of spillage from the gastrointestinal tract. Contaminated wounds show evidence of inflammation.

TABLE 24–1	**Types of Wounds**	
TYPE	CAUSE	DESCRIPTION AND CHARACTERISTICS
Incision	Sharp instrument (e.g., knife or scalpel)	Open wound; deep or shallow
Contusion	Blow from a blunt instrument	Closed wound, skin appears ecchymotic (bruised) because of damaged blood vessels
Abrasion	Surface scrape, either unintentional (e.g., scraped knee from a fall) or intentional (e.g., dermal abrasion to remove pockmarks)	Open wound involving the skin
Puncture	Penetration of the skin and often the underlying tissues by a sharp instrument, either intentional or unintentional	Open wound
Laceration	Tissues torn apart, often from accidents (e.g., with machinery)	Open wound; edges are often jagged
Penetrating wound	Penetration of the skin and the underlying tissues, usually unintentional (e.g., from a bullet or metal fragments)	Open wound

- *Dirty* or *infected wounds* include wounds containing dead tissue and wounds with evidence of a clinical infection, such as purulent drainage.

Wounds, excluding pressure ulcers and burns, are classified by depth, that is, the tissue layers involved in the wound.

PRESSURE ULCERS

Pressure ulcers were previously called **decubitus ulcers**, *pressure sores,* or *bedsores.* A pressure ulcer is any lesion caused by unrelieved pressure (a compressing downward force on a body area) that results in damage to underlying tissue, as defined by the U.S. Public Health Service's Panel for the Prediction and Prevention of Pressure Ulcers in Adults (PPPPUA, 1992b).

Pressure ulcers are a problem in both acute care settings and long-term care settings, including homes. The best estimate of the incidence of pressure ulcers in hospital settings between 2000 and 2004 was 7% to 9% (Whittington & Briones, 2004). *Healthy People 2010* has established the objective of reducing the prevalence of pressure ulcers in nursing homes by 50%—from 16 per 1000 residents reported in 1997 to 8 per 1000.

Etiology of Pressure Ulcers

Pressure ulcers are due to localized **ischemia**, a deficiency in the blood supply to the tissue. The tissue is compressed between two surfaces, usually the surface of the bed and the bony skeleton, with greater than 32 mm Hg pressure. When blood cannot reach the tissue, the cells are deprived of oxygen and nutrients, the waste products of metabolism accumulate in the cells, and the tissue consequently dies. Prolonged, unrelieved pressure also damages the small blood vessels.

After the skin has been compressed, it appears pale, as if the blood had been squeezed out of it. When pressure is relieved, the skin takes on a bright red flush, called **reactive hyperemia**. The flush is due to vasodilation, a process in which extra blood floods to the area to compensate for the preceding period of impeded blood flow. Reactive hyperemia usually lasts one-half to three-quarters as long as the duration of impeded blood flow to the area (PPPPUA, 1992a). If the redness disappears in that time, no tissue damage can be anticipated. If, however, the redness does not disappear, then tissue damage has occurred.

Risk Factors

Several factors contribute to the formation of pressure ulcers: immobility and inactivity, inadequate nutrition, fecal and urinary incontinence, decreased mental status, diminished sensation, excessive body heat, advanced age, and the presence of certain chronic conditions.

FRICTION AND SHEARING Two other factors frequently act in conjunction with pressure to produce pressure ulcers: friction and shearing force. Friction is a force acting parallel to the skin surface. Friction can abrade the skin, that is, remove the superficial layers, making it more prone to breakdown.

Shearing force is a combination of friction and pressure. It occurs commonly when a client assumes a Fowler's position in bed. In this position, the body tends to slide downward toward the foot of the bed. This downward movement is transmitted to the sacral bone and the deep tissues. At the same time, the skin over the sacrum tends not to move because of the adherence between the skin and the bed linens. The skin and superficial tissues are thus relatively unmoving in relation to the bed surface, whereas the deeper tissues are firmly attached to the skeleton and move downward. This causes a shearing force in the area where the deeper tissues and the superficial tissues meet. The force damages the blood vessels and tissues in this area.

IMMOBILITY Immobility refers to a reduction in the amount and control of movement a person has. Normally people move when they experience discomfort due to pressure on an area of the body. Healthy people rarely exceed their tolerance to pressure. However, paralysis, extreme weakness, pain, or any cause of decreased activity can hinder a person's ability to change positions independently and relieve the pressure, even if the person can perceive the pressure.

INADEQUATE NUTRITION Prolonged inadequate nutrition causes weight loss, muscle atrophy, and the loss of subcutaneous tissue. These three reduce the amount of padding between the skin and the bones, thus increasing the risk of pressure ulcer development. More specifically, inadequate intake of protein, carbohydrates, fluids, zinc, and vitamin C contributes to pressure ulcer formation.

Hypoproteinemia (abnormally low protein content in the blood), due either to inadequate intake or abnormal loss, predisposes the client to dependent edema. Edema (the presence of excess interstitial fluid) makes skin more prone to injury by decreasing its elasticity, resilience, and vitality. Edema increases the distance between the capillaries and the cells, thereby slowing the diffusion of oxygen to the tissue cells and of metabolites away from the cells.

FECAL AND URINARY INCONTINENCE Moisture from incontinence promotes skin **maceration** (tissue softened by prolonged wetting or soaking) and makes the epidermis more easily eroded and susceptible to injury. Digestive enzymes in feces, gastric tube drainage, and urea in urine also contribute to skin **excoriation** (area of loss of the superficial layers of the skin also known as *denuded* area). Any accumulation of secretions or excretions (including blood) is irritating to the skin, harbors microorganisms, and makes an individual prone to skin breakdown and infection.

DECREASED MENTAL STATUS Individuals with a reduced level of awareness are at risk for pressure ulcers because they are less able to recognize and respond to pain associated with prolonged pressure.

DIMINISHED SENSATION Loss of sensation reduces a person's ability to respond to trauma, to injurious heat and cold, and to the tingling ("pins and needles") that signals loss of circulation. Sensory loss also impairs the body's ability to recognize and provide healing mechanisms for a wound.

EXCESSIVE BODY HEAT Body heat is another factor in the development of pressure ulcers. An elevated body temperature increases the metabolic rate, thus increasing the cells' need for oxygen. This increased need is particularly severe in the cells of an area under pressure, which are already oxygen deficient. Severe infections with accompanying elevated body temperatures may affect the body's ability to deal with the effects of tissue compression.

ADVANCED AGE The aging process brings about several changes in the skin and its supporting structures, making the older person more prone to impaired skin integrity. These changes include the following:

- Loss of lean body mass
- Generalized thinning of the epidermis
- Decreased strength and elasticity of the skin due to changes in the collagen fibers of the dermis
- Increased dryness due to a decrease in the amount of oil produced by the sebaceous glands
- Diminished pain perception due to a reduction in the number of cutaneous end organs responsible for the sensation of pressure and light touch
- Diminished venous and arterial flow due to aging vascular walls

CHRONIC MEDICAL CONDITIONS Certain chronic conditions such as diabetes and cardiovascular disease are risk factors for skin breakdown and delayed healing. These conditions compromise oxygen delivery to tissues by poor perfusion and thus cause poor and delayed healing and increase risk of pressure sores.

OTHER FACTORS Other factors contributing to the formation of pressure ulcers are poor lifting and transferring techniques, incorrect positioning, hard support surfaces, and incorrect application of pressure-relieving devices.

Stages of Pressure Ulcers

The four recognized stages of pressure ulcers related to observable tissue damage are shown in Figure 24–1.

RISK ASSESSMENT TOOLS Although clients may be at risk for developing a number of different alterations in skin integrity, the most common and most preventable are pressure ulcers. Several risk assessment tools are available that provide the nurse with systematic means of identifying clients at high risk for pressure ulcer development. The PPPPUA (1992a) has recommended that the tool include data collection in the areas of immobility, incontinence, nutrition, and level of consciousness.

In 1987, Bergstrom, Braden, Laguzza, and Holman published the Braden Scale for Predicting Pressure Sore Risk. Their scale consists of six subscales: sensory percep-

tion, moisture, activity, mobility, nutrition, and friction and shear (see Figure 24–2). A total of 23 points is possible. An adult who scores below 18 points is considered at risk (Folkedahl & Frantz, 2002b). For best results, nurses should be trained in proper use of the scale.

Norton's Pressure Area Risk Assessment Form Scale (Table 24–2) includes the categories of general physical condition, mental state, activity, mobility, and incontinence. A category of medications was added in 1987, resulting in a possible score of 24. Scores of 15 or 16 should be viewed as indicators, not predictors, of risk. The Braden and Norton tools should be used when the client first enters the health care agency and whenever the client's condition changes. In some long-term care facilities, a risk assessment scale such as the Braden or Norton scale is done on admission and then on a regular basis, usually weekly. This increases awareness of specific risk factors and serves as assessment data from which to plan goals and interventions to either maintain or improve skin integrity.

> ### CLINICAL ALERT
>
> The two validated assessment tools supported by the PPPPUA are the Braden scale and the Norton scale.

WOUND HEALING

Healing is a quality of living tissue; it is also referred to as **regeneration** (renewal) of tissues. Healing can be considered in terms of *types of healing,* having to do with the caregiver's decision on whether to allow the wound to seal itself or to purposefully close the wound, and *phases of healing,* which refer to the steps in the body's natural processes of tissue repair. The phases are the same for all wounds, but the rate of healing depends on factors such as the type of healing, the location and size of the wound, and the health of the client.

Types of Wound Healing

There are two types of healing, influenced by the amount of tissue loss. **Primary intention healing** occurs where the tissue surfaces have been **approximated** (closed) and there is minimal or no tissue loss; it is characterized by the formation of minimal granulation tissue and scarring. It is also called *primary union* or *first intention healing.* An example of wound healing by primary intention is a closed surgical incision.

A wound that is extensive and involves considerable tissue loss, and in which the edges cannot or should not be approximated, heals by **secondary intention healing**. An example of wound healing by secondary intention is a pressure ulcer. Secondary intention healing differs from primary intention healing in three ways: (a) The repair time is longer, (b) the scarring is greater, and (c) the susceptibility to infection is greater.

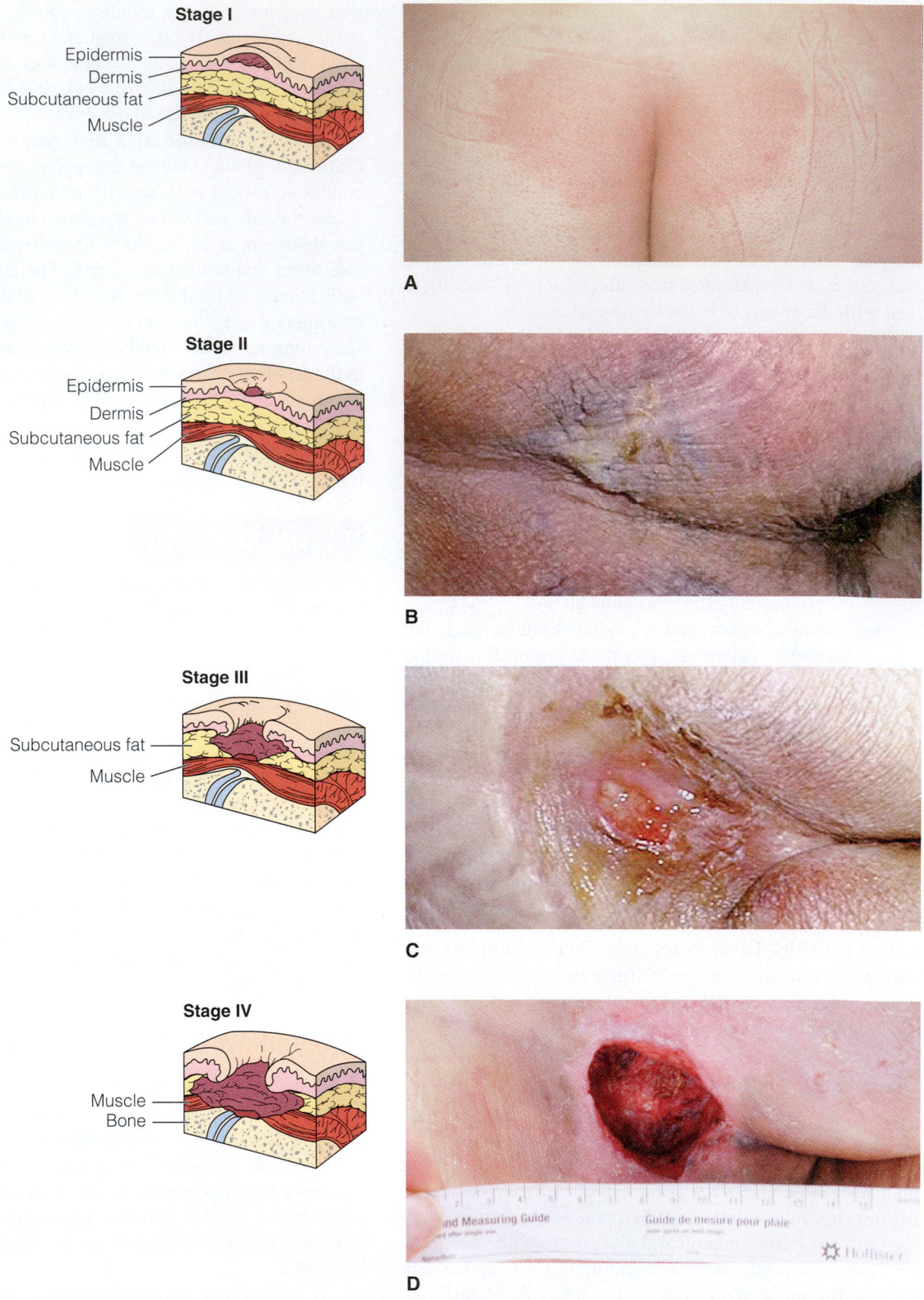

Figure 24–1 ○ Four stages of pressure ulcers. **A,** stage I: nonblanchable erythema signaling potential ulceration; **B,** stage II: partial-thickness skin loss (abrasion, blister, or shallow crater) involving the epidermis and possibly the dermis; **C,** stage III: full-thickness skin loss involving damage or necrosis of subcutaneous tissue that may extend down to, but not through, underlying fascia. The ulcer presents clinically as a deep crater with or without undermining of adjacent tissue; **D,** stage IV: full-thickness skin loss with tissue necrosis or damage to muscle, bone, or supporting structures, such as a tendon or joint capsule. Undermining and sinus tracts may also be present.

Source: Line art from "Clinical Practice Guideline, Pressure Ulcers in Adults: Prediction and Prevention," by U.S. Department of Health and Human Services, PPPPUA Pub. No. 92-0047, pp. 16–17, 1992, Rockville, MD: Public Health Service. Photos from Cory Patrick Hartley, RN.

BRADEN SCALE FOR PREDICTING PRESSURE SORE RISK

Patient's Name _____   Evaluator's Name _____   Date of Assessment _____

SENSORY PERCEPTION Ability to respond meaningfully to pressure-related discomfort	**1. Completely Limited:** Unresponsive (does not moan, flinch, or grasp) to painful stimuli, due to diminished level of consciousness or sedation, OR limited ability to feel pain over most of body surface.	**2. Very Limited:** Responds only to painful stimuli. Cannot communicate discomfort except by moaning or restlessness, OR has a sensory impairment which limits the ability to feel pain or discomfort over 1/2 of body.	**3. Slightly Limited:** Responds to verbal commands but cannot always communicate discomfort or need to be turned, OR has some sensory impairment which limits ability to feel pain or discomfort in 1 or 2 extremities.	**4. No Impairment:** Responds to verbal commands. Has no sensory deficit which would limit ability to feel or voice pain or discomfort.
MOISTURE Degree to which skin is exposed to moisture	**1. Constantly Moist:** Skin is kept moist almost constantly by perspiration, urine, etc. Dampness is detected every time patient is moved or turned.	**2. Moist:** Skin is often but not always moist. Linen must be changed at least once a shift.	**3. Occasionally Moist:** Skin is occasionally moist, requiring an extra linen change approximately once a day.	**4. Rarely Moist:** Skin is usually dry; linen requires changing only at routine intervals.
ACTIVITY Degree of physical activity	**1. Bedfast:** Confined to bed.	**2. Chairfast:** Ability to walk severely limited or nonexistent. Cannot bear own weight and/or must be assisted into chair or wheelchair.	**3. Walks Occasionally:** Walks occasionally during day but for very short distances, with or without assistance. Spends majority of each shift in bed or chair.	**4. Walks Frequently:** Walks outside the room at least twice a day and inside room at least once every 2 hours during waking hours.
MOBILITY Ability to change and control body position	**1. Completely Immobile:** Does not make even slight changes in body or extremity position without assistance.	**2. Very Limited:** Makes occasional slight changes in body or extremity position but unable to make frequent or significant changes independently.	**3. Slightly Limited:** Makes frequent though slight changes in body or extremity position independently.	**4. No Limitations:** Makes major and frequent changes in position without assistance.
NUTRITION Usual food intake pattern	**1. Very Poor:** Never eats a complete meal. Rarely eats more than 1/3 of any food offered. Eats 2 servings or less of protein (meat or dairy products) per day. Takes fluids poorly. Does not take a liquid dietary supplement, OR is NPO and/or maintained on clear liquids or IV's for more than 5 days.	**2. Probably Inadequate:** Rarely eats a complete meal and generally eats only about 1/2 of any food offered. Protein intake includes only 3 servings of meat or dairy products per day. Occasionally will take a dietary supplement, OR receives less than optimum amount of liquid diet or tube feeding.	**3. Adequate:** Eats over half of most meals. Eats a total of 4 servings of protein (meat, dairy products) each day. Occasionally will refuse a meal, but will usually take a supplement if offered, OR is on a tube feeding or TPN regimen, which probably meets most of nutritional needs.	**4. Excellent:** Eats most of every meal. Never refuses a meal. Usually eats a total of 4 or more servings of meat and dairy products. Occasionally eats between meals. Does not require supplementation.
FRICTION AND SHEAR	**1. Problem:** Requires moderate to maximum assistance in moving. Complete lifting without sliding against sheets is impossible. Frequently slides down in bed or chair, requiring frequent repositioning with maximum assistance. Spasticity, contractures, or agitation leads to almost constant friction.	**2. Potential Problem:** Moves feebly or requires minimum assistance. During a move skin probably slides to some extent against sheets, chair, restraints, or other devices. Maintains relatively good position in chair or bed most of the time but occasionally slides down.	**3. No Apparent Problem:** Moves in bed and in chair independently and has sufficient muscle strength to lift up completely during move. Maintains good position in bed or chair at all times.	

Total Score _____

Figure 24-2 ● Braden Scale for Predicting Pressure Sore Risk.

Source: From "Clinical Practice Guideline, Pressure Ulcers in Adults: Prediction and Prevention," by U.S. Department of Health and Human Services, PPPPUA Pub No. 92-0047, pp. 16–17, 1992, Rockville, MD: Public Health Service. Copyright © Barbara Braden and Nancy Bergstrom, 1988. Reprinted with permission.

TABLE 24–2 Norton's Pressure Area Risk Assessment Form (Scoring System)

A. GENERAL PHYSICAL CONDITION		B. MENTAL STATE		C. ACTIVITY		D. MOBILITY		E. INCONTINENCE	
Good	4	Alert	4	Ambulatory	4	Full	4	Absent	4
Fair	3	Apathetic	3	Walks with help	3	Slightly limited	3	Occasional	3
Poor	2	Confused	2	Chairbound	2	Very limited	2	Usually urinary	2
Very bad	1	Stuporous	1	Bedfast	1	Immobile	1	Double	1

Note: Reprinted from *An Investigation of Geriatric Nursing Problems in Hospital,* by D. Norton, R. McLaren, and A. N. Exton-Smith, Copyright © 1975, with permission from Elsevier.

Those wounds that are left open for 3 to 5 days to allow edema or infection to resolve or exudate to drain and are then closed with sutures, staples, or adhesive skin closures, heal by **tertiary intention**. This is also called delayed primary intention.

Phases of Wound Healing

Wound healing can be broken down into three phases: inflammatory, proliferative, and maturation or remodeling.

INFLAMMATORY PHASE The inflammatory phase is initiated immediately after injury and lasts 3 to 6 days. Two major processes occur during this phase: hemostasis and phagocytosis.

Hemostasis (the cessation of bleeding) results from vasoconstriction of the larger blood vessels in the affected area, retraction (drawing back) of injured blood vessels, the deposition of **fibrin** (connective tissue), and the formation of blood clots in the area. The blood clots, formed from blood platelets, provide a matrix of fibrin that becomes the framework for cell repair. A scab also forms on the surface of the wound. Consisting of clots and dead and dying tissue, this scab serves to aid hemostasis and inhibit contamination of the wound by microorganisms. Below the scab, epithelial cells migrate into the wound from the edges. The epithelial cells serve as a barrier between the body and the environment, preventing the entry of microorganisms.

The inflammatory phase also involves vascular and cellular responses intended to remove any foreign substances and dead and dying tissues. The blood supply to the wound increases, bringing with it oxygen and nutrients needed in the healing process. The area appears reddened and edematous as a result. Exudate of fluid and cell debris is a normal accumulation and helps cleanse the wound. Overproduction of this exudate and other factors can impair wound healing, especially in chronic wounds (Hanson, Langemo, Thompson, Anderson, & Hunter, 2005).

During cell migration, leukocytes (specifically, neutrophils) move into the interstitial space. These are replaced about 24 hours after injury by macrophages, which arise from the blood monocytes. These macrophages engulf microorganisms and cellular debris by a process known as phagocytosis. The macrophages also secrete an angiogenesis factor (AGF), which stimulates the formation of epithelial buds at the end of injured blood vessels. The microcirculatory network that results sustains the healing process and the wound during its life. This inflammatory response is essential to healing. Measures that impair inflammation, such as steroid medications, can place the healing process at risk.

PROLIFERATIVE PHASE The proliferative phase, the second phase in healing, extends from day 3 or 4 to about day 21 postinjury. Fibroblasts (connective tissue cells), which migrate into the wound starting about 24 hours after injury, begin to synthesize collagen. **Collagen** is a whitish protein substance that adds tensile strength to the wound. As the amount of collagen increases, so does the strength of the wound; thus the chance that the wound will remain closed progressively increases. If the wound is sutured, a raised "healing ridge" appears under the intact suture line. In a wound that is not sutured, the new collagen is often visible.

Capillaries grow across the wound, increasing the blood supply. Fibroblasts move from the bloodstream into the wound, depositing fibrin. As the capillary network develops, the tissue becomes a translucent red color. This tissue, called **granulation tissue**, is fragile and bleeds easily.

When the skin edges of a wound are not sutured, the area must be filled in with granulation tissue. When the granulation tissue matures, marginal epithelial cells migrate to it, proliferating over this connective tissue base to fill the wound. If the wound does not close by epithelialization, the area becomes covered with dried plasma proteins and dead cells. This is called **eschar**. Initially, wounds healing by secondary intention seep blood-tinged (serosanguineous) drainage. Later, if they are not covered by epithelial cells, they become covered with thick, gray, fibrinous tissue that is eventually converted into dense scar tissue.

MATURATION PHASE The maturation phase begins about day 21 and can extend 1 or 2 years after the injury. Fibroblasts continue to synthesize collagen. The collagen fibers themselves, which were initially laid in a haphazard fashion, reorganize into a more orderly structure. During maturation, the wound is remodeled and contracted. The scar becomes stronger but the repaired area is never as strong as the original tissue. In some individuals, particularly dark-skinned persons, an abnormal amount of collagen is laid down. This can result in a hypertrophic scar, or **keloid**.

One method of documenting the progress of healing in pressure ulcers is to use the Pressure Ulcer Scale for Healing (PUSH) tool (National Pressure Ulcer Advisory Panel

[NPUAP], 2003). This well-validated tool assigns scores to the ulcer length, width, amount of exudate, and tissue type. The change in the total score over time can be used as an indication of healing.

Types of Wound Exudate

Exudate is material, such as fluid and cells, which have escaped from blood vessels during the inflammatory process and is deposited in tissue or on tissue surfaces. The nature and amount of exudate vary according to the tissue involved, the intensity and duration of the inflammation, and the presence of microorganisms.

There are three major types of exudate: serous, purulent, and sanguineous (hemorrhagic). A **serous exudate** consists chiefly of serum (the clear portion of the blood) derived from blood and the serous membranes of the body, such as the peritoneum. It looks watery and has few cells. An example is the fluid in a blister from a burn.

A **purulent exudate** is thicker than serous exudate because of the presence of pus, which consists of leukocytes, liquefied dead tissue debris, and dead and living bacteria. The process of pus formation is referred to as **suppuration**, and the bacteria that produce pus are called **pyogenic bacteria**. Not all microorganisms are pyogenic. Purulent exudates vary in color, some acquiring tinges of blue, green, or yellow. The color may depend on the causative organism.

A **sanguineous (hemorrhagic) exudate** consists of large amounts of red blood cells, indicating damage to capillaries that is severe enough to allow the escape of red blood cells from plasma. This type of exudate is frequently seen in open wounds. Mixed types of exudates are often observed. A **serosanguineous** (consisting of clear and blood-tinged drainage) exudate is commonly seen in surgical incisions. A *purosanguineous* discharge (consisting of pus and blood) is often seen in a new wound that is infected.

> ### CLINICAL ALERT
>
> A bright sanguineous exudate indicates fresh bleeding, whereas dark sanguineous exudate denotes older bleeding.

Complications of Wound Healing

Several untoward events can interfere with the healing of a wound. These include hemorrhage, infection, and dehiscence and evisceration.

HEMORRHAGE Some escape of blood from a wound is normal. Hemorrhage (massive bleeding), however, is abnormal. A dislodged clot, a slipped stitch, or erosion of a blood vessel may cause severe bleeding.

Internal hemorrhage may be detected by swelling or distention in the area of the wound and, possibly, by sanguineous drainage from a surgical drain. A primary indicator of internal hemorrhage is the complete blood count, specifically the hemoglobin, hematocrit, and red blood cell count. Some clients will have a **hematoma**, a localized collection of blood underneath the skin that may appear as a reddish blue swelling (bruise). A large hematoma may be dangerous in that it places pressure on blood vessels and can thus obstruct blood flow.

The risk of hemorrhage is greatest during the first 48 hours after surgery. Hemorrhage is an emergency; the nurse should apply pressure dressings to the area and monitor the client's vital signs. In many instances, the client must be taken to the operating room for surgical intervention.

INFECTION Contamination of a wound surface with microorganisms (colonization) is an inevitable result. Because the colonizing organisms compete with new cells for oxygen and nutrition, and because their by-products can interfere with a healthy surface condition, the presence of contamination can impair wound healing and lead to infection. When the microorganisms colonizing the wound multiply excessively or invade tissues, infection occurs. Infection suggested by the presence of a change in wound color, pain, or drainage is confirmed by performing a culture of the wound (see Chapter 20 ∞). Severe infection causes fever and elevated white blood cell count. Clients who are immunosuppressed, such as those with HIV or receiving myelosuppressive treatment for cancer, are especially susceptible to wound infections.

A wound can be infected with microorganisms at the time of injury, during surgery, or postoperatively. Wounds that occur as a result of injury are most likely to be contaminated at the time of injury. Surgery involving the intestines can also result in infection from the microorganisms inside the intestine. Surgical infection is most likely to become apparent 2 to 11 days postoperatively.

DEHISCENCE WITH POSSIBLE EVISCERATION **Dehiscence** is the partial or total rupturing of a sutured wound. Dehiscence usually involves an abdominal wound in which the layers below the skin also separate. **Evisceration** is the protrusion of the internal viscera through an incision. A number of factors, including obesity, poor nutrition, multiple trauma, failure of suturing, excessive coughing, vomiting, and dehydration, heighten a client's risk of wound dehiscence. Wound dehiscence is more likely to occur 4 to 5 days postoperatively before extensive collagen is deposited in the wound.

Sudden straining, such as coughing or sneezing, may precede dehiscence. It is not unusual for a client to feel that "something has given away." When dehiscence or evisceration occurs, the wound should be quickly supported by large sterile dressings soaked in sterile normal saline. Place the client in bed with knees bent to decrease pull on the incision. The surgeon must be notified because immediate surgical repair of the area may be necessary.

Factors Affecting Wound Healing

Characteristics of the individual such as age, nutritional status, lifestyle, and medications influence the speed of wound healing.

BOX 24–1	Factors Inhibiting Wound Healing in Older Adults

- Vascular changes associated with aging, such as atherosclerosis and atrophy of capillaries in the skin, can impair blood flow to the wound.
- Collagen tissue is less flexible, which increases the risk of damage from pressure, friction, and shearing.
- Scar tissue is less elastic.
- Changes in the immune system may reduce the formation of the antibodies and monocytes necessary for wound healing.

- Nutritional deficiencies may reduce the numbers of red blood cells and leukocytes, thus impeding the delivery of oxygen and the inflammatory response essential for wound healing. Oxygen is needed for the synthesis of collagen and the formation of new epithelial cells.
- Having diabetes or cardiovascular disease increases the risk of delayed healing due to impaired oxygen delivery to these tissues.
- Cell renewal is slower, leading to delayed healing.

DEVELOPMENTAL CONSIDERATIONS Healthy children and adults often heal more quickly than older adults, who are more likely to have chronic diseases that hinder healing. Box 24–1 lists factors inhibiting wound healing in older adults.

NUTRITION Wound healing places additional demands on the body. Clients require a diet rich in protein, carbohydrates, lipids, vitamins A and C, and minerals, such as iron, zinc, and copper. Malnourished clients may require time to improve their nutritional status before surgery, if this is possible. Obese clients are at increased risk of wound infection and slower healing because adipose tissue usually has a minimal blood supply.

LIFESTYLE People who exercise regularly tend to have good circulation and because blood brings oxygen and nourishment to the wound, they are more likely to heal quickly. Smoking reduces the amount of functional hemoglobin in the blood, thus limiting the oxygen-carrying capacity of the blood, and constricts arterioles.

MEDICATIONS Anti-inflammatory drugs and antineoplastic agents interfere with healing. Prolonged use of antibiotics may make a person susceptible to wound infection by resistant organisms.

NURSING MANAGEMENT

ASSESSING

Assessment of Skin Integrity

The nurse conducts an examination of the integument as part of a routine assessment and during regular care. Removing barriers to assessment is very important. Antiembolic stockings, braces, or devices must be removed to assess the skin condition underneath.

NURSING HISTORY AND PHYSICAL ASSESSMENT During the review of systems as part of the nursing history, information regarding skin diseases, previous bruising, general skin condition, skin lesions, and usual healing of sores is elicited. Inspection and palpation of the skin focus on determination of skin color distribution, skin turgor, presence of edema, and characteristics of any lesions that are present. Particular attention is paid to skin condition in areas most

likely to break down: in skin folds such as under the breasts, in areas that are frequently moist such as the perineum, and in areas that receive extensive pressure such as the bony prominences. Refer to Chapter 17 ∞ for further detail regarding skin assessment.

Assessment of Wounds

Nurses commonly assess both untreated and treated wounds. Although a pressure ulcer can be categorized as an untreated or treated wound, the specific assessment of pressure ulcers is discussed separately.

UNTREATED WOUNDS Untreated wounds usually are seen shortly after an injury. Guidelines for care follow:

- Control severe bleeding by (a) applying direct pressure over the wound and (b) elevating the involved extremity.
- Prevent infection by (a) cleaning or flushing abrasions or lacerations with normal saline and (b) covering the wound with a clean dressing, if possible (a sterile dressing is preferred). When applying a dressing, wrap the wound tightly enough to apply pressure and approximate the wound edges, if possible. If the first layer of dressing becomes saturated with blood, apply a second layer. Do so without removing the first layer of dressing, because blood clots might be disturbed, resulting in more bleeding.
- Control swelling and pain by applying ice over the wound and surrounding tissues.
- If bleeding is severe or if internal bleeding is suspected, and if emergency equipment is available, assess the client for signs of shock (rapid thready pulse, cold clammy skin, pallor, lowered blood pressure).

TREATED WOUNDS Treated wounds, or sutured wounds, are usually assessed to determine the progress of healing. These wounds may be inspected during changing of a dressing. If the wound itself cannot be directly inspected, the dressing is inspected and other data regarding the wound are assessed.

Assessment of a treated wound involves observation of its appearance, size, drainage, and the presence of swelling, pain, and status of drains or tubes. In some long-term facilities, home care situations, and outpatient clinics, photographs are taken weekly for a visual record of the progress of pressure ulcers and wounds. Other assessments are documented and dated along with the photograph. Details about these assessments and signs of healing for a surgical incision are discussed with surgical wounds in Chapter 25 ∞.

Estimating the amount of wound drainage can be difficult. One recommendation is to describe the degree to which the dressing is saturated. Minimal drainage only stains the dressing, moderate drainage saturates the dressing without leakage prior to scheduled dressing changes, and heavy drainage overflows the dressing prior to scheduled changes (Brown, 2006). These terms, plus the description of the drainage and the amount and type of dressing material used, should be well understood by all care providers.

Sometimes, the wound reaches under the skin surface (called undermining). The edges of the wound around an open center may be raw or appear healed, but the undermining can result in a sinus tract or tunnel that extends the wound many centimeters beyond the main wound surface. To fully assess the size of the wound, the nurse gently explores the undermined area with a thin, flexible probe. Do not use a cotton-tipped swab since it can leave fibers behind in the wound. Once the end of the tract is reached, gently raise the probe so that the bulge created by the end can be seen and its length measured on the skin surface. Sinus tracts are often caused by infection and have significant drainage. They may be treated using antibiotics, irrigation, surgical incision to open and drain the tract, or vacuum therapy for large tracts.

PRESSURE ULCERS When a pressure ulcer is present, the nurse notes the following:

- Location of the ulcer, related to a bony prominence
- Size of ulcer in centimeters (Measure length, width, and depth, beginning with length [head to toe] and then width [side to side]. To measure depth, insert a sterile applicator swab at the deepest part of the wound, and then measure it against a measuring guide.)
- Presence of undermining or sinus tracts, assessed as face on a clock, 12 o'clock as the client's head
- Stage of the ulcer (see Figure 24–1)
- Color of the wound bed and location of necrosis or eschar
- Condition of the wound margins
- Integrity of surrounding skin
- Clinical signs of infection, such as redness, warmth, swelling, pain, odor, and exudate (note color of exudate)

Document the status of the client's skin and wounds on the standard agency form. It is important to be able to determine how these change over time.

LABORATORY DATA Laboratory data can often support the nurse's clinical assessment of the wound's progress in healing. A decreased leukocyte count can delay healing and increase the possibility of infection. A hemoglobin level below normal range indicates poor oxygen delivery to the tissues. Blood coagulation studies are also significant. Prolonged coagulation times can result in excessive blood loss and prolonged clot absorption. Hypercoagulability can lead to intravascular clotting. Intra-arterial clotting can result in a deficient blood supply to the wound area. Serum protein analysis provides an indication of the body's nutritional reserves for rebuilding cells. Albumin is an important indicator of nutritional status. A value below 3.5 g/dL indicates poor nutrition and may increase the risk of poor healing and infection. Wound cultures can either confirm or rule out the presence of infection. Sensitivity studies are helpful in the selection of appropriate antibiotic therapy. The nurse obtains a wound culture whenever an infection is suspected.

DIAGNOSING

The NANDA nursing diagnoses (2009) that relate to clients who have skin wounds or who are at risk for skin breakdown are

- *Risk for Impaired Skin Integrity:* At risk for skin being adversely altered.
- *Impaired Skin Integrity:* Altered epidermis and/or dermis.
- *Impaired Tissue Integrity:* Damage to mucous membrane, corneal, integumentary, or subcutaneous tissues.

Impaired Skin Integrity commonly applies to pressure ulcers and to wounds extending through the epidermis but not through the dermis. *Impaired Tissue Integrity* applies to pressure ulcers and to wounds extending into subcutaneous tissue, muscle, or bone. Examples of clinical applications of these diagnoses using NANDA, NIC, and NOC designations are shown in Identifying Nursing Diagnoses, Outcomes, and Interventions.

Additional nursing diagnoses may be appropriate for clients with existing impaired skin or tissue integrity. Examples of these diagnoses include:

- *Risk for Infection* if the skin impairment is severe, the client is immunosuppressed, or the wound is caused by trauma.
- *Pain* related to nerve involvement within the tissue impairment or as a consequence of procedures used to treat the wound.

PLANNING

The major goals for clients at *Risk for Impaired Skin Integrity* (pressure ulcer development) are to maintain skin integrity and to avoid potential associated risks. Clients with *Impaired Skin Integrity* need goals to demonstrate progressive wound healing and regain intact skin within a specified time frame (see Identifying Nursing Diagnoses, Outcomes, and Interventions).

IMPLEMENTING

Nursing interventions for maintaining skin integrity and wound care involve supporting wound healing, preventing pressure ulcers, treating pressure ulcers, dressing and cleaning wounds, applying heat and cold, and supporting and immobilizing wounds.

IDENTIFYING NURSING DIAGNOSES, OUTCOMES, AND INTERVENTIONS — Clients at Risk for or with Impaired Skin Integrity

Data Cluster Juanita Perez, an 85-year-old, is pale, emaciated, and listless. Weight 90 lb. is incontinent of urine and stool, and is bedridden.

NURSING DIAGNOSIS/DEFINITION	SAMPLE DESIRED OUTCOMES*/ *DEFINITION*	INDICATORS	SELECTED INTERVENTIONS*/ *DEFINITION*	SAMPLE NIC ACTIVITIES
Risk for Impaired Skin Integrity related to incontinence and immobility/*At risk for skin being adversely altered*	Tissue Integrity: Skin and Mucous Membranes [1101]/ *Structural intactness and normal physiological function of skin and mucous membranes*	Mildly compromised • Elasticity None • Skin lesions	Positioning [0840]/*Deliberative placement of the patient or a body part to promote physiological and/or psychological well-being.* Pressure Ulcer Prevention [3540]/ *Prevention of pressure ulcers for an individual at high risk for developing them*	• Explain to the client that she is going to be turned (and how often) • Position in proper body alignment • Place on an appropriate therapeutic mattress or bed • Document skin status at least each shift • Remove moisture from the skin caused by urinary and fecal incontinence • Apply protective barriers such as creams or pads to absorb excess moisture

Data Cluster Matthew Brown, an obese 70-year-old hemiplegic, complains of discomfort in his left heel after attempting to move in bed. Superficial skin abrasion 1.2 cm in diameter present at base of left heel.

Impaired Skin Integrity (stage II pressure ulcer) related to friction/*Altered epidermis and/or dermis*	Wound Healing: Secondary Intention [1103]/*Extent of regeneration of cells and tissues in an open wound*	Substantial • Granulation • Decreased wound size	Pressure Ulcer Care [3520]/*Facilitation of healing in pressure ulcers*	• Cleanse the skin around the ulcer with mild soap and water at least daily • Note characteristics of any drainage • Ensure adequate nutrition • Apply a transparent wound barrier • Use devices on the bed that protect the individual

*The NOC # for desired outcomes and the NIC # for nursing interventions are listed in brackets following the appropriate outcome or intervention. Outcomes, indicators, interventions, and activities selected are only a sample of those suggested by NOC and NIC and should be further individualized for each client.

Supporting Wound Healing

The four major areas in which nurses can help clients develop optimal conditions for wound healing are maintaining moist wound healing, providing sufficient nutrition and hydration, preventing wound infections, and proper positioning.

MOIST WOUND HEALING The dressing and frequency of change should support moist wound bed conditions. Wound beds that are too dry or disturbed too often fail to heal.

NUTRITION AND FLUIDS Clients should be assisted to take in at least 2500 mL of fluids a day unless conditions contraindicate this amount. Although there is no evidence that excessive doses of vitamins or minerals enhance wound healing, adequate amounts are extremely important. The nurse should ensure that clients receive sufficient protein, vitamins C, A, B_1, and B_5, and zinc. Obtaining a registered dietitian consultation for wound healing nutrition is helpful for ensuring that correct supplementation needs are met.

Maintaining Intact Skin

- Discuss relationship between adequate nutrition (especially fluids, protein, vitamins B and C, iron, and calories) and healthy skin.
- Demonstrate appropriate positions for pressure relief.
- Establish a turning or repositioning schedule.
- Demonstrate application of appropriate skin protection agents and devices.
- Instruct to report persistent reddened areas.
- Identify potential sources of skin trauma and means of avoidance.

Promoting Wound Healing

- Discuss importance of adequate nutrition (especially fluids, protein, vitamins B and C, iron, and calories).
- Instruct in wound assessment and provide mechanism for documenting.
- Emphasize principles of asepsis, especially hand hygiene and proper methods of handling used dressings.
- Provide information about signs of wound infection and other complications to report.
- Reinforce appropriate aspects of pressure ulcer prevention.
- Demonstrate wound care techniques such as wound cleansing and dressing changing.
- Discuss pain control measures, if needed.

PREVENTING INFECTION There are two main aspects to controlling wound infection: preventing microorganisms from entering the wound, and preventing the transmission of bloodborne pathogens to or from the client to others. See Chapter 19 ∞ for more information about infection control.

POSITIONING To promote wound healing, clients must be positioned to keep pressure off the wound (sometimes referred to as *off-loading*). Changes of position and transfers can be accomplished without shear or friction damage. In addition to proper positioning, the client should be assisted to be as mobile as possible because activity enhances circulation. If the client cannot move independently, range-of-motion exercises and a turning schedule are implemented.

Preventing Pressure Ulcers

To reduce the likelihood of pressure ulcer development in all clients, the nurse employs a variety of preventive measures to maintain the skin integrity and instructs the client, support people, and caregivers in how to prevent pressure ulcers.

PROVIDING NUTRITION Because an inadequate intake of calories, protein, vitamins, and iron is believed to be a risk factor for pressure ulcer development, nutritional supplements should be considered for nutritionally compromised clients. The diet should be similar to that which supports

wound healing, as discussed earlier. Monitor weight regularly to help assess nutritional status. Pertinent lab work should also be monitored including lymphocyte count, protein (especially albumin), and hemoglobin.

MAINTAINING SKIN HYGIENE Obtain baseline data using the established tool and then reassess the skin at least daily in the hospital and weekly at home. When bathing the client, the nurse should minimize the force and friction applied to the skin, using mild cleansing agents that minimize irritation and dryness and that do not disrupt the skin's "natural barriers." Also, avoid using hot water, which increases skin dryness and irritation. Nurses can minimize dryness by avoiding exposure to cold and low humidity. Dry skin is best treated with moisturizing lotions applied while the skin is moist after bathing. The client's skin should be kept clean and dry and free of irritation and maceration by urine, feces, sweat, or incomplete drying after a bath. Apply skin protection if indicated. Dimethicone-based creams or alcohol-free barrier films are available in liquid, spray, and moist wipe format and are very effective in preventing moisture or drainage from collecting on the skin. In most cases, the nurse can apply these without a primary care provider's order. Petroleum-based creams and ointments are no longer advised related to poor overall skin protection and interference with diaper/ incontinence product absorption.

In addition, massage over bony prominences should be avoided. Traditionally, nurses have used massage to stimulate blood circulation, with the intention of preventing pressure ulcers. However, scientific evidence does not support this belief. In fact, vigorous massage may lead to deep tissue trauma (Folkedahl & Frantz, 2002a; NPUAP, 2001).

AVOIDING SKIN TRAUMA Providing the client with a smooth, firm, and wrinkle-free foundation on which to sit or lie helps prevent skin trauma. To prevent injury due to friction and shearing forces, clients must be positioned, transferred, and turned correctly. For bedridden clients, shearing force can be reduced by elevating the head of the bed to no more than 30 degrees, if this position is not contraindicated by the client's condition. (For example, clients with respiratory disorders may find it easier to breathe in Fowler's position.) When the head of the bed is raised, the skin and superficial fascia stick to the bed linen while the deep fascia and skeleton slide down toward the bottom of the bed. As a result, blood vessels in the sacral area become twisted, and the tissues in the area can become ischemic and necrotic. Baby powder and cornstarch are never used as friction or moisture prevention. These powders create harmful abrasive grit damaging to tissues and are considered a respiratory hazard when airborne. Instead, use moisturizing creams and protective films, such as transparent dressings and alcohol-free barrier films.

Frequent shifts in position, even if only slight, effectively change pressure points. The client should shift weight 10 to 15 degrees every 15 to 30 minutes and, whenever possible, exercise or ambulate to stimulate blood circulation.

When lifting a client to change position, nurses should use a lifting device such as a trapeze rather than dragging the client across or up in bed. The friction that results from dragging the skin against a sheet can cause blisters and abrasions, which may contribute to more extensive tissue damage. Therefore, using devices that lift the client's weight off the bed surface is the method of choice.

Any at-risk client confined to bed—even when a special support mattress is used—should be repositioned at least every 2 hours, depending on the client's need, to allow another body surface to bear the weight. Six body positions can usually be used: prone, supine, right and left lateral (side-lying), and right and left Sims' positions. When a lateral position is used, the nurse should avoid positioning the client directly on the trochanter and instead position the client on a 30-degree angle. A written schedule should be established for turning and repositioning.

PROVIDING SUPPORTIVE DEVICES In order for circulation to remain uncompromised, pressure on the bony prominences should remain below capillary pressure for as much time as possible through a combination of turning, positioning, and use of pressure-relieving surfaces. Mean capillary pressure can be estimated at 20 mm Hg although this varies. Although some research has been conducted evaluating the effectiveness of pressure-reducing support surfaces in preventing pressure ulcers in clients at low, intermediate, or high risk, the results are often inconclusive (Cullum, McInnes, Bell-Syer, & Legood, 2005). The nurse should review the manufacturer's product descriptions that report the amount of time that the pressure between the surface and the bony prominence is above or below specified levels and determine if this is adequate to protect a particular client.

For clients confined to bed, three types of support surfaces can be used to relieve pressure. The overlay mattress is applied on top of the standard bed mattress. A replacement mattress is used instead of the standard mattress; most are made of foam and gel combinations. Specialty beds replace hospital beds. They provide pressure relief, eliminate shearing and friction, and decrease moisture. Examples are high-air-loss beds, low-air-loss beds, and beds that provide kinetic therapy. Kinetic beds provide continuous passive motion or oscillation therapy, which is intended to counteract the effects of a client's immobility. Table 24–3 lists selected mechanical devices for reducing pressure on body parts.

When a client is confined to bed or to a chair, pressure-reducing devices, such as pillows made of foam, gel, air, or a combination of these, can be used. When the client is sitting, weight should be distributed over the entire seating surface so that pressure does not center on just one area. To protect a client's heels in bed, supports such as wedges or pillows can be used to raise the heels completely off the bed. Doughnut-type devices should not be used since they limit blood flow and can cause tissue damage to the areas in direct contact with the device.

Treating Pressure Ulcers

Pressure ulcers are a challenge for nurses because of the number of variables involved and the numerous treatment measures advocated. Existing and potential infections are the most serious complications of pressure ulcers. In treating pressure ulcers, nurses should follow the agency protocols and the primary care provider's orders, if any. Prompt treatment can prevent further tissue damage and pain and facilitate wound healing. See the accompanying Practice Guidelines.

THE RYB COLOR CODE To guide wound care, the nurse can use the RYB color code of wounds. This concept is based on the color of an open wound—red, yellow, or black (RYB)—rather than the depth or size of a wound. On this scheme, the goals of wound care are to protect red, cleanse yellow, and debride black.

Wounds that are red are usually in the late regeneration phase of tissue repair. They need to be protected to avoid disturbance to regenerating tissue. The nurse protects red wounds by (a) gentle cleansing, (b) protecting periwound skin with alcohol-free barrier film, (c) filling dead space with hydrogel or alginate, (d) covering with an appropriate dressing such as transparent film, hydrocolloid dressing, or a clear absorbent acrylic dressing, and (e) changing the dressing as infrequently as possible.

Yellow wounds are characterized primarily by liquid to semiliquid "slough" that is often accompanied by purulent drainage or previous infection. The nurse cleanses yellow

---

PRACTICE GUIDELINES

Treating Pressure Ulcers

- Minimize direct pressure on the ulcer. Reposition the client at least every 2 hours. Make a schedule, and record position changes on the client's chart. Provide devices to minimize or float pressure areas.
- Clean the pressure ulcer with every dressing change. The method of cleaning depends on the stage of the ulcer, products available, and agency protocol. Skill 24–1 details the steps involved in irrigating a wound.

- Clean and dress the ulcer using surgical asepsis. Never use alcohol or hydrogen peroxide as they are cytotoxic to tissue beds.
- If the pressure ulcer is infected, obtain a sample of the drainage for culture and sensitivity to antibiotic agents.
- Teach the client to move, even if only slightly, to relieve pressure.
- Provide range-of-motion (ROM) exercises and mobility out of bed as the client's condition permits.

| TABLE 24–3 | **Mechanical Devices for Reducing Pressure on Body Parts** |

DEVICE	DESCRIPTION/COMMENTS
Gel flotation pads	Polyvinyl, silicone, or Silastic pads filled with a gelatinous substance similar to fat.
Pillows and wedges (foam, gel, air, fluid)	Supports positioning and offloads bone on bone contact.
Heel protectors (sheepskin boots, padded splints, off-loading inflatable boots, foam blocks)	Can raise or "float" a body part (e.g., heels) off the surface. Prevent shearing and limit pressure on heel area. (Figure 24–3).

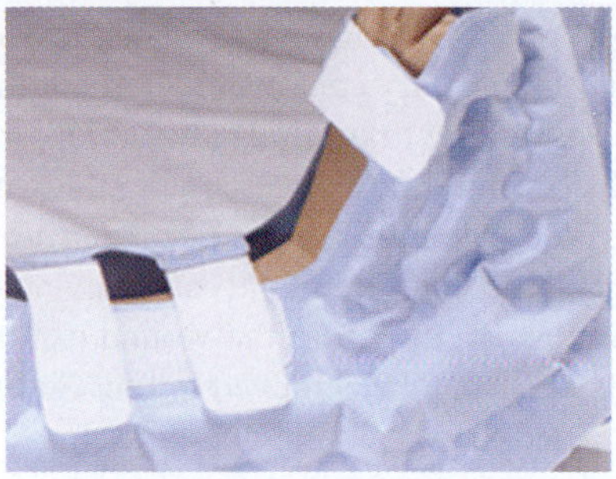

Figure 24–3 ◯ Heel protector.
(Courtesy of Gaymar Industries, Inc.)

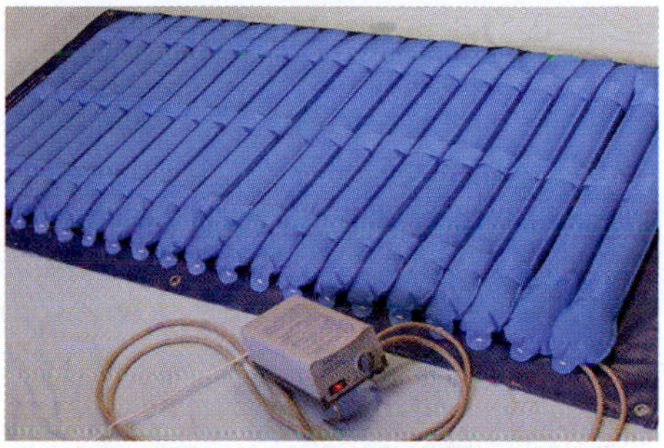

Memory foam mattress/ chair pad	Polyurethane foam mattress distributes weight over bony areas evenly. Foam molds to the body.
Alternating pressure mattress	Composed of a number of cells in which the pressure alternately increases and decreases; uses a pump (see Figure 24–4).
Water bed	Support surface filled with water. Water temperature can be controlled.

Figure 24–4 ◯ Alternating pressure mattress.
(Courtesy of Ease)

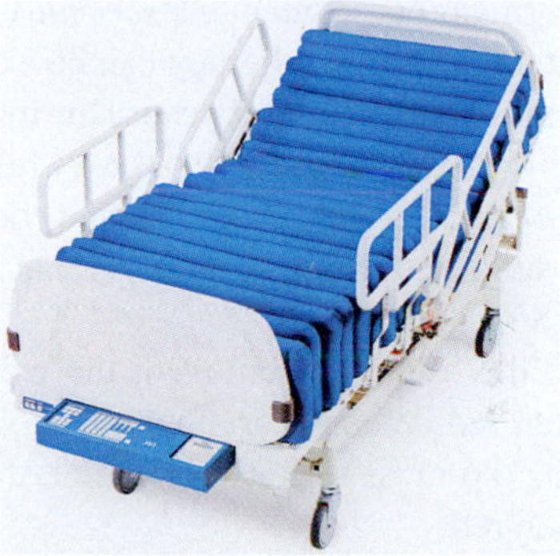

Static low-air-loss (LAL) bed	Consists of many air-filled cushions divided into four or five sections. Separate controls permit each section to be inflated to a different level of firmness; thus pressure can be reduced on bony prominences but increased under other body areas for support (see Figure 24–5).
Active or second-generation LAL bed	Like the static LAL, but in addition gently pulsates or rotates from side to side, thus stimulating capillary blood flow and facilitating movement of pulmonary secretions.

Figure 24–5 ◯ Low-air-loss bed.
(KinAir MedSurg® Courtesy of KCI Licensing, Inc., San Antonio, TX).

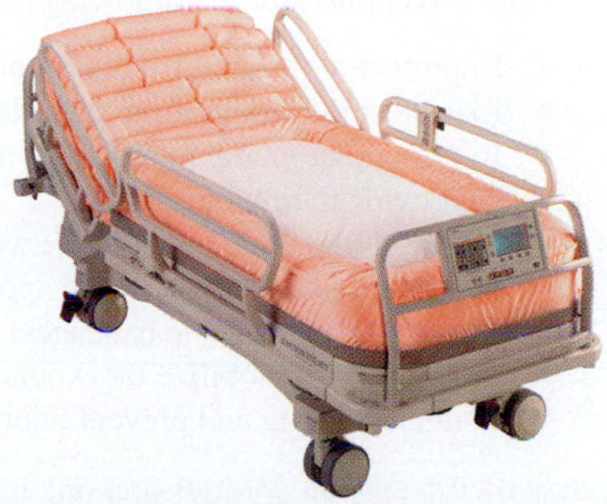

Air-fluidized (AF) bed (static high-air-loss bed)	Forced temperature-controlled air is circulated around millions of tiny silicone-coated beads, producing a fluid-like movement. Provides uniform support to body contours. Decreases skin maceration by its drying effect. Moisture from the client penetrates the linens and soaks the beads. Air flow forces the beads away from the client and rapidly dries the sheet. A major disadvantage is that the head of the bed cannot be elevated.
	Some beds are a unique combination of air fluidized therapy and low air loss therapy on an articulating frame. These are used with patients who require head elevation (see Figure 24–6).

Figure 24–6 ◯ Low-air-loss and air-fluidized combo bed (Clinitron/Rite Hite).
(Courtesy of Hill-Rom Services, Inc. Reprinted with permission. All rights reserved.)

wounds to remove nonviable tissue. Methods used may include applying moist-to-moist normal saline dressings, irrigating the wound, using absorbent dressing materials such as impregnated hydrogel or alginate dressings, and consulting with the primary care provider about the need for a topical antimicrobial to minimize bacterial growth.

Black wounds are covered with thick necrotic tissue, or eschar. Black wounds require **debridement** (removal of the necrotic material). Removal of nonviable tissue from a wound must occur before the wound can be staged or heal. Debridement may be achieved in four different ways: sharp, mechanical, chemical, and autolytic. In *sharp debridement,* a scalpel or scissors is used to separate and remove dead tissue. In many settings, specially trained nurses, physical therapists, and physician's assistants are permitted to perform sharp debridement. *Mechanical debridement* is accomplished through scrubbing force or moist-to-moist dressings. *Chemical debridement* is more selective than sharp or mechanical techniques. Collagenase enzyme agents such as papain-urea are currently most recommended for this use. In *autolytic debridement,* dressings that contain wound moisture, such as hydrocolloid and clear absorbent acrylic dressings, trap the wound drainage against the eschar. The body's own enzymes in the drainage break down the necrotic tissue. Although this method takes longer than the other three, it is the most selective and therefore causes the least damage to healthy surrounding and healing tissues. Recently, the use of fly larvae (maggots, *Phaenicia sericata*) has received increased attention. Larval therapy can be extremely effective in cleansing chronic wounds because the maggots secrete enzymes that break down necrotic tissue (while leaving healthy tissue untouched), eat bacteria, and decrease bacterial growth through the rise in surface pH that results from their presence (Sosin, 2005).

When the eschar is removed, the wound is treated as yellow, then red. When more than one color is present, the nurse treats the most serious color first, that is, black, then yellow, then red.

Dressing Wounds

Dressings are applied for the following purposes:

- To protect the wound from mechanical injury
- To protect the wound from microbial contamination
- To provide or maintain moist wound healing
- To provide thermal insulation
- To absorb drainage or debride a wound or both
- To prevent hemorrhage (when applied as a pressure dressing or with elastic bandages)
- To splint or immobilize the wound site and thereby facilitate healing and prevent injury

TYPES OF DRESSINGS Various dressing materials are available to cover wounds. The type of dressing used depends on (a) the location, size, and type of the wound; (b) the amount of exudate; (c) whether the wound requires debridement or is infected; and (d) such considerations as frequency of

dressing change, ease or difficulty of dressing application, and cost (Table 24–4).

Transparent dressings are often applied to wounds including ulcerated or burned skin areas. These dressings offer several advantages:

- They act as temporary skin.
- They are nonporous, nonabsorbent, self-adhesive dressings that do not require changing as other dressings do. They are often left in place until healing has occurred or as long as they remain intact.
- Because they are transparent, the wound can be assessed through them.
- Because they are semi-occlusive, the wound remains moist and can retain a small amount of serous exudate, which promotes epithelial growth, hastens healing, and reduces the risk of infection.
- Because they are elastic, they can be placed over a joint without disrupting the client's mobility.
- They adhere only to the skin area around the wound and not to the wound itself because they keep the wound moist.
- They allow the client to shower or bathe without removing the dressing.

Hydrocolloid dressings (see Table 24–4) are frequently used over pressure ulcers. These dressings offer several advantages:

- They last 3 to 7 days.
- They do not need a "cover" dressing and are water resistant, so the client can shower or bathe.
- They can be molded to uneven body surfaces.
- They act as temporary skin and provide an effective bacterial barrier.
- They decrease pain and thus reduce the need for analgesics.
- They absorb moderate drainage and therefore can be used on slowly draining wounds.
- They contain wound odor.

These dressings have certain limitations, however:

- They are occlusive, are opaque, and obscure wound visibility.
- They have a limited absorption capacity.
- They can facilitate anaerobic bacterial growth.
- They can soften and wrinkle at the edges with wear and movement.
- They can be difficult to remove and may leave a residue on the skin.

Because of these limitations, hydrocolloid dressings should not be used for infected wounds or those with deep tracts or *fistulas* (abnormal passage that develops between a hollow organ and the skin or between two hollow organs).

SECURING DRESSINGS The nurse tapes the dressing over the wound, ensuring that the dressing covers the entire wound and does not become dislodged. The correct type of

TABLE 24–4   **Selected Types of Wound Dressings**

DRESSING	DESCRIPTION	PURPOSE	INDICATIONS	EXAMPLES
Transparent film	Adhesive plastic, semipermeable, nonabsorbent dressings allow exchange of oxygen between the atmosphere and wound bed. They are impermeable to bacteria and water.	To provide protection against contamination and friction; to maintain a clean moist surface that facilitates cellular migration; to provide insulation by preventing fluid evaporation; and to facilitate wound assessment	IV dressing Central line dressing Superficial wounds Pressure ulcers Stage I	Tegaderm, Bioclusive. Op-Site
Impregnated nonadherent	Woven or nonwoven cotton or synthetic materials are impregnated with petrolatum, saline, zinc-saline, antimicrobials, or other agents. Require secondary dressings to secure them in place, retain moisture, and provide wound protection.	To cover, soothe, and protect partial- and full-thickness wounds without exudate	Postoperative dressing over staple/sutures Superficial burns	Adaptic, Carrasyn, Xeroform dressings
Hydrocolloids	Waterproof adhesive wafers, pastes, or powders. Wafers, designed to be worn for up to 7 days, consist of two layers. The inner adhesive layer has particles that absorb exudates and form a hydrated gel over the wound; the outer film provides an occlusive seal.	To absorb exudate; to produce a moist environment that facilitates healing but does not cause maceration of surrounding skin; to protect the wound from bacterial contamination, foreign debris, and urine or feces; and to prevent shearing	Pressure ulcers Stage II–IV Autolytic debridement of eschar Partial-thickness wounds	Tegasorb DuoDerm, Comfeel, Restore, Replicare
Clear absorbent acrylic	Transparent absorbent wafer designed to be worn 5–7 days. The acrylic layer absorbs exudates and evaporates the excess off the transparent membrane.	Maintains a transparent membrane for easy wound bed assessment, provides bacterial and shearing protection. Maintains moist wound healing. Can be used with alginates to provide packing to deeper wound beds.	Pressure ulcers Skin tears Venous stasis ulcers Surgical wounds Wounds undergoing chemical debridement agents	Tegaderm
Hydrogels	Glycerin or water-based nonadhesive jellylike sheets, granules, or gels are oxygen permeable, unless covered by a plastic film. Requires secondary occlusive dressing.	To liquefy necrotic tissue or slough, rehydrate the wound bed, and fill in dead space	Pressure ulcers Skin tears Partial-thickness wounds	Curosol, Tegaderm Hydrogel Elasto-Gel, Vigilon
Polyurethane foams	Nonadherent hydrocolloid dressings; these need to have their edges taped down or sealed. Require secondary dressings to obtain an occlusive environment. Surrounding skin must be protected to prevent maceration.	Absorbs up to heavy amounts of exudate; provides and maintains moist wound healing	Light to highly exudating wounds Pressure ulcers Skin tears Venous stasis ulcers Surgical wounds Wounds undergoing chemical debridement agents	Tegaderm Foam Lyofoam, Allevyn, Vigifoam, Flexzan
Alginates (exudate absorbers)	Nonadherent dressings of powder, beads or granules, ropes, sheets, or paste conform to the wound surface and absorb up to 20 times their weight in exudate; require a secondary dressing.	To provide a moist wound surface by interacting with exudate to form a gelatinous mass; to absorb exudate; to eliminate dead space or pack wounds; and to support debridement	Pressure ulcers Skin tears Venous stasis ulcers Surgical wounds Wounds undergoing chemical debridement agents	Debrisan, Sorbsan, Kaltostat, Algiderm

tape must be selected for the purpose. The nurse follows these steps:

1. Place the tape so that the dressing cannot be folded back to expose the wound. Place strips at the ends of the dressing, and space tapes evenly in the middle.
2. Ensure that the tape is long and wide enough to adhere to several inches of skin on each side of the dressing, but not so long or wide that the tape loosens with activity.
3. Place the tape in the opposite direction from the body action, for example, across a body joint or crease, not lengthwise.

Montgomery straps (tie tapes) are used for wounds requiring frequent dressing changes (see Figure 24–7). These straps prevent skin irritation and discomfort caused by removing the adhesive each time the dressing is changed.

Medical tapes can cause injuries if used incorrectly. Blisters will form if too much tension is applied while placing the tape, when edema has collected after the tape was placed, and when alcohol or benzoic-based prep solutions are used under the tape. Medical tape manufacturers issue safety guidelines for specific tape products. Before using medical tapes read the safety guidelines for indications of use and safe application and removal.

Cleaning Wounds

Wound cleaning involves the removal of debris. The choices of cleaning agent and method depend largely on agency protocol and the primary care provider's preference. Recommended guidelines for cleaning wounds are shown in the accompanying Practice Guidelines.

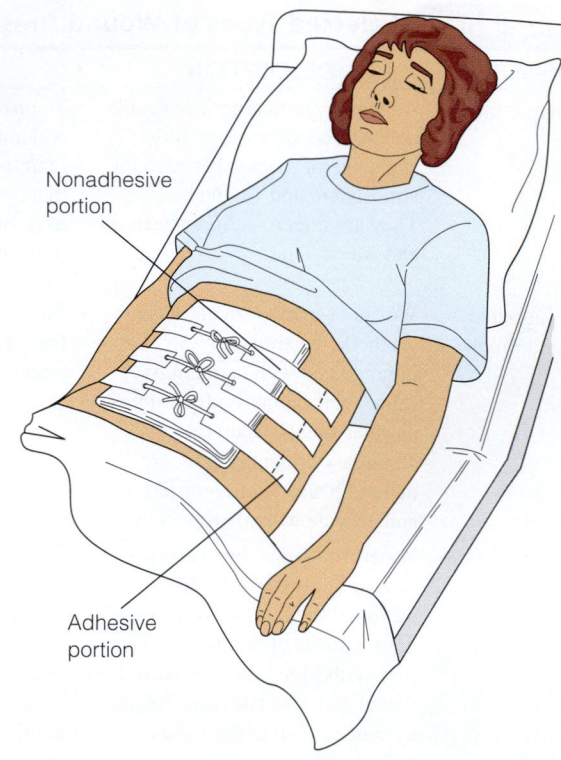

Nonadhesive portion

Adhesive portion

Figure 24–7 ◉ Montgomery straps, or tie tapes, are used to secure large dressings that require frequent changing.

Commonly used methods to clean a surgical wound and drain site are shown in Chapter 25 ∞.

An irrigation (lavage) is the washing or flushing out of an area. Sterile technique is required for a wound irrigation because there is a break in the skin integrity.

PRACTICE GUIDELINES	**Cleaning Wounds**

- Follow standard precautions for personal protection. Wear gloves, gown, goggles, and mask as indicated.
- Use solutions such as isotonic saline or wound cleansers to clean or irrigate wounds. If antimicrobial solutions are used, make sure they are well diluted.
- Microwave heating is not recommended. When possible, warm the solution to body temperature before use. *This prevents lowering the wound temperature, which slows the healing process. Microwave heating could cause the solution to become too hot.*
- If a wound is grossly contaminated by foreign material, bacteria, slough, or necrotic tissue, clean the wound at every dressing change. *Foreign bodies and devitalized tissue act as a focus for infection and can delay healing.*
- If a wound is clean, has little exudate, and reveals healthy granulation tissue, avoid repeated cleaning. *Unnecessary cleaning can delay wound healing by traumatizing newly produced, delicate tissues, reducing the surface temperature of the wound, and removing exudate which itself may have bactericidal properties.*

- Use gauze squares. Avoid using cotton balls and other products that shed fibers onto the wound surface. *The fibers become embedded in granulation tissue and can act as foci for infection. They may also stimulate "foreign body" reactions, prolonging the inflammatory phase of healing and delaying the healing process.*
- Clean superficial noninfected wounds by irrigating them with normal saline. *The hydraulic pressure of an irrigating stream of fluid dislodges contaminating debris and reduces bacterial colonization.*
- *To retain wound moisture,* avoid drying a wound after cleaning it.
- Hold cleaning sponges with forceps or with a sterile gloved hand.
- Clean from the wound in an outward direction to avoid transferring organisms from the surrounding skin into the wound.
- Consider not cleaning the wound at all if it appears to be clean.

Using piston syringes instead of bulb syringes to irrigate a wound reduces the risk of aspirating drainage and provides safe, effective pressure. For deep wounds with small openings, a sterile straight catheter may also be necessary. Irrigation pressures should range from 4 to 15 pounds per square inch (psi). Below 4 psi, the irrigation may not be effective, and above 15 psi it may damage tissues. A 35-mL syringe with a 19-gauge needle or catheter provides approximately 8 psi (Bergstrom et al., 1994). Some providers advocate the use of a commercial oral water jet for wound cleansing. This can be effective if kept at the lowest setting that provides the desired pressure. Frequently used irrigation solutions are sterile normal saline, lactated Ringer's solution, and antibiotic solutions. Skill 24–1 details the steps involved in irrigating a wound.

SKILL 24–1

IRRIGATING A WOUND

PURPOSES
- To clean the area
- To apply heat and hasten the healing process
- To apply an antimicrobial solution

ASSESSMENT
Assess
- The client's record to determine previous appearance and size of the wound
- The character of the exudate
- Presence of pain and the time of the last pain medication
- Clinical signs of systemic infection
- Allergies to the wound irrigation agent or tape

PLANNING
- Before irrigating a wound, determine (a) the type of irrigating solution to be used, (b) the frequency of irrigations, and (c) the temperature of the solution.
- If possible, schedule the irrigation at a time convenient for the client. Some irrigations require only a few minutes and others can take much longer.

> **Delegation**
> Due to the need for aseptic technique and assessment skills, wound irrigations are not delegated to UAP. However, UAP may observe the wound and dressing during usual care and must report abnormal findings to the nurse. Abnormal findings must be validated and interpreted by the nurse.

EQUIPMENT
- Sterile dressing equipment and dressing materials
- Sterile irrigation set or individual supplies that include
  - Sterile syringe (e.g., a 30- to 60-mL syringe) with a catheter of an appropriate size (e.g., #18 or #19) or an irrigating (catheter) tip syringe
  - Sterile graduated container for irrigating solution
  - Basin for collecting the used irrigating solution
  - Moisture-proof sterile drape
- Moisture-proof bag
- Irrigating solution, usually 200 mL (6.5 oz) of solution warmed to body temperature, according to the agency's or primary care provider's choice
- Goggles, gown, and mask
- Clean gloves
- Sterile gloves

Although a wound may already be contaminated, sterile equipment is usually used during irrigation to prevent the possibility of adding new nonresident microorganisms to the site. In settings outside of hospitals, some reusable supplies such as irrigating syringes or basins may be cleaned and used again for a specific wound.

IMPLEMENTATION
Preparation
Check that the irrigating fluid is at the proper temperature.

Performance
1. Prior to performing the procedure, introduce self and verify the client's identity using agency protocol. Explain to the client what you are going to do, why it is necessary, and how he or she can participate. Discuss how the results will be used in planning further care or treatments.
2. Perform hand hygiene and observe appropriate infection control procedures.
3. Provide for client privacy.
4. Prepare the client.
   - Assist the client to a position in which the irrigating solution will flow by gravity from the upper end of the wound to the lower end and then into the basin.
- Place the waterproof drape under the wounds and over the bed.
- Apply clean gloves and remove and discard the old dressing. **Rationale:** *Because the nurse is not touching the wound, clean gloves are appropriate when removing a soiled dressing.*
- If indicated, clean the wound from the center of the wound outward, using circular strokes. **Rationale:** *The goal is to push the debris from the center of the wound out and away from the wound.*
- Use a separate swab for each stroke, and discard each swab after use. **Rationale:** *This prevents the introduction of microorganisms to other wound areas.*
- Assess the wound and drainage. **Rationale:** *The wound should be assessed before and after irrigating to note differences and no procedure should be performed without assessing for continuing need.*
- Remove and discard gloves.

(continued)

IRRIGATING A WOUND (continued)

5. Prepare the equipment.
   - Open the sterile dressing set and supplies.
   - Pour the ordered solution into the solution container.
   - Position the basin below the wound to receive the irrigating fluid. **Rationale:** *This prevents wetting of the client's clothes or bed linens.*
6. Irrigate the wound.
   - Apply clean gloves.
   - Instill a steady stream of irrigating solution into the wound. Make sure all areas of the wound are irrigated. **Rationale:** *The flow of solution helps to move debris within the wound.*
   - Use either a syringe with a catheter attached or with an irrigating tip to flush the wound. **Rationale:** *Allows for greater accuracy in flushing the correct area.*
   - If you are using a catheter to reach tracks or crevices, insert the catheter into the wound until resistance is met. Do not force the catheter. **Rationale:** *Forcing the catheter can cause tissue damage.*
   - Continue irrigating until the solution becomes clear (no exudate is present). **Rationale:** *Until the solution clears the irrigation process is continuing to remove debris.*

   - Dry the area around the wound. **Rationale:** *Moisture left on the skin promotes the growth of microorganisms and can cause skin irritation and breakdown.*
7. Assess and dress the wound.
   - Assess the appearance of the wound again, noting in particular the type and amount of exudate still present and the presence and extent of granulation tissue. **Rationale:** *Assessing the wound after irrigation helps the nurse to note change resulting from irrigation.*
   - Using sterile technique, apply a dressing to the wound based on the amount of drainage expected (see Table 24–4). **Rationale:** *Sterile technique will reduce the risk of introducing pathogens into the wound.*
8. Document the irrigation and the client's response in the client record using forms or checklists supplemented by narrative notes when appropriate. Many agencies use a designated wound/skin documentation sheet.

SAMPLE DOCUMENTATION

1/5/2010 1530 Midline abdominal wound 7 cm c̄ intact sutures except for center 3 cm. Open area draining moderate amt. thin serosang. Irrigated c̄ NS until clear. Redressed c̄ sterile technique. ———————————— N. Jamaghani, RN

EVALUATION

- Perform follow-up based on findings that deviate from expected or normal for the client. Relate findings to previous assessment data if available.
- Report significant deviations to the primary care provider.

Gauze packing using the damp-to-damp technique has been used to pack wounds that require debridement. In this technique, moist 4 × 4 non-cotton–filled gauzes are packed in the wound to absorb exudate but they are not allowed to dry before removal. However, newer advanced dressing materials have significant advantages over the use of gauze.

See the accompanying Practice Guidelines for issues related to using damp-to-damp dressings.

Many of the techniques described here for dressing wounds may be combined depending on the specific type of wound. In addition, therapies are constantly being designed and evaluated. One example is *vacuum-assisted closure*

PRACTICE GUIDELINES   Issues Related to the Use of Damp Gauze versus Advanced Dressings

- To keep the gauze damp, it must be changed or remoistened with saline frequently. *If the gauze is allowed to dry out, removal results in pain and disruption of wound healing through drying of the surface and tissue adherence to the gauze.*
- A wound requires moisture and warmth for optimal healing. Evaporation of the saline causes wound cooling, vasoconstriction, and dehydration.
- Moistened gauze cannot prevent introduction of bacteria into the wound.
- Gauze is easy to use and can be manipulated to fit almost any wound.
- The diversity of advanced dressings may be confusing for clients and health care providers.

- Although gauze is much less expensive than advanced dressings (e.g., polymers, alginates, collagens), the cost per week can be higher due to the number of dressing changes required. Including the price of the dressing, gloves, saline, and tape, the materials cost for a gauze dressing change twice per day versus an advanced dressing three times per week is very similar. However, at approximately $100 per nurse home visit, the gauze dressing is almost five times as expensive.
- Wounds have been shown to heal twice as quickly with advanced dressings compared to gauze.

Conclusions: Practitioners should become familiar with the range and uses of advanced dressing materials. The selection of dressing materials must consider time, material cost, client comfort, and speed of wound healing.

LIFESPAN CONSIDERATIONS   Pressure Ulcer and Wound Care

Infants

- The skin of infants is more fragile than that of older children and adults, and more susceptible to infection, shearing from friction, and burns.

Children

- Staphylococcus and fungus are two major infectious agents affecting the skin of children. Abrasions or small lacerations, commonly experienced by children, provide an entry in the skin for these organisms. Minor wounds should be cleansed with warm, soapy water, and covered with a sterile bandage. Children should be instructed not to touch the wound.
- With more serious skin lesions, remind the child not to touch the wound, drains, or dressing. Cover with an appropriate bandage that will remain intact during the child's usual activities. Cover a transparent dressing with opaque material if viewing the site is distressing to the child. Restrain only when all alternatives have been tried and when absolutely necessary.

- For younger children, demonstrate wound care on a doll. Reassure that the wound will not be permanent and that nothing will fall out of the body.

Older Adults

- Hold wrinkled skin taut during application of a transparent dressing. Obtain assistance if needed.
- Skin is more fragile and can easily tear with removal of tape (especially adhesive tape). Use paper tape and tape remover as indicated, keeping tape use to the minimum required. Use extreme caution during tape removal.
- Older adults who are in long-term care facilities often have the following factors: immobility, malnutrition, and incontinence—all of which increase the risk for development of skin breakdown.
- Skin breakdown can occur as quickly as within 2 hours, so assessments should be done with each repositioning of the client.
- A thorough assessment of a client's heels should be done every shift. The skin can break down quickly from friction of movement in bed.

(VAC), which refers to the use of suction equipment to apply negative pressure to a variety of wound types. This therapy has been shown to speed tissue generation, reduce swelling around the wound, and enhance wound healing by providing a moist and protected environment. Sterile foam sponges are placed into a clean wound and covered with a transparent adhesive drape, and then a hole is cut in the drape to allow insertion of the vacuum tubing. For maximum effectiveness the vacuum is applied for almost 24 hours each day (Mendez-Eastman, 2005) and portable systems are available for ambulatory clients. VAC has also been shown to heal pressure ulcers better than alginate or hydrocolloid dressings (Smith, 2004).

Supporting and Immobilizing Wounds

Bandages and binders serve various purposes:

- Supporting a wound (e.g., a fractured bone)
- Immobilizing a wound (e.g., a strained shoulder)
- Applying pressure (e.g., elastic bandages on the lower extremities to improve venous blood flow)
- Securing a dressing (e.g., for an extensive abdominal surgical wound)
- Retaining warmth (e.g., a flannel bandage on a rheumatoid joint)

There are several types of bandages and binders and several ways in which they are applied. When correctly applied, they promote healing, provide comfort, and can prevent injury (see accompanying Practice Guidelines).

A **bandage** is a strip of cloth used to wrap some part of the body. Bandages are available in various widths, most commonly 1.5 to 7.5 cm (0.5 to 3 in.). They are usually supplied in rolls for easy application to a body part.

PRACTICE GUIDELINES

Assessing before Applying Bandages or Binders

- Inspect and palpate the area for swelling.
- Inspect for the presence of and status of wounds (open wounds will require a dressing before a bandage or binder is applied).
- Note the presence of drainage (amount, color, odor, viscosity).
- Inspect and palpate for adequacy of circulation (skin temperature, color, and sensation). Pale or cyanotic skin, cool temperature, tingling, and numbness can indicate impaired circulation.
- Ask the client about any pain experienced (location, intensity, onset, quality).
- Assess the ability of the client to reapply the bandage or binder when needed.
- Assess the capabilities of the client regarding activities of daily living (e.g., to eat, dress, comb hair, bathe) and assess the assistance required during the convalescence period.

Many types of materials are used for bandages. Gauze is one of the most commonly used, because it is light and porous and readily molds to the body. It is also relatively inexpensive, so it is generally discarded when soiled. Gauze is used to retain dressings on wounds and to bandage the fingers, hands, toes, and feet. It supports dressings and at the same time permits air to circulate; it can be impregnated with petroleum jelly or other medications for application to wounds.

Elasticized bandages are applied to provide pressure to an area. They are commonly used as tensor bandages or as

<table>
<tr><td>

PRACTICE GUIDELINES   Bandaging

- Whenever possible, bandage the part in its normal position, with the joint slightly flexed *to avoid putting strain on the ligaments and the muscles of the joint.*
- Pad between skin surfaces and over bony prominences *to prevent friction from the bandage and consequent abrasion of the skin.*
- Always bandage body parts by working from the distal to the proximal end *to aid the return flow of venous blood.*
- Bandage with even pressure *to prevent interference with blood circulation.*
- Whenever possible, leave the end of the body part (e.g., the toe) exposed *so that you will be able to assess the adequacy of the blood circulation to the extremity.*
- Cover dressings with bandages at least 5 cm (2 in.) beyond the edges of the dressing *to prevent the dressing and wound from becoming contaminated.*

</td></tr>
</table>

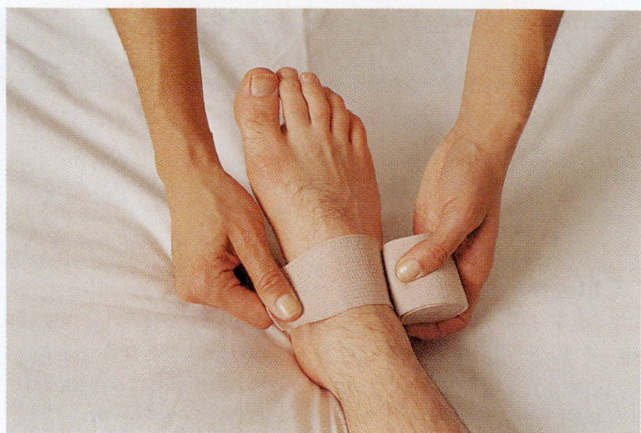

Figure 24–8 ● Starting a bandage with two circular turns.

partial stockings to provide support and improve the venous circulation in the legs.

The width of the bandage used depends on the size of the body part to be bandaged. For example, a 2.5-cm (1-in.) bandage is used for a finger, a 5-cm (2-in.) bandage for an arm, and a 7.5-cm or 10-cm (3-in. or 4-in.) bandage for a leg. Padding (e.g., abdominal pads and gauze squares) is frequently used to cover bony prominences (e.g., the elbow) or to separate skin surfaces (e.g., the fingers).

Before applying a bandage, the nurse needs to know its purpose and to assess the area requiring support (see accompanying Practice Guidelines). When bandages are used to secure dressings, the nurse wears gloves to prevent contact with body fluids.

BASIC TURNS FOR ROLLER BANDAGES Applying bandages to various parts of the body involves one or more of five basic bandaging turns: circular, spiral, spiral reverse, recurrent, and figure-eight. *Circular* turns are used to anchor bandages and to terminate them. Circular turns usually are not applied directly over a wound because of the discomfort the bandage would cause.

Spiral turns are used to bandage parts of the body that are fairly uniform in circumference, for example, the upper arm or upper leg. *Spiral reverse* turns are used to bandage cylindrical parts of the body that are not uniform in circumference, for example, the lower leg or forearm. *Recurrent* turns are used to cover distal parts of the body, for example, the end of a finger, the skull, or the stump of an amputation. *Figure-eight* turns are used to bandage an elbow, knee, or ankle, because they permit some movement after application.

Circular Turns

- Hold the bandage in your dominant hand, keeping the roll uppermost, and unroll the bandage about 8 cm

(3 in.). This length of unrolled bandage allows good control for placement and tension.

- Apply the end of the bandage to the part of the body to be bandaged. Hold the end down with the thumb of the other hand (Figure 24–8).
- Encircle the body part a few times or as often as needed, making sure that each layer overlaps one-half to two-thirds of the previous layer. This provides even support to the area.
- The bandage should be firm, but not too tight. Ask the client if the bandage feels comfortable. A tight bandage can interfere with blood circulation, whereas a loose bandage does not provide adequate protection.
- Secure the end of the bandage with tape or a safety pin over an uninjured area. Pins can cause discomfort when situated over an injured area.

Spiral Turns

- Make two circular turns. Two circular turns anchor the bandage.
- Continue spiral turns at about a 30-degree angle, each turn overlapping the preceding one by two-thirds the width of the bandage (Figure 24–9).

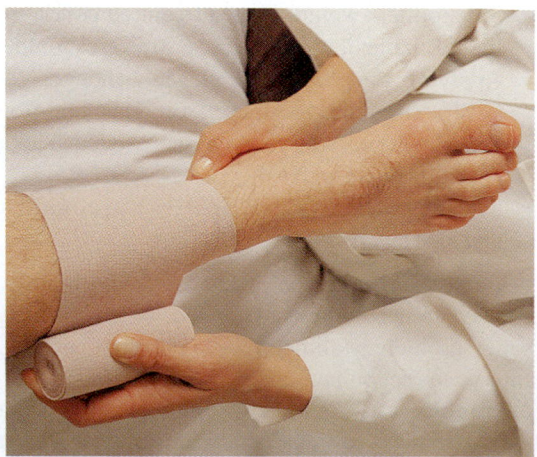

Figure 24–9 ● Applying spiral turns.

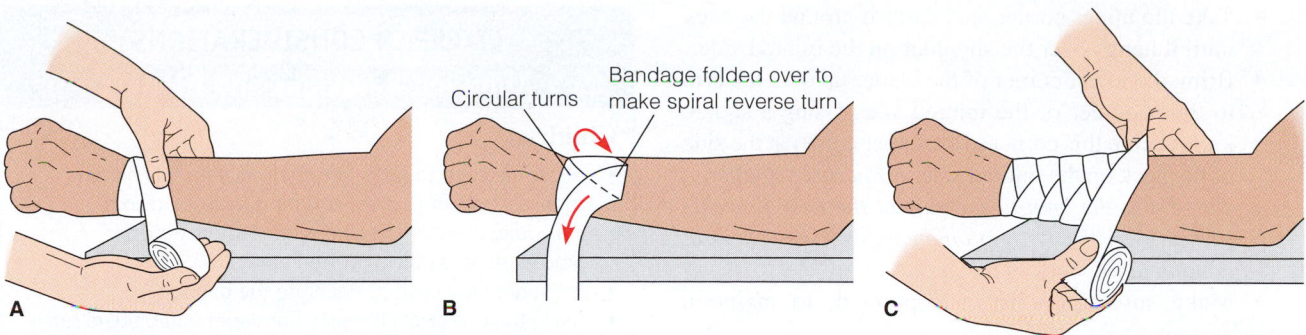

A   B   C

Figure 24–10 ⬤ Applying spiral reverse turns.

- Terminate the bandage with two circular turns, and secure the end as described for circular turns.

Spiral Reverse Turns
- Anchor the bandage with two circular turns, and bring the bandage upward at about a 30-degree angle.
- Place the thumb of your free hand on the upper edge of the bandage (Figure 24–10, A). The thumb will hold the bandage while it is folded on itself.
- Unroll the bandage about 15 cm (6 in.), and then turn your hand so that the bandage falls over itself (Figure 24–10, B).
- Continue the bandage around the limb, overlapping each previous turn by two-thirds the width of the bandage. Make each bandage turn at the same position on the limb so that the turns of the bandage will be aligned (Figure 24–10, C).
- Terminate the bandage with two circular turns, and secure the end as described for circular turns.

Recurrent Turns
- Anchor the bandage with two circular turns.
- Fold the bandage back on itself, and bring it centrally over the distal end to be bandaged.
- Holding it with the other hand, bring the bandage back over the end to the right of the center bandage but overlapping it by two-thirds the width of the bandage.
- Bring the bandage back on the left side, also overlapping the first turn by two-thirds the width of the bandage.
- Continue this pattern of alternating right and left until the area is covered. Overlap the preceding turn by two-thirds the bandage width each time.
- Terminate the bandage with two circular turns. Secure the end appropriately.

Figure-Eight Turns
- Anchor the bandage with two circular turns.
- Carry the bandage above the joint, around it, and then below it, making a figure-eight (Figure 24–11).
- Continue above and below the joint, overlapping the previous turn by two-thirds the width of the bandage.
- Terminate the bandage above the joint with two circular turns, and then secure the end appropriately.

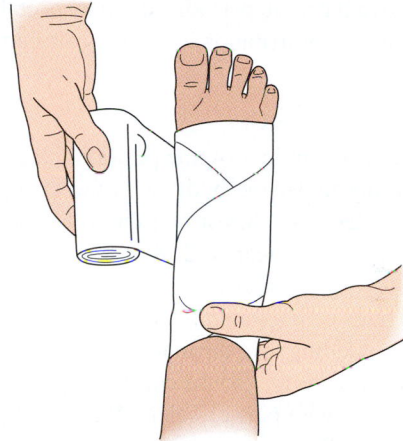

Figure 24–11 ⬤ Applying a figure-eight bandage.

BINDERS A **binder** is a type of bandage designed for a specific body part; for example, the triangular binder (sling) fits the arm. Binders are used to support large areas of the body, such as the abdomen, arm, or chest. Binders can be simple, inexpensive, and customizable by using plain material such as the triangular sling described below. Or, they can be of commercial design which are often easier to use, more expensive, and slightly less modifiable such as the hook-and-loop (Velcro) binder which is also described below.

Triangular Arm Sling
- Ask the client to flex the elbow to an 80-degree angle or less, depending on the purpose. The thumb should be facing upward or inward toward the body. *An 80-degree angle is sufficient to support the forearm, to prevent swelling of the hand, and to relieve pressure on the shoulder joint (e.g., to support the paralyzed arm of a stroke client whose shoulder might otherwise become dislocated). A more acute angle is preferred if there is swelling of the hand (see how to apply a sling for maximum hand elevation, below).*
- Place one end of the unfolded triangular binder over the shoulder of the uninjured side so that the binder falls down the front of the chest of the client with the point of the triangle (apex) under the elbow of the injured side.

- Take the upper corner, and carry it around the neck until it hangs over the shoulder on the injured side.
- Bring the lower corner of the binder up over the arm to the shoulder of the injured side. Using a square knot, secure this corner to the upper corner at the side of the neck on the injured side. *A square knot will not slip. Tying the knot at the side of the neck prevents pressure on the bony prominences of the vertebral column at the back of the neck.*
- Make sure the wrist is supported, to maintain alignment.
- Fold the sling neatly at the elbow, and secure it with safety pins or tape. It may be folded and fastened at the front.
- Remove the sling periodically to inspect the skin for indications of irritation, especially around the site of the knot.

Straight Abdominal Binder
- With the client in a supine position, place the binder smoothly under the body, with the upper border of the binder at the waist and the lower border at the level of the gluteal fold. *A binder placed over the waist interferes with respiration; one placed too low interferes with elimination and walking.*
- Apply padding over the iliac crests if the client is thin.
- Bring the ends around the client, overlap them, and secure them with pins or Velcro. Place the top pin horizontally at the waist to allow for comfort when moving.

SECURING PERINEAL DRESSINGS Previously, T-binders were used to secure dressings to the perineal area. T-binders have been replaced with sanitary disposable garments that fit like briefs. Placing an appropriate sized abdominal pad or sanitary napkin in the garment allows the wound to be protected and drainage to be collected for either males or females.

Heat and Cold Applications

Heat and cold are applied to the body for local and systemic effects. Table 24–5 lists the physiologic effects of heat and cold.

LOCAL EFFECTS OF HEAT AND COLD Heat is an old remedy for aches and pains, and people often equate heat with comfort and relief. Heat causes vasodilation and increases blood flow to the affected area, bringing oxygen, nutrients, antibodies, and leukocytes.

Application of heat promotes soft tissue healing and increases suppuration. A possible disadvantage of heat is that it increases capillary permeability, which allows extracellular fluid and substances such as plasma proteins to pass through the capillary walls and may result in edema or an increase in preexisting edema. Heat is often used for clients with musculoskeletal problems such as joint stiffness from arthritis, contractures, and low back pain.

Generally, the physiologic effects of cold are opposite to the effects of heat. Cold lowers the temperature of the skin and underlying tissues and causes vasoconstriction. Vaso-

<table>
<tr><td colspan="2">
LIFESPAN CONSIDERATIONS
Applying Bandages and Binders
</td></tr>
</table>

Children
- Allow the child to help with the procedure by holding supplies, opening boxes, counting turns, and so on.
- If a young client is apprehensive, demonstrate the procedure on a doll or stuffed animal.
- Encourage the child to decorate the bandage.
- Teach the caregivers to apply bandages and binders safely.

Older Adults
- Older clients may need extra support during the procedure, especially if arthritis, contractures, or tremors are present.
- Avoid constricting the client's circulation with a tight bandage or binder. Observe skin and bony prominences frequently for signs of impaired circulation. The risk for skin breakdown increases with age.

TABLE 24–5	Physiologic Effects of Heat and Cold

HEAT	COLD
Vasodilation	Vasoconstriction
Increases capillary permeability	Decreases capillary permeability
Increases cellular metabolism	Decreases cellular metabolism
Increases inflammation	Slows bacterial growth, decreases inflammation
Sedative effect	Local anesthetic effect

constriction reduces blood flow to the affected area and thus reduces the supply of oxygen and metabolites, decreases the removal of wastes, and produces skin pallor and coolness. Prolonged exposure to cold results in impaired circulation, cell deprivation, and subsequent damage to the tissues from lack of oxygen and nourishment. The signs of tissue damage due to cold are a bluish purple mottled appearance of the skin, numbness, and sometimes blisters and pain. Cold is most often used for sports injuries (e.g., sprains, strains, fractures) to limit postinjury swelling and bleeding.

SYSTEMIC EFFECTS OF HEAT AND COLD Heat applied to a localized body area, particularly a large body area, may cause excessive peripheral vasodilation, which produces a drop in blood pressure. A significant drop in blood pressure can cause fainting. Clients who have heart or pulmonary disease and who have circulatory disturbances such as arteriosclerosis are more prone to this effect than healthy people are. With extensive cold applications and vasoconstriction, a client's blood pressure can increase because blood is shunted from the cutaneous circulation to the internal blood

BOX 24–2	Variables Affecting Physiologic Tolerance to Heat and Cold

Body part. The back of the hand and foot are not very temperature sensitive. In contrast, the inner aspect of the wrist and forearm, the neck, and the perineal area are temperature sensitive.

Size of the exposed body part. The larger the area exposed to heat and cold, the lower the tolerance.

Individual tolerance. The very young and the very old generally have the lowest tolerance. Persons who have neurosensory impairments may have a high tolerance, but the risk of injury is greater.

Length of exposure. People feel hot and cold applications most while the temperature is changing. After a period of time, tolerance increases.

Intactness of skin. Injured skin areas are more sensitive to temperature variations.

TABLE 24–6	Temperatures for Hot and Cold Applications	
DESCRIPTION	**TEMPERATURE**	**APPLICATION**
Very cold	Below 15°C (59°F)	Ice bags
Cold	15–18°C (59–65°F)	Cold pack
Cool	18–27°C (65–80°F)	Cold compresses
Tepid	27–37°C (80–98°F)	Alcohol sponge bath
Warm	37–40°C (98–105°F)	Warm bath, aquathermia pads
Hot	40–46°C (105–115°F)	Hot soak, irrigations, hot compresses
Very hot	Above 46°C (above 115°F)	Hot water bags for adults

vessels. Shivering, a generalized effect of prolonged cold, is a normal response as the body attempts to warm itself.

THERMAL TOLERANCE   Various parts of the body differ in tolerance to heat and cold. The physiologic tolerance of individuals also varies (see Box 24–2). Specific conditions necessitate precautions in the use of hot or cold applications:

- *Neurosensory impairment.* People with sensory impairments are unable to perceive that heat is damaging the tissues and are at risk for burns or are unable to perceive discomfort from cold and prevent tissue injury.
- *Impaired mental status.* People who are confused or have an altered level of consciousness need monitoring during applications to ensure safe therapy.
- *Impaired circulation.* People with peripheral vascular disease, diabetes, or congestive heart failure lack the normal ability to dissipate heat via the blood circulation, which puts them at risk for tissue damage with heat and cold applications.
- *Immediately after injury or surgery.* Heat increases bleeding and swelling.
- *Open wounds.* Cold can decrease blood flow to the wound, thereby inhibiting healing.

ADAPTATION OF THERMAL RECEPTORS   Heat and cold receptors adapt to temperature changes. When they are subjected to an abrupt change in temperature, the receptors are strongly stimulated initially. This strong stimulation declines rapidly during the first few seconds and then more slowly during the next half hour or more as the receptors adapt to the new temperature.

Nurses and clients need to understand this adaptive response when applying heat and cold. Clients may be tempted to change the temperature of a thermal application because of the change in thermal sensation following adaptation. Increasing the temperature of a hot application after adaptation can result in serious burns. Decreasing the tem-

perature of a cold application can result in pain and serious impairment of circulation to the body part. Table 24–6 lists temperatures of hot and cold applications.

REBOUND PHENOMENON   The rebound phenomenon occurs at the time the maximum therapeutic effect of the hot or cold application is achieved and the opposite effect begins. For example, heat produces maximum vasodilation in 20 to 30 minutes; continuation of the application beyond 30 to 45 minutes brings tissue congestion, and the blood vessels then constrict for reasons unknown. If the heat application is continued, the client is at risk for burns because the constricted blood vessels are unable to dissipate the heat adequately via the blood circulation.

With cold applications, maximum vasoconstriction occurs when the involved skin reaches a temperature of 15°C (60°F). Below 15°C, vasodilation begins. This mechanism is protective: It helps to prevent freezing of body tissues normally exposed to cold, such as the nose and ears. It also explains the ruddiness of the skin of a person who has been walking in cold weather.

An understanding of the rebound phenomenon is essential for the nurse and client. Thermal applications must be halted before the rebound phenomenon begins.

APPLYING HEAT AND COLD   Heat can be applied to the body in both dry and moist forms. Dry heat is applied locally by means of a hot water bottle, aquathermia pad, disposable heat pack, or electric pad. Moist heat can be provided by compress, hot pack, soak, or sitz bath. Selected indications for the use of heat and cold are found in Table 24–7.

Dry cold is generally applied locally by means of a cold pack, ice bag, ice glove, or ice collar. Moist cold can be provided by compress or a cooling sponge bath.

For all local applications of heat or cold, the nurse needs to follow these guidelines:

- Determine the client's ability to tolerate the therapy.
- Identify conditions that might contraindicate treatment (e.g., bleeding, circulatory impairment).
- Explain the application to the client.

TABLE 24–7 Selected Indications for Heat and Cold Applications

INDICATION	EFFECT OF HEAT	EFFECT OF COLD
Muscle spasm	Relaxes muscles and increases their contractility.	Relaxes muscles and decreases muscle contractility.
Inflammation	Increases blood flow, softens exudates.	Vasoconstriction decreases capillary permeability, decreases blood flow, slows cellular metabolism.
Pain	Relieves pain, possibly by promoting muscle relaxation, increasing circulation, and promoting psychologic relaxation and a feeling of comfort; acts as a counterirritant.	Decreases pain by slowing nerve conduction rate and blocking nerve impulses; produces numbness, acts as a counterirritant, increases pain threshold.
Contracture	Reduces contracture and increases joint range of motion by allowing greater distention of muscles and connective tissue.	
Joint stiffness	Reduces joint stiffness by decreasing viscosity of synovial fluid and increasing tissue distensibility.	
Traumatic injury		Decreases bleeding by constricting blood vessels; decreases edema by reducing capillary permeability.

- Assess the skin area to which the heat or cold will be applied.
- Ask the client to report any discomfort.
- Return to the client 15 minutes after starting the heat or cold, and observe the local skin area for any untoward signs (e.g., redness). Stop the application if any problems occur.
- Remove the equipment at the designated time, and dispose of it appropriately.
- Examine the area to which the heat or cold was applied, and record the client's response.

For contraindications to the use of heat or cold, see Box 24–3.

Hot Water Bag A hot water bag or bottle has been a common source of dry heat used in the home. It is convenient and relatively inexpensive. However, because of the danger of burning from improper use, many agencies now use other devices.

The following temperatures of the water in the bag are considered safe in most situations and provide the desired effect: normal adult and child over 2 years, 46°C to 52°C (115°F to 125°F); debilitated or unconscious adult, or child under 2 years, 40.5°C to 46°C (105°F to 115°F).

To apply a hot water bag:

- Measure the temperature of the water using a bath thermometer.

BOX 24–3 Contraindications to the Use of Heat and Cold

Determine the presence of any conditions contraindicating the use of heat:

- *The first 24 hours after traumatic injury.* Heat increases bleeding and swelling.
- *Active hemorrhage.* Heat causes vasodilation and increases bleeding.
- *Noninflammatory edema.* Heat increases capillary permeability and edema.
- *Localized malignant tumor.* Because heat accelerates cell metabolism and cell growth and increases circulation, it may accelerate metastases (secondary tumors).
- *Skin disorder that causes redness or blisters.* Heat can burn or cause further damage to the skin.

Determine the presence of any conditions contraindicating the use of cold:

- *Open wounds.* Cold can increase tissue damage by decreasing blood flow to an open wound.
- *Impaired circulation.* Cold can further impair nourishment of the tissues and cause tissue damage. In clients with Raynaud's disease, cold increases arterial spasm.

- *Allergy or hypersensitivity to cold.* Some clients have an allergy to cold that may be manifested by an inflammatory response, for example, erythema, hives, swelling, joint pain, and occasional muscle spasm. Some react with a sudden increase in blood pressure, which can be hazardous if the person is hypersensitive.

Determine the presence of any conditions indicating the need for special precautions during heat and cold therapy:

- *Neurosensory impairment.* Persons with sensory impairments are unable to perceive that heat is damaging the tissues and are at risk for burns, or they are unable to perceive discomfort from cold and are unable to prevent tissue injury.
- *Impaired mental status.* Persons who are confused or have an altered level of consciousness need monitoring and supervision during applications to ensure safe therapy.
- *Impaired circulation.* Persons with peripheral vascular disease, diabetes, or congestive heart failure lack the normal ability to dissipate heat via the blood circulation, which puts them at risk for tissue damage with heat applications. Cold applications are contraindicated for these people.
- *Open wounds.* Tissues around an open wound are more sensitive to heat and cold.

- Fill the bag about two-thirds full.
- Expel the remaining air and secure the top. With the air removed, the bag can be molded to the body part.
- Dry the bag and hold it upside down to test for leakage.
- Wrap the bag in a towel or cover and place it on the body site.
- Remove after 30 minutes or in accordance with agency protocol.

Aquathermia Pad   The aquathermia or aquamatic pad (also referred to as a K-pad) is a pad constructed with tubes containing water. The pad is attached by tubing to an electrically powered control unit that has an opening for water and a temperature gauge. Some aquathermia pads have an absorbent surface through which moist heat can be applied. The other surface of the pad is waterproof. These pads are disposable.

To apply an aquathermia pad, the nurse carries out the following steps:

- Fill the reservoir of the unit two-thirds full of distilled water.
- Set the desired temperature. Check the manufacturer's instructions. Most units are set at 40.5°C (105°F) for adults.
- Cover the pad and plug in the unit. Some manufacturers suggest warming the pad before applying it.
- Apply the pad to the body part. The treatment is usually continued for 30 minutes. Check orders and agency protocol.

Hot and Cold Packs   Commercially prepared hot and cold packs provide heat or cold for a designated time. Directions on the package tell how to initiate the heating or cooling process, for example, by striking, squeezing, or kneading the pack.

Electric Pads   Electric pads provide a constant, even heat, are lightweight, and can be molded to a body part. Electric pads, however, can burn if the setting is too high. Some models have waterproof covers for use when the pad is placed over a moist dressing.

In applying electric pads, the nurse follows these guidelines:

- Do not insert sharp objects (e.g., pins) into the pad. The pin could damage a wire and cause an electric shock.
- Ensure that the body area is dry unless there is a waterproof cover on the pad. Electricity in the presence of water can cause a shock.
- Use pads with a preset heating switch so a client cannot increase the heat.
- Do not place the pad under the client. Heat will not dissipate, and the client may be burned.

Ice Bags, Ice Gloves, and Ice Collars   Ice bags, ice gloves, and ice collars are filled either with ice chips or with an alcohol-based solution. They are applied to the body to provide cold to a localized area (e.g., a collar is often applied to

the throat following a tonsillectomy). Always wrap the container in a towel or cover.

Compresses   Compresses can be either warm or cold. A **compress** is a moist gauze dressing applied to a wound. When hot compresses are ordered, the solution is heated to the temperature indicated by the order or according to agency protocol, for example, 40.5°C (105°F). When there is a break in the skin or when the body part (e.g., an eye) is vulnerable to microbial invasion, sterile technique is necessary; therefore, sterile gloves are needed to apply the compress and all materials must be sterile.

Soak   A soak refers to immersing a body part (e.g., an arm) in a solution or to wrapping a part in gauze dressings and then saturating the dressing with a solution. Sterile technique is generally indicated for open wounds, such as a burn or an unhealed surgical incision. Determine agency protocol regarding the temperature of the solution. Hot soaks are frequently done to soften and remove encrusted secretions and dead tissue.

Sitz Bath   A sitz bath, or hip bath, is used to soak a client's pelvic area. The client sits in a special tub or chair and is usually immersed from the midthighs to the iliac crests or umbilicus. Special tubs or chairs are preferred because when the legs are also immersed, as in a regular bathtub, blood circulation to the perineum or pelvic area is decreased. Disposable sitz baths are also available.

The temperature of the water should be from 40°C to 43°C (105°F to 110°F), unless the client is unable to tolerate the heat. Determine agency protocol. Some sitz tubs have temperature indicators attached to the water taps. The duration of the bath is generally 15 to 20 minutes, depending on the client's health. To provide a sitz bath:

- Assist the client into the tub. Provide support for the client's feet; a footstool can prevent pressure on the backs of the thighs.
- Provide a bath blanket for the client's shoulders, and eliminate drafts to prevent chilling.
- Observe the client closely during the bath for signs of faintness, dizziness, weakness, accelerated pulse rate, and pallor.
- Maintain the water temperature.
- Following the sitz bath, assist the client out of the tub. Help the client to dry.

Cooling Sponge Bath   The purpose of a cooling sponge bath is to reduce a client's fever by promoting heat loss through conduction and vaporization. Cool sponge baths are used with extreme caution, and only for clients with very high temperatures such as over 40°C (104°F), because rapid skin temperature drop can cause chills that actually increase heat production. The bath is accompanied by antipyretic medication that acts to reset the hypothalamus set point. The temperatures for cooling sponge baths range from 18°C to 32°C (65°F to 93°F).

To provide a cooling sponge bath, the nurse should:

- Sponge the face, arms, legs, back, and buttocks. The chest and abdomen are not usually sponged. Each area is sponged slowly and gently. Rubbing may increase heat production.
- Leave each area wet and cover with a damp towel.
- Place ice bags and cold packs, if used, or a cool cloth on the forehead for comfort and in each axilla and at the groin. These areas contain large superficial blood vessels that help the transfer of heat.
- Sponge one body part and then another. The sponge bath should take about 30 minutes. A bath given more quickly tends to increase the body's heat production by causing shivering.
- Discontinue the bath if the client becomes pale or cyanotic or shivers, or if the pulse becomes rapid or irregular.
- Reassess the vital signs at 15 minutes and after completing the sponge bath.

EVALUATING

The goals established during the planning phase are evaluated according to specific desired outcomes also established in that phase (see Identifying Nursing Diagnoses, Outcomes, and Interventions earlier). To judge whether client outcomes have been achieved, the nurse uses data collected during care, such as skin status over bony prominences, nutritional and fluid intake, mental status, signs of healing if an ulcer is present, and so on. If outcomes are not achieved, the nurse should explore the reasons why:

- Has the client's physical condition changed?
- Were risk factors correctly identified?
- Were appropriate devices and techniques used?
- Did the client fail to comply with instructions about moving and turning? Why?
- Were appropriate pressure-relieving devices used, and were they applied correctly?
- Was the repositioning schedule adhered to?
- Are the client's nutritional and fluid intake adequate?
- Were appropriate measures used to control incontinence and protect the client's skin?
- Was the wound supported and immobilized effectively?
- Were stringent aseptic practices implemented when cleaning and changing dressings to prevent infection?
- Was the client receiving antineoplastic or antiinflammatory medications that interfere with healing?
- Was nonviable tissue removed by autolytic, chemical, mechanical, or surgical debridement?
- Was the appropriate dressing applied to maintain moist wound healing?

CHAPTER HIGHLIGHTS

- Maintaining skin integrity is an important independent function of nursing.
- Wounds are described as intentional or unintentional, closed or open, and clean, clean-contaminated, contaminated, or dirty (infected). Wounds are also classified by depth as partial thickness or full thickness. In addition, wounds are classified according to how they are acquired, as incisions, contusions, abrasions, punctures, lacerations, and penetrating wounds.
- A pressure ulcer is any lesion caused by unrelieved pressure that results in damage to underlying tissues. Pressure ulcers usually occur over bony prominences.
- Two other factors that act in conjunction with pressure to produce a pressure ulcer are friction and shearing forces.
- Several factors increase the risk for the development of pressure ulcers: immobility and inactivity, inadequate nutrition, fecal and urinary incontinence, decreased mental status, diminished sensation, excessive body heat, and advanced age.
- Several risk assessment tools are available to identify clients at risk for pressure ulcer development. They include scoring systems to evaluate a person's degree of risk.

- There are four stages of pressure ulcers, which vary according to the degree of tissue damage.
- There are two types of wound healing, which are distinguished by the amount of tissue loss: primary intention healing and secondary intention healing.
- The wound-healing process has three phases: inflammatory, proliferative, and maturation.
- Major types of wound exudate are serous, purulent, and sanguineous (hemorrhagic). Exudate can be a combination of two or three of these types (e.g., serosanguineous). The process of pus formation is referred to as suppuration.
- The main complications of wound healing are hemorrhage, infection, dehiscence, and evisceration, each of which is identifiable by specific clinical signs and symptoms.
- Factors affecting wound healing include developmental stage, nutritional status, lifestyle, medications, underlying disease processes, and the presence of infection.
- Meticulous skin assessment of common pressure ulcer sites by the nurse is an important ongoing assessment activity for clients at risk.
- When a pressure ulcer is present, the nurse describes the ulcer in terms of location, size, depth, stage, color, status

of wound bed and surrounding skin, and specific signs of infection, if present.
- Wound assessment is an ongoing process to evaluate healing. The nurse assesses wounds by visual inspection, palpation, measurements, and the sense of smell. Essential data for assessing wounds include wound appearance, size, exudate, swelling, pain, and the presence of tubes and drains.
- Laboratory data that may be used to assess the progress of wound healing include leukocyte count, hemoglobin, blood coagulation studies, serum protein analysis, and wound cultures. Nurses are usually responsible for obtaining specimens of wound drainage for culture.
- The NANDA nursing diagnoses *Risk for Impaired Skin Integrity, Impaired Skin Integrity,* and *Impaired Tissue Integrity* apply to clients at risk for developing and to those with pressure ulcers.
- Nursing diagnoses related to clients with wounds may include *Risk for Infection* and *Pain.*
- Major goals for clients at risk for developing pressure ulcers are to maintain skin integrity and to avoid potential associated risks.
- Nursing interventions to prevent the formation of pressure ulcers include conducting ongoing assessment of risk factors and skin status, providing skin care to maintain skin integrity, ensuring adequate nutrition, implementing measures to avoid skin trauma, providing supportive devices, and client teaching.
- Treatment for pressure ulcers varies according to the stage of the ulcer and agency protocol.
- Major nursing responsibilities related to wound care include assisting the client in obtaining sufficient nutrition and fluids, preventing wound infections, and proper positioning.

- Wound care may involve cleaning/irrigating, protecting, filling/hydrating, and covering wounds; applying heat and cold; and applying bandages and binders.
- Various dressing materials are available to protect wounds, absorb exudate, and keep the wound bed moist, thus facilitating healing.
- Synthetic dressings have been developed for use with specific types of wounds. These include transparent adhesive films, impregnated nonadherent dressings, hydrocolloids, hydrogels, polyurethane foams, clear acrylic dressings, and alginates. The nurse must be aware of the specific purposes of each and their indications for use.
- The type of dressing used depends on (a) location, size, and type of the wound; (b) amount of exudate; (c) whether or not the wound requires debridement, is infected, or has sinus tracts; and (d) such considerations as frequency of dressing change, ease or difficulty of dressing applications, and cost.
- The RYB color code of wounds can assist nurses to provide appropriate nursing interventions for wounds that heal by secondary intention. In this scheme, the nurse protects red, cleanses yellow, and debrides black.
- Heat and cold produce specific local physiologic and systemic responses that account for their therapeutic effects.
- Various parts of the body differ in tolerance to heat and cold. The physiologic tolerance of individuals also varies. Specific conditions such as neurosensory and circulatory impairments necessitate precautions when applying heat or cold.
- When applying heat or cold, clients and nurses need to be aware of the effects of thermal receptor adaptation and the rebound phenomenon.

THINK ABOUT IT

Refer to the chapter-opening scenario and answer these questions.

1. What factors placed Ms. Cassidy at increased risk for poor wound healing?

2. What orders do you anticipate the nurse will receive from the provider when the client's symptoms are reported to the provider?

3. What interventions would you plan for this client's care to improve wound healing?

∞ *See suggested responses to Think About It on MyNursingKit.*

TEST YOUR KNOWLEDGE

1. The nurse is caring for a client with a Braden scale score of 17. The appropriate nursing action is to:
1. Assess the client again in 24 hours; the score is within normal limits.
2. Implement a turning schedule; the client is at increased risk of skin breakdown.
3. Apply a transparent wound barrier to major pressure sites; the client is at moderate risk of skin breakdown.
4. Request an order for a special low-air-loss bed; the client is at very high risk of skin breakdown.

2. The nurse, functioning as the charge nurse on a long-term care skilled unit, would identify which of the following clients at greatest risk for pressure ulcers?
1. The 34-year-old client in a chronic vegetative state following a diving accident
2. The 84-year-old client with hemiplegia on the left side attending rehabilitation daily
3. The 59-year-old client in the end stages of terminal bowel cancer with a draining lower abdominal wound
4. The 94-year-old woman diagnosed with Alzheimer's disease who often wanders

3. A client has a pressure ulcer with a shallow, partial skin thickness eroded area but no necrosis. The most appropriate dressing for the nurse to use to treat the area would be which of the following?
   1. Alginate
   2. Dry gauze
   3. Hydrocolloid
   4. No dressing is indicated

4. Thirty (30) minutes after application is initiated, the client requests that the nurse leave the heating pad in place. The nurse explains to the client that:
   1. Heat application for longer than 30 minutes can actually cause the opposite effect (constriction) of the one desired (dilation).
   2. It will be acceptable to leave the pad in place if the temperature is reduced.
   3. It will be acceptable to leave the pad in place for another 30 minutes if the site appears satisfactory when assessed.
   4. It will be acceptable to leave the pad in place as long as it is moist heat.

5. Which statement, if made by the client or family member, would the nurse evaluate as indicating the need for further teaching?
   1. "If a skin area gets red but then the red goes away after turning, I should report it to the nurse."
   2. "Putting foam pads under the heels or other bony areas can help decrease pressure."
   3. "If a person cannot turn himself or herself in bed, someone should help the person change position every 4 hours."
   4. "The skin should be washed with only warm water (not hot) and lotion put on while it is still a little wet."

6. The nurse is caring for a client who is only comfortable lying on the left or right side. What four areas should the nurse assess as potential sites of pressure ulcers?

   _____

7. An appropriate nursing diagnosis for a client with large areas of skin excoriation resulting from scratching an allergic rash is:
   1. *Risk for Impaired Skin Integrity*
   2. *Impaired Skin Integrity*
   3. *Impaired Tissue Integrity*
   4. *Risk for Infection*

8. The nurse anticipates which of the following could place the client at increased risk for pressure ulcers? Select all that apply.
   1. Low-protein diet
   2. Insomnia
   3. Lengthy surgical procedures
   4. Fever
   5. Sleeping on a waterbed.

9. When performing a wound irrigation the nurse would use which of the following? Select all that apply.
   1. Clean gloves
   2. Sterile gloves
   3. Refrigerated irrigating solution
   4. 60-mL syringe
   5. Microwaved irrigating solution

10. When the nurse applies a triangle arm sling which of the following would indicates proper technique?
    1. The elbow is kept flexed at 90 degrees or more.
    2. The knot is placed on either side of the vertebrae of the neck.
    3. The sling extends to just proximal of the hand.
    4. Remove the sling every 2 hours to check for circulation and skin integrity.

∞ *See answers to Test Your Knowledge in Appendix A.*

REFERENCES AND SELECTED BIBLIOGRAPHY

Anderson, I. (2006). Debridement methods in wound care. *Nursing Standard, 20*(24), 65–66, 68, 70.

Ankrom, M. A., Bennett, R. G., Sprigle, S., Langemo, D., Black, J. M., Berlowitz, D. R., et al. (2005). Pressure related deep tissue injury under intact skin and the current pressure ulcer staging systems. *Advances in Skin and Wound Care, 18*(1), 35–42.

Baldwin, K. M. (2006). Damage control: Preventing and treating pressure ulcers. *Nursing Made Incredibly Easy, 4*(1), 12–15, 17–23, 25–27.

Baranoski, S., & Ayello, E. A. (2005). Wound & skin care. Using a wound assessment form. *Nursing, 35*(3), 14–15.

Bergstrom, N., Allman, R. M., Alvarez, A. M., Bennett, M. A., Carlson, C. E., Frantz, R. A., et al. (1994). *Pressure Ulcer Treatment: Clinical Practice Guideline Number 15. Quick Reference Guide for Clinicians* (Publication No. 95-0653). Rockville, MD: Agency for Health Care Policy and Research, Public Health Service, U.S. Department of Health and Human Services.

Braden, B. J., & Maklebust, J. (2005). Preventing pressure ulcers with the Braden Scale. *American Journal of Nursing, 105*(6), 70–72.

Brown, G. (2006). Wound documentation: Managing risk. *Advances in Skin and Wound Care, 19*, 155–165.

Bulechek, G. M., Butcher, H. K., & Dochterman, J. M., (Eds.). (2008). *Nursing interventions: Classification (NIC)* (5th ed.). St. Louis: Mosby.

Coulthard, P., Worthington, H., Esposito, M., van der Elst, M., & van Waes, O. J. F. (2005). Tissue adhesives for closure of surgical incisions. *The Cochrane Library* (ID #CD004287).

Cullum, N., McInnes, E., Bell-Syer, S. E. M., & Legood, R. (2005). Support surfaces for pressure ulcer prevention. *The Cochrane Library* (ID #CD001735).

Duimel-Peeters, I. (2005). Preventing pressure ulcers with massage? *American Journal of Nursing, 105*(8), 31, 33.

Fernandez, R., Griffiths, R., & Ussia, C. (2006). Water for wound cleansing (Cochrane Review). In *The Cochrane Library*, Issue 1, 2006. Oxford: Update Software.

Folkedahl, B. A., & Frantz, R. (2002a). *Prevention of pressure ulcers.* Iowa City, IA: University of Iowa Gerontological Nursing Interventions Research Center, Research Dissemination Core; 2002. Retrieved December 5, 2009, from http://www.rnao.org/Storage/29/2371_BPG_Pressure_Ulcers_I_to_IV.pfg

Folkedahl, B. A., & Frantz, R. (2002b). *Treatment of pressure ulcers.* Iowa City; IA: University of Iowa Gerontological Nursing Interventions Research Center, Research Dissemination Core. Retrieved December 5, 2009, from http://www.rnao.org/Storage/29/2371_BPG_Pressure_Ulcers_I_to_IV.pdf

Frantz, R. A., Tang, J. H., & Titler, M. G. (2004). Evidence-based protocol: Prevention of pressure ulcers. *Journal of Gerontological Nursing, 30*(5), 4–11.

Hanson, D., Langemo, D., Thompson, P., Anderson, J., & Hunter, S. (2005). Understanding wound fluid and the phases of healing. *Advances in Skin & Wound Care, 18*, 360–362.

Keefe, S. (2004). Healing severe wounds. *Advance for Nurses, 1*(12), 32, 40.

Langemo, D., & Hanson, D. (2005). Sizing up wounds accurately, *Nursing, 35*(4), 70–71.

Mendez-Eastman, S. (2005). Using negative-pressure for positive results. *Nursing, 35*(5), 48–50.

Moorhead, S., Johnson, M., Maas, M. L., & Swanson, E. (Eds.). (2008). *Nursing outcomes classification (NOC)* (4th ed.). St. Louis: Mosby.

Moz, T. (2004). Action Stat: Wound dehiscence and evisceration. *Nursing, 34*(5), 88.

National Pressure Ulcer Advisory Panel. (2001). *Pressure ulcer prevention: RN competency-based curriculum.* Reston, VA: Author.

National Pressure Ulcer Advisory Panel. (2003). *PUSH Tool 3.0.* Retrieved June 9, 2006, from http://www.npuap.org/PDF/push3.pdf

NANDA International. (2009). *NANDA Nursing diagnoses: Definitions and classification 2009–2011.* West Sussex, U.K.: Wiley-Blackwell.

Norton, D., McLaren, R., & Exton-Smith, A. N. (1975). *An investigation of geriatric nursing problems in hospital.* Edinburgh, UK: Churchill Livingstone.

Ousey, K. (2005). *Pressure area care.* Oxford, UK: Blackwell.

Panel for the Prediction and Prevention of Pressure Ulcers in Adults. (1992a). *Clinical practice guideline, pressure ulcers in adults: Prediction and prevention* (Publication No. 92–0047). Rockville, MD: Agency for Health Care Policy and Research, Public Health Service, U.S. Department of Health and Human Services.

Panel for the Prediction and Prevention of Pressure Ulcers in Adults. (1992b). *Pressure ulcers in adults: Prediction and prevention. Quick reference guide for clinicians* (AHCPR Publication No. 92-0050). Rockville, MD: Agency for Health Care Policy and Research, Public Health Service, U.S. Department of Health and Human Services.

Sarvis, C. (2004). Wound and skin care: The role of bacterial toxins in wounds. *Nursing, 34*(7), 68.

Smith, N. (2004). The benefits of VAC therapy in the management of pressure ulcers. *British Journal of Nursing, 13*, 1359–60, 1362, 1364–5.

Sosin, J. (2005). Ancient remedy heals today's wounds. *Nursing Spectrum, 14*(6), 32–33.

U.S. Department of Health and Human Services. (2000). *Healthy people 2010: Understanding and improving health* (2nd ed.). Washington, DC: U.S. Government Printing Office.

Verdu, J. (2003). Can a decision tree help nurses to grade and treat pressure ulcers? *Journal of Wound Care, 12*(2), 45–50.

Whittington, K. T. (2005). Cost-saving wound assessments. *Advance for Nurses, 2*(2), 25–26.

Whittington, K. T., & Briones, R. (2004). National prevalence and incidence study, 6 year sequential acute care data. *Advances in Skin and Wound Care, 17*, 490–494.

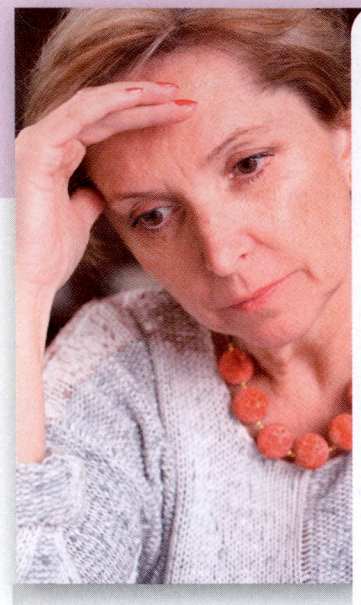

Cheryl Klein, 54 years old, is admitted to the surgical center at 6 AM for repair of a torn rotator cuff. The nurse obtains vital signs and notes the client is mildly hypertensive, her blood pressure being elevated from the baseline vital signs obtained at the provider's office several days ago. Her heart rate is within normal limits at 92 beats per minute, which is also higher than her baseline. Cheryl tells the nurse she has never had surgery before and will be glad when it is over. When the nurse questions her about specific concerns, Cheryl says she's afraid she'll talk and say something stupid while she's anesthetized or that the surgeon will make a mistake and operate on the wrong body part. She reports that a friend told her the pain after this particular surgery is excruciating, and she's worried she won't be able to stand the discomfort.

LEARNING OUTCOMES

After completing this chapter, you will be able to:

1. Describe how surgery can be classified based on urgency, risk, and purpose.

2. Apply the nursing process to nursing care in the preoperative phase, the intraoperative phase, and the postoperative phase.

3. Describe client teaching that is important in each stage of perioperative nursing.

4. Contrast various types of anesthesia and their indications.

5. Identify nursing interventions that can reduce the risk of common postoperative complications.

6. Describe the essential care for clients with gastrointestinal suction and wound care needs in the postoperative period.

KEY TERMS

Atelectasis p763
Bier block p755
Circulating nurse p755
Closed-wound drainage systems p770
Conscious sedation p755
Elective surgery p743

Emergency surgery p743
Epidural anesthesia p755
General anesthesia p754
Intraoperative phase p743
Intravenous block p755
Local anesthesia p755

Nerve block p755
Penrose drain p770
Peridural anesthesia p755
Perioperative period p743
Postoperative phase p743
Preoperative phase p743

Regional anesthesia p754
Scrub person p755
Spinal anesthesia p755
Surface anesthesia p754
Thrombophlebitis p763
Topical anesthesia p754

Surgery is a unique experience of a planned physical alteration encompassing three phases: preoperative, intraoperative, and postoperative. These three phases are together referred to as the **perioperative period**. Perioperative nursing is the delivery of nursing care through the framework of the nursing process. It also includes collaborating with members of the health care team, making nursing referrals, and delegating and supervising nursing care.

The **preoperative phase** begins when the decision to have surgery is made; it ends when the client is transferred to the operating table. The nursing activities associated with this phase include assessing the client, identifying potential or actual health problems, planning specific care based on the individual's needs, and providing preoperative teaching for the client, the family, and significant others.

The **intraoperative phase** begins when the client is transferred to the operating table and ends when the client is admitted to the postanesthesia care unit (PACU), also called the postanesthetic room or recovery room. The nursing activities related to this phase include a variety of specialized procedures designed to create and maintain a safe therapeutic environment for the client and the health care personnel. These activities include interventions that provide for the client's safety, maintaining an aseptic environment, ensuring proper functioning of equipment, and providing the surgical team with the instruments and supplies needed during the procedure.

The **postoperative phase** begins with the admission of the client to the postanesthesia area and ends when healing is complete. During the postoperative phase, nursing activities include assessing the client's response to surgery, performing interventions to facilitate healing and prevent complications, teaching and providing support to the client and support people, and planning for home care. The goal is to assist the client to achieve the most optimal health status possible.

Perioperative nursing is practiced in hospital-based inpatient and outpatient surgical/laser/endoscopy suites, physician office-based surgical suites (outpatient), and/or freestanding outpatient/ ambulatory surgical centers. Outpatient procedures do not require an overnight hospital stay. The client goes to the outpatient site the day of surgery, has the procedure, and leaves the same day. The perioperative nurse's role is underscored by the nursing process and all the care activities inherent in that process regardless of the health care setting in which it is operationalized.

TYPES OF SURGERY

Surgical procedures are commonly grouped according to (a) purpose, (b) degree of urgency, and (c) degree of risk.

Purpose

Surgical procedures may be categorized according to their purpose (see Box 25–1).

BOX 25–1	**Purposes of Surgical Procedures**
Diagnostic	Confirms or establishes a diagnosis; for example, biopsy of a mass in a breast.
Palliative	Relieves or reduces pain or symptoms of a disease; it does not cure; for example, resection of nerve roots.
Ablative	Removes a diseased body part; for example, removal of a gallbladder (cholecystectomy).
Constructive	Restores function or appearance that has been lost or reduced; for example, breast implant.
Transplant	Replaces malfunctioning structures; for example, kidney transplant.

Degree of Urgency

Surgery is classified by its urgency and necessity to preserve the client's life, body part, or body function. **Emergency surgery** is performed immediately to preserve function or the life of the client. Surgeries to control internal hemorrhage or repair a fracture are examples of emergency surgeries. **Elective surgery** is performed when surgical intervention is the preferred treatment for a condition that is not imminently life threatening (but may ultimately threaten life or well-being) or to improve the client's life. Examples of elective surgeries include cholecystectomy for chronic gallbladder disease, hip replacement surgery, and plastic surgery procedures such as breast reduction surgery.

Degree of Risk

Surgery is also classified as major or minor according to the degree of risk to the client. Major surgery involves a high degree of risk, for a variety of reasons: It may be complicated or prolonged, large losses of blood may occur, vital organs may be involved, or postoperative complications may be likely. Examples are organ transplant, open heart surgery, and removal of a kidney. In contrast, minor surgery normally involves little risk, produces few complications, and is often performed in an outpatient setting. Examples are breast biopsy, removal of tonsils, and knee surgery.

The degree of risk involved in a surgical procedure is affected by the client's age, general health, nutritional status, use of medications, and mental status.

AGE Neonates/infants and older adults are greater surgical risks than children and adults. Age and developmental status affect a child's ability to cope with the physiologic and psychologic stresses of surgery. Neonates and infants have a higher metabolic rate and a different physiologic makeup than adults. These differences cause a substantially different response to a surgical procedure. Because of the infant's relatively large body surface area and immature temperature regulatory mechanisms, the risk of hypothermia during surgery is significant. Other organ systems, such as the kidneys, liver, and immune system, also have not achieved maturity in infants, affecting their ability to metabolize and eliminate drugs and resist infection.

Toddlers and older children are better able to withstand surgery physiologically, but they often fear separation from their parents, strangers, bodily injury/mutilation, and death. The child's developmental level and age-appropriate communication are important in implementing the pediatric plan of care. The parent–child relationship, the parents' coping abilities, and the preoperative teaching and support will affect how well the child is able to deal with these surgical fears and the level of anxiety experienced.

The older adult (65 years and older) often has fewer physiologic reserves to meet the extra demands caused by surgery. The physiologic deficits of aging increase the surgical risk for the older adult. Many older adults demonstrate changes in liver and kidney function, both of which can affect response to anesthesia and other medications that may be administered during the perioperative period. The older adult may be poorly nourished, which can impair healing. Declines in sensory function (hearing in particular) or the presence of dementia make it more difficult to understand directions and teaching. In addition, the older adult is more likely to have a chronic disease, such as cardiovascular disease, chronic lung disease, or diabetes, that affects healing and responses to medication and surgery.

GENERAL HEALTH   Surgery is least risky when the client's general health is good. Any infection or pathophysiology increases the risk. Of particular concern are upper respiratory tract infections, which together with a general anesthetic can adversely affect respiratory function. Where there is a high risk of infection, antibiotics may be administered parenterally within 1 hour of surgery and continued for 24 to 72 hours after surgery. This practice allows time for drugs to reach therapeutic levels in the tissues but does not permit bacterial resistance to develop. Common health problems that increase surgical risk and may lead to the decision to postpone or cancel surgery are listed in Box 25–2.

NUTRITIONAL STATUS   Adequate nutrition is required for normal tissue repair. Surgery increases the body's need for nutrients for the needed tissue healing and prevention of infection required during the postoperative period. Obesity and malnutrition increase surgical risk.

Obesity contributes to postoperative complications such as pneumonia, wound infections, and wound separation. Both obese and underweight clients are vulnerable to pressure ulcer formation due to positioning required for surgery. The perioperative nurse provides padding and other measures to protect the client's skin over pressure points during surgery.

Many vitamins and minerals are essential in wound healing. A malnourished client is at risk for delayed wound healing, wound infection, and fluid and electrolyte alterations. If a client has serious malnutrition, the surgery may be postponed to improve the nutritional status. If the surgery cannot be delayed, parenteral or enteral nutrition may be initiated.

MEDICATIONS   The regular use of certain medications can increase surgical risk. Consider these examples:

- *Anticoagulants* increase blood coagulation time.
- *Tranquilizers* may interact with anesthetics, increasing the risk of respiratory depression.
- *Corticosteroids* may interfere with wound healing and increase the risk of infection.
- *Diuretics* may affect fluid and electrolyte balance.

Clients may be unaware of the potential adverse interactions of medications and may fail to report the use of medications for conditions unrelated to the indication for surgery. The astute nurse interviewer should question the client and family about the use of commonly prescribed medications, over-the-counter preparations, and any herbal remedies for specific conditions mentioned during the nursing history.

MENTAL STATUS   Disorders that affect cognitive function, such as mental illness, mental retardation, or developmental delay, affect the client's ability to understand and cope with the stresses of surgery. These clients also may require medication such as anticonvulsants or antipsychotic drugs that can interact with anesthetic and analgesic medications used during and after surgery.

| **BOX 25–2** | **Health Problems that Increase Surgical Risk** |

- Malnutrition can lead to delayed wound healing, infection, and reduced energy. Protein and vitamins are needed for wound healing; vitamin K is essential for blood clotting.
- Obesity leads to hypertension, impaired cardiac function, and impaired respiratory ventilation. Obese clients are also more likely to have delayed wound healing and wound infection because adipose tissue impedes blood circulation and its delivery of nutrients, antibodies, and enzymes required for wound healing.
- Cardiac conditions such as angina pectoris, recent myocardial infarction, hypertension, and heart failure weaken the heart. Well-controlled cardiac problems generally pose minimal operative risk.
- Blood coagulation disorders may lead to severe bleeding, hemorrhage, and subsequent shock.
- Upper respiratory tract infections or chronic obstructive lung diseases such as emphysema adversely affect pulmonary function, especially when exacerbated by the effects of general anesthesia. They also predispose the client to postoperative lung infections.
- Renal disease impairs regulation of the body's fluids and electrolytes and excretion of drugs and other toxins.
- Diabetes mellitus predisposes the client to wound infection and delayed healing.
- Liver disease (e.g., cirrhosis) impairs the liver's abilities to detoxify medications used during surgery, produce the prothrombin necessary for blood clotting, and metabolize nutrients essential for healing.
- Uncontrolled neurologic disease such as epilepsy may result in seizures during surgery or recovery.

Clients with dementia may have difficulty understanding proposed surgical procedures and may respond unpredictably to anesthetics. Manifestations of dementia such as confusion, disorientation, and agitation also may be aggravated by the change of environment in the hospital, interfering with the client's ability to cooperate with pre- and postoperative care.

Extreme anxiety also increases surgical risk and interferes with the client's ability to process information and respond appropriately to instructions. In some instances, professional counseling is indicated prior to surgery. It is also important to determine whether clients have coping skills and support systems to help them.

PREOPERATIVE PHASE

Preoperative Consent

Prior to any surgical procedure, informed consent is required from the client or legal guardian. Informed consent implies that the client has been informed and involved in decisions affecting his or her health. The surgeon is responsible for obtaining the informed consent by providing the following information to the client or legal guardian:

- The nature of and the reason for the surgery
- All available options and the risks associated with each option
- The risks of the surgical procedure and its potential outcomes
- Name and qualifications of the surgeon performing the procedure
- The right to refuse consent or later withdraw consent

The surgeon documents the informed consent conversation with the client or legal guardian in the preoperative progress note.

The surgical consent form, provided by the agency, protects the client from incorrect/unwanted procedures and the surgeon and agency from litigation related to unauthorized surgeries or uninformed clients. This consent form becomes part of the client's medical record and goes to the operating room with the client.

Although the surgeon maintains legal responsibility for ensuring that the client is giving informed consent, the nurse may witness the client's signature on the agency consent form. In doing so, the nurse ensures that the consent form is signed and serves as a witness to the signature, not to the fact that the client is informed. If the nurse assesses that the client does not understand the procedure to be performed, the surgeon is contacted and requested to speak with the client before surgery can proceed.

Informed consent is possible only when the client understands the provided information, that is, speaks the language and is conscious, mentally competent, and not sedated. Informed consent may not be given by a minor. Specific guidelines regarding consent for minors vary among the states. Nurses must be aware of their responsibilities regarding consent and of the particular hospital's policies (see Chapter 2 ∞).

NURSING MANAGEMENT

ASSESSING

Preoperative assessment includes collecting and reviewing physical, psychologic, and social client data to determine the client's needs throughout the three perioperative phases. The perioperative nurse collects the data by interviewing the client in the presurgical care unit or by telephone prior to the day of surgery. When data cannot be collected directly, the perioperative nurse uses other data sources such as the nursing admission assessment. Although forms vary considerably among agencies, Box 25–3 summarizes essential preoperative information that should be included.

Physical Assessment

Preoperatively, the nurse performs a brief but complete physical assessment, paying particular attention to systems that could affect the client's response to anesthesia or surgery. A brief or "mini" mental status examination provides valuable baseline data for evaluating the client's mental status and alertness after surgery. It is also important to evaluate the client's ability to understand what is happening. For example, assessment of hearing and vision help guide perioperative teaching. Respiratory and cardiovascular assessments provide baseline data for not only evaluating the client's postoperative status but also may alert care providers to a problem (e.g., a respiratory infection or irregular pulse rate) that may affect the client's response to surgery and anesthesia. Other systems (gastrointestinal, genitourinary, and musculoskeletal) are examined to provide baseline data (see Chapter 17 ∞).

Screening Tests

The surgeon and/or anesthesiologist orders preoperative diagnostic tests. Abnormalities may warrant treatment prior to surgery. The nurse's responsibility is to check the orders carefully, to see that they are carried out, and to ensure that the results are obtained and in the client's record prior to surgery. Table 25–1 lists routine preoperative screening tests. In addition to these routine tests, diagnostic tests directly related to the client's disease are usually appropriate.

DIAGNOSING

Nursing diagnoses that may be appropriate for the preoperative client include the following:

- *Deficient Knowledge* related to
  - A lack of education about the perioperative process
  - A lack of exposure to the specific perioperative experience

BOX 25-3 Preoperative Assessment Data

- *Current health status.* Essential information includes general health status and the presence of any chronic diseases, such as diabetes or asthma, that may affect the client's response to surgery or anesthesia. Note any physical limitations that may affect the client's mobility or ability to communicate after surgery, as well as any prostheses such as hearing aids or contact lenses.
- *Allergies.* Include allergies to prescription and nonprescription drugs, food allergies, and allergies to tape, latex, soaps, or antiseptic agents. Some food allergies may indicate a potential reaction to drugs or substances used during surgery or diagnostic procedures; for example, an allergy to seafood alerts the nurse to a potential allergy to iodine-based dyes or soaps commonly used in hospitals.
- *Medications.* List all current medications (prescribed and OTC). It may be vital to maintain a blood level of some medications (e.g., anticonvulsants) throughout the surgical experience; others, such as anticoagulants or aspirin, increase the risks of surgery and anesthesia and need to be discontinued several days prior to surgery. It is important to include in the list any herbal remedies the client currently takes.
- *Previous surgeries.* Previous surgical experiences may influence the client's physical and psychologic responses to surgery or may reveal unexpected responses to anesthesia.
- *Mental status.* The client's mental status and ability to understand and respond appropriately can affect the entire perioperative experience. Note any developmental disabilities, mental illness, history of dementia, or excessive anxiety related to the procedure.
- *Understanding of the surgical procedure and anesthesia.* The client should have a good understanding of the planned procedure and what to expect during and after surgery as well as the expected outcome of the procedure.
- *Smoking.* Smokers may have more difficulty clearing respiratory secretions after surgery, increasing the risk of postoperative complications such as pneumonia and atelectasis and delayed wound healing.
- *Alcohol and other mind-altering substances.* Use of substances that affect the central nervous system, liver, or other body systems can affect the client's response to anesthesia and surgery, and postoperative recovery.
- *Coping.* Clients with a healthy self-concept who have successfully employed appropriate coping mechanisms in the past are better able to deal with the stressors associated with surgery.
- *Social resources.* Determine the availability of family or other caregivers as well as the client's social support network. These resources are important to the client's recovery, particularly for the client undergoing same-day or short-stay surgery.
- *Cultural and spiritual considerations.* Culture and spirituality influence the client's response to surgery; respecting cultural and spiritual beliefs and practices can reduce preoperative anxiety and improve recovery.

TABLE 25-1 Routine Preoperative Screening Tests

TEST	RATIONALE
Complete blood count (CBC)	RBCs, hemoglobin (Hgb), and hematocrit (Hct) are important to the oxygen-carrying capacity of the blood; WBCs are an indicator of immune function
Blood grouping and cross-matching	Determined in case blood transfusion is required during or after surgery
Serum electrolytes (Na^+, K^+, Ca^{2+}, Mg^{2+}, Cl^-, HCO_3^-)	To evaluate fluid and electrolyte status
Fasting blood glucose	High levels may indicate undiagnosed diabetes mellitus
Blood urea nitrogen (BUN) and creatinine	To evaluate renal function
ALT, AST, LDH, and bilirubin	To evaluate liver function
Serum albumin and total protein	To evaluate nutritional status
Urinalysis	To determine urine composition and possible abnormal components (e.g., protein or glucose) or infection
Chest x-ray	To evaluate respiratory status and heart size
Electrocardiogram (ECG) (all clients over 40 years of age and/or clients with preexisting cardiac conditions)	To identify preexisting cardiac problems or disease
Pregnancy test (all female clients of childbearing age)	To identify if the client is pregnant

- *Anxiety* related to
  - Effects of surgery on ability to function in usual roles
  - Outcome of exploratory surgery for malignancy
  - Risk of death
  - Loss of control during anesthesia or waking up during anesthesia
  - Perceived inadequate postoperative analgesia
  - Change in health status and/or body image
- *Disturbed Sleep Pattern* related to
  - Hospital routines
  - Psychologic stress
- *Anticipatory Grieving* related to
  - Perceived loss of body part associated with planned surgery
- *Ineffective Coping* related to
  - Conflicting values
  - Lack of clear outcomes of surgery
  - Unresolved past negative experience with surgery

Examples of clinical application of some of these diagnoses using NANDA, NIC, and NOC designations are shown in Identifying Nursing Diagnoses, Outcomes, and Interventions.

PLANNING

The overall goal in the preoperative period is to ensure that the client is mentally and physically prepared for surgery. Examples of nursing activities to meet this goal are discussed in the "Implementing" section that follows. Planning should involve the client, the family, and/or significant others. Preoperative care planning and teaching interventions are usually done on an outpatient basis either in person or via a telephone interview by the perioperative nurse. Examples of clinical application of NOC outcomes and NIC interventions are shown in Identifying Nursing Diagnoses, Outcomes, and Interventions.

Discharge Planning

For the perioperative client, discharge planning begins before admission for the planned procedure. Early planning to meet the discharge needs of the client is particularly important for outpatient procedures, as generally these clients are discharged within hours after the procedure is performed. Discharge planning incorporates an assessment of the client's, family's, and significant others' abilities and resources for care, their financial resources, and the need for referrals and home health services. However, the extent of

---

IDENTIFYING NURSING DIAGNOSES, OUTCOMES, AND INTERVENTIONS — The Preoperative Client

DATA CLUSTER Mr. Taylor, 62 years old, has disabling osteoarthritis and is scheduled for a total knee replacement tomorrow. This is his first surgical experience and he is asking many questions about what to expect before and after surgery. He says, "The more I know, the less anxious I feel."

NURSING DIAGNOSIS/ DEFINITION	SAMPLE DESIRED OUTCOME*/*DEFINITION*	INDICATORS	SELECTED INTERVENTIONS/ *DEFINITION*	SAMPLE NIC ACTIVITIES
Deficient Knowledge (Surgery)/Absence or deficiency of cognitive information related to a specific topic	Knowledge: Treatment Procedure(s) [1814]/ *Extent of understanding conveyed about procedure(s) required as part of a treatment regimen*	Substantial: • Description of steps of procedure (e.g., preoperative process) • Description of treatment procedures (e.g., deep breathing and coughing, leg exercises)	Teaching: Preoperative [5610]/ *Assisting a patient to understand and mentally prepare for surgery and the postoperative recovery period*	• Provide time for the client to ask questions and discuss concerns • Describe the preoperative routines (e.g., anesthesia, diet, tests/lab, voiding, IV therapy, family waiting area) as appropriate • Instruct the client on the technique of splinting his/her incision, coughing, and deep breathing • Evaluate the client's ability to return demonstrate leg exercise

*The NOC # for desired outcomes and the NIC # for nursing interventions are listed in brackets following the appropriate outcome or intervention. Outcomes, indicators, interventions, and activities selected are only a sample of those suggested by NOC and NIC and should be further individualized for each client.

discharge planning and home care will vary significantly for clients having different types of surgery.

IMPLEMENTING

The major nursing activity to ensure that the client is prepared for surgery is preoperative teaching.

Preoperative Teaching

Preoperative teaching is a vital part of nursing care. Studies have shown that preoperative teaching reduces clients' anxiety and postoperative complications and increases their satisfaction with the surgical experience. Good preoperative teaching also facilitates the client's successful and early return to work and other activities of daily living. Four dimensions of preoperative teaching have been identified as important to clients:

- *Information, including what will happen to the client, when, and what the client will experience, such as expected sensations and discomfort.* The nurse needs to listen carefully and attentively to the client to identify specific concerns and fears. Typical questions are: "What will happen during surgery? How will I feel after the operation? What will the surgeon find? How long will I be in the hospital?"
- *Psychosocial support to reduce anxiety.* The nurse provides support by actively listening and providing accurate information. It is important to rectify any misperceptions the client may have.

- *The roles of the client and support people in preoperative preparation, the surgical procedure, and during the postoperative phase.* Understanding his or her role during the perioperative experience increases the client's sense of control and reduces anxiety. This includes what will be expected of the client, desired behaviors, self-care activities, and what the client can do to facilitate recovery.
- *Skills training.* This includes moving, deep breathing, coughing, splinting incisions with the hands or a pillow, and using an incentive spirometer.

If the client is scheduled for outpatient surgery, preoperative teaching is often provided before the day of surgery using some combination of videos and verbal and written instructions. The client may have an appointment with the outpatient perioperative nurse (usually scheduled to coincide with preoperative diagnostic testing) to discuss preoperative concerns and implement the teaching plan. Written instructions are always provided to reinforce verbal teaching. Teaching is further reinforced on admission the day of surgery and before discharge from the postanesthesia unit. Preoperative instructions are summarized in Box 25–4.

When the client is a child, addressing the fears and anxieties of both the child and the family is vital. Parents need to know what to expect and to be able to express their concerns. Parents should be considered members of the perioperative team and allowed to participate in providing as much care as possible.

Skill 25–1 provides guidelines for teaching clients about moving, leg exercises, deep breathing, and coughing.

BOX 25–4   Preoperative Instructions

Preoperative Regimen

- Explain the need for preoperative tests.
- Discuss bowel preparation, if required.
- Discuss skin preparation, including operative area and preoperative bath or shower.
- Discuss preoperative medications, if ordered.
- Explain individual therapies ordered by the primary care provider.
- Discuss the visit by the anesthetist.
- Explain the need to restrict food and oral fluids. (Note that recent research indicates less time NPO may be required than in the past.)
- Provide a general timetable for perioperative events, including the time of surgery.
- Discuss the need to remove jewelry, makeup, and all prostheses immediately before surgery.
- Inform client about the preoperative holding area, and give the location of the waiting room for support people.
- Teach deep-breathing and coughing exercises, leg exercises, ways to turn and move, and splinting techniques.
- Complete the preoperative checklist.

Postoperative Regimen

- Discuss the postanesthesia recovery room's routines and emergency equipment.
- Review type and frequency of assessment activities.

- Discuss pain management.
- Explain usual activity restrictions and precautions related to getting up for the first time postoperatively.
- Describe usual dietary alterations.
- Discuss postoperative dressings and drains.
- Provide an explanation and tour of the intensive care unit if client is to be transferred there postoperatively.

Outpatient Surgical Clients

- Review all instructions in the preoperative and postoperative regimen.
- Confirm place and time of surgery, including when to arrive and where to register.
- Discuss what to wear.
- Explain the need for a responsible adult to drive or accompany the client home.
- Discuss discharge criteria and how long the client should expect to stay postoperatively.
- Discuss medications, including specific preoperative medications and the client's current medication regimen.
- Communicate by telephone the evening before surgery to confirm time of surgery and arrival time.
- Communicate by telephone within 48 hours postoperatively to evaluate surgical outcomes and identify any problems or complications.

SKILL 25–1

TEACHING MOVING, LEG EXERCISES, DEEP BREATHING, AND COUGHING

PURPOSES

Moving
- To promote venous return
- To enhance lung expansion and mobilize secretions
- To stimulate gastrointestinal motility
- To facilitate early ambulation

Leg exercises
- To promote venous return, thereby preventing thrombophlebitis and thrombus formation

Deep breathing and coughing
- To enhance lung expansion and mobilize secretions, thereby preventing atelectasis and pneumonia

ASSESSMENT

Assess
- Vital signs
- Discomfort
- Temperature and color of feet and legs
- Breath sounds
- Presence of dyspnea or cough
- Learning needs of the client
- Anxiety level of the client
- Client experience with previous surgeries and anesthesia

PLANNING

Before commencing to teach moving, leg exercises, deep-breathing exercises, and coughing, determine (a) the type of surgery, (b) the time of the surgery, (c) the name of the surgeon, (d) the preopera-tive orders, and (e) the agency's practices for preoperative care. Also, verify that the primary care provider has completed the medical history and physical examination and that the client or the family has signed the consent form.

> **Delegation**
> Assessment of the learning needs of the client and his or her support people and determining the teaching content and appropriate strategies for teaching requires application of professional knowledge and critical thinking. Preoperative teaching is conducted by the nurse and is not delegated to unlicensed assistive personnel (UAP). The UAP, however, can reinforce teaching, assist the client with the exercises, and report to the nurse if the client is unable to perform the exercises.

EQUIPMENT
- Pillow
- Teaching materials (e.g., videotape, written materials) if available at the agency

IMPLEMENTATION

Preparation
Ensure that potential distracters (e.g., pain, TV, visitors) to teaching are not present. Family and/or significant others should be included in the teaching plan, if appropriate.

Performance

1. Prior to performing the procedure, introduce self and verify the client's identity using agency protocol. Explain to the client what you are going to teach and the importance of the client's participation in the exercises he or she is going to be taught.
2. Perform hand hygiene and observe appropriate infection control procedures.
3. Provide for client privacy.
4. Show the client ways to turn in bed and to get out of bed.
   - Instruct a client who will have a right abdominal incision or a right-sided chest incision to turn to the left side of the bed and sit up as follows:
     a. Flex the knees.
     b. Splint the wound by holding the left arm and hand or a small pillow against the incision.
     c. Turn to the left while pushing with the right foot and grasping a partial side rail on the left side of the bed with the right hand.
     d. Come to a sitting position on the side of the bed by using the right arm and hand to push down against the mattress and swinging the feet over the edge of the bed.

- Teach a client with a left abdominal or left-sided chest incision to perform the same procedure but splint with the right arm and turn to the right.
- For clients with orthopedic surgery, use special aids, such as a trapeze, to assist with movement.

5. Teach the client the following three leg exercises:
   - Alternate dorsiflexion and plantar flexion of the feet. **Rationale:** *This exercise is sometimes referred to as calf pumping, because it alternately contracts and relaxes the calf muscles, including the gastrocnemius muscles.*
   - Flex and extend the knees, and press the backs of the knees into the bed while dorsiflexing the feet. ❶ Instruct clients who cannot raise their legs to do isometric exercises that contract and relax the muscles.
   - Raise and lower the legs alternately from the surface of the bed. Flex the knee of the stable leg and extend the knee of the moving leg. ❷ **Rationale:** *This exercise contracts and relaxes the quadriceps muscles.*

6. Demonstrate deep-breathing (diaphragmatic) exercises as follows:
   - Place your hands palms down on the border of your rib cage, and inhale slowly and evenly through the nose until the greatest chest expansion is achieved.
   - Hold your breath for 2 to 3 seconds.
   - Then exhale slowly through the mouth.
   - Continue exhalation until maximum chest contraction has been achieved.

(continued)

SKILL 25–1

TEACHING MOVING, LEG EXERCISES, DEEP BREATHING, AND COUGHING *(continued)*

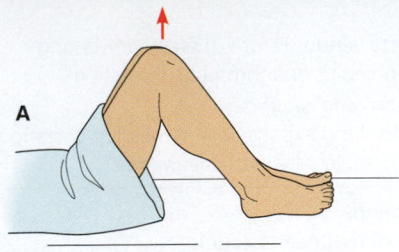

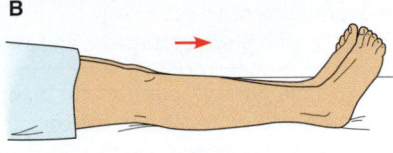

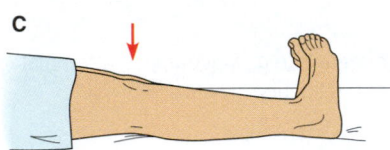

1 Flexing and extending the knees

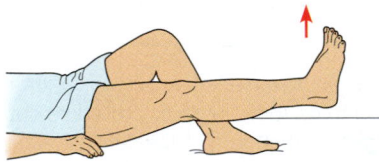

2 Raising and lowering the legs.

7. Help the client perform deep-breathing exercises.
   - Ask the client to assume a sitting position.
   - Place the palms of your hands on the border of the client's rib cage to assess respiratory depth.
   - Ask the client to perform deep breathing, as described in step 6.

8. Instruct the client to cough voluntarily after five deep inhalations.
   - Ask the client to inhale deeply, hold the breath for a few seconds, and then cough once or twice.
   - Ensure that the client coughs deeply and does not just clear the throat.

9. If the incision will be painful when the client coughs, demonstrate techniques to splint the abdomen.
   - Show the client how to support the incision by placing the palms of the hands on either side of the incision site or directly over the incision site, holding the palm of one hand over the other. **Rationale:** *Coughing uses the abdominal and other accessory respiratory muscles. Splinting the incision may reduce pain while coughing if the incision is near any of these muscles.*
   - Show the client how to splint the abdomen with clasped hands and a firmly rolled pillow held against the client's abdomen.

10. Inform the client about the expected frequency of these exercises.
    - Instruct the client to start the exercises as soon after surgery as possible.
    - Encourage clients to carry out deep breathing and coughing at least every 2 hours, taking a minimum of five breaths at each session. Note, however, that the number of breaths and frequency of deep breathing varies with the client's condition. People who are susceptible to pulmonary problems may need deep-breathing exercises every hour. People with chronic respiratory disease may need special breathing exercises (e.g., pursed-lip breathing, abdominal breathing, exercises using various kinds of incentive spirometers). See Chapter 35 ∞.

11. Document the teaching and all assessments. Some agencies may have a preoperative teaching flow sheet. Check agency policy.

SAMPLE DOCUMENTATION

2/1/2010 0900 Instructed how to splint abdomen while deep breathing and coughing. Able to perform correctly. Stated that he will use this technique after surgery. ———— A. Moore, RN

EVALUATION

Document the outcome of the teaching plan such as:

- Client's demonstrated ability to perform moving, leg exercises, deep-breathing, and coughing exercises.
- Client's verbalization of key information presented.

LIFESPAN CONSIDERATIONS   Preoperative Teaching

Children

- Parents need to know what to expect and to be able to express their concerns.
- Separation from parents often is the child's greatest fear; the time of separation should be minimized and parents allowed to interact with the child both immediately preceding and following the surgery.
- Teaching/communicating with children (both timing and content) should be geared to the child's developmental level and cognitive abilities (e.g., "You will have a sore tummy").
- Play is an effective teaching tool with children (e.g., the child can put a bandage on an incision on a doll).

Older Adults

- Assess hearing ability to ensure the older adult hears the necessary information.
- Assess short-term memory. Presenting one focused idea at a time and repeating or reinforcing information may be necessary.

- Older adults are at greater risk for postoperative complications, such as pneumonia. Reinforce moving and deep-breathing and coughing exercises.
- Assess potential postoperative needs at this time. Arrangements can be made preoperatively to obtain necessary items. Examples are medical equipment, such as walkers, raised toilet seats, and bed trapezes; Meals on Wheels; and help with transportation.
- If the older adult client will need to be in extended care for a period of time after surgery, this is the time to initiate these plans.
- Assess the client for risk of pressure ulcer development postoperatively and be extra attentive to use of proper paddings and support devices to prevent injury during positioning and transfers in the operating room. Risks are:
  - Older age.
  - Poor nutritional status.
  - History of diabetes or cardiovascular problems.
  - History of taking steroids, which cause increased bruising and skin breakdown.

Physical Preparation

Preoperative preparation includes the following areas: nutrition and fluids, elimination, hygiene, medications, rest, care of valuables and prostheses, special orders, and surgical skin preparation. In many agencies a preoperative checklist is used on the day of surgery. The nurse completes the agency's preoperative checklist following appropriate documenting procedures. It is essential that all pertinent records (laboratory records, x-ray films, consents) be available for perioperative personnel to refer to them and that all physical preparation is completed to ensure client safety.

NUTRITION AND FLUIDS Adequate hydration and nutrition promote healing. Nurses need to identify and record any signs of malnutrition or fluid imbalance. If the client is on intravenous fluids or on measured fluid intake, nurses must ensure that the fluid intake and output is accurately measured and recorded.

The order "NPO after midnight" has been a long-standing tradition because it was believed that anesthetics depress gastrointestinal functioning and there was a danger the client would vomit and aspirate during the administration of a general anesthetic. Reevaluation and research, however, do not support this tradition. As a result, the American Society of Anesthesiology (ASA) revised its practice guidelines for preoperative fasting in healthy clients undergoing elective procedures. According to Crenshaw and Winslow (2002, p. 38), the revised guidelines allow for:

- The consumption of clear liquids up to 2 hours before elective surgery requiring general anesthesia, regional anesthesia, or sedation-analgesia.

- A light breakfast (e.g., tea and toast) 6 hours before the procedure.
- A heavier meal 8 hours or more before surgery.

ELIMINATION Enemas before surgery are no longer routine, but cleansing enemas may be ordered if bowel surgery is planned. The enemas help prevent postoperative constipation and contamination of the surgical area (during surgery) by feces. After surgery involving the intestines, peristalsis often doesn't return for 24 to 48 hours.

Prior to surgery an in-and-out/straight catheterization or an indwelling Foley catheter may be ordered to ensure that the bladder remains empty. This helps prevent inadvertent injury to the bladder, particularly during pelvic surgery. If the client does not have a catheter, it is important to empty the bladder prior to receiving preoperative medications.

HYGIENE In some settings, clients are asked to bathe or shower the evening or morning of surgery (or both). The purpose of hygienic measures is to reduce the risk of wound infection by reducing the amount of bacteria on the client's skin. The bath includes a shampoo whenever possible.

The client's nails should be trimmed and free of polish, and all cosmetics should be removed so that the nail beds, skin, and lips are visible when circulation is assessed during the perioperative phases.

Intraoperatively the client will be required to wear a surgical cap. The surgical cap contains the client's hair and any microorganisms on the hair and scalp.

Before going into the operating room the client should remove all hair pins and clips as they may cause pressure or accidental damage to the scalp when the client is unconscious. The client also removes personal clothing and puts on an operating room gown.

MEDICATIONS The anesthetist or anesthesiologist may order routinely taken medications be held the day of surgery. In some settings preoperative medications are given to the client prior to going to the operating room. Commonly used preoperative medications include the following:

- *Sedatives* and *tranquilizers* such as secobarbital and diazepam (Valium) to reduce anxiety and ease anesthetic induction
- *Narcotic analgesics* such as morphine and meperidine (Demerol) to provide client sedation and reduce the required amount of anesthetic
- *Anticholinergics* such as atropine, scopolamine, and glycopyrrolate (Robinul) to reduce oral and pulmonary secretions and prevent laryngospasm
- *Histamine-receptor antihistamines* such as cimetidine (Tagamet) and ranitidine (Zantac) to reduce gastric fluid volume and gastric acidity
- *Neuroleptanalgesic* agents such as Innovar to induce general calmness and sleepiness

Preoperative medications must be given at a scheduled time or "on call," that is, when the operating room notifies the nurse to give the medication.

REST AND SLEEP Nurses should do everything to help the client sleep the night before surgery. Often a sedative is ordered. Adequate rest helps the client manage the stress of surgery and helps healing.

VALUABLES Valuables such as jewelry and money should be sent home with the client's family or significant other. If valuables/money cannot be sent home, they need to be labeled and placed in a locked storage area per the agency's policy. Removing jewelry also means removing body-piercing jewelry; there is a risk of injury from burns if an electrosurgical unit is used (Larkin, 2004). If a client wishes not to remove a wedding band, the nurse can tape it in place. Wedding bands must be removed, however, if there is danger of the fingers swelling after surgery. Situations warranting removal include surgery on or cast application to an arm, or a mastectomy that involves removal of the lymph nodes. (Mastectomies may cause edema of the arm and hand.)

PROSTHESES All prostheses (artificial body parts, such as partial or complete dentures, contact lenses, artificial eyes, and artificial limbs) and eyeglasses, wigs, and false eyelashes must be removed before surgery. Hearing aids are often left in place and the operating room personnel notified.

In some hospitals, dentures are placed in a locked storage area; in others they are placed in labeled containers and kept at the client's bedside. Partial dentures can become dislodged and obstruct an unconscious client's breathing. The nurse also checks for the presence of chewing gum or loose teeth. Loose teeth are a common problem with 5- or 6-year-olds undergoing tonsillectomy because they can become dislodged and/or aspirated during anesthesia.

SPECIAL ORDERS The nurse checks the surgeon's orders for special requirements (e.g., the insertion of a nasogastric tube prior to surgery, the administration of medications,

---

> **CULTURALLY COMPETENT CARE**   **Body Piercing**
>
> With the increasing number of people with body piercings, it is important for the perioperative nurse to deliver culturally sensitive care to clients with body piercings. Understanding the cultural and social meanings of body piercing helps provide cultural sensitivity while ensuring client safety.
>
> The nurse needs to ensure that this jewelry is removed in addition to the more traditional jewelry. Safety issues that can occur if the body-piercing jewelry is not removed include alternate site burns when using electrosurgery, pressure injuries from the jewelry, dislocation and aspiration of the jewelry during tracheal intubation, and possible inability to insert a urinary catheter because of genitalia piercings.
>
> The perioperative nurse may need to help the client remove the jewelry. It is important that the jewelry not be damaged or the client harmed (physically or psychologically) when removing the jewelry. Certain tools may need to be available for removal of the jewelry.
>
> *Note:* Reprinted from *AORN Journal*, vol. 79, B. G. Larkin, "The Ins and Outs of Body Piercing," pp. 333–334. Copyright 2004, with permission from AORN, Inc.

such as insulin, or the application of antiemboli stockings). For the technique of inserting a nasogastric tube, see Skill 32-1 in Chapter 32 ∞.

SKIN PREPARATION In most agencies, skin preparation is carried out during the intraoperative phase. The surgical site is cleansed with an antimicrobial to remove soil and reduce the resident microbial count to subpathogenic levels.

SAFETY PROTOCOLS The Joint Commission on Accreditation of Healthcare Organizations (The Joint Commission) established, effective July 2004, the Universal Protocol for Preventing Wrong Site, Wrong Procedure, Wrong Person Surgery (Joint Commission, 2003; Steefel, 2004). This protocol involves three steps. The first step requires preoperative verification. Client verification used to be a one-time procedure. The protocol requires client verification at the time surgery is scheduled, during admission, and whenever the client is transferred to another caregiver.

The second step involves marking of the operative site in an unambiguous manner. The protocol does not specify the type of mark; however, the Joint Commission does require that the surgical site marking method be consistent throughout the facility and encourages client involvement. The facility chooses its own surgical site method. An "X" is considered ambiguous and cannot be used for marking the site. The mark must be permanent and visible after the client has been prepped and draped for surgery.

The third step is called "time-out." Before surgery begins the surgical team takes a time-out to conduct a final verification of the correct client, procedure, and site. Any questions or concerns must be resolved before the procedure can begin.

VITAL SIGNS Preoperatively assess and document vital signs for baseline data. Report any abnormal findings, such as elevated blood pressure or elevated temperature.

ANTIEMBOLI STOCKINGS Antiemboli (elastic) stockings are firm elastic hose that compress the veins of the legs and thereby facilitate the return of venous blood to the heart. They also improve arterial circulation to the feet and prevent edema of the legs and feet. These stockings are frequently applied to surgical clients.

There are several types of stockings. One type extends from the foot to the knee and another from the foot to midthigh. These stockings usually have a partial foot that exposes the heel or toes so that extremity circulation can be assessed. Elastic stockings usually come in small, medium, and large sizes. Skill 25–2 details the steps required to apply antiemboli stockings.

SKILL 25–2

APPLYING ANTIEMBOLI STOCKINGS

PURPOSES
- To facilitate venous return from the lower extremities
- To prevent venous stasis and venous thrombosis
- To reduce peripheral edema

ASSESSMENT
Assess both lower extremities for
- Rates, volumes, and rhythms of posterior tibial and dorsalis pedis pulses
- Skin color (note pallor, cyanosis, or other pigmentation)

- Skin temperature
- Presence of distended veins or edema
- Skin condition (e.g., thickened, shiny, taut)
- Homans' sign (pain in calf with passive dorsiflexion of the foot)

PLANNING
Before applying antiemboli stockings, determine any potential or present circulatory problems and the surgeon's orders involving the lower extremities.

> **Delegation**
> UAP frequently remove and apply antiemboli stockings as part of morning and evening hygiene care. The nurse should stress the importance of removing and reapplying the stockings and reporting any changes in the client's skin to the nurse.

EQUIPMENT
- Tape measure
- Clean antiemboli stockings of appropriate size and of the type ordered

IMPLEMENTATION

Preparation

Take measurements as needed to obtain the appropriate size stockings.

- Measure the length of both legs from the heel to the gluteal fold (for thigh-length stockings) or from the heel to the popliteal space (for knee-length stockings).
- Measure the circumference of each calf and each thigh at the widest point.
- Compare the measurements to the size chart to obtain stockings of correct size. Obtain two sizes if there is a significant difference. **Rationale:** *Stockings that are too large for the client do not place adequate pressure on the legs to facilitate venous return, and may bunch, increasing the risk of pressure and skin irritation. Stockings that are too small may impede blood flow to the feet and cause skin breakdown.*

Performance

1. Prior to performing the procedure, introduce self and verify the client's identity using agency protocol. Explain to the client what you are going to do, why it is necessary, and how he or she can participate.
2. Perform hand hygiene and observe other appropriate infection control procedures.
3. Provide for client privacy.

4. Select an appropriate time to apply the stockings.
   - Apply stockings in the morning, if possible, before the client arises. **Rationale:** *In sitting and standing positions, the veins can become distended so that edema occurs; the stockings should be applied before this occurs.*
   - Assist the client who has been ambulating to lie down and elevate the legs for 15 to 30 minutes before applying the stockings. **Rationale:** *This facilitates venous return and reduces swelling.*
5. Prepare the client.
   - Assist the client to a lying position in bed.
   - Wash and dry the legs as needed.
6. Apply the stockings.
   - Reach inside the stocking from the top, and grasping the heel, turn the upper portion of the stocking inside out so the foot portion is inside the stocking leg. **Rationale:** *Firm elastic stockings are easier to fit over the foot and calf when inverted in this manner rather than bunching up the stocking.*
   - Ask the client to point his or her toes, then position the stocking on the client's foot. With the heel of the stocking down and stretching each side of the stocking, ease the stocking over the toes taking care to place the toe and heel portions of the stocking appropriately. **Rationale:** *Pointing the toes makes application easier.*

(continued)

APPLYING ANTIEMBOLI STOCKINGS *(continued)*

- Grasp the loose portion of the stocking at the ankle and gently pull the stocking over the leg, turning it right side out in the process.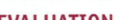
- Inspect the client's leg and stocking, smoothing any folds or creases. Ensure that the stocking is not rolled down or bunched at the top or ankle. **Rationale:** *Folds and creases can cause skin irritation under the stocking; bunching of the stocking can further impair venous return.*
- Remove the stockings per agency policy, inspecting the legs and skin while the stockings are off.
- Soiled stockings may be laundered by hand with warm water and mild soap. Hang to dry.
7. Document the procedure. Record the procedure, your assessment data, and when the stockings are removed and reapplied.

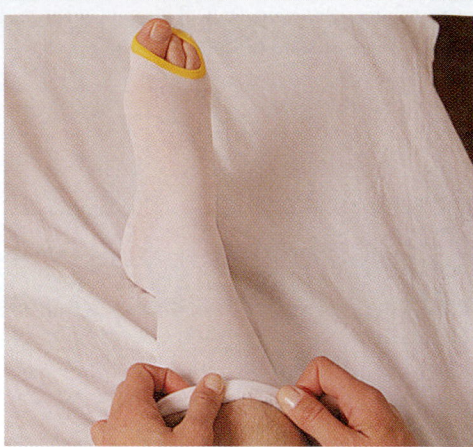

❶ Pulling the stocking snugly over the leg.

EVALUATION

- Remove antiembolism stockings one to three times a day for 30 minutes for skin care and inspection.
- Note the appearance of the legs and skin integrity, any edema, peripheral pulses, and skin color and temperature. Compare to previous assessment data.

- If complications occur, remove the stockings and report findings to the primary care provider.

SEQUENTIAL COMPRESSION DEVICES Clients who are undergoing surgery may benefit from a sequential compression device (SCD) to promote venous return from the legs. SCDs inflate and deflate plastic sleeves wrapped around the legs to promote venous flow. SCDs are discussed in Chapter 35 ∞ (see Skill 35–5).

EVALUATING

The goals established during the planning phase are evaluated according to specific desired outcomes, also established in that phase. An example of client outcomes and related indicators was shown earlier in Identifying Nursing Diagnoses, Outcomes, and Interventions.

INTRAOPERATIVE PHASE

The intraoperative nurse uses the nursing process to design, coordinate, and deliver care to meet the identified needs of clients whose protective reflexes or self-care abilities are potentially compromised because they are having operative or other invasive procedures.

Types of Anesthesia

Anesthesia is classified as *general*, *regional*, or *local*. Anesthetic agents usually are administered by an anesthesiolo-

gist or a certified registered nurse anesthetist (CRNA). **General anesthesia** is the loss of all sensation and consciousness. Under general anesthesia, protective reflexes such as cough and gag reflexes are lost. A general anesthetic acts by blocking awareness centers in the brain so that amnesia (loss of memory), analgesia (insensibility to pain), hypnosis (artificial sleep), and relaxation (rendering a part of the body less tense) occur. General anesthetics are usually administered by intravenous infusion or by inhalation of gases through a mask or through an endotracheal tube inserted into the trachea.

General anesthesia has certain advantages. Because the client is unconscious rather than awake and anxious, respiration and cardiac function are readily regulated. Also, the anesthesia can be adjusted to the length of the operation and the client's age and physical status. Its chief disadvantage is that it depresses the respiratory and circulatory systems. Some clients become more anxious about a general anesthetic than about the surgery itself. Often this is because they fear losing the capacity to control their own bodies.

Regional anesthesia is the temporary interruption of the transmission of nerve impulses to and from a specific area or region of the body. The client loses sensation in an area of the body but remains conscious. Several techniques are used.

- **Topical (surface) anesthesia** is applied directly to the skin and mucous membranes, open skin surfaces, wounds, and burns. The most commonly used topical agents are lidocaine (Xylocaine) and benzocaine. Topical anesthetics are readily absorbed and act rapidly.

- **Local anesthesia** (infiltration) is injected into a specific area and is used for minor surgical procedures such as suturing a small wound or performing a biopsy. Lidocaine or tetracaine 0.1% may be used.
- A **nerve block** is a technique in which the anesthetic agent is injected into and around a nerve or small nerve group that supplies sensation to a small area of the body. Major blocks involve multiple nerves or a plexus; minor blocks involve a single nerve.
- An **intravenous block** (**Bier block**) is used most often for procedures involving the arm, wrist, and hand. An occlusion tourniquet is applied to the extremity to prevent infiltration and absorption of the injected intravenous agent beyond the involved extremity.
- **Spinal anesthesia** is also referred to as subarachnoid block (SAB). It requires a lumbar puncture through one of the interspaces between lumbar disc 2 (L_2) and the sacrum (S_1). An anesthetic agent is injected into the subarachnoid space surrounding the spinal cord. Spinal anesthesia is often categorized as a low, mid, or high spinal. Low spinals (saddle or caudal blocks) are primarily used for surgeries involving the perineal or rectal areas. Mid-spinals (below the level of the umbilicus—T_{10}) can be used for hernia repairs or appendectomies, and high spinals (reaching the nipple line—T_4) can be used for surgeries such as cesarean sections.
- **Epidural (peridural) anesthesia** is an injection of an anesthetic agent into the epidural space, the area inside the spinal column but outside the dura mater.

Conscious sedation may be used alone or in conjunction with regional anesthesia for some diagnostic tests and surgical procedures. **Conscious sedation** refers to minimal depression of the level of consciousness in which the client retains the ability to maintain a patent airway and respond appropriately to commands. Intravenous narcotics such as morphine or fentanyl (Sublimaze) and antianxiety agents such as diazepam (Valium) or midazolam (Versed) are commonly used to induce and maintain conscious sedation. Conscious sedation increases the client's pain threshold and induces a degree of amnesia but allows for prompt reversal of its effects and a rapid return to normal activities of daily living. Procedures such as endoscopies, incision and drainage of abscesses, and even balloon angioplasty may be performed under conscious sedation.

NURSING MANAGEMENT

ASSESSING

On the client's admission to the surgical suite or procedure room, the perioperative nurse confirms the client's identity and assesses the client's physical and emotional status. The nurse

verifies the information on the preoperative checklist and evaluates the client's knowledge about the surgery and events to follow. The client's response to preoperative medications is assessed, as well as the placement and patency of tubes such as IV lines, nasogastric tubes, and urinary catheters.

Assessment continues throughout surgery, as the anesthesiologist and/or the CRNA continuously monitor the client's vital signs, ECG, and oxygen saturation. Fluid intake and urinary output are monitored throughout surgery, and blood loss is estimated. In addition, arterial and venous pressures, pulmonary artery pressures, and laboratory values such as blood glucose, hemoglobin, hematocrit, serum electrolytes, and arterial blood gases may be evaluated during surgery. Continual assessment is necessary to rapidly identify adverse responses to surgery or anesthesia and intervene promptly to prevent complications.

DIAGNOSING

NANDA nursing diagnoses that may be appropriate for the intraoperative client include the following:

- *Risk for Aspiration*
- *Ineffective Protection*
- *Impaired Skin Integrity*
- *Risk for Perioperative Positioning Injury*
- *Risk for Imbalanced Body Temperature*
- *Ineffective Tissue Perfusion*
- *Risk for Deficient Fluid Volume*

PLANNING

The overall goals of care in the intraoperative period are to maintain the client's safety and to maintain homeostasis. Examples of nursing activities to achieve these goals include the following:

- Position the client appropriately for surgery.
- Perform preoperative skin preparation.
- Assist in preparing and maintaining the sterile field.
- Open and dispense sterile supplies during surgery.
- Provide medications and solutions for the sterile field.
- Monitor and maintain a safe, aseptic environment.
- Manage catheters, tubes, drains, and specimens.
- Perform sponge, sharp, and instrument counts.
- Document nursing care provided and the client's response to interventions.

IMPLEMENTING

Intraoperative interventions are carried out by the circulating nurse and the scrub person. The **circulating nurse** coordinates activities and manages client care by continually assessing client safety, aseptic practice, and the environment. The **scrub person** is usually a UAP but can be an RN or LPN. Their role is to assist the surgeons. They wear sterile gowns, gloves, caps, and eye protection. Their responsibilities include draping the client with sterile drapes and handling sterile instruments and supplies. The circulating nurse and scrub person are responsible for accounting of all sponges, needles, and instruments at the close of surgery. This precaution avoids leaving any foreign bodies inside the client.

Surgical Skin Preparation

Surgical skin preparation involves cleaning the surgical site, removing hair only if necessary, and applying an antimicrobial agent. In most surgery centers, skin preparation is done by surgery personnel near the time of surgery. The purpose of a surgical skin preparation is to reduce the risk of postoperative wound infection. This is done by:

- Removing transient microbes from the skin.
- Reducing the resident microbial count to subpathogenic amounts in a short time and with the least amount of tissue irritation.
- Inhibiting rapid rebound growth of microbes.

The Association of Operating Room Nurses (AORN) recommends the following skin preparation practices to reduce the risk of postoperative wound infections:

- Clean the surgical site and surrounding areas. This can be accomplished before the surgical prep by having the client shower and shampoo or wash the surgical site before arriving in the surgical setting, or by washing the surgical site in the surgical setting immediately before applying an antimicrobial agent.
- Assess the surgical site before skin preparation. The nurse assesses the site for moles, warts, rashes, or other skin conditions such as pustules, abrasions, or exudate, and documents their presence before skin preparation.
- Remove hair from the surgical site only when necessary or according to the primary care provider's orders or institutional policies and procedures. Personnel skilled in hair removal should remove hair using techniques that preserve skin integrity. Electric clippers or a depilatory cream should be used to reduce the risk of traumatizing the skin during hair removal. If a depilatory is used, hypersensitivity testing is performed prior to applying it to the surgical site. Skin trauma and abrasions increase the risk of microorganisms colonizing the surgical site. If hair is to be removed, it is done as close to the time of surgery as possible and not in the vicinity of the sterile field to avoid dispersal of loose hair and potential contamination of the sterile field.
- Prepare the surgical site and surrounding area with an antimicrobial agent when indicated. A nontoxic antimicrobial agent with a broad range of germicidal action is used to inhibit the growth of microorganisms during and following the surgical procedure. The agent selected depends on the client's history of hypersensitivity reactions, the location of the surgical site, and the skin condition. The area prepared needs to be large enough to accommodate an extension of the incision and any potential drain sites or additional incisions if needed.

- Document surgical skin preparation in the client's record. Documentation should include the skin condition, including any growths, abrasions, or rashes; hair removal and the techniques used, if performed; the skin preparation, including cleansing and antimicrobial agent applied; who performed the preoperative skin preparation; and any adverse or hypersensitivity responses noted (Anonymous, 2002).

Positioning

The perioperative nurse, surgeon, and anesthesiologist/CRNA work as a team to minimize the risk of perioperative complications related to positioning (AORN, 2005).

The client's position should provide:

- Optimal visualization of and access to the surgical site.
- Optimal access to IV lines and monitoring devices.
- Protection of the client from harm.

Positioning is performed after anesthesia is induced and before surgical draping of the client. The client is lifted into position to prevent shearing forces on the skin from sliding or rolling. The exact position for the client depends on the operation, that is, the surgical approach. For example, a lithotomy position is usually used for vaginal surgery.

Positions on the operating table are maintained by straps, and body prominences are frequently padded. The position should consider normal joint range of motion and good body alignment, thereby avoiding strain or injury to muscles, bones, and ligaments.

CLINICAL ALERT

Be especially aware of the intraoperative position required for older adults. Because older adults are vulnerable to pressure ulcer formation, check the appropriate pressure points of that surgical position on the client.

EVALUATING

The intraoperative nurse uses the goals developed during the planning stage and collects data to evaluate whether the desired outcomes have been achieved.

DOCUMENTATION

The intraoperative nurse documents the perioperative plan of care including assessment, diagnosis, outcome identification, planning, implementation, and evaluation.

POSTOPERATIVE PHASE

Nursing during the postoperative phase is especially important for the client's recovery because anesthesia impairs the ability of clients to respond to environmental stimuli and to help themselves, although the degree of consciousness of clients will vary. Moreover, surgery itself traumatizes the body by disrupting protective mechanisms and homeostasis.

Immediate Postanesthetic Phase

Recovery/PACU nurses have specialized skills to care for clients recovering from anesthesia and surgery. Once the health status has stabilized, the client is returned to the nursing unit or, in the case of an outpatient, to the outpatient surgery area before discharge. Assessment of the client in the immediate postanesthetic period is summarized in Box 25–5.

During the immediate postanesthetic stage, an unconscious client is positioned on the side, with the face slightly down. A pillow is not placed under the head. In this position, gravity keeps the tongue forward, preventing occlusion of the pharynx and allowing drainage of mucus or vomitus out of the mouth rather than down the respiratory tree.

The nurse ensures maximum chest expansion by elevating the client's upper arm on a pillow. The upper arm is supported because the pressure of an arm against the chest reduces chest expansion potential. An artificial airway is maintained in place, and the client is suctioned as needed until cough and swallowing reflexes return. Generally the client spits out an oropharyngeal airway when coughing returns. Endotracheal tubes are not removed until clients are awake

---

BOX 25–5 | Clinical Assessment

Immediate Postanesthetic Phase

- Adequacy of airway
- Oxygen saturation
- Adequacy of ventilation
  - Respiratory rate, rhythm, and depth
  - Use of accessory muscles
  - Breath sounds
- Cardiovascular status
  - Heart rate and rhythm
  - Peripheral pulse amplitude and equality
  - Blood pressure
  - Capillary filling
- Level of consciousness
  - Not responding
  - Arousable with verbal stimuli
  - Fully awake
  - Oriented to time, person, and place
- Presence of protective reflexes
- Activity, ability to move extremities
- Skin color
- Fluid status
  - Intake and output
  - Status of IV infusions
  - Signs of dehydration or fluid overload (see Chapter 36 ∞)
- Condition of operative site
  - Status of dressing
  - Drainage (amount, type, and color)
- Patency of and character and amount of drainage from catheters, tubes, and drains
- Discomfort, nausea, vomiting
- Safety

---

and able to maintain their own airway. The client is then helped to turn, cough, and take deep breaths, provided that vital signs are stable. When spinal anesthesia is used, the client may be required to remain flat for a specified period. See Chapter 35 ∞ for information about artificial airways.

The return of the client's reflexes, such as swallowing and gagging, indicates that anesthesia is ending. Time of recovery from anesthesia varies with the kind of anesthetic agent used, its dosage, and the individual's response to it. Nurses should arouse clients by calling them by name, and in a normal tone of voice repeatedly telling them that the surgery is over and that they are in the PACU.

Once the health status has stabilized, the client is returned to the nursing unit or the outpatient surgery discharge area.

Clients are usually discharged from the PACU when:

- They are conscious and oriented.
- They are able to maintain a clear airway and deep breathe and cough freely.
- Vital signs have been stable or consistent with preoperative vital signs for at least 30 minutes.
- Protective reflexes are active.
- They are able to move all extremities.
- Intake and urinary output is adequate.
- They are afebrile or a febrile condition has been attended to.
- Dressings are dry and intact; there is no overt drainage.

Preparing for Ongoing Care of the Postoperative Client

While the client is in the operating room, the client's bed and room are prepared for the postoperative phase. In some agencies, the client is brought back to the unit on a stretcher and transferred to the bed in the room. In other agencies, the client's bed is brought to the surgery suite, and the client is transferred there. In the latter situation, the bed needs to be made with clean linens as soon as the client goes to surgery so that it can be taken to the operating room when needed. In addition, the nurse must obtain and set up any special equipment, such as an intravenous pole, suction, oxygen equipment, and orthopedic appliances (e.g., traction). If these are not requested on the client's record, the nurse should consult with the perioperative nurse or surgeon.

NURSING MANAGEMENT

ASSESSING

As soon as the client returns to the nursing unit, the nurse conducts an initial assessment. The sequence of these activities varies with the situation. For example, the nurse may need to check the primary care provider's stat orders before conducting the initial assessment; in such a case, nursing interventions to implement the orders can be carried out at the same time as assessment.

The nurse consults the surgeon's postoperative orders to learn the following:

- Food and fluids permitted by mouth
- Intravenous solutions and intravenous medications
- Position in bed
- Medications ordered (e.g., analgesics, antibiotics)
- Laboratory tests
- Intake and output, which in some agencies are monitored for all postoperative clients
- Activity permitted, including ambulation.

The nurse also checks the PACU record for the following data:

- Operation performed
- Presence and location of any drains
- Anesthetic used
- Postoperative diagnosis
- Estimated blood loss
- Medications administered in the recovery room

Many hospitals have postoperative protocols for regular assessment of clients. In some agencies, assessments are made every 15 minutes until vital signs stabilize, every hour for the next 4 hours, then every 4 hours for the next 2 days. It is important that the assessments be made as often as the client's condition requires. The nurse assesses the following:

- *Level of consciousness.* Assess orientation to time, place, and person. Most clients are fully conscious but drowsy when returned to their unit. Assess reaction to verbal stimuli and ability to move extremities.
- *Vital signs.* Take the client's vital signs (pulse, respiration, blood pressure, and oxygen saturation level) every 15 minutes until stable or in accordance with agency protocol. Compare initial findings with PACU data. In addition, assess the client's lung sounds and assess for signs of common circulatory problems such as postoperative hypotension, hemorrhage, or shock. Hypovolemia due to fluid losses during surgery is a common cause of postoperative hypotension. Hemorrhage can result from insecure ligation of blood vessels or disruption of sutures. Massive hemorrhage or cardiac insufficiency can lead to shock postoperatively. Common postoperative complications with their manifestations and preventive measures are listed in Table 25–2.
- *Skin color and temperature,* particularly that of the lips and nail beds. The color of the lips and nail beds is an indicator of tissue perfusion (passage of blood through the vessels). Pale, cyanotic, cool, and moist skin may be a sign of circulatory problems.

CLINICAL ALERT

Older adults may not show the classic signs of infection (e.g., fever, tachycardia, increased WBC); instead there may be an abrupt change in their mental status.

- *Comfort.* Assess pain with the client's vital signs and as needed between vital sign measurements. Assess the location and intensity of the pain. Do not assume that reported pain is incisional; other causes may include muscle strains, flatus, and angina. Ask the client to rate pain on a scale of 0 to 10, with 0 being no pain and 10 the worst pain imaginable. Evaluate the client for objective indicators of pain: pallor, perspiration, muscle tension, and reluctance to cough, move, or ambulate. Determine when and what analgesics were last administered, and assess the client for any side effects of medication such as nausea and vomiting.
- *Fluid balance.* Assess the type and amount of intravenous fluids, flow rate, and infusion site. Monitor the client's fluid intake and output. In addition to watching for shock, assess the client for signs of circulatory overload, and monitor serum electrolytes. Anesthetics and surgery affect the hormones regulating fluid and electrolyte balance (aldosterone and anti-diuretic hormone in particular), placing the client at risk for decreased urine output and fluid and electrolyte imbalances.
- *Dressing and bedclothes.* Inspect the client's dressings and bedclothes underneath the client. Excessive bloody drainage on dressings or on bedclothes, often appearing underneath the client, can indicate hemorrhage. The amount of drainage on dressings is recorded by describing the diameter of the stains or by denoting the number and type of dressings saturated with drainage.
- *Drains and tubes.* Determine color, consistency, and amount of drainage from all tubes and drains. All tubes should be patent, and tubes and suction equipment should be functioning. Drainage bags must be hanging properly.

Document the client's time of arrival and all assessments. Many agencies have progress flow records for this purpose. Alter the frequency, parameters, and priorities to meet the individual needs of the client.

DIAGNOSING

Because surgery can involve many body systems both directly and indirectly and is a complex experience for the client, the nursing diagnoses focus on a wide variety of actual, potential, and collaborative problems.

Actual and potential NANDA diagnoses for the postoperative client include the following:

- *Acute Pain*
- *Risk for Infection*
- *Risk for Injury*
- *Risk for Deficient Fluid Volume*
- *Ineffective Airway Clearance*
- *Ineffective Breathing Pattern*
- *Self-Care Deficit: Bathing/Hygiene, Dressing/Grooming, Toileting*
- *Delayed Surgical Recovery*
- *Disturbed Body Image*

TABLE 25–2   Potential Postoperative Problems

PROBLEM	DESCRIPTION	CAUSE	CLINICAL SIGNS	PREVENTIVE INTERVENTIONS
Respiratory				
Pneumonia	Inflammation of the alveoli	Infection, toxins, or irritants causing inflammatory process Immobility and impaired ventilation result in atelectasis and promote growth of pathogens	Elevated temperature, cough, expectoration of blood-tinged or purulent sputum, dyspnea, chest pain	Deep-breathing exercises and coughing, moving in bed, early ambulation
Atelectasis	A condition in which alveoli collapse and are not ventilated	Mucous plugs blocking bronchial passageways, inadequate lung expansion, analgesics, immobility	Dyspnea, tachypnea, tachycardia; diaphoresis, anxiety; pleural pain, decreased chest wall movement; dull or absent breath sounds; decreased oxygen saturation (SpO_2)	Deep-breathing exercises and coughing, moving in bed, early ambulation
Pulmonary embolism	Blood clot that has moved to the lungs and blocks a pulmonary artery, thus obstructing blood flow to a portion of the lung	Stasis of venous blood from immobility, venous injury from fractures or during surgery, use of oral contraceptives high in estrogen, preexisting coagulation or circulatory disorder	Sudden chest pain, shortness of breath, cyanosis, shock (tachycardia, low blood pressure)	Turning, ambulation, antiemboli stockings, sequential compression devices
Circulatory				
Hypovolemia	Inadequate circulating blood volume	Fluid deficit, hemorrhage	Tachycardia, decreased urine output, decreased blood pressure	Early detection of signs; fluid and/or blood replacement
Hemorrhage	Internal or external bleeding	Disruption of sutures, insecure ligation of blood vessels	Overt bleeding (dressings saturated with bright blood; bright, free-flowing blood in drains or chest tubes), increased pain, increasing abdominal girth, swelling or bruising around incision	Early detection of signs
Hypovolemic shock	Inadequate tissue perfusion resulting from markedly reduced circulating blood volume	Severe hypovolemia from fluid deficit or hemorrhage	Rapid weak pulse, dyspnea, tachypnea; restlessness and anxiety; urine output less than 30 mL/hr; decreased blood pressure; cool, clammy skin, thirst, pallor	Maintain blood volume through adequate fluid replacement, prevent hemorrhage; early detection of signs
Thrombophlebitis	Inflammation of the veins, usually of the legs and associated with a blood clot	Slowed venous blood flow due to immobility or prolonged sitting; trauma to vein, resulting in inflammation and increased blood coagulability	Aching, cramping pain; affected area is swollen, red, and hot to touch; vein feels hard; discomfort in calf when foot is dorsiflexed or when client walks (Homans' sign)	Early ambulation, leg exercises, antiemboli stockings, SCDs, adequate fluid intake

(continued)

TABLE 25–2 | **Potential Postoperative Problems** *(continued)*

PROBLEM	DESCRIPTION	CAUSE	CLINICAL SIGNS	PREVENTIVE INTERVENTIONS
Thrombus	Blood clot attached to wall of vein or artery (most commonly the leg veins)	As for thrombophlebitis for venous thrombi; disruption or inflammation of arterial wall for arterial thrombi	*Venous:* same as thrombophlebitis *Arterial:* pain and pallor of affected extremity; decreased or absent peripheral pulses	*Venous:* same as thrombophlebitis *Arterial:* maintain prescribed position; early detection of signs
Embolus	Foreign body or clot that has moved from its site of formation to another area of the body (e.g., the lungs, heart, or brain)	Venous or arterial thrombus; broken intravenous catheter, fat, or amniotic fluid	In venous system, usually becomes a pulmonary embolus (see pulmonary embolism); signs of arterial emboli may depend on the location	Turning, ambulation, leg exercises, sequential compression devices; careful maintenance of IV catheters
Urinary				
Urinary retention	Inability to empty the bladder, with excessive accumulation of urine in the bladder	Depressed bladder muscle tone from narcotics and anesthetics; handling of tissues during surgery on adjacent organs (rectum, vagina)	Fluid intake larger than output; inability to void or frequent voiding of small amounts, bladder distention, suprapubic discomfort, restlessness	Monitoring of fluid intake and output, interventions to facilitate voiding, urinary catheterization as needed
Urinary tract infection	Inflammation of the bladder, ureters, or urethra Infrequent or no stool passage for abnormal length of time (e.g., within 48 hours after solid diet started)	Immobilization and limited fluid intake, instrumentation of the urinary tract	Burning sensation when voiding, urgency, cloudy urine, lower abdominal pain	Adequate fluid intake, early ambulation, aseptic straight catheterization only as necessary, good perineal hygiene
Gastrointestinal				
Nausea and vomiting		Pain, abdominal distention, ingesting food or fluids before return of peristalsis, certain medications, anxiety	Complaints of feeling sick to the stomach, retching or gagging	IV fluids until peristalsis returns; then clear fluids, full fluids, and regular diet; antiemetic drugs if ordered; analgesics for pain
Constipation	Infrequent or no stool passage for abnormal length of time (e.g., within 48 hours after solid diet started)	Lack of dietary roughage, analgesics (decreased intestinal motility), immobility	Absence of stool elimination, abdominal distention, and discomfort	Adequate fluid intake, high-fiber diet, early ambulation
Tympanites	Retention of gases within the intestines	Slowed motility of the intestines due to handling of the bowel during surgery and the effects of anesthesia	Obvious abdominal distention, abdominal discomfort (gas pains), absence of bowel sounds	Early ambulation; avoid using a straw, provide ice chips or water at room temperature
Postoperative ileus	Intestinal obstruction characterized by lack of peristaltic activity	Handling the bowel during surgery, anesthesia, electrolyte imbalance, wound infection	Abdominal pain and distention; constipation; absent bowel sounds; vomiting	
Wound				
Wound infection	Inflammation and infection of incision or drain site	Poor aseptic technique; laboratory analysis of wound swab identifies causative microorganism	Purulent exudate, redness, tenderness, elevated body temperature, wound odor	Keep wound clean and dry, use surgical aseptic technique when changing dressings

| TABLE 25–2 | Potential Postoperative Problems *(continued)* | | | |

PROBLEM	DESCRIPTION	CAUSE	CLINICAL SIGNS	PREVENTIVE INTERVENTIONS
Wound dehiscence	Separation of a suture line before the incision heals	Malnutrition (emaciation, obesity), poor circulation, excessive strain on suture line	Increased incision drainage, tissues underlying skin become visible along parts of the incision	Adequate nutrition, appropriate incisional support and avoidance of strain
Wound evisceration	Extrusion of internal organs and tissues through the incision	Same as for wound dehiscence	Opening of incision and visible protrusion of organs	Same as for wound dehiscence
Psychologic				
Postoperative depression	Mental disorder characterized by altered mood	Weakness, surprise nature of emergency surgery, news of malignancy, severely altered body image, other personal matter; may be a physiologic response to some surgeries	Anorexia, tearfulness, loss of ambition, withdrawal, rejection of others, feelings of dejection, sleep disturbances (insomnia or excessive sleeping)	Adequate rest, physical activity, opportunity to express anger and other negative feelings

Collaborative problems that may be experienced by the postoperative client are summarized in Table 25–2. Examples of clinical application of some of these diagnoses using NANDA, NIC, and NOC designations are shown in Identifying Nursing Diagnoses, Outcomes, and Interventions.

PLANNING

Postoperative care planning and discharge planning begin in the preoperative phase when preoperative teaching is implemented. Examples of clinical application of NOC outcomes and NIC interventions are shown in Identifying Nursing Diagnoses, Outcomes, and Interventions.

Discharge Planning

To provide for continuity of care for the surgical client after discharge, the nurse needs to consider the client's needs for assistance with care in the home setting. Discharge planning for both the day-surgery client and the client who has been hospitalized for several days following surgery incorporates an assessment of the client's and family's abilities for self-care, financial resources, and the need for referrals and home health services. It is important to remember that surgical clients have diverse needs, and additional assessment data may be required.

IMPLEMENTING

Nursing interventions designed to promote client recovery and prevent complications include (a) pain management, (b) appropriate positioning, (c) incentive spirometry and deep-breathing and coughing exercises, (d) leg exercises, (e) early ambulation, (f) adequate hydration, (g) diet, (h) promoting uri-nary and bowel elimination, (i) suction maintenance, and (j) wound care.

Pain Management

Although pain is a sensory and emotional experience that serves to alert us to harm and initiate responses to avoid or minimize harm, pain in the surgical client has little protective value. It can, in fact, have detrimental effects, leading to stimulation of the sympathetic nervous system, tachycardia, shallow breathing, atelectasis, altered gas exchange, immobility, and immunosuppression. Chapter 18 ∞ provides a more in-depth discussion of pain and pain management. Pain is usually greatest 12 to 36 hours after surgery, decreasing after the second or third postoperative day.

An anti-inflammatory agent such as ibuprofen or ketorolac (Toradol) is often administered in conjunction with a narcotic analgesic to enhance pain relief. Clients need to be reminded that analgesics are most effective when taken on a regular basis or before pain becomes severe. Because muscle tension increases pain perception and responses, nurses need to use nonpharmacologic measures in addition to prescribed analgesia. These include ensuring that the client is warm and providing back rubs, position changes, diversional activities, and adjunctive measures such as imagery.

Positioning

Position the client as ordered. Clients who have had spinal anesthetics usually lie flat for 8 to 12 hours. An unconscious or semiconscious client is placed on one side with the head slightly elevated, if possible, or in a position that allows fluids to drain from the mouth. Unless contraindicated, elevation of affected extremities with the distal extremity higher than the heart promotes venous drainage and reduces swelling.

IDENTIFYING NURSING DIAGNOSES, OUTCOMES, AND INTERVENTIONS   **The Postoperative Client**

DATA CLUSTER Mrs. Polk, 65 years old, was scheduled for a right total hip replacement and has returned to her room. Her VS are stable. She is NPO with an IV infusing at 100 cc/hr. Her right hip dressing is dry and intact. A Hemovac drain is in place and draining a small to moderate amount of bloody drainage. Her respirations are 30/min and shallow. Breath sounds are clear but diminished throughout. She is awake and c/o right hip pain which she rates as "8" on a 0–10 scale. She guards her right hip and flinches when someone touches her.

NURSING DIAGNOSIS/DEFINITION	SAMPLE DESIRED OUTCOME*/DEFINITION	INDICATORS	SELECTED INTERVENTIONS*/DEFINITION	SAMPLE NIC ACTIVITIES
Acute Pain/Unpleasant sensory and emotional experience arising from actual or potential tissue damage (International Association for the Study of Pain); sudden or slow onset of any intensity from mild to severe with an anticipated or predictable end and a duration of less than 6 months	Pain Control [1605]/*Personal actions to control pain*	Often demonstrated: • Describes causal factors • Recognizes pain onset • Uses analgesics appropriately • Reports changes in pain symptoms or sites to health care professional • Reports pain controlled	Pain Management [1400]/*Alleviation of pain or a reduction in pain to a level of comfort that is acceptable to the patient*	• Perform a comprehensive assessment of pain to include location, characteristics, onset/duration, intensity or severity of pain and precipitating factors • Assure client of attentive analgesic care • Consider cultural influences on pain response • Monitor client satisfaction with pain management at specified intervals
Ineffective Breathing Pattern/Inspiration and/or expiration that does not provide adequate ventilation	Respiratory Status: Ventilation [0403]/*Movement of air in and out of the lungs*	Not compromised: • Respiratory rate in expected range • Respiratory rhythm in expected range • Ease of breathing No: • Adventitious breath sounds	Respiratory Monitoring [3350]/*Collection and analysis of patient data to ensure airway patency and adequate gas exchange*	• Monitor rate, rhythm, depth, and effort of respirations • Auscultate breath sounds, noting areas of decreased/absent ventilation and presence of adventitious sounds • Monitor client's ability to cough effectively
Risk for Infection/At increased risk for being invaded by pathogenic organisms	Wound Healing: Primary Intention [1102]/*Extent of regeneration of cells and tissues following intentional closure*	Extensive: • Skin approximation No: • Sanguineous drainage • Surrounding skin erythema	Infection Control [6540]/*Minimizing the acquisition and transmission of infectious agents*	• Wash hands before and after each client activity • Institute standard precautions • Ensure appropriate wound care technique

*The NOC # for desired outcomes and the NIC # for nursing interventions are listed in brackets following the appropriate outcome or intervention. Outcomes, indicators, interventions, and activities selected are only a sample of those suggested by NOC and NIC and should be further individualized for each client.

Deep-Breathing and Coughing Exercises

Deep-breathing exercises help remove mucus, which can form and remain in the lungs due to the effects of general anesthetic and analgesics. These drugs depress the action of both the cilia of the mucous membranes lining the respiratory tract and the respiratory center in the brain. By increasing lung expansion and preventing the accumulation of secretions, deep breathing helps prevent pneumonia and **atelectasis** (collapse of the alveoli), which may result from stagnation of fluid in the lungs.

An incentive spirometer is often ordered for the postoperative client to encourage deep breathing. This device measures the flow of air inhaled through a mouthpiece (see Chapter 35 ∞). The client is instructed to breathe in through the mouthpiece until a certain level is achieved. Inhalation and ventilation are enhanced using the incentive spirometer. Deep breathing frequently initiates the coughing reflex. Voluntary coughing in conjunction with deep breathing facilitates the movement and expectoration of respiratory tract secretions.

Encourage the client to do deep-breathing and coughing exercises hourly, or at least every 2 hours, during waking hours for the first few days. Assist the client to a sitting position in bed or on the side of the bed. The client can splint the incision with a pillow when coughing, or the nurse can splint the incision for the client to reduce discomfort.

Leg Exercises

Encourage the client to do leg exercises taught in the preoperative period every 1 to 2 hours during waking hours. Muscle contractions compress the veins, preventing the stasis of blood in the veins, a cause of thrombus (stationary clot adhered to the wall of a vessel) formation and subsequent **thrombophlebitis** (inflammation of a vein followed by formation of a blood clot) and emboli (a blood clot that has moved). Contractions also promote arterial blood flow.

RESEARCH NOTES
Is Postoperative Surgical Pain an Adverse Effect of Surgery or an Accepted Consequence?

Evidenced-based guidelines for the monitoring and management of pain have been widely distributed by the American Pain Society, the Agency for Healthcare Research and Quality, and the Oncology Nursing Society. A recent research study (Sherwood et al., 2003) indicates that these widely distributed guidelines have not altered practice. Reports from acute care hospitals reveal no improvement in client-rated pain or client satisfaction with pain management. Clients accept pain as part of hospitalization, indicating that acute pain continues to be problematic. Barriers to effective pain management include inadequate knowledge, beliefs, and attitudes of both clients and clinicians. Postoperative pain should be treated as an adverse effect of surgery, not as an accepted consequence. Preoperative teaching is key to successful pain management. Best practice calls for an interactive partnership of clinician and client. Both are responsible for assessing, implementing, and evaluating the pain management plan. Preoperative teaching helps the client understand how to communicate about pain and enhances comfort and satisfaction.

Implications

Clinicians and clients working together can change practice for more effective pain management outcomes.

Note: Reprinted from *AORN Journal*, vol. 77, G. D. Sherwood, J. A. McNeil, P. L. Starck, & G. Disnard, "Changing Acute Pain Management Outcomes in Surgical Patients," pp. 374–395. Copyright 2003, with permission from AORN, Inc.

Moving and Ambulation

Encourage the client to turn from side to side at least every 2 hours. Turning alternates which lung can achieve maximum expansion; this occurs in the uppermost lung that is not in contact with the bed. Avoid placing pillows or rolls under the client's knees because pressure on the popliteal blood vessels can interfere with blood circulation to and from the lower extremities. Clients who practice turning before surgery usually find it easier to do after surgery.

The client should ambulate as soon as possible after surgery in accordance with the surgeon's orders. Generally clients begin ambulation the evening of the day of surgery or the first day after surgery, unless contraindicated. Early ambulation prevents respiratory, circulatory, urinary, and gastrointestinal complications. It also prevents general muscle weakness. Schedule ambulation for periods after the client has taken an analgesic or when the client is comfortable. Ambulation should be gradual, starting with the client sitting on the bed and dangling the feet over the side. A client who cannot ambulate is periodically assisted to a sitting position in bed, if allowed, and turned frequently. The sitting position permits the greatest lung expansion.

Hydration

Maintain intravenous infusions as ordered to replace body fluids lost either before or during surgery. When oral intake is permitted, initially offer only small sips of water. Large amounts of water can induce vomiting because anesthetics and narcotic analgesics temporarily inhibit the motility of the stomach. The client who cannot take fluids by mouth may be allowed by the surgeon's orders to suck ice chips. Provide mouth care and place a mouthwash at the client's bedside. Postoperative clients often complain of thirst and a dry, sticky mouth. These discomforts are a result of the preoperative fasting period, preoperative medications (such as atropine), and loss of body fluid.

Measure the client's fluid intake and output for at least 2 days or until fluid balance is stable without an intravenous infusion. Ensuring adequate fluid balance is important. Sufficient fluids keep the respiratory mucous membranes and secretions moist, thus facilitating the expectoration of mucus during coughing. Also, an adequate fluid balance is important to maintain renal and cardiovascular function.

Diet

The surgeon orders the client's postoperative diet. Depending on the extent of surgery and the organs involved, the client may be allowed nothing by mouth for several days or may be able to resume oral intake when nausea is no longer present. When "diet as tolerated" is ordered, offer clear liquids initially. If the client tolerates these with no nausea, the diet can often progress to full liquids and then to a regular diet, provided that gastrointestinal functioning is normal. Assess the return of peristalsis by auscultating the abdomen. Gurgling and rumbling sounds indicate peristalsis. Anesthetic agents, narcotics, handling of the intestines during abdominal surgery, fasting, and inactivity all inhibit peristalsis. Therefore, bowel sounds should be carefully assessed every 4 to 6 hours. Oral fluids and food are usually started after the return of peristalsis. Assist very weak clients to eat.

Observe the client's tolerance of the food and fluids ingested and note and report the passage of flatus or abdominal distention.

Urinary Elimination

Provide measures that promote urinary elimination. For example, help male clients stand at the bedside, or female clients to a bedside commode if allowed, and ensure that fluid intake is adequate. Determine whether the client has any difficulties voiding and assess the client for bladder distention. Report to the surgeon if a client does not void within 8 hours following surgery, unless another time frame is specified.

Anesthetic agents temporarily depress urinary bladder tone, which usually returns within 6 to 8 hours after surgery. Surgery in the pubic area, vagina, or rectum, during which the surgeon may manipulate the bladder, often causes urinary retention. If all measures to promote voiding fail, a urinary catheterization is often ordered (see Chapter 33 ∞). Measure the fluid intake and output (I&O) of all new postoperative clients. Generally I&O records are kept for at least 2 days or until the client reestablishes fluid balance without an IV or catheter in place.

Suction

Some clients return from surgery with a gastric or intestinal tube in place and orders to connect the tube to suction. For more information about gastrointestinal tubes, see Chapter 32 ∞. The suction ordered can be continuous or intermittent. Intermittent suction is applied when a single-lumen gastric tube is used to reduce the risk of damaging the mucous membrane near the distal port of the tube. Continuous suction may be applied if a double-lumen tube is in place. Fluids and electrolytes must be replaced intravenously when gastric suction or continuous drainage is ordered. Nasogastric tubes may be irrigated if the lumen becomes clogged. They are generally irrigated before and after tube feedings or the instillation of medications. Nasogastric irrigation may require a primary care provider's order, particularly following gastrointestinal surgery. Skill 25–3 describes the management of gastrointestinal suction.

MANAGING GASTROINTESTINAL SUCTION

PURPOSES
- To relieve abdominal distention
- To maintain gastric decompression after surgery
- To remove blood and secretions from the gastrointestinal tract
- To relieve discomfort (e.g., when a client has a bowel obstruction)
- To maintain the patency of the nasogastric tube

ASSESSMENT

Assess
- Presence of abdominal distention on palpation
- Bowel sounds
- Abdominal discomfort
- Vital signs for baseline data
- Amount and characteristics of drainage

PLANNING
Before initiating gastric suction, determine (a) whether the suction is continuous or intermittent; (b) the ordered suction pressure (a low suction pressure is between 80 and 100 mm Hg, and a high pressure is between 100 and 120 mm Hg); and (c) whether there is an order to irrigate the gastrointestinal tube and, if so, the type of solution to use.

> **Delegation**
> Managing gastrointestinal suction requires application of knowledge and problem solving and is not delegated to UAP. The UAP, however, can assist with emptying the drainage receptacle and reporting changes in amount and/or color of the drainage to the nurse.

- 50-mL syringe with an adapter
- Stethoscope
- Suction device for either continuous or intermittent suction
- Connector and connecting tubing
- Clean gloves

Maintaining Suction
- Graduated container as required to measure gastric drainage
- Basin of water
- Cotton-tipped applicators
- Ointment or lubricant
- Clean gloves

Irrigation
- Clean gloves
- Stethoscope
- Disposable irrigating set containing a sterile 50-mL syringe, moisture-resistant pad, basin, and graduated container
- Sterile normal saline (500 mL) or the ordered solution

EQUIPMENT

Initiating Suction
- Gastrointestinal tube in place in the client
- Basin

IMPLEMENTATION

Performance
1. Prior to performing the procedure, introduce self and verify the client's identity using agency protocol. Explain to the client what you are going to do, why it is necessary, and how he or she can participate. Discuss the purpose(s) for the gastrointestinal suction.
2. Perform hand hygiene and observe other appropriate infection control procedures (e.g., clean gloves).
3. Provide for client privacy.

INITIATING SUCTION
4. Position the client appropriately.
   - Assist the client to a semi-Fowler's position if it is not contraindicated. **Rationale:** *In the semi-Fowler's position, the tube is not as likely to lie against the wall of the stomach and will therefore suction most efficiently. The semi-Fowler's position also prevents reflux of gastric contents, which could lead to aspiration.*
5. Confirm that the tube is in the stomach.
   - Apply clean gloves.
   - Aspirate stomach contents and check the acidity using a pH test strip.
   - Insert air into the tube with the syringe and listen with a stethoscope over the stomach (just below the xiphoid process) for a swish of air.
   - Use other methods in accordance with agency protocol. See Chapter 32 ∞, Skill 32–1.
   - Remove and discard gloves. Perform hand hygiene.

6. Set and check the suction.
   - Connect the appropriate suction regulator to the wall suction outlet and the collection device to the regulator. Intermittent suction regulators generally are used with single-lumen tubes and apply suction for a set interval (15 to 60 seconds), followed by an interval of no suction. Intermittent suction is set at 80 to 100 mm Hg or as ordered by the primary care provider. Check the suction level by occluding the drainage tube and observing the regulator dial during a suction cycle. Continuous suction regulators are used with double-lumen (e.g., Salem sump) nasogastric tubes. Set continuous suction as ordered by the primary care provider, or at 60 to 120 mm Hg.
   - If using a portable suction machine, turn on the machine and regulate the suction as above. The Gomco pump has two settings: low intermittent for single-lumen tubes, and high for double-lumen tubes.
   - Test for proper suctioning by holding the open end of the suction tube to the ear and listening for a sucking noise or by occluding the end of the tube with a thumb.
7. Establish gastric suction.
   - Connect the gastrointestinal tube to the tubing from the suction by using the connector.
   - If a Salem sump tube is in place, connect the larger lumen to the suction equipment. This double-lumen tube has a smaller tube running inside the primary suction tube. **Rationale:** *The smaller tube provides a*

(continued)

MANAGING GASTROINTESTINAL SUCTION *(continued)*

continuous flow of atmospheric air through the drainage tube at its distal end and prevents excessive suction force on the gastric mucosa at the drainage outlets. Damage to the gastric mucosa is thus avoided.

- Always keep the air vent tube of a Salem sump tube open and above the level of the stomach when suction is applied. **Rationale:** *Closing the vent would stop the sump action and cause mucosal damage. Keeping the end of the air vent tube higher than the stomach prevents reflux of gastric contents into the air lumen of the tube.*
- After suction is applied, watch the tubing for a few minutes until the gastric contents appear to be running through the tubing into the receptacle. A Salem sump tube makes a soft, hissing sound when it is functioning correctly.
- If the suction is not working properly, check that all connections are tight and that the tubing is not kinked.
- Coil and pin the tubing to the client's gown so that it does not loop below the suction bottle. **Rationale:** *If the tubing falls below the suction bottle, the suction may be obstructed because of the pressure required to push the fluid against gravity.*

8. Assess the drainage.
   - Observe the amount, color, odor, and consistency of the drainage. Normal gastric drainage has a mucoid (resembling mucus) consistency and is either colorless or yellow-green because of the presence of bile. A coffee-ground color and consistency may indicate bleeding.
   - Test the gastric drainage for pH and blood when indicated. A person who has had gastrointestinal surgery can be expected to have some blood in the drainage.

MAINTAINING SUCTION

9. Assess the client and the suction system regularly.
   - Assess the client every 30 minutes until the system is running effectively and then every 2 hours, or as the client's health indicates, to ensure that the suction is functioning properly. If the client complains of fullness, nausea, or epigastric pain or if the flow of gastric secretions is absent in the tubing or in the collection bottle, ineffective suctioning or blockage of the nasogastric tube is likely.
   - Inspect the suction system for patency of the system (e.g., kinks or blockages in the tubing) and tightness of the connections. **Rationale:** *Loose connections can permit air to enter and thus decrease the effectiveness of the suction by decreasing the negative pressure.*

10. Relieve blockages if present.
    - Apply clean gloves.
    - Check the suction equipment. To do this, disconnect the nasogastric tube from the suction over a collecting basin (to collect gastric drainage), and then, with the suction on, place the end of the suction tubing in a basin of water. If water is drawn into the drainage bottle, the suction equipment is functioning properly, but the nasogastric tube is either blocked or positioned incorrectly.
    - Reposition the client (e.g., to the other side) if permitted. **Rationale:** *This may facilitate drainage.*

- Rotate the nasogastric tube and reposition it. This step is contraindicated for clients with gastric surgery. **Rationale:** *Moving the tube may interfere with gastric sutures.*
- Irrigate the nasogastric tube as agency protocol states or on the order of the primary care provider (see steps 14 to 16).

11. Prevent reflux into the vent lumen of a Salem sump tube. **Rationale:** *Reflux of gastric contents into the vent lumen may occur when stomach pressure exceeds atmospheric pressure. In this situation, gastric contents follow the path of least resistance and flow out the vent lumen rather than the drainage lumen.*

TO PREVENT REFLUX

- Place the vent tubing higher than the client's stomach to prevent gastric fluid backup into the blue lumen air vent.
- Keep the drainage lumen free of particulate matter that may obstruct the lumen (see steps 14 to 16 for irrigating a nasogastric tube).

12. Ensure client comfort.
    - Clean the client's nostrils as needed, using the cotton-tipped applicators and water. Apply a water-soluble lubricant or ointment.
    - Provide mouth care every 2 to 4 hours and as needed. Some postoperative clients are permitted to suck ice chips or a moist cloth to maintain the moisture of the oral mucous membranes.

13. Change the drainage receptacle according to agency policy.
    - Clamp the nasogastric tube and turn off the suction.
    - Apply clean gloves.
    - If the receptacle is graduated, determine the amount of drainage.
    - Disconnect the receptacle.
    - Inspect the drainage carefully for color, consistency, and presence of substances.
    - Replace a full receptacle and attach it to the suction. Check agency policy.
    - Turn on the suction and unclamp the nasogastric tube.
    - Observe the system for several minutes to make sure function is reestablished.
    - Remove and discard gloves. Perform hand hygiene.
    - Go to step 17.

IRRIGATING A GASTROINTESTINAL TUBE

14. Prepare the client and the equipment.
    - Place the moisture-resistant pad under the end of the gastrointestinal tube.
    - Turn off the suction.
    - Apply clean gloves.
    - Disconnect the gastrointestinal tube from the connector.
    - Determine that the tube is in the stomach. See step 5. **Rationale:** *This ensures that the irrigating solution enters the client's stomach.*

15. Irrigate the tube.
    - Draw up the ordered volume of irrigating solution in the syringe; 30 mL of solution per instillation is usual, but up to 60 mL may be given per instillation if ordered.
    - Attach the syringe to the nasogastric tube and slowly inject the solution.

- Gently aspirate the solution. **Rationale:** *Forceful withdrawal could damage the gastric mucosa.*
- If you encounter difficulty in withdrawing the solution, inject 20 mL of air and aspirate again, and/or reposition the client or the nasogastric tube. **Rationale:** *Air and repositioning may move the end of the tube away from the stomach wall.* If aspirating difficulty continues, reattach the tube in intermittent low suction, and notify the nurse in charge.
- Repeat the preceding steps until the ordered amount of solution is used.
- *Note:* A Salem sump tube can also be irrigated through the vent lumen without interrupting suction. However, only small quantities of irrigant can be injected via this lumen compared to the drainage lumen.
- After irrigating a Salem sump tube, inject 10 to 20 mL of air into the vent lumen while applying suction to the drainage lumen. **Rationale:** *This tests the patency of the vent and ensures sump functioning.*

16. Reestablish suction.
- Reconnect the nasogastric tube to suction.
- If a Salem sump tube is used, inject the air vent lumen with 10 mL of air after reconnecting the tube to suction.

- Observe the system for several minutes to make sure it is functioning.
- Remove and discard gloves. Perform hand hygiene.

17. Document all relevant information.
- Record the time suction was started. Also record the pressure established, the color and consistency of the drainage, and nursing assessments.
- During maintenance, record assessments, supportive nursing measures, and data about the suction system.
- When irrigating the tube, record verification of tube placement; the time of the irrigation; the amount and type of irrigating solution used; the amount, color, and consistency of the returns; the patency of the system following the irrigation; and nursing assessments.

SAMPLE DOCUMENTATION

2/1/2010 1300 Returned from PACU. Salem sump tube in place and connected to low continuous suction. Checked for correct placement. Draining small to moderate amount of tannish fluid. —————————————R. Martinez, RN

EVALUATION

- Conduct appropriate follow-up such as relief of abdominal distention or discomfort, bowel sounds, character and amount of gastric drainage, integrity of nares, hydration of oral mucous membranes, patency of tube, and system functioning.

- Compare to previous findings if available.
- Report significant deviations from normal to the primary care provider.

Suction may also be applied to other drainage tubes such as chest tubes or a wound drain. The type and amount of suction is ordered by the primary care provider. Most agencies have wall suction units available (Figure 25–1). A suction regulator with a drainage receptacle connects to a wall outlet that provides negative pressure. Check the receptacle frequently to prevent excess drainage from interfering with the suction apparatus; empty or change the receptacle according to agency policy. Portable electric suction units or pumps (e.g., the Gomco pump) may be used in the home or when wall suction is not available.

Wound Care

Most clients return from surgery with a sutured wound covered by a dressing, although in some cases the wound may be left unsutured. Dressings are inspected regularly to ensure that they are clean, dry, and intact. Excessive drainage may indicate hemorrhage, infection, or an open wound.

When dressings are changed, the nurse assesses the wound for appearance, size, drainage, swelling, pain, and the status of a drain or tubes.

Because surgical incisions heal by primary intention, the nurse can expect the following sequential signs of healing:

1. *Absence of bleeding and the appearance of a clot binding the wound edges.* The wound edges are well approximated and bound by fibrin in the clot within the first few hours after surgical closure.
2. *Inflammation (redness and swelling) at the wound edges for 1 to 3 days.*

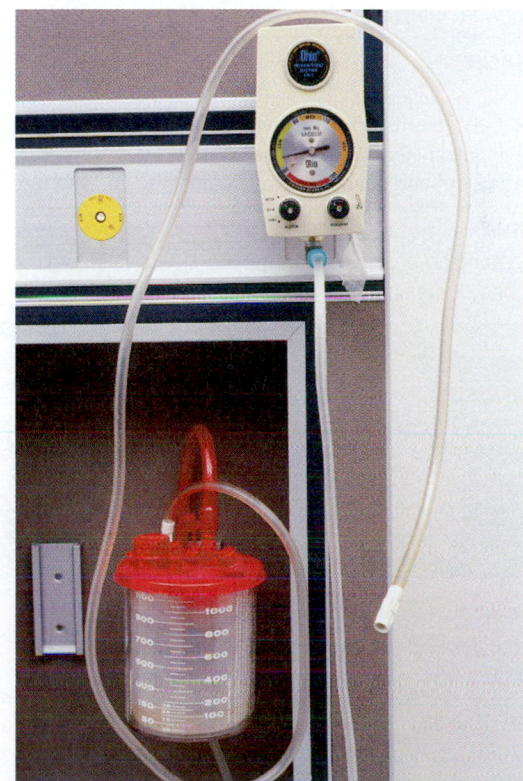

Figure 25–1 ◯ Wall suction unit for generating negative pressure for nasogastric suction.

3. *Reduction in inflammation when the clot diminishes,* as granulation tissue starts to bridge the area. The wound is bridged and closed within 7 to 10 days. Increased inflammation associated with fever and drainage is indicative of wound infection; the wound edges then appear brightly inflamed and swollen.
4. *Scar formation.* Collagen synthesis starts 4 days after injury and continues for 6 months or longer.
5. *Diminished scar size over a period of months or years.* An increase in scar size indicates keloid formation.

See Chapter 24 ∞ for information about wound drainage, cleaning wounds, wound irrigation, hot and cold applications, and supporting and immobilizing wounds.

CLINICAL ALERT

Assess the client immediately if he or she reports a "giving" or "popping" sensation in the incisional area. The client may be experiencing dehiscence or evisceration of the wound.

SURGICAL DRESSINGS Not all surgical dressings require changing. Sometimes surgeons in the operating room apply a dressing that remains in place until the sutures are removed, and no further dressings are required. In many situations, however, surgical dressings are changed regularly to prevent the growth of microorganisms.

In some instances a client may have a Penrose drain inserted (see the next section). In this situation the main surgical incision is considered cleaner than the surgical stab wound made for the drain insertion, because there is usually considerable drainage. The main incision is therefore cleaned first, and under no circumstances are materials that were used to clean the stab wound used subsequently to clean the main incision. In this way, the main incision is kept free of the microorganisms around the stab wound. Cleaning a wound and applying a sterile dressing are detailed in Skill 25–4.

SKILL 25–4

CLEANING A SUTURED WOUND AND APPLYING A STERILE DRESSING

PURPOSES
- To promote wound healing by primary intention
- To prevent infection
- To assess the healing process
- To protect the wound from mechanical trauma

ASSESSMENT
Assess
- Client allergies to wound cleaning agents
- The appearance and size of the wound
- The amount and character of exudates
- Client complaints of discomfort
- The time of the last pain medication
- Signs of systemic infection (e.g., elevated body temperature, diaphoresis, malaise, leukocytosis)

PLANNING
Before changing a dressing, determine any specific orders about the wound or dressing.

> **Delegation**
> Cleaning a newly sutured wound, especially one with a drain, requires application of knowledge, problem solving, and aseptic technique. As a result, this procedure is not delegated to UAP. The nurse can ask the UAP to report soiled dressings that need to be changed or if a dressing has become loose and needs to be reinforced. The nurse is responsible for the assessment and evaluation of the wound.

EQUIPMENT
- Bath blanket (if necessary)
- Moisture-proof bag

- Mask (optional)
- Acetone or another solution (if necessary to loosen adhesive)
- Clean gloves
- Sterile gloves
- Sterile dressing set; if none is available, gather the following sterile items:
  - Drape or towel
  - Gauze squares
  - Container for the cleaning solution
  - Cleaning solution (e.g., normal saline)
  - Two pairs of forceps
  - Gauze dressings and surgipads
  - Applicators or tongue blades to apply ointments
- Additional supplies required for the particular dressing (e.g., extra gauze dressings and ointment, if ordered)
- Tape, tie tapes, or binder

IMPLEMENTATION
Preparation
Prepare the client and assemble the equipment.
- Acquire assistance for changing a dressing on a restless or confused adult. **Rationale:** *The person might move and contaminate the sterile field or the wound.*

- Assist the client to a comfortable position in which the wound can be readily exposed. Expose only the wound area, using a bath blanket to cover the client, if necessary.
  Rationale: *Undue exposure is physically and psychologically distressing to most people.*

- Make a cuff on the moisture-proof bag for disposal of the soiled dressings, and place the bag within reach. It can be taped to the bedclothes or bedside table. **Rationale:** *Making a cuff helps keep the outside of the bag free from contamination by the soiled dressings and prevents subsequent contamination of the nurse's hands or of sterile instrument tips when discarding dressing or sponges. Placement of the bag within reach prevents the nurse from reaching across the sterile field and the wound and potentially contaminating these areas.*
- Apply a face mask, if required. **Rationale:** *Some agencies require that a mask be worn for surgical dressing changes to prevent contamination of the wound by droplet spray from the nurse's respiratory tract.*

Performance

1. Prior to performing the procedure, introduce self and verify the client's identity using agency protocol. Explain to the client what you are going to do, why it is necessary, and how he or she can participate. Discuss how the results will be used in planning further care or treatments.
2. Perform hand hygiene and observe other appropriate infection control procedures.
3. Provide for client privacy.
4. Remove binders and tape.
   - Remove binders, if used, and place them aside. Untie tie tapes, if used. Montgomery straps (tie tapes) are commonly used for wounds requiring frequent dressing changes. **Rationale:** *These straps prevent skin irritation and discomfort caused by removing the adhesive each time the dressing is changed.*
   - If adhesive tape was used, remove it by holding down the skin and pulling the tape gently but firmly toward the wound. **Rationale:** *Pressing down on the skin provides countertraction against the pulling motion. Tape is pulled toward the incision to prevent strain on the sutures or wound.*
   - Use a solvent to loosen tape, if required. **Rationale:** *Moistening the tape with acetone or a similar solvent lessens the discomfort of removal, particularly from hairy surfaces.*

5. Remove and dispose of soiled dressings appropriately.
   - Apply clean gloves and remove the outer abdominal dressing or surgipad.
   - Lift the outer dressing so that the underside is *away* from the client's face. **Rationale:** *The appearance and odor of the drainage may be upsetting to the client.*
   - Place the soiled dressing in the moisture-proof bag without touching the outside of the bag. **Rationale:** *Contamination of the outside of the bag is avoided to prevent the spread of microorganisms to the nurse and subsequently to others.*
   - Remove the under dressings, taking care not to dislodge any drains. If the gauze sticks to the drain, support the drain with one hand and remove the gauze with the other.
   - Assess the location, type (color, consistency), and odor of wound drainage, and the number of gauzes saturated or the diameter of drainage collected on the dressings.
   - Discard the soiled dressings in the bag as before.
   - Remove and discard gloves in the moisture-proof bag, and perform hand hygiene.
6. Set up the sterile supplies.
   - Open the sterile dressing set, using surgical aseptic technique.
   - Place the sterile drape beside the wound.
   - Open the sterile cleaning solution and pour it over the gauze sponges in the plastic container.
   - Apply sterile gloves.
7. Clean the wound, if indicated.
   - Clean the wound, using your gloved hands or forceps and gauze swabs moistened with cleaning solution.
   - If using forceps, keep the forceps tips lower than the handles at all times. **Rationale:** *This prevents their contamination by fluid traveling up to the handle and nurse's wrist and back to the tips.*
   - Use the cleaning methods illustrated and described in ❶ or one recommended by agency protocol.
   - Use a separate swab for each stroke and discard each swab after use. **Rationale:** *This prevents the introduction of microorganisms to other wound areas.*

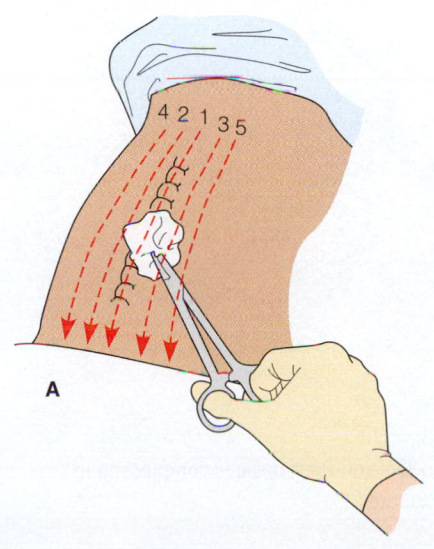
A

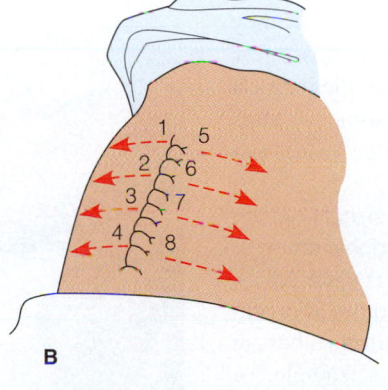
B

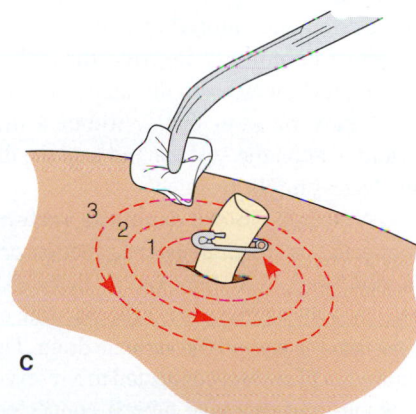
C

❶ Methods of cleaning surgical wounds: **A**, cleaning the wound from top to bottom, starting at the center; **B**, cleaning a wound outward from the incision; **C**, cleaning around a Penrose drain site. For all methods, a clean sterile swab is used for each stroke.

(continued)

SKILL 25–4

CLEANING A SUTURED WOUND AND APPLYING A STERILE DRESSING *(continued)*

- If a drain is present, clean it next, taking care to avoid reaching across the cleaned incision. Clean the skin around the drain site by swabbing in half or full circles from around the drain site outward, using separate swabs for each wipe ❶ C.
- Support and hold the drain erect while cleaning around it. Clean as many times as necessary to remove the drainage.
- Dry the surrounding skin with dry gauze swabs as required. Do not dry the incision or wound itself. Moisture facilitates wound healing.

8. Apply dressings to the drain site and the incision.
   - Place a precut 4 × 4 in. gauze snugly around the drain ❷, or open a 4 × 4 in. gauze to 4 in. × 8 in., fold it lengthwise to 2 × 8 in., and place the 2 × 8 in. gauze around the drain so that the ends overlap. **Rationale:** *This dressing absorbs the drainage and helps prevent it from excoriating the skin. Using precut gauze or folding it as described, instead of cutting the gauze, prevents any threads from coming loose and getting into the wound, where they could cause inflammation and provide a site for infection.*
   - Apply the sterile dressings one at a time over the drain and the incision. Place the bulk of the dressings over the drain area and below the drain, depending on the client's

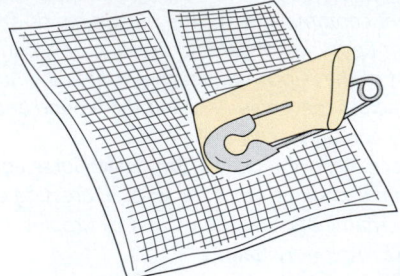

❷ Precut gauze in place around a drain.

usual position. **Rationale:** *Layers of dressings are placed for best absorption of drainage, which flows by gravity.*
   - Apply the final surgipad, remove gloves, and dispose of them. Secure the dressing with tape or ties.

9. Document the procedure and all nursing assessments.

SAMPLE DOCUMENTATION

2/1/2010 1100 Abdominal dressing changed. Small amount of sero-sanguinous drainage – size of a half dollar in middle of dressing. Incision approximated with slight redness at edges. Sutures intact. —————————————S. Jones, RN

EVALUATION
- Conduct appropriate follow-up, such as amount of granulation tissue or degree of healing; amount of drainage and its color, consistency, and odor; presence of inflammation; and degree of discomfort associated with the incision or drain site.
- Compare to previous findings, if available.
- Report significant deviations from normal to the primary care provider.

WOUND DRAINS AND SUCTION Surgical drains, for example a **Penrose drain**, are inserted to permit the drainage of excessive serosanguineous fluid and purulent material and to promote healing of underlying tissues. These drains may be inserted and sutured through the incision line, but they are most commonly inserted through stab wounds a few centimeters away from the incision line so that the incision itself may be kept dry. Without a drain, some wounds would heal on the surface and trap the discharge inside, and an abscess might form.

A **closed-wound drainage system** consists of a drain connected to either an electric suction or a portable drainage suction, such as a Hemovac or Jackson-Pratt (Figure 25–2). The closed system reduces the possible entry of microorganisms into the wound through the drain. The drainage tubes are sutured in place and connected to a reservoir. For example, the Jackson-Pratt drainage tube is connected to a reservoir that maintains constant low suction. These portable wound suctions also provide for accurate measurement of the drainage.

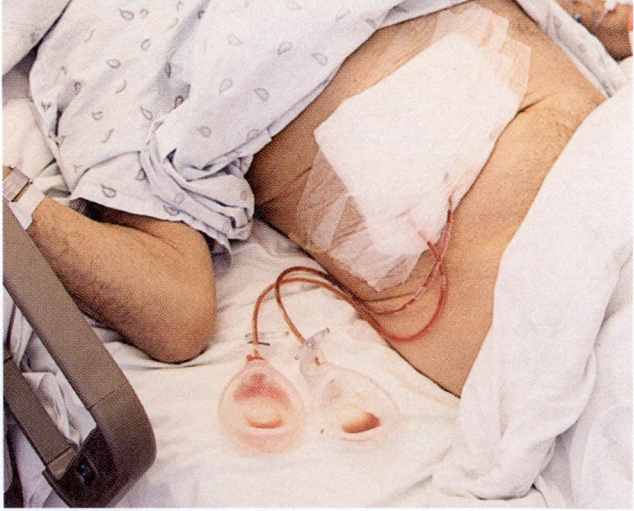

Figure 25–2 ◯ Two Jackson-Pratt devices compressed to facilitate collection of exudates.

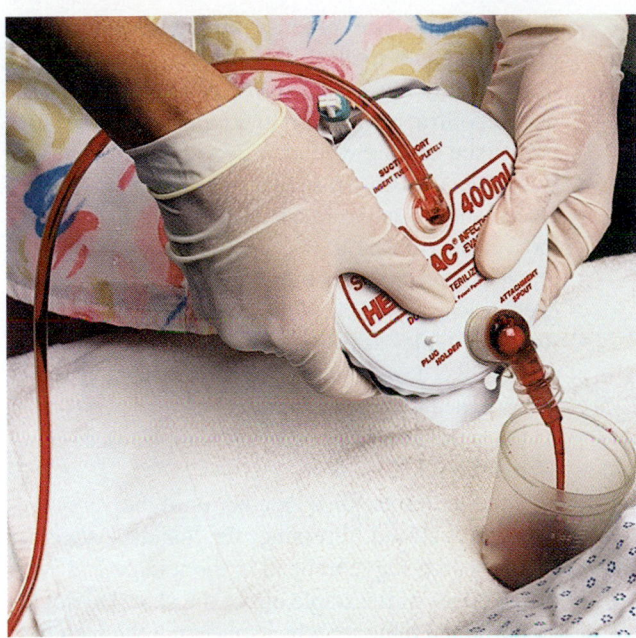

Figure 25–3 ⬤ Emptying drainage from Hemovac drainage system.

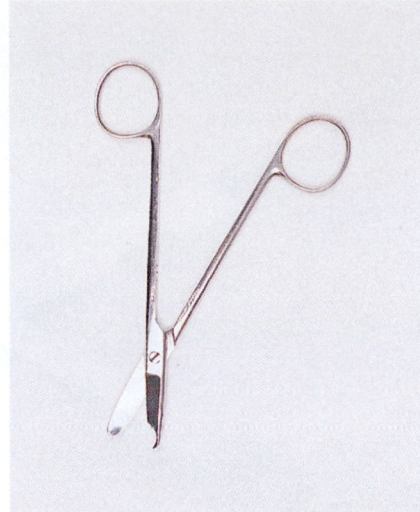

Figure 25–4 ⬤ Suture scissors.

The surgeon inserts the wound drainage tube during surgery. Generally the suction is discontinued from 3 to 5 days postoperatively or when the drainage is minimal. Nurses are responsible for maintaining the wound suction, which hastens the healing process by draining excess exudate that might otherwise interfere with the formation of granulation tissue.

Closed-wound drainage systems have directions for use printed on the drainage container. When emptying the container, the nurse should wear gloves and avoid touching the drainage port (Figure 25–3). To reestablish suction, the nurse places the container on a solid, flat surface with the port open. The palm of one hand presses the top and bottom together while the other hand cleanses the opening and plug with an alcohol swab. Replace the drainage plug before releasing hand pressure to reestablish the vacuum necessary for the closed drainage system to work.

SUTURES A suture is a thread used to sew body tissues together. Sutures used to attach tissues beneath the skin are often made of an absorbable material that disappears in several days. Skin sutures, by contrast, are made of a variety of nonabsorbable materials, such as silk, cotton, linen, wire, nylon, and Dacron. Silver wire clips or staples are also available. Usually skin sutures are removed 7 to 10 days after surgery. Retention sutures are very large sutures used in addition to skin sutures for some incisions. They are frequently left in place longer than skin sutures (14 to 21 days) but in some instances are removed at the same time as the skin sutures. To prevent these large sutures from irritating the incision, the surgeon may place rubber tubing over them or a roll of gauze under them extending down the incision line.

The primary care provider orders the removal of sutures. In some agencies, only primary care providers remove sutures; in others, registered nurses and nursing students with appropriate supervision may do so. Agency policies about removal of retention sutures vary. The nurse should verify whether they are to be removed and who may remove them.

Sterile technique and special suture scissors are used in suture removal. The scissors have a short, curved cutting tip that readily slides under the suture (Figure 25–4). Wire clips or staples are removed with a special instrument that squeezes the center of the clip to remove it from the skin (Figure 25–5). Guidelines for removing sutures and staples follow:

- Before removing skin sutures, verify (a) the orders for suture removal (in many instances, only *alternate* interrupted sutures are removed one day, and the remaining sutures are removed a day or two later) and (b) whether a dressing is to be applied following the suture removal. Some primary care providers prefer no dressing; others prefer a small, light gauze dressing to prevent friction by clothing.
- Inform the client that suture removal may produce slight discomfort, such as a pulling or stinging sensation, but should not be painful.
- Remove dressings and clean the incision in accordance with agency protocol. Cleaning the suture line with an antimicrobial solution before and after suture removal may help prevent infection.
- Put on sterile gloves.
- Remove plain interrupted sutures as follows:
  a. Grasp the suture at the knot with a pair of forceps.
  b. Place the curved tip of the suture scissors under the suture as close to the skin as possible, either on the side opposite the knot or directly under the

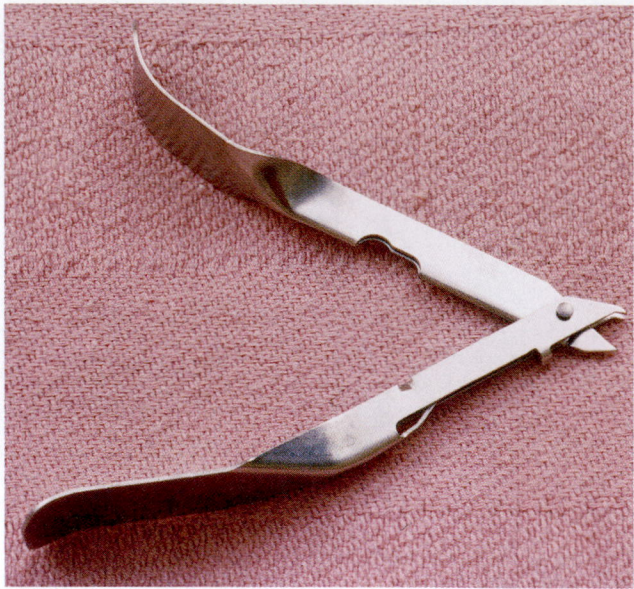

Figure 25–5 ○ Staple remover.

knot. Cut the suture. Sutures are cut as close to the skin as possible on one side of the visible part because the suture material that is visible to the eye is in contact with resident bacteria of the skin and must not be pulled beneath the skin during removal. Suture material that is beneath the skin is considered free from bacteria.

   c. With the forceps, pull the suture out in one piece. Inspect the suture carefully to make sure that all suture material is removed. Suture material left beneath the skin acts as a foreign body and causes inflammation.

- Remove mattress interrupted sutures as follows:
   a. When possible, cut the visible part of the suture close to the skin, opposite the knot, and remove this small visible piece. Discard it as described in the following bullet. The visible part opposite the knot may be so small in some sutures that it can be cut only once.
   b. Grasp the knot with forceps. Remove the remainder of the suture beneath the skin by pulling out in the direction of the knot.

- Discard the suture onto a piece of sterile gauze or into the moisture-proof bag, being careful not to contaminate the forceps tips.

- Continue to remove alternate sutures, that is, the third, fifth, seventh, and so forth. Alternate sutures are removed first so that remaining sutures keep the skin edges in close approximation and prevent any dehiscence from becoming large.

- If no dehiscence occurs, remove the remaining sutures. If dehiscence does occur, do not remove the remaining sutures, and report the dehiscence to the nurse in charge.

- If Steri-Strips are ordered by the primary care provider, apply them to the wound after removing the sutures or clips. Some primary care providers order Steri-Strip application to provide additional support to the healing wound.

- Reapply a dressing, if indicated.

- Document the suture removal; number of sutures removed; appearance of the incision; application of a dressing, Steri-Strips, or butterfly tapes (if appropriate); client teaching; and client tolerance of the procedure.

- Remove staples as follows:
   a. Remove dressings and clean the incision in accordance with agency protocol.
   b. Place the lower tips of a sterile staple remover under the staple.
   c. Squeeze the handles together until they are completely closed. Pressing the handles together causes the staple to bend in the middle and pulls the edges of the staple out of the skin. Do not lift the staple remover when squeezing the handles.
   d. When both ends of the staple are visible, gently move the staple away from the incision site.
   e. Hold the staple remover over a disposable container, release the staple remover handles, and release the staple.

Discharge Teaching

To ensure continuity of care and restoration of the client's health, nurses must meet the learning needs of clients and their support people. Teaching should focus on actions to maintain comfort, to promote healing and restore wellness, and to make use of appropriate community agencies and other sources of help.

MAINTAINING COMFORT

- Instruct the client to use pain medications as ordered, not allowing pain to become severe before taking the prescribed dose.

- If not contraindicated, discuss the use of over-the-counter analgesics such as aspirin or acetaminophen as postoperative pain becomes less severe or if the client is reluctant to use prescription drugs due to side effects.

- Teach the client to avoid using alcohol or other central nervous system depressants while taking narcotic analgesics.

- Discuss the importance of gradually resuming activities, avoiding overexertion.

- Emphasize the importance of paying attention to increasing pain or discomfort. Instruct the client to contact the primary care provider if pain increases after a period of decreasing discomfort.

- Teach the client to use nonpharmacologic measures to help manage pain, such as conscious relaxation, distraction, meditation, or visualization.

PROMOTING HEALING

- If indicated, teach the client how to change wound dressings and perform wound care.
- Emphasize the importance of hygiene and hand washing to prevent infections.
- Instruct the client to report promptly to the primary care provider any increasing redness, swelling, pain, or discharge from the incision or drain sites.
- Discuss any prescribed activity restrictions such as avoiding lifting.
- Discuss the importance of keeping follow-up appointments to monitor healing and recovery after surgery.

RESTORING WELLNESS

- Discuss the relationship of increasing activities to restoring wellness and promoting a sense of well-being.
- Teach the client that surgery and stressors can depress immune function and to avoid exposure to illness (e.g., crowded areas and people with upper respiratory illnesses) whenever possible.
- Emphasize the importance of adequate rest for healing and immune function.
- If appropriate, discuss lifestyle changes to promote wellness, such as smoking cessation, increasing activity level, reducing stress, and consuming a healthy diet high in fruits, vegetables, and whole grains with adequate protein to promote healing.

COMMUNITY AGENCIES AND OTHER SOURCES OF HELP

- Provide information about where durable medical equipment can be purchased, rented, or obtained free of charge; how to access home health and other services; and where to obtain supplies such as dressings or nutritional supplements.

- Suggest additional sources of information, such as the National Rehabilitation Information Center, Reach to Recovery, and United Ostomy Association.

REFERRALS The nurse needs to consider appropriate referrals for the client, such as:

- Home health agencies for wound care and assessment and for assistance with ADLs if necessary.
- Community social services for assistance in obtaining medical and assistive equipment.
- Respiratory, physical, or occupational therapy services as indicated.

EVALUATING

Using the goals developed during the planning stage, the nurse collects data to evaluate whether the identified goals and desired outcomes have been achieved. Examples of client outcomes and related indicators are shown in the earlier Identifying Nursing Diagnoses, Outcomes, and Interventions boxes.

If the desired outcomes are not achieved, the nurse and client, and support people, if appropriate, need to explore the reasons before modifying the care plan. For example, if the outcome "Pain control" is not met, questions to be considered include:

- What is the client's perception of the problem?
- Does the client understand how to use PCA?
- Is the prescribed analgesic dose adequate for the client?
- Is the client allowing pain to become intense prior to requesting medication or using PCA?
- Where is the client's pain? Could it be due to a problem unrelated to surgery (e.g., chronic arthritis, anginal pain)?
- Is there evidence of a complication that could cause increased pain (an infection, abscess, or hematoma)?

CHAPTER HIGHLIGHTS

- Surgery is a unique experience that creates stress and necessitates physical and psychologic changes.
- The perioperative period includes three phases: preoperative, intraoperative, and postoperative.
- Surgical procedures are categorized by degree of urgency, purpose, and degree of risk.
- Factors such as age, general health, nutritional status, medication use, and mental status affect a client's risk during surgery.
- Clients must agree to surgery via informed consent and sign a consent form.

- Nursing history and physical assessment data are important sources for planning preoperative and postoperative care.
- The overall goal of nursing care during the preoperative phase is to prepare the client mentally and physically for surgery.
- Preoperative teaching includes situational information and psychosocial support, the role of the client throughout the perioperative period, expected sensations and discomfort, and training for the postoperative period.

- Preoperative teaching should include moving, leg exercises, and coughing and deep-breathing exercises. Many aspects of preoperative teaching are intended to prevent postoperative complications.
- Physical preparation includes the following areas: nutrition and fluids, elimination, hygiene, rest, medications, care of valuables and prostheses, special orders, and surgical skin preparation.
- Antiemboli stockings or sequential compression devices may be ordered for some clients to facilitate venous return.
- A preoperative checklist provides a guide to and documentation of a client's preparation before surgery.
- Maintaining the client's safety is the overall goal of nursing care during the intraoperative phase.
- Anesthesia may be general or regional. Regional anesthesia includes topical, local, nerve block, intravenous block, spinal anesthesia (subarachnoid block), and epidural.
- A surgical skin preparation should be carried out as close to the time of surgery as possible and is commonly performed during the intraoperative phase.
- Positioning of the client during surgery is important to reduce the risk of tissue and nerve damage.
- Immediate postanesthetic care focuses on assessment and monitoring parameters to prevent complications from anesthesia or surgery.

- Initial and ongoing assessment of the postoperative client includes level of consciousness, vital signs, oxygen saturation, skin color and temperature, comfort, fluid balance, dressings, drains, and tubes.
- The overall goals of nursing care during the postoperative period are to promote comfort and healing, restore the highest possible level of wellness, and prevent associated risks such as infection or respiratory and cardiovascular complications.
- Ongoing postoperative nursing interventions include (a) managing pain, (b) appropriate positioning, (c) encouraging incentive spirometry and deep-breathing and coughing exercises, (d) promoting leg exercises and early ambulation, (e) maintaining adequate hydration and nutritional status, (f) promoting urinary elimination, (g) continuing gastrointestinal suction, and (h) providing wound care.
- Surgical aseptic technique (sterile technique) is used when changing dressings on surgical wounds to promote healing and reduce the risk of infection.
- Penrose drains and Hemovac drainage systems are examples of drains that may be placed in or near surgical wounds to promote drainage of excess serosanguineous or purulent exudate.
- Sutures, wire clips, or staples are used to approximate skin and underlying tissues after surgery. These are generally removed 7 to 10 days after surgery.

THINK ABOUT IT

Refer to the chapter-opening scenario and answer these questions.

1. If you were the nurse caring for Ms. Klein, how would you respond to her concern regarding the possibility of the surgeon operating on the wrong body part?

2. How would you respond to the client's concern regarding postoperative pain?

3. The surgeon and anesthesiologist speak with Ms. Klein to explain the procedure and assess her physical condition. Afterwards, the surgeon writes an order to administer preoperative medications and obtain a signature on the operative consent. In what order would you perform these two interventions? What acts would you perform before administering the preoperative medication?

∞ *See suggested responses to Think About It on MyNursingKit.*

TEST YOUR KNOWLEDGE

1. Which of the following tests is the best resource for determing the status of a client's preoperative liver function?
   1. Serum electrolytes
   2. Blood urea nitrogen (BUN), creatinine
   3. Alanine amino transferase (ALT) and bilirubin
   4. Serum albumin and hematocrit

2. A client who is having a mastectomy expresses sadness about losing her breast. Based on this information, the nurse would identify that the client is at risk for which nursing diagnosis?
   1. *Body Image Disturbance*
   2. *Anticipatory Grieving*
   3. *Fear*
   4. *Ineffective Coping*

3. Which of the following statements by the client indicates that the preoperative teaching regarding gallbladder surgery has been effective?
   1. "I cannot eat or drink anything after midnight."
   2. "I'm not going to cough after surgery because it might open my incision."
   3. "I might have a stroke if I stop taking my anticoagulant."
   4. "The nurse showed me how to contract and relax my calf muscles."

4. The nurse assesses a postoperative client who has a rapid, weak pulse; urine output less than 30 mL/hr; and decreased blood pressure. The client's skin is cool and clammy. What complication should the nurse suspect?
   1. Thrombophlebitis
   2. Hypovolemic shock
   3. Aspiration pneumonia
   4. Wound dehiscence

5. The nurse anticipates needing to administer the greatest amount of analgesia for pain to the client during which of the following time periods?
   1. Immediately after surgery
   2. 4 hours after surgery
   3. 12 to 36 hours after surgery
   4. 48 to 60 hours after surgery

6. A postop client who had abdominal surgery is holding a pillow against his abdomen during deep breathing and coughing. What term does the nurse use to describe this procedure? _____

7. A semiconscious client in the post-anesthesia care unit (PACU) is experiencing dyspnea (difficulty breathing). Which of the following nursing interventions takes greatest priority?
   1. Place a pillow under the client's head.
   2. Remove the oropharyngeal airway.
   3. Apply oxygen by mask.
   4. Reposition the client to keep the tongue forward.

8. The client's postop orders state "diet as tolerated." The client has been NPO. The nurse will advance the client's diet to clear liquids based on which of the following assessments? Select all that apply.
   1. No complaints of nausea or vomiting.
   2. Pain level is maintained at a rating of 2–3/10.
   3. States passing flatus.
   4. Ambulates with minimal assistance.
   5. Expresses feeling "hungry."

9. The overall goal of nursing care during the intraoperative phase is the client's _____.

10. The nurse plans to remove the client's sutures. Which of the following actions demonstrate appropriate standards of care? Select all that apply.
   1. Use clean technique.
   2. Grasp the suture at the knot with a pair of forceps.
   3. Place the curved tip of the suture scissors under the suture as close to the skin as possible.
   4. Pull the suture material that is visible beneath the skin during removal.
   5. Remove alternate sutures first.

∞ *See answers to Test Your Knowledge in Appendix A.*

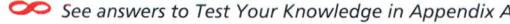

EXPLORE PEARSON **mynursingkit**™

MyNursingKit is your one stop for online chapter review materials and resources. Prepare for success with additional NCLEX®-style practice questions, interactive assignments and activities, web links, animations and videos, and more!

Register your access code from the front of your book at
www.mynursingkit.com.

REFERENCES AND SELECTED BIBLIOGRAPHY

Amella, E. J. (2006). Presentation of illness in older adults. *AORN Journal, 83*(2), 373–391.

American Society of PeriAnesthesia Nurses. (2006). *Standards, recommended practices and guidelines.* Denver, CO: Author.

Anonymous. (2002). Recommended practices for skin preparation of patients. *AORN Journal, 75*(1), 184–187.

Anonymous. (2005). AORN guidance statement: Preoperative patient care in the ambulatory surgery setting. *AORN Journal, 81*(4), 871–878.

Anonymous. (2005). AORN guidance statement: Postoperative patient care in the ambulatory surgery setting. *AORN Journal, 81*(4), 881–888.

Association of Operating Room Nurses. (2005). Recommended practices for positioning the patient in the perioperative practice setting. *2005 standards, recommended practices, and guidelines.* Denver, CO: Author.

Bulechek, G. M., Butcher, H. K., & Dochterman, J. M. (Eds.). (2008). *Nursing interventions: classification (NIC)* (5th ed.). St. Louis, MO: Mosby.

Cofer, M. J. (2005). Unwelcome companion to older patients: Postoperative delirium. *Nursing, 35*(1), 32hn1–32hn3.

Connor, R. (2001). *Ambulatory surgery principles and practices: Standards and recommended practices for ambulatory surgery* (2nd ed.). Denver, CO: AORN.

Crenshaw, J. T., & Winslow, E. H. (2002). Preoperative fasting: Old habits die hard. *American Journal of Nursing, 102*(5), 36–44.

Ebersole, P., Hess, P., & Luggen, A. (2004). *Towards healthy aging: Human needs and nursing response* (6th ed.). St. Louis: Mosby.

Golembiewski, J., & O'Brien, D. (2003). Morphine and hydromorphone for post-operative analgesia: Focus on safety. *Journal of PeriAnesthesia Nursing, 18*(2), 120–122.

Halliday, A.B. (2006). Shades of sedation. *Nursing, 36*(4), 36–41.

Her, C., & Culhane-Pera, K. A. (2004). Culturally responsive care for Hmong patients. *Postgraduate Medicine, 116*(6), 39–45.

Joint Commission on Accreditation of Healthcare Organizations. (2003). *Universal protocol for preventing wrong site, wrong procedure, wrong person surgery.* Retrieved December 5, 2009, from http://www.jointcommission.org/PatientSafety/Universal_Protocol.pdf

Larkin, B. G. (2004). The ins and outs of body piercing. *AORN Journal, 79*(2), 333–342.

Meeker, M. H., & Rothrock, J. C. (2003). *Alexander's care of the patient in surgery* (12th ed.). St. Louis: Mosby.

Meltzer, B. (2003). Seven keys to fast-track anesthesia. *Outpatient Surgery, IV*(3), 52–62.

Meyer, M., & Driscoll, E. (2004). Perioperative surgery in the twenty-first century. *AORN Journal, 80*(4), 725–733.

Millsaps, C. C. (2006). Pay attention to patient positioning! *RN, 69*(1), 59–63.

Moorhead, S., Johnson, M., Maas, M. L., & Swanson, E. (Eds.). (2008). *Nursing outcomes classification (NOC)* (4th ed.). St. Louis: Mosby.

Moz, T. (2004). Wound dehiscence and evisceration. *Nursing, 34*(5), 88.

Murphy, E. K. (2004). Negligence cases concerning positioning injuries. *AORN Journal, 30*(2), 311–314.

NANDA International. (2009). *NANDA nursing diagnoses: Definitions & classification 2009–2011.* West Sussex, U.K.: Wiley-Blackwell.

Pullen, R. (2003). Removing sutures and staples. *Nursing, 33*(10), 18.

Seal, L., & Paul-Cheadle, D. (2004). A systems approach to preoperative surgical patient skin preparation. *American Journal of Infection Control, 32*(2), 57–62.

Sherwood, G. D., McNeil, J. A., Starck, P. L., & Disnard, G. (2003). Changing acute pain management outcomes in surgical patients. *AORN Journal, 77*(2), 374–393.

Squires, A. (2003). Documenting surgical incision site care. *Nursing, 33*(1), 74.

Steefel, L. (2004). Marks of safety. Preop safety protocols help teams check blind spots that will prevent surgical errors. *Nurse Week MountainWest Edition, 5*(20), 17–18.

Tittle, M., McMillan, S., & Hagan, S. (2003). Validating the Brief Pain Inventory for use with surgical patients with cancer. *Oncology Nursing Forum, 30*(2), 325–330.

Warnock, K. (2003). Preventing surgical errors: The role of the surgical technologist. *Surgical Technologist, 35*(6), 15–29.

Sensory Perception

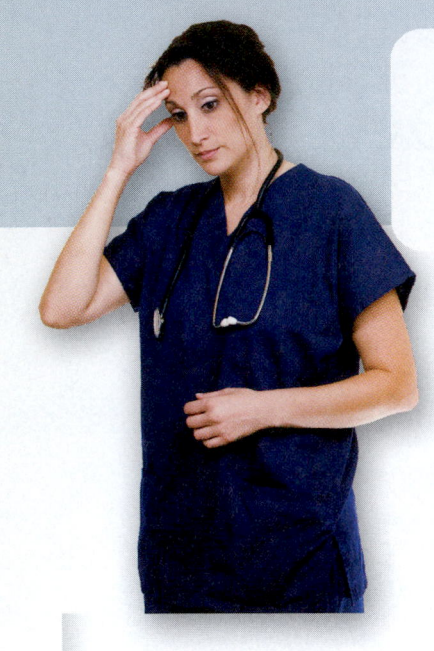

Susan is a senior nursing student beginning her first clinical day in the intensive care unit of a local acute care facility. She is a bit nervous about working in a high acuity unit, even though she is well prepared, having researched her client's medical record, and has prepared a nursing care plan for the day. When she enters the unit, she hears two client call bells ringing and sees the staff is involved in a cardiac resuscitation in one of the rooms—not her assigned client. The bank of monitors at the desk is alarming, due to the resuscitated client's asystole, and family members are sitting in the waiting room crying. The phone is ringing. She learns the unit clerk has taken some STAT specimens to the laboratory. Oncoming nursing staff are talking at the nurse's desk, and she learns that her client, who is calling for her dog to come home, is experiencing ICU psychosis. Student nurses who arrived before Susan are talking quietly with their instructor near the nurse's desk, and doctors and other hospital persons are moving in and out of the unit. The unit is very brightly lit with sunlight streaming through the windows and all of the overhead florescent lights on. Susan finds herself feeling completely overwhelmed by what seems to be chaos in the department, and she wonders how she will be able to concentrate enough to deliver good care to her client.

LEARNING OUTCOMES

After completing this chapter, you will be able to:

1. Discuss anatomic and physiologic components of the sensory-perception process.

2. Describe factors influencing sensory function.

3. Identify clinical signs and symptoms of sensory overload and deprivation.

4. Describe essential components in assessing a client's sensory-perception function.

5. Discuss factors that place a client at risk for sensory disturbances.

6. Develop nursing diagnoses and outcome criteria for clients with impaired sensory function.

7. Discuss nursing interventions to promote and maintain sensory function.

8. Identify strategies to promote and maintain orientation to person, place, time, and situation for the client with acute confusion/delirium.

9. Promote structured sensory stimulation for the unconscious client.

An individual's senses are essential for growth, development, and survival. Sensory stimuli give meaning to events in the environment. Any alteration in people's sensory functions can affect their ability to function within the environment. For example, many clients have impaired sensory functions that put them at risk in the health care setting; nurses can help them find ways to function safely in this often confusing environment.

COMPONENTS OF THE SENSORY EXPERIENCE

The sensory process involves two components: reception and perception. **Sensory reception** is the process of receiving stimuli or data. These stimuli are either external or internal to the body. External stimuli are visual (sight), auditory (hearing), olfactory (smell), tactile (touch), and gustatory (taste). Gustatory stimuli can be internal as well. Other types of internal stimuli are kinesthetic or visceral. **Kinesthetic** refers to awareness of the position and movement of body parts. For example, a person walking is aware of which leg is forward. A related sense is **stereognosis**, the ability to perceive and understand an object through touch by its size, shape, and texture. For example, a person holding a tennis ball is aware of its size, round shape, and soft surface without seeing it. Visceral refers to any large organ within the body. Visceral organs may produce stimuli that make a person aware of them (e.g., a full stomach). **Sensory perception** involves the conscious organization and translation of the data or stimuli into meaningful information.

For an individual to be aware of the surroundings, four aspects of the sensory process must be present: a stimulus, a receptor, impulse conduction, and perception.

- *Stimulus.* This is an agent or act that stimulates a nerve receptor.
- *Receptor.* A nerve cell acts as a receptor by converting the stimulus to a nerve impulse. Most receptors are specific, that is, sensitive to only one type of stimulus, such as visual, auditory, or touch.
- *Impulse conduction.* The impulse travels along nerve pathways to the spinal cord or directly to the brain (see Figure 26–1). For example, auditory impulses travel to the organ of Corti in the inner ear. From there the impulses travel along the eighth cranial nerve to the temporal lobe of the brain.

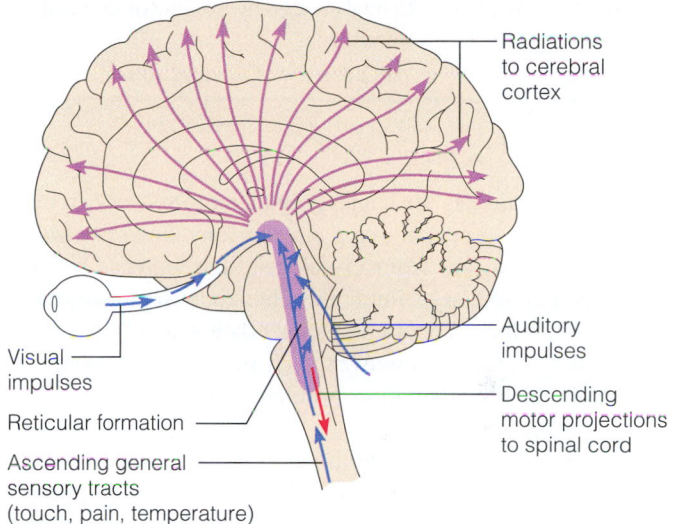

Figure 26–1 ⬤ The nerve impulses run along the ascending sensory tracts to reach the reticular activating system (RAS); then certain impulses reach the cerebral cortex where they are perceived. (From *Human Anatomy & Physiology,* 7th ed., by Elaine N. Marieb and Katja Hoehn. Copyright © 2007 (p. 455) by Benjamin Cummings Publishing Company. Reprinted by permission of Pearson Education, Inc.)

- *Perception.* Perception, or awareness and interpretation of stimuli, takes place in the brain, where specialized brain cells interpret the nature and the quality of the sensory stimuli. The level of consciousness affects the perception of the stimuli.

Arousal Mechanism

For the person to receive and interpret stimuli, the brain must be alert. The *reticular activating system* (RAS) in the brainstem is thought to mediate the arousal mechanism. There are two components of the reticular activating system, the *reticular excitatory area* (REA) and the *reticular inhibitory area* (RIA). The REA is responsible for stimulus arousal and wakefulness.

People have their own zone of optimum arousal, the level at which the person feels comfortable. **Sensoristasis** is the term used to describe when a person is in optimal arousal. Beyond this comfort zone people must adapt to the increased or decreased sensory stimuli. An absence of stimuli from the RAS to the cerebrum results in the brain's becoming inactive or useless.

TABLE 26–1   States of Awareness

STATE	DESCRIPTION
Full consciousness	Alert; oriented to time, place, person; understands verbal and written words
Disoriented	Not oriented to time, place, or person
Confused	Reduced awareness, easily bewildered; poor memory, misinterprets stimuli; impaired judgment
Somnolent	Extreme drowsiness but will respond to stimuli
Semicomatose	Can be aroused by extreme or repeated stimuli
Coma*	Will not respond to verbal stimuli

*See Glasgow Coma Scale, Table 17-5 in Chapter 17 ∞.

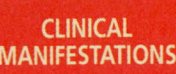

CLINICAL MANIFESTATIONS   Sensory Deprivation

- Excessive yawning, drowsiness, sleeping
- Decreased attention span, difficulty concentrating, decreased problem solving
- Impaired memory
- Periodic disorientation, general confusion, or nocturnal confusion
- Preoccupation with somatic complaints, such as palpitations
- Hallucinations or delusions
- Crying, annoyance over small matters, depression
- Apathy, emotional lability

The brain has the capacity to adapt to sensory stimuli. For example, a person living in a city may not notice traffic noise that someone from a rural area finds loud and disturbing. Not all sensory stimuli are acted upon; some are stored by the memory to be used at a later date. Cognition is cerebral functioning. It involves such processes as conscious thought, reality orientation, problem solving, judgment, and comprehension.

Awareness is the ability to perceive environmental stimuli and body reactions and to respond appropriately through thought and action. The normal, alert person can assimilate many kinds of information at one time. There are several states of awareness (see Table 26–1).

SENSORY ALTERATIONS

People become accustomed to certain sensory stimuli, and when these change markedly the individual may experience discomfort. For example, when clients enter a hospital they usually experience stimuli that differ in quantity and quality from those to which they are accustomed. These changes may cause clients to become confused and disoriented (see Table 26–1).

Nurses are aware of the behaviors that often result from different stimuli. They now pay more attention to color, sound, privacy, and social interaction for clients so that the stimuli more closely resemble those in the home environment. Factors that contribute to alterations in behavior include sensory deprivation, sensory overload, and sensory deficits.

Sensory Deprivation

Sensory deprivation is generally thought of as a decrease in or lack of meaningful stimuli. When a person experiences sensory deprivation, the balance in the reticular activating system is disturbed. The RAS is unable to maintain normal stimulation to the cerebral cortex. Because of this reduced stimulation, a person becomes more acutely aware of the remaining stimuli and often perceives these in a distorted manner. Thus the person often experiences alterations in

perception, cognition, and emotion. The Clinical Manifestations box lists clinical signs of sensory deprivation.

Sensory Overload

Sensory overload generally occurs when a person is unable to process or manage the amount or intensity of sensory stimuli. Three factors contribute to sensory overload:

- Increased quantity or quality of internal stimuli, such as pain, dyspnea, anxiety
- Increased quantity or quality of external stimuli, such as a noisy health care setting, intrusive diagnostic studies, contacts with many strangers
- Inability to disregard stimuli selectively, perhaps as a result of nervous system disturbances or medications that stimulate the arousal mechanism

Sensory overload can prevent the brain from ignoring or responding to specific stimuli. Because of the many stimuli, the individual has difficulty perceiving the environment in a way that makes sense. As a result the individual's thoughts race in many directions and restlessness occurs. The person usually feels overwhelmed and does not feel in control. It is important for nurses to remember that sights and sounds that are familiar to them often represent overload to clients. People who have sensory overload may appear fatigued. They often cannot internalize new information and experience cognitive overload as a result of everything that is happening to them. Such factors as pain, lack of sleep, and worry can also contribute to sensory overload. See the Clinical Manifestations box for common signs of sensory overload.

Sensory Deficits

A **sensory deficit** is impaired reception, perception, or both, of one or more of the senses. Blindness and deafness are sensory deficits. When only one sense is affected, other senses may become more acute to compensate for the loss. However, sudden loss of eyesight can result in disorientation.

When the loss of sensory function is gradual, individuals often develop behaviors to compensate for the loss;

Sensory Overload

- Complaints of fatigue, sleeplessness
- Irritability, anxiety, restlessness
- Periodic or general disorientation
- Reduced problem-solving ability and task performance
- Increased muscle tension
- Scattered attention and racing thoughts

sometimes these behaviors are unconscious. For example, a person with gradual hearing loss in the right ear may unconsciously turn the left ear toward a speaker. When the loss is sudden, however, compensatory behavior often takes days or weeks to develop.

Some neurologic diseases cause changes in the kinesthetic sense and tactile perceptions. Diseases of the inner ear, for example, can cause loss of kinesthetic sense.

Clients with sensory deficits are at risk for both sensory deprivation and sensory overload. Persons with visual problems may be unable to read, watch television, or recognize nurses by sight. An unfamiliar environment can add to their confusion. Blind people often have highly structured home environments, and the diversity and unfamiliarity of the hospital environment can create sensory overload. At the same time, impaired vision often results in an inability to move around readily or socialize with others.

FACTORS AFFECTING SENSORY FUNCTION

A number of factors affect the amount and quality of sensory stimulation, including a person's developmental stage, culture, level of stress, medications and illness, and lifestyle.

Developmental Stage

Perception of sensation is critical to the intellectual, social, and physical development of infants and children. Infants learn to recognize the face of the mother or caregiver and establish bonding essential to later emotional development. Young children respond to music by singing and dancing as they begin to interact with their peers in groups. As children grow, they learn to interpret visual and auditory signals when preparing to cross the street. Adults have many learned responses to sensory cues. The sudden loss or impairment of any sense, therefore, has a profound effect on both the child and the adult.

Normal physiologic changes in older adults put them at higher risk for altered sensory function. The diminishing of sensory perception that may come with chronic disease or aging is generally gradual. For example, hearing loss is the third most common condition reported by older adults. Approximately 40% to 45% of people over age 65 and more than 83% over the age of 70 have a hearing impairment (Gordon-Salant, 2005).

Culture

An individual's culture often determines the amount of stimulation that a person considers usual or "normal." For example, a child reared in a big-city Latino neighborhood where extended families share responsibilities for all the children may be accustomed to more stimulation than a child reared in a European American suburb of scattered single-family homes. In addition, the normal amount of stimulation associated with ethnic origin, religious affiliation, and income level, for example, also affects the amount of stimulation an individual desires and believes to be meaningful. A sudden change in cultural surroundings experienced by immigrants or visitors to a new country, especially where there are differences in language, dress, and cultural behaviors, may also result in sensory overload or cultural shock.

Cultural deprivation, or **cultural care deprivation**, is a lack of culturally assistive, supportive, or facilitative acts. It is important that nurses be sensitive to what stimulation is culturally acceptable to a client. For example, in some cultures touching is comforting, whereas in others it is offensive. Some clients find the presence of cultural or religious symbols reassuring and their absence a source of anxiety. Nurses should encourage clients who want to have culturally related symbols present and to follow practices with which they are comfortable, provided that these practices do not endanger health.

Stress

During times of increased stress, people may find their senses already overloaded and thus seek to decrease sensory stimulation. For example, a client dealing with physical illness, pain, hospitalization, and diagnostic tests may wish to have only close support people visit. In addition, the client may need the nurse's help to decrease unnecessary stimuli (e.g., noise) as much as possible. On the other hand, clients may seek sensory stimulation during times of low stress.

Medications and Illness

Certain medications can alter an individual's awareness of environmental stimuli. Narcotics and sedatives, for example, can decrease awareness of stimuli. Some antidepressants can alter perceptions of stimuli. Anyone taking several medications concurrently may show alterations in sensory function; older adults are especially at risk and need to be monitored carefully. Certain medications, if taken over a long period of time, become ototoxic, injuring the auditory nerve and causing hearing loss that may be irreversible. Some of these medications are aspirin, furosemide (Lasix), the aminoglycosides, and certain drugs given for cancer chemotherapy.

Certain diseases, such as atherosclerosis, restrict blood flow to the receptor organs and the brain, thereby decreasing awareness and slowing responses. Uncontrolled diabetes mellitus can impair vision and is a leading cause of blindness in the United States. Some central nervous system diseases cause varying degrees of paralysis and sensory loss.

Lifestyle and Personality

Lifestyle influences the quality and quantity of stimulation to which an individual is accustomed. A client who is employed in a large company may be accustomed to many diverse stimuli, whereas a client who is self-employed and works in the home is exposed to fewer, less diverse stimuli. People's personalities also differ in terms of the quantity and quality of stimuli with which they are comfortable. Some people delight in constantly changing stimuli and excitement, whereas others prefer a more structured life with few changes.

NURSING MANAGEMENT

ASSESSING

Nursing assessment of sensory-perceptual functioning includes six components: (a) nursing history, (b) mental status examination, (c) physical examination, (d) identification of clients at risk, (e) the client's environment, and (f) social support network.

Nursing History

During the nursing history the nurse assesses present sensory perceptions, usual functioning, sensory deficits, and potential problems. In some instances, significant others can provide data the client cannot. For example, support people may reveal signs of recent changes in the client's hearing ability, such as inattention to others, recent mood swings, difficulty following clear instructions, frequent requests to have something repeated, and unusually loud radio or television volumes. Examples of interview questions to elicit data about the client's sensory-perceptual functioning are shown in the Assessment Interview box.

Mental Status

Mental status is critical to any evaluation of the sensory-perceptual process. Usually data on mental status including level of consciousness, orientation, memory, and attention span can be obtained during the nursing history (see Chapter 17 ∞). It is important to note that sensory alterations can cause changes in cognitive functioning (Wahl & Heyl, 2003).

Physical Examination

Physical assessment determines whether the senses are impaired. During the physical examination the nurse assesses vision and hearing, and the olfactory, gustatory, tactile, and kinesthetic senses. The examination should reveal the client's specific visual and hearing abilities; perception of heat, cold, light touch, and pain in the limbs; and awareness of the position of the body parts. Specific sensory tests include the following:

- Visual acuity, using a Snellen chart or other reading material such as a newspaper, and visual fields

---

ASSESSMENT INTERVIEW — Sensory-Perceptual Functioning

Visual

- How would you rate your vision (excellent, good, fair, or poor)?
- Do you wear eyeglasses or contact lenses?
- Describe any recent changes in your vision.
- Do you have any difficulty seeing near or far objects?
- Do you have any difficulty seeing at night? Have you ever experienced blurred vision, double vision, spots moving in front of your eyes, blind spots, light sensitivity, flashing lights, or halos around objects?
- When did you last visit an eye doctor?

Auditory

- How would you rate your hearing (excellent, good, fair, or poor)?
- Do you wear a hearing aid?
- Describe any recent changes in your hearing.
- Can you locate the direction of sounds and distinguish various voices?
- Do you experience any dizziness or vertigo? Do you experience any ringing, buzzing, humming, crackling noises, or fullness in the ears?

Gustatory

- Have you experienced any changes in taste (e.g., difficulty in differentiating sweet, sour, salty, and bitter tastes)?
- Do you enjoy the taste of foods as you did previously?

Olfactory

- Have you experienced any changes in smell?
- Do things (foods, flowers, perfumes, and so on) smell the same as previously?
- Can you distinguish foods by their odors and tell when something is burning?
- Have you experienced any changes in appetite? (Changes in appetite may be related to an impaired sense of smell.)

Tactile

- Are you experiencing any pain or discomfort?
- Have you experienced any decrease in your ability to perceive heat, cold, or pain in your limbs?
- Do you have any numbness or tingling in your extremities?

Kinesthetic

- Have you noticed any difficulty in perceiving the position of parts of your body?

- Hearing acuity, by observing the client's conversation with others and by performing the whisper test and the Weber and Rinne tuning fork tests
- Olfactory sense, by identifying specific aromas
- Gustatory sense, by identifying three tastes such as lemon, salt, and sugar
- Tactile sense, by testing light touch, sharp and dull sensation, two-point discrimination, hot and cold sensation, vibration sense, position sense, and stereognosis

These tests are described in detail in Chapter 17 ∞. The nurse should also determine whether sensory adaptive devices that the client uses, such as eyeglasses or hearing aids, function properly.

Clients at Risk for Sensory Deprivation or Overload

Clients at risk for sensory-perceptual alterations need to be identified to ensure that preventive measures can be initiated. Box 26–1 describes clients at risk.

Client Environment

The nurse assesses the client's environment for quantity, quality, and type of stimuli. The client's environment may produce insufficient stimuli, placing the client at risk for sensory deprivation, or excessive stimuli, placing the client at risk for sensory overload (Figure 26–2). Nonstimulating environments include those that (a) severely restrict physical activity and (b) limit social contact with family and friends. Because appropriate or meaningful stimuli decrease the incidence of sensory deprivation, the nurse must consider the client's health care environment for the presence of the following stimuli:

- Radio or other auditory device (e.g., cassette or CD player), television
- Clock or calendar
- Reading material (or toys for children)
- Number and compatibility of roommates
- Number of visitors

In the client's home, the nurse may also note the presence of a video/DVD recorder, pets, bright colors, adequate lighting, and so on.

To assess a health care environment that produces excessive stimuli, the nurse considers, for example, bright lights, noise, therapeutic measures, and frequency of assessments and procedures.

CLINICAL ALERT

Are you aware of the noise level around you or the noise level you create while providing nursing care? The standard of 45 decibels (dB) for rest and sleep is often not met. For example, studies have shown that sounds in critical care units range from 60 to 83 dB, thereby suggesting sensory overload.

Social Support Network

The degree of isolation a person feels is significantly influenced by the quality and quantity of support from family members and friends. The nurse assesses (a) whether the client lives alone, (b) who visits and when, and (c) any signs indicating social deprivation, such as withdrawal from contact with others to avoid embarrassment or dependence on others, negative self-image, reports of lack of meaningful communication with others, and absence of opportunities to discuss fears or concerns that facilitate coping mechanisms.

DIAGNOSING

The North American Nursing Diagnosis Association (NANDA International, 2009) includes the following diagnostic labels for sensory perception alterations:

- *Disturbed Sensory Perception (Specify: Visual, Auditory, Kinesthetic, Gustatory, Tactile, Olfactory):* Change in the amount or patterning of incoming stimuli accompanied by a diminished, exaggerated,

---

BOX 26–1   Clients at Risk for Sensory Deprivation and Overload

Sensory Deprivation: Clients who
- are confined in a nonstimulating or monotonous environment in the home or health care agency
- have impaired vision or hearing
- have mobility restrictions such as quadriplegia or paraplegia with bed rest, traction apparatus
- are unable to process stimuli (e.g., clients who have brain damage or who are taking medications that affect the central nervous system)
- have emotional disorders (e.g., depression) and withdraw within themselves
- have limited social contact with family and friends (e.g., clients from a different culture)

Sensory Overload: Clients who
- have pain or discomfort
- are acutely ill and have been admitted to an acute care facility
- are being closely monitored in an intensive care unit (ICU) (Figure 26–2) and have intrusive tubes such as IVs, catheters, or nasogastric or endotracheal tubes
- have decreased cognitive ability (e.g., head injury)

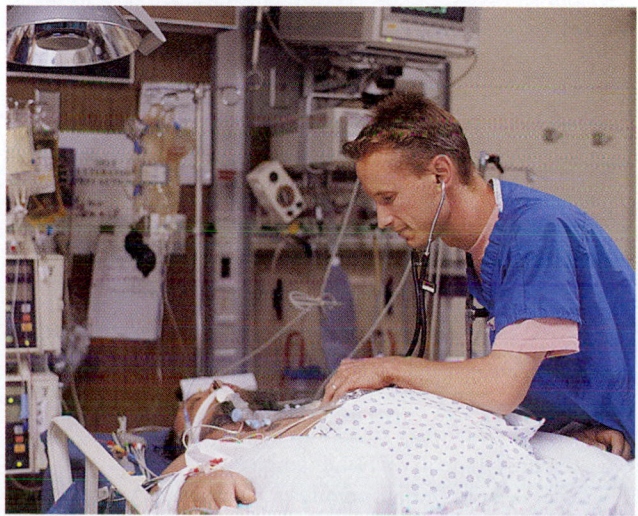

Figure 26–2 ◉ A client in an ICU may experience sensory overload.

distorted, or impaired response to such stimuli (NANDA International, 2009). This diagnostic label is used to describe clients whose perception has been altered by physiologic factors such as pain, sleep deprivation, immobility, and excessive or decreased meaningful environmental stimuli (Carpenito-Moyet, 2009).

Other diagnostic labels that can relate to sensory perception alterations include

- *Acute Confusion:* Abrupt onset of a cluster of global, transient changes and disturbances in attention, cognition, psychomotor activity level of consciousness, and/or sleep/wake cycle (NANDA International, 2009).
- *Chronic Confusion:* Irreversible, long-standing, and/or progressive deterioration of intellect and personality characterized by decreased ability to interpret environmental stimuli; and decreased capacity for intellectual thought processes; and manifested by disturbances of memory, orientation, and behavior (NANDA International, 2005, p. 39).
- *Impaired Memory:* Inability to remember or recall bits of information or behavior skills. Impaired memory may be attributed to pathophysiological or situational causes that are either temporary or permanent (NANDA International, 2009).

CLINICAL ALERT

It is easy to confuse the two nursing diagnoses *Disturbed Sensory Perception* and *Disturbed Thought Processes*. You may find it helpful to remember that the diagnosis *Disturbed Sensory Perception* refers to sensory input—the person's ability to accurately interpret stimuli. In contrast, when a person's cognitive abilities (because of mental disorders, i.e., dementia) interfere with the ability to interpret stimuli accurately, the diagnosis is more likely *Disturbed Thought Processes*. Double-check your assessment data to see if the primary problem is one of sensory input or cognitive ability.

Sensory-Perception Problem as the Etiology

Depending on the data obtained, alterations in sensory-perception function may affect other areas of human functioning and indicate other diagnoses. In these instances the sensory-perception problem becomes the etiology.

Examples of nursing diagnoses for which sensory-perception disturbances are the etiology include the following:

- *Risk for Injury* related to sensory-perception disturbance (specify). For example,
  a. Visual impairment (e.g., decreased depth perception)
  b. Reduced tactile sensation secondary to neurologic or circulatory alterations

c. Decreased sense of smell
d. Hearing impairment
e. Decreased kinesthetic sense

- *Impaired Home Maintenance* related to sensory-perception disturbance (declining visual abilities)
- *Risk for Impaired Skin Integrity* related to sensory-perception disturbance (altered tactile sensation)
- *Impaired Verbal Communication* related to sensory-perception disturbance (specify). For example,
  a. Altered level of consciousness
  b. Hearing impairment
  c. Sensory overload
  d. Sensory deprivation
- *Self Care Deficit: Bathing/Hygiene* related to sensory-perception disturbance (specify). For example,
  a. Visual impairment
  b. Diminished kinesthetic sense
  c. Inability to perceive body part or spatial relationship
- *Social Isolation* related to sensory-perception disturbance (specify). For example,
  a. Impaired vision
  b. Impaired hearing

PLANNING

Planning includes goals associated with the care of clients independent of setting and those specific to the home environment.

Planning Independent of Setting

The overall outcome criteria for clients with sensory-perception alterations are to:

- Prevent injury.
- Maintain the function of existing senses.
- Develop an effective communication mechanism.
- Prevent sensory overload or deprivation.
- Reduce social isolation.
- Perform activities of daily living independently and safely.

The NIC developed by the Iowa Intervention Project can be a guide when planning care (Bulechek, Butcher, & Dochterman, 2008). Appropriate nursing activities may be selected from the following nursing interventions:

- Cognitive Stimulation
- Communication Enhancement: Hearing Deficit
- Communication Enhancement: Visual Deficit
- Nutrition Management
- Environmental Management
- Fall Prevention
- Body Mechanics Promotion
- Peripheral Sensation Management
- Emotional Support
- Surveillance: Safety

Planning for Home Care

To provide for continuity of care, the nurse must consider the client's needs for assistance with care in the home or residential treatment setting. Some clients with severe alterations in sensory-perception functioning may be discharged to an assisted living facility that provides the specific support the client requires. Discharge planning incorporates a reassessment of the client's abilities for self-care, the availability and skills of support people, financial resources, and the need for referrals and home health services. A major aspect of discharge planning involves the instructional needs of the client and family. The next section provides strategies to support visual and auditory function and maintain a safe environment for clients.

IMPLEMENTING

Nurses can assist clients with sensory alterations by promoting healthy sensory function, by adjusting environmental stimuli, and by helping clients to manage acute sensory deficits.

Promoting Healthy Sensory Function

Detecting sensory problems early is one step toward preventing serious problems. The arousal mechanism for sensation is normally present at birth; however, it is undifferentiated. The special senses are also present at birth, although some changes in function occur during the growth process.

Early screening to detect problems in the visual and hearing functions is essential. All infants should be screened for hearing loss by 1 month of age, preferably before hospital discharge. Infants identified with a hearing loss should get follow-up evaluation before 3 months; those who are deaf or hard of hearing should be enrolled in an intervention program by 6 months of age (Centers for Disease Control and Prevention, 2004). In addition, children with chronic ear infections and people who live or work in an environment where there is a high noise level should receive routine auditory testing. Women who are considering pregnancy should be advised of the importance of testing for syphilis and rubella, which can cause hearing impairments in newborns. Periodic vision screening of all newborns and children is recommended to detect congenital blindness, strabismus, and refractive errors. A child's visual acuity develops during early childhood. Children often have 20/20 vision by 6 years of age (Ball & Bindler, 2010).

Healthy sensory function can be promoted with environmental stimuli that provide appropriate sensory input. This input should vary and be neither excessive nor too limited. As many senses as possible should be stimulated. Various colors, sounds, textures, smells, and body positions can provide various sensations. Nurses can teach parents to stimulate infants and children, and teach family members to stimulate an older adult and others in the home with sensory deficits. Social activities often help stimulate the mind and the senses.

CLIENT TEACHING — Preventing Sensory Disturbances

- Have regular health examinations.
- Have regular eye examinations as recommended by the primary care provider to screen for eye problems. For clients ages 40 and over, a medical eye examination is generally recommended every 3 to 5 years, or every 1 to 2 years if there is a family history of glaucoma.
- Seek early medical attention (a) if signs suggesting visual impairment arise, for example, failure to react to light, or reduced eye contact from an infant; (b) if the child complains of an earache or has an ear infection; and (c) for persistent eye redness, discharge or increased tearing, growths on or near the eye, pupil asymmetry or other irregularity, or any pain or discomfort.
- Obtain regular immunizations of children against diseases capable of causing hearing loss (e.g., rubella, mumps, and measles).
- Avoid giving infants and toddlers toys with long pointed handles and keep pointed instruments (e.g., scissors and screwdrivers) out of reach. Supervise preschoolers when they use scissors.
- Make sure that toddlers do not walk or run with a pointed object in hand; teach preschoolers to walk carefully when carrying such objects as sticks or toy weapons.
- Teach school-age children and adolescents the proper use of sports equipment (e.g., hockey sticks) and power tools.
- Wear protective eye goggles when using power tools, riding motorcycles, spraying chemicals, and so on.
- Wear ear protectors when working in an environment with high noise levels or brief loud impulse noises (e.g., blasting).
- Wear dark glasses with UV protection to avoid damage from ultraviolet rays and never look directly into the sun.

Nurses should also teach clients at risk of sensory loss how to prevent or reduce the loss and should teach general health measures, such as getting regular eye examinations and controlling chronic diseases such as diabetes (see the Client Teaching box).

ENSURING CLIENT SAFETY. Nurses must implement safety precautions in health care settings for clients with sensory deficits. Examples of precautions include, keeping the bed in the lowest position and placing the call light within reach.

Adjusting Environmental Stimuli

The client functions best when the environment is somewhat similar to that of the individual's ordinary daily life. Sometimes nurses need to take steps to adjust the client's environment to prevent either sensory overload or sensory deprivation.

PREVENTING SENSORY OVERLOAD. For clients who are at risk of overstimulation, nurses should reduce the number and type of environmental stimuli. The nurse can counteract

---

BOX 26–2   **Preventing Sensory Overload**

- Minimize unnecessary light, noise, and distraction. Provide dark glasses and earplugs as needed.
- Control pain as indicated at the level desired by the client, on a scale of 0 to 10.
- Introduce yourself by name, and address the client by name.
- Provide orienting cues, such as clocks, calendars, equipment, and furniture in the room.
- Provide a private room.
- Limit visitors.
- Plan care to allow for uninterrupted periods for rest or sleep.
- Schedule a routine of care so the client knows when and what to expect (post the schedule for the client wherever possible).

- Speak in a low tone of voice and in an unhurried manner.
- Provide new information gradually to enable the client to process the meaning. When providing information, ask the client to repeat it so that there are no misunderstandings.
- Describe any tests and procedures to the client beforehand.
- Reduce noxious odors. Empty a commode or bedpan immediately after use, keep wounds clean and covered, use a room deodorizer when indicated, and provide good ventilation.
- Take time to discuss the client's problems and to correct misinterpretations.
- Assist the client with stress-reducing techniques.

---

sensory overload by blocking stimuli and by helping the client organize the stimuli and alter responses to the stimuli.

Dark glasses with UV protection can partially block light rays, and a window shade or drape can reduce visual stimulation. Earplugs reduce auditory stimuli, as do soft background music and earphones. The odor from a draining wound can be minimized by keeping the dressing dry and clean and applying a liquid deodorant on a gauze near the wound.

Another method of blocking stimuli is to reduce novelty and surprise and provide rest intervals free of interruptions. Sometimes the number of visitors and the length of visits must be restricted. Also, if the nurse carries out several nursing measures together, the client can have a scheduled quiet period before the next activity.

By explaining sounds in the environment, the nurse can help the client organize them mentally: A bell signals a change of shift; a beep, an IV alarm. When clients understand their meaning, stimuli are frequently less confusing and more easily ignored. People can also learn through practice and feedback to alter their responses to the stimuli. Clients can employ relaxation techniques to reduce anxiety and stress despite continual sensory stimulation (see Chapter 30 ∞). Box 26–2 provides nursing measures for clients with sensory overload.

PREVENTING SENSORY DEPRIVATION. For clients who are at risk for sensory deprivation, nurses can increase environ-

mental stimuli in a number of ways. For example, newspapers, books, music, and television can stimulate the visual and auditory senses. Providing objects that are pleasant to touch, such as a pet to stroke, can provide tactile and interactive stimulation. Clocks that differentiate night from day by color can help orient a client to time. The olfactory sense can be stimulated by the presence of fresh flowers or plants.

Arrangements should also be made for people to visit and talk with the client regularly. Many church and community groups provide visitors to "shut-ins," that is, people who are confined to their homes or who reside in nursing homes. Box 26–3 provides measures to prevent sensory deprivation.

Managing Acute Sensory Deficits

When assisting clients who have a sensory deficit, the nurse needs to (a) encourage the use of sensory aids to support residual sensory function, (b) promote the use of other senses, (c) communicate effectively, and (d) ensure client safety.

Sensory Aids

Many sensory aids are available for clients who have visual and hearing deficits. Sensory aids can be used in the health care setting as well as in the home. In all situations, the assistance of support people needs to be enlisted whenever possible to help the client deal with the deficit.

BOX 26–3   **Preventing Sensory Deprivation**

- Encourage the client to use eyeglasses and hearing aids.
- Address the client by name and touch the client while speaking if this is not culturally offensive.
- Communicate frequently with the client and maintain meaningful interactions (e.g., discuss current events).
- Provide a telephone, radio and/or TV, clock, and calendar.
- Provide murals, pictures, sculptures, and wall hangings. Many libraries and museums will lend artwork free of charge, or a local school may provide art projects developed by their students.
- Have family and friends bring freshly cut flowers and plants.
- Consider having a resident pet such as fish, a cat, or a bird or make arrangements for pets to visit on a regular basis.

- Include different textured objects to feel such as a sheepskin pillow, silk scarf, soft blanket, or other inanimate object.
- Increase tactile stimulation through physical care measures such as back massages, hair care, and foot soaks.
- Encourage social interaction through activity groups or visits by family and friends.
- Encourage the use of crossword puzzles or games to stimulate mental function.
- Encourage environment changes such as a walk through a mall, or for an immobilized client, sitting near a window or at a place on the nursing unit where the client can watch local traffic.
- Encourage the use of self-stimulation techniques such as singing, humming, whistling, or reciting.

Promoting the Use of Other Senses

When one sense is lost, the nurse can teach the client to use other senses to supplement the loss. This stimulation is similar to that provided to prevent sensory deprivation, discussed earlier. However, the type of stimulation needs to be adapted in accordance with the client's specific deficit. For example, for the visually impaired client, stimulation of hearing, taste, smell, and touch can be encouraged. A radio, audiotapes of music or books, clocks that chime, music boxes, and wind chimes can be used for auditory stimulation. Diets that include a variety of flavors, temperatures, and textures can be planned to stimulate the taste buds. Taking sips of water between foods and eating foods separately can emphasize the taste sensation. Fresh flowers, scented candles (safely used), room fragrances, brewing coffee, and baking can stimulate the sense of smell. Clients can also be encouraged to remember pleasant or familiar odors such as the perfume of sweet peas. Measures such as providing a hug, massage, hair brushing, grooming, different textures in clothing and upholstery fabrics, and pets can be used to stimulate touch receptors.

Communicating Effectively

Communication with clients who have sensory deficits should convey respect, enhance the person's self-esteem, and ensure the exchange of correct information. A person with a hearing impairment has to concentrate more than other people and therefore tires more readily. Fatigue compounded by an illness can further reduce the person's ability to hear. A person with a visual impairment is unable to observe most nonverbal cues during communication and relies largely on the spoken word and tone of voice. Guidelines for communicating with people who are visually or hearing impaired are shown in Box 26–4.

Impaired Vision

For clients with visual impairments, nurses need to do the following in a health care setting:

- Orient the client to the arrangement of room furnishings and maintain an uncluttered environment.
- Keep pathways clear and do not rearrange furniture without orienting the client. Ensure that housekeeping personnel are informed about this.
- Organize self-care articles within the client's reach and orient the client to his or her location.
- Keep the call light within easy reach and place the bed in the low position.
- Assist with ambulation by standing at the client's side, walking about 1 foot ahead, and allowing the person to grasp your arm. Confirm whether the client prefers grasping your arm with the dominant or nondominant hand.

Research has established an association between vision impairment and greater disability in activities of daily living (e.g., bathing, dressing, eating) and instrumental

---

MyNursingKit | Lighthouse International

| BOX 26–4 | **Communicating with Clients Who Have a Visual or Hearing Deficit** |

Visual Deficit

- Always announce your presence when entering the client's room and identify yourself by name.
- Stay in the client's field of vision if the client has a partial vision loss.
- Speak in a warm and pleasant tone of voice. Some people tend to speak louder than necessary when talking to a blind person.
- Always explain what you are about to do before touching the person.
- Explain the sounds in the environment.
- Indicate when the conversation has ended and when you are leaving the room.

Hearing Deficit

- Before initiating conversation, convey your presence by moving to a position where you can be seen or by gently touching the person.
- Decrease background noises (e.g., television) before speaking.
- Talk at a moderate rate and in a normal tone of voice. Shouting does not make your voice more distinct and in some instances makes understanding more difficult.
- Address the person directly. Do not turn away in the middle of a remark or story. Make sure the person can see your face easily and that it is well lighted.

- Avoid talking when you have something in your mouth, such as chewing gum. Avoid covering your mouth with your hand.
- Keep your voice at about the same volume throughout each sentence, without dropping the voice at the end of each sentence.
- Always speak as clearly and accurately as possible. Articulate consonants with particular care.
- Do not "overarticulate"; mouthing or overdoing articulation is just as troublesome as mumbling. Pantomime or write ideas, or use sign language or finger spelling as appropriate.
- Use longer phrases, which tend to be easier to understand than short ones. For example, "Would you like a drink of water?" presents much less difficulty than "Would you like a drink?" Word choice is important: "Fifteen cents" and "fifty cents" may be confused, but "half a dollar" is clear.
- Pronounce every name with care. Make a reference to the name for easier understanding, for example, "Joan, the girl from the office" or "Sears, the big downtown store."
- Change to a new subject at a slower rate, making sure that the person follows the change to the new subject. A key word or two at the beginning of a new topic is a good indicator.

CULTURALLY COMPETENT CARE
Vision Impairment and Older Adults

The most common vision diseases affecting older adults are macular degeneration, glaucoma, cataract, and diabetic retinopathy.

- Age-related macular degeneration (ARMD) is the most common cause of new cases of vision impairment in people older than 65. It is the leading cause of vision impairment in adults 75 and older. The prevalence of ARMD is the same for African Americans and Caucasians up to age 75, with rates higher for Caucasians after 75.
- African Americans are 3 to 4 times more likely to have open-angle glaucoma.
- People of Asian descent and Eskimos are more likely to have closed-angle glaucoma.
- Diabetic retinopathy is more prevalent among African Americans, Hispanics, and Native Americans, than among Caucasians.

Note: From "The Prevalence and Consequences of Vision Impairment in Later Life," by A. Horowitz, 2004, *Topics in Geriatric Rehabilitation, 20*(3), pp. 185–195. Reprinted with permission.

tasks (e.g., shopping, housekeeping) (Horowitz, 2004). Studies have also shown that visual impairment increases the risk of depression among older adults living in the community (Horowitz, 2003, 2004). Explanations for this relationship vary. One explanation is that vision loss leads to increased disability which leads to depression. Another explanation states that loss of vision causes fear—a fear of losing one's autonomy and becoming dependent on another or others. Visual loss also affects how a person obtains information (e.g., reading the newspaper). In addition, reading is often a leisure activity and its loss can affect a person's quality of life. It is important for the nurse to be aware of and assess for signs of depression and intervene as appropriate if an older adult is experiencing depression as a result of a visual impairment.

Impaired Hearing

Clients with hearing impairments who are unable to hear the alarms of IV pumps and cardiac monitors need to be assessed frequently. They can be taught to use their visual sense to identify kinks in the IV tubing or a loose ECG lead, and so on. For home safety, clients with impaired hearing need to obtain devices that either amplify sounds or respond with flashing lights to sounds such as a doorbell or smoke detector, a baby crying, or a burglar alarm. The sounds of doorbells and alarm clocks may be amplified or changed to a lower frequency or buzzerlike sound. These devices can be obtained from hearing aid dealers, telephone companies, and appliance stores.

An important consequence of a decline in hearing as a person ages is difficulty understanding speech. Factors that influence this difficulty are the environment, rate of speech, and presence of an accent. Environments that are noisy and

reverberant (echoing, hollow sounds) cause difficulty for older adult listeners. Older adults with a hearing loss have difficulty understanding fast speech. Research indicates that the older adult's ability to process the fast verbal information is slower and that rapid speech allows for less time for the older adult to recognize the acoustic or auditory cues of the speech (Gordon-Salant, 2005). A person who speaks with an accent can also affect speech understanding by the older person. Non-native English speakers may vary their pronunciation of syllables and/or words, making it challenging for the older adult.

Impaired Olfactory Sense

Clients with an impaired sense of smell need to be taught about the dangers of cleaning with chemicals such as ammonia. Because a gas leak can go undetected, clients need to keep gas stoves and heaters in good working order. Strong chemicals such as ammonia used in confined spaces such as a bathroom may affect the client before they are smelled. Food poisoning is a concern with clients who have difficulty detecting spoiled meat or dairy products. These clients need to carefully inspect food for freshness (check its color and texture) and check expiration dates on food packages.

Impaired Tactile Sense

Clients with an impaired sense of touch may not be aware of hot temperatures, which can cause burns, or pressure on bony prominences, which can produce pressure ulcers. Clients with decreased sensation to temperature should have the temperature adjusted on their hot water heater and test water temperature with a thermometer before bathing. Clients with decreased sensation to pressure must change their position frequently.

The Confused Client

Confusion can occur in clients of all ages, but it is most commonly seen in older people. The terms *acute confusion* and *delirium* are used interchangeably by most health professionals, with nurses tending to favor the use of *acute confusion* and physicians using the term *delirium* (McCurren & Cronin, 2003, p. 319). Delirium occurs in 6% to 30% of the general hospital population and 7% to 52% of postsurgical clients (Edwards, 2003, p. 347). Delirium in the intensive care unit (ICU) setting is a common problem and has been described as sundown syndrome, ICU psychosis, and ICU syndrome. Unfortunately, delirium is unrecognized or misdiagnosed by both the physician and the nurse in up to two-thirds of cases (Hanley, 2004, p. 218).

There are numerous reasons for the older adult being at risk for delirium when hospitalized. They often have other chronic medical problems (e.g., dementia, chronic obstructive pulmonary disease, hypertension, stroke) that place them at risk. Many older adults take numerous medications with anticholinergics, narcotics, and sedatives often increasing the risk for delirium. Undertreating pain can also contribute to the

RESEARCH NOTES

What Is the Impact of Hearing Loss on the Quality of Life for Older Adults?

The researchers investigated the impact of hearing loss on communication, activities of daily living (ADLs), instrumental activities of daily living (IADLs) and health-related quality of life issues in a large population (i.e., 2,800) of older adults ranging from 57 to 97 years of age. Standardized audiometric testing procedures and self-reported surveys were used.

The study resulted in the following findings:

- Fifty-two percent of the participants self-reported having problems with communication.
- Severity of hearing loss was associated with reduced functioning of ADLs and IADLs. The researchers noted that hearing loss was not a direct cause of ADL functioning (e.g., toileting, ambulation) but an indication that hearing loss accompanies the general decline of aging. On the other hand, the IADLs (e.g., shopping, managing finances,

preparing meals, and talking on the telephone) are directly affected by hearing loss as communication is needed for IADL activities.

- Severity of hearing loss and self-report of communication problems were associated with reduced quality of life.

Implications

Hearing loss is often dismissed as not being important or as a part of the aging process. It is important to realize how it can affect quality of life for the older person. Identifying hearing loss, supplying adaptive equipment, and teaching coping strategies may have a positive effect on quality of life for older adults.

Note: Based on "The Impact of Hearing Loss on Quality of Life in Older Adults," by D. Dalton, K. Cruickshanks, B. Klein, R. Klein, T. Wiley, and D. Nondahl, *The Gerontologist,* 2003.

risk. Many older adults have a vision or hearing loss. All of these risks plus the unfamiliar surroundings and routine of a hospital, possible sleep deprivation, stress, and sensory overload compound the older adult's risk for developing delirium.

Confusion often presents with subtle symptoms, but an attempt should be made to differentiate between **acute confusion (delirium)** and chronic confusion (*dementia*). Delirium is often called acute confusion; it has an abrupt onset and a cause which, when treated, reverses the confusion. Dementia is often called chronic confusion with symptoms that are gradual and irreversible (e.g., Alzheimer's disease). It is often difficult to differentiate between the two conditions, but it is important to treat causes, if possible, in order

to be able to reverse the condition. See Table 26–2. Clients who are confused often know something is wrong and want help. Box 26–5 lists nursing interventions to help promote a therapeutic environment for the client with acute confusion/delirium (see Figure 26–3).

The Unconscious Client

The number of people surviving with traumatic brain injury is increasing, and most experience some form of coma and significant deficits. Coma is a deep state of unconsciousness that lasts for a period more than 2 to 4 weeks following a traumatic brain injury (Gerber, 2005, p. 98). Previously, the

TABLE 26–2   Differentiating between Delirium and Dementia

CHARACTERISTIC	DELIRIUM	DEMENTIA
Distinguishing feature	Acute, fluctuating change in mental status.	Memory impairment.
Onset	Sudden, acute onset.	Slow, insidious.
Duration	Temporary. May last hours to days.	Chronic, gradual, irreversible.
Time of day	Worsens at night.	No change with time of day.
Sleep–wake cycles	Disturbed. Cycles often reversed.	Disturbed. Fragmented. Awakens often during the night.
Alertness	Fluctuates. May be alert and oriented during the day but become confused and disoriented at night.	Generally normal.
Thinking	Disorganized, distorted. Impaired attention. Alterations in memory.	Judgment impaired. Difficulty with abstraction and word finding.
Delusions/hallucinations	May have visual, auditory, and tactile hallucinations. Misinterpretation of real sensory experiences.	Delusions. Usually no hallucinations.
Causative and risk factors	Cerebral and cardiovascular disease, infections, reduced hearing and vision, environmental change, stress, sleep deprivation, polypharmacy, dehydration.	Alzheimer's disease. Multiple infarct dementia.

BOX 26–5   **Promoting a Therapeutic Environment for a Client with Acute Confusion/Delirium**

- Wear a readable name tag.
- Address the person by name and introduce yourself frequently: "Good morning, Mr. Richards. I am Betty Brown. I will be your nurse today."
- Identify time and place as indicated: "Today is December 5, and it is 8:00 in the morning."
- Ask the client, "Where are you?" and orient the client to place (e.g., nursing home) if indicated.
- Place a calendar and clock in the client's room. Mark holidays with ribbons, pins, or other means.
- Speak clearly and calmly to the client, allowing time for your words to be processed and for the client to give a response.
- Encourage family to visit frequently except if this activity causes the client to become hyperactive.

- Provide clear, concise explanations of each treatment procedure or task.
- Eliminate unnecessary noise.
- Reinforce reality by interpreting unfamiliar sounds, sights, and smells; correct any misconceptions of events or situations.
- Schedule activities (e.g., meals, bath, activity and rest periods, treatments) at the same time each day to provide a sense of security. If possible, assign the same caregivers.
- Provide adequate sleep.
- Keep glasses and hearing aid within reach.
- Ensure adequate pain management.
- Keep familiar items in the client's environment (e.g., photographs), and keep the environment uncluttered. A disorganized, cluttered environment increases confusion.
- Keep room well lit during waking hours.

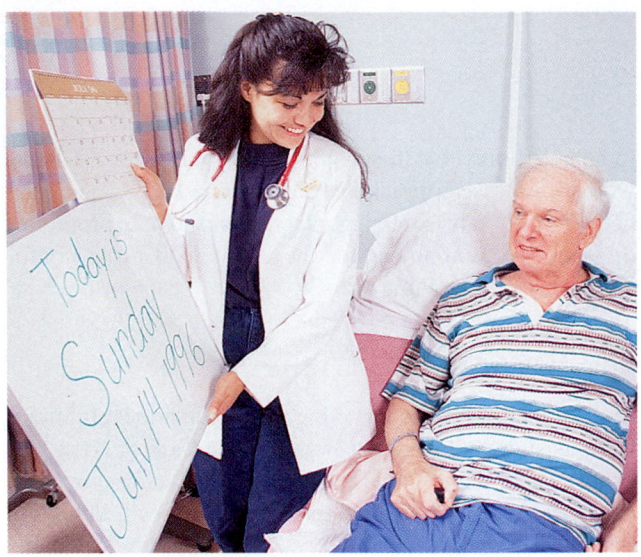

Figure 26–3 ● Promoting orientation to time and date is essential for clients who are confused or have a memory loss.

client would be medically stabilized and approximately 6 months later transferred to a rehabilitation setting for coma stimulation. It is thought that unconscious clients suffer from sensory deprivation because they are in a cold, sterile environment, immobilized, and without the usual stimulation humans need (Gerber, 2005, p. 104). As a result, the current trend is to begin a coma stimulation program earlier, while the client is in the acute care setting. Coma stimulation consists of providing sensory stimulation to promote brain recovery by waking up the reticular activating system (RAS). Box 26–6 provides examples of sensory stimulation that a nurse and/or family member may provide for the unconscious client. It is important that the stimulation be delivered in a quiet environment (to prevent sensory overload) and done slowly to allow time for a response to occur. Sensory stimulation sessions are of a certain time duration (e.g., 30 to 45 minutes), and the number of sessions will vary in a 12-hour day. It is also important to provide the client with sleep/rest periods that alternate with the structured sensory stimulation sessions.

BOX 26–6   **Promoting Sensory Stimulation for the Unconscious Client**

Auditory

- Introduce yourself to the client.
- Orient the client to time, month, year, location, and what happened.
- Inform client beforehand the care to be provided.
- Read literature aloud to the client.
- Play a tape recording of a familiar voice.
- Converse directly to the client.

Visual

- Sit client upright in a chair or bed (provides normal visual orientation).

Olfactory

- Provide aromatic stimuli that may include client's favorites (e.g., coffee, lemon, cologne or perfume).

Gustatory

- Provide mouth care using mint-flavored cleaning agent.
- Place different tastes on tongue.

Tactile

- Incorporate during bath activities (e.g., temperature and texture of washcloth, back massage, brushing hair, rubbing lotion on extremities).

Kinesthetic

- Perform range-of-motion exercises.
- Change client's position.

Note: From C. Gerber, "Understanding and Managing Coma Stimulation: Are We Doing Everything We Can?" *Critical Care Nursing Quarterly, 2005* vol. 28, issue number 2, pp. 94–108. Copyright © 2005 Lippincott, Williams & Wilkins. Reprinted with permission.

LIFESPAN CONSIDERATIONS   Sensory Perception

Children

Newborns should be screened for hearing loss prior to hospital discharge. Universal screening of all newborns is mandated in at least 30 states, and in all states screening is done for children who are at high risk (e.g., have a history of infection during gestation, or are born with anomalies of the head or face). If a hearing loss is detected early, treatment can begin early and complications such as speech loss can be prevented. If an infant is found to have a hearing loss, it is recommended that treatment begin before 6 months of age (Joint Committee on Infant Hearing, 2000).

Older Adults

Normal changes of aging often result in varying degrees of impairments in sensory perception of the senses—hearing, vision,

smell, taste, and touch. Diseases and conditions that are more common in older adults and which also alter sensory perception are diabetes, strokes, and other neurologic disorders such as Parkinson's disease. Nursing interventions need to be very specific and individualized and may be directed to either increase or decrease sensory stimuli.

The goals of nursing care should be focused on maintaining safety and communication with clients who have these impairments. Clients with dementia may have problems that fit more appropriately under "altered thought processes," but the goals should be similar—to maximize their potential, maintain their quality of life and dignity, and at the same time, be aware of safety and communication issues.

EVALUATING

Using the measurable desired outcomes developed during the planning stage as a guide, the nurse collects data needed to judge whether client goals and outcomes have been achieved. Examples of client outcomes and related indica-

tors are shown in the earlier Identifying Nursing Diagnoses, Outcomes, and Interventions and in the Nursing Care Plan. If outcomes are not achieved, the nurse and client, and support people if appropriate, need to explore the reasons before modifying the care plan.

Nursing Care Plan   Sensory-Perception Disturbance

ASSESSMENT DATA	NURSING DIAGNOSIS	DESIRED OUTCOMES*
Nursing Assessment Julia Hagstrom is an 80-year-old widow who has recently become a resident of an extended care facility. Just prior to her admission she underwent surgery for the removal of cataracts and also experienced more difficulty with hearing. Her children were concerned about her physical safety and lack of socialization and urged her to enter a nursing home. Mrs. Hagstrom had cared for herself independently for 15 years in her own home. Three days after admission the nurse finds the client somewhat confused and disoriented to place and time. She appears restless and withdrawn. She states, "I'm afraid of all of these strange creatures in this orphanage."	*Disturbed Sensory Perception (Sensory Overload)* related to change in environment, and hearing loss (as evidenced by disorientation to time and place; restlessness; and altered behavior)	**Cognitive Orientation** [0901] as evidenced by not compromised: • Identifies significant other(s) • Identifies current place • Identifies correct season **Hearing Compensation Behavior** [1610] as evidenced by often demonstrated: • Positions self to advantage hearing • Reminds others to use techniques that advantage hearing • Eliminates background noise • Uses hearing supportive devices

Physical Examination

Height: 160 cm (5'3")
Weight: 55.3 kg (122 lb)
Temperature: 37°C (98.6°F)
Pulse: 72 BPM
Respirations: 18/minute
Blood Pressure: 128/74 mm Hg
Rinne test: negative

Diagnostic Data

Chest x-ray, CBC, and urinalysis all negative

(continued)

Nursing Care Plan   Sensory-Perception Disturbance *(continued)*

NURSING INTERVENTIONS*/SELECTED ACTIVITIES	RATIONALE
Reality Orientation [4820]	
Provide a consistent physical environment and a daily routine.	*Routine eliminates the element of surprise, overstimulation, and further confusion.*
Provide access to familiar objects, when possible.	*Familiarity helps reduce confusion.*
Provide a low-stimulation environment for Mrs. Hagstrom because disorientation may be increased by overstimulation.	*A disruption in the quality or quantity of incoming stimuli can affect a person's cognitive status. Sensory overload blocks out meaningful stimuli.*
Provide for adequate rest, sleep, and daytime naps.	*Reduces overstimulation and fatigue, which may be contributing factors to confusion.*
Use a calm and unhurried approach when interacting with Mrs. Hagstrom.	*Promotes communication that enhances the person's sense of dignity.*
Speak to the client in a slow, distinct manner with appropriate volume.	*The client who has difficulty hearing will be better able to lip read and comprehend speech.*
Engage Mrs. Hagstrom in concrete "here and now" activities (that is, ADLs) that focus on something outside the self that is concrete and reality oriented.	*Assists the individual to differentiate between own thoughts and reality.*
Communication Enhancement: Hearing Deficit [4974]	
• Facilitate use of hearing aids, as appropriate.	*Hearing can be enhanced if the volume is appropriate and the hearing aid is consistently used.*
• Listen attentively.	*Effective listening is essential in a nurse–client relationship. Poor listening skills can undermine trust and block therapeutic communication.*
• Use simple words and short sentences, as appropriate.	*Using simple terms and short sentences facilitates understanding and minimizes anxiety.*
• Obtain Mrs. Hagstrom's attention through touch.	*Gaining the attention of a client with a hearing impairment is an essential first step toward effective communication. However, the client's personal space should be respected and permission to touch should be obtained.*
Evaluation	

Outcomes met. Mrs. Hagstrom identifies her primary nurse by sight and name on the third day. She is aware that Christmas is 3 weeks away and is anxious to go shopping with the group. Her daughter has brought new batteries for her hearing aid, which she wears during the day.

The NOC # for desired outcomes and the NIC # for nursing interventions are listed in brackets following the appropriate outcome or intervention. Outcomes, interventions, and activities selected are only a sample of those suggested by NOC and NIC and should be further individualized for each client.

CONCEPT MAP   Sensory-Perception Disturbance

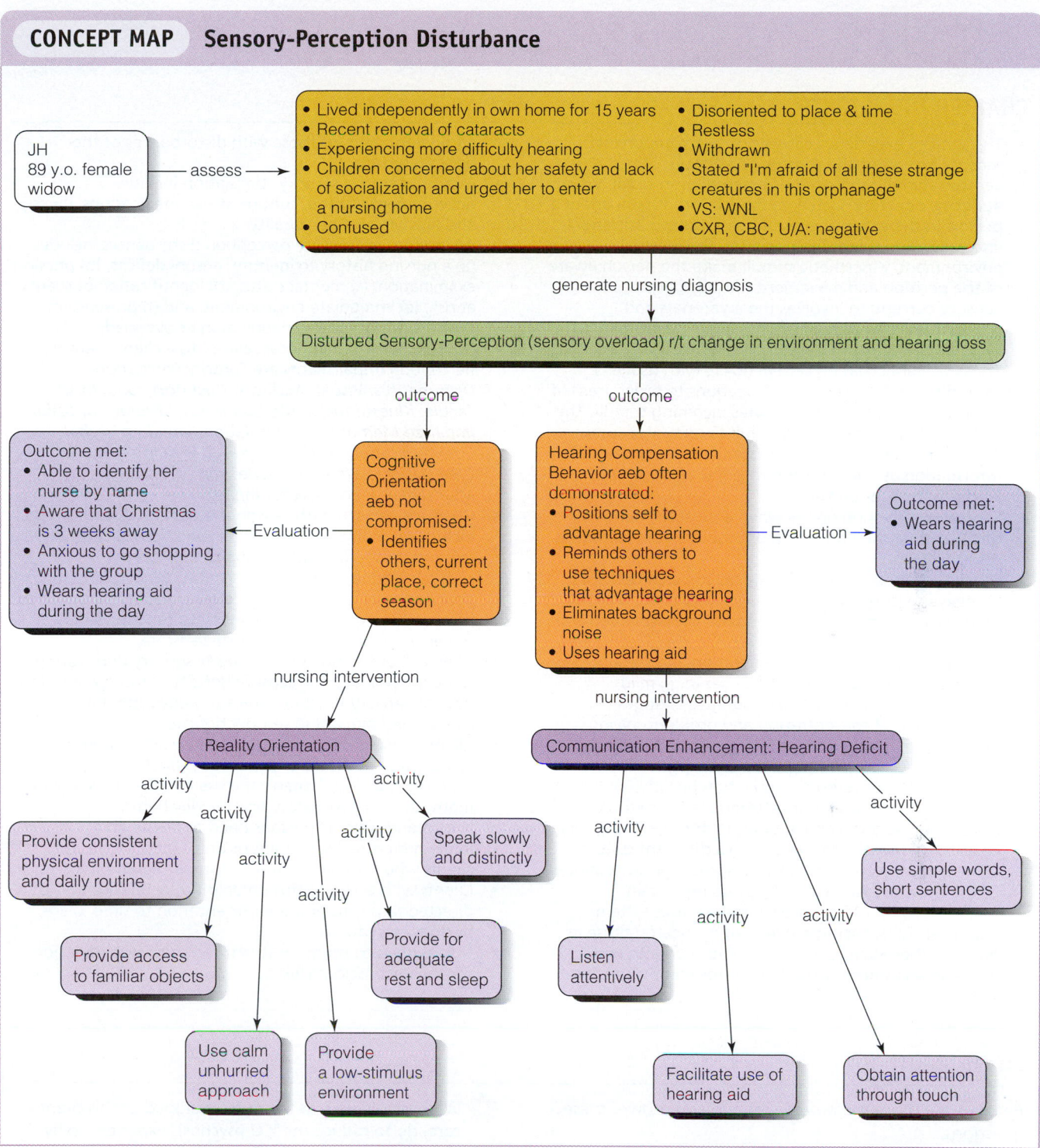

CHAPTER HIGHLIGHTS

- The sensory experience consists of two components: sensory reception and sensory perception.
- Sensory stimuli can be either external or internal. Visual, auditory, olfactory, tactile, and gustatory stimuli orient a person to the external environment. Kinesthetic and visceral stimuli orient the person to the internal environment. Kinesthetic stimuli make the person aware of the position and movement of body parts.
- Sensory perception involves the awareness and interpretation of stimuli into meaningful information. This process occurs in the cerebral cortex.
- The reticular activating system (RAS), with its many ascending and descending connections to other areas of the brain, monitors and regulates incoming stimuli. The RAS maintains, enhances, or inhibits cortical arousal.
- The normal, alert person can assimilate many kinds of information at one time and respond appropriately through thought and action.
- Sensory deprivation occurs when a person receives decreased sensory input or monotonous or meaningless sensory input.
- Sensory overload occurs when a person experiences excessive sensory input and is unable to process or manage the stimuli. The person feels overwhelmed and not in control.
- Responses to both sensory deprivation and sensory overload include perceptual changes (e.g., mild distortions or hallucinations), cognitive changes (e.g., decreased concentration and problem-solving ability), and affective changes (e.g., apathy, anxiety, anger, depression, and rapid mood swings).
- Clients at risk for sensory deprivation include (a) those who are homebound or institutionalized, (b) those on bed rest or isolation precautions, (c) those with sensory deficits, (d) those who come from a different culture, (e) those with certain affective disorders or disturbances of the nervous system, and (f) those on certain medications that affect the central nervous system.
- Clients at risk for sensory overload include (a) those in pain, (b) those in intensive care units, (c) those with intrusive and uncomfortable monitoring or treatment equipment, and (d) those with disturbances of the nervous system.
- Factors affecting sensory stimulation include developmental stage, culture, stress, medications, illness, and lifestyle and personality.
- Assessment for sensory-perception disturbances includes (a) a nursing history to identify sensory deficits, (b) physical examination, (c) mental status, (d) identification of clients at risk, (e) immediate environment, and (f) presence of clinical signs of sensory deprivation or overload.
- NANDA nursing diagnoses related to a client's sensory-perception impairments are *Sensory Perception Disturbances: Visual, Auditory, Gustatory, Olfactory, Tactile, Kinesthetic; Acute Confusion; Chronic Confusion; Impaired Memory; Social Isolation; Impaired Verbal Communication; Risk for Impaired Skin Integrity; Self-Care Deficit: Bathing/Hygiene; Impaired Home Maintenance;* and *Risk for Injury.*
- Goals for persons with sensory-perception disturbances include (a) maintaining or promoting the function of existing senses, (b) maintaining or improving communication, (c) preventing injury, (d) avoiding sensory deprivation or overload, (e) reducing social isolation, and (f) maintaining or restoring ability to function safely in the environment and to perform self-care.
- Interventions to prevent or modify sensory deprivation, sensory overload, and sensory deficits include promoting healthy sensory function, adjusting environmental stimuli, and managing sensory deficits.
- Clients with sensory deficits need instruction about sensory aids available to support residual sensory function, ways to promote the use of other senses, and methods to ensure safety from bodily harm.
- Nurses and support persons need to devise and implement effective communication mechanisms for clients who have visual and hearing impairments.
- Clients with acute confusion/delirium need care that is directed to promoting their orientation to time, place, person, and situation.
- Nurses need to promote structured sensory stimulation for the unconscious client.

THINK ABOUT IT

Refer to the chapter-opening scenario and answer these questions.

1. How would you describe Susan's perception as she begins her first clinical day in the ICU?

2. What might Susan do to help her to concentrate on delivering client care?

3. If you were the nurse manger of this unit, what changes might you make to reduce the amount of stimuli and create a calmer environment?

4. What would you, as the nurse assigned to this client's care, do to reduce the ICU psychosis experienced by the client calling for her dog?

∞ *See suggested responses to Think About It on MyNursingKit.*

TEST YOUR KNOWLEDGE

1. The nurse would identify which of the following clients as being at greatest risk for sensory overload?
1. A 40-year-old client in isolation with no family
2. A 28-year-old quadriplegic client in a private room
3. A 16-year-old listening to loud music
4. An 80-year-old client admitted for emergency surgery

2. An alert 80-year-old client is transferred to a long-term care facility. On the second night he becomes confused and agitated. What is the most appropriate nursing diagnosis?
1. *Chronic Confusion*
2. *Impaired Memory*
3. *Disturbed Sensory Perception*
4. *Disturbed Thought Processes*

3. The nursing diagnosis *Risk for Impaired Skin Integrity* related to sensory-perception disturbance would best fit a client who:
1. Cut his foot by stepping on broken glass.
2. Uses a wheelchair due to paraplegia.
3. Wears glasses because of poor vision.
4. Is legally blind and smokes in bed.

4. The nurse is performing a home visit and identifies a client in need of a sensory aid when the client makes which of the following statements?
1. "I tripped over that throw rug again."
2. "I can't hear the doorbell."
3. "My eyesight is good if I wear my glasses."
4. "I can hear the TV if I turn the volume up high enough."

5. A hospitalized client is disoriented and believes she is in a train station. Which of the following is the most appropriate response by the nurse?
1. "You wouldn't be getting a bath at the train station."
2. "Let's finish your bath before the train arrives."
3. "Don't you know where you are?"
4. "It may seem like a train station sometimes, but this is Valley Hospital."

6. A client with impaired vision is admitted to the hospital. Which nursing interventions are most appropriate to meet the client's needs? Select all that apply.
1. Identify yourself by name.
2. Decrease background noise before speaking.
3. Stay in the client's field of vision.
4. Explain the sounds in the environment.
5. Keep your voice at the same level throughout the conversation.

7. A client is exhibiting signs and symptoms of acute confusion/delirium. The nurse implements which of the following strategies to promote a therapeutic environment?
1. Keep lights in the room dimmed to reduce stimulation.
2. Keep the environmental noise level high to increase stimulation.
3. Keep the room organized and clean.
4. Use restraints for client safety.

8. The nurse identifies a client as being at risk for sensory deprivation. Which of the following clinical signs are most likely to contribute? Select all that apply.
1. Sleeplessness
2. Decreased attention span
3. Irritability
4. Excessive sleeping
5. Crying, depression

9. When assessing the client for sensory-perceptual functioning, the nurse includes which of the following components? Select all that apply.
1. Nursing history
2. Discharge planning
3. Physical examination
4. Client's environment and social network
5. Risk assessment

10. An 85-year-old client has impaired hearing. When creating the care plan, which of the following should have the highest nursing priority?
1. Obtaining an amplified telephone
2. Teaching the importance of changing his position
3. Providing reading material with large print
4. Checking expiration dates on food packages

∞ *See answers to Test Your Knowledge in Appendix A.*

REFERENCES AND SELECTED BIBLIOGRAPHY

Allen, N. H., Burns, A., Newton, V., Hickson, F., Ramsden, R., Rogers, J., et al. (2003). The effects of improving hearing in dementia. *Age and Ageing, 32*(2), 189–193.

Arditi, A. (2005). Enhancing the visual environment for older and visually impaired persons. *Alzheimer's Care Quarterly, 6*(4), 294–299.

Arnold, E. (2005). Sorting out the 3 D's: Delirium, dementia, depression: Learn how to sift through overlapping signs and symptoms so you can help improve an older patient's quality of life. *Holistic Nursing Practice, 19*(3), 99.

Bakker, R. (2003). Sensory loss, dementia, and environments. *Generations, 27*(1), 46–51.

Ball, J. W., Bindler, R. C., & Cowen, K. J. (2010). *Child health nursing.* (2nd ed.). Upper Saddle River, NJ: Pearson Education.

Ball, J., & Haight, B. K. (2005). Creating a multisensory environment for dementia: The goals of a Snoezelen® room. *Journal of Gerontological Nursing, 31*(10), 4–10.

Boyd-Monk, H. (2005). The eyes have it: Understanding problems of the aging eye. *Nursing Made Incredibly Easy, 3*(5), 34–45.

Bulechek, G. M., Butcher, H. K., & Dochterman, J. M. (Eds.). (2008). *Nursing interventions: Classification (NIC)* (5th ed.). St. Louis, MO: Mosby.

Carpenito-Moyet, L. J. (2009). *Nursing diagnosis: Application to clinical practice* (13th ed.). Philadelphia: Lippincott Williams & Wilkins.

Celik, S., Oztekin, D., Akyolcu, N., & Issever, H. (2005). Sleep disturbance: The patient care activities applied at the night shift in the intensive care unit. *Journal of Clinical Nursing, 14*(1), 102–106.

Centers for Disease Control and Prevention, Developmental Disabilities. (2004). *Hearing loss: Screening.* Retrieved June 28, 2006, from http://www.cdc.gov/ncbddd/dd/ddhi.htm

Cimarolli, V. R., & Boerner, K. (2005). Social support and well-being in adults who are visually impaired. *Journal of Visual Impairment & Blindness, 99*(9), 521–534.

Cohen, A. S., & Ayello, E. A. (2005). Diabetes has taken a toll on your patient's vision—how can you help? *Nursing, 35*(5), 44–47.

Connolly, J. L., Carron, J. D., & Roark, S. D. (2005). Universal newborn hearing screening: Are we achieving the Joint Committee on Infant Hearing (JCIH) objectives? *Laryngoscope, 115*(2), 232–236.

Crews, J. E., & Campbell, V. A. (2004). Vision impairment and hearing loss among community-dwelling older Americans: Implications for health and functioning. *American Journal of Public Health, 94*(5), 823–829.

Dalton, D. S., Cruickshanks, K. J., Klein, B. E., Klein, R., Wiley, T. L., & Nondahl, D. M. (2003). The impact of hearing loss on quality of life in older adults. *Gerontologist, 43*(5), 661–668.

Ebersole, P., & Hess, P. (2003). *Toward healthy aging: Human needs and nursing response.* New York: Elsevier.

Edwards, N. (2003). Differentiating the three D's: Delirium, dementia, and depression. *Medsurg Nursing, 12*(6), 347–357.

Eliopoulos, C. (2009). *Gerontological nursing* (7th ed.). Philadelphia: Lippincott.

Gerber, C. (2005). Understanding and managing coma stimulation: Are we doing everything we can? *Critical Care Nursing Quarterly, 28*(2), 94–108.

Gerdner, L. A., Xiong, S. V., & Cha, D. (2006). Chronic confusion and memory impairment in Hmong elders. *Journal of Gerontological Nursing, 32*(3), 23–31.

Gordon-Salant, S. (2005). Hearing loss and aging: New research findings and clinical implications. *Journal of Rehabilitation Research & Development, 42*(4), 9–24.

Halvorson, P. (2005). The silent thief. *RN, 68*(3), 41–45.

Hanley, C. (2004). Delirium in the acute care setting. *Medsurg Nursing, 13*(4), 217–225.

Hertz, J., Koren, M., Rossetti, J., Monroe, D., Berent, G., & Plonczynski, D. (2005). Collaboration to promote best practices in care of older adults. *Medsurg Nursing, 14*(5), 311–315.

Horowitz, A. (2003). Depression and vision and hearing impairment in later life. *Generations, 27*(1), 32–38.

Horowitz, A. (2004). The prevalence and consequences of vision impairment in later life. *Topics in Geriatric Rehabilitation, 20*(3), 185–195.

Joint Committee on Infant Hearing. (2000). Joint Committee on Infant Hearing year 2000 position statement: Principles and guidelines for early hearing detection and intervention programs. *Pediatrics, 106*(4), 798–817.

Marieb, E., & Hoehn, K. (2007). *Anatomy and physiology* (7th ed.). San Francisco: Pearson Benjamin Cummings.

Marshall, M. C., & Soucy, M. D. (2003). Delirium in the intensive care unit. *Critical Care Nursing Quarterly, 26*(3), 172–178.

McCurren, C., & Cronin, S. N. (2003). Delirium: Elders tell their stories and guide nursing practice. *Medsurg Nursing, 12*(5), 318–323.

Moorhead, S., Johnson, M., Maas, M. L., & Swanson, E. (Eds.). (2008). *Nursing outcomes classification (NOC)* (4th ed.). St. Louis: Mosby.

Munson, B. L. (2006). Now, listen up! Understanding hearing loss and deafness. *Nursing Made Incredibly Easy, 4*(2), 38–47.

NANDA International. (2005). *NANDA nursing diagnoses: Definitions and classification 2005–2006.* Philadelphia: Author.

NANDA International. (2009). *NANDA nursing diagnoses: Definitions and classification 2009–2011.* West Sussex, U.K.: Wiley-Blackwell.

Pankow, L., Luchins, D., Studebaker, J., & Chettleburgh, D. (2004). Evaluation of a vision rehabilitation program for older adults with visual impairment. *Topics in Geriatric Rehabilitation, 20*(3), 223–232.

Pitkala, K. H., Laurila, J. V., Strandberg, T. E., & Tilvis, R. S. (2006). Multicomponent geriatric intervention for elderly inpatients with delirium: A randomized, controlled trial. *Journal of Gerontology, 61A*(2), 176–181.

Pullen, R. L. (2006). Spin control: Caring for a patient with inner ear disease. *Nursing, 36*(5), 48–51.

Ricketts, T. A. (2005). Directional hearing aids: Then and now. *Journal of Rehabilitation Research and Development, 42*(4), 133–145.

Smith, M., & Buckwalter, K. (2005). Behaviors associated with dementia: Whether resisting care or exhibiting apathy, an older adult with dementia is attempting communication. Nurses and other caregivers must learn to "hear" this language. *American Journal of Nursing, 105*(7), 40–52.

Spires, R. (2006). How you can help when older eyes fail. *RN, 69*(2), 38–43.

Twedell, D. (2005). Delirium. *Journal of Continuing Education in Nursing, 36*(3), 102–103.

Wahl, H., & Heyl, V. (2003). Connection between vision, hearing, and cognitive function. *Generations, 27*(1), 39–47.

Wahl, H., Becker, S., Burmedi, D., & Schilling, O. (2004). The role of primary and secondary control in adaptation to age-related vision loss: A study of older adults with macular degeneration. *Pschology and Aging, 19*(1), 235–239.

Wold, G. H. (2008). *Basic geriatric nursing* (4th ed.). New York: Elsevier.

Zeng, F. (2004). Trends in cochlear implants. *Trends in Amplification, 8*(1), 1–34.

Self-Concept

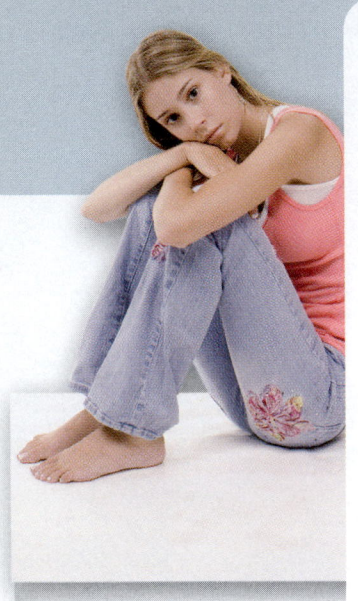

Briana, 22 years old, is admitted to the hospital in diabetic ketoacidosis and is newly diagnosed with type 1 diabetes. When asked, she says she has no family, but the truth is that her father is probably still alive somewhere. Her mother was killed by a drunk driver when Briana was only 5 years old, and she was raised by her father, who was physically abusive, especially when he was drunk. The state intervened when Briana was taken to the emergency room after her father broke her arm, and she lived in a series of foster homes until she turned 18. She moved into an apartment that she shared with another girl while she attended school and obtained a license as a beautician. She currently lives in her own apartment and works full-time at a high-priced salon. She dreams of opening her own shop but doesn't have enough money to do that.

LEARNING OUTCOMES

After completing this chapter, you will be able to:

1. Identify four dimensions of self-concept.

2. Give Erikson's explanation of the effects of psychosocial tasks on self-concept and self-esteem.

3. Describe the four components of self-concept.

4. Identify common stressors affecting self-concept and coping strategies.

5. Describe the essential aspects of assessing role relationships.

6. Identify nursing diagnoses related to altered self-concept.

7. Describe nursing interventions designed to achieve identified outcomes for clients with altered self-concept.

8. Describe ways to enhance client self-esteem.

KEY TERMS

Body image p801
Core self-concept p800
Global self p799
Global self-esteem p802

Ideal self p801
Role ambiguity p802
Role conflicts p802
Role development p802

Role mastery p802
Role performance p802
Role strain p802
Self-awareness p799

Self-concept p799
Self-esteem p802
Specific self-esteem p802

Self-concept is one's mental image of oneself. A positive self-concept is essential to a person's mental and physical health. Individuals with a positive self-concept are better able to develop and maintain interpersonal relationships and resist psychologic and physical illness. An individual possessing a strong self-concept should be better able to accept or adapt to changes that may occur over the lifespan. How one views oneself affects one's interaction with others.

Nurses have a responsibility to assess clients for a negative self-concept and to identify the possible causes in order to help them develop a more positive view of themselves. Individuals who have a poor self-concept may express feelings of worthlessness, self-dislike, or even self-hatred. They may feel sad or hopeless, and may state they lack energy to perform even the simplest of tasks.

SELF-CONCEPT

Self-concept involves all of the self-perceptions—appearance, values, and beliefs—that influence behavior and are referred to when using the words *I* or *me*. Self-concept is a complex idea that influences the following:

- How one thinks, talks, and acts
- How one sees and treats another person
- Choices one makes
- Ability to give and receive love
- Ability to take action and to change things

There are four dimensions of self-concept:

- *Self-knowledge:* the knowledge that one has about oneself, including insights into one's abilities, nature, and limitations
- *Self-expectation:* what one expects of oneself; may be a realistic or unrealistic expectation
- *Social self:* how a person is perceived by others and society
- *Social evaluation:* the appraisal of oneself in relationship to others, events, or situations

People who value "how I perceive me" above "how others perceive me" can be termed *me-centered.* They try hard to live up to their own expectations and compete only with themselves, not others. In contrast, strongly *other-centered* people have a high need for approval from others and try hard to live up to the expectations of others, comparing, competing, and evaluating themselves in relation to others. They tend not to deal with their personal shortcomings, are unable to assert themselves, and fear disapproval. The positive self-concept, therefore, is me-centered and is formed with minimal reference to others' opinions.

Assessing and promoting a positive self-concept is not limited to the nurse acting on the client. A nurse's own self-concept is also important. Nurses who understand the different dimensions of themselves are better able to understand the needs, desires, feelings, and conflicts of their clients. Nurses who feel positive about themselves are more likely to help clients meet their needs.

Self-awareness refers to the relationship between one's perception of himself or herself and others' perceptions of him or her. Thus, a nurse who is very self-aware has perceptions that are very congruent. Becoming more self-aware is a process that requires time and energy and is never complete. One important component of the process is introspection, which involves the nurse considering his or her own beliefs, attitudes, motivations, strengths, and limitations (Donnelly, 2004). In addition to using individual reflective exercises, the nurse gains insight into the self through working with other nurses who serve as mentors and by taking seriously and acting on the feedback obtained during regular performance reviews.

Once the nurse has developed a clear understanding and awareness of self, the nurse can respect and avoid projecting his or her own beliefs onto others. While in the caregiver role, the self-aware nurse is able to suspend judgment and focus on the needs of the client, even if they differ from those of the nurse. When conflicts arise, the nurse can analyze his or her reactions through introspection and by asking:

- "What is there in me that produces this kind of reaction in the client?"
- "Why do I react this way (fear, anger, anxiety, annoyance, worry)?"
- "Can I change the way I respond to this situation to affect the client's reaction in a helpful way?"

FORMATION OF SELF-CONCEPT

A person is not born with a self-concept; rather, it develops as a result of social interactions with others. Chapter 9 ∞ discusses the development of self-concept, including Erikson's stages of development, Piaget's cognitive developmental stages, and Havighurst's developmental tasks.

According to Erikson (1963), throughout life people face developmental tasks associated with eight psychosocial stages that provide a theoretical framework. The success with which a person copes with these developmental tasks largely determines the development of self-concept. Difficulty in coping results in self-concept problems at the time and, often, later in life. Table 27–1 lists examples of behaviors indicating successful and unsuccessful resolution of these developmental tasks.

There are three broad steps in the development of one's self-concept:

- The infant learns that the physical self is separate and different from the environment.
- The child internalizes others' attitudes toward self.
- The child and adult internalize the standards of society.

The term **global self** refers to the collective beliefs and images one holds about oneself. It is the most complete description that individuals can give of themselves at any one time. It is also a person's frame of reference for experiencing

TABLE 27–1 **Examples of Behaviors Associated with Erikson's Stages of Psychosocial Development**

STAGE: DEVELOPMENTAL TASK	BEHAVIORS INDICATING POSITIVE RESOLUTION	BEHAVIORS INDICATING NEGATIVE RESOLUTION
Infancy: trust vs. mistrust	Requesting assistance and expecting to receive it Expressing belief of another person Sharing time, opinions, and experiences	Restricting conversation to superficialities Refusing to provide a person with personal information Being unable to accept assistance
Toddlerhood: autonomy vs. shame and doubt	Accepting the rules of a group but also expressing disagreement when it is felt Expressing one's own opinion Easily accepting deferment of a wish fulfillment	Failing to express needs Not expressing one's own opinion when opposed Overconcern about being clean
Early childhood: initiative vs. guilt	Starting projects eagerly Expressing curiosity about many things Demonstrating original thought	Imitating others rather than developing independent ideas Apologizing and being very embarrassed over small mistakes Verbalizing fear about starting a new project
Early school years: industry vs. inferiority	Completing a task once it has been started Working well with others Using time effectively	Not completing tasks started Not assisting with the work of others Not organizing work
Adolescence: identity vs. role confusion	Asserting independence Planning realistically for future roles Establishing close interpersonal relationships	Failing to assume responsibility for directing one's own behavior Accepting the values of others without question Failing to set goals in life
Early adulthood: intimacy vs. isolation	Establishing a close, intimate relationship with another person Making a commitment to that relationship, even in times of stress and sacrifice Accepting sexual behavior as desirable	Remaining alone Avoiding close interpersonal relationships
Middle-aged adults: generativity vs. stagnation	Being willing to share with another person Guiding others Establishing a priority of needs, recognizing both self and others	Talking about oneself instead of listening to others Showing concern for oneself in spite of the needs of others Being unable to accept interdependence
Older adults: integrity vs. despair	Using past experience to assist others Maintaining productivity in some areas Accepting limitations	Crying and being apathetic Not accepting changes Demanding unnecessary assistance and attention from others

and viewing the world. Some of these beliefs and images represent statements of fact, for example, "I am a woman"; "I am a father"; "I am short." Others refer to less tangible aspects of self, for instance, "I am competent"; "I am shy."

Each separate image and belief one holds about oneself has a bearing on self-concept. However, self-concept is not simply a sum of its parts. The various images and beliefs people hold about themselves are not given equal weight and prominence. Each person's self-concept is like a piece of art. At the center of the art are the beliefs and images that are most vital to the person's identity. They constitute **core self-concept**. For example: "I am very smart/of average intelligence"; "I am male/female." Images and beliefs that are less important to the person are on the periphery. For example: "I am left-/right-handed"; "I am athletic/unathletic."

People are thought to base their self-concept on how they perceive and evaluate themselves in these areas:

- Vocational performance
- Intellectual functioning
- Personal appearance and physical attractiveness
- Sexual attractiveness and performance
- Being liked by others
- Ability to cope with and resolve problems
- Independence
- Particular talents

Self-concept in these areas also extends to the choices people make and perceptions they have about their health. Persons with strong positive self-concept about appearance are likely to value healthy behaviors and take action to maintain the health of their skin, hair, and body tone, for example. Persons with negative self-concepts may be less proactive about health promotion and illness prevention activities.

Maintaining and evaluating one's self-concept is an on-going process. Events or situations may change the level of self-concept over time. Having a basic self-concept includes how we see ourselves and how we are seen by others. There is also the **ideal self**, which is how we should be or would prefer to be. The ideal self is the individual's perception of how one should behave based on certain personal standards, aspirations, goals, and values. Sometimes this ideal self is realistic; sometimes it is not. When perceived self is close to ideal self, people do not wish to be much different from what they believe they already are. A discrepancy between ideal self and perceived self can be an incentive to self-improvement. However, when the discrepancy is great, low self-esteem can result.

Nurses, like other adults, view themselves based on both internal and external inputs acquired over many years. The ability to appraise one's own strengths, the desire to fol-low in the steps of role models, and the feedback received from colleagues and clients are some of the influences on the nurse's self-concept.

COMPONENTS OF SELF-CONCEPT

There are four components of self-concept: personal iden-tity, body image, role performance, and self-esteem.

Personal Identity

Personal identity is the conscious sense of individuality and uniqueness that is continually evolving throughout life. Peo-ple often view their identity in terms of name, sex, age, race, ethnic origin or culture, occupation or roles, talents, and other situational characteristics (e.g., marital status and education).

Personal identity also includes beliefs and values, per-sonality, and character. For instance, is the person outgoing, friendly, reserved, generous, selfish? Personal identity thus encompasses both the tangible and factual, such as name and sex, and the intangible, such as values and beliefs. Iden-tity is what distinguishes self from others.

A person with a strong sense of identity has integrated body image, role performance, and self-esteem into a complete self-concept. This sense of identity provides a person with a feeling of continuity and a unity of personality. Furthermore, the individual sees himself or herself as a unique person.

Body Image

The image of physical self, or **body image**, is how a person perceives the size, appearance, and functioning of the body and its parts. Body image has both cognitive and affective aspects. The cognitive is the knowledge of the material body; the affective includes the sensations of the body, such as pain, pleasure, fatigue, and physical movement. Body im-age is the sum of these attitudes, conscious and unconscious, that a person has toward his or her body.

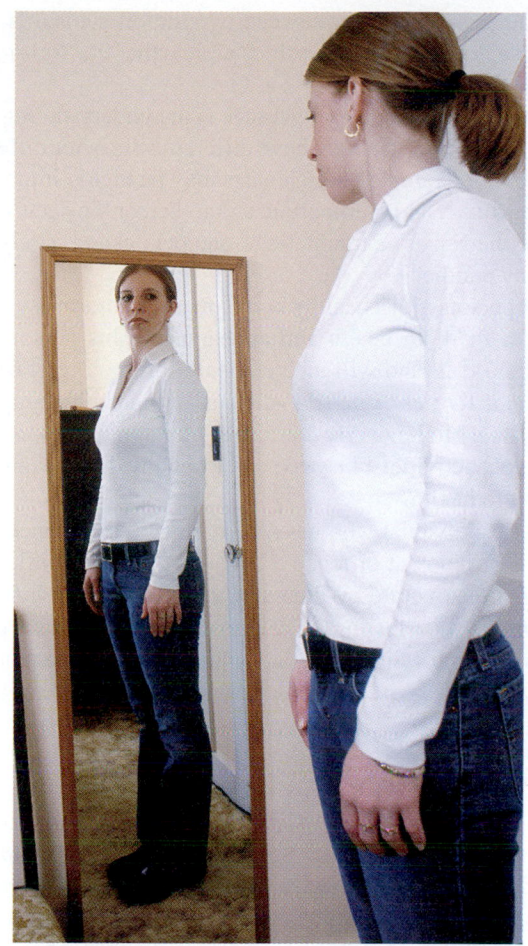

Figure 27–1 ◉ Body image is the sum of a person's conscious and unconscious attitudes about his or her body.

Body image includes clothing, makeup, hairstyle, jew-elry, and other things intimately connected to the person (Figure 27–1). It also includes body prostheses, such as ar-tificial limbs, dentures, and hairpieces, as well as devices re-quired for functioning, such as wheelchairs, canes, and eyeglasses. Past as well as present perceptions and how the body has evolved over time are part of one's body image.

A person's body image develops partly from others' at-titudes and responses to that person's body and partly from the individual's own exploration of the body. For example, body image develops in infancy as the parents or caregivers respond to the child with smiles, holding, and touching, and as the child explores its own body sensations during breast-feeding, thumb sucking, and bathing. Cultural and societal values also influence a person's body image.

The various information and entertainment media have played a part over the years in how individuals view them-selves and others. During adolescence, concerns related to body image are of paramount concern. The "ideal" person portrayed by the media is really an unrealistic goal for many.

If a person's body image closely resembles one's body ideal, the individual is more likely to think positively about the physical and nonphysical components of the self. The body ideal is greatly influenced by cultural standards. For example, currently in North America the fit, well-toned body is admired.

Another aspect of body image is the understanding that different parts of the body have different values for different people. For example, large breasts may be highly important to one woman and unimportant to another, or the occurrence of gray hair may be traumatic to one person and barely noticed by another.

A person with a healthy body image will normally show concern for both health and appearance. This person will seek help if ill and will include health-promoting practices in daily activities. A person who has an unhealthy body image is likely to be overly concerned about minor illness and to neglect activities like sleep and a healthy diet that are important to health.

The individual who has a body image disturbance may hide or not look at or touch a body part that is significantly changed in structure by illness or trauma. Some individuals may also express feelings of helplessness, hopelessness, powerlessness, and vulnerability, and may exhibit self-destructive behavior such as over- or undereating or suicide attempts.

Role Performance

Throughout life people undergo numerous role changes. A role is a set of expectations about how the person occupying one position behaves. **Role performance** relates what a person in a particular role does to the behaviors expected of that role. **Role mastery** means that the person's behaviors meet social expectations. Expectations, or standards of behavior of a role, are set by society, a cultural group, or a smaller group to which a person belongs. Each person usually has several roles, such as husband, parent, brother, son, employee, friend, nurse, and church member. Some roles are assumed for only limited periods, such as client, student, and ill person. **Role development** involves socialization into a particular role. For example, nursing students are socialized into nursing through exposure to their instructors, clinical experience, classes, laboratory simulations, and seminars.

To act appropriately, people need to know who they are in relation to others and what society expects for the positions they hold. **Role ambiguity** occurs when expectations are unclear, and people do not know what to do or how to do it and are unable to predict the reactions of others to their behavior. Failure to master a role creates frustration and feelings of inadequacy, often with consequent lowered self-esteem.

Self-concept is also affected by role strain and role conflicts. People undergoing **role strain** are frustrated because they feel or are made to feel inadequate or unsuited to a role. Role strain is often associated with sex role stereotypes. For example, women in occupations traditionally held by men might be treated as having less knowledge and competence than men in the same roles.

Role conflicts arise from opposing or incompatible expectations. In an interpersonal conflict, people have different expectations about a particular role. For example, a grandparent may have different expectations than the mother about how she should care for her children. In an interrole conflict, one person's or group's role expectations differ from the expectations of another person or group. For example, a woman who has little flexibility in her full-time job schedule has a role conflict if her husband expects her to handle all childcare problems. In a person-role conflict, role expectations violate the beliefs or values of the role occupant. For example, a nurse in a family planning clinic may be expected to advise couples about birth control methods that are not consistent with the nurse's belief system regarding prevention or management of unwanted pregnancy. Role conflict can lead to tension, decrease in self-esteem, and embarrassment if needs for achievement, independence, and recognition are unmet.

CLINICAL ALERT

If Maslow's level of love and belonging needs are met, the needs for self-esteem are next higher on the hierarchy. When the need for self-esteem is satisfied, the individual strives for self-actualization.

Self-Esteem

Self-esteem is one's judgment of one's own worth, that is, how that person's standards and performances compare to others and to one's ideal self. If a person's self-esteem does not match with the ideal self, then low self-concept results.

There are two types of self-esteem: global and specific. **Global self-esteem** is how much one likes oneself as a whole. **Specific self-esteem** is how much one approves of a certain part of oneself. Global self-esteem is influenced by specific self-esteem. For example, if a man values his looks, then how he looks will strongly affect his global self-esteem. By contrast, if a man places little value on his cooking skills, then how well or badly he cooks will have little influence on his global self-esteem.

Self-esteem is derived from self and others. In infancy, self-esteem is related to the caregiver's evaluations and acceptances. Later the child's self-esteem is affected by competition with others. As an adult, a person who has high self-esteem has feelings of significance, of competence, of the ability to cope with life, and of control over one's destiny.

The foundation for self-esteem is established during early life experiences, usually within the family structure. However, an adult's level of overall self-esteem may change markedly from day to day and moment to moment. Severe stress—for example, stress related to prolonged illness or unemployment—can substantially lower a person's self-esteem. In health care, persons who believe that their condition is viewed negatively by society may have lower self-esteem (Berge & Ranney, 2005). People frequently focus on their negative aspects and spend less time on their positive aspects. It is important that both strengths and weaknesses be identified.

FACTORS THAT AFFECT SELF-CONCEPT

Many factors affect a person's self-concept. Major factors are stage of development, family and culture, stressors, resources, history of success and failure, and illness.

Stage of Development

As an individual develops, the conditions that affect the self-concept change. For example, an infant requires a supportive, caring environment, while a child requires freedom to explore and learn. Older adults' self-concept is based on their experiences in progressing through life's stages.

Family and Culture

A young child's values are largely influenced by the family and culture. Later on, peers influence the child and thereby affect the sense of self. When the child is confronted by differing expectations from family, culture, and peers, the child's sense of self is often confused. For example, a child may realize that his parents expect he will not drink alcohol and that he will attend religious services each Saturday evening. At the same time, his peers drink beer and encourage him to spend Saturday evenings with them.

Stressors

Stressors can strengthen the self-concept as an individual copes successfully with problems. On the other hand, overwhelming stressors can cause maladaptive responses including substance abuse, withdrawal, and anxiety. The ability of a person to handle stressors will largely depend on personal resources.

Resources

An individual's resources are internal and external. Examples of internal resources include confidence and values, whereas external resources include support network, sufficient finances, and organizations. Generally the greater the number of resources a person has and uses, the more positive the effect on the self-concept.

History of Success and Failure

People who have a history of failures come to see themselves as failures, whereas people with a history of successes will have a more positive self-concept. Likewise, persons with a positive self-concept tend to find contentment in their level of success while a negative self-concept can lead to viewing one's life situation as negative.

Illness

Illness and trauma can also affect the self-concept. A woman who has a mastectomy may see herself as less attractive, and the loss may affect how she acts and values herself. People respond to stressors such as illness and alterations in function related to aging in a variety of ways. Acceptance, denial, withdrawal, and depression are common reactions.

It is sometimes difficult to determine the direction of the relationship between self-concept and health. Some research has shown that persons with a positive self-concept may enhance their health because they are more likely to follow the health care plan (Burkhart & Rayens, 2005). Other research shows that health conditions, including psychosocial situations such as loss and grieving, have an impact on self-concept (see Montpetit, Bisconti, & Bergeman, 2004). Thus, self-concept and health-related behavior are intertwined.

NURSING MANAGEMENT

ASSESSING

A thorough assessment includes a psychosocial assessment of the client and the family or support person because this provides clues to actual or potential problems. The nurse assessing

---

RESEARCH NOTES

Can Assertiveness Training Improve Nursing Students' Self-Esteem?

These researchers' objective was to evaluate a training program on nursing and medical students' assertiveness, self-esteem, and interpersonal communication satisfaction. They followed 69 participants who had been identified as having low assertiveness assigned to either an experimental or comparison group. Participants in the experimental group received assertiveness training once a week. Data were collected before and after training and again one month after the end of the training. The assertiveness and self-esteem of the experimental group were significantly improved in nursing and medical students after assertiveness training, although interpersonal communication satisfaction of the experimental group was not significantly improved after the training program.

Implications

This study shows that it is possible to improve both self-esteem and assertiveness through educational intervention if the initial level of assertiveness is low. It is unknown for how long the improvement might last. The details regarding the training, and the meaning of the failure to improve satisfaction with communication, need to be evaluated for influence of culture. Communication styles differ significantly among ethnic groups and it is important to determine whether the ethnicity of health care providers is similar to or different from that of the dominant society (see Chapter 4 ∞).

Note: Based on "Evaluation of an Assertiveness Training Program on Nursing and Medical Students' Assertiveness, Self Esteem, and Interpersonal Communication Satisfaction," by Y. Lin, I. Shiah, T. Lai, K. Wang, and K. Chou, 2004, *Nurse Education Today, 24*(8), pp. 656–665.

self-concept focuses on the four components: (a) personal identity, (b) body image, (c) role performance, and (d) self-esteem.

Before conducting a psychosocial assessment, the nurse must establish trust and a working relationship with the client. Guidelines for conducting a psychosocial assessment include the following:

- Create a quiet, private environment.
- Minimize interruptions if possible.
- Maintain appropriate eye contact.
- Sit at eye level with the client.
- Demonstrate an interest in the client's concerns.
- Indicate acceptance of the client by not criticizing, frowning, or demonstrating shock.
- Ask open-ended questions to encourage the client to talk rather than close-ended questions that tend to block free sharing.
- Avoid asking more personal questions than are actually needed.
- Minimize writing detailed notes during the interview because this can create client concern that confidential material is being "recorded" as well as interfere with your ability to focus on what the client is saying.
- Determine whether the family can provide additional information.
- Maintain confidentiality.
- Be aware of your own biases and discomforts that could influence the assessment.
- Consider how the client's behavior is influenced by culture.

It is also important that the nurse identify any stressors that may affect aspects of a client's self-concept. See Box 27–1 for examples of stressors that may place a client at risk for problems with self-concept.

When stressors are identified, the nurse needs to determine how the client perceives the stressor. A positive, growth-oriented perception of stressful events reinforces self-worth; a negative, hopeless, defeatist perception leads to decreased self-esteem. The nurse should also identify the

CULTURALLY COMPETENT CARE | Assessing Self-Concept

It is the nurse's responsibility to use therapeutic communication and to remain sensitive to the effect that cultural influences will have on the client's behaviors and needs. Cultural background is not only assessed directly but is also considered as a factor in the areas of self-perception, role relationships, major stressors, and coping strategies. In the area of behaviors that may suggest low self-esteem, nurses need to ask themselves the following question: Is this really a behavior that would suggest a low self-esteem or is it part of the cultural behavior(s) of the client? In addition, might the client be experiencing cultural dissonance, a situation in which there are conflicting beliefs and attitudes between the client's culture and the one in which the client is living?

BOX 27–1 Stressors Affecting Self-Concept

Identity Stressors

- Change in physical appearance (e.g., facial wrinkles)
- Declining physical, mental, or sensory abilities
- Inability to achieve goals
- Relationship concerns
- Sexuality concerns
- Unrealistic ideal self

Body Image Stressors

- Loss of body parts (e.g., amputation, mastectomy, hysterectomy)
- Loss of body functions (e.g., from stroke, spinal cord injury, neuromuscular disease, arthritis, declining mental or sensory abilities)
- Disfigurement (e.g., through pregnancy, severe burns, facial blemishes, colostomy, tracheostomy)
- Unrealistic body ideal (e.g., a muscular configuration that cannot be achieved)

Self-Esteem Stressors

- Lack of positive feedback from significant others
- Repeated failures
- Unrealistic expectations
- Abusive relationship
- Loss of financial security

Role Stressors

- Loss of parent, spouse, child, or close friend
- Change or loss of job or other significant role
- Divorce
- Illness
- Ambiguous or conflicting role expectations
- Inability to meet role expectations

CLINICAL ALERT

The degree to which a stressor is perceived to affect self-concept varies from person to person. For example, whereas some people may respond to repeated failures by trying harder, others may give up.

---

client's coping style and determine whether this style is effective by asking the client such questions as these:

- When you have a problem or face a stressful situation, how do you usually deal with it?
- Do these methods work?

Personal Identity

When assessing self-concept, the information the nurse first needs is about the client's personal identity. This involves who the client believes he or she is. See the accompanying Assessment Interview for examples of questions to ask.

Body Image

If there are indications of a body image disturbance, the nurse should assess the client carefully for possible functional or

ASSESSMENT INTERVIEW Personal Identity

* How would you describe your personal characteristics? *or,* How do you see yourself as a person?
* How do others describe you as a person?
* What do you like about yourself?
* What do you do well?
* What are your personal strengths, talents, and abilities?
* What would you change about yourself if you could?
* Does it bother you a great deal if you think someone doesn't like you?

physical problems. The disturbance may be a result of a present deformity or malfunction or an anticipated one. In addition to the stated responses about the problem, it is important to assess related behavior. See the accompanying Assessment Interview for examples of questions to ask about body image.

Role Performance

The nurse assesses the client's satisfactions and dissatisfactions associated with role responsibilities and relationships: family roles, work roles, student roles, and social roles. Family roles are especially important to people because family relationships are particularly close. Relationships can be supportive and growth producing or, at the opposite extreme, highly stressful if there is violence or abuse. Assessment of family role relationships may begin with structural aspects such as the number in the family group, ages, and residence location. To obtain data related to the client's family relationships and satisfaction or dissatisfaction with work roles and social roles, the nurse might ask some of the questions shown in the accompanying Assessment Interview. Keep in mind, however, that questions need to be tailored to the individuals and their culture, age, and situation.

Self-Esteem

A nurse can ask the following questions to determine a client's self-esteem:

* Are you satisfied with your life?
* How do you feel about yourself?

ASSESSMENT INTERVIEW Body Image

* Is there any part of your body you would like to change?
* Are you comfortable discussing your surgery?
* Do you feel different or inferior to others?
* How do you feel about your appearance?
* What changes in your body do you expect following your surgery?
* How have significant others in your life reacted to changes in your body?

ASSESSMENT INTERVIEW Role Performance

Family Relationships

* Tell me about your family.
* What is home like?
* How is your relationship with your spouse/partner/significant other (if appropriate)?
* What are your relationships like with your other relatives?
* How are important decisions made in your family?
* What are your responsibilities in the family?
* How well do you feel you accomplish what is expected of you?
* What about your role or responsibilities would you like changed?
* Are you proud of your family members?
* Do you feel your family members are proud of you?

Work Roles and Social Roles

* Do you like your work?
* How do you get along at work?
* What about your work would you like to change if you could?
* How do you spend your free time?
* Are you involved in any community groups?
* Are you most comfortable alone, with one other person, or in a group?
* Who is most important to you?
* Whom do you seek out for help?

* Are you accomplishing what you want?
* What goals in life are important to you?

It is important for the nurse to determine the client's cultural background first in order to not misinterpret specific behaviors. The following behaviors might reflect low self-esteem or may be misinterpreted due to the client's cultural background:

* Avoids eye contact.
* Stoops in posture and moves slowly.
* Is poorly groomed and has an unkempt appearance.
* Is hesitant or halting in speech.
* Is overly critical of self (e.g., "I'm no good," "I'm ugly," or "People don't like me.").
* May be overly critical of others.
* Is unable to accept positive remarks about self.
* Apologizes frequently.
* Verbalizes feelings of hopelessness, helplessness, and powerlessness, such as "I really don't care what happens," "I'll do whatever anyone wants," "Whatever is destined will happen."

DIAGNOSING

Three of the NANDA nursing diagnostic labels relating specifically to the domain of self-perception and the classes of self-concept, self-esteem, and body image include the following:

* *Disturbed Body Image*
* *Ineffective Role Performance*

- *Chronic Low Self-Esteem*
- *Situational Low Self-Esteem*

Additional nursing diagnoses that may apply to clients with problems of self-concept include the following:

- *Disturbed Personal Identity*
- *Anxiety* related to changed physical appearance (e.g., amputation, mastectomy)

- *Impaired Adjustment* to changed physical functioning or appearance
- *Ineffective Coping* with role change related to death of spouse
- *Grieving* or *Complicated Grieving* related to change in physical appearance
- *Hopelessness*
- *Powerlessness*

IDENTIFYING NURSING DIAGNOSES, OUTCOMES, AND INTERVENTIONS   Clients with Self-Concept and Role Problems

DATA CLUSTER Frank Sawyers had a permanent colostomy 7 days ago for cancer of the sigmoid colon. When the nurse was changing the colostomy appliance, Frank said, "I am really repulsed by this." He avoided looking at the stoma and put his arm over his eyes.

NURSING DIAGNOSIS/DEFINITION	SAMPLE DESIRED OUTCOMES*/DEFINITION	INDICATORS	SELECTED INTERVENTIONS*/DEFINITION	SAMPLE NIC ACTIVITIES
Disturbed Body Image/Confusion in mental picture of one's physical self	Body Image [1200]/*Perception of own appearance and body functions*	Often positive • Willingness to touch affected body part • Adjustment to changes in body function	Body Image Enhancement [522]/*Improving a patient's conscious and unconscious perceptions and attitudes toward his/her body* Self-Care Assistance [1800]/*Assisting another to perform activities of daily living*	• Assist patient to discuss changes caused by illness/surgery • Assist patient in identifying parts of his body that have positive perceptions associated with them • Facilitate contact with individuals with similar changes in body image • Encourage independence but intervene when patient is unable to perform

DATA CLUSTER Sophie Ferraro, a 73-year-old with right-sided (dominant) hemiplegia, says, "Although the Rehabilitation Center taught me so much about how to manage in my home, my poor husband has to do a lot to help me with cooking meals and cleaning the house."

Ineffective Role Performance/Patterns of behavior and self-expression that do not match the environmental context, norms, and expectations	Caregiver–Patient Relationship [2204]/*Positive interactions and connections between the caregiver and the care recipient*	Not compromised • Effective communication • Companionship • Collaborative problem solving	Role Enhancement [5370]/*Assisting a patient, significant other, and/or family to improve relationships by clarifying and supplementing specific role relationships*	• Assist patient to identify positive strategies for managing role changes • Facilitate discussion of expectations between patient and significant other in reciprocal role

DATA CLUSTER George Kawazi, a first-year college student, is studying liberal arts and the sciences. George states that even though he attends all his classes and studies every day and on weekends, his grades do not please his father, who expects straight A's. "I've always had trouble measuring up to Father's expectations. He never thought I was as good as my older brother."

Chronic Low Self-Esteem/Long-standing negative self-evaluation/feelings about self or self-capabilities	Self-Esteem [1205]/*Personal judgment of self-worth*	Often positive • Acceptance of self-limitations • Willingness to confront others • Description of success in school	Self-Esteem Enhancement [5400]/*Assisting a patient to increase his/her personal judgment of self-worth*	Determine patient's confidence in own judgment • Reinforce strengths the patient identifies • Assist in setting realistic goals • Explore previous experiences of success

*The NOC # for desired outcomes and the NIC # for nursing interventions are listed in brackets following the appropriate outcome or intervention. Outcomes, indicators, interventions, and activities selected are only a sample of those suggested by NOC and NIC and should be further individualized for each client.

- *Parental Role Conflict*
- *Readiness for Enhanced Self-Concept*
- *Disturbed Sleep Pattern*
- *Social Isolation*
- *Spiritual Distress*
- *Disturbed Thought Processes*

PLANNING

The nurse develops plans in collaboration with the client and support people when possible, according to the client's state of health, level of anxiety, resources, coping mechanisms, and sociocultural and religious affiliation. The nurse who has little experience in intervening with clients with altered self-concept may wish to consult with a more experienced nurse to develop effective plans. The nurse and client set goals to enhance the client's self-concept.

The goals established will vary according to the diagnoses and defining characteristics related to each individual. Examples of desired outcomes, interventions, and activities are shown in Identifying Nursing Diagnoses, Outcomes, and Interventions. Specific nursing orders associated with each of these activities can be selected to meet the individual needs of the client.

IMPLEMENTING

Nursing interventions to promote a positive self-concept include helping a client to identify areas of strength. In addition, for clients who have an altered self-concept, nurses should establish a therapeutic relationship and assist clients to evaluate themselves and make behavioral changes.

Identifying Areas of Strength

Healthy people often perceive their problems and weaknesses more easily than their assets and strengths. People with low self-esteem tend to focus even more on their limitations and to be aware of fewer strengths and many more problems. When a client has difficulty identifying personality strengths and assets, the nurse provides the client with a set of guidelines or a framework for identifying personality strengths (Box 27–2).

Nurses can employ the following specific strategies to reinforce strengths:

- Stress positive thinking rather than self-negation.
- Notice and verbally reinforce client strengths.
- Encourage the setting of attainable goals.
- Acknowledge goals that have been attained.
- Provide honest, positive feedback.

Enhancing Self-Esteem

Nurses assisting clients who have an altered self-concept must establish a therapeutic relationship. To do this the nurse must have self-awareness and effective communication skills. The following nursing techniques may help clients analyze the problem and enhance the self-concept:

- Encourage clients to appraise the situation and express their feelings.
- Encourage clients to ask questions.
- Provide accurate information.
- Become aware of distortions, inappropriate or unrealistic standards, and faulty labels in clients' speech.
- Explore clients' positive qualities and strengths.
- Encourage clients to express positive self-evaluation more than negative self-evaluation.
- Avoid criticism.
- Teach clients to substitute negative self-talk ("I can't walk to the store anymore") with positive self-talk ("I can walk half a block each morning"). Negative self-talk reinforces a negative self-concept.

Certain strategies vary depending on the age of the client (see Lifespan Considerations box).

BOX 27–2 **Framework for Identifying Personality Strengths**

Note past, present, and anticipated future participation in:

- Hobbies and crafts.
- Expressive arts such as writing, painting, sketching, or music appreciation.
- Sports and outdoor activities, including spectator sports.
- Education, training, and related areas (including self-education).
- Work, vocation, job, or position.

In addition, determine:

- Sense of humor and the ability to laugh at oneself and take kidding.
- Health status including healthy aspects of body function and good health maintenance practices.

- Special aptitudes such as sales or mechanical ability; a "green thumb"; ability to recognize and enjoy beauty; ability to solve problems; a liking for adventure or pioneering; having perseverance and the drive needed to get things done.
- Relationship strengths including the ability to make people feel comfortable, the capacity to enjoy being with people, being aware of people's needs and feelings, and being able to listen.
- Emotional strengths including the capacity to give and receive warmth, affection, and love; the ability to "take" anger and to feel and express a wide range of emotions; and the capacity for empathy.
- Spiritual strengths such as religious faith or love of God, membership and participation in church and related activities.

LIFESPAN CONSIDERATIONS   Enhancing Self-Esteem

Children

- Children build strong self-esteem if they develop five basic attitudes: (a) security and trust, (b) identity, (c) belonging, (d) purpose, and (e) personal competence.
  - Security and trust are developed early in life; infants should not be left "to cry it out," for example, but should learn that they can rely on their parents to meet their needs promptly and consistently. With older children, trust and security are strengthened when adults spend time with them: listening, playing, reading, or just being there. Both emotional and physical contact, such as a hug, convey warmth and caring.
  - Identity is developed when children are allowed to explore and experiment with the world around them and to express themselves as unique individuals in that world. They should be given opportunities to "practice" who they are. Preschoolers, for example, love to dress themselves and should be allowed to wear outlandish outfits (within limits of weather and safety) if they choose. Teenagers who try new hair colors and styles, some of which may "offend" their parents, are engaging in a crucial developmental step.
  - Belonging is essential for all humans, and having a sense that others in your social network care about you, want you there, and benefit by your contribution is important to healthy self-esteem. Children gain this sense of belonging by being included in activities, by being praised for their efforts and achievements, and by being valued by parents, siblings, caregivers, and other adults. Parents should make an effort to "catch their children doing well" and praise them for it (e.g., "I like the way you share with your brother"). Children should also hear that they are valued just for being themselves (e.g., "I like doing things with you. Remember when we went to the park? Wasn't that fun?").
  - Purpose and belonging are closely related. Children need opportunities to participate in the family and their community in order to discover what they can best contribute based on their strengths and skills. One mother, for example, stated "Leo (age 4) is our actor. He is wonderful with costumes and can make any of us smile when he starts his routine." Leo may never become an actor, but he knows he makes a significant contribution to his family's well-being. He brings them joy.
  - Personal competence grows as children identify and refine their skill sets. Children develop competence as they confront and solve problems, face challenges, expand their thinking, and are asked to do more than they think they can do. Adults must, however, provide children with support, guidance, appropriate assistance, and constructive feedback (including praise) in order to prevent the child from being overwhelmed. Too much frustration or uncertainty can lead to giving up, avoidance, lying, bullying, and other antisocial behaviors. If adults help children to accomplish goals that are important to them, children are more likely to develop a sense of personal competence and independence.
- Key ingredients for helping children develop high self-esteem are love, acceptance, firmness, consistency, and the establishment of expectations. Such qualities provide children with a safe, loving, supportive, and predictable world in which to live.

Adolescents

- Provide increasing levels of responsibility. Adolescents need to experience successes and failures and the consequences of their own behavior.
- Encourage discussion about issues including problems and mistakes.
- Show appreciation for effort and contributions. Emphasize the process, not just the result.
- Ask for their opinions and suggestions.
- Encourage participation in decision making in areas that affect the adolescent. Show confidence in the teen's judgments.
- Avoid comparison with or ridicule or punishment in front of others.
- Assist in the creation of realistic goals and standards.
- Adolescents often engage in volunteer activities in their schools or communities, helping them to identify their strengths and find meaning in their activities. Knowing that they have a purpose and make a difference gives children strong self-esteem.

Adults

- Explore the meaning of self-esteem and how his or her self-esteem has influenced past behaviors and actions (and can influence present and future plans and decisions).
- Assist the client in assessing the internal and external forces contributing to or retarding his or her self-esteem.
- Act in ways that demonstrate belief that the person can cope with the realities and demands of life and is worthy of experiencing joy and happiness.
- Avoid comparisons with other people.
- Discourage statements about the self that are negative.
- Encourage the use of affirmations to enhance self-esteem: statements such as "I like myself" or "I am a valuable person."
- Encourage associations with positive, supportive people.
- Make positive statements about the person's past successes (major or minor).
- Assist the person to make a list of his or her positive qualities and to review this list often.
- Suggest the person do things for others. Making a positive contribution enhances positive feelings of self-worth.

Older Adults

Older adults who become increasingly dependent can develop low self-esteem. Old age is frequently accompanied by changes such as reduced income, decline in physical health, loss of friends and family, and retirement. In addition to those actions listed above for use with adults, nurses can use the following techniques to help older adults enhance their self-esteem:

- Encourage clients to participate in planning their own care.
- Listen carefully to their concerns.
- Assist clients to identify and use their own strengths.
- Encourage them to participate in activities in which they can be successful.
- Communicate that the client is valued. Use the client's name and ask for advice.

- Encourage older adults to stay connected with their memories. Reminiscing by writing or recording an autobiography or storytelling are excellent ways to do this.
- For older adults who are in hospitals or nursing homes, make sure that they are always shown respect and dignity and are provided privacy.
- Encourage creative activities to tap their resources. Examples are music, art, storytelling, quilting, and photography.
- Work with clients to establish goals in small steps that are achievable—this, in itself, can bolster self-esteem.

EVALUATING

To determine whether client outcomes have been achieved, the nurse uses data collected during interactions with the client and significant others (see earlier Identifying Nursing Diagnoses, Outcomes, and Interventions). If outcomes are not achieved, the nurse should explore the reasons, considering questions such as the following:

- Have old situations recurred, triggering feelings or behaviors associated with low self-esteem?
- Have new stressful situations occurred with which the client feels unable to cope, resulting in continuing or recurrent low self-esteem?
- Are new or additional roles causing increased stress in adapting?
- Are significant others supporting the client adequately in attempts to improve self-esteem?

- Did the client follow through on referrals to appropriate agencies? Did the agencies provide the expected services?
- Were the client's expectations too high in relation to the time needed for successful resolution of self-esteem problems?

The nurse, client, and significant others need to understand that to change beliefs, feelings, and behaviors affecting self-esteem requires time and ongoing effort. Unlike many physical problems (e.g., wounds) where healing can be quickly observed, improving one's self-concept can be a continuing concern and is not so easily evaluated. New crises can cause clients to doubt themselves and revert to former feelings of inadequacy. People can learn from each new situation and gain new strategies for feeling satisfied with themselves.

CHAPTER HIGHLIGHTS

- A positive self-concept is essential to a person's physical and psychologic well-being.
- A person's self-perception can differ from the person's perception of how others see him or her and from the ideal self, that is, how the person would like to be.
- Interactions with significant others create the conditions that influence self-concept throughout life.
- When individuals are able to conceptualize the self, they begin a lifelong process of deciding whether and to what extent they are valuable and worthy.
- Individuals who grow up in families whose members value each other are likely to feel good about themselves.

- Factors affecting self-concept include development, family and culture, stressors, resources, history of success and failure, and illness.
- The nurse assesses four areas of self-concept: personal identity, body image, self-esteem, and role performance and relationships.
- Because a positive self-concept is basic to health, one of the nurse's major responsibilities is to assist clients whose self-concept is disturbed to develop a more positive and realistic image of themselves.
- A trusting client–nurse relationship is essential for the effective assessment of a client's self-concept, for providing help and support, and for motivating client behavior change.

THINK ABOUT IT

Refer to the chapter-opening scenario and answer these questions.

1. The nurse, beginning to teach Briana how to administer subcutaneous insulin injections, notices that Briana constantly apologizes for making even the simplest of mistakes, such as not inserting the needle directly into the center of the medication vial. Briana tells the nurse, "I'm so stupid. I'll never be able to learn this!" The nurse interprets Briana's behavior as indicating lack of success in which of Erikson's stages of development?

2. What stressors and resources does the nurse identify in Briana's life?

3. What actions might the nurse take to build Briana's self-esteem and improve her success in learning diabetes self-care activities?

∞ *See suggested responses to Think About It on MyNursingKit.*

TEST YOUR KNOWLEDGE

1. Sally is 5'7", weighs 105 lb, and believes she's fat. The nurse recognizes this perception as which of the following?
   1. Altered body image
   2. Altered personal identity
   3. Excessive self-expectation
   4. Altered core self-concept

2. The nursing student who is juggling the responsibilities of work, school, and family is most likely to experience which of the following?
   1. Role ambiguity
   2. Role strain
   3. Role conflict
   4. Role enhancement

3. The nurse is caring for a client experiencing situational low self-esteem and sets which of the following as an appropriate desired outcome?
   1. Restored self-esteem
   2. Consistently verbalizes self-acceptance
   3. Teaches adaptive skills
   4. Describes preoccupation with altered self

4. An 89-year-old client states, "I'm a lost cause. I can't even stand long enough to cook my own meals anymore." Which of the following is the most appropriate nursing response?
   1. "That must be difficult. What things are you still able to do?"
   2. "Well, that is to be expected at your age."
   3. "Do you have someone else who can cook for you?"
   4. "Are you a good cook?"

5. The nurse recognizes which of the following behaviors as indicating an adult who failed to resolve the developmental tasks of adolescence?
   1. Asserts independence
   2. Is unable to express personal desires
   3. Has difficulty working as a member of a team
   4. Goes along with the crowd in all activities

6. During an annual performance review, which statement by the nurse indicates insight into self-awareness?
   1. "I rarely make any medication errors."
   2. "I am willing to mentor new nurses."
   3. "My client satisfaction reports agree that I am friendly and helpful."
   4. "All of my clients have recovered quickly from their health problems."

7. When asked to describe herself, a client newly diagnosed with a chronic illness describes only those roles involving others (e.g., wife, mother, medical assistant) and no personal hobbies or interests. In planning her care, the nurse should include which of the following?
   1. How her treatment will affect her ability to perform those roles
   2. How to set goals for her to develop personal hobbies or interests
   3. Including the family in developing the treatment plan
   4. Need for psychologic counseling regarding role performance in addition to her medical treatment needs

8. The nurse is caring for a client who has a nursing diagnosis of *Chronic Low Self-Esteem*. Which behaviors does the nurse consider consistent with this diagnosis? Select all that apply.
   1. Confronts authority.
   2. Verbalizes own weaknesses.
   3. Is unable to perform consistent with their role in the family (e.g., mother, father).
   4. Sets unrealistic goals.
   5. Has difficulty making positive observations about self.

9. Which of the following nursing interventions are appropriate for a client with low/poor self-concept? Select all that apply.
   1. Encourage the client to compare self with others.
   2. Suggest the client not say negative things about self.
   3. Suggest the client say positive things about self.
   4. Recommend the client avoid situations of having to care for others.
   5. Communicate very low-level expectations of the client's behavior.

10. The nurse recognizes that even appropriate nursing interventions are not likely to alter which of the following?
    1. Resources
    2. Self-knowledge
    3. Core self-concept
    4. Social self

∞ *See answers to Test Your Knowledge in Appendix A.*

REFERENCES AND SELECTED BIBLIOGRAPHY

Benjamin, O., & Kamin-Shaaltiel, S. (2004). It's not because I'm fat: Perceived overweight and anger avoidance in marriage. *Health Care for Women International, 25*, 853–871.

Berge, M., & Ranney, M. (2005). Self-esteem and stigma among persons with schizophrenia: Implications for mental health. *Journal of Long Term Home Health Care, 6*, 139–144.

Boston Women's Health Book Collective. (2005). *Our bodies, our selves: A new edition for a new era.* New York: Touchstone.

Bulechek, G. M., Butcher, H. K., & Dochterman, J. M. (Eds.). (2008). *Nursing interventions: classification (NIC)* (5th ed.). St. Louis, MO: Mosby.

Burkhart, P. V., & Rayens, M. K. (2005). Self-concept and health locus of control: Factors related to children's adherence to recommended asthma regimen. *Pediatric Nursing, 31*, 404–409.

Donnelly, G. (2004). Thinking about feeling: The value of introspection. *Holistic Nursing Practice, 18*, 275.

Erikson, E. H. (1963). *Childhood and society* (2nd ed.). New York: Norton.

Gordon, A. (2004). Maintaining an older person's concept of self. *Nursing and Residential Care, 6*, 536–538.

Heidrich, S. M., & Wells, T. J. (2004). Effects of urinary incontinence, psychological well being and distress in older community dwelling women. *Journal of Gerontological Nursing, 30*(5), 47–54.

Larner, S. (2005). Common psychological challenges for patients with newly acquired disability. *Nursing Standard, 19*(28), 33–39.

Limb, M. K. (2004). An evaluation survey of self concept issues in adult clients undergoing limb reconstruction procedures. *Journal of Orthopaedic Nursing, 8*(1), 34–40.

Lin, Y., Shiah, I., Chang, Y., Lai, T., Wang, K., & Chou, K. (2004). Evaluation of an assertiveness training program on nursing and medical students' assertiveness, self esteem, and interpersonal communication satisfaction. *Nurse Education Today, 24*(8), 656–665.

Montpetit, M., Bisconti, T., & Bergeman, C. (2004). Self-concept in bereavement: Evidence for structural change. *Gerontologist, 44*, 572–573.

Moorhead, S., Johnson, M., Maas, M. L., & Swanson, E. (Eds.). (2008). *Nursing outcomes classification (NOC)* (4th ed.). St. Louis: Mosby.

NANDA International. (2009). *NANDA nursing diagnoses: Definitions and classification 2009–2011.* West Sussex, U.K.: Wiley-Blackwell.

Patterson, C. (2006). Measuring changes in self-concept: A qualitative evaluation of outcome questionnaires in people having acupuncture for their chronic health problems. *BMC Complementary and Alternative Medicine, 6*(7), 1–11.

Stewart, J. (2004). *Self-esteem.* John D. and Catherine T. MacArthur Research Network on Socioeconomic Status and Health. Retrieved December 16, 2009, from http://www.macses.ucsf.edu/ Research/Psychosocial/notebook/ selfesteem.html

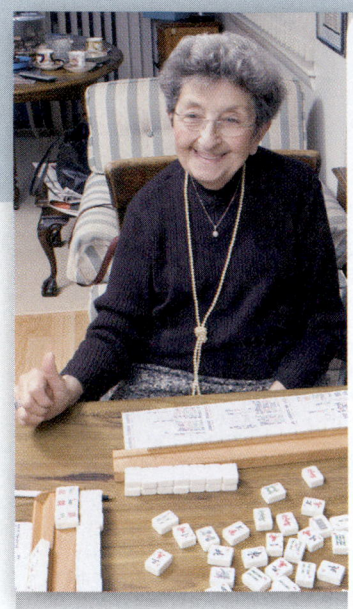

Meredith O'Leary is a 72-year-old woman living in an assisted care facility. While she has her own apartment and manages to meet most of her ADLs, she appreciates having a communal cafeteria where she goes for meals and to socialize with other residents. She describes herself as a devout Catholic and was married for 51 years to her high school sweetheart. They raised two children who are now living within a few miles of the assisted living facility and visit their mother regularly with their spouses and children. Ms. O'Leary has recently formed an intimate relationship with a man who also lives in the same facility and often has dinner with him. At her annual examination she mentions her new "beau" and says how happy having someone in her life has made her.

LEARNING OUTCOMES

After completing this chapter, you will be able to:

1. Describe sexual development and concerns across the life span.

2. Define sexual health.

3. Discuss the varieties of sexuality.

4. Give examples of how the family, culture, religion, and personal ethics influence one's sexuality.

5. Describe physiologic changes in males and females during the sexual response cycle.

6. Identify the forms of male and female sexual dysfunction.

7. Identify basic sexual questions the nurse should ask during client assessment.

8. Formulate nursing diagnoses and interventions for the client experiencing sexual problems.

9. Recognize health promotion teaching related to reproductive structures.

KEY TERMS

Androgyny p817
Cross-dressers p818
Desire phase p821
Dissatisfaction problems p824
Dyspareunia p824
Excitement phase p821
Female orgasmic disorder p824

Female sexual arousal disorder p824
Gender-role behavior p817
Genital intercourse p819
Hypoactive sexual desire disorder p823
Intersex p818

Male erectile disorder p824
Male orgasmic disorder p824
Orgasmic phase p822
Resolution phase p822
Sexual aversion disorder p824
Sexual health p816

Sexual orientation p818
Sexual self-concept p817
Transgenderism p818
Transsexuals p818
Vaginismus p824
Vestibulitis p824
Vulvodynia p824

All humans are sexual beings. Regardless of gender, age, race, socioeconomic status, religious beliefs, physical and mental health, or other demographic factors, we express our sexuality in a variety of ways throughout our lives.

Human sexuality is difficult to define. Sexuality is an individually expressed and highly personal phenomenon whose meaning evolves from life experiences. Physiologic, psychosocial, and cultural factors influence a person's sexuality and lead to the wide range of attitudes and behaviors seen in humans. There are no normal, universal sexual behaviors. Satisfying or "normal" sexual expression can generally be described as whatever behaviors give pleasure and satisfaction to those adults involved, without threat of coercion or injury to self or others. What constitutes "normal" sexual expression, however, varies among cultures and religions.

DEVELOPMENT OF SEXUALITY

The development of sexuality begins with conception and continues throughout the life span. Table 28–1 outlines characteristics of sexual development through the life span, with nursing interventions and teaching guidelines for each developmental stage.

Birth to 12 Years

The ability of the human body to experience a sexual response is present before birth. As evidenced by ultrasound, males have erections several months before birth. They continue to experience erections after birth. Since females have vaginal lubrication at birth, it is assumed that lubrication also occurs prior to birth. When babies find their fingers and toes, they also find their genitals. They seem to experience a pleasurable sensation from the touch but one would not call this a sexual experience. By the age of 3 more purposeful masturbation begins and the orgasmic response is quite common, although males do not ejaculate until after puberty. By age 2 1/2 or 3, children know what gender they are and have beginning awareness of genital differences between males and females.

Around age 9 or 10, the first physical changes of puberty begin—the development of breast buds in girls and the growth of pubic hair. As the adrenal glands mature they produce more testosterone and estradiol, which contributes to the first experiences of sexual attraction to another person. Girls need to be taught about menstruation (monthly uterine bleeding) and related self-care.

Adolescence

During early adolescence (12 to 13 years), primary and secondary sex characteristics continue to develop, necessitating more information about body changes. For boys, the testes and scrotum increase in size, the skin over the scrotum becomes darker, pubic hair grows, and axillary sweating begins. Development of the genitals to adult size takes about 5 to 6 years. For girls, the pelvis and hips broaden, the breast tissue develops (see Chapter 17 ∞), pubic hair grows, axillary sweating begins, and vaginal secretions become milky and change from an alkaline to an acid pH.

Although it is difficult to apply statistical data on large populations to local populations, it is generally accepted that sexual experimentation is currently occurring at ages younger than in previous decades. One study showed first sexual experience reported occurring within ages 10 to 16 for one-third of the sample of almost 10,000 young adults (Kaestle, Halpern, Miller, & Ford, 2005).

Teenagers may have irregular menstruation initially, which can lead to embarrassment because of stained clothing. They can be taught to be aware of subtle signs of impending menstruation, such as tender breasts, water retention or bloating, or the appearance of skin eruptions or pimples. Girls should also be counseled regarding the variety of feminine hygiene products available (e.g., sanitary pads and tampons) so that they can make intelligent choices. Parents, family members, and nurses should advise teenage girls to wash their hands thoroughly before inserting a tampon, to change tampons frequently, to alternate them with sanitary pads, and to use pads at night. These measures will help to decrease infection, including the risk of "toxic shock," a particular type of *Staphylococcus aureus* infection. Thorough cleaning of the genital area and wiping from front to back will also decrease infection and prevent odors.

Dysmenorrhea (painful menstruation) is prevalent among adolescent females. Cramping, lower abdominal pain radiating to the back and upper thighs, nausea, vomiting, diarrhea, and headaches may occur for a few hours up to 3 days. Dysmenorrhea results from powerful uterine contractions, which cause ischemia and, in turn, cramping pain. The symptoms of dysmenorrhea are treated with bed rest, administration of analgesics such as aspirin, application of heat to the abdomen, certain exercises such as abdominal muscle strengthening, biofeedback, and nonsteroidal anti-inflammatory medications, such as ibuprofen. Masturbation to orgasm also eases cramping through the associated uterine contractions and increased blood flow.

All adolescents want to know about sexual behaviors but are often uneasy about discussing these concerns with their parents. Nurses, the schools, and the family need to provide accurate information. During the nursing assessment, teenagers should be asked directly what they know about sex, contraception, and reproduction. Sometimes a lot of the teenager's information is based on popular myths and little, if any, on fact. The nurse should discuss factual information about sex, sexual actions and their consequences, the

TABLE 28–1   Sexual Development throughout Life

STAGE	CHARACTERISTICS	NURSING INTERVENTIONS AND TEACHING GUIDELINES
Infancy Birth to 18 months	Given gender assignment of male or female. Differentiates self from others gradually. External genitals are sensitive to touch. Male infants have penile erections; females, vaginal lubrication.	Self-manipulation of the genitals is normal. Caregivers need to recognize these behaviors as common in children.
Toddler 1–3 years	Continues to develop gender identity. Able to identify own gender.	Body exploration and genital fondling is normal. Use names for body parts. Children from single-parent homes should have contact with adults of both sexes.
Preschooler 4–5 years	Becomes increasingly aware of self. Explores own and playmates' body parts. Learns correct names for body parts. Learns to control feelings and behavior. Focuses love on parent of the other sex.	Answer questions about "where babies come from" honestly and simply. Parental overreaction to exploration of genitals and masturbation can lead to feelings that sex is "bad."
School Age 6–12 years	Has strong identification with parent of same gender. Tends to have friends of the same gender. Has increasing awareness of self. Increased modesty, desire for privacy. Continues self-stimulating behavior. Learns the role and concepts of own gender as part of the total self-concept. At about 8 or 9 years becomes concerned about specific sex behaviors and often approaches parents with explicit concerns about sexuality and reproduction.	Provide parents and children with opportunities to express their concerns and ask questions regarding sex. Answer all questions with factual data and perhaps follow up with appropriate books and other material. Advise parents to discuss basic information about sexual intercourse, menstruation, and reproduction with children at about 10 years of age. Give children reading material and then discuss it with them.
Adolescence 12–18 years	Primary and secondary sex characteristics develop. Menarche usually takes place. Develops relationships with interested partners. Masturbation is common. May participate in sexual activity. May experiment with homosexual relationships. Are at risk for pregnancy and sexually transmitted diseases.	Adolescents require information about body changes. Peer groups have great importance at this time and assist in forming gender roles. Dating helps adolescents prepare for adult roles. Parents influence values and beliefs regarding behavior. Teenagers require information about contraceptive measures and precautions to take in regard to STIs.
Young Adulthood 18–40 years	Sexual activity is common. Establishes own lifestyle and values. Homosexual identity usually established by mid-20s. Many couples share financial obligations and household tasks.	Young adults often require information about measures to prevent unwanted pregnancies (i.e., abstinence or contraceptive devices). Require information to prevent STIs. Regular communication is required to understand partner's sexual needs and to work through problems and stresses.
Middle Adulthood 40–65 years	Men and women experience decreased hormone production. The menopause occurs in women, usually anywhere between 40 and 55 years. The climacteric occurs gradually in men. Quality rather than the number of sexual experiences becomes important. Individuals establish independent moral and ethical standards.	Women and men may need help adjusting to new roles. People may require counseling to help them reevaluate and direct their energies. Encourage couples to look at the positive aspects of this time of life.

TABLE 28–1	Sexual Development throughout Life *(continued)*	
STAGE	CHARACTERISTICS	NURSING INTERVENTIONS AND TEACHING GUIDELINES
Late Adulthood 65 years and over	Interest in sexual activity often continues. Sexual activity may be less frequent. Women's vaginal secretions diminish, and breasts atrophy. Men produce fewer sperm and need more time to achieve an erection and to ejaculate.	Older adults often continue to be sexually active. Couples may require counseling about adapting their affection and sexual needs to physical limitations.

individual's right to make a decision regarding ways to express oneself sexually, and the responsibilities of each person with respect to sexual activity. See Table 28–2.

Sexually transmitted infections (STIs) are the most common bacterial infections among adolescents. Teens need education about these diseases, preventive measures, and early treatment. The Clinical Manifestations feature lists the common types and symptoms of STIs for which teenagers should seek medical care. The nurse should also inform teens about the various methods of birth control: abstinence, pills, timed-release transdermal patches and implants, diaphragms, intrauterine devices, the rhythm method, and condoms to prevent an unplanned pregnancy. These are discussed later in this chapter.

Young and Middle Adulthood

In young adulthood, many people begin to form intimate relationships with long-term implications. These relationships may take the form of dating, cohabitation, or marriage.

Note, however, that some people do not form intimate relationships until late adulthood and that some never form these types of relationships.

Young adult men and women are often concerned about normal sexual response, for both themselves and their partners. In heterosexual relationships, problems may arise because of basic differences in male and female expectations and responses. Gay and lesbian couples often fare better in this respect. Couples need to communicate their needs to one another early in their courtship so that a successful intimate relationship can develop and grow. Young adults should also be aware that because sexual needs and responses may change, each partner should listen and respond to the needs of the other.

During middle adulthood both men and women experience decreased hormone production resulting in climacteric, commonly called menopause in women and andropause in men. These events often affect the individual's sexual self-concept, body image, and sexual identity. See Chapter 10 ∞ for further information on menopause.

TABLE 28–2	Common Sexual Misconceptions	
MISCONCEPTION	FACT	
Nearly all men over 70 years old have erectile dysfunction.	Sexual ability is not lost due to age. Changes are commonly due to disease or medication.	
Masturbation causes certain mental instabilities.	Masturbation is a common and healthy behavior.	
Sexual activity weakens a person.	There is no evidence that sexual activity weakens a person.	
Women who have experienced orgasm are more likely to become pregnant.	Conceiving is not related to experiencing orgasm.	
Nice girls shouldn't feel entitled to their own sexual satisfaction.	As women become more comfortable with their own sexuality, they advocate for their own sexual fulfillment.	
A large penis provides greater sexual satisfaction to women than a small penis.	There is no evidence that a large penis provides greater satisfaction.	
Alcohol is a sexual stimulant.	Alcohol is a relaxant and central nervous system depressant. Chronic alcoholism is associated with erectile dysfunction.	
Intercourse during menstruation is dangerous (i.e., it will cause vaginal tissue damage).	There is no physiologic basis for abstinence during menses.	
The face-to-face coital position is the moral or proper one.	The position that offers the most pleasure and is acceptable to both partners is the correct one.	

CLINICAL MANIFESTATIONS   Sexually Transmitted Infections

Infection	Male	Female
Gonorrhea	Painful urination; urethritis with watery white discharge, which may become purulent.	May be asymptomatic; or vaginal discharge, pain, and urinary frequency may be present.
Syphilis	Chancre, usually on glans penis, which is painless and heals in 4–6 weeks; secondary symptoms—skin eruptions, low-grade fever, inflammation of lymph glands—in 6 weeks to 6 months after chancre heals.	Chancre on cervix or other genital areas, which heals in 4–6 weeks; symptoms same as for male.
Genital warts (condyloma acuminatum)	The infection is caused by the human papilloma virus (HPV). Single lesions or clusters of lesions growing beneath or on the foreskin, at external meatus, or on the glans penis. On dry skin areas, lesions are hard and yellow-gray. On moist areas, lesions are pink or red and soft with a cauliflower-like appearance.	Certain strains of HPV have been linked to cervical cancer. Lesions appear at the bottom part of the vaginal opening, on the perineum, the vaginal lips, inner walls of the vagina, and the cervix.
Chlamydial urethritis	Urinary frequency; watery, mucoid urethral discharge.	Commonly a carrier; vaginal discharge, dysuria, urinary frequency.
Trichomoniasis	Slight itching; moisture on top of penis; slight, early morning urethral discharge. Many males are asymptomatic.	Itching and redness of vulva and skin inside thighs; copious watery, frothy vaginal discharge.
Candidiasis	Itching, irritation, discharge, plaque of cheesy material under foreskin.	Red and excoriated vulva; intense itching of vaginal and vulvar tissues; thick, white, cheesy or curd-like discharge.
Acquired immune deficiency syndrome (AIDS)	Symptoms can appear anytime from several months to several years after acquiring the virus. The person has reduced immunity to other diseases. Symptoms include any of the following for which there is no other explanation: persistent heavy night sweats; extreme fatigue; severe weight loss; enlarged lymph glands in neck, axillae, or groin; persistent diarrhea; skin rashes; blurred vision or chronic headache; harsh, dry cough; thick gray-white coating on tongue or throat.	
Herpes genitalis (herpes simplex of the genitals)	Primary herpes involves the presence of painful sores or large, discrete vesicles that last for weeks; vesicles rupture. Recurrent herpes is itchy rather than painful; it lasts for a few hours to 10 days.	

Older Adulthood

Older adults may define sexuality far more broadly and include in their definition such things as touching, hugging, romantic gestures (e.g., giving or receiving roses), comfort, warmth, dressing up, joy, spirituality, and beauty. Interest in sexual activity is not lost as people age. For men, however, more time is needed to achieve an erection and to ejaculate (the erection may last longer than at a younger age); more direct genital stimulation is required to achieve an erection; the volume of ejaculated fluid decreases; and the intensity of contractions with orgasm may decrease. The refractory period after orgasm is longer.

Older women remain capable of multiple orgasms and may, in fact, experience an increase in sexual desire after menopause; vaginal lubrication and elasticity decrease with menopause and decreased estrogen, and phases of the sexual response cycle may take longer to occur. There is a possibility of pain during sexual activity and intercourse (dyspareunia) related to vaginal dryness or chronic health conditions (e.g., diabetes or arthritis). Lack of privacy may be a concern for older adults who live with family or in a rehabilitation or nursing home facility.

Many products are available to assist older adults with enhancing their sexual experiences. These range from simple lubricants to surgically implanted devices that enable penile erections. Although older adults' technique may require modification, the nurse should never assume that they are less interested or motivated to have an active sex life.

SEXUAL HEALTH

Sexual health is an individual and constantly changing phenomenon falling within the wide range of human sexual thoughts, feelings, needs, and desires. For most people, sexual health is not considered until its absence or an impairment is noticed. A person's degree of sexual health is best determined by that individual, sometimes with the assistance of a qualified professional. The World Health Organization defined **sexual health** in 1975 as "the integration of the somatic, emotional, intellectual, and social aspects of sexual being, in ways that are positively enriching and that enhance personality, communication, and love" (p. 6). This definition recognizes the biologic, psychologic, and socio-cultural dimensions of sexuality. Characteristics of sexual health are listed in Box 28–1.

Components of Sexual Health

Five critical components of sexual health are sexual self-concept, body image, gender identity, gender role behavior, and freedoms and responsibilities.

BOX 28–1   Characteristics of Sexual Health

- Knowledge about sexuality and sexual behavior
- Ability to express one's full sexual potential, excluding all forms of sexual coercion, exploitation, and abuse
- Ability to make autonomous decisions about one's sexual life within a context of personal and social ethics
- Experience of sexual pleasure as a source of physical, psychologic, cognitive, and spiritual well-being
- Capability to express sexuality through communication, touch, emotional expression, and love
- Right to make free and responsible reproductive choices
- Ability to access sexual health care for the prevention and treatment of all sexual concerns, problems, and disorders

Note: From Declaration of Sexual Rights, by the World Association of Sexology, 1999, Adopted at the 14th World Congress of Sexology, Hong Kong and People's Republic of China. Reprinted with permission from the World Association for Sexual Health (WAS). All rights reserved.

One's **sexual self-concept** (how one values oneself as a sexual being) determines with whom one will have sex, the gender and kinds of people a person is attracted to, and the values about when, where, with whom, and how one expresses sexuality. A positive sexual self-concept enables people to form intimate relationships throughout life. A negative sexual self-concept may impede the formation of relationships.

Body image, a central part of the sense of self, is constantly changing. Pregnancy, aging, trauma, disease, and therapies can alter an individual's appearance and function, which can affect body image. How a person feels about his or her body is related to one's sexuality. People who feel good about their bodies are likely to be comfortable with and enjoy sexual activity. People who have a poor body image may respond negatively to sexual arousal. A major influence on body image for women is the media focus on physical attractiveness and large breasts. Likewise, many men worry about penis size. The myth that "larger is better," particularly if it is erect and has staying power, is pervasive in North America. A person's body image can suffer when unable to achieve these expectations.

Gender identity is one's self-image as a female or male. More than just the biologic component, it also includes social and cultural norms. Gender identity is the result of a long series of developmental events that may or may not conform to one's apparent biologic sex. Once gender identity is established, it cannot be easily changed.

Gender-role behavior is the outward expression of a person's sense of maleness or femaleness as well as the expression of what is perceived as gender-appropriate behavior. Each society defines its roles for males and females; boys are given reinforcement for behaving in a "masculine" way, and girls receive reinforcement for exhibiting "feminine" behaviors.

Physical structure, variations in the internal sense of what is male or female, family values, and cultural values all influence gender-role behavior. In North America, expected adult male roles include breadwinner, heterosexual lover, father, and athlete. Expected male behaviors include wearing trousers, demonstrating physical strength, and expressing feelings in a controlled fashion. Women are expected to express their emotions more freely and to be gentler in their physical responses; they also have a broader choice of clothing than men do.

Androgyny, or flexibility in gender roles, is the belief that most characteristics and behaviors are human qualities that should not be limited to one specific gender or the other. Being androgynous does not mean being sexually neutral or imply anything about one's sexual orientation. Rather, it describes the degree of flexibility a person has regarding gender-stereotypic behaviors. Adults who can behave flexibly regarding their sexual roles may be able to adapt better than those who adopt rigid stereotyped gender roles.

Sexual health includes both *freedoms* and *responsibilities.* Sexually healthy people engage in activities that are freely chosen, including both self-pleasuring and shared-pleasuring activities. Individuals also have freedom of their sexual thoughts, feelings, and fantasies. Sexually healthy people are ethically motivated to exercise behavioral, emotional, economic, and social responsibility for themselves ("Vision of Sexual Health," 2004).

VARIETIES OF SEXUALITY

There are many varieties of sexuality. There is a tremendous range of variation in how people experience and express their sexuality. There are also many differences in the priority people place on sexuality in their lives. Sexual varieties include sexual orientation, gender identity, erotic preferences, and sexual lifestyles.

Sexual Orientation

One's attraction to people of the same sex, other sex, or both sexes is referred to as **sexual orientation.** Sexual orientation lies along a continuum with a wide range between the two extremes of exclusively heterosexual attraction and exclusively homosexual attraction. Individuals who are attracted to people of both genders are referred to as *bisexuals.*

The origins of sexual orientation are still not well understood. Some biologic theories describe sexual orientation in terms of the genetic composition of the individual. Psychologic theories stress the role of early learning experiences and cognitive processes. Other theories acknowledge the confluence of genetics and the environment in the development of sexual orientation.

Estimates of the percentage of the population with a homosexual orientation vary, although the usual figure is 5% to 10% of men and 2% to 4% of women (McCammon, Knox, & Schacht, 2004). Because these individuals grow up acutely aware of the discrimination they face in North America, many do not disclose their sexual orientation; thus actual figures are not available.

Gender Identity

Western culture is deeply committed to the idea that there are only two sexes. Biologically speaking, however, there are many gradations running from female to male; this is known as **transgenderism.** In some cases gender is clear, in other cases there is a blending of both genders within the same individual, and in some it is unclear.

INTERSEX   About 1 in every 2,000 babies is born with an **intersex** condition in which there are contradictions among chromosomal gender, gonadal gender, internal organs, and external genital appearance. The gender of such an infant is ambiguous. What this means is that an intersexed person has some parts usually associated with males and some parts usually associated with females. Intersex anatomy may not be apparent at birth. Sometimes it is undetected until puberty, until the person is identified as an infertile adult, or until the person dies and is autopsied. For more information, see the Intersex Society of North America.

TRANSSEXUALS   The medical profession considers **transsexuals** to have a condition called *gender dysphoria* (strong and persistent feelings of discomfort with one's assigned gender) or *gender identity disorder.* For the transsexual person, sexual anatomy is not consistent with gender identity. Those who are born physically male but are emotionally and psychologically female are called male-to-female (MTF) transsexuals. Those who are born female but are emotionally and psychologically male are called female-to-male (FTM) transsexuals.

Most transsexuals report that they have felt gender dysphoria since early childhood. They often suffer for many years and try to hide the situation from family and friends for fear of being considered "crazy." Being transgendered puts women and men at extreme risk of being:

- Ridiculed and humiliated.
- In constant jeopardy over getting and keeping a job.
- Evicted without cause from restaurants and stores.
- Denied housing.
- Refused medical treatment, even to save a life (Lips, 2005).

As self-understanding and acceptance increase, many transsexuals live part or full time as members of the other sex. Cross-dressing (dressing in the clothing of the other sex) not only makes their outward appearance consistent with their inner identity and gender role, but also increases their comfort with themselves. Their sexual orientation may be heterosexual, homosexual, or bisexual.

CROSS-DRESSERS   **Cross-dressers** are typically males who cross-dress to express the feminine side of their personality. In most instances cross-dressers are not interested in permanently altering their bodies through surgical means, especially since the majority of them are comfortable with their original birth identity and behavior in their public and professional lives.

Cross-dressing is a conscious choice and may occur at home or in public settings. The frequency of the activity ranges from rarely to often. It is not unusual for cross-dressers to have a female name to go with the female personality and wardrobe. Cross-dressing occurs more frequently in cultures where males are expected to be strong, independent, and unemotional protectors. If the social climate is considered to be one with rigid gender roles, some men may need to express their gentleness and dependence by creating a separate world and female persona within that social climate (Barnett & Rivers, 2004).

Erotic Preferences

Over a lifetime, sexual fantasies and single-partner sex are the most common sexual outlets for women and men, single and coupled persons, and heterosexual, gay/lesbian, and bisexual persons. Masturbation is the ongoing love affair that each of us has with ourselves throughout our lifetime. It is the way we discover our erotic feelings and learn about our sexual response. Mutual masturbation can provide sexual pleasuring and intimacy without hurrying to genital interaction before both partners are ready. Masturbation shared with a partner is a safe alternative to unprotected genital sex.

Male-to-female or female-to-female oral–genital sex is known technically as *cunnilingus*. This involves kissing, licking, or sucking of the female genitals including the mons pubis, vulva, clitoris, labia, and vagina. *Fellatio* is oral stimulation of the penis by licking and sucking. *Sixty-nine* is simultaneous oral–genital stimulation by two persons. Preconceptions and myths are a major deterrent for those who have not tried oral sex. However, like most sexual practices, oral–genital sex is not completely free of the potential for STI transmission, and safer sex practices must be used.

Anal stimulation can be a source of sexual pleasure because the anus has a rich nerve supply. Stimulation may be applied with fingers, mouth, or sex toys such as vibrators. The anus is surrounded by strong muscles, and the rectum contains no natural lubrication. Thus inserting a finger or penis in the rectum requires relaxation and water-soluble lubricant.

A common form of sexual activity for heterosexual couples is **genital intercourse.** Penile–vaginal intercourse (coitus) can be both physically and emotionally satisfying. There are varieties of positions for this kind of intercourse; the most common is lying face to face (with female or male on top). Side-lying, standing, sitting, and rear-entry positions are also used. Side-lying, female-on-top, and rear-entry positions facilitate clitoral stimulation, either by penile or manual contact. The choice of intercourse positions and activities depends on physical comfort and beliefs, values, and attitudes about different practices.

During intercourse, the man moves the penis back and forth along the vaginal walls by rhythmic thrusting movements of his hips. At the same time the woman may move her own body to match the partner's hip movements. Movements continue until orgasm is achieved by one or both partners. Simultaneous orgasm can be difficult to achieve. After coitus, caressing, hugging, and kissing can increase the shared intimacy and should be encouraged.

The other form of genital intercourse is *anal intercourse,* during which the penis is inserted into the anus and rectum of the partner. Anal intercourse is commonly practiced by gay men, but a number of heterosexual couples engage in it as well. Positions for anal intercourse are similar to those for penile–vaginal intercourse, with minor differences due to the position of the anus.

Current practice dictates the use of a condom in both forms of intercourse to prevent the transmission of disease. Because anorectal tissue is not self-lubricating, a lubricant must be used on the condom. Also, since normal bacterial flora from the bowel can produce infection in other parts of the body, the used condom should be removed and another applied before inserting the penis into other body orifices.

There are many other varieties of sexuality that are beyond the scope of this chapter. These include several or many partners, nudism, swinging, group sex, fetishism, sexual sadism, and sexual masochism.

FACTORS INFLUENCING SEXUALITY

Many factors influence a person's sexuality. Discussed here are family, culture, religion, and personal expectations and ethics.

Family

For the majority of us, the family is the earliest and most enduring social relationship. Families are the fabric of our day-to-day lives and shape the quality of our lives by influencing our outlooks on life, our motivations, our strategies for achievement, and our styles for coping with adversity. It is within our families that we develop our gender identity, body image, sexual self-concept, and capacity for intimacy. Through family interactions we learn about relationships and gender roles and our expectations of others and ourselves.

From earliest beginnings, children observe their parents and model themselves after these role models. If parents are able to share affection with one another and other family members, children will most likely become adults who are able to give and receive affection. If parents seldom hug, hold hands, or kiss each other, their children may become adults who are very uncomfortable with romantic touch. If family gender role behavior is very rigid, arguments and hurt feelings will abound if a person from this system is partnered with a person who grew up in an androgynous family system. Family messages about sex range from "sex is so shameful it shouldn't be talked about" to "sex is a joyful part of adult relationships." The following are some common sexual messages children get from their families:

- Sex is dirty.
- Premarital sex is sinful.
- Good girls don't do it.
- Masturbation is disgusting.
- Men should be the sexual experts.
- Sex is mainly for procreating.
- Bodies, including genitals, are beautiful.
- Sex should be fun for both women and men.
- Sexual thoughts and feelings are natural.
- Masturbation is a common, pleasurable activity.
- There is great variety in sexual behaviors.

Culture

Sexuality is regulated by the individual's culture. For example, culture influences the sexual nature of dress, rules about marriage, expectations of role behavior and social responsibilities, and specific sex practices. Societal attitudes vary widely. Attitudes about childhood sexual play with self or children of the same gender or other gender may be restrictive or permissive. Premarital and extramarital sex and homosexuality may be unacceptable or tolerated. Polygamy (several marriage partners) or monogamy (one marriage partner) may be the norm. Gender role behavior also varies from culture to culture. Culture is so much a part of everyday life that it is taken for granted. We tend to assume that others share our own perspective, including those for whom we provide care. It is impossible to provide sensitive nursing care if we believe that our own culture is more important than, and preferable to, any other culture.

Cultures differ with regard to which body parts they find to be erotic. In some cultures, legs are erotic and breasts are not. Body weight may also be a determinant of sexual attractiveness. There is a great deal of pressure in American culture to be very thin. Women who would be considered to be obese in America are found highly attractive in other cultures. The degree of public nudity ranges from women's entire bodies and faces being covered in Islamic societies to complete nudity in some cultures in New Guinea and Australia.

Female circumcision, also known as female genital mutilation, female ritual cutting (FRC), or *female genital cutting* (FGC), is a dangerous practice in parts of Africa. Some of the cultural beliefs behind the practice include the following: female genitals are offensive to men, if not removed the clitoris will become the size of a penis, the labia get in the way of in-

---

TABLE 28–3   **Physiologic Changes Associated with the Sexual Response Cycle**

PHASE OF THE SEXUAL RESPONSE CYCLE	SIGNS PRESENT IN BOTH SEXES	SIGNS PRESENT IN MALES ONLY	SIGNS PRESENT IN FEMALES ONLY
Excitement/Plateau	Muscle tension increases as excitement increases. Sex flush, usually on chest. Nipple erection.	Penile erection; glans size increases as excitement increases. Appearance of a few drops of lubricant, which may contain sperm.	Erection of the clitoris. Vaginal lubrication. Labia may increase 2 to 3 times in size. Breasts enlarge. Inner two-thirds of vagina widens and lengthens; outer third swells and narrows. Uterus elevates.
Orgasmic	Respirations may increase to 40 breaths per minute. Involuntary spasms of muscle groups throughout the body. Diminished sensory awareness. Involuntary contractions of the anal sphincter. Peak heart rate (110–180 BPM), respiratory rate (40/min or greater), and blood pressure (systolic 30–80 mm Hg and diastolic 20–50 mm Hg above normal).	Rhythmic, expulsive contractions of the penis at 0.8-sec intervals. Emission of seminal fluid into the prostatic urethra from contraction of the vas deferens and accessory organs (stage 1 of the expulsive process). Closing of the internal bladder sphincter just before ejaculation to prevent retrograde ejaculation into bladder. Orgasm may occur without ejaculation. Ejaculation of semen through the penile urethra and expulsion from the urethral meatus. The force of ejaculation varies from man to man and at different times but diminishes after the first two to three contractions (stage 2 of the expulsive process).	Approximately 5–12 contractions in the orgasmic platform at 0.8-sec intervals. Contraction of the muscles of the pelvic floor and the uterine muscles. Varied pattern of orgasms, including minor surges and contractions, multiple orgasms, or a simple intense orgasm similar to that of the male.
Resolution	Reversal of vasocongestion in 10–30 min; disappearance of all signs of myotonia within 5 min. Genitals and breasts return to their preexcitement states. Sex flush disappears in reverse order of appearance. Heart rate, respiratory rate, and blood pressure return to normal. Other reactions include sleepiness, relaxation, and emotional outbursts such as crying or laughing.	A refractory period during which the body will not respond to sexual stimulation; varies, depending on age and other factors, from a few moments to hours or days.	

tercourse, the cutting enhances fertility, and it prepares the woman for childbirth. Removal of the clitoris may or may not be accompanied by removal of the labia and closure of the vaginal entrance except for a small opening. Long-term medical complications include urinary incontinence, chronic urinary tract infections, vaginal scarring, pain syndromes, infertility, and sexual dysfunctions. FGC is illegal in several African and European countries and in Canada and the United States. In 1980, the World Health Organization and the United Nations Children's Fund (UNICEF) unanimously recommended that all forms of female circumcision be abolished (Elwood, 2005).

Male circumcision is controversial. The American Academy of Pediatrics Committee on the Fetus and Newborn stated in 1971 that there were no valid medical indications for circumcision for newborns. The Academy's current policy is that "Existing scientific evidence demonstrates potential medical benefits of newborn male circumcision; however, these data are not sufficient to recommend routine neonatal circumcision" (American Academy of Pediatrics Task Force on Circumcision, 1999). They support informed decision making on the part of parents. The change in the rate of circumcisions is variably reported. Some studies show an increase (Nelson, Dunn, Wan, & Wei, 2005), while the U.S. National Center for Health Statistics (2005) indicates little change in the overall rate of about 65% in the past 20 years. All studies show highest rates in the Midwest segment of the country (81%) and lowest rates in the West (37%).

Religion

Religion influences sexual expression. It provides guidelines for sexual behavior and acceptable circumstances for the behavior, as well as prohibited sexual behavior and the consequences of breaking the sexual rules. The guidelines or rules may be detailed and rigid or broad and flexible. For example, some religions view forms of sexual expression other than male–female intercourse as unnatural and hold virginity before marriage to be the rule.

Many religious values conflict with the more flexible values of society that have developed during the last few decades (often labeled the "sexual revolution") such as the acceptance of premarital sex, unwed parenthood, homosexuality, and abortion. These conflicts create marked anxiety and potential sexual dysfunctions in some individuals. See Chapter 29 ∞ for additional information about religious values.

Personal Expectations and Ethics

Although ethics is integral to religion, ethical thought and ethical approaches to sexuality can be viewed separately from religion. Cultures have developed written or unwritten codes of conduct based on ethical principles. Personal expectations concerning sexual behavior come from these cultural norms. What one person or culture views as bizarre, perverted, or wrong may be completely natural and right to another. Examples include values regarding masturbation, oral or anal intercourse, and cross-dressing. Many people accept a variety of sexual expressions if they are performed by consenting adults, are practiced in private, and are not harmful. Couples need to explore and communicate clearly about various types of acceptable sexual expression to prevent domination of sexual decision making by one member of the couple.

SEXUAL RESPONSE CYCLE

Commonly occurring phases of the human sexual response follow a similar sequence in both females and males regardless of sexual orientation. It does not matter if the motive for being sexually active is true love or passionate lust. Table 28–3 provides a summary of the physiologic changes associated with each of the phases of the cycle.

The response cycle starts in the brain, with conscious sexual desires called the **desire phase.** Sexually arousing stimuli, often called erotic stimuli, may be real or symbolic. Sight, hearing, smell, touch, and imagination (sexual fantasy) can all invoke sexual arousal. Sexual desire fluctuates within each person and varies from person to person. If people suppress or block out conscious sexual desires, they may not experience any physiologic response. Although psychologic issues are the more common causes of lack of sexual desire, medications, drugs, and hormone imbalances can also interfere.

The **excitement phase** involves two primary physiologic changes (see Figure 28–1). *Vasocongestion* is an increase in the blood flow to various body parts resulting in erection of the penis and clitoris and swelling of the labia, testes, and breasts. Vasocongestion stimulates sensory receptors within these body parts that in turn transmit messages to the conscious brain where they are usually interpreted as pleasurable sensations. When stimulation is continued, vasocongestion increases until it either is released by orgasm or fades away. Likewise, *myotonia,* an increase of tension in

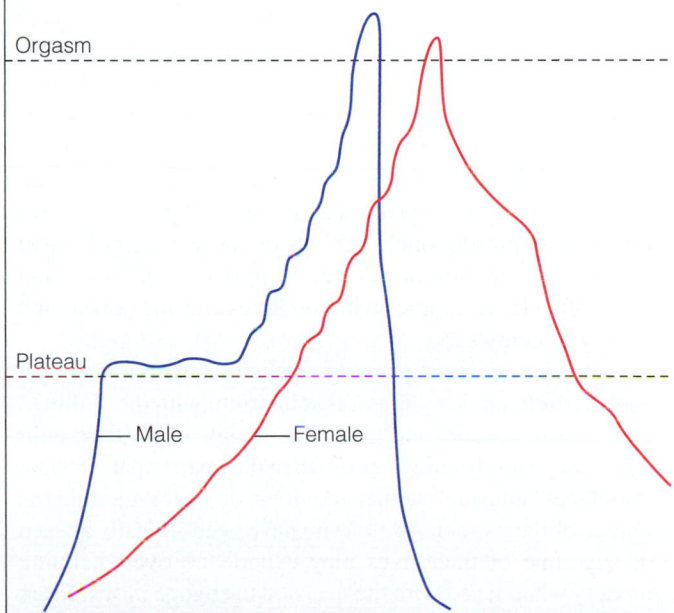

Figure 28–1 ○ Phases of the sexual response cycle.

muscles, may increase until released by orgasm, or it may also simply fade away.

The **orgasmic phase** is the involuntary climax of sexual tension, accompanied by physiologic and psychologic release. This phase is considered the measurable peak of the sexual experience. Although the entire body is involved, the major focus of the orgasm is felt in the pelvic region. Male orgasms usually last 10 to 30 seconds while female orgasms last 10 to 50 seconds. Men usually have an *ejaculation* and expel semen as part of their orgasm. Before puberty and in later years, males experience orgasms without ejaculation.

The **resolution phase,** the period of return to the unaroused state, may last 10 to 15 minutes after orgasm, or longer if there is no orgasm. This phase in females is quite varied as some women experience multiple successive orgasms followed by a longer period of resolution.

ALTERED SEXUAL FUNCTION

The ability to engage in sexual behavior is of great importance to most people. Many individuals experience transient problems with their ability to respond to sexual stimulation or to maintain the response. A smaller percentage of individuals experience problems that are lifelong in duration. The problems may be generalized to all sexual interactions and settings, or they may be situational, occurring in a specific setting or with specific types of sexual activity. It is often difficult to sort out the multiple factors contributing to an individual's or a couple's sexual problems. Generally a number of past and current factors are involved.

Past and Current Factors

Sociocultural factors interfering in sexual function include a very restrictive upbringing accompanied by inadequate sex education. Rigid gender role socialization may inhibit exploration of sexual activities, positions, toys, and other lovemaking behaviors. If people's religious affiliations believe that sex is only for procreation, there may be great difficulty in celebrating the pleasure and fun of a loving sexual relationship. Another factor may be parental punishment for normally exploring one's genitals or for normal childhood sex play. In our current culture, the pressures of family and work often leave couples with too little time and not enough energy to enjoy sex.

Psychologic factors may include negative feelings, such as guilt, anxiety, or fear that interfere with the ability to experience pleasure and joy. Some people experience guilt when they simply enjoy sex or when they participate in what they label "unusual" sexual activities, or guilt regarding the choice of the partner. Adults who have been sexually abused at any time of their lives may experience overwhelming anxiety when faced with the decision to engage in sex. Fears may include pregnancy, sexually transmitted infections, or pain. Because vulnerability and intimacy are inherent in most sexual relationships, fear of these may lead to an avoidance of sex. Fear of failure in sexual performance often becomes a vicious cycle; that is, fear of failure creates actual failure, which in turn produces more fear. Spectatoring is the detached appraisal of sexual performance or the body during a sexual act: "Am I going to lose my erection?" "Am I going to have an orgasm this time?" "My stomach is too flabby." "When did his thighs get that fat?" Depressed people lose interest in sexual activity and often experience a complete loss of sexual desire and fulfillment.

Cognitive factors include the internalization of negative expectations and beliefs. Those with low self-esteem may not understand how another person could value and love them and also find them sexually attractive. For those who have not yet accepted their sexual orientation or gender identity, this cognitive conflict may interfere with sexual relationships.

Sexual problems may also be symptomatic of *relationship* problems. Conflict and anger with one's partner are not conducive to positive sexual interaction. Some persons lose the physical attraction to another or feel more attracted to someone else.

Lack of intimacy and feeling like a sex object inhibit the feeling of communion and connection that is an important part of making love. Another factor is expecting one's partner to read one's mind about sexual needs. Failure to communicate may result in one or both partners not knowing how to please the other. Unless the partners experiment, sex may, in time, become boring. Disagreements in sexual frequency and/or sexual activities may lead to further relationship conflict.

Health factors can interfere with people's expression of sexuality. Physical changes brought on by illness, injury, or surgery may inhibit full sexual expression. Throughout your program of nursing education, you will learn about the sexual side effects of a number of diseases such as heart disease, diabetes mellitus, joint disease, cancer, and mental disorders. You will also study the impact of surgeries such as hysterectomy, prostate surgery, and radical surgeries that alter a person's body image. Spinal cord injuries, traumatic amputations, or disfiguring accidents negatively affect sexual functioning. The presence of an STI in one partner induces fear of transmission in the other, often resulting in abstinence of sexual contact. In some situations, the presence of an STI is unknown and transmission occurs.

Many prescription medications have side effects that affect sexual functioning beyond those intended for that purpose. Most frequently, the impact is negative, but sometimes there is a positive impact. Table 28–4 provides an overview of the effects of medications on sexual function. For example, antidepressants may slow ejaculation. This may be a problem for the man who finds himself suddenly feeling unable to ejaculate. If the man is suffering from rapid ejaculation, however, the antidepressant may "cure" this problem. Some street drugs such as marijuana, amphetamines, and cocaine enhance sexual functioning. Others, such as opioids and anabolic steroids, interfere with sexual functioning.

TABLE 28–4 Effects of Medications on Sexual Function

MEDICATION	POSSIBLE EFFECTS*
Alcohol	Moderate amounts: increased sexual functioning; chronic use: decreased sexual desire, orgasmic dysfunction, and erectile dysfunction
Alpha-blockers	Inability to ejaculate
Amphetamines	Increased sex drive, delayed orgasm
Amyl nitrate	Reported enhanced orgasm; vasodilation, fainting
Anabolic steroids	Decreased sex drive, shrinking of testicles and infertility in men
Antianxiety agents	Decreased sexual desire; orgasmic dysfunction in women; delayed ejaculation
Anticonvulsants	Decreased sexual desire; reduced sexual response
Antidepressants	Decreased sexual desire; orgasmic delay or dysfunction in women; delayed or failed ejaculation; painful erection
Antihistamines	Decreased vaginal lubrication; decreased desire
Antihypertensives	Decreased sexual desire; erectile failure; ejaculation dysfunction
Antipsychotics	Decreased sexual desire; orgasmic dysfunction in women; delayed ejaculation; ejaculatory failure
Barbiturates	In low doses, increased sexual pleasure; in large doses, decreased sexual desire, orgasmic dysfunction, and erectile dysfunction
Beta-blockers	Decreased sexual desire
Cardiotonics	Decreased sexual desire
Cocaine	Increased intensity of sexual experience; with chronic use, decreased sexual desire and sexual dysfunction
Diuretics	Decreased vaginal lubrication; decreased sexual desire; erectile dysfunction
Marijuana	As above for cocaine, but prolonged use reduces testosterone levels and reduces sperm production
Narcotics	Inhibited sexual desire and response; erectile and ejaculatory dysfunctions

*Nurses and clients must familiarize themselves with the specific medication prescribed or used, because effects vary in each category of drug.

Sexual Desire Disorders

For most people, sexual desire varies from day to day as well as over the years. Some people, however, report a deficiency in or absence of sexual fantasies and persistently low interest or a total lack of interest in sexual activity; these clients suffer from **hypoactive sexual desire disorder.** If both individuals in a relationship are similarly uninterested in sex, there really is no problem. More typically, there is a disparity of sexual needs, and the person with the greater desire

---

DRUG CAPSULE

The Client Taking Medication for Erectile Dysfunction (ED) phosphodiesterase type 5 (PDE5) inhibitor *sildenafil citrate* (Viagra); *tadalafil* (Cialis); *vardenafil* (Levitra)

In erectile dysfunction (ED) the sexually stimulated penis does not achieve or maintain an erection, often due to restricted blood flow to the penis. These medications inhibit the breakdown of the enzymes and products that allow the muscle relaxation which, in turn, facilitates adequate blood flow to the penis. Thus, the medications do not enhance sexual desire or cure the ED but allow the stimulated penis to obtain and sustain an erection.

Nursing Responsibilities

- ED medications are contraindicated for men with uncontrolled high or low blood pressure, stroke, renal or liver problems, vision loss, or bleeding disorders.
- Men with an anatomically deformed penis should consult with the primary care provider prior to taking these medications.
- Medications come in different dose strengths and may require adjustment.

Client and Family Teaching

- General safety in using these medications is the same as for engaging in sexual activity overall. The risk of adverse outcomes of sexual activity after taking these medications is not increased.

- Explain that men who take medications that are nitrates—those that are prescribed (e.g., nitroglycerin) or those that are recreational (e.g., amyl nitrate–"poppers")—should not take these medications.
- The client should take the medication about 1 hour prior to sexual activity (up to 4 hours prior) and not more than once per day.
- Teach side effects to immediately report to the primary care provider: loss of vision, or erection that lasts more than 4 hours.
- Other common side effects may include headache, muscle pain, flushing, or stuffy nose.
- These medications do not prevent pregnancy or STIs.

Note: Prior to administering any medication, review all aspects with a current drug handbook or other reliable source.

becomes dissatisfied with the sexual relationship. The key issue in the relationship is not frequency but rather the dovetailing of partners' needs.

Sexual aversion disorder is a severe distaste for sexual activity or the thought of sexual activity, which then leads to a phobic avoidance of sex. It occurs in both women and men. Intense emotional dread of an impending sexual interaction also can trigger the physiologic symptoms of anxiety: sweating, increased heart rate, and extreme muscle tension. The person then stops the sexual interaction or prevents it from even beginning. The most common cause of sexual aversion disorder is childhood sexual abuse or adult rape. The severe trauma can lead to a phobic response to sexual activity (McCammon et al., 2004).

Sexual Arousal Disorders

Sexual arousal refers to the physiologic responses and subjective sense of excitement experienced during sexual activity. Lack of lubrication and failure to attain or maintain an erection are the major disorders of the arousal phase. In **female sexual arousal disorder,** the lack of vaginal lubrication causes discomfort or pain during sexual intercourse. The diagnosis of **male erectile disorder** is usually made when the man has erection problems during 25% or more of his sexual interactions. Some men cannot attain a full erection, and others lose their erection prior to orgasm. The term commonly applied to this condition, *impotency,* implies that the man is feeble, inadequate, and incompetent. The accurate term is *erectile dysfunction (ED),* which is objectively descriptive and not judgmental. Arousal disorder may also be diagnosed even when lubrication and erection are adequate if individuals report a persistent or recurring lack of subjective sexual excitement or pleasure.

Orgasmic Disorders

The term commonly applied in the past to women who did not experience orgasm, *frigid,* implied that the woman was totally incapable of responding sexually. The more accurate and objective term is **female orgasmic disorder,** which simply means that the sexual response stops before orgasm occurs. *Preorgasmic* women have never experienced an orgasm. Studies indicate that 10% to 15% of women are preorgasmic, and another 20% to 22% report irregular orgasms. Compounding the orgasmic difficulty is the associated anxiety. In the preoccupation with orgasm, the real goal of being sexual—mutual pleasuring and intimacy—is lost, and the interchange becomes one of anxiety, frustration, and anger (McCammon et al., 2004).

Some men suffer from **male orgasmic disorder.** Men with this disorder can maintain an erection for long periods (an hour or more) but have extreme difficulty ejaculating, referred to as *retarded ejaculation.* In heterosexual intercourse, the difficulty may be limited to ejaculation in the vagina. Some men ejaculate after self-stimulation or manual or oral stimulation by the partner, whereas others have great difficulty ejaculating with any type of stimulation. This disorder is much less common than rapid ejaculation.

Rapid ejaculation is one of the most common sexual dysfunctions among men. There are many definitions, with descriptions ranging from ejaculating before being touched, ejaculating before penetration, ejaculating with one internal thrust, to ejaculating within a minute or two of penetration. A more helpful description is the *absence of voluntary control of ejaculation.* The problem is best self-defined as when a man is concerned about his ejaculatory control, or the couple agrees that ejaculation is too rapid for mutual satisfaction.

Sexual Pain Disorders

Both women and men can experience **dyspareunia,** pain during or immediately after intercourse. It is associated with many physiologic causes, especially those that inhibit lubrication. Thus skin irritations, vaginal infections, estrogen deficiencies, and use of medications that dry vaginal secretions can cause women to experience discomfort with intercourse.

Pelvic disorders, such as infections, lesions, endometriosis, scar tissue, or tumors, can result in painful intercourse. Similarly, in males, infection or inflammation of the glans penis or other genitourinary organs can cause pain with intercourse. Also, some contraceptive foams, creams, sponges, or latex products can irritate either the vagina or penis.

Vaginismus is the involuntary spasm of the outer one-third of the vaginal muscles, making penetration of the vagina painful and sometimes impossible. The woman often experiences desire, excitement, and orgasm with stimulation of the external sexual structures. Attempts at intercourse, however, elicit the involuntary spasm. She may have similar difficulty undergoing pelvic exams and inserting tampons or a diaphragm.

Vulvodynia is constant, unremitting burning that is localized to the vulva with an acute onset. The girl or woman has problems in sitting, standing, and sleeping related to the intensity of pain. **Vestibulitis** causes severe pain only on touch or attempted vaginal entry. Half of the women with vestibulitis report lifelong dyspareunia. Women with either of these disorders report a negative impact on their sexual functioning and partner relationship, as well as their self-esteem and mental health (Metzger, 2004).

Problems with Satisfaction

Some people experience sexual desire, arousal, and orgasm and yet feel dissatisfied with their sexual relationships. These sexual problems are more commonly related to the emotional tone of the relationship than to the physiologic response. Since giving and receiving pleasure in a mutually intimate relationship are the primary goals of sex for most people, **dissatisfaction problems** may be more disturbing than other types of sexual dysfunctions.

At times, satisfaction problems may be situational. For example, one partner may choose an inconvenient time, or a partner may feel anxious and therefore cannot experience much pleasure or joy. Some people describe their problems as related to lack of extragenital satisfaction. These people describe how much they miss and continue to need all the touching and caressing of their earlier lovemaking experiences. Unfortunately, people who have been relating sexually for a long time often become genitally focused and neglect the rest of the body. One or both partners may feel touch starved, long for more extragenital loving, and become dissatisfied with sex.

Satisfaction problems are often related to relationship difficulties. The inability to communicate effectively in other relationship areas frequently results in sexual frustration. Partners who are angry with each other and make love without resolving the conflict may feel unhappy about the relationship despite having experienced arousal and orgasm. Couples who define their relationship in terms of rigid, unequal power and gender roles may have difficulty negotiating and compromising about sexual issues. Not infrequently, the person with the least amount of power feels helpless and dissatisfied with the sexual interchanges.

Lack of intimacy or a feeling of connectedness is understandably related to satisfaction problems. If one has sex with a stranger, the body may function well, but there is often a sense of something missing after the sexual experience. Making love to one person while feeling more attracted to or in love with another person can result in feelings of emptiness or disconnection. Even couples in a committed relationship may complain of lack of intimacy. Dissatisfaction issues include lack of romance, love, tenderness, and nurturance. Fulfillment of sexuality, then, depends on the ability to relate with a partner in an intimate and mutually pleasing manner that is compatible with values and chosen lifestyle.

NURSING MANAGEMENT

ASSESSING

Because sexuality and sexual functioning are aspects of health and well-being, they are a part of nursing care and need to be assessed. Clients are often hesitant to introduce the topic of sex with their primary health care providers. They may be too embarrassed, they may think that they should not have sexual problems in our liberated times, or they may think they are too old or too young to have these problems. When health care professionals do not introduce the topic, these individuals are unrecognized and unserved.

Information about a client's sexual health status should always be an integral part of a nursing assessment. The amount and kind of data collected depend on the context of the assessment, that is, the client's reason for seeking health care and how the client's sexuality interacts with other problems.

Generally, the nurse conducts a sexual history on the following categories of clients:

- Those receiving care for pregnancy, infertility, contraception, or an STI
- Those whose illness or therapy will affect sexual functioning (e.g., clients with diabetes, gynecologic problems, or heart disease)
- Those currently experiencing a sexual problem

Nursing History

Including a sexual history as part of the general nursing history is important for some clients and not important for other clients. It is critical, however, to introduce the topic of sexuality to all clients in order to give them permission to bring up any concerns or problems. All nursing histories should at least include a question such as "What changes, if any, have you experienced in your sexual functioning that might be related to your illness or the medications you take?" Nurses might also facilitate communication by saying, "As a nurse, I'm concerned about all aspects of your health. People often have questions about sexual matters, both when they are well and when they are ill. When I take your history, sexual concerns are included to help plan a comprehensive treatment approach."

It is critical that nurses not make assumptions about clients because assumptions interfere with accurate history taking. If you assume that all people do all things you will be more open to clients than if you make assumptions about who is and who is not sexually active and what activities they perform. Imposing personal values on others is detrimental to the nurse–client relationship.

Interviewing a client regarding sexual health may be uncomfortable for some nurses (and for the client). Nurses must be aware of their own feelings and beliefs so that they can prepare approaches for gathering data and creating the nursing care plan. The nurse sets aside personal values about sexual practices and uses a culturally competent, nonjudgmental, nonthreatening, and reassuring approach. It is extremely important to create an atmosphere that facilitates open communication and comfort for the client. Remind the client that all personal health information is handled in a confidential manner. Also see Chapter 2 ∞ for a review of values clarification and Chapter 7 ∞ for more information on the health history.

The accompanying Assessment Interview: Sexual Health History provides questions that nurses may ask as part of the health history. These questions typically are asked in the assessment process after a rapport has been established.

Physical Examination

Physical examination of the female genitals and reproductive tract and the male genitals is part of a routine physical examination in some agencies. Check agency protocol. See Chapter 17 ∞ for details of the examination. If the client has not been examined in the past year or if data from the recent nursing history indicate a need, the nurse performs a physical examination. Nursing history data indicating the need for a physical examination include the following:

- Suspicion of infertility, pregnancy, or an STI
- Reports of discharge, presence of a lump or sore, or change in color, size, and shape of a genital organ
- Changes in urinary function
- Need for Papanicolaou test
- Request for birth control

ASSESSMENT INTERVIEW — Sexual Health History

- Are you currently sexually active? With men, women, or both?
- With one or more than one partner?
- Describe the positive and negative aspects of your sexual functioning.
- Do you have difficulty with sexual desire? Arousal? Orgasm? Satisfaction?
- Do you experience any pain with sexual interaction?
- If there are problems, how have they influenced how you feel about yourself? How have they affected your partner? How have they affected the relationship?
- Do you expect your sexual functioning to be altered because of your illness?
- What are your partner's concerns about your future sexual functioning?
- Do you have any other sexual questions or concerns that I have not addressed?

Identifying Clients at Risk

Clients at risk for altered sexual patterns include those experiencing the following:

- Altered body structure or function due to trauma, pregnancy, recent childbirth, anatomic abnormalities of the genitals, or a variety of diseases
- Physical, psychosocial, emotional, or sexual abuse; sexual assault
- Disfiguring conditions, such as burns, skin conditions, birthmarks, scars (e.g., mastectomy), and ostomies
- Specific medication therapy that causes sexual problems (see Table 28–4)
- Temporary or long-term impaired physical ability to perform grooming and maintain sexual attractiveness

- Value conflicts between personal beliefs and religious doctrine
- Loss of a partner
- Lack of knowledge or misinformation about sexual functioning and expression

DIAGNOSING

The NANDA nursing diagnoses relating specifically to sexuality include the following:

- *Ineffective Sexuality Pattern*
- *Sexual Dysfunction*

Sexual problems can also be the etiology of other diagnoses, including the following:

- *Deficient Knowledge* (e.g., about conception, STIs, contraception, or normal sexual changes over the life span) related to misinformation and sexual myths
- *Pain* related to inadequate vaginal lubrication or effects of genital surgery
- *Anxiety* related to loss of sexual desire or functioning
- *Fear* related to history of sexual abuse or dyspareunia
- *Disturbed Body Image* (e.g., mastectomy) related to perceived sexual rejection by spouse

PLANNING

Overall goals to meet clients' sexual needs include the following:

- Maintain, restore, or improve sexual health.
- Increase knowledge of sexuality and sexual health.
- Prevent the occurrence or spread of STIs.
- Prevent unwanted pregnancy.
- Increase satisfaction with the level of sexual functioning.
- Improve sexual self-concept.

RESEARCH NOTES — How Is Sexual Orientation Related to Sexual Health Risks in Homeless Adolescents?

In this study, 248 homeless males and 177 homeless females (total 425 teens) were surveyed regarding their sexual health risks and protective resources. Previous studies grouped gay, lesbian, and bisexual (GLB) youth in a single category of sexual minorities. The purpose of this study was to compare similarities and differences between GLB youth and heterosexual youth in the homeless population. A further goal was to determine if there were differences between the gay, lesbian, and bisexual subgroups.

Heterosexual youth were more likely to be homeless because of their parents' disapproval of their drug/alcohol use. Gay and lesbian youth were more likely to be homeless because of their parents' disapproval of their sexual orientation, and bisexual youth identified physical abuse at home as the cause of their homelessness. GLB youth reported higher incidence rates for all sexually transmitted infections. The order of childhood sexual abuse history is as follows: gay/lesbian, 77.6%; bisexual, 62.5%; and heterosexual, 37.1%.

There was no significant relationship between sexual orientation and receiving immunizations for hepatitis B. There were no significant differences between the use of condoms or the measure of risky sexual behaviors.

Implications

Nurses must ensure that their histories and assessments do not presume heterosexuality. An example of this is: "Are you sexually active? If so, with males, females, or both?" Youth who are homeless as the result of disapproval and abuse have difficulty trusting adults. Nurses must be nonjudgmental and ensure confidentiality for these young people.

Note: From "Sexual Health Risks and Protective Resources in Gay, Lesbian, Bisexual, and Heterosexual Homeless Youth," by L. Rew, T. A. Whittaker, M. A. Taylor-Seehafer, and L. R. Smith, 2005, *Journal for Specialists in Pediatric Nursing, 10*(1), pp. 11–19.

Nursing interventions to promote sexual health and function focus largely on the nurse's teaching role. For example, clients need to be taught about normal sexual function, the effects of medications on sexual function, preventing sexually transmitted diseases, and performing breast and testicular self-examinations. In addition to teaching, nurses can do the following to help clients maintain a healthy sexual self-concept:

- Provide privacy during intimate body care.
- Involve the client's partner in physical care.
- Give attention to the client's appearance and dress.
- Give clients privacy to meet their sexual needs alone or with a partner within physically safe limits.

Remember that clients' comfort in discussing sex-related topics and being examined is culturally influenced. For example, Latina women prefer to establish a comfortable rapport with providers by discussing casual topics before discussing intimate issues (Katz, 2003). Culture and age interact in determining some sexual practices. For example, one study showed that sexually active African American adolescents with demanding mothers were more likely to use condoms, and sexually active white adolescents with demanding mothers were less likely to use condoms (Cox, 2006). Asian American adolescents receive very little sex education from their parents since this is a culturally unmentionable subject. However, although they believe themselves to be at low risk, Asian American women have among the highest rates of certain STIs (Kao, 2006). Thus, planning for these clients must include using culturally sensitive communication techniques implemented with both clients and culturally appropriate family members.

IMPLEMENTING

The interventions the nurse selects are based on the data obtained from the client and the identified nursing diagnoses. Many interventions are directed at providing information about sexual health and counseling for altered sexual function.

Nurses require six basic skills to help clients in the area of sexuality:

- Self-knowledge and comfort with their own sexuality
- Acceptance of sexuality as an important area for nursing intervention and a willingness to work with clients who express their sexuality in a variety of ways
- Knowledge of sexual growth and development throughout the life cycle
- Knowledge of basic sexuality, including how certain health problems and treatments may affect sexuality and sexual function and which interventions facilitate sexual expression and functioning
- Therapeutic communication skills
- Ability to recognize the need for all clients and family members to have the topic of sexuality introduced not only in written or audiovisual materials but also in a verbal discussion.

> ### CLINICAL ALERT
>
> As a result of culture, age, gender, and personal characteristics, not every nurse will be comfortable discussing sex with every client. However, it is the nurse's responsibility to ensure that someone introduces the topic with the client.

Providing Sexual Health Teaching

Providing education for sexual health is an important component of nursing implementation. Many sexual problems exist because of sexual ignorance; many others can be prevented with effective sexual health teaching. Examples of important areas of teaching are sex education (including self-examination) and responsible sexual behavior.

SEX EDUCATION Nurses can assist clients to understand their anatomy and how their body functions. For example, understanding the anatomy of the genitals may help women learn how their body responds to sexual stimulation. Both men and women need to learn the kind of stimulation that is pleasing and causes arousal. The importance of open communication between partners should also be encouraged. Women may also benefit from learning Kegel exercises. These exercises involve contraction and relaxation of the pubococcygeal muscle, the muscle that contracts when a person prevents urine flow. The benefits of Kegel exercises include increased pelvic floor muscle tone; increased vaginal lubrication during sexual arousal; increased sensation during intercourse; increased genital sensitivity; stronger gripping of the base of the penis; earlier postpartum recovery of the pelvic floor muscle; and increased flexibility of episiotomy scars (Berman & Berman, 2005). The steps to perform Kegel exercises are discussed in Chapter 33 ∞ because these exercises are also used in bladder retraining.

Details about physiologic changes that occur during major developmental crises should be provided as part of general health care. For example, the nurse needs to discuss the effects of puberty, pregnancy, menopause, and the male climacteric on sexual function. When clients experience illness or surgery that may alter sexual function, the nurse needs to discuss effects of treatment (e.g., medications) and any changes that need to be undertaken to ensure safe sex (e.g., position changes or a safe time to resume sexual intercourse after a heart attack).

Parents often need assistance to learn ways to answer questions and what information to provide for their children starting in the preschool years. Parents need to be the primary educators of children at an early age; however, peers, teachers, media, and toys also teach about sexual issues.

Although there is an increasing awareness today of sexuality and sexual functioning, some people still hold certain myths and misconceptions about sexuality. Many of these are handed down in families and are part of the beliefs in a particular culture. It is highly important that nurses learn about the beliefs clients hold and provide up-to-date information. The website of the Sexuality Information and Education

Council of the United States has a wealth of information on various aspects of sexuality.

TEACHING SELF-EXAMINATION Monthly breast self-examination (BSE) for women and monthly testicular self-examination (TSE) for men can play an important role in early detection of disease, resulting in a greater chance of cure and less complex treatment. Clients need to be assured that most lumps discovered are not cancerous, but it is essential that all lumps or other detected abnormalities be checked by the client's primary care provider for accurate diagnosis. All nursing history assessments of clients need to include the client's understanding and practice of BSE or TSE. Self-examination involves both inspection and palpation procedures and should be conducted once a month.

Although 99% of the more than 200,000 new breast cancers in the United States each year occur in women (Jemal et al., 2005), men with an increased risk of breast cancer due to high estrogen levels or strong family history of breast cancer should also learn BSE (Smith, Cokkinides, & Eyre, 2006). For BSE a regular time is best—such as 1 week following menstruation, when breast tenderness and fullness caused by fluid retention have subsided, or on the same day of the month for men or postmenopausal women. People who examine themselves regularly become familiar with the shape and texture of their breasts. The steps of BSE are very similar to those used when the nurse performs breast examination (see Skill 17–13 Chapter 17 ∞). For specific techniques of breast self-examination, see Client Teaching.

Testicular cancer occurs in more than 8,000 American men each year (Jemal et al., 2005). Starting at age 15, monthly self-exams of the testicles are an effective way for men to get to know this area of their body and thus detect testicular cancer at an early and very curable stage. The best time for TSE is after a warm bath or shower when the scrotal sac is relaxed. For specific techniques of self-examination, see the Client Teaching feature.

RESPONSIBLE SEXUAL BEHAVIOR Responsible sexual behavior involves the prevention of sexually transmitted diseases, the prevention of unwanted pregnancy, and the avoidance of sexual harassment or abuse.

STI Prevention The prevention of STIs is an essential part of sexual health teaching. Increases in these diseases are due to two factors: (a) changing sexual morality that has permitted increased sexual activity and (b) an increase in the number of sexual partners. Because the term *sexually transmitted disease* elicits feelings of guilt, shame, and fear, people frequently do not seek medical help as early as they should. Clients need education about these diseases, preventive measures, and early treatment. Many STIs can be treated quickly and effectively. Others may have serious consequences. For example, women may develop pelvic inflammatory disease (PID) resulting in damage to the reproductive structures and possible infertility. AIDS has no cure. The anxiety about HIV transmission has caused many individuals to alter their sexual behavior, such as using a condom during intercourse.

CLIENT TEACHING — Breast Self-Examination

Inspection before a Mirror

Look for any change in size or shape; lumps or thickenings; any rashes or other skin irritations; dimpled or puckered skin; any discharge or change in the nipples (e.g., position or asymmetry). Inspect the breasts in all of the following positions:

- Stand and face the mirror with your arms relaxed at your sides or hands resting on the hips; then turn to the right and the left for a side view (look for any flattening in the side view).
- Bend forward from the waist with arms raised over the head.
- Stand straight with the arms raised over the head and move the arms slowly up and down at the sides. (Look for free movement of the breasts over the chest wall.)
- Press your hands firmly together at chin level while the elbows are raised to shoulder level.

Palpation: Lying Position

- Place a pillow under your right shoulder and place the right hand behind your head. This position distributes breast tissue more evenly on the chest.
- Use the finger pads (tips) of the three middle fingers (held together) on your left hand to feel for lumps.
- Press the breast tissue against the chest wall firmly enough to know how your breast feels. A ridge of firm tissue in the lower curve of each breast is normal.
- Use small circular motions systematically all the way around the breast as many times as necessary until the entire breast is covered. (Review Skill 17–13 in Chapter 17 ∞ for patterns that the client may use.)
- Bring your arm down to your side and feel under your armpit, where breast tissue is also located.
- Repeat the exam on your left breast, using the finger pads of your right hand.

Palpation: Standing or Sitting

- Repeat the examination of both breasts while upright with one arm behind your head. This position makes it easier to check the area where a large percentage of breast cancers are found, the upper outer part of the breast and toward the armpit.
- *Optional:* Do the upright BSE in the shower. Soapy hands glide more easily over wet skin. Report any changes to your health care provider promptly.

The Clinical Manifestations feature, earlier in this chapter, lists common signs of STIs for which people should seek medical care. Methods for decreasing exposure to STIs are described in the Client Teaching feature.

CLINICAL ALERT

It may be wise for both male and female nurses to request permission from a parent or guardian before teaching testicular self-examination to teenage boys. Although the nurse need not touch the boy during the teaching, the boy must touch himself during TSE and parents may prefer the nurse not instruct him to do so.

Testicular Self-Examination

- Choose one day of each month (e.g., the first or last day of each month) to examine yourself.
- Examine yourself when you are taking a warm shower or bath.
- Support the testicle underneath with one hand. Place the fingers of the other hand under the testicle and the thumb on top (this may be easier to do if the leg on that side is raised).
- Roll each testicle between the thumb and fingers of your hand, feeling for lumps, thickening, or a hardening in consistency (Figure 28–2). The testes should feel smooth.
- Palpate the epididymis, a cordlike structure on the top and back of the testicle. The epididymis feels soft and not as smooth as a testicle.
- Locate the spermatic cord, or vas deferens, which extends upward from the scrotum toward the base of the penis. It should feel firm and smooth.

- Using a mirror, inspect your testicles for swelling, any enlargement, or lumps in the skin of the testicle.
- Report any lumps or other changes to your health care provider promptly.

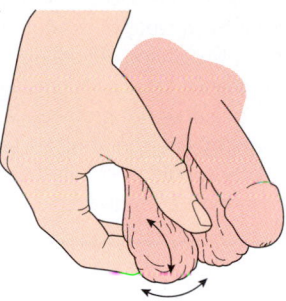

Figure 28–2 ● Rolling the testicle between the thumb and fingers.

Preventing Transmission of STIs and HIV

- Limit the number of sexual partners.
- Use condoms in nonmonogamous and homosexual relationships or other relationships that have the potential for STI transmission.
- Follow safer sex practices during oral sex including the use of a latex dental dam during cunnilingus or oral anal contact to prevent STI transmission.
- Talk openly with sexual partners about how to have "safer sex" and be honest about any history of an STI.
- Abstain from high-risk sexual activity with a partner known to have or suspected of having an STI.
- Report to a health care facility for examination whenever in doubt about possible exposure or when signs of an STI are evident.
- When an STI is diagnosed, notify all partners and encourage them to seek treatment.
- Avoid transfusions of banked blood or blood products. Use autologous transfusions (donation of own blood before surgery) for elective surgery whenever possible.

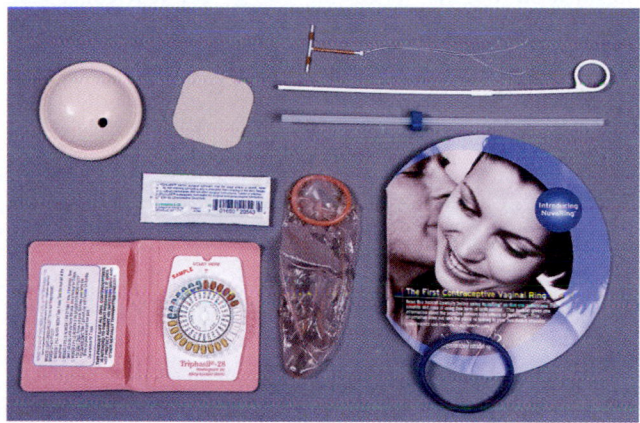

Figure 28–3 ● Methods of contraception.

Prevention of Unwanted Pregnancies Prevention of unwanted pregnancies must be addressed not only with adolescents but also with couples who are planning the time of births and want to space children and limit family size. Nurses need to be familiar with various contraceptive methods and their advantages, disadvantages, contraindications, effectiveness, safety, and cost (Figure 28–3). The various methods are outlined in Box 28–2. It is beyond the scope of this text to discuss contraceptives in detail.

Counseling for Altered Sexual Function

One technique nurses can use to help clients with altered sexual function is the PLISSIT model, developed by Annon

(1974) for this purpose. The model involves four progressive levels represented by the acronym PLISSIT:

P	Permission giving
LI	Limited information
SS	Specific suggestions
IT	Intensive therapy

At each level, the nurse provides additional guidance and information to the client and therefore requires more specialized and specific knowledge and skill. All professional nurses should be able to function at the first three levels. At the levels of limited information, specific suggestions, and intensive therapy, the nurse can also refer the client to a health care provider more skilled to assist the client with the particular issues identified during the first level.

PERMISSION GIVING Clients may feel that they need permission to be sexual beings, to ask questions, to show affection, and to express themselves sexually. Giving

---

BOX 28–2 Methods of Pregnancy Avoidance

- Abstinence
- Withdrawal of the penis before ejaculation (coitus interruptus)
- Fertility awareness (identification of the days of the month when conception is most likely to occur and abstaining during that time)
- Mechanical barriers: vaginal diaphragm, cervical cap, condom (*Note*: There are three types of condom materials: latex, lambskin, and polyurethane. All are equally effective at preventing pregnancy. Latex condoms are the least expensive. Lambskin pore size does not protect against STIs as well as the others. Polyurethane condoms are recommended if contact with latex should be avoided. Polyurethane is the material used in female condoms.)

- Chemical barriers: insertion of spermicidal foams, creams, jellies, or suppositories into the vagina before intercourse
- Intrauterine devices (IUDs)
- Hormonal: oral contraceptives (birth control pills), subdermal implants of synthetic progestin, transdermal patches (*Note*: Certain antibiotics decrease the effectiveness of oral contraceptives and patches. Women on these antibiotics must use an alternative method of contraception until their antibiotic treatment is completed. Other drug interactions can occur with implants.)
- Surgical sterilization: tubal ligation and vasectomy
- Abortion

---

permission means that the nurse by attitude or word lets the client know that sexual thoughts, fantasies, and behaviors between informed consenting adults are allowed. Giving permission begins when the nurse acknowledges the client's spoken and unspoken sexual concerns and conveys the attitude that sexual concerns and needs are important to health and recovery.

For example, the nurse might ask a client recuperating from a heart attack the following questions:

"Now that you're recuperating and you've had some time to sort out your feelings, have you thought about how your heart attack might alter your sex life?"

"Have you and your partner discussed how you both feel about it?"

LIMITED INFORMATION Clients need accurate but concise information. The nurse might explain what is normal; how some medical conditions, treatments, injuries, or surgeries may affect sexuality and sexual functioning; or how aging may affect sexuality and functioning.

Continuing with the preceding example, the nurse shares information and informs the client about how the heart attack might affect the client's sex life, including the following:

"Your heart attack will not change your sexual responsiveness. Most people can resume intercourse in 4 to 6 weeks, but this should be confirmed by your doctor. If you can climb a flight of stairs without having chest pain you should be able to resume having sex since it takes about the same amount of energy."

"Many postcoronary clients fear sexual intercourse because of the physical exertion associated with it. However, your prescribed program of progressive physical activity will also increase your tolerance for sexual activity."

Many clients recuperating from childbirth, for example, or specific illness or disease (e.g., heart attack) need in-

struction about safer sexual activities and the effects that therapy may have on sexual functioning. The following topics need to be considered:

- When sexual activity is safe
- Specific sexual activities that are unsafe, and why
- Adaptations needed for resuming a satisfactory sexual life
- The side effects of prescribed medications on sexual functioning, and the need to notify the primary care provider for possible dose or medication adjustment should problems develop

SPECIFIC SUGGESTIONS At this level, the nurse requires specialized knowledge and skill about how sexuality and functioning may be affected by a disease process or therapy and what interventions might be effective. The nurse offers suggestions to help the client adapt sexual activity to promote optimal functioning, such as what measures might be used to alleviate vaginal dryness, safe positions for intercourse following a total hip replacement, safer and unsafe sexual practices following a heart attack, and ways to handle ostomy appliances, urinary catheters, casts, or other devices (e.g., prostheses) during sexual activity. Similarly, nurses who work on a cardiac unit need specialized knowledge about sexual readjustment during cardiac rehabilitation, and nurses working with clients with spinal cord injuries need information about the sexual consequences of spinal injuries at various levels.

Using the example of the client recuperating from a heart attack, the nurse may offer the following suggestion:

"Many people express concern about the stress of certain positions for intercourse, but you may use whatever position is comfortable for you and your partner, or try side-lying or partner-on-top positions."

INTENSIVE THERAPY At this level of intervention, nurses must have specialized preparation and knowledge of sexual and gender identity disorders. Nurses who function in the sex therapist role should meet the qualifications for practice identified by the American Association of Sexuality Educators, Counselors, and Therapists (AASECT), which differentiate sex counseling from sex therapy. *Sex counseling* helps clients incorporate their sexual knowledge into satisfying lifestyles and socially responsible behavior. *Sex therapy* is a highly specialized, in-depth treatment to help clients resolve serious sexual problems. AASECT publishes a national directory of professionals certified to provide sex education, counseling, or therapy.

Dealing with Inappropriate Sexual Behavior

Nurses, both male and female, may encounter a variety of sexually inappropriate behaviors for a number of reasons. The behavior may be either aggressive or nonaggressive. Clients may act out sexually by:

- Exposing themselves.
- Asking the nurse to provide intimate physical care, such as bathing genital areas, when they are capable of doing this themselves.
- Touching or grabbing the nurse's genitals or buttocks.
- Making blatant sexual statements to the nurse.
- Offering the nurse sex.
- Whistling; making comments about the nurse's attractiveness or desirability.
- Making sexual comments to another client in the same room or to visitors about the "sexy" nurse or what they would like to do sexually with the nurse.

Possible reasons for this inappropriate behavior are:

- Fear or anxiety over future ability to function sexually.
- Unmet needs for intimacy and sexual closeness because of hospitalization, injury, illness, treatment, lack of a partner, or lack of privacy.
- Misinterpretation of the nurse's behavior as sexual or provocative.
- Need for reassurance that they are still sexual beings and still sexually attractive.
- Need for attention.
- Confusion: Neurologic impairment or trauma can lead clients to use profane sexual language, engage in masturbation, expose themselves, or inappropriately touch or grab at the nurse.
- Need to control: Clients may be experiencing loss of control over their lives because of hospitalization, injury, or illness.
- Need for power.
- Belief that flirtatious behavior is expected due to media portrayal of nurses as sexy, available, and experienced.

Before implementing any nursing interventions, the nurse should first ensure that the behavior is inappropriate and not an attempt to communicate a physical need. For example, clients may expose themselves if they are febrile, pull at the penis if a catheter is uncomfortable or irritating, or reach for the nurse if unable to communicate verbally. Nursing strategies to deal with inappropriate sexual behavior are listed in Box 28–3.

| **BOX 28–3** | **Nursing Strategies for Inappropriate Sexual Behavior** |

- Communicate that the behavior is not acceptable by saying, for example, "I really do not like the things you are saying," or "I see you are not dressed. I will be back in 10 minutes and will help you with breakfast when you get your clothes on."
- Tell the client how the behavior makes you feel: "When you act like that toward me, I am very uncomfortable. It embarrasses me and makes it hard for me to give you the kind of nursing care you need."
- Identify the behavior you expect: "Please call me by my name, not 'honey,'" or "I expect you to keep yourself covered when I am in the room. If you are feeling hot or something is uncomfortable, let me know, and I will try to make you more comfortable."
- Set firm limits: Take the client's hand and move it away, use direct eye contact, and say, "Don't do that!"

- Try to refocus clients from the inappropriate behavior to their real concerns and fears; offer to discuss sexuality concerns: "All morning you have been making very personal sexual comments about yourself. Sometimes people talk like that when they are concerned about the sexual part of their life and how their illness will affect them. Are there things that you have questions about or would like to talk about?"
- Report the incident to your nursing instructor, charge nurse, or clinical nurse specialist. Discuss the incident, your feelings, and possible interventions.
- Assign a nurse who will confront the behavior and relate to the client in a consistent manner.
- Clarify the consequences of continued inappropriate behavior (avoidance, withdrawal of services, no chance to help resolve underlying concerns of client).

EVALUATING

The goals established during the planning phase are evaluated according to specific desired outcomes also established during that phase. If any outcomes have not been achieved, the nurse should explore the reasons with questions such as the following:

- Were risk factors correctly identified?
- Did the client convey all significant fears and concerns about sexuality?

- Was the client more comfortable following discussions about sexual matters?
- Did the client understand the nurse's teaching?
- Was the health teaching compatible with the client's culture and religious values?
- Was the client ready to deal with sexuality problems?

CHAPTER HIGHLIGHTS

- Sexuality is important in developing self-identity, interpersonal relationships, intimacy, and love.
- There is a tremendous range of variation in how people express their sexuality including sexual orientation, gender identity, erotic preferences, and sexual lifestyles.
- Factors that affect sexuality include developmental level, family, culture, religious values, personal expectations and ethics, disease processes, medications, and relationship problems.
- Sexual problems include desire disorders, arousal disorders, orgasmic disorders, problems with satisfaction, and sexual pain disorders.
- Assessing risk for or actual sexual problems is part of the initial nursing assessment. Assessment should also be carried out when clients or support people present cues that problems exist or when clients have an illness that could cause sexual problems.
- Nurses assess attitudes toward sexuality, including factors that affect attitudes and behaviors.

- Before assisting clients with sexual problems, nurses must acquire accurate information about sexuality, identify and accept their own sexual values and behaviors as well as those of others, and be comfortable acquiring and disseminating information about sexuality.
- Nursing diagnoses for clients with sexual problems are related to many contributing factors, including altered body structure or function, lack of knowledge or misinformation about sexual matters, physical or psychologic abuse, value conflicts, and loss or lack of a partner.
- Nursing interventions focus largely on teaching clients about sexual function and sexuality, responsible sexual behavior that includes the prevention of STIs and unwanted pregnancies, and self-examination of the breasts and testicles.
- Counseling clients with altered sexual functions can be facilitated by using the PLISSIT model: permission giving (P), limited information (LI), and specific suggestions (SS). Intensive therapy (IT) requires intervention by clinical nurse specialists or sex therapists.

THINK ABOUT IT

Refer to the chapter-opening scenario and answer these questions.

1. Assuming the nurse caring for Mrs. O'Leary is much younger than she, how might the nurse increase the client's comfort level when discussing sexual and intimate matters?

2. When conducting a nursing interview related to sexual matters, what questions might you want to ask?

3. What teaching would you anticipate appropriate for this client?

∞ *See suggested responses to Think About It on MyNursingKit.*

TEST YOUR KNOWLEDGE

1. The nursing student asks if clients ever introduce the topic of sex. The nursing instructor explains that clients are not likely to introduce the topic of sex because:
   1. They assume that sexual functioning is not something nurses would be knowledgeable about.
   2. Most clients have few, if any, questions or problems regarding sexual function.
   3. Clients prefer to discuss problems with health care providers of the same sex.
   4. They are too embarrassed.

2. A nurse receives information that a client is a transsexual. Appropriate care is based on the knowledge that which of the following is most representative of this client?
   1. Gonadal gender, internal organs, and external genitals are contradictory.
   2. Sexual anatomy is not consistent with gender identity.
   3. Sexual attraction is to individuals of both genders.
   4. Gender identity is altered by acute psychosis.

3. In conducting client teaching the nurse bases content on knowing that which of the following is true regarding masturbation?
   1. People who masturbate are psychologically disturbed.
   2. Teenage masturbation interferes with academic achievement.
   3. Most people do not masturbate past the teenage years.
   4. Masturbation is a way people learn about their sexual response.

4. A male client is beginning an antidepressant medication. Which of the following should the nurse include in the teaching plan?
   1. "Your partner will be pleased because your sexual functioning is going to improve."
   2. "You may find that your desire for sex will decrease while on this medication."
   3. "Retrograde ejaculation is a common problem when taking antidepressants."
   4. "Your skin will probably become supersensitive to touch, so you may need to change your activity during sex."

5. A client who had a hysterectomy 3 days ago says to the nurse, "I no longer feel like a real woman." What is the nurse's best response?
   1. "Don't worry about that. The feeling will probably go away."
   2. "You should talk to your doctor about how you feel."
   3. "I don't blame you but sex isn't that important anymore is it?"
   4. "You feel like the loss of your uterus affected your sexuality? Tell me more about your feelings."

6. Because a client reports having dyspareunia, it is most appropriate for the nurse to ask which of the following questions?
   1. "Have you talked with your partner about this discomfort?"
   2. "Have you had these spasms since you became sexually active?"
   3. "Do you have pain before your period begins?"
   4. "Do your breasts swell large enough to need a larger bra?"

7. It is most important for the nurse to include at least some sexual health history questions for clients taking:
   1. Anti-inflammatories (such as aspirin or ibuprofen).
   2. Hypnotics (sleeping pills).
   3. Antihypertensives (blood pressure medications).
   4. Antihistamines (cold medications).

8. A nurse informs a client who is 8 1/2 months pregnant that it is best to abstain from intercourse until after the birth of the baby. This communication is most representative of which component of the PLISSIT model?
   1. Permission giving (P)
   2. Limited information (LI)
   3. Specific suggestions (SS)
   4. Intensive therapy (IT)

9. A 75-year-old male client reports decreased frequency of sexual intercourse although he does not express dissatisfaction or difficulty. He seems a little embarrassed by the discussion but is engaged and asks some questions. An appropriate nursing diagnosis would be which of the following?
   1. *Sexual Dysfunction*
   2. *Disturbed Body Image*
   3. *Sedentary Lifestyle*
   4. *Readiness for Enhanced Knowledge*

10. Which of the following outcomes may indicate to the nurse a need for a referral to a more highly skilled therapist?
    1. The client verbalizes methods of modifying sexual activity according to physical limitations.
    2. The client requests the phone number of a sex education support group.

3. Suggestions given by the nurse are ineffective in reaching the desired goals.
4. The client reports experimenting with new sexual activities.

∞ *See answers to Test Your Knowledge in Appendix A.*

REFERENCES AND SELECTED BIBLIOGRAPHY

American Academy of Pediatrics Task Force on Circumcision. (1999). Circumcision policy statement. *Pediatrics, 103,* 686–693.

Annon, J. (1974). *The behavioral treatment of sexual problems. Vol. 1. Brief therapy.* New York: Harper & Row.

Barnett, R., & Rivers, C. (2004). *Same difference.* New York: Basic Books.

Berman, L., & Berman, J. (2005). *Secrets of the sexually satisfied woman: Ten keys to unlocking ultimate pleasure.* New York: Hyperion Press.

Bulechek, G. M., Butcher, H. K., & Dochterman, J. M. (Eds.). (2008). *Nursing interventions: classification (NIC)* (5th ed.). St. Louis: Mosby.

Butler, S. S. (2004). Gay, lesbian, bisexual, and transgender (GLBT) elders: The challenges and resilience of this marginalized group. *Journal of Human Behavior in the Social Environment, 9*(4), 25–44.

Cornog, M. (2003). *The BIG book of masturbation.* San Francisco: Down There Press.

Cox, M. F. (2006). Racial differences in parenting dimensions and adolescent condom use at sexual debut. *Public Health Nursing, 23*(1), 2–10.

Elson, J. (2004). *Am I still a woman? Hysterectomy and gender identity.* Philadelphia: Temple University Press.

Elwood, A. (2005). Female genital cutting, 'circumcision' and mutilation. *Contemporary Sexuality, 39*(1), i–vii.

Givson, M. C. (2004). Sexual health: The neglected component of care. *Perspectives, 27*(4), 5–7.

Hammoud, M. M., White, C. B., & Fetters, M. D. (2005). Opening cultural doors: Providing culturally sensitive healthcare to Arab American and American Muslim patients. *American Journal of Obstetrics and Gynecology, 193,* 1307–1311.

Higgins, A., Barker, P., & Begley, C. M. (2004). Hypersexuality and dementia: Dealing with inappropriate sexual expression. *British Journal of Nursing, 13,* 1330–1334.

Jemal, A., Tiwari, R. C., Murray, T., Ghafoor, A., Samuels, A., Ward, E., et al. (2005). Cancer statistics, 2004. *CA: A Cancer Journal for Clinicians, 54,* 8–29, 57–59.

Joannides, P. (2004). *The guide to getting it on* (3rd ed.). West Hollywood, CA: Goofy Foot Press.

Kaestle, C. E., Halpern, C. T., Miller, W. C., & Ford, C. A. (2005). Young age at first sexual intercourse and sexually transmitted infections in adolescents and young adults. *American Journal of Epidemiology, 161,* 774–780.

Kao, T. S. (2006). Sexual health education disparities in Asian American adolescents. *Journal for Specialists in Pediatric Nursing, 11,* 57–60.

Katz, A. (2003). Culturally competent care. "Where I come from, we don't talk about that": Exploring sexuality & culture among Blacks, Asians and Hispanics. *AWHONN-Lifelines, 6*(6), 533–536.

Katz, A. (2005a). Cultural diversity. "Caregiving" is cultural. *Journal of Professional Nursing, 21,* 139–140.

Katz, A. (2005b). Sexually speaking. Do ask, do tell: Why do so many nurses avoid the topic of sexuality? *American Journal of Nursing, 105*(7), 66–68.

Katz, A. (2005c). Sexually speaking. Sexuality and hysterectomy: Finding the right words: Responding to patients' concerns about the potential effects of surgery. *American Journal of Nursing, 105*(12), 65–68.

Katz, A. (2005). The sounds of silence: Sexuality information for cancer patients. *Journal of Clinical Oncology, 23,* 238–241.

Kaufman, M., Silverberg, C., & Odette, F. (2003). *The ultimate guide to sex and disability: For all of us who live with disabilities, chronic pain and illness.* San Francisco: Cleis Press.

Lewis, J. H., Rosen, R., Goldstein, I., & the Consensus Panel on Health Care Clinician Management of Erectile Dysfunction. (2003). Erectile dysfunction: A panel's recommendations for management. *American Journal of Nursing, 102*(10), 48–57.

Lips, H. M. (2005). *Sex and gender* (5th ed.). Columbus, OH: McGraw-Hill.

Lund-Nielsen, B., Muller, K., & Adamsen, L. (2005). Malignant wounds in women with breast cancer: Feminine and sexual perspectives. *Journal of Clinical Nursing, 14,* 56–64.

McCammon, S. L., Knox, D., & Schacht, C. (2004). *Choices in sexuality* (2nd ed.). Cincinnati, OH: Atomic Dog Publishing.

Metzger, D. A. (2004). New advances in the diagnosis and treatment of vulvar/vestibular pain disorders. *Conference proceedings: Women's Sexual Health.* The Berman Center and Northwestern University, Feinberg School of Medicine, Department of Obstetrics and Gynecology, Chicago.

Mick, J., Hughes, M., & Cohen, M. Z. (2004). Using the BETTER model to assess sexuality. *Clinical Journal of Oncology Nursing, 8,* 84–86.

Moorhead, S., Johnson, M., Maas, M. L., & Swanson, E. (Eds.). (2008). *Nursing outcomes classification (NOC)* (4th ed.). St. Louis: Mosby.

Morrison, T. (1992). *Jazz.* New York: Alfred A. Knopf.

NANDA International. (2009). *NANDA nursing diagnoses: Definitions and classification 2009–2011.* West Sussex, U.K.: Wiley-Blackwell.

Nelson, C. P., Dunn, R., Wan, J., & Wei, J. T. (2005). The increasing incidence of newborn circumcision: Data from the nationwide inpatient sample. *Journal of Urology, 173,* 978–981.

Rew, L., Whittaker, T. A., Taylor-Seehafer, M. A., & Smith, L. R. (2005). Sexual health risks and protective resources in gay, lesbian, bisexual, and heterosexual homeless youth. *Journal for Specialists in Pediatric Nursing, 10*(1), 11–19.

Smith, R. A., Cokkinides, V., & Eyre, H. J. (2006). American Cancer Society recommendations for the early detection of cancer, 2006. *CA: A Cancer Journal for Clinicians, 56,* 11–25.

Snow, J. (2004). *How it feels to have a gay or lesbian parent.* Binghamton, NY: Haworth Press.

U.S. National Center for Health Statistics. (2005). *Trends in circumcisions among newborns.* Retrieved December 5, 2009, from http://www.cdc.gov/nchs/data/hestat/circumcisions/circumcisions.htm

van Daalen, C. (2005). Girls' experiences in physical education, competition, evaluation, & degradation. *Journal of School Nursing, 21*(2), 115–121.

Vision of sexual health. (2004). *Contemporary Sexuality, 38*(7), 1–5.

World Association of Sexology. (1999). *Declaration of sexual rights.* Adopted at the 14th World Congress of Sexology, Hong Kong and People's Republic of China.

World Health Organization. (1975). *Education and treatment in human sexuality: The training of health professionals.* Geneva: Author.

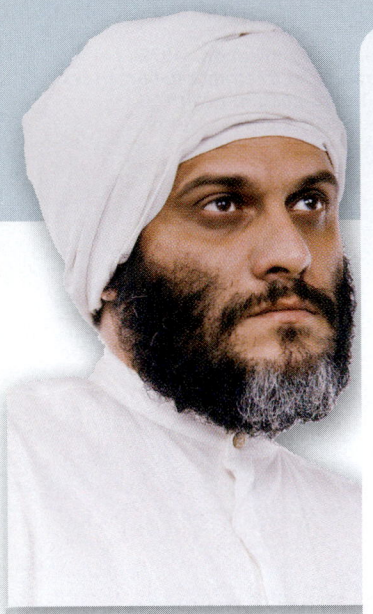

Felix Kamarra is a 41-year-old Muslim admitted to the acute care facility follow-ing a severe episode of rectal bleeding. After several diagnostic tests, Mr. Kamarra is diagnosed with anal cancer with metastasis to the liver, bone, and brain. He meets with the oncologist, who informs him they will treat the disease aggressively but pro-vides a poor prognosis for success. Mr. Kamarra tells the nurse, "I have done many things in my life that I am not proud of, and I guess this is my punishment for sins against Allah."

LEARNING OUTCOMES

After completing this chapter, you will be able to:

1. Define the concepts of spirituality and religion as they relate to nursing and health care.

2. Identify characteristics of spiritual health.

3. Identify factors associated with spiritual distress and manifestations of it.

4. Describe the spiritual development of the individual across the life span.

5. Describe the influence of spiritual and religious beliefs about diet, dress, prayer and meditation, and birth and death on health care.

6. Assess the spiritual needs of clients and plan nursing care to assist clients with spiritual needs.

7. Describe nursing interventions to support clients' spiritual beliefs and religious practices.

8. Identify desired outcomes for evaluating the client's spiritual health.

KEY TERMS

Agnostic p839
Atheist p839
Faith p839
Holy day p840

Hope p839
Kosher p842
Meditation p842
Monotheism p839

Polytheism p839
Prayer p841
Presencing p845
Spiritual distress p838

Spiritual health p837
Spiritual well-being p837
Spirituality p837
Transcendence p839

Because nurses provide holistic care, they care not only for the physical body and mind, but also for the client's spirit. Meeting the client's spiritual needs can decrease suffering and aid in physical and mental healing. To implement spiritual care, nurses need to be skilled in establishing trusting nurse–client relationships. Such spiritual caregiving skill requires that the nurse possess a healthy spiritual self-awareness. This personal spirituality inevitably influences nursing care. In particular, this spiritual self-awareness will help the nurse to identify and be empathic toward the spiritual concerns of clients.

In addition to spiritual self-awareness, nurses need some awareness of the diverse spiritual beliefs and practices that their clients may possess. Because spiritual beliefs and practices are coping resources for persons, understanding how such beliefs and practices help or hinder a client's health is vital. A client's experience with what is seen as sacred or divine is complex and individual. Thus, each client needs to be approached in light of these unique needs. In addition to distressing spiritual or religious needs, many clients have spiritual strengths that the nurse can nurture. Whether the client presents with a need to relieve spiritual distress or to enhance spiritual health, nurses can implement spiritual care therapeutics that promote spiritual and emotional health, help with coping and adjustment, or assist one to face a more peaceful death.

SPIRITUALITY DESCRIBED

Spirituality, faith, and religion are separate entities, yet the words are often used interchangeably. The word *spiritual* derives from the Latin word *spiritus,* which means "to blow" or "to breathe," and has come to connote that which gives life or essence to being human. **Spirituality** refers to that part of being human that seeks meaningfulness through intra-, inter-, and transpersonal connection (Reed, 1992). Spirituality generally involves a belief in a relationship with some higher power, creative force, divine being, or infinite source of energy. For example, a person may believe in "God," "Allah," the "Great Spirit," or a "Higher Power." Spirituality includes the following aspects (Martsolf & Mickley, 1998):

- Meaning (having purpose, making sense of life)
- Value (having cherished beliefs and standards)
- Transcendence (appreciating a dimension that is beyond the self)
- Connecting (relating to others, nature, Ultimate Other)
- Becoming (which involves reflection, allowing life to unfold, and knowing who one is)

Words or concepts reflective of spirituality, such as faith, courage, cheer, and hope, may be used in ordinary speech when discussing spirituality.

Spirituality can be described by measuring it, so to speak, on a "spirit titer" (Jourard, 1971). One's spirit titer is

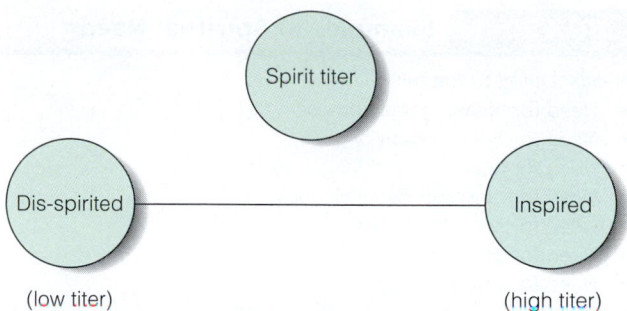

Figure 29–1 ● Spirit titer.

influenced by numerous factors, such as life experiences, coping skills, social supports, and individual belief systems. Individuals experience multiple changes and losses over their life span, and if their spirit titer is low they may become dis-spirited, or depressed. If they have a high spirit titer, they will lean toward being inspired and becoming an inspiration to others in spite of hardships they experience (Figure 29–1). Nurses need to direct their goals and planning to assist clients in attaining and maintaining a high spirit titer.

Spiritual Needs

Just as everybody has a spiritual dimension, all clients have needs that reflect their spirituality. These needs are often accentuated by an illness or other health crisis. Clients who have well-defined spiritual beliefs may find that their beliefs are challenged by their health situation, or may cling to their beliefs more firmly and appreciatively. Clients who have no defined beliefs may suddenly come face to face with challenging questions such as "why me?" and others related to the meaning and purpose of life. Nurses need to be sensitive to indications of the client's spiritual needs and respond appropriately, as discussed later. Examples of spiritual needs are listed in Box 29–1.

Spiritual Well-Being

Spiritual health, or **spiritual well-being,** is manifested by a feeling of being "generally alive, purposeful, and fulfilled" (Ellison, 1983, p. 332). According to Pilch (1998), spiritual wellness is "a way of living, a lifestyle that views and lives life as purposeful and pleasurable, that seeks out life-sustaining and life-enriching options to be chosen freely at every opportunity, and that sinks its roots deeply into spiritual values and/or specific religious beliefs" (p. 31). Spiritual health, as defined by the Nursing Outcomes Classification project (Moorhead, Johnson, & Maas, 2004, p. 519) is the "connectedness with self, others, higher power, all life, nature and the universe that transcends and empowers the self." Indicators of spiritual health are shown in Box 29–2.

People nurture or enhance their spirituality in many ways. Some focus on development of the inner self; others focus on the expression of their spiritual energy with others or the outer world. Relating to one's inner self or soul may be achieved by conducting an inner dialogue with a higher

---

BOX 29–1   **Examples of Spiritual Needs**

Needs related to the self:
- Need for meaning and purpose
- Need to express creativity
- Need for hope
- Need to transcend life challenges
- Need for personal dignity
- Need for gratitude
- Need for vision
- Need to prepare for and accept death

Needs related to others:
- Need to forgive others
- Need to cope with loss of loved ones

Needs related to the Ultimate Other:
- Need to be certain there is a God or Ultimate Power in the universe
- Need to believe that God is loving, and personally present
- Need to worship

Needs among and within groups:
- Need to contribute or improve one's community
- Need to be respected and valued
- Need to know what and when to give and take

Note: From *Spiritual Care: Nursing Theory, Research, and Practice* by E. J. Taylor, 2002, Upper Saddle River, NJ: Prentice Hall. Reprinted by permission of Pearson Education, Inc., Upper Saddle River, New Jersey.

BOX 29–2   **Indicators of Spiritual Health**

Uncompromised . . .

faith

hope

meaning and purpose in life

achievement of spiritual world

feelings of peacefulness

ability to love

ability to forgive

ability to pray

ability to worship

spiritual experiences

participation in spiritual rites and passages

participation in meditation

participation in spiritual reading

interaction with spiritual leaders

expression through song/music

expression through art

expression through writing

connectedness with inner-self

connectedness with others

interaction with others to share thoughts, feelings, and beliefs

Note: Reprinted from *Iowa Intervention Project: Nursing Outcome Classification* by S. Moorhead, M. Johnson, & M. Maas. Copyright © 2008, with permission from Elsevier.

---

power or with oneself through prayer or meditation, by analyzing dreams, by communing with nature, or by experiencing the inspiration of art (e.g., drama, music, dance). The expression of a person's spiritual energy to others is manifested in loving relationships with and service to others, joy and laughter, participation in religious services and associated fellowship gatherings and activities, and expression of compassion, empathy, forgiveness, and hope. Nurses who attend to their own spirituality are better able to work with clients who have spiritual needs (Taylor, 2005). Therefore, it is important to be comfortable with one's own spirituality.

Spiritual Distress

Spiritual distress refers to a challenge to the spiritual well-being or to the belief system that provides strength, hope, and meaning to life. Some factors that may be associated with or contribute to a person's spiritual distress include physiologic problems, treatment related concerns, and situational concerns. Physiologic problems include having a medical diagnosis of a terminal or debilitating disease, ex-

periencing pain, experiencing the loss of a body part or function, or experiencing a miscarriage or stillbirth. Treatment-related factors include recommendation for blood transfusions, abortion, surgery, dietary restrictions, amputation of a body part, or isolation. Situational factors include the death or illness of a significant other, inability to practice one's spiritual rituals, or feelings of embarrassment when practicing them (Carpenito-Moyet, 2009).

NANDA International (2009) offers the following as defining characteristics of spiritual distress:

- Expresses lack of hope, meaning and purpose in life, forgiveness of self
- Expresses being abandoned by or having anger toward God
- Refuses interaction with friends, family
- Sudden changes in spiritual practices
- Requests to see a religious leader
- No interest in nature, reading spiritual literature

No list could be complete, however, considering the complexity and variability of people and their spiritual dimensions.

RELATED CONCEPTS

Because spirituality is a reflection of an inner experience that is expressed individually, it includes as many representations as there are human beings. Concepts related to spirituality include religion, faith, hope, transcendence, and forgiveness.

Religion

Religion is an organized system of beliefs and practices. It offers a way of spiritual expression that provides guidance for believers in responding to life's questions and challenges. According to Vardey (1996, p. xv), the organized religions offer (a) a sense of community bound by common beliefs; (b) the collective study of scripture (the Torah, Bible, Koran, or others); (c) the performance of ritual; (d) the use of disciplines and practices, commandments, and sacraments; and (e) ways of taking care of the person's spirit (such as fasting, prayer, and meditation). Many traditional religious practices and rituals are related to such life events as birth, transition from childhood to adulthood, marriage, illness, and death (Figure 29–2). Religious rules of conduct, typically influenced concurrently by culture, may also apply to matters of daily life such as dress, food, social interaction, menstruation, and sexual relationships.

Religious development of an individual refers to the acceptance of specific beliefs, values, rules of conduct, and rituals. Religious development may or may not parallel spiritual development. For example, a person may follow certain religious practices and yet not internalize the symbolic meaning behind the practices. Often religious development undergirds and enhances spirituality by providing a system of belief that can suggest areas of growth to the believer. For example, the daily prayers of the Muslims bring the believers into direct relationship with the profound questions of life several times per day.

An **agnostic** is a person who doubts the existence of God or a supreme being or believes the existence of God has not been proved. An **atheist** is one without belief in a God. **Monotheism** is the belief in the existence of one God, while **polytheism** is the belief in more than one god.

Faith

Faith is to believe in or be committed to something or someone. Fowler (1981) described faith as being present in both religious and nonreligious people. Faith gives life meaning, providing the individual with strength in times of difficulty. For the client who is ill, faith—whether in a higher authority (e.g., God, Allah, Jehovah), in oneself, in the health care team, or in a combination of all—provides strength and hope.

Hope

Hope is a concept that incorporates spirituality. Stephenson (1991) suggested this definition: "a process of anticipation that involves the interaction of thinking, acting, feeling, and relating, and is directed toward a future fulfillment that is personally meaningful" (p. 1459). In the absence of hope, the client gives up, losing spirit, and illness is likely to progress more rapidly.

Transcendence

The term **transcendence** is often used interchangeably with self-transcendence, which Coward (1990) defined as: "the capacity to reach out beyond oneself, to extend oneself beyond personal concerns and to take on broader life perspectives, activities, and purposes" (p. 162). Transcendence is also thought to involve a person's recognition that there is something other or greater than the self and a seeking and valuing of that greater other, whether it is an ultimate being, force, or value.

Forgiveness

The concept of forgiveness is receiving increased attention among health care professionals. For many clients, illness or disability brings a sense of shame or guilt. The health problem is interpreted as a punishment for past sins (e.g., "Having sex before I got married is why I have breast cancer"). Clients facing imminent death may seek forgiveness from others as well as from God. Mickley and Cowles's (2001) research suggested that nurses can play a pivotal role in assisting clients to understand the process of forgiveness and to persevere through it.

SPIRITUAL DEVELOPMENT

Just as individuals develop physically, cognitively, and morally, they also develop spiritually. Several theologians have identified specific linear stages through which individuals may progress while maturing spiritually. Westerhoff (1976), for example, described faith as a way of behaving that evolves from a faith guided by parents and others during infancy and childhood to an owned faith that is internalized in adulthood and serves as a directive for

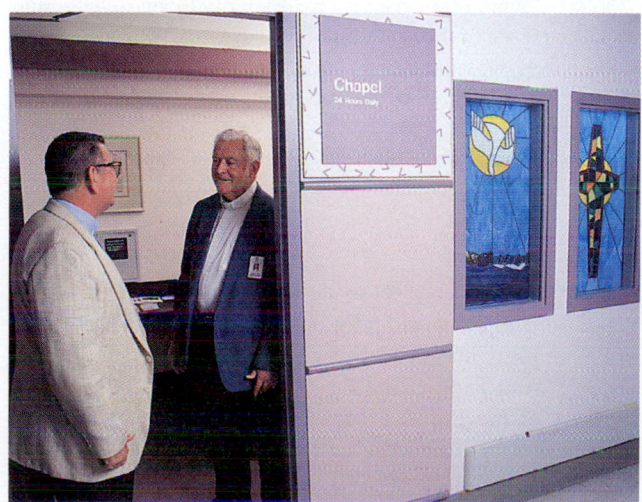

Figure 29–2 ⬤ Hospital chaplains minister to clients and their families.

TABLE 29–1	Stages of Spiritual Development
DEVELOPMENTAL STAGE	CHARACTERISTICS
0–3 years	Neonates and toddlers are acquiring fundamental spiritual qualities of trust, mutuality (shared beliefs among the group), courage, hope, and love. Transition to next stage of faith begins when child's language and thought begin to allow use of symbolism.
3–7 years	Fantasy-filled, imitative phase when child can be influenced by examples, moods, actions. Child relates intuitively to ultimate conditions of existence through stories and images, the fusion of facts and feelings. Make-believe is experienced as reality (Santa Claus, God as grandfather in the sky).
7–12 years, even into adulthood	Child attempting to sort fantasy from fact by demanding proofs or demonstrations of reality. Stories are important for finding meaning and organizing experience. Child accepts stories and beliefs literally. Ability to learn the beliefs and practices of the culture, religion.
Adolescence	Experience of the world now beyond the family unit and spiritual beliefs can aid understanding of extended environment. Generally conform to the beliefs of those around them; begin to examine beliefs objectively, especially in late adolescence.
Young adulthood	Development of a self-identity and world view differentiated from those of others. The individual forms independent commitments, lifestyle, beliefs, and attitudes. Begins to develop personal meaning for symbols of religion and faith.
Mid-adulthood	Newfound appreciation for the past; increased respect for inner voice; more awareness of myths, prejudices, and images that exist because of social background. Attempts to reconcile contradictions in mind and experience and to remain open to others' truths.
Mid- to late adulthood	Able to believe in, and live with a sense of participation in, a nonexclusive community. May work to resolve social, political, economic, or ideological problems in society. Able to embrace life, yet hold it loosely. (Martin Luther King, Jr., Mahatma Gandhi, and Mother Teresa illustrate this stage.)

Note: Adapted from content from *Stages of Faith Development: The Psychology of Human Development and the Quest for Meaning,* by James W. Fowler. Copyright © 1981, by James W. Fowler. Reprinted with permission of HarperCollins Publishers.

action. Table 29–1 describes some of the aspects of spiritual development and healthful religious behaviors during different life stages.

SPIRITUAL PRACTICES AFFECTING NURSING CARE

Clients frequently identify religious practices such as prayer as important strategies for coping with illness (Mauk & Schmidt, 2004; Taylor, 2003b). The most common practices affecting the nursing care of clients include holy days, sacred writings, sacred symbols, prayer, meditation, and those associated with diet, nutrition, healing, dress, birth, and death.

It is possible for nurses to unethically impose personal spiritual beliefs on clients, whose circumstances inherently leave them vulnerable. Observing guidelines for ethical conduct in spiritual caregiving is essential. The following guidelines for nurses were offered by Winslow and Winslow (2003):

- First seek a basic understanding of clients' spiritual needs, resources, and preferences (i.e., assess).
- Follow the client's expressed wishes regarding spiritual care.
- Do not prescribe or urge clients to adopt certain spiritual beliefs or practices, and do not pressure them to relinquish such beliefs or practices.

- Strive to understand personal spirituality and how it influences caregiving.
- Provide spiritual care in a way that is consonant with personal beliefs.

CLINICAL ALERT

While some clients are eager for nurses' overt offers of "spiritual care," others may be uncertain or opposed to such offers (Taylor, 2003a). Clients often confuse religiosity with spirituality; this may contribute to their uncertainty about receiving spiritual care from nurses. Observing and using the client's language for spirituality (e.g., "being at peace" or "faith"), as well as large measures of sensitivity and respect, will help nurses to converse therapeutically with clients to provide spiritual care.

Holy Days

A **holy day** is a day set aside for special religious observance, and all the world religions observe certain holy days. For example, Christians observe Easter and Christmas, Jews observe Yom Kippur and Passover, Buddhists observe the birthday of the Buddha, Muslims observe the month-long holy period of Ramadan, and Hindus observe Mahashivarathri, a celebration of Lord Shiva. Many religions require fasting, extended prayer, and reflection or ritual observances on sacred (or high holy) days. Believers who are seriously ill are often exempted from such requirements.

The concept of the Sabbath is common to both Christians and Jews, in response to the biblical commandment "Remember the Sabbath day to keep it holy." Most Christians observe the Sabbath on Sunday, whereas Jews and sabbatarian Christians (e.g., Seventh-Day Adventists) observe Saturday as their Sabbath. Clients who are devout in their religious practices may want to avoid any special treatments or other intrusions on their day of rest and reflection.

Muslims follow the practice of prayer fives times a day, and the Muslim client may need assistance to maintain this commitment. In addition, Muslims traditionally gather on Friday at noon to worship and learn about their faith. Both Hindus and Buddhists practice meditation, and the nurse may create a quiet time for them to meditate.

Solemn religious observances throughout the year may be referred to as *high holy days* and may include fasting, reflection, and prayer. Examples of such holy days are Rosh Hashanah and Yom Kippur (Jewish), Good Friday (Christian), and the month-long Ramadan (Islam). Many hospitals and health organizations facilitate ritual observances for clients and staff on holy days. Because many religions follow different calendars, a multifaith calendar can be used to identify the holy days of the various religious groups (Griffith, 1996).

Sacred Writings

Each religion has sacred and authoritative scriptures that provide guidance for its adherents' beliefs and behaviors; in addition, sacred writings frequently tell instructive stories of the religion's leaders, kings, and heroes. In most religions, these scriptures are thought to be the word of the Supreme Being as written down by prophets or other human representatives. Christians rely on the Bible, Jews on the Torah and Talmud, and Muslims on the Koran; Hindus have several holy texts, or Vedas, and Buddhists value the teachings of the Tripitakas. Scriptures generally set forth religious law in the form of admonitions and rules for living (e.g., the Ten Commandments). This religious law may be interpreted in various ways by subgroups of a religion's adherents and may affect a client's willingness to accept treatment suggestions; for example, blood transfusions are in conflict with the religious admonitions of Jehovah's Witnesses.

People often gain strength and hope from reading religious writings when they are ill or in crisis. Examples of scriptural stories that may give comfort to clients are Job's suffering, in both the Jewish and Christian scriptures, and Jesus's healing of people who were physically or mentally ill, in the New Testament.

Sacred Symbols

Sacred symbols include jewelry, medals, amulets, icons, totems, or body ornamentation (e.g., tattoos) that carry religious or spiritual significance. They may be worn to pronounce one's faith, to remind the practitioner of the faith, to provide spiritual protection, or to be a source of comfort or strength. People may wear religious medals at all times, and they may wish to wear them when they are undergoing di-

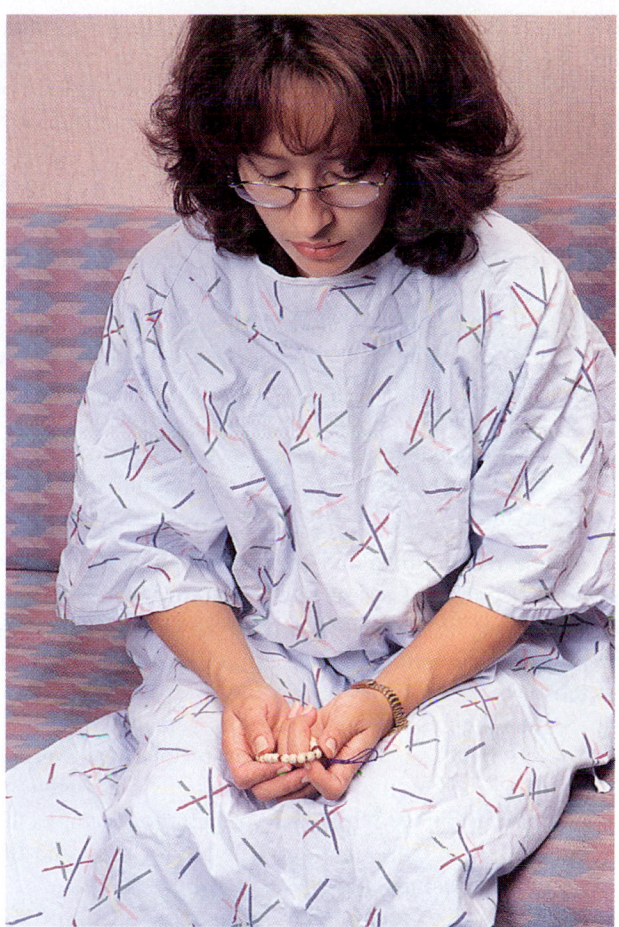

Figure 29–3 ● Clients may bring objects to the hospital to use in prayer or other religious rituals. Caregivers should respect such objects, because they usually have great significance for clients.

agnostic studies, medical treatment, or surgery. People who are Roman Catholic may carry a rosary for prayer; a person who is Muslim may carry a mala, or string of prayer beads (Figure 29–3).

People may have religious icons or statues in their home, car, or place of work as a personal reminder of their faith or as part of a personal place of worship or meditation. Hospitalized clients or long-term care residents may wish to have their spiritual icons or statues with them as a source of comfort.

Prayer and Meditation

Prayer is a spiritual practice; for many, it is also a religious practice. An encyclopedia of religion defines **prayer** simply as "human communication with divine and spiritual entities" (Gill, 1987, p. 489). Some argue that because prayer requires a belief in a divine or spiritual entity not all people pray, while others consider prayer a universal phenomenon that does not require such belief. Ulanov and Ulanov (1983), for example, proposed that everyone prays: "People pray whether or not they call it prayer. We pray every time we ask for help, understanding, or strength, in or out of religion . . . who and what we are speak out of us. . . . To pray is to listen to and hear this self who is speaking" (p. 1). Prayer is intention plus love, often communicated with "the Absolute," according to Dossey (1999); that is, prayer is a loving wish or thought for oneself or another, and not an invocation of positive or negative forms of magic.

There are different types of prayer experience. Poloma and Gallup (1991) categorized prayer experiences as follows:

- Ritual (e.g., Hail Mary, memorized prayers that can be repeated)
- Petitionary (e.g., "God, cure me!" or intercessory prayers when one is requesting something of the divine)
- Colloquial (i.e., conversational prayers)
- Meditational (e.g., moments of silence focused on nothing, a meaningful phrase, or a certain aspect of the divine)

While meditational and colloquial prayer experiences have been found to be associated with spiritual well-being and quality of life in healthy adults, ritual and petitionary prayer experiences may be most comforting and appropriate for those who are ill.

Some religions have prescribed prayers that are printed in a prayer book, such as the Anglican/Episcopal *Book of Common Prayer* or the Catholic *Missal*. Some religious prayers are attributed to the source of faith; for example, the Lord's Prayer for Christians is attributed to Jesus, and the first sutra for Muslims is attributed to Mohammed.

Some religions require daily prayers or dictate specific times for prayer and worship: the five daily prayers, or Salat, of the Muslims (performed while facing east toward Mecca at dawn, noon, midafternoon, sunset, and evening), the daily Kaddish of the Jews, or the seven canonical prayers of the Roman Catholics. People who are ill may want to continue or increase their prayer practices (Moschella, Pressman, Pressman, & Weissman, 1997). They may need uninterrupted quiet time during which they have their prayer books, rosaries, malas, or other icons available to them.

Meditation is the act of focusing one's thoughts or engaging in self-reflection or contemplation. Some people believe that, through deep meditation, one can influence or control physical and psychologic functioning and the course of illness.

Beliefs Affecting Diet and Nutrition

Many religions have proscriptions regarding diet. There may be rules about which foods and beverages are allowed and which are prohibited. For example, Orthodox Jews are not to eat shellfish or pork, and Muslims are not to drink alcoholic beverages or eat pork. Members of the Church of Jesus Christ of Latter-Day Saints (Mormons) are not to drink caffeinated or alcoholic beverages. Older Catholics may choose not to eat meat on Fridays because it was proscribed in years past. Buddhists and Hindus are generally vegetarian, not wanting to take life to support life. Religious law may also dictate how food is prepared; for example, many Jewish people require **kosher** food, which is food prepared according to Jewish law.

Some solemn religious observances are marked by fasting, which is the abstinence from food for a specified period of time. Some religions also restrict beverages; others allow drinking of water or other sustaining beverages on fast days. Examples of religions that observe fasting include Islam, Judaism, and Catholicism. During the month of Ramadan, devout Muslims eat no food and avoid beverages during daylight hours; the fast is broken after sunset. Members of Jewish synagogues fast on Yom Kippur, and devout Catholics may fast on Good Friday. Most religions lift the fasting requirements for seriously ill believers for whom fasting may be a detriment to health (e.g., diabetic clients). Some religions may exempt nursing mothers or menstruating women from fasting requirements.

It is important that health care providers prescribe diet plans with an awareness of the client's dietary and fasting beliefs.

Beliefs Related to Healing

Clients may have religious beliefs that attribute illness to a spiritual disruption. Healing for such clients may appear to be unrelated to current treatment practices. The nurse needs to assess the client's beliefs and, if possible, include some aspects of healing that are part of the client's belief system in the planning of care.

Beliefs Related to Dress

Many religions have laws or traditions that dictate dress. For example, Orthodox and Conservative Jewish men believe that it is important to have their heads covered at all times and therefore wear yarmulkes. Orthodox Jewish women cover their hair with a wig or scarf as a sign of respect to God. Many Muslim women also cover their hair in accordance with their particular ethnic or national background. Mormons may wear temple undergarments in compliance with religious law.

Some religions require that women dress in a conservative manner, which may include wearing sleeves and modestly cut tops, and skirts that cover the knees. Some religions, for example, Islam, may require that the body (torso, arms, and legs) be covered. Hindu women accustomed to wearing saris prefer to cover all of the body except arms and feet (Figure 29–4). Hospital gowns may make women wishing to comply with religious dress codes uneasy and uncomfortable. Clients may be especially disconcerted when undergoing diagnostic tests or treatments, such as mammography, that require body parts to be bared.

Beliefs Related to Birth

For all religions the birth of a child is an important event giving cause for celebration. Many religions have specific ritual ceremonies that consecrate the new child to God. When a Muslim child is born, "someone recites the call to prayer in the infant's ear." On the seventh day after birth, the child is named, and a tuft of hair is shaved from the head (Denny, 1993, p. 682).

In the Christian faith, baptism and christening ceremonies may take place after the birth of a child to confirm

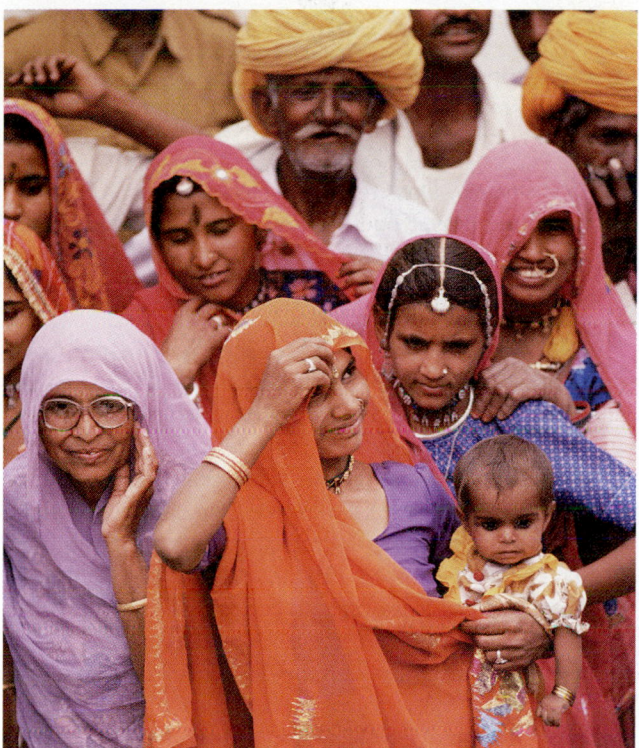

Figure 29–4 ● Hindu women dressed in saris.
(Charlie Westerman/Getty Images.)

that the "infant [was] born into a Christian family as part of the organism of the church" (Frankiel, 1993, p. 556). Christian parents of seriously ill infants may want baptism performed at birth by the nurse or primary care provider, if a chaplain or clergy person is not present.

In the Jewish religion, the ritual circumcision conducted on male children on the eighth day after birth is an expression of the religious bond between the prophet Abraham, his descendants, and their God. Following the ritual circumcision by the trained person, called a *mohel,* the child is named. Girls are named in the synagogue on the Sabbath after the birth (Fishbane, 1993).

When nurses are aware of the religious needs of families and their infants, they can assist families in fulfilling their religious obligations. This is especially important when the newborn infant is seriously ill or in danger of dying because some people believe that if religious obligations are not fulfilled the infant will not be accepted into the community of the faithful after death.

Beliefs Related to Death

Spiritual and religious beliefs play a significant role in the believer's approach to death just as they do in other major life events. Many believe that the person who dies transcends this life for a better place or state of being.

Some religions have special rituals surrounding dying and death that must be observed by the faithful. Observance of these rituals provides comfort to the dying person and their loved ones. Some rituals are carried out while the per-

son is still alive, and can include special prayers, singing or chants, and reading of sacred scriptures. Roman Catholic priests perform the Sacrament of the Sick (previously referred to as the Last Rites) when clients are very ill or near death. Muslims who are dying want their body or head turned toward Mecca (Denny, 1993).

Jews have a tradition of burial within 24 hours following death, except on the Sabbath, and they "sit Shiva" (gather to pay respects), draping any mirrors in black to ensure that guests are focused on memory of the deceased rather than on themselves. Tibetan Buddhists read the *Tibetan Book of the Dead* within 7 days of the death to release the soul of the deceased from the Bardos, or nether worlds. Hindus cremate the body within 24 hours to release the soul from any earthly attachment.

Griffith (1996) suggested that during a terminal illness the client and family should be queried about observances or rituals that follow death. Some religions require that the body of the deceased be touched only by members of that faith. In both the Muslim (Denny, 1993) and the Jewish (Fishbane, 1993) religions, believers may require that a ritual bath be done after death by a family member or by a ritual burial society. Religious symbols or objects should be treated with respect and kept with the body (Griffith, 1996). The nurse can support the family of the deceased by providing an environment conducive to the performance of their traditional death rituals.

CLINICAL ALERT

Before sharing personal beliefs or practices, a nurse must consider questions such as the following:

- For what purpose am I sharing my beliefs or practices? By doing so, am I meeting my needs or my client's?
- Is my spiritual care reflecting a spiritual assessment?
- Am I preying on a vulnerable client?
- Am I offering my beliefs or practices in a manner that allows my client comfortably to refuse?
- Does my spiritual care hurt or contribute to a therapeutic relationship with the client?

SPIRITUAL HEALTH AND THE NURSING PROCESS

The nursing process, which includes assessing, diagnosing, planning, implementing, and evaluating, can be applied to the area of spiritual health.

NURSING MANAGEMENT

ASSESSING

Data about a client's spiritual beliefs are obtained from the client's general history (religious preferences or orientation); through a nursing history; and by clinical observations of the client's behavior, verbalizations, mood, and so on. Nurses should never assume that a client follows all the practices of the client's stated religion.

Nursing History

The Joint Commission on Accreditation of Healthcare Organizations (2000) mandates that each client admitted to an institution's care must be assessed for spiritual beliefs and practices. Several experts (Cole, Benore, & Pargament, 2004; Koenig, 2002; Massey, Fitchett, & Roberts, 2004; Taylor, 2002) recommend a two-tiered approach to spiritual assessment. All clients can be asked a general question or two (e.g., "What spiritual beliefs or practices are important to you now while you live with illness?" "How would you like your health care team to support you spiritually?"). Only those who manifest some type of unhealthful spiritual need or are at risk for spiritual distress need be subjected to a more thorough spiritual assessment. Even this assessment can be streamlined to hone in on the particular spiritual concern present.

Although the nurse will continually be assessing, the initial spiritual assessment is best taken at the end of the assessment process, or following the psychosocial assessment, after the nurse has developed a relationship with the client and/or support person. A nurse who has demonstrated sensitivity and personal warmth, earning some rapport, will be more successful during a spiritual assessment.

The questions provided in the accompanying Assessment Interview may be suitable. Remembering an acronym such as FICA can also help the nurse to ask appropriate questions:

F   (faith or beliefs)—for example, What spiritual beliefs are most important to you?

I   (implications or influence)—for example, How is your faith affecting the way you cope now?

C   (community)—for example, Is there a group of like-minded believers with which you regularly meet?

A   (address)—for example, How would you like your health care team to support you spiritually? (Dameron, 2005; Massey et al., 2004).

ASSESSMENT INTERVIEW   **Spirituality**

- Are any particular religious practices important to you? If so, could you please tell me about them?
- How will being sick interfere with your religious practices?
- How is your faith helpful to you? In what ways is it important to you right now?
- In what ways can I support your spirit? For example, would you like me to read your prayer book to you?
- Would you like a visit from your spiritual counselor or the hospital chaplain?
- What are your hopes and your sources of strength right now? What comforts you during hard times?

Clinical Assessment

Cues to spiritual and religious preferences, strengths, concerns, or distress may be revealed by one or more of the following (Taylor, 2002):

1. *Environment.* Does the client have a Bible, Torah, Koran, other prayer book, devotional literature, religious medals, a rosary, cross, Star of David, or religious get-well cards in the room? Does a church send altar flowers or Sunday bulletins?
2. *Behavior.* Does the client appear to pray before meals or at other times or read religious literature? Does the client have nightmares and sleep disturbances or express anger at religious representatives or at a deity?
3. *Verbalization.* Does the client mention God or a higher power, prayer, faith, the church, synagogue, temple, a spiritual or religious leader, or religious topics? Does the client ask about a visit from the clergy? Does the client express fear of death, concern with the meaning of life, inner conflict about religious beliefs, concern about a relationship with the deity, questions about the meaning of existence or the meaning of suffering, or about the moral or ethical implications of therapy?
4. *Affect and attitude.* Does the client appear lonely, depressed, angry, anxious, agitated, apathetic, or preoccupied?
5. *Interpersonal relationships.* Who visits? How does the client respond to visitors? Does a minister come? How does the client relate to other clients and nursing personnel?

See also specific manifestations of spiritual health and spiritual distress on page 838.

DIAGNOSING

In diagnosing spiritual health, the nurse may find that spiritual problems provide the diagnostic label, or that spiritual distress is the etiology of the problem.

Spiritual Issues as the Diagnostic Label

The North American Nursing Diagnosis Association (NANDA International, 2009) recognizes three diagnoses related to spirituality:

- *Spiritual Distress* is "impaired ability to experience and integrate meaning and purpose in life through a person's connectedness with self, others, art, music, literature, nature, or a power greater than oneself" (p. 186).
- *Readiness for Enhanced Spiritual Well-Being* recognizes that spiritual well-being is the "ability to experience and integrate meaning and purpose in life through a person's connectedness with self, others, art, music, literature, nature, or a power greater than oneself" (p. 189). This wellness diagnosis describing spiritual health acknowledges that some people

respond to adversity with an increased sensitivity to spirituality or spiritual maturation.

- *Risk for Spiritual Distress* is defined by NANDA (2009) as being "at risk for an impaired ability to experience and integrate meaning and purpose in life through connectedness with self, others, art, music, literature, nature, and/or a power greater than oneself" (p. 303). This diagnosis may be appropriate for a client who presently shows no indication of this disruption of spirit yet may if a nurse fails to intervene.

Religious Issues as the Diagnostic Label

There are three nursing diagnoses that reflect client religious issues. These include the following (Burkhart, 2005, p. 10):

Impaired Religiosity "Impaired ability to exercise reliance on religious beliefs and/or participate in rituals of a particular faith tradition"

Risk for Impaired Religiosity "At risk for an impaired ability to exercise reliance on religious beliefs and/or participate in rituals of a particular faith tradition"

Readiness for Enhanced Religiosity "Ability to increase reliance on religious beliefs and/or participate in rituals of a particular faith tradition"

Spiritual or Religious Distress as the Etiology

Spiritual distress may affect other areas of functioning and indicate other diagnoses. In these instances, spiritual distress becomes the etiology. Examples include the following:

- *Fear* related to apprehension about the soul's future after death and unpreparedness for death
- *Chronic* or *Situational Low Self-Esteem* related to failure to live within the precepts of one's faith
- *Disturbed Sleep Pattern* related to spiritual distress
- *Ineffective Coping* related to feelings of abandonment by God and loss of religious faith
- *Decisional Conflict* related to conflict between treatment plan and religious beliefs

PLANNING

In the planning phase, the nurse identifies interventions to help the client achieve the overall goal of maintaining or restoring spiritual well-being so that spiritual strength, serenity, and satisfaction are realized.

Planning in relation to spiritual needs should be designed to do one or more of the following:

- Help the client fulfill religious obligations.
- Help the client draw on and use inner resources more effectively to meet the present situation.
- Help the client maintain or establish a dynamic, personal relationship with a supreme being in the face of unpleasant circumstances.

- Help the client find meaning in existence and the present situation.
- Promote a sense of hope.
- Provide spiritual resources otherwise unavailable.

IMPLEMENTING

Numerous nursing actions are available to help clients meet their spiritual needs (Cole et al., 2004; Mauk & Schmidt, 2004; Taylor, 2002). Spiritual care includes actions as diverse as recognizing and validating inner resources of an individual, such as coping methods, humor, motivation, self-determination, positive attitude, and optimism. It can also include assisting the client to leave a legacy by storytelling and/or recording life stories for family and friends, and encouraging creative expression through art, music, and writing. (This keeps the imagination alive and serves to regenerate the body, mind, and spirit.) Fostering ways for clients to keep in touch with nature and maintain a sense of wonder are also forms of spiritual care. Recognizing the seasons, the emergence of flowers in spring, the phases of the moon, the migrations of birds, and the unchanging stars provides examples of orderliness in the universe, even in the midst of chaos and loss. A client with a good measure of spiritual health will find hope, meaning, purpose, and value in existence. Although nursing therapeutics that enhance spiritual health are diverse, some of the most common and most desired include (a) providing presence, (b) supporting religious practices, (c) assisting clients with prayer, and (d) referring clients for spiritual counseling (Taylor & Mamier, 2005).

Providing Presence

Presencing, which is defined as being present, being there, or just being with a client, is a term that identifies one of the competencies incorporated by expert nurses (Zerwekh, 1997). Pettigrew (1990) identified four distinguishing features of presencing:

- Giving of self in the present moment
- Being available with all of the self
- Listening, with full awareness of the privilege of doing so
- Being there in a way that is meaningful to another person

Fredriksson (1999) noted that presencing is a "gift of self" given by the nurse who maintains an attitude of attentiveness toward the client. Thus, nurses who listen attentively to clients yet fail to give of self (i.e., inwardly "make room") diminish their effectiveness.

There are multiple levels of presencing. Osterman and Schwartz-Barcott (1996) identified four ways of being present for clients:

- Presence (when a nurse is physically present but not focused on the client)
- Partial presence (when a nurse is physically present and attending to some task on the client's behalf but not relating to the client on any but the most superficial level)

PRACTICE GUIDELINES

Supporting Religious Practices

- Create a trusting relationship with the client so that any religious concerns or practices can be openly discussed and addressed.
- If unsure of client religious needs, ask how nurses can assist in having these needs met. Avoid relying on personal assumptions when caring for clients.
- Do not discuss personal spiritual beliefs with a client unless the client requests it. Be sure to assess whether such self-disclosure contributes to a therapeutic nurse–client relationship.
- Inform clients and family caregivers about spiritual support available at your institution (e.g., chapel or meditation room, chaplain services).
- Allow time and privacy for, and provide comfort measures prior to, private worship, prayer, meditation, reading, or other spiritual activities.
- Respect and ensure safety of the client's religious articles (e.g., icons, amulets, clothing, jewelry).

- If desired by client, facilitate clergy or spiritual care specialist visitation. Collaborate with chaplain (if available).
- Prepare client's environment for spiritual rituals or clergy visitations as needed (e.g., have chair near bedside for clergy, create private space).
- Make arrangements with dietitian so that dietary needs can be met. If institution cannot accommodate client's needs, ask family to bring food. (Most religions have some recommendations about diet, such as espousing vegetarianism, rejecting alcohol.)
- Acquaint yourself with the religions, spiritual practices, and cultures of the area in which you are working.
- Remember the difference between facilitating/supporting a client's religious practice and participating in it yourself.
- Ask another nurse to assist you if a particular religious practice makes you uncomfortable.
- All spiritual interventions must be done within agency guidelines.

- Full presence (when a nurse is mentally, emotionally, and physically present; intentionally focusing on the client)
- Transcendent presence (when a nurse is physically, mentally, emotionally, and spiritually present for a client; involves a transpersonal and transforming experience)

Presencing is often the best and sometimes the only intervention to support a client who suffers under circumstances that medical interventions cannot address. When a client is helpless, powerless, and vulnerable, a nurse's presencing can be most beneficial. Rather than worrying about saying or doing "the right thing," nurses should focus on being fully present (Taylor, 2002).

Supporting Religious Practices

During the assessment of the client, the nurse will have obtained specific information about the client's religious preference and practices. Nurses need to consider specific religious practices that will affect nursing care, such as the client's beliefs about birth, death, dress, diet, prayer, sacred symbols, sacred writings, and holy days as discussed earlier in this chapter. See Practice Guidelines for ways the nurse can help clients to continue their usual spiritual practices. Box 29–3 provides health-related information about specific religions.

Assisting Clients with Prayer

Prayer involves a sense of love and connection, as well as a reaching out. It has many health benefits and healing properties (Dossey, 1996). It offers a means for someone to talk to, a mechanism for expressing care, and a sense of serenity and connection with something greater.

Clients may choose to participate in private prayer or want group prayer with family, friends, or clergy. In such situations the nurse's major responsibility is to ensure a quiet environment and privacy. Nursing care may need to be adjusted to accommodate periods for prayer.

Illness can interfere with some clients' ability to pray (Taylor, 2003a). Feelings such as anxiety, fear, guilt, grief, despair, and isolation can produce barriers to relationships in general and to the relationship the person has with the Divine. In these instances the client may ask the nurse to pray with him or her. Prayers with clients should be done only when there is mutual agreement between the clients and those praying with them. Nurses who are unaccustomed to praying aloud or in public may find it helpful to have a formal prayer or a scriptural passage readily available. Because prayer can evoke deep feelings, the nurse needs to spend time with the client following a prayer to enable the client to express these feelings. The Practice Guidelines on page 848 provide clinical suggestions for praying with clients.

Referring Clients for Spiritual Counseling

There are times when spiritual care is best referred to other members of the health care team. Referrals can be made for hospitalized clients and their families through the hospital chaplain's office if one is available. Nurses in home and community health settings can identify spiritual resources by checking directories of community service agencies, telephone directories, or religious directories that describe available spiritual counselors and the services provided through the religious community. Many religious counselors will provide assistance to members of their faith who are not members of their specific religious community. For example, a priest may attend a client in the

| BOX 29–3 | Health-Related Information about Specific Religions: A Sampler |

Amish, Mennonite—Likely will not have insurance coverage; rely on religious community for support.

Anglicans, Episcopalians, Roman Catholics—Appreciate receiving Eucharist (Holy Communion), a ritual of ingesting bread and wine (or grape juice) led by clergy or lay leaders to commemorate death of Jesus. Forehead may be marked by priest with ashes on Ash Wednesday (40 days before Easter); no need to wash off. Lenten season (Ash Wednesday to Easter) may involve some degree of abstention from food.

Buddhist—May be vegetarian. Facilitate meditation (may desire incense, visual focal point, use breathing or chanting, etc.).

Christian Scientist—Typically oppose Western medical interventions, relying instead on lay and professional Christian Science practitioners.

Hindu—Most eat no beef; many are vegetarian. Cleanliness highly valued. Many food preferences (e.g., foods fresh or cooked in oil).

Jehovah's Witnesses—Abstain from most blood products; need to discuss alternative treatments such as blood conservation strategies, autologous techniques, hematopoietic agents, nonblood volume expanders, and so on; contact local Jehovah's Witness hospital liaison committee.

Jews—Some observe kosher diet to varying degrees (e.g., avoid pork and shellfish, do not mix dairy and meat). Sabbath observance varies (e.g., Orthodox Jews avoid traveling in vehicles, writing, turning on electric appliances and lights, etc.).

Latter-Day Saints (LDS or Mormons)—Avoid alcohol, caffeine, smoking. Prefer to wear temple undergarments. Arrange for priestly blessing if requested.

Muslim—Respect modesty, avoid nakedness. Provide same-gender nurse if possible. Support prayers five times daily (may need to assist with ritual washing and positioning beforehand). Allow for family and imam (religious leader) to follow Islamic guidelines for burial when client dies. Eat no pork. Children, pregnant, older adults, and sick exempt from daytime fast during month of Ramadan.

Roman Catholics—Sacrament of the Sick (previously known as Last Rites) appropriate for the ill. Be aware that some may think rite means they are dying.

Seventh-Day Adventists—Avoid unnecessary treatments on Saturday (Sabbath). Sabbath begins Friday sundown, ends Saturday sundown. Adventists prefer restful, spirit-nurturing, family activities on Sabbaths. Likely to be vegetarian and abstain from caffeinated beverages. Do not smoke or drink alcohol.

RESEARCH NOTES

Spiritual Care Nursing: What Do Cancer Clients and Family Caregivers Want?

A convenience sample of 156 adult cancer clients and 68 family caregivers self-completed the Nurse Spiritual Therapeutics Scale, which measured how much these clients would want a nurse to provide different spiritual care therapeutics—for example, how much they would want a nurse to help them have quiet time or space, listen to them talk about spiritual concerns, ask them about religious practices, arrange for a minister or chaplain to visit, pray, and so forth.

Findings from these data indicated that while some cancer clients and family members are eager for a nurse to provide some spiritual care "therapeutics," others do not want it. Therapeutics that did not involve much intimacy, are traditional, and are not overtly religious are those most desired by clients. To illustrate, these participants *most wanted* the nurse to provide:

- humor,
- private prayer,
- and help to find quiet time or space.

Least wanted therapeutics included instruction about writing or drawing their spirituality, discussion about the difficulties of praying when sick, and help with understanding dreams. No differences were observed between client and family member preferences. A modest, positive correlation was also found between frequency of attending religious services and greater desire for nurse-provided spiritual care.

Implications

The researchers concluded that nurses must be sensitive to providing spiritual care in ways that are welcomed by clients.

Note: From "Spiritual Care Nursing: What Cancer Patients and Family Caregivers Want," by E. J. Taylor and I. Mamier, 2005, *Journal of Advanced Nursing. 49*(3), pp. 260–267. Copyright © 2005 Blackwell Publishing. Reprinted with permission.

---

hospital or at home even though the person is not a member of the priest's parish.

Referrals may be necessary when the nurse makes a diagnosis of spiritual distress. In this situation the nurse and religious counselor can work together to meet the client's needs. One situation the nurse may encounter is client refusal of necessary medical intervention because of religious tenets. In this case the nurse encourages the client, primary care provider, and spiritual adviser to discuss the conflict and consider alternative methods of therapy. The nurse's major role is to provide information the client needs to make an informed decision, and to support the client's decision. See the Practice Guidelines on page 846.

EVALUATING

Using the measurable desired outcomes developed during the planning stage, the nurse collects data needed to judge whether client goals and outcomes have been achieved. See the accompanying Nursing Care Plan.

PRACTICE GUIDELINES   **Praying with Clients**

- Clients' preferences for prayer reflect their personalities. That is, introverts may prefer being alone to pray, and their prayers will reflect their capacity for introspection. In contrast, extroverts' prayers may revolve around their relationships with others and be expressed in creative, verbal ways. Similarly, a prayer of a feeling type of client may be emotion filled, whereas the prayer of a thinking-type client may be based on ideas and logic. Structure prayer interventions accordingly.
- When assessing whether a client would like you to pray, ask to pray in a way that allows both of you to feel comfortable if the answer is no. ("Some people tell me prayer helps them to cope with rough times like this. Would you feel comfortable if I prayed with you?")
- Assess how the client approaches the addressee of prayer. For example, a Baptist may pray to Jesus, whereas a Jew would pray directly to God, or Yahweh. This assessment can usually be made while listening to a client talk about religious beliefs.
- Before praying, assess what they would like for you to pray. Listen carefully. The answer may provide greater insight into their fears and concerns.
- Personalize the prayer. Present your client's name and personal concerns to the Divine.
- Prayer can be used to summarize a conversation. This lets the client know you have heard what was said. It may also help the client to view circumstances more objectively.
- Prayer may be the springboard to further discussion or catharsis. Stay with the client after a prayer until there has been time for conversation.
- Follow a prayer with nonverbal communication (e.g., eye contact or touch) to convey "See, I am me, a person, and you are you, and we have returned from our brief journey inward."

- Remember some clients would like to pray aloud with you, just as you may with them. This can be a beautiful experience that nurtures both the client and nurse. It allows the client to reciprocate caring.
- Be mindful of one difference between magic and prayer. Magic invokes a greater power for personal gain. Prayer allows the greater power to do the greater good ("Thy will be done").
- Praying with a client may not involve verbalization. You may feel it will be more comfortable or appropriate if you remain quiet and fully present, praying silently.
- Facilitate the clients' prayer practices. Schedule time for them when they will be undisturbed, palliate distressing symptoms that interfere with praying, help with articles that accompany prayers (e.g., rosaries, prayer garments, books of prayers).
- In times of distress, a client or loved one may not be able to construct a prayer spontaneously. You may want to teach a centering prayer that is very brief (e.g., "Lord, have mercy/healing"). Nurses can discuss with care recipients what prayer would benefit them most and encourage them to use it while alone. These prayers may be more beneficial when they are framed in a positive sense. To illustrate, "Jesus loves me" or "The Lord has mercy."
- Encourage clients to think (privately or with you) about what prayer means to them. Offer questions like these: Why do you pray? What do you expect from your praying? Are these expectations appropriate? How content are you with your prayer experiences? Is there a yearning for something more in your prayer experience?

Note: From "Caring for the Spirit," by E. J. Taylor. In *Psychosocial Dimensions of Oncology Nursing Care,* by C. C. Burke (Ed.), 1998, pp. 55–75. Pittsburgh, PA: Oncology Nursing Press. Adapted with permission.

PRACTICE GUIDELINES   **When Nurse–Client Spiritual Values Conflict**

When the nurse's spiritual beliefs conflict with the client's, the nurse must remember his or her role is as a health care provider and not a spiritual counselor. If the conflict is minor, the nurse may be able to support the client's beliefs and help the client to resolve issues of concern. However, if the conflict is great and the nurse cannot support the client in an objective manner, it is most appropriate for the nurse to find a spiritual counselor who shares the client's beliefs. The client's permission is needed before seeking an outside counselor in order to protect the client's right to confidentiality.

LIFESPAN CONSIDERATIONS   **Spiritual Development**

Children

The development of spirituality in children parallels their cognitive and psychosocial development. As children mature, they are increasingly capable of understanding spiritual matters, stating spiritual beliefs, and incorporating spirituality into their lives.

A developing spirituality includes:

- A sense of wholeness, having internal resources and identity.

- Being attached to others, being a part of a greater, even transcendent world.
- Having a sense of meaning and purpose in one's life.
- Being able to express hope, even in the face of fear, uncertainty, and serious illness (Howden, 1992).

Nurses should help ill children and their parents identify and express these qualities. This can be done by actively listening, by offering opportunities to practice religious rituals, and by providing materials for nonverbal expression (e.g., painting, play, music).

Older Adults

Many older adults frequently use and highly value religious coping strategies such as prayer. Evidence shows spiritual well-being to be directly correlated with mental health and less medical illness among older adults (Koenig, 2002). It is, therefore, important to address the spiritual issues of older adults. Older adults may be especially concerned about living a purposeful life, about maintaining loving relationships to avoid social isolation, and about preparing for a good death. Nursing care for older adults that attends to such spiritual issues includes:

- Supporting meaning-making activities (e.g., conducting a life review or reminiscence therapy; allowing the client to weave together the strands of lived life; encouraging the client to become dedicated to some social, political, religious, or artistic cause; supporting the client to leave a legacy or do an altruistic deed). Such activities provide older adults with a sense of purpose for their life and assist them to make sense of the life that they have lived.

- Allowing open discussions about suffering and dying, encouraging client disclosure by asking open-ended questions, and providing responses that are respectful and compassionate. Do not avoid discomforting topics and questions older adults raise by imposing positivity, giving "pat" answers, and otherwise minimizing or avoiding their spiritual pain.

- As appropriate, supporting older adults to reframe the "losses" of aging as "liberations." For example, older adults possess great wisdom and are in a season of life that promotes spiritual growth.

Older adults with dementia present special circumstances for spiritual caregiving. Nurses can help those with early stages of dementia to focus on the positives, the "haves" rather than the losses. Allowing older adults with dementia to tell their stories allows them to maintain some identity (amidst a disease that threatens the very sense of self), and allows the nurse a window into their world. Older adults with dementia can also worship and express their hope and creativity through various art forms (e.g., movement, painting, music). It is also possible for them to experience the compassion of others when they feel their caring touch or hear their soothing voice.

Nursing Care Plan   Spiritual Distress

ASSESSMENT DATA	NURSING DIAGNOSIS	DESIRED OUTCOMES*
Nursing Assessment Mrs. Sally Horton is a 60-year-old hospitalized homemaker who is recovering from a right radical mastectomy. Her primary care provider told her yesterday that due to metastases of the cancer, her prognosis is poor. This morning her nurse finds her tearful, stating she slept poorly and has no appetite. She asks the nurse, "Why has God done this to me? Perhaps it's because I have sinned in my life. I've not gone to church or spoken to a minister in several years. Is there a chapel in the hospital where I could go and pray? I'm terribly afraid of dying and what awaits me."	*Spiritual Distress* related to feelings of guilt and alienation from God as evidenced by questioning why "God has done this"; inquiries about praying in a chapel; insomnia; no appetite	Spiritual Health [2001] as evidenced by - Interacts with spiritual leader of her religion - Uses a type of spiritual experience that provides her comfort - Connects with others to share thoughts, feelings, and beliefs

Physical Examination
Height: 165.1 cm (5′ 5″)
Weight: 54.0 kg (199 lb)
Temperature: 36.6°C (98°F)
Pulse: 88 BPM
Respirations: 22/minute
Blood Pressure: 146/86 mm Hg

Diagnostic Data
RBC: 3.5 million/μl $\times$ 10^{12}/I
Hgb: 10.5 g/L
Hct: 35%

Large surgical dressing right chest wall and axillary region, dry and intact. Slight edema right hand and arm.

NURSING INTERVENTIONS*/SELECTED ACTIVITIES	RATIONALE
Spiritual Support [5420]	
Be open to Mrs. Horton's feelings about illness and death.	*Encourages expression of inner fears and concerns and teaches the client the value of confronting issues.*
Assist her to properly express and relieve anger in appropriate ways.	*Anger can be a source of energy and its release a source of freedom when expressed in a constructive manner.*
Observe and listen empathetically to her communication.	*The nature of spiritual care may directly affect the speed and quality of recovery and/or redefining hope and finding meaning in death.*
Encourage the use of spiritual resources, if desired.	*Spiritual needs may sometimes be overlooked or ignored. Recognizing and respecting the individual's spiritual needs is an important advocacy role for nurses.*

(continued)

Nursing Care Plan Spiritual Distress (continued)

NURSING INTERVENTIONS*/SELECTED ACTIVITIES	RATIONALE (continued)
Coping Enhancement [5230]	
Create an accepting, nonjudgmental atmosphere.	*Establishes rapport and the therapeutic relationship, which promotes communication and open expression.*
Encourage verbalization of feelings, perceptions, and fears. Allow time for grieving.	*Being with the person who is suffering gives meaning to his or her experience.*
Encourage her to list values that guide behavior in times of tragedy.	*Helps the client clarify values and beliefs by reflecting on past behaviors. Experience is a major source for values development.*

EVALUATION

Outcome met. Mrs. Horton has been visited on several occasions by her minister. She reads scripture each day and has found consolation in reading the Book of Psalms. She states "God is merciful and will help me bear my suffering."

The NOC # for desired outcomes and the NIC # for nursing interventions are listed in brackets following the appropriate outcome or intervention. Outcomes, indicators, interventions, and activities selected are only a sample of those suggested by NOC and NIC and should be further individualized for each client.

CONCEPT MAP Spiritual Distress

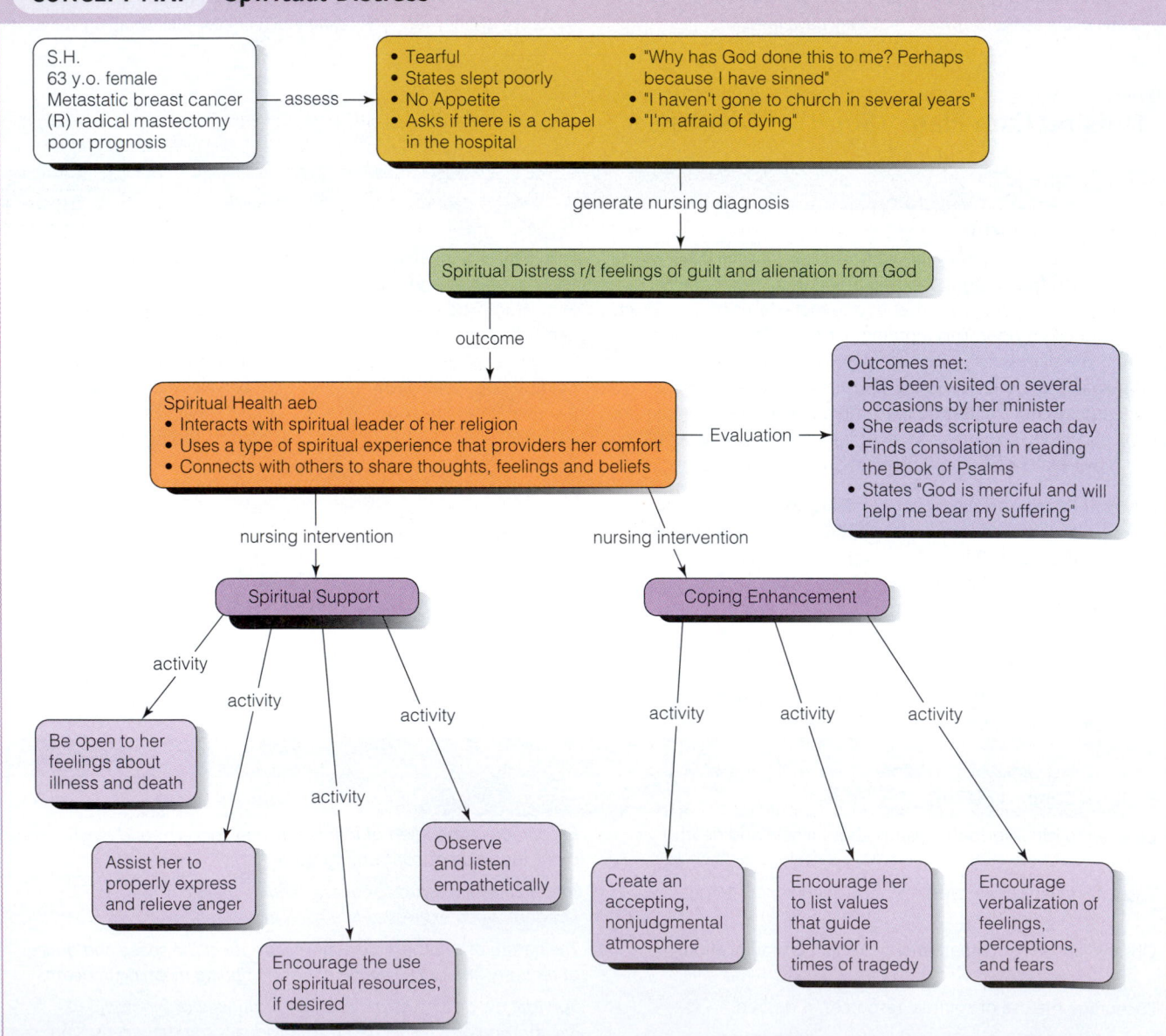

CHAPTER HIGHLIGHTS

- To implement spiritual care, nurses need to be skilled in establishing a trusting nurse–client relationship.
- Clients have a right to receive care that respects their individual spiritual and religious values.
- Nurses must follow ethical guidelines for providing spiritual care, and not impose personal beliefs or practices on clients.
- Nurses need to be aware of their own spiritual beliefs in order to be comfortable assisting others.
- The spiritual needs of clients and support persons often come into focus at a time of illness. Spiritual beliefs can help people accept illness and plan for what lies ahead.
- Spiritual distress refers to a disturbance in or a challenge to a person's belief or value system that provides strength, hope, and meaning to life. Possible factors in spiritual distress include physiologic problems, treatment-related concerns, and situational concerns. Spiritual distress may be reflected in a number of behaviors,

including depression, anxiety, verbalizations of unworthiness, and fear of death.
- Nurses can support clients' religious practices if they understand needs related to holy days, sacred writings, sacred symbols, prayer and meditation, dietary practices, dress requirements or prohibitions, healing, birth rituals, and death rituals.
- Spiritual assessment can follow a two-tiered approach. While all clients should be screened for spiritual needs, only those who indicate needs require a pertinent, in-depth assessment. The initial spiritual assessment should collect information not only about spiritual beliefs and practices affecting health, but also about how the client desires spiritual care from the health care team.
- Nursing interventions that promote spiritual health include offering one's presence, supporting the client's religious practices, praying with a client, and referring the client to a religious counselor.

THINK ABOUT IT

Refer to the chapter-opening scenario and answer these questions.

1. What nursing diagnosis might the nurse apply to Mr. Kamarra based on his comment that his cancer diagnosis is a punishment for sins against Allah?

2. As the nurse caring for Mr. Kamarra, what nursing interventions might you include in his plan of care?

3. If the nurse providing care to Mr. Kamarra is unfamiliar with the traditions of the Muslim religion, how would the nurse obtain more information in order to meet his spiritual needs?

∞ *See suggested responses to Think About It on MyNursingKit.*

TEST YOUR KNOWLEDGE

1. The nurse, working in a skilled nursing facility, is caring for an older adult who is searching to make life meaningful. Which of the following would be a priority nursing intervention?
1. Assess for depression.
2. Diagnose and document that the client has "spiritual distress."
3. Keep the client busy with social activities.
4. Assist the client to explore his or her desired legacy.

2. A client's wife asks the nurse to pray for her husband. The nurse, who believes in prayer, would best respond by saying:
1. "May I call the chaplain to come and pray with you?"
2. "I know your faith is important to you. It is to me, too."
3. "What should I pray for?"
4. "Isn't it wonderful that we have a God with whom we can share our concerns?"

3. A client is experiencing severe pain that cannot be controlled by analgesics. An appropriate nursing intervention is full presencing, which involves which of the following?
1. Physical presence
2. Physical presence with mental awareness of the client
3. Physical, mental, and emotional presence
4. Physical, mental, emotional, and spiritual presence

4. A client reports, "Cancer was the best thing that happened to me! It is making me appreciate life so much more." This statement would indicate that which of the following would be the best nursing diagnosis for this client?
1. *Spiritual Distress*
2. *Risk for Spiritual Distress*
3. *Readiness for Enhanced Spiritual Well-Being*
4. *Cognitive Denial*

5. A dying client states, "Part of what makes dying so hard is that I don't know for sure where I'm going. Nurse, what do you believe happens in the hereafter?" What ethical guideline should guide the nurse's response?
1. Never share personal spiritual beliefs.
2. Share all spiritual beliefs, favoring none.
3. Share only your strongest beliefs.
4. Assess the client's beliefs first.

6. Nursing research that supports providing spiritual care to older adults suggests that:
1. Older adults are not very religious, but are very spiritual.
2. Older adults who are more religious have more illness.
3. Spiritual health and mental health are correlated.
4. Increased spiritual well-being is found among older adults with depression.

7. A client in the emergency department, who needs red blood cells, is a Jehovah's Witness who believes it would be medical rape for the nurse to give the prescribed blood transfusion. Which of the following statements would most likely lead to a resolution for this conflict?
1. "You must accept the transfusion or else leave."
2. "Don't worry, you can ask for pardon after you receive the blood."
3. "May I call a representative from your church to help you explore other options to a blood transfusion?"
4. "I understand your position; I'll be here with you as you die."

8. An 88-year-old woman has just been admitted to a skilled nursing facility. She tells the nurse that she has been a Sunday school teacher and volunteers for many of her church's projects. Which of the following NANDA diagnoses is most appropriate?
1. *Risk for Spiritual Distress*
2. *Risk for Impaired Religiosity*
3. *Readiness for Enhanced Spiritual Well-Being*
4. *Impaired Religiosity*

9. Which of the following is an appropriate question for the nurse performing a spiritual screening or assessment?
1. "Tell me more about your religion."
2. "How can we support your spiritual beliefs and practices?"
3. "How has your prayer experience been affected by your illness?"
4. "What do you see as the purpose or mission for your life?"

10. The mother of a pediatric client states, "I can't understand why God would allow this to happen to my innocent child!" Which NANDA diagnosis is most appropriate?
1. *Spiritual Distress* related to search for meaning of child's illness
2. *Impaired Religiosity* related to anger at God
3. *Ineffective Coping* related to anger
4. *Risk for Spiritual Distress* related to threatened sense of hope

∞ *See answers to Test Your Knowledge in Appendix A.*

EXPLORE PEARSON **mynursingkit™**

MyNursingKit is your one stop for online chapter review materials and resources. Prepare for success with additional NCLEX®-style practice questions, interactive assignments and activities, web links, animations and videos, and more!

Register your access code from the front of your book at
www.mynursingkit.com.

REFERENCES AND SELECTED BIBLIOGRAPHY

Andrews, M. M., & Hanson, P. A. (2008). Religion, culture, and nursing. In M. M. Andrews & J. S. Boyle (Eds.), *Transcultural concepts in nursing care* (5th ed.). Philadelphia: Lippincott.

Bulechek, G. M., Butcher, H. K., & Dochterman, J. M. (Eds.). (2008). *Nursing interventions: classification (NIC).* (5th ed.). St. Louis: Mosby.

Burkhardt, M. A. (1989). Spirituality: An analysis of the concept. *Holistic Nursing Practice, 3*(3), 69–77.

Burkhardt, M. A., & Nagai-Jacobson, M. G. (2002). *Spirituality: Living our connectedness.* Albany, NY: Delmar.

Burkhart, L. (2005). A click away: Documenting spiritual care. *Journal of Christian Nursing, 22*(1), 6–12.

Butcher, H. K., & McGonigal-Kenney, M. (2005). Depression & dispiritedness in later life. *American Journal of Nursing, 105*(12), 52–61.

Carpenito-Moyet, L. J. (2009). *Nursing diagnosis: Application to clinical practice* (13th ed.). Philadelphia: Lippincott Williams & Wilkins.

Carson, V. B., & Koenig, H. G. (2004). *Spiritual caregiving: Healthcare as ministry.* Philadelphia: Templeton Foundation Press.

Cole, B., Benore, E., & Pargament, K. I. (2004). Spirituality and coping with trauma. In S. Sorajjakool & H. Lamberton (Eds.), *Spirituality, health, and wholeness* (pp. 49–76). New York: Haworth Press.

Coward, D. D. (1990). The lived experience of self-transcendence in women with advanced breast cancer. *Nursing Science Quarterly, 3*(4), 162–169.

Dameron, C. M. (2005). Spiritual assessment made easy . . . with acronyms! *Journal of Christian Nursing, 22*(1), 14–16.

Denny, F. M. (1993). Islam and the Muslim community. In H. Byron Earhart (Ed.), *Religious traditions of the world* (pp. 603–713). New York: HarperSanFrancisco.

Dossey, L. (1996). *Prayer is good medicine. How to reap the benefits of prayer.* New York: HarperCollins.

Dossey, L. (1999). Healing and the nonlocal mind: Interview by Bonnie Horrigan. *Alternative Therapies in Health and Medicine, 5*(6), 85–93.

Ellison, C. W. (1983, April). Spiritual well-being: Conceptualization and measurement. *Journal of Psychology and Theology, 11,* 330–340.

Fishbane, M. (1993). Judaism: Revelation and traditions. In H. Byron Earhart (Ed.), *Religious traditions of the world* (pp. 373–484). New York: HarperSanFrancisco.

Fowler, J. W. (1981). *Stages of faith development: The psychology of human development and the quest for meaning.* San Francisco: Harper & Row.

Frankiel, S. S. (1993). Christianity: A way of salvation. In H. Byron Earhart (Ed.), *Religious traditions of the world* (pp. 484–601). New York: HarperSanFrancisco.

Fredriksson, L. (1999). Modes of relating in a caring conversation: A research synthesis on presence, touch, and listening. *Journal of Advanced Nursing, 30,* 1167–1176.

Gill, S. D. (1987). Prayer. In M. Eliade (Ed.), *The encyclopedia of religion* (pp. 489–492). New York: Macmillan.

Griffith, J. K. (1996). *The religious aspects of nursing care.* Vancouver, BC: Author.

Halstead, M. T., & Hull, M. (2001). Struggling with paradoxes: The process of spiritual development in women with cancer. *Oncology Nursing Forum, 28,* 1534–1544.

Howden, J. W. (1992). *Development and psychometric characteristics of the Spirituality Assessment Scale.* Unpublished doctoral dissertation, Texas Women's University, Denton.

Joint Commission on Accreditation of Healthcare Organizations. (2000). *Hospital accreditation standards.* Oakbrook, IL: Author.

Jourard, S. (1971). *The transparent self.* London: Van Nostrand.

Knestrick, J., & Lohri-Posey, B. (2005). Spirituality and health: Perceptions of older women in a rural senior high rise. *Journal of Gerontological Nursing, 31*(10), 44–50.

Kociszewski, C. (2004). Spiritual care: A phenomenologic study of critical care nurses. *Heart & Lung, 33,* 401–411.

Koenig, H. G. (2002). *Spirituality in patient care: Why, how, when, and what.* Radnor, PA: Templeton Press.

Martsolf, D. S., & Mickley, J. R. (1998). The concept of spirituality in nursing theories: Differing world-views and extent of focus. *Journal of Advanced Nursing, 27,* 294–303.

Massey, K., Fitchett, G., & Roberts, P. A. (2004). In K. L. Mauk & N. K. Schmidt (Eds.), *Spiritual care in nursing practice. Assessment and diagnosis in spiritual care* (Chapter 14, pp. 209–242). Philadelphia: Lippincott Williams & Wilkins.

Mauk, K. L., & Schmidt, N. K. (2004). *Spiritual care in nursing practice.* Philadelphia: Lippincott Williams & Wilkins.

Mickley, J. R., & Cowles, K. (2001). Ameliorating the tension: Use of forgiveness for healing. *Oncology Nursing Forum, 28,* 31–38.

Moorhead, S., Johnson, M., & Maas, M. L., & Swanson, E. (Eds.). (2008). *Nursing outcomes classification (NOC)* (4th ed.). St. Louis: Mosby.

Moschella, V. D., Pressman, K. R., Pressman, P., & Weissman, D. E. (1997). The problem of theodicy and religious responses to cancer. *Journal of Religion & Health, 36*(1), 17–20.

Murray, C. K. (1998). Say a little prayer. *Nursing, 28*(6), 55.

NANDA International. (2009). *NANDA nursing diagnoses: Definitions and classification 2009–2011.* West Sussex, U.K.: Wiley-Blackwell.

Osterman, P., & Schwartz-Barcott, D. (1996). Presence: Four ways of being there. *Nursing Forum, 31*(2), 23–30.

Pettigrew, J. (1990). Intensive nursing care: The ministry of presence. *Critical Care Nursing Clinics of North America, 2,* 503–508.

Pilch, J. J. (1998, May/June). Wellness spirituality. *Health Values, 12,* 28–31.

Plotnikoff, G. A. (2000). Should medicine reach out to the spirit? Understanding a patient's spiritual foundation can guide appropriate care. *Postgraduate Medicine, 108*(6), 19–21.

Poloma, M. M., & Gallup, G. H., Jr. (1991). *Varieties of prayer: A survey report.* Philadelphia: Trinity Press International.

Reed, P. G. (1992). An emerging paradigm for the investigation of spirituality in nursing. *Research in Nursing and Health, 15,* 349–357.

Sherwood, G. D. (2000). The power of nurse-client encounters: Interpreting spiritual themes. *Journal of Holistic Nursing, 18*(2), 159–175.

Sorajjakool, S., & Lamberton, H. (Eds.). (2004). *Spirituality, health, and wholeness: An introductory guide for health care professionals.* New York: Haworth Press.

Stephenson, C. (1991). The concept of hope revisited for nursing. *Journal of Advances in Nursing, 16,* 1456–1461.

Sulmasy, D. P. (2001). Addressing the religious and spiritual needs of dying patients. *Western Journal of Medicine, 175*(4), 251–254.

Taylor, E. J. (1998). Caring for the spirit. In C. C. Burke (Ed.), *Psychosocial dimensions of oncology nursing care.* Pittsburgh: Oncology Nursing Press.

Taylor, E. J. (2001). Spirituality, culture, and cancer care. *Seminars in Oncology Nursing, 17*(3), 197–205.

Taylor, E. J. (2002). *Spiritual care: Nursing theory, research, and practice.* Upper Saddle River, NJ: Prentice Hall.

Taylor, E. J. (2003a). Nurses caring for the spirit: Patients with cancer and family caregiver expectations. *Oncology Nursing Forum, 30,* 585–594.

Taylor, E. J. (2003b). Prayer's clinical issues and implications. *Holistic Nursing Practice, 17*(4), 179–188.

Taylor, E. J. (2005). What have we learned from spiritual care research? *Journal of Christian Nursing, 22*(1), 22–28.

Taylor, E. J., & Mamier, I. (2005). Spiritual care nursing: what cancer patients and family caregivers want. *Journal of Advanced Nursing, 49*(3), 260–267.

Taylor, E. J., & Outlaw, F. H. (2002). Use of prayer among persons with cancer. *Holistic Nursing Practice, 16*(3), 46–60.

Taylor, E. J., Outlaw, F. H., Bernardo, T., & Roy, A. (1999). Spiritual conflicts associated with praying about cancer. *Psycho-Oncology, 8,* 386–414.

Ulanov, A., & Ulanov, B. (1983). *Primary speech: A psychology of prayer.* Atlanta: John Knox Press. (Classic.)

Van Dover, L. J., & Bacon, J. M. (2001). Spiritual care in nursing practice: A close-up view. *Nursing Forum, 36*(3), 18–28.

Van Leeuwen, R., & Cusveller, B. (2004). Nursing competencies for spiritual care. *Journal of Advanced Nursing, 48,* 234–246.

Vardey, L. (1996). *God in all worlds.* Toronto: Vintage Canada.

Westerhoff, J. (1976). *Will our children have faith?* New York: Seabury Press.

Winslow, G. R., & Winslow, B. W. (2003). Examining the ethics of praying with patients. *Holistic Nursing Practice, 17*(4), 170–177.

Zerwekh, J. V. (1997). The practice of presencing. *Seminars in Oncology Nursing, 13,* 260–262.

CHAPTER 30

Coping with Stress, Loss, and Death

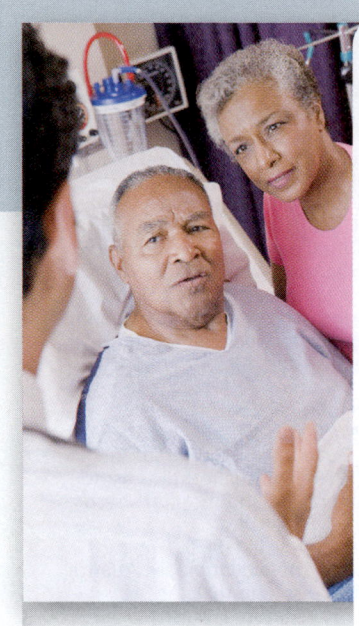

Bob (age 65) and Boots (age 62) McGhee were married 41 years ago and have a very close relationship. They have fun going out to dinner, playing duplicate bridge, and spending time with their family. They retired in their late 50s after selling their business and moved to a beach community and have many plans for traveling. They are looking forward to their oldest granddaughter's graduation in August from nursing school.

They have both generally been healthy, although both of them smoke cigarettes. In early July Bob developed a fever and felt like he had the flu. After three days with no improvement, he went to his doctor and was diagnosed with right bacterial lobar pneumonia. He took his antibiotics as prescribed and returned to the doctor for a follow-up x-ray. The doctor found a spot on the x-ray that became apparent when the consolidation from the pneumonia cleared. Following an MRI of the chest and abdomen, biopsy of the involved area of lung, and blood tests, the doctor confirmed the diagnosis of lung cancer, specifically oat cell carcinoma. They were referred to an oncologist and learned the prognosis is poor, but planned to treat the cancer as aggressively as possible.

Bob does not tolerate chemotherapy, with thrombocytopenia (platelet count 11,000/mL) requiring numerous transfusions. His weight decreases with noticeable muscle wasting, and he becomes progressively weaker, needing increasing assistance from his wife. He repeatedly apologizes to her for the pain he knows she'll experience when he dies. Boots says she feels like she's walking through a nightmare and is waiting to wake up. She wants to stay strong for her children and grandchildren but confides in the nurse that she's frightened about the prospect of life without her husband.

LEARNING OUTCOMES

After completing this chapter, you will be able to:

1. Differentiate the concepts of stress as a stimulus, a response, and as a transaction.

2. Describe physiologic, psychologic, and cognitive indicators of stress.

3. Compare four levels of anxiety.

4. Identify behaviors related to specific ego defense mechanisms.

5. Contrast different types of coping, and coping strategies.

6. Demonstrate nursing care that helps clients minimize and cope with stress, including thorough assessment,

diagnosing, planning, intervening, and evaluation of care.

7. Identify types, sources, factors affecting, and clinical symptoms of grief.

8. Describe measures that facilitate the grieving process.

9. List clinical signs of impending and actual death.

10. Describe the role of the nurse in helping clients die with dignity while supporting the family and caregivers.

11. Describe nursing care of the client after death.

KEY TERMS

Algor mortis p882
Anticipatory grief p871
Anticipatory loss p867
Anxiety p857
Bereavement p869
Burnout p866
Caregiver burden p862
Cerebral death p877

Closed awareness p878
Complicated grief p871
Coping p860
Coping mechanism p860
Coping strategy p860
Crisis counseling p865
Crisis intervention p865

Ego defense
   mechanisms p860
Fear p858
General adaptation
   syndrome p856
Grief p869
Livor mortis p882
Loss p867

Mourning p869
Mutual pretense p878
Open awareness p878
Palliative care p881
Perceived loss p867
Rigor mortis p882
Stressor p855

STRESS AND COPING

Stress is a universal phenomenon. Stress can result from both positive and negative experiences. The concept of stress is important because it provides a way of understanding the person as a being who responds in totality to a variety of changes that take place in daily life. Stress is a condition in which the person experiences changes in the normal balanced state. A **stressor** is any event or stimulus that causes an individual to experience stress. When a person faces stressors, responses are referred to as *coping strategies, coping responses,* or *coping mechanisms.*

Sources of Stress

There are many sources of stress. They can be broadly classified as internal or external stressors, or developmental or situational stressors. *Internal stressors* originate within a person, for example, infection or feelings of depression. *External stressors* originate outside the individual, for example, a move to another city, a death in the family, or pres-

sure from peers. *Developmental stressors* occur at predictable times throughout an individual's life (Table 30–1). *Situational stressors* are unpredictable and may occur at any time during life. Situational stress may be positive or negative and may include death of a loved one, marriage, divorce, birth of a child, or a new job. The degree to which these events have a positive or negative effect can impact an individual's developmental stage and coping strategies.

Effects of Stress

Stress can have physical, emotional, intellectual, social, and spiritual consequences. Usually the effects are mixed, because stress affects the whole individual. Physically, stress can threaten a person's physiologic homeostasis. Emotionally, stress can produce negative or nonconstructive feelings about the self. Intellectually, stress can influence a person's perceptual and problem-solving abilities. Socially, stress can alter a person's relationships with others. Spiritually, stress can challenge one's beliefs and values. Many health conditions have been linked to stress (Box 30–1).

TABLE 30–1	Selected Stressors Associated with Developmental Stages

DEVELOPMENTAL STAGE	STRESSORS
Child	Beginning school
	Establishing peer relationships
	Peer competition
Adolescent	Changing physique
	Relationships involving sexual attraction
	Exploring independence
	Choosing a career
Young adult	Marriage
	Leaving home
	Managing a home
	Getting started in an occupation
	Continuing one's education
	Children
Middle adult	Physical changes of aging
	Maintaining social status and standard of living
	Helping teenage children to become independent
	Aging parents
Older adult	Decreasing physical abilities and health
	Changes in residence
	Retirement and reduced income
	Death of spouse and friends

Models of Stress

Models of stress assist nurses to identify the stressor in a particular situation and to predict the individual's responses. Nurses can use these models to assist clients in strengthening healthy coping responses and in adjusting unhealthy, unproductive responses. Three main models of stress are stimulus based, response based, and transaction based.

STIMULUS-BASED MODELS In stimulus-based stress models, stress is defined as a stimulus, a life event, or a set of circumstances that arouses physiologic and/or psychologic reactions that may increase the individual's vulnerability to illness. In their classic work, Holmes and Rahe (1967) assigned a numeric value to 43 life changes or events. The most recent version of that scale includes 77 items (Miller & Rahe, 1997). The scale of stressful life events is used to document a person's relatively recent experiences, such as divorce, pregnancy, and retirement. In this view, both positive and negative events are considered stressful. Similar scales have since been developed, but all scales should be used with caution because the degree of stress an event presents is highly individual.

BOX 30–1	Disorders Caused or Aggravated by Stress

Cancer

Accident proneness

Decreased immune response

Metabolic disorders
- Hyperthyroidism
- Hypothyroidism
- Diabetes

Skin disorders
- Eczema
- Pruritus
- Urticaria
- Psoriasis

Respiratory disorders
- Asthma
- Hay fever
- Tuberculosis

Cardiovascular disorders
- Coronary artery disease
- Essential hypertension
- Congestive heart failure

Gastrointestinal disorders
- Constipation
- Diarrhea
- Duodenal ulcer
- Anorexia nervosa (severe loss of appetite)
- Obesity
- Ulcerative colitis

Menstrual irregularities

Musculoskeletal disorders
- Rheumatoid arthritis
- Low back pain
- Migraine headache
- Muscle tension

RESPONSE-BASED MODELS Stress may also be considered as a response. This definition was developed and described by Selye (1956, 1976) as "the nonspecific response of the body to any kind of demand made upon it" (1976, p. 1).

Selye's stress response is characterized by a chain or pattern of physiologic events called the **general adaptation syndrome (GAS)** or *stress syndrome*. Because stress is a state of the body, it can be observed only by the changes it produces in the body. This response of the body, the stress syndrome, or GAS, occurs with the release of certain adaptive hormones and subsequent changes in the structure and chemical composition of the body. Parts of the body particularly affected by stress are the gastrointestinal tract, the adrenal glands, and the lymphatic structures. With prolonged stress, the adrenal glands enlarge considerably; the lymphatic structures, such as the thymus, spleen, and lymph nodes, atrophy (shrink); and deep ulcers appear in the lining of the stomach. The three stages of adaptation to stress in this model are shown in Figure 30–1.

TRANSACTION-BASED MODELS Transactional theories of stress are based on the work of Lazarus (1966), who stated that the stimulus theory and the response theory do not consider individual differences. Neither theory explains the factors that lead some people and not others to respond effectively nor interprets why some people are able to adapt for longer periods than are others.

Although Lazarus recognizes that certain environmental demands and pressures produce stress in substantial numbers of people, he emphasizes that people and groups differ in their sensitivity and vulnerability to certain types of events, as well as in their interpretations and reactions. To explain variations among individuals under comparable conditions, the Lazarus model takes into account cognitive processes that intervene between the encounter and the reaction, and the factors that affect

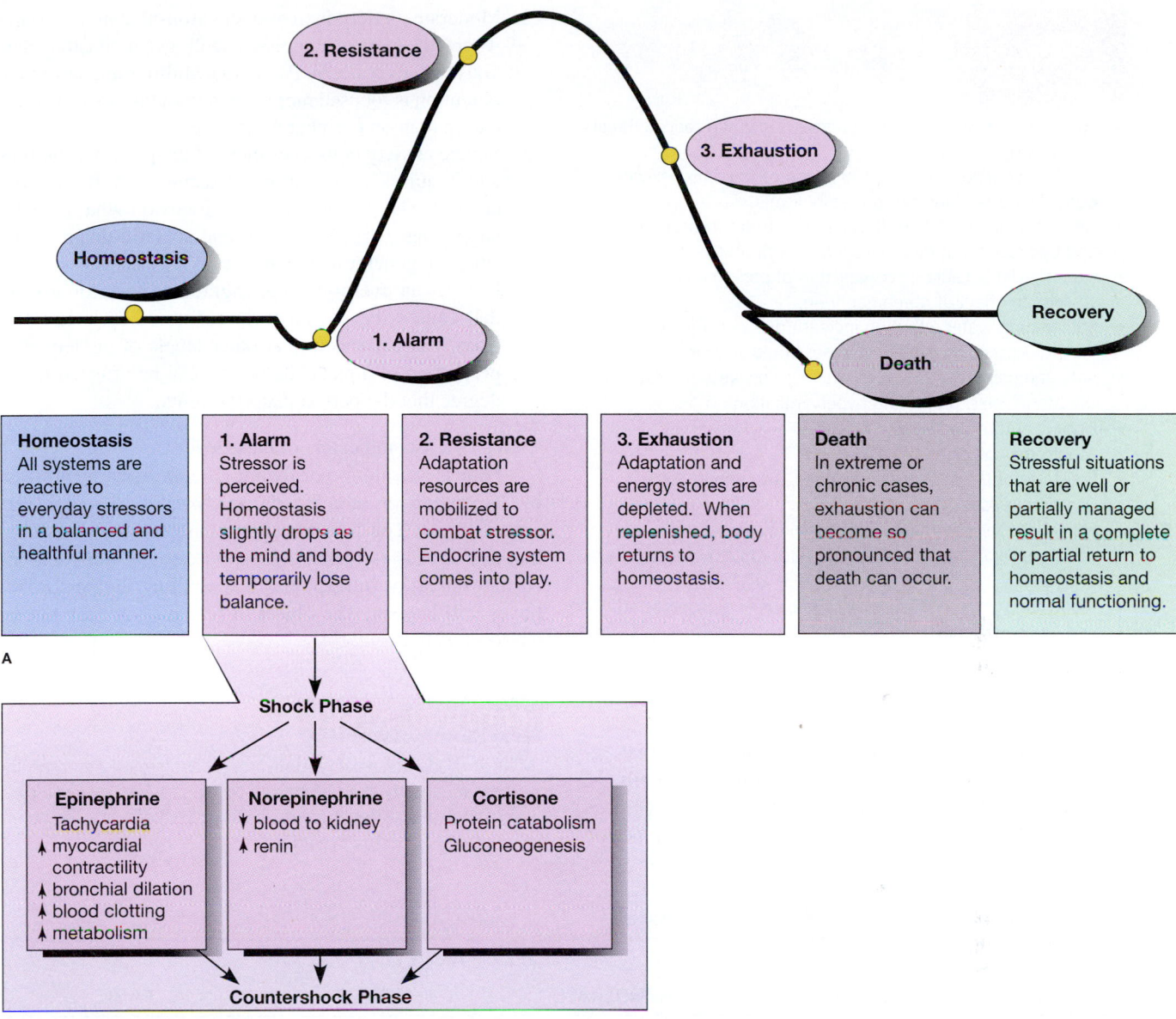

Figure 30–1 ⬤ The three stages of adaptation to stress: The alarm reaction, the stage of resistance, and the stage of exhaustion.

Note: "A" is from *Wellness: Concepts and Application*, 6th ed. (p. 298), by D. J. Anspaugh, M. Hamrick, and F. D. Rosato, 2005, New York: McGraw-Hill. Reprinted with permission.

the nature of this process. In contrast to Selye, who focuses on physiologic responses, Lazarus includes mental and psychologic components or responses as part of his concept of stress.

Indicators of Stress

Indicators of an individual's stress may be physiologic, psychologic, or cognitive.

PHYSIOLOGIC INDICATORS   Responses to stress vary depending on the individual's perception of events. The physiologic signs and symptoms of stress result from activation of the sympathetic and neuroendocrine systems of the body. The Clinical Manifestations box lists physiologic indicators of stress.

PSYCHOLOGIC INDICATORS   Psychologic manifestations of stress include anxiety, fear, anger, depression, and unconscious ego defense mechanisms. Some of these coping patterns are helpful; others are a hindrance, depending on the situation and the length of time they are used or experienced.

A common reaction to stress is **anxiety,** a state of mental uneasiness, apprehension, dread, or foreboding or a feeling of helplessness related to an impending or anticipated unidentified threat to self or significant relationships. Anxiety can be experienced at the conscious, subconscious, or unconscious level. As many as one-fourth of Americans experience an anxiety disorder sometime in their lifetime, over half of which are debilitating (Antai-Otong, 2003).

CLINICAL MANIFESTATIONS **Stress**

- Pupils dilate to increase visual perception when serious threats to the body arise.
- Sweat production (diaphoresis) increases to control elevated body heat due to increased metabolism.
- Heart rate and cardiac output increase to transport nutrients and by-products of metabolism more efficiently.
- Skin is pallid because of constriction of peripheral blood vessels, an effect of norepinephrine.
- Sodium and water retention increase due to release of mineralocorticoids, which increases blood volume.
- Rate and depth of respirations increase because of dilation of the bronchioles, promoting hyperventilation.
- Urinary output decreases.
- Mouth may be dry.
- Peristalsis of the intestines decreases, resulting in possible constipation and flatus.
- For serious threats, mental alertness improves.
- Muscle tension increases to prepare for rapid motor activity or defense.
- Blood sugar increases because of release of glucocorticoids and gluconeogenesis.

Anxiety may be manifested on four levels:

1. Mild anxiety produces a slight arousal state that enhances perception, learning, and productive abilities. Most healthy people experience mild anxiety, perhaps as a feeling of mild restlessness that prompts a person to seek information and ask questions.

2. Moderate anxiety increases the arousal state to a point where the person expresses feelings of tension, nervousness, or concern. Perceptual abilities are narrowed. Attention is focused more on a particular aspect of a situation than on peripheral activities.

3. Severe anxiety consumes most of the person's energies and requires intervention. Perception is further decreased. The person, unable to focus on what is really happening, focuses on only one specific detail of the situation generating the anxiety.

4. Panic is an overpowering, frightening level of anxiety that causes the person to lose control. It is less frequently experienced than other levels of anxiety. The perception of a panicked person can be affected to the degree that the person distorts events.

Table 30–2 lists indicators of these levels.

Fear is an emotion or feeling of apprehension aroused by impending or seeming danger, pain, or another perceived threat. The fear may be in response to something that has already occurred, in response to an immediate or current threat, or in response to something the person believes will happen. The object of fear may or may not be based in reality.

CLINICAL ALERT

Mild or moderate anxiety motivates goal-directed behavior. In this sense, anxiety is an effective coping strategy. For example, mild anxiety motivates students to study. Excessive anxiety, however, often has destructive effects.

TABLE 30–2 **Indicators of Levels of Anxiety**

CATEGORY	LEVEL OF ANXIETY			
	MILD	MODERATE	SEVERE	PANIC
Verbalization changes	Increased questioning	Voice tremors and pitch changes	Communication difficult to understand	Communication may not be understandable
Motor activity changes	Mild restlessness	Tremors, facial twitches, and shakiness	Increased motor activity, inability to relax	Increased motor activity, agitation
	Sleeplessness	Increased muscle tension	Fearful facial expression	Unpredictable responses
Perception and attention changes	Feelings of increased arousal and alertness	Narrowed focus of attention	Inability to focus or concentrate	Trembling, poor motor coordination
		Able to focus but selectively inattentive	Easily distracted	Perception distorted or exaggerated
	Uses learning to adapt	Learning slightly impaired	Learning severely impaired	Unable to learn or function
Respiratory and circulatory changes	None	Slightly increased respiratory and heart rates	Tachycardia, hyperventilation	Dyspnea, palpitations, choking, chest pain, or pressure
Other changes	None	Mild gastric symptoms (e.g., "butterflies in the stomach")	Headache, dizziness, nausea	Feeling of impending doom
				Paresthesia, sweating

Note: From *Nursing Diagnosis: Application to Clinical Practice*, 11th ed. (pp. 97–109), by L. J. Carpenito-Moyet, 2006, Philadelphia: Lippincott; *Mental Health Nursing*, 6th ed. (p. 227), by K. L. Fontaine, Upper Saddle River, NJ: Pearson Education. Adapted with permission.

Anxiety and fear differ in four ways:

- The source of anxiety may not be identifiable; the source of fear is identifiable.
- Anxiety is related to the future, that is, to an anticipated event. Fear is related to the present.
- Anxiety is vague, whereas fear is definite.
- Anxiety is the result of psychologic or emotional conflict; fear is the result of a discrete physical or psychologic entity.

Anger is an emotional state consisting of a subjective feeling of animosity or strong displeasure. People may feel guilty when they feel anger because they have been taught that to feel angry is wrong. However, anger can be expressed in a nonalienating verbal manner; it is then considered a positive emotion and a sign of emotional maturity because growth and beneficial interactions result from it.

A verbal expression of anger can be considered a signal to others of one's internal psychologic discomfort and a call for assistance to deal with perceived stress. In contrast, hostility is usually marked by overt antagonism and harmful or destructive behavior; aggression is an unprovoked attack or a hostile, injurious, or destructive action or outlook; and violence is the exertion of physical force to injure or abuse. Verbally expressed anger differs from hostility, aggression, and violence, but it can lead to destructiveness and violence if the anger persists unabated.

A clearly expressed verbal communication of anger, when the angry person tells the other person about the anger and carefully identifies the source, is constructive. This clarity of communication gets the anger out into the open so that the other person can deal with it and help to alleviate it. The angry person "gets it off the chest" and prevents an emotional buildup.

Depression is a common reaction to events that seem overwhelming or negative. Depression, an extreme feeling of sadness, despair, dejection, lack of worth, or emptiness, affects millions of Americans a year. The signs and symptoms of depression and the severity of the problem vary with the client and the significance of the precipitating event. Emotional symptoms can include feelings of tiredness, sadness, emptiness, or numbness. Behavioral signs of depression include irritability, inability to concentrate, difficulty making decisions, loss of sexual desire, crying, sleep disturbance, and social withdrawal. Physical signs of depression may include loss of appetite, weight loss, constipation, headache, and dizziness. Many people experience short periods of depression in response to overwhelming stressful events, such as the death of a loved one or loss of a job; prolonged depression, however, is a cause for concern and may require treatment.

DRUG CAPSULE | **Selective Serotonin Reuptake Inhibitor (SSRI)** *Sertraline HCl (Zoloft)*

The Client Taking Anti-Anxiety Medication

Sertraline is approved to treat depression, social anxiety disorder, posttraumatic stress disorder (PTSD), panic disorder, obsessive compulsive disorder (OCD), and premenstrual dysphoric disorder (PMDD) in adults over age 18. It is also approved for OCD in children and adolescents age 6 to 17 years. Sertaline acts by inhibiting serotonin reabsorption by the nerve cells. An elevated level of serotonin is closely related to depression, bipolar disorder, and anxiety. Reducing levels of serotonin provides the client relief from symptoms.

Nursing Responsibilities

- Sertraline may be given with or without meals but with sufficient water. The concentrate must be diluted after measurement.
- Setraline is available as oral concentrate or tablets. It is taken once per day.
- This medication should not be taken if the client is already taking monoamine oxidase inhibitors (MAOI) or pimozide. Use with caution in clients taking anticoagulant medications. Always check the list of client medications for possible interactions.
- Adverse effects may include dry mouth, insomnia, sexual side effects, diarrhea, nausea, and sleepiness.
- There is a warning from the U.S. Food and Drug Administration (FDA) on all materials related to antidepressants due to an increased risk of suicidal thoughts and behavior from 2% to 4% in people under age 18. This risk must be balanced with the medical need. Those starting medication should be watched closely for suicidal thoughts, worsening of depression, or unusual changes in behavior.

- This is an expensive medication. It can cost more than $2.50 per day. Explore insurance and other forms of the client's ability to manage this cost.

Client and Family Teaching

- This medication is not habit forming and does not cause weight gain (as do some medications prescribed for similar purposes).
- Do not stop taking this medication without consulting the primary care provider. Some symptoms might start to improve within 1 to 2 weeks, but it could take up to 8 weeks, depending on the person. Treatment may last 6 months to 1 year.
- Sertraline comes in different dose strengths, and the primary care provider may need to adjust the dosage to find the correct amount.
- Avoid alcohol while taking sertraline.
- Take at the same time every day.
- Store at room temperature.
- Use caution when driving, operating machinery, or performing other hazardous activities. Sertraline may cause dizziness or drowsiness.

Note: Prior to administering any medication, review all aspects with a current drug handbook or other reliable source.

Ego defense mechanisms are unconscious psychologic adaptive mechanisms or, according to Sigmund Freud (1946), mental mechanisms that develop as the personality attempts to defend itself, establish compromises among conflicting impulses, and calm inner tensions. Defense mechanisms are the unconscious mind working to protect the person from anxiety. They can be considered precursors to conscious cognitive coping mechanisms that will ultimately solve the problem. Like some verbal and motor responses, defense mechanisms release tension. Table 30–3 describes these mechanisms and lists examples of their adaptive and maladaptive use.

COGNITIVE INDICATORS Cognitive indicators of stress are thinking responses that include problem solving, structuring, self-control or self-discipline, suppression, and fantasy. *Problem solving* involves thinking through the threatening situation, using specific steps to arrive at a solution. The person assesses the situation or problem, analyzes or defines it, chooses alternatives, carries out the selected alternative, and evaluates whether the solution was successful.

Structuring is the arrangement or manipulation of a situation so that threatening events do not occur. For example, a nurse can structure or control an interview with a client by asking only direct, closed questions. Structuring can be productive in certain situations. A person who schedules a dental examination semiannually to prevent severe dental disease is using productive structuring.

Self-control (*discipline*) is assuming a manner and facial expression that convey a sense of being in control or in charge. When self-control prevents panic and harmful or nonproductive actions in a threatening situation, it is a helpful response that conveys strength. Self-control carried to an extreme, however, can delay problem solving and prevent a person from receiving the support of others, who may perceive the person as handling the situation well, as cold, or as unconcerned.

Suppression is consciously and willfully putting a thought or feeling out of mind: "I won't deal with that today. I'll do it tomorrow." This response relieves stress temporarily but does not solve the problem. A man who keeps ignoring a toothache, pushing it out of his mind because he fears the pain of having a filling, will not obtain relief of his symptoms.

Fantasy or *daydreaming* is likened to make-believe. Unfulfilled wishes and desires are imagined as fulfilled, or a threatening experience is reworked or replayed so that it ends differently from reality. Experiences can be relived, everyday problems solved, and plans for the future made. The outcome of current problems may also be fantasized. For example, a client who is awaiting the results of a breast biopsy may fantasize the surgeon as saying, "You do not have cancer." Fantasy responses can be helpful if they lead to problem solving. For example, the client awaiting breast biopsy results might say to herself, "Even if the doctor says, 'You have cancer,' as long as he also says it can be treated, I can accept that." Fantasies can be destructive and nonproductive if a person uses them to excess and retreats from reality.

Coping

Coping may be described as dealing with change—successfully or unsuccessfully. A **coping strategy** (or **coping mechanism**) is a natural or learned way of responding to a changing environment or specific problem or situation. According to Folkman and Lazarus (1991), coping is "the cognitive and behavioral effort to manage specific external and/or internal demands that are appraised as taxing or exceeding the resources of the person" (p. 210).

Two types of coping strategies have been described: problem-focused and emotion-focused coping. *Problem-focused coping* refers to efforts to improve a situation by making changes or taking some action. *Emotion-focused coping* includes thoughts and actions that relieve emotional distress. Emotion-focused coping does not improve the situation, but the person often feels better. Both types of strategies usually occur together (Lazarus, 2000).

Coping strategies are also viewed as long term or short term. *Long-term coping strategies* can be constructive and realistic. For example, in certain situations, talking with others and trying to find out more about the situation are long-term strategies. Other long-term strategies include a change in lifestyle patterns such as eating a healthy diet, exercising regularly, balancing leisure time with working, or using problem solving in decision making instead of anger or other nonconstructive responses.

Short-term coping strategies can reduce stress to a tolerable limit temporarily but are ineffective ways to permanently deal with reality. They may even have a destructive or detrimental effect on the person. Examples of short-term strategies are using alcoholic beverages or drugs, daydreaming and fantasizing, relying on the belief that everything will work out, and giving in to others to avoid anger.

Coping strategies vary among individuals and are often related to the individual's perception of the stressful event. Three approaches to coping with stress are to alter the stressor, adapt to the stressor, or avoid the stressor. A person's coping strategies often change with a reappraisal of a situation. There is never only one way to cope. Some people choose avoidance; others confront a situation as a means of coping. Still others seek information or rely on religious beliefs.

Coping can be adaptive or maladaptive. *Adaptive coping* helps the person to deal effectively with stressful events and minimizes distress associated with them. *Maladaptive coping* can result in unnecessary distress for the person and others associated with the person or stressful event. In nursing literature, effective and ineffective coping are often differentiated. *Effective coping* results in adaptation; *ineffective coping* results in maladaptation.

Although the coping behavior may not always seem appropriate, the nurse needs to remember that coping is always

TABLE 30–3   Defense Mechanisms

DEFENSE MECHANISM	EXAMPLE(S)	USE/PURPOSE
Compensation Covering up weaknesses by emphasizing a more desirable trait or by overachievement in a more comfortable area.	A high school student too small to play football becomes the star long-distance runner for the track team.	Allows a person to overcome weakness and achieve success.
Denial An attempt to screen or ignore unacceptable realities by refusing to acknowledge them.	A woman, though told her father has metastatic cancer, continues to plan a family reunion 18 months in advance.	Temporarily isolates a person from the full impact of a traumatic situation.
Displacement The transferring or discharging of emotional reactions from one object or person to another object or person.	A husband and wife are fighting, and the husband becomes so angry he hits a door instead of his wife.	Allows for feelings to be expressed through or to less dangerous objects or people.
Intellectualization A mechanism by which an emotional response that normally would accompany an uncomfortable or painful incident is evaded by the use of rational explanations that remove from the incident any personal significance and feelings.	The pain over a parent's sudden death is reduced by saying, "He wouldn't have wanted to live with a disability."	Protects a person from pain and traumatic events.
Introjection A form of identification that allows for the acceptance of others' norms and values into oneself, even when contrary to one's previous assumptions.	A 7-year-old tells his little sister, "Don't talk to strangers." He has introjected this value from the instructions of parents and teachers.	Helps a person avoid social retaliation and punishment; particularly important for the child's development of superego.
Projection A process in which blame is attached to others or the environment for unacceptable desires, thoughts, shortcomings, and mistakes.	A mother is told her child must repeat a grade in school, and she blames this on the teacher's poor instruction. A husband forgets to pay a bill and blames his wife for not giving it to him earlier.	Allows a person to deny the existence of shortcomings and mistakes; protects self-image.
Rationalization Justification of certain behaviors by faulty logic and ascribing motives that are socially acceptable but did not in fact inspire the behavior.	A mother spanks her toddler too hard and says it was all right because he couldn't feel it through the diapers anyway.	Helps a person cope with the inability to meet goals or certain standards.
Reaction formation A mechanism that causes people to act exactly opposite to the way they feel.	An executive resents his bosses for calling in a consulting firm to make recommendations for change in his department but verbalizes complete support of the idea and is exceedingly polite and cooperative.	Aids in reinforcing repression by allowing feelings to be acted out in a more acceptable way.
Regression Resorting to an earlier, more comfortable level of functioning that is characteristically less demanding and responsible.	An adult throws a temper tantrum when he does not get his own way. A critically ill client allows the nurse to bathe and feed him.	Allows a person to return to a point in development when nurturing and dependency were needed and accepted with comfort.
Repression An unconscious mechanism by which threatening thoughts, feelings, and desires are kept from becoming conscious; the repressed material is denied entry into consciousness.	A teenager, seeing his best friend killed in a car accident, becomes amnesic about the circumstances surrounding the accident.	Protects a person from a traumatic experience until he or she has the resources to cope.
Sublimation Displacement of energy associated with more primitive sexual or aggressive drives into socially acceptable activities.	A person with excessive sexual drives invests psychic energy into a well-defined religious value system.	Protects a person from behaving in irrational, impulsive ways.

Note: From Mental Health Nursing, *6th ed. (pp. 12–13), by K. L. Fontaine, 2009, Upper Saddle River, NJ: Pearson Education. Reprinted with permission.*

purposeful. The effectiveness of an individual's coping is influenced by a number of factors, including:

- The number, duration, and intensity of the stressors.
- Past experiences of the individual.
- Support systems available to the individual.
- Personal qualities of the person.

If the duration of the stressors is extended beyond the coping powers of the individual, that person becomes exhausted and may develop increased susceptibility to health problems. Reaction to long-term stress is seen in family members who undertake the care of a person in the home for a long period. This stress is called **caregiver burden** and produces responses such as chronic fatigue, sleeping difficulties, and high blood pressure. Prolonged stress can also result in mental illness. As coping strategies or defense mechanisms become ineffective, the individual may have interpersonal problems, work difficulties, and a significant decrease in abilities to meet basic human needs.

NURSING MANAGEMENT

ASSESSING

Nursing assessment of a client's stress and coping patterns includes (a) nursing history and (b) physical examination of the client for indicators of stress (e.g., nail biting, nervousness, weight changes) or stress-related health problems (e.g., hypertension, dyspnea). When obtaining the nursing history, the nurse poses questions about client-perceived stressors or stressful incidents, manifestations of stress, and past and present coping strategies. During the physical examination, the nurse observes for verbal, motor, cognitive, or other physical manifestations of stress. Remember, however, that clinical signs and symptoms may not occur when cognitive coping is effective.

In addition, the nurse should be aware of expected developmental transitions (predictable tasks that must be accomplished if the person is to grow psychologically as well as physically; see Chapters 9 and 10 ∞). Persons go through different developmental stages from infancy to old age when certain tasks are expected to be completed or resolved. When these tasks are carried over and not resolved, stress increases as they become older. For example, if an infant does not learn to trust those around him during infancy, this mistrust may accompany him through life, influencing his relationships and possibly being the root of dysfunction, stress, and ineffective coping. This knowledge helps the nurse identify additional stressors that are present and the client's response to them (see Table 30–1).

DIAGNOSING

NANDA diagnostic labels related to stress, adaptation, and coping include (in alphabetical order):

- *Anxiety:* Vague, uneasy feeling of discomfort or dread accompanied by an autonomic response (the source often nonspecific or unknown to the individual); a feeling of apprehension caused by the anticipation of danger. It is an alerting signal that warns of impending danger and enables the individual to take measures to deal with a threat.
- *Caregiver Role Strain:* Difficulty in performing the caregiver role.
- *Compromised Family Coping:* Usually supportive primary person (family member or close friend) provides insufficient, ineffective, or compromised support, comfort, assistance, or encouragement that may be needed by the client to manage or master adaptive tasks related to his or her health challenge.
- *Decisional Conflict (Specify):* Uncertainty about course of action to be taken when the choice among competing actions involves risk, loss, or challenge to personal life values.
- *Defensive Coping:* Repeated projection of falsely positive self-evaluation based on a self-protective pattern that defends against underlying perceived threats to positive self-regard.
- *Disabled Family Coping:* Behavior of significant person (family member or other primary person) that disables his/her capacities and the client's capacities to effectively address tasks essential to either person's adaption to the health challenge.
- *Fear:* Response to perceived threat that is consciously recognized as a danger.
- *Impaired Adjustment:* Inability to modify lifestyle/behavior in a manner consistent with a change in health status.
- *Ineffective Coping:* Inability to form a valid appraisal of the stressors, inadequate choices of practiced responses, and/or inability to use resources.
- *Ineffective Denial:* Conscious or unconscious attempt to disavow the knowledge or meaning of an event to reduce anxiety/fear, but leading to the detriment of health.
- *Posttrauma Syndrome:* Sustained maladaptive response to a traumatic, overwhelming event.
- *Relocation Stress Syndrome:* Physiologic and/or psychosocial disturbance following transfer from one environment to another.

Examples of clinical applications of these diagnoses using NANDA, NIC, and NOC designations are shown in the accompanying Identifying Nursing Diagnoses, Outcomes, and Interventions, "Clients with Stress and Coping Challenges."

PLANNING

The nurse develops plans in collaboration with the client and significant support people when possible, according to the client's state of health (e.g., ability to return to work), level of anxiety, support resources, coping mechanisms, and sociocultural and religious affiliation. The nurse with little experience intervening with clients undergoing stress may wish to consult with a more experienced nurse to develop ef-

Clients with Stress and Coping Challenges

DATA CLUSTER: Darryl Johnson, a 67-year-old accountant, was diagnosed with a heart attack. "I'm scared about this. My dad died of a heart attack when he was 68 years old. But, I don't think I can give up smoking, take up exercising, and change my diet."

NURSING DIAGNOSIS/DEFINITION	SAMPLE DESIRED OUTCOMES*/ *DEFINITION*	INDICATORS	SELECTED INTERVENTIONS*/ *DEFINITION*	SAMPLE NIC ACTIVITIES
Impaired Adjustment/Inability to modify lifestyle behavior in a manner consistent with a change in health status	Psychosocial Adjustment: Life Change [1305]/ *Adaptive psychosocial response of an individual to a significant life change*	Substantial • Recognition of reality of current health situation • Demonstration of positive self-regard • Clarification of values	Counseling [5240]/ *Use of an interactive helping process focusing on the needs, problems, or feelings of the patient and significant others to enhance or support coping, problem solving, and interpersonal relationships*	• Demonstrate empathy, warmth, and genuineness • Provide factual information as appropriate • Use techniques of reflection and clarification to facilitate expression of feelings

*The NOC # for desired outcomes and the NIC # for nursing interventions are listed in brackets following the appropriate outcome or intervention. Outcomes, indicators, interventions, and activities selected are only a sample of those suggested by NOC and NIC and should be further individualized for each client.

fective plans. The nurse and client set goals to change the existing client responses to the stressor or stressors.

The overall client goals for persons experiencing stress-related responses are to:

- Decrease or resolve anxiety.
- Increase ability to manage or cope with stressful events or circumstances.
- Improve role performance.

Examples of clinical applications of NOC outcomes and NIC interventions are shown in Identifying Nursing Diagnoses, Outcomes, and Interventions. A sample nursing care plan and concept map using NIC interventions and selected activities are shown on pages 868–870.

IMPLEMENTING

Although stress is part of daily life, it is also highly individual; a situation that to one person is a major stressor may not affect another. Some methods to help reduce stress will be effective for one person; other methods will be appropriate for a different person. A nurse who is sensitive to clients' needs and reactions can choose those methods of intervention that will be most effective for each individual.

Encouraging Health Promotion Strategies

Several health promotion strategies are often appropriate as interventions for clients with stress-related nursing diagnoses. Among these are physical exercise, optimal nutrition, adequate rest and sleep, and time management.

EXERCISE Regular exercise promotes both physical and emotional health. Physiologic benefits include improved muscle tone, increased cardiopulmonary function, and weight control. Psychologic benefits include relief of tension, a feeling of well-being, and relaxation. In 2005, the federal Dietary Guidelines Advisory Committee recommended 30 minutes of daily exercise (United States Department of Agriculture, 2005).

NUTRITION Optimal nutrition is essential for health and in increasing the body's resistance to stress. To minimize the negative effects of stress (e.g., irritability, hyperactivity, anxiety), people need to avoid excesses of caffeine, salt, sugar, and fat, and deficiencies in vitamins and minerals. Guidelines for a well-balanced, healthy diet are detailed in Chapter 32 ∞.

CLINICAL ALERT

Many persons have "comfort foods"— things they like to eat that actually make them feel better emotionally.

SLEEP Sleep restores the body's energy levels and is an essential aspect of stress management. To ensure adequate sleep, clients may need help to attain comfort (such as pain management) and to learn techniques that promote peace of mind and relaxation. (See "Using Relaxation Techniques" on page 865.)

TIME MANAGEMENT People who manage their time effectively usually experience less stress because they feel more in control of their circumstances. Clients who feel overwhelmed often need help to prioritize tasks and to consider whether modifications can be made to decrease role demands. Working mothers, for example, may need to consider delegating tasks to family members or hiring part-time help. Controlling the demands of others is also an important aspect of effective time management because requests made by others cannot always be met. Clients may need to learn to develop an awareness of which requests they can meet without undue stress, which ones can be negotiated, and which ones need to be declined. Feelings of control can be enhanced when clients schedule a daily or weekly period of time to deal with specific tasks. Time management must address both what is important to the client and what can realistically be achieved. For example, clients need to consider whether a clean house and time spent with the children can both be accomplished satisfactorily and, if not, which is more important. Clients who are feeling overwhelmed need to reexamine the "should do," "ought to do," and "must do" situations in their lives and develop realistic self-expectations.

Minimizing Anxiety

Nurses carry out measures to minimize clients' anxiety and stress. For example, nurses encourage clients to take deep breaths before an injection, explain procedures before they are implemented including sensations likely to be experienced during the procedure, administer a massage to help the client relax, and offer support to clients and families during times of illness. The nurse recognizes that quick action may be necessary to avoid the contagious nature of anxiety. That is, the anxious feeling of one person tends to make others around him or her also anxious. This can include family members, other clients nearby, or health care providers. General guidelines for helping clients who are stressed and feeling anxious are outlined in Box 30–2.

Mediating Anger

Often nurses find clients' anger difficult to handle. Caring for the client who is angry is difficult for two reasons:

- Clients seldom state, "I feel angry or frustrated," or indicate the reason for their anger. Instead, they may refuse treatment, become verbally abusive or demanding, threaten violence, or become overly critical. Their complaints rarely reflect the cause of their anger.
- Anger from clients can elicit fear and anger in the nurse, who may respond in a manner that intensifies the client's anger, even to the point of violence. Nurses tend to respond in a way that reduces their own stress rather than the client's stress.

Fontaine (2009) recommends the following strategies for dealing with clients' anger:

- Know and understand your own response to the feelings and expressions of anger.
- Accept the client's right to be angry; feelings are real and cannot be discounted or ignored.
- Try to understand the meaning of the client's anger.
- Ask the client what contributed to the anger.
- Help the client "own" the anger—do not assume responsibility for her or his feelings.
- Let clients talk about their anger.
- Listen to the client, and act as calmly as possible.
- After the interaction is completed, take time to process your feelings and your responses to the client with your colleagues.

Always ensure the safety of the client and others. Know the agency procedures to call for assistance from other staff or security personnel if you believe someone (including yourself) is in danger.

BOX 30–2   Minimizing Stress and Anxiety

- Listen attentively; try to understand the client's perspective on the situation.
- Provide an atmosphere of warmth and trust; convey a sense of caring and empathy.
- Determine if it is appropriate to encourage clients' participation in the plan of care; give them choices about some aspects of care but do not overwhelm them with choices.
- Stay with clients as needed to promote safety and feelings of security and to reduce fear.
- Control the environment to minimize additional stressors such as reducing noise, limiting the number of persons in the room, and providing care by the same nurse as much as possible.
- Implement suicide precautions if indicated.
- Communicate in short, clear sentences.
- Help clients to:
  a. Determine situations that precipitate anxiety and identify signs of anxiety.

  b. Verbalize feelings, perceptions, and fears as appropriate. Some cultures discourage the expression of feelings.
  c. Identify personal strengths.
  d. Recognize usual coping patterns and differentiate positive from negative coping mechanisms.
  e. Identify new strategies for managing stress (e.g., exercise, massage, progressive relaxation).
  f. Identify available support systems.
- Teach clients about:
  a. The importance of adequate exercise, a balanced diet, and rest and sleep to energize the body and enhance coping abilities.
  b. Support groups available such as Alcoholics Anonymous, Weight Watchers or Overeaters Anonymous, and parenting and child abuse support groups.
  c. Educational programs available such as time management, assertiveness training, and meditation groups.

CLINICAL ALERT

A nurse who is concerned for his or her own safety while working with an angry client should withdraw from the situation or obtain support from another individual.

Using Relaxation Techniques

Several relaxation techniques can be used to quiet the mind, release tension, and counteract the fight or flight responses of GAS discussed earlier in this chapter. Nurses can teach these techniques to clients. Nurses should also encourage clients to use these techniques when they encounter stressful health situations. Examples of these situations are (a) during childbirth, (b) postoperatively to cope with pain, and (c) before and during a painful procedure. Many agencies now have relaxation tapes available that the client can borrow or purchase. Some clients make their own recordings. Specific relaxation techniques are discussed in Chapter 5 ∞ and include the following:

- Breathing exercises
- Massage
- Progressive relaxation
- Imagery
- Biofeedback
- Yoga
- Meditation
- Therapeutic touch
- Music therapy
- Humor and laughter

Crisis Intervention

A *crisis* is an acute, time-limited state of disequilibrium resulting from situational, developmental, or societal sources of stress. A person in crisis is temporarily unable to cope with or adapt to the stressor by using previous methods of problem solving. People in crisis generally have a distorted perception of the event and do not have adequate situational support or coping mechanisms. Common characteristics of crises are shown in Box 30–3.

Crisis intervention is a short-term helping process of assisting clients to (a) work through a crisis to its resolution and (b) restore their precrisis level of functioning. It is a process that includes not only the client in crisis but also various members of the client's support network. Crisis intervention is not the specialty of any one professional group. People who intervene in crises come from the fields of nursing, medicine, psychology, social work, and theology. Police officers, teachers, school guidance counselors, and rescue workers, among others, are often on the spot in moments of crisis.

Because a state of disequilibrium is so uncomfortable, a crisis is self-limiting. However, a person experiencing a crisis alone is more vulnerable to unsuccessful negotiation than is a person working through a crisis with help. Working with another person increases the likelihood that the person in crisis will resolve it in a positive way. Often a state of crisis offers the individual or family great potential for growth and change.

The traditional steps of the nursing process correspond closely to the steps of crisis intervention. In assessment, the nurse or helper must focus on the person and the problem, collecting data about the client, the client's coping style, the precipitating event, the situational supports, the client's perception of the crisis, and the client's ability to handle the problem. This information is the basis for later decisions about how and when to intervene and whom to call. An individual's perception of the event and personal response will determine the nursing diagnoses. The most common nursing diagnoses for people in crisis are similar to those cited earlier in this chapter. In addition, diagnoses such as *Risk for Self-Directed Violence, Risk for Other-Directed Violence, Rape Trauma Syndrome,* and *Hopelessness* may be appropriate.

Effective planning for crisis intervention must be based on careful assessment and developed in active collaboration with the person in crisis and the significant people in that person's life.

Implementation involves crisis counseling and home crisis visits. **Crisis counseling** focuses on solving immediate problems and it involves individuals, groups, or families. Crisis intervention centers rely heavily on telephone counseling by volunteers who have professional consultation available to them. Also known as hotlines and often available around the clock, they allow callers to remain anonymous. The volunteers usually work within a protocol that indicates what information they need from the client to assess the crisis. Their goal is to plan steps to provide immediate relief and then long-term follow-up if necessary.

Crisis home visits are made when telephone counseling does not suffice or when the crisis workers need to

BOX 30–3 Common Characteristics of Crises

- All crises are experienced as sudden. The person is usually not aware of a warning signal, even if others could "see it coming." The individual or family may feel that they had little or no preparation for the event or trauma.
- The crisis is often experienced as ultimately life threatening, whether this perception is realistic or not.
- Communication with significant others is often decreased or cut off.

- There may be perceived or real displacement from familiar surroundings or loved ones.

  All crises have an aspect of loss, whether actual or perceived. The losses can include an object, a person, a hope, a dream, or any significant factor for that individual.

obtain additional information by direct observation or to reach a client who is unobtainable by telephone. Home visits are appropriate when crisis workers need to initiate contacts rather than waiting for clients to come to them; for example, when a telephone caller is assessed to be highly suicidal or when a concerned neighbor, primary care provider, or clergy member informs the agency of clients in potential crisis.

Stress Management for Nurses

Nurses, like clients, are susceptible to experiencing anxiety and stress. Nursing practice involves many stressors related to both clients and the work environment—understaffing, increasing severity of client illnesses, adjusting to various work shifts, being expected to assume responsibilities for which one is not prepared, inadequate support from supervisors and peers, visiting homes that are depressing, caring for dying clients, and so on. Although most nurses cope effectively with the physical and emotional demands of nursing, in some situations nurses become overwhelmed and develop **burnout,** a complex syndrome of behaviors that can be likened to the exhaustion stage of the general adaptation syndrome. The nurse with burnout manifests physical and emotional depletion, a negative attitude and self-concept, and feelings of helplessness and hopelessness.

Nurses can prevent burnout by using the techniques to manage stress discussed for clients. Nurses must first recognize their stress and become attuned to such responses as feelings of being overwhelmed, fatigue, angry outbursts, physical illness, and increases in coffee drinking, smoking, or substance abuse. Once attuned to stress and personal reactions, it is necessary to identify which situations produce the most pronounced reactions so that steps may be taken to reduce the stress. Suggestions include:

- Plan a daily relaxation program with meaningful quiet times to reduce tension (e.g., read, listen to music, soak in a tub, or meditate).
- Establish a regular exercise program to direct energy outward.
- Study assertiveness techniques to overcome feelings of powerlessness in relationships with others. Learn to say no.
- Learn to accept failures—your own and others—and make it a constructive learning experience. Recognize that most people do the best they can. Learn to ask for help, to show your feelings with colleagues, and to support your colleagues in times of need.
- Accept what cannot be changed. There are certain limitations in every situation. Get involved in constructive change efforts if organizational policies and procedures cause stress.
- Develop collegial support groups to deal with feelings and anxieties generated in the work setting.
- Participate in professional organizations to address workplace issues.
- Seek counseling if indicated to help clarify concerns.

EVALUATING

Using the desired outcomes developed during the planning stage as a guide, the nurse collects data needed to determine whether client goals and outcomes have been achieved. Examples of client goals and related outcomes are shown in Identifying Nursing Diagnoses, Outcomes, and Interventions earlier and in the accompanying Nursing Care Plan.

If outcomes are not achieved, the nurse, client, and support people, if appropriate, need to explore the reasons before modifying the care plan. Questions such as the following need to be considered:

- How does the client perceive the problem?
- Is there an underlying problem that has not been identified?
- Have new stressors occurred that interfere with successful coping?
- Were existing coping strategies sufficient to meet intended outcomes?
- How does the client perceive the effectiveness of new coping strategies?
- Did the client implement new coping strategies properly?
- Did the client access and use available resources?
- Have family members and significant others provided effective support?

LOSS AND GRIEF

Everyone experiences loss, grieving, and death at some time during his or her life. People may suffer the loss of valued relationships through life changes, such as moving from one city to another, separation, divorce, or the death of a parent, spouse, or friend. People may grieve changing life roles as they watch grown children leave home or they retire from their lifelong work. The loss of valued material objects through theft or natural disaster can evoke feelings of grief and loss. When people's lives are affected by civil or national strife, they may grieve the loss of valued ideals such as safety, freedom, or democracy.

In the clinical setting, the nurse encounters clients who may be experiencing grief related to declining health, loss of a body part, terminal illness, or the impending death of self or a significant other. The nurse may also work with clients in community settings who are grieving losses related to personal crisis (e.g., divorce, separation) or disaster (e.g., war, earthquakes, terrorism, or hurricanes). Therefore, it is important for the nurse to understand the significance of loss and develop the ability to assist clients as they work through the grieving process.

Nurses may interact with dying clients and their families or caregivers in a variety of settings, from a fetal demise (death of an unborn child), to the adolescent victim of an accident, to an elderly client who finally succumbs to a chronic illness. Nurses must recognize the various influences on the dying process—legal, ethical, religious and

LIFESPAN CONSIDERATIONS   Stress and Coping

Infants and Children

- Children's perceptions of and responses to stress are dependent on their developmental stage. Infants sense stressors in their environment and respond in a diffuse way, often crying and clinging. Toddlers and preschool-age children may be frightened and react by withdrawing or losing control. School-age children and adolescents are more capable of thinking about incidents that cause stress (e.g., a catastrophic accident) and talking about it with adults.
- Temperament is a factor that influences how children respond to stress. An outgoing, low-sensitivity child, for example, is less likely than a timid, intense child to be upset by a family move to a different state.
- Anxiety disorders are the most common psychiatric disorders in children but are frequently unrecognized (Antai-Otong, 2003).
- As children grow, they are able to develop more coping skills to manage stressful situations. Nurses have an important role in teaching parents to recognize stress in their children and to help their children cope.

Middle-Aged Adults

- Middle-aged adults are often called the "sandwich generation." They find themselves caring for children and grandchildren and often caring for aging parents at the same time. When these activities become time and energy consuming, there is often not enough time left for attention to self. Nurses need to be aware of this and assist in suggesting resources and effective planning to ease the strain.

Older Adults

- Older adults experience many losses and changes in their lives. They may be incremental and, over time, become stressful and possibly overwhelming. Changes in health, decreased functional ability and independence, need for relocation, loss of family and friends, and becoming a caregiver for a spouse or friend are a few of the stresses often experienced by older adults. Many of them have survived significant challenges in their earlier lives and have learned effective coping skills. Nurses can help them plan, evaluate their strategies, and learn new strategies, if needed. Informal and formal social supports are very important in learning to successfully live with these changes and stress.
- Some effective coping methods for older adults are exercise, learning different relaxation techniques, participation in activities, adequate nutrition and rest, and engaging in expressive creative activities, such as art, music, and journaling. Referral to community resources and supports should be done when appropriate. It is most important to see older adults as unique individuals, with unique past experiences and very specific needs as they age.

---

spiritual, biologic, personal—and be prepared to provide sensitive, skilled, and supportive care to all those affected.

Loss is an actual or potential situation in which something that is valued is changed or no longer available. People can experience the loss of body image, a significant other, a sense of well-being, a job, personal possessions, or beliefs. Illness and hospitalization often produce losses.

Death is a fundamental loss, both for the dying person and for those who survive. Although death is inevitable, it can stimulate people to grow in their understanding of themselves and others. Death can be viewed as the dying person's final opportunity to experience life in ways that bring significance and fulfillment. People experiencing loss often search for the meaning of the event, and it is generally accepted that finding meaning is needed in order for healing to occur. However, persons can be well adjusted without searching for meaning, and even those who find meaning may not see it as an end point but rather an ongoing process.

Types and Sources of Loss

There are two general types of loss, actual and perceived. An actual loss can be recognized by others. A **perceived loss** is experienced by one person but cannot be verified by others. Psychologic losses are often perceived losses in that they are not directly verifiable. For example, a woman who leaves her employment to care for her children at home may perceive a loss of independence and freedom. Both losses can be anticipatory. An **anticipatory loss** is experienced before the loss actually occurs. For example, a woman whose husband is dying may experience actual loss in anticipation of his death.

Loss can be viewed as situational or developmental. The loss of one's job, the death of a child, or the loss of functional ability because of acute illness or injury are *situational losses*. Losses that occur in the process of normal development—such as the departure of grown children from the home, retirement from a career, and the death of aged parents—are *developmental losses* that can to some extent be anticipated and prepared for.

There are many sources of loss: (a) loss of an aspect of oneself—a body part, a physiologic function, or a psychologic attribute; (b) loss of an object external to oneself; (c) separation from an accustomed environment; and (d) loss of a loved or valued person.

ASPECT OF SELF   The loss of an aspect of self changes a person's body image, even though the loss may not be obvious. A face scarred from a burn is generally obvious to people; loss of part of the stomach or loss of ability to feel emotion may not be as obvious. The degree to which these

Nursing Care Plan   Ineffective Coping

ASSESSMENT DATA	NURSING DIAGNOSIS	DESIRED OUTCOMES*
Nursing Assessment Ruby Smithson is a 55-year-old mother of four children who is hospitalized with breast cancer. She is scheduled for a modified radical mastectomy. Ruby was relatively healthy until she found a lump in her right breast 1 week ago. She and her husband are extremely anxious about the surgery. Ruby confides to the admitting nurse that "I can't stand the idea of having one of my breasts cut off; I don't know how I'm going to be able to even look at myself." Mr. Smithson informs the nurse that Ruby has been abusing alcohol since her diagnosis and neglecting her responsibilities as a mother. She is tearful and doesn't see how she will be able to continue her work as a dress designer.	*Ineffective Coping* related to personal vulnerability secondary to mastectomy (as evidenced by verbalization of inability to cope, substance abuse, inability to meet role expectations)	**Coping** [1302], as evidenced by often demonstrating ability to • Identify effective and ineffective coping patterns • Verbalize sense of control • Report decrease in negative feelings • Modify lifestyle as needed **Social Support** [1504], as evidenced by substantial reports of • Willingness to call on others for help • Emotional assistance provided by others
Physical Examination Height: 164 cm (5'5") Weight: 58 kg (158 lb) Temperature: 37°C (98.6°F) Pulse rate: 88 BPM Respirations: 16/minute Blood pressure: 142/88 mm Hg	**Diagnostic Data** Chest x-ray negative, CBC, and urinalysis within normal limits	

NURSING INTERVENTIONS*/ SELECTED ACTIVITIES	RATIONALE
Coping Enhancement [5230]	
Provide an atmosphere of acceptance.	*Establishing rapport is essential to a therapeutic relationship and supports the client in self-reflection. Recognizing problems and sharing feelings is best brought about in an atmosphere of warmth and trust.*
Provide factual information concerning the diagnosis, treatment, and prognosis.	*Factual information serves as a foundation for Ruby to explore feelings and alternative coping strategies. Stressed clients often misunderstand facts and require frequent clarification so that appropriate conclusions can be drawn. Having valid information helps relieve stress.*
Appraise Ruby's adjustment to changes in body image.	*Alteration in body image may be a major issue for Ruby and should be explored to facilitate therapeutic intervention. Coping strategies often change with a reappraisal of the situation.*
Arrange situations that encourage her autonomy. Give her as many opportunities as possible to make decisions/choices for herself.	*Enhances a sense of control, personal achievement, and self-esteem.*
Explore with her previous methods of dealing with life problems.	*Present and past coping status assists both Ruby and her husband in capitalizing on successful methods, identifying ineffective strategies, and developing new skills more appropriate to the present situation. Also determines risk for inflicting self-harm.*
Encourage verbalization of feelings, perceptions, and fears.	*Open, nonthreatening discussions facilitate the identification of causative and contributing factors.*
Encourage Ruby to identify her own strengths and abilities.	*Assists Ruby to develop appropriate strategies for coping based on personal strengths and previous experiences. Improves self-concept and sense of ability to manage stress.*
Encourage Ruby to realistically describe changes in her role.	*Individuals experiencing stress may have unrealistic perceptions or reality distortions. Helping Ruby clearly describe her role would be beneficial in developing realistic goals for role achievement.*
Foster constructive outlets for anger and hostility.	*Assists the individual in channeling potentially harmful emotions and physical energy into constructive behavior.*

Support System Enhancement [5440]

Observe the degree of family support.	*Assessing family interaction serves as a basis for identifying Ruby's support systems or lack thereof.*
Determine barriers to using support systems.	*Although adequate support systems may be available, Ruby may not be using them or may be using them ineffectively.*
Involve husband, family, and friends in the care and planning.	*Supporting Ruby in acknowledging changes in her appearance conveys acceptance and provides a foundation for her to begin to adjust.*
Discuss with concerned others how they can help.	*Family and friends are often willing but unsure how to help. Identifying specific strategies such as praise and encouragement during rehabilitation and healing will promote acceptance of change.*
Refer Ruby to a community-based breast cancer support group.	*Community support is beneficial in helping to meet unresolved needs, decreasing feelings of social isolation, and facilitating a positive self-image.*

EVALUATION

The coping outcome was not met. Following surgery, Ruby was withdrawn. During bathing, she would not assist and turned her head away when the dressing was removed. She refused to learn how to manage the wound drain or to discuss her feelings or plans for the future. Because clients having a mastectomy are often hospitalized for only a few days, it may be that she requires more time to reach the desired outcome. Continue to offer information and demonstrate availability for when she is ready to verbalize feelings. Social support outcome partly met. Ruby allows her husband to provide direct care and emotional support for her. A social worker was consulted and discharge was delayed for 24 hours. Ruby has agreed that the social worker can contact a breast cancer support group and ask the group to call her.

The NOC # for desired outcomes and the NIC # for nursing interventions are listed in brackets following the appropriate outcome or intervention. Outcomes, indicators, interventions, and activities selected are only a sample of those suggested by NOC and NIC and should be further individualized for each client.

CRITICAL THINKING QUESTIONS

1. If Ruby had been able to choose a lumpectomy rather than a mastectomy (less visible, smaller, potentially less "meaningful" tissue removal), would the nursing diagnosis and expected outcomes remain the same? Why or why not?

2. Does Ruby's situation reflect more of a stimulus-based model or a response-based model? Why?

3. While working with Ruby, she becomes very angry and says to you "You don't understand. You've never had to go through this." How would you respond?

4. Based on the evaluation above, do you believe that Ruby is in crisis? What factors led to your decision? How does your view change the modifications indicated in her care?

5. Give one example of how Ruby might use the defense mechanisms described on page 861. Explain whether this is adaptive or maladaptive.

∞ *See Answers in MyNursingKit.*

losses affect a person largely depends on the integrity of the person's body image.

During old age, changes occur in physical and mental capabilities. Again the self-image is vulnerable. Old age is the stage in life when people may experience many losses: of employment, of usual activities, of independence, of health, of friends, and of family.

EXTERNAL OBJECTS Loss of external objects includes (a) loss of inanimate objects that have importance to the person, such as the loss of money or the burning down of a family's house; and (b) loss of animate (live) objects such as pets that provide love and companionship.

FAMILIAR ENVIRONMENT Separation from an environment and people who provide security can result in a sense of loss. The 6-year-old is likely to feel loss when first leaving the home environment to attend school. The university student who moves away from home for the first time also experiences a sense of loss.

LOVED ONES The loss of a loved one or valued person through illness, divorce, separation, or death can be very disturbing. In some illnesses (such as Alzheimer's dementia), a person may undergo personality changes that make friends and family feel they have lost that person.

The death of a loved one is a permanent and complete loss. In contemporary American society, people may be uncomfortable talking about death and being around people who are dying. There is a tendency to consider using extraordinary measures to prolong and preserve life.

Grief, Bereavement, and Mourning

Grief is the total response to the emotional experience related to loss. Grief is manifested in thoughts, feelings, and behaviors associated with overwhelming distress or sorrow. **Bereavement** is the subjective response experienced by the surviving loved ones after the death of a person with whom they have shared a significant relationship. **Mourning** is the behavioral process through which grief

CONCEPT MAP   Ineffective Coping

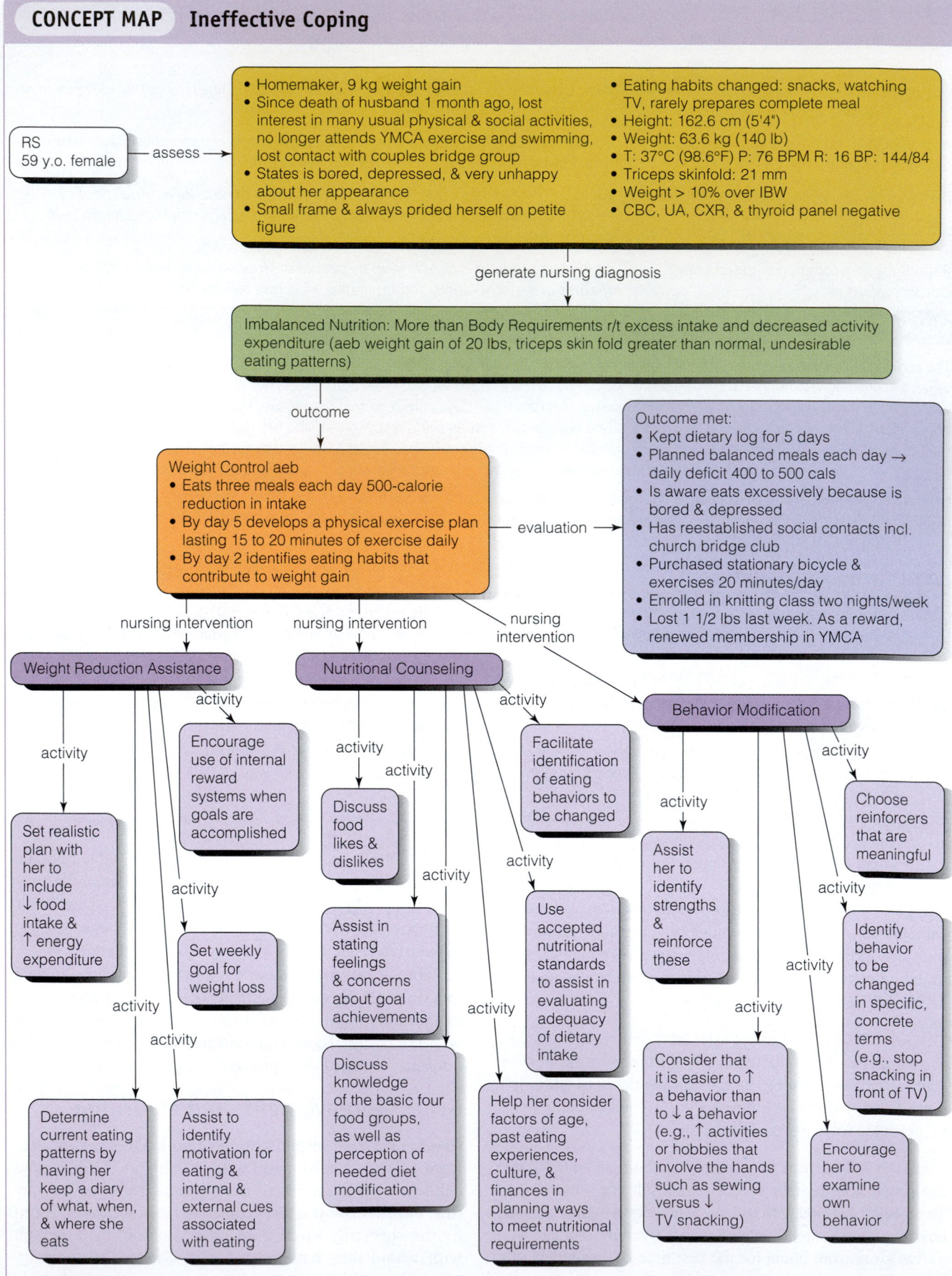

RS
59 y.o. female

→ assess →

- Homemaker, 9 kg weight gain
- Since death of husband 1 month ago, lost interest in many usual physical & social activities, no longer attends YMCA exercise and swimming, lost contact with couples bridge group
- States is bored, depressed, & very unhappy about her appearance
- Small frame & always prided herself on petite figure
- Eating habits changed: snacks, watching TV, rarely prepares complete meal
- Height: 162.6 cm (5'4")
- Weight: 63.6 kg (140 lb)
- T: 37°C (98.6°F) P: 76 BPM R: 16 BP: 144/84
- Triceps skinfold: 21 mm
- Weight > 10% over IBW
- CBC, UA, CXR, & thyroid panel negative

generate nursing diagnosis

Imbalanced Nutrition: More than Body Requirements r/t excess intake and decreased activity expenditure (aeb weight gain of 20 lbs, triceps skin fold greater than normal, undesirable eating patterns)

outcome

Weight Control aeb
- Eats three meals each day 500-calorie reduction in intake
- By day 5 develops a physical exercise plan lasting 15 to 20 minutes of exercise daily
- By day 2 identifies eating habits that contribute to weight gain

→ evaluation →

Outcome met:
- Kept dietary log for 5 days
- Planned balanced meals each day → daily deficit 400 to 500 cals
- Is aware eats excessively because is bored & depressed
- Has reestablished social contacts incl. church bridge club
- Purchased stationary bicycle & exercises 20 minutes/day
- Enrolled in knitting class two nights/week
- Lost 1 1/2 lbs last week. As a reward, renewed membership in YMCA

nursing intervention

Weight Reduction Assistance

activity → Encourage use of internal reward systems when goals are accomplished

activity → Set realistic plan with her to include ↓ food intake & ↑ energy expenditure

activity → Set weekly goal for weight loss

activity → Determine current eating patterns by having her keep a diary of what, when, & where she eats

activity → Assist to identify motivation for eating & internal & external cues associated with eating

nursing intervention

Nutritional Counseling

activity → Discuss food likes & dislikes

activity → Facilitate identification of eating behaviors to be changed

activity → Assist in stating feelings & concerns about goal achievements

activity → Discuss knowledge of the basic four food groups, as well as perception of needed diet modification

activity → Use accepted nutritional standards to assist in evaluating adequacy of dietary intake

activity → Help her consider factors of age, past eating experiences, culture, & finances in planning ways to meet nutritional requirements

nursing intervention

Behavior Modification

activity → Assist her to identify strengths & reinforce these

activity → Choose reinforcers that are meaningful

activity → Identify behavior to be changed in specific, concrete terms (e.g., stop snacking in front of TV)

activity → Consider that it is easier to ↑ a behavior than to ↓ a behavior (e.g., ↑ activities or hobbies that involve the hands such as sewing versus ↓ TV snacking)

activity → Encourage her to examine own behavior

is eventually resolved or altered; it is often influenced by culture, spiritual beliefs, and custom. Grief and mourning are experienced not only by the person who faces the death of a loved one but also by the person who suffers other kinds of losses. Grieving is essential for good mental and physical health. It permits the individual to cope with the loss gradually and to accept it as part of reality. Grief is a social process; it is best shared and carried out with the assistance of others.

Working through one's grief is important because bereavement may have potentially devastating effects on health. Among the symptoms that can accompany grief are anxiety, depression, weight loss, difficulties in swallowing, vomiting, fatigue, headaches, dizziness, fainting, blurred vision, skin rashes, excessive sweating, menstrual disturbances, palpitations, chest pain, and dyspnea. The bereaved may also experience alterations in libido, concentration, and patterns of eating, sleeping, activity, and communication.

Although bereavement can threaten health, a positive resolution of the grieving process can enrich the individual with new insights, values, challenges, openness, and sensitivity. For some, the pain of loss, though diminished, recurs for the rest of their lives.

TYPES OF GRIEF RESPONSES   A normal grief reaction may be abbreviated or anticipatory. *Abbreviated grief* is brief but genuinely felt. This can occur when the lost object is not significantly important to the grieving person or may have been replaced immediately by another, equally esteemed object. **Anticipatory grief** is experienced in advance of the event such as the wife who grieves before her ailing husband dies. A young girl may grieve in advance of an operation that will leave a scar on her body. Because many of the normal symptoms of grief will have already been expressed in anticipation, the reaction when the loss actually occurs is sometimes quite abbreviated.

Disenfranchised grief occurs when a person is unable to acknowledge the loss to other persons. Situations in which this may occur often relate to a socially unacceptable loss that cannot be spoken about, such as suicide, abortion, or giving a child up for adoption. Other examples include losses of relationships that are socially unsanctioned and may not be known to other people (such as homosexuality or extramarital relationships).

Unhealthy grief—that is, pathologic or **complicated grief**—exists when the strategies to cope with the loss are maladaptive. Many factors can contribute to complicated grief, including a prior traumatic loss, family or cultural barriers to the emotional expression of grief, sudden death, strained relationships between the survivor and the deceased, and lack of adequate support for the survivor (Egan & Arnold, 2003).

Complicated grief may take several different forms. *Unresolved or chronic grief* is extended in length and severity. The same signs are expressed as with normal grief, but the bereaved may also have difficulty expressing the grief, may deny the loss, or may grieve beyond the expected time.

With *inhibited grief,* many of the normal symptoms of grief are suppressed, and other effects, including somatic, are experienced instead. *Delayed grief* occurs when feelings are purposely or subconsciously suppressed until a much later time. A survivor who appears to be using dangerous activities as a method to lessen the pain of grieving may be experiencing *exaggerated grief.*

Complicated grief after a death may be inferred from the following data or observations:

- The client fails to grieve; for example, a husband does not cry at, or absents himself from, his wife's funeral.
- The client avoids visiting the grave and refuses to participate in memorial services, even though these practices are a part of the client's culture.
- The client becomes recurrently symptomatic on the anniversary of a loss or during holidays.
- The client develops persistent guilt and lowered self-esteem.
- Even after a prolonged period, the client continues to search for the lost person. Some may consider suicide to effect reunion.
- A relatively minor event triggers symptoms of grief.
- Even after a period of time, the client is unable to discuss the deceased with composure; for example, the client's voice cracks and quivers, and eyes become moist.
- After the normal period of grief, the client experiences physical symptoms similar to those of the person who died.
- The client's relationships with friends and relatives worsen following the death.

Many factors contribute to unresolved grief after a death:

- Ambivalence (intense feelings, both positive and negative) toward the lost person
- A perceived need to be brave and in control; fear of losing control in front of others
- Endurance of multiple losses, such as the loss of an entire family, which the bereaved finds too overwhelming to contemplate
- Extremely high emotional value invested in the dead person; failure to grieve in this instance helps the bereaved avoid the reality of the loss
- Uncertainty about the loss—for example, when a loved one is "missing in action"
- Lack of support systems

Stages of Grieving

Many authors have described stages or phases of grieving, perhaps the most well known of them being Kübler-Ross (1969), who described five stages: denial, anger, bargaining, depression, and acceptance (Table 30–4). Engel (1964) identified six stages of grieving: shock and disbelief, developing awareness, restitution, resolving the loss, idealization, and outcome. Sanders (1998) described five phases of bereavement: shock, awareness, conservation/withdrawal, healing, and renewal.

TABLE 30–4   Client Responses and Nursing Implications in Kübler-Ross's Stages of Grieving

STAGE	BEHAVIORAL RESPONSES	NURSING IMPLICATIONS
Denial	Refuses to believe that loss is happening.	Verbally support client but do not reinforce denial.
	Is unready to deal with practical problems, such as prosthesis after the loss of a leg.	Examine your own behavior to ensure that you do not share in client's denial.
	May assume artificial cheerfulness to prolong denial.	
Anger	Client or family may direct anger at nurse or staff about matters that normally would not bother them.	Help client understand that anger is a normal response to feelings of loss and powerlessness.
		Avoid withdrawal or retaliation; do not take anger personally.
		Deal with needs underlying any angry reaction.
		Provide structure and continuity to promote feelings of security.
		Allow clients as much control as possible over their lives.
Bargaining	Seeks to bargain to avoid loss. May express feelings of guilt or fear of punishment for past sins, real or imagined.	Listen attentively, and encourage client to talk to relieve guilt and irrational fear.
		If appropriate, offer spiritual support.
Depression	Grieves over what has happened and what cannot be.	Allow client to express sadness.
	May talk freely (e.g., reviewing past losses such as money or job), or may withdraw.	Communicate nonverbally by sitting quietly without expecting conversation.
		Convey caring by touch.
Acceptance	Comes to terms with loss.	Help family and friends understand client's decreased need to socialize.
	May have decreased interest in surroundings and support people.	Encourage client to participate as much as possible in the treatment program.
	May wish to begin making plans (e.g., will, prosthesis, altered living arrangements).	

Martocchio (1985) described five clusters of grief—shock and disbelief; yearning and protest; anguish, disorganization, and despair; identification in bereavement; and reorganization and restitution—and maintained that there is no single correct way, nor a correct timetable, by which a person progresses through the grief process. Whether a person can succeed in integrating the loss and how this is accomplished are related to that person's individual development and personal makeup. In addition, individuals responding to the very same loss cannot be expected to follow the same pattern or schedule in resolving their grief, even while they support each other.

Rando (1991, 1993, 2000) has written extensively on the subject of grief, describing three categories of responses: avoidance, confrontation, and accommodation. Avoidance is similar to Kübler-Ross's phases of denial, anger, and bargaining and Engel's phase of shock and disbelief. Confrontation is the most upsetting phase for the grieving person facing the loss. Accommodation is the phase in which the person begins to resume more usual activities, feels better, and places the loss in perspective.

The nurse assesses the grieving client or family members following a loss to determine the phase or stage of grieving. Physiologically, the body responds to a current or anticipated loss with a stress reaction. The nurse can assess the clinical signs of this response.

Manifestations of grief that would be considered normal include verbalization of the loss, crying, sleep disturbance, loss of appetite, and difficulty concentrating. Complicated grieving may be characterized by extended time of denial, depression, severe physiologic symptoms, or suicidal thoughts.

Factors Influencing the Loss and Grief Responses

A number of factors affect a person's response to a loss or death. These factors include age, significance of the loss, culture, spiritual beliefs, gender, socioeconomic status, support systems, and the cause of the loss or death. Nurses can learn general concepts about the influence of these factors of the grieving experience, but the constellation of these factors and their significance will vary from individual to individual.

AGE   Age affects a person's understanding of and reaction to loss. With familiarity, people usually increase their understanding and acceptance of life, loss, and death.

People do not usually experience the loss of loved ones at regular intervals. As a result, preparation for these experiences is difficult. Coping with other of life's losses, such as the loss of a pet, the loss of a friend, and the loss of youth or a job, can help people anticipate the more severe loss of death of loved ones by teaching them successful coping strategies.

Childhood   Children differ from adults not only in their understanding of loss and death but also in how they are affected by the loss of others. The loss of a parent or other significant person can threaten the child's ability to develop, and regression sometimes results. Assisting the child with the grief experience includes helping the child regain the normal continuity and pace of emotional development.

Some adults may assume that children do not have the same need as an adult to grieve the loss of others. In situations of crisis and loss, children are sometimes pushed aside or protected from the pain. They can feel afraid, abandoned, and lonely. Careful work with bereaved children is especially necessary because experiencing a loss in childhood can have serious effects later in life.

Early and Middle Adulthood   As people grow, they come to experience loss as part of normal development. By middle age, for example, the loss of a parent through death seems a more normal occurrence compared to the death of a younger person. Coping with the death of an aged parent has even been viewed as an essential developmental task of the middle-aged adult.

The middle-aged adult can experience losses other than death. For example, losses resulting from impaired health or body function and losses of various role functions can be difficult for the middle-aged adult. How the middle-aged adult responds to such losses is influenced by previous experiences with loss, the person's sense of self-esteem, and the strength and availability of support.

Late Adulthood   Losses experienced by older adults include loss of health, mobility, independence, and work role. Limited income and the need to change one's living accommodations can also lead to feelings of loss and grieving.

For older adults, the loss through death of a longtime mate is profound. Although individuals differ in their ability to deal with such a loss, research suggests that health problems for widows and widowers increase following the death of the spouse (Caserta, Lund, & Obray, 2004). Because the majority of deaths occur among older adults, and because the number of older adults is increasing in North America, nurses will need to be especially alert to the potential problems of older grieving adults.

SIGNIFICANCE OF THE LOSS   The significance of a loss depends on the perceptions of the individual experiencing the loss. One person may experience a great sense of loss over a divorce; another may find it only mildly disrupting. A number of factors affect the significance of the loss:

- Importance of the lost person, object, or function
- Degree of change required because of the loss
- The person's beliefs and values

For older people who have already encountered many losses, an anticipated loss such as their own death may not be viewed as highly negative, and they may be apathetic about it instead of reactive. More than fearing death, some may fear loss of control or becoming a burden.

CULTURE   Culture influences an individual's reaction to loss. How grief is expressed is often determined by the customs of the culture. Unless an extended family structure exists, grief is handled by the nuclear family. The death of a family member in a typical nuclear family leaves a great void because the same few individuals fill most of the roles. In cultures where several generations and extended family members either reside in the same household or are physically close, the impact of a family member's death may be softened because the roles of the deceased are quickly filled by other relatives.

Some persons have adopted the belief that grief is a private matter to be endured internally. Therefore, feelings tend to be repressed and may remain unidentified. People who have been socialized to "be strong" and "make the best of the situation" may not express deep feelings or personal concerns when they experience a serious loss.

Some cultural groups value social support and the expression of loss. In some groups, expressions of grief through wailing, crying, physical prostration, and other outward demonstrations are acceptable and encouraged. Other groups may frown on this demonstration as a loss of control, favoring a more quiet and stoic expression of grief. In cultural groups where strong kinship ties are maintained, physical and emotional support and assistance are provided by family members.

SPIRITUAL BELIEFS   Spiritual beliefs and practices greatly influence both a person's reaction to loss and subsequent behavior. Most religious groups have practices related to dying, and these are often important to the client and support people. To provide support at a time of death, nurses need to understand the client's particular beliefs and practices.

GENDER   The gender roles into which many people are socialized in the United States and Canada affect their reactions at times of loss. Men are frequently expected to "be strong" and show very little emotion during grief, whereas it is acceptable for women to show grief by crying. Often when a wife dies, the husband, who is the chief mourner, is expected to repress his own emotions and to comfort sons and daughters in their grieving.

Gender roles also affect the significance of body image changes to clients. A man might consider his facial scar to be "macho," but a woman might consider hers ugly. Thus the woman, but not the man, would see the change as a loss.

SOCIOECONOMIC STATUS   The socioeconomic status of an individual often affects the support system available at the time of a loss. A pension plan or insurance, for example, can offer a widowed or disabled person a choice of ways to deal with a loss; a person who is confronted with both severe loss and economic hardship may not be able to cope with either.

SUPPORT SYSTEM   The people closest to the grieving individual are often the first to recognize and provide needed emotional, physical, and functional assistance. However, because many people are uncomfortable or inexperienced in dealing with losses, the usual support people may instead withdraw from the grieving individual. In addition, support may be available when the loss is first recognized, but as the support people return to their usual activities, the need for ongoing support may be unmet. Sometimes, the grieving individual is unable or unready to accept support when it is offered.

CAUSE OF LOSS OR DEATH Individual and societal views on the cause of a loss or death may significantly influence the grief response. Some diseases are considered "clean," such as cardiovascular disorders, and engender compassion, whereas others may be viewed as repulsive and less unfortunate. A loss or death that is beyond the control of those involved may be more acceptable than one that is preventable, such as a drunk driving accident. Injuries or deaths occurring during respected activities, such as "in the line of duty," are considered honorable, whereas those occurring during illicit activities may be considered the individual's just rewards.

NURSING MANAGEMENT

ASSESSING

Nursing assessment of the client experiencing a loss includes three major components: (a) nursing history, (b) assessment of personal coping resources, and (c) physical assessment. During the routine health assessment of every client, the nurse poses questions regarding previous and current losses. The nature of the loss and the significance of such losses to the client must be explored.

If there is a current or recent loss, greater detail is needed in the assessment. Because clients do not always associate physical ailments with emotional responses such as grief, the nurse may need to probe to identify possible loss-related stresses. If the client reports significant losses, it is important to examine how the client usually copes with loss and what resources are available to assist the client in coping. Data regarding general health status; other personal stressors; cultural and spiritual traditions, rituals, and beliefs related to loss and grieving; and the person's support network will be needed in order to determine a plan of care. In assessing the client's response to a current loss, the nurse may identify complicated grief best treated by a health care professional who is expert in assisting such clients. If the nursing assessment reveals severe physical or psychologic signs and symptoms, the client should be referred to an appropriate care provider.

DIAGNOSING

Nursing diagnoses (NANDA International, 2009) relating specifically to grieving include the following:

- *Grieving:* A normal complex process that includes emotional, physical, spiritual, social, and intellectual responses and behaviors by which individuals,

families, and communities incorporate an actual, anticipated, or perceived loss into their daily lives.
- *Complicated Grieving:* A disorder that occurs after the death of a significant other, in which the experience of distress accompanying bereavement fails to follow normative expectations and manifests in functional impairment. *Risk for Complicated Grieving* replaced *Risk for Dysfunctional Grieving* in 2007, which had been added as a new diagnosis in 2005.

Other nursing diagnoses may include:

- *Interrupted Family Processes* if the loss has such impact on the individual and family that usual effective roles and interactions are negatively affected.
- *Risk-prone Health Behavior* if the client has great difficulty placing the loss in appropriate perspective to his or her other life activities.
- *Risk for Loneliness* related to the loss of relationships with others.

Examples of clinical applications of some of these diagnoses using NANDA, NIC, and NOC designations are shown in the accompanying Identifying Nursing Diagnoses, Outcomes, and Interventions, "Clients Who Are Grieving."

PLANNING

The overall goals for clients who are grieving the loss of body function or a body part are to adjust to the changed ability and to redirect both physical and emotional energy into rehabilitation. The goals for clients who are grieving the loss of a loved one or thing are to remember them without feeling intense pain and to redirect emotional energy into one's own life and adjust to the actual or impending loss.

Examples of clinical applications of NOC outcomes and NIC interventions are shown in the accompanying Identifying Nursing Diagnoses, Outcomes, and Interventions, "Clients Who Are Grieving."

Planning for Home Care

Clients who have sustained or anticipate a loss may require ongoing nursing care to assist them in adapting to the loss. The determination of how much and what type of home care follow-up is needed is based in great part on the nurse's knowledge of how the client and family have coped with previous losses. In preparation for home care, the nurse reassesses the client's abilities and needs.

IMPLEMENTING

The skills most relevant to situations of loss and grief are attentive listening, silence, open and closed questioning, paraphrasing, clarifying and reflecting feelings, and summarizing. Less helpful to clients are responses that give advice and evaluation, those that interpret and analyze, and those that give unwarranted reassurance. To ensure effective

IDENTIFYING NURSING DIAGNOSES, OUTCOMES, AND INTERVENTIONS   Clients Who Are Grieving

DATA CLUSTER: Teresa Jimenez's son Ramon, age 15, has cystic fibrosis of the lungs. Mother and son are waiting for an appropriate donor for a heart-lung transplant. She says, "We've been called to the transplant unit twice, but things didn't work out. Ramon gets his hopes all geared up, and then he's deflated. I can't eat or sleep worrying. I don't know what I'll do if he doesn't get that transplant. He's all I've got since my husband left us six years ago."

NURSING DIAGNOSIS/DEFINITION	SAMPLE DESIRED OUTCOMES*/ DEFINITION	INDICATORS	SELECTED INTERVENTIONS*/ DEFINITION	SAMPLE NIC ACTIVITIES
Grieving/A normal complex process that includes emotional, physical, spiritual, social, and intellectual responses and behaviors by which individuals, families, and communities incorporate an actual, anticipated, or perceived loss into their daily lives	Grief Resolution [1304]/*Adjustment to actual or impending loss*	Often demonstrated: • Maintains living environment • Seeks social support • Progresses through stages of grief	Grief Work Facilitation [5290]/*Assistance with the resolution of a significant loss*	• Encourage discussion of previous loss experiences (e.g., husband leaving) • Communicate acceptance of discussing loss • Identify sources of community support • Reinforce progress made in the grieving process

*The NOC # for desired outcomes and the NIC # for nursing interventions are listed in brackets following the appropriate outcome or intervention. Outcomes, indicators, interventions, and activities selected are only a sample of those suggested by NOC and NIC and should be further individualized for each client.

communication, the nurse must make an accurate assessment of what is appropriate for the client.

Communication with grieving clients needs to be relevant to their stage of grief. Whether the client is angry or depressed affects how the client hears messages and how the nurse interprets the client's statements.

In addition to using effective communication skills, the nurse implements a plan to provide client and family teaching and to help the client work through the stages of grief.

Facilitating Grief Work

- Explore and respect the client's and family's ethnic, cultural, religious, and personal values in their expressions of grief.
- Teach the client or family what to expect in the grief process, such as that certain thoughts and feelings are normal (acceptable) and that labile emotions, feelings of sadness, guilt, anger, fear, and loneliness will stabilize or lessen over time. Knowing what to expect may lessen the intensity of some reactions.
- Encourage the client to express and share grief with support people. Sharing feelings reinforces relationships and facilitates the grief process.
- Teach family members to encourage the client's expression of grief, not to push the client to move on or enforce his or her own expectations of appropriate reactions. If the client is a child, encourage fam-

ily members to be truthful and to allow the child to participate in the grieving activities of others.
- Encourage the client to resume normal activities on a schedule that promotes physical and psychologic health. Some clients may try to return to normal activities too quickly. However, a prolonged delay in return may indicate complicated grieving.

Providing Emotional Support

- Use silence and personal presence along with techniques of therapeutic communication. These techniques enhance exploration of feelings and let clients know that the nurse acknowledges their feelings.
- Acknowledge the grief of the client's family and significant others. Family support persons are part of the grieving client's world.
- Offer choices that promote client autonomy. Clients need to have a sense of some control over their own lives at a time when much control may not be possible.
- Provide appropriate information regarding how to access community resources: clergy, support groups, and counseling services.
- Suggest additional sources of information and help such as:
  a. Grief Recovery Institute.
  b. Partnership of Caring: America's Voice for the Dying.

    c. American Association of Retired Persons.

    d. Compassionate Friends (for those who have lost a child).

Examples of nursing actions appropriate for clients in various stages of the grief process are shown in the Concept Map at the end of the chapter.

EVALUATING

Evaluating the effectiveness of nursing care of the grieving client is difficult because of the long-term nature of the life transition. Criteria for evaluation must be based on goals set by the client and family.

Client goals and related desired outcomes for a grieving client will depend on the characteristics of the loss and the client. Examples of client goals and related outcomes are shown in the accompanying Identifying Nursing Diagnoses, Outcomes, and Interventions.

If outcomes are not achieved, the nurse needs to explore why the plan was unsuccessful. Such exploration begins with reassessing the client in case the nursing diagnoses were inappropriate. Examples of questions guiding the exploration include:

- Do the client's grieving behaviors indicate dysfunctional grieving or another nursing diagnosis?
- Is the expected outcome unrealistic for the given time frame?
- Does the client have additional stressors previously not considered that are affecting grief resolution?
- Have nursing orders been implemented consistently, compassionately, and genuinely?

DEATH AND DYING

The concept of death is developed over time, as the person grows, experiences various losses, and thinks about concrete and abstract concepts. In general, humans move from a childhood belief in death as a temporary state, to adulthood in which death is accepted as very real but also very frightening, to older adulthood in which death may be viewed as more desirable than living with a poor quality of life. Table 30–5 describes some of the specific beliefs common to different age groups. The nurse's knowledge of these developmental stages helps in understanding some of the client's responses to a life-threatening situation.

Responses to Dying and Death

The reaction of any person to another person's impending or real death, or to the potential reality of his or her own death, depends on all the factors regarding loss and the development of the concept of death. In spite of the individual variations in a person's views about the cause of death, spiritual beliefs, availability of support systems, or any other factor, responses tend to cluster in the phases described by Kübler-Ross (see Table 30–4).

Both the client who is dying and the family members grieve as they recognize the loss. Defining characteristics for the nursing diagnosis of *Grieving* include denial, guilt, anger, despair, feelings of worthlessness, crying, and inability to concentrate. They may extend to thoughts of suicide, delusions, and hallucinations. *Fear,* the feeling of disruption that is related to an identifiable source (in this case someone's death), may also be present. Many of the characteristics seen in a fearful person are similar to those of grieving and include crying, immobility, increased pulse and respirations, dry mouth, anorexia, difficulty sleeping, and nightmares. *Hopelessness* occurs when the person perceives no solutions to a problem—when the death becomes inevitable and the person is unable to see how to move beyond the death. The nurse may observe apathy, pessimism, and inability to make decisions. A person who does perceive a solution to the problem but does not believe that it is possible to implement the solution may be said to experience *Powerlessness.* This loss of control may be manifested by anger, violence, acting out, or depression and passive behavior.

> ### CLINICAL ALERT
> Persons who have experienced the deaths of multiple significant others, such as members of the AIDS community, do not necessarily feel the loss or grieve any more or less than those who have experienced fewer deaths.

Caregivers, both professionals and support persons, also respond to the impending death. The NANDA diagnosis *Risk for Caregiver Role Strain* may be applied to this group. The ongoing responsibilities for providing physical, economic, psychologic, and social support to a dying person can create extreme stress for the provider. Often, the length of time between a terminal diagnosis and when death will occur is unknown and the people supporting the dying person become fatigued and depressed. There may be anger due to loss of time and resources for personal activities or attention to other people. Within a family that usually functions effectively, death of a member may result in *Interrupted Family Processes.* In this situation, the family may be unable to meet the physical, emotional, or spiritual needs of the members and may have difficulty communicating and problem solving.

Professional caregivers, including nurses, may experience role strain due to repeated interactions with dying clients and their families. Although most nurses who work in oncology, hospice, intensive care, emergency, or other areas where client deaths are common have chosen such assignments, there can still be a sense of failure when clients die. Just as there must be support systems for grieving clients, there must also be support systems for grieving health care professionals.

Some people may think of death as the worst occurrence in life and do their best to avoid thinking or talking about death—especially their own. Nurses are not immune to such attitudes. They need to take time to analyze their own feelings about death before they can effectively help

TABLE 30–5	**Development of the Concept of Death**
AGE	BELIEFS/ATTITUDES
Infancy to 5 years	Does not understand concept of death.
	Infant's sense of separation forms basis for later understanding of loss and death.
	Believes death is reversible, a temporary departure, or sleep.
	Emphasizes immobility and inactivity as attributes of death.
5 to 9 years	Understands that death is final.
	Believes own death can be avoided.
	Associates death with aggression or violence.
	Believes wishes or unrelated actions can be responsible for death.
9 to 12 years	Understands death as the inevitable end of life.
	Begins to understand own mortality, expressed as interest in afterlife or as fear of death.
12 to 18 years	Fears a lingering death.
	May fantasize that death can be defied, acting out defiance through reckless behaviors (e.g., dangerous driving, substance abuse).
	Seldom thinks about death, but views it in religious and philosophic terms.
	May seem to reach "adult" perception of death but be emotionally unable to accept it.
	May still hold concepts from previous developmental stages.
18 to 45 years	Has attitude toward death influenced by religious and cultural beliefs.
45 to 65 years	Accepts own mortality.
	Encounters death of parents and some peers.
	Experiences peaks of death anxiety.
	Death anxiety diminishes with emotional well-being.
65+ years	Fears prolonged illness.
	Encounters death of family members and peers.
	Sees death as having multiple meanings (e.g., freedom from pain, reunion with already deceased family members).

others with a terminal illness. Nurses who are uncomfortable with dying clients tend to impede the clients' attempts to discuss dying and death in these ways:

- Change the subject (e.g., "Let's think of something more cheerful" or "You shouldn't say things like that").
- Offer false reassurance (e.g., "You are doing very well").
- Deny what is happening (e.g., "You don't really mean that" or "You're going to live until you're a hundred").
- Be fatalistic (e.g., "Everyone dies sooner or later" or "What's meant to be, will be").
- Block discussion (e.g., "I don't think things are really that bad") and convey an attitude that stops further discussion of the subject.
- Be aloof and distant or avoid the client.
- "Manage" the client's care and make the client feel increasingly dependent and powerless.

Caring for the dying and the bereaved is one of the nurse's most complex and challenging responsibilities, bringing into play all the skills needed for holistic physiologic and psychosocial care. To be effective, nurses must come to grips with their own attitudes toward loss, death, and dying, because these attitudes will directly affect their ability to provide care.

Definitions and Signs of Death

The traditional clinical signs of death were cessation of the apical pulse, respirations, and blood pressure, also referred to as heart-lung death. However, since the advent of artificial means to maintain respirations and blood circulation, identifying death is more difficult. In 1968, the World Medical Assembly adopted the following guidelines for physicians as indications of death:

- Total lack of response to external stimuli
- No muscular movement, especially breathing
- No reflexes
- Flat encephalogram (brain waves)

In instances of artificial support, absence of brain waves for at least 24 hours is an indication of death. Only then can a physician pronounce death, and only after this pronouncement can life-support systems be shut off.

Another definition of death is **cerebral death** or higher brain death, which occurs when the higher brain center, the cerebral cortex, is irreversibly destroyed. In this case, there is "a clinical syndrome characterized by the permanent loss of cerebral and brainstem function, manifested by absence of responsiveness to external stimuli, absence of cephalic reflexes, and apnea. An isoelectric electroencephalogram for at least 30 minutes in the absence of hypothermia and poisoning by central nervous system depressants supports the diagnosis" (Stedman's Medical Dictionary, 2005). People who support this definition of death believe the cerebral cortex, which holds the capacity for thought, voluntary action, and movement, is the individual.

Death-Related Religious and Cultural Practices

Various cultural and religious traditions and practices associated with death, dying, and the grieving process help people cope with these experiences. Nurses are often present through the dying process and at the moment of death. Knowledge of the client's religious and cultural heritage helps nurses provide individualized care to clients and their families, even though they may not participate in the rituals associated with death.

In many cultures, people prefer a peaceful death at home rather than in the hospital. Members of some ethnic groups may request that health professionals not reveal the prognosis to dying clients. They believe the person's last days should be free of worry. People in other cultures prefer that a family member (preferably a male in some cultures) be told the diagnosis so that the client can be tactfully informed by a family member in gradual stages or not be told at all. Nurses also need to determine whom to call, and when, as the impending death draws near.

Beliefs and attitudes about death, its cause, and the soul also vary among cultures. Unnatural deaths, or "bad deaths," are sometimes distinguished from "good deaths." In addition, the death of a person who has behaved well in life may be considered less threatening based on the belief that the person will be reincarnated into a good life.

Beliefs about preparation of the body, autopsy, organ donation, cremation, and prolonging life are closely allied to the person's religion. Autopsy, for example, may be prohibited, opposed, or discouraged by Eastern Orthodox religions, Muslims, Jehovah's Witnesses, and Orthodox Jews. Some religions prohibit the removal of body parts or dictate that all body parts be given appropriate burial. Organ donation is prohibited by Jehovah's Witnesses and Muslims, whereas Buddhists in America consider it an act of mercy and encourage it. Cremation is discouraged, opposed, or prohibited by the Mormon, Eastern Orthodox, and Islamic faiths. Hindus, in contrast, prefer cremation and cast the ashes in a holy river. Prolongation of life is generally encouraged; however, some religions, such as Christian Science, are unlikely to recommend medical means to prolong life, and the Jewish faith generally opposes prolonging life after irreversible brain damage. In hopeless illness, Buddhists may permit euthanasia.

Nurses also need to be knowledgeable about the client's death-related rituals, such as last rites, chanting at the bedside, and other practices, such as special procedures for washing, dressing, positioning, shrouding, and attending the dead. For example, certain cultures retain their native customs in which family members of the same sex wash and prepare the body for burial and cremation. Muslims also customarily turn the body toward Mecca. In several religions, the body cannot be left unattended until burial and persons may be hired to sit with the body if family members do not perform this duty. Nurses need to ask family members about their preference and verify who will carry out these activities. Burial clothes and other cultural or religious items are often important symbols for the funeral. For example, Mormons are often dressed in their "temple clothes." Some Native Americans may be dressed in elaborate apparel and jewelry and wrapped in new blankets with money. The nurse must ensure that any ritual items present in the health care agency be returned to the family or to the funeral home.

NURSING MANAGEMENT

ASSESSING

To gather a complete database that allows accurate analysis and identification of appropriate nursing diagnoses for dying clients and their families, the nurse first needs to recognize the states of awareness manifested by the client and family members.

In cases of terminal illness, the state of awareness shared by the dying person and the family affects the nurse's ability to communicate freely with clients and other health care team members and to assist in the grieving process. Three types of awareness that have been described are closed awareness, mutual pretense, and open awareness (Glaser & Strauss, 1965).

In **closed awareness,** the client is not made aware of impending death. The family may choose this because they do not completely understand why the client is ill or they believe the client will recover. The primary care provider may believe it is best not to communicate a diagnosis or prognosis to the client. Nursing personnel are confronted with an ethical problem in this situation. See Chapter 2 ∞ for further information on ethical dilemmas.

With **mutual pretense,** the client, family, and health personnel know that the prognosis is terminal but do not talk about it and make an effort not to raise the subject. Sometimes the client refrains from discussing death to protect the family from distress. The client may also sense discomfort on the part of health personnel and therefore not bring up the subject. Mutual pretense permits the client a degree of privacy and dignity, but it places a heavy burden on the dying person, who then has no one in whom to confide.

With **open awareness,** the client and others know about the impending death and feel comfortable discussing it, even though it is difficult. This awareness provides the client an opportunity to finalize affairs and even participate in planning funeral arrangements.

Not all people are comfortable with open awareness. Some believe that terminal clients acquire knowledge of their condition even if they are not directly informed. Others believe that clients remain unaware of their condition until the end. It is difficult, however, to distinguish what clients know from what they are willing to accept or acknowledge.

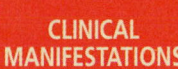

Impending Clinical Death

Loss of Muscle Tone

- Relaxation of the facial muscles (e.g., the jaw may sag)
- Difficulty speaking
- Difficulty swallowing and gradual loss of the gag reflex
- Decreased activity of the gastrointestinal tract, with subsequent nausea, accumulation of flatus, abdominal distention, and retention of feces, especially if narcotics or tranquilizers are being administered
- Possible urinary and rectal incontinence due to decreased sphincter control
- Diminished body movement

Slowing of the Circulation

- Diminished sensation
- Mottling and cyanosis of the extremities
- Cold skin, first in the feet and later in the hands, ears, and nose (the client, however, may feel warm if there is a fever)
- Slower and weaker pulse
- Decreased blood pressure

Changes in Respirations

- Rapid, shallow, irregular, or abnormally slow respirations
- Noisy breathing, referred to as the death rattle, due to collecting of mucus in the throat
- Mouth breathing, dry oral mucous membranes

Sensory Impairment

- Blurred vision
- Impaired senses of taste and smell

Nursing care and support for the dying client and family include making an accurate assessment of the physiologic signs of approaching death. In addition to signs related to the client's specific disease, certain other physical signs are indicative of impending death. The four main characteristic changes are loss of muscle tone, slowing of the circulation, changes in respirations, and sensory impairment. Clinical Manifestations lists indications of impending clinical death.

Various consciousness levels may exist just before death. Some clients are alert, whereas others are drowsy, stuporous, or comatose. Hearing is thought to be the last sense lost.

As death approaches, the nurse assists the family and other significant people to prepare. Depending in part on knowledge of the person's state of awareness, the nurse asks questions that help identify ways to provide support during the period before and after death. In particular, the nurse needs to know what the family expects to happen when the person dies so accurate information can be given at the appropriate depth. When the family members know what to expect, they may be better able to support the dying person and others who are grieving. In addition, they may be able to make certain decisions about events surrounding the death such as whether they will want to view the body after death.

DIAGNOSING

A range of nursing diagnoses, addressing both physiologic and psychosocial needs, can be applied to the dying client, depending on the assessment data. Diagnoses that may be particularly appropriate for the dying client are *Fear, Hopelessness,* and *Powerlessness.* In addition, *Risk for Caregiver Role Strain* and *Interrupted Family Processes* are not uncommon diagnoses for caregivers and family members.

Examples of clinical applications of some of these diagnoses using NANDA, NIC, and NOC designations are shown in the accompanying Identifying Nursing Diagnoses, Outcomes, and Interventions, "Clients Who Are Dying."

PLANNING

Major goals for dying clients are (a) maintaining physiologic and psychologic comfort and (b) achieving a dignified and peaceful death, which includes maintaining personal control and accepting declining health status. When planning care with these clients, the "Dying Person's Bill of Rights" (Box 30–4) can be a useful guide.

BOX 30–4 | **The Dying Person's Bill of Rights**

I have the right to be treated as a living human being until I die.

I have the right to maintain a sense of hopefulness however changing its focus may be.

I have the right to express my feelings and emotions about my approaching death in my own way.

I have the right to participate in decisions concerning my care.

I have the right to expect continuing medical and nursing attention even though cure goals must be changed to comfort goals.

I have the right not to die alone.

I have the right to be free from pain.

I have the right to have my questions answered honestly.

I have the right not to be deceived.

I have the right to have help from and for my family in accepting my death.

I have the right to die in peace and with dignity.

I have the right to retain my individuality and not be judged for my decisions which may be contrary to the beliefs of others.

I have the right to be cared for by caring, sensitive, knowledgeable people who will attempt to understand my needs and will be able to gain some satisfaction in helping me face my death.

Note: From "The Dying Person's Bill of Rights," by A. J. Barbus, 1975, created at the workshop *The Terminally Ill Patient and the Helping Person,* Lansing, MI: South Western Michigan Inservice Education Council.

DATA CLUSTER: Keisha Washington, who has multiple sclerosis and is paralyzed from the neck down, has appealed for someone to help her commit suicide. Her mind and speaking ability appear unimpaired. "I don't want to end up like my sister, who also had MS and had severe pain and became blind and mute before she died."

NURSING DIAGNOSIS/DEFINITION	SAMPLE DESIRED OUTCOMES*/DEFINITION	INDICATORS	SELECTED INTERVENTIONS*/DEFINITION	SAMPLE NIC ACTIVITIES
Hopelessness/Subjective state in which an individual sees limited or no alternatives or personal choices available and is unable to mobilize energy on own behalf	Quality of Life [2000]/*Extent of positive perception of current life circumstances*	Moderately satisfied: • Ability to cope • Pervasive mood	Hope Instillation [5310]/*Facilitation of the development of a positive outlook in a given situation*	• Assist Keisha to identify areas of hope in life • Expand her repertoire of coping mechanisms • Facilitate her reliving and savoring past achievements and experiences • Provide her opportunity to be involved with support groups

*The NOC # for desired outcomes and the NIC # for nursing interventions are listed in brackets following the appropriate outcome or intervention. Outcomes, indicators, interventions, and activities selected are only a sample of those suggested by NOC and NIC and should be further individualized for each client.

Examples of clinical applications of NOC outcomes and NIC interventions are shown in the Identifying Nursing Diagnoses, Outcomes, and Interventions chart.

A major factor in determining whether a person will die in a health care facility or at home is the availability of willing and able caregivers. If the dying person wishes to be at home, and family or others can provide care to maintain symptom control, the nurse should facilitate a referral to outpatient hospice services. Hospice staff and nurses will then conduct a full assessment of the home and care providers' skills.

IMPLEMENTING

The major nursing responsibility for clients who are dying is to assist the client to a peaceful death. More specific responsibilities are the following:

- To minimize loneliness, fear, and depression
- To maintain the client's sense of security, self-confidence, dignity, and self-worth
- To help the client accept losses
- To provide physical comfort

Helping Clients Die with Dignity

Nurses need to ensure that the client is treated with dignity, that is, with honor and respect. Dying clients often feel they have lost control over their lives and over life itself. Helping clients die with dignity involves maintaining their humanity, consistent with their values, beliefs, and culture. By introducing options available to the client and significant others, nurses can restore and support feelings of control. Some choices that clients can make are the location of care (e.g., hospital, home, or hospice facility), times of appointments with health professionals, activity schedule, use of health resources, and times of visits from relatives and friends.

Clients want to be able to manage the events preceding death so they can die peacefully. Nurses can help clients to determine their own physical, psychologic, and social priorities. Dying people often strive for self-fulfillment more than for self-preservation, and may need to find meaning in continuing to live while suffering. Part of the nurse's challenge, then, is to support the client's will and hope.

Although it is natural for people to be uncomfortable discussing death, steps can be taken to make such discussions easier for both the nurse and the client. Strategies include the following:

- Identify your personal feelings about death and how they may influence interactions with clients. Acknowledge personal fears about death, and discuss them with a friend or colleague.
- Focus on the client's needs. The client's fears and beliefs may be different from the nurse's. It is im-

portant that the nurse avoid imposing personal fears and beliefs on the client or family.

- Talk to the client or the family about how the client usually copes with stress. Clients will use their usual coping strategies for dealing with impending death. For example, if they are usually quiet and reflective, they will become more quiet and withdrawn when facing terminal illness.
- Establish a communication relationship that shows concern for and commitment to the client. Communication strategies that let the client know you are available to talk about death include the following:
  a. Describe what you see, for example, "You seem sad. Would you like to talk about what's happening to you?"
  b. Clarify your concern, for example, "I'd like to know better how you feel and how I may help you."
  c. Acknowledge the client's struggle, for example, "It must be difficult to feel so uncomfortable. I would like to help you be more comfortable."
  d. Provide a caring touch. Holding the client's hand or offering a comforting massage can encourage the client to verbalize feelings.
- Determine what the client knows about the illness and prognosis.
- Respond with honesty and directness to the client's questions about death.
- Make time to be available to the client to provide support, listen, and respond.

Hospice and Palliative Care

The hospice movement was founded by the physician Cecily Saunders (who died in 2005) in London, England, in 1967. It was later extended to the United States by Sylvia Lack, also a medical doctor. Hospice care focuses on support and care of the dying person and family, with the goal of facilitating a peaceful and dignified death. Hospice care is based on holistic concepts, emphasizes care to improve quality of life rather than cure, supports the client and family through the dying process, and supports the family through bereavement. Assessing the needs of the client's family is just as important as caring for the client who is receiving hospice care. The condition of the client usually deteriorates, and attention needs to be focused on the caregivers to ensure that they are receiving support and resources as these changes occur. If the hospice team meets regularly, these needs can be discussed and interventions initiated. Physical needs are usually apparent, but emotional and behavioral signs are often more subtle. A good assessment and ongoing evaluation can help indicate when modifications or changes are needed.

The principles of hospice care can be carried out in a variety of settings, the most common being home and the hospital (or nursing home)-based unit. Services focus on symptom control and pain management. Commonly, clients

are eligible for hospice care or hospice insurance benefits when certified by a physician to be likely to die within 6 months. Hospice care is always provided by a team of both health professionals and nonprofessionals to ensure a full range of care services. The National Hospice and Palliative Care Organization reports that over 1 million Americans access hospice services each year.

Palliative care, as described by the World Health Organization, is an approach that improves the quality of life of clients and their families facing the problem associated with life-threatening illness, through the prevention and relief of suffering by means of early identification and impeccable assessment and treatment of pain and other problems, physical, psychosocial and spiritual. Palliative care:

- Provides relief from pain and other distressing symptoms;
- Affirms life and regards dying as a normal process;
- Intends neither to hasten nor postpone death;
- Integrates the psychological and spiritual aspects of client care;
- Offers a support system to help clients live as actively as possible until death;
- Offers a support system to help the family cope during the client's illness and in their own bereavement;
- Uses a team approach to address the needs of clients and their families, including bereavement counselling, if indicated;
- Will enhance quality of life, and may also positively influence the course of illness;
- Is applicable early in the course of illness, in conjunction with other therapies that are intended to prolong life, such as chemotherapy or radiation therapy, and includes those investigations needed to better understand and manage distressing clinical complications (n.d.).

This care may differ from hospice in that the client is not necessarily believed to be imminently dying. Both hospice and palliative care can include end-of-life care, that is, the care provided in the final weeks before death.

There are more than 9,000 nurses in the United States who are nationally certified in hospice and palliative care (National Board for Certification of Hospice and Palliative Nurses, 2006). Beginning in 2005, advanced hospice and palliative care certification is also available for master's-prepared nurses.

Meeting the Physiologic Needs of the Dying Client

The physiologic needs of people who are dying are related to a slowing of body processes and to homeostatic imbalances. Interventions include providing personal hygiene measures; controlling pain; relieving respiratory difficulties; assisting with movement, nutrition, hydration, and elimination; and providing measures related to sensory changes.

Pain control is essential to enable clients to maintain some quality in their life and their daily activities, including eating, moving, and sleeping. Many drugs have been used to control the pain associated with terminal illness: morphine, heroin, methadone, and alcohol. Usually the primary care provider determines the dosage, but the client's opinion should be considered; the client is the one ultimately aware of personal pain tolerance and fluctuations of internal states. Because primary care providers usually prescribe dosage ranges for pain medication, nurses use their own judgment as to the amount and frequency of pain medication in providing client relief. Because of decreased blood circulation, if analgesics cannot be administered orally, they are given by intravenous infusion, sublingually, or rectally, rather than subcutaneously or intramuscularly. Clients on narcotic pain medications also require implementation of a protocol to treat opioid-induced constipation. See Chapter 18 ∞ for more on pain management.

Providing Spiritual Support

Spiritual support is of great importance in dealing with death. Although not all clients identify with a specific religious faith or belief, most have a need for meaning in their lives, particularly as they experience a terminal illness.

The nurse has a responsibility to ensure that the client's spiritual needs are attended to, either through direct intervention or by arranging access to individuals who can provide spiritual care. Nurses need to be aware of their own comfort with spiritual issues and be clear about their own ability to interact supportively with the client. Nurses have a responsibility to not impose their own religious or spiritual beliefs on a client but to respond to the client in relation to the client's own background and needs. Communication skills are most important in helping the client articulate needs and in developing a sense of caring and trust.

Specific interventions may include facilitating expressions of feeling, prayer, meditation, reading, and discussion with appropriate clergy or a spiritual adviser. It is important for nurses to establish an effective interdisciplinary relationship with spiritual support specialists. For a further discussion of spiritual issues, see Chapter 29 ∞.

Supporting the Family

The most important aspects of providing support to the family members of a dying client involve using therapeutic communication to facilitate their expression of feelings. When nothing can reverse the inevitable dying process, the nurse can provide an empathetic and caring presence. The nurse also serves as a teacher, explaining what is happening and what the family can expect. Due to the stress of moving through the grieving process, family members may not absorb what they are told and may need to have information provided repeatedly. The nurse must have a calm and patient demeanor.

Family members should be encouraged to participate in the physical care of the dying person as much as they wish to and are able. The nurse can suggest that they assist with bathing, speak or read to the client, and hold hands. The nurse must not, however, have specific expectations for family members' participation. Those who feel unable to care for or be with the dying person also require support from the nurse and from other family members. They should be shown an appropriate waiting area if they wish to remain nearby.

Sometimes, it seems as if the client is "holding on," possibly out of concern for the family not being ready. It may be therapeutic for both the client and the family for the family to verbally give permission to the client to "let go," to die when he or she is ready. This is a painful process, and the nurse must be prepared to encourage and support the family through saying their last good-byes.

After the client dies, the family should be encouraged to view the body, because this has been shown to facilitate the grieving process (Rich, 2005). They may wish to clip a lock of hair as a remembrance. Children should be included in the events surrounding the death if they wish to.

Postmortem Care

Rigor mortis is the stiffening of the body that occurs about 2 to 4 hours after death. It results from a lack of adenosine triphosphate (ATP), which causes the muscles to contract, which in turn immobilizes the joints. Rigor mortis starts in the involuntary muscles (heart, bladder, and so on), then progresses to the head, neck, and trunk, and finally reaches the extremities.

Because the deceased person's family often wants to view the body, and because it is important that the deceased appear natural and comfortable, nurses need to position the body, place dentures in the mouth, and close the eyes and mouth before rigor mortis sets in. Rigor mortis usually leaves the body about 96 hours after death.

Algor mortis is the gradual decrease of the body's temperature after death. When blood circulation terminates and the hypothalamus ceases to function, body temperature falls about 1°C (1.8°F) per hour until it reaches room temperature. Simultaneously, the skin loses its elasticity and can easily be broken when removing dressings and adhesive tape.

After blood circulation has ceased, the red blood cells break down, releasing hemoglobin, which discolors the surrounding tissues. This discoloration, referred to as **livor mortis,** appears in the lowermost or dependent areas of the body.

Tissues after death become soft and eventually liquefied by bacterial fermentation. The hotter the temperature, the more rapid the change. Therefore, bodies are often stored in cool places to delay this process. Embalming prevents the process through injection of chemicals into the body to destroy the bacteria.

Nursing personnel may be responsible for care of a body after death. Postmortem care should be carried out according to the policy of the hospital or agency. Because care of the body may be influenced by religious law, the nurse should check the client's religion and make every attempt to comply. If the deceased's family or friends wish to view the body, it is important to make the environment as clean and pleasant as possible and to make the body appear natural and comfortable. All equipment, soiled linen, and supplies should be removed from the bedside. Some agencies require that all tubes in the body remain in place; in other agencies, tubes may be cut to within 2.5 cm (1 in.) of the skin and taped in place; in others, all tubes may be removed.

Normally the body is placed in a supine position with the arms either at the sides, palms down, or across the abdomen. One pillow is placed under the head and shoulders to prevent blood from discoloring the face by settling in it. The eyelids are closed and held in place for a few seconds so they remain closed. Dentures are usually inserted to help give the face a natural appearance. The mouth is then closed.

Soiled areas of the body are washed; however, a complete bath is not necessary, because the body will be washed by the mortician (also referred to as an undertaker), a person trained in care of the dead. Absorbent pads are placed under the buttocks to take up any feces and urine released because of relaxation of the sphincter muscles. A clean gown is placed on the client, and the hair is brushed and combed. All jewelry is removed, except a wedding band in some instances, which is taped to the finger. The top bed linens are adjusted neatly to cover the client to the shoulders. Soft lighting and chairs are provided for the family.

In the hospital, after the body has been viewed by the family, the deceased's wrist identification tag is left on and additional identification tags are applied. The body is wrapped in a shroud, a large piece of plastic or cotton material used to enclose a body after death. Identification is then applied to the outside of the shroud. The body is taken to the morgue if arrangements have not been made to have a mortician pick it up from the client's room. Nurses have a duty to handle the deceased with dignity and to label the corpse appropriately. Mishandling can cause emotional distress to survivors. Mislabeling can create legal problems if the body is inappropriately identified and prepared incorrectly for burial or a funeral.

EVALUATING

To evaluate the achievement of client goals, the nurse collects data in accordance with the desired outcomes estab-

lished in the planning phase. Evaluation activities may include the following:

- Listening to the client's reports of feeling in control of the environment surrounding death, such as control over pain relief, visitation of family and support people, or treatment plans
- Observing the client's relationship with significant others
- Listening to the client's thoughts and feelings related to hopelessness or powerlessness

Examples of desired outcomes for dying clients are shown in Identifying Nursing Diagnoses, Outcomes, and Interventions on page 880. Some of the special needs of older adults and their families during death and dying are found in Lifespan Considerations.

LIFESPAN CONSIDERATIONS
Responses to Death

Children

- Children's response to death or loss depends on the messages they get from adults and others around them as well as their understanding of death. When adults are able to cope effectively with a death, they are more likely to be able to support children through the process.
- As children develop, they will "reprocess" their grieving around a loss or death. Preschoolers who have lost a parent, for example, often reconceptualize their understanding of that loss when they reach school age and adolescence and have greater cognitive and emotional skills. The same process occurs with parents who have lost a child to death; as the years pass and the child "would have been in first grade," for example, parents must cope with the added dimensions of the loss.

Older Adults

Older adults who are dying often have a need to know that their lives had meaning. An excellent way to assure them of this is to make audiotapes or videotapes of them telling stories of their lives. This gives the client a sense of value and worth and also lets him or her know that family members and friends will also benefit from it. Doing this with children and grandchildren often eases communication and support during this difficult time.

Caregivers of a dying person need ongoing support and ongoing teaching as the client's condition changes. Some of these needs are teaching:

- ways to feed the client when swallowing becomes difficult.
- ways to transfer and reposition the client safely.
- ways to communicate if verbalization becomes more difficult.
- nonpharmacological methods of pain control.
- comfort measures, such as frequent oral care and frequent repositioning.

CONCEPT MAP The Grieving Client

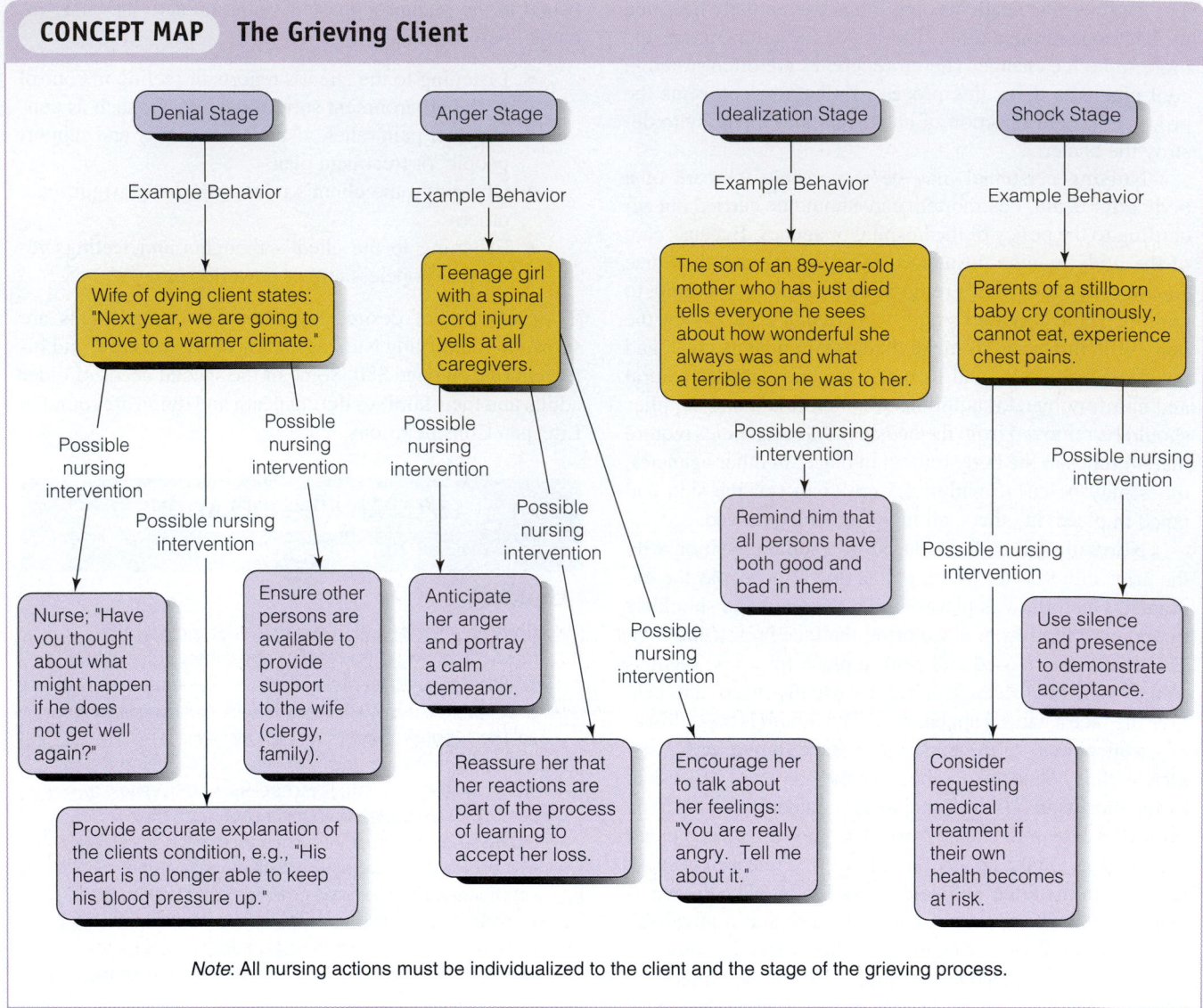

Note: All nursing actions must be individualized to the client and the stage of the grieving process.

CHAPTER HIGHLIGHTS

- Stress is a state of physiologic and psychologic tension that affects the whole person—physically, emotionally, intellectually, socially, and spiritually.
- Models view stress as a stimulus, stress as a response, and stress as a transaction.
- General adaptation syndrome (GAS) is a multisystem response to stress and involves three steps: alarm reaction, stage of resistance, and stage of exhaustion.
- Local adaptation syndrome (LAS) is a localized physiologic response that also expresses the three stages of GAS. An example of LAS is the inflammatory response.
- There are physiologic, psychologic, and cognitive indicators of stress. Physiologic indicators are the result of increased activity of the sympathetic and neuroendocrine systems.

- Common psychologic indicators are anxiety, fear, anger, and depression. Anxiety, the most common response, has four levels: mild, moderate, severe, and panic. Ego defense mechanisms such as denial, rationalization, compensation, and sublimation protect individuals from anxiety.
- Cognitive indicators or thinking responses to stress include problem solving, structuring, self-control (discipline), suppression, and fantasy.
- Coping strategies to deal with stress vary significantly among individuals. Strategies may be problem focused or emotion focused, long term or short term, and effective or ineffective.
- The effectiveness of individual coping depends on the number, duration, and intensity of the stressors; past

experience; support systems available; and the personal qualities of the person.

- Prolonged stress and ineffective coping interfere with the meeting of basic needs and can affect physical and mental health.
- Nursing assessment of a client experiencing stress involves a nursing history to identify perceptions of and duration of stressors and coping strategies and also a physical examination for physical indicators of stress.
- Nursing interventions for clients who are stressed are aimed at encouraging health promotion strategies (exercise, healthy diet, adequate rest, and time management), minimizing anxiety, mediating anger, teaching about specific relaxation techniques, and implementing crisis interventions as needed.
- Because nursing practice involves many stressors related to both clients and the work environment, nurses are susceptible to anxiety and burnout. Like clients, they need to implement stress reduction measures.
- Nurses help clients deal with all kinds of losses, including loss of body image, loss of a loved one, loss of a sense of well-being, and loss of a job.
- Loss, especially loss of a loved one or a valued body part, can be viewed as either a situational or a developmental loss and as either an actual or a perceived loss (both of which can be anticipatory).
- Grieving is a normal, subjective emotional response to loss; it is essential for mental and physical health. Grieving allows the bereaved person to cope with loss gradually and to accept it as part of reality.
- Knowledge of different stages or phases of grieving and factors that influence the loss reaction can help the nurse understand the responses and needs of clients.
- How an individual deals with loss is closely related to the individual's stage of development, personal resources, and social support system.
- Caring for the dying and the bereaved is one of the nurse's most complex and challenging responsibilities.
- Nurses' attitudes about death and dying directly affect their ability to provide care.
- Nurses must consider the entire family as requiring care in situations involving loss, especially death.
- Dying clients require open communication, physical help, and emotional and spiritual support to ensure a peaceful and dignified death. They need to maintain a sense of control in managing the events preceding death.

THINK ABOUT IT

Refer to the chapter-opening scenario and answer these questions.

1. If you were the nurse assigned to care for Mr. McGhee when he is admitted to the hospital, how would you help both the client and his wife meet their psychosocial needs?

2. How do the stressors faced by Mr. McGhee differ from the stressors his wife is facing?

3. Mrs. McGhee tells you that one of their daughters lives on the other side of the state and their other daughter lives several states away. She says they feel guilty because they can't spend more time with their father, whom they adore. What recommendations or strategies might you suggest to help the daughters cope with their father's illness?

∞ *See suggested responses to Think About It on MyNursingKit.*

TEST YOUR KNOWLEDGE

1. The nurse helps a 50-year-old diabetic client who is to begin giving insulin injections identify previously successful coping strategies that may be useful in the current situation. Which of the following stressors is closely related to the new stressor?
   1. Interviewing for a new job
   2. Death of a pet while the person was a teenager
   3. The person's partner filing for a divorce
   4. Starting to wear eyeglasses at age 30

2. A client who was informed of a cancer diagnosis assures the nurse he is fine. Which of the following is the most indicative physical evidence to the nurse of the client's stress?
   1. Constricted pupils
   2. Dilated peripheral blood vessels (flush)
   3. Hyperventilation
   4. Decreased heart rate

3. Immediately after the parents of a hospitalized child are informed that the child has leukemia, the father responds by continuing his usual work schedule, rarely visiting, and asking when the child can return to school. Of the following, which is the **least** likely to be an appropriate nursing diagnosis at this time?
   1. *Ineffective Denial*
   2. *Caregiver Role Strain*
   3. *Fear*
   4. *Compromised Family Coping*

4. Which of the following may be considered normal or "healthy" types of grief? Select all that apply.
   1. Abbreviated grief
   2. Anticipatory grief
   3. Disenfranchised grief
   4. Unresolved grief
   5. Inhibited grief

5. A client's family tells the nurse that their culture does not permit a dead person to be alone before burial. Hospital policy states that after 6:00 PM when mortuaries are closed, bodies are to be stored in the hospital morgue refrigerator until the next day. How would the nurse best manage this situation?

1. Gently explain the policy to the family and then implement it.
2. Inquire of the nursing supervisor how an exception to the policy could be made.
3. Call the client's primary care provider for advice.
4. Move the deceased to an empty room and assign an aide to stay with the body.

6. The shift changed while the nursing staff was waiting for the adult children of a deceased client to arrive. The oncoming nurse has never met the family. Which of the following greetings is most appropriate?

1. "I'm very sorry for your loss."
2. "I'll take you in to view the body."
3. "I didn't know your father but I am sure he was a wonderful person."
4. "How long will you want to stay with your father?"

7. An 82-year-old man has been told by his primary care provider that it is no longer safe for him to drive a car. Which statement by the client would indicate beginning positive adaptation to this loss?

1. "I told the doctor I would stop driving, but I am not going to yet."
2. "I always knew this day would come, but I hoped it wouldn't be now."
3. "What does he know? I'm a better driver than he will ever be."
4. "Well, at least I have friends and family who can take me places."

8. The student nurse is preparing to take a final examination. What level of anxiety will improve the student's performance on the exam?

1. Mild anxiety
2. Moderate anxiety
3. Severe anxiety
4. Panic

9. The nurse, working on a hospice unit, identifies which of the following clients as being closest to death?

1. The 85-year-old female who is incontinent of urine
2. The 58-year-old man with diminished sensation in the right lower leg
3. The 28-year-old client with a slow weak pulse and irregular breathing
4. The 47-year-old client with absent gag reflex

10. The nurse is caring for a terminally ill client who anticipates dying while hospitalized. During routine care the client often laments not being able to say good-bye to his dog but recognizes that hospital regulations prevent animals from visiting. A priority nursing action is to:

1. Find alternate means for the client to say good-bye to his dog such as talking to the dog over the phone or via a picture.
2. Encourage the family to sneak the dog into the client's room and assure them the nurses will look the other way.
3. Obtain permission from the physician to place the client onto a stretcher and wheel him outside where his family can be waiting with his dog.
4. Tell the client, "I am so sorry you can't see your dog. That must be very difficult for you. Would you like me to put pictures of your dog on the wall so you can at least see him?"

∞ *See answers to Test Your Knowledge in Appendix A.*

REFERENCES AND SELECTED BIBLIOGRAPHY

Anspaugh, D. J., Hamrick, M., & Rosato, F. D. (2008). *Wellness: Concepts and applications* (7th ed.). New York: McGraw-Hill.

Antai-Otong, D. (2003). Anxiety disorders: Helping your patient conquer her fears. *Nursing, 33*(12), 36–41.

Barbus, A. J. (1975). *The dying person's bill of rights.* Created at the workshop *The terminally ill patient and the helping person,* Lansing, MI: South Western Michigan Inservice Education Council.

Bulechek, G. M., Butcher, H. K. & Dochterman, J. M., (Eds.). (2008). *Nursing interventions: classification (NIC)* (5th ed.). St. Louis: Mosby.

Carpenito-Moyet, L. J. (2009). *Nursing diagnosis: Application to clinical practice* (13th ed.). Philadelphia: Lippincott Williams & Wilkins.

Caserta, M. S., Lund, D. A., & Obray, S. J. (2004). Promoting self-care and daily living skills among older widows and widowers: Evidence from the Pathfinders demonstration project. *OMEGA: The Journal of Death and Dying, 49,* 217–236.

Clements, P. T., & Stenerson, H. J. (2004). Surviving sudden loss: When life, death, and technology collide. *Journal of Vascular Nursing, 22,* 134–137.

Cooke, M., Chaboyer, W., & Hiratos, M. A. (2005). Music and its effect on anxiety in short waiting periods: A critical appraisal. *Journal of Clinical Nursing, 14,* 145–155.

Cote, J. K., & Pepler, C. (2005). Cognitive coping intervention for acutely ill HIV positive men. *Journal of Clinical Nursing, 14,* 321–326.

Cox, S. (2004). Curing fixer-pleaser syndrome. *Nursing, 34*(5), 64.

Dobbins, E. H. (2005). Helping your patient to a "good death." *Nursing, 35*(2), 43–45.

Dunne, K. (2004). Grief and its manifestations. *Nursing Standard, 18*(45), 45–53.

Edlin, G., & Golanty, E. (2007). *Health and wellness: A holistic approach* (9th ed.). Boston: Jones & Bartlett.

Egan, K. A., & Arnold, R. L. (2003). Grief and bereavement care. *American Journal of Nursing, 103*(9), 42–53.

Engel, G. L. (1964). Grief and grieving. *American Journal of Nursing, 64,* 93–98.

Ferrell, B. R., & Coyle, N. (Eds.). (2006). *Textbook of palliative care nursing* (2nd ed.). Oxford, England: Oxford University Press.

Folkman, S., & Lazarus, R. S. (1991). Coping and emotion. In A. Monat & R. S. Lazarus (Eds.), *Stress and coping* (3rd ed.). New York: Columbia University Press.

Fontaine, K. L. (2009). *Mental health nursing* (6th ed.). Upper Saddle River, NJ: Pearson Education.

Freud, S. (1946). *The ego and the mechanisms of defense.* New York: International Universities Press.

Furman, J. (2004). Healing the mind and spirit as the body fails. *Nursing, 34*(4), 50–51.

Glaser, B., & Strauss, A. (1965). *Awareness of dying.* Chicago: Aldine.

Griffie, J., Nelson-Marten, P., & Muchka, S. (2004). Acknowledging the 'elephant': Communication in palliative care. *American Journal of Nursing, 104*(1), 48–57.

Hoffman, R. L. (2005). The evolution of hospice in America: Nursing's role in the movement. *Journal of Gerontological Nursing, 31,* 26–34.

Holmes, T. H., & Rahe, R. H. (1967). The social readjustment rating scale. *Journal of Psychosomatic Research, 11,* 213–218.

Kübler-Ross, E. (1969). *On death and dying.* New York: Macmillan.

Kübler-Ross, E. (1974). *Questions and answers on death and dying.* New York: Macmillan.

Kübler-Ross, E. (1975). *Death: The final stage of growth.* Englewood Cliffs, NJ: Prentice Hall.

Kübler-Ross, E. (1978). *To live until we say good-bye.* Englewood Cliffs, NJ: Prentice Hall.

Larner, S. (2005). Common psychological challenges for patients with newly acquired disability. *Nursing Standard, 19*(28), 33–39.

Lazarus, R. S. (1966). *Psychological stress and the coping process.* New York: McGraw-Hill.

Lazarus, R. S. (2000). Toward better research on stress and coping. *American Psychologist, 55,* 665–673.

LeSergent, C. M., & Haney, C. J. (2005). Rural hospital nurse's stressors and coping strategies: A survey. *International Journal of Nursing Studies, 42,* 315–324.

Lunney, J. R., Lynn, J., Foley, D. J., Lipson, S., & Guralnik, J. M. (2003). Patterns of functional decline at the end of life. *Journal of the American Medical Association, 289,* 2387–2392.

Lyons, K. S., Stewart, B. J., Archbold, P. G., Carter, J. H., & Perrin, N. A. (2004). Pessimism and optimism as early warning signs for compromised health for caregivers of patients with Parkinson's disease. *Nursing Research, 53,* 354–362.

Martocchio, B. C. (1985). Grief and bereavement: Healing through hurt. *Nursing Clinics of North America, 20,* 327–341.

Mathes, M. M. (2004). Assisted suicide and nursing ethics. *Medsurg Nursing, 13,* 261–264.

Matzo, M., & Sherman, D. W. (Eds.). (2005). *Palliative care nursing: Quality care to the end of life* (2nd ed.). New York: Springer.

Mazanec, P., & Tyler, M. K. (2003). Cultural considerations in end-of-life care. *American Journal of Nursing, 103*(3), 50–58.

McClement, S. E., Chochinov, H. M., Hack, T. F., Kristjanson, L. J., & Harlos, M. (2004). Dignity-conserving care: Application of research findings to practice. *International Journal of Palliative Nursing, 10,* 173–179.

Miller, M. A., & Rahe, R. H. (1997). Life changes scaling for the 1990s. *Journal of Psychosomatic Research, 43,* 279–292.

Mitchell, M. L., & Courtney, M. (2004). Reducing family members' anxiety and uncertainty in illness around transfer from intensive care, an intervention study. *Intensive and Critical Care Nursing, 20,* 223–231.

Monat, A., & Lazarus, R. S. (Eds.). (1991). *Stress and coping* (3rd ed.). New York: Columbia University Press.

Moorhead, S., Johnson, M., & Maas, M. L., & Swanson, E. (Eds.). (2008). *Nursing outcomes classification (NOC)* (4th ed.). St. Louis: Mosby.

NANDA International. (2009). *NANDA nursing diagnoses: Definitions and classification 2009–2011.* West Sussex, U.K.: Wiley-Blackwell.

National Board for Certification of Hospice and Palliative Nurses. (2006). Certificants. Retrieved December 5, 2009, from http://www.nbchpn.org/DisplayPage .aspx?Title=Welcome!

National Consensus Project for Quality Palliative Care. (2004). *Clinical practice guidelines for quality palliative care.* Retrieved December 5, 2009, from http:// www.nationalconsensusproject.org/ AboutGuidelines.asp

Rahe, R. H., & Tolles, R. L. (2002). The brief stress and coping inventory: A useful stress management instrument. *International Journal of Stress Management, 9,* 61–70.

Rando, T. A. (1991). *How to go on living when someone you love dies.* New York: Bantam.

Rando, T. A. (1993). *Treatment of complicated mourning.* Champaign, IL: Research Press.

Rando, T. A. (2000). *Clinical dimensions of anticipatory mourning: Theory and practice in working with the dying, their loved ones, and their caregivers.* Champaign, IL: Research Press.

Resnik, D. (2005). *Dying declarations: Notes from a hospice volunteer.* Binghamton, NY: Haworth Press.

Rich, S. (2005). Providing quality end-of-life care. *Journal of Cardiovascular Nursing, 20,* 141–145.

Sanders, C. M. (1998). *Grief: The mourning after: Dealing with adult bereavement* (2nd ed.). New York: Wiley.

Scanlon, C. (2003). Ethical concerns in end-of-life care. *American Journal of Nursing, 103*(1), 48–55.

Selye, H. (1956). *The stress of life.* New York: McGraw-Hill.

Selye, H. (1976). *The stress of life* (Rev. ed.). New York: McGraw-Hill.

Sharpe, L., Butow, P., Smith, C., McConnell, D., & Clarke, S. (2005).The relationship between available support, unmet needs and caregiver burden in patients with advanced cancer and their carers. *Psycho-Oncology, 14*, 102–114.

Shear, K., Frank, E., Houck, P. R., & Reynolds, C. F. (2005). Treatment of complicated grief: A randomized controlled trial. *Journal of the American Medical Association, 293*, 2601–2608.

Sheehan, D. K., & Schirm, V. (2003). End-of-life care of older adults: Debunking some common misconceptions about dying in old age. *American Journal of Nursing, 103*(11), 48–58.

Stedman's medical dictionary for the health professions and nursing (5th ed.). (2005). Philadelphia: Lippincott Williams & Wilkins.

United States Department of Agriculture. (2005). *Nutrition and your health: Dietary guidelines for Americans.* Retrieved June 18, 2006, from http://www.health.gov/dietaryguidelines/dga2000/document/aim.htm#physical_top

Virani, R., & Sofer, D. (2003). Improving the quality of end-of-life care. *American Journal of Nursing, 103*(5), 52–61.

Wanzer, M., Booth-Butterfield, M. M., & Booth-Butterfield, S. (2005). "If we didn't use humor, we'd cry": Humorous coping communication in health care settings. *Journal of Health Communication, 10*, 105–125.

Westley, C., & Briggs, L. A. (2004). Using the stages of change model to improve communication about advance care planning. *Nursing Forum, 39*(3), 5–12.

World Health Organization. (n.d.). *WHO definition of palliative care.* Retrieved June 24, 2006, from http://www.who.int/cancer/palliative/definition/en/

Promoting Physiologic Health

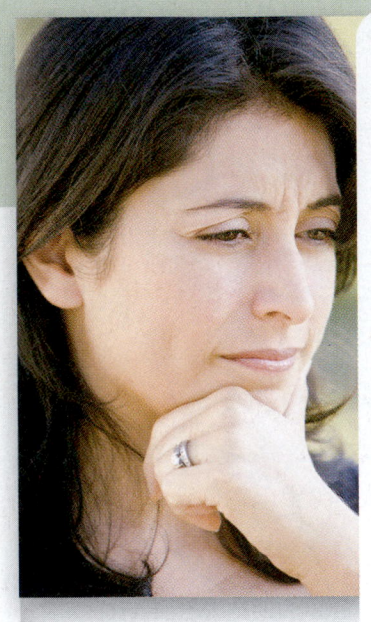

Mathew and Miriam Burt have no children but had two dogs that are like children to them. One afternoon a teenager in the neighborhood shot one of their dogs, killing it. Both Mathew and Miriam were devastated, but Miriam was particularly impacted because she no longer felt safe in her home. The adolescent denied responsibility, and no police action resulted because they could not prove he was responsible.

Miriam has a history of borderline hypertension that she has controlled through diet, and she quit smoking 3 months ago. However, with the trauma of losing her dog, her blood pressure (which she monitors at home) is elevated, and she has returned to her 1 pack a day smoking habit. She is having trouble sleeping at night and wakes frequently believing she heard something and feels her heart pounding. After several weeks of this, she realizes she must see her health care provider to help her control her blood pressure and seek help for her ongoing disordered sleep.

LEARNING OUTCOMES

After completing this chapter, you will be able to:

1. Differentiate the basic elements of normal movement and types of exercise.

2. Compare the effects of exercise and immobility on the body systems.

3. Describe factors influencing a person's body alignment and activity.

4. Predict potential problems related to immobility.

5. Apply the nursing process to clients with immobility or at risk for immobility concerns.

6. Describe safe practices for positioning, moving, lifting, and ambulating clients.

7. Identify the function, physiology, and characteristics of sleep.

8. Summarize variations in sleep patterns and factors that affect normal sleep.

9. Distinguish among common sleep disorders and their manifestations, and describe nursing considerations for each.

10. Apply the nursing process to planning care for a client with sleep problems.

KEY TERMS

Active ROM exercises p918
Activity tolerance p892
Aerobic exercise p893
Anaerobic exercise p893
Atrophy p896
Basal metabolic rate p930
Base of support p891
Biological rhythms p929
Center of gravity p891
Contracture p892
Foot drop p904
Functional strength p892

Our ability to move is an essential aspect of our well-being. Psychophysiologic self-regulation and overall health are affected by our activities. At the 2005–2006 North American Nursing Diagnosis Association (NANDA) Conference, the new diagnosis *Sedentary Lifestyle* was approved, underscoring the role of exercise and activity as an essential component of health. Many *Healthy People 2010* objectives pertain to exercise and activity. Evidence shows that exercise can prevent and even reverse many of the chronic diseases experienced by aging adults. According to researchers at Harvard's School of Public Health (HSPH), a mixture of healthy eating and regular physical activity is the best form of health promotion and maintenance. Recent data from the large Nurses' Health Study conducted through HSPH suggest that weight and exercise are both important predictors of longevity (Hu et al., 2004). During 24 years of data collection, mortality rates have been lowest for women who are lean *and* active, moderate for women who are one or the other, and highest for women who are obese *and* sedentary.

An activity-exercise pattern refers to a person's routine of exercise, activity, leisure, and recreation. **Mobility**, the ability to move freely, easily, rhythmically, and purposefully in the environment, is an essential part of living. People often define their health and physical fitness by their activity because mental well-being and the effectiveness of body functioning depend largely on their mobility status. The ability to move without pain also influences self-esteem and body image. For those with impaired mobility, movement must be fostered to the full extent of capability to facilitate a satisfying life.

NORMAL MOVEMENT

Normal movement and stability are the result of an intact musculoskeletal system, an intact nervous system, and intact inner ear structures responsible for equilibrium. Body movement requires coordinated muscle activity and neurologic integration. It involves four basic elements: body alignment (posture), joint mobility, balance, and coordinated movement.

Alignment and Posture

Proper body alignment and posture bring body parts into position in a manner that promotes optimal balance and maximal body function whether the client is standing, sitting, or lying down. A person maintains balance as long as the **line of gravity** (an imaginary vertical line drawn through the body's center of gravity) passes through the **center of gravity** (the point at which all of the body's mass is centered) and the **base of support** (the foundation on which the body rests). In humans, the usual line of gravity begins at the top of the head and falls between the shoulders, through the trunk, slightly anterior to the sacrum, and between the weight-bearing joints and base of support (Figure 31–1).

When the body is well aligned, strain on the joints, muscles, tendons, or ligaments are minimized and internal structures and organs are supported. Proper body alignment enhances lung expansion and promotes efficient circulatory, renal, and gastrointestinal functions. A person's posture is one criterion for assessing general health, physical fitness, and attractiveness. Posture reflects the mood, self-esteem, and personality of an individual, and vice versa.

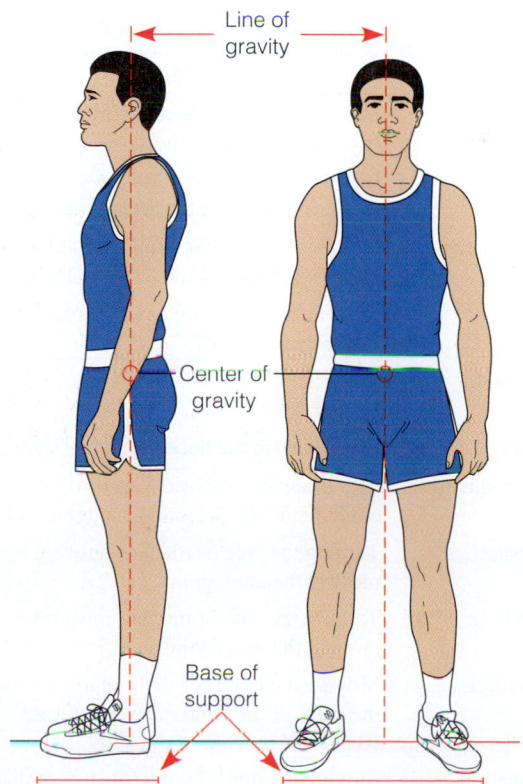

Figure 31–1 ⊙ The center of gravity and the line of gravity influence standing alignment.

Joint Mobility

Joints are the functional units of the musculoskeletal system. The bones of the skeleton articulate at the joints, and most of the skeletal muscles attach to the two bones at the joint. These muscles are categorized according to the type of joint movement they produce on contraction. The flexor muscles are stronger than the extensor muscles. Thus, when a person is inactive, the joints are pulled into a flexed (bent) position. If this tendency is not counteracted with exercise and position changes, the muscles permanently shorten, and the joint becomes fixed in a flexed position (**contracture**). Types of joint movement are shown in Table 31–1.

The **range of motion (ROM)** of a joint is the maximum movement that is possible for that joint. Joint range of motion varies from individual to individual and is determined by genetic makeup, developmental patterns, the presence or absence of disease, and the amount of physical activity in which the person normally engages.

Balance

The mechanisms involved in maintaining balance and posture are complex and involve informational inputs from the labyrinth (inner ear), from vision (vestibulo-ocular input), and from stretch receptors of muscles and tendons (vestibulospinal input). Mechanisms of equilibrium (sense of balance) respond, frequently without our awareness, to various head movements. Under normal conditions the equilibrium receptors in the semicircular canals and vestibule, collectively called the vestibular apparatus, send signals to the brain that initiate reflexes needed to make required changes in position. This enables fast reflexive responses to body imbalance. **Proprioception** is the term used to describe awareness of posture, movement, and changes in equilibrium and the knowledge of position, weight, and resistance of objects in relation to the body.

Coordinated Movement

Balanced, smooth, purposeful movement is the result of proper functioning of the cerebral cortex, cerebellum, and basal ganglia. The cerebral cortex initiates voluntary motor activity, the cerebellum coordinates the motor activities of movement, and the basal ganglia maintain posture. The cerebral cortex operates movements, not muscles. The cerebellum, which operates below the level of consciousness, blends and coordinates the muscles involved in voluntary movement. When a client's cerebellum is injured, movements become clumsy, unsure, and uncoordinated.

EXERCISE

The U.S. Department of Health and Human Services defines exercise and physical activity as follows (Edelman & Mandle, 2010):

- **Physical activity** is bodily movement produced by skeletal muscle contraction that increases energy expenditure.
- **Exercise** is a type of physical activity defined as a planned, structured, and repetitive bodily movement performed to improve or maintain one or more components of physical fitness.

Activity tolerance is the type and amount of exercise or daily living activities an individual is able to perform without experiencing adverse effects. **Functional strength** is another goal of exercise, and defined as the ability of the body to perform work.

Types of Exercise

Exercise involves the active contraction and relaxation of muscles. Exercises can be classified according to the type of muscle contraction (isotonic, isometric, or isokinetic) and according to the source of energy (aerobic or anaerobic).

Isotonic (dynamic) exercises are those in which the muscle shortens to produce muscle contraction and active movement. Most physical conditioning exercises are isotonic, as are ADLs and active ROM exercises (those initiated by the client). Isotonic exercises increase muscle tone, mass, and strength and maintain joint flexibility and circulation. During isotonic exercise, both heart rate and cardiac output quicken to increase blood flow to all parts of the body.

Isometric (static or setting) exercises are those in which there is muscle contraction without moving the joint

TABLE 31–1	Types of Joint Movements
MOVEMENT	**ACTION**
Flexion	Decreasing the angle of the joint (e.g., bending the elbow)
Extension	Increasing the angle of the joint (e.g., straightening the arm at the elbow)
Hyperextension	Further extension or straightening of a joint (e.g., bending the head backward)
Abduction	Movement of the bone away from the midline of the body
Adduction	Movement of the bone toward the midline of the body
Rotation	Movement of the bone around its central axis
Circumduction	Movement of the distal part of the bone in a circle while the proximal end remains fixed
Eversion	Turning the sole of the foot outward by moving the ankle joint
Inversion	Turning the sole of the foot inward by moving the ankle joint
Pronation	Moving the bones of the forearm so that the palm of the hand faces downward when held in front of the body
Supination	Moving the bones of the forearm so that the palm of the hand faces upward when held in front of the body

(muscle length does not change). These exercises involve exerting pressure against a solid object and are useful for strengthening abdominal, gluteal, and quadriceps muscles used in ambulation; for maintaining strength in immobilized muscles in casts or traction; and for endurance training. Isometric exercises produce a mild increase in heart rate and cardiac output, but no appreciable increase in blood flow to other parts of the body.

Isokinetic (resistive) exercises involve muscle contraction or tension against resistance; thus, they can be either isotonic or isometric. During isokinetic exercises, the person moves (isotonic) or tenses (isometric) against resistance. Special machines or devices provide the resistance to the movement. These exercises are used in physical conditioning and are often done to build up certain muscle groups. An increase in blood pressure and blood flow to muscles occurs with resistance training (Burke & Laramie, 2004).

Aerobic exercise is activity during which the amount of oxygen taken into the body is greater than that used to perform the activity. Aerobic exercises use large muscle groups that move repetitively. Aerobic exercises improve cardiovascular conditioning and physical fitness. Assessment of physical fitness is discussed in Chapter 5 ∞. The accompanying Client Teaching feature describes frequency, duration, and types of activity recommended for healthy adults.

Intensity of exercise can be measured in three ways:

1. *Target heart rate.* The goal is to work up to and sustain a target heart rate during exercise, based on the person's age. To determine target heart rate, first calculate the person's maximum heart rate by subtracting his or her current age in years from 220. Then obtain the target heart rate by taking 60% to 85% of the maximum. Because heart rates vary among individuals, the tests that follow are replacing this measure.
2. *Talk test.* When exercising, the person should experience labored breathing, yet still be able to carry on a conversation which keeps most people at 60% of maximum heart rate or more.
3. *Borg scale of perceived exertion* (Borg, 1998). This scale measures "how difficult" the exercise feels to the person in terms of heart and lung exertion. The scale progresses from 1 to 20 with the following markers: 7 = very, very light; 9 = very light; 11 = fairly light; 13 = somewhat hard; 15 = hard; 17 = very hard; and 19 = very, very hard. "Very, very hard" corresponds closely to 100% of maximum heart rate. "Very light" is close to 40%. Most people need to strive for the "somewhat hard" level (13/20), which corresponds to 75% of maximum heart rate.

Anaerobic exercise involves activity in which the muscles cannot draw out enough oxygen from the bloodstream, and anaerobic pathways are used to provide additional energy for a short time. This type of exercise is used in endurance training for athletes.

Benefits of Exercise

In general, regular exercise is essential for maintaining mental and physical health of all body systems. The size, shape, tone, and strength of muscles (including the heart muscle) are maintained with mild exercise and increased with strenuous exercise. With strenuous exercise, muscles **hypertrophy** (enlarge), and the efficiency of muscular contraction increases. Exercise increases joint flexibility, stability, and range of motion and improve blood supply to the joint. Bone density and strength is maintained through weight bearing.

The American Heart Association's most recent guidelines for primary prevention of stroke and cardiovascular disease (Freeman, 2004) placed great emphasis on physical activity. Adequate moderate-intensity exercise (40% to 60% of maximum capacity such as walking a mile in 15 to 20 minutes) increases the heart rate, the strength of heart muscle contraction, and the blood supply to the heart and muscles

---

CLIENT TEACHING

Guidelines and Minimal Requirements for Physical Activity

Frequency and Duration

- *Aerobic:* Cumulative 30 minutes or more daily (can be divided throughout the day) of "moderate intensity" movement as measured by talk test and perceived exertion scale.
- *Stretching:* Should be added onto that minimum requirement so that all parts of the body are stretched each day.
- *Strength training:* Should be added onto these minimum requirements so that all muscle groups are addressed at least three times a week, with a day of rest after training.

Type of Exercise

- *Aerobic:* Elliptical exercisers, walking, biking, gardening, dancing, and swimming are recommended for all persons,

including beginners and older adults. Activities that are more strenuous include jogging, running, Spinning®, power yoga, bouncing, boxing, and jumping rope.
- *Stretching:* Yoga, Pilates, qi gong, and many other flexibility programs are effective.
- *Strength training:* Resistance can be provided with weights, bands, balls, apparatus, and body weight.

Safety

- Stress the importance of balance and prevention of falls, proper clothing to ensure thermal safety, checking equipment for proper function, wearing a helmet and other protective gear, using reflective devices at night, and carrying identification and emergency information.

CULTURALLY COMPETENT CARE

Therapeutic Movement Modalities from Eastern Cultures

Therapeutic movement modalities from eastern cultures are finding a place in evidence-based health care. In particular, hatha yoga, qigong, and t'ai chi are receiving wide attention for improving strength and balance as well as treating a wide variety of health problems. The beauty of yoga is that it can be fully practiced by those who must use a wheelchair or remain in bed. The regular practice of qigong is intended to generate as well as conserve energy to maintain health or treat illness.

In several studies investigating immune effects of qigong practice, levels of white blood cells, monocytes, and lymphocytes increased significantly after training. In an investigation with hypertension clients, both systolic and diastolic blood pressure, norepinephrine, metanephrine, and epinephrine levels were significantly reduced in the group given qigong training versus those in the control group. In this same study, ventilatory functions were also improved in the qigong group. In a randomized study it was found that older adults practicing t'ai chi had an increase in varicella zoster virus cell-mediated immunity and thus, decreased risk for the virus (Freeman, 2004). A quasi-experimental, randomized controlled study of 54 persons with hypertension revealed significant decreases in both systolic and diastolic blood pressure, self-reported stress, heart rate, and body mass index after 8 weeks of yoga practice (McCaffrey et al., 2005).

Nurses can independently recommend that clients who are able to do so consider initiating these movement modalities. Through appropriate referrals to group classes in the community as well as the use of videotapes in homes and long-term care facilities, clients can take charge of their own health in ways that are empowering, holistic, and free of negative side effects. Nurses should assess each individual for readiness, safety issues, balance, and ability to engage in any physical activity.

through increased cardiac output. The types of exercise that will provide cardiac benefit vary. They include aerobic exercise such as walking and cycling (Freeman, 2004).

Ventilation and oxygen intake increase during exercise, thereby improving gas exchange. More toxins are eliminated with deeper breathing, and problem solving and emotional stability are enhanced due to increased oxygen to the brain. Adequate exercise also prevents pooling of secretions in the bronchi and bronchioles, decreasing breathing effort and risk of infection (Freeman, 2004).

Exercise improves the appetite and increases gastrointestinal tract tone, facilitating peristalsis. Exercise elevates the metabolic rate, thus increasing the production of body heat and waste products and calorie use. During strenuous exercise, the metabolic rate can increase to as much as 20 times the normal rate. This elevation lasts after exercise is completed. Exercise increases the use of triglycerides and fatty acids, resulting in a reduced level of serum triglycerides and cholesterol.

As respiratory and musculoskeletal effort increase with exercise and as gravity is enlisted with postural changes, lymph fluid is more efficiently pumped from tissues into lymph capillaries and vessels throughout the body. Circulation through lymph nodes where destruction of pathogens and removal of foreign antigens can occur is also improved. While moderate exercise seems to enhance immunity, strenuous exercise may reduce immune function, leaving a window of opportunity for infection during the recovery phase. Adequate rest is important after vigorous training to allow the body to recover (Edelman & Mandle, 2010).

A strong and growing body of evidence supports the role of exercise in elevating mood and relieving stress and anxiety across the life span. Solid data examining relationships between both aerobic and nonaerobic styles of exercise support the use of this modality to relieve symptoms of depression. The mechanism of action is thought to be a result of one or more of the following: exercise increases levels of metabolites for neurotransmitters such as norepinephrine and serotonin; exercise releases endogenous opioids, thus increasing levels of endorphins; exercise increases levels of oxygen to the brain and other body systems, inducing euphoria; and through muscular exertion (especially with movement modalities such as yoga and t'ai chi) the body releases stored stress associated with accumulated emotional demands. Regular exercise also improves quality of sleep for most individuals (Freeman, 2004).

By eliciting the relaxation response (RR), exercise is beneficial for counteracting some of the harmful effects of stress on the body and mind. The RR is a healthful physiologic state that can be elicited through deep relaxation breathing with emphasis on a prolonged exhalation phase (Edelman & Mandle, 2010). Emphasis on the exhalation recruits parasympathetic nervous system response, the "rest and digest" reflex. Progressive muscle relaxation techniques involve contracting and then releasing groups of muscles throughout the body until all parts of the body feel relaxed. These movements are subtle and, along with relaxation breathing, can be done by almost anyone at any time, regardless of mobility or fitness status, providing potent stress relief and neurocardiovascular health benefits.

Current research supports the positive effects of exercise on cognitive functioning, in particular decision-making and problem-solving processes, planning, and paying attention. Physical exertion induces cells in the brain to strengthen and build neuronal connections. Jackson (2003) found that a program of Pilates and yoga-style exercise significantly enhanced students' experiences of mind-body-spirit connection and relationship with God.

FACTORS AFFECTING BODY ALIGNMENT AND ACTIVITY

A number of factors affect an individual's body alignment, mobility, and daily activity level. These include growth and development, nutrition, personal values and attitudes, certain external factors, and prescribed limitations.

Growth and Development

A person's age and musculoskeletal and nervous system development affect posture, body proportions, body mass, body movements, and reflexes. Newborn movements are reflexive and random. All extremities are generally flexed but can be passively moved through a full range of motion. As the neurologic system matures, control over movement progresses during the first year. From ages 1 to 5 years, both gross and fine motor skills are refined. From 6 to 12 years, refinement of motor skills continues and exercise patterns for later life are generally determined. In adolescence, growth spurts and behaviors may result in postural changes that often persist into adulthood. Adults between 20 and 40 years of age generally have few physical changes affecting mobility, with the exception of pregnant women. Pregnancy alters center of gravity and affects balance. Studies support the long-term benefits of exercise during pregnancy to control excess weight gain, thus preventing long-term obesity after delivery. Leaner babies may also be at lower risk for obesity later in life.

As age advances, muscle tone and bone density decrease, joints lose flexibility, reaction time slows, and bone mass decreases, particularly in women who have osteoporosis (bones become brittle and fragile due to calcium depletion). All of these changes affect older adults' posture, gait, and balance. Posture becomes forward leaning and stooped, which shifts the center of gravity forward. To compensate for this shift, the knees flex slightly for support and the base of support is widened. **Gait** becomes wide based, short stepped, and shuffling. A strong body of research supports the benefits of regular activity for older adults to maintain and regain strength, flexibility, cardiovascular fitness, and bone density.

Nutrition

Both undernutrition and overnutrition can influence body alignment and mobility. Poorly nourished people may have muscle weakness and fatigue. Vitamin D deficiency causes bone deformity during growth. Inadequate calcium intake and vitamin D synthesis and intake increase the risk of osteoporosis. Obesity can distort movement and stress joints, adversely affecting posture, balance, and joint health.

Personal Values and Attitudes

The value placed on regular exercise is often the result of family influences. In families that incorporate regular exercise in their daily routine or spend time together in activities, children learn to value physical activity. Sedentary families, on the other hand, participate in sports only as spectators, and this lifestyle is often transmitted to their children. Values about physical appearance also influence some people's participation in regular exercise. People who value a muscular build or physical attractiveness may participate in regular exercise programs to produce the appearance they desire. Choice of physical activity or type of exercise is also influenced by values, geographic location, and cultural role expectations. Motivational states influence our behavior and choices, and vary widely from day to day. To design individualized exercise prescriptions that tailor exercise mode and dose and address these varying states with each person will ensure greater adherence to an exercise program (Burke & Laramie, 2004; Edelman & Mandle, 2010). Prescriptions should include frequency of the activity, intensity, and time (the FIT model).

Nurses must assess each client for potentially motivating factors such as the following: degree of fun or challenge of any given activity; use of music; opportunities for socializing and group cohesion and having an exercise partner; positive sensations of the exercise experience; pleasurable feelings associated with increased stress reduction; increased energy and fitness; mastering the activity; goal setting and progress; daily logs or weekly written schedules; competition with oneself or others; promotion of a sense of accomplishment; weight management; emphasis on self-talk about how exercise will prevent fatigue, depression, weight gain, or anxiety; and the need to explore less intense and challenging, noncompetitive activities (Keele-Smith & Leon, 2003). Nurses, taking into account motivation to participate, medical conditions and level of fitness, and safety issues, can use individualized exercise prescriptions to encourage exercise and activity in all of their clients. Clients who experience orthostatic hypotension, impaired equilibrium, and gait disturbance should begin exercising in supervised environments.

External Factors

Many external factors affect a person's mobility. Excessively high temperatures and high humidity discourage activity, whereas comfortable temperatures and low humidity are conducive to activity. Proper hydration needs vary according to the individual, health status, activity levels, and environment. The IOM recommends that men consume 3 liters (12 cups) of beverage a day, and women 2.2 liters (about 9 cups). Quality water is the best fluid to replace loss incurred through metabolic processes and exercise. Drinking 1 to 2 cups of water is usually adequate for shorter bouts of exercise. For longer bouts such as marathons, drinking 2 cups of water 2 hours prior to the event and then replacing fluids with a sports drink that contains sodium during and after can be beneficial. The availability of recreational facilities also influences activity.

Prescribed Limitations

Limitations to movement may be medically prescribed for some health problems. The term bed rest varies in meaning to some extent. In some agencies bed rest means strict confinement to bed or "complete" bed rest. Others may allow the client to use a bedside commode or have bathroom privileges. Nurses need to familiarize themselves with the meaning of bed rest in their practice setting. In any case, the effects of limiting activity are immediate and negative

EFFECTS OF IMMOBILITY

Mobility and activity tolerance are affected by any disorder that impairs the ability of the nervous system, musculoskeletal system, cardiovascular system, respiratory system, and vestibular apparatus. Individuals who have inactive lifestyles or who are faced with inactivity because of illness or injury are at risk for many problems that can affect major body systems. Whether immobility causes any problems often depends on the duration of the inactivity, the client's health status, and the client's sensory awareness. The most obvious signs of prolonged immobility are often manifested in the musculoskeletal system, and the deconditioning effects can be observed even after a matter of days. Clients experience a significant decrease in muscular strength and agility whenever they do not maintain a moderate amount of physical activity. In addition, immobility adversely affects the cardiovascular, respiratory, metabolic, urinary, and psychoneurologic systems. Nurses need to understand these effects and encourage client movement as much as possible. Early ambulation after illness or surgery is an essential measure to prevent complications (Box 31–1).

BOX 31–1   Effects of Immobility on Body Systems

Musculoskeletal System

- Disuse osteoporosis
- Disuse **atrophy** (Fig. 31–2)
- Contractures
- Stiffness and pain in the joints

Cardiovascular System

- Diminished cardiac reserve
- Increased use of the **Valsalva maneuver** (holding the breath and straining against a closed glottis)
- Orthostatic (postural) hypotension
- Venous vasodilation and stasis (Fig. 31–3)
- Dependent edema
- Thrombus formation

Respiratory System

- Decreased respiratory movement
- Pooling of respiratory secretions
- Atelectasis
- Hypostatic pneumonia

Metabolic System

- Decreased metabolic rate
- Negative nitrogen balance
- Anorexia
- Negative calcium balance

Urinary System

- Urinary stasis
- Renal calculi
- Urinary retention
- Urinary infection

Gastrointestinal System

- Constipation

Integumentary System

- Reduced skin turgor
- Skin breakdown

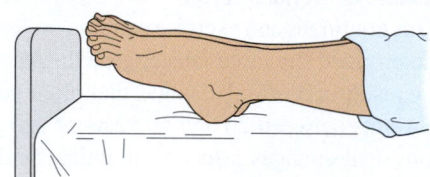

Figure 31–2 ○ Plantar flexion contracture (foot drop).

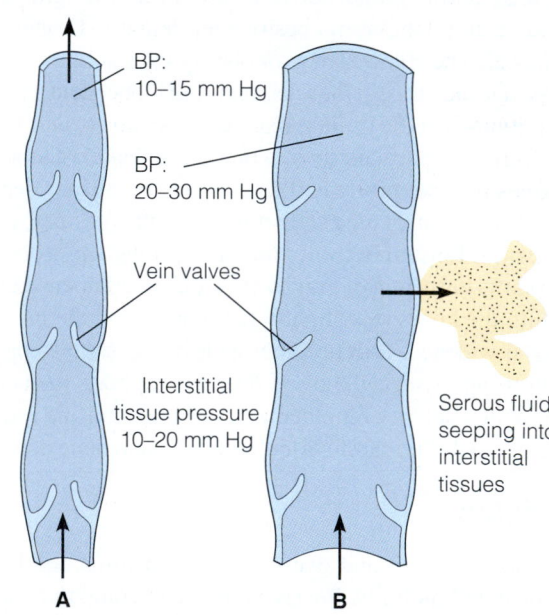

BP: 10–15 mm Hg

BP: 20–30 mm Hg

Vein valves

Interstitial tissue pressure 10–20 mm Hg

Serous fluid seeping into interstitial tissues

A   B

Figure 31–3 ○ Leg veins: **A**, in a mobile person; **B**, in an immobile person.

Psychoneurologic System

- Negative effects on mood
- Lower self-esteem
- Frustration and decreased self-esteem may provoke exaggerated emotional reactions
- Perception of time intervals deteriorates
- Problem-solving and decision-making abilities may deteriorate
- Loss of control over events can cause anxiety

CLINICAL ALERT

A review of 39 studies on effects of bed rest in clients with 15 different disorders revealed that bed rest for treatment of medical conditions is associated with worse outcomes than early mobilization. In general, there are few indications for bed rest, and bed rest may delay recovery or actually harm clients (NANDA, 2005).

NURSING MANAGEMENT

ASSESSING

Assessment relative to a client's activity and exercise should be routinely addressed and includes a nursing history and physical examination of body alignment, gait, appearance and movement of joints, capabilities and limitations for movement, muscle mass and strength, activity tolerance, problems related to immobility, and physical fitness. The nurse collects information from the client, from other nurses, and from the client's records.

Nursing History

An activity and exercise history is usually part of the comprehensive nursing history. Examples of interview questions to elicit these data are shown in the accompanying Assessment Interview. If the client indicates a recent pattern change or difficulties with mobility, a more detailed history is required. This detailed history should include the specific nature of the problem, when it first began, its frequency, its causes if known, how the problem affects daily living, what the client is doing to cope with the problem, and whether these methods have been effective.

Physical Examination

Conduct of the physical examination focusing on activity and exercise emphasizes body alignment, gait, appearance and movement of joints, capabilities and limitations for movement, muscle mass and strength, and activity tolerance (Box 31–2).

Problems Related to Immobility

When collecting data pertaining to the problems of immobility, the nurse uses the assessment methods of inspection, palpation, and auscultation; checks results of laboratory tests; and takes measurements, including body weight, fluid intake, and fluid output. Specific techniques for assessing immobility problems and abnormal assessment findings related to the complications of immobility are listed in Table 31–2. It is extremely important to obtain and record baseline assessment data soon after the client first becomes immobile. These baseline data serve as the standard against which all data collected throughout the period of immobilization are compared. Because a major nursing responsibility is to prevent the compli-

cations of immobility, the nurse needs to identify clients at risk of developing such complications before problems arise.

CLINICAL ALERT

Prolonged inactivity (such as bed rest or sleeping during a long plane ride) in combination with oral contraceptive use can lead to dangerous clot formation in deep leg veins, even in otherwise healthy young women. Smoking increases this risk. Regular movement, stretching, and keeping legs uncrossed are recommended. Monitor for tenderness, redness or discoloration, warmth, and/or swelling in the legs.

DIAGNOSING

Mobility problems may be appropriate as the diagnostic label or as the etiology for other nursing diagnoses.

NANDA includes the following nursing diagnostic labels for activity and exercise problems:

- *Activity Intolerance:* Insufficient physiological or psychological energy to endure or complete required or desired daily activities. Four levels that can be used after the diagnostic label include:
  Level I: Walk, regular pace, on level ground indefinitely; climb one flight of stairs or more but more short of breath than normally.
  Level II: Walk one city block or 500 feet on level ground; climb one flight slowly without stopping.
  Level III: Walk no more than 50 feet on level ground without stopping; unable to climb one flight of stairs without stopping.
  Level IV: Dyspnea and fatigue at rest.
- *Risk for Activity Intolerance:* At risk for experiencing insufficient physiological or psychological energy to endure or complete required or desired daily activities.
- *Impaired Physical Mobility:* Limitation in independent, purposeful physical movement of the body or of one or more extremities.
    More specific versions of this diagnosis are
    Impaired Bed Mobility
    Impaired Walking
    Impaired Wheelchair Mobility
    Impaired Transfer Ability
- *Sedentary Lifestyle:* Reports a habit of life that is characterized by a low physical activity level.
- *Risk for Disuse Syndrome:* At risk for deterioration of body systems as the result of prescribed or unavoidable musculoskeletal inactivity.

A clinical example of this nursing diagnosis is shown in the Nursing Care Plan and the Concept Map on pages 926–928.

Depending on the data obtained, problems with mobility often affect other areas of human functioning and indicate other diagnoses. In these instances, the mobility problem

BOX 31–2	Assessment Focus during the Physical Examination

Body Alignment

Assessment includes an inspection of the client while the client stands from lateral, anterior, and posterior perspectives.

- Normal developmental variations in posture.
- Posture and learning needs to maintain good posture.
- Factors contributing to poor posture, such as fatigue or low self-esteem.
- Muscle weakness or other motor impairments.
- The shoulders and hips are level.
- The toes point forward.
- The spine is straight, not curved to either side.

Gait

- Chin is level, gaze is straight ahead, sternum is lifted, and shoulders are down and back, relaxed away from the ears.
- Heel strikes the ground before the toe. It is here, where both feet are taking some body weight, that the spine is most rotated.
- Feet are dorsiflexed in the swing phase.
- Arm opposite the swing-through foot moves forward at the same time.
- Gait is smooth, coordinated, and rhythmic, with even weight borne on each foot. Hips gently sway with spinal rotation; the body moves forward smoothly, stopping and starting with ease.

Pace

Pace is the number of steps taken per minute, which often slows with age and disability.

- A normal walking pace is 70 to 100 steps per minute.
- The pace of an older person may slow to about 40 steps per minute.
- Need for a prosthesis or assistive device

Appearance and Movement of Joints

- Any joint swelling or redness, which could indicate the presence of an injury or an inflammation.
- Any deformity, such as a bony enlargement or contracture, and symmetry of involvement.
- The muscle development associated with each joint and the relative size and symmetry of the muscles on each side of the body.
- Any reported or palpable tenderness.
- Crepitation
- Increased temperature over the joint.
- Degree of joint movement.

Capabilities and Limitations of Movement

- How the client's illness influences the ability to move and whether the client's health contraindicates any exertion, position, or movement.
- Encumbrances to movement.
- Mental alertness and ability to follow directions.
- Balance and coordination.
- Presence of orthostatic hypotension before transfers.
- Degree of comfort.
- Vision.
- Moving in the bed.
  a. From a supine position to a lateral position.
  b. From a lateral position on one side to a lateral position on the other.
  c. From a supine position to a sitting position in bed.
- Rising from a lying position to a sitting position on the edge of the bed.
- Rising from a chair to a standing position.
- Coordination and balance.
- Muscle mass and strength.

Activity Tolerance

The most useful measures in predicting activity tolerance are heart rate, strength, and rhythm; respiratory rate, depth, and rhythm; and blood pressure. These data are obtained at the following times:

- Before the activity starts (baseline data), while the client is at rest
- During the activity
- Immediately after the activity stops
- Three minutes after the activity has stopped and the client has rested

The activity should be stopped immediately in the event of any physiologic change indicating the activity is too strenuous or prolonged for the client. These changes include the following:

- Sudden facial pallor
- Feelings of dizziness or weakness
- Change in level of consciousness
- Heart rate or respiratory rate that significantly exceeds baseline or preestablished levels
- Change in heart or respiratory rhythm from regular to irregular
- Weakening of the pulse
- Dyspnea, shortness of breath, or chest pain
- Diastolic blood pressure change of 10 mm Hg or more

If the client tolerates the activity well, and if the client's heart rate returns to baseline levels within 5 minutes after the activity ceases, the activity is considered safe. This activity can then serve as a standard for predicting the client's tolerance for similar activities.

Daily Activity Level

- What activities do you carry out during a routine day?
- Are you able to carry out the following tasks independently?
  a. Eating
  b. Dressing/grooming
  c. Bathing
  d. Toileting
  e. Ambulating
  f. Using a wheelchair
  g. Transferring in and out of bed, bath, and car
  h. Cooking
  i. House cleaning
  j. Shopping
- Where problems exist in your ability to carry out such tasks:
  a. Would you rate yourself as partially or totally dependent?
  b. How is the task achieved (by family, friend, agency, or use of specialized equipment)?

Activity Tolerance

- What types of activities make you tired?

- Do you ever experience dizziness, shortness of breath, marked increase in respiratory rate, or other problems following mild or moderate activity?

Exercise

- What type of exercise do you carry out to enhance your physical fitness?
- What is the frequency and length of this exercise session?
- Do you believe exercise is beneficial to your health? Explain.

Factors Affecting Mobility

- Environmental factors. Do stairs, lack of railings or other assistive devices, or an unsafe neighborhood impede your mobility or exercise regimen?
- Health problems. Do any of the following health problems affect your muscle strength or endurance: heart disease, lung disease, stroke, cancer, neuromuscular problems, musculoskeletal problems, visual or mental impairments, trauma, or pain?
- Financial factors. Are your finances adequate to obtain equipment or other aids that you require to enhance your mobility?

TABLE 31–2   **Assessing Problems of Immobility**

ASSESSMENT	PROBLEM
Musculoskeletal System	
Measure arm and leg circumferences	Decreased circumference due to decreased muscle mass
Palpate and observe body joints	Stiffness or pain in joints
Take goniometric measurements of joint ROM	Decreased joint ROM, joint contractures
Cardiovascular System	
Auscultate the heart	Increased heart rate
Measure blood pressure	Orthostatic hypotension
Palpate and observe sacrum, legs, and feet	Peripheral dependent edema, increased peripheral vein engorgement
Palpate peripheral pulses	Weak peripheral pulses
Measure calf muscle circumferences	Edema
Observe calf muscle for redness, tenderness, and swelling	Thrombophlebitis
Respiratory System	
Observe chest movements	Asymmetric chest movements, dyspnea
Auscultate chest	Diminished breath sounds, crackles, wheezes, and increased respiratory rate
Metabolic System	
Measure height and weight	Weight loss due to muscle atrophy and loss of subcutaneous fat
Palpate skin	Generalized edema due to low blood protein levels
Urinary System	
Measure fluid intake and output	Dehydration
Inspect urine	Cloudy, dark urine; high specific gravity
Palpate urinary bladder	Distended urinary bladder due to urinary retention
Gastrointestinal System	
Observe stool	Hard, dry, small stool
Auscultate bowel sounds	Decreased bowel sounds due to decreased intestinal motility
Integumentary System	
Inspect skin	Break in skin integrity
Psychoneurologic System	
Observe behaviors, affect, and cognition	Anger, flat affect, crying, confusion, anxiety, decline in cognitive function, or vegetative signs such as sleep and appetite disturbances
Monitor developmental skills in children	warrant further evaluation

becomes the etiology. Examples in which *Impaired Physical Mobility* is the etiology follow. The etiology needs to be described more explicitly in terms such as reduced ROM, neuromuscular impairment or musculoskeletal impairment of upper and lower extremities, or joint pain.

- *Fear* (of falling)
- *Ineffective Coping*
- *Low Self-Esteem*
- *Powerlessness*
- *Risk for Falls*
- *Self-Care Deficit*

When problems associated with prolonged immobility arise, many other diagnoses may be necessary. Examples include, but are not limited to, the following:

- *Ineffective Airway Clearance* if there is stasis of pulmonary secretions
- *Risk for Infection* if there is stasis of urinary or pulmonary secretions
- *Risk for Injury* if orthostatic hypotension is present
- *Risk for Disturbed Sleep Pattern* if there is a lack of daytime physical activity
- *Risk for Situational Low Self-Esteem* if there is functional impairment and/or role disturbance

PLANNING

When planning for desired outcomes, Nursing Outcomes Classification (NOC) labels that pertain to exercise and activity can be helpful and include the following: activity tolerance; anxiety level and self-control; body image; body positioning; bowel elimination; caregiver physical health; coordinated movement; depression self-control; diabetes self-management; endurance; fall prevention behavior; immobility consequences, both physiological and psychocognitive; joint movement; mobility; mood equilibrium; personal well-being; physical fitness; play participation; quality of life; respiratory status, ventilation and gas exchange; role performance; self-care; sleep; stress level; and weight control (Moorhead, Johnson, & Maas, 2008).

Positioning, transferring, and ambulating clients are almost always independent nursing functions. The primary care practitioner usually orders specific body positions only after surgery, anesthesia, or trauma involving the nervous and musculoskeletal systems. All clients should have an activity order written by their primary care practitioner when they are admitted to the agency for care.

As part of planning, the nurse is responsible for identifying those clients who need assistance with body alignment and determining the degree of assistance they need. The nurse must be sensitive to the client's need to function as independently as possible yet provide assistance when the client needs it.

Most clients require some nursing guidance and assistance to learn about, achieve, and maintain proper body mechanics. The nurse should also plan to teach clients applicable skills. For example, a client with a back injury needs to learn how to get out of bed safely and comfortably,

a client with an injured leg needs to learn how to transfer from bed to wheelchair safely, and a client with a newly acquired walker needs to learn how to use it safely. Nurses often teach family members or caregivers safe moving, lifting, and transfer techniques in the home setting.

The goals established for clients will vary according to the diagnosis and defining characteristics related to each individual. Examples of overall goals for clients with actual or potential problems related to mobility or activity follow.

The client will have:

- Increased tolerance for physical activity.
- Restored or improved capability to ambulate and/or participate in ADLs.
- Absence of injury from falling or improper use of body mechanics.
- Enhanced physical fitness.
- Absence of any complications associated with immobility.
- Improved social, emotional, and intellectual well-being.

Examples of desired outcomes, interventions, and activities are provided in the Nursing Care Plan and Concept Map on pages 926–928.

IMPLEMENTING

Nurses can initiate and apply a wide variety of exercise and activity interventions as needed to address a multitude of client concerns. Nursing Interventions Classification (NIC) labels that pertain to exercise and activity include the following: activity therapy; calming technique; cardiac care; rehabilitation; cognitive stimulation; constipation management; distraction; exercise promotion (strength and stretching); exercise therapy (ambulation, balance, joint mobility, muscle control); fall prevention; health education; infection prevention; memory training; mood management; pelvic muscle exercise; pressure ulcer prevention; progressive muscle relaxation; recreation therapy; religious ritual enhancement; self-care assistance; self-esteem enhancement; simple relaxation therapy; sleep enhancement; spiritual growth facilitation; sports-injury prevention; teaching; prescribed activity/exercise; therapeutic play; and weight management and weight reduction (Bulechek, Butcher, & Dochterman, 2008).

Nursing strategies to maintain or promote body alignment and mobility involve positioning clients appropriately, moving and turning clients in bed, transferring clients, providing ROM exercises, ambulating clients with or without mechanical aids, and strategies to prevent the complications of immobility. Whenever positioning, moving, lifting, and ambulating clients, nurses must use proper body mechanics to avoid musculoskeletal strain and injury.

Using Body Mechanics

Body mechanics is the term used to describe the efficient, coordinated, and safe use of the body to move objects and carry out the activities of daily living. Until recently, it was thought that using good body mechanics reduced energy requirements, fatigue, and risk of injury for both nurses and clients, especially during lifting, transferring, and repositioning. In reality, 35 years of body mechanics (ergonomics) research show that:

- Training nurses in body mechanics alone will not prevent job-related injuries.
- Back belts are likely *not* effective in reducing back injury.
- Nurses who are physically fit are at no less risk of injury.
- The average nurse should not lift more than 51 pounds and only under very controlled circumstances.
- Long-term benefits of proper equipment far outweigh costs related to injuries.
- Staff will use equipment when they participate in the decision-making process for purchasing the equipment (American Nurses Association, n.d.).

Even with careful attention to body mechanics, nursing is ranked as the sixth most at-risk occupation for back injuries. The development of assistive client handling equipment and devices has rendered strict "manual" client handling unnecessary. It is also thought to provide greater client safety, dignity, and comfort. Costs of equipment appear to be less than the costs of work-related injury (Nelson, Fragala, & Menzel, 2003). The equipment recommendations include full sling mechanical lift devices for totally dependent or extensive assistance level clients; full sling, stand assist lift, or full sling mechanical lifts for dependent lifts from the floor; and transfer or gait belts for client-assisted lifts from the floor.

Until all work settings provide safe environments in which nurses have the equipment they need, content pertaining to body mechanics will be included here. Readers are encouraged to support "No Manual Lift" and "No Solo Lift" policies in their workplaces, and to become involved

in legislation and equipment purchase initiatives. Nurses must participate in this shift in ergonomic awareness, and are encouraged to visit the American Nurses Association website to read more about the "Handle with Care" campaign to prevent workplace injuries.

When a person moves, the center of gravity shifts continuously in the direction of the moving body parts. Balance depends on the interrelationship of the center of gravity, the line of gravity, and the base of support. The closer the line of gravity is to the center of the base of support, the greater the person's stability (Figure 31–4, *A*). Conversely, the closer the line of gravity is to the edge of the base of support, the more precarious the balance (Figure 31–4, *B*). If the line of gravity falls outside the base of support, the person falls (Figure 31–4, *C*).

CLINICAL ALERT

The American Federation of State, County, and Municipal Employees (AFSCME) reports that back injuries are caused by force, repetition, and awkward positions. The most common injuries among health care workers are low back pain, herniated discs, strained muscles, pulled and/or torn ligaments, and disc degradation (AFSCME, 2002).

The broader the base of support and the lower the center of gravity, the greater the stability and balance. Body balance, therefore, can be greatly enhanced by (a) widening the base of support and (b) lowering the center of gravity, bringing it closer to the base of support. The base of support is easily widened by spreading the feet farther apart. The center of gravity is readily lowered by flexing the hips and knees until a squatting position is achieved. The importance of these alterations cannot be overemphasized for nurses.

Two movements to avoid because of their potential for causing back injury are twisting (rotation) of the

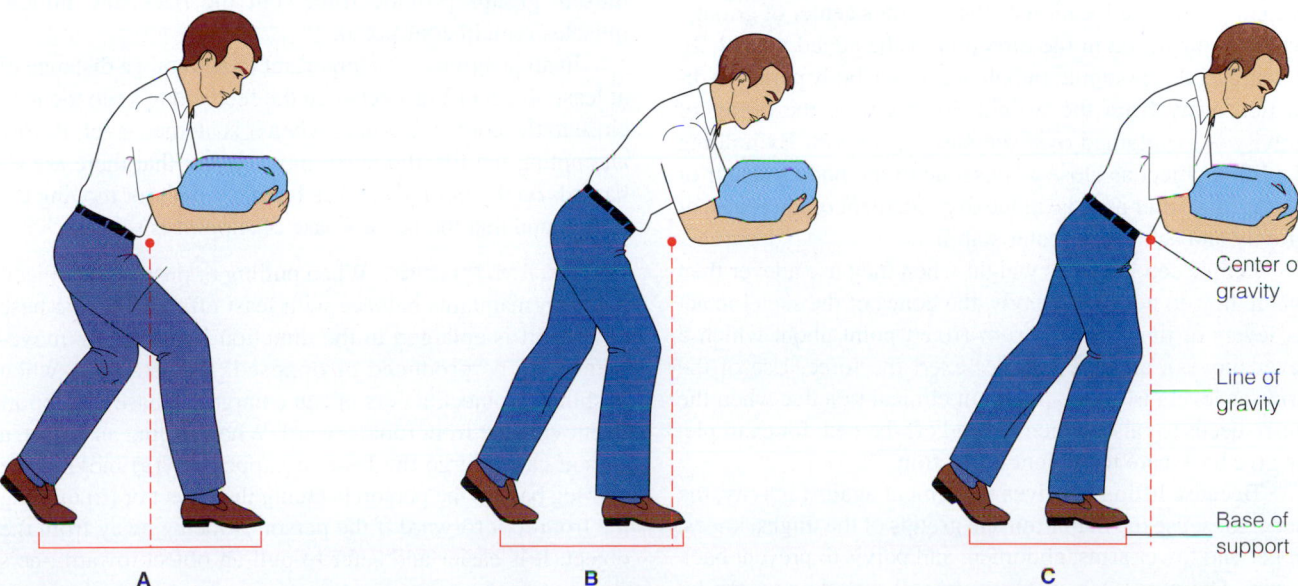

Figure 31–4 ⬤ *A*, Balance is maintained when the line of gravity falls close to the base of support. *B*, Balance is precarious when the line of gravity falls at the edge of the base of support. *C*, Balance cannot be maintained when the line of gravity falls outside the base of support.

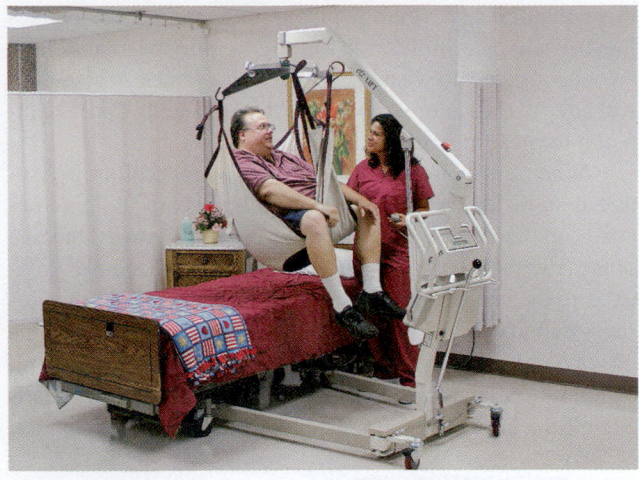

Figure 31–5 ⬤ EZ Lift is an electric client lift that functions to lift clients from bed, chair, toilet, and floor.
(EZ Way, Inc.)

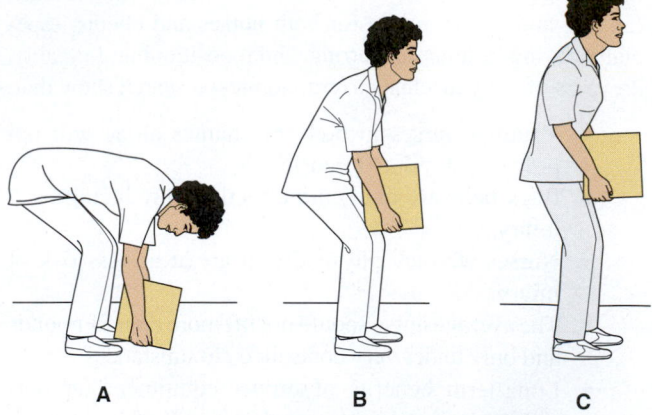

Figure 31–6 ⬤ Lifting heavy objects from the floor to waist level. **A,** Stand close to the load and flex the back and the knees, lowering the body to grasp the load. **B,** Begin lifting with the back flexed, and gradually straighten the knees so that the leg muscles bear most of the burden. **C,** To hold or walk with the object, maintain a less flexed but not a completely straight position.

thoracolumbar spine and acute flexion of the back with hips and knees straight (stooping). Undesirable twisting of the back can be prevented by squarely facing the direction of movement, whether pushing, pulling, or sliding, and moving the object directly toward or away from one's center of gravity.

LIFTING It is important to remember that nurses should not lift more than 51 pounds without assistance from proper equipment and/or other persons. See Figure 31–5. At times it may be necessary to lift under less than ideal circumstances. It is always wise to use proper body mechanics, even though they do not guarantee freedom from injury.

When a person lifts or carries an object, the weight of the object becomes part of the person's body weight. This weight affects the location of the person's center of gravity, which is displaced in the direction of the added weight. To counteract this potential imbalance, move body parts in a direction away from the weight. In this way, the center of gravity is maintained over the base of support. By holding the lifted object as close as possible to the body's center of gravity, the lifter avoids undue displacement of the center of gravity and achieves greater stability.

People can lift more weight when they use a lever than when they do not. In the body, the bones of the skeleton act as levers, a joint is a fulcrum (fixed point about which a lever moves), and the muscles exert the force. Use of the arms as levers is often applied in clinical practice when the nurse needs to raise a client's head off the bed, for example, or give back care to a client in traction.

Because lifting involves movement against gravity, the nurse must use the major muscle groups of the thighs, knees, upper and lower arms, abdomen, and pelvis to prevent back strain. The nurse can increase overall muscle strength by synchronized use of as many muscle groups as possible during an activity.

Another technique based on the principle of leverage can be used when lifting objects from the floor to waist level. In this technique, the back and knees are flexed until the load is at thigh level, at which point the knees remain flexed to provide thrust as the back begins to straighten (Figure 31–6). This technique provides for balance, leverage, and synchronized use of muscles, which help avoid back pain and injury. When one lifts an object to knee level, the shoulder and arm muscles pull, the abdominal and lumbar muscles contract for leverage and pull, and the thigh and leg muscles exert the upward thrust to bring the object off the floor. When one lifts an object from midthigh to waist level, essentially the leg and thigh muscle groups provide force, but the back and lumbar muscles remain contracted.

In all positions, it is important to maintain a distance of at least 30 cm (12 in.) between the feet and to keep the load close to the body, especially when it is at knee level. Before attempting the lift, the nurse must ensure that there are no hazards on the floor, that there is a clear path for moving the object, and that the nurse's base of support is secure.

PULLING AND PUSHING When pulling or pushing an object, a person maintains balance with least effort when the base of support is enlarged in the direction in which the movement is to be produced or opposed. For example, when pushing an object, a person can enlarge the base of support by moving the front foot forward. When pulling an object, a person can enlarge the base of support by (a) moving the rear leg back if the person is facing the object or (b) moving the front foot forward if the person is facing away from the object. It is easier and safer to pull an object toward one's own center of gravity than to push it away, because a person can exert more control of the object's movement when pulling it.

CLINICAL ALERT

Lateral-assist devices such as horizontal air transfer mattresses and transfer chairs are essential equipment for most client care areas to prevent acute and chronic back pain and disability. Observing principles of body mechanics is recommended even when using assistive equipment, as any lifting and forceful movement is potentially injurious, especially when repeated over time.

PIVOTING Pivoting is a technique in which the body is turned in a way that avoids twisting of the spine. To pivot, place one foot ahead of the other, raise the heels very slightly, and put the body weight on the balls of the feet. When the weight is off the heels, the frictional surface is decreased and the knees are not twisted when turning. Keeping the body aligned, turn (pivot) about 90 degrees in the desired direction. The foot that was forward will now be behind.

Preventing Back Injury

Many factors increase the potential for lower back injuries. A major contributor is habitually poor standing and sitting posture, which produces lordosis. Overweight individuals who carry their extra weight over their abdomen, pregnant women, and women who consistently wear high-heeled shoes are at risk because of the exaggerated lumbar curvature these situations produce. Sedentary persons are at greater risk because of weak back and abdominal muscles. Guidelines for preventing back injuries are presented in Box 31–3.

Positioning Clients

Positioning a client in good body alignment and changing the position regularly (every 2 hours) and systematically are essential aspects of nursing practice. Clients who can move easily automatically reposition themselves for comfort. Such people generally require minimal positioning assistance from nurses, other than guidance about ways to maintain body alignment and to exercise their joints. However, people who are weak, frail, in pain, paralyzed,

or unconscious rely on nurses to provide or assist with position changes. For all clients, it is important to assess the skin and provide skin care before and after a position change.

Any position, correct or incorrect, can be detrimental if maintained for a prolonged period. Frequent change of position helps to prevent muscle discomfort, undue pressure resulting in pressure ulcers, damage to superficial nerves and blood vessels, and contractures. Position changes also maintain muscle tone and stimulate postural reflexes.

When the client is not able to move independently or assist with moving, the preferred method is to use appropriate assistive equipment, as well as to have two or more people move or turn the client. Appropriate assistance reduces the risk of muscle strain and body injury to both the client and nurse, and is likely to protect the dignity and comfort of the client.

When positioning clients in bed, the nurse can do a number of things to ensure proper alignment and promote client comfort and safety:

- Make sure the mattress is firm and level yet has enough give to fill in and support natural body curvatures. A sagging mattress, a mattress that is too soft, or an underfilled waterbed used over a prolonged period can contribute to the development of hip flexion contractures and low back strain and pain. Bed boards made of plywood and placed beneath a sagging mattress are increasingly recommended for clients who have back problems or are prone to them. Some bed boards are hinged across the middle so that they will bend as the head of the bed is raised. It is particularly important in the home setting to inspect the mattress for support.
- Ensure that the bed is clean and dry. Wrinkled or damp sheets increase the risk of pressure ulcer formation. Make sure extremities can move freely whenever possible. For example, the top bedclothes need to be loose enough for clients to move their feet.

BOX 31–3	**Preventing Back Injuries**

- Understand that the use of body mechanics will not necessarily prevent injury if manually handling a load greater than 51 pounds without the use of assistive devices.
- Avoid lifting anything greater than 51 pounds. Use assistive equipment, get help from co-workers, and participate in the purchasing/ordering process of appropriate assistive equipment for your work setting.
- Become consciously aware of your posture and body mechanics.
- When standing for a period of time, periodically move legs and hips, and flex one hip and knee and rest your foot on an object if possible.
- When sitting, keep your knees slightly higher than your hips.
- Use a firm mattress and soft pillow that provide good body support at natural body curvatures.

- Exercise regularly to maintain overall physical condition and regulate weight; include exercises that strengthen the pelvic, abdominal, and spinal muscles.
- Avoid movements that cause pain or require spinal flexion with straight legs (e.g., toe-touching and sit-ups) or spinal rotation (twisting).
- When moving an object, spread your feet apart to provide a wide base of support.
- When lifting an object, distribute the weight between large muscles of the legs and arms, limiting the load to 15 to 25 pounds held at elbow height.
- Wear comfortable low-heeled shoes that provide good foot support and reduce the risk of slipping, stumbling, or turning your ankle.

BOX 31–4   Support Devices

- *Pillows.* Different sizes are available. Used for support or elevation of a body part (e.g., an arm). Specially designed dense pillows can be used to elevate the upper body.
- *Mattresses.* There are two types of mattresses: ones that fit on the bed frame (e.g., standard bed mattress) and mattresses that fit on the standard bed mattress (e.g., egg crate mattress). Mattresses should be periodically rotated and evenly supportive.
- *Bed boards.* The boards are usually made of wood and are placed under the mattress to provide support.

- *Chair beds.* These beds can be placed into the position of a chair for clients who cannot move from the bed but require a sitting position.
- *Foot boot.* These are made of a variety of substances. They usually have a firm exterior and padding of foam to protect the skin. They provide support to the feet in a natural position and keep the weight of covers off the toes. Clients who are able to sit may benefit from high-top shoes to maintain foot alignment.
- *Footboard.* A flat panel often made of plastic or wood. It keeps the feet in dorsiflexion to prevent plantar flexion.

- Place support devices in specified areas according to the client's position. Box 31–4 lists commonly used support devices. Use only those support devices needed to maintain alignment and to prevent stress on the client's muscles and joints. If the person is capable of movement, too many devices limit mobility and increase the potential for muscle weakness and atrophy.
- Avoid placing one body part, particularly one with bony prominences, directly on top of another body part. Excessive pressure can damage veins and predispose the client to thrombus formation. Pressure against the popliteal space may damage nerves and blood vessels in this area. Pillows can provide needed cushioning.
- Plan a systematic 24-hour schedule for position changes.

Sometimes a person who appears well aligned may be experiencing real discomfort. Both appearance, in relation to alignment criteria, and comfort are important in achieving effective alignment.

Fowler's position, or a semisitting position, is a bed position in which the head and trunk are raised 45 to 90 degrees. In low Fowler's or semi-Fowler's position, the head and trunk are raised 15 to 45 degrees; in high Fowler's position, the head and trunk are raised 90 degrees (see Table 31–3). Fowler's position is the position of choice for people who have difficulty breathing and for some people with heart problems. When the client is in this position, gravity pulls the diaphragm downward, allowing greater chest expansion and lung ventilation.

In the orthopneic position, the client sits either in bed or on the side of the bed with an overbed table across the lap

TABLE 31–3   Positions

Fowler's Position

UNSUPPORTED POSITION	PROBLEM TO BE PREVENTED	CORRECTIVE MEASURE*
Bed-sitting position with upper part of body elevated 30–90° commencing at hips	Posterior flexion of lumbar curvature	Pillow at lower back (lumbar region) to support lumbar region
Head rests on bed surface	Hyperextension of neck	Pillows to support head, neck, and upper back
Arms fall at sides	Shoulder muscle strain, possible dislocation of shoulders, edema of hands and arms with flaccid paralysis, flexion contracture of the wrist	Pillow under forearms to eliminate pull on shoulder and assist venous blood flow from hands and lower arms
Legs lie flat and straight on lower bed surface	Hyperextension of knees	Small pillow under thighs to flex knees
Heels rest on bed surface	Pressure on heels	Pillow under lower legs
Feet are in plantar flexion	Plantar flexion of feet (**foot drop**)	Footboard to provide support for dorsal flexion

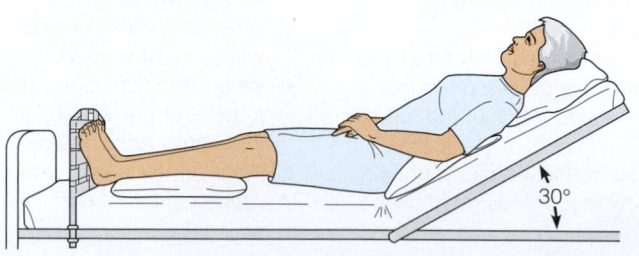

30°

TABLE 31–3   Positions *(continued)*

Dorsal Recumbent Position

UNSUPPORTED POSITION	PROBLEM TO BE PREVENTED	CORRECTIVE MEASURE*
Head is flat on bed surface	Hyperextension of neck in thick-chested person	Pillow of suitable thickness under head and shoulders if necessary for alignment
Lumbar curvature of spine is apparent	Posterior flexion of lumbar curvature	Roll or small pillow under lumbar curvature
Legs may be externally rotated	External rotation of legs	Roll or sandbag placed laterally to trochanter of femur (optional)
Legs are extended	Hyperextension of knees	Small pillow under thigh to flex knee slightly
Feet assume plantar flexion position	Plantar flexion (foot drop)	Footboard or rolled pillow to support feet in dorsal flexion
Heels on bed surface	Pressure on heels	Pillow under lower legs

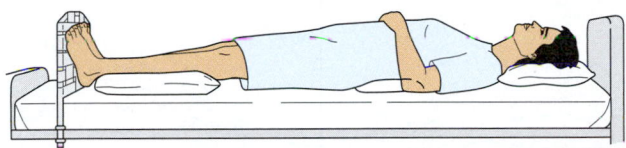

Prone Position

UNSUPPORTED POSITION	PROBLEM TO BE PREVENTED	CORRECTIVE MEASURE*
Head is turned to side and neck is slightly flexed	Flexion or hyperextension of neck	Small pillow under head unless contraindicated because of promotion of mucous drainage from mouth
Body lies flat on abdomen accentuating lumbar curvature	Hyperextension of lumbar curvature; difficulty breathing; pressure on breasts (women); pressure on genitals (men)	Small pillow or roll under abdomen just below diaphragm
Toes rest on bed surface; feet are in plantar flexion	Plantar flexion (foot drop)	Allow feet to fall naturally over end of mattress, or support lower legs on a pillow so that toes do not touch the bed

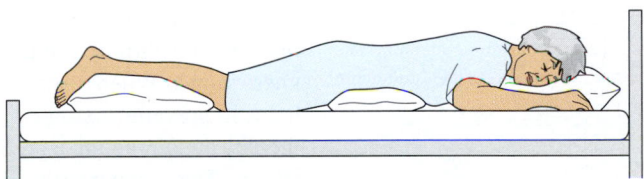

Lateral Position

UNSUPPORTED POSITION	PROBLEM TO BE PREVENTED	CORRECTIVE MEASURE*
Body is turned to side, both arms in front of body, weight resting primarily on lateral aspects of scapula and ilium	Lateral flexion and fatigue of sternocleidomastoid muscles	Pillow under head and neck to provide good alignment
Upper arm and shoulder are rotated internally and adducted	Internal rotation and adduction of shoulder and subsequent limited function; impaired chest expansion	Pillow under upper arm to place it in good alignment; lower arm should be flexed comfortably
Upper thigh and leg are rotated internally and adducted	Internal rotation and adduction of femur; twisting of the spine	Pillow under leg and thigh to place them in good alignment; shoulders and hips should be aligned

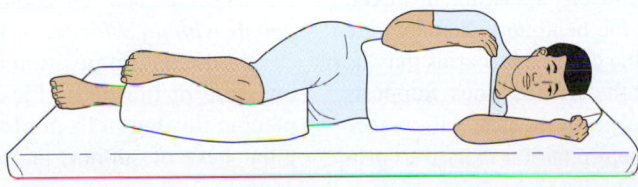

(continued)

TABLE 31–3   Positions *(continued)*

Sims' (Semiprone) Position

UNSUPPORTED POSITION	PROBLEM TO BE PREVENTED	CORRECTIVE MEASURE*
Head rests on bed surface; weight is borne by lateral aspects of cranial and facial bones	Lateral flexion of neck	Pillow supports head, maintaining it in good alignment unless drainage from the mouth is required
Upper shoulder and arm are internally rotated	Internal rotation of shoulder and arm; pressure on chest, restricting expansion during breathing	Pillow under upper arm to prevent internal rotation
Upper leg and thigh are adducted and internally rotated	Internal rotation and adduction of hip and leg	Pillow under upper leg to support it in alignment
Feet assume plantar flexion	Foot drop	Sandbags to support feet in dorsal flexion

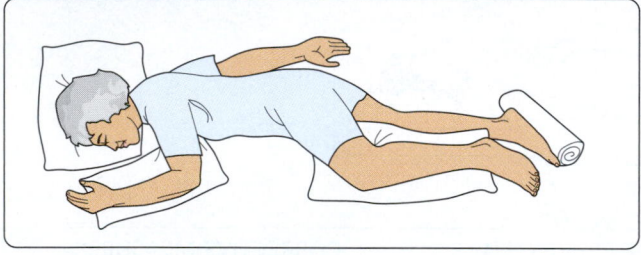 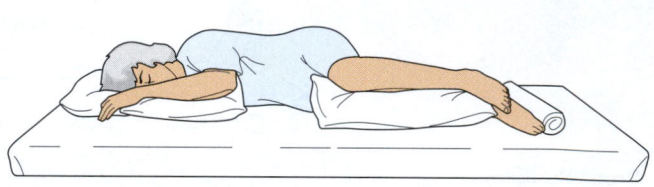

*The amount of correction depends on the needs of the individual client.

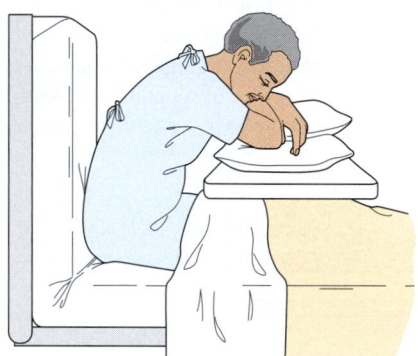

Figure 31–7 ● Orthopneic position.

(Figure 31–7). This position facilitates respiration by allowing maximum chest expansion. It is particularly helpful to clients who have problems exhaling, because they can press the lower part of the chest against the edge of the overbed table.

In the dorsal recumbent (back-lying) position, the client's head and shoulders are slightly elevated on a small pillow. In some agencies, the terms *dorsal recumbent* and *supine* are used interchangeably; strictly speaking, however, in the supine or dorsal position the head and shoulders are not elevated. In both positions, the client's forearms may be elevated on pillows or placed at the client's sides. Supports are similar in both positions, except for the head pillow (see Table 31–3). The dorsal recumbent position is used to pro-

vide comfort and to facilitate healing following certain surgeries or anesthetics (e.g., spinal).

In the prone position, the client lies on the abdomen with the head turned to one side. The hips are not flexed. Both children and adults often sleep in this position, sometimes with one or both arms flexed over their heads. It is the only bed position that allows full extension of the hip and knee joints. When used periodically, the prone position helps to prevent flexion contractures of the hips and knees, thereby counteracting a problem caused by all other bed positions. The prone position also promotes drainage from the mouth and is especially useful for unconscious clients or those clients recovering from surgery of the mouth or throat (see Table 31–3). The prone position poses some distinct disadvantages. The pull of gravity on the trunk produces a marked lordosis in most people, and the neck is rotated laterally to a significant degree. For this reason, the prone position may not be recommended for people with problems of the cervical or lumbar spine. This position also causes plantar flexion. Some clients with cardiac or respiratory problems find the prone position confining and suffocating because chest expansion is inhibited during respirations. *The prone position should be used only when the client's back is correctly aligned, only for short periods, and only for people with no evidence of spinal abnormalities.*

In the lateral position (side-lying), the person lies on one side of the body. Flexing the top hip and knee and placing this leg in front of the body creates a wider, triangular base of support and achieves greater stability. The greater the flexion of the top hip and knee, the greater the stability and balance in this position. This flexion reduces lordosis and promotes good back alignment. For this reason, the lateral position is good for resting and sleeping clients. The lateral position helps to relieve pressure on the sacrum and heels in people who sit for much of the day or who are confined to bed and rest in Fowler's or dorsal recumbent positions much of the time. In the lateral position, most of the body's weight is borne by the lateral aspect of the lower scapula, the lateral aspect of the ilium, and the greater trochanter of the femur. People who have sensory or motor deficits on one side of the body usually find that lying on the uninvolved side is more comfortable (see Table 31–3).

In Sims' (semiprone) position, the client assumes a posture halfway between the lateral and the prone positions. The lower arm is positioned behind the client, and the upper arm is flexed at the shoulder and the elbow. Both legs are flexed in front of the client. The upper leg is more acutely flexed at both the hip and the knee than is the lower one. Sims' position may be used for unconscious clients because it facilitates drainage from the mouth and prevents aspiration of fluids. It is also used for paralyzed clients because it reduces pressure over the sacrum and greater trochanter of the hip. It is often used for clients receiving enemas and occasionally for clients undergoing examinations or treatments of the perineal area. Many people, especially pregnant women, find Sims' position comfortable for sleeping. People with sensory or motor deficits on one side of the body usually find that lying on the uninvolved side is more comfortable (see Table 31–3).

Moving and Turning Clients in Bed

Although healthy people usually take for granted that they can change body position and go from one place to another with little effort, ill people may have difficulty moving, even in bed. How much assistance clients require depends on their own ability to move and their health status. Nurses should be sensitive to both the need of people to function independently and their need for assistance to move.

When a nurse assists a person to move, correct body mechanics need to be employed so that the nurse is not injured. Correct body alignment for the client must also be maintained so that undue stress is not placed on the musculoskeletal system.

Actions and rationales applicable to moving and lifting clients include these:

- Before moving a client, assess the degree of exertion permitted, the client's physical abilities (e.g., muscle strength, presence of paralysis) and ability to assist with the move, ability to understand instructions, degree of comfort or discomfort when moving, client's weight, presence of orthostatic hypotension (particularly important when client will be standing), and your own strength and ability to move the client.
- If indicated, use pain relief modalities or medication prior to moving the client.
- Prepare any needed assistive devices and supportive equipment.
- Plan around encumbrances to movement.
- Be alert to the effects of any medications the client takes that may impair alertness, balance, strength, or mobility.
- Obtain required assistance from other persons.
- Explain the procedure to the client and listen to any suggestions the client or support people have.
- Provide privacy.
- Wash hands.
- Raise the height of the bed *to bring the client close to your center of gravity.*
- Lock the wheels on the bed, and raise the rail on the side of the bed opposite you *to ensure client safety.*
- Face in the direction of the movement *to prevent spinal twisting.*
- Assume a broad stance *to increase stability and provide balance.*
- Lean your trunk forward, and flex your hips, knees, and ankles *to lower your center of gravity, increase stability, and ensure use of large muscle groups during movements.*
- Tighten your gluteal, abdominal, leg, and arm muscles *to prepare them for action and prevent injury.*
- Rock from the front leg to the back leg when pulling or from the back leg to the front leg when pushing *to overcome inertia, counteract the client's weight, and help attain a balanced, smooth motion.*
- After moving the client, determine and document the client's comfort (presence of anxiety, dizziness, or pain), body alignment, tolerance of the activity (e.g., check pulse rate, blood pressure), ability to assist, use of support devices, and safety precautions required (e.g., side rails).

See Skills 31–1 through 31–4 on moving and turning clients in bed and helping them sit up on the edge of the bed.

Note: The Assessment, Planning, Delegation, and Equipment sections as listed in Skill 31–1 are the same for each of these four procedures and are not repeated. The Evaluation section at the end of Skill 31–4 is also the same for all four procedures and, hence, is not repeated.

MOVING A CLIENT UP IN BED

ASSESSMENT

Before moving a client, assess the following:

- The client's physical abilities (e.g., muscle strength, presence of paralysis)
- Ability to understand instructions

- Degree of comfort or discomfort when moving. If needed, administer analgesics or perform other pain relief measures (see Chapter 18 ∞).
- Client's weight
- The availability of equipment and other personnel to assist you

PLANNING

Review the client record to determine if previous nurses have recorded information about the client's ability to move. Use proper assistive equipment and additional personnel whenever needed.

Delegation

The skills of moving and turning clients in bed can be delegated to unlicensed assistive personnel (UAP). The nurse should make sure that any needed equipment and additional personnel are available to reduce risk of injury to the health care personnel. Emphasize the need for the UAP to report changes in the client's condition that require assessment and intervention by the nurse.

EQUIPMENT

- Assistive devices such as overhead trapeze, pull and/or turn sheet, and transfer or sliding bar

Purpose

- Clients who have slid down in bed from the Fowler's position or been pulled down by traction often need assistance to move up in bed.

IMPLEMENTATION

Preparation

Determine:

- Assistive devices that will be required.
- Encumbrances to movement such as an IV or a heavy cast on one leg.
- Medications the client is receiving, because certain medications may hamper movement or alertness of the client.
- Assistance required from other health care personnel.

Performance

1. Prior to performing the procedure, introduce self and verify the client's identity using agency protocol. Explain to the client what you are going to do, why it is necessary, and how he or she can participate. Listen to any suggestions made by the client or support people. Discuss how the results will be used in planning further care or treatments.
2. Perform hand hygiene and observe other appropriate infection control procedures.
3. Provide for client privacy.
4. Adjust the bed and the client's position.
   - Adjust the head of the bed to a flat position or as low as the client can tolerate. **Rationale:** *Moving the client upward against gravity requires more force and can cause back strain.*
   - Raise the bed to the height of your center of gravity.
   - Lock the wheels on the bed and raise the rail on the side of the bed opposite you.
   - Remove all pillows, then place one against the head of the bed. **Rationale:** *This pillow protects the client's head from inadvertent injury against the top of the bed during the upward move.*
5. Elicit the client's help in lessening your workload.
   - Ask the client to flex the hips and knees and position the feet so that they can be used effectively for pushing.

Rationale: *Flexing the hips and knees keeps the entire lower leg off the bed surface preventing friction during movement, and ensures use of the large muscle groups in the client's legs when pushing, thus increasing the force of movement.*

- Ask the client to
  a. Grasp the head of the bed with both hands and pull during the move

     or

  b. Raise the upper part of the body on the elbows and push with the hands and forearms during the move

     or

  c. Grasp the overhead trapeze with both hands and lift and pull during the move. **Rationale:** *Client assistance provides additional power to overcome inertia and friction during the move. These actions also keep the client's arms partially off the bed surface, reducing friction during movement, and make use of the large muscle groups of the client's arms to increase the force during movement.*

6. Position yourself appropriately, and move the client.
   - Face the direction of the movement, and then assume a broad stance with the foot nearest the bed behind the forward foot and weight on the forward foot. Lean your trunk forward from the hips. Flex hips, knees, and ankles.
   - Place your near arm under the client's thighs. ❶ **Rationale:** *This supports the heaviest part of the body (the buttocks).* Push down on the mattress with the far arm. **Rationale:** *The far arm acts as a lever during the move.*
   - Tighten your gluteal, abdominal, leg, and arm muscles and rock from the back leg to the front leg and back again. Then, shift your weight to the front leg as the client pushes with the heels and pulls with the arms so that the client moves toward the head of the bed.

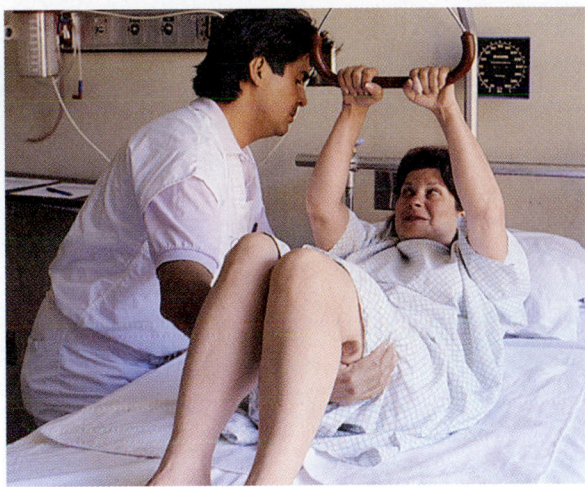

① Moving a client up in bed.

7. Ensure client comfort.
   • Elevate the head of the bed and provide appropriate support devices for the client's new position.
   • See the sections on positioning clients earlier in this chapter.

VARIATION: A CLIENT WHO HAS LIMITED STRENGTH OF THE UPPER EXTREMITIES

   • Assist the client to flex the hips and knees as in step 5 previously. Place the client's arms across the chest. **Rationale:** *This keeps the client off the bed surface and minimizes friction during movement.* Ask the client to flex the neck during the move and keep the head off the bed surface.

• Position yourself as in step 6 and place one arm under the client's back and shoulders and the other arm under the client's thighs. **Rationale:** *This placement of the arms distributes the client's weight and supports the heaviest part of the body (the buttocks).* Shift your weight as in step 6.

VARIATION: TWO NURSES USING A TURN SHEET

Two nurses can use a turn sheet to move a client up in bed. **Rationale:** *A turn sheet distributes the client's weight more evenly, decreases friction, and exerts a more even force on the client during the move. In addition, it prevents injury of the client's skin, because the friction created between two sheets when one is moved is less than that created by the client's body moving over the sheet.*

   • Place a drawsheet or a full sheet folded in half under the client, extending from the shoulders to the thighs. Each person rolls up or fanfolds the turn sheet close to the client's body on either side.
   • Both individuals grasp the sheet close to the shoulders and buttocks of the client. **Rationale:** *This draws the weight closer to the nurse's center of gravity and increases the nurse's balance and stability, permitting a smoother movement.* Follow the method of moving clients with limited upper extremity strength as described earlier.

8. Document all relevant information.
   Record:
   • Time and change of position moved from and position moved to.
   • Any signs of pressure areas.
   • Use of support devices.
   • Ability of client to assist in moving and turning.
   • Response of client to moving and turning (e.g., anxiety, discomfort, dizziness).

SKILL 31–2

TURNING A CLIENT TO THE LATERAL OR PRONE POSITION IN BED

PURPOSES
• Movement to the lateral (side-lying) position may be necessary when placing a bedpan beneath the client, when changing the client's bed linen, or when repositioning the client.

IMPLEMENTATION

Preparation
Determine:
• Assistive devices that will be required.
• Encumbrances to movement such as an IV or a heavy cast on one leg.
• Medications the client is receiving, because certain medications may hamper movement or alertness of the client.
• Assistance required from other health care personnel.

Performance
1. Prior to performing the procedure, introduce self and verify the client's identity using agency protocol. Explain to the client what you are going to do, why it is necessary, and how he or she can participate. Discuss how the results will be used in planning further care or treatments.

2. Perform hand hygiene and observe other appropriate infection control procedures.
3. Provide for client privacy.
4. Position yourself and the client appropriately before performing the move.
   • Move the client closer to the side of the bed opposite the side the client will face when turned. **Rationale:** *This ensures that the client will be positioned safely in the center of the bed after turning.* Use a pull sheet beneath the client's trunk and thighs to pull the client to the side of the bed. Roll up the sheet as close as possible to the client's body and pull the client to the side of the bed. Adjust the client's head and reposition the legs appropriately.
   • While standing on the side of the bed nearest the client, place the client's near arm across the chest. Abduct the

(continued)

client's far shoulder slightly from the side of the body and externally rotate the shoulder. **Rationale:** *Pulling the one arm forward facilitates the turning motion. Pulling the other arm away from the body and externally rotating the shoulder prevents that arm from being caught beneath the client's body during the roll.*

- Place the client's near ankle and foot across the far ankle and foot. **Rationale:** *This facilitates the turning motion. Making these preparations on the side of the bed closest to the client helps prevent unnecessary reaching.*

- Raise the side rail next to the client before going to the other side of the bed. **Rationale:** *This ensures that the client, who is close to the edge of the mattress, will not fall.*

- Position yourself on the side of the bed toward which the client will turn, directly in line with the client's waistline and as close to the bed as possible.

- Lean your trunk forward from the hips. Flex your hips, knees, and ankles. Assume a broad stance with one foot forward and the weight placed on this forward foot.

5. Pull or roll the client toward you to the lateral position.
   - Place one hand on the client's far hip and the other hand on the client's far shoulder. ❶ **Rationale:** *This position of the hands supports the client at the two heaviest parts of the body, providing greater control in movement during the roll.*

   - Tighten your gluteal, abdominal, leg, and arm muscles; rock backward, shifting your weight from the forward to the backward foot, and roll the client onto the side of the body to face you. **Rationale:** *Turning the client toward you promotes the client's sense of security.*

   - Position the client on his or her side with arms and legs positioned and supported properly (see Table 31–3).

VARIATION: TURNING THE CLIENT TO A PRONE POSITION

To turn a client to the prone position, follow the preceding steps, with two exceptions:

- Instead of abducting the far arm, keep the client's arm alongside the body for the client to roll over. **Rationale:** *Keeping the arm alongside the body prevents it from being pinned under the client when the client is rolled.*

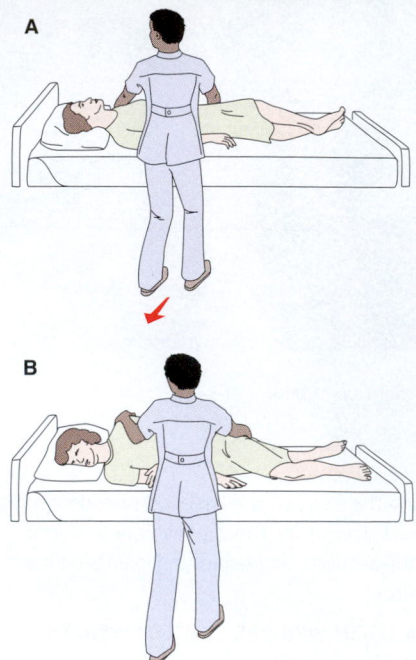

❶ Moving a client to a lateral position.

- Roll the client completely onto the abdomen. **Rationale:** *It is essential to move the client as close as possible to the edge of the bed before the turn so that the client will be lying on the center of the bed after rolling.* Never pull a client across the bed while the client is in the prone position. **Rationale:** *Doing so can injure a woman's breasts or a man's genitals.*

6. Document all relevant information.
   Record:
   - Time and change of position moved from and position moved to.
   - Any signs of pressure areas.
   - Use of support devices.
   - Ability of client to assist in moving and turning.
   - Response of client to moving and turning (e.g., anxiety, discomfort, dizziness).

PURPOSES

- **Logrolling** is a technique used to turn a client whose body must at all times be kept in straight alignment (like a log). An example is the client with a spinal injury. Considerable care

must be taken to prevent additional injury. This technique requires two nurses or, if the client is large, three nurses. For the client who has a cervical injury, one nurse must maintain the client's head and neck alignment.

IMPLEMENTATION

Preparation

Determine:
- Assistive devices that will be required.
- Encumbrances to movement such as an IV or a heavy cast on one leg.

- Medications the client is receiving, because certain medications may hamper movement or alertness of the client.
- Assistance required from other health care personnel.

Performance

1. Prior to performing the procedure, introduce self and verify the client's identity using agency protocol. Explain to the

client what you are going to do, why it is necessary, and how he or she can participate.

2. Perform hand hygiene and observe other appropriate infection control procedures.

3. Provide for client privacy.

4. Position yourselves and the client appropriately before the move.
   - Stand on the same side of the bed, and assume a broad stance with one foot ahead of the other.
   - Place the client's arms across the chest. **Rationale:** *Doing so ensures that the arms will not be injured or become trapped under the body when the body is turned.*
   - Lean your trunk, and flex your hips, knees, and ankles.
   - Place your arms under the client. **Rationale:** *Each staff member then has a major weight area of the client centered between the arms.*
   - Tighten your gluteal, abdominal, leg, and arm muscles.

5. Pull the client to the side of the bed.
   - One nurse counts: One, two, three, go. Then, at the same time, all staff members pull the client to the side of the bed by shifting their weight to the back foot. **Rationale:** *Moving the client in unison maintains the client's body alignment.*
   - Elevate the side rail on this side of the bed. **Rationale:** *This prevents the client from falling while lying so close to the edge of the bed.*

6. Move to the other side of the bed, and place supportive devices for the client when turned.
   - Place a pillow where it will support the client's head after the turn. **Rationale:** *The pillow prevents lateral flexion of the neck and ensures alignment of the cervical spine.*
   - Place one or two pillows between the client's legs to support the upper leg when the client is turned. **Rationale:** *This pillow prevents adduction of the upper leg and keeps the legs parallel and aligned.*

7. Roll and position the client in proper alignment.
   - All nurses flex their hips, knees, and ankles and assume a broad stance with one foot forward.
   - All nurses reach over the client and place hands as shown in. ❶ **Rationale:** *Doing so centers a major weight area of the client between each nurse's arms.*
   - One nurse counts: One, two, three, go. Then, at the same time, all nurses roll the client to a lateral position.
   - Support the client's head, back, and upper and lower extremities with pillows.
   - Raise the side rails and place the call bell within the client's reach.

VARIATION: USING A TURN OR LIFT SHEET
   - Use a turn sheet to facilitate logrolling. First, stand with another nurse on the same side of the bed. Assume a broad stance with one foot forward, and grasp half of

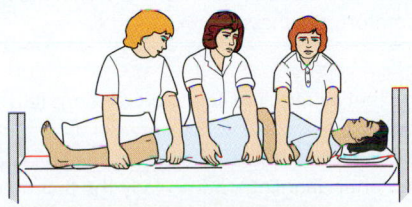

❶ Correct hand placement for logrolling a client.

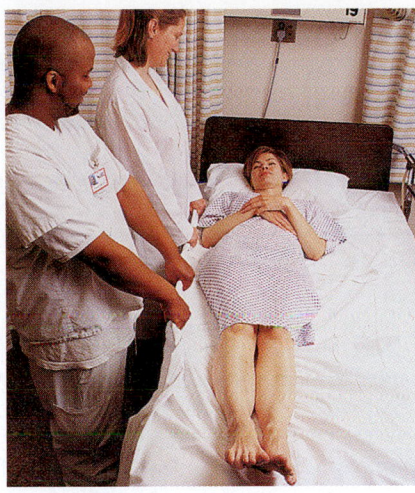

❷ Using a turn sheet, the nurses pull the sheet with the client on it to the edge of the bed.

the fanfolded or rolled edge of the turn sheet. On a signal, pull the client toward both of you. ❷
   - Before turning the client, place pillow supports for the head and legs, as described in step 6. This helps maintain the client's alignment when turning. Then, go to the other side of the bed (farthest from the client), and assume a stable stance. Reaching over the client, grasp the far edges of the turn sheet, and roll the client toward you. ❸ The second nurse (behind the client) helps turn the client and provides pillow supports to ensure good alignment in the lateral position.

8. Document all relevant information.
   Record:
   - Time and change of position moved from and position moved to.
   - Any signs of pressure areas.
   - Use of support devices.
   - Ability of client to assist in moving and turning.
   - Response of client to moving and turning (e.g., anxiety, discomfort, dizziness).

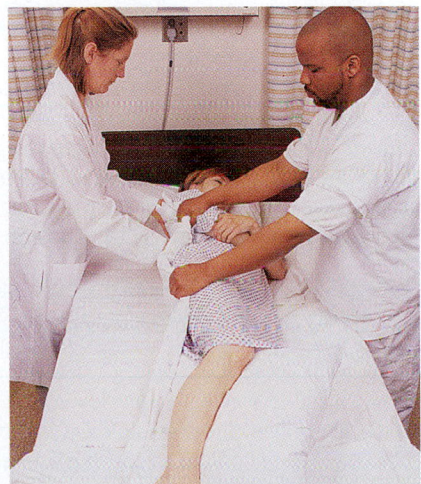

❸ The nurse on the right uses the far edge of the sheet to roll the client toward him; the nurse on the left remains behind the client and assists with turning.

SKILL 31–4

ASSISTING THE CLIENT TO SIT ON THE SIDE OF THE BED (DANGLING)

PURPOSES
- The client assumes a sitting position on the edge of the bed before walking, moving to a chair or wheelchair, eating, or performing other activities.

IMPLEMENTATION

Preparation
Determine:
- Assistive devices that will be required.
- Encumbrances to movement such as an IV or a heavy cast on one leg.
- Medications the client is receiving, because certain medications may hamper movement or alertness of the client.
- Assistance required from other health care personnel.

Performance
1. Prior to performing the procedure, introduce self and verify the client's identity using agency protocol. Explain to the client what you are going to do, why it is necessary, and how he or she can participate.
2. Perform hand hygiene and observe other appropriate infection control procedures.
3. Provide for client privacy.
4. Position yourself and the client appropriately before performing the move.
   - Assist the client to a lateral position facing you.
   - Raise the head of the bed slowly to its highest position. **Rationale:** *This decreases the distance that the client needs to move to sit up on the side of the bed.*
   - Position the client's feet and lower legs at the edge of the bed. **Rationale:** *This enables the client's feet to move easily off the bed during the movement, and the client is aided by gravity into a sitting position.*
   - Stand beside the client's hips and face the far corner of the bottom of the bed (the angle in which movement will occur). Assume a broad stance, placing the foot nearest the client forward. Lean your trunk forward from the hips. Flex your hips, knees, and ankles. ❶
5. Move the client to a sitting position.
   - Place one arm around the client's shoulders and the other arm beneath both of the client's thighs near the knees. **Rationale:** *Supporting the client's shoulders prevents the client from falling backward during the movement. Supporting the client's thighs reduces friction of the thighs against the bed surface during the move and increases the force of the movement.*
   - Tighten your gluteal, abdominal, leg, and arm muscles.
   - Lift the client's thighs slightly. **Rationale:** *This reduces the friction of the client's thighs and the nurse's arm against the bed surface.*

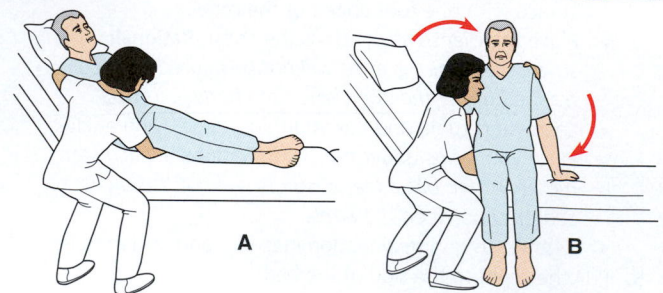

❶ Assisting a client to a sitting position on the edge of the bed.

- Pivot on the balls of your feet in the desired direction facing the foot of the bed while pulling the client's feet and legs off the bed (Figure ❶, *B*). **Rationale:** *Pivoting prevents twisting of the nurse's spine. The weight of the client's legs swinging downward increases downward movement of the lower body and helps make the client's upper body vertical.*
- Keep supporting the client until the client is well balanced and comfortable. **Rationale:** *This movement may cause some clients to faint.*
- Assess vital signs (e.g., pulse, respirations, and blood pressure) as indicated by the client's health status.

VARIATION: TEACHING A CLIENT HOW TO SIT ON THE SIDE OF THE BED INDEPENDENTLY

A client who has had recent abdominal surgery or who is weak may have too much abdominal pain or too little strength to sit straight up in bed. This person can be taught to assume a dangle position without assistance. Instruct the client to:
- Roll to the side and lift the far leg over the near leg.
- Grasp the mattress edge with the lower arm and push the fist of the upper arm into the mattress.
- Push up with the arms as the heels and legs slide over the mattress edge.
- Maintain the sitting position by pushing both fists into the mattress behind and to the sides of the buttocks.
6. Document all relevant information.
   Record:
   - Ability of client to assist in moving and turning.
   - Response of client to moving and turning (e.g., anxiety, discomfort, dizziness).

EVALUATION
- Check the skin integrity of the pressure areas from the previous position. Relate findings to previous assessment data if available. Conduct follow-up assessment for previous and/or new skin breakdown areas.
- Check for proper alignment after the position change. Do a visual check and ask the client for a comfort assessment.
- Determine that all required safety precautions (e.g., side rails) are in place.
- Determine client's tolerance of the activity (e.g., vital signs before and after dangling), particularly the first time the client changes position.
- Report significant changes to the primary care practitioner.

Positioning, Moving, and Turning Clients

Infants
- Position infants on their back for sleep, even after feeding. There is little risk of regurgitation and choking, and the rate of sudden infant death syndrome (SIDS) is significantly lower in infants who sleep on their backs.
- The skin of newborns can be fragile and may be abraded or torn (sheared) if the infant is pulled across a bed.

Children
- Carefully inspect the dependent skin surfaces of all infants and children confined to bed at least three times in each 24-hour period.

Older Adults
- In clients who have had cerebrovascular accidents (strokes), there is a risk of shoulder displacement on the paralyzed side from improper moving or repositioning techniques. Use care when moving, positioning in bed, and transferring. Pillows or foam devices are helpful to support the affected arm and shoulder and prevent injury.
- Decreased subcutaneous fat and thinning of the skin place older adults at risk for skin breakdown. Repositioning approximately every 2 hours (more or less, depending on the unique needs of the individual client) helps reduce pressure on bony prominences and avoid tissue trauma.

Transferring Clients

Many clients require some assistance in transferring between bed and chair or wheelchair, between wheelchair and toilet, and between bed and stretcher. Before transferring any client, however, the nurse must determine the client's physical and mental capabilities to participate in the transfer technique. In addition, the nurse must analyze and organize the activity. General guidelines for transfer techniques include these:

- Plan what to do and how to do it. Determine the space in which the transfer is maneuvered (bathrooms, for instance, are usually cramped); the number of assistants (one or two) needed to accomplish the transfer safely; the skill and strength of the nurse(s); and the client's capabilities.
- Obtain essential equipment before starting, and check its function.
- Remove obstacles from the area used for the transfer.
- Explain the transfer to the client, including what the client should do.
- Explain the transfer to the nursing personnel who are helping; specify who will give directions (one person needs to be in charge).
- Always support or hold the client rather than the equipment and ensure the client's safety and dignity.
- During the transfer, explain step by step what the client should do, for example, "Move your right foot forward."
- Make a written plan of the transfer, including the client's tolerance.

Because wheelchairs and stretchers are unstable, they can predispose the client to falls and injury. Guidelines for the safe use of wheelchairs and stretchers are shown in the accompanying Practice Guidelines.

Transfer (walking) belts provide the greatest safety. The nurse grasps the belt to control movement of the client during the transfer. Hospitals and nursing homes should require that personnel use the transfer belt to ambulate or move clients. See Skill 31–5 for transferring a client between a bed and a chair, and Skill 31–6 for transferring a client between a bed and a stretcher. The Evaluation section at the end of Skill 31–6 also applies to Skill 31–5.

SKILL 31–5

TRANSFERRING BETWEEN BED AND CHAIR

PURPOSES
- A client may need to be transferred between the bed and a wheelchair or chair, the bed and the commode, or a wheelchair and the toilet. There are numerous variations in the technique. Which variation the nurse selects depends on factors related to the client, the environment, and the health care provider that are assessed prior to beginning the transfer.

ASSESSMENT
Before transferring a client, assess the following:
- The client's body size
- Ability to follow instructions
- Activity tolerance
- Muscle strength
- Joint mobility
- Presence of paralysis
- Level of comfort
- Presence of orthostatic hypotension
- The technique with which the client is familiar
- The space in which the transfer will need to be maneuvered (bathrooms, for example, are usually cramped)
- The number of assistants (one or two) needed to accomplish the transfer safely
- The skill and strength of the nurse(s)

(continued)

SKILL 31–5

TRANSFERRING BETWEEN BED AND CHAIR *(continued)*

PLANNING

Review the client record to determine if previous nurses have recorded information about the client's ability to transfer. Implement pain-relief measures so that they are effective when the transfer begins.

Delegation

The skill of transferring a client can be delegated to UAP who have demonstrated safe transfer technique for the involved client. It is important for the nurse to assess the client's capabilities and communicate specific information about what the UAP should report back to the nurse.

EQUIPMENT

- Robe or appropriate clothing
- Slippers or shoes with nonskid soles
- Transfer (walking) belt
- Chair, commode, wheelchair, or stretcher as appropriate to client need
- Sliding board

IMPLEMENTATION

Preparation

- Plan what to do and how to do it.
- Obtain essential equipment before starting (e.g., transfer belt, wheelchair), and check that it is functioning correctly.
- Remove obstacles from the area used for the transfer.

Performance

1. Prior to performing the procedure, introduce self and verify the client's identity using agency protocol. Explain the transfer process to the client. During the transfer, explain step by step what the client should do, for example, "Move your right foot forward."
2. Perform hand hygiene and observe other appropriate infection control procedures.
3. Provide for client privacy.
4. Position the equipment appropriately.
   - Lower the bed to its lowest position so that the client's feet will rest flat on the floor. Lock the wheels of the bed.
   - Place the wheelchair parallel to the bed as close to the bed as possible. ❶ Put the wheelchair on the side of the bed that allows the client to move toward his or her stronger side. Lock the wheels of the wheelchair and raise the footplate.

❶ The wheelchair is placed parallel to the bed as close to the bed as possible. Note that placement of the nurse's feet mirrors that of the client's feet.

5. Prepare and assess the client.
   - Assist the client to a sitting position on the side of the bed (see Skill 31–4).
   - Assess the client for orthostatic hypotension before moving the client from the bed.
   - Assist the client in putting on a bathrobe and nonskid slippers or shoes.
   - Place a transfer belt snugly around the client's waist. Check to be certain that the belt is securely fastened.
6. Give explicit instructions to the client.
   Ask the client to:
   - Move forward and sit on the edge of the bed. **Rationale:** *This brings the client's center of gravity closer to the nurse's.*
   - Lean forward slightly from the hips. **Rationale:** *This brings the client's center of gravity more directly over the base of support and positions the head and trunk in the direction of the movement.*
   - Place the foot of the stronger leg beneath the edge of the bed and put the other foot forward. **Rationale:** *In this way, the client can use the stronger leg muscles to stand and power the movement. A broader base of support makes the client more stable during the transfer.*
   - Place the client's hands on the bed surface or on your shoulders so that the client can push while standing. **Rationale:** *This provides additional force for the movement and reduces the potential for strain on the nurse's back. The client should not grasp your neck for support.* **Rationale:** *Doing so can injure the nurse.*
7. Position yourself correctly.
   - Stand directly in front of the client. Lean the trunk forward from the hips. Flex the hips, knees, and ankles. Assume a broad stance, placing one foot forward and one back. Mirror the placement of the client's feet, if possible. **Rationale:** *This helps prevent loss of balance during the transfer.*
   - Encircle the client's waist with your arms, and grasp the transfer belt at the client's back with thumbs pointing downward. **Rationale:** *The belt provides a secure handle for holding on to the client and controlling the movement. Downward placement of the thumbs prevents potential wrist injury as the nurse lifts. By supporting the client in this manner, you keep the client from tilting backward during the transfer.*
   - Tighten your gluteal, abdominal, leg, and arm muscles.

8. Assist the client to stand, and then move together toward the wheelchair.
   - On the count of three, ask the client to push with the back foot, rock to the forward foot, and extend (straighten) the joints of the lower extremities. Push or pull up with the hands, while pushing with the forward foot, rock to the back foot, extend the joints of the lower extremities, and pull the client (directly toward your center of gravity) into a standing position.
   - Support the client in an upright standing position for a few moments. **Rationale:** *This allows the nurse and the client to extend the joints and provides the nurse with an opportunity to ensure that the client is stable before moving away from the bed.*
   - Together, pivot or take a few steps toward the wheelchair.
9. Assist the client to sit.
   - Ask the client to:
     a. Back up to the wheelchair and place the legs against the seat. **Rationale:** *Having the client place the legs against the wheelchair seat minimizes the risk of the client falling when sitting down.*
     b. Place the foot of the stronger leg slightly behind the other. **Rationale:** *This supports body weight during the movement.*
     c. Keep the other foot forward. **Rationale:** *This provides a broad base of support.*
     d. Place both hands on the wheelchair arms or on your shoulders. **Rationale:** *This increases stability and lessens the strain on the nurse.*
   - Stand directly in front of the client. Place one foot forward and one back.
   - Tighten your grasp on the transfer belt, and tighten your gluteal, abdominal, leg, and arm muscles.
   - On the count of three, have the client shift the body weight by rocking to the back foot. Lower the body onto the edge of the wheelchair seat by flexing the joints of the legs and arms. Place some body weight on the arms, while shifting your body weight by stepping back with the forward foot and pivoting toward the chair while lowering the client onto the wheelchair seat.
10. Ensure client safety.
    - Ask the client to push back into the wheelchair seat. **Rationale:** *Sitting well back on the seat provides a broader base of support and greater stability and minimizes the risk of falling from the wheelchair. A wheelchair can topple forward when the client sits on the edge of the seat and leans far forward.*
    - Lower the footplates, and place the client's feet on them.
    - Apply a seat belt as required.

VARIATION: ANGLING THE WHEELCHAIR

For clients who have difficulty walking, place the wheelchair at a 45-degree angle to the bed. **Rationale:** *This enables the client to pivot into the chair and lessens the amount of body rotation required.*

VARIATION: TRANSFERRING WITHOUT A BELT

- For clients who need minimal assistance, place the hands against the sides of the client's chest (not at the axillae) during the transfer. For clients who require more assistance, reach through the client's axillae and place the hands on the client's scapulae during the transfer. Avoid placing hands or pressure on the axillae, especially for clients who have upper extremity paralysis or paresis.
- Follow the steps described previously.

VARIATION: TRANSFERRING WITH A BELT AND TWO NURSES

- When the client is able to stand, position yourselves on both sides of the client, facing the same direction as the client. Flex your hips, knees, and ankle. Grasp the client's transfer belt with the hand closest to the client, and with the other hand support the client's elbows.
- Coordinating your efforts, all three of you stand simultaneously, pivot, and move to the wheelchair. Reverse the process to lower the client onto the wheelchair seat.

VARIATION: TRANSFERRING A CLIENT WITH AN INJURED LOWER EXTREMITY

When the client has an injured lower extremity, movement should always occur toward the client's unaffected (strong) side. For example, if the client's right leg is injured and the client is sitting on the edge of the bed preparing to transfer to a wheelchair, position the wheelchair on the client's left side. In this way, the client can use the unaffected leg most effectively and safely.

VARIATION: USING A SLIDING BOARD

- For clients who cannot stand, use a sliding board to help them move without nursing assistance. This method not only promotes clients' sense of independence but also preserves your energy.
11. Document relevant information:
    - Client's ability to bear weight and pivot
    - Number of staff needed for transfer
    - Length of time up in chair
    - Client response to transfer and being up in chair or wheelchair

TRANSFERRING BETWEEN BED AND STRETCHER

PURPOSES

- The stretcher, or gurney, is used to transfer supine clients from one location to another. Whenever the client is capable of accomplishing the transfer from bed to stretcher independently, either by lifting onto it or by rolling onto it, the client should be encouraged to do so. If the client cannot move onto the stretcher independently, at least two nurses are needed to assist with the transfer; more are needed if the client is totally helpless or is heavy.

ASSESSMENT

Before transferring a client, assess the following:
- The client's body size
- Ability to follow instructions
- Activity tolerance
- Level of comfort
- The space in which the transfer is maneuvered
- The number of assistants (one or two others) needed to accomplish the transfer safely
- The skill and strength of the nurses

PLANNING

Review the client record to determine if previous nurses have recorded information about how the client tolerated similar transfers. If indicated, implement pain-relief measures so that they are effective when the transfer begins.

EQUIPMENT

- Stretcher
- Optional: sliding board

Delegation

The skill of transferring a client can be delegated to UAP who have demonstrated good body mechanics and safe transfer technique for the involved client. It is important for the nurse to assess the client's capabilities and communicate specific information about what the UAP should report to the nurse.

IMPLEMENTATION

Preparation

Obtain the necessary equipment and nursing personnel to assist in the transfer.

Performance

1. Prior to performing the procedure, introduce self and verify the client's identity using agency protocol. Explain to the client what you are going to do, why it is necessary, and how he or she can participate. Explain the transfer to the nursing personnel who are helping and specify who will give directions (one person needs to be in charge).
2. Perform hand hygiene and observe other appropriate infection control procedures.
3. Provide for client privacy.
4. Adjust the client's bed in preparation for the transfer.
   - Lower the head of the bed until it is flat or as low as the client can tolerate.
   - Raise the bed so that it is slightly higher than the surface of the stretcher. **Rationale:** *It is easier for the client to move down a slant.*
   - Ensure that the wheels on the bed are locked.
   - Pull the drawsheet out from both sides of the bed.
5. Move the client to the edge of the bed and position the stretcher.
   - Roll the drawsheet as close to the client's side as possible.
   - Pull the client to the edge of the bed and cover the client with a sheet or bath blanket to maintain comfort.
   - Place the stretcher parallel to the bed next to the client and lock the stretcher wheels.
   - Fill the gap that exists between the bed and the stretcher loosely with the bath blankets (optional).
6. Transfer the client securely to the stretcher.
   - In unison with the other staff members, press your body tightly against the stretcher. **Rationale:** *This prevents the stretcher from moving.*
   - Roll the pull sheet tightly against the client. **Rationale:** *This achieves better control over client movement.*
   - Flex your hips and pull the client on the pull sheet in unison directly toward you and onto the stretcher. **Rationale:** *Pulling downward requires less force than pulling along a flat surface.*
   - Ask the client to flex the neck during the move, if possible, and place the arms across the chest. **Rationale:** *This prevents injury to these body parts.*
7. Ensure client comfort and safety.
   - Make the client comfortable, unlock the stretcher wheels, and move the stretcher away from the bed.
   - Immediately raise the stretcher side rails and/or fasten the safety straps across the client. **Rationale:** *Because the stretcher is high and narrow, the client is in danger of falling unless these safety precautions are taken.*

VARIATION: USING A TRANSFER BOARD

The transfer board is a lacquered or smooth polyethylene board measuring 45 to 55 cm (18 to 22 in.) by 182 cm (72 in.) with handholds along its edges. Transfer mattresses are also available, as are mechanical assistive devices. It is imperative to have enough people assisting with the transfer to prevent injury to staff as well as clients. Turn the client to a lateral position away from you, position the board close to the client's back, and roll the client onto the board. Pull the client and board across the bed to the stretcher. Safety belts may be placed over the chest, abdomen, and legs.

8. Document relevant information:
   • Equipment used

- • Number of people needed for transfer
- • Destination if reason for transfer is transport from one location to another

EVALUATION

- • Compare client capabilities such as weight-bearing, pivoting ability, and strength and control to previous transfers.
- • Report any significant deviations from normal to the primary care practitioner.

- • NOTE USE OF APPROPRIATE SAFETY MEASURES (E.G.,TRANSFER BELT, LOCKING WHEELS OF BED, AND WHEELCHAIR) BY UAP DURING TRANSFER PROCESS.

PRACTICE GUIDELINES   **Wheelchair Safety**

- • Always lock the brakes on both wheels of the wheelchair when the client transfers in or out of it.
- • Raise the footplates before transferring the client into the wheelchair.
- • Lower the footplates after the transfer, and place the client's feet on them.
- • Ensure the client is positioned well back in the seat of the wheelchair.
- • Use seat belts that fasten behind the wheelchair to protect confused clients from falls. *Note:* Seat belts are a form of restraint and must be used in accordance with policies and procedures that apply to the use of restraints (see Chapter 21 ∞).

- • Back the wheelchair into or out of an elevator, rear large wheels first.
- • Place your body between the wheelchair and the bottom of an incline.

CLINICAL ALERT

Air, foam, and gel cushions that distribute weight evenly (not doughnut-type cushions) are essential for clients confined to a wheelchair and must be checked frequently to ensure they are intact. Strict continence management is also important for preventing skin breakdown. Maintaining tire pressure will prevent added resistance and energy expenditure. Periodically monitor the client's upper extremities for pain and overuse syndromes.

PRACTICE GUIDELINES   **Safe Use of Stretchers**

- • Lock the wheels of the bed and stretcher before the client transfers in or out of them.
- • Fasten safety straps across the client on a stretcher, and raise the side rails.
- • Never leave a client unattended on a stretcher unless the wheels are locked and the side rails are raised on both sides and/or the safety straps are securely fastened across the client.
- • Always push a stretcher from the end where the client's head is positioned. This position protects the client's head in the event of a collision.

- • If the stretcher has two swivel wheels and two stationary wheels:
  a. Always position the client's head at the end with the stationary wheels and
  b. Push the stretcher from the end with the stationary wheels. The stretcher is maneuvered more easily when pushed from this end.
- • Maneuver the stretcher when entering the elevator so that the client's head goes in first.

LIFESPAN CONSIDERATIONS   Transferring Clients

Infants

- The infant who is lying down, on the side or supine, can be placed in either a bassinet or crib for transport. If the bassinet has a bottom shelf, it can be used for carrying the IV pump or monitor.

Children

- The toddler should be transported in a high-top crib with the side rails up and the protective top in place. Stretchers should not be used because the mobile toddler may roll or fall off.

Older Adults

- Since conditions of older adults can change from day to day, always assess the situation to ensure that you have the right equipment and enough people to assist when transferring a client.
- Use special caution with older clients to prevent skin tears or bruising during a transfer or when using a hydraulic lift.
- Write the method used to transfer each client—equipment used, best position, and number of people needed to assist in transfer. This can be part of the care plan and also be available in the client's room as a guide to all personnel caring for the client.
- Avoid sudden position changes. They can cause orthostatic hypotension and increase the risk of fainting and falls.

Using a Hydraulic Lift

Hydraulic lifts, such as the Hoyer lift, are an example of assistive equipment to take the place of manual lifts and transfers. The lift can be used in transferring the client between the bed and a wheelchair, the bed and the bathtub, and the bed and a stretcher. The Hoyer lift consists of a base on casters, a hydraulic mechanical pump, a mast boom, and a sling. The sling may consist of a one-piece or two-piece canvas seat. The one-piece seat stretches from the client's head to the knees. The two-piece seat has one canvas strap to support the client's buttocks and thighs and a second strap extending up to the axillae to support the back. It is important to be familiar with the model used and the practices that accompany use. Before using the lift, the nurse ensures that it is in working order and that the hooks, chains, straps, and canvas seat are in good repair. Most agencies recommend that two nurses operate a lift. Check agency policy. See Figure 31–5 for an example of the use of a hydraulic lift.

Providing ROM Exercises

When people are ill, they may need to perform ROM exercises until they can regain their normal activity levels. **Active ROM exercises** are isotonic exercises in which the client moves each joint in the body through its complete range of movement, maximally stretching all muscle groups within each plane over the joint. These exercises maintain or increase muscle strength and endurance and help to maintain cardiorespiratory function in an immobilized client. They also prevent deterioration of joint capsules, ankylosis, and contractures.

Full ROM does not occur spontaneously in the immobilized individual who independently achieves ADLs, moves about in bed, transfers between bed and wheelchair or chair, or ambulates a short distance, because only a few muscle groups are maximally stretched during these activities. Although the client may successfully achieve some active ROM movements of the upper extremities while combing the hair, bathing, and dressing, the immobilized client is very unlikely to achieve any active ROM movements of the lower extremities when these are not used in the normal functions of standing and walking about. For this reason, most clients who use a wheelchair and many ambulatory clients need active ROM exercises until they regain their normal activity levels.

At first, the nurse may need to teach the client to perform the needed ROM exercises; eventually, the client may be able to accomplish these independently. Instructions for the client performing active ROM exercises are shown in the accompanying Client Teaching feature.

During **passive ROM exercises**, another person moves each of the client's joints through its complete range of movement, maximally stretching all muscle groups within each plane over each joint. Because the client does not contract the muscles, passive ROM exercises are of no value in maintaining muscle strength but are useful in maintaining joint flexibility. For this reason, passive ROM exercises should be performed only when the client is unable to accomplish the movements actively.

Passive ROM exercises should be accomplished for each movement of the arms, legs, and neck that the client is unable to achieve actively. As with active ROM exercises, passive ROM exercises should be accomplished to the point of slight resistance, but not beyond, and never to the point of discomfort. The movements should be systematic, and the same sequence should be followed during each exercise session. Each exercise should consist of three repetitions, and the series of exercises should be done twice daily. Performing one series of exercises along with the bath is helpful. Passive ROM exercises are accomplished most effectively when the client lies supine in bed. General guidelines for providing passive exercises are shown in the accompanying Practice Guidelines.

During active-assistive ROM exercises, the client uses a stronger, opposite arm or leg to move each of the joints of a limb incapable of active motion. The client learns to sup-

Active ROM Exercises

- Perform each ROM exercise as taught to the point of slight resistance, but not beyond, and never to the point of discomfort.
- Perform the movements systematically, using the same sequence during each session.
- Perform each exercise three times.
- Perform each series of exercises twice daily.

Older Adults

- For older adults, it is not essential to achieve full range of motion in all joints. Instead, emphasize achieving a sufficient range of motion to carry out ADLs, such as walking, dressing, combing hair, showering, and preparing a meal.

port and move the weak arm or leg with the strong arm or leg as far as possible. Then the nurse continues the movement passively to its maximal degree. This activity increases active movement on the strong side of the client's body and maintains joint flexibility on the weak side. Such exercise is especially useful for clients who have had a stroke and are hemiplegic.

CLINICAL ALERT

Clients who require passive ROM exercises after a disability should have a goal of progressing to active-assistive ROM exercises and, finally, to active ROM exercises.

PRACTICE GUIDELINES **Providing Passive ROM Exercises**

- Ensure that the client understands the reason for doing ROM exercises.
- If there is a possibility of hand swelling, make sure rings are removed.
- Clothe the client in a loose gown, and cover the body with a bath blanket.
- Use correct body mechanics when providing ROM exercise to avoid muscle strain or injury to both yourself and the client.
- Position the bed at an appropriate height.
- Expose only the limb being exercised to avoid embarrassing the client.
- Support the client's limbs above and below the joint as needed to prevent muscle strain or injury. This may also be done by cupping joints in the palm of your hand or cradling limbs along your forearm. If a joint is painful (e.g., arthritic), support the limb in the muscular areas above and below the joint.
- Use a firm, comfortable grip when handling the limb.
- Move the body parts smoothly, slowly, and rhythmically. Jerky movements cause discomfort and, possibly, injury. Fast movements can cause spasticity or rigidity.

- Avoid moving or forcing a body part beyond the existing range of motion. Muscle strain, pain, and injury can result. This is particularly important for people with flaccid paralysis, whose muscles can be stretched and joints dislocated without their awareness.
- If muscle spasticity occurs during movement, stop the movement temporarily, but continue to apply slow, gentle pressure on the part until the muscle relaxes; then proceed with the motion.
- If a contracture is present, apply slow firm pressure, without causing pain, to stretch the muscle fibers.
- If rigidity occurs, apply pressure against the rigidity, and continue the exercise slowly.
- Teach client's caregiver the purposes and technique of performing passive ROM at home if appropriate.
- Avoid hypertension of joints in older adults if joints are arthritic.
- Use the exercises as an opportunity to also assess skin condition.

Ambulating Clients

Ambulation (the act of walking) is a function that most people take for granted. However, when people are ill they are often confined to bed and are thus nonambulatory. The longer clients are in bed, the more difficulty they have walking.

Even 1 or 2 days of bed rest can make a person feel weak, unsteady, and shaky when first getting out of bed. A client who has had surgery, is an older adult, or has been immobilized for a longer time will feel more pronounced weakness. The potential problems of immobility are far less likely to occur when clients become ambulatory as soon as possible. The nurse can assist clients to prepare for ambulation by helping them become as independent as possible while in bed. Nurses should encourage clients to perform ADLs, maintain good body alignment, and carry out active ROM exercises to the maximum degree possible yet within the limitations imposed by their illness and recovery program.

PREAMBULATORY EXERCISES Clients who have been in bed for long periods often need a plan of muscle tone exercises to strengthen the muscles used for walking before attempting to walk. One of the most important muscle groups is the quadriceps femoris, which extends the knee and flexes the thigh. This group is also important for elevating the legs. To strengthen these muscles, the client consciously tenses them, drawing the kneecap upward and inward. The client pushes the popliteal space of the knee against the bed surface, relaxing the heels on the bed surface. On the count of 1, the muscles are tensed; they are held during the counts of 2, 3, 4; and they are relaxed at the count of 5. The exercise should be done within the client's tolerance. Carried out several times an hour during waking hours, this simple exercise significantly strengthens the muscles used for walking.

ASSISTING CLIENTS TO AMBULATE Clients who have been immobilized for even a few days may require assistance with ambulation. The amount of assistance will depend on the client's condition, including age, health status, and length of inactivity. Assistance may mean walking alongside the client while providing physical support (see Skill 31–7) or providing instruction to the client about the use of assistive devices such as a cane, walker, or crutches.

Some clients experience postural (orthostatic) hypotension on assuming a vertical position from a lying position and may need information about ways to control this problem (see Client Teaching). The client may exhibit some or all of the following symptoms: pallor, diaphoresis, nausea, tachycardia, and dizziness. If any of these are present, the client should be assisted to a supine position in bed and closely assessed.

SKILL 31–7

ASSISTING THE CLIENT TO AMBULATE

PURPOSE
- To provide a safe condition for the client to walk with whatever support is needed.

ASSESSMENT
Assess the following:
- Length of time in bed and time up previously
- Baseline vital signs
- Range of motion of joints needed for ambulating (e.g., hips, knees, ankles)
- Muscle strength of lower extremities
- Need for ambulation aids (e.g., cane, walker, crutches)

- Client's intake of medications (e.g., narcotics, sedatives, tranquilizers, and antihistamines) that may cause drowsiness, dizziness, weakness, and orthostatic hypotension and seriously hinder the client's ability to walk safely
- Presence of joint inflammation, fractures, muscle weakness, or other conditions that impair physical mobility
- Ability to understand directions
- Level of comfort

PLANNING
Implement pain-relief measures so that they are effective when the transfer begins.

The amount of assistance needed while ambulating will depend on the client's condition, for example, age, health status, length of inactivity, and emotional readiness. Review any previous experiences with ambulation and the success of such efforts. Plan the length of the walk with the client, in light of the nursing or primary care practitioner's orders. Be prepared to shorten the walk according to the person's activity tolerance.

> **Delegation**
> Ambulation of clients is frequently delegated to UAP. However, the nurse should conduct an initial assessment of the client's abilities in order to direct other personnel in providing appropriate assistance. Any unusual events that arise from assisting the client in ambulation must be validated and interpreted by the nurse.

EQUIPMENT
- Transfer belt if the client is known to be unsteady
- Wheelchair for following client, or chairs along the route if the client needs to rest

---

IMPLEMENTATION
Preparation
Be certain that others are available to assist you if needed. Also, plan the route of ambulation that has the fewest hazards.

Performance
1. Prior to performing the procedure, introduce self and verify the client's identity using agency protocol. Explain to the client how you are going to assist, why ambulation is necessary, and how he or she can participate. Discuss how this activity relates to the overall plan of care.
2. Perform hand hygiene and observe appropriate infection control procedures.
3. Ensure that the client is appropriately dressed to walk and has shoes or slippers with nonskid soles.
4. Prepare the client for ambulation.
   - Have client sit up in bed for at least 1 minute prior to preparing to dangle legs.
   - Apply elastic (antiemboli) stockings as required.
   - Assist the client to sit on the edge of the bed and allow dangling for at least 1 minute.
   - Assess the client carefully for signs and symptoms of orthostatic hypotension (dizziness, light-headedness, or a sudden increase in heart rate) prior to leaving the bedside.

   - Assist the client to stand by the side of the bed for at least 1 minute or until he or she feels secure.
5. Ensure client safety while assisting the client to ambulate.
   - Encourage the client to ambulate independently if he or she is able, but walk beside the client's weak side, if appropriate.
   - Remain physically close to the client in case assistance is needed at any point.
   - Use a transfer or walking belt if the client is slightly weak and unstable. Make sure the belt is pulled snugly around the client's waist and fastened securely. Grasp the belt at the client's back, and walk behind and slightly to one side of the client. ❶
   - If it is the client's first time out of bed following surgery, injury, or an extended period of immobility, or if the client is quite weak or unstable, have an assistant follow you and the client with a wheelchair in the event that it is needed quickly.
   - If the client is moderately weak and unstable, walk on the client's weaker side and interlock your forearm with the client's closest forearm. Encourage the client to press the forearm against your hip or waist for stability if desired. In addition, have the client wear a transfer or walking belt. **Rationale:** *You can quickly grab the belt and prevent a fall if the client feels faint.*

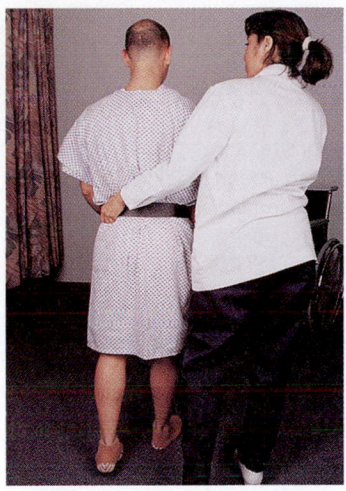

❶ Using a transfer (walking) belt to support the client.

- If the client is very weak and unstable, place your near arm around the client's waist, and with your other arm support the client's near arm at the elbow. Walk on the client's stronger side. Again, have the client wear a transfer or walking belt in case of an emergency. Encourage the client to assume a normal walking stance and gait as much as possible.

6. Protect the client who begins to fall while ambulating.
   - If a client begins to experience the signs and symptoms of orthostatic hypotension or extreme weakness, quickly assist the client into a nearby wheelchair or other chair, and help the client to lower the head between the knees.
   - Stay with the client. **Rationale:** *A client who faints while in this position could fall head first out of the chair.*
   - When the weakness subsides, assist the client back to bed.
   - If a chair is not close by, assist the client to a horizontal position on the floor before fainting occurs.
     a. Assume a broad stance with one foot in front of the other. **Rationale:** *A broad stance widens your base of support. Placing one foot behind the other allows you to rock backward and use the femoral muscles when supporting the client's weight and lowering the center of gravity (see the next step), thus preventing back strain.*

b. Bring the client backward so that your body supports the person. **Rationale:** *Clients who faint or start to fall usually pitch slightly forward because of the momentum of ambulating. Bringing the client's weight backward against your body allows gradual movement to the floor without injury to the client.*

c. Allow the client to slide down your leg, and lower the person gently to the floor, making sure the client's head does not hit any objects.

VARIATION: TWO NURSES

- After the client stands, assume a position with one nurse at either side. Grasp the inferior aspect of the client's upper arm with your nearest hand and the client's lower arm or hand with your other hand. **Rationale:** *This provides a secure grip for each nurse.*
- *Optional:* Place a walking belt around the client's waist. Each nurse grasps the side handle with the near hand and the lower aspect of the client's upper arm with the other hand.
- Walk in unison with the client, using a smooth, even gait, at the same speed and with steps the same size as the client's. **Rationale:** *This gives the client a greater feeling of security.*
- If the client starts to fall and cannot regain strength or balance, slip your arms under the client's axillae, grasp the client's hands, and lower the person gently to the floor or to a nearby chair. **Rationale:** *Placing the nurse's arms under the client's axillae evenly balances the client's weight between the two nurses, preventing injury to both the nurses and the client.*

7. Document distance and duration of ambulation in the client record using forms or checklists supplemented by narrative notes when appropriate. Include description of the client's gait (including body alignment) when walking; pace; activity tolerance when walking (e.g., pulse rate, facial color, any shortness of breath, feelings of dizziness, or weakness); degree of support required; and respiratory rate and blood pressure after initial ambulation to compare with baseline data.

EVALUATION

- Establish a plan for continued ambulation based on expected or normal ability for the client.

Controlling Postural Hypotension

- Rest with the head of the bed elevated 8 to 12 inches. This position makes the position change on rising less severe.
- Avoid sudden changes in position. Arise from bed in three stages:
  a. Sit up in bed for 1 minute.
  b. Sit on the side of the bed with legs dangling for 1 minute.
  c. Stand with care, holding onto the edge of the bed or another nonmovable object for 1 minute.
- Never bend down all the way to the floor or stand up too quickly after stooping.
- Postpone activities such as shaving and hair grooming for at least 1 hour after rising.
- Wear elastic stockings at night to inhibit venous pooling in the legs.

- Be aware that the symptoms of hypotension are most severe at the following times:
  a. 30 to 60 minutes after a heavy meal
  b. 1 to 2 hours after taking an antihypertension medication
- Get out of a hot bath very slowly, because high temperatures can lead to venous pooling.
- Use a rocking chair to improve circulation in the lower extremities. Even mild leg conditioning can strengthen muscle tone and enhance circulation.
- Refrain from any strenuous activity that results in holding the breath and bearing down. This Valsalva maneuver slows the heart rate, leading to subsequent lowering of blood pressure.

LONG-TERM CARE CONSIDERATIONS

Assisting the Client to Ambulate

Older Adults

- Inquire how the client has ambulated previously and modify assistance accordingly.
- Take into account a decrease in speed, strength, resistance to fatigue, reaction time, and coordination due to a decrease in nerve conduction.
- Be cautious when using a transfer belt with a client with osteoporosis. Too much pressure from the belt can increase the risk of vertebral compression fractures.
- If assistive devices such as a walker or cane are used, make sure clients are supervised in the beginning to learn the proper method of using them. Crutches may be much more difficult for older adults due to decreased upper body strength.

- Be alert to signs of activity intolerance, especially in older adults with cardiac and lung problems.
- Set small goals and increase slowly to build endurance, strength, and flexibility.
- Be aware of any fall risks the older adult may have, such as the following:
  - Effects of medications
  - Neurological disorders
  - Environmental hazards
  - Orthostatic hypotension
  - In older adults, the body's responses return to normal more slowly. For instance, an increase in heart rate from exercise may stay elevated for hours before returning to normal.

Using Mechanical Aids for Walking

Mechanical aids for ambulation include canes, walkers, and crutches.

CANES Two types of canes are used today: the standard straight-legged cane and the quad cane, which has four feet and provides the most support (Figure 31–8). Cane tips should have rubber caps to improve traction and prevent slipping. The length should permit the elbow to be slightly flexed. Clients may use either one or two canes, depending on how much support they require.

WALKERS Walkers are mechanical devices for ambulatory clients who need more support than a cane provides. The standard type has four legs with rubber tips and plastic hand grips. Many walkers have adjustable legs. The standard walker needs to be picked up to be used. The client therefore requires partial strength in both hands and wrists, strong elbow extensors, and strong shoulder depressors. The client also needs the ability to bear at least partial weight on both legs.

Four-wheeled and two-wheeled models of walkers (roller walkers, Figure 31–9) do not need to be picked up to be moved, but they are less stable than the standard walker.

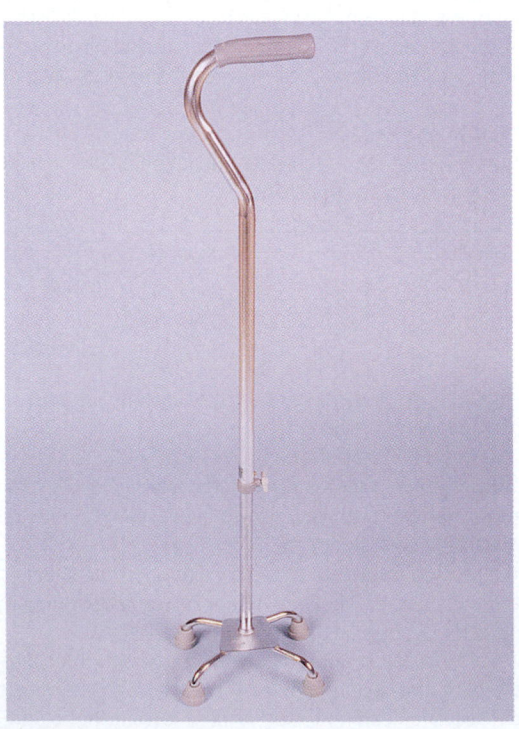

Figure 31–8 ❍ A quad cane.

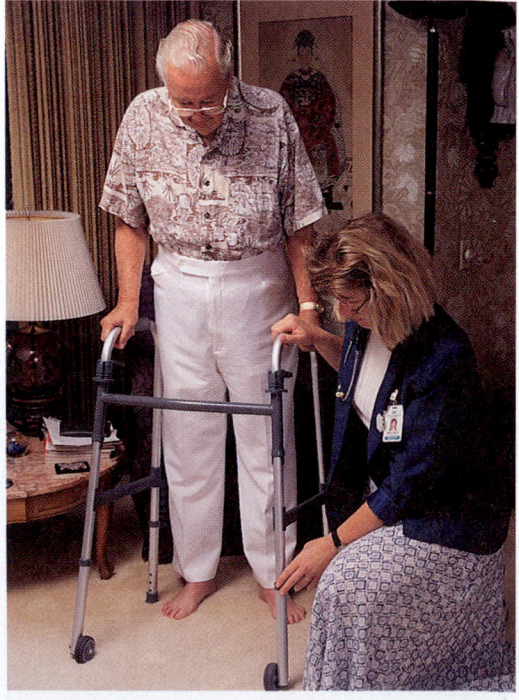

Figure 31–9 ❍ Two-wheeled walker.

Using Canes

- Hold the cane with the hand on the stronger side of the body to provide maximum support and appropriate body alignment when walking.
- Position the tip of a standard cane (and the nearest tip of other canes) about 15 cm (6 in.) to the side and 15 cm (6 in.) in front of the near foot, so that the elbow is slightly flexed.

When Maximum Support Is Required

- Move the cane forward about 30 cm (1 ft), or a distance that is comfortable while the body weight is borne by both legs (Figure 31–10, A).
- Then move the affected (weak) leg forward to the cane while the weight is borne by the cane and stronger leg (Figure 31–10, B).

- Next, move the unaffected (stronger) leg forward ahead of the cane and weak leg while the weight is borne by the cane and weak leg (Figure 31–10, C).
- Repeat the steps. This pattern of moving provides at least two points of support on the floor at all times.

As You Become Stronger and Require Less Support

- Move the cane and weak leg forward at the same time, while the weight is borne by the stronger leg (Figure 31–11, A).
- Move the stronger leg forward, while the weight is borne by the cane and the weak leg (Figure 31–11, B).

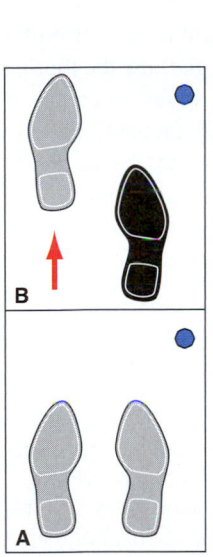
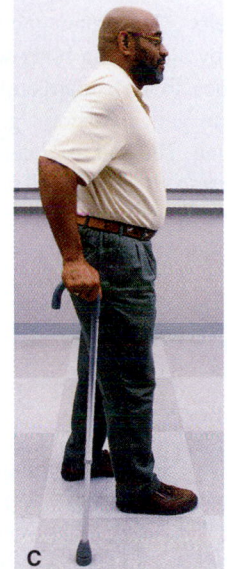

Figure 31–10 ○ Steps involved in using a cane to provide maximum support.

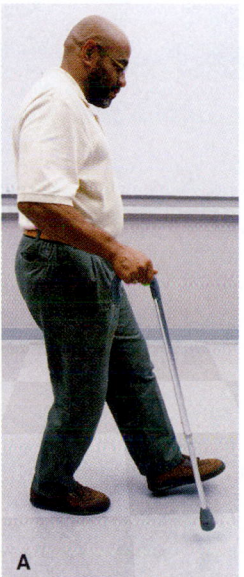
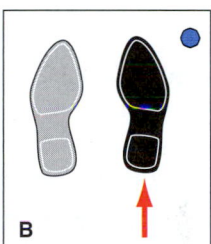

Figure 31–11 ○ Steps involved in using a cane when less than maximum support is required.

They are used by clients who are too weak or unstable to pick up and move the walker with each step. Some roller walkers have a seat at the back so the client can sit down to rest when desired. An adaptation of the standard and four-wheeled walker is one that has two tips and two wheels. This type provides more stability than the four-wheeled model yet still permits the client to keep the walker in contact with the ground all the time. The client tilts the walker toward the body, lifting the tips while the wheels remain on the ground, and then pushes the walker forward.

The nurse may need to adjust the height of a client's walker so that the hand bar is just below the client's waist and the client's elbows are slightly flexed. This position helps the client assume a more normal stance. A walker that is too low causes the client to stoop; one that is too high makes the client stretch and reach.

CRUTCHES Crutches may be a temporary need for some people and a permanent one for others. Clients realize that they can no longer take balance for granted when they must cope with the weight of a heavy cast or a paralyzed limb. Frequently, progress may be slower than the client anticipated. Encouragement from the nurse and the setting of realistic goals are especially important.

There are several kinds of crutches. The most frequently used are the underarm crutch, or axillary crutch with hand bars, and the Lofstrand crutch, which extends only to the forearm (Figure 31–12). On the Lofstrand crutch, the metal cuff around the forearm and the metal bar stabilize the wrists and thus make walking safer and easier. The platform, or elbow extensor, crutch also has a cuff for the upper arm. All crutches require suction tips, usually made of rubber, which help to prevent slipping on a floor surface.

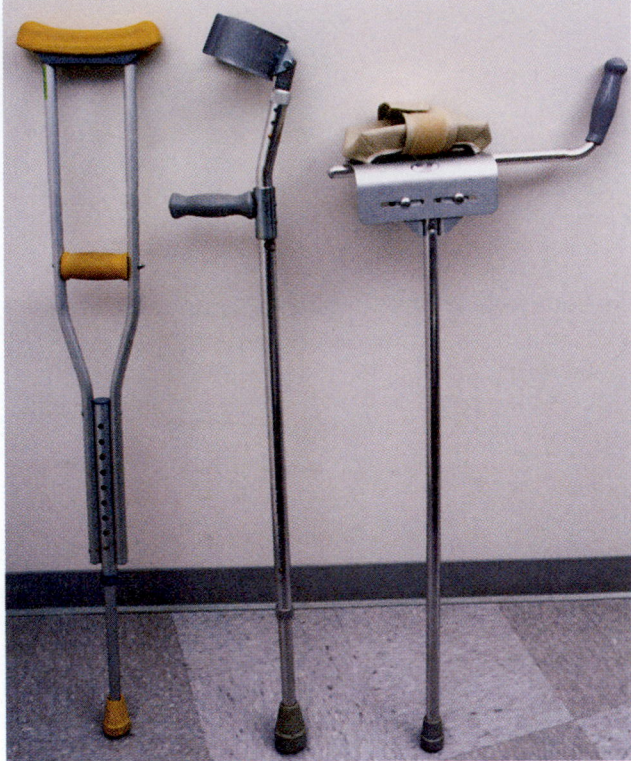

Figure 31–12 ● Types of crutches: axillary, Lofstrand, and platform.

of the hand piece. There are two methods of measuring crutch length:

1. The client lies in a supine position and the nurse measures from the anterior fold of the axilla to the heel of the foot and adds 2.5 cm (1 in.).
2. The client stands erect and positions the crutch as shown in Figure 31–13. The nurse makes sure the shoulder rest of the crutch is at least three finger widths, that is, 2.5 to 5 cm (1 to 2 in.), below the axilla.

To determine the correct placement of the hand bar:

1. The client stands upright and supports the body weight by the hand grips of the crutches.
2. The nurse measures the angle of elbow flexion. It should be about 30 degrees. A goniometer may be used to verify the correct angle.

Crutch Gaits The crutch gait is the gait a person assumes on crutches by alternating body weight on one or both legs and the crutches. Five standard crutch gaits are the four-point gait, three-point gait, two-point gait, swing-to gait, and swing-through gait. The gait used depends on the following individual factors: (a) the ability to take steps, (b) the ability to bear weight and keep balance in a standing position on both legs or only one, and (c) the ability to hold the body erect.

In crutch walking, the client's weight is borne by the muscles of the shoulder girdle and the upper extremities. Before beginning crutch walking, exercises that strengthen the upper arms and hands are recommended.

Measuring Clients for Crutches When nurses measure clients for axillary crutches, it is most important to obtain the correct length for the crutches and the correct placement

---

CLIENT TEACHING — Using Walkers

When Maximum Support Is Required

- Move the walker ahead about 15 cm (6 in.) while your body weight is borne by both legs.
- Then move the right foot up to the walker while your body weight is borne by the left leg and both arms.
- Next, move the left foot up to the right foot while your body weight is borne by the right leg and both arms.

If One Leg Is Weaker than the Other

- Move the walker and the weak leg ahead together about 15 cm (6 in.) while your weight is borne by the stronger leg.
- Then move the stronger leg ahead while your weight is borne by the affected leg and both arms.

CLIENT TEACHING — Using Crutches

- Follow the plan of exercises developed for you to strengthen your arm muscles before beginning crutch walking.
- Have a health care professional establish the correct length for your crutches and the correct placement of the handpieces. Crutches that are too long force your shoulders upward and make it difficult for you to push your body off the ground. Crutches that are too short will make you hunch over and develop an improper body stance.
- The weight of your body should be borne by the arms rather than the axillae (armpits). Continual pressure on the axillae can injure the radial nerve and eventually cause crutch palsy, a weakness of the muscles of the forearm, wrist, and hand.
- Maintain an erect posture as much as possible to prevent strain on muscles and joints and to maintain balance.
- Each step taken with crutches should be a comfortable distance for you. It is wise to start with a small rather than large step.
- Inspect the crutch tips regularly, and replace them if worn.
- Keep the crutch tips dry and clean to maintain their surface friction. If the tips become wet, dry them well before use.
- Wear a shoe with a low heel that grips the floor. Rubber soles decrease the chances of slipping. Adjust shoelaces so they cannot come untied or reach the floor where they might catch on the crutches. Consider shoes with alternative forms of closure (e.g., Velcro), especially if you cannot easily bend to tie laces. Slip-on shoes are acceptable only if they are snug and the heel does not come loose when the foot is bent.

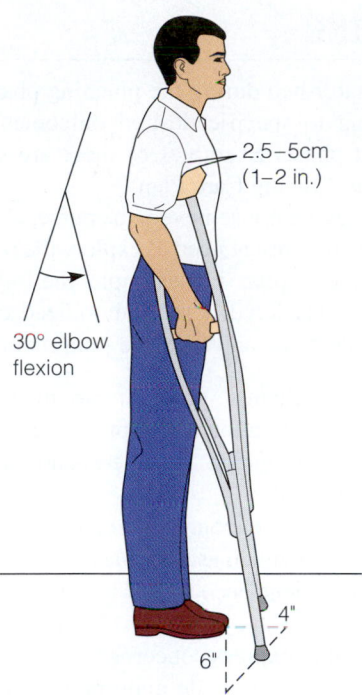

2.5–5cm
(1–2 in.)

30° elbow
flexion

4"

6"

Figure 31–13 ● The standing position for measuring the correct length for crutches.

Clients also need instruction about how to get into and out of chairs and go up and down stairs safely. All of these crutch skills are best taught before the client is discharged and preferably before the client has surgery.

Crutch Stance (Tripod Position) Before crutch walking is attempted, the client needs to learn facts about posture and balance. The proper standing position with crutches is called the tripod (triangle) position. The crutches are placed about 15 cm (6 in.) in front of the feet and out laterally about 15 cm (6 in.), creating a wide base of support. The feet are slightly apart. A tall person requires a wider base than a short person does. Hips and knees are extended, the back is straight, and the head is held straight and high. There should be no hunch to the shoulders and thus no weight borne by the axillae. The elbows are extended sufficiently to allow weight bearing on the hands. If the client is unsteady, the nurse places a walking belt around the client's waist and grasps the belt from above, not from below. A fall can be prevented more effectively if the belt is held from above.

Four-Point Alternate Gait This is the most elementary and safest gait, providing at least three points of support at all times, but it requires coordination. Clients can use it when walking in crowds because it does not require much space. To use this gait, the client needs to be able to bear weight on both legs. The nurse asks the client to:

1. Move the right crutch ahead a suitable distance, such as 10 to 15 cm (4 to 6 in.).
2. Move the left front foot forward, preferably to the level of the left crutch.

3. Move the left crutch forward.
4. Move the right foot forward.

Three-Point Gait To use this gait, the client must be able to bear the entire body weight on the unaffected leg. The two crutches and the unaffected leg bear weight alternately. The nurse asks the client to:

1. Move both crutches and the weaker leg forward.
2. Move the stronger leg forward.

Two-Point Alternate Gait This gait is faster than the four-point gait. It requires more balance because only two points support the body at one time; it also requires at least partial weight bearing on each foot. In this gait, arm movements with the crutches are similar to the arm movements during normal walking. The nurse asks the client to:

1. Move the left crutch and the right foot forward together.
2. Move the right crutch and the left foot ahead together.

Swing-to Gait The swing gaits are used by clients with paralysis of the legs and hips. Prolonged use of these gaits results in atrophy of the unused muscles. The swing-to gait is the easier of these two gaits. The nurse asks the client to:

1. Move both crutches ahead together.
2. Lift body weight by the arms and swing to the crutches.

Swing-through Gait This gait requires considerable skill, strength, and coordination. The nurse asks the client to:

1. Move both crutches forward together.
2. Lift body weight by the arms and swing through and beyond the crutch.

Getting into a Chair Chairs that have armrests and are secure or braced against a wall are essential for clients using crutches. For this procedure, the nurse instructs the client to:

1. Stand with the back of the unaffected leg centered against the chair. The chair helps support the client during the next steps.
2. Transfer the crutches to the hand on the affected side and hold the crutches by the hand bars. The client grasps the arm of the chair with the hand on the unaffected side. This allows the client to support the body weight on the arms and the unaffected leg.
3. Lean forward, flex the knees and hips, and lower into the chair.

Getting out of a Chair For this procedure, the nurse instructs the client to:

1. Move forward to the edge of the chair and place the unaffected leg slightly under or at the edge of the chair. This position helps the client stand up from the chair and achieve balance, since the unaffected leg is supported against the edge of the chair.
2. Grasp the crutches by the hand bars in the hand on the affected side, and grasp the arm of the chair by the hand on the unaffected side. The body weight is placed on the

crutches and the hand on the armrest to support the un-affected leg when the client rises to stand.
3. Push down on the crutches and the chair armrest while elevating the body out of the chair.
4. Assume the tripod position before moving.

Going Up Stairs   For this procedure, the nurse stands behind the client and slightly to the affected side if needed. The nurse instructs the client to:

1. Assume the tripod position at the bottom of the stairs.
2. Transfer the body weight to the crutches and move the unaffected leg onto the step.
3. Transfer the body weight to the unaffected leg on the step and move the crutches and affected leg up to the step. The affected leg is always supported by the crutches.
4. Repeat steps 2 and 3 until the client reaches the top of the stairs.

Going Down Stairs   For this procedure, the nurse stands one step below the client on the affected side if needed. The nurse instructs the client to:

1. Assume the tripod position at the top of the stairs.
2. Shift the body weight to the unaffected leg, and move the crutches and affected leg down onto the next step.
3. Transfer the body weight to the crutches, and move the unaffected leg to that step. The affected leg is always supported by the crutches.
4. Repeat steps 2 and 3 until the client reaches the bottom of the stairs.

EVALUATING

The goals established during the planning phase are evaluated according to specific desired outcomes, also established in that phase. Examples of these are shown in the accompanying Nursing Care Plan.

If outcomes are not achieved, the nurse, client, and support person if appropriate need to explore the reasons before modifying the care plan. For example, the following questions may be considered if an immobilized client fails to maintain muscle mass and tone and joint mobility:

- Has the client's physical or mental condition changed motivation to perform required exercise?
- Were appropriate range-of-motion exercises implemented?
- Was the client encouraged to participate in self-care activities as much as possible?
- Was the client encouraged to make as many decisions as possible when developing a daily activity plan and to express concerns?
- Did the nurse provide appropriate supervision and monitoring?
- Was the client's diet adequate to provide appropriate nourishment for energy requirements?

Nursing Care Plan   Risk for Disuse Syndrome

ASSESSMENT DATA	NURSING DIAGNOSIS	DESIRED OUTCOMES*
Nursing Assessment		
Peter Chan, a 69-year-old, unmarried accountant being treated for congestive heart failure, states he has dyspnea with mild activity. ("I cannot climb a flight of stairs without stopping and resting and become breathless even when walking on level ground.") Prefers the orthopneic position. He works at home and sits at a table for most of the day.	*Risk for Disuse Syndrome* related to decreased activity resulting from inadequate balance between oxygen supply and demand associated with decreased cardiac output and obesity.	**Immobility Consequences:** Physiological [0204], as evidenced by no • Pressure ulcers • Decreased muscle strength **Immobility Consequences:** Psycho-cognitive [0205], as evidenced by no • Apathy • Sleep disturbances • Negative body image **Mobility [0208],** as evidenced by mildly compromised • Walking • Balance

Physical Examination
Height: 178 cm (5′10″)
Weight: 102 kg (225 lb)
Temperature: 37.8°C (100.4°F)
Pulse rate: 94 BPM
Respirations: 20/minute
Blood pressure: 174/92 mm Hg
Rales present in both lungs.
Respirations slightly labored. Color pale.
3+ (5 mm) edema both feet and ankles

Diagnostic Data
CBC, and urinalysis within normal limits.
CXR reveals an enlarged heart.

NURSING INTERVENTIONS*/SELECTED ACTIVITIES	RATIONALE
Positioning [0840]	
Position to alleviate dyspnea, e.g., high Fowler's.	*Clients with increased pulmonary secretions are able to breathe better when upright because abdominal organs are lower and there is greater room for lung and diaphragmatic excursion.*
Provide support to edematous areas, e.g., elevate feet on foot stool when sitting.	*Elevating the dependent area assists with decreasing tissue pressure and promoting fluid return to the venous system and the heart.*
Encourage active range of motion exercises.	*Active ROM helps keep muscles in current strength and promotes circulation. Mild activity also helps burn unneeded calories.*
Exercise Therapy: Muscle Control [0226]	
Collaborate with physical, occupational, and recreational therapists in developing and executing an individually tailored exercise program.	*This client will need a multidisciplinary approach to his care. Each member contributes from his or her area of expertise. Research supports efficacy of individually tailored exercise plans. Factors such as having an exercise partner, using music, and type of activity can motivate client and enhance adherence to the plan over time.*
Offer options, explain rationale for type of exercise and protocol to client, and allow him to make choices that appeal to him and that address his needs.	*If the client understands what the reasons are for activity, he can make good choices.*
Provide step-by-step cuing for each motor activity during exercise or ADLs.	*As-needed reminders help the client recall what to do next.*
Use visual aids to facilitate learning how to perform exercises.	*Some people have better visual memory than auditory memory.*

EVALUATION

Outcomes met. Mr. Chan did not develop any skin breakdown or other evidence of the complications of immobility to date. However, since the risk factors remain, the care plan will be ongoing.

The NOC # for desired outcomes and the NIC # for nursing interventions are listed in brackets following the appropriate outcome or intervention. Outcomes, indicators, interventions, and activities selected are only a sample of those suggested by NOC and NIC and should be further individualized for each client.

CRITICAL THINKING QUESTIONS

1. What assessment findings alert you that Mr. Chan is developing problems associated with his current state of decreased mobility?

2. Mr. Chan may benefit from using a walker to assist with ambulation at home. What teaching should be done in regard to use of a walker?

3. The care plan does not address one of Mr. Chan's risk factors—obesity. Would you add this to the plan?

4. What assumptions has the nurse made in assigning the desired outcome of "Immobility Consequences: Psycho-Cognitive"?

5. How are the choices of outcomes influenced by the cause of his nursing diagnosis (a chronic illness)?

∞ **See Answers in MyNursingKit.**

CONCEPT MAP   Client at Risk for Disuse Syndrome

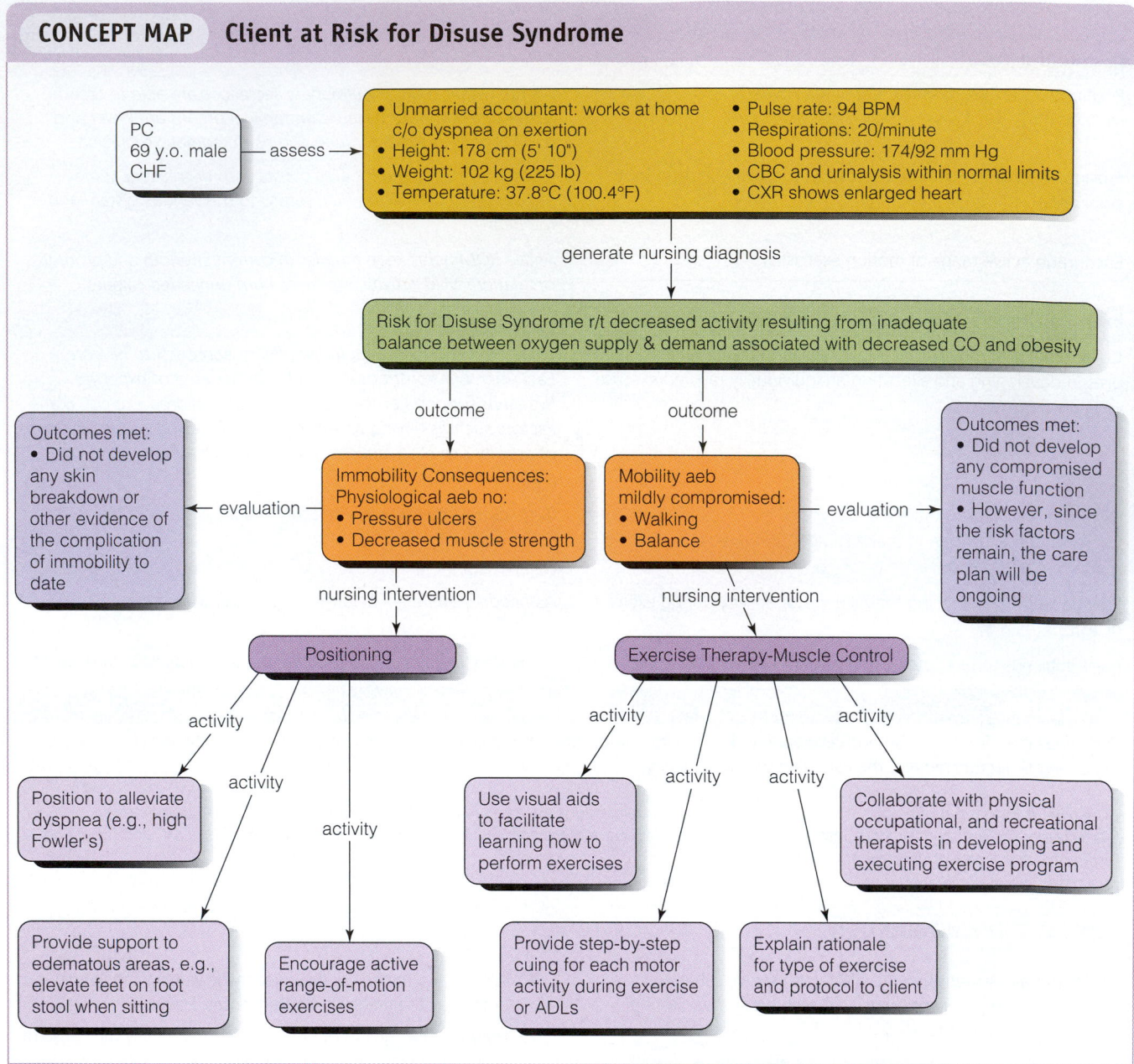

SLEEP

Sleep is a basic human need; it is a universal biological process common to all people. Humans spend about one-third of their lives asleep. We require sleep for many reasons: to cope with daily stresses, to prevent fatigue, to conserve energy, to restore the mind and body, and to enjoy life more fully. Sleep enhances daytime functioning. It is vital for not only optimal psychological functioning but also physiological functioning as the rate of healing of damaged tissue is greatest during sleep (Robinson, Weitzel, & Henderson, 2005, p. 263). Sleep is an important factor in a person's quality of life. And yet, a 2006 report from the Institute of Medicine (IOM) states that sleep disorders and sleep deprivation are unmet public health problems. It is estimated that 50 mil-

lion to 70 million Americans suffer from a chronic disorder of sleep and wakefulness that hinders daily functioning and adversely affects health (IOM, 2006, p. 24). Numerous *Sleep in America* polls by the National Sleep Foundation reflect that Americans, from infants to older adults, need more sleep.

Furthermore, many members of the general public and health professionals are unaware of the consequences of chronic sleep loss. Almost 20% of all serious car crash injuries are associated with driver sleepiness (IOM, 2006, p. 25). As a result, the IOM report made a number of recommendations, including: (a) increasing financial investments in interdisciplinary **somnology** (the study of sleep) and sleep medicine research training; (b) increasing public awareness by establishing a multimedia public education campaign; (c) increasing education and training of health care professionals in somnology and sleep medicine; (d) developing new technologies for the diagnosis and treatment of sleep disorders; and (e) monitoring the American population's sleep patterns and the prevalence and health outcomes associated with sleep disorders (IOM, 2006).

Physiology of Sleep

Historically, sleep was considered a state of unconsciousness. More recently, sleep has come to be considered an altered state of consciousness in which the individual's perception of and reaction to the environment are decreased. Sleep is characterized by minimal physical activity, variable levels of consciousness, changes in the body's physiologic processes, and decreased responsiveness to external stimuli. Some environmental stimuli, such as a smoke detector alarm, will usually awaken a sleeper, whereas many other noises will not. It appears that individuals respond to meaningful stimuli while sleeping and selectively disregard nonmeaningful stimuli.

The cyclic nature of sleep is thought to be controlled by centers located in the lower part of the brain. Neurons within the reticular formation, located in the brain stem, integrate sensory information from the peripheral nervous system and relay the information to the cerebral cortex. The upper part of the reticular formation consists of a network of ascending nerve fibers called the reticular activating system (RAS), which is involved with the sleep–wake cycle. An intact cerebral cortex and reticular formation are necessary for the regulation of sleep and waking states.

Neurotransmitters, located within neurons in the brain, affect the sleep–wake cycles. Another key factor to sleep is exposure to darkness. Darkness and preparing for sleep causes a decrease in stimulation of the RAS. During this time, the pineal gland in the brain begins to actively secrete the natural hormone melatonin, and the person feels less alert. During sleep, the growth hormone is secreted and cortisol is inhibited.

With the beginning of daylight, melatonin is at its lowest level in the body and the stimulating hormone, cortisol, is at its highest. Wakefulness is also associated with high levels of acetylcholine, dopamine, and noradrenaline. Acetylcholine is released in the reticular formation, dopamine in the midbrain, and noradrenaline in the pons. These neurotransmitters are localized within the reticular formation and influence cerebral cortical arousal.

CIRCADIAN RHYTHMS **Biological rhythms** exist in plants, animals, and humans. In humans, these are controlled from within the body and synchronized with environmental factors, such as light and darkness. The most familiar biological rhythm is the circadian rhythm. The term *circadian* is from the Latin *circa dies,* meaning "about a day." Although sleep and waking cycles are the best known of the circadian rhythms, body temperature, blood pressure, and many other physiologic functions also follow a circadian pattern.

Sleep is a complex biological rhythm. When a person's biological clock coincides with the sleep–wake cycles, the person is said to be in circadian synchronization; that is, the person is awake when the body temperature is highest, and asleep when the body temperature is lowest. Circadian regularity begins to develop by the sixth week of life, and by 3 to 6 months most infants have a regular sleep–wake cycle.

TYPES OF SLEEP **Sleep architecture** refers to the basic organization of normal sleep. There are two types of sleep: **NREM** (non-rapid-eye-movement) **sleep** and **REM** (rapid-eye-movement) **sleep**. During sleep, NREM and REM sleep alternate in cycles. Irregular cycling and/or absent sleep stages are associated with sleep disorders (IOM, 2006, p. 42).

NREM Sleep   NREM sleep occurs when activity in the RAS is inhibited. About 75% to 80% of sleep during a night is NREM sleep. NREM sleep is divided into four stages, each associated with distinct brain activity and physiology. *Stage I* is the stage of very light sleep and lasts only a few minutes. During this stage, the person feels drowsy and relaxed, the eyes roll from side to side, and the heart and respiratory rates drop slightly. The sleeper can be readily awakened and may deny that he or she was sleeping.

Stage II is the stage of light sleep during which body processes continue to slow down. The eyes are generally still, the heart and respiratory rates decrease slightly, and body temperature falls. Stage II lasts only about 10 to 15 minutes but constitutes 44% to 55% of total sleep (IOM, 2006, p. 44). An individual in stage II requires more intense stimuli than in stage I to awaken.

Stages III and IV are the deepest stages of sleep, differing only in the percentage of delta waves recorded during a 30-second period. During *deep sleep* or *delta sleep,* the sleeper's heart and respiratory rates drop 20% to 30% below those exhibited during waking hours. The sleeper is difficult to arouse. The person is not disturbed by sensory stimuli, the skeletal muscles are very relaxed, reflexes are diminished, and snoring is most likely to occur. Even swallowing and saliva production are reduced during delta sleep (Orr, 2000). These stages are essential for restoring energy and releasing important growth hormones. See Box 31–5.

CLINICAL ALERT

In a sleep-deprived client, the loss of NREM sleep causes immunosuppression, slows tissue repair, lowers pain tolerance, triggers profound fatigue, and increases susceptibility to infection (Lower, Bonsack, & Guion, 2003, p. 40D).

REM Sleep   REM sleep usually recurs about every 90 minutes and lasts 5 to 30 minutes. Most dreams take place during REM sleep but usually will not be remembered unless the person arouses briefly at the end of the REM period.

During REM sleep, the brain is highly active, and brain metabolism may increase as much as 20%. For example, during REM sleep, levels of acetylcholine and dopamine increase, with the highest levels of acetylcholine release occurring during REM sleep. Since both of these neurotransmitters are

BOX 31–5	Physiologic Changes during NREM Sleep

- Arterial blood pressure falls.
- Pulse rate decreases.
- Peripheral blood vessels dilate.
- Cardiac output decreases.
- Skeletal muscles relax.
- **Basal metabolic rate** decreases 10% to 30%.
- Growth hormone levels peak.
- Intracranial pressure decreases.

associated with cortical activation, it makes sense that their levels would be high during dreaming sleep. This type of sleep is also called paradoxical sleep because electroencephalogram (EEG) activity resembles that of wakefulness. Distinctive eye movements occur, voluntary muscle tone is dramatically decreased, and deep tendon reflexes are absent. In this phase, the sleeper may be difficult to arouse or may wake spontaneously, gastric secretions increase, and heart and respiratory rates often are irregular. It is thought that the regions of the brain that are used in learning, thinking, and organizing information are stimulated during REM sleep.

CLINICAL ALERT

In a sleep-deprived client, the loss of REM sleep causes psychologic disturbances such as apathy, depression, irritability, confusion, disorientation, hallucinations, impaired memory, and paranoia (Lower, Bonsack, & Guion, 2003, p. 40D).

SLEEP CYCLES During a sleep cycle, people typically pass through NREM and REM sleep, the complete cycle usually lasting about 90 to 110 minutes in adults. In the first sleep cycle, a sleeper usually passes through all of the first three NREM stages in a total of about 20 to 30 minutes. Then, stage IV may last about 30 minutes. After stage IV NREM, the sleep passes back through stages III and II over about 20 minutes. Thereafter, the first REM stage occurs, lasting about 10 minutes, completing the first sleep cycle. It is not unusual for the first REM period to be very brief or even skipped entirely. The healthy adult sleeper usually experiences four to six cycles of sleep during 7 to 8 hours. The sleeper who is awakened during any stage must begin anew at stage I NREM sleep and proceed through all the stages to REM sleep.

The duration of NREM stages and REM sleep varies throughout the sleep period. During the early part of the night, the deep sleep periods are longer. As the night progresses, the sleeper spends less time in stages III and IV of NREM sleep. REM sleep increases and dreams tend to lengthen. Before sleep ends, periods of near wakefulness occur, and stages I and II NREM sleep and REM sleep predominate.

Functions of Sleep

The effects of sleep on the body are not completely understood. Sleep exerts physiologic effects on both the nervous system and other body structures. Sleep in some way restores normal levels of activity and normal balance among parts of the nervous system. Sleep is also necessary for protein synthesis, which allows repair processes to occur.

The role of sleep in psychological well-being is best noticed by the deterioration in mental functioning related to sleep loss. Persons with inadequate amounts of sleep tend to become emotionally irritable, have poor concentration, and experience difficulty making decisions.

Sleep Patterns throughout the Lifespan

Although it used to be believed that maintaining a regular sleep–wake rhythm is more important than the number of hours actually slept, recent research has shown that sleep deprivation is associated with significant cognitive and health problems. Although reestablishing the sleep–wake rhythm is an important aspect of nursing, it is not appropriate to curtail or decrease daytime napping in hospitalized clients.

Newborns sleep 16 to 18 hours a day, on an irregular schedule with periods of 1 to 3 hours spent awake. Unlike older children and adults, newborns enter REM sleep (called *active sleep* during the newborn period) immediately. Rapid eye movements are observable through closed lids, and the body movements and irregular respirations may be observed. NREM sleep (also called *quiet sleep* during the newborn period) is characterized by regular respirations, closed eyes, and the absence of body and eye movements. Newborns spend nearly 50% of their time in each of these states, and the sleep cycle is about 50 minutes.

At first, infants awaken every 3 or 4 hours, eat, and then go back to sleep. Periods of wakefulness gradually increase during the first months. By 6 months, most infants sleep through the night (from midnight to 5 AM) and begin to establish a pattern of daytime naps. At the end of the first year, an infant usually takes two naps per day and should get about 14 to 15 hours of sleep in 24 hours. About half of the infant's sleep time is spent in light sleep. Putting infants to bed when they are drowsy but not asleep helps them to become "self-soothers."

Between 12 and 14 hours of sleep are recommended for children 1 to 3 years of age. Most still need an afternoon nap, but the need for midmorning naps gradually decreases. The toddler may exhibit a great deal of resistance to going to bed and may awaken during the night. Nighttime fears and nightmares are also common. A security object such as a blanket or stuffed animal may help. Parents need assurance that if the child has had adequate attention from them during the day, maintaining a daily sleep schedule and consistent bedtime routine will promote good sleep habits for the entire family.

The preschool child (3 to 5 years of age) requires 11 to 13 hours of sleep per night, particularly if the child is in preschool. Sleep needs fluctuate in relation to activity and growth spurts. Many children of this age dislike bedtime and resist by requesting another story, game, or television program. The 4- to 5-year-old may become restless and irritable if sleep requirements are not met. Parents can help children who resist bedtime by maintaining a regular and consistent sleep schedule with a relaxing bedtime routine. Preschool children wake up frequently at night, and they may be afraid of the dark or experience night terrors or nightmares.

The school-age child (5 to 12 years of age) needs 10 to 11 hours of sleep, but most receive less because of increasing demands. They may also be spending more time at the computer and watching TV. Some may be drinking caffeinated beverages. All of these activities can lead to difficulty falling asleep and fewer hours of sleep. Nurses can teach parents and school-age children about healthy sleep habits. A regular and consistent sleep schedule and bedtime routine need to be continued.

CLINICAL ALERT

Children who have a TV and/or computer in their bedroom are more likely to get less sleep.

Adolescents (12 to 18 years of age) require 9 to 10 hours of sleep each night; however, few actually get that much sleep (IOM, 2006, p. 56). Lack of sleep can result in lower grades, negative moods, and increased potential for car accidents. Nurses can teach parents to recognize signs and symptoms that indicate their teen is not getting enough sleep. As children reach adolescence, their circadian rhythms tend to shift. Research in the 1990s found that later sleep and wake patterns among adolescents are biologically determined; the natural tendency for teenagers is to stay up late at night and wake up later in the morning (National Sleep Foundation, n.d.a). Many schools, however, start at 7 AM, which is in conflict with the adolescent's sleep patterns and contributes to their sleep deprivation. During adolescence, boys begin to experience nocturnal emissions (orgasm and emission of semen during sleep), known as "wet dreams," several times each month. See the Clinical Manifestations box.

Most healthy adults need 7 to 9 hours of sleep a night (National Sleep Foundation, n.d.b). However, there is individual variation as some adults may be able to function well with 6 hours of sleep and others may need 10 hours to function optimally. Signs that may indicate that a person is not getting enough sleep include falling asleep or becoming drowsy during a task that is not fatiguing, not being able to concentrate or remember information, and being unreasonably irritable with others. The National Sleep Foundation (n.d.b) reports that certain adults are particularly vulnerable for not getting enough sleep: students, shift workers, travelers, and persons suffering from acute stress, depression, or chronic pain. Nurses need to teach adults the importance of obtaining sufficient sleep and tips on how to promote sleep that results in the client waking up feeling restored or refreshed.

A hallmark change with age is a tendency toward earlier bedtime and wake times. Older adults may show an increase in disturbed sleep that can create a negative impact on their quality of life, mood, and alertness. Although the ability to sleep becomes more difficult, the need to sleep does not decrease with age (IOM, 2006, pp. 57–59). It is im-

---

| CLINICAL MANIFESTATIONS | **Sleep Deprivation and Sleep Problems in Teens** |

The teen:

- Has difficulty waking in the morning for school and yawns frequently throughout the day.
- Is continuously late for class and has trouble getting out the door in the morning.
- Can't seem to get through the day without drinking caffeinated beverages like coffee or cola.
- Is having difficulty in school, or a teacher notices that the student falls asleep in class periodically.
- Is irritable, is anxious, and gets angry easily on days when he or she gets less sleep.
- Runs from one activity to the next—he or she participates in extra-curricular activities, has a job, and stays up late doing homework every night, cutting into sleep time.
- Takes naps during the week for more than 45 minutes and "sleeps in" for 2 hours or longer on the weekends than during the week.

Note: From "Parents of Teens: Recognize the Signs & Symptoms of Sleep Deprivation and Sleep Problems," by National Sleep Foundation (n.d.e). Retrieved from http://www.sleepfoundation.org/_content/hottopics/teensigns.pdf. Used with permission of the National Sleep Foundation. For further information, please visit http://www.sleepfoundation.org.

---

portant for the nurse to teach about the connection between sleep, health, and aging. See the Client Teaching box about sleep promotion later in this chapter.

Some older adult clients with dementia may experience *sundown syndrome*. Although not a sleep disorder directly, it refers to a pattern of symptoms (e.g., agitation, anxiety, aggression, and sometimes delusions) that occur in the late afternoon (thus the name). These symptoms can last through the night, further disrupting sleep (Arnold, 2004).

Factors Affecting Sleep

Both the quality and the quantity of sleep are affected by a number of factors. *Sleep quality* is a subjective characteristic and is often determined by whether a person wakes up feeling energetic or not. *Quantity of sleep* is the total time the individual sleeps.

ILLNESS Illness that causes pain or physical distress can result in sleep problems. People who are ill require more sleep than normal, and the normal rhythm of sleep and wakefulness is often disturbed. People deprived of REM sleep subsequently spend more sleep time than normal in this stage.

Respiratory conditions can disturb an individual's sleep. Shortness of breath often makes sleep difficult, and people who have nasal congestion or sinus drainage may have trouble breathing and hence may find it difficult to sleep. People who have gastric or duodenal ulcers may find their sleep disturbed because of pain, often a result of the increased gastric secretions that occur during REM sleep. Certain endocrine disturbances can also affect

LIFESPAN CONSIDERATIONS   Sleep Disturbances

Children

Learning to sleep alone without the parent's help is a skill that all children need to master. Regular bedtime routines and rituals such as reading a book help children learn this skill and can prevent sleep disturbance. Some sleep disturbances seen in children include the following:

- Trained night feeder. Infants who are fed during the night, who are fed until they fall asleep and then put in bed, or who have a bottle left with them in their bed learn to expect and demand middle-of-the-night feedings. Infants who are growing well do not need night feeding after about 4 months of age. Infants who are failing to thrive may need feeding at night.
- Sleep refusal. Many toddlers and young children are resistant to settling down to sleep. This sleep refusal may be due to not being tired, anxiety about separation from the parent, stress (e.g., a recent move), lack of a regular sleep routine, the child's temperament, or changes in sleep arrangements (e.g., move from a crib to a "big" bed).
- Night terrors. Night terrors are partial awakenings from non-REM, stage III or IV sleep. They are usually seen in children 3 to 6 years of age. The child may sleepwalk, or may sit up in bed screaming and thrashing about. They usually cannot be wakened, but should be protected from injury, helped back to bed, and soothed back to sleep. Babysitters should be alerted to the possibility of a night terror occurring. Children do not remember the incident the next day, and there is no indication of a neurological or emotional problem. Excessive fatigue and a full bladder may contribute to the problem. Having the child take an afternoon nap and empty the bladder before going to sleep at night may be helpful.

Adults

- New jobs, pregnancy, and babies are common examples that often disrupt the sleep of a young adult.
- The sleep patterns of middle-aged adults can be disrupted by taking care of older adult parents and/or chronically ill partners in the home.

- See the Client Teaching box on page 940 for healthy sleep tips for the adult.

Older Adults

The quality of sleep is often diminished in older adults. Some of the leading factors that often are influential in sleep disturbances include the following:

- Side effects of medications
- Gastric reflux disease
- Respiratory and circulatory disorders, which may cause breathing problems or discomfort
- Pain from arthritis, increased stiffness, or impaired immobility
- Nocturia
- Depression
- Loss of life partner and/or close friends
- Confusion related to delirium or dementia

Interventions to promote sleep and rest can help enhance the rejuvenation and renewal that sleep provides. The following interventions can help promote sleep:

- Reduce or eliminate the consumption of caffeine and nicotine.
- Be sure their environment is warm and safe, especially if they get out of bed during the night.
- Provide comfort measures, such as analgesics if indicated, and proper positioning.
- Enhance the sense of safety and security by checking on clients frequently and making sure that the call light is within reach.
- If lack of sleep is caused by medications or certain health conditions, interventions should focus on resolving the underlying problem.
- Evaluate the situation and find out what the rest and sleep disturbances mean to the client. They may not perceive sleeplessness to be a serious problem, but will just do other activities and sleep when tired.

---

sleep. Elevated body temperatures can cause some reduction in delta sleep and REM sleep. The need to urinate during the night also disrupts sleep, and people who awaken at night to urinate sometimes have difficulty getting back to sleep.

ENVIRONMENT Environment can promote or hinder sleep. Any change can inhibit sleep. The absence of usual stimuli or the presence of unfamiliar stimuli can prevent people from sleeping. Hospital environments can be quite noisy, and special care needs to be taken to reduce noise in the hallways and nursing care units. In fact, some hospitals have instituted "quiet times" in the afternoon on nursing units where the lights are lowered and activity and noise are purposefully decreased so clients can rest or nap.

Discomfort from environmental temperature and lack of ventilation can affect sleep. Light levels can be another factor. A person accustomed to darkness while sleeping may find it difficult to sleep in the light. Another influence includes the comfort and size of the bed. A person's partner who has different sleep habits, snores, or has other sleep difficulties may become a problem for the person also.

LIFESTYLE Following an irregular morning and nighttime schedule can affect sleep. Moderate exercise in the morning or early afternoon usually is conducive to sleep, but exercise late in the day can delay sleep. The person's ability to relax before retiring is an important factor affecting the ability to fall asleep. It is best, therefore, to avoid doing homework or office work before or after getting into bed.

| RESEARCH NOTES | Can Clients Sleep in a Hospital? |

Nurses know the importance of sleep. However, the researchers believe that sleep has been undervalued by nursing practice. For example, noise is a major disturbance in the hospital setting, making it difficult for clients to sleep. Clients are often awakened early for obtaining lab specimens, weights, assessments, and medication administration. Using a conceptual model developed by Dreher, the researchers implemented a nonpharmacologic intervention to promote sleep on a 36-bed medical unit.

Guided by a nurse manager, clinical nurse IV, and gerontological clinical nurse specialist, the certified nursing assistants (CNAs) completed an educational program about how to implement nonpharmacological interventions that promote sleep. The program used "sleep baskets," which held materials needed for the interventions and a list of possible interventions to help remind the CNA (e.g., back rub, warm drink, aromatherapy, a warmed blanket, relaxation music, earplugs, and closed doors).

In preparation for bedtime, the CNA used the sleep basket and asked the client to select sleep interventions. In addition, other noise reduction strategies were used. Staff were reminded to use "quiet voices" after 10 PM and to avoid hallway discussions on the night shift. Doors to client rooms were closed when bedtime routines were completed (unless the client required close monitoring). And, the intercom was not used at night.

To evaluate the effectiveness of the project, the CNA who used a sleep basket on the evening shift completed a form as to which interventions were performed. The next morning, the day CNA asked the client to rate the quality and quantity of sleep, to identify which interventions were the most helpful, and if the nonpharmacological interventions helped them sleep. During the evaluation period, 40 clients (average age of 75) were evaluated. The warmed blanket was their favorite intervention. Seventy-five percent of the clients stated that the interventions helped them sleep, and 60% rated their sleep quality as "good."

Implications

Project interventions appear helpful for sleep improvement, especially during the retiring phase of sleep. The researchers state that the program is now being used on four nursing units. Nurses and CNAs are more aware of clients who have had an exhausting day and try to help these clients take a 45-minute nap by posting signs that say: "Do not disturb. Client napping between the hours of _____ and _____."

Note: From "The Sh-h-h-h Project. Nonpharmacological Interventions" by S. B. Robinson, T. Weitzel, & L. Henderson. (2005). *Holistic Nursing Practice, 19*(6), 263–266. Copyright Lippincott, Williams & Wilkins. Reprinted with permission.

Night shift workers frequently obtain less sleep than other workers and have difficulty falling asleep after getting off work. Wearing dark wrap-around sunglasses during the drive home and light-blocking shades can minimize the alerting effects of exposure to daylight, thus making it easier to fall asleep when body temperature is rising.

EMOTIONAL STRESS Stress is considered by most sleep experts to be the number one cause of short-term sleeping difficulties (National Sleep Foundation, n.d.b). A person preoccupied with personal problems may be unable to relax sufficiently to get to sleep. Anxiety increases the norepinephrine blood levels through stimulation of the sympathetic nervous system. These chemical changes can result in less deep sleep and REM sleep and more stage changes and awakenings.

STIMULANTS AND ALCOHOL Caffeine-containing beverages act as stimulants of the central nervous system. Drinking beverages containing caffeine in the afternoon or evening may interfere with sleep. People who drink an excessive amount of alcohol often find their sleep disturbed. Alcohol disrupts REM sleep, although it may hasten the onset of sleep. While making up for lost REM sleep after some of the effects of the alcohol have worn off, people often experience nightmares. The alcohol-tolerant person may be unable to sleep well and become irritable as a result.

DIET Weight gain has been associated with reduced total sleep time as well as broken sleep and earlier awakening.

Weight loss, on the other hand, seems to be associated with an increase in total sleep time and less broken sleep. Dietary L-tryptophan—found, for example, in cheese and milk—may induce sleep, a fact that might explain why warm milk helps some people get to sleep.

SMOKING Nicotine has a stimulating effect on the body, and smokers often have more difficulty falling asleep than nonsmokers do. Smokers are usually easily aroused and often describe themselves as light sleepers. By refraining from smoking after the evening meal, the person usually sleeps better; moreover, many former smokers report that their sleeping patterns improved once they stopped smoking.

MOTIVATION Motivation can increase alertness in some situations. Motivation alone, however, is usually not sufficient to overcome the normal circadian drive to sleep during the night. Nor is motivation sufficient to overcome sleepiness due to insufficient sleep. Boredom alone is not sufficient to cause sleepiness, but when insufficient sleep combines with boredom, sleep is likely to occur.

MEDICATIONS Some medications affect the quality of sleep. Most hypnotics can interfere with deep sleep and suppress REM sleep. Beta-blockers have been known to cause insomnia and nightmares. Narcotics, such as meperidine hydrochloride (Demerol) and morphine, are known to suppress REM sleep and to cause frequent awakenings and drowsiness. Tranquilizers interfere with REM sleep. Although antidepressants suppress REM sleep, this effect is

---

BOX 31–6	**Drugs that Disrupt Sleep**

These drugs may disrupt REM sleep, delay onset of sleep, or decrease sleep time:

- Alcohol
- Amphetamines
- Antidepressants
- Beta-blockers
- Bronchodilators
- Caffeine
- Decongestants
- Narcotics
- Steroids

CLINICAL MANIFESTATIONS **Insomnia**

- Difficulty falling asleep
- Waking up frequently during the night
- Difficulty returning to sleep
- Waking up too early in the morning
- Unrefreshing sleep
- Daytime sleepiness
- Difficulty concentrating
- Irritability

Note: From "Insomnia Symptoms" by National Sleep Foundation, 2005b. Retrieved from http://www.sleepfoundation.org/article/sleep-related-problems/insomnia-and-sleep. Used with permission of the National Sleep Foundation. For further information, please visit http://www.sleepfoundation.org

---

considered a therapeutic action. In fact, selectively depriving a depressed client of REM sleep will result in an immediate but transient improvement in mood. Clients accustomed to taking hypnotic medications and antidepressants may experience a REM rebound (increased REM sleep) when these medications are discontinued. Warning clients to expect a period of more intense dreams when these medications are discontinued may reduce their anxiety about this symptom. Boxes 31–6 and 31–7 list drugs that can disrupt sleep or cause excessive daytime sleepiness.

Common Sleep Disorders

A knowledge of common sleep disorders can help nurses assess the sleep complaints of their clients and, when appropriate, make a referral to a specialist in sleep disorders medicine. Although sleep disorders are typically categorized for the purpose of research as dysomnias, parasomnias, and disorders associated with medical or psychiatric illness, it is usually more appropriate for clinicians to focus on the client's symptoms occurring during sleep (parasomnias).

INSOMNIA Insomnia is described as the inability to fall asleep or remain asleep. Persons with insomnia awaken not feeling rested. Insomnia is the most common sleep complaint in America. Acute insomnia lasts one to several nights and is often caused by personal stressors and/or worry. If the insomnia persists for longer than a month, it is considered chronic insomnia. More often, people experience chronic-intermittent insomnia, which means difficulty sleeping for a few nights, followed by a few nights of adequate sleep before the problem returns (National Sleep Foundation, 2005a). See Clinical Manifestations for symptoms of insomnia. The two main risk factors of insomnia are older age and female gender (IOM, 2006, p. 91). Women suffer sleep loss in connection with hormonal

changes. The incidence of insomnia increases with age, but it is thought that this is caused by some other medical condition. Treatment for insomnia frequently requires the client to develop new behavior patterns that induce sleep and maintain sleep. Examples of behavioral treatments include the following:

- Stimulus control: creating a sleep environment that promotes sleep
- Cognitive therapy: learning to develop positive thoughts and beliefs about sleep
- Sleep restriction: following a program that limits time in bed in order to get to sleep and stay asleep throughout the night (National Sleep Foundation, 2005a).

The long-term efficacy of hypnotic medications is questionable. Such medications do not deal with the cause of the problem, and their prolonged use can create drug dependencies. Although antihistamines such as diphenhydramine (Benadryl) are thought to be safer for older adult clients than hypnotics, their side effects (i.e., atropine-like effects, dizziness, sedation, and hypotension) make them extremely hazardous. In fact, antihistamines should not be recommended for any client with a history of asthma, increased intraocular pressure, hyperthyroidism, cardiovascular disease, or hypertension.

EXCESSIVE DAYTIME SLEEPINESS Clients may experience excessive daytime sleepiness as a result of hypersomnia, narcolepsy, sleep apnea, and insufficient sleep.

Hypersomnia **Hypersomnia** refers to conditions where the affected individual obtains sufficient sleep at night but still cannot stay awake during the day. Hypersomnia can be caused by medical conditions, for example, central nervous system damage and certain kidney, liver, or metabolic disorders, such as diabetic acidosis and hypothyroidism. Rarely does hypersomnia have a psychological origin.

Narcolepsy **Narcolepsy** is a disorder of excessive daytime sleepiness caused by the lack of the chemical hypocretin in the

---

BOX 31–7	**Drugs that May Cause Excessive Daytime Sleepiness**

These drugs may be associated with excessive daytime sleepiness:

- Antidepressants
- Antihistamines
- Beta-blockers
- Narcotics

---

area of the central nervous system that regulates sleep. Clients with narcolepsy have sleep attacks or excessive daytime sleepiness, and their sleep at night usually begins with a sleep-onset REM period. The majority of clients also have cataplexy or the sudden onset of muscle weakness or paralysis in association with strong emotion, sleep paralysis (transient paralysis when falling asleep or waking up), hypnagogic hallucinations (visual, auditory, or tactile hallucinations at sleep onset or when waking up), and/or fragmented nighttime sleep. Their fragmented nocturnal sleep is not the cause of their excessive daytime sleepiness; many clients, particularly younger clients, have sound restorative nocturnal sleep but still cannot stay awake during the daytime. Onset of symptoms tends to occur between ages 15 and 30, and symptom severity usually stabilizes within the first 5 years of onset. Central nervous system stimulants such as methylphenidate (Ritalin) or amphetamines have been used to reduce excessive daytime sleepiness. Antidepressants, both older MAO inhibitors and the newer sertonergic antidepressants, are usually quite effective for controlling cataplexy. In 1999, the U.S. Food and Drug Administration (FDA), approved modafinil (Provigil) for control of excessive daytime sleepiness in narcoleptic clients. Although its exact mechanism of action is unknown, it has fewer side effects, and a lower potential for abuse. A second drug, sodium oxybate (Xyrem), approved in 2002 for the treatment of cataplexy, has also been shown to reduce excessive daytime sleepiness in clients with narcolepsy. Because Xyrem is difficult to administer (it is available only as a liquid and taken at bedtime and then again 2.5 to 4 hours after sleep onset) and its use is tightly controlled by the FDA, only those clients whose symptoms are not controlled by other medications are usually offered Xyrem. Only one pharmacy in the United States is allowed to dispense Xyrem. As a result, clients need to allow adequate time for obtaining their medications from the central pharmacy.

CLINICAL ALERT

Sodium oxybate is also known as gamma hydroxybutyrate or GHB—one of the drugs frequently associated with "date rapes."

Sleep Apnea   **Sleep apnea** is characterized by frequent short breathing pauses during sleep. Although all individuals have occasional periods of apnea during sleep, more than five apneic episodes or five breathing pauses longer than 10 seconds/hour is considered abnormal and should be evaluated by a sleep medicine specialist. Symptoms suggestive of sleep apnea include loud snoring, frequent nocturnal awakenings, excessive daytime sleepiness, difficulties falling asleep at night, morning headaches, memory and cognitive problems, and irritability. Although sleep apnea is most frequently diagnosed in men and postmenopausal women, it may occur during childhood.

The periods of apnea, which last from 10 seconds to 2 minutes, occur during REM or NREM sleep. Frequency of episodes ranges from 50 to 600 per night. Because these apneic pauses are usually associated with an arousal, clients frequently report that their sleep is nonrestorative and that they regularly fall asleep when engaging in sedentary activities during the day.

Three common types of sleep apnea are obstructive apnea, central apnea, and mixed apnea. Obstructive apnea occurs when the structures of the pharynx or oral cavity block the flow of air. The person continues to try to breathe; that is, the chest and abdominal muscles move. The movements of the diaphragm become stronger and stronger until the obstruction is removed. Enlarged tonsils and adenoids, a deviated nasal septum, nasal polyps, and obesity predispose the client to obstructive apnea. An episode of obstructive sleep apnea usually begins with snoring; thereafter, breathing ceases, followed by marked snorting as breathing resumes. Toward the end of each apneic episode, increased carbon dioxide levels in the blood cause the client to wake.

Central apnea is thought to involve a defect in the respiratory center of the brain. All actions involved in breathing, such as chest movement and airflow, cease. Clients who have brain stem injuries and muscular dystrophy, for example, often have central sleep apnea. At this time, there is no available treatment. Mixed apnea is a combination of central apnea and obstructive apnea.

Treatment for sleep apnea is directed at the cause of the apnea. For example, enlarged tonsils may be removed. Other surgical procedures, including laser removal of excess tissue in the pharynx, reduce or eliminate snoring and may be effective in relieving the apnea. In other cases, the use of a nasal continuous positive airway pressure (CPAP) device at night is effective in maintaining an open airway. Weight loss may also help decrease the severity of symptoms.

Sleep apnea profoundly affects a person's work or school performance. In addition, prolonged sleep apnea can cause a sharp rise in blood pressure and may lead to cardiac arrest. Over time, apneic episodes can cause cardiac arrhythmias, pulmonary hypertension, and subsequent left-sided heart failure.

Insufficient Sleep   Healthy individuals who obtain less sleep than they need will experience sleepiness and fatigue during the daytime hours. Depending on the severity and

CLINICAL ALERT

Partners of clients with sleep apnea may become aware of the problem because they hear snoring that stops during the apneic period and then restarts. Surgical removal of tonsils or other tissue in the pharynx, if not the cause of the sleep apnea, can actually worsen the situation by removing the snoring and, thus, the warning that apnea is occurring.

chronicity of this voluntary, albeit unintentional sleep deprivation, individuals may develop attention and concentration deficits, reduced vigilance, distractibility, reduced motivation, fatigue, malaise, and occasionally diplopia and dry mouth. The cause of these symptoms may or may not be attributed to insufficient sleep, since many Americans believe that 6.8 hours of sleep is sufficient to maintain optimal daytime performance. In fact, the sleep times of Americans have decreased dramatically over the past decade, with adults averaging only 6.8 hours of sleep on weekdays and 7.4 hours on weekends. All age groups, not just adults and adolescents, are getting less than the recommended amounts of sleep. Even 4- to 5-year-old children now average less than 9.5 hours of sleep, approximately 1.5 to 2.5 hours less than recommended.

Although the effects of obtaining less than optimal amounts of sleep are generally considered benign, there is growing evidence that insufficient sleep can have significant deleterious effects. Staying awake 19 consecutive hours produces the same impairments in reaction times and cognitive function as a blood alcohol level of 0.05, and staying awake for 24 consecutive hours has the same effects on reaction times and cognitive function as being legally drunk (with a blood alcohol level of 0.1). Nurses who report reduced hours of sleep are more likely to make an error, to have difficulty staying awake on duty, and to have difficulty staying awake while driving home from work than those who obtained more sleep.

When clients report obtaining more sleep on weekends or days off, it usually indicates that they are not obtaining sufficient sleep. Convincing the client to obtain more sleep may be difficult, but it can result in the resolution of their daytime symptoms.

PARASOMNIAS A **parasomnia** is behavior that may interfere with sleep and may even occur during sleep. The *International Classification of Sleep Disorders* (American Sleep Disorders Association, 2005) subdivides parasomnias into arousal disorders (e.g., sleepwalking, sleep terrors), sleep–wake transition disorders (e.g., sleep talking), parasomnias associated with REM sleep (e.g., nightmares), and others (e.g., bruxism). Box 31–8 describes examples of parasomnias.

NURSING MANAGEMENT

ASSESSING

A complete assessment of a client's sleep difficulty includes a sleep history, health history, physical exam, and, if warranted, a sleep diary and diagnostic studies. Only nurse practitioners with specialized training should investigate a complaint of excessive daytime sleepiness, investigate a sleep complaint lasting more than 6 months, or order and interpret diagnostic studies. All nurses, however, can take a brief sleep history and educate their clients about normal sleep.

Sleep History

A brief sleep history, which is usually part of the comprehensive nursing history, should be obtained for all clients entering a health care facility. It should, however, be deferred or omitted if the client is critically ill. Key questions to ask include the following:

- When do you usually go to sleep? And when do you wake up? Do you nap? If so, when? If the client is a child, it is also important to ask about bedtime rituals. This information provides the nurse with information about the client's usual sleep duration and preferred sleep times, and allows for the incorporation of the client's preferences in the plan of care.
- Do you have any problems with your sleep? Has anyone ever told you that you snore loudly or thrash around a lot at night? Are you able to stay awake at work, when driving, or engaging in your usual activities?

These questions elicit information about sleep complaints including the possibility of excessive daytime sleepiness. Loud snoring suggests the possibility of obstructive sleep apnea, and any client replying yes to this question should be referred to a specialist in sleep disorders medi-

---

BOX 31–8   Parasomnias

- *Bruxism.* Usually occurring during stage II NREM sleep, this clenching and grinding of the teeth can eventually erode dental crowns, cause teeth to come loose, and lead to deterioration of the temporomandibular joint and TMJ syndrome.
- *Enuresis.* Bed-wetting during sleep can occur in children over 3 years old. More males than females are affected. It often occurs 1 to 2 hours after falling asleep, when rousing from NREM stages III and IV.
- *Periodic limb movements (PLMs) disorder.* In this condition, the legs jerk twice or three times per minute during sleep. It is most common among older adults. This kicking motion can wake the client and result in poor sleep. The condition may

be treated with medications such as those otherwise used for Parkinson's disease. PLMs differ from restless leg syndrome (RLS), which occurs whenever the person is at rest, not just at night when sleeping. RLS may occur during pregnancy or be due to other medical problems that can be treated.
- *Sleeptalking.* Talking during sleep occurs during NREM sleep before REM sleep. It rarely presents a problem to the person unless it becomes troublesome to others.
- *Somnambulism.* Somnambulism (sleepwalking) occurs during stages III and IV of NREM sleep. It is episodic and usually occurs 1 to 2 hours after falling asleep. Sleepwalkers tend not to notice dangers (e.g., stairs) and often need to be protected from injury.

cine. Referrals should also be made if clients indicate they have difficulty staying awake during the day or that their movements disturb the sleep of their bed partners.

- Do you take any prescribed medications, over-the-counter medications, or herbal remedies to help you sleep? Or to stay awake?

This information alerts the nurse to the use of prescription hypnotics and stimulants as well as the use of over-the-counter sleep aids and herbal remedies.

- Is there anything else I need to know about your sleep?

This allows the client to voice any concerns or bring up topics that the nurse may not have asked about.

If the client is being admitted to a long-term care facility, it is also appropriate to ask about preferred room temperature, lighting (complete darkness versus using a night-light), and preferred bedtime routine.

A more detailed assessment is required if the client indicates any difficulty sleeping, difficulty remaining awake during the day, and/or recent changes in sleep pattern. This detailed history should explore the exact nature of the problem and its cause, when it first began and its frequency, how it affects daily living, what the client is doing to cope with the problem, and whether these methods have been effective. Questions the nurse might ask the client with a sleeping disturbance are shown in the accompanying Assessment Interview.

Health History

A health history is obtained to rule out medical or psychiatric causes of the client's difficulty sleeping. It is important to note that the presence of a medical or psychiatric illness (e.g., depression, Parkinson's disease, Alzheimer's disease, arthritis, or other disorders) does not preclude the possibility that a second problem (e.g., obstructive sleep apnea) may be contributing to the difficulty sleeping. Since medications can frequently cause or exacerbate sleep disturbances, information should be obtained about all of the prescribed and nonprescription medications, including herbal remedies that a client consumes.

Physical Examination

Rarely are sleep abnormalities noted during the physical exam unless the client has obstructive sleep apnea or some other health problem. Common findings among clients with sleep apnea include an enlarged and reddened uvula and soft palate, enlarged tonsils and adenoids (in children), obesity (in adults), and in male clients a neck size greater than 17.5 inches. Occasionally a deviated septum may be noted, but it is rarely the cause of obstructive sleep apnea.

Sleep Diary

A sleep specialist may ask clients to keep a sleep diary or log for 1 to 2 weeks in order to get a more complete picture of their sleep complaints. A sleep diary may include all or se-

ASSESSMENT INTERVIEW — Sleep Disturbances

- How would you describe your sleeping problem? What changes have occurred in your sleeping pattern? How often does this happen?
- How many cups of coffee, tea, or caffeinated beverages do you drink per day? Do you drink alcohol? If so, how much?
- Do you have difficulty falling asleep?
- Do you wake up often during the night? If so, how often?
- Do you wake up earlier in the morning than you would like and have difficulty falling back to sleep?
- How do you feel when you wake up in the morning?
- Do you sleep more than usual? If so, how often do you sleep?
- Do you have periods of overwhelming sleepiness? If so, when does this happen?
- Have you ever suddenly fallen asleep in the middle of a daytime activity? Does anything unusual happen when you laugh or get angry?
- Has anyone ever told you that you snore, walk in your sleep, or stop breathing for a while when sleeping?
- What have you been doing to deal with this sleeping problem? Does it help?
- What do you think might be causing this problem? Do you have any medical condition that might be causing you to sleep more (or less)? Are you receiving medications for an illness that might alter your sleeping pattern? Are you experiencing any stressful or upsetting events or conflicts that may be affecting your sleep?
- How is your sleeping problem affecting you?

lected aspects of the following information that pertain to the client's specific problem:

- Time of (a) going to bed, (b) trying to fall asleep, (c) falling asleep (approximate time), (d) any instances of waking up and duration of these periods, (e) waking up in the morning, and (f) any naps and their duration
- Activities performed 2 to 3 hours before bedtime (type, duration, and time)
- Consumption of caffeinated beverages and alcohol and amounts of those beverages
- Any prescribed medications, over-the-counter medications, and herbal remedies taken during the day
- Bedtime rituals before sleep
- Any difficulties remaining awake during the day and times when difficulties occurred
- Any worries that the client believes may affect sleep
- Factors that the client believes have a positive or negative effect on sleep

If the client is a child, the sleep diary or log may be completed by a parent.

Diagnostic Studies

Sleep is measured objectively in a sleep disorder laboratory by **polysomnography:** An electroencephalogram

(EEG), electromyogram (EMG), and electro-oculogram (EOG) are recorded simultaneously. Electrodes are placed on the scalp to record brain waves (EEG), on the outer canthus of each eye to record eye movement (EOG), and on the chin muscles to record the structural electromyogram (EMG). The electrodes transmit electric energy from the cerebral cortex and muscles of the face to pens that record the brain waves and muscle activity on graph paper. Respiratory effort and airflow, ECG, leg movements, and oxygen saturation are also monitored. Oxygen saturation is determined by monitoring with a pulse oximeter, a light-sensitive electric cell that attaches to the ear or a finger. Oxygen saturation and ECG assessments are of particular importance if sleep apnea is suspected. Through polysomnography, the client's activity (movements, struggling, noisy respirations) during sleep can be assessed. Such activity of which the client is unaware may be the cause of arousal during sleep.

DIAGNOSING

Insomnia, the NANDA (2009) diagnosis given to clients with sleep problems, is usually made more explicit with descriptions such as "difficulty falling asleep" or "difficulty staying asleep;" for example, "*Insomnia* (delayed onset of sleep) related to overstimulation prior to bedtime."

Various factors or etiologies may be involved and must be specified for the individual. These include physical discomfort or pain; anxiety about actual or anticipated loss of a loved one, loss of a job, loss of life due to serious disease process, or worry about a family member's behavior or illness; frequent changes in sleep time due to shift work or overtime; and changes in sleep environment or bedtime rituals (e.g., noisy environment, alcohol or other drug dependency, drug withdrawal, misuse of sedatives prescribed for insomnia, and effects of medications such as steroids or stimulants). Examples of clinical applications of this diagnosis using NANDA, NIC, and NOC designations are shown in Identifying Nursing Diagnoses, Outcomes, and Interventions.

Sleep pattern disturbances may also be stated as the etiology of another diagnosis, in which case the nursing interventions are directed toward the sleep disturbance itself. Examples include the following:

- *Risk for Injury* related to somnambulism
- *Ineffective Coping* related to insufficient quality and quantity of sleep
- *Fatigue* related to insufficient sleep
- *Risk for Impaired Gas Exchange* related to sleep apnea
- *Deficient Knowledge* (Nonprescription remedies for sleep) related to misinformation
- *Anxiety* related to sleep apnea and/or the diagnosis of a sleep disorder
- *Activity Intolerance* related to sleep deprivation or excessive daytime sleepiness

PLANNING

The major goal for clients with sleep disturbances is to maintain (or develop) a sleeping pattern that provides sufficient energy for daily activities. Other goals may relate to enhancing the client's feeling of well-being or improving the quality and quantity of the client's sleep. The nurse plans specific nursing interventions to reach the goal based on the etiology of each nursing diagnosis. These interventions may include reducing environmental distractions, promoting bedtime rituals, providing comfort measures, scheduling nursing care to provide for uninterrupted sleep periods, and teaching stress reduction, relaxation techniques, or good sleep hygiene.

Examples of NOC outcomes and NIC interventions to assist clients with sleep disturbances are shown in Identifying Nursing Diagnoses, Outcomes, and Interventions. Specific nursing activities associated with each of these interventions can be selected to meet the individual needs of the client. See the Nursing Care Plan and Concept Map on pages 943–945.

IMPLEMENTING

Sleep hygiene is a term referring to interventions used to promote sleep. Nursing interventions to enhance the quantity and quality of clients' sleep involve largely nonpharmacologic measures. These involve health teaching about sleep habits, support of bedtime rituals, the provision of a restful environment, specific measures to promote comfort and relaxation, and appropriate use of hypnotic medications.

For hospitalized clients, sleep problems are often related to the hospital environment or their illness. Assisting the client to sleep in such instances can be challenging to a nurse, often involving scheduling activities, administering analgesics, and providing a supportive environment. Explanations and a supportive relationship are essential for the fearful or anxious client. Different types of hypnotics may be prescribed depending on the type of sleep problem (e.g., difficulties falling asleep or difficulties maintaining sleep). Drugs with longer half-lives are often prescribed for difficulties maintaining sleep, but must be used with caution in older adults.

Client Teaching

Healthy individuals need to learn the importance of sleep in maintaining active and productive lifestyles. They need to learn (a) the conditions that promote sleep and those that interfere with sleep, (b) safe use of sleep medications, (c) effects of other prescribed medications on sleep, and (d) effects of their disease states on sleep. Client teaching for promoting sleep is shown in Client Teaching.

Supporting Bedtime Rituals

Most people are accustomed to bedtime rituals or presleep routines that are conducive to comfort and relaxation. Altering or eliminating such routines can affect a client's

Clients with Sleep Problems

DATA CLUSTER Gillian Marks, 51, states she has had a problem falling asleep since her mastectomy 2 months ago. Says fears of prognosis become prominent when she is not active and busy. Has tried reading or watching TV but neither makes her sleepy or relaxed. Appears agitated and restless.

NURSING DIAGNOSIS/DEFINITION	SAMPLE DESIRED OUTCOMES*/ DEFINITION	INDICATORS	SELECTED INTERVENTIONS*/ DEFINITION	SAMPLE NIC ACTIVITIES
Insomnia/A disruption in amount and quality of sleep that impairs functioning	Personal Well-Being [2002]/Extent of positive perception of one's own health status and life circumstances	Very satisfied with • Ability to relax • Ability to express emotions	Coping Enhancement [5230]/Assisting a patient to adapt to perceived stressors, changes, or threats that interfere with meeting life demands and roles	• Appraise adjustment to changes in body image • Explore previous methods of dealing with life problems • Encourage verbalization of feelings, perceptions, and fears • Instruct on the use of relaxation techniques

DATA CLUSTER Thomas Strep states that a recent shortage of paramedics has resulted in extensive overtime and frequent "double shifts" and rotations from his usual two weekly 7–3 and 3–7 shifts. States, "All I want to do is go to sleep when I get home, but I can't. I guess I'm too riled up."

| Sleep Deprivation/Prolonged periods of time without sleep (sustained natural, periodic suspension of relative consciousness) | Rest [0003]/Quantity and pattern of diminished activity for mental and physical rejuvenation | Not compromised • Amount of rest • Rest pattern • Mentally rested | Progressive Muscle Relaxation [1460]/Facilitating the tensing and releasing of successive muscle groups while attending to the resulting differences in sensation Simple Guided Imagery [6000]/Purposeful use of imagination to achieve relaxation and/or direct attention away from undesirable sensations | • Choose quiet, comfortable setting • Have the client tense, for 5 to 10 seconds, each of 8 to 16 major muscle groups • Instruct client to focus on the sensations in the muscles when tensed and when relaxed • Discuss an image the client has experienced that is pleasurable and relaxing, such as lying on a beach, watching a snowfall, floating on a raft • Choose a scene that involves as many of the senses as possible • Have the client travel mentally to the scene and report how it smells, looks, feels, etc. • Assist the client to develop a method of ending the imagery such as counting while breathing deeply |

*The NOC # for desired outcomes and the NIC # for nursing interventions are listed in brackets following the appropriate outcome or intervention. Outcomes, indicators, interventions, and activities selected are only a sample of those suggested by NOC and NIC and should be further individualized for each client.

sleep. Common prebedtime activities of adults include listening to music, reading, taking a soothing bath, and praying. Children need to be socialized into a presleep routine such as a bedtime story, holding onto a favorite toy or blanket, and kissing everyone goodnight. Sleep is also usually preceded by hygienic routines, such as washing the face and hands (or bathing), brushing the teeth, and voiding.

In institutional settings, nurses can provide similar bedtime rituals—assisting with a hand and face wash, providing a massage or hot drink, plumping of pillows, and providing extra blankets as needed. Conversing about accomplishments of the day or enjoyable events such as visits from friends can also help to relax clients and bring peace of mind.

CLIENT TEACHING   Promoting Sleep

Sleep Pattern

- If you have difficulty falling asleep or staying asleep, it is important to establish a regular bedtime and wake-up time for all days of the week to enhance your biological rhythm. A short daytime nap (e.g., 15 to 30 minutes), particularly among older adults, can be restorative and not interfere with nighttime sleep. A younger person with insomnia should not nap.
- Establish a regular, relaxing bedtime routine before sleep such as reading, listening to soft music, taking a warm bath, or doing some other quiet activity you enjoy.
- Avoid dealing with office work or family problems before bedtime.
- Get adequate exercise during the day to reduce stress, but avoid excessive physical exertion at least 3 hours before bedtime.
- Use the bed for sleep or sexual activity, so that you associate it with sleep. Take work material, computers, and TVs out of the bedroom. Lying awake, tossing and turning, will strengthen the association between wakefulness and lying in bed (many people with insomnia report falling asleep in a chair or in front of the TV but having trouble falling asleep in bed).
- When you are unable to sleep, get out of bed, go into another room, and pursue some relaxing activity until you feel drowsy.

Environment

- Create a sleep-conducive environment that is dark, quiet, comfortable, and cool.

- Keep noise to a minimum; block out extraneous noise as necessary with white noise from a fan, air conditioner, or white noise machine. Music is not recommended as studies have shown that music will promote wakefulness (it is interesting and people will pay attention to it).
- Sleep on a comfortable mattress and pillows.

Diet

- Avoid heavy meals 2 to 3 hours before bedtime.
- Avoid alcohol and caffeine-containing foods and beverages (e.g., coffee, tea, chocolate) at least 4 hours before bedtime. Caffeine can interfere with sleep. Both caffeine and alcohol act as diuretics, creating the need to void during sleep time.
- If a bedtime snack is necessary, consume only light carbohydrates or a milk drink. Heavy or spicy foods can cause gastrointestinal upsets that disturb sleep.

Medications

- Use sleeping medications only as a last resort. Use over-the-counter medications sparingly because many contain antihistamines that cause daytime drowsiness.
- Take analgesics before bedtime to relieve aches and pains.
- Consult with your health care provider about adjusting other medications that may cause insomnia.

Creating a Restful Environment

All people need a sleeping environment with minimal noise, a comfortable room temperature, appropriate ventilation, and appropriate lighting. Although most people prefer a darkened environment, a low light source may provide comfort for children or those in a strange environment. Infants and children need a quiet room usually separate from the parents' room, a light or warm blanket as appropriate, and a location away from open windows or drafts.

Environmental distractions such as environmental noises and staff communication noise are particularly trou-
blesome for hospitalized clients. Environmental noises include the sound of paging systems, telephones, and call lights; doors closing; elevator chimes; furniture squeaking; and linen carts being wheeled through corridors. Staff communication is a major factor creating noise, particularly at staff change of shift.

To create a restful environment, the nurse needs to reduce environmental distractions, reduce sleep interruptions, ensure a safe environment, and provide a room temperature that is satisfactory to the client. Some interventions to reduce environmental distractions, especially noise, are listed in Box 31–9.

BOX 31–9   **Reducing Environmental Distractions in Hospitals**

- Close window curtains if street lights shine through.
- Close curtains between clients in semiprivate and larger rooms.
- Reduce or eliminate overhead lighting; provide a night-light at the bedside or in the bathroom.
- Use a flashlight to check drainage bags, etc., without turning on the overhead lights.
- Ensure a clear pathway around the bed to avoid bumping the bed and jarring the client during sleeping hours.
- Close the door of the client's room.
- Adhere to agency policy about times to turn off communal televisions or radios.

- Lower the ring tone of nearby telephones.
- Discontinue use of the paging system after a certain hour (e.g., 2100 hours) or reduce its volume.
- Keep required staff conversations at low levels; conduct nursing reports or other discussions in a separate area away from client rooms.
- Wear rubber-soled shoes.
- Ensure that all cart wheels are well oiled.
- Perform only essential noisy activities during sleeping hours.

The environment must also be safe so that the client can relax. People who are unaccustomed to narrow hospital beds may feel more secure with side rails.

Additional safety measures include:

- Placing beds in low positions.
- Using night-lights.
- Placing call bells within easy reach.

Promoting Comfort and Relaxation

Comfort measures are essential to help the client fall asleep and stay asleep, especially if the effects of the person's illness interfere with sleep. A concerned, caring attitude, along with the following interventions, can significantly promote client comfort and sleep:

- Provide loose-fitting nightwear.
- Assist clients with hygienic routines.
- Make sure the bed linen is smooth, clean, and dry.
- Assist or encourage the client to void before bedtime.
- Offer to provide a back massage before sleep.
- Position dependent clients appropriately to aid muscle relaxation, and provide supportive devices to protect pressure areas.
- Schedule medications, especially diuretics, to prevent nocturnal awakenings.
- For clients who have pain, administer analgesics 30 minutes before sleep.
- Listen to the client's concerns and deal with problems as they arise.

People of any age, but especially older adults, are unable to sleep well if they feel cold. Changes in circulation, metabolism, and body tissue density reduce the older person's ability to generate and conserve heat. To compound this problem, hospital gowns have short sleeves and are made of thin polyester. Bed sheets also are often made of polyester rather than a warm fabric, such as cotton flannel. The following interventions can be used to keep older adults warm during sleep:

- Before the client goes to bed, warm the bed with prewarmed bath blankets.
- Use 100% cotton flannel sheets or apply thermal blankets between the sheet and bedspread.
- Encourage the client to wear own clothing, such as flannel nightgown or pajamas, socks, leg warmers, long underwear, sleeping cap (if scalp hair is sparse), or sweater, or use extra blankets.

Emotional stress obviously interferes with a person's ability to relax, rest, and sleep, and inability to sleep further aggravates feelings of tension. Sleep rarely occurs until a person is relaxed. Relaxation techniques can be encouraged as part of the nightly routine. Slow, deep breathing for a few minutes followed by slow, rhythmic contraction and relaxation of muscles can alleviate tension and induce calm. Imagery, meditation, and yoga can also be taught. These techniques are discussed in Chapter 5 ∞.

Enhancing Sleep with Medications

Sleep medications often prescribed on a prn (as-needed) basis for clients include the sedative-hypnotics, which induce sleep, and antianxiety drugs or tranquilizers, which decrease anxiety and tension. When prn sleep medications are ordered in institutional settings, the nurse is responsible for making decisions with the client about when to administer them. These medications should be administered only with complete knowledge of their actions and effects and only when indicated.

Both nurses and clients need to be aware of the actions, effects, and risks of the specific medication prescribed. Although medications vary in their activity and effects, considerations include the following:

- Sedative-hypnotic medications produce a general central nervous system (CNS) depression and an unnatural sleep; REM or NREM sleep is altered to some extent and daytime drowsiness and a morning hangover effect may occur. Some of the new hypnotics, such as zolpidem (Ambien), do not alter REM sleep or produce rebound insomnia when discontinued.
- Antianxiety medications decrease levels of arousal by facilitating the action of neurons in the CNS that suppress responsiveness to stimulation. These medications are contraindicated in pregnant women because of their associated risk of congenital anomalies, and in breast-feeding mothers because the medication is excreted in breast milk.
- Sleep medications vary in their onset and duration of action and will impair waking function as long as they are chemically active. Some medication effects can last many hours beyond the time that the client's perception of daytime drowsiness and impaired psychomotor skills have disappeared. Clients need to be cautioned about such effects and about driving or handling machinery while the drug is in their system.
- Sleep medications affect REM sleep more than NREM sleep. Clients need to be informed that one or two nights of increased dreaming (REM rebound) are usual after the drug is discontinued after long-term use.
- Initial doses of medications should be low and increases added gradually, depending on the client's response. Older adults, in particular, are susceptible to side effects because of their metabolic changes; they need to be closely monitored for changes in mental alertness and coordination. Clients need to be instructed to take the smallest effective dose and then only for a few nights or intermittently as required.
- Regular use of any sleep medication can lead to tolerance over time (e.g., 4 to 6 weeks) and rebound insomnia. In some instances, this may lead clients to increase the dosage. Clients must be cautioned about developing a pattern of drug dependency.

- Abrupt cessation of barbiturate sedative-hypnotics can create withdrawal symptoms such as restlessness, tremors, weakness, insomnia, increased heart rate, seizures, convulsions, and even death. Long-term users need to taper their medications under the supervision of a specialist.

About half of the clients who seek medical intervention for sleep problems are treated with sedative-hypnotics (Vitiello, 1999). Sometimes the prescription of hypnotics can be appropriate. For example, women with chronic difficulties maintaining sleep or nonrestorative sleep associated with menopausal symptoms often benefit by the prescription of 10 mg of zolpidem, a low dose that was documented to be both safe and efficacious in this population. Hypnotics are not appropriate if clients have any symptoms suggestive of sleep-related breathing disorders, or decreased renal and/or hepatic function.

Table 31–4 presents some of the common medications used for enhancing sleep and the half-life of these medications. The half-life represents how long it takes for half of the medication to be metabolized and eliminated by the body; hence, those with shorter half-lives are less likely to cause residual drowsiness after administration, but may be less effective for the treatment of sleep maintenance insomnia.

EVALUATING

Using data collected during care and the desired outcomes developed during the planning stage as a guide, the nurse judges whether client goals and outcomes have been achieved. Data collection may include (a) observations of the duration of the client's sleep, (b) questions about how the client feels on awakening, or (c) observations of the client's level of alertness during the day. Examples of client goals

---

| DRUG CAPSULE | The Client with Medications that Affect Sleep or Alertness *zolpidem* (Ambien) |

Zolpidem is used for the short-term management of insomnia. The medication is used to reduce sleep latency and awakenings, and to lengthen sleep durations. Unlike traditional benzodiazepine sedative-hypnotics, zolpidem does not reduce REM sleep durations or cause rebound insomnia when the drug is discontinued. At therapeutic doses, it causes little or no respiratory depression, and it has a low potential for abuse. Clients using it for short periods have not demonstrated tolerance, physical dependence, or withdrawal symptoms. It has a rapid onset of action and a half-life of 2.6 hours.

Nursing Responsibilities

- The drug has a rapid onset of action, so it should not be given until just prior to bedtime in order to minimize sedation while awake.

- Clients should be monitored for side effects (e.g., daytime drowsiness and dizziness). Older clients and those with hepatic insufficiency should start with a lower dose (e.g., 5 mg).

Client and Family Teaching

- Clients should be cautioned that zolpidem can intensify the actions of other CNS depressants and warned against combining zolpidem with alcohol and all other drugs that depress CNS function.
- Clients should be cautioned not to take this medication until they are ready to go to bed because of its rapid onset of action.

---

modafinil (Provigil)

Modafinil has recently been approved by the FDA for the treatment of narcolepsy, excessive daytime sleepiness associated with obstructive sleep apnea, and shift work sleep disorder. Because the drug does not alter the function of the dopamine neurotransmitter system, modafinil lacks the addictive potential of traditional stimulants. It has a long half-life (approximately 15 hours) and thus can usually be administered only once a day (in the morning). It does not interfere with sleep at night.

Nursing Responsibilities

- Monitor the client for side effects, particularly if the client is an older adult or has hepatic dysfunction. Side effects are rare and usually consist of headache, nausea, and nervousness.
- If the client has obstructive sleep apnea, ensure that the client continues to use nasal CPAP.

Client and Family Teaching

- Explain that modafinil is not a substitute for obtaining adequate amounts of sleep. Any client with the diagnosis of narcolepsy, obstructive sleep apnea, or shift work sleep disorder needs to obtain adequate amounts of sleep in addition to taking prescribed medications.
- Caution clients with obstructive sleep apnea that it is very important to continue using nasal CPAP and that modafinil is being prescribed only to reduce excessive daytime sleepiness and will not reduce the number of apneic episodes during sleep.
- Modafinil may accelerate the metabolism of oral contraceptives, leading to lower plasma levels. Women using low-dose birth control pills may want to consider switching birth control methods or adding a second type of birth control.

Note: Prior to administering any medication, review all aspects with a current drug handbook or other reliable source.

TABLE 31–4 Selected Sedative-Hypnotic Medications Used for Insomnia

MEDICATION	HALF-LIFE
Chloral hydrate (Noctec)	7–10 hours
Eszopiclone (Lunesta)	6 hours
Ethchlorvynol (Placidyl)	10–20 hours
Flurazepam (Dalmane)	47–100 hours
Glutethimide (Doriden)	1–12 hours
Lorazepam (Ativan)	10–20 hours
Melatonin	1 hour
Temazepam (Restoril)	9–15 hours
Triazolam (Halcion)	1.5–5.5 hours
Zaleplon (Sonata)	1 hour
Zolpidem (Ambien)	2.6 hours

and related outcomes are shown in Identifying Nursing Diagnoses, Outcomes, and Interventions earlier in this chapter.

If the desired outcomes are not achieved, the nurse and client should explore the reasons, which may include answers to the following questions:

- Were etiologic factors correctly identified?
- Has the client's physical condition or medication therapy changed?
- Did the client comply with instructions about establishing a regular sleep–wake pattern?
- Did the client avoid ingesting caffeine?
- Did the client participate in stimulating daytime activities to avoid excessive daytime naps?
- Were all possible measures taken to provide a restful environment for the client?
- Were the comfort and relaxation measures effective?

Nursing Care Plan Sleep

ASSESSMENT DATA	NURSING DIAGNOSIS	DESIRED OUTCOMES*
Nursing Assessment		
Jack Harrison is a 36-year-old police officer assigned to a high-crime police precinct. One week ago he received a surface bullet wound to his arm. Today he arrives at the outpatient clinic to have the wound redressed. While speaking with the nurse, Mr. Harrison mentions that he has recently been promoted to the rank of detective and has assumed new responsibilities. He states that since his promotion, he has experienced increasing difficulty falling asleep and sometimes staying asleep. He expresses concern over the danger of his occupation and his desire to do well in his new position. He complains of waking up feeling tired and irritable.	*Insomnia* related to anxiety (as evidenced by difficulty falling and remaining asleep, fatigue, and irritability)	Sleep [0004] as evidenced by: • Sleeps through the night consistently • Feels rejuvenated after sleep • No dependence on sleep aids
Physical Examination Height: 185.4 cm (6′2″) Weight: 85.7 kg (189 lb) Temperature: 37.0°C (98.6°F) Pulse: 80 BPM Respirations: 18/minute Blood pressure: 144/88 mm Hg **Diagnostic Data** CBC within normal range, x-ray left arm: evidence of superficial soft tissue injury		

NURSING INTERVENTIONS*/SELECTED ACTIVITIES	RATIONALE
Sleep Enhancement [1850]	
Determine the client's sleep and activity pattern.	*The amount of sleep an individual needs varies with lifestyle, health, and age.*
Encourage Mr. Harrison to establish a bedtime routine to facilitate transition from wakefulness to sleep.	*Rituals and routines induce comfort, relaxation, and sleep.*
Encourage him to eliminate stressful situations before bedtime.	*Stress interferes with a person's ability to relax, rest, and sleep.*
Instruct Mr. Harrison and significant others about factors (e.g., physiologic, psychologic, lifestyle, frequent work shift changes, excessively long work hours, and other environmental factors) that contribute to sleep pattern disturbances.	*Knowledge of causative factors can enable the client to begin to control factors that inhibit sleep.*

(continued)

Nursing Care Plan   Sleep *(continued)*

NURSING INTERVENTIONS*/SELECTED ACTIVITIES	RATIONALE
Sleep Enhancement [1850]	
Discuss with Mr. Harrison and his family comfort measures, sleep-promoting techniques, and lifestyle changes that can contribute to optimal sleep.	*Knowledge of factors that affect sleep enables the client to implement changes in lifestyle and prebedtime activities.*
Monitor bedtime food and beverage intake for items that facilitate or interfere with sleep.	*Milk and protein foods contain tryptophan, a precursor of serotonin, which is thought to induce and maintain sleep. Stimulants should be avoided because they inhibit sleep.*
Security Enhancement [5380]	
Discuss specific situations or individuals that threaten Mr. Harrison or his family.	*Fear is reduced when the reality of a situation is confronted in a safe environment. Awareness of factors that cause intensification of fears enhances control.*
Assist him to use coping responses that have been successful in the past.	*Feelings of safety and security increase when an individual identifies previously successful ways of dealing with anxiety-provoking or fearful situations.*
Anxiety Reduction [5820]	
Create an atmosphere to facilitate trust.	*Trust is an essential first step in the therapeutic relationship.*
Seek to understand Mr. Harrison's perspective of a stressful situation.	*Anxiety is a feeling aroused by a vague, nonspecific threat. Identifying the client's perspective will facilitate planning for the best approach to anxiety reduction.*
Encourage verbalization of feelings, perceptions, and fears.	*Open expression of feelings facilitates identification of specific emotions such as anger or helplessness, distorted perceptions, and unrealistic fears.*
Determine the client's decision-making ability.	*Maladaptive coping mechanisms are characterized by an inability to make decisions and choices.*

EVALUATION

Outcome met. Mr. Harrison acknowledges his insomnia is a somatic expression of his anxiety regarding job promotion and fear of failing. He states that talking with the police department counselor has been helpful. He is practicing relaxation techniques each night and sleeps an average of 7 hours a night. Mr. Harrison expresses a feeling of being rested upon awakening.

The NOC # for desired outcomes and the NIC # for nursing interventions are listed in brackets following the appropriate outcome or intervention. Outcomes, interventions, and activities selected are only a sample of those suggested by NOC and NIC and should be further individualized for each client.

CRITICAL THINKING QUESTIONS

1. What further information would be helpful to obtain from Mr. Harrison about his sleep problem?

2. What suggestions can you make that may help him develop better sleep habits?

3. What are the most common problems that interfere with clients' ability to sleep?

∞ *See Answers in MyNursingKit.*

CONCEPT MAP   Sleep

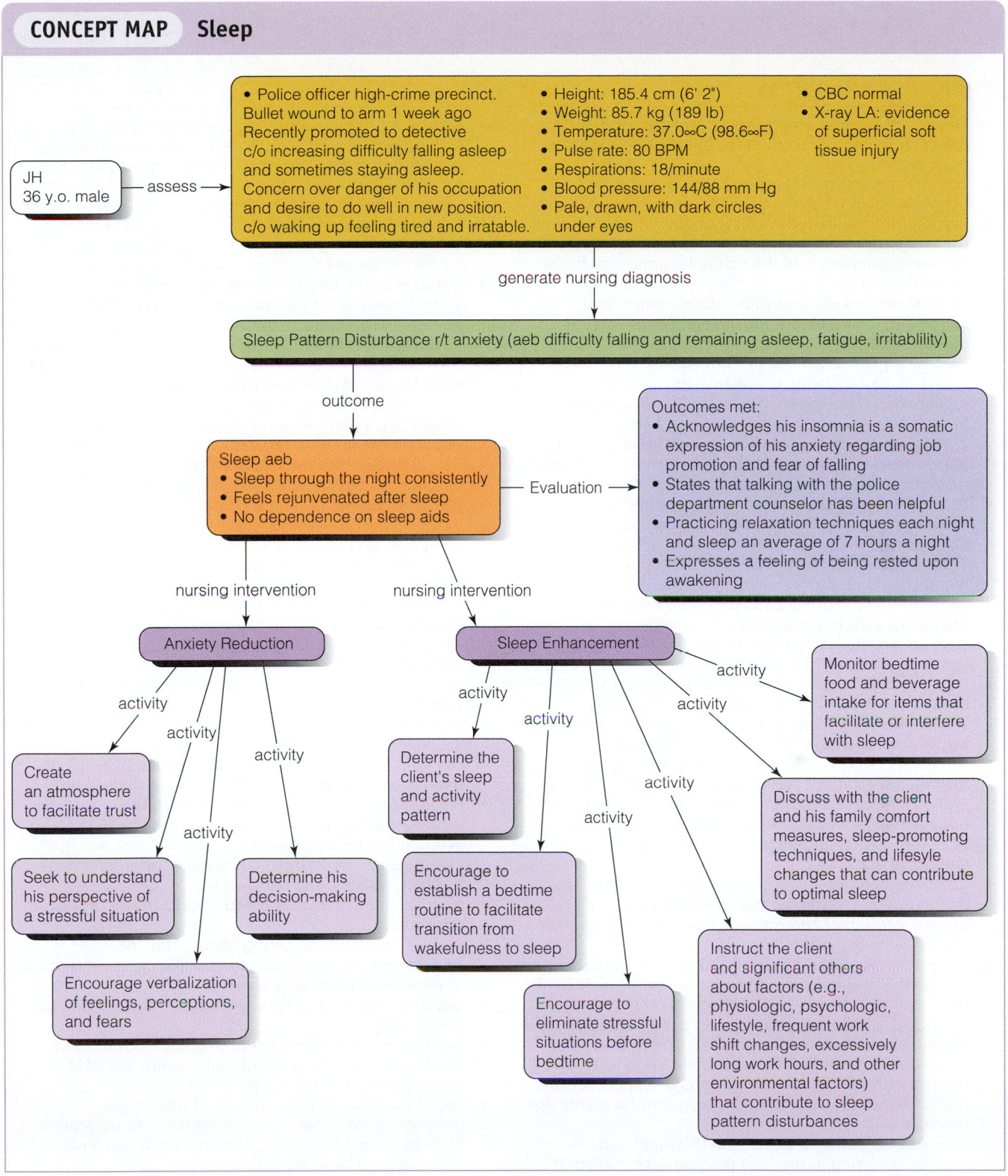

JH
36 y.o. male

→ assess →

• Police officer high-crime precinct.
  Bullet wound to arm 1 week ago
  Recently promoted to detective
  c/o increasing difficulty falling asleep
  and sometimes staying asleep.
  Concern over danger of his occupation
  and desire to do well in new position.
  c/o waking up feeling tired and irratable.

• Height: 185.4 cm (6' 2")
• Weight: 85.7 kg (189 lb)
• Temperature: 37.0∞C (98.6∞F)
• Pulse rate: 80 BPM
• Respirations: 18/minute
• Blood pressure: 144/88 mm Hg
• Pale, drawn, with dark circles
  under eyes

• CBC normal
• X-ray LA: evidence
  of superficial soft
  tissue injury

↓ generate nursing diagnosis

Sleep Pattern Disturbance r/t anxiety (aeb difficulty falling and remaining asleep, fatigue, irritablility)

↓ outcome

Sleep aeb
• Sleep through the night consistently
• Feels rejunvenated after sleep
• No dependence on sleep aids

— Evaluation →

Outcomes met:
• Acknowledges his insomnia is a somatic
  expression of his anxiety regarding job
  promotion and fear of falling
• States that talking with the police
  department counselor has been helpful
• Practicing relaxation techniques each night
  and sleep an average of 7 hours a night
• Expresses a feeling of being rested upon
  awakening

nursing intervention ↓   nursing intervention ↓

Anxiety Reduction   **Sleep Enhancement**

activity ↓   activity ↓   activity   activity   activity →

Create
an atmosphere
to facilitate trust

Monitor bedtime
food and beverage
intake for items that
facilitate or interfere
with sleep

activity   activity

Seek to understand
his perspective of
a stressful situation

Determine his
decision-making
ability

Determine the
client's sleep
and activity
pattern

Discuss with the client
and his family comfort
measures, sleep-promoting
techniques, and lifesyle
changes that can contribute
to optimal sleep

activity

Encourage verbalization
of feelings, perceptions,
and fears

Encourage to
establish a bedtime
routine to facilitate
transition from
wakefulness to sleep

Instruct the client
and significant others
about factors (e.g.,
physiologic, psychologic,
lifestyle, frequent work
shift changes, excessively
long work hours, and other
environmental factors)
that contribute to sleep
pattern disturbances

Encourage to
eliminate stressful
situations before
bedtime

CHAPTER HIGHLIGHTS

- The ability to move freely, easily, and purposefully in the environment is essential for people to meet their basic needs.
- Exercise and activity are essential components for maintaining and regaining health and wellness.
- Purposeful coordinated movement of the body relies on the integrated functioning of the musculoskeletal system, the nervous system, and the vestibular apparatus of the inner ear.
- Body movement involves four basic elements: body alignment, joint mobility, balance, and coordinated movement.
- Exercise is physical activity performed to maintain muscle tone and joint mobility, to enhance physiologic functioning of body systems, and to improve physical fitness. Activity tolerance is the type and amount of exercise or daily living activities an individual is able to perform without experiencing adverse effects. Functional strength is the ability to do work.
- Exercise is classified as either isotonic, isometric, or isokinetic and as either aerobic or anaerobic.
- Many factors influence body alignment and activity. These include growth and development, physical health, mental health, personal values and attitudes, medications, and prescribed limitations to movement.
- Immobility affects almost every body organ and system adversely; complications also include psychosocial problems. Exercise, by contrast, provides many benefits to the same body organs and systems, and can actually be used to prevent and treat many disease processes.
- Problems of immobility include disuse osteoporosis and atrophy; contractures; diminished cardiac reserve; orthostatic hypotension; venous stasis, edema, and thrombus formation; decreased respiratory movement and pooling of secretions; decreased metabolic rate and negative nitrogen balance; urinary stasis, retention, infection, and calculi; constipation; and varying emotional reactions.
- Complete bed rest is almost never required, and is usually dangerous due to the hazards of immobility. A risk-benefit assessment and ongoing assessment of rationale for complete bed rest is essential.
- The nurse has responsibilities (a) to determine root causes of immobility and address these whenever possible (with the client) with the goal of getting the client moving as much and as soon as possible, (b) to prevent the complications of immobility and reduce the severity of any problems resulting from immobility, and (c) to partner with the client and appropriate support persons to design individualized exercise programs for clients that promote wellness.
- Assessment relative to a client's activity and exercise includes a nursing history and physical examination of body alignment, gait, joint appearance and movement, capabilities and limitations for movement, muscle mass and strength, activity tolerance, and problems related to immobility.
- An activity and exercise history includes daily activity level, activity tolerance, type and frequency of exercise, and factors affecting mobility.
- NANDA nursing diagnoses that relate to activity and mobility problems include *Activity Intolerance, Risk for Activity Intolerance, Impaired Physical Mobility,* and *Risk for Disuse Syndrome.* Other relevant diagnoses are *Self-Care Deficit, Risk for Injury, Fear* (of falling), *Powerlessness, Low Self-Esteem, Ineffective Coping,* and, if the client is immobilized, many other potential problems such as *Ineffective Airway Clearance* and *Risk for Infection.*
- Nurses must use good body mechanics in their daily work and especially when moving and turning clients in bed and assisting clients to make transfers. Proper body mechanics do not ensure protection from injury, however, and nurses and caregivers are encouraged to avoid manual lifting and repositioning of clients. At the very least, they should avoid solo lifting, repositioning, and transferring.
- Positioning a client in good body alignment and changing the position regularly and systematically are essential aspects of nursing practice.
- Before positioning dependent clients, the nurse should plan a systematic 24-hour schedule for position changes, including positions that provide for full extension of the neck, hips, and knees. The nurse also uses appropriate supportive devices to maintain alignment and prevent strain on the client's muscles and joints.
- Before moving, turning, or transferring a client, the nurse must consider the client's health status and degree of exertion permitted, physical ability to assist, ability to comprehend instruction, degree of discomfort, client's weight, and whether to use assistive devices or another caregiver to assist.
- Ambulating techniques that facilitate normal walking gait yet provide needed supports are most effective. The nurse can assist clients to prepare for ambulation by helping them become as independent as possible while in bed.
- Preambulatory exercises that strengthen the muscles for walking are essential for clients who have been immobilized for a prolonged period.
- Clients need specific instructions about appropriate use of canes, walkers, and crutches.
- Insufficient sleep is widespread among all age groups in this country.
- Sleep is a naturally occurring altered state of consciousness in which a person's perception and reaction to the environment are decreased.
- Sleep is needed for optimal physiologic and psychologic functioning.
- During a normal night's sleep, an adult has four to six sleep cycles, each with NREM (quiet sleep) and REM (rapid-eye-movement) sleep.
- NREM (slow-wave) sleep consists of four stages, progressing from stage I, very light sleep, to stages III and IV, deep sleep. NREM sleep predominates during naps and nocturnal sleep periods.
- REM sleep recurs about every 90 minutes and is often associated with dreaming.
- Many factors can affect sleep, including illness, environment, lifestyle, emotional stress, stimulants and alcohol, diet, smoking, motivation, and medications.
- Assessment of a client's sleep includes obtaining a sleep history, obtaining a health history, and

conducting a physical examination to detect signs suggestive of sleep apnea.
- Nursing responsibilities to help clients sleep include (a) teaching clients ways to enhance sleep, (b) supporting bedtime rituals, (c) creating a restful environment,

(d) promoting comfort and relaxation, and (e) using prescribed sleep medications.
- Nonpharmacologic interventions to induce and maintain sleep are always the preferred interventions.

THINK ABOUT IT

Refer to the chapter-opening scenario and answer these questions.

1. As the nurse admitting Miriam to the provider's office, what impact would you associate with Miriam's sleep deprivation and her symptoms of hypertension? Explain your answer.

2. What recommendations would you make in order to help Miriam sleep soundly through the night?

3. What referrals may be required for Miriam to help her to return to normal sleep behaviors?

∞   *See suggested responses to Think About It on MyNursingKit.*

TEST YOUR KNOWLEDGE

1. To increase stability during client transfer, the nurse increases the base of support by performing which of the following?
1. Leaning slightly backward
2. Spacing the feet farther apart
3. Tensing the abdominal muscles
4. Bending the knees

2. The nurse promotes isotonic exercises such as walking in order to achieve which of the following? Select all that apply.
1. Increase muscle tone and improve circulation
2. Increase blood pressure
3. Increase muscle mass and strength
4. Decrease heart rate and cardiac output
5. Maintain joint range of motion

3. Five minutes after the client's first postoperative exercise, the client's vital signs have not yet returned to baseline. An appropriate nursing diagnosis might be
1. *Activity Intolerance.*
2. *Risk for Activity Intolerance.*
3. *Impaired Physical Mobility.*
4. *Risk for Disuse Syndrome.*

4. The nurse receives an order for each of the following drugs for an older adult client at risk for falling. Which would the nurse question?
1. Sinemet
2. Benzodiazepines
3. Elavil
4. Lasix

5. The client is ambulating for the first time after surgery. The client tells the nurse, "I feel faint." The best action by the nurse includes which of the following?
1. Find another nurse for help.
2. Return the client to her room as quickly as possible.
3. Tell the client to take rapid, shallow breaths.
4. Assist the client to a nearby chair.

6. The nurse is performing an assessment of an immobilized client. Which of the following assessments causes the nurse to take action?
1. Heart rate 86
2. Reddened area on sacrum
3. Nonproductive cough
4. Urine output of 50 mL/hour

7. A client is admitted for a sleep disorder. The nurse is explaining the role of the RAS in regulating sleep and wake sites and demonstrates its location at which of the following locations in the figure?

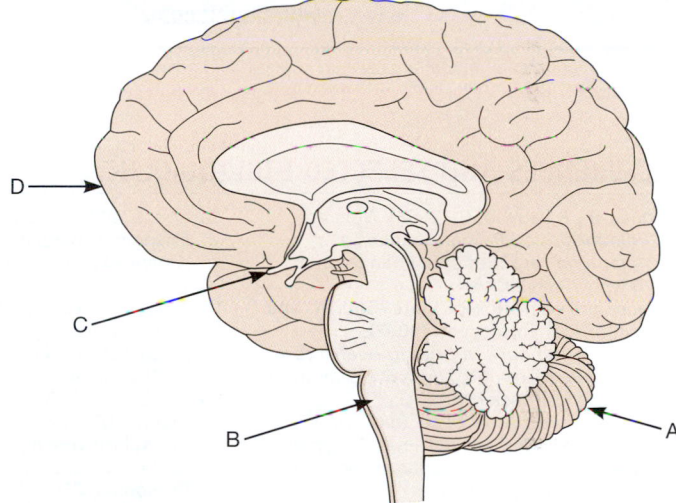

1. A
2. B
3. C
4. D

8. A client has a history of sleep apnea. A priority nursing interview question is which of the following?
1. "Do you have a history of cardiac irregularities?"
2. "Do you have a history of any kind of nasal obstruction?"
3. "Have you had chest pain with or without activity?"
4. "Do you have difficulty with daytime sleepiness?"

9. A client reports to the nurse that she has been taking barbiturate sleeping pills every night for several months and wants to stop taking them. The nurse advises the client to:
1. Take the last pill on a Friday night so disrupted sleep can be compensated on the weekend.
2. Continue to take the pills since sleeping without them after such a long time will be difficult and perhaps impossible.

3. Discontinue taking the pills.

4. Continue taking the pills and discuss tapering the dose with the primary care provider.

10. During a well-child visit, a mother tells the nurse that her 4-year old daughter typically goes to bed at 10:30 PM and awakens each morning at 7 AM. She does not take a nap in the afternoon. Which of the following is the best response?

1. Encourage the mother to consider putting her daughter to bed between 8 and 9 PM.

2. Reassure the mother that it is normal for 4-year-olds to resist napping, but encourage her to insist that she rest quietly each afternoon.

3. Recommend that her daughter be allowed to sleep later in the morning.

4. Reassure her that her daughter's sleep pattern is normal and that she has outgrown her need for an afternoon nap.

∞ *See answers to Test Your Knowledge in Appendix A.*

EXPLORE PEARSON **mynursingkit™**

MyNursingKit is your one stop for online chapter review materials and resources. Prepare for success with additional NCLEX®-style practice questions, interactive assignments and activities, web links, animations and videos, and more!

Register your access code from the front of your book at
www.mynursingkit.com.

REFERENCES AND SELECTED BIBLIOGRAPHY

Ackley, B., & Ladwig, G. (2008). *Nursing diagnosis handbook: A guide to planning care* (8th ed.). Philadelphia: Mosby/Elsevier.

American Federation of State, County, and Municipal Employees. (2002). *Preventing back injuries in health care.* Retrieved from http://www.afscme.org/health/faq-back.htm

American Nurses Association. (n.d.). *Handle with care fact sheet.* Retrieved December 5, 2009, from http://www.nursingworld.org/MainMenuCategories/OccupationalandEnvironmental/occupationahealth/handlewithcare/Resources/Factsheet.aspx

American Sleep Disorders Association. (2005). *The international classification of sleep disorders: Diagnostic and coding manual.* Lawrence, KS: Allen Press.

Arnold, E. (2004). Sorting out the 3 D's: Delirium, dementia, and depression. *Nursing, 34*(6), 36–42.

Bephage, G. (2005). Promoting quality sleep in older people: The nursing care role. *British Journal of Nursing, 14*(4), 205–210.

Blocks, M. (2005). Practical solutions for safe patient handling. *Nursing, 35*(10), 44–45.

Borg, G. (1998). *Borg's perceived exertion and pain scales.* Champaign, IL: Human Kinetics.

Bulechek, G. M., Butcher, H. K., & Dochterman, J. M. (Eds.). (2008). *Nursing interventions: classification (NIC)* (5th ed.). St. Louis, MO: Mosby.

Burke, M., & Laramie, J. (2004). *Primary care of the older adult: A multidisciplinary approach* (2nd ed.). Philadelphia: Mosby/Elsevier.

Carlson, B. W., & Mascarella, J. J. (2005). Changes in sleep patterns in COPD. *American Journal of Nursing, 103*(12), 71–74.

Centers for Disease Control and Prevention. (n.d.). *Introducing the youth media campaign.* Retrieved from http://www.cdc.gov/youthcampaign/index.htm

Clements, P. T., DeRanieri, J. T., Clark, K., Manno, M. S., & Kuhn, D. W. (2005). Workplace violence and corporate policy for health care settings. *Nursing Economics, 23*(3), 119–124.

Cmiel, C. A., Gasser, D. M., Oliphant, L. M., & Neveau, A. J. (2004). Noise control: A nursing team's approach to sleep promotion. *American Journal of Nursing, 104*(2), 40–48.

Cole, C., & Richards, K. C. (2006). Sleep in persons with dementia: Increasing quality of life by managing sleep disorders. *Journal of Gerontological Nursing, 32*(3), 48–53.

Colson, E. R., McCabe, L. K., Fox, K., Levenson, S., Colton, T., Lister, G., et al. (2005). Barriers to following the back-to-sleep recommendations: Insights from focus groups with inner-city caregivers. *Ambulatory Pediatrics, 5*(6), 349–354.

Converso, A., & Murphy, C. (2004). Winning the battle against back injuries. *RN, 67*(2), 52–57.

Cummings, R., & Couteur, D. (2003). Benzodiazepines and risk of hip fractures in older people: A review of the evidence. *CNS Drugs, 17*(11), 825–837.

Doenges, M. E., Moorhouse, M. F., & Geissler-Murr, A. C. (2005). *Nursing diagnosis manual: Planning, individualizing and documenting client care.* Philadelphia: Davis.

Dulak, S. B. (2005). Dangerous bedfellows. *RN, 68*(4), 33–37.

Edelman, C., & Mandle, C. (2010). *Health promotion throughout the lifespan* (7th ed.). Philadelphia: Mosby/Elsevier.

Fontaine, K. (2005). *Complementary and alternative therapies for nursing practice* (2nd ed.). Upper Saddle River, NJ: Pearson/Prentice Hall.

Freeman, L. (2004). *Mosby's complementary & alternative medicine: A research-based approach* (2nd ed.). Philadelphia: Mosby/Elsevier.

French, D., Campbell, R., Spehar, A., & Angaran, D. (2004). Benzodiazepines and injury: A risk adjusted model. *Pharmacoepidemiology and Drug Safety, 14*(1), 17–24.

Gangwisch, J. E., Malaspina, D., Boden-Albala, B., & Heymsfield, S. B. (2005). Inadequate sleep as a risk factor for obesity: Analysis of the NHANES I. *Sleep, 28,* 1289–1296.

Harvard School of Public Health. (2006). *Exercise.* Retrieved from http://www.hsph.harvard.edu/nutritionsource/Exercise.htm

Hoffman, S. (2003). Sleep in older adults. *Geriatric Nursing, 24,* 210–216.

Honkus, V. L. (2003). Sleep deprivation in critical care units. *Critical Care Nursing Quarterly, 26*(3), 179–189.

Hu, F. B., Willett, W. C., Li, T., Stampfer, M. J., Colditz, G. A., & Manson, J. E. (2004). Adiposity as compared with physical activity in predicting mortality among women. *New England Journal of Medicine, 351*(26), 2649–2703.

Hughes, R. G., & Rogers, A. E. (2004). Are you tired? Sleep deprivation compromises nurses' health—and jeopardizes patients. *American Journal of Nursing, 104,* 36–37.

Institute of Medicine (IOM). (2006). *Sleep disorders and sleep deprivation: An unmet public health problem.* Washington, DC: Author.

International Osteoporosis Foundation. (2005). *Invest in your bones. Move it or lose it.* Retrieved from http://www .osteofound.org/publications/ move_it_or_lose_it.html

Jackson, C. (2003). Movement, breathing and Christian meditation: Catalysts for spiritual growth. *International Journal of Healing and Caring On-Line, 3*(2), 1–24.

Joanna Briggs Institute. (2004). Strategies to manage sleep in residents of aged care facilities. *Best Practice. Evidence Based Practice Information Sheets for Health Professionals, 8*(3), 1–5.

Keele-Smith, R., & Leon, T. (2003). Evaluation of individually tailored interventions on exercise adherence. *Western Journal of Nursing Research, 25*(6), 623–640.

Kennedy, M. (2004). Back to sleep. Many nurses don't follow the recommended sleep guidelines for infants. *American Journal of Nursing, 104*(6), 17.

Kreiger, A. C., & Redeker, N. S. (2002). Obstructive sleep apnea syndrome: Its relationship with hypertension. *Journal of Cardiovascular Nursing, 17,* 1–11.

Liu, B. (2003). Relationship between antidepressants and the risk of falls. *Geriatrics and Aging, 6*(7), 45–47.

Lower, J., Bonsack, C., & Guion, J. (2003). Peace and quiet. *Nursing Management, 34*(4), 40A–40D.

McCaffrey, R., Ruknui, P., Hatthakit, U., & Kasetsomboon, P. (2005). The effects of yoga on hypertensive persons in Thailand. *Holistic Nursing Practice, 19*(4), 173–180.

Maindonald, E. (2005). Helping parents reduce the risk of SIDS. *Nursing, 35*(7), 50–53.

Mauk, K. L. (2005). Promoting sound sleep habits in older adults. *Nursing, 35*(2), 22, 25.

McKibbin, C. L., Ancoli-Isreal, S., Dimsdale, J., Archuleta, C., von Kanel, R., Mills, P., et al. (2005). Sleep in spousal caregivers of people with Alzheimer's disease. *Sleep, 28,* 1245–1250.

Micozzi, M. (2006). *Fundamentals of complementary and alternative medicine* (3rd ed.). Philadelphia: Mosby/Elsevier.

Moorhead, S., Johnson, M., & Maas, M. (Eds.). (2008). *Nursing outcomes classification (NOC)* (4th ed.). St. Louis: Mosby.

Morgan, R., Virnig, B., Duque, M., Abdel-Moty, E., & DeVito, C. (2004). Low-intensity exercise and reduction of the risk for falls among at-risk elders. *Journals of Gerontology Series A: Biological and Medical Sciences, 59,* M 1062–M 1067.

Nagel, C. L., Markie, M. B., Richards, K. C., & Taylor, J. L. (2003). Sleep promotion in hospitalized elders. *Medsurg Nursing, 12*(5), 279–289.

NANDA International. (2005). *Nursing diagnoses: Definitions and classification 2005–2006.* Philadelphia: Author.

NANDA International. (2009). *NANDA nursing diagnoses: Definitions and classification 2009–2011.* West Sussex, U.K.: Wiley-Blackwell.

National Sleep Foundation. (n.d.a). *A look at the school start times debate.* Retrieved from http://www .sleepfoundation.org/hottopics/index .php?secid=18&id=206

National Sleep Foundation. (n.d.b). *ABCs of ZZZZ—When you can't sleep.* Retrieved from http://www.sleepfoundation .org/sleeplibrary/index.php?secid=id=53

National Sleep Foundation. (n.d.c). *Aging gracefully and sleeping well.* Retrieved from http://www.sleepfoundation.org/ hottopics/index.php?secid=12&id=225

National Sleep Foundation. (n.d.d). *Children's sleep habits.* Retrieved from http://www.sleepfoundation.org/ hottopics/index.php?secid=11&id=39

National Sleep Foundation. (n.d.e). *Parents of teens: Recognize the signs and symptoms of sleep deprivation and sleep problems.* Retrieved from http://www .sleepfoundation.org/_content/hottopics/ teensigns.pdf

National Sleep Foundation. (2005a). *Insomnia.* Retrieved from http://www.sleepfoundation.org/ sleeptionary/index.php?id=19

National Sleep Foundation. (2005b). *Insomnia symptoms.* Retrieved from http://www.sleepfoundation.org/ sleeptionary/index.php?id= 19&subsection=symptoms

National Sleep Foundation. (2006). *National Sleep Foundation 2006 Sleep in America poll highlights and key findings.* Retrieved from http://www .sleepfoundation.org/_content/hottopics/ Highlights_facts_06.pdf

Nelson, A., Fragala, G., & Menzel, N. (2003). Myths and facts about back injuries in nursing. *American Journal of Nursing, 103*(2), 32–40.

Nelson, A., Owen, B., Lloyd, J. D., Fragala, G., Matz, M. W., Amato, M., et al. (2003). Safe patient handling & move-

ment. *American Journal of Nursing, 103*(3), 32–43.

Oken, B., Zajdel, D., Kishiyama, S., Flegal, K., Dehen, C., Haas, M., et al. (2006). Randomized, controlled, six-month trial of yoga in healthy seniors: Effects on cognition and quality of life. *Alternative Therapies, 12*(1), 40–47.

Orr, W. C. (2000). Editorial: Sleep and functional bowel disorders: Can bad bowels cause bad dreams? *American Journal of Gastroenterology, 95,* 1118–1121.

Powers, S., & Dodd, S. (2003). *Total fitness and wellness.* New York: Benjamin Cummings.

Quillen, T. F. (2005). Sounding the alarm for narcolepsy. *Nursing, 35*(6), 74–75.

Rice, J., Kaliszer, M., Walsh, M., Jenkinson, A., & O'Brien, T. (2004). Movements at the low back during normal walking. *Clinical Anatomy, 17*(8), 662–666.

Robinson, S. B., Weitzel, T., & Henderson, L. (2005). The sh-h-h project. Nonpharmacological interventions. *Holistic Nursing Practice, 19*(6), 263–266.

Rogers, A. E., & Dreher, H. M. (2002). Narcolepsy. *Nursing Clinics of North America, 37,* 1–18.

Smith, B. K. (2004). Test your stamina for workplace fatigue. *Nursing Management, 35*(10), 38–40.

Smyth, C. (2003). The Pittsburgh sleep quality index. *Medsurg Nursing, 12*(4), 261–262.

Thompson, D. G. (2005). Safe sleep practices for hospitalized infants. *Pediatric Nursing, 31*(5), 400–403.

Vitiello, M. V. (1999). Effective treatments for age-related sleep disturbances. *Geriatrics, 54,* 47–52.

Westley, C. (2004). Sleep: Geriatric self-learning module. *Medsurg Nursing, 13*(5), 291–295.

Williams, J. (2004). Gerontologic nurse practitioner care guidelines: Sleep in the elderly. *Geriatric Nursing, 25,* 310–312.

Wilson, B., Shannon, M., & Stang, C. (2006). *Nurse's drug guide 2006.* Upper Saddle River, NJ: Prentice Hall.

Yantis, M. A. (2002). Obstructive sleep apnea. *American Journal of Nursing, 102*(6), 83, 85.

Young, M. (2003). *A review on postural realignment and its muscular and neural components.* Retrieved December 5, 2009, from http://www.elitetrack.com/ articles/read/2301/

Zielinski, K. (2004). The healing power of the labyrinth. *Real Living with Multiple Sclerosis, 11*(8), 6–7.

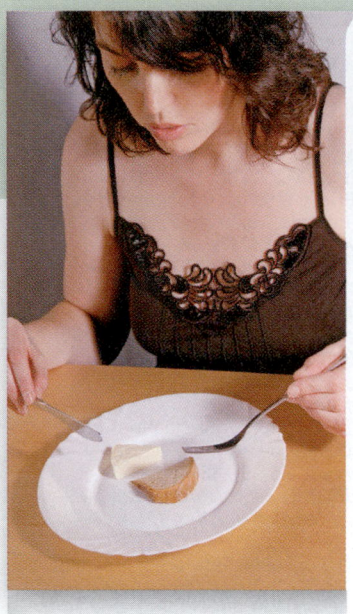

Melissa Markum, 17, hopes to be a fashion model. She gets together with friends to look through fashion magazines, and they try to copy those styles within their limited clothing allowance. When she's alone in her room Melissa pretends she's a famous runway model and practices how she will walk, turn, and show off the latest style in important cities like Paris and New York. Melissa is very diet conscious and doesn't understand how those models in the magazines stay so thin because no matter what she does, when she looks in the mirror she sees fat. She decides to limit her caloric intake to no more than 1,000 calories per day and to exercise strenuously at least 2 hours every day. She weighs herself every morning and is disgusted that at 5 feet 10 inches tall she weighs what she calls a "pudgy" 120 pounds.

LEARNING OUTCOMES

After completing this chapter you will be able to:

1. Define key terms.

2. Identify essential nutrients and their dietary sources, and describe how they are digested, absorbed, and metabolized.

3. Identify the essential components required to maintain energy balance.

4. Explain the importance of body weight and body mass standards, how to calculate them, and how ideals are maintained.

5. Identify factors influencing nutrition, and describe each factor.

6. Identify specific considerations for nutrition in each stage of the lifespan.

7. List the dietary guidelines for Americans and evaluate a diet based on the food guide pyramid.

8. Demonstrate the ability to read a food label and analyze significance of nutrient content.

9. List types of, risk factors for, and clinical signs of malnutrition.

10. Identify components of a nursing assessment for nutritional screening.

11. List four potential nursing diagnoses and nursing outcomes that could be used for clients with nutritional problems.

12. Describe nursing interventions to treat clients with nutritional problems.

13. Demonstrate the skills of inserting and discontinuing enteral tubes, administering tube feedings, and administering medications through enteral tubes.

14. List the nutrients found in, conditions requiring the use of, risk factors associated with, and nursing actions required for the client receiving parenteral nutrition.

15. List strategies the nurse could use to evaluate and document nursing care associated with nursing diagnoses related to nutritional problems.

KEY TERMS

Anabolism p952

Basal metabolic rate p953

Body mass index p953

Caloric value p953

Calorie p953

Catabolism p952

Cholesterol p952

Complete proteins p952

Demand feeding p956

Diet history p965

Disaccharides p951

Enteral p971

Enzymes p951

Essential amino acids p952

Fat-soluble vitamins p953

Fats p952

Fatty acids p952

Food diary p965

Glycerides p952

Glycogen p952

Glycogenesis p952

Ideal body weight p953

Incomplete protein p952

Kilocalorie p953

Kilojoule p953

Large calorie p953

Lipids p952

Lipoprotein p953

Macrominerals p953

Macronutrients p951

Malnutrition p963

Metabolism p953

Microminerals p953

Micronutrients p951

Mid-arm circumference p966

Mid-arm muscle circumference p966

Minerals p953

Monosaccharide p951

Monounsaturated fatty acid p952

Nonessential amino acids p952

Nutrients p951

Nutrition p951

Nutritive value p951

Obese p963

Oils p952

Overnutrition p963

Overweight p963

Parenteral p981

Partially complete proteins p952

Polysaccharides p951

Polyunsaturated fatty acid p952

Protein-calorie malnutrition p963

Pureed diet p969

Resting energy expenditure p953

Saturated fatty acids p952

Small calorie p953

Triglycerides p952

Undernutrition p963

Unsaturated fatty acid p952

Vitamin p953

Water-soluble vitamin p953

Nutrition is what a person eats and how the body uses the nutrients provided. **Nutrients** are organic and inorganic substances found in foods that are required for body functioning. Adequate food intake consists of a balance of nutrients: water, carbohydrates, proteins, fats, vitamins, and minerals. Foods differ greatly in their **nutritive value** (the nutrient content of a specified amount of food), and no one food provides all essential nutrients. Nutrients have three major functions: providing energy for body processes and movement, providing structural material for body tissues, and regulating body processes.

ESSENTIAL NUTRIENTS

The body's most basic nutrient need is water. Every cell requires a continuous supply of fuel so the next most important nutrients are those that provide energy. Energy providing nutrients are carbohydrates, fats, and proteins. Hunger compels people to eat enough energy providing nutrients to satisfy their energy needs. Carbohydrates, fats, and protein are referred to as **macronutrients,** because they are needed in large amounts (e.g., hundreds of grams) to provide energy. **Micronutrients,** vitamins and minerals, are those required in small amounts (e.g., milligrams or micrograms) to metabolize the energy-providing nutrients.

Carbohydrates

Carbohydrates, composed of carbon (C), hydrogen (H), and oxygen (O), are of two basic types: simple carbohydrates

(sugars) and complex carbohydrates (starches and fiber). As with all nutrients, carbohydrates must be ingested, digested, and metabolized.

TYPES OF CARBOHYDRATES Sugars are the simplest of all carbohydrates, are water soluble and produced naturally by plants and animals. Sugars may be **monosaccharides** (single molecules) or **disaccharides** (double molecules). Of the three monosaccharides (glucose, fructose, and galactose), glucose is by far the most abundant simple sugar. Lactose is a combination of glucose and galactose and is found in animal milk.

Starches are the insoluble form of carbohydrate that is not sweet. They are **polysaccharides** because they have branched chains of dozens to hundreds of glucose molecules. Starches exist naturally in plants such as grains, legumes, and potatoes.

Fiber is a complex carbohydrate derived from plants and they supply roughage (or bulk) to the diet because they cannot be digested by humans. Fiber helps to satisfy the appetite and helps the digestive tract function effectively to eliminate waste. Fiber is present in the outer layer of grains, bran and in the skin, seeds, and pulp of many vegetables and fruits.

Natural sources of carbohydrates are essential to the diet because they contain vital nutrients. Processed carbohydrate foods are relatively low in nutrients and high in calories so they are often called "empty calories." Examples of processed carbohydrates include alcoholic beverages.

CARBOHYDRATE DIGESTION AND METABOLISM All carbohydrates are normally broken down to monosaccharides by **enzymes**, biologic catalysts that speed up chemical reactions, and absorbed by the small intestine. Major enzymes of carbohydrate digestion include ptyalin (salivary amylase), pancreatic amylase, and the disaccharidases (maltase, sucrose, and lactase). Some simple sugars are already monosaccharides, or glucose.

Carbohydrate metabolism is a major source of body energy. Glucose circulates in the blood to provide a ready source of energy. The remainder is stored. Insulin enhances the transport of glucose into the cells. Glucose is stored as either glycogen or fat. **Glycogen** is a compound molecule of glucose formed by the process called **glycogenesis.** While most cells are capable of storing glycogen, most is stored in the liver and skeletal muscles so it is easily converted back to glucose. When glucose cannot be stored as glycogen it is converted to fat.

Proteins

Amino acids, or proteins, are a combination of molecules containing carbon, hydrogen, oxygen, and nitrogen. Every cell in the body contains some protein.

TYPES OF PROTEIN Amino acids are categorized as **essential amino acids** (those that cannot be manufactured by the body) and **nonessential amino acids** (those the body can manufacture). Nine essential amino acids—histidine, isoleucine, leucine, lysine, methionine, phenylalanine, tryptophan, threonine, and valine—are necessary for tissue growth and maintenance. A tenth, arginine, appears to have a role in the immune system. Nonessential amino acids include alanine, aspartic acid, cystine, glutamic acid, glycine, hydroxyproline, proline, serine, and tyrosine. The body takes amino acids derived from the diet and reconstructs new ones from their basic elements.

Proteins are further classified as **complete proteins** (containing all of the essential amino acids plus many nonessential ones), **partially complete proteins** (containing less than the required amount of one or more essential amino acids), or **incomplete proteins** (lack one or more essential amino acids). Most proteins that come from animals are complete proteins, and incomplete proteins are usually derived from vegetables. A balanced ratio of amino acids can be achieved if an appropriate mixture of plant proteins is provided in the diet. The combination of two or more vegetables to provide all essential amino acids is called complementary proteins.

PROTEIN DIGESTION AND METABOLISM Pepsin, an enzyme in the mouth, breaks protein down into smaller units but most protein digestion occurs in the small intestine. The pancreas secretes the proteolytic enzymes trypsin, chymotrypsin, and carboxypeptidase; glands in the intestinal wall secrete aminopeptidase and dipeptidase. These enzymes break protein down into smaller molecules and eventually into amino acids. Amino acids are absorbed by active transport through the small intestine into the portal blood circulation. The liver uses some amino acids to synthesize specific proteins. Plasma proteins are a storage medium that can rapidly be converted back into amino acids. Other amino acids are transported to tissues and cells throughout the body to make protein for cell structures. The body cannot store excess amino acids for future use but a limited amount is available because of the constant breakdown and buildup of protein in body tissues.

Protein metabolism includes three activities: **anabolism** (building tissue), **catabolism** (breaking down tissue), and nitrogen balance. All body cells synthesize proteins from amino acids (anabolism). Excess amino acids are degraded for energy or converted to fat, primarily in the liver (catabolism). Nitrogen is the element that distinguishes proteins from other macronutrients; nitrogen balance reflects the status of protein nutrition in the body because it measures the degree of protein anabolism and catabolism and is the net result of intake and loss of nitrogen.

Lipids

Lipids are organic substances that are greasy and insoluble in water but soluble in alcohol or ether. **Fats** are lipids that are solid at room temperature; **oils** are lipids that are liquid at room temperature. Lipids have the same elements (carbon, hydrogen, and oxygen) as carbohydrates, but they contain a higher proportion of hydrogen.

TYPES OF LIPIDS The basic structural unit of most lipids is carbon chains and hydrogen called **fatty acids.** The number of hydrogen atoms contained in the fatty acid determines if it is a **saturated fatty acid** (all carbon atoms are filled to capacity with hydrogen) or an **unsaturated fatty acid** (fatty acid that could accommodate more hydrogen atoms because it has at least two carbon atoms not attached to a hydrogen atom and forms a double bond between the two carbon atoms). Fatty acids with one double bond are **monounsaturated fatty acids** while those with more than one double bond are **polyunsaturated fatty acids. Glycerides** are the simplest and most common form of lipids consisting of a glycerol molecule with up to three fatty acids attached. **Triglycerides** have three fatty acids and account for more than 90% of lipids found in food and the body. Triglycerides may be saturated or unsaturated. Saturated triglycerides are solid at room temperature and are found in animal products while unsaturated triglycerides are liquid at room temperature and are found in plant products. **Cholesterol** is a fatlike substance found in foods of animal origin and synthesized in the liver. Cholesterol is needed to create bile acids, to synthesize steroid hormones, and large quantities are present in cell membranes and other cell structures.

LIPID DIGESTION AND METABOLISM Lipid digestion begins in the stomach but lipids are mainly digested in the small intestine by bile, pancreatic lipase, and enteric lipase. The end products of lipid digestion are glycerol, fatty acids, and cholesterol, which are reassembled inside the intestinal cells into triglycerides and cholesterol esters (cholesterol with a fatty acid attached to it), which are not water soluble. The small intestine and the liver must convert them into soluble compounds called **lipoproteins** (made up of various lipids and a protein) so they can be transported and used.

The enzyme lipase breaks down triglycerides in adipose cells, releasing glycerol and fatty acids into the blood to be used for energy production. Only glycerol can be converted to glucose, an essential ingredient for brain, nerve, and red blood cells.

Micronutrients

Vitamins are compounds that cannot be manufactured by the body and are needed in small quantities to catalyze metabolic processes. Vitamins are categorized as **water-soluble vitamins** (vitamins C and B–complex) or **fat-soluble vitamins** (vitamins A, D, E, and K). The body cannot store water-soluble vitamins so they must be supplied daily and are affected by food processing, storage, and preparation. Fat-soluble vitamins can be stored in the body although vitamins E and K can be stored only in limited amounts. Vitamin content is highest in fresh foods that are consumed soon after harvest.

Minerals are found in organic compounds, as inorganic compounds, and as free ions. Calcium and phosphorus make up 80% of all mineral elements in the body. The two categories of minerals are **macrominerals** (required in amounts over 100 mg and include calcium, phosphorus, sodium, potassium, magnesium, chloride, and sulfur) and **microminerals** (required in amounts less than 100 mg and include iron, zinc, manganese, iodine, fluoride, copper, cobalt, chromium, and selenium). Inadequate intake can result in problems such as anemia (inadequate iron intake) or osteoporosis (loss of bone calcium). Additional information on fluid and electrolyte balance can be found in Chapter 36. ∞

ENERGY BALANCE

Energy balance is the relationship between the energy derived from food and the energy used by the body. The body obtains energy from macronutrients and uses energy for voluntary and involuntary activities. A person's energy balance is determined by comparing energy intake with energy output.

Energy Intake

The amount of energy that nutrients or foods supply to the body is their **caloric value**. A **calorie (c, cal, kcal)** is a unit of heat energy. A **small calorie** is the amount of heat required to raise the temperature of 1 gram of water 1 degree Celsius. This unit of measure is used in chemistry and physics. A **large calorie (Calorie, kilocalorie [Kcal])** is the amount of heat energy required to raise the temperature of 1 gram of water 15 to 16 degrees Celsius and is the unit used in nutrition. It was recommended in 1970 that the unit kilojoule (kJ), a metric measurement, replace the kilocalorie. However, to date, the United States and Canada have not made the change. A

kilojoule (kJ) is the amount of work energy required when a force of 1 newton (N) moves 1 kilogram of weight 1 meter distance. One Calorie (Kcal) equals 4.18 kilojoules. Carbohydrates and protein produce 4 Calories/gram (17 kJ), fat produces 9 Calories/gram (38 kJ), and alcohol produces 7 Calories/gram (29 kJ).

Energy Output

Metabolism refers to all biochemical and physiologic processes by which the body grows and maintains itself. Metabolic rate is normally expressed in terms of the rate of heat liberated during these chemical reactions. The **basal metabolic rate (BMR)** is the rate at which the body metabolizes food to maintain the energy requirements of a person who is awake and at rest. The energy in food maintains the basal metabolic rate of the body and provides energy for activities such as running and walking.

Resting energy expenditure (REE) is the amount of energy required to maintain basic body functions; in other words, the calories required to maintain life. The REE of healthy persons is generally about 1 cal/kg of body weight/hr for men and 0.9 cal/kg/hr for women, although there is great variation among individuals. BMR is calculated by measuring the REE in the early morning, 12 hours after eating. The actual daily expenditure of energy depends on the degree of activity of the individual.

BODY WEIGHT AND BODY MASS STANDARDS

Maintaining a healthy or ideal body weight requires a balance between the expenditure of energy and the intake of nutrients. Generally, when energy requirements of an individual equate with the daily caloric intake, the body weight remains stable. **Ideal body weight (IBW)** is the optimal weight recommended for optimal health. To determine an individual's approximate IBW, the nurse can consult standardized tables or can quickly calculate a value using the Rule of 5 for women and the Rule of 6 for men (see Box 32–1). The nurse should use great caution in suggesting that these weights apply to all clients.

Many health professionals consider the body mass index to be a more reliable indicator of a person's healthy weight. For people older than 18 years, the **body mass index (BMI)** is an indicator of changes in body fat stores and whether a person's weight is appropriate for height, and may provide a useful estimate of malnutrition. Use results with caution in people who have fluid retention, athletes, or older adults. To calculate the BMI:

1. Measure the person's height in meters, e.g., 1.7 m (1 meter = 3.3 ft, or 39.6 in)
2. Measure the weight in kilograms, e.g., 72 kg (1 kg = 2.2 pounds)

BOX 32–1	Approximating Ideal Body Weight

Rule of 5 for females:
100 lb for 5 ft of height
+ 5 lb for each inch over 5 ft
±10% for body-frame size*

Rule of 6 for males:
106 lb for 5 ft of height
+ 6 lb for each inch over 5 ft
±10% for body-frame size*

*Determine body-frame size by measuring the client's wrist circumference and applying to the table below. Add 10% for large body-frame size, and subtract 10% for small body-frame size.

	Female Wrist Measurements			Male Wrist Measurements
	Height less than 5' 2" (less than 155 cm)	Height 5' 2" – 5' 5" (155 cm – 163 cm)	Height more than 5' 5" (more than 163 cm)	Height more than 5' 5" (More than 163 cm)
Small	Less than 5.5" (140 mm)	Less than 6.0" (152 mm)	Less than 6.25" (159 mm)	5.5"–6.5" (140–165 mm)
Medium	5.5"–5.75" (140–146 mm)	6"–6.25" (152–159 mm)	6.25"–6.5" (159–165 mm)	6.5"–7.5" (165–191 mm)
Large	More than 5.75" (146 mm)	More than 6.25" (159 mm)	More than 6.5" (165 mm)	More than 7.5" (191 mm)

BOX 32–2	Classification of Overweight and Obesity

	BMI (kg/m²)	Obesity Class	Disease Risk* Relative to Normal Weight and Waist Circumference	
			Men 102 cm (40 in) or less Women 88 cm (35 in) or less	Men > 102 cm (40 in) Women > 88 cm (35 in)
Underweight	<18.5		-	-
Normal+	18.5–24.9		-	-
Overweight	25.0–29.9		Increased	High
Obesity	30.0–34.9 35.0–39.9	I II	High Very high	Very high Very high
Extreme obesity	40.0+	III	Extremely high	Extremely high

From *Clinical Guidelines on the Identification, Evaluation, and Treatment of Overweight and Obesity in Adults: The Evidence Report,* by the National Heart, Lung, and Blood Institute, 1998, p. xvii, Washington, DC: U.S. Department of Health & Human Services. Retrieved from http://www.nhlbi.nih.gov/guidelines/obesity/ob_gdlns.htm

* Disease risk for type 2 diabetes, hypertension, and cardiovascular disease.

+ Increased waist circumference can also be a marker for increased risk even in persons of normal weight.

3. Calculate the BMI using the following formula

$$BMI = \frac{\text{Weight in kilograms}}{(\text{Height in meters})^2}$$

or

$$\frac{72 \text{ kilograms}}{1.7 \times 1.7 \text{ (meters)}^2} = 24.9$$

Box 32–2 provides an interpretation of the results.

Another measure of body mass is percent body fat. Because BMI uses only height and weight, it can give misleading results for certain groups of clients such as athletes, frail older adults, and children. Percent of body fat can be measured by underwater weighing and dual-energy x-ray absorptiometry (DEXA), but these methods are time consuming and expensive. Other indirect, but more practical measures include waist circumference (see Box 32–2), skinfold testing, and near-infrared interactance.

FACTORS AFFECTING NUTRITION

An individual's food preferences and habits are often a major factor affecting what a person eats. Eating habits are influenced by developmental considerations, gender, ethnicity and culture, beliefs about food, personal preferences, religious practices, lifestyle, economics, medications and therapies, health, alcohol consumption, advertising, and psychological factors.

Development People in rapid periods of growth have increased needs for nutrients. Older adults need fewer calories and dietary changes may be required in view of the risk for coronary heart disease, osteoporosis, and hypertension.

Gender Nutrient requirements are different for men and women because of differences in body composition and reproductive functions. Men, with larger muscle mass, require more calories and proteins while women require more iron during childbearing years. Pregnant and lactating women have increased caloric and fluid needs.

Ethnicity and Culture Ethnicity and culture often determines food preferences. Traditional foods are eaten long after other customs are abandoned. Nurses' should realize that variations of intake are acceptable under different circumstances with universally accepted guidelines eating a wide variety of foods to furnish adequate nutrients and eat moderately to maintain correct body weight. Food preferences probably differ as much among individuals of the same cultural background as it does between cultures.

Beliefs about Food Beliefs about effects of foods on health and well-being can affect food choices. Many people acquire their beliefs about food from television, magazines, and other media. Food fads (a widespread but short-lived interest or practice followed with considerable zeal) that involve nontraditional food practices are relatively common. Fads may be based on the belief that certain foods have special powers or on the notion that certain foods are harmful. Some fads are harmless while others are potentially danger-

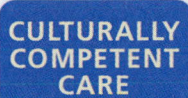

Variations in Nutritional Practices and Preferences among Different Cultures

African American Heritage

Gifts of food are common and should never be rejected, diets are often high in fat, cholesterol and sodium, being overweight is viewed as positive, and most persons are lactose intolerant.

Arab Heritage

Use many spices and herbs, meats are often skewer roasted or slow simmered (lamb and chicken are common), bread is served at all meals, Muslims do not eat pork and all meats must be well done, food is eaten (and clients are fed) with the right hand, beverages are consumed after meals, and Muslims fast during daylight hours during the month of Ramadan.

Chinese Heritage

Foods are served at meals in a specific order, each region in China has its own traditional diet, traditional Chinese may not want ice in their drinks, and foods are chosen to balance *yin* and *yang* in order to avoid indigestion.

Jewish Heritage

Dietary laws govern killing, preparing, and eating of foods, meat and milk are not eaten at the same time although dietary substitutes are permitted, pork is forbidden, all blood must be drained from meats (Kosher), and always wash hands before eating.

Mexican Heritage

Rice, beans, and tortillas are essential foods, many persons are lactose intolerant, being overweight is viewed as positive, sweet fruit drinks are popular, the main meal is at noontime, and foods are chosen according to hot and cold theory.

Navajo Heritage

Rites of passage and ceremonies are celebrated with food, herbs are used to treat many illnesses, sheep are the major source of meat, squash and corn are major vegetables, and most persons are lactose intolerant.

---

ous (Daniels, 2004). Determining the needs a fad diet fills for the client enables the nurse both to support these needs and to suggest a more nutritious diet.

Personal Preferences People develop likes and dislikes based on associations with a typical food. Individual likes and dislikes can also be related to familiarity. Some adults are very adventuresome and eager to try new foods while others prefer to eat the same foods repeatedly. Preferences in the tastes, smells, flavors (blends of taste and smell), temperatures, colors, shapes, texture, and sizes of food influence a person's food choices.

Religious Practices Religious practice also affects diet. Some Roman Catholics avoid meat on certain days, and some Protestant faiths prohibit meat, tea, coffee, or alcohol. Both Orthodox Judaism and Islam prohibit pork. Orthodox Jews observe kosher customs, eating certain foods only if they are inspected by a rabbi and prepared according to dietary laws. The nurse must plan care with consideration of such religious dietary practices.

Lifestyle Certain lifestyles are linked to food-related behaviors. People who are always in a hurry may buy convenience items or eat at fast food chains. People who spend many hours at home may take time to prepare more meals "from scratch." Individual differences also influence lifestyle patterns (e.g., cooking skills, concern about health). Some people work at different times, such as evening or night shifts and may need to adapt their eating habits to this, as well as making changes in their medication schedules if they are related to food intake. The type of work performed also affects food intake. Physically active work requires more calories than mentally active work, which requires only about 4 Kcal per hour.

Economics People with limited income may not be able to afford meat and fresh vegetables while people with higher incomes may purchase more proteins and fats and fewer complex carbohydrates. Not all persons have the financial resources for extensive food preparation and storage facilities. The nurse should not assume that clients have their own stove, refrigerator, or freezer.

Medications and Therapy The effects of drugs on nutrition vary considerably. They may alter appetite, disturb taste perception, or interfere with nutrient absorption or excretion. Nurses need to be aware of the nutritional effects of specific drugs when evaluating a client for nutritional problems. Conversely, nutrients can affect drug utilization. Older adults are at particular risk for drug–food interactions due to the number of medications they may take, age-related physiologic changes affecting medication actions (e.g., decrease in lean-to-fat ratio, decrease in renal or hepatic function), and disease-restricted diets (Leibovitch, Deamer, & Sanderson, 2004). Normal cells of the bone marrow and the gastrointestinal mucosa are naturally very active and particularly susceptible to antineoplastic agents. Oral ulcers, intestinal bleeding, or diarrhea resulting from the toxicity of antineoplastic agents used in chemotherapy can seriously diminish a person's nutritional status and must be monitored by the nurse.

Health An individual's health status greatly affects eating habits and nutritional status. Disease processes and surgery of the gastrointestinal tract can affect digestion, absorption, metabolism, and excretion of essential nutrients. Gastrointestinal and other diseases also create nausea, vomiting, and diarrhea, all of which can adversely affect a person's appetite and nutritional status. Gallstones, which can block the flow of bile, are a common cause of impaired lipid digestion.

Metabolic processes can be impaired by diseases of the liver. Diseases of the pancreas can affect glucose metabolism or fat digestion.

Alcohol Consumption   The calories contained in alcoholic drinks include both those of the alcohol and any mixers that may be used. This can constitute large numbers of calories. Drinking alcohol can lead to weight gain through the addition of these calories to the regular diet plus the effect of alcohol on fat metabolism. A small amount of the alcohol is converted directly to fat. However, the greater effect is that the remainder of the alcohol is converted into acetate by the liver. The acetate released to the bloodstream is used for energy instead of fat and the fat is then stored. Excessive alcohol use contributes to nutritional deficiencies in a number of ways. Alcohol may replace food in a person's diet, and it can depress the appetite. Excessive alcohol can have a toxic effect on the intestinal mucosa, thereby decreasing the absorption of nutrients. The need for vitamin B increases, because it is used in alcohol metabolism. Alcohol can impair the storage of nutrients and increase nutrient catabolism and excretion.

Advertising   Through the use of popular actors and strong persuasion, advertising can alter food choices. Products such as alcoholic beverages, coffee, frozen foods, and soft drinks are more heavily advertised than such products as bread, vegetables, and fruits. Convenience foods and take-out foods are heavily advertised. Commercials during children's television shows often promote snack foods, candy, soda, and sugared cereals over fresh, healthy foods. There has been an increase in advertising that targets older adults in particular and encourages use of herbs and supplements.

Psychologic Factors   Although some people overeat when stressed, depressed, or lonely, others eat very little under the same conditions. Anorexia and weight loss can indicate severe stress or depression. Anorexia nervosa and bulimia are severe psychophysiologic conditions seen most frequently in female adolescents.

NUTRITIONAL VARIATIONS THROUGHOUT THE LIFE CYCLE

Nutritional requirements vary throughout the life cycle. Guidelines follow for the major developmental stages.

Neonates to 1 Year

The neonate's fluid and nutritional needs are met by breast milk or formula. It is recommended that infants be breast-fed until 1 year of age (American Academy of Pediatrics, 2005). Fluid needs of infants are proportionately greater than those of adults because of a higher metabolic rate, immature kidneys, and greater water losses through the skin and the lungs. The last is largely due to rapid respirations. The total daily nutritional requirement of the newborn is about 80 to 100 mL of breast milk or formula per kilogram of body weight. The newborn infant's stomach capacity is about 90 mL, and feedings are required every 2½ to 4 hours.

The newborn infant is usually fed "on demand." **Demand feeding** means that the child is fed when hungry, which decreases the risk of overfeeding or underfeeding. Regurgitation, or spitting up, during or after a feeding is a common occurrence during the first year. Although this may be of concern to parents, it does not usually result in nutritional deficiency. Demonstration of adequate weight gain should reassure parents that the infant is receiving adequate nutrition. Once satisfaction has been demonstrated, infants should not be coaxed into finishing the feeding to prevent discomfort or overfeeding.

The addition of solid food to the diet usually takes place between 4 and 6 months of age. Six-month-old infants can consume solid food more readily because they can sit up, can hold a spoon, and have decreased sucking and tongue protrusion reflexes. Solid foods (strained or pureed) are generally introduced in the following order: cereals (rice), fruits, vegetables (yellow before green), and strained meats. Foods are introduced one at a time, usually with only one new food introduced every 5 days to ensure that the infant tolerates the food and demonstrates no allergy. This sequence can vary according to cultural preferences. With the eruption of teeth at about 7 to 9 months, the infant is ready to chew and can begin to experience different textures of food. At this time, the infant enjoys finger foods, such as skinless fruit cut into small pieces to prevent choking, dry cereal, or toast. At about 6 months of age, infants require iron supplementation to prevent iron deficiency anemia. Because honey can contain spores of *Clostridium botulinuma*, a source of infection (and death) for infants, children less than 12 months old should not be fed honey. According to the Centers for Disease Control (2005), honey is safe for persons 1 year of age and older. By the age of 1, most infants can be completely fed on table food, and milk intake is about 20 ounces per day.

Toddler

Toddlers can eat most foods and adjust to three meals a day. Toddlers' fine motor skills are sufficiently well developed for them to learn how to feed themselves. Before the age of 20 months, most toddlers require help with glasses and cups because their wrist control is limited. By age 3, when most of the deciduous teeth have emerged, the toddler is able to bite and chew adult table food.

Developing independence may be exhibited through the toddler's refusal of certain foods. Meals should be short because of the toddler's brief attention span and environmental distractions. Often toddlers display their liking of rituals by eating foods in a certain order, cutting foods a specific way, or accompanying certain foods with a particular drink.

During the toddler stage, the caloric requirement is 900 to 1,800 Kcal per day with fluid needs for a child weighing 15 kg (33 lb) about 1,250 mL of fluid per 24 hours. From 1 to 2 years of age, the toddler may be eating a combination of prepared toddler foods and some table foods. Parents should be instructed to read labels carefully and be aware that table foods offer more variety and are less expensive and more nutritious than prepared toddler foods. The need for adequate iron, calcium, and vitamins C and A, which are common toddler deficiencies, should also be discussed.

The following suggestions may help parents meet the child's nutritional needs and promote effective parent–child interactions: (a) Make mealtime a pleasant time by avoiding tensions at the table and discussions of bad behavior; (b) offer a variety of simple, attractive foods in small portions, and avoid meals that combine foods into one dish, such as a stew; (c) do not use food as a reward or punish a child who does not eat; (d) schedule meals, sleep, and snack times that will allow for optimum appetite and behavior; and (e) avoid the routine use of sweet desserts.

Preschooler

The preschooler eats adult foods. Children at this age are very active and may rush through meals to return to play. The 4-year-old still requires parents' help in cutting meat and may spill milk when pouring from a large container. Parents also need to teach the preschooler how to use utensils and should provide them with the opportunity to practice. However, 4- and 5-year-olds often use their fingers to pick food up. Table manners are marginal at best. Active children often require snacks between meals. Cheese, fruits, yogurt, raw vegetables, and milk are good choices. Children at this age may enjoy helping in the kitchen, and both girls and boys should be encouraged to do so. The average 5-year-old weighing 20 kg (45 lb) requires at least 75 mL of liquid per kilogram of body weight per day, or 1,500 mL every 24 hours.

School-Age Child

School-age children require a balanced diet including 2,400 Kcal per day. School-age children eat three meals a day and one or two nutritious snacks. Children need a protein-rich food at breakfast to sustain the prolonged physical and mental effort required at school. Children who skip breakfast become inattentive and restless by late morning and have decreased problem-solving ability. Undernourished children become fatigued easily and face a greater risk of infection, resulting in frequent absences from school.

The average healthy 8-year-old weighing 30 kg (66 lb) requires about 1,750 mL of fluid per day. Eating a balanced diet should be the norm for both parent and child. Poor eating habits may result in obesity. Childhood obesity is an increasing problem.

Adolescent

The adolescent's need for nutrients and calories increases, particularly during the growth spurt. In particular, the need for protein, calcium, vitamin D, iron, and B vitamins increases during adolescence. An adequate diet for an adolescent is 1 quart of milk per day as well as appropriate amounts of meat, vegetables, fruits, breads, and cereals. Calcium intake during adolescent years (1,200 to 1,500 mg/day) may help decrease osteoporosis (a decrease in bone density) in later life (Schettler & Gustafson, 2004). Common problems related to nutrition and self-esteem among adolescents includes obesity, anorexia nervosa, and bulimia.

Many parents may observe that teenagers, particularly boys, seem to be eating all the time. Teenagers tend to diet or snack frequently, often eating high-calorie foods. Parents and nurses can promote better lifelong eating habits by encouraging teenagers to eat healthy snacks. The teenager's food choices relate to physical, social, emotional factors and impulses and may not be influenced by teaching. Nurses need to advise parents that adolescents must take responsibility for their decisions in many areas of life, and parents should avoid conflicts that relate to food.

Young Adult

The nutritional habits established during young adulthood often lay the foundation for the patterns maintained throughout a person's life. Many young adults are aware of food groups but may not be knowledgeable about how many servings of each group they need or how much a serving constitutes. The nurse should provide the young adult client with resources such as a chart or list that contains the foods and the amounts needed in each category.

Young adult females need to maintain adequate iron intake (18 mg of iron daily). The nurse should instruct the female client to include iron-rich foods, such as organ meats (liver and kidneys), eggs, fish, poultry, leafy vegetables, and dried fruits, in her daily diet. Calcium is needed in young adulthood to maintain bones and help decrease the chances of developing osteoporosis in later life. Along with calcium, the person must have adequate vitamin D, necessary for the calcium to enter the bloodstream.

Obesity may occur during the young adult years as the active teen becomes the sedentary adult but does not decrease caloric intake. The overweight or obese young adult is at risk for hypertension, a major health problem for this age group.

Middle-Aged Adult

The middle-aged adult should continue to eat a healthy diet, following the recommended portions of the food groups, with special attention to protein, calcium, and limiting cholesterol and caloric intake. Two or three liters of fluid should be included in the daily diet. Postmenopausal women need to ingest sufficient calcium and vitamin D to reduce osteoporosis, and antioxidants such as vitamins A, C, and E may be helpful in reducing the risks of heart disease in women. Although iron supplements are no longer needed, the amount in a multivitamin is not harmful and may be beneficial for postmenopausal women taking estrogen supplements (Maurer et al., 2005).

Medications for Weight Loss

Meridia (sibutramine) may be used with a reduced calorie diet and an exercise plan to help clients lose weight. Normal dosage ranges from 5–15 mg every day. It is classified as an appetite suppressant. Because of the side effect of increased blood pressure and heart rate, it should not be used by people with uncontrolled hypertension, a history of heart disease, congestive heart failure, irregular heartbeat, or strokes. Contraindications include MAO inhibitors. It is important to get a complete drug history from the client as many medication dosages may need to be adjusted for the client taking Meridia. Common side effects include headache, change in appetite, heartburn, dry mouth, constipation, and insomnia.

Xenical (orlistat), 120 mg taken TID with meals, works by reducing the body's ability to absorb dietary fat by about 1/3. Side effects include flatus with discharge, fecal urgency, fatty stools, in-creased defecation, and fecal incontinence. Increased gastrointestinal complaints have been associated with clients who take Xenical while eating a high-fat diet. Clients should be encouraged to take a fat-soluble vitamin supplement while on Xenical. Research indicates it is safe for use in obese adolescents as well as adults.

Xenical and Meridia are the only medications currently approved for longer-term use in significantly obese people, although the safety and effectiveness have not been established for use beyond 2 years.

Other FDA medications available to reduce appetite include Didrex, Tenuate, Sanorex, Mazanor, Adipex-P, Lonamin, and Bontril. These medications are only to be used short-term, meaning for a few weeks or months and should not be used long-term.

Middle-aged adults have decreased metabolic activity and decreased physical activity resulting in a decrease in caloric need. The nurse's role in nutritional health promotion is to counsel clients to prevent obesity by reducing caloric intake and participating in regular exercise. Clients should also be warned that being overweight is a risk factor for many chronic diseases. Clients should seek medical advice before considering any major changes in their diets.

During late middle age, gastric juice secretions and free acid gradually decline. As a result, some individuals may complain of "heartburn" (acid indigestion) or an increase in belching. They may determine that certain foods disagree with them. Clients should be advised to develop sensible eating habits and avoid fried or fatty foods.

Older Adults

The older adult requires the same basic nutrition as the younger adult. However, fewer calories are needed by older adults because of the lower metabolic rate and the decrease in physical activity. Some older adults may need more carbohydrates for fiber and bulk, but most nutrient require-

Nutrition for Older Adults

- *Include each group on the Food Pyramid.* For example, a 65-year-old female who performs less than 30 minutes of exercise per day requires 1,600 Kcalories consisting of the following:

Grains	5 ounces
Vegetables	2 cups
Fruits	1.5 cups
Milk, yogurt, and cheese	3 cups
Meat and beans	5 ounces

- *Reduce caloric intake.* Caloric needs generally decrease in older adults often because of decreased activity. Older adults need to consume nutrient-dense foods and avoid foods that are high in calories but have few nutrients.
- *Reduce fat consumption.* Use leaner cuts of meat, and limit portions to 4 to 6 oz per day. (But be sure intake of meat is sufficient, because older adults often consume inadequate amounts of these foods.) Broil, boil, or bake foods instead of frying them. Use low-fat milk and cheese; limit intake of butter, margarine, and salad dressings.
- *Reduce consumption of empty calories.* Substitute fruit or puddings made with low-fat milk in place of pastry, cookies, and rich desserts.

- *Reduce sodium consumption for clients who have hypertension or other cardiac problems.* Avoid canned soups, ketchup, and mustard. Avoid salted, smoked, cured, and pickled meats (e.g., ham and bacon), poultry, and fish. Do not add salt when cooking foods or at the table.
- *Ensure adequate calcium intake (at least 800 mg) to prevent bone loss.* Milk, cheese, yogurt, cream soups, puddings, and frozen milk products are good sources.
- *Ensure adequate vitamin D intake.* Vitamin D is essential to maintain calcium homeostasis. Include some milk, because other dairy products are not usually fortified with vitamin D. If milk cannot be tolerated because of a lactose deficiency, provide vitamin supplements.
- *Ensure adequate iron intake.* Iron intake in older people may be compromised by such factors as increased incidence of gastrointestinal disturbance, chronic diarrhea, regular aspirin use, and possible reduction in meat consumption.
- *Consume fiber-rich foods to prevent constipation and minimize use of laxatives.* Because fiber-rich foods provide bulk and a feeling of fullness, they help people control their appetites and lose weight.

LIFESPAN CONSIDERATIONS Nutrition

Children

- Children learn eating habits from their parents. It is the parents' responsibility to be good nutritional role models, both in terms of what they eat and how they incorporate food into their lifestyle.
- During the preschool and early school-age years children learn lifelong eating habits. It is the parents' responsibility to provide the child with adequate amounts of nutritious foods in an environment that is relaxed and comfortable for eating. It is the child's responsibility to decide what and how much of the nutritious foods to eat. Parents should be counseled that eating can become a source of conflict if the parent tries to tell the child what and how much to eat, or if the child tries to tell the parent what foods should be eaten. Children's access to "junk food" should be limited, but completely forbidding a food may also create conflict.
- Although adolescents who are vegetarians are at risk for some nutritional deficits, the diet of adolescents who eat eggs, milk products, and, on occasion, non-red meat is more healthful than that of their red-meat-eating peers (Haddad & Tanzman, 2003).

Older Adults

Most older adults take several medications as a result of having an increase in the number of chronic illnesses. Considerations for potential problems include:

- Some foods interact adversely or decrease the effectiveness of certain medications, such as foods high in vitamin K and the anticoagulant Coumadin. Older adults should not change their diet significantly without consulting the

health care provider since drug dosage may have been based on the older adult's previous dietary intake.
- Some medications increase appetite, such as glucocorticoids.
- Some medications decrease appetite by their actions or by causing an unpleasant taste.
- Certain tablets should not be crushed to be given by mouth or by gastric tubes, such as enteric-coated or slow-release medications.

Conditions such as neuromuscular disorders and dementia can make it difficult for older adults to eat or to be fed. Safety should always be a priority concern with attention paid to prevent aspiration. All health care personnel and family caregivers should be taught proper techniques to reduce this risk. Effective techniques include:

- Use the chin-tuck method when feeding clients with dysphagia. Having them flex the head toward the chest when swallowing decreases the risk of aspiration into the lungs.
- Use foods of prescribed consistency. Many older adults can swallow foods with thicker consistency more easily than thin liquids.
- Try to focus on food preferences—the family can help provide this information.
- Try to maintain mealtime as a positive social occasion with conversations and extra attention to having a pleasant environment.

Economic factors may influence older adults' nutritional status if they cannot afford food, especially if a prescribed diet requires expensive supplements. Inexpensive or convenience foods such as canned soups are often high in fat and sodium.

---

ments remain relatively unchanged. Such physical changes as tooth loss and impaired sense of taste and smell may affect eating habits. Decreased saliva and gastric juice secretion may also affect a person's nutrition.

Psychosocial factors may also contribute to nutritional problems. Some older adults who live alone do not want to cook for themselves or eat alone. As a result, they may adopt poor dietary habits. Other factors, such as lack of transportation, poor access to stores, and inability to prepare the food also affect nutritional status. Loss of spouse, anxiety, depression, dependence on others, and lowered income all affect eating habits. Guidelines for the inclusion of high-nutrient foods that are compatible with the nutritional needs of older adults are summarized in Client Teaching: "Nutrition for Older Adults" and Lifespan Considerations.

STANDARDS FOR A HEALTHY DIET

Various daily food guides have been developed to help healthy people meet the daily requirements of essential nutrients and to facilitate meal planning. Food group plans emphasize the general types or groups of foods rather than the

specific foods, because related foods are similar in composition and often have similar nutrient values.

Dietary Guidelines for Americans

This guide is published by the U.S. Department of Agriculture (USDA) every 5 years, and the 2005 revision contains recommendations for food choices to help reduce calorie consumption and increase physical activity. Key points of the dietary guidelines follow:

- Consume nutrient-dense foods within caloric needs.
- Maintain weight in a healthy range.
- Engage in regular physical activity.
- Consume recommended amounts of fruit, vegetables, whole grains, and milk each day.
- Keep total fat intake within 20% to 35% of total calories and less than 10% from saturated fatty acids. (See also Client Teaching for ways to reduce fat intake.)
- Consume less than 2,300 mg of sodium per day and add potassium-rich foods.
- If you drink alcohol, do so in moderation (one drink per day for women and two drinks per day for men).

<table>
<tr><td>

CLIENT TEACHING   Reducing Dietary Fat

- Cook meat by grilling, baking, broiling, or microwaving rather than frying.
- Substitute popcorn or pretzels for such snacks as potato chips, cheese puffs, and corn chips.
- Read labels. Some crackers, for example, are high in fat; others are not.
- Limit desserts high in fat, such as candy, ice cream, cake, and cookies.
- Substitute hard candies for chocolate bars.
- Use skim or reduced-fat milk instead of whole milk, for drinking as well as in recipes.
- Use less butter or margarine on breads.
- Remove fat from meat and skin from chicken before cooking.
- Eat less meat; eat more fish.
- Use less dressing, or use low-fat dressings, on salads.
- Eat plant sources of protein (e.g., kidney, lima, and navy beans).
- Use nuts as a source of protein, but since they are high in fat, use to replace meat rather than in addition.

</td></tr>
</table>

These dietary recommendations are intended to help achieve the nutritional goals stated in *Healthy People 2010*. In that report, the U.S. surgeon general identified 25 specific nutritional objectives, such as the following (U.S. Department of Health and Human Services, 2000):

- Reduce the incidence of overweight adults (target = 15%) and children (target = 5%).
- Reduce growth retardation among low-income children aged 5 and younger to less than 5%.
- Increase the proportion of persons aged 2 years and older who consume no more than 30% of calories from total fat to 75%.
- Increase the proportion of persons aged 2 years and older who consume no more than 2,400 mg of sodium daily to 65%.

The Food Guide Pyramid

The Food Guide Pyramid is a graphic aid that was developed by the USDA as a guide in making daily food choices. Previously, one pyramid was intended for use by all persons. In 2005, the USDA issued a new pyramid in a food guidance

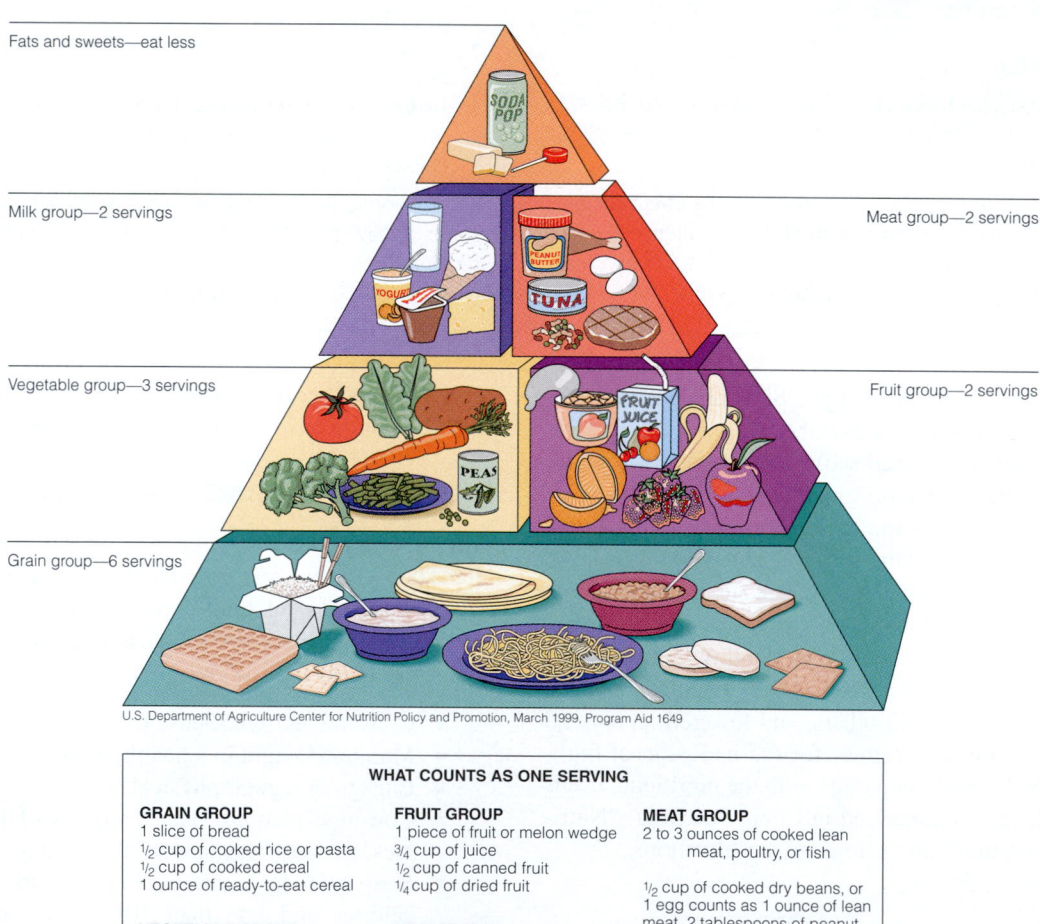

Fats and sweets—eat less

Milk group—2 servings   Meat group—2 servings

Vegetable group—3 servings   Fruit group—2 servings

Grain group—6 servings

U.S. Department of Agriculture Center for Nutrition Policy and Promotion, March 1999, Program Aid 1649

WHAT COUNTS AS ONE SERVING

GRAIN GROUP
1 slice of bread
½ cup of cooked rice or pasta
½ cup of cooked cereal
1 ounce of ready-to-eat cereal

VEGETABLE GROUP
½ cup of chopped raw
   or cooked vegetables
1 cup of raw leafy vegetables

FRUIT GROUP
1 piece of fruit or melon wedge
¾ cup of juice
½ cup of canned fruit
¼ cup of dried fruit

MILK GROUP
1 cup of milk or yogurt
2 ounces of cheese

MEAT GROUP
2 to 3 ounces of cooked lean
   meat, poultry, or fish

½ cup of cooked dry beans, or
1 egg counts as 1 ounce of lean
meat. 2 tablespoons of peanut
butter count as 1 ounce of
meat.

FATS AND SWEETS
Limit calories from these.

Four- to 6-year-olds can eat these serving sizes. Offer 2- to 3-year-olds less, except for milk.
Two- to 6 year-old children need a total of 2 servings from the milk group each day.

Figure 32–1 ● Food guide pyramid for young children.

system on the Internet to allow people to customize their pyramid based on a variety of characteristics. On the new pyramid, the food groups—grains, vegetables, fruits, milk, and meat and beans—are drawn from the base of the pyramid to the apex. This indicates that activity, moderation, personalization, proportionality, variety, and gradual improvement are the keys to good nutrition.

There are many variations of the standard food pyramid, not all of which have been modified following issuance of the new general pyramid. Examples include the pyramid for young children (Fig. 32–1) and the pyramid for older adults (Fig. 32–2).

Using and following this guide does not guarantee that a person will consume the necessary levels of all essential nutrients. However, the food guide is easy to follow, and people who eat a variety of foods from each group, in the suggested amounts, are likely to come close to recommended nutrient levels. The Food Guide Pyramid does not address fluid intake or provide guidelines about combina-

tion foods (such as chili, which contains meat, beans, and a vegetable) or about convenience foods (such as hamburgers, milk shakes, and pizzas), which are a large part of the North American diet, although a chart with some of this information is found on the website.

Recommended Dietary Intake

The Committee on the Scientific Evaluation of Dietary Reference Intakes of the Institute of Medicine publishes the Dietary Reference Intakes (DRIs) tables, which contain four sets of reference values: estimated average requirements (EARs), recommended dietary allowances (RDAs), adequate intakes (AIs), and tolerable upper intake levels (ULs). Definitions of these terms are found on the companion website that comes with this textbook. The values for RDAs and AIs in the tables are modified for different age groups and according to gender. The Canadian Department of National Health and Welfare also adopted the DRIs in 2003. The effect of illness or injury

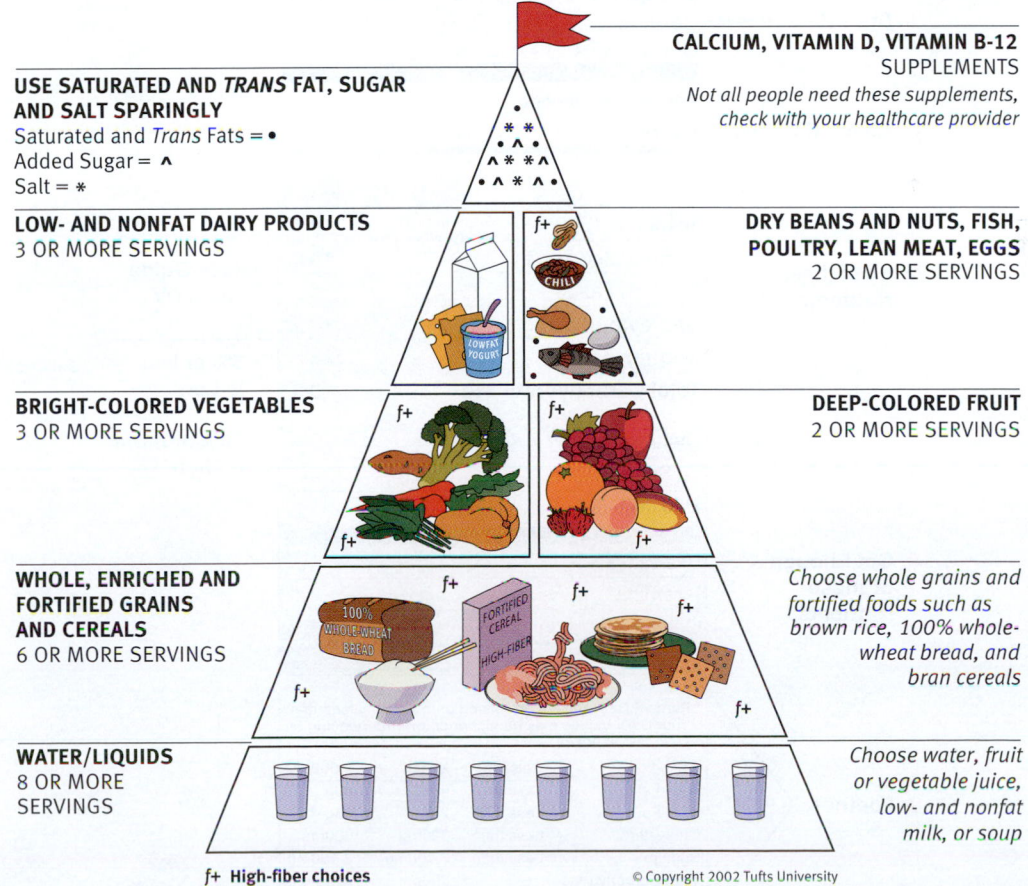

TUFTS
Food Guide Pyramid for Older Adults

CALCIUM, VITAMIN D, VITAMIN B-12
SUPPLEMENTS
Not all people need these supplements, check with your healthcare provider

USE SATURATED AND *TRANS* FAT, SUGAR AND SALT SPARINGLY
Saturated and *Trans* Fats = •
Added Sugar = ∧
Salt = *

LOW- AND NONFAT DAIRY PRODUCTS
3 OR MORE SERVINGS

DRY BEANS AND NUTS, FISH, POULTRY, LEAN MEAT, EGGS
2 OR MORE SERVINGS

BRIGHT-COLORED VEGETABLES
3 OR MORE SERVINGS

DEEP-COLORED FRUIT
2 OR MORE SERVINGS

WHOLE, ENRICHED AND FORTIFIED GRAINS AND CEREALS
6 OR MORE SERVINGS

Choose whole grains and fortified foods such as brown rice, 100% whole-wheat bread, and bran cereals

WATER/LIQUIDS
8 OR MORE SERVINGS

Choose water, fruit or vegetable juice, low- and nonfat milk, or soup

f+ **High-fiber choices**   © Copyright 2002 Tufts University

For additional copies visit us on the web at **http://nutrition.tufts.edu**

Figure 32–2 ● Food guide pyramid for older adults.

and the variability among individuals within any given subgroup are not taken into account in the DRIs.

Consumers most commonly learn recommended dietary intake information from the U.S. Food and Drug Administration (FDA) nutrition labels called Nutrition Facts. Food labeling is required for most prepared foods, such as breads, cereals, canned and frozen foods, snacks, desserts, and drinks. Nutrition labeling for raw produce (fruits and vegetables) and fish is voluntary.

Reading Food Labels

The section at the top of the label ❶ indicates serving size and number of servings in the container (Fig. 32–3). The remaining information on the label indicates the values for *each serving*. Thus, if the person consumes a container that has more than one serving, the person must multiply the values in order to know the real nutrient content. The next section ❷ indicates the number of total calories and calories from fat per serving. Based on a 2,000-calorie diet, a serving with 40 calories is considered low, 100 calories moderate, and 400 calories high. Section ❸ has those nutrients that should be minimized: fats, cholesterol, and sodium. A % Daily Value (DV) of 5% or less is low, and 20% or more is high. When adding the % DV from all foods eaten in one day, the goal is to keep the total below 100%. Effective January 1, 2006, packaged foods must list *trans*-fat content. *Trans*-fats are created when unsaturated oils are hydrogenated to create a solid form and are used in frying foods, margarine, and many snack products. They are also present in meat and dairy fats. *Trans*-fats have been shown to increase cholesterol and contribute to heart disease. The next section ❹ includes fiber, vitamins, and minerals commonly insufficient in American diets. When adding the percent values from all foods eaten in one day, the goal is to keep the total DV of each of these at least at 100%. Again, a % DV of 5 or less is low and 20% or more is high. The footnote ❺ indicates the approximate DVs for fat, cholesterol, sodium, total carbohydrate, and fiber in 2,000- and 2,500-calorie diets. The 2,000-calorie values are used for the % DV numbers in the upper sections.

If the label on a food is missing, consumers can retrieve the information from several websites. It is important to

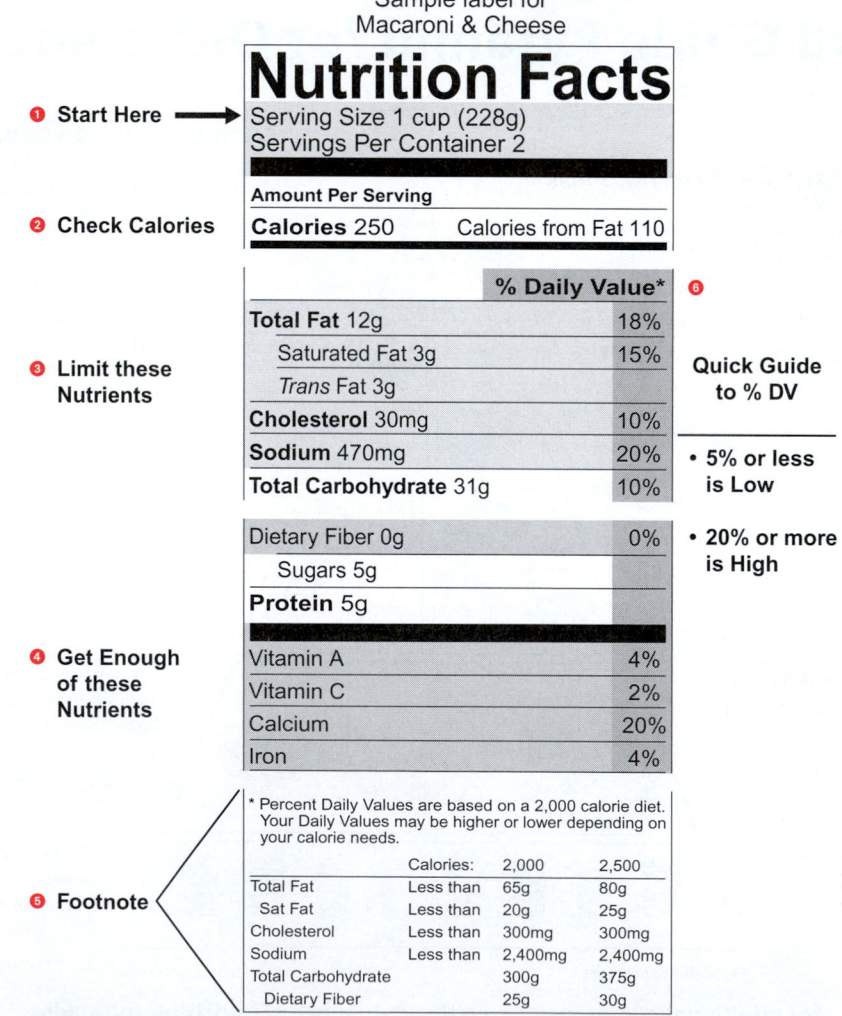

Figure 32–3 ● The nutrition facts label.

teach clients how to choose foods using food labels in order to follow prescribed diets. The Student Navigation Guide that is available with this book has exercises on using food labels to compare quality of food choices.

Vegetarian Diets

People may become vegetarians for economic, health, religious, ethical, or ecologic reasons. There are two basic vegetarian diets: those that use only plant foods (vegan) and those that include milk, eggs, or dairy products. Some people eat fish and poultry but not beef, lamb, or pork; others eat only fresh fruit, juices, and nuts; and still others eat plant foods and dairy products but not eggs. Vegetarian diets can be nutritionally sound if they include a wide variety of foods and if proper protein and vitamin and mineral supplementation are provided (Anonymous, 2003). Because the proteins found in plant foods are incomplete proteins, vegetarians must eat complementary protein foods to obtain all the essential amino acids. A plant protein can be complemented by combining it with a different plant protein in order to produce a complete protein. Obtaining complete proteins is especially important for growing children and pregnant and lactating women, whose protein needs are high. Generally, legumes (starchy beans, peas, lentils) have complementary relationships with grains, nuts, and seeds. Complementary foods must be eaten in the same meal. Diets such as the fruitarian diet do not provide sufficient amounts of essential nutrients and are not recommended for long-term use.

Foods of animal origin are the best source of vitamin B_{12}. Therefore, vegans need to obtain this vitamin from other sources. Because iron from plant sources is not absorbed as efficiently as iron from meat, vegans should eat iron-rich foods and iron-enriched foods. They should eat a food rich in vitamin C at each meal to enhance iron absorption. Calcium deficiency is a concern only for strict vegetarians. It can be prevented by including soybean milk and tofu fortified with calcium and leafy green vegetables in the diet.

ALTERED NUTRITION

Malnutrition is commonly defined as the lack of necessary or appropriate food substances, but in practice includes both undernutrition and overnutrition. **Overnutrition** refers to a caloric intake in excess of daily energy requirements, resulting in storage of energy in the form of adipose tissue. As the amount of stored fat increases, the individual becomes overweight or obese. A person is said to be **overweight** when BMI is between 25 and 29.9 kg/m² and **obese** when BMI is > 30 kg/m² (National Heart, Lung, and Blood Institute, 1998).

Excess body weight increases the stress on body organs and predisposes people to chronic health problems. Obesity that interferes with mobility or breathing is referred to as morbid obesity. Obese people may also manifest undernourishment in important nutrients even though excess calories are ingested.

Undernutrition refers to an intake of nutrients insufficient to meet daily energy requirements because of inadequate food intake or improper digestion and absorption of food. An inadequate food intake may be caused by the inability to acquire and prepare food, inadequate knowledge about essential nutrients and a balanced diet, discomfort during or after eating, or many medical concerns. Improper digestion and absorption of nutrients may be caused by an inadequate production of hormones or enzymes or by medical conditions resulting in inflammation or obstruction of the gastrointestinal tract.

Inadequate nutrition is associated with marked weight loss, generalized weakness, altered functional abilities, delayed wound healing, increased susceptibility to infection, decreased immunocompetence, impaired pulmonary function, and prolonged length of hospitalization. In response to undernutrition, carbohydrate reserves, stored as liver and muscle glycogen, are mobilized. However, these reserves can only meet energy requirements for a short time (e.g., 24 hours) and then body protein is mobilized.

Protein-calorie malnutrition (PCM), once associated with the manifestation of undernutrition seen in starving children of third world countries, is now recognized as a significant problem of clients with long-term deficiencies in caloric intake. Characteristics of PCM are depressed visceral proteins, weight loss, and visible muscle and fat wasting.

Protein stores in the body are generally divided into two compartments: somatic and visceral. Somatic protein consists largely of skeletal muscle mass; it is assessed most commonly by conducting anthropometric measurements such as the mid-arm circumference (MAC) and the mid-arm muscle circumference (MAMC). Visceral protein includes plasma protein, hemoglobin, several clotting factors, hormones, and antibodies. It is usually assessed by measuring serum protein levels such as albumin and transferrin.

LONG-TERM CARE CONSIDERATIONS
Involuntary Weight Loss

Involuntary weight loss is a major problem among residents of long-term care facilities, with malnutrition found in 23%–85% of clients. Malnutrition is associated with poor clinical outcomes and is an indicator of risk for increased mortality in older adults. Early identification of malnutrition should lead to early intervention, which may correct reversible nutritional deficits. The Omnibus Budget Reconciliation Act of 1987 and the Balanced Budget Act of 1997 state that a facility must ensure that a resident maintains acceptable parameters of nutritional status, such as body weight and protein levels and that a therapeutic diet be supplied when there are nutritional problems. It is the nurse's responsibility to monitor the client's nutritional status and report involuntary weight loss to the physician so that the proper dietary referrals can be ordered. (Thomas et al., 2000)

NURSING MANAGEMENT

ASSESSING

The purpose of a nutritional assessment is to identify clients at risk for malnutrition and those with poor nutritional status. In most health care facilities, the responsibility for nutritional assessment and support is shared by the primary care provider, the dietitian, and the nurse. Because a comprehensive nutritional assessment is time consuming and expensive, various levels and types of assessment are available. Generally, nurses perform a nutritional screen. A comprehensive nutritional assessment is often performed by a nutritionist or a dietitian, and the primary care provider. Components of a nutritional assessment, and the opportunity to practice performing one, are found in the student navigation guide and may be remembered as ABCD data: anthropometric, biochemical, clinical, and dietary.

Nutritional Screening

A nutritional screen is an assessment performed to identify clients at risk for malnutrition or those who are malnourished. Clients who are found to be at moderate or high risk are followed with a comprehensive assessment by a dietitian. Medicare standards for nursing homes require that any resident whose percent of meals eaten falls below 75% receive a full nutritional assessment by a nurse.

Nurses carry out nutritional screens through routine nursing histories and physical examinations. Custom-designed screens for a particular population (e.g., older adults and pregnant women) and specific disorders (e.g., cardiac disease) are available.

Screening tools such as the Patient-Generated Subjective Global Assessment (PG-SGA) and the Nutrition Screening Initiative (NSI) can be incorporated into the nursing history. The PG-SGA is a method of classifying clients as either well nourished, moderately malnourished, or severely malnourished based on a dietary history and physical examination. It was established primarily for use with cancer patients but has been widely tested and is appropriate for both inpatient and outpatient clients with various diagnoses (Green & Watson, 2005). A version of the instrument can be completed and analyzed online by the client without a health care provider.

The NSI is an ongoing project of the American Academy of Family Physicians, the American Dietetic Association, the National Council on Aging, and other organizations to promote nutrition screening and improved nutritional care for older adults. The NSI estimates that approximately half of hospitalized, nursing home, and home care older adults are malnourished. The NSI screens older adults using a nutrition checklist that contains nine warning signs of conditions that can interfere with good nutrition. Older adults can also complete the tool online and have a risk score calculated.

Nursing History

Nurses obtain considerable nutrition-related data in the routine admission nursing history. Data to obtain, specific to

nutritional assessment, include condition of the oral cavity, difficulty eating, activity level, change in appetite or weight, difficulty purchasing, preparing, or eating food, cultural and religious beliefs affecting food choices, living arrangements and economic status, and medication history.

Physical Examination

Physical examination may reveal some nutritional deficiencies and excesses in addition to obvious weight changes. Assessment focuses on rapidly proliferating tissues such as skin, hair, nails, eyes, and mucosa but also includes a systematic review comparable to any routine physical examination. See Clinical Manifestations for signs associated with malnutrition. These signs must be viewed as suggestive of malnutrition because the signs are nonspecific. For example, red conjunctiva may indicate an infection rather than a nutritional deficit, and dry, dull hair may be related to excessive exposure to the sun rather than severe protein-energy malnutrition. To confirm malnutrition, clinical findings need to be substantiated with laboratory tests and dietary data.

Calculating Percentage of Weight Loss

Accurate assessment of the client's height, current body weight (CBW), and usual body weight (UBW) is essential. Although the client's CBW can be compared with an ideal body weight discussed earlier, the IBW is based on healthy people and does not account for changes in the client's body composition that accompany illness or reflect any changes in weight. The client's UBW better indicates weight change and the possibility of malnutrition. Calculation and interpretation of the percent of deviation from UBW and the percent of weight loss are shown in Box 32–3. An important aspect of weight assessment, obtained in the nursing history, is a description of weight change. The nurse should describe any weight loss or gain, the duration of the change, and whether the weight change was intentional or unintentional.

Diet History

A dietary history includes data about the client's usual eating patterns and habits; food preferences, allergies, and intolerances; frequency, types, and quantities of foods consumed; and social, economic, ethnic, or religious factors

CLINICAL MANIFESTATIONS — Malnutrition

Area of Examination (possible cause)	Signs Associated with Malnutrition
General appearance and vitality	Apathetic, listless, looks tired, easily fatigued
Weight	Overweight or underweight
Skin	Dry, flaky, or scaly; pale or pigmented; presence of petechiae or bruises; lack of subcutaneous fat; edema
Nails	Brittle, pale, ridged, or spoon shaped (iron)
Hair	Dry, dull, sparse, loss of color, brittle
Eyes	Pale or red conjunctiva, dryness, soft cornea, dull cornea, night blindness (vitamin A deficiency)
Lips	Swollen, red cracks at side of mouth, vertical fissures (B vitamins)
Tongue	Swollen, beefy red or magenta colored (B vitamins); smooth appearance (B vitamins deficiency); decrease or increase in size
Gums	Spongy, swollen, inflamed; bleed easily (vitamin C deficiency)
Muscles	Underdeveloped, flaccid, wasted, soft
Gastrointestinal system	Anorexia, indigestion, diarrhea, constipation, enlarged liver, protruding abdomen
Nervous system	Decreased reflexes, sensory loss, burning and tingling of hands and feet (B vitamins), mental confusion or irritability

typical 24-hour period when at home. The data obtained are then generally evaluated according to the Food Guide Pyramid to judge overall adequacy.

A food frequency record is a checklist that indicates how often general food groups or specific foods are eaten. Frequency may be categorized as times/day, times/week, times/month, or frequently, seldom, never. This record, like the 24-hour food recall, provides information about the types of foods eaten but not the quantities. When specific foods or nutrients are suspected of being deficient or excessive, the health care professional may use a selective food frequency that focuses, for example, on fat, fruit, vegetable, or fiber intake.

A **food diary** is a detailed record of measured amounts (portion sizes) of all food and fluids a client consumes during a specified period, usually 3 to 7 days. The client is asked to record their intake at the time they consume it with the amount consumed.

A **diet history** is a comprehensive time-consuming assessment of a client's food intake that involves an extensive interview by a nutritionist or dietitian. It includes characteristics of foods usually eaten as well as the frequency and amount of food consumed. Thus, it may include a 24-hour recall, a food frequency record, and a food diary. Medical and psychosocial factors are also assessed to evaluate their impact on nutritional requirements, food habits, and choices. Data obtained are analyzed by computer and translated into caloric and nutrient intake. Results are compared with the DRIs that are appropriate for the client's age, sex, and condition.

Anthropometric Measurements

Anthropometric measurements are noninvasive techniques that aim to quantify body composition. A skinfold measurement is performed to determine fat stores. The most common site for measurement is the triceps skinfold (TSF). The fold of skin measured includes subcutaneous tissue but not the underlying muscle. It is measured in millimeters using special calipers. To measure the TSF, locate the midpoint of the upper arm (halfway between the acromion process and the olecranon process), then grasp the skin on the back of the upper arm along the long axis of the humerus (Figure 32–4). Placing the calipers 1 cm (0.4 in.) below the nurse's fingers, measure the thickness of the fold to the nearest millimeter.

influencing nutrition. Four possible methods for collecting dietary data are a 24-hour food recall, a food frequency record, a food diary, and a diet history. All four methods rely on subjective data and are only as accurate as the information supplied by the client.

For a 24-hour food recall, the nurse asks the client to recall all the food and beverages the client consumes during a

BOX 32–3 — Calculating and Interpreting the Percent of Deviation from Usual Body Weight and the Percent of Weight Loss

Calculating Percent of Usual Body Weight

$$\% \text{ usual body weight} = \frac{\text{Current weight}}{\text{Usual body weight}} \times 100$$

Mild malnutrition	85%–90%
Moderate malnutrition	75%–84%
Severe malnutrition	Less than 74%

Calculating Percent of Weight Loss

$$\% \text{ weight loss} = \frac{\text{Usual weight} - \text{current weight}}{\text{Usual weight}}$$

Significant Weight Loss	Severe Weight Loss
5% over 1 mo	> 5% over 1 mo
7.5% over 3 mo	> 7.5% over 3 mo
10% over 6 mo	> 10% over 6 mo

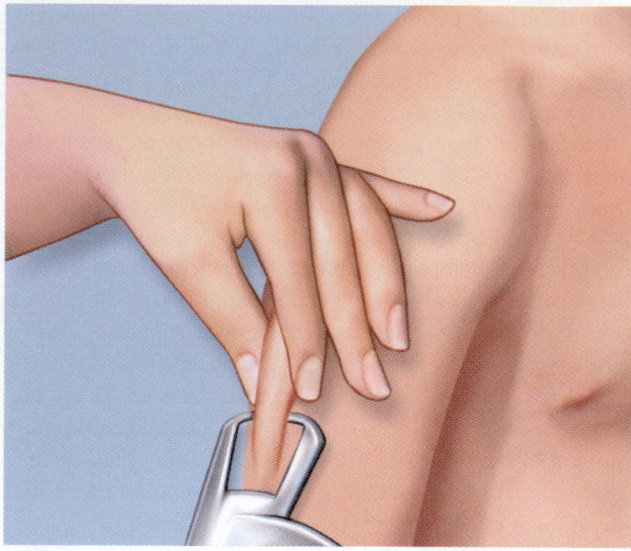

Figure 32–4 ● Measuring the triceps skinfold.

The **mid-arm circumference (MAC)** is a measure of fat, muscle, and skeleton. To measure the MAC, ask the client to sit or stand with the arm hanging freely and the forearm flexed to horizontal. Measure the circumference at the midpoint of the arm, recording the measurement in centimeters, to the nearest millimeter (e.g., 24.6 cm) (Figure 32–5).

The **mid-arm muscle circumference (MAMC)** is then calculated by using reference tables or by using a formula that incorporates the TSF and the MAC. The MAMC is an estimate of lean body mass, or skeletal muscle reserves. If tables are not available, the nurse uses the following formula to calculate the MAMC from the triceps skinfold and MAC direct measurements:

$$\text{MAMC cm} = \frac{\text{MAC (cm)} - 3.143\ \text{TSF (mm)}}{10}$$

Standard values for anthropometric measurements for adults are shown in Table 32–1.

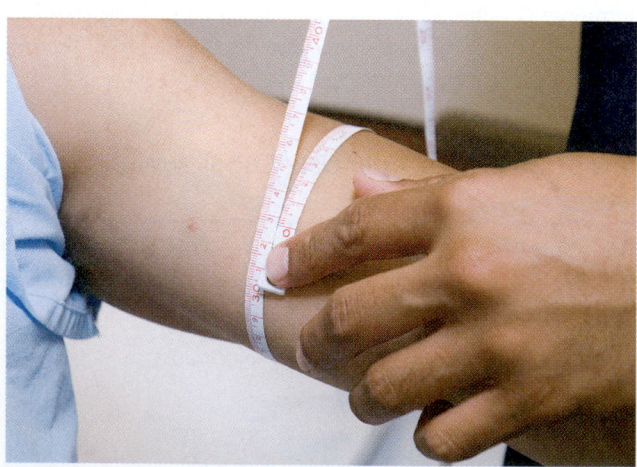

Figure 32–5 ● Measuring the mid-arm circumference.

TABLE 32–1	Standard Values for Anthropometric Measurements for Adults	
MEASUREMENT	MALE	FEMALE
Triceps skinfold (mm)	12	20
Mid-arm circumference (cm)	32	28
Mid-arm muscle circumference (cm²)	54	30

From *The Merck Manual of Diagnosis and Therapy*, 18th ed., M. H. Beers and R. Berkow (Eds.), 2006. Copyright John Wiley & Sons. Reprinted with permission.

Changes in anthropometric measurements often occur slowly and reflect chronic rather than acute changes in nutritional status. They are, therefore, used to monitor the client's progress for months to years rather than days to weeks. Ideally, initial and subsequent measurements need to be taken by the same clinician. Measurements obtained need to be interpreted with caution because fluctuations in hydration status often occur during illness and can influence accuracy. Normal standards may not account for normal changes in body composition such as those that occur with aging.

Laboratory Data

Laboratory tests can provide objective data to assessed nutritional status but many factors can influence test results so no single test specifically predicts risk or measures the degree of nutritional problems. The most common tests used are serum proteins, urinary urea nitrogen and creatinine, and total lymphocyte count.

Serum proteins include hemoglobin, albumin, transferrin, total iron-binding capacity, and prealbumin. Low hemoglobin may indicate iron deficiency anemia but can also be due to blood loss. Albumin is one of the most common visceral proteins evaluated but albumin levels change slowly because it is not broken down quickly (half life of 18–20 days). A low serum albumin level indicates prolonged protein depletion. Altered liver function, hydration status, and losses from open wounds or burns can also impact albumin levels. Transferrin is a protein that binds and carries iron from the intestine through the serum and has a shorter half-life than albumin (8–9 days) so it responds more quickly to protein depletion. Transferrin can be measured directly or by a total iron-binding capacity (TIBC) test, which indicates the amount of iron in the blood available to bind to transferrin. Low serum transferrin levels indicate protein loss, iron deficiency anemia, pregnancy, hepatitis, or liver dysfunction. An increase indicates iron deficiency anemia. Prealbumin, or thyroxine-binding albumin, has the shortest half-life and smallest body pool so it shows changes in nutritional status more quickly. It is considered the "gold standard" for assessing possible protein malnutrition (Kuszajewski & Clontz, 2005). It should be measured twice a week with normal values of 15–35 mg/dl. A level below 15 indicates a client at risk and a level below 11 indicates a need for aggressive nutritional intervention.

Urinary tests include urinary urea nitrogen and urinary creatinine, which measures protein catabolism and the state of nitrogen balance. Urea is the chief end product of amino acid metabolism and directly reflects the intake and breakdown of dietary protein, rate of urea production in the liver, and rate of urea removal by the kidneys. Urinary creatinine reflects a person's total muscle mass because creatinine is the chief end product of the creatine produced when energy is released during skeletal muscle metabolism. The rate of creatinine formation is directly proportional to the total muscle mass so high urine creatinine means greater muscle mass. As skeletal muscle atrophies during malnutrition, creatinine excretion decreases. The state of nitrogen balance is determined by comparing nitrogen intake to nitrogen output over a 24-hour period. A positive nitrogen balance exists when intake exceeds nitrogen output while a negative nitrogen balance occurs when output exceeds intake.

Total lymphocyte count decreases as protein depletion occurs. Some nutritional deficiencies and forms of PCM can depress the immune system.

DIAGNOSING

NANDA (2009) includes the following diagnostic labels for nutritional problems:

- *Imbalanced Nutrition: More Than Body Requirements*
- *Imbalanced Nutrition: Less Than Body Requirements*
- *Readiness for Enhanced Nutrition*
- *Risk for Imbalanced Nutrition: More Than Body Requirements*

Clinical examples of assessment data clusters and related nursing diagnoses are shown in Identifying Nursing Diagnoses, Outcomes, and Interventions.

Many other NANDA nursing diagnoses may apply to certain individuals, because nutritional problems often affect other areas of human functioning. In this case, the nutritional diagnostic label may be used as the etiology of other diagnoses. Examples include:

- *Activity Intolerance* related to inadequate intake of iron-rich foods resulting in iron-deficiency anemia

IDENTIFYING NURSING DIAGNOSES, OUTCOMES, AND INTERVENTIONS — Clients with Nutritional Disorders

DATA CLUSTER Dedra Bronsky, a 63-year-old, has chronic rheumatoid arthritis. Her husband died 8 months ago. She says, "It's just no fun to cook anymore. There's no one to share meals with and so many things connected to cooking hurts my hands. I just never seem to feel hungry and I am not interested in food." She is 5′ 5″ (165 cm) tall and weighs 88 lb (40 kg). Her TSF is 11.0 mm; MAMC is 13.4 mm; UBW is 125 lb (56.8 kg). Dietary assessment indicates that she eats mostly bread, cereal, whole milk, and canned fish. She eats almost no fruits and vegetables.

NURSING DIAGNOSIS/DEFINITION	SAMPLE DESIRED OUTCOMES*/*DEFINITION*	INDICATORS	SELECTED INTERVENTIONS*/*DEFINITION*	SAMPLE NIC ACTIVITIES
Imbalanced Nutrition: Less Than Body Requirements/Intake of nutrients insufficient to meet metabolic needs	Nutritional Status: Nutrient Intake [1009]/*Adequacy of usual pattern of nutrient intake*	Substantially adequate • Caloric intake • Vitamin intake	Nutrition Therapy [1120]/*Administration of food and fluids to support metabolic processes of a client who is malnourished or at high risk of becoming malnourished*	• Determine food preferences with consideration of cultural and religious preferences • Determine—in collaboration with the dietitian—the number of calories and type of nutrients needed • Provide needed nourishment within limits of prescribed diet • Structure the environment to create a pleasant and relaxing atmosphere • Arrange for appropriate referrals to community resources that provide meals

*The NOC # for desired outcomes and the NIC # for nursing interventions are listed in brackets following the appropriate outcome or intervention. Outcomes, indicators, interventions, and activities selected are only a sample of those suggested by NOC and NIC and should be further individualized for each client.

- *Constipation* related to inadequate fluid intake and fiber intake
- *Low Self-Esteem* related to obesity
- *Risk for Infection* related to immunosuppression secondary to insufficient protein intake

PLANNING

Major goals for clients with or at risk for nutritional problems include:

- Maintain or restore optimal nutritional status.
- Promote healthy nutritional practices.
- Prevent complications associated with malnutrition.
- Decrease weight.
- Regain specified weight.

Examples of NOC outcomes and NIC interventions related to some of these goals are shown in Identifying Nursing Diagnoses, Outcomes, and Interventions (page 967). Specific nursing activities associated with each of these interventions can be selected to meet the individual needs of the client. See the Nursing Care Plan and Concept Map at the end of this chapter.

Planning for Home Care

Planning for discharge and home care begins at admission and the nurse must consider the client's need for assistance with nutrition. Home care planning begins with an assessment of the client and family's abilities for self-care, financial resources, and the need for referrals and home health services. A major aspect of discharge planning involves instructional needs of the client and family (see Client Teaching).

CLIENT TEACHING   Healthy Nutrition

- Instruct clients about the content of a healthy diet based on the Food Guide Pyramid and *Dietary Guidelines for Americans.*
- Encourage clients, particularly older clients, to reduce dietary fat (see Client Teaching on reducing dietary fat, page 960).
- Instruct strict vegetarians about proper protein complementation and additional vitamin and mineral supplementation.
- Discuss foods high in specific nutrients required such as protein, iron, calcium, vitamin C, and fiber.
- Discuss importance of properly fitted dentures and dental care.
- Discuss safe food preparation and preservation techniques as appropriate.

Dietary Alterations

- Explain the purpose of the diet.
- Discuss allowed and excluded foods.
- Explain the importance of reading food labels when selecting packaged foods.
- Include family or significant others.
- Reinforce information provided by the dietitian or nutritionist as appropriate.
- Discuss herbs and spices as alternatives to salt and substitutes for sugar.

For Overweight Clients

- Discuss physiologic, psychologic, and lifestyle factors that predispose to weight gain.
- Provide information about desired weight range and recommended calorie intake.
- Discuss principles of a well-balanced diet and high- and low-calorie foods.
- Encourage intake of low-calorie, caffeine-free beverages and plenty of water.
- Discuss ways to adapt eating practices by using smaller plates, taking smaller servings, chewing each bite a specified number of times, and putting fork down between bites.
- Discuss ways to control the desire to eat by taking a walk, drinking a glass of water, or doing slow deep-breathing exercises.
- Discuss the importance of exercise and help the client plan an exercise program.

- Discuss stress reduction techniques.
- Provide information about available community resources (e.g., weight-loss groups, dietary counseling, exercise programs, self-help groups).

For Underweight Clients

- Discuss factors contributing to inadequate nutrition and weight loss.
- Discuss recommended calorie intake and desired weight range.
- Provide information about the content of a balanced diet.
- Provide information about ways to increase calorie intake (e.g., high-protein or high-calorie foods and supplements).
- Discuss ways to manage, minimize, or alter the factors contributing to malnourishment.
- If appropriate, discuss ways to purchase low-cost nutritious foods.
- Provide information about community agencies that can assist in providing food (e.g., Meals on Wheels).

Preventing Foodborne Illness

- Reinforce hygienic handling of food and dishes.
  - Wash hands before preparing foods.
  - Wash hands and all dishes and utensils with hot water and soap after contact with raw meats.
  - Defrost frozen foods in the refrigerator.
  - Cook beef, poultry, and eggs thoroughly. Use a cooking thermometer.
  - Refrigerate leftovers promptly (at 40°F [5°C] or less) and keep no more than 3 to 5 days.
  - Wash or peel raw fruits and vegetables.
  - Do not use foods from containers that have been damaged or have opened seals.
  - Follow the rules "keep hot foods hot and cold foods cold" and "when in doubt, throw it out."
- Recommend the client consider a preventive vaccination for hepatitis A.
- Instruct clients to seek medical attention for prolonged vomiting, fever, abdominal pain, or severe diarrhea following a meal.

IMPLEMENTING

Nursing interventions to promote optimal nutrition for hospitalized clients are often provided in collaboration with the primary care provider who writes the diet orders and the dietitian who informs clients about special diets. The nurse reinforces these instructions, creates an atmosphere that encourages eating, provides assistance with eating, monitors the client's appetite and food intake, administers enteral and parenteral feedings, and consults with the primary care provider and dietitian about nutritional problems that arise.

Assisting with Special Diets

Alterations in the client's diet are often needed to treat a disease process such as diabetes mellitus, to prepare for a special examination or surgery, to increase or decrease weight, to restore nutritional deficits, or to allow an organ to rest and promote healing. Diets may be modified in texture, kilocalories, specific nutrients, seasonings, or consistency.

Hospitalized clients who do not have special needs eat the regular (standard or house) diet, a balanced diet that supplies the metabolic requirements of a sedentary person (about 2,000 Kcal). Most agencies offer clients a daily menu from which to select their meals for the next day; others provide standard meals to each client on the general diet.

A variation of the regular diet is the light diet, designed for postoperative and other clients who are not ready for the regular diet. Foods in the light diet are plainly cooked and fat is usually minimized, as are bran and foods containing a great deal of fiber.

Diets that are modified in consistency are often given to clients before and after surgery or to promote healing in clients with gastrointestinal distress. These diets include clear liquid, full liquid, soft, and diet as tolerated. In some agencies, gastrointestinal surgery clients are not permitted red-colored liquids or candy since, if vomited, the color may be confused with blood.

The clear liquid diet is limited to water, tea, coffee, clear broths, ginger ale, or other carbonated beverages, strained and clear juices, and plain gelatin. Note that "clear" does not necessarily mean "colorless" but can generally be seen through. This diet provides the client with fluid and carbohydrate but does not supply adequate protein, fat, vitamins, minerals, or calories. It is a short-term diet (24–36 hours). The major objectives of this diet are to relieve thirst, prevent dehydration, and minimize stimulation of the gastrointestinal tract.

The full liquid diet contains only liquids or foods that turn to liquid at body temperature, such as ice cream. Full liquid diets are often eaten by clients who are unable to tolerate solid or semisolid foods. This diet is not recommended for long-term use because it is low in iron, protein, and calories and high in cholesterol. Clients requiring long-term liquid diets are usually given a nutritionally balanced oral supplement, such as Ensure or Sustacal. The full liquid diet is monotonous and difficult for clients to accept. Planning six or more feedings per day may encourage a more adequate intake.

The soft diet is easily chewed and digested. It is often ordered for clients who have difficulty chewing and swallowing. It is a low-residue (low-fiber) diet containing very few uncooked foods; however, restrictions vary among agencies and according to individual tolerance. The **pureed diet** is a modification of the soft diet. Liquid may be added to the food, which is then blended to a semisolid consistency.

Diet as tolerated is ordered when the client's appetite, ability to eat, and tolerance for certain foods may change. The nurse orders the type of diet the client is most able to tolerate.

Many special diets may be prescribed to meet requirements for disease process or altered metabolism. For example, a client with diabetes mellitus may need a diet recommended by the American Diabetes Association, an obese client may need a calorie-restricted diet, a cardiac client may need sodium and cholesterol restrictions, and a client with allergies will need a hypoallergenic diet. Some clients follow these diets for a lifetime and must understand the diet and develop a positive attitude about it. Assisting clients and support persons with special diets is a function shared by the dietitian or nutritionist and the nurse. See Box 32–4.

Some clients may have no difficulty with choosing a healthy diet, but be at risk for nutritional problems due to dysphagia (difficulty swallowing). These clients may have inadequate solid or fluid intake, be unable to swallow their medications, or aspirate food or fluids into the lungs—causing pneumonia. Nurses may be the first persons to detect dysphagia and are in an excellent position to recommend further evaluation; implement specialized feeding techniques and diets; and work with clients, family members, and other health care professionals to develop a plan to assist the client with difficulties. If the client condition suggests dysphagia, the nurse should review the history in detail; interview the client or family; assess the mouth, throat, and chest; and observe the client swallowing. Presence of the gag reflex, often thought to indicate that the client can swallow safely, has not been shown to be a reliable indicator (Zagaria, 2005). Confirmation of the tendency for food to divert to the trachea is best done through x-ray. A multidisciplinary group has developed the National Dysphagia Diet (NDD) delineating standards of food textures (American Dietetic Association, 2003). In consultation with the dietician, occupational therapist, swallowing specialist, speech-language pathologist, and/or primary care provider these standards can be used to determine a consistent approach to a particular client's dysphagia.

BOX 32–4   Physician's Office Considerations

The nurse, working in the physician's office, will treat clients requiring special diets. If the client does not require hospitalization, the office nurse may be the client's only contact with a health care provider who can help them comply with their prescribed diet. It is important for the nurse to question what foods they are eating, problems they are encountering, and provide additional teaching on dietary compliance.

All dietary instructions must be individually designed to meet the client's intellectual ability, motivation level, lifestyle, culture, and economic status. Both nutritionists and dietitians help to adapt a diet to suit the client. Simple verbal instructions need to be given and reinforced with written material. Family and support persons must be included in the dietary instruction.

Stimulating the Appetite

Physical illness, unfamiliar or unpalatable food, environmental and psychological factors, and physical discomfort or pain may depress the appetites of many clients. A short-term decrease in food intake usually is not a problem for adults; over time it leads to weight loss, decreased strength and stamina, and other nutritional problems. A decreased food intake is often accompanied by a decrease in fluid intake, which may cause fluid and electrolyte problems. Stimulating a person's appetite requires the nurse to determine the reason for the lack of appetite and then deal with the problem. Some general interventions for improving the client's appetite are summarized in Box 32–5.

Assisting Clients with Meals

Even clients who normally eat independently may require some assistance when attempting to eat in bed. Long-term care facilities and some hospitals serve meals to mobile clients in a special dining area. Guidelines for providing meals to clients are summarized in Box 32–6.

Certain clients frequently require help with their meals: older adults who are weakened, persons with disabilities, those who must remain in a back-lying position, or those who cannot use their hands. The client's nursing care plan should indicate that assistance is required with meals.

BOX 32–5   **Improving Appetite**

- Provide familiar food that the person likes. Often the relatives of clients are pleased to bring food from home but may need some guidance about special diet requirements.
- Select small portions so as not to discourage the anorexic client.
- Avoid unpleasant or uncomfortable treatments immediately before or after a meal.
- Provide a tidy, clean environment that is free of unpleasant sights and odors. A soiled dressing, a used bedpan, an uncovered irrigation set, or even used dishes can negatively affect the appetite.
- Encourage or provide oral hygiene before mealtime. This improves the client's ability to taste.
- Relieve illness symptoms that depress appetite before mealtime; for example, give an analgesic for pain or an antipyretic for a fever or allow rest for fatigue.
- Reduce psychologic stress. A lack of understanding of therapy, the anticipation of an operation, and fear of the unknown can cause anorexia. Often, the nurse can help by discussing feelings with the client, giving information and assistance, and allaying fears.

BOX 32–6   **Providing Client Meals**

- Offer the client assistance with hand washing and oral hygiene before a meal.
- If it is permitted, assist the client to a comfortable position in bed or in a chair, whichever is appropriate.
- Clear the over-bed table so that there is space for the tray. If the client must remain in a lying position in bed, arrange the over-bed table close to the bedside so that the client can see and reach the food.
- Check each tray for the client's name, the type of diet, and completeness. Do not leave an incorrect diet for a client to eat.
- Assist the client as required.
- For a blind person, identify the placement of the food as you would describe the time on a clock.
- After the client has completed the meal, observe how much and what the client has eaten and the amount of fluid taken. Use a standard tool to estimate the amount eaten in relation to a typical meal. For example, if served a donut and hot chocolate for breakfast, although the client may have eaten all of these, they certainly do not represent 100% of a nutritious breakfast.
- If the client is on a special diet or is having problems eating, record the amount of food eaten and any pain, fatigue, or nausea experienced.
- If the client is not eating, document this so that changes can be made, such as rescheduling the meals, providing smaller, more frequent meals, or obtaining special self-feeding aids.

The nurse must be sensitive to clients' feelings of embarrassment, resentment, and loss of autonomy. Whenever possible, the nurse should help incapacitated clients feed themselves as much as possible. Some clients become depressed because they feel dependent and burdensome. Although feeding a client is time consuming, nurses should try to appear unhurried and convey that they have ample time. Sitting at the bedside is one way to convey this impression. If the client is to be fed by unlicensed assistive personnel, the nurse must ensure that the same standards are met.

When feeding a client, ask in which order the client would like to eat the food. If the client cannot see, tell the client which food is being given. Always allow ample time for the client to chew and swallow the food before offering more. Provide fluids as requested, or, if the client is unable to communicate, offer fluids after every three or four mouthfuls of solid food. It is important to make the time a pleasant one, choosing topics of conversation that are of interest to clients who want to talk.

Although normal utensils should be used whenever possible, special utensils may be needed to assist a client to eat. For clients who have difficulty drinking from a cup or glass, a straw often permits them to obtain liquids with less effort and less spillage. Special drinking cups are also available. A standard eating utensil with a built-up or widened handle helps clients who cannot grasp objects easily. Handles may be bent or angled to compensate for limited motion. Clients requiring pureed or liquid diets

BOX 32–7 **Supervision**

Feeding the client or delivering the client's meal tray may be delegated to unlicensed assistive personnel (UAP). However, it remains the responsibility of the nurse to assure that the client receives the proper diet and is fed properly. Nurses should supervise the UAP and provide feedback as needed. Taking the time to teach the UAP to improve performance will benefit both the nurse and the client.

are sometimes fed with a feeding syringe. Plates with rims and plastic or metal plate guards enable the client to pick up the food by first pushing it against this raised edge. A suction cup or damp sponge or cloth may be placed under the dish to keep it from moving while the client is eating. See Box 32–7.

Special Community Nutritional Services

In many places, community programs have been developed to help clients meet nutritional needs. For older adults who cannot prepare meals or leave their homes, ready-to-eat meals or frozen dinners are delivered to the home by local organizations like Meals on Wheels. For people who can prepare meals but have physical disabilities and are unable to shop for groceries, there are grocery delivery services. The USDA funds a food stamp program for the poor.

Enteral Nutrition

An alternative feeding method to ensure adequate nutrition includes **enteral** (through the gastrointestinal system) methods. Enteral nutrition (EN), also referred to as total enteral nutrition (TEN), is provided when the client is unable to ingest foods or the upper gastrointestinal tract is impaired and the transport of food to the small intestine is interrupted. Enteral feedings are administered through nasogastric and small-bore feeding tubes, or through gastrostomy or jejunostomy tubes.

A nasogastric tube is inserted through one of the nostrils, past the nasopharynx, and into the alimentary tract. Traditional firm, large-bore nasogastric tubes (i.e., those larger than 12 Fr in diameter) are placed in the stomach. The larger lumen of the Salem sump tube allows delivery of liquids to the stomach or removal of gastric contents. When the Salem tube is used for suction of gastric contents, the smaller vent lumen (the proximal port is often referred to as the *blue pigtail*) allows for an inflow of atmospheric air, which prevents a vacuum if the gastric tube adheres to the wall of the stomach. Irritation of the gastric mucosa is thereby avoided. Softer, more flexible and less irritating small-bore tubes (smaller than 12 Fr in diameter) are frequently used. Nasogastric tubes are used to feed clients with adequate gastric emptying requiring short-term feedings. They are not advised for feeding clients without intact gag and cough reflexes since the risk of accidental placement of the tube into the lungs is much higher. Skill 32–1 provides guidelines for inserting a nasogastric tube. Skill 32–2 outlines the steps for removing a nasogastric tube.

SKILL 32–1

INSERTING A NASOGASTRIC TUBE

PURPOSES
- To administer tube feedings and medications to clients unable to eat by mouth or swallow a sufficient diet without aspirating food or fluids into the lungs

- To establish a means for suctioning stomach contents to prevent gastric distention, nausea, and vomiting
- To remove stomach contents for laboratory analysis
- To lavage (wash) the stomach in case of poisoning or overdose of medications

ASSESSMENT
Assess the following:
- Check for history of nasal surgery or deviated septum. Assess patency of nares.

- Determine presence of gag reflex.
- Assess mental status or ability to cooperate with procedure.

PLANNING
Before inserting a nasogastric tube, determine the size of tube to be inserted and whether the tube is to be attached to suction.

Delegation
Insertion of a nasogastric tube is an invasive procedure requiring application of knowledge (e.g., anatomy and physiology, risk factors) and problem solving. In some agencies, only health care providers with advanced training are permitted to insert nasogastric tubes that require use of a stylet. Delegation of this skill to unlicensed assistive personnel (UAP) is not appropriate. The UAP, however, can assist with the oral hygiene needs of a client with a nasogastric tube.

EQUIPMENT
- Large- or small-bore tube (nonlatex preferred)
- Nonallergenic adhesive tape, 2.5 cm (1 in.) wide

- Clean gloves
- Water-soluble lubricant
- Facial tissues
- Glass of water and drinking straw
- 20- to 50-mL syringe with an adapter
- Basin
- pH test strip or meter
- Bilirubin dipstick
- Stethoscope
- Disposable pad or towel
- Clamp or plug (optional)
- Antireflux valve for air vent if Salem sump tube is used
- Suction apparatus
- Safety pin and elastic band
- CO_2 detector (optional)

(continued)

SKILL 32–1

INSERTING A NASOGASTRIC TUBE *(continued)*

IMPLEMENTATION

Preparation

Assist the client to a high Fowler's position if his or her health condition permits, and support the head on a pillow. **Rationale:** *It is often easier to swallow in this position and gravity helps the passage of the tube.*

Place a towel or disposable pad across the chest.

Performance

1. Prior to performing the insertion, introduce self and verify the client's identity using agency protocol. Explain to the client what you are going to do, why it is necessary, and how he or she can participate. The passage of a gastric tube is unpleasant because the gag reflex is activated during insertion. Establish a method for the client to indicate distress and a desire for you to pause the insertion. Raising a finger or hand is often used for this.

2. Perform hand hygiene and observe other appropriate infection control procedures (e.g., clean gloves).

3. Provide for client privacy.

4. Assess the client's nares.
   - Ask the client to hyperextend the head, and, using a flashlight, observe the intactness of the tissues of the nostrils, including any irritations or abrasions.
   - Examine the nares for any obstructions or deformities by asking the client to breathe through one nostril while occluding the other.
   - Select the nostril that has the greater airflow.

5. Prepare the tube.
   - If a small-bore tube is being used, ensure stylet or guidewire is secured in position. **Rationale:** *An improperly positioned stylet or guidewire can traumatize the nasopharynx, esophagus, and stomach.*

6. Determine how far to insert the tube.
   - Use the tube to mark off the distance from the tip of the client's nose to the tip of the earlobe and then from the tip of the earlobe to the tip of the xiphoid. ❶ **Rationale:** *This length approximates the distance from the nares to the stomach. This distance varies among individuals.*

   - Mark this length with adhesive tape if the tube does not have markings.

7. Insert the tube.
   - Put on gloves.
   - Lubricate the tip of the tube well with water-soluble lubricant or water to ease insertion. **Rationale:** *A water-soluble lubricant dissolves if the tube accidentally enters the lungs. An oil-based lubricant, such as petroleum jelly, will not dissolve and could cause respiratory complications if it enters the lungs.*
   - Insert the tube, with its natural curve toward the client, into the selected nostril. Ask the client to hyperextend the neck, and gently advance the tube toward the nasopharynx. **Rationale:** *Hyperextension of the neck reduces the curvature of the nasopharyngeal junction.*
   - Direct the tube along the floor of the nostril and toward the ear on that side. **Rationale:** *Directing the tube along the floor avoids the projections (turbinates) along the lateral wall.*
   - Slight pressure and a twisting motion are sometimes required to pass the tube into the nasopharynx, and some client's eyes may water at this point. **Rationale:** *Tears are a natural body response.* Provide the client with tissues as needed.
   - If the tube meets resistance, withdraw it, re-lubricate it, and insert it in the other nostril. **Rationale:** *The tube should never be forced against resistance because of the danger of injury.*
   - Once the tube reaches the oropharynx (throat), the client will feel the tube in the throat and may gag and retch. Ask the client to tilt the head forward, and encourage the client to drink and swallow. **Rationale:** *Tilting the head forward facilitates passage of the tube into the posterior pharynx and esophagus rather than into the larynx; swallowing moves the epiglottis over the opening to the larynx.* ❷

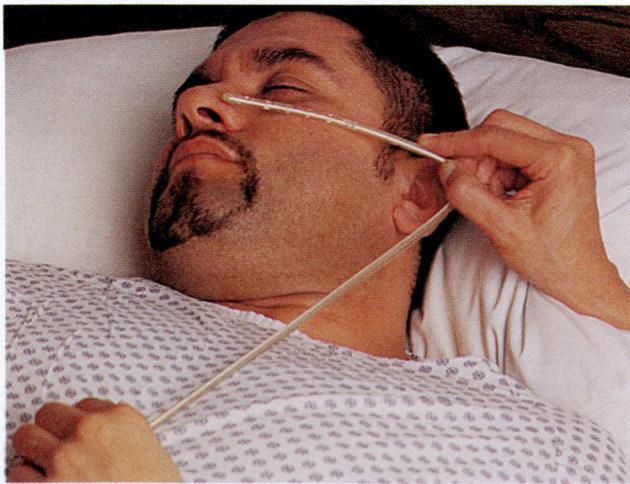

❶ Measuring the appropriate length to insert a nasogastric tube.

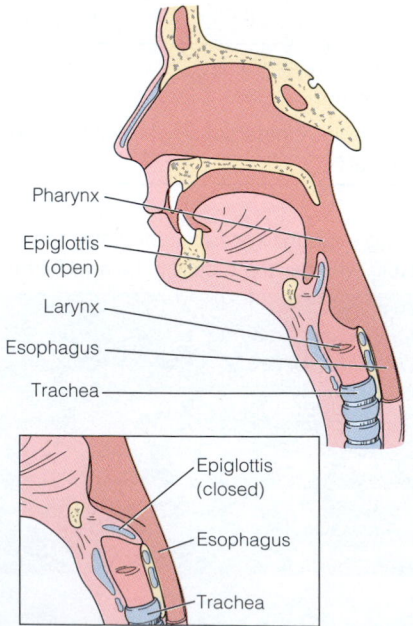

❷ Swallowing closes the epiglottis.

- If the client gags, stop passing the tube momentarily. Have the client rest, take a few breaths, and take sips of water to calm the gag reflex.
- In cooperation with the client, pass the tube 5 to 10 cm (2 to 4 in.) with each swallow, until the indicated length is inserted.
- If the client continues to gag and the tube does not advance with each swallow, withdraw it slightly, and inspect the throat by looking through the mouth. **Rationale:** *The tube may be coiled in the throat.* If so, withdraw it until it is straight, and try again to insert it.
- If a CO_2 detector is used, after the tube has been advanced approximately 30 cm (12 in.), draw air through the detector. Any change in color of the detector indicates placement of the tube in the respiratory tract. Immediately withdraw the tube and reinsert.

8. Ascertain correct placement of the tube.
   - Aspirate stomach contents, and check the pH, which should be acidic. **Rationale:** *Testing pH is a reliable way to determine location of a feeding tube. Gastric contents are commonly pH 1 to 5; 6 or greater would indicate the contents are from lower in the intestinal tract or in the respiratory tract. Some researchers suggest that a pH of greater than 5 should be followed by further confirmation of tube location* (Huffman, Jarczyk, O'Brien, Pieper, & Bayne, 2004).
   - Aspirate can also be tested for bilirubin. Bilirubin levels in the lungs should be almost zero, while levels in the stomach will be approximately 1.5 mg/dL and in the intestine over 10 mg/dL.
   - Almost all nasogastric tubes are radiopaque, and position can be confirmed by x-ray. Check agency policy. If a small-bore tube is used, leave the stylet or guidewire in place until correct position is verified by x-ray. If the stylet has been removed, never reinsert it while the tube is in place. **Rationale:** *The stylet is sharp and could pierce the tube and injure the client or cut off the tube end.*
   - Place a stethoscope over the client's epigastrium and inject 10 to 20 mL of air into the tube while listening for a whooshing sound. Although still one of the methods used, do not use this method as the *primary* method for determining placement of the feeding tube. **Rationale:** *This method does not guarantee tube position.*
   - If the signs indicate placement in the lungs, remove the tube and begin again.
   - If the signs do not indicate placement in the lungs or stomach, advance the tube 5 cm (2 in.), and repeat the tests.

9. Secure the tube by taping it to the bridge of the client's nose.
   - If the client has oily skin, wipe the nose first with alcohol to defat the skin.
   - Cut 7.5 cm (3 in.) of tape, and split it lengthwise at one end, leaving a 2.5-cm (1-in.) tab at the end.
   - Place the tape over the bridge of the client's nose, and bring the split ends either under and around the tubing, or under the tubing and back up over the nose. ❸ **Rationale:** *Taping in this manner prevents the tube*

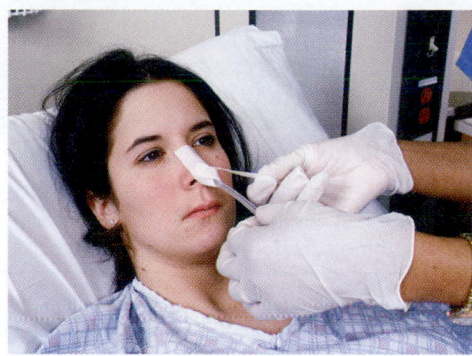

❸ Taping a nasogastric tube to the bridge of the nose.

from pressing against and irritating the edge of the nostril.

10. Once correct position has been determined, attach the tube to a suction source or feeding apparatus as ordered, or clamp the end of the tubing.

11. Secure the tube to the client's gown.
    - Loop an elastic band around the end of the tubing, and attach the elastic band to the gown with a safety pin.
      or
    - Attach a piece of adhesive tape to the tube, and pin the tape to the gown. **Rationale:** *The tube is attached to prevent it from dangling and pulling.*
    If a Salem sump tube is used, attach the antireflux valve to the vent port (if used) and position the port above the client's waist *so gastric contents do not flow into the vent lumen.*

12. Document relevant information: the insertion of the tube, the means by which correct placement was determined, and client responses (e.g., discomfort or abdominal distention).

13. Establish a plan for providing daily nasogastric tube care.
    - Inspect the nostril for discharge and irritation.
    - Clean the nostril and tube with moistened, cotton-tipped applicators.
    - Apply water-soluble lubricant to the nostril if it appears dry or encrusted.
    - Change the adhesive tape as required.
    - Give frequent mouth care. Due to the presence of the tube, the client may breathe through the mouth.

14. If suction is applied, ensure that the patency of both the nasogastric and suction tubes is maintained.
    - Irrigations of the tube may be required at regular intervals. In some agencies, irrigations must be ordered by the primary care provider.
    - If a Salem sump tube is used, follow agency policies for irrigating the vent lumen with air to maintain patency of the suctioning lumen. Often, a sucking sound can be heard from the vent port if it is patent.
    - Keep accurate records of the client's fluid intake and output, and record the amount and characteristics of the drainage.

15. Document the type of tube inserted, date and time of tube insertion, type of suction used, color and amount of gastric contents, and the client's tolerance of the procedure.

(continued)

SKILL 32–1

INSERTING A NASOGASTRIC TUBE *(continued)*

SAMPLE DOCUMENTATION

1/5/10 1030 #8 Fr feeding tube inserted s— difficulty through R nare c— stylet in place. To x-ray to check placement. Radiologist reports tube tip in stomach. Stylet removed. Aspirate pH 4. Tube secured to nose. Pt. verbalizes understanding of need to not pull on tube ———————————— M. Marshall, RN

EVALUATION

Conduct appropriate follow-up, such as degree of client comfort, client tolerance of the nasogastric tube, correct placement of na-sogastric tube in stomach, client understanding of restrictions, color and amount of gastric contents if attached to suction, or stomach contents aspirated.

SKILL 32–2

REMOVING A NASOGASTRIC TUBE

ASSESSMENT

Assess

- For the presence of bowel sounds.
- For the absence of nausea or vomiting when tube is clamped.

PLANNING

> **Delegation**
> Due to the need for assessment of client status, the skill of re-moving a nasogastric tube is not delegated to UAP.

EQUIPMENT

- Disposable pad or towel
- Tissues
- Clean gloves
- 50-mL syringe (optional)
- Plastic trash bag

IMPLEMENTATION

Preparation

- Confirm the primary care provider's order to remove the tube.
- Assist the client to a sitting position if health permits.
- Place the disposable pad or towel across the client's chest to collect any spillage of secretions from the tube.
- Provide tissues to the client to wipe the nose and mouth after tube removal.

Performance

1. Prior to performing the removal, introduce self and verify the client's identity using agency protocol. Explain to the client what you are going to do, why it is necessary, and how he or she can participate.
2. Perform hand hygiene and observe other appropriate infection control procedures (e.g., clean gloves).
3. Provide for client privacy.
4. Detach the tube.
   - Apply clean gloves.
   - Disconnect the nasogastric tube from the suction apparatus, if present.
   - Unpin the tube from the client's gown.
   - Remove the adhesive tape securing the tube to the nose.
5. Remove the nasogastric tube.
   - (Optional) Instill 50 mL of air into the tube. **Rationale:** *This clears the tube of any contents such as feeding or gastric drainage.*
   - Ask the client to take a deep breath and to hold it. **Rationale:** *This closes the glottis, thereby preventing accidental aspiration of any gastric contents.*
   - Pinch the tube with the gloved hand. **Rationale:** *Pinching the tube prevents any contents inside the tube from draining into the client's throat.*
   - Smoothly, withdraw the tube.
   - Place the tube in the plastic bag. **Rationale:** *Placing the tube immediately into the bag prevents the transference of microorganisms from the tube to other articles or people.*
   - Observe the intactness of the tube.
6. Ensure client comfort.
   - Provide mouth care if desired.
   - Assist the client as required to blow the nose. **Rationale:** *Excessive secretions may have accumulated in the nasal passages.*
7. Dispose of the equipment appropriately.
   - Place the pad, bag with tube, and gloves in the receptacle designated by the agency. **Rationale:** *Correct disposal prevents the transmission of microorganisms.*
8. Document all relevant information.
   - Record the removal of the tube, the amount and appearance of any drainage if connected to suction, and any relevant assessments of the client.

SAMPLE DOCUMENTATION

1/8/10 1500 NG tube removed intact s— difficulty. Oral & nasal care given. No bleeding or excoriation noted. Pt. states he is hungry & thirsty. 60 mL apple juice given. No c/o nausea. ———————————— B. Martin, RN

EVALUATION

- Perform a follow-up examination, such as presence of bowel sounds, absence of nausea or vomiting when tube is removed, and intactness of tissues of the nares.
- Relate findings to previous assessment data if available.
- Report significant deviations from normal to the primary care provider.

Nasogastric tubes may be inserted for reasons other than to provide a route for feeding the client, including prevention of nausea, vomiting, and gastric distention following surgery; removing stomach contents for laboratory analysis, and lavaging the stomach in cases of poisoning or medication overdosage.

A nasoenteric (or nasointestinal) tube, a longer tube than the nasogastric tube (at least 40 inches for an adult), is inserted through one nostril into the upper small intestine. Some agencies may require that specially trained nurses or primary care providers perform the procedure. Nasoenteric tubes are used for clients who are at risk for aspiration. Clients at risk for aspiration are those who manifest decreased levels of consciousness, poor cough or gag reflex, endotracheal intubation, recent extubation, inability to cooperate, or restlessness or agitation.

Gastrostomy and jejunostomy devices are used for long-term nutritional support, generally more than 6 to 8 weeks. Tubes are placed surgically or by laparoscopy through the abdominal wall into the stomach (Figure 32–6)

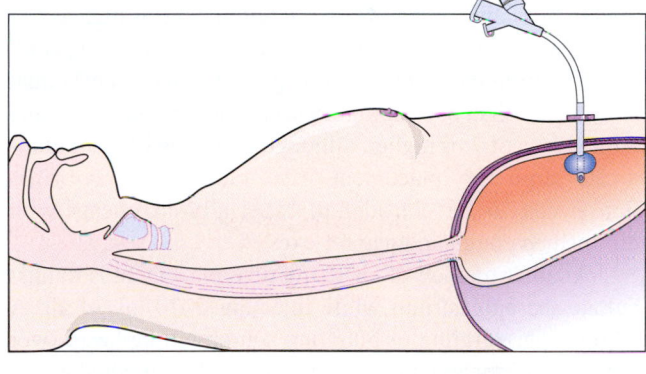

Figure 32–6 ⬤ Percutaneous endoscopic gastrostomy tube.

and/or into the jejunum (Figure 32–7). A percutaneous endoscopic gastrostomy (PEG) or percutaneous endoscopic jejunostomy (PEJ) is created by using an endoscope to visualize the inside of the stomach, making a puncture through the skin and subcutaneous tissues of the abdomen into the stomach, and inserting the PEG or PEJ catheter through the puncture. The surgical opening is sutured tightly around the tube or catheter to prevent leakage. Care of this opening before it heals requires surgical asepsis. The catheter has an external bumper and an internal inflatable retention balloon to maintain placement. After approximately one month the tract is established and the tube or catheter can be removed and reinserted for each feeding.

Before feedings are introduced, tube placement is confirmed by radiography, particularly when a small-bore tube has been inserted or when the client is at risk for aspiration.

LIFESPAN CONSIDERATIONS
Inserting a Nasogastric Tube

Infants and Young Children

- Restraints may be necessary during tube insertion and throughout therapy. *Restraints will prevent accidental dislodging of the tube.*
- Place the infant in an infant seat or position the infant with a rolled towel or pillow under the head and shoulders.
- When assessing the nares, obstruct one of the infant's nares and feel for air passage from the other. If the nasal passageway is very small or is obstructed, an orogastric tube may be more appropriate.
- Measure appropriate nasogastric tube length from the nose to the tip of the earlobe and then to the point midway between the umbilicus and the xiphoid process.
- If an orogastric tube is used, measure from the tip of the earlobe to the corner of the mouth to the xiphoid process.
- Do not hyperextend or hyperflex an infant's neck. *Hyperextension or hyperflexion of the neck could occlude the airway.*
- Tape the tube to the area between the end of the nares and the upper lip as well as to the cheek.

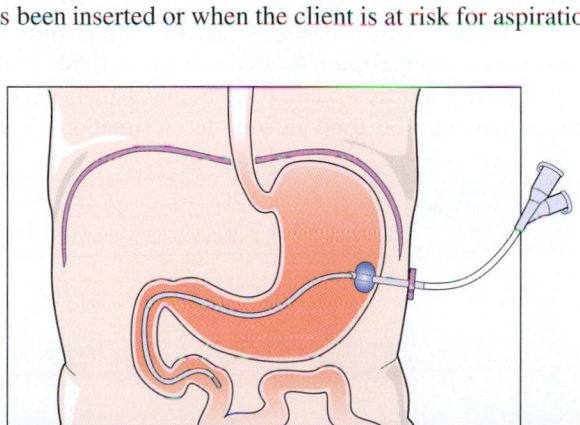

Figure 32–7 ⬤ Percutaneous endoscopic jejunostomy tube.

This is the most effective method of confirming tube placement but repeated x-ray studies are not feasible in terms of cost. After placement is confirmed, the nurse marks the tube with indelible ink or places a piece of tape at its exit point from the nose and documents the length of visible tubing for baseline data.

The nurse is responsible for verifying tube placement before each intermittent feeding and at regular intervals, usually at least once per shift, when continuous feedings are being administered. Tube placement can be verified by aspirating gastrointestinal secretions and measuring the pH of aspirated fluid (recommended method). Gastric aspirates tend to be acidic with a pH of 1–4 but may be as high as 6 if the client is receiving medications that control gastric acid. Aspirate from the small intestine generally have a pH equal to or higher than 6. Respiratory secretions are more alkaline with values of 7 or higher, although a reading of 6 could indicate respiratory placement. Also, radiological confirmation needs to be considered, especially in clients with diminished cough and gag reflexes.

Another method of checking tube placement is to auscultate the epigastrium while injecting 5–20 mL of air. A whooshing, gurgling or bubbling sound will be heard over the epigastrium and upper left quadrant. This method is less reliable than pH testing.

Finally, the nurse can check tube placement by confirming the length of tube insertion with the insertion mark. If more tube is visible the placement should be questioned. This is useful in conjunction with other methods but is not reliable by itself.

ENTERAL FEEDINGS The type and frequency of feedings and amounts to be administered are ordered by the primary care provider. Liquid feeding mixtures are available commercially or may be prepared by the dietary department in accordance with the primary care provider's orders. A standard formula provides 1 Kcal per milliliter of solution with protein, fat, carbohydrate, minerals, and vitamins in specified proportions.

Enteral feedings can be given intermittently or continuously. Intermittent feedings are the administration of 300 to 500 mL of enteral formula several times per day over at least 30 minutes using a syringe to deliver formula into the stomach as the preferred site. Because the formula is delivered rapidly by this method, it is not usually recommended but may be used in long-term situations if the

client tolerates it. These feedings must be given only into the stomach; the client must be monitored closely for distention and aspiration.

Continuous feedings are generally administered over a 24-hour period using an infusion pump that guarantees a constant flow rate. Continuous feedings are essential when feedings are administered in the small bowel. They are also used when smaller bore gastric tubes are in place or when gravity flow is insufficient to instill the feeding.

Cyclic feedings are continuous feedings that are administered in less than 24 hours (e.g., 12 to 16 hours). These feedings, often administered at night, allow the client to attempt to eat regular meals through the day. Because nocturnal feedings may use higher nutrient densities and higher infusion rates than the standard continuous feeding, particular attention needs to be given to monitoring fluid status and circulating volume.

Enteral feedings are administered to clients through open or closed systems. Open systems use an open-top container or a syringe for administration. Enteral feedings for use with open systems are provided in flip-top cans or powdered formulas that are reconstituted with sterile water. Sterile water, rather than tap water, reduces the risk of microbial contamination. Open systems should have no more than 8 to 12 hours of formula poured at one time. At the completion of this time, remaining formula should be discarded and the container rinsed before new formula is poured. The bag and tubing should be replaced every 24 hours (Rolfes et al., 2009). Closed systems consist of a prefilled container that is spiked with enteral tubing and attached to the enteral access device. Prefilled containers can hang safely for 48 hours if sterile technique is used.

Skill 32–3 provides the essential steps involved in administering a tube feeding, and Skill 32–4 indicates the steps involved in administering a gastrostomy or jejunostomy tube feeding.

SKILL 32–3

ADMINISTERING A TUBE FEEDING

PURPOSES
- To restore or maintain nutritional status
- To administer medications

ASSESSMENT

Assess
- For any clinical signs of malnutrition or dehydration.
- For allergies to any food in the feeding. If the client is lactose intolerant, check the tube feeding formula. Notify the primary care provider if any incompatibilities exist.
- For the presence of bowel sounds.
- For any problems that suggest lack of tolerance of previous feedings (e.g., delayed gastric emptying, abdominal distention, diarrhea, cramping, or constipation).

PLANNING
Before commencing a tube feeding, determine the type, amount, and frequency of feedings and tolerance of previous feedings.

> **Delegation**
> Administering a tube feeding requires application of knowledge and problem solving and it is not usually delegated to UAP. Some agencies, however, may allow a trained UAP to administer a feeding. In this case, it is the responsibility of the nurse to assess tube placement and determine that the tube is patent. The nurse should reinforce major points, such as making sure the client is sitting upright, and instruct the UAP to report any difficulty administering the feeding or any complaints voiced by the client.

EQUIPMENT
- Correct type and amount of feeding solution
- 60-mL catheter-tip syringe
- Emesis basin
- Clean gloves
- pH test strip or meter
- Large syringe or calibrated plastic feeding bag with label and tubing that can be attached to the feeding tube or prefilled bottle with a drip chamber, tubing, and a flow-regulator clamp
- Measuring container from which to pour the feeding (if using open system)
- Water (60 mL unless otherwise specified) at room temperature
- Feeding pump as required

IMPLEMENTATION

Preparation

Assist the client to a Fowler's position (at least 30 degrees elevation) in bed or a sitting position in a chair, the normal position for eating. If a sitting position is contraindicated, a slightly elevated right side-lying position is acceptable. **Rationale:** *These positions enhance the gravitational flow of the solution and prevent aspiration of fluid into the lungs.*

Performance

1. Prior to performing the feeding, introduce self and verify the client's identity using agency protocol. Explain to the client what you are going to do, why it is necessary, and how he or she can participate. Inform the client that the feeding should not cause any discomfort but may cause a feeling of fullness.
2. Perform hand hygiene and observe appropriate infection control procedures (e.g., clean gloves).
3. Provide privacy for this procedure if the client desires it. Tube feedings are embarrassing to some people.
4. Assess tube placement.
   - Apply clean gloves.
   - Attach the syringe to the open end of the tube and aspirate. Check the pH.
   - Allow 1 hour to elapse before testing the pH if the client has received a medication.
   - Use a pH meter rather than pH paper if the client is receiving a continuous feeding. Follow agency policy if the pH is equal to or greater than 6.
5. Assess residual feeding contents.
   - If the tube is placed in the stomach, aspirate all contents and measure the amount before administering the feeding. **Rationale:** *This is done to evaluate absorption of the last feeding; that is, whether undigested formula from a previous feeding remains. If the tube is in the small intestine, residual contents cannot be aspirated.*
   - If 100 mL (or more than half the last feeding) is withdrawn, check with the nurse in charge or refer to agency policy before proceeding. The precise amount is usually determined by the primary care provider's order or by agency policy. **Rationale:** *At some agencies, a feeding is delayed when the specified amount or more of formula remains in the stomach.*
     or
   - Reinstill the gastric contents into the stomach if this is the agency policy or primary care provider's order. **Rationale:** *Removal of the contents could disturb the client's electrolyte balance.*
   - If the client is on a continuous feeding, check the gastric residual every 4 to 6 hours or according to agency protocol.
6. Administer the feeding.
   - Before administering feeding:
     Check the expiration date of the feeding.
     Warm the feeding to room temperature. **Rationale:** *An excessively cold feeding may cause abdominal cramps.*
   - When an open system is used, clean the top of the feeding container with alcohol before opening it. **Rationale:** *This minimizes the risk of contaminants entering the feeding syringe or feeding bag.*

FEEDING BAG (OPEN SYSTEM)
- Hang the labeled bag from an infusion pole about 30 cm (12 in.) above the tube's point of insertion into the client.
- Clamp the tubing and add the formula to the bag.

(continued)

SKILL 32–3

ADMINISTERING A TUBE FEEDING *(continued)*

- Open the clamp, run the formula through the tubing, and reclamp the tube. **Rationale:** *The formula will displace the air in the tubing, thus preventing the instillation of excess air into the client's stomach or intestine*
- Attach the bag to the feeding tube ❶ and regulate the drip by adjusting the clamp to the drop factor on the bag (e.g., 20 drops/mL) if not placed on a pump.

SYRINGE (OPEN SYSTEM)

- Remove the plunger from the syringe and connect the syringe to a pinched or clamped nasogastric tube. **Rationale:** *Pinching or clamping the tube prevents excess air from entering the stomach and causing distention.*
- Add the feeding to the syringe barrel. ❷
- Permit the feeding to flow in slowly at the prescribed rate. Raise or lower the syringe to adjust the flow as needed. Pinch or clamp the tubing to stop the flow for a minute if the client experiences discomfort. **Rationale:** *Quickly administered feedings can cause flatus, cramps, and/or vomiting.*

PREFILLED BOTTLE WITH DRIP CHAMBER (CLOSED SYSTEM)

- Remove the screw-on cap from the container and attach the administration set with the drip chamber and tubing. ❸
- Close the clamp on the tubing.
- Hang the container on an intravenous pole about 30 cm (12 in.) above the tube's insertion point into the client. **Rationale:** *At this height, the formula should run at a safe rate into the stomach or intestine.*
- Squeeze the drip chamber to fill it to one-third to one-half of its capacity.
- Open the tubing clamp, run the formula through the tubing, and reclamp the tube. **Rationale:** *The formula will displace the air in the tubing, thus preventing the instillation of excess air.*
- Attach the feeding set tubing to the feeding tube and regulate the drip rate to deliver the feeding over the desired length of time or attach to a feeding pump.

7. If another bottle is not to be immediately hung, flush the feeding tube before all of the formula has run through the tubing.
   - Instill 50 to 100 mL of water through the feeding tube or medication port. **Rationale:** *Water flushes the lumen of the tube, preventing future blockage by sticky formula.*
   - Be sure to add the water before the feeding solution has drained from the neck of a syringe or from the tubing of an administration set. **Rationale:** *Adding the water before the syringe or tubing is empty prevents the instillation of air into the stomach or intestine and thus prevents unnecessary distention.*

8. Clamp the feeding tube.
   - Clamp the feeding tube before all of the water is instilled. **Rationale:** *Clamping prevents leakage and air from entering the tube if done before water is instilled.*

9. Ensure client comfort and safety.
   - Secure the tubing to the client's gown. **Rationale:** *This minimizes pulling of the tube, thus preventing discomfort and dislodgment.*

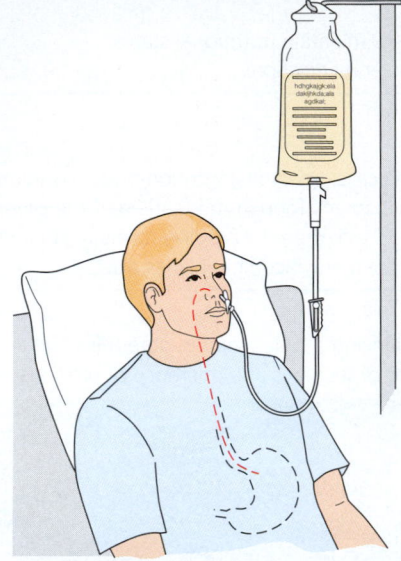

❶ Using a calibrated plastic bag to administer a tube feeding.

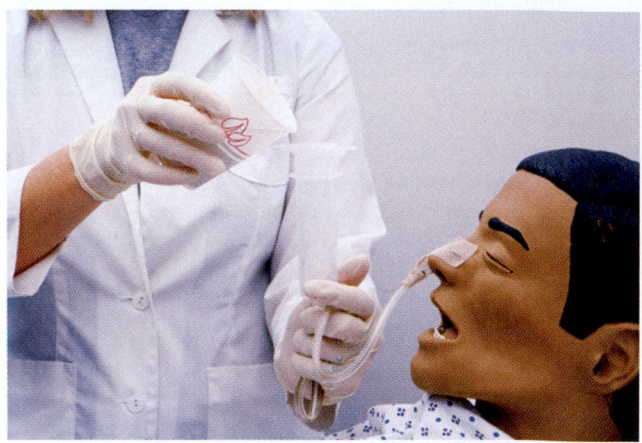

❷ Using the barrel of a syringe to administer a tube feeding.

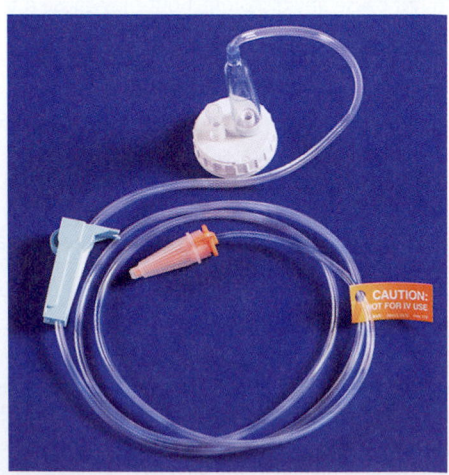

❸ Feeding set tubing with drip chamber. (Ross Products Division, Abbot Laboratories. Used with permission.)

(continued)

- Ask the client to remain sitting upright in Fowler's position or in a slightly elevated right lateral position for at least 30 minutes. **Rationale:** *These positions facilitate digestion and movement of the feeding from the stomach along the alimentary tract, and prevent the potential aspiration of the feeding into the lungs.*
- Check the agency's policy on the frequency of changing the nasogastric tube and the use of smaller lumen tubes if a large-bore tube is in place. **Rationale:** *These measures prevent irritation and erosion of the pharyngeal and esophageal mucous membranes.*

10. Dispose of equipment appropriately.
    - If the equipment is to be reused, wash it thoroughly with soap and water so that it is ready for reuse.
    - Change the equipment every 24 hours or according to agency policy.

11. Document all relevant information.
    - Document the feeding, including amount and kind of solution taken, duration of the feeding, and assessments of the client.
    - Record the volume of the feeding and water administered on the client's intake and output record.

SAMPLE DOCUMENTATION

1/5/10 1330 Aspirated 20 mL pale yellow fluid from NG tube, pH 5. Pt. in Fowler's position. 1 L room-temperature ordered formula begun @ 60 mL/hour on pump. No nausea reported. ———————————————— R. Orr, RN

EVALUATION

Perform a follow-up examination of the following:

- Tolerance of feeding (e.g., nausea, cramping)
- Bowel sounds
- Regurgitation and feelings of fullness after feedings
- Weight gain or loss

12. Monitor the client for possible problems.
    - Carefully assess clients receiving tube feedings for problems.
    - To prevent dehydration, give the client supplemental water in addition to the prescribed tube feeding as ordered.

VARIATION: CONTINUOUS-DRIP FEEDING

- Clamp the tubing at least every 4 to 6 hours, or as indicated by agency protocol or the manufacturer, and aspirate and measure the gastric contents. Then flush the tubing with 30 to 50 mL of water. **Rationale:** *This determines adequate absorption and verifies correct placement of the tube. If placement of a small-bore tube is questionable, a repeat x-ray should be done.*
- Determine agency protocol regarding withholding a feeding. Many agencies withhold the feeding if more than 75 to 100 mL of feeding is aspirated.
- To prevent spoilage or bacterial contamination, do not allow the feeding solution to hang longer than 4 to 8 hours. Check agency policy or manufacturer's recommendations regarding time limits.
- Follow agency policy regarding how frequently to change the feeding bag and tubing. Changing the feeding bag and tubing every 24 hours reduces the risk of contamination.

- Fecal elimination pattern (e.g., diarrhea, flatulence, constipation)
- Skin turgor
- Urine output and specific gravity
- Glucose and acetone in urine

Relate findings to previous assessment data if available. Report significant deviations from normal to the primary care provider.

SKILL 32–4

ADMINISTERING A GASTROSTOMY OR JEJUNOSTOMY FEEDING

PURPOSES

See Skill 32–3.

ASSESSMENT

See Skill 32–3.

PLANNING

Before commencing a gastrostomy or jejunostomy feeding, determine the type and amount of feeding to be instilled, frequency of feedings, and any pertinent information about previous feedings (e.g., the positioning in which the client best tolerates the feeding).

Delegation

See Skill 32–3.

EQUIPMENT

- Correct amount of feeding solution
- Graduated container and tubing with clamp to hold the feeding
- 60-mL catheter-tip syringe

For a Tube that Remains in Place

- Mild soap and water
- Clean gloves
- Petrolatum, zinc oxide ointment, or other skin protectant
- Precut 4 × 4 in. gauze squares
- Uncut 4 × 4 in. gauze squares

For Tube Insertion

- Clean gloves
- Moisture-proof bag
- Water-soluble lubricant
- Feeding tube (if needed)

(continued)

SKILL 32–4

ADMINISTERING A GASTROSTOMY OR JEJUNOSTOMY FEEDING *(continued)*

IMPLEMENTATION

Preparation
See Skill 32–3.

Performance

1. Prior to performing the feeding, introduce self and verify the client's identity using agency protocol. Explain to the client what you are going to do, why it is necessary, and how he or she can participate.

2. Perform hand hygiene and observe other appropriate infection control procedures (e.g., clean gloves).

3. Provide for client privacy.

4. Assess and prepare the client.
   - Apply clean gloves.
   - See Skill 32–3.

5. Insert a feeding tube, if one is not already in place.
   - Wearing gloves, remove the dressing. Then discard the dressing and gloves in the moisture-proof bag.
   - Apply new clean gloves.
   - Lubricate the end of the tube, and insert it into the ostomy opening 10 to 15 cm (4 to 6 in.).

6. Check the location and patency of a tube that is already in place.
   - Determine correct placement of the tube by aspirating secretions and checking the pH.
   - Follow agency policy for amount of residual formula. This may include withholding the feeding, rechecking in 3 to 4 hours, or notifying the primary care provider if a large residual remains.
   - For continuous feedings, check the residual every 4 to 6 hours and hold feedings according to agency policy.
   - Remove the syringe plunger. Pour 15 to 30 mL of water into the syringe, remove the tube clamp, and allow the water to flow into the tube. **Rationale:** *This determines the patency of the tube. If water flows freely, the tube is patent.*
   - If the water does not flow freely, notify the nurse in charge and/or primary care provider.

7. Administer the feeding.
   - Hold the barrel of the syringe 7 to 15 cm (3 to 6 in.) above the ostomy opening.
   - Slowly pour the solution into the syringe and allow it to flow through the tube by gravity.

   - Just before all the formula has run through and the syringe is empty, add 30 mL of water. **Rationale:** *Water flushes the tube and preserves its patency.*
   - If the tube is to remain in place, hold it upright, remove the syringe, and then clamp or plug the tube to prevent leakage.
   - If a catheter was inserted for the feeding, remove it.

8. Ensure client comfort and safety.
   - After the feeding, ask the client to remain in the sitting position or a slightly elevated right lateral position for at least 30 minutes. **Rationale:** *This minimizes the risk of aspiration.*
   - Assess status of peristomal skin. **Rationale:** *Gastric or jejunal drainage contains digestive enzymes that can irritate the skin.* Document any redness and broken skin areas.
   - Check orders about cleaning the peristomal skin, applying a skin protectant, and applying appropriate dressings. Generally, the peristomal skin is washed with mild soap and water at least once daily. The tube may be rotated between thumb and forefinger to release any sticking and promote tract formation. Petrolatum, zinc oxide ointment, or other skin protectant may be applied around the stoma, and precut 4 × 4 in. gauze squares may be placed around the tube. The precut squares are then covered with regular 4 × 4 in. gauze squares, and the tube is coiled over them.
   - Observe for common complications of enteral feedings: aspiration, hyperglycemia, abdominal distention, diarrhea, and fecal impaction. Report findings to primary care provider. Often, a change in formula or rate of administration can correct problems.
   - When appropriate, teach the client how to administer feedings and when to notify the health care provider concerning problems.

9. Document all assessments and interventions.

SAMPLE DOCUMENTATION

1/24/10 2045 No fluid aspirated from gastrostomy tube. Pt. in Fowler's position. 30 mL water flowed freely by gravity through tube. 250 mL room-temperature Ensure formula given over 20 minutes. No complaints of discomfort. —————————— J. Poole, RN

EVALUATION

See Skill 32–3.

Before administering a tube feeding, the nurse must determine any food allergies of the client and assess tolerance to previous feedings. The nurse must also check the expiration date on a commercially prepared formula or the preparation date and time of agency-prepared solution, discarding any formula that has passed the expiration date or that was prepared more than 24 hours previously.

Feedings are usually administered at room temperature unless the order specifies otherwise. The nurse warms the specified amount of solution in a basin of warm water or leaves it to stand for a while until it reaches room temperature. Because a formula that is warmed can grow microorganisms, it should not hang longer than the manufacturer recommends. Continuous-feeding formulas should be kept cold; excessive heat coagulates feedings of milk and egg, and hot liquids can irritate the mucous membranes. However, excessively cold feedings can reduce the flow of digestive juices by causing vasoconstriction and may cause cramps.

LIFESPAN CONSIDERATIONS   Administering a Tube Feeding

Infants

- Feeding tubes may be reinserted at each feeding to prevent irritation of the mucous membrane, nasal airway obstruction, and stomach perforation that may occur if the tube is left in place continuously. Check agency practice.

Children

- Position a small child or infant in your lap, provide a pacifier, and hold and cuddle the child during feedings. This promotes comfort, supports the normal sucking instinct of the infant, and facilitates digestion.

Older Adults

- Physiologic changes associated with aging may make the older adult more vulnerable to complications associated with enteral feedings. Decreased gastric emptying may necessitate checking frequently for gastric residual. Diarrhea from administering the feeding too fast or at too high a concentration may cause dehydration. If the feeding has a high concentration of glucose, assess for hyperglycemia because with aging, the body has a decreased ability to handle increased glucose levels.

- Conditions such as hiatal hernia and diabetes mellitus may cause the stomach to empty more slowly. This increases the risk of aspiration in a client receiving a tube feeding. Checking for gastric residual more frequently can help document this if it is an ongoing problem. Changing the formula or the rate of administration, repositioning the client, or obtaining a primary care provider's order for a medication to increase stomach emptying may resolve this problem.

Managing Clogged Feeding Tubes   Even if feeding tubes are flushed with water before and after feedings and medications, they can still become clogged. This can occur when the feeding container runs dry, solid medication is not adequately crushed, or medications are mixed with formula. Even the important practice of aspirating to check residual volume increases the incidence of clogging (Reising & Neal, 2005). To avoid the necessity of removing the tube and reinserting a new tube, both prevention and intervention strategies must be used.

To prevent clogged feeding tubes, flush liberally (at least 30 mL water) before, between, and after each separate medication is instilled, using a 60-mL piston syringe. The larger the barrel of the syringe, the less pressure exerted. High pressure can rupture the tube—especially small-bore feeding tubes. Do not add medications to formula or to other medications.

Many strategies have been used to try to unclog feeding tubes. Strategies that have shown inconsistent effectiveness include instilling meat tenderizer, carbonated beverages, or cranberry juice, or flushing with small barrel syringes with or without digestive enzymes such as papain or chymotrypsin. Soda has actually been found to make the clog worse (Novartis, 2003).

The first strategy that should be tried is to reposition the client (this may allow a kink to straighten). Alternately flush and aspirate the tube with water. One institution has had success with a hollow catheter that allows unclogging solution to be delivered as the catheter is advanced down the clogged tube (Smith & Myers, 2005).

Parenteral Nutrition

Parenteral nutrition (PN), also referred to as total parenteral nutrition (TPN) or intravenous hyperalimentation (IVH), is provided when the gastrointestinal tract is nonfunctional. **Parenteral** nutrition is administered intravenously. TPN is a means of achieving an anabolic state in clients who are unable to maintain a normal nitrogen balance.

Parenteral feedings are solutions of 10% to 50% dextrose, water, fat, proteins, electrolytes, vitamins, and trace elements;

CLIENT TEACHING   Tube Feedings

Clients and caregivers need the following instructions to manage these feedings:

- Preparation of the formula. Include name of the formula and how much and how often it is to be given; the need to inspect the formula for expiration date and leaks and cracks in bags or cans; how to mix or prepare the formula, if needed; and aseptic techniques such as swabbing the container's top with alcohol before opening it, and changing the syringe administration set and reservoir every 24 hours.
- Proper storage of the formula. Include the need to refrigerate diluted or reconstituted formula and formula that contains additives.
- Administration of the feeding. Include proper hand washing technique, how to fill and hang the feeding bag, operation of an infusion pump if indicated, the feeding rate, and client positioning during and after the feeding.
- Management of the enteral or parenteral access device. Include site care, aseptic precautions, dressing change, as indicated, how the site should look normally, and flushing protocols (e.g., type of irrigant and schedule).
- Daily monitoring needs. Include temperature, weight, and intake and output.
- Signs and symptoms of complications to report. Include fever, increased respiratory rate, decrease in urine output, increased stool frequency, and altered level of consciousness.
- Whom to contact about questions or problems. Include emergency telephone numbers of home care agency, nursing clinician and/or primary care provider, or other 24-hour on-call emergency service.

they provide all needed calories. Additives are modified to each client's nutritional needs. Fat emulsions may be given to provide essential fatty acids to correct and/or prevent essential fatty acid deficiency or to supplement the calories for clients who have high calorie needs or cannot tolerate glucose as the only calorie source. Note that 1,000 mL of 5% glucose or dextrose contains 50 grams of sugar providing less than 200 calories. Because TPN solutions are hypertonic (highly concentrated in comparison to the solute concentration of blood), they are injected only into high-flow central veins, where they are diluted by the client's blood.

TPN is not risk-free. Infection control is of utmost importance during TPN therapy. The nurse must always observe surgical aseptic technique when changing solutions, tubing, dressings, and filters. Clients are at increased risk of fluid, electrolyte, and glucose imbalances and require frequent evaluation and modification of the TPN mixture.

Because TPN solutions are high in glucose, infusions are started gradually to prevent hyperglycemia with gradually increasing glucose concentrations to allow the pancreas to increase insulin output. Glucose levels are monitored during the infusion.

When TPN therapy is to be discontinued, the TPN infusion rates are decreased slowly to prevent hyperinsulinemia and hypoglycemia. Weaning a client from TPN may take up to 48 hours but can occur in 6 hours as long as the client receives adequate carbohydrates either orally or intravenously. Enteral or parenteral feedings may be continued beyond hospital care in the client's home or may be initiated in the home.

EVALUATING

The goals established in the planning phase are evaluated according to specific desired outcomes, also established in that phase (see Identifying Nursing Diagnoses, Outcomes, and Interventions on page 967).

If the outcomes are not achieved, the nurse should explore how the plan of care may need to be changed. The nurse might consider the following questions:

- Was the cause of the problem correctly identified?
- Was the family included in the teaching plan? Are family members supportive?
- Is the client experiencing symptoms that cause loss of appetite?
- Were the outcomes unrealistic for this person?
- Were the client's food preferences considered?
- Is anything interfering with digestion or absorption of nutrients?

Nursing Care Plan	The Client with Imbalanced Nutrition

ASSESSMENT DATA	NURSING DIAGNOSIS	DESIRED OUTCOMES*
Nursing Assessment Mrs. Maryann Gardner, a 59-year-old homemaker, attends a community hospital–sponsored health fair. She approaches the nutrition information booth, and the clinical specialist in nutritional support gathers a nutritional history. Mrs. Gardner is very upset about her 9-kg (20-lb) weight gain. She relates to the nurse clinician that since the death of her husband 1 month ago she has lost interest in many of her usual physical and social activities. She no longer attends YMCA exercise and swimming sessions and has lost contact with her couple's bridge group. Mrs. Gardner states she is bored, depressed, and very unhappy about her appearance. She has a small frame and has always prided herself on her petite figure. She says her eating habits have changed considerably. She snacks while watching TV and rarely prepares a complete meal.	*Imbalanced Nutrition: More than body requirements* related to excess intake and decreased activity expenditure (as evidenced by weight gain of 20 lb, triceps skin fold greater than normal, undesirable eating patterns).	**Weight Control [1612]** as evidenced by demonstrating • Eats three meals each day that result in a 500-calorie reduction in intake. • Develops a physical exercise plan that engages her in 15 to 20 minutes of exercise by day 5. • Identifies eating habits that contribute to weight gain by day 2.

Physical Examination
Height: 162.6 cm (5′ 4″)
Weight: 63.6 kg (140 lb)
Temperature: 37°C (98.6°F)
Pulse: 76 BPM
Respirations: 16/minute
Blood pressure: 144/84 mm Hg
Triceps skinfold: 21 mm
Small frame, weight in excess of
10% over ideal for height and frame

Diagnostic Data
CBC normal, urinalysis negative, chest x-ray negative, thyroid profile within normal limits

NURSING INTERVENTIONS*/SELECTED ACTIVITIES	RATIONALE
Weight Reduction Assistance [1280]	
Determine current eating patterns by having Mrs. Gardner keep a diary of what, when, and where she eats.	*Increases awareness of activities and foods that contribute to excessive intake.*
Set a weekly goal for weight loss.	*The desirable weight loss rate is 1–2 pounds per week.*
Encourage use of internal reward systems when goals are accomplished.	*Goal setting provides motivation, which is essential for a successful weight-loss program.*
Set a realistic plan with Mrs. Gardner to include reduced food intake and increased energy expenditure.	*A combined plan of calorie reduction and exercise can enhance weight loss since exercise increases caloric utilization.*
Assist client to identify motivation for eating and internal and external cues associated with eating.	*Awareness of factors that contribute to overeating will assist the individual in planning behavior modification techniques to avoid situations that prompt excess food consumption.*
Encourage attendance at support groups for weight loss and/or refer to a community weight control program.	*Overweight people are often nutritionally deprived. Intake must be reduced by 500 calories per day to obtain a one-pound-per-week weight loss.*
Develop a daily meal plan with a well-balanced diet, reduced calories, and reduced fat.	*Support groups can provide companionship, increase motivation, and offer practical solutions to problems associated with dieting.*
Nutritional Counseling [5246]	
Facilitate identification of eating behaviors to be changed.	*Increases individual's awareness of those actions that contribute to excessive intake.*
Use accepted nutritional standards to assist Mrs. Gardner in evaluating adequacy of dietary intake.	*Comparing the individual's dietary history with nutritional standards will facilitate identification of nutritional deficiencies and/or excesses.*
Help Mrs. Gardner to consider factors of age, past eating experiences, culture, and finances in planning ways to meet nutritional requirements.	*Social, economic, physical, and psychologic factors play a role in nutrition and/or malnutrition.*
Discuss Mrs. Gardner's knowledge of the basic four food groups, as well as perceptions of the needed diet modification.	*Helps to determine the client's knowledge base and identify misconceptions and/or gaps in understanding.*
Discuss food likes and dislikes.	*Incorporating Mrs. Gardner's food preferences into the dietary plan will promote adherence to the weight loss program.*
Assist Mrs. Gardner in stating her feelings and concerns about goal achievement.	*Fear of success, failure, or other concerns may block goal achievement.*
Behavior Modification [4360]	
Assist Mrs. Gardner to identify strengths and reinforce these.	*Reinforcing strengths enhances self-esteem and encourages the individual to draw on these assets during the weight-loss program.*
Encourage her to examine her own behavior.	*Involving Mrs. Gardner in self-appraisal will promote identification of behaviors that may be contributing to excessive caloric intake.*
Identify the behavior to be changed in specific, concrete terms (e.g., stop snacking in front of the TV).	*Identification of specific behaviors is essential for planning behavior modification.*
Consider that it is easier to increase a behavior than to decrease a behavior (e.g., increase activities or hobbies that involve the hands such as sewing versus decreasing TV snacking).	*Habitual behaviors are difficult to change. Breaking old habits may be easier if viewed from the standpoint of increasing an enjoyable, healthy activity.*
Choose reinforcers that are meaningful to Mrs. Gardner.	*Positive reinforcement is not likely to be an effective part of behavior modification if the reinforcer is meaningless to the individual.*

EVALUATION

Outcome met. Mrs. Gardner kept a dietary log for 5 days and has eaten balanced meals each day, resulting in a daily deficit of 400 to 500 calories. She is aware that she eats excessively because she is bored and depressed. She has reestablished her former social contacts, including her church bridge club. Mrs. Gardner has purchased a stationary bicycle and exercises 20 minutes daily. She enrolled in a knitting class that meets two nights per week. She has lost 1 1/2 lb in the past week. As a reward, Mrs. Gardner renewed her membership to the YMCA.

The NOC # for desired outcomes and the NIC # for nursing interventions are listed in brackets following the appropriate outcome or intervention. Outcomes, interventions, and activities selected are only a sample of those suggested by NOC and NIC and should be further individualized for each client.

(continued)

CRITICAL THINKING QUESTIONS

1. How do Mrs. Gardner's personal characteristics influence her nutritional needs?

2. What further information do you need regarding Mrs. Gardner's present diet?

3. Offer suggestions for ways to modify Mrs. Gardner's tendency to snack.

4. Mrs. Gardner asks what her weight should be. How do you respond?

∞ *See Answers in MyNursingKit.*

CONCEPT MAP   Nutrition

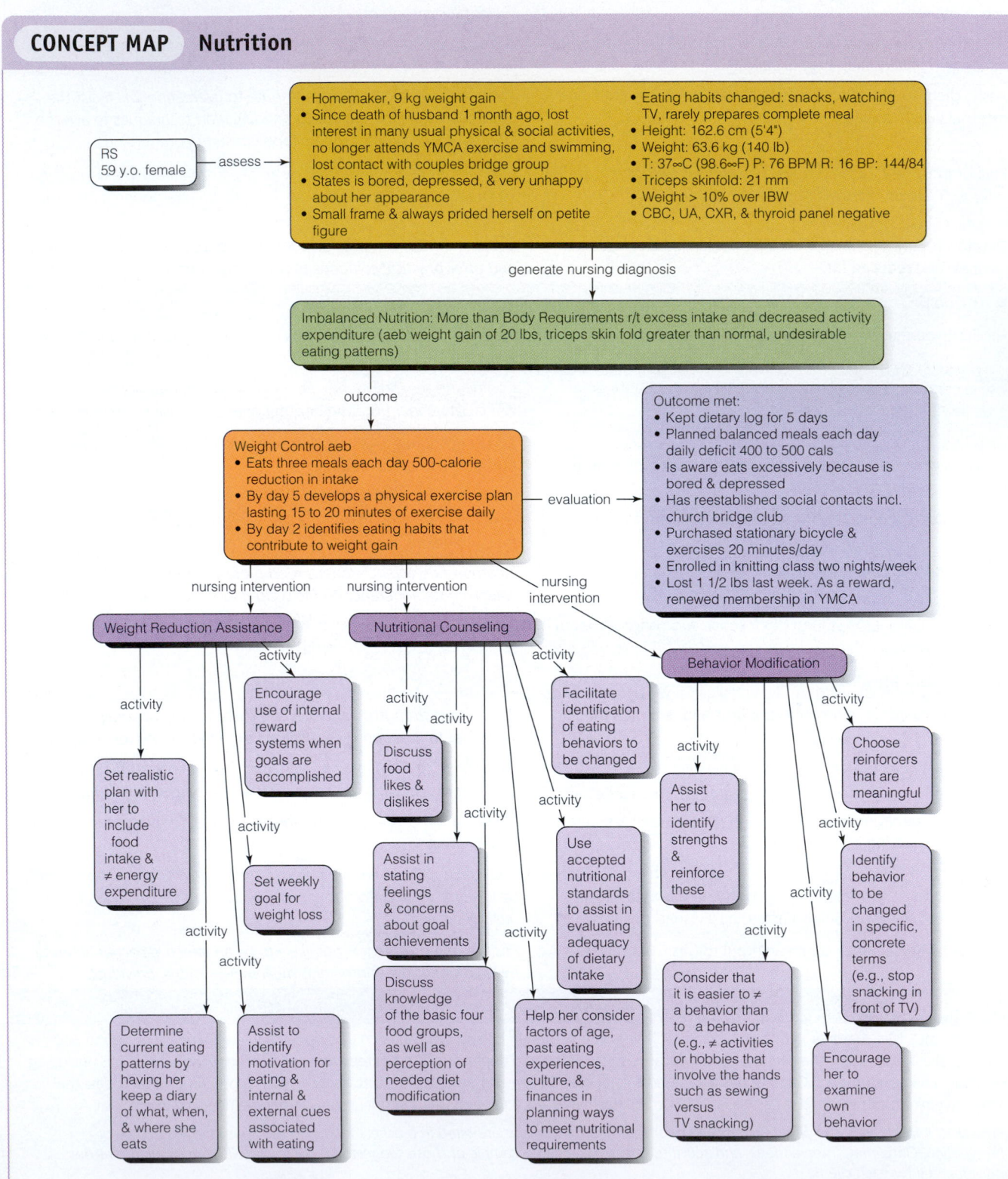

RS
59 y.o. female

→ assess →

• Homemaker, 9 kg weight gain
• Since death of husband 1 month ago, lost interest in many usual physical & social activities, no longer attends YMCA exercise and swimming, lost contact with couples bridge group
• States is bored, depressed, & very unhappy about her appearance
• Small frame & always prided herself on petite figure

• Eating habits changed: snacks, watching TV, rarely prepares complete meal
• Height: 162.6 cm (5'4")
• Weight: 63.6 kg (140 lb)
• T: 37∞C (98.6∞F) P: 76 BPM R: 16 BP: 144/84
• Triceps skinfold: 21 mm
• Weight > 10% over IBW
• CBC, UA, CXR, & thyroid panel negative

generate nursing diagnosis

Imbalanced Nutrition: More than Body Requirements r/t excess intake and decreased activity expenditure (aeb weight gain of 20 lbs, triceps skin fold greater than normal, undesirable eating patterns)

outcome

Weight Control aeb
• Eats three meals each day 500-calorie reduction in intake
• By day 5 develops a physical exercise plan lasting 15 to 20 minutes of exercise daily
• By day 2 identifies eating habits that contribute to weight gain

evaluation →

Outcome met:
• Kept dietary log for 5 days
• Planned balanced meals each day daily deficit 400 to 500 cals
• Is aware eats excessively because is bored & depressed
• Has reestablished social contacts incl. church bridge club
• Purchased stationary bicycle & exercises 20 minutes/day
• Enrolled in knitting class two nights/week
• Lost 1 1/2 lbs last week. As a reward, renewed membership in YMCA

nursing intervention — Weight Reduction Assistance

nursing intervention — Nutritional Counseling

nursing intervention — Behavior Modification

Weight Reduction Assistance

activity → Set realistic plan with her to include food intake & ≠ energy expenditure

activity → Encourage use of internal reward systems when goals are accomplished

activity → Set weekly goal for weight loss

activity → Determine current eating patterns by having her keep a diary of what, when, & where she eats

activity → Assist to identify motivation for eating & internal & external cues associated with eating

Nutritional Counseling

activity → Discuss food likes & dislikes

activity → Assist in stating feelings & concerns about goal achievements

activity → Discuss knowledge of the basic four food groups, as well as perception of needed diet modification

activity → Facilitate identification of eating behaviors to be changed

activity → Use accepted nutritional standards to assist in evaluating adequacy of dietary intake

activity → Help her consider factors of age, past eating experiences, culture, & finances in planning ways to meet nutritional requirements

Behavior Modification

activity → Assist her to identify strengths & reinforce these

activity → Consider that it is easier to ≠ a behavior than to a behavior (e.g., ≠ activities or hobbies that involve the hands such as sewing versus TV snacking)

activity → Choose reinforcers that are meaningful

activity → Identify behavior to be changed in specific, concrete terms (e.g., stop snacking in front of TV)

activity → Encourage her to examine own behavior

CHAPTER HIGHLIGHTS

- Essential nutrients are grouped into categories: carbohydrates, proteins, lipids, vitamins, and minerals.
- Nutrients serve three basic purposes: forming body structures (such as bones and blood), providing energy, and helping to regulate the body's biochemical reactions.
- The amount of energy that nutrients or foods supply to the body is their caloric value. The amount of energy required to maintain basic body functions is referred to as the resting energy expenditure (REE). The basal metabolic rate (BMR) is the rate at which the body metabolizes food to maintain the energy and requirements of a person who is awake and at rest.
- A person's state of energy balance can be determined by comparing caloric intake with caloric expenditure.
- Ideal body weight (IBW) is the optimal weight recommended for optimal health.
- Body mass index (BMI) and percent body fat are indicators of changes in body fat stores. They indicate whether a person's weight is appropriate for height and may provide a useful estimate of nutrition.
- Factors influencing a person's nutrition include development, gender, ethnicity and culture, beliefs about foods, personal preferences, religious practices, lifestyle, economics, medications and therapy, health, alcohol consumption, advertising, and psychologic factors.
- Nutritional needs vary considerably according to age, growth, and energy requirements. Adolescents have high energy requirements due to their rapid growth; a diet plentiful in milk, meats, green and yellow vegetables, and fresh fruits is required. Middle-aged adults and older adults often need to reduce their caloric intake because of decreases in metabolic rate and activity levels.
- Various daily food guides have been developed to help healthy people meet the daily requirements of essential nutrients and to facilitate meal planning. These include the *Dietary Guidelines for Americans* and the Food Guide Pyramid.
- Both inadequate and excessive intakes of nutrients result in malnutrition. The effects of malnutrition can be general or specific, depending on which nutrients and what level of deficiency or excess are involved.
- Assessment of nutritional status may involve all or some of the following: nursing history data, nutritional screening, physical examination, calculation of the percentage of weight loss, a dietary history, anthropometric measurements, and laboratory data.
- Nursing diagnoses for clients with nutritional problems may be broadly stated as *Imbalanced Nutrition: Less Than Body Requirements* or *More Than Body Requirements*. Because nutritional problems may affect many other areas of human functioning, the nutritional problem may be the etiology of other diagnoses, such as *Activity Intolerance* and *Low Self-Esteem*.
- Major goals for clients with or at risk for nutritional problems include the following: maintain or restore optimal nutritional status, decrease or regain specified weight, promote healthy nutritional practices, and prevent complications associated with malnutrition.
- Assisting clients and support persons with therapeutic diets is a function shared by the nurse and the dietitian. The nurse reinforces the dietitian's instructions, assists the client to make beneficial changes, and evaluates the client's response to planned changes.
- Because many hospitalized clients have poor appetites, a major responsibility of the nurse is to provide nursing interventions that stimulate their appetites.
- Whenever possible, the nurse should help incapacitated clients to feed themselves; a number of self-feeding aids help clients who have difficulty handling regular utensils.
- The nurse can refer clients to various community programs that help special subgroups of the population meet their nutritional needs.
- Enteral feedings, administered through nasogastric, nasointestinal, gastrostomy, or jejunostomy tubes, are provided when the client is unable to ingest foods or the upper gastrointestinal tract is impaired.
- A nasogastric or nasointestinal tube is used to provide enteral nutrition for short-term use. A gastrostomy or jejunostomy tube can be used to supply nutrients via the enteral route for long-term use.
- The two most accurate methods of confirming gastrointestinal tube placement are radiographs and pH testing of aspirate.
- Aseptic technique is required during tube feedings.
- Parenteral nutrition (PN), provided when the gastrointestinal tract is nonfunctional (e.g., absorptive capacity impaired), is given intravenously into a large central vein (e.g., the superior vena cava).

THINK ABOUT IT

Refer to the chapter-opening scenario and answer these questions.

1. Melissa Markum is displaying signs of anorexia nervosa. Based on her body weight, what calorie count would you suggest, without taking her exercise plan into consideration?

2. If you were the nurse caring for Melissa, what nursing diagnoses would be appropriate for her plan of care?

3. Linking your knowledge of psychosocial development with nutrition, what form of therapy would be most effective for this client?

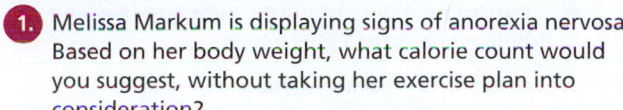 *See suggested responses to Think About It on MyNursingKit.*

TEST YOUR KNOWLEDGE

1. Which of the following nursing diagnoses is most appropriate for a client with a body mass index (BMI) of 35?
1. *Imbalanced Nutrition: Less Than Body Requirements*
2. *Imbalanced Nutrition: More Than Body Requirements*
3. *Risk for Imbalanced Nutrition*
4. *Deficient Knowledge*

2. An adult reports eating, on average, the following each day: 3 cups dairy, 2 cups fruit, 2 cups vegetables, 5 ounces grains, and 5 ounces meat. The nurse would counsel the client to:
1. Maintain the diet; the servings are adequate.
2. Increase the number of servings of dairy.
3. Decrease the number of servings of vegetables.
4. Increase the number of servings of grains.

3. Which of the following foods would the nurse find acceptable on a full liquid diet? Select all that apply.
_____ 1. Scrambled eggs
_____ 2. Chocolate pudding
_____ 3. Tomato juice
_____ 4. Hard candy
_____ 5. Mashed potatoes
_____ 6. Cream of wheat cereal
_____ 7. Oatmeal cereal
_____ 8. Fruit "smoothies"

4. Which of the following would the nurse consider the best indication of proper placement of a nasogastric tube in the stomach?
1. Client is able to speak normally.
2. Client does not gag during insertion.
3. pH of the aspirate is less than 5.
4. Fluid flows easily into the tube.

5. The nurse would do which of the following when delivering a gravity tube feeding via gravity flow?
1. Bag with feeding tube is hung 1 foot higher than the tube's insertion point into the client.
2. Nurse administers the next feeding only if there is less than 25 mL of residual volume from the previous feeding.
3. Place client in the left lateral position.
4. Feeding is administered directly from the refrigerator.

6. A 55-year-old female is about 20 lb over her desired weight. She has been on a "low calorie" diet with no improvement. The nurse would consider which of the following statements as reflecting a healthy approach to the desired weight loss? "I need to:
1. Increase my exercise to at least 30 minutes every day."
2. Switch to a low-carbohydrate diet."
3. Refer to a list of my forbidden foods with every meal."
4. Buy more organic and less processed foods."

7. An older adult Asian client has mild dysphagia from a recent stroke. The nurse plans the client's meals based on the need to:
1. Have at least one serving of thick dairy (e.g., pudding, ice cream) per meal.
2. Eliminate the beer usually ingested every evening.
3. Include as many of the client's favorite foods as possible.
4. Increase the calories from lipids to 40%.

8. Two (2) months ago a client weighed 195 pounds. The client's current weight is 182 pounds. Calculate the client's percent weight loss and determine its significance.

_____ % weight loss

_____ Not significant

_____ Significant weight loss

_____ Severe weight loss

9. The nurse, viewing an X-ray, would consider the tube properly placed if the tip of a small-bore nasally placed feeding tube was in which area? Indicate site on the diagram below.

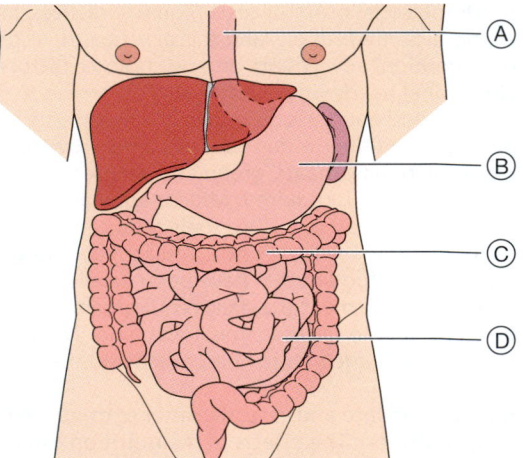

10. Which of the following meals would the nurse recommend to the client as highest in calcium, iron, and fiber?
1. 3 ounces cottage cheese with 1/3 cup raisins and 1 banana
2. 1/2 cup broccoli with 3 ounces chicken and 1/2 cup peanuts
3. 1/2 cup spaghetti with 2 ounces ground beef and 1/2 cup lima beans plus 1/2 cup ice cream
4. 3 ounces tuna plus 1 ounce cheese sandwich on whole wheat bread plus a pear

∞ *See answers to Test Your Knowledge in Appendix A.*

EXPLORE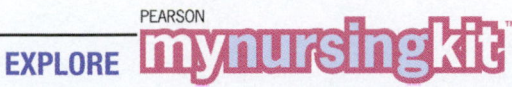

MyNursingKit is your one stop for online chapter review materials and resources. Prepare for success with additional NCLEX®-style practice questions, interactive assignments and activities, web links, animations and videos, and more!

Register your access code from the front of your book at
www.mynursingkit.com.

REFERENCES AND SELECTED BIBLIOGRAPHY

American Academy of Pediatrics Section on Breastfeeding. (2005). Policy statement: Breastfeeding and the use of human milk. *Pediatrics, 115*(2), 496–506.

American Dietetic Association. (2003). *National dysphagia diet: Standardization for optimal care.* Chicago: Author.

Anonymous. (2003). Position of the American Dietetic Association and Dieticians of Canada. *Journal of the American Dietetic Association, 103,* 748–765.

Centers for Disease Control and Prevention, National Center for Infectious Diseases, Division of Bacterial and Mycotic Diseases. (2005). *Botulism.* Retrieved December 11, 2009, from http://www.cdc.gov/ncidod/dbmd/disaseinfo/botulism_g.htm

Daniels, J. (2004). Fad diets: Slim on good nutrition. *Nursing, 34*(12), 22–23.

Green, S. M., & Watson, R. (2005). Nutritional screening and assessment tools for use by nurses: Literature review. *Journal of Advanced Nursing, 50,* 69–83.

Haddad, E. H., & Tanzman, J. S. (2003). What do vegetarians in the United States eat? *American Journal of Clinical Nutrition, 78,* 626S–632S.

Huffman, S., Jarczyk, K. S., O'Brien, E., Pieper, P., & Bayne, A. (2004). Methods to confirm feeding tube placement: Application of research to practice. *Pediatric Nursing, 30,* 10–13.

Kuszajewski, M. L., & Clontz, A. S. (2005). Prealbumin is best for nutritional monitoring. *Nursing, 35*(5), 70–71.

Leibovitch, E. R., Dreamer, R. L., & Sanderson, L. A. (2004). Food-drug interactions: Care, drug selection and patient counseling can reduce the risk in older patients. *Geriatrics, 59,* 19–33.

Maurer, J., Harris, M. M., Stanford, V. A., Lohman, T. G., Cussler, E. B., Going, S. B., et al. (2005). Dietary iron positively influences bone mineral density in postmenopausal women on hormone replacement therapy. *Journal of Nutrition, 135,* 863–869.

NANDA International. (2009). *NANDA nursing diagnoses: Definitions and classification 2009–2011.* West Sussex, U.K.: Wiley-Blackwell.

National Heart, Lung, and Blood Institute. (1998). *Clinical guidelines on the identification, evaluation, and treatment of overweight and obesity in adults: The evidence report.* Washington, DC: U.S. Department of Health & Human Services. Retrieved December 11, 2009, from http://www.nhlbi.nih.gov/guidelines/obesity/ob_gdlns.htm

Novartis Nutrition Corporation. (2003). *Nasogastric tube care and maintenance procedures.* New York: Author. Retrieved from http://www.novartisnutrition.com/us/productDetail?id=42

Reising, D. L., & Neal, R. S. (2005). Enteral tube flushing: What you think are the best practices may not be. *American Journal of Nursing, 105*(3), 58–64.

Rolfes, S. R., Pinna, K., & Whitney, E. (2009). *Understanding normal and clinical nutrition* (8th ed.). Belmont, CA: Thomson Wadsworth.

Schettler, A. E., & Gustafson, E. M. (2004). Osteoporosis prevention starts in adolescence. *Journal of the American Academy of Nurse Practitioners, 16,* 274–282.

Smith, R. M., & Myers, S. A. (2005). Two devices that unclog feeding tubes. *RN, 68*(1), 36–41.

Thomas, D. R., Ashmen, W., Morley, J. E., & Evans, W. J., et al. (2000). Nutritional management in long-term care: Development of a clinical guideline. *The Journals of Gerontology, 55A*(12), M725–735. doi:10795006

U.S. Department of Health and Human Services. (2000). *Healthy people 2010: Understanding and improving health* (2nd ed.). Washington, DC: U.S. Government Printing Office.

Zagaria, M. A. (2005). Implications of dysphagia in the elderly. *U.S. Pharmacist, 30*(1), 30–39. Retrieved from http://www.uspharmacist.com/index.asp?show=article&page=8_1410.htm

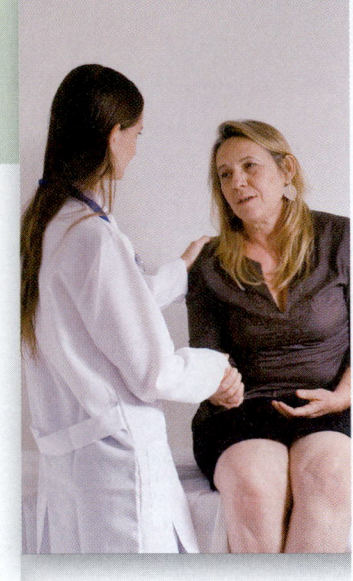

Lisa Jordan is a 46-year-old woman with two adolescent children ages 15 and 19. Her 15-year-old son has always been a big boy, weighing 13 pounds 4 ounces at birth. Lisa comes to the provider's office today reporting worsening urinary incontinence. She says she used to experience a few drops of urine expelled when she sneezed or coughed, but now the amount of urine expelled is increasing, and when her bladder is full the sense of urgency is acute because if she doesn't get to the bathroom quickly she wets her pants and has to change her clothes.

The provider orders a routine urinalysis, which rules out the possibility of a urinary tract infection. Upon examination, a mild prolapse of the bladder into the vaginal wall is noted. The provider explains the situation to Lisa and recommends against surgery, saying that the problem can be managed medically. Lisa says she'll do whatever is necessary because the condition is impacting her social life, as she's afraid she'll be embarrassed and she doesn't even want to have sexual relations with her husband for fear of uncontrollable incontinence. She says she's been trying to limit the problem by reducing her intake of fluid, especially when planning to go out with friends. She has considered wearing some type of "adult diaper" but avoids that choice because they are bulky and worries that others will be able to tell she's wearing them.

LEARNING OUTCOMES

After completing this chapter, you will be able to:

1. Describe factors that influence urinary elimination.

2. Contrast common problems with urine production and elimination.

3. Apply the nursing process when meeting clients' needs for urinary elimination.

4. Describe the steps required in the application or insertion of external, straight, and indwelling catheters including client care following the procedure.

5. Describe the care of clients requiring bladder irrigations, suprapubic catheter care, and urinary diversions.

Elimination from the urinary tract is usually taken for granted. Only when a problem arises do most people become aware of their urinary habits and any associated symptoms. A person's urinary habits depend on social culture, personal habits, and physical abilities. Personal habits regarding urination are affected by the social propriety of leaving to urinate, the availability of a private clean facility, and initial bladder training. Urinary elimination is essential to health, and voiding can be postponed for only so long before the urge normally becomes too great to control.

PHYSIOLOGY OF URINARY ELIMINATION

Urinary elimination depends on effective functioning of the upper urinary tract (kidneys and ureters) and the lower urinary tract (urinary bladder, urethra, and pelvic floor).

The paired kidneys are situated on either side of the spinal column, behind the peritoneal cavity. They are the primary regulators of fluid and acid–base balance in the body. The functional units of the kidneys, the nephrons, filter the blood and remove metabolic wastes. In the average adult 1,200 mL of blood, or about 21% of the cardiac output, passes through the kidneys every minute. Each nephron has a glomerulus, a tuft of capillaries surrounded by Bowman's capsule (Figure 33–1). The endothelium of glomerular capillaries is porous, allowing fluid and solutes to readily move across this membrane into the capsule. Plasma proteins and blood cells, however, are too large to cross the membrane normally. Glomerular filtrate is similar in composition to plasma, made up of water, electrolytes, glucose, amino acids, and metabolic wastes.

From Bowman's capsule the filtrate moves into the tubule of the nephron. In the proximal convoluted tubule, most of the water and electrolytes are reabsorbed. Solutes such as glucose are reabsorbed in the loop of Henle, but in the same area, other substances are secreted into the filtrate, concentrating the urine. In the distal convoluted tubule, additional water and sodium are reabsorbed under the control of hormones such as antidiuretic hormone (ADH) and aldosterone. This controlled reabsorption al-

lows fine regulation of fluid and electrolyte balance in the body. When fluid intake is low or the concentration of solutes in the blood is high, ADH is released from the anterior pituitary, more water is reabsorbed in the distal tubule, and less urine is excreted. By contrast, when fluid intake is high or the blood solute concentration is low, ADH is suppressed. Without ADH, the distal tubule becomes impermeable to water, and more urine is excreted. Aldosterone also affects the tubule. When aldosterone is released from the adrenal cortex, sodium and water are

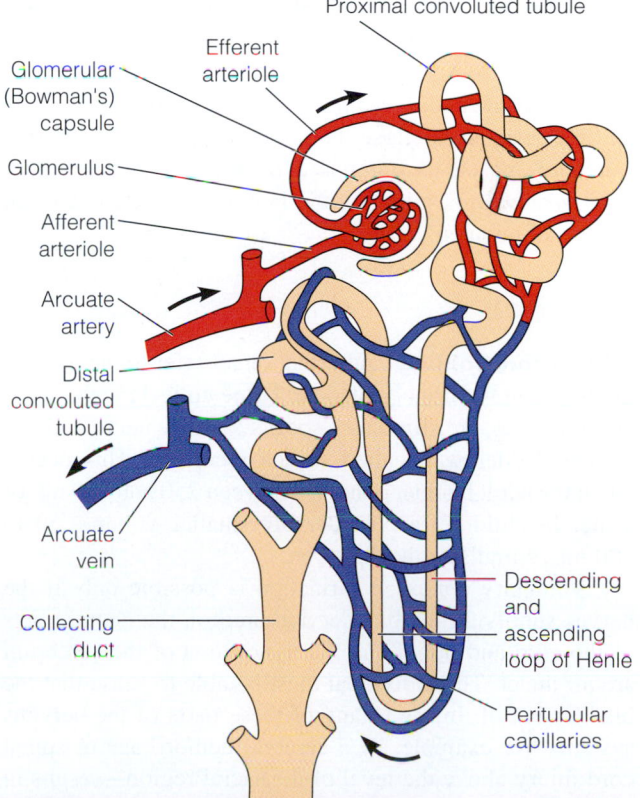

Figure 33–1 ● The nephrons of the kidney are composed of six parts: the glomerulus, Bowman's capsule, proximal convoluted tubule, loop of Henle, distal convoluted tubule, and collecting duct.

reabsorbed in greater quantities, increasing the blood volume and decreasing urinary output.

Once the urine is formed in the kidneys, it moves through the collecting ducts into the calyces of the renal pelvis and from there into the ureters. The lower ends of the ureters enter the bladder at the posterior corners of the floor of the bladder. At the junction between the ureter and the bladder, a flaplike fold of mucous membrane acts as a valve to prevent **reflux** (backflow) of urine up the ureters.

The urinary bladder (vesicle) is a hollow, muscular organ that serves as a reservoir for urine and as the organ of excretion. When empty, it lies behind the symphysis pubis. In men, the bladder lies in front of the rectum and above the prostate gland; in women it lies in front of the uterus and vagina. The wall of the bladder is made up of four layers: (a) an inner mucous layer, (b) a connective tissue layer, (c) three layers of smooth muscle fibers, some of which extend lengthwise, some obliquely, and some more or less circularly, and (d) an outer serous layer.

The urethra extends from the bladder to the urinary meatus (opening). The male urethra is longer than the female urethra and serves as a passageway for semen as well as urine. The urethra has a mucous membrane lining that is continuous with the bladder and the ureters.

The vagina and the urethra and rectum pass through the pelvic floor which consists of sheets of muscles and ligaments that provide support to the viscera of the pelvis. They extend from the symphysis pubis to the coccyx, forming a sling. Specific sphincter muscles contribute to the continence mechanism. The internal sphincter muscle situated in the proximal urethra and the bladder neck is composed of smooth muscle under *involuntary* control. It provides active tension designed to close the urethral lumen. The external sphincter muscle is composed of skeletal muscle under *voluntary* control, allowing the individual to choose when urine is eliminated.

Urination

Micturition, voiding, and urination all refer to the process of emptying the urinary bladder. Urine collects in the bladder until pressure stimulates special sensory nerve endings in the bladder wall called stretch receptors. This occurs when the adult bladder contains between 250 and 450 mL of urine. In children, a considerably smaller volume, 50 to 200 mL, stimulates these nerves.

Voluntary control of urination is possible only if the nerves supplying the bladder and urethra, the neural tracts of the cord and brain, and the motor area of the cerebrum are all intact. The individual must be able to sense that the bladder is full. Injury to any of these parts of the nervous system—for example, by a cerebral hemorrhage or spinal cord injury above the level of the sacral region—results in intermittent involuntary emptying of the bladder. Older adults whose cognition is impaired may not be aware of the need to urinate or able to respond to this urge by seeking toilet facilities.

FACTORS AFFECTING VOIDING

Numerous factors affect the volume and characteristics of the urine produced and the manner in which it is excreted.

Developmental Factors

INFANTS   Urine output varies according to fluid intake but gradually increases to 250 to 500 mL a day during the first year. An infant may urinate as often as 20 times a day. The urine of the neonate is colorless and odorless and has a specific gravity of 1.008. Because newborns and infants have immature kidneys, they are unable to concentrate urine very effectively. Infants are born without urinary control. Most will develop this between the ages of 2 and 5 years. Control during the daytime normally precedes nighttime control.

PRESCHOOLERS   The preschooler is able to take responsibility for independent toileting. Parents need to realize that accidents do occur and the child should never be punished or chastised for this. Children often forget to wash their hands or flush the toilet and need instruction in wiping themselves. Girls should be taught to wipe from front to back to prevent contamination of the urinary tract by feces.

SCHOOL-AGE CHILDREN   The school-age child's elimination system reaches maturity during this period. The kidneys double in size between ages 5 and 10 years. During this period, the child urinates six to eight times a day. **Enuresis,** which is defined as the involuntary passing of urine when control should be established (about 5 years of age), can be a problem for some school-age children. About 10% of all 6-year-olds experience difficulty controlling the bladder. Nocturnal enuresis, or bed-wetting, is the involuntary passing of urine during sleep. It has many causes but basically it occurs because the client fails to awaken when the bladder empties (Nield & Kamat, 2004, p. 409). Bed-wetting should not be considered a problem until after the age of 6. Nocturnal enuresis may be referred to as primary when the child has never achieved nighttime urinary control. The incidence of nocturnal enuresis declines as the child matures. Secondary enuresis is that which appears after the child has achieved dryness for a period of 6 consecutive months. It is often related to another problem such as constipation, stress, or illness and may resolve when the cause is eliminated. Recent research indicates that primary and secondary nocturnal enuresis may both be related to poor daytime voiding habits, and children should be taught to be aware of the sensation to void (Robson, Leung, & Van Howe, 2005).

OLDER ADULTS   The excretory function of the kidney diminishes with age, but usually not significantly below normal levels unless a disease process intervenes. Blood flow can be reduced by arteriosclerosis, impairing renal function. With age, the number of functioning nephrons decreases to some degree, impairing the kidney's filtering abilities. Conditions that alter normal fluid intake and output, such as having influenza or having surgery, can compromise the kidney's ability to filter, maintain acid–base balance, and maintain electrolyte balance in older adults. It also takes a much longer time for these processes to return to normal functioning. The decrease in kidney function also places the older adult at higher risk for toxicity from medications if excretion rates are longer.

The more noticeable changes with age are those related to the bladder. Complaints of urinary urgency and urinary frequency are common. In men these changes are often due to an enlarged prostate gland, and in women they may be due to weakened muscles supporting the bladder or weakness of the urethral sphincter. The capacity of the bladder and its ability to completely empty diminish with age. This explains the need for older adults to arise during the night to void (**nocturnal frequency**) and the retention of residual urine, predisposing the older adult to bladder infections.

See Table 33–1 for a summary of the developmental changes affecting urinary output and the Lifespan Considerations feature.

Psychosocial Factors

For many people, a set of conditions helps stimulate the micturition reflex. These conditions include privacy, normal position, sufficient time, and, occasionally, running water. Circumstances that do not allow for the client's accustomed conditions may produce anxiety and muscle tension. As a result, the person is unable to relax abdominal and perineal muscles and the external urethral sphincter, and voiding is inhibited. People also may voluntarily suppress urination because of perceived time pressures; for example, nurses often ignore the urge to void until they are able to take a break. This behavior can increase the risk of urinary tract infections.

Fluid and Food Intake

The healthy body maintains a balance between the amount of fluid ingested and the amount of fluid eliminated. When the amount of fluid intake increases, therefore, the output normally increases. Certain fluids, such as alcohol, increase fluid output by inhibiting the production of antidiuretic hormone. Fluids that contain caffeine also increase urine production. By contrast, food and fluids high in sodium can cause fluid retention because water is retained to maintain the normal concentration of electrolytes.

Some foods and fluids can change the color of urine. For example, beets can cause urine to appear red; foods containing carotene can cause the urine to appear yellower than usual.

Medications

Many medications, particularly those affecting the autonomic nervous system, interfere with the normal urination

TABLE 33–1	Changes in Urinary Elimination through the Life Span
STAGE	**VARIATIONS**
Fetuses	The fetal kidney begins to excrete urine between the 11th and 12th week of development.
Infants	Ability to concentrate urine is minimal; therefore, urine appears light yellow.
	Because of neuromuscular immaturity, voluntary urinary control is absent.
Children	Kidney function reaches maturity between the first and second year of life; urine is concentrated effectively and appears a normal amber color.
	Between 18 and 24 months of age, the child starts to recognize bladder fullness and is able to hold urine beyond the urge to void.
	At approximately 2 1/2 to 3 years of age, the child can perceive bladder fullness, hold urine after the urge to void, and communicate the need to urinate.
	Full urinary control usually occurs at age 4 or 5 years; daytime control is usually achieved by age 3 years.
	The kidneys grow in proportion to overall body growth.
Adults	The kidneys reach maximum size between 35 and 40 years of age.
	After 50 years, the kidneys begin to diminish in size and function. Most shrinkage occurs in the cortex of the kidney as individual nephrons are lost.
Older adults	An estimated 30% of nephrons are lost by age 80.
	Renal blood flow decreases because of vascular changes and a decrease in cardiac output.
	The ability to concentrate urine declines.
	Bladder muscle tone diminishes, causing increased frequency of urination and nocturia (awakening to urinate at night).
	Diminished bladder muscle tone and contractility may lead to residual urine in the bladder after voiding, increasing the risk of bacterial growth and infection.
	Urinary incontinence may occur due to mobility problems or neurologic impairments.

LIFESPAN CONSIDERATIONS   Factors Affecting Voiding

Infants and Children

- Urinary tract infections (UTIs) are the second most common infection in children, after respiratory infections. They are seen more frequently in newborn and young infant boys than girls and are most often due to obstructions or malformations of the urinary system in these children (Ball & Bindler, 2006). In older infants and children, girls have more UTIs than boys, usually due to contamination of the urethra with stool (Cavagnaro, 2005).
- Teaching proper perineal hygiene can reduce infection. Girls should learn to wipe from front to back and wear cotton underwear.
- Teach children and parents that they should go to the bathroom as soon as the sensation to void is felt and not try to hold the urine in.

Older Adults

Many changes of aging cause specific problems in urinary elimination in the older adult. Many conditions can be treated and interventions can be used to either resolve or decrease the problem. Some of the following conditions are etiological factors in problems with urinary elimination:

- Many older men have enlarged prostate glands, which can inhibit complete emptying of the bladder resulting in urinary retention and urgency, which sometimes causes incontinence.
- Women past menopause have decreased estrogen, which results in a decrease in perineal tone and support of bladder, vagina, and supporting tissues. This often results in urgency and stress incontinence and can even increase the incidence of urinary tract infections.
- Increased stiffness and pain in joints, previous joint surgery, and neuromuscular problems can impair mobility and often make it difficult to get to the bathroom.
- Cognitive impairment, such as in dementia, often prevents the person from understanding the need to urinate and the actions needed to perform the activity.

Interventions that may improve these conditions include:

- Medications or surgery to relieve obstructions in men and strengthen support in the urogenital area in women.
- Behavioral training for better bladder control.
- Providing safe, easy access to the bathroom or bedside commode, whether at home or in an institution. Make sure the room is well lit, the environment is safe, and the proper assistive devices are within reach (such as walkers, canes).
- Habit training, such as taking the person to the bathroom at a regular, scheduled time. This can often work very well with cognitively impaired persons.

---

process and may cause retention (see Box 33–1). Diuretics (e.g., chlorothiazide and furosemide) increase urine formation by preventing the reabsorption of water and electrolytes from the tubules of the kidney into the bloodstream. Some medications may alter the color of the urine.

Muscle Tone

Good muscle tone is important to maintain the stretch and contractility of the **detrusor muscle** so the bladder can fill adequately and empty completely. Clients who require a retention catheter for a long period may have poor bladder muscle tone because continuous drainage of urine prevents the bladder from filling and emptying normally. Pelvic muscle tone also contributes to the ability to store and empty urine.

Pathologic Conditions

Some diseases and pathologies can affect the formation and excretion of urine. Diseases of the kidneys may affect the ability of the nephrons to produce urine. Abnormal amounts of protein or blood cells may be present in the urine, or the kidneys may virtually stop producing urine altogether, a condition known as renal failure. Heart and circulatory disorders such as heart failure, shock, or hypertension can affect blood flow to the kidneys, interfering with urine production. If abnormal amounts of fluid are lost through another route (e.g., vomiting or high fever), water is retained by the kidneys and urinary output falls.

Processes that interfere with the flow of urine from the kidneys to the urethra affect urinary excretion. A urinary stone (calculus) may obstruct a ureter, blocking urine flow from the kidney to the bladder. Hypertrophy of the prostate gland, a common condition affecting older men, may obstruct the urethra, impairing urination and bladder emptying.

Surgical and Diagnostic Procedures

Some surgical and diagnostic procedures affect the passage of urine and the urine itself. The urethra may swell follow-

BOX 33–1   Medications that May Cause Urinary Retention

- Anticholinergic and antispasmodic medications, such as atropine and papaverine
- Antidepressant and antipsychotic agents, such as phenothiazines and MAO inhibitors
- Antihistamine preparations, such as pseudoephedrine (Actifed and Sudafed)
- Antihypertensives, such as hydralazine (Apresoline) and methyldopate (Aldomet)
- Antiparkinsonism drugs, such as levodopa, trihexyphenidyl (Artane), and benztropine mesylate (Cogentin)
- Beta-adrenergic blockers, such as propranolol (Inderal)
- Opioids, such as hydrocodone (Vicodin)

ing a cystoscopy, and surgical procedures on any part of the urinary tract may result in some postoperative bleeding; as a result, the urine may be red or pink tinged for a time.

Spinal anesthetics can affect the passage of urine because they decrease the client's awareness of the need to void. Surgery on structures adjacent to the urinary tract (e.g., the uterus) can also affect voiding because of swelling in the lower abdomen.

ALTERED URINE PRODUCTION

Although people's patterns of urination are highly individual, most people void about 5 to 6 times a day. People usually void when they first awaken in the morning, before they go to bed, and around mealtimes. Table 33–2 shows the average urinary output per day at different ages.

Polyuria

Polyuria (or **diuresis**) refers to the production of abnormally large amounts of urine by the kidneys, often several liters more than the client's usual daily output. Polyuria can follow excessive fluid intake, a condition known as **polydipsia,** or may be associated with diseases such as diabetes mellitus, diabetes insipidus, and chronic nephritis. Polyuria can cause excessive fluid loss, leading to intense thirst, dehydration, and weight loss.

Oliguria and Anuria

The terms *oliguria* and *anuria* are used to describe decreased urinary output. **Oliguria** is low urine output, usually less than 500 mL a day or 30 mL an hour for an adult. Although oliguria may occur because of abnormal fluid losses or a lack of fluid intake, it often indicates impaired blood flow to the kidneys or impending renal failure and should be promptly reported to the primary care provider. Restoring renal blood flow and urinary output promptly can prevent renal failure and its complications. **Anuria** refers to a lack of urine production.

TABLE 33–2	Average Daily Urine Output by Age
AGE	**AMOUNT (ML)**
1 to 2 days	15–60
3 to 10 days	100–300
10 days to 2 months	250–450
2 months to 1 year	400–500
1 to 3 years	500–600
3 to 5 years	600–700
5 to 8 years	700–1,000
8 to 14 years	800–1,400
14 years through adulthood	1,500
Older adulthood	1,500 or less

Should the kidneys become unable to adequately function, some mechanism of filtering the blood is necessary to prevent illness and death. This filtering is done though the use of renal **dialysis,** a technique by which fluids and molecules pass through a semipermeable membrane according to the rules of osmosis. The two most common methods of dialysis are hemodialysis and peritoneal dialysis. In hemodialysis, the client's blood flows through vascular catheters, passes by the dialysis solution in an external machine, and then returns to the client. In peritoneal dialysis, the dialysis solution is instilled into the abdominal cavity through a catheter, allowed to rest there while the fluid and molecules exchange, and then removed through the catheter. Both hemodialysis and peritoneal dialysis must be performed at frequent intervals until the client's kidneys can resume the filtering function.

ALTERED URINARY ELIMINATION

Despite normal urine production, a number of factors or conditions can affect urinary elimination. Frequency, nocturia, urgency, and dysuria often are manifestations of underlying conditions such as a urinary tract infection. Enuresis, incontinence, retention, and neurogenic bladder may be either a manifestation or the primary problem affecting urinary elimination. Selected factors associated with altered patterns of urine elimination are identified in Table 33–3.

Frequency and Nocturia

Urinary frequency is voiding at frequent intervals, that is, more than 4 to 6 times per day. An increased intake of fluid causes some increase in the frequency of voiding. Conditions such as urinary tract infection, stress, and pregnancy can cause frequent voiding of small quantities (50 to 100 mL) of urine. Total fluid intake and output may be normal.

Nocturia is voiding two or more times at night. Like frequency, it is usually expressed in terms of the number of times the person gets out of bed to void, for example, "nocturia X 4."

Urgency

Urgency is the sudden strong desire to void. There may or may not be a great deal of urine in the bladder, but the person feels a need to void immediately. Urgency accompanies psychologic stress and irritation of the trigone and urethra. It is also common in people who have poor external sphincter control and unstable bladder contractions. It is not a normal finding.

Dysuria

Dysuria means voiding that is either painful or difficult. It can accompany a stricture (decrease in caliber) of the urethra, urinary infections, and injury to the bladder and urethra. Often clients will say they have to push to void or that

TABLE 33–3	Selected Factors Associated with Altered Urinary Elimination
PATTERN	**SELECTED ASSOCIATED FACTORS**
Polyuria	Ingestion of fluids containing caffeine or alcohol
	Prescribed diuretic
	Presence of thirst, dehydration, and weight loss
	History of diabetes mellitus, diabetes insipidus, or kidney disease
Oliguria, anuria	Decrease in fluid intake
	Signs of dehydration
	Presence of hypotension, shock, or heart failure
	History of kidney disease
	Signs of renal failure such as elevated blood urea nitrogen (BUN) and serum creatinine, edema, hypertension
Frequency or nocturia	Pregnancy
	Increase in fluid intake
	Urinary tract infection
Urgency	Presence of psychologic stress
	Urinary tract infection
Dysuria	Urinary tract inflammation, infection, or injury
	Hesitancy, hematuria, pyuria (pus in the urine), and frequency
Enuresis	Family history of enuresis
	Difficult access to toilet facilities
	Home stresses
Incontinence	Bladder inflammation or other disease
	Difficulties in independent toileting (mobility impairment)
	Leakage when coughing, laughing, sneezing
	Cognitive impairment
Retention	Distended bladder on palpation and percussion
	Associated signs, such as pubic discomfort, restlessness, frequency, and small urine volume
	Recent anesthesia
	Recent perineal surgery
	Presence of perineal swelling
	Medications prescribed
	Lack of privacy or other factors inhibiting micturition

burning accompanies or follows voiding. The burning may be described as severe, like a hot poker, or more subdued, like a sunburn. Often, **urinary hesitancy** (a delay and difficulty in initiating voiding) is associated with dysuria.

Enuresis

Enuresis is involuntary urination in children beyond the age when voluntary bladder control is normally acquired, usually 4 or 5 years of age. Nocturnal enuresis often is irregular in occurrence and affects boys more often than girls. Diurnal (daytime) enuresis may be persistent and pathologic in origin. It affects women and girls more frequently.

Urinary Incontinence

Urinary incontinence, or involuntary urination, is a symptom, not a disease. It can have a significant impact on the client's life, creating physical problems such as skin breakdown and possibly leading to psychosocial problems such as embarrassment, isolation, and social withdrawal. Common causes of incontinence include urinary tract infections, urethritis, pregnancy, hypercalcemia, volume overload, delirium, restricted mobility, stool impaction, and psychologic causes (Morantz, 2005, p. 175). Urinary incontinence can be broken into two categories: acute and chronic.

ACUTE Many factors can contribute to acute or reversible incontinence, including polyuria, exposure to irritants, infection, urinary retention, use of pharmaceuticals, stool impaction or constipation, atrophic urethritis or vaginitis, restricted mobility or dexterity, psychologic conditions, and delirium or acute confused state. Some of these factors are readily reversible with a lessening of syptoms if not complete resolution of urinary incontinence.

CHRONIC There are different types of chronic incontinence, each having a different etiology, including stress, urge, reflex, retention with overflow, and functional incontinence. NANDA categorizes five types of incontinence (see "Diagnosing" on page 997). Although incontinence is experienced in some older adults, it is *not* a normal consequence of aging and can often be treated.

The preliminary assessment and identification of the symptom of urinary incontinence is truly within the scope of nursing practice. All clients should be asked about their voiding patterns. Older adults who are incontinent while in their home or who manage to contain or conceal their incontinence from others do not consider themselves incontinent. Therefore, if asked if they are incontinent, they may deny it. However, asking if they lose urine when they don't want to may provide more accurate information (Palmer & Newman, 2006). If incontinence is described, a thorough history and assessment is indicated. Treatment may include surgery, medication, or behavioral therapies. Nursing management of incontinence includes implementing individualized bladder programs, containment of urine, and meticulous skin care.

Urinary Retention

When emptying of the bladder is impaired, urine accumulates and the bladder becomes overdistended, a condition known as **urinary retention.** Overdistention of the bladder causes poor contractility of the detrusor muscle, further impairing urination. Common causes of urinary retention include prostatic hypertrophy (enlargement), surgery, and some medications (see Box 33–1).

Clients with urinary retention may experience overflow voiding or incontinence, eliminating 25 to 50 mL of urine at frequent intervals. The bladder is firm and distended on palpation and may be displaced to one side of midline.

Neurogenic Bladder

Impaired neurologic function can interfere with the normal mechanisms of urine elimination, resulting in a **neurogenic bladder.** The client with a neurogenic bladder does not perceive bladder fullness and is unable to control the urinary sphincters. The bladder may become flaccid and distended or spastic, with frequent involuntary urination.

NURSING MANAGEMENT

ASSESSING

Nursing History

The nurse determines the client's normal voiding pattern and frequency, appearance of the urine and any recent changes, any past or current problems with urination, the presence of an ostomy, and factors influencing the elimination pattern.

The specific assessment interview questions asked of the client depend on the individual and his or her responses.

Physical Assessment

Complete physical assessment of the urinary tract usually includes percussion of the kidneys to detect areas of tenderness. Palpation and percussion of the bladder are also performed. If the client's history or current problems indicate a need for it, the urethral meatus of both male and female clients is inspected for swelling, discharge, and inflammation.

Because problems with urination can affect the elimination of wastes from the body, it is important that the nurse assess the skin for color, texture, and tissue turgor as well as the presence of edema. If incontinence, dribbling, or dysuria is noted in the history, the skin of the perineum should be inspected for irritation because contact with urine can excoriate the skin.

Assessing Urine

Normal urine consists of 96% water and 4% solutes. Organic solutes include urea, ammonia, creatinine, and uric acid. Urea is the chief organic solute. Inorganic solutes include sodium, chloride, potassium, sulfate, magnesium, and phosphorus. Sodium chloride is the most abundant inorganic salt. Variations in color can occur. Characteristics of normal and abnormal urine are shown in Table 33–4.

MEASURING URINARY OUTPUT Normally, the kidneys produce urine at a rate of approximately 60 mL per hour or about 1,500 mL per day. Urine output is affected by many factors, including fluid intake, body fluid losses through other routes such as perspiration and breathing or diarrhea, and the cardiovascular and renal status of the individual.

Urine outputs below 30 mL per hour may indicate low blood volume or kidney malfunction and must be reported. To measure fluid output the nurse follows these steps:

- Wear clean gloves to prevent contact with microorganisms or blood in urine.
- Ask the client to void in a clean urinal, bedpan, commode, or toilet collection device ("hat").
- Instruct the client to keep urine separate from feces and to avoid putting toilet paper in the urine collection container.
- Pour the voided urine into a calibrated container.
- Holding the container at eye level, read the amount in the container. Containers usually have a measuring scale on the inside.
- Record the amount on the fluid intake and output sheet, which may be at the bedside or in the bathroom.
- Rinse the urine collection and measuring containers with cool water and store appropriately.
- Remove gloves and perform hand hygiene.
- Calculate and document the total output at the end of each shift and at the end of 24 hours on the client's chart.

Many clients can measure and record their own urine output when the procedure is explained to them.

When measuring urine from a client who has a urinary catheter, the nurse follows these steps:

- Put on clean gloves.
- Take the calibrated container to the bedside.
- Place the container under the urine collection bag so that the spout of the bag is above the container but

TABLE 33–4   Characteristics of Normal and Abnormal Urine

CHARACTERISTIC	NORMAL	ABNORMAL	NURSING CONSIDERATIONS
Amount in 24 hours (adult)	1,200–1,500 mL	Under 1,200 mL A large amount over intake	Urinary output normally is approximately equal to fluid intake. Output of less than 30 mL/hr may indicate decreased blood flow to the kidneys and should be immediately reported.
Color, clarity	Straw, amber Transparent	Dark amber Cloudy Dark orange Red or dark brown Mucous plugs, viscid, thick	Concentrated urine is darker in color. Dilute urine may appear almost clear, or very pale yellow. Some foods and drugs may color urine. Red blood cells in the urine (hematuria) may be evident as pink, bright red, or rusty brown urine. Menstrual bleeding can also color urine but should not be confused with hematuria. White blood cells, bacteria, pus, or contaminants such as prostatic fluid, sperm, or vaginal drainage may cause cloudy urine.
Odor	Faint aromatic	Offensive	Some foods (e.g., asparagus) cause a musty odor; infected urine can have a fetid odor; urine high in glucose has a sweet odor.
Sterility	No microorganisms present	Microorganisms present	Urine in the bladder is sterile. Urine specimens, however, may be contaminated by bacteria from the perineum during collection.
pH	4.5–8	Over 8 Under 4.5	Freshly voided urine is normally somewhat acidic. Alkaline urine may indicate a state of alkalosis, urinary tract infection, or a diet high in fruits and vegetables. More acidic urine (low pH) is found in starvation, with diarrhea, or with a diet high in protein foods or cranberries.
Specific gravity	1.010–1.025	Over 1.025 Under 1.010	Concentrated urine has a higher specific gravity; diluted urine has a lower specific gravity.
Glucose	Not present	Present	Glucose in the urine indicates high blood glucose levels (>180 mg/dL) and may be indicative of undiagnosed or uncontrolled diabetes mellitus.
Ketone bodies (acetone)	Not present	Present	Ketones, the end product of the breakdown of fatty acids, are not normally present in the urine. They may be present in the urine of clients who have uncontrolled diabetes mellitus, who are in a state of starvation, or who have ingested excessive amounts of aspirin.
Blood	Not present	Occult (microscopic) Bright red	Blood may be present in the urine of clients who have urinary tract infection, kidney disease, or bleeding from the urinary tract.

not touching it. The calibrated container is not sterile, but the inside of the collection bag is sterile.

- Open the spout and permit the urine to flow into the container.
- Close the spout, then proceed as described in the previous list.

MEASURING RESIDUAL URINE **Residual urine** (urine remaining in the bladder following the voiding) is normally 50 to 100 mL. However, a bladder outlet obstruction (e.g., enlargement of the prostate gland) or loss of bladder muscle tone may interfere with complete emptying of the bladder during urination. Manifestations of urine retention may include frequent voiding of small amounts (e.g., less than 100 mL in an adult). Urinary stasis and urinary tract infection are possible consequences of incomplete bladder emptying. Residual urine is measured to assess the amount of retained urine after voiding and determine the need for interventions (e.g., medications to promote detrusor muscle contraction).

To measure residual urine, the nurse catheterizes or bladder scans the client after voiding. The amount of urine voided and the amount obtained by catheterization or bladder scan are measured and recorded. An indwelling catheter may be inserted if the residual urine exceeds a specified amount.

Diagnostic Tests

Blood levels of two metabolically produced substances, urea and creatinine, are routinely used to evaluate renal function. Both are normally eliminated by the kidneys through filtration and tubular secretion. Urea, the end product of protein metabolism, is measured as blood urea nitrogen (BUN). Creatinine is produced in relatively constant quantities by the muscles. The creatinine clearance test uses 24-hour urine and serum creatinine levels to determine the glomerular filtration rate, a sensitive indicator of renal function. Other tests related to urinary functions such as collecting urine specimens, measuring specific gravity, and visualization procedures are described in Chapter 20 ∞.

DIAGNOSING

NANDA (2009) includes one general diagnostic label for urinary elimination problems and several labels that are more specific:

- *Impaired Urinary Elimination:* dysfunctional in urine elimination

Other NANDA nursing diagnoses related to urinary elimination are subcategories of this diagnosis, and include the following:

- *Functional Urinary Incontinence*
- *Reflex Urinary Incontinence*
- *Stress Urinary Incontinence*
- *Total Urinary Incontinence*
- *Urge Urinary Incontinence*
- *Overflow Urinary Incontinence*
- *Urinary Retention*

See Box 33–2 for definitions of NANDA diagnoses related to incontinence.

Clinical examples of assessment data clusters and related nursing diagnoses, outcomes, and interventions are shown in Identifying Nursing Diagnoses, Outcomes, and Interventions on page 998 and in the Nursing Care Plan and Concept Map at end of this chapter.

Problems of urinary elimination also may become the etiology for other problems experienced by the client. Examples include the following:

- *Risk for Infection* if the client has urinary retention or undergoes an invasive procedure such as catheterization or cystoscopic examination.
- *Low Self-Esteem* or *Social Isolation* if the client is incontinent. Incontinence can be physically and emotionally distressing to clients because it is considered socially unacceptable. Often the client is em-

barrassed about dribbling or having an accident and may restrict normal activities for this reason.
- *Risk for Impaired Skin Integrity* if the client is incontinent. Bed linens and clothes saturated with urine irritate and macerate the skin. Prolonged skin dampness leads to dermatitis (inflammation of the skin) and subsequent formation of dermal ulcers.
- *Self-Care Deficit: Toileting* if the client has functional incontinence.
- *Risk for Deficient Fluid Volume* or *Excess Fluid Volume* if the client has impaired urinary function associated with a disease process.
- *Disturbed Body Image* if the client has a urinary diversion ostomy.
- *Deficient Knowledge* if the client requires self-care skills to manage (e.g., a new urinary diversion ostomy).
- *Risk for Caregiver Role Strain* if the client is incontinent and being cared for by a family member for extended periods.
- *Risk for Social Isolation* if the client is incontinent.

PLANNING

The goals established will vary according to the diagnosis and defining characteristics. Examples of overall goals for clients with urinary elimination problems may include the following:

- Maintain or restore a normal voiding pattern.
- Regain normal urine output.
- Prevent associated risks such as infection, skin breakdown, fluid and electrolyte imbalance, and lowered self-esteem.
- Perform toilet activities independently with or without assistive devices.
- Contain urine with the appropriate device, catheter, ostomy appliance, or absorbent product.

Appropriate preventive and corrective nursing interventions that relate to these must be identified. Specific nursing activities associated with each of these interventions can be selected to meet the client's individual needs. Examples of clinical applications of these using NANDA, NIC, and NOC designations are shown in Identifying Nursing Diagnoses, Outcomes, and Interventions and in the Nursing Care Plan and Concept Map at the end of the chapter.

IMPLEMENTING

Maintaining Normal Urinary Elimination

Most interventions to maintain normal urinary elimination are independent nursing functions. These include promoting adequate fluid intake, maintaining normal voiding habits, and assisting with toileting.

BOX 33–2 **Definitions of NANDA Incontinence Diagnoses**

- *Functional Urinary Incontinence*—Inability of usually continent person to reach toilet in time to avoid unintentional loss of urine.
- *Reflex Urinary Incontinence*—Involuntary loss of urine at somewhat predictable intervals when a specific bladder volume is reached.
- *Stress Urinary Incontinence*—Sudden leakage of urine occurring with activities that increase abdominal pressure.
- *Total Urinary Incontinence*—Continuous and unpredictable passage of urine.
- *Urge Urinary Incontinence*—Involuntary passage of urine occurring soon after a strong sense of urgency to void.

Note: Reprinted from *Nursing Outcomes Classification* (NOC), 3rd ed., by S. Moorhead, M. Johnson, & M. Meridean, Copyright © 2004 with permission from Elsevier.

DRUG CAPSULE   Anticholinergic Agents *oxybutynin ER (Ditropan XL)*

The Client with Medications for Urge Urinary Incontinence

Anticholinergic agents reduce urgency and frequency by blocking muscarinic receptors in the detrusor muscle of the bladder, thereby inhibiting contractions and increasing storage capacity. They are useful in relieving symptoms associated with voiding in clients with neurogenic bladder and reflex neurogenic bladder, and urge urinary incontinence.

Nursing Responsibilities

- Monitor for constipation, dry mouth, urinary retention, blurred vision, and mental confusion in older adults; symptoms may be dose related.
- Keep primary care provider informed of expected responses to therapy (e.g., effect on urinary frequency, urge incontinence, nocturia, and bladder emptying).
- Start with small doses to clients over the age of 75.

- Try using intermittently.
- Oxybutynin is contraindicated in clients with urinary retention, gastrointestinal motility problems (partial or complete GI obstruction, paralytic ileus), or uncontrolled narrow-angle glaucoma.

Client and Family Teaching

- Explain the reason for taking oxybutynin.
- Explain the side effects and the importance of reporting them to the health care provider.
- Exercise caution in hot environments. By suppressing sweating, oxybutynin can cause fever and heat stroke.
- Provide strategies for managing dry mouth.
- Instruct and advise regarding behavioral therapies for urge suppression.

Note: Prior to administering any medication, review all aspects with a current drug handbook or other reliable source.

IDENTIFYING NURSING DIAGNOSES, OUTCOMES, AND INTERVENTIONS   Clients with Urinary Elimination Disorders

DATA CLUSTER Mrs. Amy Brown, 75, reports accidental loss of urine before she is able to reach the toilet. She is aware of the urge to void but states, "Because of my stroke I sometimes can't get there soon enough."

NURSING DIAGNOSIS/DEFINITION	SAMPLE DESIRED OUTCOMES*/*DEFINITION*	INDICATORS	SELECTED INTERVENTIONS*/*DEFINITION*	SAMPLE NIC ACTIVITIES
Functional Urinary Incontinence/Inability of usually continent person to reach toilet in time to avoid unintentional loss of urine	Urinary Continence [0502]/*Control of the elimination of urine from the bladder*	Consistently demonstrated: • Responds to urge in timely manner • Gets to toilet between urge and passage of urine • Voids > 150 mL each time	Prompted Voiding [0640]/*Promotion of urinary continence through the use of timed verbal toileting reminders and positive social feedback for successful toileting*	• Determine client awareness of continence status by asking if wet or dry • Prompt up to three times to use toilet or substitute, regardless of continence status • Give positive feedback by praising desired toileting behavior • Document outcomes of toileting session

DATA CLUSTER Tammy Tyndale reports dribbling whenever she laughs, coughs, or sneezes. She is 8 months pregnant.

Stress Urinary Incontinence/Sudden loss of urine occurring with activities that increase abdominal pressure	Symptom Control [1608]/*Personal actions to minimize perceived adverse changes in physical and emotional functioning*	Consistently demonstrated: • Uses preventive measures • Uses available resources	Pelvic Muscle Exercise [0560]/*Strengthening and training the levator ani and urogenital muscles through voluntary repetitive contraction to decrease stress, urge, or mixed types of urinary incontinence*	• Instruct client to tighten, then relax, the ring of muscle around urethra and anus, as if trying to prevent urination or bowel movement • Provide positive feedback for doing exercises as prescribed

*The NOC # for desired outcomes and the NIC # for nursing interventions are listed in brackets following the appropriate outcome or intervention. Outcomes, indicators, interventions, and activities selected are only a sample of those suggested by NOC and NIC and should be further individualized for each client.

PROMOTING FLUID INTAKE Increasing fluid intake increases urine production, which in turn stimulates the micturition reflex. A normal daily intake averaging 1,500 mL of measurable fluids is adequate for most adult clients.

Many clients have increased fluid requirements, necessitating a higher daily fluid intake. For example, clients who are perspiring excessively (have diaphoresis) or who are experiencing abnormal fluid losses through vomiting, gastric suction, diarrhea, or wound drainage require fluid to replace these losses in addition to their normal daily intake requirements.

Clients who are at risk for urinary tract infection or urinary calculi (stones) should consume 2,000 to 3,000 mL of fluid daily. Dilute urine and frequent urination reduce the risk of urinary tract infection as well as stone formation.

Increased fluid intake may be contraindicated for some clients such as people with kidney failure or heart failure. For these clients, a fluid restriction may be necessary to prevent fluid overload and edema.

MAINTAINING NORMAL VOIDING HABITS Prescribed medical therapies often interfere with a client's normal voiding habits. When a client's urinary elimination pattern is adequate, the nurse helps the client adhere to normal voiding habits as much as possible (see Practice Guidelines).

ASSISTING WITH TOILETING Clients who are weakened by a disease process or impaired physically may require assistance with toileting. The nurse should assist these clients to the bathroom and remain with them if they are at risk for falling. The bathroom should contain an easily accessible call signal to summon help if needed. Clients also need to be encouraged to use handrails placed near the toilet.

For clients unable to use bathroom facilities, the nurse provides urinary equipment close to the bedside (e.g., urinal, bedpan, commode) and provides the necessary assistance to use them.

Preventing Urinary Tract Infections

The incidence of urinary tract infection (UTI) is greater in women than men because of the short urethra and its proximity to the anal and vaginal areas (Anonymous, 2004). UTIs are the most common type of nosocomial infection found in long-term care facilities (Midthun, 2004). Most UTIs are caused by bacteria common to the intestinal environment (e.g., *Escherichia coli*). These gastrointestinal bacteria can colonize in the perineal area and move into the urethra, especially when there is urethral trauma, irritation, or manipulation. Women are particularly at risk.

For women who have experienced a UTI, nurses need to provide instructions about ways to prevent a recurrence. The following guidelines are useful for anyone:

- Drink eight 8-ounce glasses of water per day to flush bacteria out of the urinary system.
- Practice frequent voiding (every 2 to 4 hours) to flush bacteria out of the urethra and prevent organisms from ascending into the bladder. Void immediately after intercourse.

PRACTICE GUIDELINES

Maintaining Normal Voiding Habits

Positioning

- Assist the client to a normal position for voiding: standing for male clients; for female clients, squatting or leaning slightly forward when sitting. These positions enhance movement of urine through the tract by gravity.
- If the client is unable to ambulate to the lavatory, use a bedside commode for females and a urinal for males standing at the bedside.
- If necessary, encourage the client to push over the pubic area with the hands or to lean forward to increase intra-abdominal pressure and external pressure on the bladder.

Relaxation

- Provide privacy for the client. Many people cannot void in the presence of another person.
- Allow the client sufficient time to void.
- Suggest the client read or listen to music.
- Provide sensory stimuli that may help the client relax. Pour warm water over the perineum of a female or have the client sit in a warm bath to promote muscle relaxation. Applying a hot water bottle to the lower abdomen of both men and women may also foster muscle relaxation.

- Turn on running water within hearing distance of the client to stimulate the voiding reflex and to mask the sound of voiding for people who find this embarrassing.
- Provide ordered analgesics and emotional support to relieve physical and emotional discomfort to decrease muscle tension.

Timing

- Assist clients who have the urge to void immediately. Delays only increase the difficulty in starting to void, and the desire to void may pass.
- Offer toileting assistance to the client at usual times of voiding, for example, on awakening, before or after meals, and at bedtime.

For Clients Who Are Confined to Bed

- Warm the bedpan. A cold bedpan may prompt contraction of the perineal muscles and inhibit voiding.
- Elevate the head of the client's bed to Fowler's position, place a small pillow or rolled towel at the small of the back to increase physical support and comfort, and have the client flex the hips and knees. This position simulates the normal voiding position as closely as possible.

- Avoid use of harsh soaps, bubble bath, powder, or sprays in the perineal area. These substances can be irritating to the urethra and encourage inflammation and bacterial infection.
- Avoid tight-fitting pants or other clothing that creates irritation to the urethra and prevents ventilation of the perineal area.
- Wear cotton rather than nylon underclothes. Accumulation of perineal moisture facilitates bacterial growth, and cotton enhances ventilation of the perineal area.
- Girls and women should always wipe the perineal area from front to back following urination or defecation in order to prevent introduction of gastrointestinal bacteria into the urethra.
- If recurrent urinary infections are a problem, take showers rather than baths. Bacteria present in bathwater can readily enter the urethra.

Managing Urinary Incontinence

It is important to remember that urinary incontinence is *not* a normal part of aging and often is treatable. Independent nursing interventions for clients with urinary incontinence (UI) include (a) a behavior-oriented continence training program that may consist of bladder training, habit training, prompted voiding, pelvic muscle exercises, and positive reinforcement; (b) meticulous skin care; and (c) for males, application of an external drainage device (condom-type catheter device).

CLINICAL ALERT

Stress incontinence in women may be successfully treated by insertion (under local anesthesia) of a transvaginal tape (TVT) sling to support the urethra.

CONTINENCE (BLADDER) TRAINING A continence training program requires the involvement of the nurse, the client, and support people. Clients must be alert and physically able or have caregivers who can assist with implementation of the plan of care in order to follow a program. A bladder training program may include the following:

- Education of the client and support people.
- **Bladder training**, which requires that the client postpone voiding, resist or inhibit the sensation of urgency, and void according to a timetable rather than according to the urge to void. The goals are to gradually lengthen the intervals between urination to correct the client's frequent urination, to stabilize the bladder, and to diminish urgency. This form of training may be used for clients who have bladder instability and urge incontinence. Delayed voiding provides larger voided volumes and longer intervals between voiding. Initially, voiding may be encouraged every 2 to 3 hours except during sleep and then every 4 to 6 hours. A vital component of bladder training is inhibiting the urge-to-void sensation. To do this, the nurse instructs the client to practice deep, slow breathing until the urge diminishes or disappears. This is performed every time the client has a premature urge to void.
- **Habit training**, also referred to as timed voiding or scheduled toileting, attempts to keep clients dry by having them void at regular intervals. With habit training, there is no attempt to motivate the client to delay voiding if the urge occurs. This approach can be effective in children who are experiencing urinary dysfunction. Biofeedback therapy in which the child is taught to relax the pelvic floor can also decrease incidents of wetting (Shei Dei Yang & Cheng Wang, 2005).
- **Prompted voiding** supplements habit training by encouraging the client to try to use the toilet (prompting) and reminding the client when to void.

PELVIC MUSCLE EXERCISES Pelvic muscle exercises (PME), or Kegel exercises, help to strengthen pelvic floor muscles

---

RESEARCH NOTES

What Are the Accuracy and Clinical Benefits of Using a Bladder Scanner?

The authors conducted a research review and synthesis as a component in the model for change to evidence-based practice. They initially identified evidence of a need for a research utilization project of urinary tract infection (UTI) and the use of bladder scanner technology. The team reviewed 12 research studies—7 pertained to accuracy of the bladder scanner and 5 investigated the clinical benefits of the technology. All of the studies used nonexperimental designs. Most of the samples were by convenience and tended to be too small to identify significant differences. Despite these limitations, the studies did demonstrate that the bladder scanners were accurate. Clinical benefits included that the bladder scanners were effective in diagnosing urinary retention without using intermittent catheterization, which decreased the costs of catheterization equipment and the risk of UTI to the client. The studies also provided beginning evidence that both clients and health care providers were satisfied with the outcomes of using the bladder scanner.

Implications

The bladder scanner is used as an assessment tool to reduce the incidence of nosocomial infections as a result of invasive urinary catheterizations. Additional research, preferably experimental with large samples, is needed before a recommendation can be made to use bladder scanning in lieu of intermittent catheterization.

Note: From "The Clinical Benefits of the Bladder Scanner: A Research Synthesis," by A. Sparks et al., *Journal of Nursing Care Quality, 19*(3), 2004, pp. 188–192. Copyright Lippincott Williams & Wilkins. Reprinted with permission.

Pelvic Muscle Exercises (Kegels)

- First, sit or lie in a comfortable, relaxed position.
- Contract your pelvic muscles whereby you pull your rectum, urethra, and vagina up inside, and hold for a count of 3 to 5 seconds. Then relax the same muscles for a count of 3 to 5 seconds.
- Initially perform each contraction 10 times, three times daily. Gradually increase the count to a full 10 seconds for both contraction and relaxation.
- Develop a schedule that will help remind you to do these exercises, for example, before getting out of bed in the morning, when working at the kitchen sink, or at scheduled times (e.g., 0700, 1200, 1800 hours).
- To control episodes of stress incontinence, perform a pelvic muscle contraction when initiating any activity that increases intra-abdominal pressure, such as coughing, laughing, sneezing, or lifting.

and can reduce or eliminate episodes of incontinence. The client can identify the perineal muscles by stopping urination midstream or by tightening the anal sphincter as if to hold a bowel movement.

The following technique is sometimes used to teach PME. Ask the client to think of the perineal muscles as an elevator. When the client relaxes, the elevator is on the first floor. To perform the exercise, contract the perineal muscles, bringing the elevator to the second, third, and fourth floors. Keep the elevator on the fourth floor for a few seconds, and then gradually relax the area. When the exercise

is properly performed, contraction of the muscles of the buttocks and thighs is avoided. PME can be performed anytime, anywhere, sitting or standing—even when voiding. Specific client instructions for performing PME are summarized in Client Teaching.

MAINTAINING SKIN INTEGRITY Skin that is continually moist becomes macerated (softened). Urine that accumulates on the skin is converted to ammonia, which is very irritating to the skin. Because both skin irritation and maceration predispose the client to skin breakdown and ulceration, the incontinent person requires meticulous skin care. To maintain skin integrity, the nurse washes the client's perineal area with mild soap and water or a commercially prepared no-rinse cleanser after episodes of incontinence, rinses it thoroughly if used soap and water, dries it gently and thoroughly, and provides clean, dry clothing or bed linen. The nurse applies barrier ointments or creams to protect the skin from contact with urine. If it is necessary to pad the client's clothes for protection, the nurse should use products that absorb wetness and leave a dry surface in contact with the skin.

Specially designed incontinence drawsheets may be used that provide significant advantages over standard drawsheets for incontinent clients confined to bed. These sheets are like a drawsheet but are double layered, with a quilted upper nylon or polyester surface and an absorbent viscose rayon layer below. The rayon soaker layer generally has a waterproof backing on its underside. Fluid (i.e., urine) passes through the upper quilted layer and is absorbed and dispersed by the viscose rayon, leaving the quilted surface dry to the touch. This absorbent sheet helps maintain skin integrity; it does not stick to the skin when wet, decreases the risk of bedsores, and reduces odor.

Bladder Training

- Determine the client's voiding pattern and encourage voiding at those times, or establish a regular voiding schedule and help the client to maintain it, whether the client feels the urge or not (e.g., on awakening, every 1 or 2 hours during the day and evening, before retiring at night, every 4 hours at night). The stretching–relaxing sequence of such a schedule tends to increase bladder muscle tone and promote more voluntary control. Encourage the client to inhibit the urge-to-void sensation when a premature urge to void is experienced. Instruct the client to practice slow, deep breathing until the urge diminishes or disappears.
- When the client finds that voiding can be controlled, the intervals between voiding can be lengthened slightly without loss of continence.
- Regulate fluid intake, particularly during evening hours, to help reduce the need to void during the night.
- Encourage fluids between the hours of 0600 and 1800.

- Avoid excessive consumption of citrus juices, carbonated beverages (especially those containing artificial sweeteners), alcohol, and drinks containing caffeine because these irritate the bladder, increasing the risk of incontinence.
- Schedule diuretics early in the morning.
- Explain to clients that adequate fluid intake is required to ensure adequate urine production that stimulates the micturition reflex.
- Apply protector pads to keep the bed linen dry and provide specially made waterproof underwear to contain the urine and decrease the client's embarrassment. Avoid using diapers, which are demeaning and also suggest that incontinence is permissible.
- Assist the client with an exercise program to increase the general muscle tone and a pelvic muscle exercise program aimed at strengthening the pelvic floor muscles.
- Provide positive reinforcements to encourage continence. Praise clients for attempting to toilet and for maintaining continence.

APPLYING EXTERNAL URINARY DRAINAGE DEVICES The application of a condom or external catheter connected to a urinary drainage system can be used for incontinent males. Use of a condom appliance is preferable to insertion of a retention catheter because the risk of urinary tract infection is minimal.

Methods of applying condoms vary. The nurse needs to follow the manufacturer's instructions when applying a condom. First the nurse determines when the client experiences incontinence. Some clients may require a condom appliance at night only, others continuously. Skill 33–1 describes how to apply and remove an external catheter.

SKILL 33–1

APPLYING AN EXTERNAL CATHETER

PURPOSES
- To collect urine and control urinary incontinence
- To permit the client physical activity while controlling urinary incontinence
- To prevent skin irritation as a result of urinary incontinence

ASSESSMENT
- Review the client record to determine a pattern to voiding and other pertinent data.

- Put on clean gloves and examine the client's penis for swelling or excoriation that would contraindicate use of the condom catheter.

PLANNING
Determine if the client has had an external catheter previously and any difficulties with it. Perform any procedures that are best completed without the catheter in place (for example, weighing the client would be easier without the tubing and bag).

Delegation
Applying a condom catheter may be delegated to unlicensed assistive personnel (UAP). However, the nurse must determine if the specific client has unique needs that would require special training of the UAP in the use of the condom catheter.

EQUIPMENT
- Leg drainage bag with tubing or urinary drainage bag with tubing
- Condom sheath
- Drape (e.g., sheet or bath blanket)
- Clean gloves
- Basin of warm water and soap
- Washcloth and towel
- Elastic tape or Velcro strap

IMPLEMENTATION

Preparation
- Assemble the leg drainage bag or urinary drainage bag for attachment to the condom sheath.
- Roll the condom outward onto itself to facilitate easier application. ❶ On some models, an inner flap will be exposed. This flap is applied around the urinary meatus to prevent the reflux of urine.
- Position the client in either a supine or a sitting position.

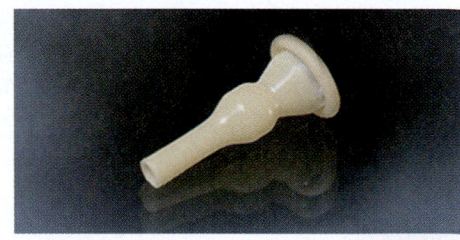

❶ Before application, roll the condom outward onto itself. (Courtesy of Bard Medical Division.)

Performance
1. Prior to performing the procedure, introduce self and verify the client's identity using agency protocol. Explain to the client what you are going to do, why it is necessary, and how he can participate.
2. Perform hand hygiene, and observe other appropriate infection control procedures. Apply clean gloves. Position the client in either a supine or sitting position.
3. Provide for client privacy.
   - Drape the client appropriately with the bath blanket, exposing only the penis.
4. Inspect and clean the penis.
   - Clean the genital area and dry it thoroughly. **Rationale:** *This minimizes skin irritation and excoriation after the condom is applied.*
5. Apply and secure the condom.
   - Roll the condom smoothly over the penis, leaving 2.5 cm. (1 in.) between the end of the penis and the rubber or plastic connecting tube. ❷ **Rationale:** *This space prevents*

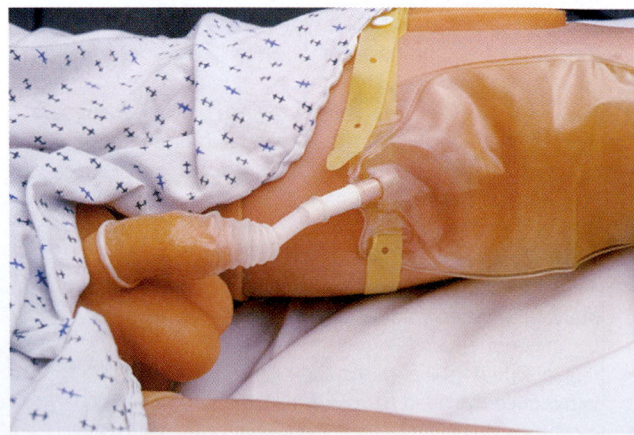

❷ The condom rolled over the penis.

irritation of the tip of the penis and provides for full drainage of urine.

- Secure the condom firmly, but not too tightly, to the penis. Some condoms have an adhesive inside the proximal end that adheres to the skin of the base of the penis. Many condoms are packaged with special tape. If neither is present, use a strip of elastic tape or Velcro around the base of the penis over the condom. Ordinary tape is contraindicated because it is not flexible and can stop blood flow.

6. Securely attach the urinary drainage system.
- Make sure that the tip of the penis is not touching the condom and that the condom is not twisted. **Rationale:** *A twisted condom could obstruct the flow of urine.*
- Attach the urinary drainage system to the condom.
- Remove the gloves and perform hand hygiene.
- If the client is to remain in bed, attach the urinary drainage bag to the bed frame.
- If the client is ambulatory, attach the bag to the client's leg. **Rationale:** *Attaching the drainage bag to the leg helps control the movement of the tubing and prevents twisting of the thin material of the condom appliance at the tip of the penis.*

7. Teach the client about the drainage system.
- Instruct the client to keep the drainage bag below the level of the condom and to avoid loops or kinks in the tubing.

8. Inspect the penis 30 minutes following the condom application, and check urine flow. Document these findings.
- Assess the penis for swelling and discoloration, *which indicates that the condom is too tight.*
- Assess urine flow if the client has voided. Normally, some urine is present in the tube if the flow is not obstructed.

9. Change the condom daily and provide skin care.
- Remove the elastic or Velcro strip, apply clean gloves, and roll off the condom.
- Wash the penis with soapy water, rinse, and dry it thoroughly.
- Assess the foreskin for signs of irritation, swelling, and discoloration.
- Reapply a new condom.

10. Document in the client record using forms or checklists supplemented by narrative notes when appropriate. Record the application of the condom, the time, and pertinent observations, such as irritated areas on the penis.

EVALUATION

- Perform a detailed follow-up based on findings that deviated from expected or normal for the client. Relate findings to previous assessment data if available.
- Report significant deviations from normal to the primary care provider.

Managing Urinary Retention

Interventions that assist the client to maintain a normal voiding pattern, discussed earlier, also apply when dealing with urinary retention. If these actions are unsuccessful, the primary care provider may order a cholinergic drug such as bethanechol chloride (Urecholine) to stimulate bladder contraction and facilitate voiding. Clients who have a flaccid bladder (weak, soft, and lax bladder muscles) may use manual pressure on the bladder to promote bladder emptying. This is known as **Credé's maneuver** or Credé's method. It is not advised without a physician or nurse practitioner's order and is used only for clients who have lost and are not expected to regain voluntary bladder control. When all measures fail to initiate voiding, urinary catheterization may be necessary to empty the bladder completely. An indwelling Foley catheter may be inserted until the underlying cause is treated. Alternatively, intermittent straight catheterization (every 3 to 4 hours) may be performed because the risk of urinary tract infection may be less than with an indwelling catheter.

Urinary Catheterization

Urinary catheterization is the introduction of a catheter into the urinary bladder. This is usually performed only when absolutely necessary, because the danger exists of introducing microorganisms into the bladder. Clients who have lowered immune resistance are at the greatest risk. Once an infection is introduced into the bladder, it can ascend the ureters and eventually involve the kidneys. The hazard of infection remains after the catheter is in place because normal defense mechanisms such as intermittent flushing of microorganisms from the urethra through voiding are bypassed. Thus, strict sterile technique is used for catheterization.

> **CLINICAL ALERT**
>
> The insertion of urinary catheters is one of the most common causes of hospital-acquired infections.

Another hazard is trauma with urethral catheterization, particularly in the male client, whose urethra is longer and more tortuous. It is important to insert a catheter along the normal contour of the urethra. Damage to the urethra can occur if the catheter is forced through strictures or at an incorrect angle. In males, the urethra is normally curved, but it can be straightened by elevating the penis to a position perpendicular to the body.

Catheters are commonly made of rubber or plastics although they may be made from latex, silicone, or polyvinyl chloride (PVC). They are sized by the diameter of the lumen using the French (Fr) scale: the larger the number, the larger the lumen. Either straight catheters, inserted to drain the bladder and then immediately removed, or retention catheters, which remain in the bladder to drain urine, may be used.

The straight catheter is a single-lumen tube with a small eye or opening about 1 1/4 cm (1/2 in.) from the insertion tip (Figure 33–2). The coudé catheter is a variation of the

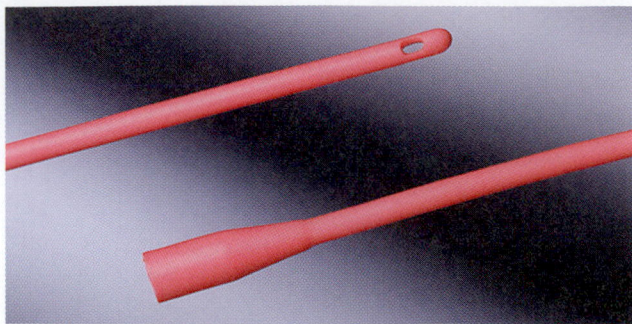

A

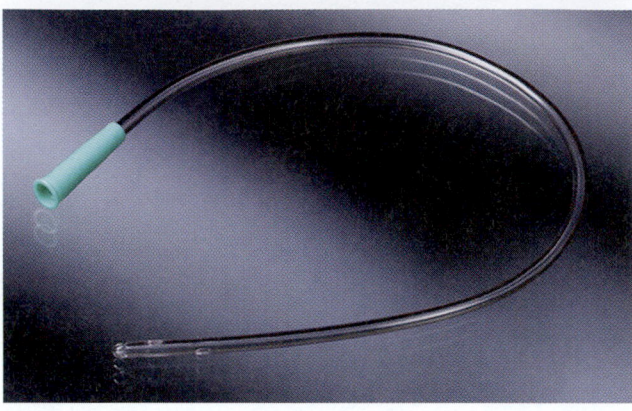

B

Figure 33–2 ○ Red-rubber or plastic Robinson straight catheters.
(Courtesy of Bard Medical Division.)

straight catheter. It is more rigid than other straight catheters and has a tapered, curved tip (Figure 33–3). This catheter may be used for men with prostatic hypertrophy because it is more easily controlled and less traumatic on insertion.

The retention, or Foley, catheter is a double-lumen catheter. The larger lumen drains urine from the bladder. A second, smaller lumen is used to inflate a balloon near the tip of the catheter to hold the catheter in place within the bladder (Figure 33–4). Clients who require continuous or

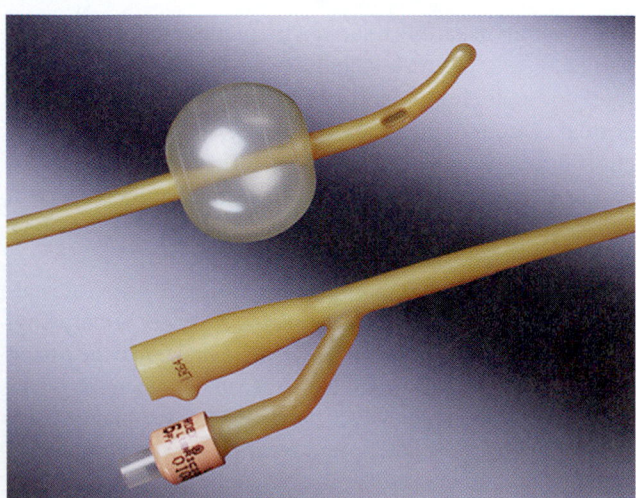

Figure 33–3 ○ A coudé catheter.
(Courtesy of Bard Medical Division.)

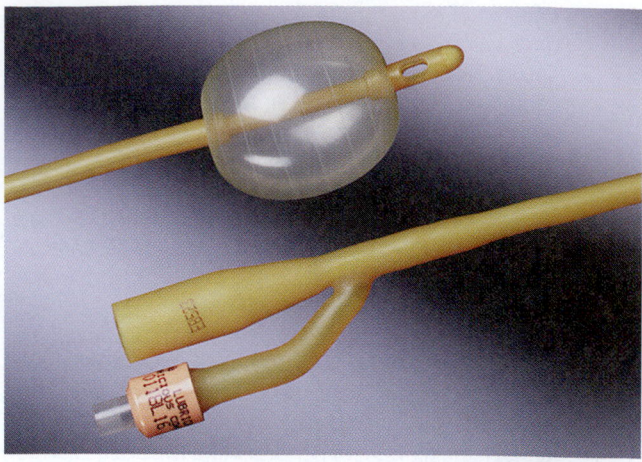

Figure 33–4 ○ An indwelling/retention (Foley) catheter with the balloon inflated.
(Courtesy of Bard Medical Division.)

intermittent bladder irrigation may have a three-way Foley catheter (Figure 33–5). The three-way catheter has a third lumen through which sterile irrigating fluid can flow into the bladder. The fluid then exits the bladder through the drainage lumen, along with the urine.

The balloons of retention catheters are sized by the volume of fluid used to inflate them. The two commonly used sizes are 10-mL and 30-mL balloons. The size of the balloon is indicated on the catheter along with the diameter, for example, "#18 Fr—10 mL." Box 33–3 provides guidelines for catheter selection.

Retention catheters usually are connected to a closed gravity drainage system. This system consists of the catheter, drainage tubing, and a collecting bag for the urine. A closed system cannot be opened anywhere along the system, from catheter to collecting bag. Closed systems reduce the risk of microorganisms entering the system and infecting the urinary tract. Urinary drainage systems typically depend on the force of gravity to drain urine from the bladder to the collecting bag.

Skill 33–2 describes catheterization of females and males, using straight and retention catheters.

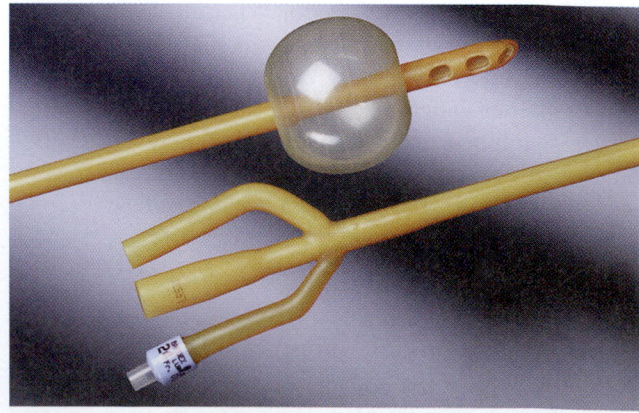

Figure 33–5 ○ A three-way Foley catheter often used for continuous bladder irrigation.
(Courtesy of Bard Medical Division.)

BOX 33–3	Selecting a Urinary Catheter

- Select the type of material in accordance with the estimated length of the catheterization period. Antimicrobial-impregnated or hydrogel/silver-coated catheters may also be used to reduce the risk of infection.
  a. Use plastic catheters for short periods only (e.g., 1 week or less), because they are inflexible.
  b. Use a rubber or Silastic catheter for periods of 2 or 3 weeks. Latex may be used for clients with no known latex allergy. However, because of these allergies, latex is being phased out of health care products.
  c. Use silicone catheters for long-term use (e.g., 2 to 3 months) because they create less encrustation at the urethral meatus. However, they are expensive.
  d. Use PVC catheters for 4- to 6-week periods. They soften at body temperature and conform to the urethra.

- Determine appropriate catheter length by the client's gender. For adult female clients, use a 22-cm catheter; for adult male clients, a 40-cm catheter.
- Determine appropriate catheter size by the size of the urethral canal. Use sizes such as #8 or #10 for children, #14 or #16 for adults. Men frequently require a larger size than women, for example, #18.
- Select the appropriate balloon size. For adults, use a 10-mL balloon to facilitate optimal urine drainage. The smaller balloons allow more complete bladder emptying because the catheter tip is closer to the urethral opening in the bladder. However, a 30-mL balloon is commonly used to achieve hemostasis of the prostatic area following a prostatectomy. Use 3-mL balloons for children.

SKILL 33–2

PERFORMING URINARY CATHETERIZATION

PURPOSES

- To relieve discomfort due to bladder distention or to provide gradual decompression of a distended bladder
- To assess the amount of residual urine if the bladder empties incompletely
- To obtain a sterile urine specimen
- To empty the bladder completely prior to surgery

- To facilitate accurate measurement of urinary output for critically ill clients whose output needs to be monitored hourly
- To provide for intermittent or continuous bladder drainage and/or irrigation
- To prevent urine from contacting an incision after perineal surgery
- To manage incontinence when other measures have failed

ASSESSMENT

- Determine the most appropriate method of catheterization based on the purpose and any criteria specified in the order such as total amount of urine to be removed or size of catheter to be used.
- Use a straight catheter if only a spot urine specimen is needed, if amount of residual urine is being measured, or if temporary decompression/emptying of the bladder is required.
- Use an indwelling/retention catheter if the bladder must remain empty or continuous urine measurement/collection is needed.

- Assess the client's overall condition. Determine if the client is able to cooperate and hold still during the procedure and if the client can be positioned supine with head relatively flat.
- Determine when the client last voided or was last catheterized.
- Percuss the bladder to check for fullness or distention.
- When possible, complete a bladder scan to assess the amount of urine present in the bladder before performing a urethral catheterization.

PLANNING

Allow adequate time to perform the catheterization. Although the entire procedure can require as little as 15 minutes, several sources of difficulty could result in a much longer time. If possible, it should not be performed just prior to or after the client eats.

Delegation

Due to the need for sterile technique and detailed knowledge of anatomy, insertion of a urinary catheter is not delegated to UAP.

EQUIPMENT

- Sterile catheter of appropriate size (An extra catheter should also be at hand.)
- Catheterization kit or individual sterile items: ❶
  - Sterile gloves
  - Waterproof drape(s)
  - Antiseptic solution

  - Cleansing balls
  - Forceps
  - Water-soluble lubricant
  - Urine receptacle
  - Specimen container
- For an indwelling catheter:
  - Syringe prefilled with sterile water in amount specified by catheter manufacturer
  - Collection bag and tubing
- 5–10 mL 2% Xylocaine gel or water-soluable lubricant for urethral injection (if agency permits)
- Clean gloves
- Supplies for performing perineal cleansing
- Bath blanket or sheet for draping the client
- Adequate lighting (Obtain a flashlight or lamp if necessary.)

(continued)

SKILL 33–2

PERFORMING URINARY CATHETERIZATION *(continued)*

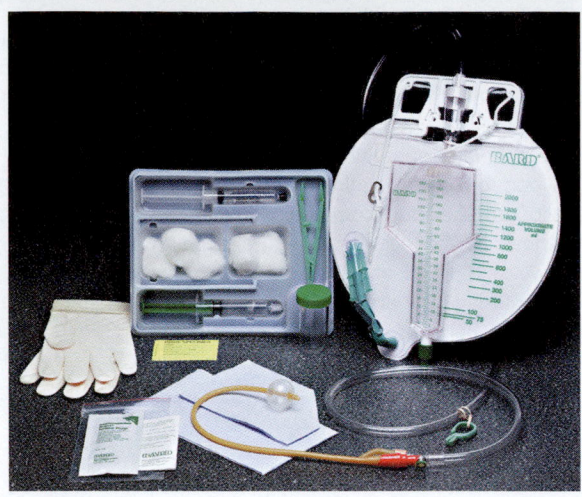

A

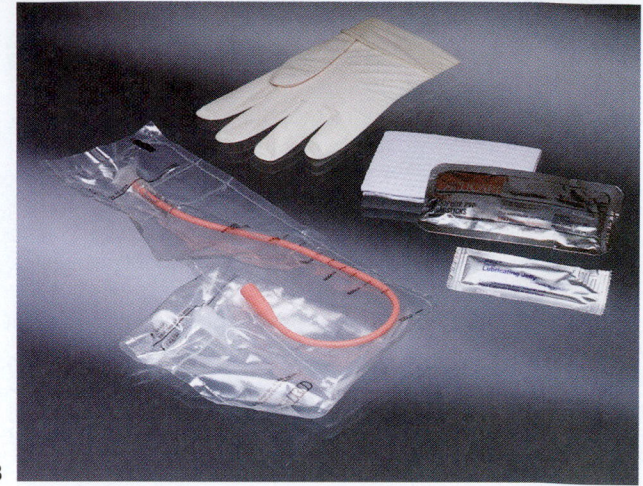

B

1 Catheter insertion kits: *A*, indwelling; *B*, straight.
(Courtesy of Bard Medical Division.)

IMPLEMENTATION

Preparation

If using a catheterization kit, read the label carefully to be sure all necessary items are included. Apply clean gloves. Perform routine perineal care to cleanse the meatus from gross contamination. For women, use this time to locate the urinary meatus relative to surrounding structures. **2**

Performance

1. Prior to performing the procedure, introduce self and verify the client's identity using agency protocol. Explain to the client what you are going to do, why it is necessary, and how he or she can participate.
2. Perform hand hygiene and observe appropriate infection control procedures.
3. Provide for client privacy.

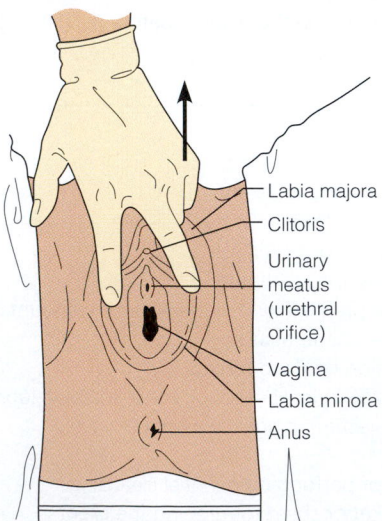

Labia majora
Clitoris
Urinary meatus (urethral orifice)
Vagina
Labia minora
Anus

2 To expose the urinary meatus, separate the labia minora and retract the tissue upward.

4. Place the client in the appropriate position and drape all areas except the perineum.
   a. Female: supine with knees flexed, feet about 2 feet apart, and hips slightly externally rotated, if possible
   b. Male: supine, thighs slightly abducted or apart
5. Establish adequate lighting. Stand on the client's right if you are right-handed, on the client's left if you are left-handed.
6. If using a collecting bag and it is not contained within the catheterization kit, open the drainage package and place the end of the tubing within reach. **Rationale:** *Since one hand is needed to hold the catheter once it is in place, open the package while two hands are still available.*
7. If agency policy permits, apply clean gloves and inject 10 to 15 mL Xylocaine gel into the urethra of both males and females (Head, 2006). In males, wipe the underside of the penile shaft to distribute the gel up the urethra. Wait at least 5 minutes for the gel to take effect before inserting the catheter. Remove and discard gloves. Perform hand hygiene.
8. Open the catheterization kit. Place a waterproof drape under the buttocks (female) or penis (male) without contaminating the center of the drape with your hands.
9. Apply sterile gloves.
10. Organize the remaining supplies:
    • Saturate the cleansing balls with the antiseptic solution.
    • Open the lubricant package.
    • Remove the specimen container and place it nearby with the lid loosely on top.
11. Attach the prefilled syringe to the indwelling catheter inflation hub and test the balloon. **Rationale:** *If the balloon malfunctions, it is important to replace it prior to use.*
12. Lubricate the catheter (1 to 2 in. for females, 6 to 7 in. for males) and place it with the drainage end inside the collection container.
13. If desired, place the fenestrated drape over the perineum, exposing the urinary meatus.

14. Cleanse the meatus. **Note:** *The nondominant hand is considered contaminated once it touches the client's skin.*
    a. Women:
    Use your nondominant hand to spread the labia. Establish a firm but gentle position. The antiseptic may make the tissues slippery but the labia must not be allowed to return over the cleaned meatus. Pick up a cleansing ball with the forceps in your dominant hand and wipe one side of the labia majora in an anteroposterior direction. ❸ Use great care that wiping the client does not contaminate this sterile hand. Use a new ball for the opposite side. Repeat for the labia minora. Use the last ball to cleanse directly over the meatus. **Note:** *Location of the urethral meatus is best identified during the cleansing process.*
    b. Men:
    Use your nondominant hand to grasp the penis just below the glans. If necessary, retract the foreskin. Hold the penis firmly upright, with slight tension. **Rationale:** *Lifting the penis in this manner helps straighten the urethra.* Pick up a cleansing ball with the forceps in your dominant hand and wipe from the center of the meatus in a circular motion around the glans. Use great care that wiping the client does not contaminate this sterile hand. Use a new ball and repeat three more times. The antiseptic may make the tissues slippery but the foreskin must not be allowed to return over the cleaned meatus nor the penis be dropped.

15. Insert the catheter.
    • Grasp the catheter firmly 2 to 3 in. from the tip. Ask the client to take a slow deep breath and insert the catheter as the client exhales. Slight resistance is expected as the catheter passes through the sphincters. If necessary, twist the catheter or hold pressure on the catheter until the sphincter relaxes.
    • Advance the catheter 2 inches farther after the urine begins to flow through it, *to be sure it is fully in the bladder.* For male clients, some agencies' policies and procedures indicate to advance the catheter to the "Y" bifurcation of the catheter. Check your agency's policy.
    • If the catheter accidentally contacts the labia or slips into the vagina, it is considered contaminated and a new, sterile catheter must be used. The contaminated catheter may be left in the vagina until the new catheter is inserted to help avoid mistaking the vaginal opening for the urethral meatus.

16. Hold the catheter with the nondominant hand. In males, lay the penis down onto the drape, being careful that the catheter does not pull out.

17. For an indwelling catheter, inflate the retention balloon with the designated volume.
    • Without releasing the catheter, hold the inflation valve between two fingers of your nondominant hand while you attach the syringe (if not left attached earlier when testing the balloon) and inflate with your dominant hand. If the client complains of discomfort, immediately withdraw the instilled fluid, advance the catheter further, and attempt to inflate the balloon again.
    • Pull *gently* on the catheter until resistance is felt to ensure that the balloon has inflated and to place it in the trigone of the bladder. ❹

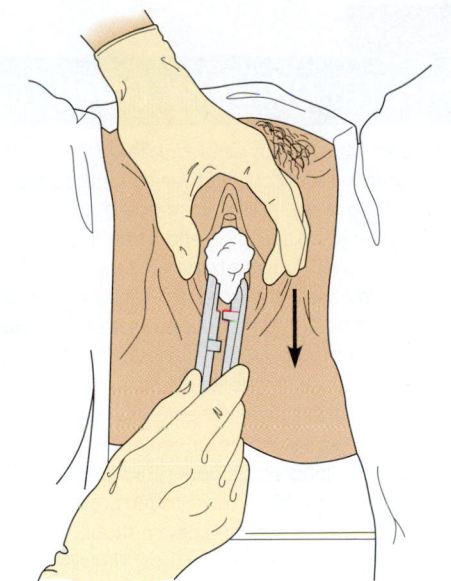

❸ When cleaning the urinary meatus, move the swab downward.

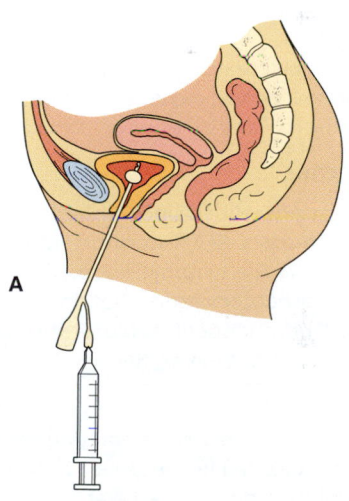

A

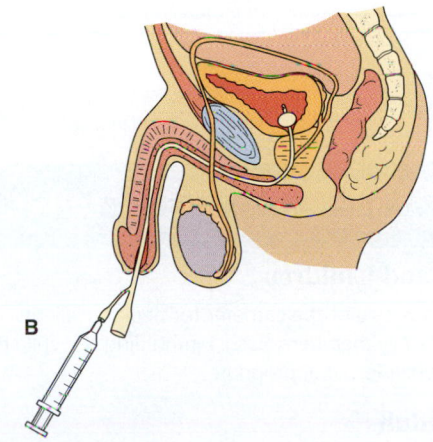

B

❹ Placement of indwelling catheter and inflated balloon in **A**, female client; and **B**, male client.

(continued)

SKILL 33–2

PERFORMING URINARY CATHETERIZATION *(continued)*

18. Collect a urine specimen if needed. Allow 20 to 30 mL to flow into the bottle without touching the catheter to the bottle.
19. Allow the straight catheter to continue draining. If necessary, attach the drainage end of an indwelling catheter to the collecting tubing and bag.
20. Examine and measure the urine. In some cases, only 750 to 1,000 mL of urine are to be drained from the bladder at one time. Check agency policy for further instructions if this should occur.
21. Remove the straight catheter when urine flow stops. For an indwelling catheter, secure the catheter tubing to the inner thigh for female clients or the upper thigh/abdomen for male clients with enough slack to allow usual movement. Tape or a manufactured catheter-securing device should be used to secure the catheter tubing to the client. This prevents unnecessary trauma to the urethra. Also secure the collecting tubing to the bed linens and hang the bag below the level of the bladder. No tubing should fall below the top of the bag. ❺
22. Wipe the perineal area of any remaining antiseptic or lubricant. Replace the foreskin if retracted earlier. Return the client to a comfortable position.
23. Discard all used supplies in appropriate receptacles and wash your hands.
24. Document the catheterization procedure including catheter size and results in the client record using forms or checklists supplemented by narrative notes when appropriate.

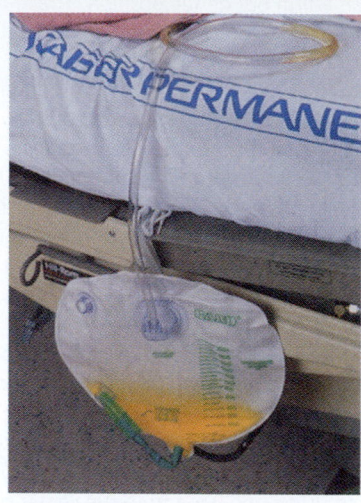

❺ Correct position for urine drainage bag and tubing.

SAMPLE DOCUMENTATION

11/24/2009 2000 Has not voided since surgery (6 hours) despite repeated attempts. C/O discomfort. Moderate distention noted above the symphysis pubis. Straight cath performed per Dr. Carpenter's order. Obtained 650 cc of clear yellow urine. Specimen sent to lab. States she "feels much better". ———— C. Chavez, RN

SAMPLE DOCUMENTATION

1/12/2010 1030 Explained that Dr. Rattigan ordered insertion of a Foley catheter. Stated that the doctor had discussed it with her previously. Explained the insertion process. Stated she understood and that she had one inserted on a previous admission. #16 Fr silicone catheter inserted without difficulty with 10 cc of solution added to balloon. Obtained 800 cc of yellow, clear urine. Specimen sent to lab. Tolerated procedure well. States she feels "comfortable and has no discomfort". ———— A. McKinney, RN

EVALUATION

Conduct appropriate follow-up such as notifying the primary care provider of the catheterization results. Perform a detailed follow-up based on findings that deviated from expected or normal for the client. Relate findings to previous assessment data if available. Teach the client how to care for the indwelling catheter, to drink more fluids, and other appropriate instructions.

LIFESPAN CONSIDERATIONS   Catheterization

Infants and Children

• Adapt the size of the catheter for pediatric clients.
• Ask a family member to assist in holding the child during catheterization, if appropriate.

Older Adults

When catheterizing older adults, be very attentive to problems of limited movement, especially in the hips. Arthritis, or previ-

ous hip or knee surgery, may limit their movement and cause discomfort. Modify the position (e.g., side-lying) as needed to perform the procedure safely and comfortably. For women, obtain the assistance of another nurse to flex and hold the client's knees and hips as necessary or place her in a modified Sims' position.

Nursing Interventions for Clients with Indwelling Catheters

Nursing care of the client with an indwelling catheter and continuous drainage is largely directed toward preventing infection of the urinary tract and encouraging urinary flow through the drainage system (Figure 33–6). It includes encouraging large amounts of fluid intake, accurately recording the fluid intake and output, changing the retention catheter and tubing, maintaining the patency of the drainage system, preventing contamination of the drainage system, and teaching these measures to the client.

FLUIDS The client with a retention catheter should drink up to 3,000 mL per day if permitted. Large amounts of fluid ensure a large urine output, which keeps the bladder flushed out and decreases the likelihood of urinary stasis and subsequent infection. Large volumes of urine also minimize the risk of sediment or other particles obstructing the drainage tubing.

DIETARY MEASURES Acidifying the urine of clients with a retention catheter may reduce the risk of urinary tract infection and calculus formation. Foods such as eggs, cheese, meat and poultry, whole grains, cranberries, plums and prunes, and tomatoes tend to increase the acidity of urine. Conversely, most fruits and vegetables, legumes, and milk and milk products result in alkaline urine.

PERINEAL CARE No special cleaning other than routine hygienic care is necessary for clients with retention catheters, nor is special meatal care recommended. Agency practices regarding catheter care vary considerably. The nurse should check agency practice in this regard.

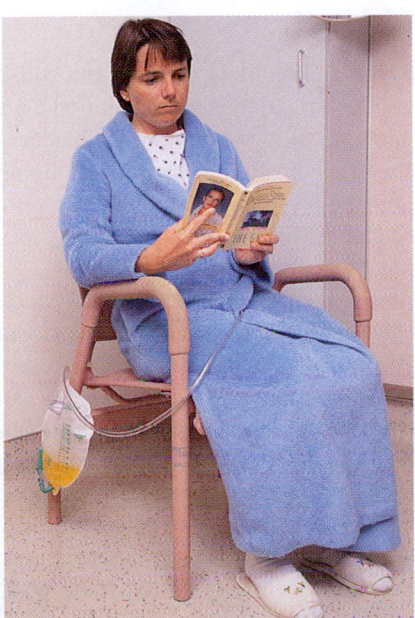

Figure 33–6 ● Positioning the collecting bag and tubing when sitting in a chair.

BOX 33–4	Ongoing Assessment of Clients with Indwelling Catheters

- Ensure that there are no obstructions in the drainage. Check that there are no kinks in the tubing, the client is not lying on the tubing, and the tubing is not clogged with mucus or blood.
- Check that there is no tension on the catheter or tubing, that the catheter is securely attached to the thigh or abdomen, and that the tubing is fastened appropriately to the bedclothes.
- Ensure that gravity drainage is maintained. Make sure there are no loops in the tubing below its entry to the drainage receptacle and that the drainage receptacle is below the level of the client's bladder.
- Ensure that the drainage system is well sealed or closed. Check that there are no leaks at the connection sites in open systems.
- Observe the flow of the urine every 2 or 3 hours, and note color, odor, and any abnormal constituents. If sediment is present, check the catheter more frequently to ascertain whether it is plugged.

CHANGING THE CATHETER AND TUBING Routine changing of catheter and tubing is not recommended. Collection of sediment in the catheter or tubing or impaired urine drainage are indicators for changing the catheter and drainage system. When this occurs the catheter and drainage system are removed and discarded, and a new sterile catheter with a closed drainage system is inserted.

Guidelines to prevent catheter-associated urinary tract infections are given in Practice Guidelines. Ongoing assessment of clients with retention catheters is a high priority (see Box 33–4).

REMOVING INDWELLING CATHETERS Indwelling catheters are removed after their purpose has been achieved, usually on the order of the primary care provider. If the catheter has been in place for a short time (e.g., a few days), the client usually has little difficulty regaining normal urinary elimination patterns. Swelling of the urethra, however, may initially interfere with voiding, so the nurse should regularly

PRACTICE GUIDELINES	Preventing Catheter-Associated Urinary Infections

- Have an established infection control program.
- Catheterize clients only when necessary, by using aseptic technique, sterile equipment, and trained personnel.
- Maintain a sterile closed-drainage system.
- Do not disconnect the catheter and drainage tubing unless absolutely necessary.
- Remove the catheter as soon as possible.
- Follow and reinforce good hand washing technique.
- Provide routine perineal hygiene, including cleansing with soap and water after defecation.
- Prevent contamination of the catheter with feces in the incontinent client.

assess the client for urinary retention until voiding is reestablished.

Clients who have had a retention catheter for a prolonged period may require bladder retraining to regain bladder muscle tone. With an indwelling catheter in place, the bladder muscle does not stretch and contract regularly as it does when the bladder fills and empties by voiding. A few days before removal, the catheter may be clamped for specified periods of time (e.g., 2 to 4 hours), then released to allow the bladder to empty. This allows the bladder to distend and stimulates its musculature. Check agency policy regarding bladder training procedures.

To remove a retention catheter, the nurse follows these steps:

- Obtain a receptacle for the catheter (e.g., a disposable basin); a clean, disposable towel; clean gloves; and a sterile syringe to deflate the balloon. The syringe should be large enough to withdraw all the solution in the catheter balloon. The size of the balloon is indicated on the label at the end of the catheter.
- Ask the client to assume a supine position as for a catheterization.
- *Optional:* Obtain a sterile specimen before removing the catheter. Check agency protocol.
- Remove the tape or catheter securing device attaching the catheter to the client, put on gloves, and then place the towel between the legs of the female client or over the thighs of the male.
- Insert the syringe into the injection port of the catheter, and withdraw the fluid from the balloon. If not all of the fluid can be removed, report this fact to the nurse in charge before proceeding.
- Do not pull the catheter while the balloon is inflated; doing so may injure the urethra.
- After all of the fluid is withdrawn from the balloon, gently withdraw the catheter and place it in the waste receptacle.
- Dry the perineal area with a towel.
- Remove gloves.
- Measure the urine in the drainage bag, and record the removal of the catheter. Include in the recording (a) the time the catheter was removed; (b) the amount, color, and clarity of the urine; (c) the intactness of the catheter; and (d) instructions given to the client.
- Provide the client with either a urinal (men), bedpan, commode, or toilet collection device ("hat") to be used with each, subsequent unassisted void.
- Following removal of the catheter, determine the time of the first voiding and the amount voided during the first 8 hours. Compare this output to the client's intake.
- Observe for dysfunctional voiding behaviors (i.e., < 100 mL per void), which might indicate urinary retention. If this occurs, perform an assessment of postvoid residuals using a bladder scanner if available. Generally postvoid residuals greater than 200 cc will require straight catheterization as needed.

Clean Intermittent Self-Catheterization

Clean intermittent self-catheterization (CISC) is performed by many clients who have some form of neurogenic bladder dysfunction, such as that caused by spinal cord injury. Clean or medical aseptic technique is used. Intermittent self-catheterization:

- Enables the client to retain independence and gain control of the bladder.
- Reduces incidence of urinary tract infection.
- Protects the upper urinary tract from reflux.
- Allows normal sexual relations without incontinence.
- Reduces the use of aids and appliances.
- Frees the client from embarrassing dribbling.

The procedure for self-catheterization is similar to that used by the nurse to catheterize a client. Essential steps are outlined in the accompanying Client Teaching feature. Because the procedure requires physical and mental preparation, client assessment is important. The client should have:

- Sufficient manual dexterity to manipulate a catheter.
- Sufficient mental ability.
- Motivation and acceptance of the procedure.
- For women, reasonable agility to access the urethra.
- Bladder capacity greater than 100 mL.

Before teaching CISC, the nurse should establish the client's voiding patterns, the volume voided, fluid intake, and residual amounts. CISC is easier for males to learn because of the visibility of the urinary meatus. Females need to learn initially with the aid of a mirror but eventually should perform the procedure by using only the sense of touch (as described in Client Teaching).

Urinary Irrigations

An **irrigation** is a flushing or washing-out with a specified solution. Bladder irrigation is carried out on a primary care provider's order, usually to wash out the bladder and sometimes to apply a medication to the bladder lining. Catheter irrigations may be performed to maintain or restore the patency of a catheter; for example, to remove pus or blood clots blocking the catheter.

The closed method is the preferred technique for catheter or bladder irrigation because it is associated with a lower risk of urinary tract infection. Closed catheter irrigations may be either continuous or intermittent. This method is most often used for clients who have had genitourinary surgery. The continuous irrigation helps prevent blood clots occluding the catheter. A three-way, or triple lumen, catheter (see Figure 33–5) is generally used for closed irrigations. The irrigating solution flows into the bladder through the irrigation port of the catheter and out through the urinary drainage lumen of the catheter.

Occasionally an open irrigation may be necessary to restore catheter patency. The risk of injecting microorgan-

CLIENT TEACHING

Clean Intermittent Self-Catheterization

- Catheterize as often as needed to maintain. At first, catheterization may be necessary every 2 to 3 hours, increasing to 4 to 6 hours.
- Attempt to void before catheterization; insert the catheter to remove residual urine if unable to void or if amount voided is insufficient (e.g., less than 100 mL).
- Assemble all needed supplies ahead of time. Good lighting is essential, especially for women.
- If a woman, remove a tampon before catheterizing. *A tampon can inhibit catheterization.*
- Wash your hands.
- Clean the urinary meatus with either a towelette or soapy washcloth, then rinse with a wet washcloth. Women should clean the area from front to back.
- Assume a position that is comfortable and that facilitates passage of the catheter, such as a semireclining position in bed or sitting on a chair or the toilet. Men may prefer to stand over the toilet; women may prefer to stand with one foot on the side of the bathtub.
- Apply lubricant to the catheter tip (1 in. [2.5 cm] for women; 2 to 6 in. [5 to 15 cm] for men).
- Insert the catheter until urine flows through.
  a. If a woman, locate the meatus using a mirror or other aid, or use the "touch" technique as follows:

- Place the index finger of your nondominant hand on your clitoris.
- Place the third and fourth fingers at the vagina.
- Locate the meatus between the index and third fingers.
- Direct the catheter through the meatus and then upward and forward.
  b. If a man, hold the penis with a slight upward tension at a 60- to 90-degree angle to insert the catheter. Return the penis to its natural position when urine starts to flow.
- Hold the catheter in place until all urine is drained.
- Withdraw the catheter slowly *to ensure complete drainage of urine.*
- Wash the catheter with soap and water; store in a clean container. Replace the catheter when it becomes difficult to clean, or too soft or hard to insert easily.
- Contact your care provider if your urine becomes cloudy or contains sediment; if you have bleeding, difficulty, or pain when passing the catheter; or if you have a fever.
- Drink at least 2,000 to 2,500 mL of fluid a day *to ensure adequate bladder filling and flushing.* To keep your urine acidic and reduce the risk of bladder infections, drink cranberry and prune juices.

isms into the urinary tract is greater with open irrigations, because the connection between the indwelling catheter and the drainage tubing is broken. Strict precautions to maintain the sterility of the drainage tubing connector and interior of the indwelling catheter must be taken to minimize this risk.

The open method of catheter or bladder irrigation is performed with double-lumen indwelling catheters. It may be necessary for clients who develop blood clots and mucous fragments that occlude the catheter and when it is undesirable to change the catheter. Techniques for catheter irrigation are outlined in Skill 33–3.

SKILL 33–3

PERFORMING BLADDER IRRIGATION

PURPOSES
- To maintain the patency of a urinary catheter and tubing (closed continuous irrigation)
- To free a blockage in a urinary catheter or tubing (open intermittent irrigation)

ASSESSMENT
- Determine the client's current urinary drainage system. Review the client record for recent intake and output and any difficulties the client has been experiencing with the system. Review the results of previous irrigations.
- Assess the client for any discomfort, bladder spasms, or distended bladder.

PLANNING
Before irrigating a catheter or bladder, check (a) the reason for the irrigation; (b) the order authorizing the continuous or intermittent irrigation (in most agencies, primary care provider's order is required); (c) the type of sterile solution, the amount, and strength to be used, and the rate (if continuous); and (d) the type of catheter in place. If these are not specified on the client's chart, check agency protocol.

Delegation

Due to the need for sterile technique, urinary irrigation is generally not delegated to UAP. If the client has continuous irrigation, the UAP may care for the client and note abnormal findings. These must be validated and interpreted by the nurse.

(continued)

SKILL 33–3

PERFORMING BLADDER IRRIGATION *(continued)*

EQUIPMENT

- Clean gloves (2 pairs)
- Retention catheter in place
- Drainage tubing and bag (if not in place)
- Drainage tubing clamp
- Antiseptic swabs
- Sterile receptacle

- Sterile irrigating solution warmed or at room temperature (Label the irrigant clearly with the words *Bladder Irrigation*, including the information about any medications that have been added to the original solution, and the date, time, and nurse's initials.)
- Infusion tubing
- IV pole

IMPLEMENTATION

Performance

1. Prior to performing the procedure, introduce self and verify the client's identity using agency protocol. Explain to the client what you are going to do, why it is necessary, and how he or she can participate. The irrigation should not be painful or uncomfortable. Discuss how the results will be used in planning further care or treatments.

2. Perform hand hygiene and observe appropriate infection control procedures.

3. Provide for client privacy.

4. Put on clean gloves.

5. Empty, measure, and record the amount and appearance of urine present in the drainage bag. Discard urine and gloves. **Rationale:** *Emptying the drainage bag allows more accurate measurement of urinary output after the irrigation is in place or completed. Assessing the character of the urine provides baseline data for later comparison.*

6. Prepare the equipment.
   - Perform hand hygiene.
   - Connect the irrigation infusion tubing to the irrigating solution and flush the tubing with solution, keeping the tip sterile. **Rationale:** *Flushing the tubing removes air and prevents it from being instilled into the bladder.*
   - Apply clean gloves and cleanse the port with antiseptic swabs.
   - Connect the irrigation tubing to the input port of the three-way catheter.
   - Connect the drainage bag and tubing to the urinary drainage port if not already in place.
   - Remove the gloves and perform hand hygiene.

7. Irrigate the bladder.
   a. For closed continuous irrigation, open the flow clamp on the urinary drainage tubing (if present). See figure. ❶ **Rationale:** *This allows the irrigating solution to flow out of the bladder continuously.*
   - Open the regulating clamp on the irrigating tubing and adjust the flow rate as prescribed by the primary care provider or to 40 to 60 drops per minute if not specified.
   - Assess the drainage for amount, color, and clarity. The amount of drainage should equal the amount of irrigant entering the bladder plus expected urine output.
   b. For closed intermittent irrigation, determine whether the solution is to remain in the bladder for a specified time.
   - If the solution is to remain in the bladder (a bladder irrigation or instillation), apply the flow clamp to the

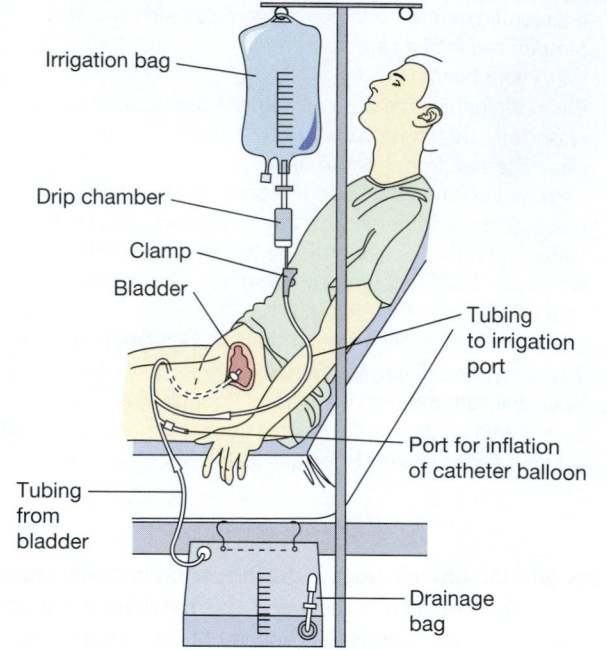

❶ A continuous bladder irrigation (CBI) setup.

urinary drainage tubing. **Rationale:** *Closing the flow clamp allows the solution to be retained in the bladder and in contact with bladder walls.*
   - If the solution is being instilled to irrigate the catheter, open the flow clamp on the urinary drainage tubing. **Rationale:** *Irrigating solution will flow through the urinary drainage port and tubing, removing mucous shreds or clots.*
   - Open the flow clamp on the irrigating tubing, allowing the specified amount of solution to infuse. Clamp the tubing.
   - After the specified period the solution is to be retained, open the drainage tubing flow clamp and allow the bladder to empty.
   - Assess the drainage for amount, color, and clarity. The amount of drainage should equal the amount of irrigant entering the bladder plus expected urine output.

8. Assess the client and the urinary output.
   - Assess the client's comfort.
   - Empty the drainage bag and measure the contents. Subtract the amount of irrigant instilled from the total volume of drainage to obtain the volume of urine output.

9. Document the procedure and results in the client record using forms or checklists supplemented by narrative notes when appropriate.
   • Note any abnormal constituents such as blood clots, pus, or mucous shreds.

VARIATION: OPEN IRRIGATION USING A TWO-WAY INDWELLING CATHETER

1. Assemble the equipment. Use an irrigation tray ❷ or assemble individual items, including
   • Clean gloves
   • Sterile gloves
   • Disposable water-resistant towel
   • Sterile irrigating solution
   • Sterile irrigation set
   • Sterile basin
   • Sterile 50-mL Asepto syringe
   • Antiseptic swabs
   • Sterile protective cap (for catheter drainage tubing)
2. Prepare the client (see steps 1–5 of main procedure for catheter irrigation).
3. Prepare the equipment.
   • Perform hand hygiene.
   • Using aseptic technique, open supplies and pour the irrigating solution into the sterile basin or receptacle. **Rationale:** *Aseptic technique is vital to reduce the risk of instilling microorganisms into the urinary tract during the irrigation.*
   • Place the disposable water-resistant towel under the catheter.
   • Put on clean gloves. Disconnect catheter from drainage tubing. Place sterile protective cap over end of drainage tubing. **Rationale:** *The end of the drainage tubing will be considered contaminated if it touches bed linens or skin surfaces.*
   • Remove clean gloves and put on sterile gloves.
   • Withdraw the prescribed amount of irrigating solution into the syringe, maintaining the sterility of the syringe and solution.

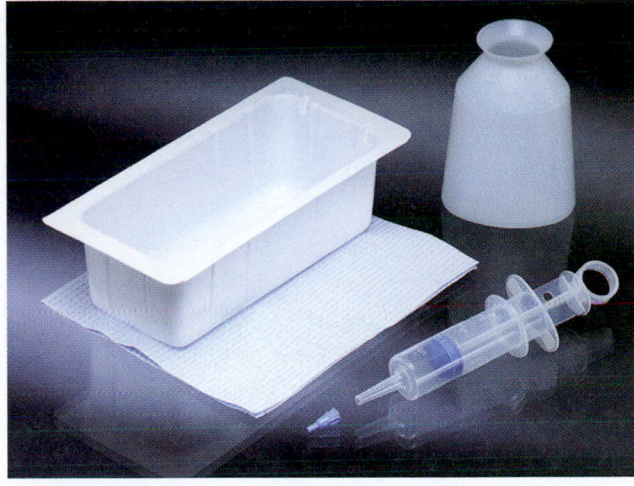

❷ An irrigation set.
(Courtesy of Bard Medical Division.)

4. Irrigate the bladder.
   • Insert the tip of the syringe into the catheter opening.
   • Gently and slowly inject the solution. In adults, about 30 to 40 mL generally is instilled for catheter irrigations; 100 to 200 mL may be instilled for bladder irrigation. **Rationale:** *Gentle instillation reduces the risks of injury to bladder mucosa and of bladder spasms.*
   • Remove syringe and allow solution to drain into basin.
   • Continue to irrigate client's bladder until fluid returns are clear and/or clots are removed.
   • Remove protective cap from drainage tube and wipe with antiseptic swab or alcohol sponge.
   • Reconnect catheter to drainage tubing.
   • Assess the drainage for amount, color, and clarity. The amount of drainage should equal the amount of irrigant entering the bladder. Determine the amount of fluid used for the irrigation and subtract from total output on the client's I&O record.
5. Assess the client and the urinary output and document the procedure as in steps 8 and 9 above.

EVALUATION
• Perform detailed follow-up based on findings that deviated from expected or normal for the client. Relate findings to previous assessment data if available.
• Report significant deviations from normal to the primary care provider.

Suprapubic Catheter Care

A **suprapubic catheter** is inserted surgically through the abdominal wall above the symphysis pubis into the urinary bladder (Figure 33–7). The physician inserts the catheter using local anesthesia or during bladder or vaginal surgery. The catheter may be secured in place with sutures if a retention balloon is not used and is then attached to a closed drainage system. The suprapubic catheter may be placed for temporary bladder drainage until the client is able to resume normal voiding (e.g., after urethral, bladder, or vaginal surgery) or it may become a permanent device (e.g., urethral or pelvic trauma).

Care of clients with a suprapubic catheter includes regular assessments of the client's urine, fluid intake, and comfort; maintenance of a patent drainage system; skin care around the insertion site; and periodic clamping of the catheter preparatory to removing it if it is not a permanent appliance. If the catheter is temporary, orders generally include leaving the catheter open to drainage for 48 to 72 hours, then clamping the catheter for 3- to 4-hour periods during the day until the client can void satisfactory amounts. Satisfactory voiding is determined by measuring the client's residual urine after voiding.

Care of the catheter insertion site involves sterile technique. Dressings around the newly placed suprapubic catheter are changed whenever they are soiled with

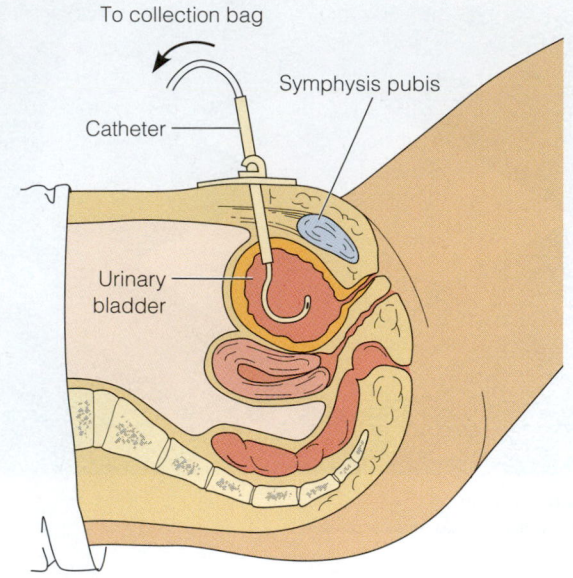

Figure 33–7 ⬤ A suprapubic catheter in place.

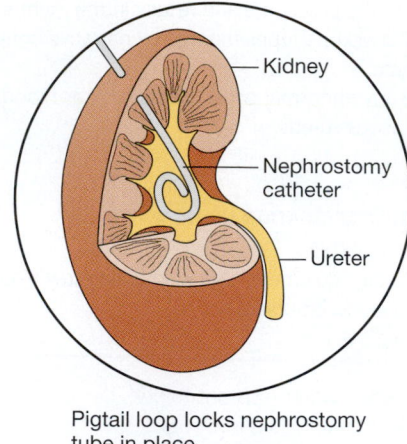

Pigtail loop locks nephrostomy
tube in place

Figure 33–8 ⬤ A nephrostomy.

drainage to prevent bacterial growth around the insertion site and reduce the potential for infection. A small amount of povidone-iodine ointment is frequently applied around the insertion site and the site covered with gauze dressings. For catheters that have been in place for an extended period, no dressing may be needed and the healed insertion tract enables removal and replacement of the catheter as needed. Securing the catheter tube to the abdomen helps to reduce tension at the insertion site. The nurse assesses the insertion area at regular intervals. If abdominal hair invades the insertion site, it may be carefully shaved. Any redness or discharge at the skin around the insertion site must be reported.

Urinary Diversions

A urinary diversion is the surgical rerouting of urine from the kidneys to a site other than the bladder. There are two categories of diversions: incontinent and continent.

INCONTINENT With incontinent diversions clients have no control over the passage of urine and require the use of an external ostomy appliance to contain the urine. Urinary diversions may or may not involve the removal of the bladder (cystectomy). Examples of incontinent diversions include ureterostomy, nephrostomy, vesicostomy, and ileal conduits. A **ureterostomy** is when one or both of the ureters may be brought directly to the side of the abdomen to form small stomas. This procedure, however, has some disadvantages in that the stomas provide direct access for microorganisms from the skin to the kidneys, the small stomas are difficult to fit with an appliance to collect the urine, and they may narrow, impairing

urine drainage. A **nephrostomy** diverts urine from the kidney to a stoma (Figure 33–8). A **vesicostomy** may be formed when the bladder is left intact but voiding through the urethra is not possible (e.g., due to an obstruction or a neurogenic bladder). The ureters remain connected to the bladder, and the bladder wall is surgically attached to an opening in the skin below the navel forming an incontinent stoma.

The most common urinary diversion is the **ileal conduit** or ileal loop (Figure 33–9). In this procedure, a segment of the ileum is removed and the intestinal ends are reattached. One end of the portion removed is closed with sutures to create a pouch, and the other end is brought out through the abdominal wall to create a stoma. The ureters are implanted into the ileal pouch. The ileal stoma is more readily fitted with an appliance than ureterostomies because of its larger size. The mucous membrane lining of the ileum also provides some protection from ascending infection. Urine drains continuously from the ileal pouch.

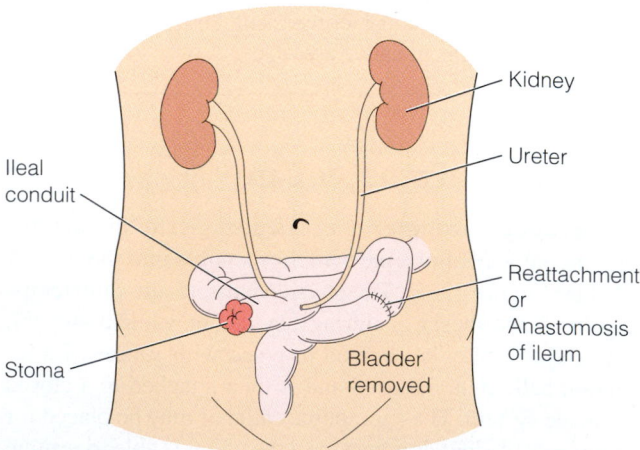

Figure 33–9 ⬤ An incontinent urinary diversion (ileal conduit).

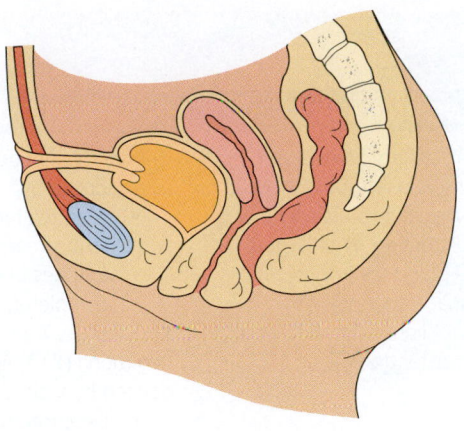

Figure 33–10 ● The Kock pouch—a continent urinary diversion.

CONTINENT With continent diversions, a continence mechanism is created giving clients control over the passage of urine, either by intermittent catheterization of the internal reservoir (e.g., Kock pouch) or by strained voiding (neobladder).

The Kock (pronounced "coke") pouch, or continent ileal bladder conduit, also uses a portion of the ileum to form a reservoir for urine (Figure 33–10). In this procedure, nipple valves are formed by doubling the tissue backward into the reservoir where the pouch connects to the skin and the ureters connect to the pouch. These valves close as the pouch fills with urine, preventing leakage and reflux of urine back toward the kidneys. The client empties the pouch by inserting a clean catheter approximately every 4 hours. Between catheterizations, a small dressing is worn to protect the stoma and clothing.

As opposed to the vesicostomy, a neobladder replaces a diseased or damaged bladder with a piece of ileum, thus making a new bladder. This new bladder is then sutured to the functional urethra. Clients with these can control voiding.

When caring for clients with a urinary diversion, the nurse must accurately assess intake and output; note any changes in urine color, odor, or clarity (mucous shreds are commonly seen in the urine of clients with an ileal diversion); and frequently assess the condition of the stoma and surrounding skin. Clients who must wear a urine collection appliance are at risk for impaired skin integrity because of irritation by urine. Well-fitting appliances are vital. The nurse should consult with the wound ostomy continence nurse (WOCN) to identify strategies for management of stoma and peristomal problems and the most appropriate appliance for the client's needs. The steps of changing a urostomy appliance are similar to those described in the procedure for changing a bowel diversion appliance (see Chapter 34 ∞). However, there are some differences, including the following: Incontinent urinary diversions drain continually. As a result the stoma must be

wicked throughout the measurement and change of the ostomy appliance. This prevents the peristomal skin from becoming wet with urine during the appliance change. Immediately following surgery, ureteral stents may be present and protruding from the stoma. They remain in place for 10 to 14 days postop and are removed by either, the surgeon or the WOCN, depending on institutional protocol. Ureteral stents are used to maintain the patency of ureters at the anastomotic sites.

Clients with urinary diversions may experience problems with their body image and sexuality and may require assistance in coping with these changes and managing the stoma. Most clients are able to resume their normal activities and lifestyle.

EVALUATING

Using the overall goals and desired outcomes identified in the planning stage, the nurse collects data to evaluate the effectiveness of nursing activities. Examples of desired outcomes for the identified goals are listed in the Identifying Nursing Diagnoses, Interventions, and Outcomes box earlier in this chapter.

If the desired outcomes are not achieved, explore the reasons before modifying the care plan. For example, if the outcome "Remains dry between voidings and at night" is not met, examples of questions that need to be considered include:

- What is the client's perception of the problem?
- Does the client understand and comply with the health care instructions provided?
- Is access to toilet facilities a problem?
- Can the client manipulate clothing for toileting? Are there adjustments that can be made to allow easier disrobing?
- Are scheduled toileting times appropriate?
- Is there adequate transition lighting for nighttime toileting?
- Are mobility aids such as a walker, elevated toilet seat, or grab bar needed? If currently used, are they appropriate or adequate?
- Is the client performing pelvic floor muscle exercises appropriately as scheduled?
- Is the client's fluid intake adequate? Does the timing of fluid intake need to be adjusted (e.g., restricted after dinner)?
- Is the client restricting caffeine, citrus juice, carbonated beverages, and artificial sweetener intake?
- Is the client taking a diuretic? If so, when is the medication taken? Do the times need to be adjusted (e.g., taking second dose no later than 4 PM)?
- Should continence aids such as a condom catheter or absorbent pads be considered or used?

Nursing Care Plan   Urinary Elimination

ASSESSMENT DATA	NURSING DIAGNOSIS	DESIRED OUTCOMES*
Nursing Assessment Mr. John Baker is a 68-year-old shopkeeper who was admitted to the hospital with urinary retention, hematuria, and fever. The admitting nurse gathers the following information when taking a nursing history. Mr. Baker states he has noticed urinary frequency during the day for the past 2 weeks, and that he doesn't feel he has emptied his bladder after urinating. He also has to get up two or three times during the night to urinate. During the past few days, he has had difficulty starting urination and dribbles afterward. He verbalizes the embarrassment his urinary problems cause in his dealings with the public. Mr. Baker is concerned about the cause of this urinary problem. He is diagnosed with benign prostatic hypertrophy (BPH) and referred to a urologist who suggests a transurethral resection of the prostate (TURP) in several months. He is placed on antibiotic therapy.	*Impaired Urinary Elimination* (retention and overflow incontinence) related to bladder neck obstruction by enlarged prostate gland (as evidenced by dysuria, frequency, nocturia, dribbling, hesitancy, and bladder distention)	Urinary Continence [0502] as evidenced by: • Able to start and stop stream • Empties bladder completely Knowledge: Treatment Regimen [1813] as evidenced by substantial: • Description of self-care responsibilities for ongoing care • Description of self-monitoring techniques
Physical Examination Height: 185.4 cm (6'2") Weight: 85.7 kg (189 lb) Temperature: 38.1°C (100.6°F) Pulse: 88 BPM Respirations: 20/minute Blood pressure: 146/86 mm Hg Catheterization for urinary retention yielded 300 mL amber urine, Foley left in place for 2 days **Diagnostic Data** CBC normal; urinalysis: amber, clear, pH 6.5, specific gravity 1.025, negative for glucose, protein, ketone, RBCs, and bacteria; IVP: evidence of enlarged prostate gland		

NURSING INTERVENTIONS*/SELECTED ACTIVITIES	RATIONALE
Urinary Incontinence Care [0610]	
Monitor urinary elimination, including consistency, odor, volume, and color.	*These parameters help determine adequacy of urinary tract function.*
Help the client select appropriate incontinence garment or pad for short-term management while more definitive treatment is designed.	*Appropriate undergarments can help diminish the embarrassing aspects of urinary incontinence.*
Instruct Mr. Baker to limit fluids for 2 to 3 hours before bedtime.	*Decreased fluid intake several hours before bedtime will decrease the incidence of urinary retention and overflow incontinence, and promote rest.*
Instruct him to drink a minimum of 1,500 mL (six 8-ounce glasses) fluids per day.	*Increased fluids during the day will increase urinary output and discourage bacterial growth.*
Limit ingestion of bladder irritants (e.g., colas, coffee, tea, and chocolate).	*Alcohol, coffee, and tea have a natural diuretic effect and are bladder irritants.*
Urinary Retention Care [0620]	
Instruct Mr. Baker or a family member to record urinary output.	*Serves as an indicator of urinary tract and renal function and of fluid balance.*
Catheterize for residual urine, as appropriate.	*An enlarged prostate compresses the urethra so that urine is retained. Checking for residual urine provides information about bladder emptying.*
Implement intermittent catheterization, as appropriate.	*Helps maintain tonicity of the bladder muscle by preventing overdistention and providing for complete emptying.*

NURSING INTERVENTIONS*/SELECTED ACTIVITIES	RATIONALE
Provide enough time for bladder emptying (10 minutes).	*In addition to the effect of an enlarged prostate on the bladder, stress or anxiety can inhibit relaxation of the urinary sphincter. Sufficient time should be allowed for micturition.*
Instruct the client in ways to avoid constipation or stool impaction.	*Impacted stool may place pressure on the bladder outlet, causing urinary retention.*
Teaching: Disease Process [5602]	
Appraise Mr. Baker's current level of knowledge about benign prostatic hypertrophy.	*Assessing the client's knowledge will provide a foundation for building a teaching plan based on his present understanding of his condition.*
Explain the pathophysiology of the disease and how it relates to urinary anatomy and function.	*In this case, urinary retention and overflow incontinence are caused by obstruction of the bladder neck by an enlarged prostate gland.*
Describe the rationale behind management, therapy, and treatment recommendations.	*Adequate information about treatment options is important to diminish anxiety, promote compliance, and enhance decision making.*
Instruct Mr. Baker on which signs and symptoms to report to the health care provider (e.g., burning on urination, hematuria, oliguria).	*In the individual with prostatic hypertrophy, urinary retention and an overdistended bladder reduce blood flow to the bladder wall, making it more susceptible to infection from bacterial growth. Monitoring for these manifestations of urinary tract infection is essential to prevent urosepsis.*

EVALUATION

Outcomes partially met. Following removal of the Foley catheter, Mr. Baker reported continued difficulty initiating a urinary stream but experienced less dribbling and nocturia. He and his wife selected an undergarment that was acceptable to Mr. Baker and he reports that he feels more confident. Intermittent catheterization not indicated. Intake is approximately 200 mL in excess of output. He is able to discuss the correlation between his enlarged prostate and urinary difficulties. A transurethral resection of the prostate is scheduled in 2 weeks.

*The NOC # for desired outcomes and the NIC # for nursing interventions are listed in brackets following the appropriate outcome or intervention. Outcomes, interventions, and activities selected are only a sample of those suggested by NOC and NIC and should be further individualized for each client.

CRITICAL THINKING QUESTIONS

1. Considering Mr. Baker's history and assessment data, what other physical conditions could explain his symptoms?

2. The primary care provider has recommended surgery. What assumptions will the nurse need to validate in helping prepare Mr. and Mrs. Baker for this surgery?

3. It does not appear that other alternatives have been considered. Why might this be so?

4. Incontinence can lead to client decisions to limit social interactions. What would be an appropriate response if Mr. Baker states that he will just stay home until he has his surgery?

∞ *See Answers in MyNursingKit.*

CONCEPT MAP Urinary Elimination

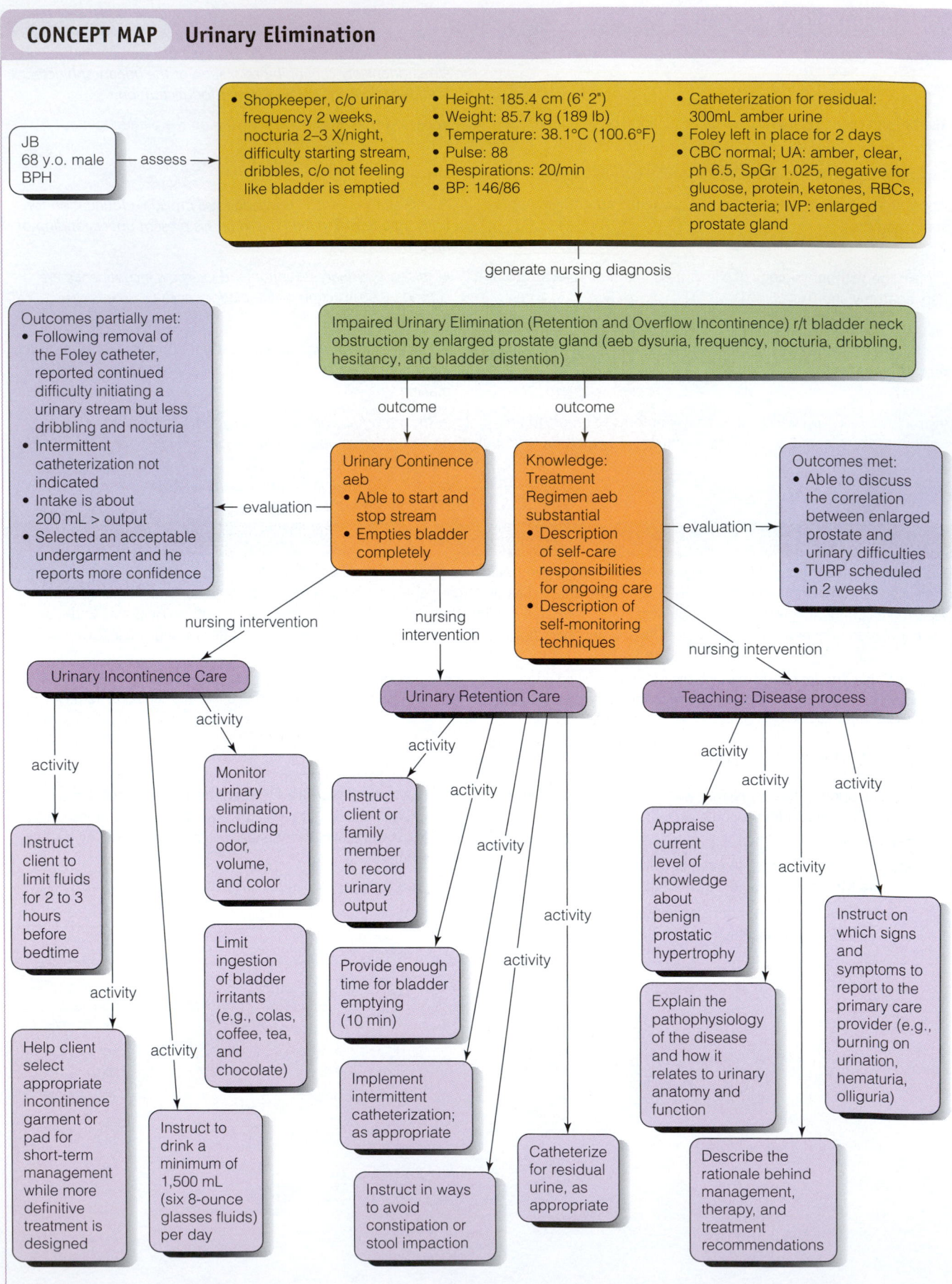

CHAPTER HIGHLIGHTS

- Urinary elimination depends on normal functioning of the urinary, cardiovascular, and nervous systems.
- Urine is formed in the nephron, the functional unit of the kidney, through a process of filtration, reabsorption, and secretion. Hormones such as antidiuretic hormone (ADH) and aldosterone affect the reabsorption of sodium and water, thus affecting the amount of urine formed.
- The normal process of urination is stimulated when sufficient urine collects in the bladder to stimulate stretch receptors. Impulses from stretch receptors are transmitted to the spinal cord and the brain, causing relaxation of the internal sphincter (unconscious control) and, if appropriate, relaxation of the external sphincter (conscious control).
- In the adult, urination generally occurs after 250 to 450 mL of urine has collected in the bladder.
- Many factors influence a person's urinary elimination, including growth and development, fluid intake, stress, activity, medications, and various diseases.
- Alterations in urine production and elimination include polyuria, oliguria, anuria, frequency, nocturia, urgency, dysuria, enuresis, hematuria, incontinence, and retention. Each may have various influencing and associated factors that need to be identified.
- Assessment of a client's urinary function includes (a) a nursing history that identifies voiding patterns, recent changes, past and current problems with urination, and factors influencing the elimination pattern; (b) a physical assessment of the genitourinary system; (c) inspection of the urine for amount, color, clarity, and odor; and, if indicated; (d) testing of urine for specific gravity, pH, and the presence of glucose, ketone bodies, protein, and occult blood.
- Many NANDA-approved nursing diagnoses may apply to clients with altered urinary elimination patterns, for example, *Functional Incontinence, Urinary Retention,* and related diagnoses such as *Risk for Infection.*
- Incontinence can be physically and emotionally distressing to clients because it is considered socially unacceptable.
- Bladder training can often reduce episodes of incontinence.

- Clients with urinary retention not only experience discomfort but also are at risk of urinary tract infection.
- The most common cause of urinary tract infection is invasive procedures such as catheterization and cystoscopic examination. Women in particular are prone to ascending urinary tract infections because of their short urethras.
- Goals for the client with problems with urinary elimination include maintaining or restoring normal elimination patterns and preventing associated risks such as skin breakdown.
- In planning for home care, the nurse considers the client's needs for teaching and assistance or assistive devices in the home.
- Nursing interventions related to urinary elimination are generally directed toward facilitating the normal functioning of the urinary system or toward assisting the client with particular problems.
- Interventions include (a) assisting the client to maintain an appropriate fluid intake, (b) assisting the client to maintain normal voiding patterns, (c) monitoring the client's daily fluid intake and output, and (d) maintaining cleanliness of the genital area.
- Urinary catheterization is frequently required for clients with urinary retention but is only performed when all other measures to facilitate voiding fail. Sterile technique is essential to prevent ascending urinary infections.
- Care of clients with indwelling catheters is directed toward preventing infection of the urinary tract and encouraging urinary flow through the drainage system.
- Clients with urinary retention may be taught to perform clean intermittent self-catheterization to enhance their independence, reduce the risk of infection, and eliminate incontinence.
- Bladder or catheter irrigations may be used to apply medication to bladder walls or maintain catheter patency.
- When the urinary bladder is removed, a urinary diversion is formed to allow urine to be eliminated from the body. The ileal conduit or ileal loop is the most common diversion and requires that the client wear a urine collection device continually over the stoma.

THINK ABOUT IT

Refer to the chapter-opening scenario and answer these questions.

1. What factors may have contributed to Lisa's development of urinary incontinence?

2. What nursing diagnoses would be appropriate for this client?

3. What strategies will you recommend to this client to help her regain bladder control?

∞ *See suggested responses to Think About It on MyNursingKit.*

TEST YOUR KNOWLEDGE

1. The nurse recognizes that urinary elimination changes may occur even in healthy older adults because:
1. The bladder distends and its capacity increases.
2. Older adults ignore the need to void.
3. Urine becomes more concentrated.
4. The amount of urine retained after voiding increases.

2. During assessment of the client with urinary incontinence, the nurse is most likely to assess which of the following? Select all that apply.
1. Perineal skin irritation
2. Fluid intake of less than 1,500 mL/day
3. History of antihistamine intake
4. History of frequent urinary tract infections
5. Childhood trauma

3. Which of the following represents the appropriate nursing management of a client wearing a condom catheter?
1. Ensure that the tip of the penis fits snugly against the end of the condom.
2. Check the penis for adequate circulation 30 minutes after applying.
3. Change the condom every 8 hours.
4. Tape the collecting tubing to the lower abdomen.

4. During the straight catheterization of a female client, if the catheter slips into the vagina, the nurse should:
1. Leave the catheter in place and get a new sterile catheter.
2. Leave the catheter in place and ask another nurse to attempt the procedure.
3. Remove the catheter and redirect it to the urinary meatus.
4. Remove the catheter, wipe it with a sterile gauze, and redirect it to the urinary meatus.

5. The nurse evaluates which of the following statements indicating a need for further teaching of the client with a long-term indwelling catheter?
1. "I will keep the collecting bag below the level of the bladder at all times."
2. "Intake of cranberry juice may help decrease the risk of infection."
3. "Soaking in a warm tub bath may ease the irritation associated with the catheter."
4. "I should use clean technique when emptying the collecting bag."

6. During shift report, the nurse learns that an older female client is unable to maintain continence after she senses the urge to void and becomes incontinent on the way to the bathroom. Which of the following nursing diagnoses is most appropriate?
1. *Stress Urinary Incontinence*
2. *Total Urinary Incontinence*
3. *Functional Urinary Incontinence*
4. *Urge Urinary Incontinence*

7. A female client has a urinary tract infection (UTI). Which of the following would be priority teaching points to include in the nurse's teaching plan? Select all that apply.
1. Limit fluids to avoid the burning sensation on urination.
2. Review symptoms of UTI with the client.
3. Wipe the perineal area from back to front.
4. Wear cotton underclothes.
5. Take baths rather than showers.

8. The nurse will need to assess the client's performance of clean intermittent self-catheterization (CISC) for a client with which of the following?
1. Ileal conduit
2. Kock pouch
3. Neobladder
4. Vesicostomy

9. Because a client has a flaccid bladder the nurse is most likely to teach which of the following?
1. Habit training: Attempt voiding at specific time periods.
2. Bladder training: Delay voiding according to a prescheduled time table.
3. Credé's maneuver: Apply gentle manual pressure to the lower abdomen.
4. Kegel exercises: Contract the pelvic muscles.

10. Which of the following behaviors does the nurse evaluate indicating that the client on a bladder training program has met the expected outcomes? Select all that apply.
1. Voids each time there is an urge.
2. Practices slow, deep breathing until the urge decreases.
3. Uses adult diapers, for "just in case."
4. Drinks citrus juices and carbonated beverages.
5. Performs pelvic muscle exercises.

∞ *See answers to Test Your Knowledge in Appendix A.*

REFERENCES AND SELECTED BIBLIOGRAPHY

Anonymous. (2004). Information from your family doctor: Urinary tract infections in adults. *American Family Physician, 69*(1), 159–160.

Ball, J. W., & Bindler, R. C. (2006). *Child health nursing.* Upper Saddle River, NJ: Prentice Hall.

Bulechek, G. M., Butcher, H. K., & Dochterman, J. M. (Eds.). (2008). *Nursing interventions: classification (NIC)* (5th ed.). St. Louis, MO: Mosby.

Cavagnaro, S. M. F. (2005). Infeccion urinaria en la infancia [Urinary infection in infancy]. *Revista Chilena de Infectologia, 22*(2), 161–168.

Colwell, C. C., Goldberg, M. T., & Carmel, J. E. (2004). *Fecal & urinary diversions: Management principles.* St. Louis: Mosby.

D'Amico, D., & Barbarito, C. (2007). *Health & physical assessment in nursing.* Upper Saddle River, NJ: Pearson Education.

Davis, K. (2004). Need urine from a catheter system? Forget the needle! *Nursing, 34*(12), 64.

Dulczak, S., & Kirk, J. (2005). Overview of the evaluation, diagnosis, and management of urinary tract infections in infants and children. *Urologic Nursing, 25*(3), 185–192.

Gray, M. (2004). Clinical practice: Stress urinary incontinence in women. *Journal of the American Academy of Nurse Practitioners, 16*(5), 188–197.

Hathaway, L. (2004). How to insert an indwelling catheter. *Nursing Made Incredibly Easy, 2*(2), 43–45.

Midthun, S. J. (2004). Criteria for urinary tract infection in the elderly: Variables that challenge nursing assessment. *Urologic Nursing, 24*(3), 157–186.

Moorhead, S., Johnson, M., Maas, M. L., & Swanson, E. (Eds.). (2008). *Nursing outcomes classification (NOC)* (4th ed.). St. Louis, MO: Mosby.

Morantz, C. A. (2005). ACOG guidelines on urinary incontinence in women. *American Family Physician, 72*(1), 175–178.

NANDA International. (2009). NANDA nursing diagnoses: Definitions and classification 2009–2011. West Sussex, U.K.: Wiley-Blackwell.

Nield, L. S., & Kamat, D. (2004). Enuresis: How to evaluate and treat. *Clinical Pediatrics, 43*(5), 409–415.

Nix, D., & Ermer-Seltun, J. (2004). A review of perineal skin care protocols and skin barrier product use. *OstomyWound Management, 50*(12), 59–67.

Palmer, M. H., & Newman, D. K. (2004). Urinary incontinence in nursing homes: Two studies show the inadequacy of care. *American Journal of Nursing, 104*(11), 57–59.

Palmer, M. H., & Newman, D. K. (2006). Bladder control: Educational needs of older adults. *Journal of Gerontological Nursing, 32*(1), 28–32.

Pomfret, I., & Tew, L. E. (2004). Urinary catheters and associated UTI's. *Journal of Community Nursing, 18*(9), 15–20.

Pullen, R. L. (2004). Inserting an indwelling urinary catheter in a male patient. *Nursing, 34*(7), 24.

Robinson, J. (2005). Clinical skills: How to remove and change a suprapubic catheter. *British Journal of Nursing, 14*(1), 30–35.

Robson, W. L. M., Leung, A. K. C., & Van Howe, R. (2005). Primary and secondary nocturnal enuresis: Similarities in presentation. *Pediatrics, 115*, 956–959.

Rushing, J. (2004). Inserting an indwelling urinary catheter in a female patient. *Nursing, 34*(8), 22.

Shei Dei Yang, S., & Cheng Wang, C. (2005). Outpatient biofeedback relaxation of the pelvic floor in treating pediatric dysfunctional voiding: A short-course program is effective. *Urologia Internationalis, 74*(2), 118–122.

Sparks, A., Boyer, D., Gambrel, A., Lovet, M., Johnson, J., Richards, T., et al. (2004). The clinical benefits of the bladder scanner: A research synthesis. *Journal of Nursing Care Quality, 19*(3), 188–192.

Toughill, E. (2005). Indwelling urinary catheters. Common mechanical and pathogenic problems. *American Journal of Nursing, 105*(5), 35–37.

Woods, A. (2005). Managing UTIs in older adults. *Nursing, 35*(3), 12.

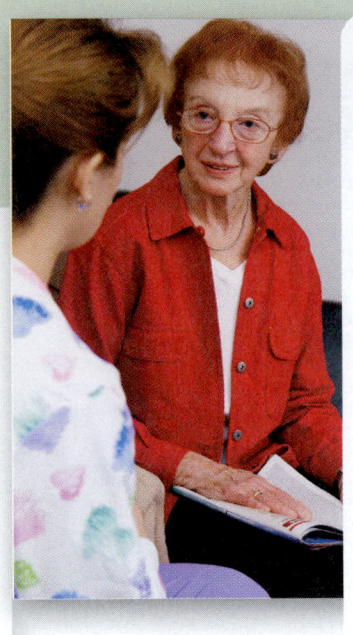

Claudette Pinnette is an 84-year-old client who presents to her primary care provider for a routine follow-up related to her chronic health problems. Ms. Pinnette has a 10-year history of congestive heart failure with hypertension and chronic renal failure. She takes several medications daily, including diuretics, and has been restricting fluids to 600 mL per day per doctor's orders. As you collect her admission data, she tells you she has been having problems with recurrent constipation and has been self-treating with over-the-counter laxatives and, when it becomes severe, oil-based cleansing enemas. She says she rarely has a bowel movement unless she uses one of these treatments and doesn't feel like she ever completely "cleans out," usually feeling the need to pass more stool. When questioned, she reports that she used to pass stool every morning within a few hours of waking but hasn't had a bowel movement for the past two days. She reports feeling uncomfortable and, on assessment, has a distended abdomen that is tender to touch.

LEARNING OUTCOMES

After completing this chapter, you will be able to:

1. Describe factors that influence fecal elimination and patterns of defecation.

2. Distinguish normal from abnormal characteristics and constituents of feces.

3. Differentiate among different types of fecal elimination problems.

4. Apply the nursing process to meeting clients' fecal elimination needs.

5. Explain nursing strategies to assist clients in maintaining normal fecal elimination patterns.

6. Differentiate the purposes and actions of commonly used enema solutions.

7. Describe essential nursing strategies for providing stoma care for clients with an ostomy.

KEY TERMS

Bowel incontinence p1028
Carminatives p1034
Cathartics p1034
Colostomy p1028
Constipation p1026
Defecation p1023

Diarrhea p1027
Enema p1034
Fecal impaction p1026
Feces p1023
Flatulence p1028
Flatus p1023

Gastrocolic reflex p1024
Gastrostomy p1028
Hemorrhoids p1023
Ileostomy p1028
Jejunostomy p1028
Laxatives p1025

Mass peristalsis p1031
Meconium p1024
Ostomy p1028
Peristalsis p1025
Stoma p1028
Suppositories p1034

Nurses are frequently consulted or involved in assisting clients with elimination problems. These problems can be embarrassing to clients and can cause considerable discomfort. Elimination of the waste products of digestion from the body is essential to health. The excreted waste products are referred to as **feces** or stool.

PHYSIOLOGY OF DEFECATION

The large intestine extends from the ileocecal valve, which lies between the small and large intestines, to the anus. The colon has seven parts: the cecum; ascending, transverse, and descending colons; sigmoid colon; rectum; and anus. The large intestine is a muscular tube lined with mucous membrane. The muscle fibers are both circular and longitudinal, permitting the intestine to enlarge and contract in both width and length.

The colon's main functions are the absorption of water and nutrients, the mucoid protection of the intestinal wall, and fecal elimination. The contents of the colon normally represent foods ingested over the previous 4 days, although most of the waste products are excreted within 48 hours of ingestion (the act of taking food). The ileocecal valve, located at the junction of the ileum of the small intestine and the first part of the large intestine, regulates the flow of chyme into the large intestine and prevents backflow into the ileum. As much as 1,500 mL of chyme passes into the large intestine daily, and all but about 100 mL is reabsorbed in the proximal half of the colon. The 100 mL of fluid is excreted in the feces.

The rectum contains folds that extend vertically and each fold contains a vein and an artery. It is believed that these folds help retain feces within the rectum. When the veins become distended, as can occur with repeated pressure, a condition known as **hemorrhoids** occurs (Figure 34–1).

The anal canal is bounded by an internal and an external sphincter muscle. The internal sphincter is under involuntary control, and the external sphincter normally is voluntarily controlled. The internal sphincter muscle is innervated by the autonomic nervous system; the external sphincter is innervated by the somatic nervous system.

Defecation is the expulsion of feces from the anus and rectum. It is also called a bowel movement. The frequency of defecation is highly individual, varying from several times per day to two or three times per week. The amount defecated also varies from person to person. When peristaltic waves move the feces into the sigmoid colon and the rectum, the sensory nerves in the rectum are stimulated and the individual becomes aware of the need to defecate.

CLINICAL ALERT

Individuals (especially children) may use very different terms for a bowel movement. The nurse may need to try several different common words before finding one the client understands.

If the defecation reflex is ignored, or if defecation is consciously inhibited by contracting the external sphincter muscle, the urge to defecate normally disappears for a few hours before occurring again. Repeated inhibition of the urge to defecate can result in expansion of the rectum to accommodate accumulated feces and eventual loss of sensitivity to the need to defecate. Constipation can be the ultimate result.

Normal feces are composed of about 75% water and 25% solid materials. They are soft but formed. If the feces are propelled very quickly along the large intestine, there is insufficient time for most of the water in the chyme to be reabsorbed and the feces will be more fluid, containing perhaps 95% water. Normal feces require a normal fluid intake; feces that contain less water may be hard and difficult to expel.

Feces are normally brown, chiefly due to the presence of stercobilin and urobilin, which are derived from bilirubin (a red pigment in bile). Another factor that affects fecal color is the action of bacteria such as *Escherichia coli* or staphylococci, which are normally present in the large intestine. The action of microorganisms on the chyme is also responsible for the odor of feces. Table 34–1 lists the characteristics of normal and abnormal feces.

An adult usually forms 7 to 10 L of **flatus** (gas) in the large intestine every 24 hours. The gases include carbon dioxide, methane, hydrogen, oxygen, and nitrogen. Some are swallowed with food and fluids taken by mouth, others are formed through the action of bacteria on the chyme in the large intestine, and other gas diffuses from the blood into the gastrointestinal tract.

FACTORS THAT AFFECT DEFECATION

Defecation patterns vary at different stages of life. Circumstances of diet, fluid intake and output, activity, psychologic factors, lifestyle, medications and medical procedures, and disease also affect defecation.

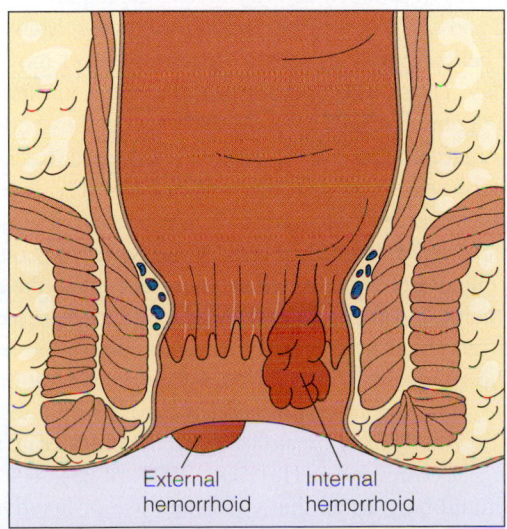

External hemorrhoid Internal hemorrhoid

Figure 34–1 ⬤ Internal and external hemorrhoids.

TABLE 34–1 Characteristics of Normal and Abnormal Feces

CHARACTERISTIC	NORMAL	ABNORMAL	POSSIBLE CAUSE
Color	Adult: brown	Clay or white	Absence of bile pigment (bile obstruction); diagnostic study using barium
	Infant: yellow	Black or tarry	Drug (e.g., iron); bleeding from upper gastrointestinal tract (e.g., stomach, small intestine); diet high in red meat and dark green vegetables (e.g., spinach)
		Red	Bleeding from lower gastrointestinal tract (e.g., rectum); some foods (e.g., beets)
		Pale	Malabsorption of fats; diet high in milk and milk products and low in meat
Consistency	Formed, soft, semisolid, moist	Orange or green	Intestinal infection
		Hard, dry	Dehydration; decreased intestinal motility resulting from lack of fiber in diet, lack of exercise, emotional upset, laxative abuse
		Diarrhea	Increased intestinal motility (e.g., due to irritation of the colon by bacteria)
Shape	Cylindrical (contour of rectum) about 2.5 cm (1 in.) in diameter in adults	Narrow, pencil-shaped, or stringlike stool	Obstructive condition of the rectum
Amount	Varies with diet (about 100–400 g per day)		
Odor	Aromatic: affected by ingested food and person's own bacterial flora	Pungent	Infection, blood
Constituents	Small amounts of undigested roughage, sloughed dead bacteria and epithelial cells, fat, protein, dried constituents of digestive juices (e.g., bile pigments, inorganic matter)	Pus	Bacterial infection
		Mucus	Inflammatory condition
		Parasites	Gastrointestinal bleeding
		Blood	Malabsorption
		Large quantities of fat	Accidental ingestion
		Foreign objects	

Development

Newborns and infants, toddlers, children, and older adults are groups within which members have similarities in elimination patterns.

Meconium is the first fecal material passed by the newborn, normally up to 24 hours after birth. It is black, tarry, odorless, and sticky. Transitional stools, which follow for about a week, are generally greenish yellow; they contain mucus and are loose. Infants pass stool frequently, often after each feeding. Because the intestine is immature, water is not well absorbed and the stool is soft, liquid, and frequent. When the intestine matures, bacterial flora increase. After solid foods are introduced, the stool becomes less frequent and firmer. Infants who are breast-fed have light yellow to golden feces, and infants who are taking formula will have dark yellow or tan stool that is more formed. Some control of defecation starts at 1 1/2 to 2 years of age. Daytime control is typically attained by age 2 1/2, after a process of toilet training. School-age children and adolescents have bowel habits similar to those of adults. Patterns of defecation vary in frequency, quantity, and consistency.

Constipation is the most common bowel-management problem in the older adult population (Mauk, 2005). This is due, in part, to reduced activity levels, inadequate amounts of fluid and fiber intake, and muscle weakness. Many older people believe that "regularity" means a bowel movement every day. Those who do not meet this criterion often seek over-the-counter preparations to relieve what they believe to be constipation. Older adults should be advised that normal patterns of bowel elimination vary considerably. Adequate roughage in the diet, adequate exercise, and 6 to 8 glasses of fluid daily are essential preventive measures for constipation. A cup of hot water or tea at a regular time in the morning is helpful for some. Responding to the **gastrocolic reflex** (increased peristalsis of the colon after food has entered the stomach) is also an important consideration. For example, toileting is recommended 5 to 15 minutes after meals, especially after breakfast when the gastrocolic reflex is strongest (Hinrichs & Huseboe, 2001, p. 23). The older adult should be warned that consistent use of laxatives inhibits natural defecation reflexes and is thought to cause rather than cure constipation.

The nurse should evaluate any complaints of constipation carefully for each individual. A change in bowel habits over several weeks with or without weight loss, pain, or fever should be referred to a primary care provider for a complete medical evaluation. See Clinical Manifestations.

Diet

Sufficient bulk (cellulose, fiber) in the diet is necessary to provide fecal volume. Bland diets and low-fiber diets are lacking in bulk and therefore create insufficient residue of waste products to stimulate the reflex for defecation. Low-residue foods move more slowly through the intestinal tract. Increasing fluid intake with such foods increases their rate of movement.

Certain foods are difficult or impossible for some people to digest. This inability results in digestive upsets and, in some instances, the passage of watery stools. Irregular eating can also impair regular defecation. Individuals who eat at the same times every day usually have a regularly timed, physiologic response to the food intake and a regular pattern of peristaltic activity in the colon.

Spicy foods can produce diarrhea and flatus in some individuals. Excessive sugar can also cause diarrhea. Other foods that may influence bowel elimination include the following:

- Gas-producing foods, such as cabbage, onions, cauliflower, bananas, and apples
- Laxative-producing foods, such as bran, prunes, figs, chocolate, and alcohol
- Constipation-producing foods, such as cheese, pasta, eggs, and lean meat

Even when fluid intake is inadequate or output is excessive for some reason, the body continues to reabsorb fluid from the chyme as it passes along the colon. The chyme becomes drier than normal, resulting in hard feces. In addition, reduced fluid intake slows the chyme's passage along the intestines, further increasing the reabsorption of fluid from the chyme. Healthy fecal elimination usually requires a daily fluid intake of 2,000 to 3,000 mL.

Activity

Activity stimulates **peristalsis**, thus facilitating the movement of chyme along the colon. Weak abdominal and pelvic muscles are often ineffective in increasing the intra-abdominal pressure during defecation or in controlling defecation. Weak muscles can result from lack of exercise, immobility, or impaired neurologic functioning. Clients confined to bed are often constipated.

Psychologic Factors

Some people who are anxious or angry experience increased peristaltic activity and subsequent nausea or diarrhea. In contrast, people who are depressed may experience slowed intestinal motility, resulting in constipation. How a person responds to these emotional states is the result of individual differences in the response of the enteric nervous system to vagal stimulation from the brain.

Defecation Habits

Early bowel training may establish the habit of defecating at a regular time. Many people defecate after breakfast, when the gastrocolic reflex causes mass peristaltic waves in the large intestine. If a person ignores this urge to defecate, water continues to be reabsorbed, making the feces hard and difficult to expel. When the normal defecation reflexes are inhibited or ignored, these conditioned reflexes tend to be progressively weakened. When habitually ignored, the urge to defecate is ultimately lost. Adults may ignore these reflexes because of the pressures of time or work. Hospitalized clients may suppress the urge because of embarrassment about using a bedpan, because of lack of privacy, or because defecation is too uncomfortable.

Medications

Some drugs have side effects that can interfere with normal elimination such as narcotics. Some medications directly affect elimination. **Laxatives** are medications that stimulate bowel activity and so assist fecal elimination. Other medications soften stool, facilitating defecation. Certain medications suppress peristaltic activity and may be used to treat diarrhea. Medications also affect the appearance of the feces.

Diagnostic Procedures

Before certain diagnostic procedures, such as visualization of the colon, the client is restricted from ingesting food or fluid. The client may also be given a cleansing enema or laxatives prior to the examination. In these instances normal defecation usually will not occur until eating resumes.

CLINICAL MANIFESTATIONS **Colorectal Cancer**

Inform clients to see their primary care provider if they have any of the following:

- A change in bowel habits such as diarrhea, constipation, or narrowing of the stool that lasts for more than a few days
- A feeling of needing to have a bowel movement that is not relieved by doing so
- Rectal bleeding or blood in the stool (often, though, the stool will look normal)
- Cramping or steady abdominal pain
- Weakness and fatigue

Note: Reprinted by permission of the American Cancer Society, Inc. from www.cancer.org. All rights reserved.

Anesthesia and Surgery

General anesthetics cause the normal colonic movements to cease or slow by blocking parasympathetic stimulation to the muscles of the colon. Clients who have regional or spinal anesthesia are less likely to experience this problem. Surgery that involves direct handling of the intestines can cause temporary cessation of intestinal movement. This condition, called ileus, usually lasts 24 to 48 hours. Listening for bowel sounds that reflect intestinal motility is an important nursing assessment following surgery.

Pathologic Conditions

Spinal cord injuries and head injuries can decrease the sensory stimulation for defecation. Impaired mobility may limit the client's ability to respond to the urge to defecate and the client may experience constipation. Or, a client may experience fecal incontinence because of poorly functioning anal sphincters.

Pain

Clients who experience discomfort when defecating often suppress the urge to defecate to avoid the pain. Such clients can experience constipation as a result.

FECAL ELIMINATION PROBLEMS

Four common problems are related to fecal elimination: constipation, diarrhea, bowel incontinence, and flatulence.

Constipation

Constipation may be defined as fewer than three bowel movements per week. This infers the passage of dry, hard stool or the passage of no stool. It occurs when the movement of feces through the large intestine is slow, thus allowing time for additional reabsorption of fluid from the large intestine. Associated with constipation are difficult evacuations of stool and increased effort or straining of the voluntary muscles of defecation. The person may also have a feeling of incomplete stool evacuation after defecation. However, it is important to define constipation in relation to the person's regular elimination pattern. Some people normally defecate only a few times a week; other people defecate more than once a day. Careful assessment of the person's habits is necessary before a diagnosis of constipation is made. Box 34–1 lists the frequent defining characteristics of constipation.

Many causes and factors contribute to constipation. Among them are the following:

- Insufficient fiber intake
- Insufficient fluid intake
- Insufficient activity or immobility
- Irregular defecation habits
- Change in daily routine

BOX 34–1	**Sample Defining Characteristics for Constipation**

- Decreased frequency of defecation
- Hard, dry, formed stools
- Straining at stool; painful defecation
- Reports of rectal fullness or pressure or incomplete bowel evacuation
- Abdominal pain, cramps, or distention
- Anorexia, nausea
- Headache

- Lack of privacy
- Chronic use of laxatives or enemas
- Irritable bowel syndrome (IBS)
- Pelvic floor dysfunction or muscle damage
- Poor motility or slow transit
- Neurological conditions (e.g., Parkinson's disease), stroke, or paralysis
- Emotional disturbances such as depression or mental confusion
- Medications such as opioids, iron supplements, antihistamines, antacids, and antidepressants

Constipation can cause health problems for some clients. In children it is often associated with urinary tract infections. Straining associated with constipation often is accompanied by holding the breath. This Valsalva maneuver can present serious problems to people with heart disease, brain injuries, or respiratory disease. Holding the breath, while bearing down, increases intrathoracic pressure and vagal tone, slowing the pulse rate (Lemone & Burke, 2007).

FECAL IMPACTION **Fecal impaction** is a mass or collection of hardened feces in the folds of the rectum. Impaction results from prolonged retention and accumulation of fecal material. In severe impactions the feces accumulate and extend well up into the sigmoid colon and beyond. Fecal impaction can be recognized by the passage of liquid fecal seepage (diarrhea) and no normal stool. The liquid portion of the feces seeps out around the impacted mass. Impaction can also be assessed by digital examination of the rectum, during which the hardened mass can often be palpated.

Along with fecal seepage and constipation, symptoms include frequent but nonproductive desire to defecate and rectal pain. A generalized feeling of illness results; the client becomes anorexic, the abdomen becomes distended, and nausea and vomiting may occur.

The causes of fecal impaction are usually poor defecation habits and constipation. The barium used in radiologic examinations of the upper and lower gastrointestinal tracts can also be a causative factor. Therefore, after these examinations, laxatives or enemas are usually taken to ensure removal of the barium.

Digital examination of the impaction through the rectum should be done gently and carefully. Although digital rectal examination is within the scope of nursing practice,

DRUG CAPSULE	**Emollient or Surfactant** *docusate calcium (Surfak)*
	docusate sodium (Colace)

The Client with Drugs for Treating the Lower Gastrointestinal Tract

Docusates lower the surface tension of fecal material, which allows water and lipids to penetrate the stool resulting in softer fecal mass. They do not stimulate peristalsis.

Docusates are commonly used for prevention of constipation and to decrease the strain of defecation in individuals who should avoid straining during bowel movements (e.g., cardiac disease [prevent Valsalva maneuver], eye surgery, rectal surgery).

Nursing Responsibilities

- Assess client for abdominal distention, bowel sounds, and usual bowel movement frequency.
- Evaluate effectiveness of medication.

Client and Family Teaching

- Advise client to drink a glass of fluid (e.g., water, juice, milk) with each dose.

- Explain that it may take 1 to 3 days to soften fecal material.
- Advise client not to take docusate within 2 hours of other laxatives, especially mineral oil, as it may cause increased absorption of the mineral oil.
- Discuss other forms of bowel regulation (e.g., increasing fiber intake, fluid intake, and activity).

Note: Prior to administering any medication, review all aspects with a current drug handbook or other reliable source.

---

some agency policies require a primary care provider's order for digital manipulation and removal of a fecal impaction.

Although fecal impaction can generally be prevented, treatment of impacted feces is sometimes necessary. When fecal impaction is suspected, the client is often given an oil retention enema, a cleansing enema 2 to 4 hours later, and daily additional cleansing enemas, suppositories, or stool softeners. If these measures fail, manual removal is often necessary.

Diarrhea

Diarrhea refers to the passage of liquid feces and an increased frequency of defecation. It is the opposite of constipation and results from rapid movement of fecal contents through the large intestine. Rapid passage of chyme reduces the time available for the large intestine to reabsorb water and electrolytes. Some people pass stool with increased frequency, but diarrhea is not present unless the stool is relatively unformed and excessively liquid. The person with

diarrhea finds it difficult or impossible to control the urge to defecate for very long. Diarrhea and the threat of incontinence are sources of concern and embarrassment. Often, spasmodic cramps are associated with diarrhea. Bowel sounds are increased. With persistent diarrhea, irritation of the anal region extending to the perineum and buttocks generally results. Fatigue, weakness, malaise, and emaciation are the results of prolonged diarrhea.

When the cause of diarrhea is irritants in the intestinal tract, diarrhea is thought to be a protective flushing mechanism. It can create serious fluid and electrolyte losses in the body, however, that can develop within frighteningly short periods of time, particularly in infants, small children, and older adults. Table 34–2 lists some of the major causes of diarrhea and the physiologic responses of the body.

The irritating effects of diarrhea stool increase the risk for skin breakdown. Therefore, the area around the anal region should be kept clean and dry and be protected with zinc oxide or other ointment. In addition, a fecal collector can be used (see page 1038).

MyNursingKit Diarrhea

TABLE 34–2   **Major Causes of Diarrhea**

CAUSE	PHYSIOLOGIC EFFECT
Psychologic stress (e.g., anxiety)	Increased intestinal motility and mucus secretion
Medications	Inflammation and infection of mucosa due to overgrowth of pathogenic intestinal microorganisms
Antibiotics	Irritation of intestinal mucosa
Iron	Irritation of intestinal mucosa
Cathartics	Incomplete digestion of food or fluid
Allergy to food, fluid, drugs	Increased intestinal motility and mucus secretion
Intolerance of food or fluid	Reduced absorption of fluids
Diseases of the colon (e.g., malabsorption syndrome, Crohn's disease)	Inflammation of the mucosa often leading to ulcer formation

Bowel Incontinence

Bowel incontinence, also called fecal incontinence, refers to the loss of voluntary ability to control fecal and gaseous discharges through the anal sphincter. The incontinence may occur at specific times, such as after meals, or it may occur irregularly. Two types of bowel incontinence are described: partial and major. Partial incontinence is the inability to control flatus or to prevent minor soiling. Major incontinence is the inability to control feces of normal consistency.

Fecal incontinence is generally associated with impaired functioning of the anal sphincter or its nerve supply, such as in some neuromuscular diseases, spinal cord trauma, and tumors of the external anal sphincter muscle.

The rate of fecal incontinence among older adults living in the community has been reported to be 4% to 17% compared to 2% in the general community population and 20% to 54% in older adult nursing home residents (Bliss, Fischer, & Savik, 2005, p. 36). Fecal incontinence is an emotionally distressing problem that can ultimately lead to social isolation. Afflicted persons withdraw into their homes or, if in the hospital, the confines of their room to minimize the embarrassment associated with soiling. Several surgical procedures are used for the treatment of fecal incontinence. These include repair of the sphincter and fecal diversion or colostomy.

Flatulence

There are three primary sources of flatus: (a) action of bacteria on the chyme in the large intestine, (b) swallowed air, and (c) gas that diffuses between the bloodstream and the intestine.

Most gases that are swallowed are expelled through the mouth by eructation (belching). However, large amounts of gas can accumulate in the stomach, resulting in gastric distention. The gases formed in the large intestine are chiefly absorbed through the intestinal capillaries into the circulation. **Flatulence** is the presence of excessive flatus in the intestines and leads to stretching and inflation of the intestines (intestinal distention). Flatulence can occur in the colon from a variety of causes, such as foods, abdominal surgery, or narcotics. If the gas is propelled by increased colon activity before it can be absorbed, it may be expelled through the anus. If excessive gas cannot be expelled through the anus, it may be necessary to insert a rectal tube to remove it.

BOWEL DIVERSION OSTOMIES

An **ostomy** is an opening for the gastrointestinal, urinary, or respiratory tract onto the skin. There are many types of intestinal ostomies. A **gastrostomy** is an opening through the abdominal wall into the stomach. A **jejunostomy** opens through the abdominal wall into the jejunum, an **ileostomy** opens into the ileum (small bowel), and a **colostomy** opens into the colon (large bowel). Gastrostomies and jejunostomies are generally performed to provide an alternate feeding route. The purpose of bowel ostomies is to divert and drain fecal material. Bowel diversion ostomies are often classified according to (a) their status as permanent or temporary, (b) their anatomic location, and (c) the construction of the **stoma**, the opening created in the abdominal wall by the ostomy. A stoma is generally red in color and moist. Initially, slight bleeding may occur when the stoma is touched and this is considered normal. A person doesn't feel the stoma because there are no nerve endings in the stoma.

Permanence

Colostomies can be either temporary or permanent. Temporary colostomies are generally performed for traumatic injuries or inflammatory conditions of the bowel. They allow the distal diseased portion of the bowel to rest and heal. Permanent colostomies are performed to provide a means of elimination when the rectum or anus is nonfunctional as a result of a birth defect or a disease such as cancer of the bowel.

CLINICAL ALERT

Surgery to reconnect the ends of the bowel of a temporary ostomy may be called a take-down.

Anatomic Location

An ileostomy generally empties from the distal end of the small intestine. A cecostomy empties from the cecum (the first part of the ascending colon). An ascending colostomy empties from the ascending colon, a transverse colostomy from the transverse colon, a descending colostomy from the descending colon, and a sigmoidostomy from the sigmoid colon (Figure 34–2).

The location of the ostomy influences the character and management of the fecal drainage. The farther along the bowel, the more formed the stool (because the large bowel reabsorbs water from the fecal mass) and the more control over the frequency of stomal discharge can be established. For example:

- An ileostomy produces liquid fecal drainage. Drainage is constant and cannot be regulated. Ileostomy drainage contains some digestive enzymes, which are damaging to the skin. For this reason, ileostomy clients must wear an appliance continuously and take special precautions to prevent skin breakdown. Compared to colostomies, however, odor is minimal because fewer bacteria are present.

- An ascending colostomy is similar to an ileostomy in that the drainage is liquid and cannot be regulated, and digestive enzymes are present. Odor, however, is a problem requiring control.

- A transverse colostomy produces a malodorous, mushy drainage because some of the liquid has been reabsorbed. There is usually no control.

- A descending colostomy produces increasingly solid fecal drainage. Stools from a sigmoidostomy are of normal or formed consistency, and the frequency of

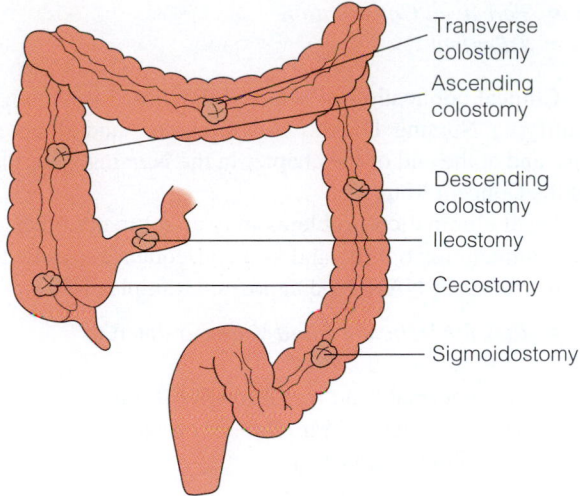

Figure 34–2 ◉ The locations of bowel diversion ostomies.

- Transverse colostomy
- Ascending colostomy
- Descending colostomy
- Ileostomy
- Cecostomy
- Sigmoidostomy

Surgical Construction of the Stoma

Stoma constructions are described as single, loop, divided, or double-barreled colostomies. The single stoma is created when one end of bowel is brought out through an opening onto the anterior abdominal wall. This is referred to as an end or terminal colostomy; the stoma is permanent.

In the loop colostomy, a loop of bowel is brought out onto the abdominal wall and supported by a plastic bridge, or a piece of rubber tubing (Figure 34–3). A loop stoma has two

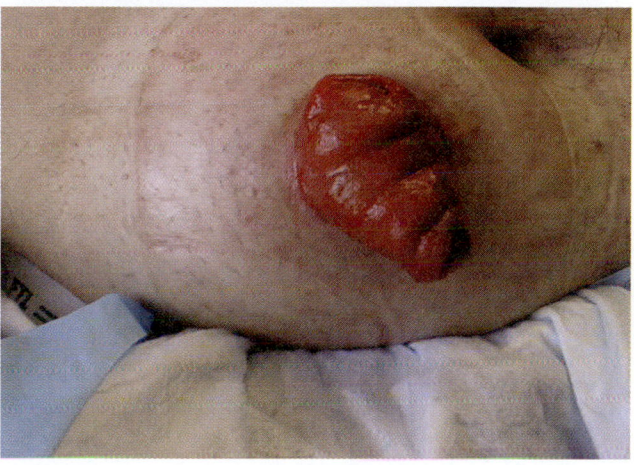

Figure 34–3 ◉ Loop colostomy.
(Courtesy of Cory Patrick Hartley, San Ramon Regional Medical Center, San Ramon, CA.)

discharge can be regulated. People with a sigmoidostomy may not have to wear an appliance at all times, and odors can usually be controlled.

The length of time that an ostomy is in place also helps to determine the consistency of the stool, particularly with transverse and descending colostomies. Over time, the stool becomes more formed because the remaining functioning portions of the colon tend to compensate by increasing water reabsorption.

LIFESPAN CONSIDERATIONS   Factors in Potential Bowel Elimination Problems

Children

- Successful toilet training can prevent many problems with elimination. The family should be assessed for "readiness to train." Assess the child's physical, cognitive, and interpersonal skills, and parental readiness. Does the child have sphincter control (usually by 18 to 24 months)? Does the child understand the meaning of toileting? Is the child able to express him- or herself and does he or she demonstrate interest in learning? Are parents ready to work with the child?
- Encourage a regular toileting routine for children. When toilet training, ensure that toddlers can rest their feet comfortably on the floor or foot stool, and are not frightened or pressured while toileting.
- An acute episode of dehydration and constipation (often related to an illness) can lead to chronic stool problems. Constipation can cause painful defecation, which causes the child to withhold stool, leading to more severe constipation, more pain on defecation, more withholding, and so on. Breaking the cycle by helping ease defecation is important to prevent long-term problems.

Older Adults

- Poor fluid intake and inability to eat a high-fiber diet, due to swallowing or chewing difficulties, are often causes of constipation.
- Medications that are commonly taken by older adults such as antacids, many antihypertensives, antidepressants, diuretics, and narcotics for pain also contribute to constipation.
- Clients receiving tube feedings can experience diarrhea. To alleviate it, they require a change of formula, a change in its strength, or a change in the speed or temperature of tube feeding administration.
- Clients receiving laxative preparation for x-rays or other procedures may experience fluid and electrolyte imbalances due to diarrhea.
- Persons with cognitive impairment, such as Alzheimer's disease, may be unaware of what and when they eat or drink or of their bowel habits. These should be monitored by the caregiver, whether the person is being cared for at home or in an institution, to note any special needs or concerns.
- Persons with impaired mobility may have difficulty getting to the bathroom or using a regular toilet. A raised toilet seat and other devices, such as bars to assist in ambulation, may be very helpful. The decrease in activity may also contribute to constipation.

openings: the proximal or afferent end, which is active, and the distal or efferent end, which is inactive. The loop colostomy is usually performed in an emergency procedure and is often situated on the right transverse colon. It is a bulky stoma that is more difficult to manage than a single stoma.

NURSING MANAGEMENT

ASSESSING

Nursing History

A nursing history for fecal elimination helps the nurse ascertain the client's normal pattern. The nurse elicits a description of usual feces and any recent changes and collects information about any past or current problems with elimination, the presence of an ostomy, and factors influencing the elimination pattern.

When eliciting data about the client's defecation pattern, the nurse needs to understand that the time of defecation and the amount of feces expelled are as individual as the frequency of defecation. Often, the patterns individuals follow depend largely on early training and on convenience.

Physical Examination

Physical examination of the abdomen in relation to fecal elimination problems includes inspection, auscultation, percussion, and palpation with specific reference to the intestinal tract. Auscultation precedes palpation because palpation can alter peristalsis. Examination of the rectum and anus includes inspection and palpation. Physical examination of the abdomen, rectum, and anus is discussed in Chapter 17 ∞.

Inspecting the Feces

Observe the client's stool for color, consistency, shape, amount, odor, and the presence of abnormal constituents. Table 34–1 earlier summarizes normal and abnormal characteristics of stool and possible causes.

Diagnostic Studies

Diagnostic studies of the gastrointestinal tract include direct visualization techniques, indirect visualization techniques, and laboratory tests for abnormal constituents (see Chapter 20 ∞).

DIAGNOSING

NANDA includes the following diagnostic labels for fecal elimination problems:

- *Bowel Incontinence*
- *Constipation*
- *Risk for Constipation*
- *Perceived Constipation*
- *Diarrhea*

Clinical application of selected diagnoses is shown in Identifying Nursing Diagnoses, Outcomes, and Interventions, and at the end of the chapter in the Nursing Care Plan and the Concept Map.

Fecal elimination problems may affect many other areas of human functioning and as a consequence may be the etiology of other NANDA diagnoses. Examples follow:

- *Risk for Deficient Fluid Volume* related to
  a. Prolonged diarrhea
  b. Abnormal fluid loss through ostomy
- *Risk for Impaired Skin Integrity* related to
  a. Prolonged diarrhea
  b. Bowel incontinence
  c. Bowel diversion ostomy
- *Low Self-Esteem* related to
  a. Ostomy
  b. Fecal incontinence
  c. Need for assistance with toileting
- *Disturbed Body Image* related to
  a. Ostomy
  b. Bowel incontinence
- *Deficient Knowledge (Bowel Training, Ostomy Management)* related to lack of previous experience
- *Anxiety* related to
  a. Lack of control of fecal elimination secondary to ostomy
  b. Response of others to ostomy

PLANNING

The major goals for clients with fecal elimination problems are to

- Maintain or restore normal bowel elimination pattern.
- Maintain or regain normal stool consistency.
- Prevent associated risks such as fluid and electrolyte imbalance, skin breakdown, abdominal distention, and pain.

Appropriate preventive and corrective nursing interventions that relate to these must be identified. Specific nursing activities associated with each of these interventions can be selected to meet the client's individual needs. Examples of clinical applications of these using NANDA, NIC, and NOC designations are shown in Identifying Nursing Diagnoses, Outcomes, and Interventions and in the Nursing Care Plan.

Discharge Planning

Clients who have bowel diversion ostomies, who wear pouches, or who have other ongoing elimination problems will need continuing care in the home setting. In preparation for discharge, the nurse needs to assess the client's and family's ability to meet specific care needs. Using the assess-

Clients with Fecal Elimination Problems

DATA CLUSTER Marvin Lombardi reports having loose, liquid, light brown stools for 2 days. Passage of stools is associated with cramping abdominal pain. Bowel sounds are hyperactive. Temperature is 38°C (100.4°F). Has not taken any medications but reports a feeling of general malaise. States he "ate at a fast-food restaurant 2 nights ago."

NURSING DIAGNOSIS/DEFINITION	SAMPLE DESIRED OUTCOMES*/DEFINITION	INDICATORS	SELECTED INTERVENTIONS*/DEFINITION	SAMPLE NIC ACTIVITIES
Diarrhea/Passage of loose, unformed stools	Bowel Elimination [0501]/*Formation and evacuation of stool*	No • Diarrhea • Painful cramps	Diarrhea Management [0460]/*Management and alleviation of diarrhea*	• Obtain stool for culture and sensitivity if diarrhea continues • Observe skin turgor • Monitor skin in perianal region for irritation or ulceration • Consult primary care provider if signs and symptoms of diarrhea persist

DATA CLUSTER Mary Kuoko has had involuntary leakage of stool. States her clothing is soiled several times a day. Says she is too embarrassed to go out with her friends because of the fecal odor. Last bowel movement was more than 3 days ago. Digital examination reveals impaction.

Bowel Incontinence/ Change in normal bowel habits, characterized by involuntary passage of stool	Bowel Continence [0500]/*Control of passage of stool from the bowel*	Consistently demonstrated • Evacuates stool at least q 3 days • Responds to urge in a timely manner • Describes relationship of food intake to stool consistency	Bowel Management [0430]/*Establishment and maintenance of a regular pattern of bowel elimination* Bowel Incontinence Care [0410]/ *Promotion of bowel continence and maintenance of perianal skin integrity*	• Instruct on foods high in fiber, as appropriate • Give warm liquids after meals, as appropriate • Initiate a bowel training program as appropriate • Wash perianal area with soap and water and dry it thoroughly after each stool • Monitor for adequate bowel evacuation • Monitor diet and fluid requirements

*The NOC # for desired outcomes and the NIC # for nursing interventions are listed in brackets following the appropriate outcome or intervention. Outcomes, indicators, interventions, and activities selected are only a sample of those suggested by NOC and NIC and should be further individualized for each client.

ment data, the nurse designs a teaching plan for the client and family (see Client Teaching).

IMPLEMENTING

Promoting Regular Defecation

The nurse can help clients achieve regular defecation by attending to (a) the provision of privacy, (b) timing, (c) nutrition and fluids, (d) exercise, and (e) positioning. See Client Teaching for healthy habits related to bowel elimination.

PRIVACY Privacy during defecation is extremely important to many people. The nurse should therefore provide as much privacy as possible for such clients but may need to

stay with those who are too weak to be left alone. Some clients also prefer to wipe, wash, and dry themselves after defecating. A nurse may need to provide water and a washcloth and towel for this purpose.

TIMING A client should be encouraged to defecate when the urge is recognized. To establish regular bowel elimination, the client and nurse can discuss when **mass peristalsis** normally occurs and provide time for defecation. Many people have well-established routines. Other activities, such as bathing and ambulating, should not interfere with the defecation time.

NUTRITION AND FLUIDS The diet a client needs for regular normal elimination varies, depending on the kind of feces the client currently has, the frequency of defecation,

CLIENT TEACHING   Fecal Elimination

Facilitating Toileting

- Ensure safe and easy access to the toilet. Make sure lighting is appropriate, scatter rugs are removed or securely fastened, and so on.
- Facilitate instruction as needed about transfer techniques.
- Suggest ways that garments can be adjusted to make disrobing easier for toileting (e.g., Velcro closing on clothing).

Monitoring Bowel Elimination Pattern

- Instruct the client, if appropriate, to keep a record of time and frequency of stool passage, any associated pain, and color and consistency of the stool.

Dietary Alterations

- Provide information about required food and fluid alterations to promote defecation or to manage diarrhea.

Medications

- Discuss problems associated with overuse of laxatives, if appropriate, and the use of alternatives to laxatives, suppositories, and enemas.
- Discuss the addition of a fiber supplement if the client is taking a constipating medication.

Measures Specific to Elimination Problem

- Provide instructions associated with specific elimination problems and treatment, such as
  a. Constipation
  b. Diarrhea
  c. Ostomy care

Community Agencies and Other Sources of Help

- Make appropriate referrals to home care or community care for assistance with resources such as installation of grab bars and raised toilet seats, structural alterations for wheelchair access, homemaker or home health aide services to assist with ADLs, and enterostomal therapy nurse for assistance with stoma care and selection of ostomy appliances.
- Provide information about companies where durable medical equipment (e.g., raised toilet seats, commodes, bedpans, urinals) can be purchased, rented, or obtained free of charge, and where medical supplies such as incontinence pads or ostomy irrigating supplies and appliances can be obtained.
- Suggest additional sources of information and help such as ostomy self-help and support groups or clubs.

CLIENT TEACHING   Healthy Defecation

- Establish a regular exercise regimen.
- Include high-fiber foods, such as vegetables, fruits, and whole grains, in the diet.
- Maintain fluid intake of 2,000 to 3,000 mL a day.
- Do not ignore the urge to defecate.
- Allow time to defecate, preferably at the same time each day.
- Avoid over-the-counter medications to treat constipation and diarrhea.

CLIENT TEACHING   Managing Diarrhea

- Drink at least 8 glasses of water per day to prevent dehydration. Consider drinking a few glasses of electrolyte replacement fluids a day.
- Eat foods with sodium and potassium. Most foods contain sodium. Potassium is found in meats and many vegetables and fruits, especially purple grape juice, tomatoes, potatoes, bananas, cooked peaches, and apricots.
- Increase foods containing soluble fiber, such as rice, oatmeal, and skinless fruits and potatoes.
- Avoid alcohol and beverages with caffeine, which aggravate the problem.
- Limit foods containing insoluble fiber, such as high-fiber whole-wheat and whole-grain breads and cereals, and raw fruits and vegetables.
- Limit fatty foods.
- Thoroughly clean and dry the perianal area after passing stool to prevent skin irritation and breakdown. Use soft toilet tissue to clean and dry the area. Apply a dimethicone-based cream or alcohol-free barrier film as needed.
- If possible, discontinue medications that cause diarrhea.
- When diarrhea has stopped, reestablish normal bowel flora by taking fermented dairy products, such as yogurt or buttermilk.
- Seek a primary care provider consultation right away if weakness, dizziness, or loose stools persist more than 48 hours.

and the types of foods that the client finds assist with normal defecation.

For constipation, increase daily fluid intake, and instruct the client to drink hot liquids and fruit juices, especially prune juice. Include fiber in the diet, that is, foods such as raw fruit, bran products, and whole-grain cereals and bread.

For diarrhea, encourage oral intake of fluids and bland food. Eating small amounts can be helpful because it is more easily absorbed. Excessively hot or cold fluids should be avoided because they stimulate peristalsis. In addition, highly spiced foods and high-fiber foods can aggravate diarrhea. See Client Teaching for details about managing diarrhea.

For flatulence, limit carbonated beverages, the use of drinking straws, and chewing gum—all of which increase the ingestion of air. Gas-forming foods, such as cabbage, beans, onions, and cauliflower, should also be avoided.

EXERCISE Regular exercise helps clients develop a regular defecation pattern. A client with weak abdominal and pelvic muscles (which impede normal defecation) may be able to strengthen them with the following isometric exercises:

- In a supine position, the client tightens the abdominal muscles as though pulling them inward, holding them for about 10 seconds and then relaxing them. This should be repeated 5 to 10 times, four times a day, depending on the client's health.
- Again in a supine position, the client can contract the thigh muscles and hold them contracted for about 10 seconds, repeating the exercise 5 to 10 times, four times a day. This helps the client confined to bed gain strength in the thigh muscles, thereby making it easier to use a bedpan.

POSITIONING Although the squatting position best facilitates defecation, on a toilet seat the best position for most people seems to be leaning forward.

For clients who have difficulty sitting down and getting up from the toilet, an elevated toilet seat can be attached to a regular toilet. Clients then do not have to lower themselves as far onto the seat and do not have to lift as far off the seat. Elevated toilet seats can be purchased for use in the home.

A bedside commode, a portable chair with a toilet seat and a receptacle beneath that can be emptied, is often used for the adult client who can get out of bed but is unable to walk to the bathroom. Some commodes have wheels and can slide over the base of a regular toilet when the waste receptacle is removed, thus providing clients the privacy of a bathroom. Some commodes have a seat and can be used as a chair. Potty chairs are available for children.

Clients restricted to bed may need to use a bedpan, a receptacle for urine and feces. Female clients use a bedpan for both urine and feces; male clients use a bedpan for feces and a urinal for urine.

There are two main types of bedpans: the regular high-back pan and the slipper, or fracture, pan. The slipper pan has a low back and is used for clients unable to raise their buttocks because of physical problems or therapy that contraindicates such movement. Many older adults benefit from the use of a slipper pan. See Practice Guidelines for the techniques of giving and removing a bedpan.

PRACTICE GUIDELINES

Giving and Removing a Bedpan

- Provide privacy.
- Wear disposable gloves.
- If the bedpan is metal, warm it by rinsing it with warm water.
- Adjust the bed to a height appropriate to prevent back strain.
- Elevate the side rail on the opposite side to prevent the client from falling out of bed.
- Ask the client to assist by flexing the knees, resting the weight on the back and heels, and raising the buttocks, or by using a trapeze bar, if present.
- Help lift the client as needed by placing one hand under the lower back, resting your elbow on the mattress, and using your forearm as a lever.
- Lubricate the back of the bedpan with a small amount of hand lotion or liquid soap to reduce tissue friction and shearing.
- Place a regular bedpan so that the client's buttocks rest on the smooth, rounded rim. Place a slipper pan with the flat, low end under the client's buttocks.
- For the client who cannot assist, obtain the assistance of another nurse to help lift the client onto the bedpan or place the client on his or her side, place the bedpan against the buttocks, and roll the client back onto the bedpan.
- To provide a more normal position for the client's lower back, elevate the client's bed to a semi-Fowler's position, if permitted. If elevation is contraindicated, support the client's back with pillows as needed to prevent hyperextension of the back.
- Cover the client with bed linen to maintain comfort and dignity.
- Provide toilet tissue, place the call light within reach, lower the bed to the low position, elevate the side rail if indicated, and leave the client alone.

- Answer the call bell promptly.
- Do not leave anyone on a bedpan longer than 15 minutes unless they are able to remove the pan themselves. Lengthy stays on a bedpan can cause pressure ulcers.
- When removing the bedpan, return the bed to the position used when giving the bedpan, hold the bedpan steady to prevent spillage of its contents, cover the bedpan, and place it on the adjacent chair.
- If the client needs assistance, don gloves and wipe the client's perineal area with several layers of toilet tissue. If a specimen is to be collected, discard the soiled tissue into a moisture-proof receptacle other than the bedpan. For female clients, clean from the urethra toward the anus to prevent transferring rectal microorganisms into the urinary meatus.
- Wash the perineal area of dependent clients with soap and water as indicated and thoroughly dry the area.
- For all clients, offer warm water, soap, a washcloth, and a towel to wash the hands.
- Assist the client to a comfortable position, empty and clean the bedpan, and return it to the bedside.
- Remove and discard your gloves and wash your hands.
- Spray the room with air freshener as needed to control odor unless contraindicated because of respiratory problems or allergies.
- Document color, odor, amount, and consistency of urine and feces, and the condition of the perineal area.

Teaching about Medications

The most common categories of medications affecting fecal elimination are cathartics and laxatives, antidiarrheals, and antiflatulents.

CATHARTICS AND LAXATIVES **Cathartics** are drugs that induce defecation. They can have a strong, purgative effect. A laxative is mild in comparison to a cathartic, and it produces soft or liquid stools that are sometimes accompanied by abdominal cramps. Examples of cathartics are castor oil, cascara, phenolphthalein, and bisacodyl.

Laxatives are contraindicated in the client who has nausea, cramps, colic, vomiting, or undiagnosed abdominal pain. Clients need to be informed about the dangers of laxative use. Continual use of laxatives to encourage bowel evacuation weakens the bowel's natural responses to fecal distention, resulting in chronic constipation. To eliminate chronic laxative use, it is usually necessary to teach the client about dietary fiber, regular exercise, taking sufficient fluids, and establishing regular defecation habits. In addition, any medication regimen should be examined to see whether it could cause constipation.

Some laxatives are given in the form of **suppositories**. These act in various ways: by softening the feces, by releasing gases such as carbon dioxide to distend the rectum, or by stimulating the nerve endings in the rectal mucosa. The best results can be obtained by inserting the suppository 30 minutes before the client's usual defecation time or when the peristaltic action is greatest, such as after breakfast.

ANTIDIARRHEAL MEDICATIONS These medications slow the motility of the intestine or absorb excess fluid in the intestine.

ANTIFLATULENT MEDICATIONS Antiflatulent agents such as simethicone do not decrease the formation of flatus but they do coalesce the gas bubbles and facilitate their passage by belching through the mouth or expulsion through the anus. These agents are frequently combined with an antacid. **Carminatives** are herbal oils known to act as agents that help expel gas from the stomach and intestines. Suppositories can also be given to relieve flatus by increasing intestinal motility.

Decreasing Flatulence

There are a number of ways to reduce or expel flatus, including avoiding gas-producing foods, exercise, moving in bed, and ambulation. Movement stimulates peristalsis and the escape of flatus and reabsorption of gases in the intestinal capillaries.

Administering Enemas

An **enema** is a solution introduced into the rectum and large intestine. The action of an enema is to distend the intestine and sometimes to irritate the intestinal mucosa, thereby increasing peristalsis and the excretion of feces and flatus. Enemas are classified into four groups: cleansing, carminative, retention, and return-flow enemas.

CLEANSING ENEMAS Cleansing enemas are intended to remove feces. They are given chiefly to:

- Prevent the escape of feces during surgery.
- Prepare the intestine for certain diagnostic tests such as x-ray or visualization tests (e.g., colonoscopy).
- Remove feces in instances of constipation or impaction.

Cleansing enemas use a variety of solutions. Table 34–3 lists commonly used solutions.

Hypertonic solutions (e.g., saline) exert osmotic pressure, which draws fluid from the interstitial space into the colon. The increased volume in the colon stimulates peristalsis and hence defecation. A commonly used hypertonic enema is the commercially prepared Fleet phosphate enema. Hypotonic solutions (e.g., tap water) exert a lower osmotic pressure than the surrounding interstitial fluid, causing water to move from the colon into the interstitial space. Before the water moves from the colon, it stimulates peristalsis and defecation. Because the water moves out of the colon, the

TABLE 34–3   **Commonly Used Enema Solutions**

SOLUTION	CONSTITUENTS	ACTION	TIME TO TAKE EFFECT	ADVERSE EFFECTS
Hypertonic	90–120 mL of solution (e.g., sodium phosphate)	Draws water into the colon	5–10 min	Retention of sodium
Hypotonic	500–1,000 mL of tap water	Distends colon, stimulates peristalsis, and softens feces	15–20 min	Fluid and electrolyte imbalance; water intoxication
Isotonic	500–1,000 mL of normal saline	Distends colon, stimulates peristalsis, and softens feces	15–20 min	Possible sodium retention
Soapsuds	500–1,000 mL (3–5 mL soap to 1,000 mL water)	Irritates mucosa, distends colon	10–15 min	Irritates and may damage mucosa
Oil (mineral, olive, cottonseed)	90–120 mL	Lubricates the feces and the colonic mucosa	1/2–3 hr	

tap water enema should not be repeated because of danger of circulatory overload when the water moves from the interstitial space into the circulatory system.

Isotonic solutions, such as physiologic (normal) saline, are considered the safest enema solutions to use. They exert the same osmotic pressure as the interstitial fluid surrounding the colon. Therefore, there is no fluid movement into or out of the colon. The instilled volume of saline in the colon stimulates peristalsis. Soapsuds enemas stimulate peristalsis by increasing the volume in the colon and irritating the mucosa. Only pure soap (i.e., castile soap) should be used in order to minimize mucosa irritation.

Some enemas are large volume (i.e., 500 to 1,000 mL) for an adult and others are small volume, including hypertonic solutions. The amount of solution administered for a high-volume enema will depend on the age and medical condition of the individual. For example, clients with certain cardiac or renal diseases would be adversely affected by significant fluid retention that might result from large-volume hypotonic enemas.

Cleansing enemas may also be described as high or low. A high enema is given to cleanse as much of the colon as possible. The client changes from the left lateral position to the dorsal recumbent position and then to the right lateral position during administration so that the solution can follow the large intestine. The low enema is used to clean the rectum and sigmoid colon only. The client maintains a left lateral position during administration.

The force of flow of the solution is governed by (a) the height of the solution container, (b) size of the tubing, (c) viscosity of the fluid, and (d) resistance of the rectum. The higher the solution container is held above the rectum, the faster the flow and the greater the force (pressure) in the rectum. During most adult enemas, the solution container should be no higher than 30 cm (12 in.) above the rectum. During a high cleansing enema, the solution container is usually held 30 to 49 cm (12 to 18 in.) above the rectum because the fluid is instilled farther to clean the entire bowel.

CARMINATIVE ENEMA A carminative enema is given primarily to expel flatus. The solution instilled into the rectum releases gas, which in turn distends the rectum and the colon, thus stimulating peristalsis. For an adult, 60 to 80 mL of fluid is instilled.

RETENTION ENEMA A retention enema introduces oil or medication into the rectum and sigmoid colon. The liquid is retained for a relatively long period (e.g., 1 to 3 hours). An oil retention enema acts to soften the feces and to lubricate the rectum and anal canal, thus facilitating passage of the feces. Antibiotic enemas are used to treat infections locally, anthelmintic enemas to kill helminths such as worms and intestinal parasites, and nutritive enemas to administer fluids and nutrients to the rectum.

RETURN-FLOW ENEMA A return-flow enema is used occasionally to expel flatus. Alternating flow of 100 to 200 mL of fluid into and out of the rectum and sigmoid colon stimulates peristalsis. This process is repeated five or six times until the flatus is expelled and abdominal distention is relieved.

Skill 34–1 describes how to administer an enema.

> ## CLINICAL ALERT
>
> Some clients may wish to administer their own enemas. If this is appropriate, the nurse validates the client's knowledge of correct technique and assists as needed.

SKILL 34–1

ADMINISTERING AN ENEMA

PURPOSES
- To achieve one or more of the following actions: cleansing, carminative, retention, or return-flow

ASSESSMENT
Assess the following:
- When the client last had a bowel movement and the amount, color, and consistency of the feces
- Presence of abdominal distention (the distended abdomen appears swollen and feels firm rather than soft when palpated)
- Whether the client has sphincter control
- Whether the client can use a toilet or commode or must remain in bed and use a bedpan

PLANNING
Before administering an enema, determine that there is a primary care provider's order. At some agencies, a primary care provider must order the kind of enema and the time to give it, for example, the morning of an examination. At other agencies, enemas are given at the nurses' discretion (i.e., as necessary on a prn order). In addition, determine the presence of kidney or cardiac disease that contraindicates the use of a hypotonic solution.

> **Delegation**
> Administration of some enemas may be delegated to unlicensed assistive personnel (UAP). However, the nurse must ensure the personnel are competent in the use of standard precautions. Abnormal findings such as inability to insert the rectal tip, client inability to retain the solution, or unusual return from the enema must be validated and interpreted by the nurse.

(continued)

SKILL 34–1

ADMINISTERING AN ENEMA *(continued)*

EQUIPMENT
- Disposable linen-saver pad
- Bath blanket
- Bedpan or commode
- Clean gloves
- Water-soluble lubricant if tubing not prelubricated
- Paper towel

LARGE-VOLUME ENEMA
- Solution container with tubing of correct size and tubing clamp
- Correct solution, amount, and temperature

SMALL-VOLUME ENEMA
- Prepackaged container of enema solution with lubricated tip

IMPLEMENTATION

Preparation
- Lubricate about 5 cm (2 in.) of the rectal tube (some commercially prepared enema sets already have lubricated nozzles). **Rationale:** *Lubrication facilitates insertion through the sphincters and minimizes trauma.*
- Run some solution through the connecting tubing of a large volume enema set and the rectal tube to expel any air in the tubing; then close the clamp. **Rationale:** *Air instilled into the rectum, although not harmful, causes unnecessary distention.*

Performance
1. Prior to performing the procedure, introduce self and verify the client's identity using agency protocol. Explain to the client what you are going to do, why it is necessary, and how he or she can participate. Discuss how the results will be used in planning further care or treatments. Indicate that the client may experience a feeling of fullness while the solution is being administered. Explain the need to hold the solution as long as possible.
2. Perform hand hygiene and observe appropriate infection control procedures. Apply clean gloves.
3. Provide for client privacy.
4. Assist the adult client to a left lateral position, with the right leg as acutely flexed as possible ❶, and the linen-saver pad under the buttocks. **Rationale:** *This position facilitates the flow of solution by gravity into the sigmoid and descending colon, which are on the left side. Having the right leg acutely flexed provides for adequate exposure of the anus.*
5. Insert the enema tube.
   - For clients in the left lateral position, lift the upper buttock *to ensure good visualization of the anus.*
   - Insert the tube smoothly and slowly into the rectum, directing it toward the umbilicus. **Rationale:** *The angle follows the normal contour of the rectum. Slow insertion prevents spasm of the sphincter.*
   - Insert the tube 7 to 10 cm (3 to 4 in.). **Rationale:** *Because the anal canal is about 2.5 to 5 cm (1 to 2 in.) long in the adult, insertion to this point places the tip of the tube beyond the anal sphincter into the rectum.*
   - If resistance is encountered at the internal sphincter, ask the client to take a deep breath, then run a small amount of solution through the tube *to relax the internal anal sphincter.*
   - Never force tube or solution entry. If instilling a small amount of solution does not permit the tube to be advanced or the solution to freely flow, withdraw the tube. Check for any stool that may have blocked the tube during insertion. If present, flush it and retry the procedure. You may also perform a digital rectal

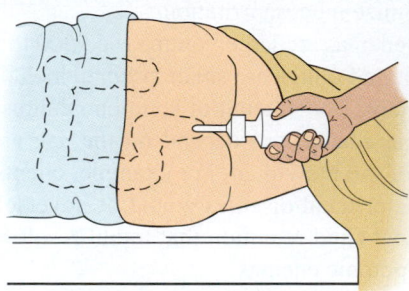

❶ Assuming a left lateral position for an enema. Note the commercially prepared enema.

examination to determine if there is an impaction or other mechanical blockage. If resistance persists, end the procedure and report the resistance to the primary care provider and nurse in charge.

6. Slowly administer the enema solution.
   - Raise the solution container, and open the clamp to allow fluid flow.
     or
   - Compress a pliable container by hand.
   - During most low enemas, hold or hang the solution container no higher than 30 cm (12 in.) above the rectum. **Rationale:** *The higher the solution container is held above the rectum, the faster the flow and the greater the force (pressure) in the rectum. During a high enema, hang the solution container about 45 cm (18 in.).* **Rationale:** *The fluid must be instilled farther to clean the entire bowel.* See agency protocol.
   - Administer the fluid slowly. If the client complains of fullness or pain, lower the container or use the clamp to stop the flow for 30 seconds, and then restart the flow at a slower rate. **Rationale:** *Administering the enema slowly and stopping the flow momentarily decreases the likelihood of intestinal spasm and premature ejection of the solution.*
   - If you are using a plastic commercial container, roll it up as the fluid is instilled. This prevents subsequent suctioning of the solution.
   - After all the solution has been instilled or when the client cannot hold any more and feels the desire to defecate (the urge to defecate usually indicates that sufficient fluid has been administered), close the clamp, and remove the enema tube from the anus.
   - Place the enema tube in a disposable towel as you withdraw it.
7. Encourage the client to retain the enema.
   - Ask the client to remain lying down. It is easier for the client to retain the enema when lying down than when

sitting or standing, because gravity promotes drainage and peristalsis.

- Request that the client retain the solution for the appropriate amount of time, for example, 5 to 10 minutes for a cleansing enema or at least 30 minutes for a retention enema.

8. Assist the client to defecate.
   - Assist the client to a sitting position on the bedpan, commode, or toilet. A sitting position facilitates the act of defecation.
   - Ask the client who is using the toilet not to flush it. The nurse needs to observe the feces.
   - If a specimen of feces is required, ask the client to use a bedpan or commode.

9. Document the type and volume, if appropriate, of enema given. Describe the results.

SAMPLE DOCUMENTATION

1/5/2010 1000. States last BM five days ago. Abdomen distended and firm. Bowel sounds hypoactive. Fleet's enema given per order resulting in large amount of firm brown stool. States he "feels better" _____ M. Lopez, RN

EVALUATION

- Perform a detailed follow-up based on findings that deviated from expected or normal for the client. Relate findings to previous assessment data if available. Report significant deviations from expected to the primary care provider.

VARIATION: ADMINISTERING AN ENEMA TO AN INCONTINENT CLIENT

Occasionally a nurse needs to administer an enema to a client who is unable to control the external sphincter muscle and thus cannot retain the enema solution for even a few minutes. In that case, after the rectal tube is inserted, the client assumes a supine position on a bedpan. The head of the bed can be elevated slightly, to 30 degrees if necessary for easier breathing, and pillows support the client's head and back.

VARIATION: ADMINISTERING A RETURN-FLOW ENEMA

For a return-flow enema, the solution (100 to 200 mL for an adult) is instilled into the client's rectum and sigmoid colon. Then the solution container is lowered so that the fluid flows back out through the rectal tube into the container, pulling the flatus with it. The inflow–outflow process is repeated five or six times (to stimulate peristalsis and the expulsion of flatus), and the solution is replaced several times during the procedure if it becomes thick with feces.

Document type of solution; length of time solution was retained; the amount, color, and consistency of the returns; and the relief of flatus and abdominal distention in the client record using forms or checklists supplemented by narrative notes when appropriate.

LIFESPAN CONSIDERATIONS Administering an Enema

Infants/Children

- Provide a careful explanation to the parents and child before the procedure.
- The enema solution should be isotonic (usually normal saline). Some hypertonic commercial solutions (e.g., Fleet phosphate enema) can lead to hypovolemia and electrolyte imbalances. In addition, the osmotic effect of the enema may produce diarrhea and subsequent metabolic acidosis.
- Infants and small children do not exhibit sphincter control and need to be assisted in retaining the enema. The nurse administers the enema while the infant or child is lying with the buttocks over the bedpan, and the nurse firmly presses the buttocks together to prevent the immediate expulsion of the solution. Older children can usually hold the solution if they understand what to do and are not required to hold it for too long a period. It may be necessary to ensure that the bathroom is available for an ambulatory child before starting the procedure or to have a bedpan ready.
- Enema temperature should be 37.7°C (100°F) unless otherwise ordered.
- Large-volume enemas consist of 50 to 200 mL in children less than 18 months old; 200 to 300 mL in children 18 months to 5 years; and 300 to 500 mL in children 5 to 12 years old.
- Careful explanation is especially important for the preschool child. An enema is an intrusive procedure and therefore threatening.

- For infants and small children, the dorsal recumbent position is frequently used. Position them on a small padded bedpan with support for the back and head. Secure the legs by placing a diaper under the bedpan and then over and around the thighs. Place the underpad under the client's buttocks to protect the bed linen, and drape the client with the bath blanket.
- Insert the tube 5 to 7.5 cm (2 to 3 in.) in the child and only 2.5 to 3.75 cm (1 to 1.5 in.) in the infant.
- For children, lower the height of the solution container appropriately for the age of the child. See agency protocol.
- To assist a small child in retaining the solution, apply firm pressure over the anus with tissue wipes, or firmly press the buttocks together.

Older Adults

- Older adults may fatigue easily.
- Older adults may be more susceptible to fluid and electrolyte imbalances. Use tap water enemas with great caution.
- Monitor the client's tolerance during the procedure, watching for vagal episodes (e.g., slow pulse) and dysrhythmias.
- Protect older adults' skin from prolonged exposure to moisture.
- Assist older clients with perineal care as indicated.

Digital Removal of a Fecal Impaction

Digital removal involves breaking up the fecal mass digitally and removing it in portions. Because the bowel mucosa can be injured during this procedure, some agencies restrict and specify the personnel permitted to conduct digital disimpactions. Rectal stimulation is also contraindicated for some people because it may cause an excessive vagal response resulting in cardiac arrhythmia. Before disimpaction it is suggested an oil retention enema be given and held for 30 minutes. After a disimpaction, the nurse can use various interventions to remove remaining feces, such as a cleansing enema or the insertion of a suppository.

Because manual removal of an impaction can be painful, the nurse may use, if the agency permits, 1 to 2 mL of lidocaine (Xylocaine) gel on a gloved finger inserted into the anal canal as far as the nurse can reach. The lidocaine will anesthetize the anal canal and rectum and should be inserted 5 minutes before the disimpaction.

For digital removal of a fecal impaction:

1. If indicated, obtain assistance from a second person who can comfort the client during the procedure.
2. Ask the client to assume a left side-lying position, with the knees flexed and the back toward the nurse.
3. Place a bedpad under the client's buttocks and a bedpan nearby to receive stool.
4. Drape the client for comfort and to avoid unnecessary exposure of the body.
5. Put on a pair of clean gloves and liberally lubricate the index finger to be inserted.
6. Gently insert the index finger into the rectum and move the finger along the length of the rectum.
7. Loosen and dislodge stool by gently massaging around it. Break up stool by working the finger into the hardened mass, taking care to avoid injury to the mucosa of the rectum.
8. Carefully work stool downward to the end of the rectum and remove it in small pieces. Continue to remove as much fecal material as possible. Periodically assess the client for signs of fatigue, such as facial pallor, diaphoresis, or change in pulse rate. Manual stimulation should be minimal.
9. Following disimpaction, assist the client to clean the anal area and buttocks. Then assist the client onto a bedpan or commode for a short time because digital stimulation of the rectum often induces the urge to defecate.

Bowel Training Programs

For clients who have chronic constipation, frequent impactions, or fecal incontinence, bowel training programs may be helpful. The program is based on factors within the client's control and is designed to help the client establish normal defecation. Such matters as food and fluid intake, exercise, and defecation habits are all considered. Before beginning such a program, clients must understand it and

want to be involved. The major phases of the program are as follows:

- Determine the client's usual bowel habits and factors that help and hinder normal defecation.
- Design a plan with the client that includes the following:
  a. Fluid intake of about 2,500 to 3,000 mL per day
  b. Increase in fiber in the diet
  c. Intake of hot drinks, especially just before the usual defecation time
  d. Increase in exercise
- Maintain the following daily routine for 2 to 3 weeks:
  a. Administer a cathartic suppository (e.g., Dulcolax) 30 minutes before the client's defecation time to stimulate peristalsis.
  b. When the client experiences the urge to defecate, assist the client to the toilet or commode or onto a bedpan. Note the length of time between the insertion of the suppository and the urge to defecate.
  c. Provide the client with privacy for defecation and a time limit; 30 to 40 minutes is usually sufficient.
  d. Teach the client to lean forward at the hips, to apply pressure on the abdomen with the hands, and to bear down for defecation. These measures increase pressure on the colon. Straining should be avoided because it can cause hemorrhoids.
- Provide positive feedback when the client successfully defecates. Refrain from negative feedback if the client fails to defecate.
- Offer encouragement to the client and convey that patience is often required. Many clients require weeks or months of training to achieve success.

Fecal Incontinence Pouch

To collect and contain large volumes of liquid feces, the nurse may place a fecal incontinence collector pouch around the anal area. The purpose of the pouch is to prevent progressive perianal skin irritation and breakdown and frequent linen changes necessitated by incontinence. In many agencies, the pouch is replacing the traditional approach to this problem, that is, inserting a large Foley catheter into the client's rectum and inflating the balloon to keep it in place—a practice that may damage the rectal sphincter and rectal mucosa. A rectal catheter also increases peristalsis and incontinence by stimulating sensory nerve fibers in the rectum.

A fecal collector is secured around the anal opening and may or may not be attached to drainage. Pouches are best applied before the perianal skin becomes excoriated. If perianal skin excoriation is present, the nurse either (a) applies a dimethicone-based moisture-barrier cream or alcohol-free barrier film to the skin to protect it from feces until it heals and then applies the pouch, or (b) applies a skin barrier or hydrocolloid barrier underneath the pouch to achieve the best possible seal.

Nursing responsibilities for clients with a rectal pouch include (a) regular assessment and documentation of the perianal skin status, (b) changing the bag every 72 hours or sooner if there is leakage, (c) maintaining the drainage system, and (d) providing explanations and support to the client and support people.

Some clients (e.g., posttrauma, quadriplegic, paraplegic, or poststroke) may be treated for fecal incontinence with surgical repair of a damaged sphincter or an artificial bowel sphincter. The artificial sphincter consists of three parts: a cuff around the anal canal, a pressure-regulating balloon, and a pump that inflates the cuff. The cuff is inflated to close the sphincter, maintaining continence. To have a bowel movement, the client deflates the cuff. The cuff automatically reinflates in 10 minutes. Management of this device is usually specific to the device; contact the manufacturing company for details.

Administering enemas and rectal medications may be harmful with this device in place. Ensure safety of these practices with the device instruction guide provided by the device manufacturer.

Ostomy Management

Clients with fecal diversions need considerable psychologic support, instruction, and physical care. This section is limited to the nurse's physical interventions of stoma assessment, application of an appliance to collect feces and protect skin, and promotion of self-care. Many agencies have access to a wound ostomy continence nurse (WOCN) to assist these clients. National organizations (e.g., United Ostomy Associations of America) have support groups whose mission is to improve the quality of life of people who have, or will have, an ostomy. Members of local chapters of such an organization have been known to meet and visit with a person who has a new ostomy. It is common for a client with a new ostomy to feel frightened and alone. Talking with another person who has gone through a similar experience may help the client realize that he or she is not alone and others are willing to listen and help.

STOMA AND SKIN CARE Care of the stoma and skin is important for all clients who have ostomies. The fecal material from a colostomy or ileostomy is irritating to the peristomal skin. This is particularly true of stool from an ileostomy, which contains digestive enzymes. It is important to assess the peristomal skin for irritation each time the appliance is changed. Any irritation or skin breakdown needs to be treated immediately. The skin is kept clean by washing off any excretion and drying thoroughly.

An ostomy appliance should protect the skin, collect stool, and control odor. The appliance consists of a skin barrier and a pouch. Some clients may prefer to also wear an adjustable ostomy belt that attaches to an ostomy pouch to hold the pouch firmly in place. Appliances can be one piece where the skin barrier is already attached to the pouch (Figure 34–4, A), or an appliance can consist of two pieces: a separate pouch with a flange and a separate skin barrier with a flange where the pouch fastens to the barrier at the flange (Figure 34–4, B). The pouch can be removed without removing the skin barrier when using a two-piece appliance. Pouches can be closed or drainable (Figure 34–5). A drain-

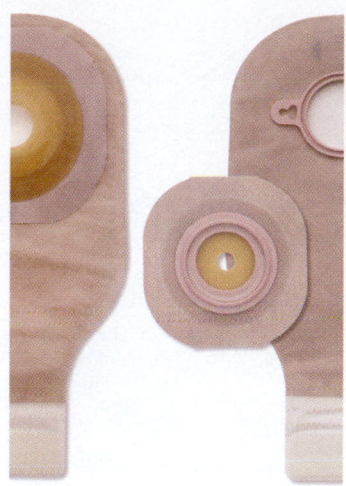

Figure 34–4 ○ *A*, A one-piece ostomy appliance or pouching system, and *B*, a two-piece ostomy appliance or pouching system. (Permission to use this copyrighted image has been granted by the owner, Hollister, Incorporated.)

able pouch usually has a clip where the end of the pouch is folded over the clamp and clipped (Figure 34–6). Newer drainable pouches have an integrated closure system instead of a clamp. The client folds up the end of the pouch three times and presses firmly to seal the pouch. Drainable pouches are usually used by people who need to empty the pouch more than twice a day.

Closed pouches are often used by people who have a regular stoma discharge (e.g., sigmoid colostomy) and only have to empty the pouch 1 or 2 times a day. Some people find it easier to change a closed pouch than emptying a drainable pouch, which requires some dexterity.

Odor control is essential to clients' self-esteem. As soon as clients are ambulatory, they can learn to work with the ostomy in the bathroom to avoid odors at the bedside. Selecting the appropriate kind of appliance promotes odor control. An intact appliance contains odors. Most pouches contain

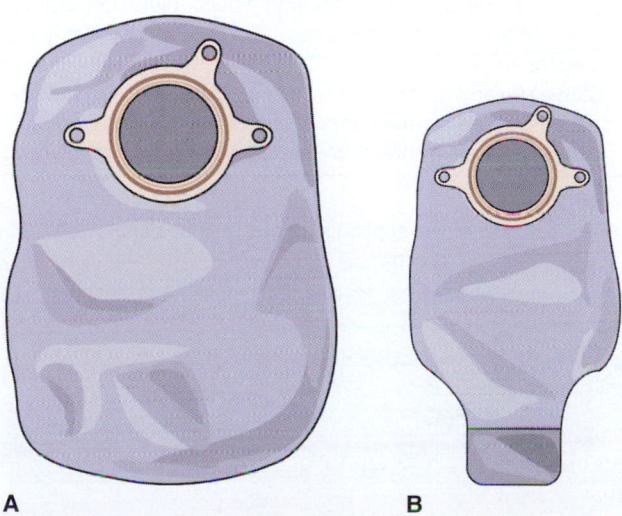

A   **B**

Figure 34–5 ○ *A*, A closed pouch, and *B*, a drainable pouch.

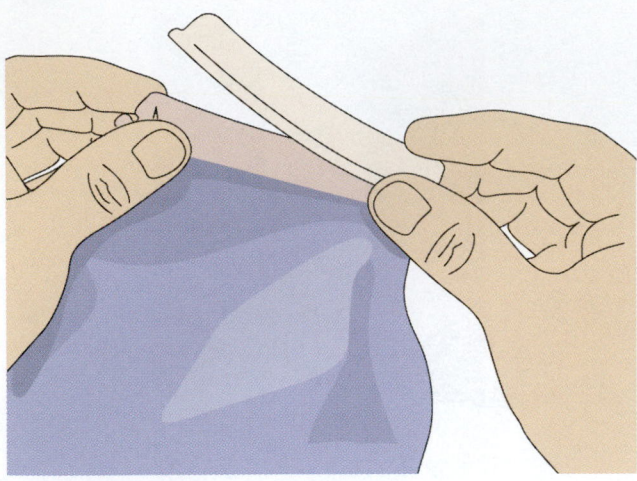

Figure 34–6 ⬤ Applying a pouch clamp.

odor-barrier material. Some pouches also have a pouch filter that allows gas out of the pouch but not the odor.

Ostomy appliances can be applied for up to 7 days. Most clinicians agree that an ostomy appliance should be changed at least once a week (Hollister, n.d.). Some manufacturers recommend removing the pouch and skin barrier twice a week to clean and inspect the peristomal skin. They require changing whenever the stool leaks onto the peristomal skin. If the skin is erythematous, eroded, denuded, or ulcerated, the pouch should be changed every 24 to 48 hours to allow appropriate treatment of the skin. More frequent changes are recommended if the client complains of pain or discomfort.

The type of ostomy and amount of ouput influences how often the pouch is emptied. The pouch is emptied when it is one-third to one-half full. If the pouch overfills, it can cause separation of the skin barrier from the skin and stool comes in contact with the skin. This results in the entire appliance needing to be removed and a new one applied.

Skill 34–2 explains how to change a bowel diversion ostomy appliance.

SKILL 34–2

CHANGING A BOWEL DIVERSION OSTOMY APPLIANCE

PURPOSES
- To assess and care for the peristomal skin
- To collect stool for assessment of the amount and type of output
- To minimize odors for the client's comfort and self-esteem

ASSESSMENT
Determine the following:
- The type of ostomy and its placement on the abdomen. Surgeons often draw diagrams when there are two stomas. If there is more than one stoma, it is important to confirm which is the functioning stoma.
- The type and size of appliance currently used and the special barrier substance applied to the skin, according to the nursing care plan.

Assess the following:
- Stoma color: The stoma should appear red, similar in color to the mucosal lining of the inner cheek and slightly moist. Very pale or darker-colored stomas with a dusky bluish or purplish hue indicate impaired blood circulation to the area. Notify the surgeon immediately.
- Stoma size and shape: Most stomas protrude slightly from the abdomen. New stomas normally appear swollen, but swelling generally decreases over 2 or 3 weeks or for as long as 6 weeks.

Failure of swelling to recede may indicate a problem, for example, blockage.
- Stomal bleeding: Slight bleeding initially when the stoma is touched is normal, but other bleeding should be reported.
- Status of peristomal skin: Any redness and irritation of the peristomal skin—the 5 to 13 cm (2 to 5 in.) of skin surrounding the stoma—should be noted. Transient redness after removal of adhesive is normal.
- Amount and type of feces: Assess the amount, color, odor, and consistency. Inspect for abnormalities, such as pus or blood.
- Complaints: Complaints of burning sensation under the skin barrier may indicate skin breakdown. The presence of abdominal discomfort and/or distention also needs to be determined.
- The client's and family members' learning needs regarding the ostomy and self-care.
- The client's emotional status, especially strategies used to cope with the body image changes and the ostomy.

PLANNING
Review features of the appliance to ensure that all parts are present and function correctly.

> **Delegation**
> Care of a *new* ostomy is not delegated to UAP. However, aspects of ostomy function are observed during usual care and may be recorded by persons other than the nurse. Abnormal findings must be validated and interpreted by the nurse. In some agencies, UAP may remove and replace well-established ostomy appliances.

EQUIPMENT
- Clean gloves
- Bedpan
- Moisture-proof bag (for disposable pouches)
- Cleaning materials, including warm water, mild soap (optional), washcloth, towel
- Tissue or gauze pad
- Skin barrier (optional)
- Stoma measuring guide
- Pen or pencil and scissors
- New ostomy pouch with optional belt
- Tail closure clamp
- Deodorant for pouch (optional)

IMPLEMENTATION

Preparation

1. Determine the need for an appliance change.
   - Assess the used appliance for leakage of stool. **Rationale:** *Stool can irritate the peristomal skin.*
   - Ask the client about any discomfort at or around the stoma. **Rationale:** *A burning sensation may indicate breakdown beneath the faceplate of the pouch.*
   - Assess the fullness of the pouch. **Rationale:** *The weight of an overly full bag may loosen the skin barrier and separate it from the skin, causing the stool to leak and irritate the peristomal skin.*
2. If there is pouch leakage or discomfort at or around the stoma, change the appliance.
3. Select an appropriate time to change the appliance.
   - Avoid times close to meal or visiting hours. **Rationale:** *Ostomy odor and stool may reduce appetite or embarrass the client.*
   - Avoid times immediately after meals or the administration of any medications that may stimulate bowel evacuation. **Rationale:** *It is best to change the pouch when drainage is least likely to occur.*

Performance

1. Prior to performing the procedure, introduce self and verify the client's identity using agency protocol. Explain to the client what you are going to do, why it is necessary, and how he or she can participate. Discuss how the results will be used in planning further care or treatments. Changing an ostomy appliance should not cause discomfort, but it may be distasteful to the client. Communicate acceptance and support to the client. It is important to change the appliance competently and quickly. Include support persons as appropriate.
2. Perform hand hygiene, and observe appropriate infection control procedures. Apply clean gloves.
3. Provide for client privacy preferably in the bathroom, where clients can learn to deal with the ostomy as they would at home.
4. Assist the client to a comfortable sitting or lying position in bed or preferably a sitting or standing position in the bathroom. **Rationale:** *Lying or standing positions may facilitate smoother pouch application, that is, avoid wrinkles.*
5. Unfasten the belt if the client is wearing one.
6. Empty the pouch and remove the ostomy skin barrier.
   - Empty the contents of a drainable pouch through the bottom opening into a bedpan or toilet. **Rationale:** *Emptying before removing the pouch prevents spillage of stool onto the client's skin.*
   - If the pouch uses a clamp, do not throw it away as it can be reused.
   - Assess the consistency, color, and amount of stool.
   - Peel the skin barrier off slowly, beginning at the top and working downward, while holding the client's skin taut. **Rationale:** *Holding the skin taut minimizes client discomfort and prevents abrasion of the skin.*
   - Discard the disposable pouch in a moisture-proof bag.
7. Clean and dry the peristomal skin and stoma.
   - Use toilet tissue to remove excess stool.
   - Use warm water, mild soap (optional), and a washcloth to clean the skin and stoma. ❶ Check agency practice on the use of soap. **Rationale:** *Soap is sometimes not advised because it can be irritating to the skin.*

If soap is allowed, do not use deodorant or moisturizing soaps **Rationale:** *They may interfere with the adhesives in the skin barrier.*
   - Dry the area thoroughly by patting with a towel. **Rationale:** *Excess rubbing can abrade the skin.*
8. Assess the stoma and peristomal skin.
   - Inspect the stoma for color, size, shape, and bleeding.
   - Inspect the peristomal skin for any redness, ulceration, or irritation. Transient redness after the removal of adhesive is normal.
9. Place a piece of tissue or gauze over the stoma, and change it as needed. **Rationale:** *This absorbs any seepage from the stoma while the ostomy appliance is being changed.*
10. Prepare and apply the skin barrier (peristomal seal).
    - Use the guide ❷ to measure the size of the stoma.
    - On the backing of the skin barrier, trace a circle the same size as the stomal opening.
    - Cut out the traced stoma pattern to make an opening in the skin barrier. ❸ Make the opening no more than 1/8 to 1/4 inch larger than the stoma (Erwin-Toth, 2003). **Rationale:** *This allows space for the stoma to expand slightly when functioning and minimizes the risk of stool contacting peristomal skin.*

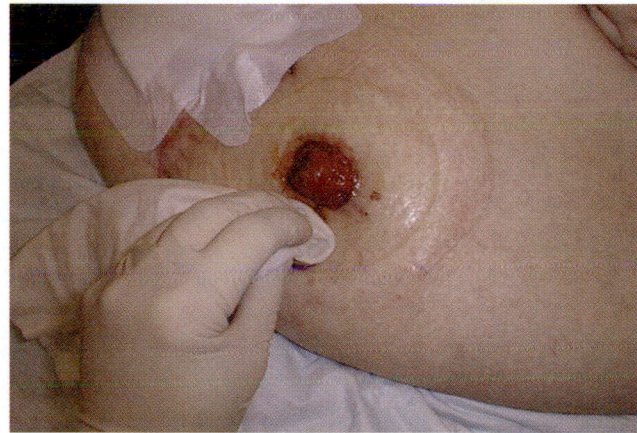

❶ Cleaning the skin.
(Cory Patrick Hartley, San Ramon Regional Medical Center, San Ramon, CA. Reprinted with permission.)

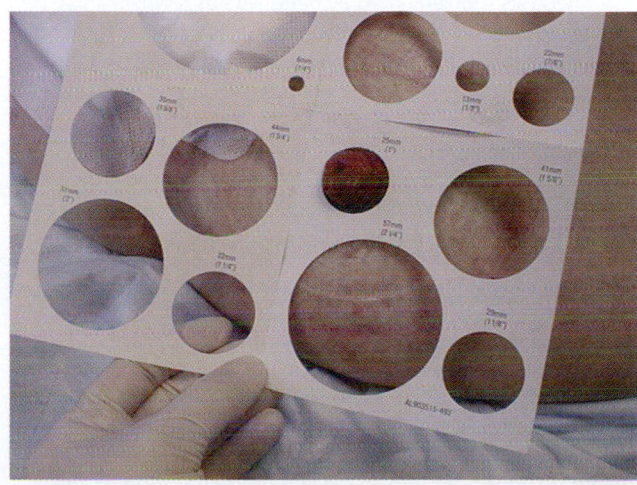

❷ A guide for measuring the stoma.
(Cory Patrick Hartley, San Ramon Regional Medical Center, San Ramon, CA. Reprinted with permission.)

(continued)

CHANGING A BOWEL DIVERSION OSTOMY APPLIANCE *(continued)*

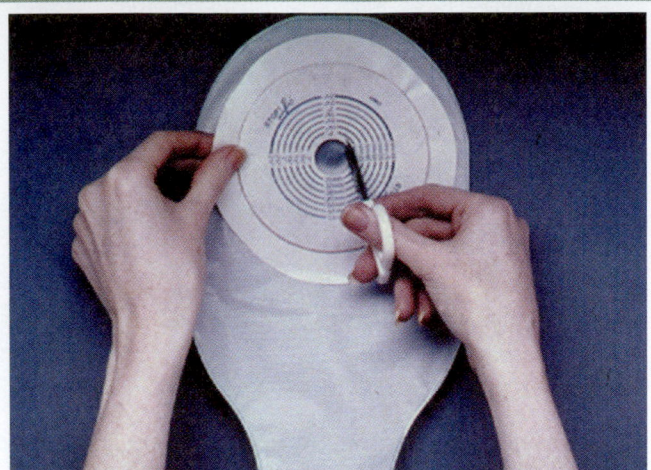

❸ The nurse is making a stoma opening on a disposable one-piece pouch.
(Courtesy of Convatec, a Bristol-Meyers Squibb Company.)

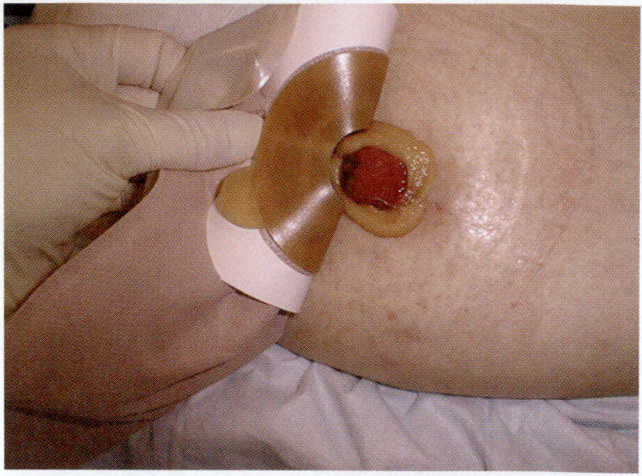

❹ Centering the skin barrier over the stoma.
(Cory Patrick Hartley, San Ramon Regional Medical Center, San Ramon, CA. Reprinted with permission.)

- Remove the backing to expose the sticky adhesive side. The backing can be saved and used as a pattern when making an opening for future skin barriers.
  For a one-piece pouching system:
- Center the one-piece skin barrier and pouch over the stoma, and gently press it onto the client's skin for 30 seconds. **Rationale:** *The heat and pressure help activate the adhesives in the skin barrier* ❹,❺.
  For a two-piece pouching system:
- Center the skin barrier over the stoma and gently press it onto the client's skin for 30 seconds.
- Remove the tissue over the stoma before applying the pouch.
- Snap the pouch onto the flange or skin barrier wafer.
- For drainable pouches, close the pouch according to the manufacturer's directions.

11. Document the procedure in the client record using forms or checklists supplemented by narrative notes when appropriate. Report and record pertinent assessments and interventions. Report any increase in stoma size, change in color indicative of circulatory impairment, and presence of skin irritation or erosion. Record on the client's chart discoloration of the stoma, the appearance of the peristomal skin, the amount and type of drainage, the client's reaction to the procedure, the client's experience with the ostomy, and skills learned by the client.

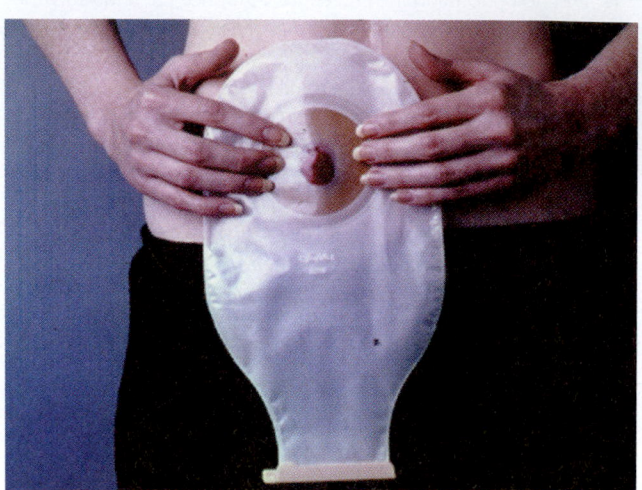

❺ Pressing the skin barrier of a disposable one-piece pouch for 30 seconds to activate the adhesives in the skin barrier.
(Courtesy of Convatec, a Bristol-Meyers Squibb Company.)

SAMPLE DOCUMENTATION

1/8/2010 0900 Colostomy bag changed. Moderate to large amount of semi-formed brown stool. Stoma reddish color. No redness or irritation around stoma. Client looked at stoma today and started asking questions as to how she will be able to change the pouch when she is home. Asked if she would like to do the next changing of the pouch. Stated "yes". ————————————————
———————————————————————— G. Hsu, RN

VARIATION: EMPTYING A DRAINABLE POUCH

- Empty the pouch when it is 1/3 to 1/2 full of stool or gas. **Rationale:** *Emptying before it is overfull helps avoid breaking the seal with the skin and stool then coming in contact with the skin.*
- Hold the pouch outlet over a bedpan or toilet. Lift the lower edge up.
- Unclamp or unseal the pouch.
- Drain the pouch.
- Clean the inside of the tail of the pouch with a tissue or a premoistened towelette.
- Apply the clamp or seal the pouch.
- Dispose of used supplies.
- Remove clean gloves. Perform hand hygiene.
- Document the amount, consistency, and color of stool.

EVALUATION

- Relate findings to previous data if available. Adjust the teaching plan and nursing care plan as needed. Reinforce the teaching each time the care is performed. Encourage and support self-care as soon as possible as clients should be able to perform self-care by discharge. **Rationale:** *Client learning is facilitated by consistent nursing interventions.*
- Perform detailed follow-up based on findings that deviated from expected or normal for the client. Report significant deviations from normal to the primary care provider.

COLOSTOMY IRRIGATION A colostomy irrigation, similar to an enema, is a form of stoma management used only for clients who have a sigmoid or descending colostomy. The purpose of irrigation is to distend the bowel sufficiently to stimulate peristalsis, which stimulates evacuation. When a regular evacuation pattern is achieved, the wearing of a colostomy pouch is unnecessary. Currently, colostomy irrigations are not routinely taught to most clients. Routine daily irrigations for control of the time of elimination ultimately become the client's decision. Some clients prefer to control the time of elimination through rigid dietary regulation and not be bothered with irrigations, which can take up to an hour to complete. When regulation by irrigation is chosen, it should be done at the same time each day. Control by irrigations also necessitates some control of the diet. For example, laxative foods that might cause an unexpected evacuation need to be avoided.

For most clients, a relatively small amount of fluid (300 to 500 mL) stimulates evacuation. For others, up to 1,000 mL may be needed because a colostomy has no sphincter and the fluid tends to return as it is instilled. This problem is reduced by the use of a cone on the irrigating catheter. The cone helps to hold the fluid within the bowel during the irrigation. Clients who have used irrigation for several years are more prone to peristomal hernias, bowel perforation, and electrolyte imbalance with large-volume irrigations (500 to 1,000 mL). Careful observation and assessment of this practice may be required in older, more fragile clients.

EVALUATING

The goals established during the planning phase are evaluated according to specific desired outcomes, also established in that phase. Examples of these are shown in Identifying Nursing Diagnoses, Outcomes, and Interventions earlier in this chapter.

If outcomes are not achieved, the nurse should explore the reasons. The nurse might consider some or all of the following questions:

- Were the client's fluid intake and diet appropriate?
- Was the client's activity level appropriate?
- Are prescribed medications or other factors affecting the gastrointestinal function?
- Do the client and family understand the provided instructions well enough to comply with the required therapy?
- Were sufficient physical and emotional support provided?

Nursing Care Plan Altered Bowel Elimination

ASSESSMENT DATA	NURSING DIAGNOSIS	DESIRED OUTCOMES
Nursing Assessment Mrs. Emma Brown is a 78-year-old widow of 9 months. She lives alone in a low-income housing complex for older adults. Her two children live with their families in a city approximately 150 miles away. She has always enjoyed cooking for her family; however, now that she is alone, she does not cook for herself. As a result, she has developed irregular eating patterns and tends to prepare soup-and-toast meals. She gets little exercise and has had bouts of insomnia since her husband's death. For the past month, Mrs. Brown has been having a problem with constipation. She states she has a bowel movement about every 3 to 4 days and her stools are hard and painful to excrete. Mrs. Brown decides to attend the health fair sponsored by the housing complex and seeks assistance from the county public health nurse.	*Constipation* related to low-fiber diet and inactivity (as evidenced by infrequent, hard stools; painful defecation; abdominal distention)	Bowel Elimination [0501], as evidenced by • Comfort of stool passage • Stool soft and formed • Passage of stool without aids

Physical Examination
Height: 162 cm (5′4″)
Weight: 65 kg (143 lb)
Temperature: 36.2°C (97.2°F)
Pulse: 82 BPM
Respirations: 20/minute
Blood pressure: 128/74 mm Hg
Active bowel sounds, abdomen slightly distended

Diagnostic Data
CBC: Hgb 10.8
Urinalysis negative

(continued)

NURSING INTERVENTIONS*/SELECTED ACTIVITIES	RATIONALE
Constipation/Impaction Management [0450]	
Identify factors (e.g., medications, bed rest, diet) that may cause or contribute to constipation.	*Assessing causative factors is an essential first step in teaching and planning for improved bowel elimination.*
Encourage increased fluid intake, unless contraindicated.	*Sufficient fluid intake is necessary for the bowel to absorb sufficient amounts of liquid to promote proper stool consistency.*
Evaluate medication profile for gastrointestinal side effects.	*Constipation is a common side effect of many drugs including narcotics and antacids.*
Teach Mrs. Brown how to keep a food diary.	*An appraisal of food intake will help identify if Mrs. Brown is eating a well-balanced diet and consuming adequate amounts of fluid and fiber. Excessive meat or refined food intake will produce small, hard stools.*
Instruct Mrs. Brown on a high-fiber diet, as appropriate.	*Fiber absorbs water, which adds bulk and softness to the stool and speeds up passage through the intestines.*
Instruct her on the relationship of diet, exercise, and fluid intake to constipation and impaction.	*Fiber without adequate fluid can aggravate, not facilitate, bowel function.*
Exercise Promotion [0200]	
Encourage verbalization of feelings about exercise or need for exercise.	*Perceptions of the need for exercise may be influenced by misconceptions, cultural and social beliefs, fears, or age.*
Determine her motivation to begin/continue an exercise program.	*Individuals who have been successful in an exercise program can assist Mrs. Brown by providing incentive and enhancing motivation. For example, a walking partner may be beneficial.*
Inform Mrs. Brown about the health benefits and physiologic effects of exercise.	*Activity influences bowel elimination by improving muscle tone and stimulating peristalsis.*
Instruct her about appropriate types of exercise for her level of health, in collaboration with a primary care provider.	*Any individual beginning an exercise program should consult a primary care provider primarily for a cardiac evaluation. Mrs. Brown's age and lack of activity should be considered in planning the level of activity.*
Assist Mrs. Brown to set short-term and long-term goals for the exercise program.	*Realistic goal setting provides direction and motivation.*

EVALUATION

Outcome not met. Mrs. Brown has kept a food diary and is able to identify the need for more fluid and fiber but has not consistently included fiber in her diet. She has started a walking program with a neighbor but is able to walk for only 10 minutes at a time twice a week. She states her last bowel movement was 3 days ago.

The NOC # for desired outcomes and the NIC # for nursing interventions are listed in brackets following the appropriate outcome or intervention. Outcomes, interventions, and activities selected are only a sample of those suggested by NOC and NIC and should be further individualized for each client.

CRITICAL THINKING QUESTIONS

1. You learn that Mrs. Brown's stools have been liquid, in very small amounts, and at infrequent intervals, generally occurring when she feels the urge to defecate. What additional data are important to obtain from her?

2. What nursing intervention is most appropriate before making suggestions to correct or prevent the problem she is experiencing?

3. What suggestions can you give her about maintaining a regular bowel pattern?

4. Explain why cathartics and laxatives are generally contraindicated for people in Mrs. Brown's situation.

∞ *See Answers in MyNursingKit.*

CONCEPT MAP   Altered Bowel Elimination

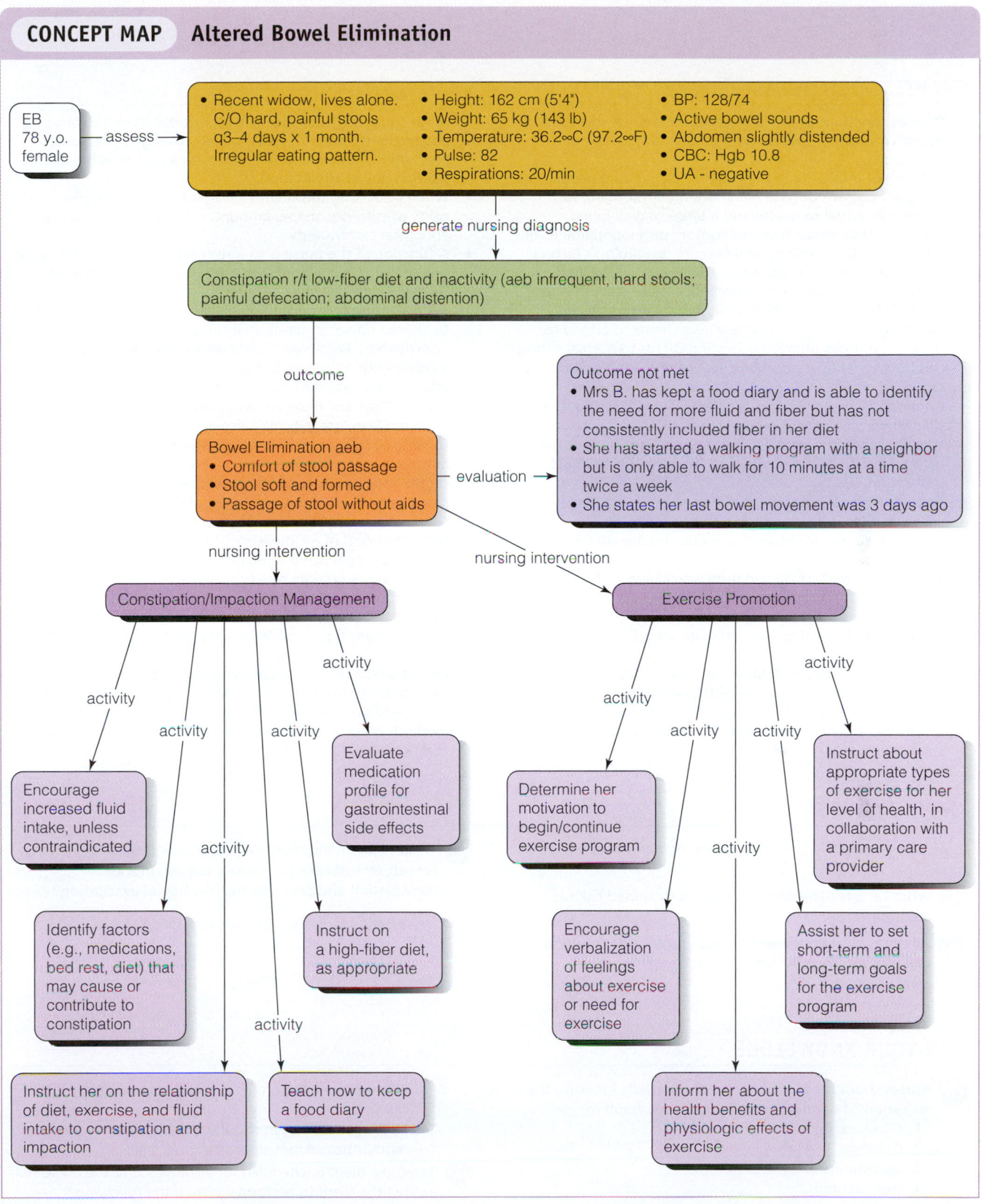

CHAPTER HIGHLIGHTS

- Primary functions of the large intestine are the excretion of digestive waste products and the maintenance of fluid balance.
- Patterns of fecal elimination vary greatly among people, but a regular pattern of fecal elimination with formed, soft stools is essential to health and a sense of well-being.
- A variety of factors affects defecation: developmental level, diet, fluid intake, activity and exercise, psychologic factors, regular defecation, medications, diagnostic procedures, anesthesia, and pathologic conditions.
- Normal defecation is often facilitated in both well and ill clients by providing privacy, teaching clients to attend to defecation urges promptly, assisting clients to normal sitting positions whenever possible, encouraging appropriate food and fluid intake, and scheduling regular exercise.
- Common fecal elimination problems include constipation, diarrhea, bowel incontinence, and flatulence. Each has specific defining characteristics and contributing causes that often relate to or are identical to the factors that affect defecation.
- Lack of exercise, irregular defecation habits, bland diets, and overuse of laxatives are all thought to contribute to constipation. Sufficient fluid and fiber intake are required to keep feces soft.
- An adverse effect of constipation is straining during defecation, during which the Valsalva maneuver may be used. Cardiac problems may ensue.
- An adverse effect of prolonged diarrhea is fluid and electrolyte imbalance.
- Assessment relative to fecal elimination includes a nursing history; physical examination of the abdomen, rectum, and anus; and in some situations, visualization studies, and inspection and analysis of stool for abnormal constituents such as blood.

- A nursing history includes data about the client's defecating pattern, description of feces and any changes, problems associated with elimination, and data about possible factors altering bowel elimination.
- When inspecting the client's stool, the nurse must observe its color, consistency, shape, amount, odor, and the presence of abnormal constituents.
- A function of the nurse is to assist clients with diet and bowel preparation before endoscopic and radiographic studies of the large intestine.
- NANDA-approved nursing diagnoses that relate specifically to altered bowel elimination include *Risk for Constipation, Constipation, Perceived Constipation, Diarrhea,* and *Bowel Incontinence.* However, because altered elimination patterns affect several areas of human functioning, diagnoses such as *Risk for Deficient Fluid Volume, Low Self-Esteem,* and *Risk for Impaired Skin Integrity* may also apply.
- Nursing strategies include administering cathartics and antidiarrheals; administering cleansing, carminative, or retention enemas; applying protective skin agents; monitoring fluid and electrolyte balance; and instructing clients in ways to promote normal defecation.
- Digital removal of an impaction should be carried out gently because of vagal nerve stimulation and subsequent depressed cardiac rate. A primary care provider's order is often necessary.
- The purpose of an enema is to increase peristalsis and the excretion of feces and flatus. Enemas are classified into four groups: cleansing, carminative, retention, and return-flow enemas.
- Clients who have bowel diversion ostomies require special care, with attention to psychologic adjustment, diet, and stoma and skin care. A variety of stoma management methods is available to these clients, depending on the type and position of the ostomy.

THINK ABOUT IT

Refer to the chapter-opening scenario and answer these questions.

1. What factors place Mrs. Pinnette at increased risk for constipation?

2. What physical assessment would you consider essential when caring for this client related to her report of constipation?

3. What recommendations would you suggest to this client for self-care at home to reduce the occurrence of constipation and promote healthy bowel evacuation?

∞ *See suggested responses to Think About It on MyNursingKit.*

TEST YOUR KNOWLEDGE

1. Nurses should teach clients that repeatedly ignoring the sensation of needing to defecate could result in
1. Constipation.
2. Diarrhea.
3. Incontinence.
4. Hemorrhoids.

2. When collecting a nursing history, which of the following statements provide evidence that an older adult who is prone to constipation is in need of further teaching?
1. "I need to drink one and a half to two quarts of liquids each day."
2. "I need to take a laxative such as milk of magnesia if I don't have a BM every day."

3. "If my bowel pattern changes on its own, I should call you."
4. "Eating my meals at regular times is likely to result in regular bowel movements."

3. Because a client is scheduled for a colonoscopy, the nurse will instruct the client to perform which of the following?
1. Oil retention enema.
2. Return flow enema.
3. High, large volume enema.
4. Low, small volume enema.

4. The nurse identifies which of the following data as indicating need to consult with the primary care

provider when caring for a client with an established colostomy?
1. The stoma extends 1/2 in. above the abdomen.
2. The skin under the appliance looks red briefly after removing the appliance.
3. The stoma color is a deep red-purple.
4. An ascending colostomy delivers liquid feces.

5. Which of the following is the most appropriate nursing goal for clients with diarrhea related to ingestion of an antibiotic for an upper respiratory infection?
1. The client will wear a medic-alert bracelet for antibiotic allergy.
2. The client will return to his or her previous fecal elimination pattern.
3. The client verbalizes the need to take an antidiarrheal medication prn.
4. The client will increase intake of insoluble fiber such as grains, rice, and cereals.

6. A client with a new stoma who has not had a bowel movement since surgery last week reports nausea. What is the appropriate nursing action?
1. Prepare to irrigate the colostomy.
2. After assessing the stoma and surrounding skin, notify the surgeon.
3. Assess bowel sounds and administer antiemetic.
4. Administer a bulk-forming laxative, and encourage increased fluids and exercise.

7. The nurse assesses a client's abdomen several days after abdominal surgery. It is firm, distended, and painful to palpate. The client reports feeling "bloated." The nurse consults with the surgeon, who orders an enema. The nurse prepares to give what kind of enema?
1. Soapsuds enema
2. Retention enema
3. Return flow enema
4. Oil retention enema

8. The nurse interprets which of the following as most likely indicating that a client is experiencing intestinal bleeding?
1. Large quantities of fat mixed with pale yellow liquid stool
2. Brown, formed stools
3. Semisoft tar-colored stools
4. Narrow, pencil-shaped stool

9. Which of the following nursing diagnoses is most applicable to a client with fecal incontinence? Select all that apply.
1. *Bowel Incontinence*
2. *Risk for Deficient Fluid Volume*
3. *Disturbed Body Image*
4. *Social Isolation*
5. *Risk for Impaired Skin Integrity*

10. A student nurse is assigned to care for a client with a sigmoidostomy. The student will assess which of the following ostomy sites?

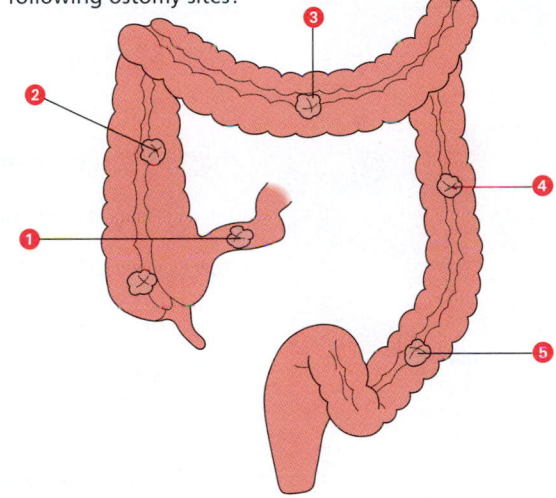

∞ *See answers to Test Your Knowledge in Appendix A.*

REFERENCES AND SELECTED BIBLIOGRAPHY

American Cancer Society (ACS). (2006). *How is colorectal cancer diagnosed?* Retrieved December 11, 2009, from http://www.cancer .org/docroot/CRI/content/CRI_2_4_3X_ How_is_colon_and_rectum_cancer_ diagnosed.asp?rnav=cri

Banks, N., & Razor, B. (2003). Preoperative stoma site assessment and marking: Trained RNs can improve ostomy outcomes. *American Journal of Nursing, 103*(3), 64A–64D.

Bliss, D. Z., Fischer, L., & Savik, K. (2005). Managing fecal incontinence: Self-care practices of older adults. *Journal of Gerontological Nursing, 31*(7), 35–44.

Bulechek, G. M., Butcher, H. K., & Dochterman, J. M. (Eds.). (2008). *Nursing interventions: classification (NIC)* (5th ed.). St. Louis, MO: Mosby.

Hinrichs, M., & Huseboe, J. (2001). Research-based protocol: Management of constipation. *Journal of Gerontological Nursing, 27*(2), 17–28.

Hollister, Inc. (n.d.). *Ostomy care FAQs.* Retrieved from http://www.hollister.com/ us/resource/faqs.asp?id=1

Hsieh, C. (2005). Treatment of constipation in older adults. *American Family Physician, 72*(11), 2277–2284.

Lemone, P., & Burke, K. (2008). *Medical-surgical nursing* (4th ed.). Upper Saddle River, NJ: Pearson Education.

Madsen, D., Sebolt, T., Cullen, L., Folkedahl, B., Mueller, T., Richardson, C., et al. (2005). Listening to bowel sounds: An evidence-based practice project. *American Journal of Nursing, 105*(12), 40–49.

Mauk, K. L. (2005). Preventing constipation in older adults. *Nursing, 35*(6), 22–23.

Moorhead, S., Johnson, M., Maas, M. L., & Swanson, E. (Eds.). (2008). *Nursing outcomes classification (NOC)* (4th ed.). St. Louis: Mosby.

NANDA International. (2009). *NANDA nursing diagnoses: Definitions and Classification 2009–2011.* West Sussex, U.K.: Wiley-Blackwell.

Peate, I. (2003). Nursing role in the management of constipation: Use of laxatives. *British Journal of Nursing, 12*(19), 1130–1136.

Ringhofer, J. (2005). Meeting the needs of your ostomy patient. *RN, 68*(8), 37–41.

Rushing, J. (2003). Administering an enema to an adult. *Nursing, 33*(11), 28.

Pullen, R. L. (2006). Teaching your patient to irrigate a colostomy. *Nursing, 36*(4), 22.

Oxygenation and Circulation

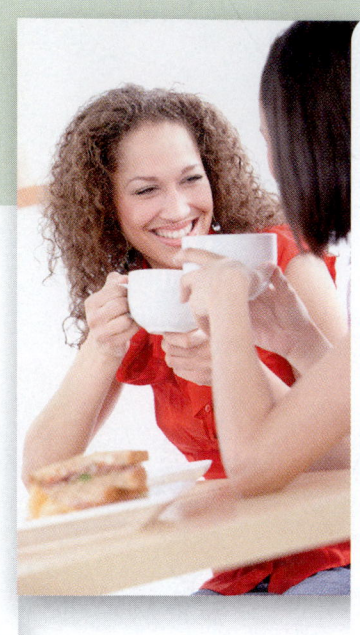

Martha Neidringhaus, 28 years old, is very excited. She and her best friend are taking a trip to Australia, and the day to leave is finally here. They plan to play card games the entire trip and keep a running score with a bet that whoever loses must pay for dinner their first night in Sydney. When the plane finally lands and Martha stands up to debark, she feels a sharp pain in her left calf. She decides it's nothing, just the result of sitting for so long, and anxiously leaves the plane looking forward to getting out of the airport and beginning their vacation.

As they are checking into the hotel in downtown Sydney, Martha suddenly feels short of breath and has a sharp right-sided pain in her chest. Since the pain is on her right chest and not her left, she doesn't think she is having a heart attack and decides she'll worry about it when she gets to her room. She finishes checking into the hotel and begins walking to the elevator but stops because the pain is so severe she can't stand it and she is so short of breath she feels like she is dying. The front desk clerk calls for emergency help, and she is rushed to a hospital emergency room where she is diagnosed with a pulmonary embolus.

LEARNING OUTCOMES

After completing this chapter, you will be able to:

1. Contrast the process of ventilation with the process of respiration.

2. Describe the impact of various factors on the function of the respiratory system and oxygenation.

3. Identify common manifestations of impaired respiratory functioning.

4. Apply the nursing process to promoting oxygenation when providing client care.

5. Contrast modifiable and nonmodifiable risk factors for impaired oxygenation and cardiovascular disease, including strategies for reducing risk.

6. Identify common manifestations and responses to alterations in cardiovascular disorders and impaired circulation.

7. Apply the nursing process to promoting circulation when providing client care.

OXYGENATION

Oxygen, a clear, odorless gas that constitutes approximately 21% of the air we breathe, is necessary for proper functioning of all living cells. The absence of oxygen can lead to cellular, tissue, and organism death. Although the delivery of oxygen to body tissues is affected at least indirectly by other body systems, the respiratory system is most directly involved in this process. Impaired function of the system can significantly affect our ability to breathe, transport gases, and participate in everyday activities.

Respiration is the process of gas exchange between the individual and the environment. The process of respiration involves three components:

1. Pulmonary ventilation or breathing; the movement of air between the atmosphere and the alveoli of the lungs as we inhale and exhale
2. Gas exchange, which involves diffusion of oxygen and carbon dioxide between the alveoli and pulmonary capillaries
3. Transport of oxygen from the lungs to the tissues, and carbon dioxide from the tissues to the lungs

Physiology of the Respiratory System

The function of the respiratory system is gas exchange. Oxygen from inspired air diffuses from alveoli in the lungs into the blood in pulmonary capillaries. Carbon dioxide produced during cell metabolism diffuses from the blood into the alveoli and is exhaled. The organs of the respiratory system facilitate this gas exchange and protect the body from foreign matter such as particulates and pathogens (Figure 35–1). The cough reflex also serves a protective function (Box 35–1).

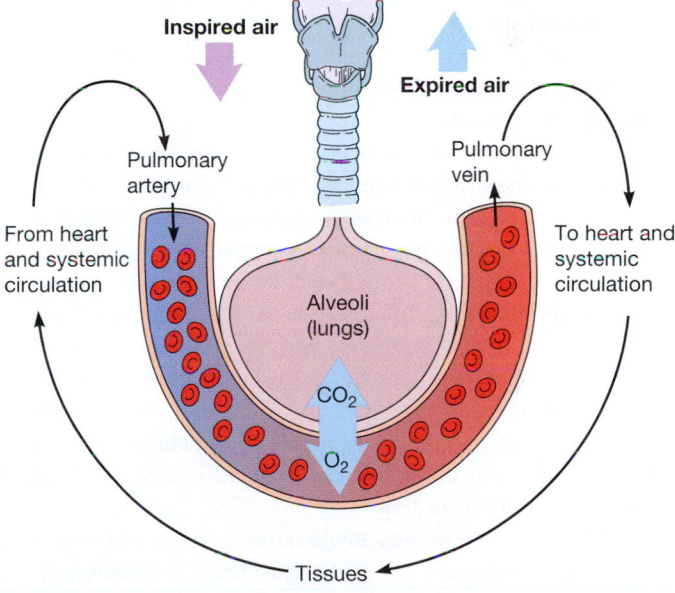

Figure 35–1 ● Gas exchange occurs between the air on the alveolar side and the blood on the capillary side.

BOX 35–1	The Cough Reflex

- Nerve impulses are sent through the vagus nerve to the medulla.
- A large inspiration of approximately 2.5 L occurs.
- The epiglottis and glottis (vocal cords) close.
- A strong contraction of abdominal and internal intercostal muscles dramatically raises the pressure in the lungs.
- The epiglottis and glottis open suddenly.
- Air rushes outward with great velocity.
- Mucus and any foreign particles are dislodged from the lower respiratory tract and are propelled up and out.

PULMONARY VENTILATION Ventilation of the lungs is accomplished through the act of breathing. Adequate ventilation depends on several factors:

- Clear airways
- An intact central nervous system and respiratory center
- An intact thoracic cavity capable of expanding and contracting
- Adequate pulmonary compliance and recoil

A number of mechanisms, including ciliary action and the cough reflex, work to keep airways open and clear in order for gas exchange to occur. In some cases, however, these defenses may be overwhelmed. The respiratory centers of the medulla and pons in the brainstem control breathing. Severe head injury or drugs that depress the central nervous system can affect the respiratory centers, impairing the drive to breathe.

Expansion and recoil of the lungs occurs passively in response to changes in pressures within the thoracic cavity and the lungs themselves. The **intrapleural pressure** (pressure in the pleural cavity surrounding the lungs) is always slightly negative in relation to atmospheric pressure. This negative pressure is essential because it creates the suction that holds the visceral pleura and the parietal pleura together as the chest cage expands and contracts. The **intrapulmonary pressure** (pressure within the lungs) always equalizes with atmospheric pressure.

The degree of chest expansion during normal breathing is minimal, requiring little energy expenditure. In adults, approximately 500 mL of air is inspired and expired with each breath. This is known as **tidal volume**. Breathing during strenuous exercise or some types of heart disease require greater chest expansion and effort. At this time, more than 1,500 mL of air may be moved with each breath. Accessory muscles of respiration, including the anterior neck muscles, intercostal muscles, and muscles of the abdomen, are employed. Active use of these muscles (retractions) and noticeable effort in breathing are frequently seen in clients with respiratory disorders.

Diseases such as muscular dystrophy or trauma such as spinal cord injury can affect the muscles of respiration impairing the ability of the thoracic cavity to expand and contract. A gunshot wound or other trauma to the chest wall may allow intrapleural pressure to equalize with the atmosphere, causing the lung to collapse.

Lung compliance, the expandability or stretchability of lung tissue, plays a significant role in the ease of ventilation. At birth, the fluid-filled lungs are stiff and resistant to expansion, much as a new balloon is difficult to inflate. With each subsequent breath, the alveoli become more compliant and easier to inflate, just as a balloon becomes easier to inflate after several tries. Lung compliance tends to decrease with aging, making it more difficult to expand alveoli and increasing risk of **atelectasis**, or collapse of a portion of the lung.

In contrast to lung compliance is **lung recoil**, the continual tendency of the lungs to collapse away from the chest wall. Just as lung compliance is necessary for normal inspiration, lung recoil is necessary for normal expiration. Although elastic fibers in lung tissue contribute to lung recoil, the surface tension of fluid lining the alveoli has the greatest effect on recoil. Fluid molecules tend to draw together, reducing the size of alveoli. **Surfactant**, a lipoprotein produced by specialized alveolar cells, acts like a detergent, reducing the surface tension of alveolar fluid. Without surfactant, lung expansion is exceedingly difficult and the lungs collapse.

ALVEOLAR GAS EXCHANGE After the alveoli are ventilated, the second phase of the respiratory process—the diffusion of oxygen from the alveoli and into the pulmonary blood vessels—begins. Diffusion is the movement of gases or other particles from an area of greater pressure or concentration to an area of lower pressure or concentration.

Pressure differences in the gases on each side of the respiratory membrane obviously affect diffusion. When the pressure of oxygen is greater in the alveoli than in the blood, oxygen diffuses into the blood. The partial pressure (the pressure exerted by each individual gas in a mixture according to its concentration in the mixture) of oxygen (PO_2) in the alveoli is about 100 mm Hg (sometimes referred to as torr, which is the same as millimeters of mercury), whereas the PO_2 in the venous blood of the pulmonary arteries is about 60 mm Hg. These pressures rapidly equalize, however, so that the arterial oxygen pressure also reaches about 100 mm Hg. By contrast, carbon dioxide in the venous blood entering the pulmonary capillaries has a partial pressure of about 45 mm Hg (PCO_2), whereas that in the alveoli has a partial pressure of about 40 mm Hg. Therefore, carbon dioxide diffuses from the blood into the alveoli, where it can be eliminated with expired air. When referring to the pressure of oxygen in the arterial blood the abbreviation is PaO_2. When referring to partial pressure in venous blood there is no "a," that is, PO_2.

TRANSPORT OF OXYGEN AND CARBON DIOXIDE The third part of the respiratory process involves the transport of respiratory gases. Oxygen needs to be transported from the lungs to the tissues, and carbon dioxide must be transported from the tissues back to the lungs. Normally most of the oxygen (97%) combines loosely with hemoglobin (oxygen-carrying red pigment) in the red blood cells and is carried to the tissues as **oxyhemoglobin** (the compound of oxygen and hemoglobin). The remaining oxygen is dissolved and transported in the fluid of the plasma and cells.

Several factors affect the rate of oxygen transport from the lungs to the tissues:

1. Cardiac output
2. Number of erythrocytes and blood hematocrit
3. Exercise

Any pathologic condition that decreases cardiac output diminishes the amount of oxygen delivered to the tissues. The heart compensates for inadequate output by increasing its pumping rate or heart rate; however, with severe damage or blood loss, this compensatory mechanism may not restore adequate blood flow and oxygen to the tissues.

The second factor influencing oxygen transport is the number of erythrocytes and the hematocrit. The hematocrit is the percentage of the blood that is erythrocytes. Excessive increases in the blood hematocrit raise the blood viscosity, reducing the cardiac output and therefore reducing oxygen transport. Excessive reductions in the blood hematocrit, such as occur in anemia, reduce oxygen transport.

Exercise also has a direct influence on oxygen transport. In well-trained athletes, oxygen transport can be increased up to 20 times the normal rate, due in part to an increased cardiac output and to increased use of oxygen by the cells.

Carbon dioxide, continually produced in the processes of cell metabolism, is transported from the cells to the lungs in three ways. The majority (about 65%) is carried inside the red blood cells as bicarbonate (HCO_3^-) and is an important component of the bicarbonate buffer system (see Chapter 36 ∞). A moderate amount of carbon dioxide (30%) combines with hemoglobin as carbhemoglobin (also known as carbaminohemoglobin) for transport. Smaller amounts (5%) are transported in solution in the plasma and as carbonic acid (the compound formed when carbon dioxide combines with water).

RESPIRATORY REGULATION Respiratory regulation includes both neural and chemical controls to maintain the correct concentrations of oxygen, carbon dioxide, and hydrogen ions in body fluids. The nervous system of the body adjusts the rate of alveolar ventilations to meet the needs of the body so that PO_2 and PCO_2 remain relatively constant. The body's "respiratory center" is actually a number of groups of neurons located in the medulla oblongata and pons of the brain.

A chemosensitive center in the medulla oblongata is highly responsive to increases in blood CO_2 or hydrogen ion concentration. By influencing other respiratory centers, this center can increase the activity of the inspiratory center and the rate and depth of respirations. In addition to this direct chemical stimulation of the respiratory center in the brain, special neural receptors sensitive to decreases in O_2 concentration are located outside the central nervous system in the carotid bodies (just above the bifurcation of the common carotid arteries) and aortic bodies located above and below the aortic arch. Decreases in arterial oxygen concentrations stimulate these chemoreceptors, and they in turn stimulate the respiratory center to increase ventilation. Of the three blood gases (hydrogen, oxygen, and carbon dioxide) that can trigger chemoreceptors, increased carbon dioxide concentration normally has the strongest effect on stimulating respiration. However, in clients with certain chronic lung ailments such as **emphysema**, oxygen concentrations, not carbon dioxide concentrations, play a major role in regulating respiration. For such clients, decreased oxygen concentrations are the main stimuli for respiration because the chronically elevated carbon dioxide levels that occur with emphysema "desensitize" the central chemoreceptors. This is sometimes called the hypoxic drive. Increasing the concentration of oxygen depresses the respiratory rate. Thus, only low concentrations of supplemental oxygen are administered to these clients.

CLINICAL ALERT

In clients with chronic obstructive lung disease, administering too much supplemental oxygen can actually cause the client to stop breathing.

Factors Affecting Respiratory Function

Factors that influence oxygenation affect the cardiovascular system as well as the respiratory system. These factors include age, environment, lifestyle, health status, medications, and stress.

AGE Developmental factors are important influences on respiratory function. At birth, profound changes occur in the respiratory systems. The fluid-filled lungs drain, the PCO_2 rises, and the neonate takes a first breath. The lungs gradually expand with each subsequent breath, reaching full inflation by 2 weeks of age. Changes of aging that affect the respiratory system of older adults become especially important if the system is compromised by changes such as infection, physical or emotional stress, surgery, anesthesia, or other procedures. Changes are:

- Chest wall and airways become more rigid and less elastic.
- The amount of exchanged air is decreased.
- The cough reflex and cilia action are decreased.
- Mucous membranes become drier and more fragile.
- Decreases in muscle strength and endurance occur.
- If osteoporosis is present, adequate lung expansion may be compromised.
- A decrease in efficiency of the immune system occurs.
- Gastroesophageal reflux disease is more common in older adults and increases the risk of aspiration. The aspiration of stomach contents into the lungs often causes bronchospasm by setting up an inflammatory response.

ENVIRONMENT Altitude, heat, cold, and air pollution affect oxygenation. The higher the altitude, the lower the PO_2 an individual breathes. As a result, the person at high altitudes has increased respiratory and cardiac rates and increased respiratory depth, which usually become most apparent when the individual exercises. Healthy people exposed to air pollution, such as smog or secondhand smoke, may experience stinging of the eyes, headache, dizziness, coughing, and choking. People who have a history of existing lung disease and altered respiratory function experience varying degrees of respiratory difficulty in a polluted environment. Some are unable to perform self-care in such an environment.

LIFESTYLE Physical exercise or activity increases the rate and depth of respirations and hence the supply of oxygen in the body. Sedentary people, by contrast, lack the alveolar expansion and deep breathing patterns of people with regular activity and are less able to respond effectively to respiratory stressors. Certain occupations predispose an individual to lung disease.

HEALTH STATUS In the healthy person, the respiratory system can provide sufficient oxygen to meet the body's needs.

LIFESPAN CONSIDERATIONS   Respiratory Development

Infants

- Respiratory rates are highest and most variable in newborns. The respiratory rate of a neonate is 40 to 80 breaths per minute.
- Infant respiratory rates average about 30 per minute.
- Because of rib cage structure, infants rely almost exclusively on diaphragmatic movement for breathing. This is seen as abdominal breathing, as the abdomen rises and falls with each breath.

Children

- The respiratory rate gradually decreases, averaging around 25 per minute in the preschooler and reaching the adult rate of 12 to 18 per minute by late adolescence.
- During infancy and childhood, upper respiratory infections are common and, fortunately, usually not serious. Infants and preschoolers also are at risk for airway obstruction by foreign objects such as coins and small toys. Cystic fibrosis is a congenital disorder that affects the lungs, causing them to become congested with thick, tenacious (sticky) mucus. Asthma is another chronic disease often identified in childhood. The airways of the asthmatic child react to stimuli such as allergens, exercise, or cold air by constricting, becoming edematous, and producing excessive mucus. Airflow is impaired, and the child may wheeze as air moves through narrowed air passages.

Older Adults

- Older adults are at increased risk for acute respiratory diseases such as pneumonia and chronic diseases such as emphysema and chronic bronchitis. Chronic obstructive pulmonary disease (COPD) may affect older adults, particularly after years of exposure to cigarette smoke or industrial pollutants.
- Pneumonia may not present with the usual symptoms of a fever, but will present with atypical symptoms, such as confusion, weakness, loss of appetite, and increase in heart rate and respirations.

Nursing interventions should be directed toward achieving optimal respiratory effort and gas exchange:

- Always encourage wellness and prevention of disease by reinforcing the need for good nutrition, exercise, and immunizations, such as for influenza and pneumonia.
- Increase fluid intake, if not contraindicated by other problems, such as cardiac or renal impairment.
- Proper positioning and frequent changing of positions allow for better lung expansion and air and fluid movement.
- Teach the client to use breathing techniques for better air exchange (see Client Teaching boxes throughout this chapter).
- Pace activities to conserve energy.
- Encourage the client to eat more frequent, smaller meals to decrease gastric distention, which can cause pressure on the diaphragm.
- Teach the client to avoid extreme hot or cold temperatures that will further tax the respiratory system.
- Teach actions and side effects of drugs, inhalers, and treatments.

Diseases of the respiratory system, however, can adversely affect the oxygenation of the blood.

MEDICATIONS A variety of medications can decrease the rate and depth of respirations. The most common medications with this effect are narcotics, benzodiazepine sedative-hypnotics, and antianxiety drugs. When administering these, the nurse must carefully monitor respiratory status, especially when the medication is begun or when the dose is increased. Although this is a safety concern, usually the importance of the medication outweighs the risk of respiratory depression.

STRESS When stress and stressors are encountered, both psychologic and physiologic responses can affect oxygenation. Some people may hyperventilate in response to stress. When this occurs, arterial PO_2 rises and PCO_2 falls. The person may experience light-headedness and numbness and tingling of the fingers, toes, and around the mouth as a result. Physiologically, the sympathetic nervous system is stimulated and epinephrine is released during stress. Epinephrine causes the bronchioles to dilate, increasing blood flow and oxygen delivery to active muscles. Although these responses are adaptive in the short term, when stress continues they can be destructive, increasing the risk of cardiovascular disease.

ALTERATIONS IN RESPIRATORY FUNCTION

Respiratory function can be altered by conditions that affect:

- The movement of air into or out of the lungs.
- The diffusion of oxygen and carbon dioxide between the alveoli and the pulmonary capillaries.
- The transport of oxygen and carbon dioxide via the blood to and from the tissue cells.

Three major alterations in respiration are hypoxia, altered breathing patterns, and obstructed or partially obstructed airway.

Hypoxia

Hypoxia is a condition of insufficient oxygen anywhere in the body, from the inspired gas to the tissues. It can be related to any of the parts of respiration—ventilation, diffusion of gases, or transport of gases by the blood—and can be caused by any condition that alters one or more parts of the process. The Clinical Manifestations box lists signs of hypoxia.

Hypoventilation, that is, inadequate alveolar ventilation, can lead to hypoxia. Hypoventilation may occur because of

> **CLINICAL MANIFESTATIONS**   **Hypoxia**
>
> - Rapid pulse
> - Rapid, shallow respirations and dyspnea
> - Increased restlessness or light-headedness
> - Flaring of the nares
> - Substernal or intercostal retractions
> - Cyanosis

diseases of the respiratory muscles, drugs, or anesthesia. With hypoventilation, carbon dioxide often accumulates in the blood, a condition called **hypercarbia (hypercapnia)**.

Hypoxia can also develop when the diffusion of oxygen from alveoli into the arterial blood decreases, as with pulmonary edema or pneumonia, or it can result from problems in the delivery of oxygen to the tissues (e.g., anemia, heart failure, and embolism). The term **hypoxemia** refers to reduced oxygen in the blood and is characterized by a low partial pressure of oxygen in arterial blood or low hemoglobin saturation.

Cyanosis (bluish discoloration of the skin, nailbeds, and mucous membranes, due to reduced hemoglobin-oxygen saturation) may be present when there is hypoxemia. Cyanosis requires these two conditions: The blood must contain about 5 g or more of unoxygenated hemoglobin per 100 mL of blood, and the surface blood capillaries must be dilated. Factors that interfere with either of these conditions (e.g., severe anemia or the administration of epinephrine) will eliminate cyanosis as a sign even if the client is experiencing hypoxia.

Adequate oxygenation is essential for cerebral functioning. The cerebral cortex can tolerate hypoxia for only 3 to 5 minutes before permanent damage occurs. The face of the acutely hypoxic person usually appears anxious, tired, and drawn. The person usually assumes a sitting position, often leaning forward slightly to permit greater expansion of the thoracic cavity.

With chronic hypoxia, the client often appears fatigued and is lethargic. The client's fingers and toes may be clubbed as a result of long-term lack of oxygen in the arterial blood supply. With clubbing, the base of the nail becomes swollen and the ends of the fingers and toes increase in size. The angle between the nail and the base of the nail increases to more than 180 degrees. See Figure 17–6 in Chapter 17 ∞.

Altered Breathing Patterns

Breathing patterns refer to the rate, volume, rhythm, and relative ease or effort of respiration. Normal respiration (**eupnea**) is quiet, rhythmic, and effortless. **Tachypnea** (rapid rate) is seen with fevers, metabolic acidosis, pain, and hypercapnia or hypoxemia. **Bradypnea** is an abnormally slow respiratory rate, which may be seen in clients who have taken drugs such as morphine, who have metabolic alkalosis, or who have increased intracranial pressure. **Apnea** is the cessation of breathing.

Hyperventilation, often called *alveolar hyperventilation,* is an increased movement of air into and out of the lungs. During hyperventilation, the rate and depth of respirations increase, and more CO_2 is eliminated than is produced. One particular type of hyperventilation that accompanies metabolic acidosis is **Kussmaul's breathing**, by which the body attempts to compensate by blowing off carbon dioxide through deep and rapid breathing. Hyperventilation can also occur in response to stress or anxiety.

Abnormal respiratory rhythms create an irregular breathing pattern. Two abnormal respiratory rhythms are

- **Cheyne-Stokes respirations.** Marked rhythmic waxing and waning of respirations from very deep to very shallow breathing and temporary apnea; common causes include congestive heart failure, increased intracranial pressure, and overdose of certain drugs. This type of breathing is frequently seen in those nearing death as well as clients with acute severe increased intracranial pressure.
- **Biot's (cluster) respirations.** Shallow breaths interrupted by apnea; may be seen in clients with central nervous system disorders.

Orthopnea is the inability to breathe except in an upright or standing position. Difficult or uncomfortable breathing is called **dyspnea**. The dyspneic person often appears anxious and may experience *shortness of breath* (SOB), a feeling of being unable to get enough air. Often the nostrils are flared because of the increased effort of inspiration. The skin may appear dusky; heart rate is increased. Dyspnea may have many causes, most of which stem from cardiac or respiratory disorders. It is a subjective feeling; that is, dyspnea may not be directly observed or measured but is reported by the client. Since treatment is aimed at removing the underlying cause, it is important for the nurse to conduct a thorough history of the onset, duration, and precipitating and relieving factors of the client's dyspnea plus a comprehensive physical examination.

Obstructed Airway

A completely or partially obstructed airway can occur anywhere along the upper or lower respiratory passageways. An upper airway obstruction—that is, in the nose, pharynx, or larynx—can arise because of a foreign object such as food, because the tongue falls back into the oropharynx when a person is unconscious, or when secretions collect in the passageways. In the latter instance, the respirations will sound gurgly or bubbly as the air attempts to pass through the secretions. Lower airway obstruction involves partial or complete occlusion of the passageways in the bronchi and lungs most often due to increased accumulation of mucus or inflammatory exudate.

Assessing for and maintaining an open (patent) airway is a nursing responsibility, one that often requires immediate action. Partial obstruction of the upper airway passages is indicated by a low-pitched snoring sound during inhalation. Complete obstruction is indicated by extreme inspiratory effort that produces no chest movement and an inability to cough or speak. Such a client, in an effort to obtain air, may also exhibit marked sternal and intercostal retractions. Lower airway obstruction is not always as easy to observe. **Stridor**, a harsh, high-pitched sound, may be heard during inspiration. The client may have altered arterial blood gas levels, restlessness, dyspnea, and **adventitious breath sounds** (abnormal breath sounds). See Table 17–9 in Chapter 17 ∞.

NURSING MANAGEMENT

ASSESSING

Nursing History

A comprehensive nursing history relevant to oxygenation status should include data about current and past respiratory problems; lifestyle; presence of cough, **sputum** (expectorated material), or pain; medications for breathing; and presence of risk factors for impaired oxygenation status. Examples of interview questions to elicit this information are shown in the Assessment Interview.

Physical Examination

In assessing a client's oxygenation status, the nurse uses all four physical examination techniques: inspection, palpation, percussion, and auscultation. The nurse first observes the rate, depth, rhythm, and quality of respirations, noting the position the client assumes for breathing. The nurse also inspects for variations in the shape of the thorax that may indicate adaptation to chronic respiratory conditions. For example, clients with emphysema frequently develop a *barrel chest.*

The nurse palpates the thorax for bulges, tenderness, or abnormal movements. Palpation is also used to detect vocal (tactile) fremitus. The thorax can be percussed for diaphragmatic excursion (the movement of the diaphragm during maximal inspiration and expiration). However, this is not commonly done in acute care and long-term care settings. And the nurse frequently auscultates the chest to assess if the client's breath sounds are normal or abnormal. See Chapter 17 ∞, Skill 17–10, "Assessing the Thorax and Lungs" for more information.

Diagnostic Studies

The primary care provider may order various diagnostic tests to assess respiratory status, function, and oxygenation. Included are sputum specimens, throat cultures, visualization procedures (see Chapter 20 ∞), venous and arterial blood specimens, and pulmonary function tests.

Measurement of arterial blood gases is an important diagnostic procedure (see Chapter 36 ∞). Specimens of arterial blood are normally taken by specialty nurses, respiratory therapists, or medical technicians. Blood for these tests is taken directly from the radial, brachial, or femoral arteries or from catheters placed in these arteries. Because of the relatively great pressure of the blood in these arteries, it is important to prevent hemorrhaging by applying pressure to the puncture site for about 5 minutes after removing the needle. Frequently the noninvasive measurement of oxygen saturation (using a device placed on the fingertip) is sufficient for attaining a measurement of oxygenation of the arterial blood.

PULMONARY FUNCTION TESTS Pulmonary function tests measure lung volume and capacity. Clients undergoing pulmonary function tests, which are usually carried out by a respiratory therapist, do not require an anesthetic. The client breathes into a machine. The tests are painless, but the client's cooperation is essential. It requires the ability to follow directions and some hand-eye coordination. Nurses need to explain the tests to clients beforehand and help them to rest afterward because the tests are often tiring. Table 35–1 describes the measurements taken, and Figure 35–2 shows their relationships and normal adult values.

TABLE 35–1	Pulmonary Volumes and Capacities
MEASUREMENT	**DESCRIPTION**
Tidal volume (V_T)	Volume inhaled and exhaled during normal quiet breathing
Inspiratory reserve volume (IRV)	Maximum amount of air that can be inhaled over and above a normal breath
Expiratory reserve volume (ERV)	Maximum amount of air that can be exhaled following a normal exhalation
Residual volume (RV)	The amount of air remaining in the lungs after maximal exhalation
Total lung capacity (TLC)	The total volume of the lungs at maximum inflation; calculated by adding the V_T, IRV, ERV, and RV
Vital capacity (VC)	Total amount of air that can be exhaled after a maximal inspiration; calculated by adding the V_T, IRV, and ERV
Inspiratory capacity	Total amount of air that can be inhaled following normal quiet exhalation; calculated by adding the V_T and IRV
Functional residual capacity (FRC)	The volume left in the lungs after normal exhalation; calculated by adding the ERV and RV
Minute volume (MV)	The total volume or amount of air breathed in 1 minute

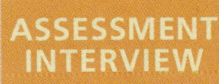

ASSESSMENT INTERVIEW

Oxygenation

Current Respiratory Problems

- Have you noticed any changes in your breathing pattern (e.g., shortness of breath, difficulty in breathing, need to be in upright position to breathe, or rapid and shallow breathing)?
- If so, which of your activities might cause these symptom(s) to occur?
- How many pillows do you use to sleep at night?

History of Respiratory Disease

- Have you had colds, allergies, asthma, tuberculosis, bronchitis, pneumonia, or emphysema?
- How frequently have these occurred? How long did they last? And how were they treated?
- Have you been exposed to any pollutants?

Lifestyle

- Do you smoke? If so, how much? If not, did you smoke previously, and when did you stop?
- Does any member of your family smoke?
- Is there cigarette smoke or other pollutants (e.g., fumes, dust, coal, asbestos) in your workplace?
- Do you use alcohol? If so, how many drinks (mixed drinks, glasses of wine, or beers) do you usually have per day or per week?
- Describe your exercise patterns. How often do you exercise and for how long?

Presence of Cough

- How often and how much do you cough?
- Is it productive, that is, accompanied by sputum, or nonproductive, that is, dry?
- Does the cough occur during certain activity or at certain times of the day?

Description of Sputum

- When is the sputum produced?
- What is the amount, color, thickness, odor?
- Is it ever tinged with blood?

Presence of Chest Pain

- How does going outside in the heat or the cold affect you?
- Do you experience any pain with breathing or activity?
- Where is the pain located?
- Describe the pain. How does it feel?
- Does it occur when you breathe in or out?
- How long does it last, and how does it affect your breathing?
- Do you experience any other symptoms when the pain occurs (e.g., nausea, shortness of breath or difficulty breathing, lightheadedness, palpitations)?
- What activities precede your pain?
- What do you do to relieve the pain?

Presence of Risk Factors

- Do you have a family history of lung cancer, cardiovascular disease (including strokes), or tuberculosis?
- The nurse should also note the client's weight, activity pattern, and dietary assessment. Risk factors include obesity, sedentary lifestyle, and diet high in saturated fats.

Medication History

- Have you taken or do you take any over-the-counter or prescription medications for breathing (e.g., bronchodilator, inhalant, narcotic)?
- If so, which ones? And what are the dosages, times taken, and results, including side effects?

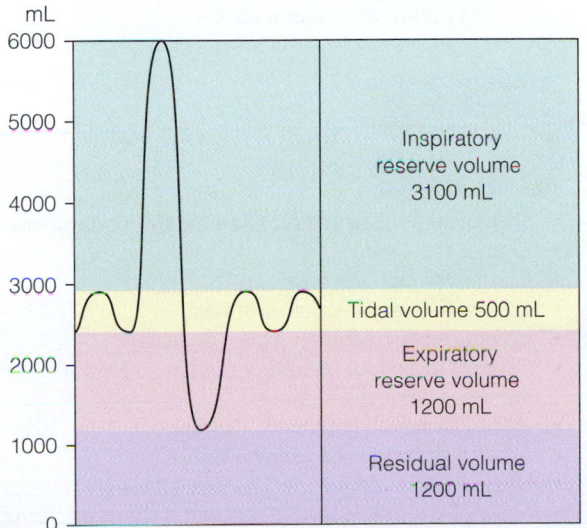
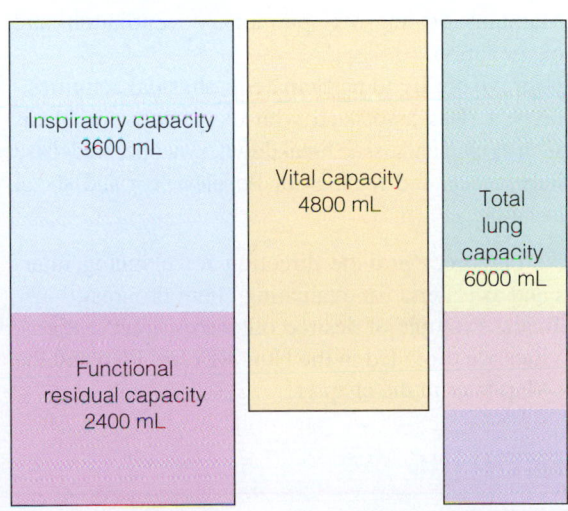

Figure 35–2 ● The relationship of lung volumes and capacities. Volumes (mL) shown are for an average adult male; female volumes are 20% to 25% smaller.

DIAGNOSING

NANDA includes the following diagnostic labels for clients with oxygenation problems:

- *Ineffective Airway Clearance:* Inability to clear secretions or obstructions from the respiratory tract to maintain a clear airway. A clinical example using this nursing diagnosis is shown in the Nursing Care Plan and the Concept Map later in the chapter.
- *Ineffective Breathing Pattern:* Inspiration and/or expiration that does not provide adequate ventilation.
- *Impaired Gas Exchange:* Excess or deficit in oxygenation and/or carbon dioxide elimination at the alveolar-capillary membrane.
- *Activity Intolerance:* Insufficient physiological or psychological energy to endure or complete required or desired daily activities.

The preceding nursing diagnoses may also be the etiology of several other nursing diagnoses. Examples follow:

- *Anxiety* related to ineffective airway clearance and feeling of suffocation
- *Fatigue* related to ineffective breathing pattern
- *Fear* related to chronic disabling respiratory illness
- *Powerlessness* related to inability to maintain independence in self-care activities because of ineffective breathing pattern
- *Insomnia* related to orthopnea and required O_2 therapy
- *Social Isolation* related to activity intolerance and inability to travel to usual social activities

PLANNING

The overall outcomes/goals for a client with oxygenation problems are to:

- Maintain a patent airway.
- Improve comfort and ease of breathing.
- Maintain or improve pulmonary ventilation and oxygenation.
- Improve ability to participate in physical activities.
- Prevent risks associated with oxygenation problems such as skin and tissue breakdown, syncope, acid–base imbalances, and feelings of hopelessness and social isolation.

These outcomes provide direction for planning interventions and as criteria for evaluating client progress.

A clinical example of desired outcomes, interventions, and activities are provided in the Nursing Care Plan and the Concept Map later in the chapter.

IMPLEMENTING

Examples of nursing interventions to facilitate pulmonary ventilation may include ensuring a patent airway, positioning, encouraging deep breathing and coughing, and ensur-

ing adequate hydration. Other nursing interventions helpful to ventilation are suctioning, lung inflation techniques, administration of analgesics before deep breathing and coughing, postural drainage, and percussion and vibration. Nursing strategies to facilitate the diffusion of gases through the alveolar membrane include encouraging coughing, deep breathing, and suitable activity. A client's nursing care plan should also include appropriate dependent nursing interventions such as oxygen therapy, tracheostomy care, and maintenance of a chest tube.

Promoting Oxygenation

Most people in good health give little thought to their respiratory function. Changing position frequently, ambulating, and exercising usually maintain adequate ventilation and gas exchange. Client Teaching lists other ways to promote healthy breathing.

When people become ill, however, their respiratory functions may be inhibited for such reasons as pain and immobility. Shallow respirations inhibit both diaphragmatic excursion and lung distensibility. The result of inadequate chest expansion is pooling of respiratory secretions, which ultimately harbor microorganisms and promote infection. Additionally, shallow respirations may potentiate alveolar collapse which may cause decreased diffusion of gases and subsequent hypoxemia. This situation is often compounded by giving narcotics for pain, because narcotics further depress the rate and depth of respiration.

Interventions by the nurse to maintain the normal respirations of clients include:

- Positioning the client to allow for maximum chest expansion.
- Encouraging or providing frequent changes in position.
- Encouraging ambulation.
- Implementing measures that promote comfort, such as giving pain medications.

CLIENT TEACHING   **Promoting Healthy Breathing**

- Sit straight and stand erect to permit full lung expansion.
- Exercise regularly.
- Breathe through the nose.
- Breathe in to expand the chest fully.
- Do not smoke cigarettes, cigars, or pipes.
- Eliminate or reduce the use of household pesticides and irritating chemical substances.
- Do not incinerate garbage in the house.
- Avoid exposure to secondhand smoke.
- Use building materials that do not emit vapors.
- Make sure furnaces, ovens, and wood stoves are correctly ventilated.
- Support a pollution-free environment.

The semi-Fowler's or high Fowler's position allows maximum chest expansion in clients who are confined to bed, particularly those with dyspnea. The nurse also encourages clients to turn from side to side frequently, so that alternate sides of the chest are permitted maximum expansion. Dyspneic clients often sit in bed and lean over their overbed tables, usually with a pillow for support. This orthopneic position is an adaptation of the high Fowler's position. It has a further advantage in that, unlike in high Fowler's, the abdominal organs are not pressing on the diaphragm. Also, a client in the orthopneic position can press the lower part of the chest against the table to help in exhaling.

Deep Breathing and Coughing

The nurse can facilitate respiratory functioning by encouraging deep breathing exercises and coughing to remove secretions from the airways. When coughing raises secretions high enough, the client may either **expectorate** (spit out) or swallow them. Swallowing the secretions is not harmful but does not allow the nurse to view the secretions for documentation purposes or to obtain a specimen for testing.

Breathing exercises are frequently indicated for clients with restricted chest expansion, such as people with chronic obstructive pulmonary disease (COPD) or clients recovering from thoracic surgery.

A commonly employed breathing exercise is *abdominal (diaphragmatic)* and pursed-lip breathing. Abdominal breathing permits deep full breaths with little effort. Pursed-lip breathing helps the client develop control over breathing. The pursed lips create a resistance to the air flowing out of the lungs, thereby prolonging exhalation and preventing airway collapse by maintaining positive airway pressure. The client purses the lips as if about to whistle and breathes out slowly and gently, tightening the abdominal muscles to exhale more effectively. The client usually inhales to a count of 3 and exhales to a count of 7.

Forceful coughing is often less effective than using controlled or huff coughing techniques. Instructions for abdominal (diaphragmatic) and pursed-lip breathing are provided in the Client Teaching.

Hydration

Adequate hydration maintains the moisture of the respiratory mucous membranes. Normally, respiratory tract secretions are thin and are therefore moved readily by ciliary action. However, when the client is dehydrated or when the environment has a low humidity, the respiratory secretions can become thick and tenacious. Fluid intake should be as great as the client can tolerate. See Chapter 36 ∞ for normal daily fluid intake.

Humidifiers are devices that add water vapor to inspired air. Room humidifiers provide cool mist to room air. Nebulizers are used to deliver humidity and medications. They may be used with oxygen delivery systems to provide moistened air directly to the client. Their purposes are to prevent mucous membranes from drying and becoming irritated and to loosen secretions for easier expectoration.

CLIENT TEACHING

Abdominal (Diaphragmatic) and Pursed-Lip Breathing

- Assume a comfortable semi-sitting position in bed or a chair or a lying position in bed with one pillow.
- Flex your knees to relax the muscles of the abdomen.
- Place one or both hands on your abdomen, just below the ribs.
- Breathe in deeply through the nose, keeping the mouth closed.
- Concentrate on feeling your abdomen rise (expand) as far as possible; stay relaxed, and avoid arching your back. If you have difficulty raising your abdomen, take a quick, forceful breath through the nose.
- Then purse your lips as if about to whistle, and breathe out slowly and gently, making a slow "whooshing" sound without puffing out the cheeks. This pursed-lip breathing creates a resistance to air flowing out of the lungs, increases pressure within the bronchi (main air passages), and minimizes collapse of smaller airways, a common problem for people with COPD.
- Concentrate on feeling the abdomen fall or sink, and tighten (contract) the abdominal muscles while breathing out to enhance effective exhalation. Count to seven during exhalation.
- Use this exercise whenever feeling short of breath, and increase gradually to 5 to 10 minutes four times a day. Regular practice will help you do this type of breathing without conscious effort. The exercise, once learned, can be performed when sitting upright, standing, and walking.

Medications

A number of types of medications can be used for clients with oxygenation problems.

Bronchodilators, anti-inflammatory drugs, expectorants, and cough suppressants are some medications that may be used to treat respiratory problems. Bronchodilators, including sympathomimetic drugs and xanthines, reduce bronchospasm, opening tight or congested airways and facilitating ventilation. These drugs may be administered orally or intravenously, but the preferred route is by inhalation to prevent many systemic side effects.

Since drugs used to dilate the bronchioles and improve breathing are usually drugs that enhance the sympathetic nervous system, clients must be monitored for side effects of increased heart rate, blood pressure, anxiety, and restlessness. This is especially important in older adults, who may also have cardiac problems. Some over-the-counter drugs for respiratory problems have these same effects, so clients should be cautioned about taking them without checking with their primary care provider. Another class of drugs used is the *anti-inflammatory drugs,* such as glucocorticoids. They can be given orally, intravenously, or by inhaler. They work by decreasing the edema and inflammation in the airways and allowing a better air exchange. If both bronchodilators and anti-inflammatory drugs are ordered by inhaler, the client should be instructed to use the bronchodilator inhaler first and then the anti-inflammatory inhaler. If the bronchioles are dilated first, more tissue is exposed for the anti-inflammatory drugs to act upon (see Drug Capsule on next page).

The beta-2 adrenergic agonists are called sympathomimetic drugs because they "mimic" the action of sympathetic stimulation to the beta-2 receptors in the smooth muscle of the lung. At therapeutic levels these drugs promote bronchodilation and so relieve bronchospasm.

Sympathomimetic agents are useful in the treatment of bronchospasm in reversible obstructive airway diseases such as asthma and bronchitis. They are also useful in preventing exercise-induced bronchospasm.

Nursing Responsibilities

- Most inhaled sympathomimetics have a very rapid onset and short duration of action, so they are useful for relief of acute attacks but not for prophylaxis.
- Monitor the client's respiratory status while administering sympathomimetics. This includes respiratory rate, lung sounds, oxygen saturation, and subjective symptoms.
- These medications should be used with caution in clients with conditions such as cardiac disease, vascular disease, hypertension, hyperthyroidism, and pregnancy.

- Monitor the client for common side effects including increased heart rate (due to sympathetic stimulation of the heart) and tremors.
- Monitor for other side effects that occur with excessive dosing, which may include central nervous system stimulation, gastrointestinal upset, hypertension, and sweating.

Client and Family Teaching

- Caution the client to use the least amount of medication needed to get relief for the shortest time period necessary. This will help prevent adverse effects.
- Counsel the client to report immediately any chest pain and/or changes in heart rate or rhythm.
- Teach the client and/or family how to use the delivery system. This will most often be a metered-dose inhaler (MDI) or dry powder inhaler (DPI) or nebulizer.
- Teach the client to record the frequency and intensity of symptoms.

Note: Prior to administering any medication, review all aspects with a current drug handbook or other reliable source.

A fairly new class of drugs is the *leukotriene modifiers*. These medications suppress the effects of leukotrienes on the smooth muscle of the respiratory tract. Leukotrienes cause bronchoconstriction, mucous production, and edema of the respiratory tract.

Expectorants help "break up" mucus, making it more liquid and easier to expectorate. Guaifenesin is a common expectorant found in many prescription and nonprescription cough syrups. When frequent or prolonged coughing interrupts sleep, a cough suppressant such as codeine may be prescribed. Adverse effects include dizziness, lightheadedness, drowsiness, nervousness, nausea, vomiting, and stomach pain. Use in children under four years of age is generally not recommended, and overdosage can result because of parental misunderstandings when administering multiple drugs all containing the same basic ingredients. Decongestants often contain pseudoephedrine, which can increase heart rate, respiratory rate, and result in insomnia due to its stimulant effects.

Other medications can be used to improve oxygenation by improving cardiovascular function. The *digitalis glycosides* act directly on the heart to improve the strength of contraction and slow the heart rate. *Beta-adrenergic blocking agents* such as propranolol affect the sympathetic nervous system to reduce the workload of the heart. These drugs, however, can negatively affect people with asthma or COPD as they may constrict airways.

CLIENT TEACHING | **Using Cough Medications**

- Do not take cough medications in excessive amounts because of adverse side effects.
- If you have diabetes mellitus, avoid cough syrups that contain sugar or alcohol; these can disturb metabolism.
- When a cough medicine does not act as expected, consult a health care professional.
- Be aware of side effects (e.g., drowsiness) that can make the operation of machinery dangerous.

Incentive Spirometry

Incentive spirometers (Figure 35–3), also referred to as *sustained maximal inspiration devices* (SMIs), measure the flow of air inhaled through the mouthpiece and are used to:

- Improve pulmonary ventilation.
- Counteract the effects of anesthesia or hypoventilation.
- Loosen respiratory secretions.
- Facilitate respiratory gaseous exchange.
- Expand collapsed alveoli.

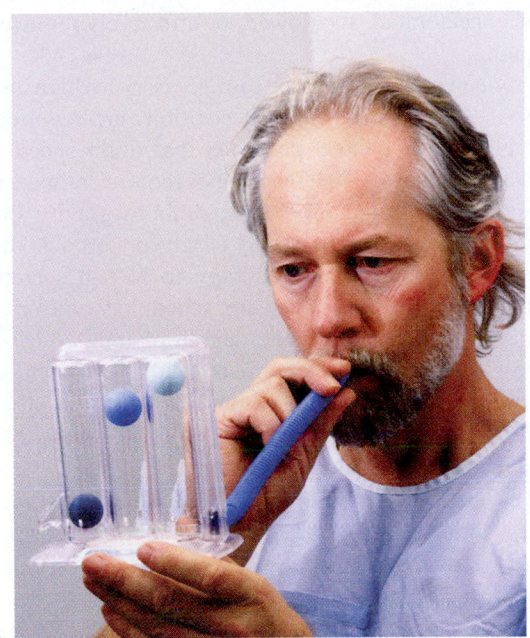
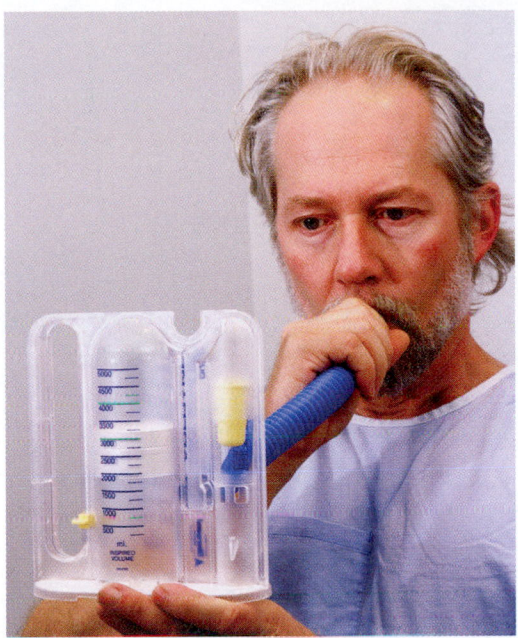

Figure 35–3 ● *A,* Flow-oriented SMI; *B,* volume-oriented SMI.

They offer an incentive to improve inhalation. When using an SMI, the client should be assisted into a position, preferably an upright sitting position in bed or a chair, that facilitates maximum ventilation. Client Teaching lists instructions for clients in the use of incentive spirometers.

Percussion, Vibration, and Postural Drainage

Percussion, vibration, and postural drainage (PVD) are dependent nursing functions performed according to a primary care provider's order. Percussion, sometimes called clapping, is forceful striking of the skin with cupped hands. Mechanical percussion cups and vibrators are also available. When the hands are used, the fingers and thumb are held together and flexed slightly to form a cup, as one would to scoop up water. Percussion over congested lung areas can mechanically dislodge tenacious secretions from the bronchial walls. Cupped hands trap the air against the chest. The trapped air sets up vibrations through the chest wall to the secretions.

To percuss a client's chest, the nurse follows these steps:

- Cover the area with a towel or gown to reduce discomfort.
- Ask the client to breathe slowly and deeply to promote relaxation.
- Alternately flex and extend the wrists rapidly to slap the chest (Figure 35–4).
- Percuss each affected lung segment for 1 to 2 minutes.

CLIENT TEACHING — **Using an Incentive Spirometer**

- Hold or place the spirometer in an upright position. A tilted *flow-oriented* device requires less effort to raise the balls or discs; a *volume-oriented* device will not function correctly unless upright.
- Exhale normally.
- Seal the lips tightly around the mouthpiece.
- Take in a slow, deep breath to elevate the balls or cylinder, and then hold the breath for 2 seconds initially, increasing to 6 seconds (optimum), to keep the balls or cylinder elevated if possible.
- For a flow-oriented device, avoid brisk, low-volume breaths that snap the balls to the top of the chamber. Greater lung expansion is achieved with a very slow inspiration than with a brisk, shallow breath, even though it may not elevate the balls or keep them elevated while you hold your breath. Sustained elevation of the balls or cylinder ensures adequate ventilation of the alveoli (lung air sacs).
- If you have difficulty breathing only through the mouth, a nose clip can be used.
- Remove the mouthpiece and exhale normally.
- Cough after the incentive effort. Deep ventilation may loosen secretions, and coughing can facilitate their removal.
- Relax and take several normal breaths before using the spirometer again.
- Repeat the procedure several times and then four or five times hourly. Practice increases inspiratory volume, maintains alveolar ventilation, and prevents atelectasis (collapse of the air sacs).
- Clean the mouthpiece with water and shake it dry.

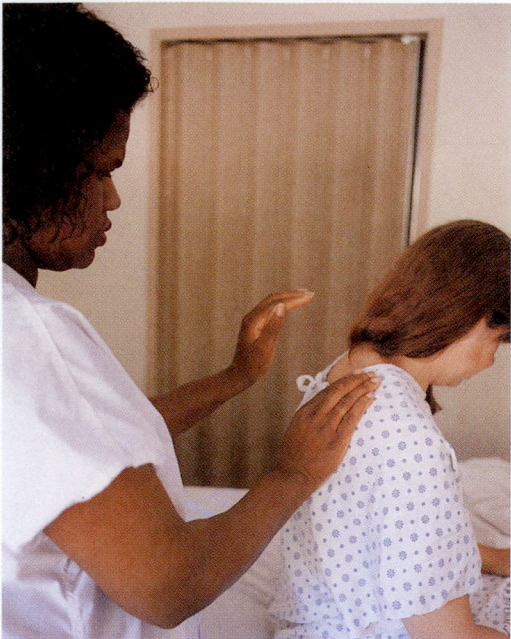

Figure 35–4 ◉ Percussing the upper posterior chest.

When done correctly, the percussion action should produce a hollow, popping sound. Percussion is avoided over the breasts, sternum, spinal column, and kidneys.

Vibration is a series of vigorous quiverings produced by hands that are placed flat against the client's chest wall. Vibration is used after percussion to increase the turbulence of the exhaled air and thus loosen thick secretions. It is often done alternately with percussion.

To vibrate the client's chest, the nurse follows these steps:

- Place hands, palms down, on the chest area to be drained, one hand over the other with the fingers together and extended. Alternatively, the hands may be placed side by side.
- Ask the client to inhale deeply and exhale slowly through the nose or pursed lips.
- During the exhalation, tense all the hand and arm muscles, and using mostly the heel of the hand, vibrate (shake) the hands, moving them downward. Stop the vibrating when the client inhales.
- Vibrate during five exhalations over one affected lung segment.
- After each vibration, encourage the client to cough and expectorate secretions into the sputum container.

Postural drainage is the drainage by gravity of secretions from various lung segments. Secretions that remain in the lungs or respiratory airways promote bacterial growth and subsequent infection. They also can obstruct the smaller airways and cause atelectasis. Secretions in the major airways, such as the trachea and the right and left main bronchi, are usually coughed into the pharynx, where they can be expectorated, swallowed, or effectively removed by suctioning.

A wide variety of positions is necessary to drain all segments of the lungs, but not all positions are required for every client. Only those positions that drain specific affected areas are used. The lower lobes require drainage most frequently because the upper lobes drain by gravity. Before postural drainage, the client may be given a bronchodilator medication or nebulization therapy to loosen secretions. Postural drainage treatments are scheduled two or three times daily, depending on the degree of lung congestion. The best times include before breakfast, before lunch, in the late afternoon, and before bedtime. It is best to avoid hours shortly after meals because postural drainage at these times can be tiring and can induce vomiting.

The nurse needs to evaluate the client's tolerance of postural drainage by assessing the stability of the client's vital signs, particularly the pulse and respiratory rates, and by noting signs of intolerance, such as pallor, diaphoresis, dyspnea, nausea, and fatigue. Some clients do not react well to certain drainage positions, and the nurse must make appropriate adjustments. For example, some become dyspneic in Trendelenburg's position and require only a moderate tilt or a shorter time in that position.

The sequence for PVD is usually as follows: positioning, percussion, vibration, and removal of secretions by coughing or suction. Each position is usually assumed for 10 to 15 minutes, although beginning treatments may start with shorter times and gradually increase.

Following PVD, the nurse should auscultate the client's lungs, compare the findings to the baseline data, and document the amount, color, and character of expectorated secretions.

Oxygen Therapy

Clients who have difficulty ventilating all areas of their lungs, those whose gas exchange is impaired, or people with heart failure may benefit from oxygen therapy to prevent hypoxia.

Oxygen therapy is prescribed by the primary care provider, who specifies the concentration, method of delivery, and depending on the method, liter flow per minute. The concentration is of more importance than the liter flow per minute. When administering oxygen is an *emergency measure*, the nurse may initiate the therapy without a primary care provider's order. For clients who have COPD, a low-flow oxygen system is essential.

Safety precautions are essential during oxygen therapy (see Box 35–2). Although oxygen by itself will not burn or explode, it does facilitate combustion. For example, a bed sheet ordinarily burns slowly when ignited in the atmosphere; however, if saturated with free-flowing oxygen and ignited by a spark, it will burn rapidly and explosively. The greater the concentration of oxygen, the more rapidly fires start and burn, and such fires are difficult to extinguish. Be-

BOX 35–2 **Oxygen Therapy Safety Precautions**

- For home oxygen use or when the facility permits smoking, teach family members and roommates to smoke only outside or in provided smoking rooms away from the client and oxygen equipment.
- Place cautionary signs reading "No Smoking: Oxygen in Use" on the client's door, at the foot or head of the bed, and on the oxygen equipment.
- Instruct the client and visitors about the hazard of smoking with oxygen in use.
- Make sure that electric devices (such as razors, hearing aids, radios, televisions, and heating pads) are in good working order to prevent the occurrence of short-circuit sparks.
- Avoid materials that generate static electricity, such as woolen blankets and synthetic fabrics. Cotton blankets should be used, and clients and caregivers should be advised to wear cotton fabrics.
- Avoid the use of volatile, flammable materials, such as oils, greases, alcohol, ether, and acetone (e.g., nail polish remover), near clients receiving oxygen.
- Be sure that electric monitoring equipment, suction machines, and portable diagnostic machines are all electrically grounded.
- Make known the location of fire extinguishers, and make sure personnel are trained in their use.

---

cause oxygen is colorless, odorless, and tasteless, people are often unaware of its presence.

Oxygen is supplied in several different ways. In hospitals and long-term care facilities, it is usually piped into wall outlets at the client's bedside, making it readily available for use at all times. Tanks or cylinders of oxygen under pressure are also frequently available for use when wall oxygen is either unavailable or impractical.

Clients who require oxygen therapy in the home may use small cylinders of oxygen, oxygen in liquid form, or an oxygen concentrator. Portable oxygen delivery systems are available to increase the client's independence. Home oxygen therapy services are readily available in most communities. These services generally supply the oxygen and delivery devices, training for the client and family, equipment maintenance, and emergency services should a problem occur.

Oxygen administered from a cylinder or wall-outlet system is dry. Dry gases dehydrate the respiratory mucous membranes. Humidifying devices that add water vapor to inspired air are thus an essential adjunct of oxygen therapy, particularly for liter flows over 2 L per minute. These devices provide 20% to 40% humidity. The oxygen passes through sterile distilled water or tap water and then along a line to the device through which the moistened oxygen is inhaled (e.g., a cannula, nasal catheter, or oxygen mask).

Humidifiers prevent mucous membranes from drying and becoming irritated and loosen secretions for easier expectoration. Oxygen passing through water picks up water

vapor before it reaches the client. The more bubbles created during this process, the more water vapor is produced. Very low liter flows (e.g., 1 to 2 L per minute by nasal cannula) do not require humidification. When a client is breathing very low flow oxygen, there is enough atmospheric air inhaled to prevent mucosal drying.

Oxygen cylinders need to be handled and stored with caution and strapped securely in wheeled transport devices or stands to prevent possible falls and outlet breakages. They should be placed away from traffic areas and heaters.

To use an oxygen wall outlet, the nurse carries out these steps:

- Attach the flow meter to the wall outlet, exerting firm pressure. The flow meter should be in the off position.
- Fill the humidifier bottle with distilled or tap water in accordance with agency protocol. This can be done before coming to the bedside. Some humidifier bottles come prefilled by the manufacturer.
- Attach the humidifier bottle to the base of the flow meter.
- Attach the prescribed oxygen tubing and delivery device to the humidifier.
- Regulate the flow meter to the prescribed level. The line for the prescribed flow rate (e.g., 2 L/min) should be in the middle of the ball of the flow meter.

OXYGEN DELIVERY SYSTEMS A number of systems are available to deliver oxygen to the client. The choice of system depends on the client's oxygen needs, comfort, and developmental considerations. With many systems, the oxygen delivered mixes with room air before being inspired. With this type of system, the amount of oxygen delivered is determined by regulating its flow rate (e.g., 2 to 6 L per minute), and precise regulation of the percentage of inspired oxygen, or fraction of inspired oxygen (FiO_2), is not possible. When it is important to regulate the percentage of oxygen received by the client more precisely, a device such as a Venturi mask may be used.

Cannula The nasal cannula (nasal prongs) is the most common and inexpensive device used to administer oxygen (Figure 35–5 *A*).

The nasal cannula is easy to apply and does not interfere with the client's ability to eat or talk. It also is relatively comfortable, permits some freedom of movement, and is well tolerated by the client. It delivers a relatively low concentration of oxygen (24% to 45%) at flow rates of 2 to 6 L per minute. Above 6 L per minute, the client tends to swallow air and the FiO_2 is not increased. Limitations of the cannula include inability to deliver higher concentrations of oxygen, and that it can be drying and irritating to mucous membranes.

Administering oxygen by cannula is detailed in Skill 35–1.

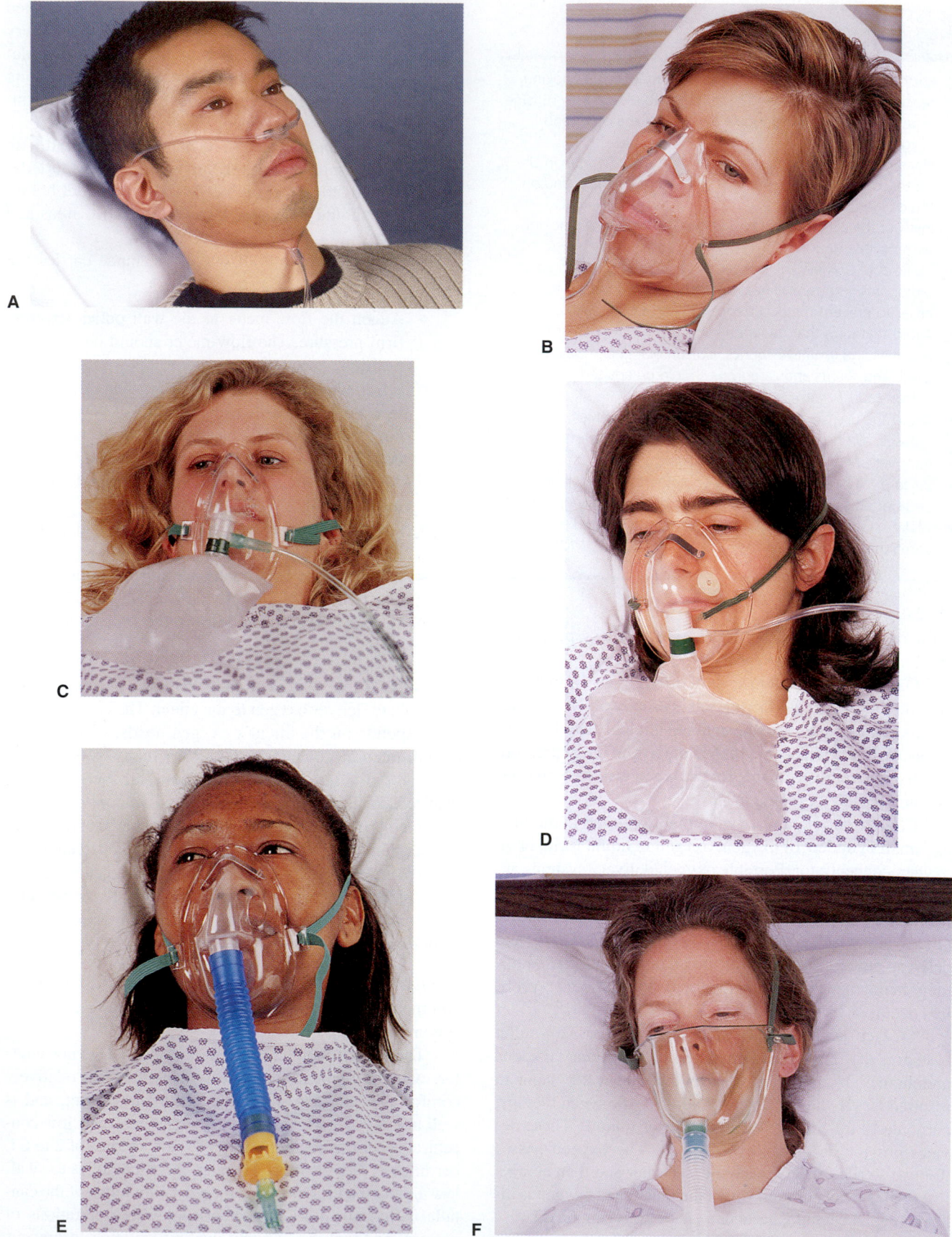

Figure 35–5 ◉ **A,** Nasal cannula; **B,** Simple face mask; **C,** Partial rebreather mask; **D,** Nonrebreather mask; **E,** Venturi mask; **F,** Oxygen face tent.

SKILL 35–1

ADMINISTERING OXYGEN BY CANNULA, FACE MASK, OR FACE TENT

Before administering oxygen, check (a) the order for oxygen, including the administering device and the liter flow rate (L/min) or the percentage of oxygen; (b) the levels of oxygen (PaO_2) and carbon dioxide ($PaCO_2$) in the client's arterial blood (PaO_2 is normally 80 to 100 mm Hg; $PaCO_2$ is normally 35 to 45 mm Hg); and (c) whether the client has COPD. NOTE: If the client has not had arterial blood gases ordered, oxygen saturation should be checked using a noninvasive oximeter.

PURPOSES

Cannula

- To deliver a relatively low concentration of oxygen when only minimal O_2 support is required
- To allow uninterrupted delivery of oxygen while the client ingests food or fluids

Face Mask

- To provide moderate O_2 support and a higher concentration of oxygen and/or humidity than is provided by cannula

Face Tent

- To provide high humidity
- To provide oxygen when a mask is poorly tolerated
- To provide a high flow of O_2 when attached to a Venturi system

ASSESSMENT

See also Skill 17–10, "Assessing the Thorax and Lungs" in Chapter 17 ∞.

Assess

- Skin and mucous membrane color: Note whether cyanosis is present.
- Breathing patterns: Note depth of respirations and presence of tachypnea, bradypnea, or orthopnea.
- Chest movements: Note whether there are any intercostal, substernal, suprasternal, supraclavicular, or tracheal retractions during inspiration or expiration.
- Chest wall configuration (e.g., kyphosis).

- Lung sounds audible by auscultating the chest and by ear.
- Presence of clinical signs of hypoxemia: tachycardia, tachypnea, restlessness, dyspnea, cyanosis, and confusion. Tachycardia and tachypnea are often early signs. Confusion is a later sign of severe oxygen deprivation.
- Presence of clinical signs of hypercarbia (hypercapnia): restlessness, hypertension, headache, lethargy, tremor.
- Presence of clinical signs of oxygen toxicity: tracheal irritation and cough, dyspnea, and decreased pulmonary ventilation.

Determine

- Vital signs, especially pulse rate and quality, and respiratory rate, rhythm, and depth.
- Whether the client has COPD. A high carbon dioxide level in the blood is the normal stimulus to breathe. However, people with COPD may have a chronically high carbon dioxide level, and their stimulus to breathe is hypoxemia. Low flows of oxygen (2 L/min) stimulate breathing for such persons by maintaining slight hypoxemia. During continuous oxygen administration, arterial blood gas levels of oxygen (PaO_2) and carbon dioxide ($PaCO_2$) are measured periodically to monitor hypoxemia.
- Results of diagnostic studies such as chest x-ray.
- Hemoglobin, hematocrit, and complete blood count.
- Oxygen saturation levels.
- Arterial blood gases levels, if available.
- Pulmonary function tests, if available.

PLANNING

Consult with a respiratory therapist as needed in the beginning and during ongoing care of clients receiving ordered oxygen therapy. In many agencies, the therapist establishes the initial equipment and client teaching.

Delegation

Initiating the administration of oxygen is considered similar to administering a medication and is not delegated to unlicensed assistive personnel (UAP). However, reapplying the oxygen delivery device may be performed by the UAP, and many aspects of the client's response to oxygen therapy are observed during usual care and may be recorded by persons other than the nurse. Abnormal findings must be validated and interpreted by the nurse. The nurse is also responsible for ensuring that the correct delivery method is being used.

EQUIPMENT

Cannula

- Oxygen supply with a flow meter and adapter
- Humidifier with distilled water or tap water according to agency protocol
- Nasal cannula and tubing
- Tape
- Padding for the elastic band

Face Mask

- Oxygen supply with a flow meter and adapter
- Humidifier with distilled water or tap water according to agency protocol
- Prescribed face mask of the appropriate size
- Padding for the elastic band

Face Tent

- Oxygen supply with a flow meter and adapter
- Humidifier with distilled water or tap water according to agency protocol
- Face tent of the appropriate size

IMPLEMENTATION

Preparation

1. Determine the need for oxygen therapy, and verify the order for the therapy.
   - Perform a respiratory assessment to develop baseline data if not already available.

2. Prepare the client and support people.
   - Assist the client to a semi-Fowler's position if possible. **Rationale:** *This position permits easier chest expansion and hence easier breathing.*

(continued)

ADMINISTERING OXYGEN BY CANNULA, FACE MASK, OR FACE TENT *(continued)*

- Explain that oxygen is not dangerous when safety precautions are observed. Inform the client and support people about the safety precautions connected with oxygen use.

Performance

1. Prior to performing the procedure, introduce self and verify the client's identity using agency protocol. Explain to the client what you are going to do, why it is necessary, and how he or she can participate. Discuss how the effects of the oxygen therapy will be used in planning further care or treatments.
2. Perform hand hygiene and observe appropriate infection control procedures.
3. Provide for client privacy, if appropriate.
4. Set up the oxygen equipment and the humidifier.
   - Attach the flow meter to the wall outlet or tank. The flow meter should be in the OFF position.
   - If needed, fill the humidifier bottle. (This can be done before coming to the bedside.)
   - Attach the humidifier bottle to the base of the flow meter.
   - Attach the prescribed oxygen tubing and delivery device to the humidifier.
5. Turn on the oxygen at the prescribed rate and ensure proper functioning.
   - Check that the oxygen is flowing freely through the tubing. There should be no kinks in the tubing, and the connections should be airtight. There should be bubbles in the humidifier as the oxygen flows through. You should feel the oxygen at the outlets of the cannula, mask, or tent.
   - Set the oxygen at the flow rate ordered.
6. Apply the appropriate oxygen delivery device.

Cannula

- Put the cannula over the client's face, with the outlet prongs fitting into the nares and the elastic band around the head (see Figure 35–5 *A*). Some models have a strap to adjust under the chin.
- If the cannula will not stay in place, tape it at the sides of the face. This can be accomplished by placing tape in front of the ears on the cheeks or by taping on either side of the nose in neonates and infants.
- Pad the tubing and band over the ears and cheekbones as needed.

Face Mask

- Guide the mask toward the client's face, and apply it from the nose downward.
- Fit the mask to the contours of the client's face (see Figure 35–5 *B*). **Rationale:** *The mask should mold to the face, so that very little oxygen escapes into the eyes or around the cheeks and chin.*
- Secure the elastic band around the client's head so that the mask is comfortable but snug.
- Pad the band behind the ears and over bony prominences. **Rationale:** *Padding will prevent irritation from the mask.*

Face Tent

- Place the tent over the client's face, and secure the ties around the head (see Figure 35–5 *F*).

7. Assess the client regularly.
   - Assess the client's vital signs, level of anxiety, color, and ease of respirations, and provide support while the client adjusts to the device.
   - Assess the client in 15 to 30 minutes, depending on the client's condition, and regularly thereafter.
   - Assess the client regularly for clinical signs of hypoxia, tachycardia, confusion, dyspnea, restlessness, and cyanosis. Review oxygen saturation or arterial blood gas results if they are available.

Nasal Cannula

- Assess the client's nares for encrustations and irritation. Apply a water-soluble lubricant as required to soothe the mucous membranes.
- Assess the top of the client's ears for any signs of irritation from the cannula strap. If present, padding with a gauze pad may help relieve the discomfort.

Face Mask or Tent

- Inspect the facial skin frequently for dampness or chafing, and dry and treat it as needed.

8. Inspect the equipment on a regular basis.
   - Check the liter flow and the level of water in the humidifier in 30 minutes and whenever providing care to the client.
   - Be sure that water is not collecting in dependent loops of the tubing.
   - Make sure that safety precautions are being followed.
9. Document findings in the client record using forms or checklists supplemented by narrative notes when appropriate.

EVALUATION

- Perform follow-up based on findings that deviated from expected or normal for the client. Relate findings to previous data if available (e.g., check oxygen saturation to evaluate adequate oxygenation).
- Report significant deviations from normal to the primary care provider.

LIFESPAN CONSIDERATIONS   Oxygen Delivery Equipment

Infants

Oxygen Hood

- An oxygen hood is a rigid plastic dome that encloses an infant's head. It provides precise oxygen levels and high humidity.
- The gas should not be allowed to blow directly into the infant's face, and the hood should not rub against the infant's neck, chin, or shoulder.

Children

Oxygen Tent

- The tent consists of a rectangular, clear, plastic canopy with outlets that connect to an oxygen or compressed air source and to a humidifier that moisturizes the air or oxygen (Figure 35–6).
- Because the enclosed tent becomes very warm, some type of cooling mechanism such as an ice chamber or a refrigeration unit is provided to maintain the temperature at 20°C to 21°C (68°F to 70°F).
- Cover the child with a gown or a cotton blanket. Some agencies provide gowns with hoods, or a small towel may be wrapped around the head. *The child needs protection from chilling and from the dampness and condensation in the tent.*

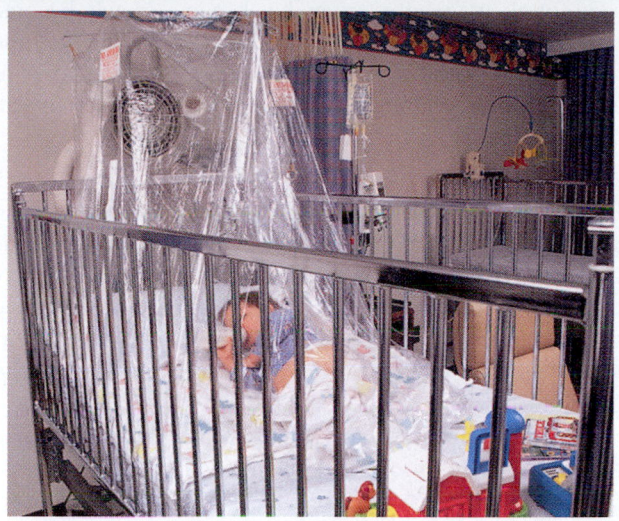

Figure 35–6 ● Pediatric oxygen tent.

- Flood the tent with oxygen by setting the flow meter at 15 L/min for about 5 minutes. Then, adjust the flow meter according to orders (e.g., 10 to 15 L/min). *Flooding the tent quickly increases the oxygen to the desired level.*
- The tent can deliver approximately 30% oxygen.

Face Mask   Face masks that cover the client's nose and mouth may be used for oxygen inhalation. Exhalation ports on the sides of the mask allow exhaled carbon dioxide to escape. A variety of oxygen masks are marketed:

- The simple face mask delivers oxygen concentrations from 40% to 60% at liter flows of 5 to 8 L per minute, respectively (Figure 35–5 *B*).
- The partial rebreather mask delivers oxygen concentrations of 60% to 90% at liter flows of 6 to 10 L per minute, respectively. The oxygen reservoir bag that is attached allows the client to rebreathe about the first third of the exhaled air in conjunction with oxygen (Figure 35–5 *C*). Thus, it increases the FiO_2 by recycling expired oxygen. The partial rebreather bag must not totally deflate during inspiration to avoid carbon dioxide buildup. If this problem occurs, the nurse increases the liter flow of oxygen.
- The nonrebreather mask delivers the highest oxygen concentration possible—95% to 100%—by means other than intubation or mechanical ventilation, at liter flows of 10 to 15 L per minute. One-way valves on the mask and between the reservoir bag and the mask prevent the room air and the client's exhaled air from entering the bag so only the oxygen in the bag is inspired (Figure 35–5 *D*). To prevent carbon dioxide buildup, the nonrebreather bag must not to-

tally deflate during inspiration. If it does, the nurse can correct this problem by increasing the liter flow of oxygen.
- The Venturi mask delivers oxygen concentrations varying from 24% to 40% or 50% at liter flows of 4 to 10 L per minute (Figure 35–5 *E*). The Venturi mask has wide-bore tubing and color-coded jet adapters that correspond to a precise oxygen concentration and liter flow. For example, a blue adapter delivers a 24% concentration of oxygen at 4 L per minute, and a green adapter delivers a 35% concentration of oxygen at 8 L per minute.

Initiating oxygen by mask is much the same as initiating oxygen by cannula, except that the nurse must find a mask of appropriate size. Smaller sizes are available for children. Administering oxygen by mask or face tent is detailed in Skill 35–1. Limitations of masks include difficulty in achieving a proper fit and poor tolerance by some clients who may complain of feeling hot or "smothering."

Face Tent   Face tents (Figure 35–5 *F*) can replace oxygen masks when masks are poorly tolerated by clients. Face tents provide varying concentrations of oxygen, for example, 30% to 50% concentration of oxygen at 4 to 8 L per minute. Frequently inspect the client's facial skin for dampness or chafing, and dry and treat as needed. As with face masks, the client's facial skin must be kept dry.

Artificial Airways

Artificial airways are inserted to maintain a patent air passage for clients whose airway has become or may become obstructed. A patent airway is necessary so that air can flow to and from the lungs. Four of the more common types of airways are oropharyngeal, nasopharyngeal, endotracheal, and tracheostomy.

OROPHARYNGEAL AND NASOPHARYNGEAL AIRWAYS

Oropharyngeal and nasopharyngeal airways are used to keep the upper air passages open when they may become obstructed by secretions or the tongue. These airways are easy to insert and have a low risk of complications. Sizes vary and should be appropriate to the size and age of the client. The airway should be well lubricated with water-soluble gel prior to inserting.

Oropharyngeal airways (Figure 35–7) stimulate the gag reflex and are only used for clients with altered levels of consciousness (e.g., because of general anesthesia, overdose, or head injury). To insert the airway:

- Place the client in a supine or semi-Fowler's position.
- Put on clean gloves.
- Hold the lubricated airway by the outer flange, with the distal end pointing up.
- Open the client's mouth and insert the airway along the top of the tongue.
- When the distal end of the airway reaches the soft palate at the back of the mouth, rotate the airway 180 degrees downward, and slip it past the uvula into the oral pharynx.
- If not contraindicated, place the client in a side-lying position or with the head turned to the side to allow secretions to drain out of the mouth.
- The oropharynx may be suctioned as needed by inserting the suction catheter alongside the airway.
- Do not tape the airway in place; remove it when the client begins to cough or gag.
- Provide mouth care at least every 2 to 4 hours, keeping suction available at the bedside.

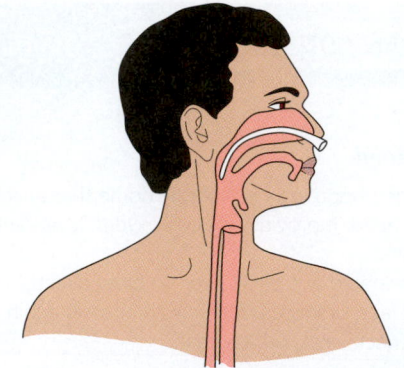

Figure 35–8 ◯ A nasopharyngeal airway in place.

- As appropriate for the client's condition, remove the airway every 8 hours to assess the mouth and provide oral care. Reinsert the airway immediately.

Nasopharyngeal airways are tolerated better by alert clients. They are inserted through the nares, terminating in the oropharynx (Figure 35–8). When caring for a client with a nasopharyngeal airway, provide frequent oral and nares care, repositioning the airway in the other naris every 8 hours or as ordered to prevent necrosis of the mucosa.

ENDOTRACHEAL TUBES

Endotracheal tubes are most commonly inserted for clients who have had general anesthetics or for those in emergency situations where mechanical ventilation is required. An endotracheal tube is inserted by the primary care provider, nurse, or respiratory therapist with specialized education. It is inserted through the mouth or the nose and into the trachea with the guide of a laryngoscope (Figure 35–9). The tube terminates just superior to the bifurcation of the trachea into the bronchi. The tube may have an air-filled cuff to prevent air leakage around it. Because an endotracheal tube passes through the epiglottis and glottis, the client is unable to speak while it is in place. Nursing interventions for clients with endotracheal tubes are shown in Box 35–3.

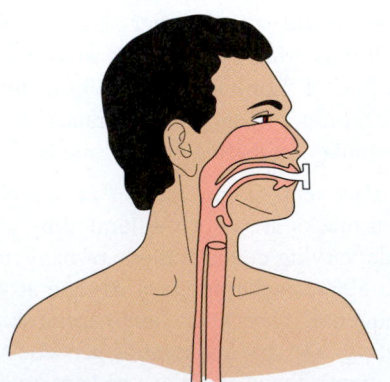

Figure 35–7 ◯ An oropharyngeal airway in place.

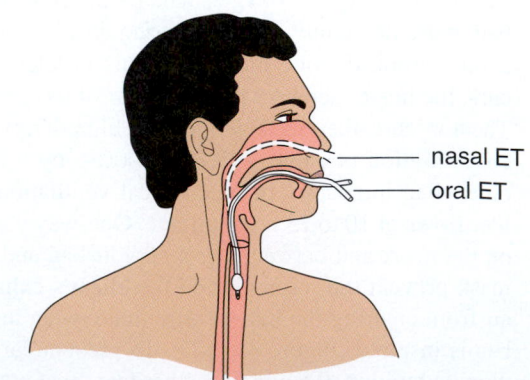

nasal ET
oral ET

Figure 35–9 ◯ An endotracheal tube (ET).

BOX 35–3	Nursing Interventions for Clients with Endotracheal Tubes

- Assess the client's respiratory status at least every 2 hours, or more frequently if indicated. Include respiratory rate, rhythm, depth, equality of chest excursion, and lung sounds; level of consciousness; and skin color in your assessment.
- Frequently assess nasal and oral mucosa for redness and irritation. Report any abnormal findings to the primary care provider.
- Secure the endotracheal tube with tape or a commercially prepared tracheostomy holder to prevent movement of the tube farther into or out of the trachea. Assess the position of the tube frequently. Notify the primary care provider immediately if the tube is dislodged out of the airway. If the tube advances into a main bronchus, it will need to be repositioned to ensure ventilation of both lungs.
- Unless contraindicated, place the client in a side-lying or semiprone position as tolerated to prevent aspiration of oral secretions.
- Using sterile technique, suction the endotracheal tube as needed to remove excessive secretions.

- Closely monitor cuff pressure, maintaining a pressure of 20 to 25 mm Hg (or as recommended by the tube manufacturer) to minimize the risk of tracheal tissue necrosis. If recommended, deflate the cuff periodically.
- Provide oral and nasal care every 2 to 4 hours. Use an oropharyngeal airway to prevent the client from biting down on an oral endotracheal tube. Move oral endotracheal tubes to the opposite side of the mouth every 8 hours or per agency protocol, taking care to maintain the position of the tube in the trachea. *This prevents irritation to the oral mucosa.*
- Provide humidified air or oxygen because the endotracheal tube bypasses the upper airways, which normally moisten the air.
- If the client is on mechanical ventilation, ensure that all alarms are enabled at all times because the client cannot call for help should an emergency occur.
- Communicate frequently with the client, providing a note pad or picture board for the client to use in communicating.

TRACHEOSTOMY Clients who need long-term airway support may have a tracheostomy. A tracheostomy is an opening into the trachea through the neck. A tube is usually inserted through this opening and an artificial airway is created. Tracheostomy is done using one of two techniques: the traditional open surgical method or a percutaneous insertion. The percutaneous method can be done at the bedside in a critical care unit. The open technique is done in the operating room, and a surgical incision is made in the trachea just below the larynx. A curved tracheostomy tube is inserted to extend through the stoma into the trachea. Tracheostomy tubes may be either plastic or metal and are available in different sizes.

Tracheostomy tubes have an outer cannula that is inserted into the trachea and a flange that rests against the neck and allows the tube to be secured in place with tape or ties (Figure 35–10). All tubes also have an obturator, which is used to insert the outer cannula and is then removed. The obturator is kept at the client's bedside in case the tube becomes dislodged and needs to be reinserted. Some tracheostomy tubes have an inner cannula that may be removed for periodic cleaning.

Cuffed tracheostomy tubes are surrounded by an inflatable cuff that produces an airtight seal between the tube and the trachea. This seal prevents aspiration of oropharyngeal secretions and air leakage between the tube and the trachea. Cuffed tubes are often used immediately after a tracheostomy and are essential when ventilating a tracheostomy client with a mechanical ventilator. Children do not require cuffed tubes, because their tracheas are resilient enough to seal the air space around the tube.

Low-pressure cuffs are commonly used to distribute a low, even pressure against the trachea, thus decreasing the risk of tracheal tissue necrosis. They do not need to be deflated periodically to reduce pressure on the tracheal wall. Foam cuffed tracheostomy tubes do not require injected air; instead, when the port is opened, ambient air enters the balloon, which then conforms to the client's trachea. Air is removed from the cuff prior to insertion or removal of the tube.

The nurse provides tracheostomy care for the client with a new or recent tracheostomy to maintain patency of the tube and reduce the risk of infection. Initially a tracheostomy may need to be suctioned (see the section on suctioning that follows) and cleaned as often as every 1 to 2 hours. After the initial inflammatory response subsides, tracheostomy care may only need to be done once or twice a day, depending on the client. Skill 35–4 later describes tracheostomy care.

When the client breathes through a tracheostomy, air is no longer filtered and humidified as it is when passing through the upper airways; therefore, special precautions are necessary. Humidity may be provided with a mist collar (Figure 35–11). Clients with long-term tracheostomies may wear a light scarf or a 4 × 4 in. gauze held in place with a cotton tie over the stoma to filter air as it enters the tracheostomy.

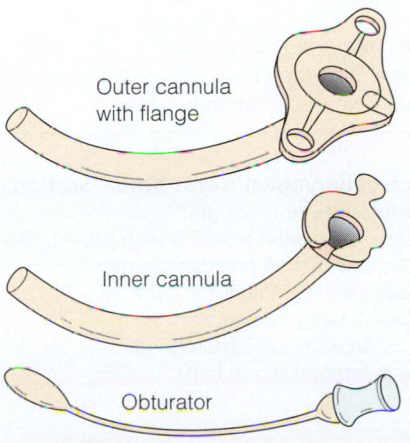

Outer cannula with flange

Inner cannula

Obturator

Figure 35–10 ⬤ Components of a tracheostomy tube.

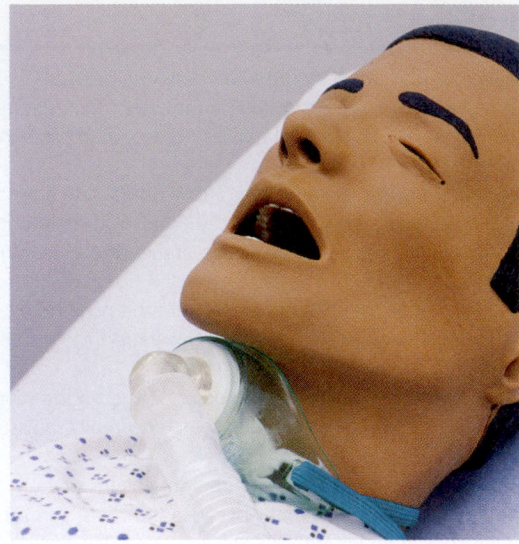

Figure 35–11 ⬤ A tracheostomy mist collar.

Suctioning

When clients have difficulty handling their secretions or an airway is in place, suctioning may be necessary to clear air passages. Suctioning is aspirating secretions through a catheter connected to a suction machine or wall suction outlet. Even though the upper airways (the oropharynx and nasopharynx) are not sterile, sterile technique is recommended for all suctioning to avoid introducing pathogens into the airways.

Suction catheters may be either open tipped or whistle tipped (Figure 35–12). The whistle-tipped catheter is less irritating to respiratory tissues, although the open-tipped catheter may be more effective for removing thick mucous

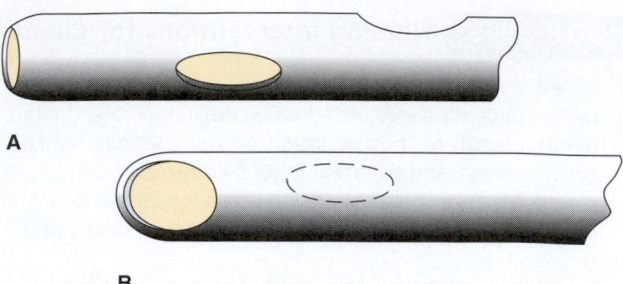

A

B

Figure 35–12 ⬤ Types of suction catheters: **A,** open tipped; **B,** whistle tipped.

plugs. An oral suction tube, or Yankauer device, is used to suction the oral cavity. Most suction catheters have a thumb port on the side to control the suction. The catheter is connected to suction tubing, which in turn is connected to a collection chamber and suction control gauge.

The nurse decides when suctioning is needed by assessing the client for signs of respiratory distress or evidence that the client is unable to cough up and expectorate secretions. Dyspnea, bubbling or rattling breath sounds, poor skin color (cyanosis), or decreased oxygen saturation (SpO_2) levels (also called O_2 sat) may indicate the need for suctioning. Good nursing judgment is necessary, because suctioning irritates mucous membranes and can increase secretions if performed too frequently. In other words, suctioning is based on clinical need versus a fixed schedule.

Oral and oropharyngeal suctioning removes secretions from the upper respiratory tract. Nasopharyngeal and nasotracheal suctioning provides closer access to the trachea and requires sterile technique. Skill 35–2 outlines oropharyngeal and nasopharyngeal suctioning.

SKILL 35–2

OROPHARYNGEAL, NASOPHARYNGEAL, AND NASOTRACHEAL SUCTIONING

PURPOSES
- To remove secretions that obstruct the airway
- To facilitate ventilation
- To obtain secretions for diagnostic purposes
- To prevent infection that may result from accumulated secretions

ASSESSMENT

Assess for clinical signs indicating the need for suctioning:

- Restlessness
- Gurgling sounds during respiration
- Adventitious breath sounds when the chest is auscultated
- Change in mental status
- Skin color
- Rate and pattern of respirations
- Pulse rate and rhythm
- Decreased oxygen saturation

PLANNING

Delegation

Oral suctioning using a Yankauer suction tube and oropharyngeal suctioning using a suction catheter can be delegated to UAP and to the client or family, if appropriate, since this is not a sterile procedure. The nurse needs to review the procedure and important points such as not applying suction during insertion of the tube to avoid trauma to the mucous membrane. In contrast, nasopharyngeal and nasotracheal suctioning uses sterile technique and requires application of knowledge and problem solving and should be performed by the nurse or respiratory therapist.

EQUIPMENT
Oral and Nasopharyngeal/Nasotracheal Suctioning
- Towel or moisture-resistant pad
- Portable or wall suction machine with tubing, collection receptacle, and suction pressure gauge
- Sterile disposable container for fluids
- Sterile normal saline or water
- Goggles or face shield, if appropriate
- Moisture-resistant disposal bag
- Sputum trap, if specimen is to be collected

Oral and Oropharyngeal Suctioning
* Yankauer suction catheter or suction catheter kit
* Clean gloves

Nasopharyngeal or Nasotracheal Suctioning
* Sterile gloves
* Sterile suction catheter kit (#12 to #18 Fr for adults, #8 to #10 Fr for children, and #5 to #8 Fr for infants)
* Water-soluble lubricant
* Y-connector

IMPLEMENTATION

Performance

1. Prior to performing the procedure, introduce self and verify the client's identity using agency protocol. Explain to the client what you are going to do, why it is necessary, and how he or she can participate. Inform the client that suctioning will relieve breathing difficulty and that the procedure is painless but may be uncomfortable and stimulate the cough, gag, or sneeze reflex. **Rationale:** *Knowing that the procedure will relieve breathing problems is often reassuring and enlists the client's cooperation.*
2. Perform hand hygiene and observe other appropriate infection control procedures.
3. Provide for client privacy.
4. Prepare the client.
   * Position a conscious person who has a functional gag reflex in the semi-Fowler's position with the head turned to one side for oral suctioning or with the neck hyperextended for nasal suctioning. **Rationale:** *These positions facilitate the insertion of the catheter and help prevent aspiration of secretions.*
   * Position an unconscious client in the lateral position, facing you. **Rationale:** *This position allows the tongue to fall forward, so that it will not obstruct the catheter on insertion. The lateral position also facilitates drainage of secretions from the pharynx and prevents the possibility of aspiration.*
   * Place the towel or moisture-resistant pad over the pillow or under the chin.
5. Prepare the equipment.
   * Turn the suction device on and set to appropriate negative pressure on the suction gauge. The amount of negative pressure should be high enough to clear secretions but not too high. **Rationale:** *Too high of a pressure can cause the catheter to adhere to the tracheal wall and cause irritation or trauma.* A rule of thumb is to use the lowest amount of suction pressure needed to clear the secretions. Wong (2007) suggests pressure be limited to 60 to 100 mm Hg for children and 40 to 80 mm Hg for premature infants. Lemone (2008) and Moore (2003) recommend suction pressures between 80 and 120 mm Hg for adults.

For Oral and Oropharyngeal Suction
* Apply clean gloves.
* Moisten the tip of the Yankauer or suction catheter with sterile water or saline. **Rationale:** *This reduces friction and eases insertion.*
* Pull the tongue forward, if necessary, using gauze.
* Do not apply suction (that is, leave your finger off the port) during insertion. **Rationale:** *Applying suction during insertion causes trauma to the mucous membrane.*

* Advance the catheter about 10 to 15 cm (4 to 6 in.) along one side of the mouth into the oropharynx. **Rationale:** *Directing the catheter along the side prevents gagging.*
* It may be necessary during oropharyngeal suctioning to apply suction to secretions that collect in the vestibule of the mouth and beneath the tongue.
* Remove and discard gloves. Perform hand hygiene.

For Nasopharyngeal and Nasotracheal Suction
* Open the lubricant.
* Open the sterile suction package.
   a. Set up the cup or container, touching only the outside.
   b. Pour sterile water or saline into the container.
   c. Apply sterile gloves, or apply a clean glove on the nondominant hand and then a sterile glove on the dominant hand. **Rationale:** *The sterile gloved hand maintains the sterility of the suction catheter, and the clean glove prevents the transmission of the microorganisms to the nurse.*
* With your sterile gloved hand, pick up the catheter and attach it to the suction connecting tubing being held in the nondominant hand. ❶
* Test the pressure of the suction and the patency of the catheter by applying your sterile gloved finger or thumb to the port or open branch of the Y-connector (the suction control) to create suction.
* If needed, apply or increase supplemental oxygen.
6. Lubricate and introduce the catheter.
   * Lubricate the catheter tip with sterile water, saline, or water-soluble lubricant. **Rationale:** *This reduces friction and eases insertion.*
   * Remove oxygen with the nondominant hand, if appropriate.
   * *Without applying suction,* insert the catheter the premeasured or recommended distance into either naris and advance it along the floor of the nasal cavity. **Rationale:** *This avoids the nasal turbinates.*
   * Never force the catheter against an obstruction. If one nostril is obstructed, try the other.
7. Perform suctioning.
   * Apply your finger to the suction control port to start suction, and gently rotate the catheter. **Rationale:** *Gentle rotation of the catheter ensures that all surfaces are*

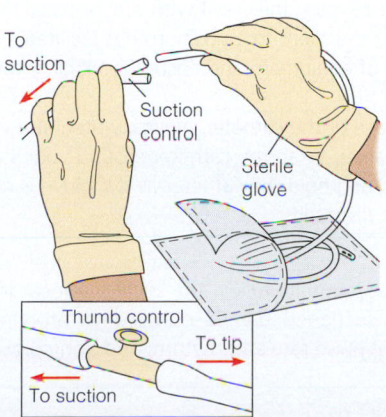

❶ Attaching the catheter to the suction unit.

(continued)

OROPHARYNGEAL, NASOPHARYNGEAL, AND NASOTRACHEAL SUCTIONING *(continued)*

reached and prevents trauma to any one area of the respiratory mucosa due to prolonged suction.

- Apply suction for 5 to 10 seconds while slowly withdrawing the catheter, then remove your finger from the control and remove the catheter.
- A suction attempt should last only 10 to 15 seconds. During this time, the catheter is inserted, the suction applied and discontinued, and the catheter removed.

8. Rinse the catheter and repeat suctioning as above.
- Rinse and flush the catheter and tubing with sterile water or saline.
- Relubricate the catheter, and repeat suctioning until the air passage is clear.
- Allow sufficient time between each suction for ventilation and oxygenation. Limit suctioning to 5 minutes in total. **Rationale:** *Applying suction for too long may cause secretions to increase or decrease the client's oxygen supply.*
- Encourage the client to breathe deeply and to cough between suctions. Use supplemental oxygen, if appropriate. **Rationale:** *Coughing and deep breathing help carry secretions from the trachea and bronchi into the pharynx, where they can be reached with the suction catheter. Deep breathing and supplemental oxygen provide oxygen to the alveoli.*

9. Obtain a specimen if required.
- Use a sputum trap ❷ as follows:
- Attach the suction catheter to the tubing of the sputum trap.
- Attach the suction tubing to the sputum trap air vent.
- Suction the client. The sputum trap will collect the mucus during suctioning.
- Remove the catheter from the client. Disconnect the sputum trap tubing from the suction catheter. Remove the suction tubing from the trap air vent.
- Connect the tubing of the sputum trap to the air vent. **Rationale:** *This retains any microorganisms in the sputum trap.*
- Connect the suction catheter to the tubing.
- Flush the catheter to remove secretions from the tubing.

10. Promote client comfort.
- Offer to assist the client with oral or nasal hygiene.
- Assist the client to a position that facilitates breathing.

11. Dispose of equipment and ensure availability for the next suction.
- Dispose of the catheter, gloves, water, and waste container. Wrap the catheter around your sterile gloved hand and hold the catheter as the glove is removed over it for disposal.

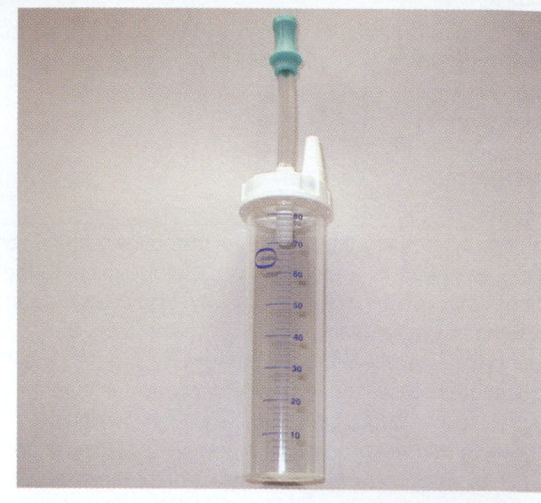

❷ A sputum collection trap.

- Rinse the suction tubing as needed by inserting the end of the tubing into the used water container. Empty and rinse the suction collection container as needed or indicated by protocol. Change the suction tubing and container daily.
- Ensure that supplies are available for the next suctioning (suction kit, gloves, water or normal saline).

12. Assess the effectiveness of suctioning.
- Auscultate the client's breath sounds to ensure they are clear of secretions. Observe skin color, dyspnea, level of anxiety, and oxygen saturation levels.

13. Document relevant data.
- Record the procedure: the amount, consistency, color, and odor of sputum (e.g., foamy, white mucus; thick, green-tinged mucus; or blood-flecked mucus) and the client's respiratory status before and after the procedure. This may include lung sounds, rate and character of breathing, and oxygen saturation.
- If the procedure is carried out frequently (e.g., every hour), it may be appropriate to record only once, at the end of the shift; however, the frequency of the suctioning must be recorded.

SAMPLE DOCUMENTATION

1/22/2010 0830 Producing large amounts of thick, tenacious white mucus to back of oral pharynx but unable to expectorate into tissue. Uses Yankauer suction tube as needed. O_2 sat increased from 89% before suctioning to 93% after suctioning. RR also decreased from 26 to 18–20 after suctioning. Continuous O_2 at 2 L/min via n/c. Will continue to reassess q hour. ─────────── L. Webb, RN

EVALUATION
- Conduct appropriate follow-up, such as appearance of secretions suctioned; breath sounds; respiratory rate, rhythm, and depth; pulse rate and rhythm; and skin color.

- Compare findings to previous assessment data if available.
- Report significant deviations from normal to the primary care provider.

Following endotracheal intubation or a tracheostomy, the trachea and surrounding respiratory tissues are irritated and react by producing excessive secretions. Sterile suctioning is necessary to remove these secretions from the trachea and bronchi to maintain a patent airway. The frequency of suctioning depends on the client's health and how recently the intubation was done. Additionally, suctioning may be necessary in clients who have increased secretions because of pneumonia or inability to clear secretions because of altered level of consciousness.

Suctioning is associated with several complications: hypoxemia, trauma to the airway, nosocomial infection, and cardiac dysrhythmia, which is related to the hypoxemia. The following techniques are used to minimize or decrease these complications:

- **Hyperinflation.** This involves giving the client breaths that are 1 to 1.5 times the tidal volume set on the ventilator through the ventilator circuit or via a manual resuscitation bag. Three to five breaths are delivered before and after each pass of the suction catheter.
- **Hyperoxygenation.** This can be done with a manual resuscitation bag or through the ventilator and is performed by increasing the oxygen flow (usually to 100%) before suctioning and between suction attempts.

For tracheostomy and endotracheal suctioning, the outer diameter of the suction catheter should not exceed one-half the internal diameter of the tracheostomy or endotracheal tube so that hypoxia can be prevented (St. John, 2004). The nurse uses sterile techniques to prevent infection of the respiratory tract (see Skill 35–3). The traditional method of suctioning an endotracheal tube or tracheostomy is sometimes referred to as the *open method*. If a client is connected to a ventilator, the nurse disconnects the client from the ventilator, suctions the airway, reconnects the client to the ventilator, and discards the suction catheter. Drawbacks to the open airway suction system include the nurse needing to wear personal protective equipment (e.g., goggles or face shield, gown) to avoid exposure to the client's sputum and the potential cost of one-time catheter use, especially if the client requires frequent suctioning.

With the *closed airway/tracheal suction system (in-line suctioning)* (Figure 35–13), the suction catheter attaches to the ventilator tubing and the client does not need to be disconnected from the ventilator. The nurse is not exposed to any secretions because the suction catheter is enclosed in a plastic sheath. The catheter can be reused as many times as necessary until the system is changed. The nurse needs to inquire about the agency's policy for changing the closed suction system.

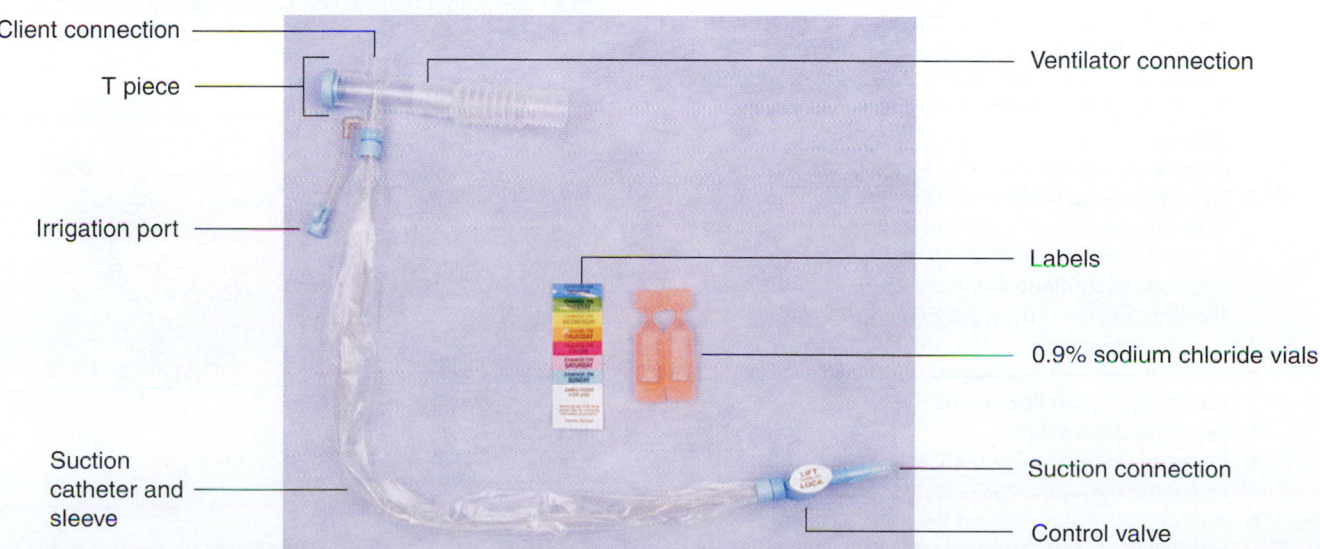

Client connection —
T piece —
Ventilator connection
Irrigation port —
Labels
0.9% sodium chloride vials
Suction catheter and sleeve —
Suction connection
Control valve

Figure 35–13 ◯ A closed airway suction (in-line) system.

SUCTIONING A TRACHEOSTOMY OR ENDOTRACHEAL TUBE

PURPOSES
- To maintain a patent airway and prevent airway obstructions
- To promote respiratory function (optimal exchange of oxygen and carbon dioxide into and out of the lungs)
- To prevent pneumonia that may result from accumulated secretions

ASSESSMENT
Assess the client for the presence of congestion on auscultation of the thorax. Note the client's ability or inability to remove the secretions through coughing.

PLANNING

> **Delegation**
>
> Suctioning a tracheostomy or endotracheal tube is a sterile, invasive technique requiring application of scientific knowledge and problem solving. This skill is performed by a nurse or respiratory therapist and is not delegated to UAP.

EQUIPMENT
- Resuscitation bag connected to 100% oxygen
- Sterile towel (optional)
- Equipment for suctioning (see Skill 35–2)
- Goggles and mask if necessary
- Gown (if necessary)
- Sterile gloves
- Moisture-resistant bag

IMPLEMENTATION

Preparation
Determine if the client has been suctioned previously and, if so, review the documentation of the procedure. This information can be very helpful in preparing the nurse for both the physiologic and psychologic impact of suctioning on the client.

Performance
1. Prior to performing the procedure, introduce self and verify the client's identity using agency protocol. Explain to the client what you are going to do, why it is necessary, and how he or she can participate. Inform the client that suctioning usually causes some intermittent coughing and that this assists in removing the secretions.
2. Perform hand hygiene and observe other appropriate infection control procedures (e.g., gloves, goggles).
3. Provide for client privacy.
4. Prepare the client.
   - If not contraindicated because of health, place the client in the semi-Fowler's position to promote deep breathing, maximum lung expansion, and productive coughing. **Rationale:** *Deep breathing oxygenates the lungs, counteracts the hypoxic effects of suctioning, and may induce coughing. Coughing helps to loosen and move secretions.*
   - If necessary, provide analgesia before suctioning. Endotracheal suctioning stimulates the cough reflex, which can cause pain for clients who have had thoracic or abdominal surgery or who have experienced traumatic injury. **Rationale:** *Premedication can increase the client's comfort during the suctioning procedure.*
5. Prepare the equipment.
   - Attach the resuscitation apparatus to the oxygen source. Adjust the oxygen flow to 100%.
   - Open the sterile supplies.
   - Place the sterile towel, if used, across the client's chest below the tracheostomy.
   - Turn on the suction, and set the pressure in accordance with agency policy. For a wall unit, a pressure setting of about 100 to 120 mm Hg is normally used for adults, 60 to 100 mm Hg for children.
   - Apply goggles, mask, and gown if necessary.
   - Apply sterile gloves. Some agencies recommend putting a sterile glove on the dominant hand and an unsterile glove on the nondominant hand to protect the nurse.
   - Holding the catheter in the dominant hand and the connector in the nondominant hand, attach the suction catheter to the suction tubing (see ❶ in Skill 35–2).
6. Flush and lubricate the catheter.
   - Using the dominant hand, place the catheter tip in the sterile saline solution.
   - Using the thumb of the nondominant hand, occlude the thumb control and suction a small amount of the sterile solution through the catheter. **Rationale:** *This determines that the suction equipment is working properly and lubricates the outside and the lumen of the catheter. Lubrication eases insertion and reduces tissue trauma during insertion. Lubricating the lumen also helps prevent secretions from sticking to the inside of the catheter.*
7. If the client does not have copious secretions, hyperventilate the lungs with a resuscitation bag before suctioning.
   - Summon an assistant, if one is available, for this step.

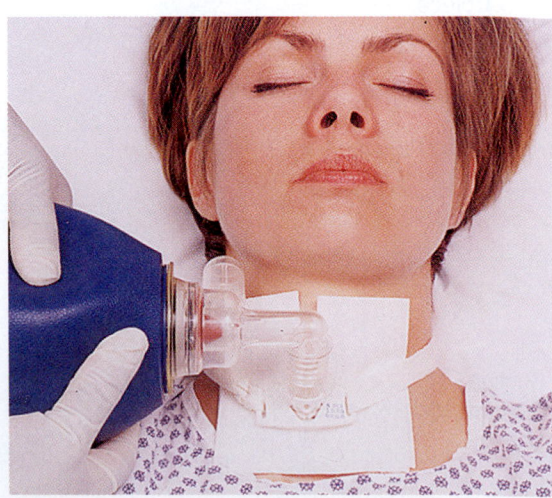

❶ Attaching the resuscitator to the tracheostomy.

- Using your nondominant hand, turn on the oxygen to 12 to 15 L/min.
- If the client is receiving oxygen, disconnect the oxygen source from the tracheostomy tube using your nondominant hand.
- Attach the resuscitator to the tracheostomy or endotracheal tube. ❶
- Compress the resuscitation bag three to five times, as the client inhales. This is best done by a second person who can use both hands to compress the bag, thus, providing a greater inflation volume.
- Observe the rise and fall of the client's chest to assess the adequacy of each ventilation.
- Remove the resuscitation device and place it on the bed or the client's chest with the connector facing up.

VARIATION: USING A VENTILATOR TO PROVIDE HYPERVENTILATION
If the client is on a ventilator, use the ventilator for hyperventilation and hyperoxygenation. Newer models have a mode that provides 100% oxygen for 2 minutes and then switches back to the previous oxygen setting as well as a manual breath or sigh button.

Rationale: The use of ventilator settings provides more consistent delivery of oxygenation and hyperinflation than a resuscitation device.

8. If the client has copious secretions, do not hyperventilate with a resuscitator. *Instead:*
   - Keep the regular oxygen delivery device on and increase the liter flow or adjust the FiO_2 to 100% for several breaths before suctioning. **Rationale:** *Hyperventilating a client who has copious secretions can force the secretions deeper into the respiratory tract.*
9. Quickly but gently insert the catheter *without* applying any suction.
   - With your nondominant thumb off the suction port, quickly but gently insert the catheter into the trachea through the tracheostomy tube. ❷ **Rationale:** *To prevent tissue trauma and oxygen loss, suction is not applied during insertion of the catheter.*
   - Insert the catheter about 12.5 cm (5 in.) for adults, less for children, or until the client coughs or you feel resistance. **Rationale:** *Resistance usually means that the catheter tip has reached the bifurcation of the trachea. To prevent damaging the mucous membranes at the*

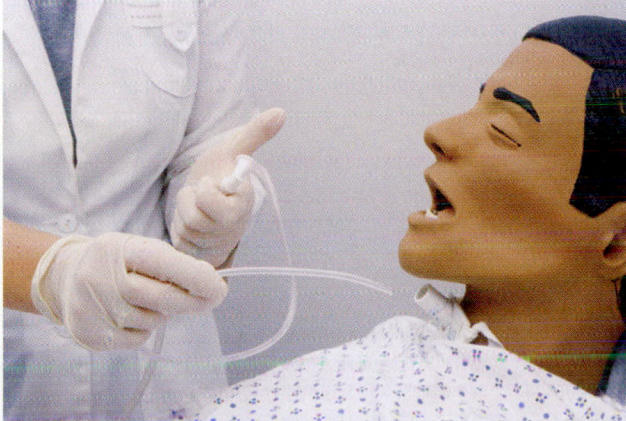

❷ Inserting the catheter into the trachea through the tracheostomy tube. Note: Suction is not applied while inserting the catheter.

bifurcation, withdraw the catheter about 1 to 2 cm (0.4 to 0.8 in.) before applying suction.
10. Perform suctioning.
   - Apply suction for 5 to 10 seconds by placing the nondominant thumb over the thumb port. **Rationale:** *Suction time is restricted to 10 seconds or less to minimize oxygen loss.*
   - Rotate the catheter by rolling it between your thumb and forefinger while slowly withdrawing it. **Rationale:** *This prevents tissue trauma by minimizing the suction time against any part of the trachea.*
   - Withdraw the catheter completely, and release the suction.
   - Hyperventilate the client.
   - Suction again, if needed.
11. Reassess the client's oxygenation status and repeat suctioning.
   - Observe the client's respirations and skin color. Check the client's pulse if necessary, using your nondominant hand.
   - Encourage the client to breathe deeply and to cough between suctions.
   - Allow 2 to 3 minutes with oxygen, as appropriate between suctions when possible. **Rationale:** *This provides an opportunity for reoxygenation of the lungs.*
   - Flush the catheter and repeat suctioning until the air passage is clear and the breathing is relatively effortless and quiet.
   - After each suction, pick up the resuscitation bag with your nondominant hand and ventilate the client with no more than three breaths.
12. Dispose of equipment and ensure availability for the next suction.
   - Flush the catheter and suction tubing.
   - Turn off the suction and disconnect the catheter from the suction tubing.
   - Wrap the catheter around your sterile hand and peel the glove off so that it turns inside out over the catheter.
   - Discard the glove and the catheter in the moisture-resistant bag.
   - Replenish the sterile fluid and supplies so that the suction is ready for use again. **Rationale:** *Clients who require suctioning often require it quickly, so it is essential to leave the equipment at the bedside ready for use.*
   - Be sure that the ventilator and oxygen settings are returned to presuctioning settings. **Rationale:** *On some ventilators this is automatic, but always check. It is very dangerous for clients to be left on 100% oxygen.*
13. Provide for client comfort and safety.
   - Assist the client to a comfortable, safe position that aids breathing. If the person is conscious, a semi-Fowler's position is frequently indicated. If the person is unconscious, Sims' position aids in the drainage of secretions from the mouth.
14. Document relevant data.
   - Record the suctioning, including the amount and description of suction returns and any other relevant assessments.

SAMPLE DOCUMENTATION

1/13/2010 1000 Coarse rales in RLL and LLL. Requires suctioning about every 1–2 hrs. Obtain large amount of pinkish tinged white thin mucous via ETT. Breath sounds clearer after suctioning. Pt. signals when he wants to be suctioned. ——————————— C. Holmes, RN

(continued)

SUCTIONING A TRACHEOSTOMY OR ENDOTRACHEAL TUBE *(continued)*

VARIATION: CLOSED SUCTION SYSTEM (IN-LINE CATHETER)

- If a catheter is not attached, put on clean gloves, aseptically open a new closed catheter set, and attach the ventilator connection on the T piece to the ventilator tubing. Attach the client connection to the endotracheal tube or tracheostomy.
- Attach one end of the suction connecting tubing to the suction connection port of the closed system and the other end of the connecting tubing to the suction device.
- Turn suction on, occlude or kink tubing, and depress the suction control valve (on the closed catheter system) to set suction to the appropriate level. Release the suction control valve.
- Use the ventilator to hyperoxygenate and hyperinflate the client's lungs.
- Unlock the suction control mechanism if required by the manufacturer.

- Advance the suction catheter enclosed in its plastic sheath with the dominant hand. Steady the T piece with the nondominant hand.
- Depress the suction control valve and apply suction for no more than 10 seconds and gently withdraw the catheter.
- Repeat as needed, remembering to provide hyperoxygenation and hyperinflation as needed.
- When completed suctioning, withdraw the catheter into its sleeve and close the access valve, if appropriate. **Rationale:** *If the system does not have an access valve on the client connector, the nurse needs to observe for the potential of the catheter migrating into the airway and partially obstructing the artificial airway.*
- Flush the catheter by instilling normal saline into the irrigation port and applying suction. Repeat until the catheter is clear.
- Close the irrigation port and close the suction valve.

EVALUATION

- Perform a follow-up examination of the client to determine the effectiveness of the suctioning (e.g., respiratory rate, depth, and character; breath sounds; color of skin and nail beds; character and amount of secretions suctioned; changes in vital signs).

- Relate findings to previous assessment data if available.
- Report significant deviations from normal to the primary care provider.

LIFESPAN CONSIDERATIONS   Suctioning a Tracheostomy or Endotracheal Tube

Infants and Children

- Have an assistant gently restrain the child to keep the child's hands out of the way. The assistant should maintain the child's head in the midline position.

Older Adults

- Do a thorough lung assessment before and after suctioning to determine effectiveness of suctioning and to be aware of any special problems.

PROVIDING TRACHEOSTOMY CARE

PURPOSES

- To maintain airway patency
- To maintain cleanliness and prevent infection at the tracheostomy site

- To facilitate healing and prevent skin excoriation around the tracheostomy incision
- To promote comfort

ASSESSMENT

Assess the following:

- Respiratory status including ease of breathing, rate, rhythm, depth, lung sounds, and oxygen saturation level
- Pulse rate

- Character and amount of secretions from tracheostomy site
- Presence of drainage on tracheostomy dressing or ties
- Appearance of incision (note any redness, swelling, purulent discharge, or odor)

PLANNING

> **Delegation**
> Tracheostomy care involves application of scientific knowledge, sterile technique, and problem solving, and therefore needs to be performed by a nurse or respiratory therapist.

EQUIPMENT

- Sterile disposable tracheostomy cleaning kit or supplies including sterile containers, sterile nylon brush and/or pipe cleaners, sterile applicators, gauze squares
- Towel or drape to protect bed linens

- Sterile suction catheter kit (suction catheter and sterile container for solution)
- Sterile normal saline (Check agency protocol for soaking solution.)
- Sterile gloves (2 pairs)
- Clean gloves

- Moisture-proof bag
- Commercially prepared sterile tracheostomy dressing or sterile 4-in. × 4-in. gauze dressing
- Cotton twill ties
- Clean scissors

IMPLEMENTATION

Performance

1. Prior to performing the procedure, introduce self and verify the client's identity using agency protocol. Explain to the client what you are going to do, why it is necessary, and how he or she can participate. Provide for a means of communication, such as eye blinking or raising a finger, to indicate pain or distress.

2. Perform hand hygiene and observe other appropriate infection control procedures.

3. Provide for client privacy.

4. Prepare the client and the equipment.
   - Assist the client to a semi-Fowler's or Fowler's position *to promote lung expansion.*
   - Suction the tracheostomy tube if needed. If suctioning required, allow client to rest and restore oxygenation.
   - Open the tracheostomy kit or sterile basins.
   - Establish a sterile field.
   - Open other sterile supplies as needed including sterile applicators, suction kit, and tracheostomy dressing.
   - Pour the soaking solution and sterile normal saline into separate containers.
   - Apply clean gloves.
   - Remove oxygen source.
   - Unlock the inner cannula (if present) and remove it by gently pulling it out toward you in line with its curvature. Place the inner cannula in the soaking solution. **Rationale:** *This moistens and loosens dried secretions.*
   - Remove the soiled tracheostomy dressing. Place the soiled dressing in your gloved hand and peel the glove off so that it turns inside out over the dressing. Remove and discard the gloves and the dressing. Perform hand hygiene.
   - Put on sterile gloves. Keep your dominant hand sterile during the procedure.

5. Clean the inner cannula. (See Variation for using a disposable inner cannula.)
   - Remove the inner cannula from the soaking solution.
   - Clean the lumen and entire inner cannula thoroughly using the brush or pipe cleaners moistened with sterile normal saline. ❶ Inspect the cannula for cleanliness by holding it at eye level and looking through it into the light.
   - Rinse the inner cannula thoroughly in the sterile normal saline.
   - After rinsing, gently tap the cannula against the inside edge of the sterile saline container. Use a pipe cleaner folded in half to dry only the inside of the cannula; do not dry the outside. **Rationale:** *This removes excess liquid from the cannula and prevents possible aspiration by the client, while leaving a film of moisture on the outer surface to lubricate the cannula for reinsertion.*

6. Replace the inner cannula, securing it in place.
   - Insert the inner cannula by grasping the outer flange and inserting the cannula in the direction of its curvature.

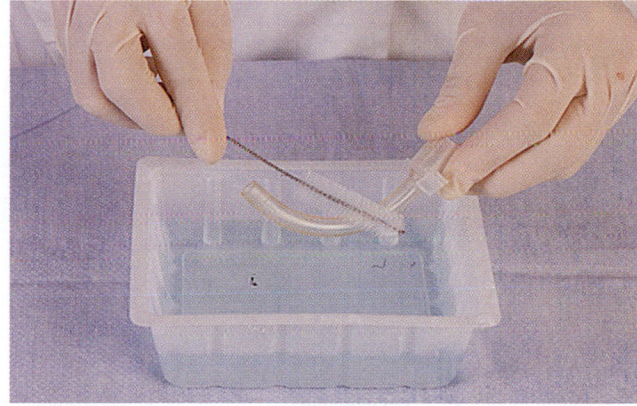

❶ Cleaning the inner cannula with a brush.

   - Lock the cannula in place by turning the lock (if present) into position to secure the flange of the inner cannula to the outer cannula.

7. Clean the incision site and tube flange.
   - Using sterile applicators or gauze dressings moistened with normal saline, clean the incision site. ❷ Handle the sterile supplies with your dominant hand. Use each applicator or gauze dressing only once and then discard. **Rationale:** *This avoids contaminating a clean area with a soiled gauze dressing or applicator.*
   - Hydrogen peroxide may be used (usually in a half-strength solution mixed with sterile normal saline; use a separate sterile container if this is necessary) to remove crusty secretions. Check agency policy. Thoroughly rinse the cleaned area using gauze squares moistened with sterile normal saline. **Rationale:** *Hydrogen peroxide can be irritating to the skin and inhibit healing if not thoroughly removed.*
   - Clean the flange of the tube in the same manner.
   - Thoroughly dry the client's skin and tube flanges with dry gauze squares.

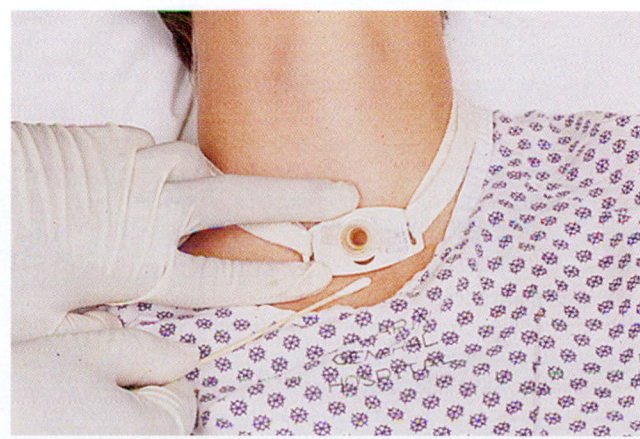

❷ Using an applicator stick to clean the tracheostomy site.

(continued)

PROVIDING TRACHEOSTOMY CARE *(continued)*

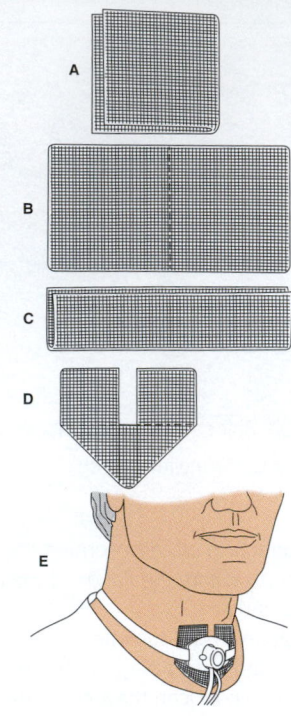

❸ Folding a 4-in. × 4-in. gauze to make a tracheostomy dressing.

8. Apply a sterile dressing.
   - Use a commercially prepared tracheostomy dressing of nonraveling material or open and refold a 4 × 4 in. gauze dressing into a V shape as shown ❸ in, *A* through *D*. Avoid using cotton-filled gauze squares or cutting the 4-in × 4-in gauze. **Rationale:** *Cotton lint or gauze fibers can be aspirated by the client, potentially creating a tracheal abscess.*
   - Place the dressing under the flange of the tracheostomy tube as shown in ❸, *E*.
   - While applying the dressing, ensure that the tracheostomy tube is securely supported. **Rationale:** *Excessive movement of the tracheostomy tube irritates the trachea.*
9. Change the tracheostomy ties.
   - Change as needed to keep the skin clean and dry.
   - Twill tape and specially manufactured Velcro ties are available. Twill tape is inexpensive and readily available; however, it is easily soiled and can trap moisture that leads to irritation of the skin of the neck. Velcro ties are becoming more commonly used. ❹ They are wider, more comfortable, and cause less skin abrasion (American Thoracic Society, 2006).

   Two-Strip Method (Twill Tape)
   - Cut two unequal strips of twill tape, one approximately 25 cm (10 in.) long and the other about 50 cm (20 in.) long. **Rationale:** *Cutting one tape longer than the other allows them to be fastened at the side of the neck for easy access and to avoid the pressure of a knot on the skin at the back of the neck.*

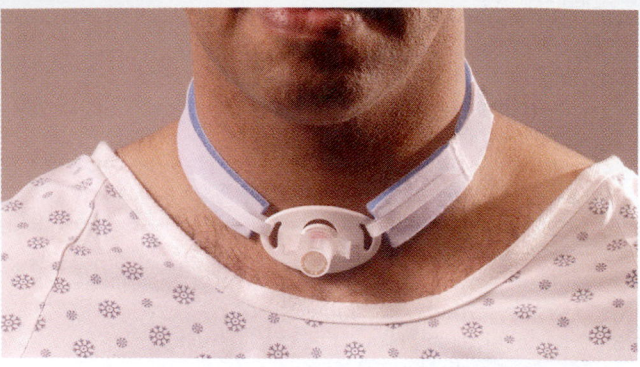

❹ A Velcro tracheostomy tie.

   - Cut a 1-cm (0.5-in.) lengthwise slit approximately 2.5 cm (1 in.) from one end of each strip. To do this, fold the end of the tape back onto itself about 2.5 cm (1 in.), then cut a slit in the middle of the tape from its folded edge.
   - Leaving the old ties in place, thread the slit end of one clean tape through the eye of the tracheostomy flange from the bottom side; then thread the long end of the tape through the slit, pulling it tight until it is securely fastened to the flange. **Rationale:** *Leaving the old ties in place while securing the clean ties prevents inadvertent dislodging of the tracheostomy tube. Securing tapes in this manner avoids the use of knots, which can come untied or cause pressure and irritation.*
   - If old ties are very soiled or it is difficult to thread new ties onto the tracheostomy flange with old ties in place, have an assistant put on a sterile glove and hold the tracheostomy in place while you replace the ties. This is very important because movement of the tube during this procedure may cause irritation and stimulate coughing. Coughing can dislodge the tube if the ties are undone.
   - Repeat the process for the second tie.
   - Ask the client to flex the neck. Slip the longer tape under the client's neck, place a finger between the tape and the client's neck ❺, and tie the tapes together at the side of the neck. **Rationale:** *Flexing the neck increases its circumference the way coughing does. Placing a finger under the tie prevents making the tie too tight, which could interfere with coughing or place pressure on the jugular veins.*
   - Tie the ends of the tapes using square knots. Cut off any long ends, leaving approximately 1 to 2 cm (0.5 in.). **Rationale:** *Square knots prevent slippage and loosening. Adequate ends beyond the knot prevent the knot from inadvertently untying.*
   - Once the clean ties are secured, remove the soiled ties and discard.

   One-Strip Method (Twill Tape)
   - Cut a length of twill tape 2.5 times the length needed to go around the client's neck from one tube flange to the other.

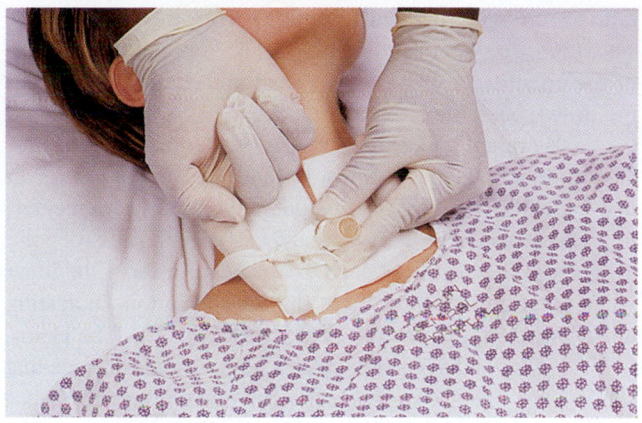

⑤ Placing a finger underneath the tie tape before tying it.

- Thread one end of the tape into the slot on one side of the flange.
- Bring both ends of the tape together. Take them around the client's neck, keeping them flat and untwisted.
- Thread the end of the tape next to the client's neck through the slot from the back to the front.
- Have the client flex the neck. Tie the loose ends with a square knot at the side of the client's neck, allowing for slack by placing two fingers under the ties as with the two-strip method. Cut off long ends.

10. Tape and pad the tie knot.
- Place a folded 4 × 4 in. gauze square under the tie knot, and apply tape over the knot. **Rationale:** *This reduces skin irritation from the knot and prevents confusing the knot with the client's gown ties.*

EVALUATION

- Perform appropriate follow-up such as determining character and amount of secretions, drainage from the tracheostomy, appearance of the tracheostomy incision, pulse rate and respiratory status compared to baseline data, and complaints of pain or discomfort at the tracheostomy site.

12. Check the tightness of the ties.
- Frequently check the tightness of the tracheostomy ties and position of the tracheostomy tube. **Rationale:** *Swelling of the neck may cause the ties to become too tight, interfering with coughing and circulation. Ties can loosen in restless clients, allowing the tracheostomy tube to extrude from the stoma.*

13. Document all relevant information.
- Record suctioning, tracheostomy care, and the dressing change, noting your assessments.

SAMPLE DOCUMENTATION

1/11/2010 0900 Respirations 18–20/min. Lung sounds clear. Able to cough up secretions requiring little suctioning. Inner cannula changed. Trach dressing changed. Minimal amount of sero-sanguinous drainage present. Trach incision area pink to reddish in color 0.2 cm around entire opening. No broken skin noted in the reddened area. ———————— J. Garcia, RN

VARIATION: USING A DISPOSABLE INNER CANNULA

- Check policy for frequency of changing inner cannula *because standards vary among institutions.*
- Open a new cannula package.
- Using a gloved hand, unlock the current inner cannula (if present) and remove it by gently pulling it out toward you in line with its curvature.
- Check the cannula for amount and type of secretions and discard properly.
- Pick up the new inner cannula touching only the outer locking portion.
- Insert the new inner cannula into the tracheostomy.
- Lock the cannula in place by turning the lock (if present).

- Relate findings to previous assessment data if available.
- Report significant deviations from normal to the primary care provider.

LIFESPAN CONSIDERATIONS

Tracheostomy Care

Infants and Children

- An assistant should *always* be present while tracheostomy care is performed.
- Always keep a sterile, packaged tracheostomy tube taped to the child's bed so that if the tube dislodges, a new one is available for immediate reintubation (Bindler & Ball, 2007).

Older Adults

- Older adult skin is more fragile and prone to breakdown. Care of the skin at the tracheostomy stoma is very important.

Chest Tubes and Drainage Systems

If the thin, double-layered pleural membrane is disrupted by lung disease, surgery, or trauma, the negative pressure between the pleural layers may be lost. The lung then collapses because it is no longer drawn outward as the diaphragm and intercostal muscles contract during inhalation. When air collects in the pleural space, it is known as a **pneumothorax**. Blood or fluid in the pleural space, a **hemothorax**, places pressure on lung tissue and interferes with lung expansion. Chest tubes may be inserted into the pleural cavity to restore negative pressure and drain collected fluid or blood. Because air rises, chest tubes for pneumothorax often are placed in the upper anterior thorax, whereas chest tubes used to drain fluid generally are placed in the lower lateral chest wall.

When chest tubes are inserted, they must be connected to a sealed drainage system or a one-way valve that allows air and fluid to be removed from the chest cavity but prevents air from entering from the outside. Sterile disposable drainage systems are used to prevent outside air from entering the chest tube. These systems typically have a suction control chamber, a water seal chamber, and a closed collection chamber, for drainage (Figure 35–14). With the water-seal system, when the client inhales, the water prevents air from entering the system from the atmosphere. During exhalation, however, air can exit the chest cavity, bubbling up through the water. Suction can be added to the system to fa-cilitate removing air and secretions from the chest cavity. The drainage system should always be kept below the level of the client's chest to prevent fluid and drainage from being drawn back into the chest cavity.

A Heimlich valve may be used for ambulatory clients. The Heimlich valve is a one-way flutter valve that allows air to escape from the chest cavity, but prevents air from reentering. The arrow on the housing of the valve should always point away from the client. At each assessment, observe the inner valve carefully for movement during exhalation, indicating airflow through the device (Carroll, 2005, p. 29). The Heimlich valve is not designed to collect fluid. Another device that can attach to the chest tube, called the Pneumostat, also has a one-way valve and a small built-in collection chamber, unlike the Heimlich valve. It is used exclusively for clients with a pneumothorax who usually have small amounts of fluid.

Nursing responsibilities regarding drainage systems include the following:

- Monitor and maintain the patency and integrity of the drainage system.
- Assess the client's vital signs, oxygen saturation, cardiovascular status, and respiratory status. Check the breath sounds bilaterally and check for symmetry of breath sounds.
- Observe the dressing site at least every 4 hours. Inspect the dressing for excessive and abnormal drainage, such as bleeding or foul-smelling discharge. Palpate around the dressing site, and listen for a crackling sound indicative of subcutaneous emphysema. *Subcutaneous emphysema, which is air in the subcutaneous tissues, can result from a poor seal at the chest tube insertion site.*
- Determine level of discomfort with and without activity and medicate the client for pain if indicated.
- Encourage deep breathing and coughing exercises every 2 hours (this may be contraindicated in clients who have had a lung removed). Have the client sit upright to perform the exercises, and splint the chest around the tube insertion site with a pillow or with a hand to minimize discomfort.
- Reposition the client every 2 hours. When the client is lying on the affected side, place rolled towels beside the tubing. *Frequent position changes promote drainage, prevent complications, and provide comfort. Rolled towels prevent occlusion of the chest tube by the client's weight.*
- Assist the client with range-of-motion exercises of the affected shoulder three times per day to maintain joint mobility.

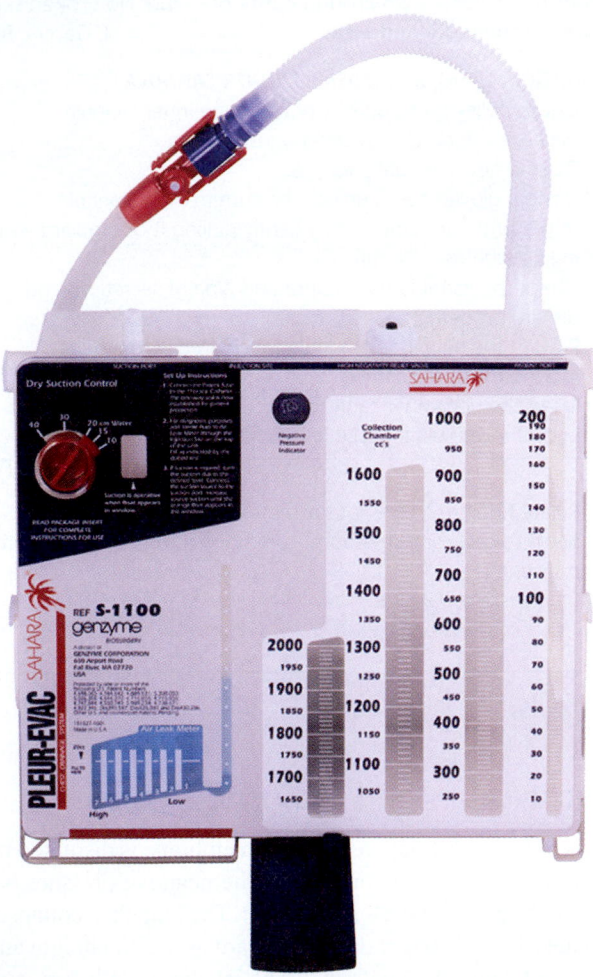

Figure 35–14 ○ A disposable chest drainage system.
(Pleur-evac® Chest Drainage System. Reprinted with permission from Genzyme Biosurgery, Cardiothoracic Division, Fall River, MA.)

- Ensure that the connections are securely taped and that the chest tube is secured to the client's chest wall.
- Keep the collection device below the client's chest level.
- Frequently check the water seal and suction control chambers. The water can evaporate and water may need to be added to the chamber. The water seal level should fluctuate with respiratory effort (Coughlin & Parchinsky, 2006).
- Assess the drainage in the tubing and collection chamber. The drainage is measured at regularly scheduled times (check the agency policy). Mark the date and time at the fluid level on the drainage chamber. The unit is not replaced until almost full.
- Avoid aggressive chest tube manipulation (e.g., milking or stripping the tube). Studies have shown that these techniques do not improve chest tube patency. If necessary, however, a gentle technique such as squeezing hand over hand along the tubing and releasing the tubing between squeezes may help improve patency (Coughlin & Parchinsky, 2006, p. 40).
- Avoid clamping the chest tube as this increases the risk of a tension pneumothorax. You can clamp the tube for a moment to replace the drainage unit or to locate the source of an air leak, but never when transporting a client or for any extended period of time (Coughlin & Parchinsky, 2006, p. 40).
- If the tube becomes disconnected from the collecting system, submerge the end in 1 in. of sterile saline or water *to maintain the seal.* If the chest tube is inadvertently pulled out, the wound should be immediately covered with a dry sterile dressing. If you can hear air leaking out the site, ensure that the dressing is not occlusive. *If the air cannot escape, this would lead to a tension pneumothorax. A tension pneumothorax occurs when there is buildup of air in the pleural space and it cannot escape, causing increased pressure. This pressure can eventually compromise cardiovascular function.*
- When transporting and ambulating the client:
  a. Keep the water-seal unit below chest level and upright.
  b. Disconnect the drainage system from the suction apparatus before moving the client and make sure the air vent is open.
- Use standard precautions and personal protective equipment while manipulating the system and assisting with insertion or removal.

Chest tube insertion and removal require sterile technique and must be done without introducing air or microorganisms into the pleural cavity. Removal of a chest tube is a brief but quite painful procedure. Medicate the client before the removal. Remove the dressing around the tube and prepare the dressing that will cover the insertion site. This will be an occlusive dressing if there is no purse-string suture around the insertion site to prevent air from entering the chest. Generally, the primary care provider performs the removal but, in some areas, specially trained nurses may be permitted to do so.

EVALUATING

Using the goals and desired outcomes identified in the planning stage of the nursing process, the nurse collects data to evaluate the effectiveness of interventions. If outcomes are not achieved, the nurse, client, and support person if appropriate need to explore the reasons before modifying the care plan. For example, if the outcome "Respirations unlabored and rate is within expected range" is not met, examples of questions that need to be considered include the following:

- What is the client's perception of the problem?
- Is the client complaining of shortness of breath or difficulty breathing?
- Is the client taking medications or performing treatments such as percussion, vibration, and postural drainage as prescribed?
- Has the client been exposed to an upper respiratory infection that is affecting breathing?
- Do other factors need to be considered, such as the client's psychologic stress level?

Examples of questions to consider if the outcome "Able to complete ADLs without fatigue" is not met include the following:

- What other factors may be affecting the client's ability to complete ADLs?
- Is the client getting adequate sleep? If not, what is interfering with the client's rest?
- Are there assistive devices (e.g., a shower chair, clothing that is easy to put on) that could help the client achieve this goal?
- Does the client need help with housework and other ADLs?
- Is the client's diet adequate to meet nutritional needs?

Nursing Care Plan   For Ineffective Airway Clearance

ASSESSMENT DATA	NURSING DIAGNOSIS	DESIRED OUTCOMES*
Nursing Assessment Johti Singh is a 39-year-old secretary who was admitted to the hospital with an elevated temperature, fatigue, rapid, labored respirations, and mild dehydration. The nursing history reveals that Ms. Singh has had a "bad cold" for several weeks that just wouldn't go away. She has been dieting for several months and skipping meals. Ms. Singh mentions that in addition to her full-time job as a secretary she is attending college classes two evenings a week. She has smoked one package of cigarettes per day since she was 18 years old. Chest x-ray confirms pneumonia.	*Ineffective Airway Clearance* related to thick sputum, secondary to pneumonia (as evidenced by rapid respirations, diminished and adventitious breath sounds, thick yellow sputum)	Respiratory Status: Airway Patency [0410] as evidenced by not compromised • Respiratory rate • Moves sputum out of airway • No adventitious breath sounds
Physical Examination Height: 167.6 cm (5'6") Weight: 54.4 kg (120 lb) Temperature: 39.4°C (103°F) Pulse: 68 BPM Respirations: 24/minute Blood pressure: 118/70 mm Hg Skin pale; cheeks flushed; chills; use of accessory muscles; inspiratory crackles with diminished breath sounds right base; expectorating thick, yellow sputum **Diagnostic Data** Chest x-ray: right lobar infiltration WBC: 14,000 pH: 7.49 $PaCO_2$: 33 mm Hg HCO_3^-: 20 mEq/L PaO_2: 80 mm Hg O_2 SAT: 88%		

NURSING INTERVENTIONS*/SELECTED ACTIVITIES	RATIONALE
Cough Enhancement [3250]	
Assist Ms. Singh to a sitting position with head slightly flexed, shoulders relaxed, and knees flexed.	*Lying flat causes the abdominal organs to shift toward the chest, crowding the lungs and making it more difficult to breathe.*
Encourage her to take several deep breaths.	*Deep breathing promotes oxygenation before controlled coughing.*
Encourage her to take a deep breath, hold for 2 seconds, and cough two or three times in succession.	*Controlled coughing is accomplished by closure of the glottis and the explosive expulsion of air from the lungs by the work of abdominal and chest muscles.*
Encourage use of incentive spirometry, as appropriate.	*Breathing exercises help maximize ventilation.*
Promote systemic fluid hydration, as appropriate.	*Adequate fluid intake enhances liquefaction of pulmonary secretions and facilitates expectoration of mucus.*
Respiratory Monitoring [3350]	
Monitor rate, rhythm, depth, and effort of respirations.	*Provides a basis for evaluating adequacy of ventilation.*
Note chest movement, watching for symmetry, use of accessory muscles, and supraclavicular and intercostal muscle retractions.	*Presence of nasal flaring and use of accessory muscles of respirations may occur in response to ineffective ventilation.*
Auscultate breath sounds, noting areas of decreased or absent ventilation and presence of adventitious sounds.	*As fluid and mucus accumulate, abnormal breath sounds can be heard including crackles and diminished breath sounds owing to fluid-filled air spaces and diminished lung volume.*
Auscultate lung sounds after treatments to note results.	*Assists in evaluating prescribed treatments and client outcomes.*
Monitor client's ability to cough effectively.	*Respiratory tract infections alter the amount and character of secretions. An ineffective cough compromises airway clearance and prevents mucus from being expelled.*
Monitor client's respiratory secretions.	*People with pneumonia commonly produce rust-colored, purulent sputum.*

NURSING INTERVENTIONS*/SELECTED ACTIVITIES	RATIONALE
Institute respiratory therapy treatments (e.g., nebulizer) as needed.	*A variety of respiratory therapy treatments may be used to open constricted airways and liquefy secretions.*
Monitor for increased restlessness, anxiety, and air hunger.	*These clinical manifestations would be early indicators of hypoxia.*
Note changes in SpO₂, tidal volume, and changes in arterial blood gas values, as appropriate.	*Evaluates the status of oxygenation, ventilation, and acid–base balance.*

EVALUATION

Outcome partially met. Ms. Singh coughs and deep breathes purposefully q1–2h during the day. Her fluid intake is approximately 1,500 mL each day. Cough continues to be productive of moderately thick, rusty-colored sputum. Inspiratory crackles remain present in right lower lobe.

*The NOC # for desired outcomes and the NIC # for nursing interventions are listed in brackets following the appropriate outcome or intervention. Outcomes, interventions, and activities selected are only a sample of those by NOC and NIC and should be further individualized for each client.

CRITICAL THINKING QUESTIONS

1. What factors may have led the medical staff to suspect that Ms. Singh had more than a very bad cold? Would you have come to the same conclusion?

2. The care plan appropriately focuses on the acute care of this client. Once she is significantly improved, the nurse will perform discharge teaching. What areas should be included?

3. The client already has some signs of respiratory distress. What signs might indicate that her condition was deteriorating into a more emergency situation? How would you handle this?

4. It appears that the client's sputum has not been cultured. In caring for this client, what infection control guidelines would be needed?

5. Ms. Singh's oxygen order is for a face mask at 6 L/minute. She repeatedly pulls it off and you find it lying in the sheets. How might you intervene?

∞ *See Answers in MyNursingKit.*

CIRCULATION

The circulatory system or cardiovascular system is responsible for transport of oxygen, fluids, electrolytes, and products of metabolism via the blood to and from tissues.

Physiology of the Cardiovascular System

The respiratory and cardiovascular systems are closely linked and dependent on one another to deliver oxygen to the tissues of the body. Alterations in function of either system can affect the other and lead to tissue hypoxia, or lack of oxygen.

The heart and the blood vessels make up the cardiovascular system. Together with blood, it is the major transport system of the body, bringing oxygen and nutrients to the cells and removing wastes for disposal. The heart serves as the system pump, moving blood through the vessels to the tissues.

THE HEART The heart is enclosed by a double layer of fibroserous membrane known as the pericardium. The parietal, or outermost, pericardium serves to protect the heart and anchor it to surrounding structures. The visceral pericardium adheres to the surface of the heart, forming the heart's outermost layer, the epicardium. The heart wall contains two additional layers: the myocardium, cardiac muscle cells that form the bulk of the heart and contract with each beat, and the endocardium, which lines the inside of the heart's chambers and great vessels.

Coronary Circulation   The heart muscle receives no oxygen or nourishment from the blood within its chambers. Instead, it is supplied by a network of vessels known as the coronary circulation or more commonly the coronary arteries. The coronary arteries originate at the base of the aorta, branching out to encircle and penetrate the myocardium. The coronary arteries fill during ventricular relaxation, bringing oxygen-rich blood to the myocardium. If these arteries become clogged with atherosclerotic plaque or are obstructed by a blood clot, the myocardium is deprived of oxygen, and the client may develop chest pain (angina) or experience a **myocardial infarction** (heart attack). The cardiac veins drain the deoxygenated blood from the myocardium into the coronary sinus, which empties into the right atrium.

Cardiac Cycle   The diastolic phase of the cardiac cycle is twice as long as the systolic phase. This is important because diastole is largely a passive process. The longer diastolic phase allows ventricular filling to occur. At the end of the diastolic phase the atria contract, adding an additional volume to the ventricles. This volume is sometimes called *atrial kick*.

CONCEPT MAP   Ineffective Airway Clearance

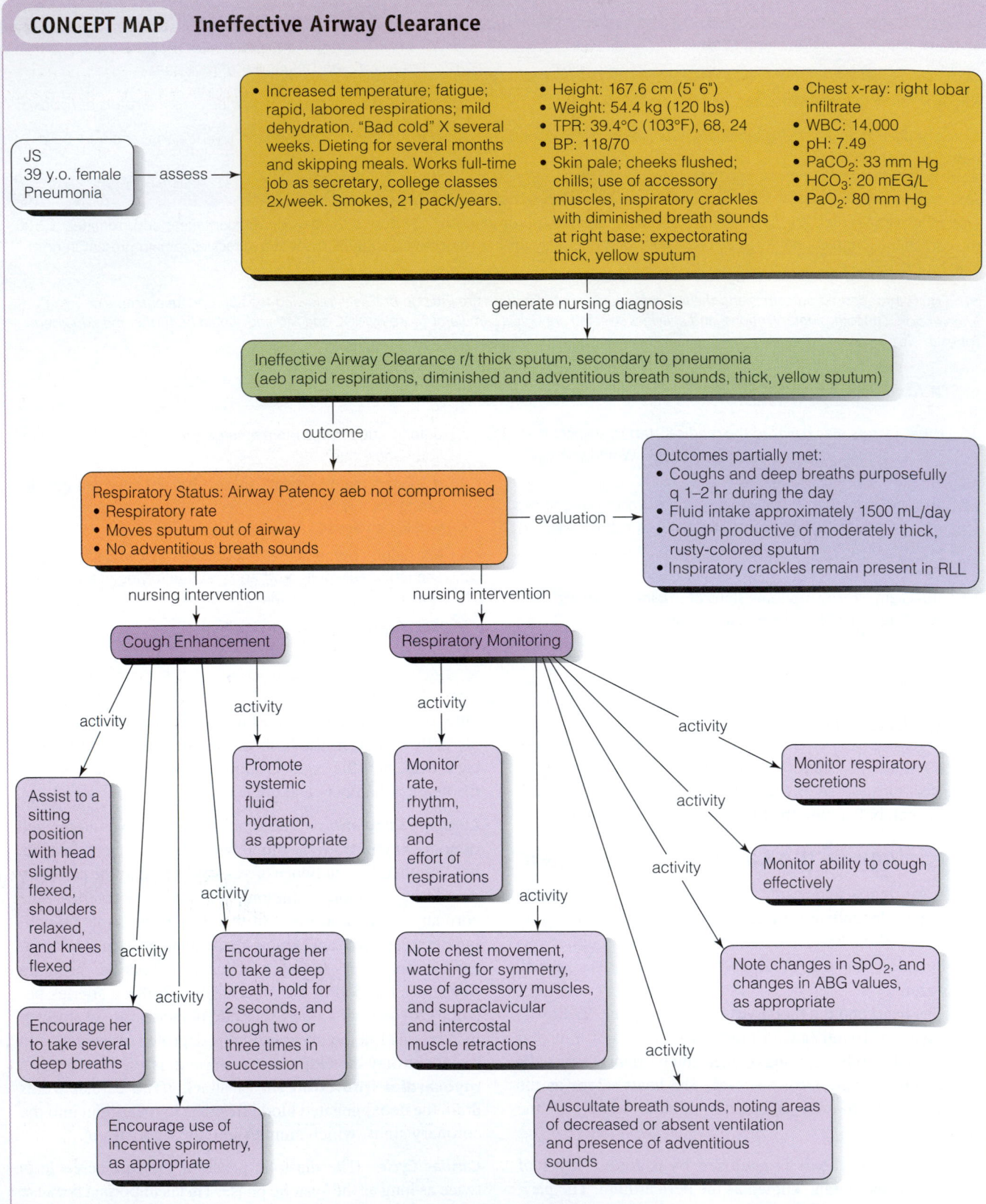

JS
39 y.o. female
Pneumonia

→ assess →

- Increased temperature; fatigue; rapid, labored respirations; mild dehydration. "Bad cold" X several weeks. Dieting for several months and skipping meals. Works full-time job as secretary, college classes 2x/week. Smokes, 21 pack/years.

- Height: 167.6 cm (5' 6")
- Weight: 54.4 kg (120 lbs)
- TPR: 39.4°C (103°F), 68, 24
- BP: 118/70
- Skin pale; cheeks flushed; chills; use of accessory muscles, inspiratory crackles with diminished breath sounds at right base; expectorating thick, yellow sputum

- Chest x-ray: right lobar infiltrate
- WBC: 14,000
- pH: 7.49
- $PaCO_2$: 33 mm Hg
- HCO_3: 20 mEG/L
- PaO_2: 80 mm Hg

↓ generate nursing diagnosis

Ineffective Airway Clearance r/t thick sputum, secondary to pneumonia (aeb rapid respirations, diminished and adventitious breath sounds, thick, yellow sputum)

↓ outcome

Respiratory Status: Airway Patency aeb not compromised
- Respiratory rate
- Moves sputum out of airway
- No adventitious breath sounds

→ evaluation →

Outcomes partially met:
- Coughs and deep breaths purposefully q 1–2 hr during the day
- Fluid intake approximately 1500 mL/day
- Cough productive of moderately thick, rusty-colored sputum
- Inspiratory crackles remain present in RLL

nursing intervention

Cough Enhancement

nursing intervention

Respiratory Monitoring

activity

Assist to a sitting position with head slightly flexed, shoulders relaxed, and knees flexed

activity

Encourage her to take several deep breaths

activity

Promote systemic fluid hydration, as appropriate

activity

Encourage her to take a deep breath, hold for 2 seconds, and cough two or three times in succession

activity

Encourage use of incentive spirometry, as appropriate

activity

Monitor rate, rhythm, depth, and effort of respirations

activity

Note chest movement, watching for symmetry, use of accessory muscles, and supraclavicular and intercostal muscle retractions

activity

Monitor respiratory secretions

activity

Monitor ability to cough effectively

activity

Note changes in SpO_2, and changes in ABG values, as appropriate

activity

Auscultate breath sounds, noting areas of decreased or absent ventilation and presence of adventitious sounds

Cardiac Conduction System Cardiac muscle contraction is a mechanical event that occurs in response to electrical stimulation. Cardiac muscle is unique in that, unlike skeletal muscle, it can generate an electrical impulse and contraction independently of the nervous system. This unique property of the heart is called **automaticity**. A network of specialized cells and pathways known as the cardiac conduction system normally controls the electrical activity and contraction of the heart.

Cardiac Output As the ventricles contract during systole, blood flows out of the ventricles through the aorta and pulmonary artery into the systemic and pulmonic circulation. The heart muscle then relaxes (the diastolic phase), allowing the ventricles to refill and cardiac muscle to be perfused. This contraction and relaxation of the heart is known as the cardiac cycle or the heartbeat. The cycle is repeated 60 to 100 times a minute in the adult, stimulated by impulses generated by the SA node.

With each contraction, a certain amount of blood, known as the stroke volume, is ejected from the ventricles into the circulation. In adults, the average stroke volume is about 70 mL per beat. **Cardiac output (CO)** is the amount of blood pumped by the ventricles in 1 minute. Cardiac output is calculated by multiplying the **stroke volume (SV)**, the amount of blood ejected with each contraction, times the heart rate (HR). Thus, SV X HR = CO. The cardiac output is an important indicator of how well the heart is functioning as a pump. If the cardiac output is poor, tissue perfusion suffers and oxygen and nutrients do not reach the cells as needed.

Cardiac output is affected by several factors:

- An increased heart rate increases cardiac output, even if the stroke volume doesn't change. Conversely, cardiac output decreases when the heart rate falls if the stroke volume remains constant. There are physiologic limits to this. For example, very rapid heart rates, more than 150 beats per minute, may not allow adequate time for the ventricles to fill, causing cardiac output to fall. The heart rate is influenced by many factors including the autonomic nervous system, blood pressure, hormones such as thyroid hormone, and some medications.
- **Preload** is the degree to which muscle fibers in the ventricle are stretched at the end of diastole. Preload largely depends on the amount of blood returning to the heart from the venous circulation: Increased volume causes increased stretch, leading to more forceful contraction of cardiac muscle fibers. This physiologic action is referred to as the Frank-Starling law of the heart. The length of the ventricular muscle fibers (stretch) at the end of diastole directly affects the strength (force) of contraction. For example, exercise increases venous return and the amount of blood in the ventricle before contraction; therefore, the heart contracts more forcefully and stroke volume and cardiac output increase during exercise.
- Contractility is the inherent ability of cardiac muscle fibers to shorten or contract. Stroke volume de-

creases if contractility is poor, reducing cardiac output. Contractility also is affected by the autonomic nervous system and certain drugs. Drugs that affect contractility are called inotropic drugs. Positive inotropic drugs increase contractility, and negative inotropic drugs decrease the contractile strength.

- **Afterload** is the resistance against which the heart must pump to eject the blood into the circulation. Blood flows from an area of higher pressure to an area of lower pressure. To move blood into the circulatory system, the ventricles must generate sufficient pressure to overcome vascular resistance or the pressure within the arteries, known as afterload. The right ventricle pumps blood into the low-pressure, low-resistance pulmonary vascular system; therefore, the pressures generated by the right ventricle are fairly low. The left ventricle, by contrast, pumps blood into the higher pressure systemic arterial system, generating much higher pressures and requiring more work. Systemic vasoconstriction increases the arterial blood pressure and afterload, increasing the cardiac workload; vasodilation, on the other hand, reduces arterial pressure and the workload of the heart. Table 35–2 summarizes the factors related to cardiac function.

THE BLOOD VESSELS With the exception of capillaries, blood vessel walls have three distinct layers, or tunics. The innermost layer, the tunica intima, is smooth endothelium that facilitates blood flow. The tunica media is made up of elastic fibers and smooth muscle cells innervated by the autonomic nervous system. This allows vessels to constrict or dilate, depending on the needs of the body. The tunica media of arteries is thicker and more muscular than in veins, a feature that helps maintain blood pressure and continuous circulation to the tissues. The outermost layer of blood vessels is the tunica adventitia, a layer of connective tissue that supports, protects, and anchors the vessel to surrounding tissues. Capillaries contain only one thin layer of tunica intima, allowing gases and molecules to diffuse between the blood and the tissues.

TABLE 35–2	**Factors Related to Cardiac Function**
INDICATOR	DEFINITION
Cardiac output (CO)	Amount of blood ejected from the heart each minute; CO = SV X HR
Stroke volume (SV)	Amount of blood ejected from the heart with each beat
Heart rate (HR)	Number of beats each minute
Contractility	Inotropic state of the myocardium, strength of contraction
Preload	Left ventricular end diastolic volume, stretch of the myocardium
Afterload	Resistance against which the heart must pump

Arterial Circulation   The arterial circulation moves blood pumped by the heart to the tissues, maintaining a constant flow to the capillary beds despite the intermittent pumping action of the heart.

Blood flow, the volume of blood flowing through a given vessel, organ, or the entire circulation over a specific period, is determined by pressure differences and resistance. Blood always moves from an area of higher pressure to an area of lower pressure. The greater the difference between pressures, the greater the blood flow. The blood pressure (BP) is the force exerted on arterial walls by the blood flowing within the vessel (see Chapter 16 ∞ for a further explanation of blood pressure). The *mean arterial pressure (MAP)* maintains blood flow to the tissues throughout the cardiac cycle. It is a product of the cardiac output times the **peripheral vascular resistance (PVR)**, or CO X PVR = MAP.

Resistance is opposition to flow; peripheral vascular resistance impedes or opposes blood flow to the tissues. PVR is determined by:

- The viscosity, or thickness, of the blood.
- Blood vessel length.
- Blood vessel diameter.

Venous Return   In contrast to the high-pressure arterial system, venous pressure is too low to adequately return blood from peripheral tissues to the heart without assistance. The fall in intrathoracic pressure that occurs with breathing draws blood upward toward the heart, an adaptation known as the respiratory pump. Skeletal muscle activity contributes to the muscular pump, as muscle contractions "milk" blood toward the heart. Venous valves are vital in making these pumps work; once blood passes a valve, it cannot flow backward away from the heart.

BLOOD   Blood serves as the transport medium within the cardiovascular system, bringing oxygen and nutrients from the environment to the cells. Blood is a complex mixture of living formed elements (the blood cells) suspended in fluid (the plasma). Its primary functions are:

- Transporting oxygen, nutrients, and hormones to the cells, and metabolic wastes from the tissues for elimination.
- Regulating body temperature, pH, and fluid volume.
- Preventing infection and blood loss.

As previously noted in this chapter, most oxygen is transported bound to hemoglobin. Hemoglobin is a major component of red blood cells (erythrocytes), the predominant cell present in blood. Hemoglobin binds easily with oxygen, releasing it in the body tissues. When all four heme groups of the hemoglobin molecule are bound to oxygen, it is said to be *fully saturated*. Oxygen binding is affected by several factors, including the PO_2, temperature, pH, and PCO_2. Up to a certain point (about 70 mm Hg), the higher the PO_2, the greater the affinity of hemoglobin for oxygen and the more saturated the hemoglobin molecules. The relationship to temperature, pH, and PCO_2 is the opposite: At higher temperatures, greater hydrogen ion concentrations (lower pH), and higher PCO_2 levels, the affinity for oxygen decreases, and hemoglobin releases its oxygen molecules. Because of hemoglobin's importance in oxygen transportation, anemia (too few red blood cells or RBCs that contain too little or abnormal hemoglobin) interferes with oxygen delivery to the tissues, leading to fatigue and activity intolerance.

Life Span Considerations

At birth, profound changes occur in the cardiovascular systems. Pulse rates are highest and most variable in newborns. The resting heart rate for a neonate ranges from 100 to 180 beats per minute immediately after birth and then stabilizes to between 120 and 160 beats per minute (Ball & Bindler, 2006, p. 303). The heart rate decreases to 80 to 130 in infants to 2 years of age and reaches the adult rate of 60 to 100 by about age 10 years. Irregular heart rates are common in infants and young children, often increasing and decreasing with each breath. This pattern of irregularity is known as sinus arrhythmia, a normal variation of the heart rate.

As the conversion from fetal circulation takes place and pressures in the left side of the heart rise, the arterial blood pressure increases. Immediately after birth (1 to 3 days of age) the blood pressure averages about 65/40. By 1 month the arterial pressure is about 90/55. It rises gradually to the adult "norm" of 120/80 by approximately 16 years of age. With aging, blood pressure may again rise as arteriosclerosis affects the blood vessels, narrowing their lumen and decreasing their compliance (ability to distend).

Congenital heart disease affects less than 1% of all live births, but is the leading cause of early death from all congenital anomalies (Hoffman, 2001). Acquired heart diseases are rare in childhood. Rheumatic fever is an inflammatory disorder that may occur following streptococcal infection (e.g., strep throat) and lead to heart valve damage. For most people, the heart continues to function effectively well into older adulthood unless the blood supply to the heart muscle is impaired by blood vessel disease. **Atherosclerosis**, the buildup of fatty plaque within the arteries, is the major contributor to cardiovascular disease, the leading cause of death in North America.

Children rarely are affected by diseases of the blood vessels. Hypertension may be associated with obesity, sedentary lifestyle, and stress in children and adolescents. During middle adulthood, the incidence of hypertension, or an elevated blood pressure, increases significantly. Hypertension, known as the silent killer because of its lack of symptoms, is a major risk factor for sudden cardiac death in middle adulthood.

FACTORS AFFECTING CARDIOVASCULAR FUNCTION

Many factors affect cardiovascular function. Some of these factors are called risk factors, because, if present, they increase the risk of cardiovascular disease. Risk factors have been identified for coronary artery disease, hypertension, and peripheral vascular disease, and the majority are the same.

LIFESPAN CONSIDERATIONS   Circulation

Children

- Blood pressure should be taken routinely on children after age 3 years.
- Heart murmurs, extra sounds detected when listening to the heart, are common in children, especially in the preschool years. The vast majority are not associated with a pathology, but are due to normal blood flow or transitional physiological processes that increase cardiac output (e.g., anemia, fever, exercise) (Blosser & Freitas-Nichols, 2004).

Older Adults

Normal changes of aging may contribute to problems of circulation in older adults, even when there is no actual pathology:

- Blood vessels become less elastic and have an increase in calcification. This results in a restricted blood flow and a decrease of oxygen and nutrients to tissues (heart, peripheral, and cerebral).
- Impaired valve function in the heart is often the result of increased stiffness and calcification and results in a decrease in cardiac output.
- A decrease of muscle tone in the heart results in a decrease in cardiac output.

- There is a decrease in baroreceptor response to blood pressure changes, making the heart and blood vessels less responsive to exercise and stress. This often results in dizziness, falls, orthostatic hypotension, and mental changes.
- A decrease in conduction ability in the heart also makes the heart less responsive to changes and stresses. This can also result in dizziness, falls, orthostatic hypotension, and mental changes.

All of these factors become important if the person is challenged by stressors, such as exercise, stress, fever, surgery, or other changes. If challenged, the circulatory system of older adults is not as effective or as quick to return to normal. Persons living with normal changes of aging and/or pathologic conditions of the circulatory system need to learn to balance diet, medications, and exercise. Nurses have a large part in working with these clients to develop appropriate interventions and provide teaching to help them maintain optimal functioning. Teaching clients to recognize any changes or worsening of their condition is very important. They need to contact the primary care provider and make any needed changes. Changing lifestyles and fine-tuning medications can be critical, and nurses can be a part of this in every phase of the nursing process.

Risk Factors

Major risk factors for cardiovascular disease in general are classified as *nonmodifiable* (cannot be altered) and *modifiable* (can be reduced) (Box 35–4).

BOX 35–4	Risk Factors for Coronary Heart Disease

Nonmodifiable Risk Factors

   Heredity
   Age
   Gender (women's risk increases at postmenopause)

Modifiable Risk Factors

   Elevated serum lipid level
   Hypertension
   Cigarette smoking
   Diabetes
   Obesity
   Sedentary lifestyle

Other Risk Factors

   Heat and cold
   Previous health status
   Stress and coping
   Dietary factors
   Alcohol intake
   Elevated homocysteine level

NONMODIFIABLE RISK FACTORS The first nonmodifiable risk factor is *heredity*. There is a genetic link for the development of coronary artery disease. The second is *age*. Coronary heart disease is mainly a disease of people over 60. It does occur in younger people as well, but generally risk increases with age. The third nonmodifiable risk factor is *gender*. Through middle adulthood (until menopause), estrogen has a protective effect in women, slowing the progress of atherosclerosis and reducing the risk of cardiovascular disease. Among people in their 40s and 50s, men have a higher incidence of hypertension than women.

The modifiable risk factors include elevated serum lipid levels, hypertension, cigarette smoking, diabetes, obesity, and sedentary lifestyle.

ELEVATED SERUM LIPID LEVELS A strong link exists between elevated serum lipid levels and the development of coronary heart disease. Lipoproteins circulate in the blood and are made up of cholesterol, triglycerides, and phospholipids. A high dietary intake of saturated fats is the most critical factor for the development of elevated serum lipids. The average American diet often contains more than 40% of its calories in fats. The American Heart Association recommends that less than 30% of total calories come from fats.

HYPERTENSION Hypertension (or increased blood pressure) increases the risk of coronary heart disease in several ways. First, it increases the workload of the heart, increasing oxygen demand and coronary blood flow. The increased workload also causes hypertrophy of the ventricles. Over time this can contribute to heart failure. Secondly, hypertension causes endothelial damage to the blood vessels, which stimulates the development of atherosclerosis.

CIGARETTE SMOKING   The cardiovascular system also is affected by cigarette smoking. Nicotine increases the heart rate, blood pressure, and peripheral vascular resistance, increasing the heart's workload. Smoking causes vasoconstriction, and in areas where vessels already are narrowed by atherosclerosis, tissue oxygenation can be impaired.

DIABETES   Diabetes mellitus increases the risk of coronary heart disease, myocardial infarction, and peripheral vascular disease. High blood sugars are linked with accelerated development of atherosclerosis as well as high levels of serum lipids and triglycerides. Closely monitoring blood sugar levels in clients with diabetes and checking blood sugar levels in all clients for the development of increased levels is an important nursing function. Control of blood sugar levels can greatly reduce risk and slow development of atherosclerosis.

OBESITY   Nearly 60% of the adult population of the United States is overweight or obese (Evangelista & Miller, 2006, p. 27). Obese people have an increased risk for the development of cardiovascular disease. Obesity is often accompanied by elevated serum lipid levels, which increase risk. Additionally, obesity places an increased workload on the heart, which increases oxygen demand. Recent research data show that obese individuals have an increased risk for heart failure and death that increases in proportion to the degree of obesity (Evangelista & Miller, 2006, p. 28).

SEDENTARY LIFESTYLE   Physical activity is associated with a reduction in the risk of death due to cardiovascular disease (Richardson, Kriska, Lantz, & Hayward, 2004, p. 192). Physical exercise or activity increases the heart rate and hence the supply of oxygen in the body. With regular vigorous exercise, the heart muscle becomes more powerful and efficient. Aerobic exercise slows the atherosclerotic process, reducing the risk of cardiovascular disease. Sedentary people, by contrast, have a higher risk of cardiovascular disease.

Other Factors Influencing Cardiovascular Function

Other factors that may influence cardiovascular function include environmental factors such as heat and cold, previous health status, stress and coping, dietary factors, alcohol intake, and an elevated homocysteine level.

HEAT AND COLD   In response to heat, the peripheral blood vessels dilate; consequently, blood flows to the skin, increasing the amount of heat lost from the body surface. With vasodilation the lumens of blood vessels enlarge, thus decreasing the resistance to the blood flow. In response the heart increases output to maintain blood pressure. The increased cardiac output requires additional oxygen, which is acquired through increased rate and depth of breathing.

In response to cold environmental temperatures, the peripheral blood vessels constrict. This mechanism helps to

---

RESEARCH NOTES   **Can the Lifetime Risk for Cardiovascular Disease Be Predicted?**

Prior to this research, the lifetime risk for cardiovascular disease (CVD) had not been estimated and the effect of possessing risk factors on lifetime risk for developing CVD was unknown.

The study included all of the Framingham Heart Study participants who were free of CVD (e.g., myocardial infarction, angina, stroke) at 50 years of age. They may have had risk factors but did not have CVD. The researchers then estimated the lifetime risk for CVD for men and women up to 95 years of age. They examined overall survival in the presence and absence of established risk factors.

During routine examinations of the Framingham Heart Study, the participants underwent standardized measurements for body mass index (BMI), diabetes, BP, cholesterol, and a self-report of smoking.

The results reflected that men free of CVD at age 50 had a 51.7% risk of developing CVD by 95 years of age and the overall survival was 30 years. Women had a 39.2% risk of developing CVD and a median overall survival of 36 years.

The study showed the following effect of individual risk factors:

- High blood pressure and total cholesterol were associated with increased lifetime risk for CVD and shorter survival.
- The highest single lifetime risk for CVD of all the risk factors was diabetes.
- Overweight and obesity resulted in modest increases in lifetime risk and reduction in survival.

On the other hand, those participants who had no established risk factors at age 50 were associated with very low lifetime risk for CVD and much longer survival.

The authors noted that CVD is the leading cause of morbidity and mortality in the United States. They also made the relevant point that in spite of this fact, most Americans perceive that cancer is their greatest health risk.

Implications

The results of this study, along with the decreased awareness of CVD risk, mandate health promotion activities to educate the public about CVD risk factors. Prevention efforts need to begin before age 50. Lifestyle activities focusing on diet and exercise in young adulthood and middle age can prevent many of the CVD risk factors such as obesity, hypertension, hyperlipidemia, and diabetes.

The authors caution that the lifetime risk estimates are based on a large population group and applying the results to an individual client should be done with caution. The results, however, can help health care providers focus on prevention and modification of CVD risk factors.

Note: From "Prediction of Lifetime Risk for Cardiovascular Disease by Risk Factor Burden at 50 Years of Age," by D. M. Lloyd-Jones, E. P. Leip, M. G. Larson, R. B. D'Agostino, A. Beiser, P. Wilson, et al., 2006, *Circulation, 113*(6), pp. 791–798. Copyright © 2006 Lippincott Williams & Wilkins.

conserve heat that is normally lost through the skin. However, the vasoconstriction also increases blood pressure which may increase the risk of a heart attack or stroke for clients with cardiac conditions.

HEALTH STATUS In the healthy person, the cardiovascular system (working together with the respiratory system) is able to provide sufficient oxygen to meet the body's needs. Diseases of the cardiovascular system will often affect the delivery of oxygen to the cells of the body, and when any system or tissue does not get the required oxygen for metabolic processes, cellular function will be altered. The body has "compensatory mechanisms" that are activated when oxygen decreases. These mechanisms include increased heart rate, increased strength of cardiac contraction, vasoconstriction, and the release of certain hormones such as aldosterone. The health status of a client may affect how the body tolerates the compensation and the decreased oxygen availability. A client with no significant health history and with good nutritional status will be more likely to tolerate short periods of decreased oxygen and the body's compensation than a client with multiple disorders and poor nutritional status.

Most cardiovascular conditions affect how the blood gets to the tissues. One cardiovascular condition that affects the oxygen-carrying capacity of the blood is anemia, described in the "Blood Alterations" section later in this chapter.

STRESS AND COPING Stress causes a neurohormonal response. The stress response involves a number of interrelated responses and effects. One of the major effects of stress is the release of adrenal medullary hormones: epinephrine and norepinephrine. Epinephrine has several effects including causing the heart to contract more forcefully, increasing heart rate, and stimulating peripheral vasoconstriction. Norepinephrine causes widespread vasoconstriction, which increases the blood pressure.

DIET Diet can also affect cardiovascular function. A healthy diet with adequate calories, protein, and other nutrients is important to maintain good immune function and increase resistance to disease. Along with certain vitamins and minerals, dietary protein is important to prevent anemia. High salt intake can affect blood pressure and contribute to the development of hypertension. High intake of sodium may contribute to hypertension in two ways. First, it may increase the release of a hormone called natriuretic hormone, which indirectly contributes to hypertension. Additionally, sodium stimulates vasopressor mechanisms, which cause vasoconstriction. There is also evidence that other factors such as low potassium, calcium, and magnesium intake may contribute to vasoconstriction and the development of hypertension. One study showed that a high consumption of dairy products and dietary calcium reduced blood pressure levels (Ruidavets et al., 2006).

ALCOHOL Recent studies suggest that moderate alcohol use (1 to 2 oz of alcohol per day) may actually reduce the risk of heart disease; however, excessive alcohol intake affects oxygenation several ways. Alcohol is a respiratory depressant, slowing respirations. Alcohol abusers often are malnourished, increasing their risk of anemia and infections. Excess alcohol intake also increases the risk of hypertension.

CULTURALLY COMPETENT CARE — Gender and Race Disparities in Clients with Cardiovascular Disease

Acute Myocardial Infarction (AMI)

Coronary heart disease is the leading cause of death in American females. Yet, they are underrepresented in the majority of cardiovascular research studies.

Women tend to have an AMI at an older age than men and are more likely to have complications. The presence of chest pain varies between men and women. More women have pain-free AMIs than men. They also tend to have more mid-back, shoulder blade, and upper-back pain than men. Research reflects that women who have an AMI have increased delays in treatment and less aggressive treatment than men. This results in increased mortality rates.

Heart Failure (HF)

Symptoms of heart failure occur earlier in African Americans, possibly because of the higher rate of uncontrolled hypertension. The rate of hypertension for both African Americans and Caucasians is greatest in the southeastern United States.

Studies reveal the following information about other risk factors for heart failure and other cardiovascular disease:

- African Americans have a higher average BMI than Caucasians. African Americans do not view obesity as a negative body image.
- African Americans have a higher incidence of diabetes than other populations.
- The incidence of HF is increasing in African American women. However, few studies have been completed in which they are the subjects of the research.

Stroke

African Americans have a greater incidence, greater mortality, and greater severity of strokes.

Implications

Research on gender differences is gradually increasing. However, research focusing on differences by race remains limited and needs to be more thoroughly investigated. In the meantime, two important areas for client education include informing women that AMI does not occur only in men, and teaching the public about how to prevent risk factors that contribute to heart failure and stroke.

ELEVATED HOMOCYSTEINE LEVEL Homocysteine is an amino acid that has been shown to be increased in many people with atherosclerosis. Clients with elevated homocysteine levels may have an increased risk of myocardial infarction, coronary artery disease, cerebrovascular accidents (stroke), and peripheral vascular disease. Individuals can reduce their homocysteine level by taking a multivitamin that provides folate, vitamin B_6, vitamin B_{12}, and riboflavin (Bergen & Compher, 2006).

ALTERATIONS IN CARDIOVASCULAR FUNCTION

Cardiovascular function can be altered by conditions that affect:

1. The function of the heart as a pump.
2. Blood flow to organs and peripheral tissues.
3. The composition of the blood and its ability to transport oxygen and carbon dioxide.

Three major alterations in cardiovascular function are decreased cardiac output, impaired tissue perfusion, and disorders that affect the composition or amount of blood available for transport of gases.

Decreased Cardiac Output

Although the heart normally is able to increase its rate and force of contraction to increase cardiac output during exercise, fever, or other times of need, some conditions interfere with these mechanisms.

The vessels that supply blood to the heart muscle may become occluded by atherosclerosis or a blood clot, shutting off the blood supply to a portion of the myocardium. When this happens, the tissue becomes necrotic and dies, a condition known as a myocardial infarction (MI) or heart attack. If a large portion of the heart muscle is affected, particularly in the left ventricle, cardiac output falls because the affected muscle no longer contracts. Signs and symptoms of myocardial infarction are variable and may include the following:

- Chest pain; substernal and/or radiating to the left arm, jaw
- Nausea
- Shortness of breath
- Diaphoresis

Heart failure may develop if the heart isn't able to keep up with the body's need for oxygen and nutrients to the tissues. Heart failure usually occurs because of myocardial infarction, but it may also result from chronic overwork of the heart, such as in clients with uncontrolled hypertension or extensive arteriosclerosis. In left-sided heart failure, the vessels of the pulmonary system become congested or engorged with blood. This may cause fluid to escape into the alveoli and interfere with gas exchange, a condition known

BOX 35–5	Examples of Conditions that May Precipitate Heart Failure

Conditions that Increase Preload

Hypervolemia
Valvular disorders such as mitral regurgitation
Congenital defects such as patent ductus arteriosus

Conditions that Increase Afterload

Hypertension

Conditions that Affect Myocardial Function

Myocardial infarction
Cardiomyopathy
Coronary artery disease

as *pulmonary edema*. Signs of heart failure may include the following:

- Pulmonary congestion; adventitious lung sounds
- Shortness of breath
- Increased heart rate
- Increased respiratory rate
- Peripheral vasoconstriction; cold, pale extremities
- Distended neck veins

Other diseases such as myocarditis and cardiomyopathy also can affect the heart muscle, impairing its ability to contract and pump. Box 35–5 gives examples of conditions which may precipitate heart failure.

Very irregular or excessively rapid or slow heart rates can decrease cardiac output. With irregular or very rapid heart rates, the ventricles may not fill adequately between beats, so the stroke volume (amount pumped with each beat) falls. If the heart rate is too slow, the heart may not be able to increase its stroke volume enough to maintain the cardiac output. Abnormalities of the heart rate and rhythm are known as dysrhythmias and can be identified on the electrocardiogram (ECG).

Alterations in the structure of the heart can affect cardiac output. Congenital heart defects result in abnormal blood flow and may even allow venous and arterial blood to mix. The oxygen supply to the tissues is affected in this case. Acquired heart diseases such as bacterial endocarditis and rheumatic fever may damage the heart valves, affecting the flow of blood within the heart and to the great vessels. For example, if the mitral (bicuspid) valve becomes scarred and stenotic (constricted), it may not open fully, impairing filling of the left ventricle. Or, if the mitral valve doesn't fully close (mitral insufficiency), blood may escape back or regurgitate into the left atrium instead of entering the aorta each time the ventricle contracts.

Impaired Tissue Perfusion

Atherosclerosis is by far the most common cause of impaired blood flow to organs and tissues. As vessels narrow and become obstructed, distal tissues receive less blood, oxygen, and nutrients. **Ischemia** is a lack of blood supply due to obstructed circulation. Any artery in the body may be affected by atherosclerosis, although the effects are often related to coronary arteries, vessels supplying blood to the brain, and arteries in peripheral tissues. Obstruction of the coronary arteries causes myocardial ischemia, often resulting in angina pectoris. If the cerebral vessels are affected, the result may be a *transient ischemic attack (TIA)* or a stroke. Peripheral vascular disease leads to ischemia of distal tissues such as the legs and feet. Gangrene and amputation may result. Signs of impaired peripheral arterial circulation may include decreased peripheral pulses, pale skin color, cool extremities, and/or decreased hair distribution.

The risk factors for peripheral atherosclerosis are similar to those for coronary artery disease and include cigarette smoking, high fat intake, obesity, and a sedentary lifestyle. Hypertension and diabetes also increase the risk for atherosclerosis, particularly if the blood pressure or blood glucose levels are not maintained at near-normal levels. Although much less common, other disorders such as vessel inflammation, arterial spasm, and blood clots also can occlude blood vessels, leading to ischemia. Tissue edema can impair flow through vessels and can increase the distance oxygen and nutrients must diffuse across to reach cells.

On the venous side, incompetent valves may allow blood to pool in veins, causing edema and decreasing venous return to the heart (Figure 35–15). Veins also can become inflamed, reducing blood flow and increasing the risk of thrombus (clot) formation. Thrombi may then break loose, becoming emboli. These emboli tend to travel as far as the pulmonary circulation where they become trapped in small vessels (pulmonary emboli), occluding blood supply to the capillary side of the alveolar-capillary-membrane. Although alveolar ventilation to the affected area often remains adequate, no gas exchange occurs there because of impaired blood flow. Signs of acute pulmonary embolism can be nonspecific and variable but may include the following:

- Sudden onset of shortness of breath
- Pleuritic chest pain

Blood Alterations

Because most oxygen is transported to the tissues in combination with hemoglobin, the problems of inadequate RBCs, low hemoglobin levels, or abnormal hemoglobin structure can affect tissue oxygenation. Anemia has several different causes: RBCs are lost along with other components because of acute or chronic bleeding; if the diet is deficient in iron or folic acid, hemoglobin and RBCs are not formed adequately; and some disorders cause RBCs to break down excessively. People with sickle-cell disease produce an abnormal form of hemoglobin and may experience tissue ischemia during exacerbations of the disease. Signs of anemia may include the following:

- Chronic fatigue
- Pallor
- Shortness of breath
- Hypotension

Blood volume also affects tissue oxygenation. If the blood volume is inadequate as in hemorrhage or severe dehydration, the blood pressure and cardiac output fall, and tissues may become ischemic. Conversely, clients with hypervolemia (excess blood volume), which can result from fluid retention or kidney failure, may develop heart failure and peripheral edema, leading to tissue ischemia.

NURSING MANAGEMENT

ASSESSING

Nursing History

A comprehensive nursing history should include data regarding:

- Current and past cardiovascular problems.
- Family history of cardiovascular problems such as high blood pressure, increased cholesterol level, and stroke.
- Other medical history including diabetes and respiratory disorders.
- Exercise program.
- History of cigarette smoking.
- Diet, including fat and salt intake, alcohol intake, caffeine intake including soft drinks, and chocolate.
- Presence of any symptoms such as pain, shortness of breath, fatigue, palpitations, cough, and fainting.

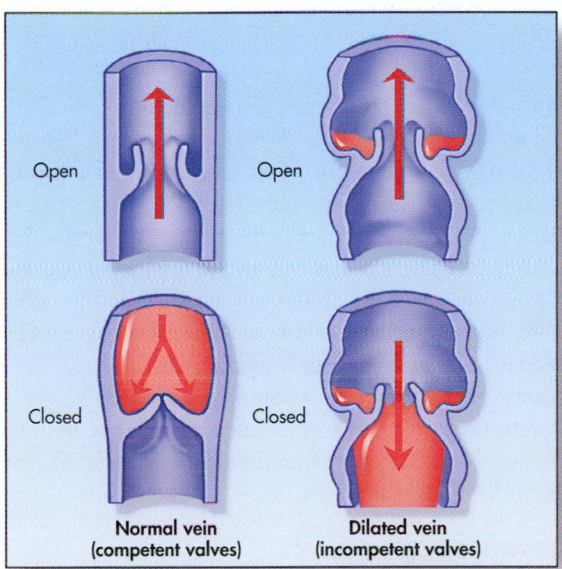

Open   Open

Closed   Closed

Normal vein
(competent valves)

Dilated vein
(incompetent valves)

Figure 35–15 ⬤ Vein with competent valve and vein with incompetent valve that allows blood to pool in the veins.

From Rice, Jane. *Medical Terminology: A Word Building Approach*, 6th. ed. © 2008. Electronically reproduced by permission of Pearson Education, Inc. Upper Saddle River, New Jersey.

- Medications for heart, blood pressure, circulation, and cholesterol.
- Lifestyle, including social support, stressors, and methods of coping (see Assessment Interview).

Physical Assessment

To examine the cardiovascular system, the nurse first evaluates the blood pressure for both arms (the results should be within 10 mm Hg of each other) and palpates peripheral pulses for their strength and equality. The apical pulse is auscultated for rate, rhythm, and the quality of heart sounds. Carotid arteries are auscultated for bruits (a sound of turbulence), which may indicate atherosclerosis and narrowing (see Chapter 17 ∞). Also important as an indicator of cardiac function is lung sounds. By auscultating the lungs for adventitious sounds, the nurse assesses for increased pulmonary vessel pressure secondary to decreased cardiac output.

Much information about the cardiovascular system is obtained by assessing the skin for color, temperature, hair distribution, lesions, and edema. Clients with extensive peripheral vascular disease may have cool feet with weak pulses and shiny, nearly hairless shins and feet. Pitting edema of the feet and ankles may be noted in clients with heart failure. See Chapter 17 ∞ for specific techniques for assessing the respiratory and cardiovascular systems.

Two methods to assess for peripheral vascular disease include the ankle/brachial index (ABI) and the toe brachial pressure index (TBPI). These measurements help determine arterial perfusion in feet and toes and help measure the severity of disease or establish a baseline. The American Diabetes Association recommends ABI screening in anyone over age 50 (Rice, 2008).

Diagnostic Studies

Many diagnostic studies are available that can help to identify the presence of cardiovascular disease. Diagnostic studies may also be used as screening tools to identify increased risk and then modifications made to reduce the risk of development of cardiovascular dysfunction. An example of this is the serum lipid level. If a client has an elevated serum lipid level, he or she should be educated about the effects of diet and the importance of reducing lipids to reduce the risk of coronary heart disease.

CARDIAC MONITORING Cardiac monitoring allows continuous observation of the client's cardiac rhythm. Cardiac monitoring is a recording of the heart's electrical activity. It is used in many instances: for clients who have known or suspected cardiovascular disease, during and after surgery, to monitor responses to drug therapy, and to monitor clients at risk for serious complications such as shock. Electrodes placed on the client's chest are attached to a monitor cable and bedside monitor. The monitor is equipped with alarms used to warn of potential problems such as very fast, very slow, or irregular heart rates. The alarm limits are set for 20 beats higher and lower than the client's baseline rate, often at 100 to 110 and

---

ASSESSMENT INTERVIEW Circulation

Current or Past Cardiovascular Problems

- Do you have high blood pressure?
- Do you have any history of heart disease such as angina, heart attack, or heart failure? Have you ever had a cardiac catheterization, angiogram, or angioplasty? Have you ever been diagnosed with rheumatic fever, endocarditis, pericarditis, or other diseases of the heart? If so, when? Have you had cardiac surgery or stent placement?
- Have you ever been told that you have peripheral vascular disease? Do you ever develop pain in the calves of your legs when walking? How far can you walk before it occurs? What do you do to relieve it? Have you had surgery on your blood vessels?
- Do your feet and ankles ever swell or feel very cold, numb, or tingling? Do you experience pain in your feet? Is the pain changed by position?
- Do you become extremely fatigued with activity? Have you ever been told that you are anemic?

Medication History

- Have you taken or do you take any over-the-counter or prescription medications for your heart or blood pressure or to increase blood flow?
- Do you take any anticoagulants or other medications to "thin" your blood?

Lifestyle

- Do you smoke?
- Do you exercise? What kind of exercise and how often?
- How often do you drink alcoholic beverages such as beer, wine, or liquor? How much do you usually drink at the time?

---

50 to 55, respectively, for adults. For ambulatory clients (in the hospital or at home), the electrodes connect to a transmitter unit (also called telemetry). This unit electronically sends the signal to a central monitor for display or may store the information to be retrieved later in the primary care provider's office. Another name for this type of ambulatory monitoring is the Holter monitor. Electrodes are attached and the client wears the monitor for 24 hours. A continuous ECG is recorded and later analyzed for irregularities.

Electrocardiography most commonly uses 12 "leads" or 12 different views of the heart. In contrast, cardiac monitoring uses 2 or 3 leads at any given time. See Chapter 20 ∞ for more information about ECGs.

CLINICAL ALERT

It is important to remember that ECG monitoring is a recording of the electrical activity of the heart; it does not reflect mechanical contraction and cardiac output. ALWAYS remember to check the client to assess for cardiac function. Just looking at the ECG does not give an assessment of the client's status.

BLOOD TESTS Specimens of venous blood are taken for several tests that may reflect some aspect of cardiovascular functioning.

Because hemoglobin is the molecule that oxygen attaches to, it gives an indication of the oxygen-carrying capacity of the blood. A decreased hemoglobin increases the risk of oxygen deficit in the tissues when cardiovascular disease is present.

Measurement of serum electrolytes is important for clients with cardiovascular problems because electrolyte abnormalities such as hyperkalemia (higher than normal potassium) and hypokalemia (lower than normal potassium) can have a critical effect on the heart. Serum levels of magnesium, calcium, sodium, and phosphorus are also important to assess.

Measurement of enzyme levels in the blood is an important part of the diagnostic evaluation of clients with chest pain. Certain enzymes such as **creatine kinase (CK)** and **troponin** are released into the blood during an MI. These enzymes are released into the blood as the cell membrane is damaged. Elevated levels of these enzymes can help differentiate between an MI (when the cells actually die) and chest pain from a different cause such as angina or pleuritic pain.

HEMODYNAMIC STUDIES Hemodynamics is the study of the forces or pressures involved in blood circulation. Hemodynamic studies or monitoring procedures may be performed to evaluate fluid status and cardiovascular function. Parameters evaluated in hemodynamic studies include heart rate, arterial blood pressure, central venous pressure, pressures in the pulmonary vascular system, and cardiac output. Some of these parameters—for example, heart rate, arterial blood pressure, and venous pressure—are measured directly using an arterial, central venous, or pulmonary artery catheter; others such as the stroke volume and cardiac output are calculated. Hemodynamic studies are performed in a diagnostic cardiac laboratory and require informed consent. Clients in intensive and cardiac care units may undergo continuous hemodynamic monitoring to evaluate cardiovascular status and the effect of interventions. Nurses in these units are responsible for maintaining accurate readings and the integrity of the system.

DIAGNOSING

NANDA includes the following diagnostic labels for clients with circulation problems:

- *Ineffective Tissue Perfusion* (Cardiopulmonary): Decrease in oxygen resulting in the failure to nourish the tissues at the capillary level
- *Decreased Cardiac Output:* Inadequate blood pumped by the heart to meet metabolic (demands) of the body
- *Activity Intolerance:* Insufficient physiological or psychological energy to endure or complete required or desired daily activities

Examples of application of these using NANDA, NIC, and NOC designations are shown in Identifying Nursing Diagnoses, Outcomes, and Interventions.

PLANNING

When planning care the nurse identifies nursing interventions that will assist the client to achieve these broad goals:

- Maintain or improve tissue perfusion.
- Maintain or restore an adequate cardiac output.

Obviously, goals will vary according to the diagnosis and defining characteristics for each individual. Appropriate preventive and corrective nursing interventions that relate to these must be identified. Specific nursing activities can be selected to meet the client's individual needs. Examples of NIC interventions related to decreased cardiac output and tissue perfusion include the following:

- Circulatory care: arterial insufficiency
- Cardiac care
- Hemodynamic regulation

To promote the transport of oxygen and carbon dioxide the nurse can optimize cardiac output by reducing stress, planning appropriate activities, and positioning the client for improved vascular blood flow (see Identifying Nursing Diagnoses, Outcomes, and Interventions).

IMPLEMENTING

Promoting Circulation

Most people in good health give little thought to their cardiovascular function. Changing position frequently, ambulating, and exercising usually maintain adequate cardiovascular functioning. See Client Teaching for other ways to promote a healthy heart.

Immobility is also detrimental to cardiovascular function. Without exercise of the calf and leg muscles, blood pools in the veins of the lower extremities. This stagnant blood flow may allow clots to develop (venous thrombosis). With time, these clots can break loose and become emboli, eventually lodging in the small vessels of the pulmonary vascular system. Blood flow and gas exchange in the lungs are then impaired.

There are many nursing interventions that can help clients maintain cardiac and vascular function. They may be classified as vascular and cardiac.

VASCULAR

- Position with the legs elevated to promote venous return to the heart. This is particularly important for clients with venous dysfunction. Care should be taken to avoid this position in clients with cardiac dysfunction because it will increase preload and may stress the dysfunctional heart.
- Avoid pillows under the knees or more than 15 degrees of knee flexion to improve blood flow to the lower extremities and reduce venous stagnation.
- Encourage leg exercises for a client on bed rest and promote ambulation as soon as possible.
- Encourage or provide frequent position changes.

Client with Decreased Cardiac Output

DATA CLUSTER Ed Wallace, a 67-year-old retired contractor, has a history of an acute myocardial infarction 1 year ago. During the last 2 weeks he has experienced a weight gain of 4 kg (9 lb). He states that he can't walk a flight of stairs without shortness of breath, and he sleeps on three pillows. His ankles are swollen, and his heart pounds at times. Physical exam reveals jugular vein distention above 3 cm; pulse (86); pitting edema in feet, ankles, and lower legs; and crackles in both lung fields.

NURSING DIAGNOSIS/DEFINITION	SAMPLE DESIRED OUTCOMES*/DEFINITION	INDICATORS	SELECTED INTERVENTIONS*/DEFINITION	SAMPLE NIC ACTIVITIES
Decreased Cardiac Output/Inadequate blood pumped by the heart to meet metabolic demands of the body	Cardiac Pump Effectiveness [0400]/*Adequacy of blood volume ejected from the left ventricle per minute to support systemic perfusion pressure*	No assessed: • Neck vein distention • Peripheral edema • Weight gain • Dyspnea	Cardiac Care [4040]/*Limitation of complications resulting from an imbalance between myocardial oxygen supply and demand for a patient with symptoms of impaired cardiac function*	• Perform a comprehensive appraisal of peripheral circulation • Monitor respiratory status for symptoms of heart failure • Monitor fluid balance (e.g., intake/output, daily weights) • Arrange exercise and rest periods to avoid fatigue • Monitor the patient's activity tolerance

*The NOC # for desired outcomes and the NIC # for nursing interventions are listed in brackets following the appropriate outcome or intervention. Outcomes, indicators, interventions, and activities selected are only a sample of those suggested by NOC and NIC and should be further individualized for each client.

CARDIAC

• Position the client in a high Fowler's position to decrease preload and reduce pulmonary congestion.
• Monitor intake and output. Fluid restriction is usually not required for clients with mild to moderate cardiac dysfunction. With severe heart failure, a fluid restriction may be ordered.

CLIENT TEACHING   **Promoting a Healthy Heart**

• Exercise regularly, participating in at least 20 minutes (40 minutes is preferred) of vigorous exercise four to five times a week.
• Do not smoke.
• Maintain your ideal weight.
• Eat a diet low in total fat, saturated fats, and cholesterol.
• Drink alcohol in moderation, if at all, consuming no more than 1 cocktail or 1 to 1 1/2 glasses of wine or beer daily.
• Reduce stress and manage anger.
• Effectively manage diabetes and hypertension, maintaining blood glucose and blood pressure levels within normal limits.
• If female, discuss with your health care provider the advantages and risks of hormone replacement therapy after menopause (or after a total hysterectomy).
• Consult your primary care provider about the advisability of low-dose aspirin therapy to further reduce the risk of cardiovascular disease.

Medications

Many classes of medications are administered to clients with cardiovascular disorders. Drugs such as nitrates, calcium channel blockers, and angiotensin-converting enzyme (ACE) inhibitors reduce the workload of the heart and prevent vasoconstriction. Various drugs are used to treat cardiac dysrhythmias. Positive inotropic drugs such as digitalis are used to increase the contractile strength of the heart. Beta adrenergic blocking agents such as propranolol or metoprolol may be given to block the sympathetic nervous system action on the heart and decrease oxygen consumption. Direct vasodilators may be used for clients with peripheral vascular disease and sometimes hypertension. Often clients are on numerous medications, and it is an important role of the nurse to help the client understand the purposes, effects, and side effects of the different medications.

Administering medications is an important nursing function. The nurse is responsible for assessing for the effects of medications and also for potential complications. Examples include:

• When diuretics are administered, the nurse assesses intake and output and potassium level (because many diuretics can lower potassium level).
• When positive inotropic medications are administered, the nurse should assess blood pressure, heart rate, peripheral pulses, and lung sounds as indicators of cardiac output.

- When antihypertensive medications are administered, it is critical for the nurse to monitor blood pressure. Additionally, many antihypertensive medications can cause postural hypotension.

Preventing Venous Stasis

When clients have limited mobility or are confined to bed, venous return to the heart is impaired and the risk of venous stasis increases. Immobility is a problem not only for ill or debilitated clients but also for some travelers who sit with legs dependent for long periods in a motor vehicle or an airplane. Venous stasis can lead to thrombus formation and edema of the extremities.

Preventing venous stasis is an important nursing intervention to reduce the risk of complications following surgery, trauma, or major medical problems. Positioning and leg exercises are discussed earlier in this chapter and antiemboli stockings are discussed in Chapter 25 ∞. Sequential compression devices are additional measures to help prevent venous stasis.

SEQUENTIAL COMPRESSION DEVICES Clients who are undergoing surgery or who are immobilized because of illness or injury may benefit from a sequential compression device (SCD) to promote venous return from the legs. SCDs inflate and deflate plastic sleeves wrapped around the legs to promote venous flow. The plastic sleeves are attached by tubing to an air pump that alternately inflates and deflates portions of the sleeve to a specified pressure. The ankle area inflates first, followed by the calf region, and then the thigh area. This sequential inflation and deflation assists the leg muscles in moving blood toward the heart.

The SCD is removed for ambulation and is usually discontinued when the client resumes activities. SCDs are useful in preventing thrombi and edema from venous stasis, but they are not used for clients who have arterial insufficiency, cellulitis, infection of the extremity, or preexisting venous thrombosis.

Skill 35–5 outlines how to apply a sequential compression device.

SKILL 35–5

SEQUENTIAL COMPRESSION DEVICES

PURPOSES
- To promote venous return from the legs
- To decrease risk of deep vein thrombosis and/or pulmonary embolism

---

ASSESSMENT
Assess for baseline data:

- Cardiovascular status, including heart rate and rhythm, peripheral pulses, and capillary refill

- Color and temperature of extremities
- Movement and sensation of feet and lower extremities and Homans' sign

---

PLANNING
Check the primary care provider's order for type of SCD sleeve. **Rationale:** *Both knee- and thigh-length sleeves are available.*

> **Delegation**
> UAP often remove and reapply the SCD when performing hygiene care. The nurse should check that the UAP knows the correct application process for the SCD. Remind the UAP that the client should not have the SCD removed for long periods of time because the purpose of the SCD is to promote circulation.

EQUIPMENT
- Measuring tape
- SCD, including disposable sleeves, air pump, and tubing

IMPLEMENTATION
Performance

1. Prior to performing the procedure, introduce self and verify the client's identity using agency protocol. Explain to the client what you are going to do, why it is necessary, and the procedure for applying the sequential compression device. **Rationale:** *The client's participation and comfort will be increased by understanding the rationale for applying the SCD.*
2. Perform hand hygiene and observe appropriate infection control procedures.
3. Provide for client privacy and drape the client appropriately.
4. Prepare the client.
   - Place the client in a dorsal recumbent or semi-Fowler's position.
   - Measure the client's legs as recommended by the manufacturer if a thigh-length sleeve is required.

Rationale: *Foot and knee-length sleeves come in just one size; the thigh circumference determines the size needed for a thigh-length sleeve.*

5. Apply the sequential compression sleeves.
   - Place a sleeve under each leg with the opening at the knee.
   - Wrap the sleeve securely around the leg, securing the Velcro tabs. Allow two fingers to fit between the leg and the sleeve. **Rationale:** *This amount of space ensures that the sleeve does not impair circulation when inflated.* ❶
6. Connect the sleeves to the control unit and adjust the pressure as needed.
   - Connect the tubing to the sleeves and control unit, ensuring that arrows on the plug and the connector are in alignment and that the tubing is not kinked or twisted. **Rationale:** *Improper alignment or obstruction of*

(continued)

SEQUENTIAL COMPRESSION DEVICES *(continued)*

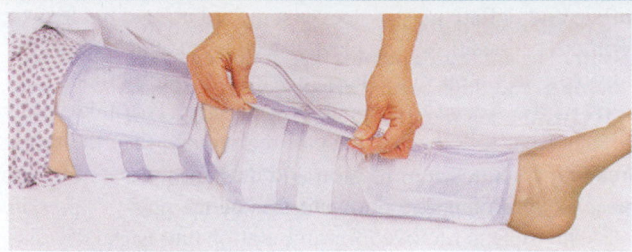

❶ Applying a sequential compression device to the leg.

the tubing by kinks or twists will interfere with operation of the SCD.
* Turn on the control unit and adjust the alarms and pressures as needed. The sleeve cooling control and

alarm should be on; ankle pressure is usually set at 35 to 55 mm Hg. **Rationale:** *It is important to have the sleeve cooling control on for comfort and to reduce the risk of skin irritation from moisture under the sleeve. Alarms warn of possible control unit malfunctions.*

7. Document the procedure.
* Record baseline assessment data and application of the SCD. Note control unit settings.
* Assess and document skin integrity and neurovascular status at least every 8 hours while the SCD is in place. Remove the unit and notify the primary care provider if the client complains of numbness and tingling or leg pain. These may be symptoms of nerve compression.

EVALUATION
* Perform appropriate follow-up assessments, such as cardiovascular status including pedal pulses, skin color and temperature, skin integrity, and neurovascular status, including movement and sensation.
* Compare to the baseline data, if available.
* Report significant deviations from normal to the primary care provider.

LIFESPAN CONSIDERATIONS   Sequential Compression Devices

Children
* As young children tend to be more active, the SCD is rarely necessary unless the child is immobile (e.g., comatose).

Older Adults
* The SCD sleeves may become loose as clients move around in bed. Check that the sleeves are secure and properly positioned.

Sequential compression therapy often complements other preventive measures. The client's risk level for DVT or pulmonary embolism often determines the preventive measures used. For example, clients at low risk may require only antiemboli stockings. Clients at moderate risk may have both antiemboli stockings and sequential therapy as part of their treatment. The primary care provider may order antiemboli stockings, sequential therapy, and anticoagulation therapy for the high-risk client.

Cardiopulmonary Resuscitation

Cardiopulmonary resuscitation (CPR) is a combination of oral resuscitation (mouth-to-mouth breathing), which supplies oxygen to the lungs, and external cardiac massage (chest compression), which is intended to reestablish cardiac function and blood circulation. CPR is also referred to as *basic life support (BLS)*.

The American Heart Association reviews resuscitation literature to evaluate their guidelines for CPR. Table 35–3 provides highlights of the American Heart Association guidelines for CPR for the health care provider.

A cardiac arrest is the cessation of cardiac function; the heart stops beating. Often a cardiac arrest is unexpected and sudden. When it occurs, the heart no longer pumps blood to any of the organs of the body. Breathing then stops, and the person becomes unconscious and limp. Within 20 to 40 seconds of a cardiac arrest the victim is clinically dead. After 4 to 6 minutes the lack of oxygen supply to the brain causes permanent and extensive damage.

The three cardinal signs of a cardiac arrest are apnea, absence of a carotid or femoral pulse, and dilated pupils. The person's skin appears pale or grayish and feels cool. Cyanosis is evident when respiratory function fails before heart failure.

A respiratory arrest (pulmonary arrest) is the cessation of breathing. It often occurs because of a blocked airway, but it can occur following a cardiac arrest and for other reasons. A respiratory arrest may occur abruptly or be preceded by short, shallow breathing that becomes increasingly labored.

It is vital that all nurses be trained to perform CPR so resuscitation measures can be initiated immediately when a cardiac or respiratory arrest occurs. Nurses can also be instrumental in increasing community awareness of the need for CPR training and ensuring its availability.

TABLE 35–3	Changes in CPR Guidelines for the Health Care Provider		
CHANGE	**NEW (2005)**	**OLD (2000)**	**RATIONALE FOR CHANGE**
Chest compressions	• "Push hard and push fast." • Compress chest at rate of 100/minute. • Allow complete chest recoil after each compression. • Minimize interruptions in chest compression.	• Quality and rate of compressions, importance of chest recoil and need to minimize interruptions were not emphasized.	• Studies showed that chest compressions were too shallow, and compressions were interrupted too often during CPR.
Compression-to-ventilation ratio	• Compression–ventilation ratio of 30:2 for single rescuer for all clients except newborns.	• Adult CPR—15:2 ratio. • Infant and child—5:1 ratio.	• Simplify training. • To ensure a longer series of uninterrupted chest compressions. • To increase blood flow to heart, brain, and vital organs.
1-second breaths	• Each rescue breath should be given over 1 second. • Chest should rise with each breath. • Avoid delivering too many breaths or breaths too large and/or too forceful.	• Different tidal volumes were recommended. • Breaths to be delivered over 1–2 seconds.	• Blood flow to the lungs is less than normal during CPR. Thus, the victim needs less ventilation than normal. • Want to reduce interruptions in compression. • Large and forceful breaths may cause gastric inflation.
Attempted defibrillation	• Deliver one shock followed by immediate CPR beginning with chest compressions. • Check rhythm after 5 cycles of CPR.	• Deliver 3 shocks without CPR between shocks. • Check rhythm before and after shocks.	• Rhythm checks resulted in delays of 37 seconds or longer before delivering compressions. • The first shock eliminates ventricular fibrillation (VF) more than 85% of the time. • Even when VF is eliminated, it takes several minutes for the heart to return to a normal rhythm. Immediate chest compressions can help deliver oxygen to the heart. • There is no evidence that compressions after a shock results in the reoccurrence of VF.

Note: From "Highlights of the 2005 American Heart Association Guidelines for Cardiopulmonary Resuscitation and Emergency Cardiovascular Care," by American Heart Association, 2005–2006, *Currents in Emergency Cardiovascular Care, 16*(4), pp. 1–27.

Each health care facility has policies and procedures for announcing cardiac/respiratory arrest and initiating interventions. In many institutions this emergency is called a Code Blue, and the announcement is referred to as "calling a code." Each health care institution has a procedure for calling a code. There may be a special Code Blue button at the head of each bed, sometimes it is a special extension on the phone, or it may be a special phone used to announce the emergency. It is critical that each member of the client care team know the procedure for announcing a code. Calling the code summons the code team to the location of the emergency. The code team is made up of specially trained staff who can handle the emer-

gency. Persons are needed to perform rescue breathing, deliver chest compressions, administer medications, and make a record of the code activities. One person must be designated as the code leader—the person who directs the activities of the other team members. Once the code is called, one member of the team should obtain the code cart which contains essential equipment and medications that will be needed during the resuscitation process.

Some clients have designated via an advance directive that, should they arrest, they not be resuscitated. It is every person's right to make an advance directive of their wishes. If it is the client's wish, the primary care provider should designate "No Code Blue," "No CPR," or "Do Not Resuscitate (DNR)" on the medical record.

EVALUATING

Using the overall goals identified in the planning stage, the nurse collects data to evaluate the effectiveness of interventions. Examples of desired outcomes for the identified goals are found in the Identifying Nursing Diagnoses, Outcomes, and Interventions box earlier in this chapter.

If desired outcomes are not achieved, the nurse, client, and support person if appropriate need to explore the reasons before modifying the care plan. For example, if the outcome "cardiac pump effectiveness" is not achieved, questions to be considered might include the following:

- Have other outcome measures for the goal of maintaining adequate cardiac output been met?
- Are prescribed medications being taken/administered as ordered?
- Are there additional factors that are placing stress on the heart?
- Is there a balance between factors that affect cardiac output, such as preload and afterload?
- Are there signs of fluid overload such as weight gain?

CHAPTER HIGHLIGHTS

- The respiratory system contributes to effective respiration through pulmonary ventilation (the movement of air between the atmosphere and the lungs), the diffusion of oxygen and carbon dioxide across the pulmonary membrane, and transport of oxygen from the lungs to the tissues and carbon dioxide from the tissues to the lungs.
- Effective pulmonary ventilation, or breathing, requires clear airways, an intact central nervous system and respiratory center, an intact thoracic cavity and musculature, and adequate pulmonary compliance (stretch) and recoil.
- Gas exchange occurs by diffusion, as gas molecules move from an area of higher concentration to an area of lower concentration. At the respiratory membrane, oxygen moves from the alveolus into the blood, while carbon dioxide moves from the blood into the alveolus.
- Most oxygen (97%) is carried to the tissues loosely combined with hemoglobin in red blood cells (RBCs). Anemia, which is too few RBCs or low hemoglobin levels, impairs oxygen transportation.
- Respiratory and pulse rates are normally highest in neonates and infants, gradually slowing to adult ranges.
- Aging affects the respiratory system: The chest wall becomes more rigid and lungs less elastic.
- Other factors affecting oxygenation include the environment, lifestyle, health status, narcotic analgesics, and stress and coping.
- Hypoxia can result from impaired ventilation or diffusion, or from impaired oxygen transportation to the tissues because of anemia or decreased cardiac output.
- Normal respirations are quiet and unlabored; altered respiratory patterns include tachypnea, bradypnea, hyperventilation, hypoventilation, and dyspnea. Shortness of breath is a subjective sensation of not getting enough air.
- Airway obstruction interferes with ventilation. A low-pitched snoring sound, stridor, and abnormal breath sounds may accompany partial airway obstruction. Extreme inspiratory effort with no chest movement indicates complete upper airway obstruction.

- The nursing history includes questions about current or past respiratory problems and about lifestyle, presence of symptoms such as cough or shortness of breath, smoking and other risk factors, and medications.
- Physical assessment should include a general assessment, as well as specific examination of the respiratory system.
- Diagnostic tests that may be performed to assess oxygenation include sputum and throat culture specimens; blood tests such as arterial blood gases; pulmonary function tests; and visualization procedures such as x-rays, lung scans, laryngoscopy, and bronchoscopy.
- Nursing diagnoses for the client with problems of oxygenation include *Ineffective Airway Clearance*, *Ineffective Breathing Pattern*, *Impaired Gas Exchange*, and *Activity Intolerance*. These problems also may be the etiology for several other nursing diagnoses, including *Anxiety*, *Fatigue*, *Fear*, *Powerlessness*, *Sleep Pattern Disturbance*, and *Social Isolation*.
- Nursing interventions to promote oxygenation include promoting healthy breathing and a healthy heart, deep breathing and coughing, and hydration; administering medications; implementing measures to clear secretions; initiating and monitoring oxygen therapy; initiating or assisting with procedures to maintain the airway; providing tracheostomy care; and monitoring chest drainage systems.
- The effectiveness of nursing interventions is evaluated by using the goals and desired outcomes identified in the planning stage of the nursing process. If a goal is not met, the nurse asks pertinent questions to assess the reason for not meeting the goal.
- Cardiac output depends on the stroke volume, or amount of blood ejected during systole, and the heart rate.
- The blood pressure rises gradually from birth to reach the adult range in adolescence.
- Atherosclerosis causes fatty plaque to develop within arteries.
- Decreased cardiac output, impaired tissue perfusion, and disorders affecting the blood are the major cardiovascular problems that may affect oxygenation.

- Cardiac output may fall with a myocardial infarction (MI), heart failure, dysrhythmias, and structural alterations of the heart (e.g., valve deformities).
- The most common cause of impaired blood flow to tissues is atherosclerosis; this can lead to tissue ischemia and pain.
- Cardiac monitoring is used for continuous observation of the heart rate and rhythm.

- Nursing interventions to promote circulation include using antiembolic stockings and sequential compression devices to prevent venous stasis and edema, and also administering cardiopulmonary resuscitation.
- Cardiopulmonary resuscitation (CPR) is used during cardiopulmonary arrest. Each nurse needs to be aware of the hospital's policies and procedures regarding emergencies.

THINK ABOUT IT

Refer to the chapter-opening scenario and answer these questions.

1. Is the problem Ms. Neidringhaus is having related to respiration or ventilation? Explain your answer.

2. What nursing diagnoses would be appropriate for this client, and of those you choose, which is the highest priority?

3. When assessing this client's lung sounds, what impact would you anticipate as a result of her disease process?

∞ *See suggested responses to Think About It on MyNursingKit.*

TEST YOUR KNOWLEDGE

1. A client with chronic obstructive pulmonary disease requires some supplemental oxygen. The nurse ensures consistent and safe delivery with which of the following?
1. 2 L/min per nasal cannula
2. 6 L/min per face mask
3. 8 L/min per partial rebreather mask
4. 10 L/min per nonrebreather mask

2. The client demonstrates knowledge of the proper use of an incentive spirometer when which of the following statements is made?
1. "I should breathe out as fast and hard as possible into the device."
2. "I should inhale slowly and steadily to keep the balls up."
3. "I should use the device three times a day, after meals."
4. "The entire device should be washed thoroughly in sudsy water once a week."

3. While a client with chest tubes is ambulating, the connection between the tube and the water seal dislodges. Which of the following actions by the nurse is most appropriate?
1. Assist the client to ambulate back to bed.
2. Reconnect the tube to the water seal.
3. Assess the client's lung sounds with a stethoscope.
4. Have the client cough forcibly several times.

4. Which of the following clients is most at risk for a problem with the transport of oxygen from the lungs to the tissues?
1. A client who has anemia
2. A client who has an infection
3. A client who has a fractured rib
4. A client who has a tumor of the medulla

5. The nurse is planning to perform percussion and postural drainage. Which of the following is an important aspect of planning the client's care?
1. Percussion and postural drainage should be done before lunch.
2. The procedure is performed in this order: coughing, percussion, positioning, and then suctioning.
3. A good time to perform percussion and postural drainage is in the morning after breakfast when the client is well rested.
4. Percussion and postural drainage should always be preceded by 3 minutes of 100% oxygen.

6. Which of the following would most likely be included in the nurse's evaluation of the client goal: "Demonstrate adequate tissue perfusion?"
1. Symmetrical chest expansion
2. Uses pursed-lip breathing
3. Brisk capillary refill
4. Activity intolerance

7. A client is admitted with acute crushing chest pain that radiates down his left arm. The nurse expects which of the following blood tests to be ordered for this client? Select all that apply.
1. Blood urea nitrogen (BUN)
2. Hemoglobin and hematocrit
3. Creatine kinase (CK)
4. Serum glucose
5. Troponin

8. The nurse monitors which of the following clients with the highest potential to experience poor cardiac output?
1. A client who has recently completed exercising
2. A client who has a stroke volume of 70 mL per beat and a heart rate of 70 beats/minute
3. A client with a sustained heart rate of 150 beats/minute
4. A client who receives a positive inotropic medication

9. Which of the following assessment findings validates that the nurse should initiate cardiopulmonary resuscitation on a comatose client?
1. Cool, pale skin; unconsciousness; absence of radial pulse
2. Cyanosis, slow pulse, dilated pupils
3. Absent pulses, flushed skin, pinpoint pupils
4. Apnea, absence of carotid or femoral pulses, dilated pupils

10. Which of the following nursing diagnoses would be most appropriate for clients with cardiovascular disease? Select all that apply.
1. Ineffective Tissue Perfusion
2. Acute Confusion
3. Decreased Cardiac Output
4. Sleep Pattern Disturbance
5. Activity Intolerance

∞ *See answers to Test Your Knowledge in Appendix A.*

PEARSON

EXPLORE **mynursingkit™**

MyNursingKit is your one stop for online chapter review materials and resources. Prepare for success with additional NCLEX®-style practice questions, interactive assignments and activities, web links, animations and videos, and more!

Register your access code from the front of your book at
www.mynursingkit.com.

REFERENCES AND SELECTED BIBLIOGRAPHY

American Heart Association. (2005–2006). Highlights of the 2005 American Heart Association guidelines for cardiopulmonary resuscitation and emergency cardiovascular care. *Currents in Emergency Cardiovascular Care, 16*(4), 1–27.

American Thoracic Society. (2006). Tracheostomy tube care. Retrieved from http://www.thoracic.org/sections/education/care-of-the-child-with-a-chronic-tracheostomy/components-of-tracheostomy-care/tracheostomy-tube-care.html

Andrs, K. (2004). Chest drainage to go. *Nursing, 34*(5), 54–55.

Anonymous. (2003). Why a drink a day may keep heart disease at bay. *Tufts University Health & Nutrition Letter, 28*(8), 2.

Astle, S. M., & Caulfield, E. V. (2003). Bedside tracheostomy: A step by step guide. *RN, 66*(10), 41–45.

Ball, J. W., & Bindler, R. C. (2006). *Child health nursing.* Upper Saddle River, NJ: Prentice Hall Health.

Bergen, C., & Compher, C. (2006). Total homocysteine concentration and associated cardiovascular and renal implications in adults. *Journal of Cardiovascular Nursing, 21*(1), 40–46.

Bindler, R. C., & Ball, J. W. (2007). *Clinical skills manual for pediatric nursing:*

Caring for children (4th ed.). Upper Saddle River, NJ: Prentice Hall Health.

Blosser, C. G., & Freitas-Nichols, J. (2004). Cardiovascular disorders. In C. E. Burns, A. M. Dunn, M. A. Brady, M. B. Starr, & C. G. Blosser, *Pediatric primary care: A handbook for nurse practitioners.* Philadelphia: Saunders/Elsevier.

Bollinger, K., & Sadar, A. M. (2003). Care and management of the patient with right heart failure secondary to diastolic dysfunction. *Critical Care Nursing Quarterly, 26*(1), 22–27.

Bolton, M. M., & Wilson, B. A. (2005). The influence of race on heart failure in African-American women. *Medsurg Nursing, 14*(1), 8–15.

Bonham, P. A. (2003). Determing the toe brachial pressure index. *Nursing, 33*(9), 54–55.

Bulechek, G. M., Butcher, H. K., & Dochterman, J. M. (Eds.). (2008). *Nursing interventions: classification (NIC)* (5th ed.). St. Louis, MO: Mosby.

Caboral, M., & Mitchell, J. (2003). B-type natriuretic peptide: A new tool in the armamentarium used to accurately diagnose heart failure. *Progress in Cardiovascular Nursing, 18*(4), 190–193.

Calver, P., Braungardt, T., Kupchik, N., Jensen, A., & Cutler, C. (2005). The big

chill: Improving the odds after cardiac arrest. *RN, 68*(5), 58–62.

Carroll, P. (2005). Keeping up with mobile chest drains. *RN, 68*(10), 26–31.

Coleman, P. R. (2004). Pneumonia in the long-term care setting: Etiology, management, and prevention. *Journal of Gerontological Nursing, 30*(4), 14–24.

Coughlin, A., & Parchinsky, C. (2006). Go with the flow of chest tube therapy. *Nursing, 36*(3), 36–42.

Covey, M. K., & Larson, J. L. (2004). Exercise and COPD. *American Journal of Nursing, 104*(5), 40–43.

Craig, K. J., & Hopkins-Pepe, L. (2006). Understanding the new AHA guidelines, part 1. *Nursing, 36*(3), 53–54.

Craig, K. J., & Hopkins-Pepe, L. (2006). Understanding the new AHA guidelines, part II. *Nursing, 36*(5), 52–53.

Duffy, J. R., Hoskins, L. M., & Chen, M. (2004). Nonpharmacological strategies for improving heart failure outcomes in the community: A systematic review. *Journal of Nursing Care Quality, 19*(4), 349–360.

Dulak, S. B. (2005). Hands-on help: Removing chest tubes. *RN, 68*(8), 28ac1–28ac4.

Dulak, S. B. (2005). Hands-on help: Sputum sample collection. *RN, 68*(10), 24ac2–24ac4.

Efre, A. J. (2004). Gender bias in acute myocardial infarction. *Nurse Practitioner, 29*(11), 42, 49–55.

Evangelista, L. S., & Miller, P. S. (2006). Overweight and obesity in the context of heart failure. Implications for practice and future research. *Journal of Cardiovascular Nursing, 21*(1), 27–33.

Fort, C. W. (2002). Get pumped to prevent DVT. *Nursing, 32*(9), 50–53.

Hockman, R. H. (2004). Pharmacologic therapy for acute exacerbations of chronic obstructive pulmonary disease: A review. *Critical Care Nursing Clinics of North America, 16*(3), 293–310.

Hoffman, J. (2001). Incidence, mortality and natural history. In R. H. Anderson, R. Anderson, E. J. Baker, F. J. McCartney, M. L. Rigby, & M. Tynan, *Paediatric cardiology* (2nd ed.). New York: Churchill Livingstone.

Hussey, L. C., & Hardin, S. (2005). Comparison of characteristics of heart failure by race and gender. *Dimensions of Critical Care Nursing, 24*(1), 41–46.

Keith, D. D., Garrett, K. M., Hickox, G., Echols, B., & Comeau, E. (2004). Ventilator-associated pneumonia: Improved clinical outcomes. *Journal of Nursing Care Quality, 19*(4), 328–344.

Konick-McMahan, J., Bixby, B., & McKenna, C. (2003). Heart failure in older adults. Providing nursing care to improve outcomes. *Journal of Gerontological Nursing, 29*(12), 35–41.

Lehne, R. A. (2010). *Pharmacology for nursing care (6th ed.).* St. Louis: Saunders.

Lippincott Williams & Wilkins. (2004). Applying antiembolism stockings isn't just pulling on socks. *Nursing, 34*(8), 48–49.

Lloyd-Jones, D. M., Leip, E. P., Larson, M. G., D'Agostino, R. B., Beiser, A., Wilson, P., et al. (2006). Prediction of lifetime risk for cardiovascular disease by risk factor burden at 50 years of age. *Circulation, 113*(6), 791–798.

Moorhead, S., Johnson, M., Maas, M. L., & Swanson, E. (Eds.). (2008). *Nursing outcomes classification (NOC)* (4th ed.). St. Louis: Mosby.

NANDA International. (2009). *NANDA nursing diagnoses: Definitions and classification 2009–2011.* West Sussex, U.K.: Wiley-Blackwell.

Nicholas, M. (2004). Heart failure: Pathophysiology, treatment and nursing care. *Nursing Standard, 19*(11), 46–51.

Puritt, B. (2005). Clear the air with closed suctioning. *Nursing, 35*(7), 4–45.

Pruitt, W. C. (2005). Teaching your patient to use a peak flowmeter. *Nursing, 35*(3), 54–55.

Pruitt, W. C., & Jacobs, M. (2003). Basics of oxygen therapy. *Nursing, 33*(10), 43–45.

Raymond, S. U., Leeder, S., & Greenberg, H. M. (2006). Obesity and cardiovascular disease in developing countries: A growing problem and an economic threat. *Current Opinion in Clinical Nutrition and Metabolic Care, 9*, 111–116.

Rice, K. L. (2005). How to measure ankle/brachial index. *Nursing, 35*(1), 56–57.

Richardson, C. R., Kriska, A. M., Lantz, P. M., & Hayward, R. A. (2004). Physical activity and mortality across cardiovascular disease risk groups. *Medicine & Science in Sports & Exercise, 36*(11), 1923–1929.

Robinson, S. L. (2004). Is it an MI? What the leads tell you. *RN, 67*(5), 48–53.

Roman, M. (2005). Tracheostomy tubes. *Medsurg Nursing, 14*(2), 143–145.

Roman, M., & Mercado, D. (2006). Review of chest tube use. *Medsurg Nursing, 15*(1), 41–43.

Ruidavets, J., Bongard, V., Simon, C., Dallongeville, J., Ducimetiere, P., Arveiler, D., et al. (2006). Independent contribution of dairy products and calcium intake to blood pressure variations at a population level. *Journal of Hypertension, 24*, 671–681.

Russell, C. (2005). Providing the nurse with a guide to tracheostomy care and management. *British Journal of Nursing, 14*(8), 428–433.

Scordo, K. A. (2005). Noninvasive diagnosis of coronary artery disease in women. *Journal of Cardiovascular Nursing, 20*(6), 420–426.

Sole, M. L., Byers, J. F., Ludy, J. E., Zhang, Y., Banta, C. M., & Brummel, K. (2003). A multisite survey of suctioning techniques and airway management practices. *American Journal of Critical Care, 12*(3), 220–230.

Stansbury, J. P., Jia, H., Williams, L. S., Vogel, W. B., & Duncan, P. W. (2005). Ethnic disparities in stroke: Epidemiology, acute care, and postacute outcomes. *Stroke, 36*, 374–386.

St. John, R. E. (2004). Airway management. *Critical Care Nurse, 24*(2), 93–96.

Warren, M. L., Jarrett, C., Senegal, R., Parker, A., Kraus, J., & Hartgraves, D. (2004). An interdisciplinary approach to transitioning ventilator-dependent patients to home. *Journal of Nursing Care Quality, 19*(1), 67–72.

Fluid, Electrolyte, and Acid–Base Balance

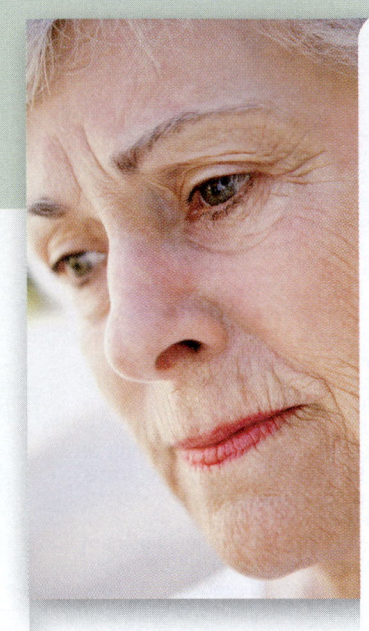

Marie LeBlanc, 62 years old, was diagnosed with type II diabetes mellitus 14 years ago and controls her blood sugar through diet and exercise. She is otherwise healthy and has no chronic health problems. She lives with her husband in a traditional two-level single family home. One evening Marie and her husband dine in a restaurant with two other couples and have a wonderful time. They come home and go to bed. At about 3 AM Marie wakes up with abdominal cramps and begins vomiting and having diarrhea.

By 9 AM she has vomited approximately 8 times and has had loose stools every 20 minutes. She checks her blood sugar and finds it is elevated at 203. She feels terrible and is too weak to climb the stairs, so she stays upstairs. Her husband brings her cold water to drink, but she only moans and says, "Get that away from me! It wouldn't stay down anyway." By 3 PM she barely has enough energy to walk to the bathroom, and her husband insists she must go to the emergency room. He wraps her in her bathrobe and helps her to the car and takes her to the local hospital emergency room.

LEARNING OUTCOMES

After completing this chapter, you will be able to:

1. Describe the function, distribution, movement, and regulation of fluids and electrolytes in the body.

2. Explain the regulation of acid–base balance in the body, including the role of the lungs, the kidneys, and the buffer systems.

3. List factors affecting normal body fluid, electrolyte, and acid–base balance.

4. Describe disturbances in body fluid volumes, electrolytes, and/or acid–base balance in terms of risk factors, causes, and effects.

5. Demonstrate an assessment of a client's fluid, electrolyte, and acid–base status.

6. Identify appropriate nursing diagnosis for clients with fluid, electrolyte, or acid–base imbalances.

7. Demonstrate appropriate nursing interventions aimed at correcting fluid, electrolyte, or acid–base imbalances, including performance of skills and client teaching.

8. Evaluate the effectiveness of nursing and collaborative interventions in correcting the client's fluid, electrolyte, or acid–base imbalances.

In good health, a delicate balance of fluids, electrolytes, and acids and bases is maintained in the body. This balance, or physiologic homeostasis, depends on multiple physiologic processes that regulate fluid intake and output, as well as the movement of water and the substances dissolved in it between body compartments. Almost every illness or injury has the potential to threaten this balance.

BODY FLUIDS AND ELECTROLYTES

Approximately 60% of the average healthy adult's weight is water. In good health this volume remains relatively constant and the person's weight varies by less than 0.2 kg (0.5 lb) in 24 hours, regardless of the amount of fluid ingested. Water is vital to health and normal cellular function, serving as a medium for metabolic reactions within cells; transport nutrients, waste products, and other substance; function as a lubricant, insulator, and shock absorber; and regulate and maintain body temperature.

Age, sex, and body fat affect total body water. Infants have the highest proportion of water, accounting for 70% to 80% of their body weight. The proportion of body water decreases with age. In people older than 60 years of age, it represents only about 50% of the total body weight. Women and older adults have reduced body water due to decreased muscle mass and a greater percentage of fat tissue, which has significantly less water than lean tissue.

Distribution of Body Fluids

The body's fluid is divided into two major compartments, intracellular and extracellular. **Intracellular fluid (ICF)** is found within the cells of the body and is vital to normal functioning of the cell. It contains solutes such as oxygen, electrolytes, and glucose, and provides a medium in which metabolic processes of the cell take place. It constitutes approximately two-thirds of the total body fluid in adults. **Extracellular fluid (ECF)** is found outside the cells and accounts for the remaining one-third of total body fluid. The two main compartments of ECF are intravascular and interstitial. **Intravascular fluid**, or **plasma**, accounts for approximately 20% of the ECF and is found within the vascular system. **Interstitial fluid** accounts for approximately 75% of the ECF and surrounds the cells. The other compartments of ECF are the lymph and transcellular fluids. Examples of **transcellular fluid** include cerebrospinal, pericardial, pancreatic, pleural, intraocular, biliary, peritoneal, and synovial fluids (Figure 36–1).

Although extracellular fluid is in the smaller of the two compartments, it is the transport system that carries nutrients to and waste products from the cells. Interstitial fluid transports wastes from the cells by way of the lymph system as well as directly into the blood plasma through capillaries.

Composition of Body Fluids

Extracellular and intracellular fluids contain oxygen from the lungs, dissolved nutrients from the gastrointestinal tract,

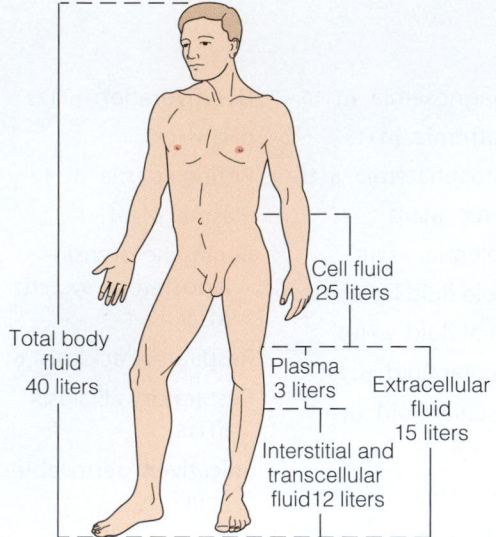

Figure 36–1 ○ Total body fluid represents 40 L in an adult male weighing 70 kg (154 lb).

excretory products of metabolism such as carbon dioxide, and charged particles called **ions**.

Many salts dissociate in water, that is, break up into electrically charged ions. The salt sodium chloride breaks up into one ion of sodium (Na^+) and one ion of chloride (Cl^-). These charged particles are called **electrolytes** because they are capable of conducting electricity. The number of ions that carry a positive charge, called **cations**, and ions that carry a negative charge, called **anions**, should be equal. Examples of cations are sodium (Na^+), potassium (K^+), calcium (Ca^{2+}), and magnesium (Mg^{2+}). Examples of anions include chloride (Cl^-), bicarbonate HCO_3^-, phosphate HPO_4^{2-}, and sulfate SO_4^{2-}.

Electrolytes generally are measured in milliequivalents per liter of water (mEq/L) or milligrams per 100 milliliters (mg/100 mL). The term **milliequivalent** refers to the chemical combining power of the ion, or the capacity of cations to combine with anions to form molecules. This combining activity is measured in relation to the combining activity of the hydrogen ion (H^+). Thus, 1 mEq of any anion equals 1 mEq of any cation. However, cations and anions may not be equal in weight: 1 mg of Na^+ does not equal 1 mg of Cl^-; rather, 3 mg of Na^+ equals 2 mg of Cl^-.

Clinically, the milliequivalent system is most often used. However, nurses need to be aware that different systems of measurement may be found when interpreting laboratory results. For example, calcium levels frequently are reported in milligrams per deciliter (1 dL = 100 mL) instead of milliequivalents per liter. It also is important to remember that laboratory tests are usually performed using blood plasma, an extracellular fluid. These results may reflect what is happening in the ECF, but it generally is not possible to directly measure electrolyte concentrations within the cell.

The composition of fluids varies from one body compartment to another. In extracellular fluid, the principal elec-

trolytes are sodium, chloride, and bicarbonate. Other electrolytes such as potassium, calcium, and magnesium are also present but in much smaller quantities. Plasma and interstitial fluid, the two primary components of ECF, contain essentially the same electrolytes and solutes, with the exception of protein. Plasma is a protein-rich fluid, containing large amounts of albumin, but interstitial fluid contains little or no protein.

The composition of intracellular fluid differs significantly from that of ECF. Potassium and magnesium are the primary cations present in ICF, with phosphate and sulfate the major anions. As in ECF, other electrolytes are present within the cell, but in much smaller concentrations (Figure 36–2).

Maintaining a balance of fluid volumes and electrolyte compositions in the fluid compartments of the body is essential to health. Normal and unusual fluid and electrolyte losses must be replaced if homeostasis is to be maintained.

Other body fluids such as gastric and intestinal secretions also contain electrolytes. This is of particular concern when these fluids are lost from the body. Fluid and electrolyte imbalances can result from excessive losses through vomiting, diarrhea, or gastric suction.

Movement of Body Fluids and Electrolytes

The body fluid compartments are separated from one another by cell membranes and the capillary membrane. While these membranes are completely permeable to water, they are considered to be **selectively permeable** to solutes as substances move across them with varying degrees of ease. Small particles such as ions, oxygen, and carbon dioxide easily move across these membranes, but larger molecules like glucose and proteins have more difficulty moving between fluid compartments. The methods by which electrolytes and other solutes move are osmosis, diffusion, filtration, and active transport.

OSMOSIS **Osmosis** is the movement of water across cell membranes, from the less concentrated solution to the more concentrated solution. In other words, water moves toward the higher concentration of solute in an attempt to equalize the concentrations.

Solutes are substances dissolved in a liquid. For example, when sugar is added to coffee, the sugar is the solute. Solutes may be **crystalloids** (salts that dissolve readily into true solutions) or **colloids** (substances such as large protein molecules that do not readily dissolve into true solutions). A **solvent** is the component of a solution that can dissolve a solute. In the previous example, coffee is the solvent for the sugar.

In the body, water is the solvent; the solutes include electrolytes, oxygen and carbon dioxide, glucose, urea, amino acids, and proteins. Osmosis occurs when the concentration of solutes on one side of a selectively permeable membrane, such as the capillary membrane, is higher than on the other side. For example, a marathon runner loses a significant amount of water through perspiration, increasing the concentration of solutes in the plasma because of water

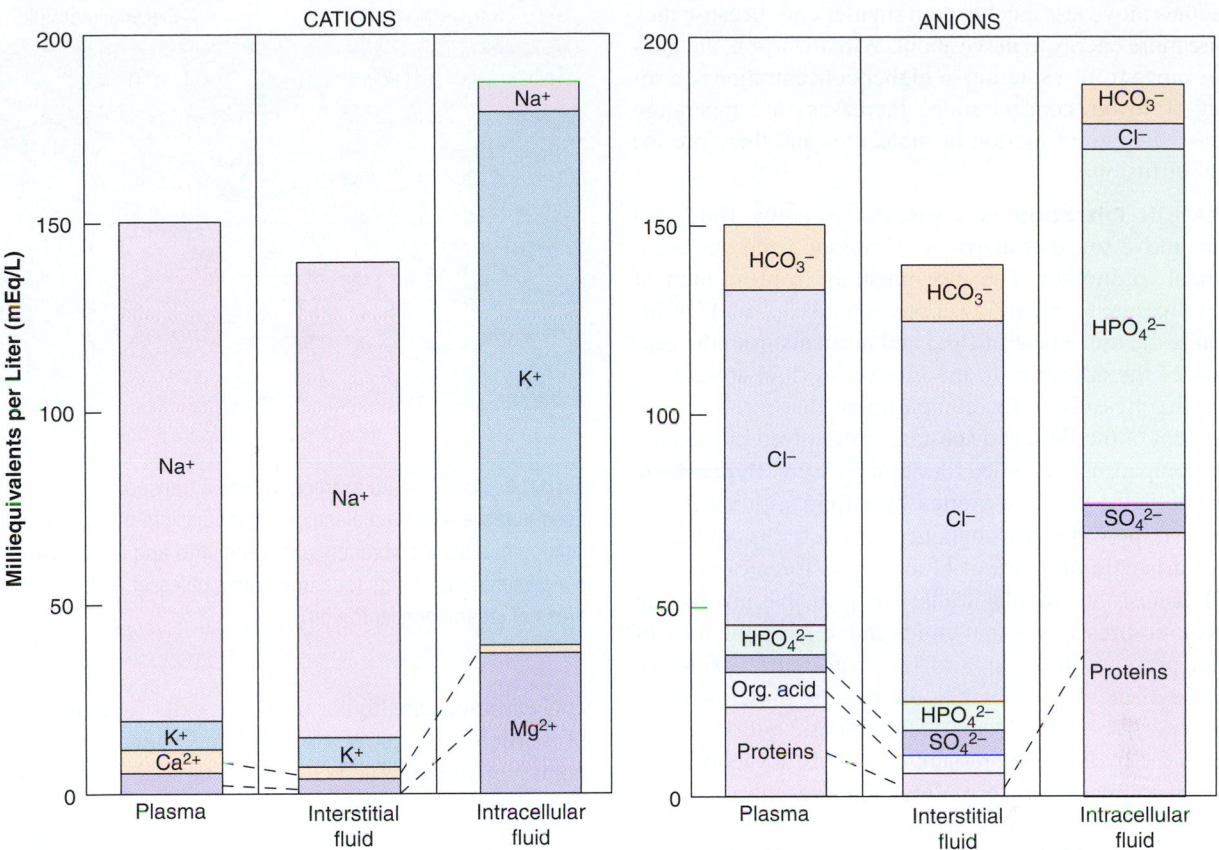

Figure 36–2 ● Electrolyte composition (cations and anions) of body fluid compartments.

Source: Martini, Fredric H., & Halyard, Rebecca A., *Fundamentals of Anatomy and Physiology Interactive,* (Media Edition), 4th ed., © 1998. Reproduced with permission of Pearson Education, Inc., Upper Saddle River, New Jersey.

loss. This higher solute concentration draws water from the interstitial space and cells into the vascular compartment to equalize the concentration of solutes in all fluid compartments. Osmosis is an important mechanism for maintaining homeostasis and fluid balance.

The concentration of solutes in body fluids is usually expressed as the **osmolality**. Osmolality is determined by the total solute concentration within a fluid compartment and is measured as parts of solute per kilogram of water. Osmolality is reported as milliosmols per kilogram (mOsm/kg).

Sodium is by far the greatest determinant of *serum osmolality,* with glucose and urea also contributing. Potassium, glucose, and urea are the primary contributors to the osmolality of intracellular fluid. The term *tonicity* may be used to refer to the osmolality of a solution. Solutions may be termed isotonic, hypertonic, or hypotonic. An **isotonic** solution has the same osmolality as body fluids. Normal saline, 0.9% sodium chloride, is an isotonic solution. **Hypertonic** solutions have a higher osmolality than body fluids; 3% sodium chloride is a hypertonic solution. **Hypotonic** solutions such as one-half normal saline (0.45% sodium chloride), by contrast, have a lower osmolality than body fluids.

Osmotic pressure is the power of a solution to draw water across a semipermeable membrane. When two solutions of different solute concentrations are separated by a semi-

permeable membrane, the solution of higher solute concentration exerts a higher osmotic pressure, drawing water across the membrane to equalize the concentrations of the solutions. For example, infusing a hypertonic intravenous solution such as 3% sodium chloride will draw fluid out of red blood cells (RBCs), causing them to shrink. On the other hand, a hypotonic solution administered intravenously will cause the RBCs to swell as water is drawn into the cells by their higher osmotic pressure. In the body, plasma proteins exert an osmotic draw called **colloidal osmotic pressure** or **oncotic pressure**, pulling water from the interstitial space into the vascular compartment. This is an important mechanism in maintaining vascular volume.

DIFFUSION Diffusion is the continual intermingling of molecules in liquids, gases, or solids brought about by the random movement of the molecules. For example, two gases become mixed by the constant motion of their molecules. The process of diffusion occurs even when two substances are separated by a thin membrane. In the body, diffusion of water, electrolytes, and other substances occurs through the "split pores" of capillary membranes.

The rate of diffusion of substances varies according to (a) the size of the molecules, (b) the concentration of the solution, and (c) the temperature of the solution. Larger molecules move less quickly than smaller ones because they require more energy to move about. With diffusion, the molecules move from a solution of higher concentration to a solution of lower concentration. Increases in temperature increase the rate of motion of molecules and therefore the rate of diffusion.

FILTRATION **Filtration** is a process whereby fluid and solutes move together across a membrane from one compartment to another. The movement is from an area of higher pressure to one of lower pressure. An example of filtration is the movement of fluid and nutrients from the capillaries of the arterioles to the interstitial fluid around the cells. The pressure in the compartment that results in the movement of the fluid and substances dissolved in fluid out of the compartment is called filtration pressure. **Hydrostatic pressure** is the pressure exerted by a fluid within a closed system on the walls of a container in which it is contained. The hydrostatic pressure of blood is the force exerted by blood against the vascular walls. The principle involved in hydrostatic pressure is that fluids move from the area of greater pressure to the area of lesser pressure. Using the example of the blood vessels, the plasma proteins in the blood exert a colloid osmotic or oncotic pressure that opposes the hydrostatic pressure and holds the fluid in the vascular compartment to maintain the vascular volume. When the hydrostatic pressure is greater than the osmotic pressure, the fluid filters out of the blood vessels. The filtration pressure in this example is the difference between the hydrostatic pressure and the osmotic pressure (Figure 36–3).

ACTIVE TRANSPORT Substances can move across cell membranes from a less concentrated solution to a more concentrated one by **active transport** (Figure 36–4). This process differs from diffusion and osmosis in that metabolic energy is expended. In active transport, a substance combines with a carrier on the outside surface of the cell membrane, and they move to the inside surface of the cell membrane. Once inside, they separate, and the substance is released to the inside of the cell. A specific carrier is required for each substance, enzymes are required for active transport, and energy is expended.

This process is of particular importance in maintaining the differences in sodium and potassium ion concentrations of ECF and ICF. Under normal conditions, sodium concentrations are higher in the extracellular fluid, and potassium

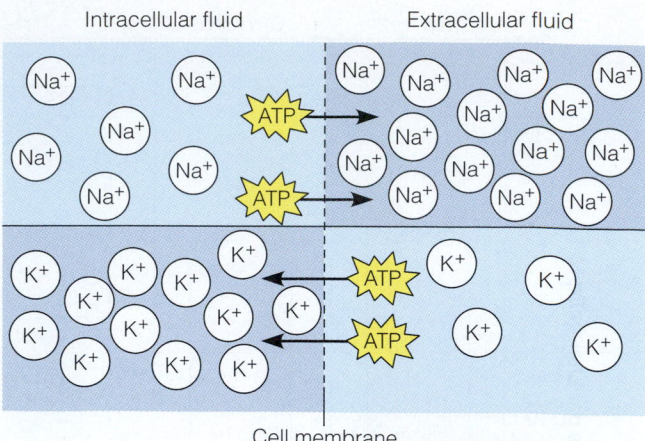

Figure 36–4 ⬤ An example of active transport. Energy (ATP) is used to move sodium molecules and potassium molecules across a semipermeable membrane against sodium's and potassium's concentration gradients (i.e., from areas of lesser concentration to areas of greater concentration).

concentrations are higher inside the cells. To maintain these proportions, the active transport mechanism (the sodium-potassium pump) is activated, moving sodium from the cells and potassium into the cells.

Regulating Body Fluids

In a healthy person, the volumes and chemical composition of the fluid compartments stay within narrow safe limits. Normally, fluid intake and fluid loss are balanced. Illness can upset this balance.

FLUID INTAKE During periods of moderate activity at moderate temperature, the average adult drinks about 1,500 mL per day but needs 2,500 mL per day, an additional 1,000 mL. This added volume is acquired from foods and from the oxidation of these foods during metabolic processes. The water content of food is relatively large, contributing about 750 mL per day. The water content of fresh vegetables is approximately 90%, of fresh fruits about 85%, and of lean meats around 60%.

Water, as a by-product of food metabolism, accounts for most of the remaining fluid volume required. This quantity is approximately 200 mL per day for the average adult. See Table 36–1.

Figure 36–3 ⬤ Schematic of filtration pressure changes within a capillary bed. On the arterial side, arterial blood pressure exceeds colloid osmotic pressure, so that water and dissolved substances move out of the capillary into the interstitial space. On the venous side, venous blood pressure is less than colloid osmotic pressure, so that water and dissolved substances move into the capillary.

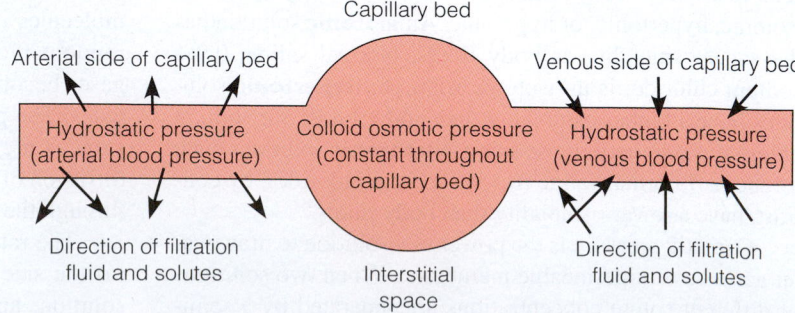

TABLE 36–1	Average Daily Fluid Intake and Output for an Adult

INTAKE	
SOURCE	AMOUNT (ML)
Oral fluids	1,200 to 1,500
Water in foods	1,000
Water as by-product of	200 food metabolism
Total	2,400 to 2,700

OUTPUT	
ROUTE	AMOUNT (ML)
Urine	1,400 to 1,500
Insensible losses	
Lungs	350 to 400
Skin	350 to 400
Sweat	100
Feces	100 to 200
Total	2,300 to 2,600

The thirst mechanism is the primary regulator of fluid intake. The thirst center is located in the hypothalamus of the brain. A number of stimuli trigger this center, including the osmotic pressure of body fluids, vascular volume, and angiotensin (a hormone released in response to decreased blood flow to the kidneys). For example, a long-distance runner loses significant amounts of water through perspiration and rapid breathing during a race, increasing the concentration of solutes and the osmotic pressure of body fluids. This increased osmotic pressure stimulates the thirst center, causing the runner to experience the sensation of thirst and the desire to drink to replace lost fluids.

Thirst is normally relieved immediately after drinking a small amount of fluid, even before it is absorbed from the gastrointestinal tract. However, this relief is only temporary, and the thirst returns in about 15 minutes. The thirst is again temporarily relieved after the ingested fluid distends the upper gastrointestinal tract. These mechanisms protect the individual from drinking too much, because it takes from 30 minutes to 1 hour for the fluid to be absorbed and distributed throughout the body.

FLUID OUTPUT Fluid losses from the body counterbalance the adult's 2,500-mL average daily intake of fluid, as shown in Table 36–1. There are four routes of fluid output:

1. Urine
2. Insensible loss
3. Noticeable loss through the skin
4. Loss through the intestines in feces

Urine Urine formed by the kidneys and excreted from the urinary bladder is the major avenue of fluid output. Normal urine output for an adult is 1,400 to 1,500 mL per 24 hours, or at least 0.5 mL per kilogram per hour. In healthy people, urine output may vary noticeably from day to day. Urine volume automatically increases as fluid intake increases. If large amounts of fluid are lost through perspiration, urine volume decreases to maintain fluid balance in the body.

Insensible Losses **Insensible fluid loss** occurs through the skin and lungs. It is called insensible because it is usually not noticeable and cannot be measured. Insensible fluid loss through the skin occurs through diffusion and perspiration (which is noticeable but not measurable). Water losses through diffusion are not noticeable but normally account for 300 to 400 mL per day. This loss can be significantly increased if the protective layer of the skin is lost as with burns or large abrasions. Perspiration varies depending on factors such as environmental temperature and metabolic activity. Fever and exercise increase metabolic activity and heat production, thereby increasing fluid losses through the skin.

Another type of insensible loss is the water in exhaled air. In an adult, this is normally 300 to 400 mL per day. When respiratory rate accelerates, this loss can increase.

Feces The chyme that passes from the small intestine into the large intestine contains water and electrolytes. The volume of chyme entering the large intestine in an adult is normally about 1,500 mL per day. Of this amount, all but about 100 mL is reabsorbed in the proximal half of the large intestine.

Certain fluid losses are required to maintain normal body function. These are known as **obligatory losses**. Approximately 500 mL of fluid must be excreted through the kidneys of an adult each day to eliminate metabolic waste products from the body. Water lost through respirations, through the skin, and in feces are also obligatory losses, necessary for temperature regulation and elimination of waste products. The total of all these losses is approximately 1,300 mL per day.

MAINTAINING HOMEOSTASIS The volume and composition of body fluids is regulated through several homeostatic mechanisms. A number of body systems contribute to this regulation, including the kidneys, the endocrine system, the cardiovascular system, the lungs, and the gastrointestinal system. Hormones such as antidiuretic hormone (ADH; also known as arginine vasopressin or AVP), the renin-angiotensin-aldosterone system, and atrial natriuretic factor are involved, as are mechanisms to monitor and maintain vascular volume.

Kidneys The kidneys are the primary regulator of body fluids and electrolyte balance. They regulate the volume and osmolality of extracellular fluids by regulating water and electrolyte excretion. The kidneys adjust the reabsorption of water from plasma filtrate and ultimately the amount excreted as urine. Although 135 to 180 L of plasma per day is normally filtered in an adult, only about 1.5 L of urine is excreted. Electrolyte balance is maintained by selective retention and excretion by the kidneys. The kidneys also play a significant role in acid–base regulation, excreting hydrogen ion (H^+) and retaining bicarbonate.

Antidiuretic Hormone Antidiuretic hormone, which regulates water excretion from the kidney, is synthesized in the anterior portion of the hypothalamus and acts on the collecting ducts of the nephrons. When serum osmolality rises, ADH is

MyNursingKit | Fluid Balance

produced, causing the collecting ducts to become more permeable to water. This increased permeability allows more water to be reabsorbed into the blood. As more water is reabsorbed, urine output falls and serum osmolality decreases because the water dilutes body fluids. Conversely, if serum osmolality decreases, ADH is suppressed, the collecting ducts become less permeable to water, and urine output increases. Excess water is excreted, and serum osmolality returns to normal. Other factors also affect the production and release of ADH, including blood volume, temperature, pain, stress, and some drugs such as opiates, barbiturates, and nicotine.

Renin-Angiotensin-Aldosterone System   Specialized receptors in the juxtaglomerular cells of the kidney nephrons respond to changes in renal perfusion. This initiates the **renin-angiotensin-aldosterone system**. If blood flow or pressure to the kidney decreases, renin is released. Renin causes the conversion of angiotensinogen to angiotensin I, which is then converted to angiotensin II by angiotensin-converting enzyme. Angiotensin II acts directly on the nephrons to promote sodium and water retention. In addition, it stimulates the release of aldosterone from the adrenal cortex. Aldosterone also promotes sodium retention in the distal nephron. The net effect of the renin-angiotensin-aldosterone system is to restore blood volume (and renal perfusion) through sodium and water retention.

Atrial Natriuretic Factor   Atrial natriuretic factor (ANF) is released from cells in the atrium of the heart in response to excess blood volume and stretching of the atrial walls. Acting on the nephrons, ANF promotes sodium wasting and acts as a potent diuretic, thus reducing vascular volume. ANF also inhibits thirst, reducing fluid intake.

Regulating Electrolytes

Electrolytes are present in all body fluids and fluid compartments. Just as maintaining the fluid balance is vital to normal body function, so is maintaining electrolyte balance. Although the concentration of specific electrolytes differs between fluid compartments, a balance of cations and anions always exists. Electrolytes are important for:

- Maintaining fluid balance.
- Contributing to acid–base regulation.
- Facilitating enzyme reactions.
- Transmitting neuromuscular reactions.

Most electrolytes enter the body through dietary intake and are excreted in the urine. Some electrolytes, such as sodium and chloride, are not stored by the body and must be consumed daily to maintain normal levels. Potassium and calcium are stored in the cells and bone, respectively. When serum levels drop, ions can shift out of the storage "pool" into the blood to maintain adequate serum levels for normal functioning. The regulatory mechanisms and functions of the major electrolytes are summarized in Table 36–2.

SODIUM (NA+)   Sodium is the most abundant cation in extracellular fluid and a major contributor to serum osmo-

lality. Normal serum sodium levels are 135 to 145 mEq/L. Sodium functions largely in controlling and regulating water balance. When sodium is reabsorbed from the kidney tubules, chloride and water are reabsorbed with it, thus maintaining ECF volume. Sodium is found in many foods, such as bacon, ham, processed cheese, and table salt.

POTASSIUM (K+)   Potassium is the major cation in intracellular fluids, with only a small amount found in plasma and interstitial fluid. ICF levels of potassium are usually 125 to 140 mEq/L while normal serum potassium levels are 3.5 to 5.0 mEq/L. The ratio of intracellular to extracellular potassium must be maintained for neuromuscular response to stimuli. Potassium is a vital electrolyte for skeletal, cardiac, and smooth muscle activity. It is involved in maintaining acid–base balance as well, and it contributes to intracellular enzyme reactions. Potassium must be ingested daily because the body can't conserve it. Many fruits and vegetables, meat, fish, and other foods contain potassium.

CALCIUM (CA²⁺)   Ninety-nine percent of calcium in the body is in the skeletal system, with a relatively small amount in extracellular fluid. It is vital in regulating muscle contraction and relaxation, neuromuscular function, and cardiac function. ECF calcium is regulated by a complex interaction of parathyroid hormone, calcitonin, and calcitriol, a metabolite of vitamin D. The normal total serum calcium levels, which range from 8.5 to 10.5 mg/dL, represent both bound and unbound calcium. The normal ionized serum calcium, which ranges from 4.0 to 5.0 mg/dL, represents calcium circulating in the plasma in free, or unbound, form (Hayes, 2004). When calcium levels in the ECF fall, parathyroid hormone and calcitriol cause calcium to be released from bones into ECF and increase the absorption of calcium in the intestines, thus raising serum calcium levels. Conversely, calcitonin stimulates the deposition of calcium in bone, reducing the concentration of calcium ions in the blood. With aging, the intestines absorb calcium less effectively and more calcium is excreted via the kidneys. Milk and milk products are the richest sources of calcium, with other foods such as dark green leafy vegetables and canned salmon containing smaller amounts. Many clients benefit from calcium supplements.

MAGNESIUM (MG²⁺)   Magnesium is primarily found in the skeleton and in intracellular fluid. It is the second most abundant intracellular cation with normal serum levels of 1.5 to 2.5 mEq/L. It is important for intracellular metabolism, being particularly involved in the production and use of ATP. Magnesium also is necessary for protein and DNA synthesis within the cells. Only about 1% of the body's magnesium is in ECF; here it is involved in regulating neuromuscular and cardiac function. Maintaining and ensuring adequate magnesium levels is an important part of care of clients with cardiac disorders. Cereal grains, nuts, dried fruit, legumes, and green leafy vegetables are good sources of magnesium in the diet, as are dairy products, meat, and fish.

TABLE 36–2	**Regulation and Functions of Electrolytes**	
ELECTROLYTE	REGULATION	FUNCTION
Sodium (Na^+)	• Renal reabsorption or excretion • Aldosterone increases Na^+ reabsorption in collecting duct of nephrons	• Regulating ECF volume and distribution • Maintaining blood volume • Transmitting nerve impulses and contracting muscles
Potassium (K^+)	• Renal excretion and conservation • Aldosterone increases K^+ excretion • Movement into and out of cells • Insulin helps move K^+ into cells; tissue damage and acidosis shift K^+ out of cells into ECF	• Maintaining ICF osmolality • Transmitting nerve and other electrical impulses • Regulating cardiac impulse transmission and muscle contraction • Skeletal and smooth muscle function • Regulating acid–base balance
Calcium (Ca^{2+})	• Redistribution between bones and ECF • Parathyroid hormone and calcitriol increase serum Ca^{2+} levels; calcitonin decreases serum levels	• Forming bones and teeth • Transmitting nerve impulses • Regulating muscle contractions • Maintaining cardiac pacemaker (automaticity)
Magnesium (Mg^{2+})	• Conservation and excretion by kidneys • Intestinal absorption increased by vitamin D and parathyroid hormone	• Blood clotting • Activating enzymes such as pancreatic lipase and phospholipase • Intracellular metabolism
Chloride (Cl^-)	• Excreted and reabsorbed along with sodium in the kidneys • Aldosterone increases chloride reabsorption with sodium	• Operating sodium-potassium pump • Relaxing muscle contractions • Transmitting nerve impulses • Regulating cardiac function
Phosphate (PO_4^-)	• Excretion and reabsorption by the kidneys • Parathyroid hormone decreases serum levels by increasing renal excretion • Reciprocal relationship with calcium: increasing serum calcium levels decrease phosphate levels; decreasing serum calcium increases phosphate	• HCl production • Regulating ECF balance and vascular volume • Regulating acid–base balance • Buffer in oxygen–carbon dioxide exchange in RBCs • Forming bones and teeth • Metabolizing carbohydrate, protein, and fat • Cellular metabolism; producing ATP and DNA
Bicarbonate (HCO_3^-)	• Excretion and reabsorption by the kidneys • Regeneration by kidneys	• Muscle, nerve, and RBC function • Regulating acid–base balance • Regulating calcium levels • Major body buffer involved in acid–base regulation

CHLORIDE (Cl^-) Chloride is the major anion of ECF, and normal serum levels are 95 to 108 mEq/L. Chloride functions with sodium to regulate serum osmolality and blood volume. The concentration of chloride in ECF is regulated secondarily to sodium; when sodium is reabsorbed in the kidney, chloride usually follows. Chloride is a major component of gastric juice as hydrochloric acid (HCl) and is involved in regulating acid–base balance. It also acts as a buffer in the exchange of oxygen and carbon dioxide in RBCs. Chloride is found in the same foods as sodium.

PHOSPHATE PO_4^- Phosphate is the major anion of intracellular fluids. It also is found in ECF, bone, skeletal muscle, and nerve tissue. Normal serum levels of phospate in adults range from 2.5 to 4.5 mg/dL. Children have much higher phosphate levels than adults, with that of a newborn nearly twice that of an adult. Higher levels of growth hormone and a faster rate of skeletal growth probably account for this difference. Phosphate is involved in many chemical actions of the cell; it is essential for functioning of muscles, nerves, and red blood cells. It is also involved in the metabolism of protein, fat, and carbohydrate. Phosphate is absorbed from the intestine and is found in many foods such as meat, fish, poultry, milk products, and legumes.

BICARBONATE HCO_3^- Bicarbonate is present in both intracellular and extracellular fluids. Its primary function is regulating acid–base balance as an essential component of the carbonic acid–bicarbonate buffering system. Extracellular bicarbonate levels are regulated by the kidneys: Bicarbonate is excreted when too much is present; if more is needed, the kidneys regenerate and reabsorb bicarbonate ions. Unlike other electrolytes that must be consumed in the diet, adequate amounts of bicarbonate are produced through metabolic processes to meet the body's needs.

ACID–BASE BALANCE

An important part of regulating the chemical balance or homeostasis of body fluids is regulating their acidity or alkalinity.

An **acid** is a substance that releases hydrogen ions (H^+) in solution. Strong acids such as hydrochloric acid release all, or nearly all, of their hydrogen ions; weak acids like carbonic acid release some hydrogen ions. **Bases**, or *alkalis*, have a low hydrogen ion concentration and can accept hydrogen ions in solution. The relative acidity or alkalinity of a solution is measured as **pH**. The pH reflects the hydrogen ion concentration of the solution: The higher the hydrogen ion concentration (and the more acidic the solution), the lower the pH. Water has a pH of 7 and is neutral; that is, it is neither acidic in nature nor is it alkaline. Solutions with a pH lower than 7 are acidic; those with a pH higher than 7 are alkaline. The pH scale is logarithmic: A solution with a pH of 5 is 10 times more acidic than one with a pH of 6.

Regulation of Acid–Base Balance

Body fluids are maintained within a narrow range that is slightly alkaline. The normal pH of arterial blood is between 7.35 and 7.45 (Figure 36–5). Acids are continually produced during metabolism. Several body systems, including buffers, the respiratory system, and the renal system, are actively involved in maintaining the narrow pH range necessary for optimal function. Buffers help maintain acid–base balance by neutralizing excess acids or bases. The lungs and the kidneys help maintain a normal pH by either excreting or retaining acids and bases.

BUFFERS **Buffers** prevent excessive changes in pH by removing or releasing hydrogen ions. If excess hydrogen ions are present in body fluids, buffers bind with the hydrogen ions, minimizing the change in pH. When body fluids become too alkaline, buffers can release hydrogen ions, again minimizing the change in pH. The action of a buffer is immediate, but limited in its capacity to maintain or restore normal acid–base balance.

The major buffer system in extracellular fluids is the bicarbonate (HCO_3^-) and carbonic acid (H_2CO_3) system. When a strong acid such as hydrochloric acid (HCl) is added, it combines with bicarbonate and the pH drops only slightly. A strong base such as sodium hydroxide combines with carbonic acid, the weak acid of the buffer pair, and the pH remains within the narrow range of normal. The amounts of bicarbonate and carbonic acid in the body vary; however, as long as a ratio of 20 parts of bicarbonate to 1 part of carbonic acid is maintained, the pH remains within its normal range of 7.35 to 7.45. Adding a strong acid to ECF can change this ratio as bicarbonate is de-

pleted in neutralizing the acid. When this happens, the pH drops, and the client has a condition called **acidosis**. The ratio can also be upset by adding a strong base to ECF, depleting carbonic acid as it combines with the base. In this case the pH rises and the client has **alkalosis**. In addition to the bicarbonate–carbonic acid buffer system, plasma proteins, hemoglobin, and phosphates also function as buffers in body fluids.

RESPIRATORY REGULATION The lungs help regulate acid–base balance by eliminating or retaining carbon dioxide (CO_2), a potential acid. Combined with water, carbon dioxide forms carbonic acid ($CO_2 + H_2O \rightarrow H_2CO_3$). This chemical reaction is reversible; carbonic acid breaks down into carbon dioxide and water. Working together with the bicarbonate–carbonic acid buffer system, the lungs regulate acid–base balance and pH by altering the rate and depth of respirations. The response of the respiratory system to changes in pH is rapid, occurring within minutes.

Carbon dioxide is a powerful stimulator of the respiratory center. When blood levels of carbonic acid and carbon dioxide rise, the respiratory center is stimulated and the rate and depth of respirations increase. Carbon dioxide is exhaled, and carbonic acid levels fall. By contrast, when bicarbonate levels are excessive, the rate and depth of respirations are reduced. This causes carbon dioxide to be retained, carbonic acid levels to rise, and the excess bicarbonate to be neutralized.

Carbon dioxide levels in the blood are measured as the PCO_2, or partial pressure of the dissolved gas in the blood. PCO_2 refers to the pressure of carbon dioxide in venous blood. $PaCO_2$ refers to the pressure of carbon dioxide in arterial blood. The normal $PaCO_2$ is 35 to 45 mm Hg.

RENAL REGULATION Although buffers and the respiratory system can compensate for changes in pH, the kidneys are the ultimate long-term regulator of acid–base balance. They are slower to respond to changes, requiring hours to days to correct imbalances, but their response is more permanent and selective than that of the other systems (Yucha, 2004).

The kidneys maintain acid–base balance by selectively excreting or conserving bicarbonate and hydrogen ions. When excess hydrogen ion is present and the pH falls (acidosis), the kidneys reabsorb and regenerate bicarbonate and excrete hydrogen ion. In the case of alkalosis and a high pH, excess bicarbonate is excreted and hydrogen ion is retained. The normal serum bicarbonate level is 22 to 26 mEq/L.

The relationship of the respiratory and renal regulation of acid–base balance is further explained in Box 36–1.

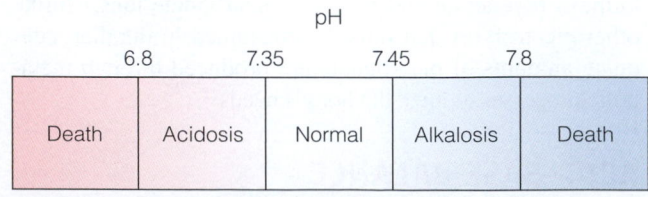

pH				
6.8	7.35	7.45	7.8	
Death	Acidosis	Normal	Alkalosis	Death

Figure 36–5 ● Body fluids are normally slightly alkaline, between a pH of 7.35 and 7.45.

BOX 36–1 Physiological Regulation of Acid–Base Balance

Lungs				Kidneys
$CO_2 + H_2O$	$\leftrightarrow$	H_2CO_3	$\leftrightarrow$	$H + HCO_3$
Carbon dioxide				Hydrogen
+		Carbonic acid		+
water				bicarbonate

LIFESPAN CONSIDERATIONS Fluid and Electrolyte Imbalance

Infants and Children

Infants are at high risk for fluid and electrolyte imbalance because:

- Their immature kidneys cannot concentrate urine.
- They have a rapid respiratory rate and proportionately larger body surface area than adults, leading to greater insensate loss through the skin and respirations.
- They cannot express thirst, nor actively seek fluids.

   Vomiting and/or diarrhea in infants and young children can lead quickly to electrolyte imbalance. Oral rehydration therapy (ORT) (e.g., electrolyte solutions such as Pedialyte) should be used to restore fluid and electrolyte balance in mild to moderate dehydration (American Medical Association et al., 2004). Prompt treatment with ORT can prevent the need for intravenous therapy and hospitalization (Spandorfer, Alessandrini, Joffe, Localio, & Shaw, 2005). Even if the child is nauseated and vomiting, small sips of ORT can be helpful.

Older Adults

Certain changes related to aging place the older adult at risk for serious problems with fluid and electrolyte imbalance, if homeostatic mechanisms are compromised. Some of the changes are:

- A decrease in thirst sensation.
- A decrease in ability of the kidneys to concentrate urine.
- A decrease in intracellular fluid and in total body water.
- A decrease in response to body hormones that help regulate fluid and electrolytes.

Other factors that may influence fluid and electrolyte balance in older adults are:

- Increased use of diuretics for hypertension and heart disease.
- Decreased intake of food and water, especially in older adults with dementia or who are dependent on others to feed them and offer them fluids.
- Preparations for certain diagnostic tests that have the client NPO for long periods of time or cause diarrhea from laxative preps.
- Clients with impaired renal function, such as older adults with diabetes.
- Those having certain diagnostic procedures. (Dyes used for some procedures, such as arteriograms and cardiac catheterizations, may cause further renal problems. Always see that the client is well hydrated before, during, and after the procedure to help in diluting and excreting the dye. If the client is NPO for the procedure, the nurse should check with the primary care provider to see if IV fluids are needed.)
- Any condition that may tax the normal compensatory mechanisms, such as a fever, influenza, surgery, or heat exposure.

   All of these conditions increase older adults' risk for fluid and electrolyte imbalance. The change can happen quickly and become serious in a short time. Astute observations and quick actions by the nurse can help prevent serious consequences. A change in mental status may be the first symptom of impairment and must be further evaluated to determine the cause.

The lungs and kidneys are the two major systems that are working on a continuous basis to help regulate the acid–base balance in the body. In the biochemical reactions above, the processes are all reversible and go back and forth as the body's needs change. The lungs can work very quickly and do their part by either retaining or getting rid of carbon dioxide by changing the rate and depth of respirations. The kidneys work much more slowly; they may take hours to days to regulate the balance by either excreting or conserving hydrogen and bicarbonate ions. Under normal conditions, the two systems work together to maintain homeostasis.

DISTURBANCES IN FLUID VOLUME, ELECTROLYTE, AND ACID–BASE BALANCES

A number of factors such as illness, trauma, surgery, and medications can affect the body's ability to maintain fluid, electrolyte, and acid–base balance. Renal disease is a significant cause of imbalances. Clients who are confused or unable to communicate their needs are at risk for inadequate fluid intake. Vomiting, diarrhea, or nasogastric suction can cause significant fluid losses. Tissue trauma, such as burns, cause fluid and electrolytes to be lost from damaged cells. Decreased blood flow to the kidneys due to im-

paired cardiac function stimulates the renin-angiotensin-aldosterone system, causing sodium and water retention. Medications such as diuretics or corticosteroids can result in abnormal losses of electrolytes and fluid loss or retention. Diseases such as diabetes mellitus or chronic obstructive lung disease may affect acid–base balance. Diabetic ketoacidosis, cancer, and head injury may also lead to electrolyte imbalances.

Factors Affecting Body Fluid, Electrolytes, and Acid–Base Balance

The ability of the body to adjust fluids, electrolytes, and acid–base balance is influenced by age, gender and body size, environmental temperature, and lifestyle.

AGE Infants and growing children have much greater fluid turnover than adults because their higher metabolic rate increases fluid loss. Infants lose more fluid through the kidneys because immature kidneys are less able to conserve water than adult kidneys. In addition, infants' respirations are more rapid and the body surface area is proportionately greater than that of adults, increasing insensible fluid losses. The more rapid turnover of fluid plus the losses produced by disease can create critical fluid imbalances in children much more rapidly than in adults.

In older adults, the normal aging process may affect fluid balance. The thirst response is often blunted. Antidiuretic hormone levels remain normal or may even be elevated, but the nephrons become less able to conserve water in response to ADH. Increased levels of atrial natriuretic factor seen in older adults may also contribute to this impaired ability to conserve water. These normal changes of aging increase the risk of dehydration. When combined with the increased likelihood of heart diseases, impaired renal function, and multiple drug regimens, the older adult's risk for fluid and electrolyte imbalance is significant. Additionally, it is important to consider that the older adult has thinner, more fragile skin and veins, which can make an intravenous insertion more difficult.

GENDER AND BODY SIZE Total body water also is affected by gender and body size. Women have proportionately more body fat and less body water than men. Water accounts for approximately 60% of an adult man's weight, but only 52% for an adult woman. In an obese individual this may be even less, with water responsible for only 30% to 40% of the person's weight.

ENVIRONMENTAL TEMPERATURE People with an illness and those participating in strenuous activity are at risk for fluid and electrolyte imbalances when the environmental temperature is high. Fluid losses through sweating are increased in hot environments as the body attempts to dissipate heat. These losses are even greater in people who have not been acclimatized to the environment. Both salt and water are lost through sweating. When only water is replaced, salt depletion is a risk. The risk of adverse effects is even greater if lost water is not replaced. Body temperature rises, and the person is at risk for heat exhaustion or heatstroke. Heatstroke may occur in older adults or ill people during prolonged periods of heat; it can also affect athletes and laborers when their heat production exceeds the body's ability to dissipate heat. Consuming adequate amounts of cool liquids reduces the risk of adverse effects from heat. Balanced electrolyte solutions and carbohydrate-electrolyte solutions such as sports drinks are recommended because they replace both water and electrolytes lost through sweat.

LIFESTYLE The intake of fluids and electrolytes is affected by the diet. People with anorexia nervosa or bulimia are at risk for severe fluid and electrolyte imbalances because of inadequate intake or purging regimens (e.g., induced vomiting, use of diuretics and laxatives). Seriously malnourished people have decreased serum albumin levels, and may develop edema because the osmotic draw of fluid into the vascular compartment is reduced. When calorie intake is not adequate to meet the body's needs, fat stores are broken down and fatty acids are released, increasing the risk of acidosis.

Regular weight-bearing physical exercise such as walking, running, or bicycling has a beneficial effect on calcium balance. The rate of bone loss that occurs in postmenopausal women and older men is slowed with regular exercise, reducing the risk of osteoporosis.

Stress can increase cellular metabolism, blood glucose concentration, and catecholamine levels. In addition, stress can increase production of ADH, which in turn decreases urine production. The overall response of the body to stress is to increase the blood volume.

Other lifestyle factors can also affect fluid, electrolyte, and acid–base balance. Heavy alcohol consumption affects electrolyte balance, increasing the risk of low calcium, magnesium, and phosphate levels. The risk of acidosis associated with breakdown of fat tissue also is greater in the person who drinks large amounts of alcohol.

Fluid Imbalances

Fluid imbalances are of two basic types: isotonic and osmolar. *Isotonic imbalances* occur when water and electrolytes are lost or gained in equal proportions, so that the osmolality of body fluids remains constant. *Osmolar imbalances* involve the loss or gain of only water, so that the osmolality of the serum is altered. Thus four categories of fluid imbalances may occur: (a) an isotonic loss of water and electrolytes, (b) an isotonic gain of water and electrolytes, (c) a hyperosmolar loss of only water, and (d) a hypo-osmolar gain of only water. These are referred to, respectively, as fluid volume deficit, fluid volume excess, dehydration (hyperosmolar imbalance), and overhydration (hypo-osmolar imbalance).

FLUID VOLUME DEFICIT Isotonic **fluid volume deficit (FVD)** occurs when the body loses both water and electrolytes from the ECF in similar proportions. Thus, the decreased volume of fluid remains isotonic. In FVD, fluid is initially lost from the intravascular compartment, so it often is called **hypovolemia**.

FVD generally occurs as a result of (a) abnormal losses through the skin, gastrointestinal tract, or kidney; (b) decreased intake of fluid; (c) bleeding; or (d) movement of fluid into a third space. See the description of third space syndrome that follows.

For the risk factors and clinical signs related to fluid volume deficit, see Table 36–3.

Third space syndrome results in fluid shifts from the vascular space into an area where it is not readily accessible as extracellular fluid. This fluid remains in the body but is essentially unavailable for use, causing an isotonic fluid volume deficit. Fluid may be sequestered in the bowel, in the interstitial space as edema, in inflamed tissue, or in potential spaces such as the peritoneal or pleural cavities.

The client with third space syndrome has an isotonic fluid deficit but may not manifest apparent fluid loss or weight loss. Careful nursing assessment is vital to effectively identify and intervene for clients experiencing third-spacing. Because the fluid shifts back into the vascular compartment after time, assessment for manifestations of fluid volume excess or hypervolemia is also vital.

FLUID VOLUME EXCESS **Fluid volume excess (FVE)** occurs when the body retains both water and sodium in similar proportions to normal ECF. This is commonly referred to as **hypervolemia** (increased blood volume). FVE is always

TABLE 36–3	Isotonic Fluid Volume Deficit	
RISK FACTORS	**CLINICAL MANIFESTATIONS**	**NURSING INTERVENTIONS**
Loss of water and electrolytes from • Vomiting • Diarrhea • Excessive sweating • Polyuria • Fever • Nasogastric suction • Abnormal drainage or wound losses Insufficient intake due to • Anorexia • Nausea • Inability to access fluids • Impaired swallowing • Confusion, depression	Complaints of weakness and thirst Weight loss • 2% loss = mild FVD • 5% loss = moderate • 8% loss = severe Fluid intake less than output Decreased tissue turgor Dry mucous membranes, sunken eyeballs, decreased tearing Subnormal temperature Weak, rapid pulse Decreased blood pressure Postural (orthostatic) hypotension (significant drop in BP when moving from lying to sitting or standing position) Flat neck veins; decreased capillary refill Decreased central venous pressure Decreased urine volume (<30 mL/h) Increased specific gravity of urine (>1.030) Increased hematocrit Increased blood urea nitrogen (BUN)	Assess for clinical manifestations of FVD. Monitor weight and vital signs, including temperature. Assess tissue turgor. Monitor fluid intake and output. Monitor laboratory findings. Administer oral and intravenous fluids as indicated. Provide frequent mouth care. Implement measures to prevent skin breakdown. Provide for safety, e.g., provide assistance for a client rising from bed.

secondary to an increase in the total body sodium content, which leads to an increase in total body water. Because both water and sodium are retained, the serum sodium concentration remains essentially normal and the excess volume of fluid is isotonic. Specific causes of FVE include (a) excessive intake of sodium chloride; (b) administering sodium-containing infusions too rapidly, particularly to clients with impaired regulatory mechanisms; and (c) disease processes that alter regulatory mechanisms, such as heart failure, renal failure, cirrhosis of the liver, and Cushing's syndrome.

The risk factors and clinical manifestations for FVE are summarized in Table 36–4.

Edema In fluid volume excess, both intravascular and interstitial spaces have an increased water and sodium content. Excess interstitial fluid is known as edema. Edema typically is most apparent in areas where the tissue pressure is low, such as around the eyes, and in dependent tissues (known as dependent edema), where hydrostatic capillary pressure is high.

Edema can be caused by several different mechanisms. The three main mechanisms are increased capillary hydrostatic pressure, decreased plasma oncotic pressure, and increased capillary permeability. It may be due to FVE that increases capillary hydrostatic pressures, pushing fluid into the interstitial tissues. This type of edema is often seen in

TABLE 36–4	Isotonic Fluid Volume Excess	
RISK FACTORS	**CLINICAL MANIFESTATIONS**	**NURSING INTERVENTIONS**
Excess intake of sodium-containing intravenous fluids Excess ingestion of sodium in diet or medications (e.g., sodium bicarbonate antacids such as Alka-Seltzer or hypertonic enema solutions such as Fleet) Impaired fluid balance regulation related to • Heart failure • Renal failure • Cirrhosis of the liver	Weight gain • 2% gain = mild FVE • 5% gain = moderate • 8% gain = severe Fluid intake greater than output Full, bounding pulse; tachycardia Increased blood pressure and central venous pressure Distended neck and peripheral veins; slow vein emptying Moist crackles (rales) in lungs; dyspnea, shortness of breath Mental confusion	Assess for clinical manifestations of FVE. Monitor weight and vital signs. Assess for edema. Assess breath sounds. Monitor fluid intake and output. Monitor laboratory findings. Place in Fowler's position. Administer diuretics as ordered. Restrict fluid intake as indicated. Restrict dietary sodium as ordered. Implement measures to prevent skin breakdown.

dependent tissues such as the feet, ankles, and sacrum because of the effects of gravity. Low levels of plasma proteins from malnutrition or liver or kidney diseases can reduce the plasma oncotic pressure so that fluid is not drawn into the capillaries from interstitial tissues, causing edema. With tissue trauma and some disorders such as allergic reactions, capillaries become more permeable, allowing fluid to escape into interstitial tissues. Obstructed lymph flow impairs the movement of fluid from interstitial tissues back into the vascular compartment, resulting in edema.

Pitting edema is edema that leaves a small depression or pit after finger pressure is applied to the swollen area. The pit is caused by movement of fluid to adjacent tissue, away from the point of pressure (Figure 36–6). Within 10 to 30 seconds the pit normally disappears.

DEHYDRATION Dehydration, or hyperosmolar imbalance, occurs when water is lost from the body leaving the client with excess sodium. Because water is lost while electrolytes, particularly sodium, are retained, the serum osmolality and serum sodium levels increase. Water is drawn into the vascular compartment from the interstitial space and cells, resulting in cellular dehydration. Older adults are at particular risk for dehydration because of decreased thirst sensation. This type of water deficit also can affect clients who are hyperventilating or have prolonged fever or are in diabetic ketoacidosis and those receiving enteral feedings with insufficient water intake.

OVERHYDRATION Overhydration, also known as hypoosmolar imbalance or water excess, occurs when water is

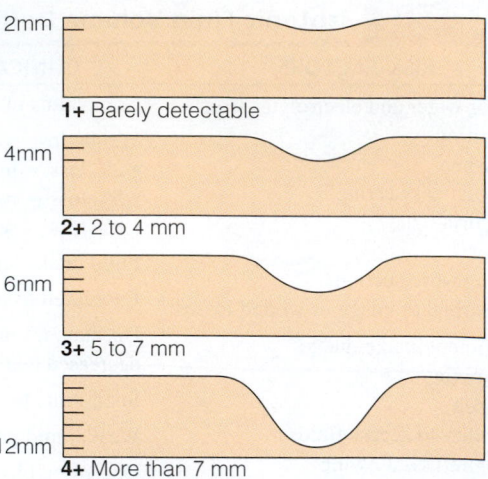

Figure 36–6 ⬤ Evaluation of edema. Four-point scale for grading edema.

gained in excess of electrolytes, resulting in low serum osmolality and low serum sodium levels. Water is drawn into the cells, causing them to swell. In the brain this can lead to cerebral edema and impaired neurologic function. Water intoxication often occurs when both fluid and electrolytes are lost, for example, through excessive sweating, but only water is replaced. It can also result from the syndrome of inappropriate antidiuretic hormone (SIADH), a disorder that can occur with some malignant tumors, AIDS, head injury, or administration of certain drugs such as barbiturates or anesthetics.

DRUG CAPSULE	**Diuretic Agent** *furosemide* (Lasix)

The Client with Fluid Volume Excess

Furosemide inhibits sodium and chloride reabsorption in the loop of Henle and the distal renal tubule. This results in significant diuresis, with renal excretion of water, sodium chloride, magnesium, hydrogen, and calcium.

Furosemide is commonly used for the clinical management of edema secondary to heart failure, treatment of hypertension, and treatment of hepatic or renal disease. Therapeutic effects include diuresis and lowering of blood pressure.

Nursing Responsibilities

- Assess the client's fluid status regularly. Assessment should include daily weights, close monitoring of intake and output, skin turgor, edema, lung sounds, and mucous membranes.
- Monitor the client's potassium levels. Furosemide is a loop diuretic which excretes potassium and may result in hypokalemia.
- Administer in the morning to avoid increased urination during hours of sleep.
- If the client is also taking digitalis glycosides, he or she should be assessed for anorexia, nausea, vomiting, muscle cramps,

paresthesia, and confusion. The potassium-depleting effect of furosemide places the client at increased risk for digitalis toxicity.

Client and Family Teaching

- Medication should be taken exactly as directed. If you miss a dose, take it as soon as possible; however, if a day has been missed, do not double the dose the next day.
- Weigh on a daily basis and report weight gain or loss of more than 3 lb in 1 day to your primary care provider.
- Contact your primary care provider immediately if you begin to experience muscle weakness, cramps, nausea, dizziness, numbness, or tingling of the extremities.
- Some form of potassium supplementation will be needed. The primary care provider may order oral potassium supplements for you; if not, you will need to consume a diet high in potassium.
- Make position changes slowly in order to minimize dizziness from orthostatic hypotension.

Note: Prior to administering any medication, review all aspects with a current drug handbook or other reliable source.

RESEARCH NOTES

How Prevalent Is Chronic Dehydration in Older Adults?

Previous research has documented that dehydration is a problem in hospitalized older adults, and low fluid intake has been documented to be a problem in nursing home residents. The authors questioned whether chronic dehydration is also a problem in older adults living in the community. The researchers conducted a descriptive, retrospective study of 185 older adults ranging from 75 to 100 years old. This group of older adults visited a hospital emergency department during a 1-month period of time. Dehydration was defined as a ratio of blood urea nitrogen to creatine (BUN:Cr) greater than 20:1. Forty-eight percent of the group were dehydrated on admission to the emergency department. The older adults from a residential facility were most likely to be dehydrated (65%); however, 44% of the older adults living in the community were dehydrated.

Implications

The results demonstrated that dehydration is a problem with both older adults living in the community as well as older adults living in residential facilities. Prevention of dehydration is an important intervention for nurses working with older adults. Nursing interventions need to include talking with older adults and their families about the dangers of dehydration and suggesting strategies to prevent dehydration.

Note: From "Unrecognized Chronic Dehydration in Older Adults. Examining Prevalence Rate and Risk Factors," by J. A. Bennett, V. Thomas, and B. Riegel, 2004, *Journal of Gerontological Nursing, 30*(1), pp. 22–28. Copyright © 2004 SLACK, Inc. Reprinted with permission.

Electrolyte Imbalances

The most common and most significant electrolyte imbalances involve sodium, potassium, calcium, magnesium, chloride, and phosphate.

SODIUM Sodium (Na^+), the most abundant cation in the extracellular fluid, not only moves into and out of the body but also moves in careful balance among the three fluid compartments. It is found in most body secretions, for example, saliva, gastric and intestinal secretions, bile, and pancreatic fluid. Continuous excretion of any of these fluids, such as seen with intestinal suction, can result in a sodium deficit. Because of its role in regulating water balance, sodium imbalances usually are accompanied by water imbalance.

Hyponatremia is a sodium deficit, or serum sodium level of less than 135 mEq/L, and is, in acute care settings, a common electrolyte imbalance. Because of sodium's role in determining the osmolality of ECF, hyponatremia typically results in a low serum osmolality. Water is drawn out of the vascular compartment into interstitial tissues and the cells, causing the clinical manifestations associated with this disorder. As sodium levels decrease, the brain and nervous system are affected by cellular edema. Severe hyponatremia, serum levels below 110 mEq/L, is a medical emergency and can lead to permanent neurological damage (Astle, 2005).

Hypernatremia is excess sodium in ECF, or a serum sodium of greater than 145 mEq/L. Because the osmotic pressure of extracellular fluid is increased, fluid moves out of the cells into the ECF. As a result, the cells become dehydrated. Like hyponatremia, the primary manifestations of hypernatremia are neurological in nature. The thirst mechanism helps to protect against hypernatremia. Clients at risk for hypernatremia are those who are unable to access water. Table 36–5 lists risk factors and clinical signs for hyponatremia and hypernatremia.

POTASSIUM Although the amount of potassium (K^+) in extracellular fluid is small, it is vital to normal neuromuscular and cardiac function. Normal renal function is important for maintenance of potassium balance as 80% of potassium is excreted by the kidneys. Potassium must be replaced daily to maintain its balance. Normally, potassium is replaced in food.

Hypokalemia is a potassium deficit or a serum potassium level of less than 3.5 mEq/L. Gastrointestinal losses of potassium through vomiting and gastric suction are common causes of hypokalemia, as are the use of potassium-wasting diuretics, such as thiazide diuretics or loop diuretics (e.g., furosemide). Symptoms of hypokalemia are usually mild until the level drops below 3 mEq/L unless the decrease in potassium was rapid. When the decrease is gradual, the body compensates by shifting potassium from the intracellular environment into the serum.

Hyperkalemia is a potassium excess or a serum potassium level greater than 5.0 mEq/L. Hyperkalemia is less common than hypokalemia and rarely occurs in clients with normal renal function. It is, however, more dangerous than hypokalemia and can lead to cardiac arrest. As with hypokalemia, symptoms are more severe and occur at lower levels when the increase in potassium is abrupt. Table 36–5 lists risk factors and clinical signs for hypokalemia and hyperkalemia.

CLINICAL ALERT

Potassium may be given intravenously for severe hypokalemia. It must ALWAYS be diluted appropriately and must NEVER be given IV push. Potassium that is to be given IV should be mixed in the pharmacy and double-checked prior to administration by two nurses. The usual concentration of IV potassium is 20 to 40 mEq/L.

CALCIUM Regulating levels of calcium (Ca^{2+}) in the body is more complex than the other major electrolytes so calcium balance can be affected by many factors. Imbalances of this electrolyte are relatively common.

TABLE 36–5   **Electrolyte Imbalances**

RISK FACTORS	CLINICAL MANIFESTATIONS	NURSING INTERVENTIONS
Hyponatremia		
Loss of sodium • Gastrointestinal fluid loss • Sweating • Use of diuretics *Gain of water* • Hypotonic tube feedings • Excessive drinking of water • Excess IV D5W (dextrose in water) administration *Syndrome of inappropriate ADH (SIADH)* • Head injury • AIDS • Malignant tumors	Lethargy, confusion, apprehension Muscle twitching Abdominal cramps Anorexia, nausea, vomiting Headache Seizures, coma *Laboratory findings:* Serum sodium below 135 mEq/L Serum osmolality below 280 mOsm/kg	Assess clinical manifestations. Monitor fluid intake and output. Monitor laboratory data (e.g., serum sodium). Assess client closely if administering hypertonic saline solutions. Encourage food and fluid high in sodium if permitted (e.g., table salt, bacon, ham, processed cheese). Limit water intake as indicated.
Hypernatremia		
Loss of water • Insensible water loss (hyperventilation or fever) • Diarrhea • Water deprivation *Gain of sodium* • Parenteral administration of saline solutions • Hypertonic tube feedings without adequate water • Excessive use of table salt (1 tsp contains 2,300 mg of sodium) Conditions such as • Diabetes insipidus • Heat stroke	Thirst Dry, sticky mucous membranes Tongue red, dry, swollen Weakness Severe hypernatremia: • Fatigue, restlessness • Decreasing level of consciousness • Disorientation • Convulsions *Laboratory findings:* Serum sodium above 145 mEq/L Serum osmolality above 300 mOsm/kg	Monitor fluid intake and output. Monitor behavior changes (e.g., restlessness, disorientation). Monitor laboratory findings (e.g., serum sodium). Encourage fluids as ordered. Monitor diet as ordered (e.g., restrict intake of salt and foods high in sodium).
Hypokalemia		
Loss of potassium • Vomiting and gastric suction • Diarrhea • Heavy perspiration • Use of potassium-wasting drugs (e.g., diuretics) • Poor intake of potassium (as with debilitated clients, alcoholics, anorexia nervosa) • Hyperaldosteronism	Muscle weakness, leg cramps Fatigue, lethargy Anorexia, nausea, vomiting Decreased bowel sounds, decreased bowel motility Cardiac dysrhythmias Depressed deep-tendon reflexes Weak, irregular pulses *Laboratory findings:* Serum potassium below 3.5 mEq/L Arterial blood gases (ABGs) may show alkalosis T wave flattening and ST segment depression on ECG	Monitor heart rate and rhythm. Monitor clients receiving digitalis (e.g., digoxin) closely, because hypokalemia increases risk of digitalis toxicity. Administer oral potassium as ordered with food or fluid to prevent gastric irritation. Administer IV potassium solutions at a rate no faster than 10–20 mEq/h; never administer undiluted potassium intravenously. For clients receiving IV potassium, monitor for pain and inflammation at the injection site. Teach client about potassium-rich foods. Teach clients how to prevent excessive loss of potassium (e.g., through abuse of diuretics and laxatives).

TABLE 36–5   **Electrolyte Imbalances—*continued***

RISK FACTORS	CLINICAL MANIFESTATIONS	NURSING INTERVENTIONS
Hyperkalemia *Decreased potassium excretion* • Renal failure • Hypoaldosteronism • Potassium-conserving diuretics *High potassium intake* • Excessive use of K$^+$ containing salt substitutes • Excessive or rapid IV infusion of potassium • Potassium shift out of the tissue cells into the plasma (e.g., infections, burns, acidosis)	Gastrointestinal hyperactivity, diarrhea Irritability, apathy, confusion Cardiac dysrhythmias or arrest Muscle weakness, areflexia (absence of reflexes) Decreased heart rate Irregular pulse Paresthesias and numbness in extremities *Laboratory findings:* Serum potassium above 5.0 mEq/L Peaked T wave, widened QRS on ECG	Closely monitor cardiac status and ECG. Administer diuretics and other medications such as glucose and insulin as ordered. Hold potassium supplements and K$^+$ conserving diuretics. Monitor serum K$^+$ levels carefully; a rapid drop may occur as potassium shifts into the cells. Teach clients to avoid foods high in potassium and salt substitutes.
Hypocalcemia *Surgical removal of the parathyroid glands* Conditions such as • Hypoparathyroidism • Acute pancreatitis • Hyperphosphatemia • Thyroid carcinoma *Inadequate vitamin D intake* • Malabsorption • Hypomagnesemia • Alkalosis • Sepsis • Alcohol abuse	Numbness, tingling of the extremities and around the mouth Muscle tremors, cramps; if severe can progress to tetany and convulsions Cardiac dysrhythmias; decreased cardiac output Positive Trousseau's and Chvostek's signs Confusion, anxiety, possible psychoses Hyperactive deep tendon reflexes *Laboratory findings:* Serum calcium less than 8.5 mg/dL or 4.5 mEq/L (total) Lengthened QT intervals Prolonged ST segments	Closely monitor respiratory and cardiovascular status. Take precautions to protect a confused client. Administer oral or parenteral calcium supplements as ordered. When administering intravenously, closely monitor cardiac status and ECG during infusion. Teach clients at high risk for osteoporosis about • Dietary sources rich in calcium. • Recommendation for 1,000–1,500 mg of calcium per day. • Calcium supplements. • Regular exercise. • Estrogen replacement therapy for postmenopausal women.
Hypercalcemia • Prolonged immobilization Conditions such as • Hyperparathyroidism • Malignancy of the bone • Paget's disease	Lethargy, weakness Depressed deep-tendon reflexes Bone pain Anorexia, nausea, vomiting Constipation Polyuria, hypercalciuria Flank pain secondary to urinary calculi Dysrhythmias, possible heart block *Laboratory findings:* Serum calcium greater than 10.5 mg/dL or 5.5 mEq/L (total) Shortened QT intervals Shortened ST segments	Increase client movement and exercise. Encourage oral fluids as permitted to maintain a dilute urine. Teach clients to limit intake of food and fluid high in calcium. Encourage ingestion of fiber to prevent constipation. Protect a confused client; monitor for pathologic fractures in clients with long-term hypercalcemia. Encourage intake of acid–ash fluids (e.g., prune or cranberry juice) to counteract deposits of calcium salts in the urine.

(continued)

TABLE 36–5   Electrolyte Imbalances—*continued*

RISK FACTORS	CLINICAL MANIFESTATIONS	NURSING INTERVENTIONS
Hypomagnesemia		
• Excessive loss from the gastrointestinal tract (e.g., from nasogastric suction, diarrhea, fistula drainage) • Long-term use of certain drugs (e.g., diuretics, aminoglycoside antibiotics)	Neuromuscular irritability with tremors Increased reflexes, tremors, convulsions Positive Chvostek's and Trousseau's signs	Assess clients receiving digitalis for digitalis toxicity. Hypomagnesemia increases the risk of toxicity.
Conditions such as • Chronic alcoholism • Pancreatitis • Burns	Tachycardia, elevated blood pressure, dysrhythmias Disorientation and confusion Vertigo Anorexia, dysphagia Respiratory difficulties *Laboratory findings:* Serum magnesium below 1.5 mEq/L Prolonged PR intervals, widened QRS complexes, prolonged QT intervals, depressed ST segments, broad flattened T waves, prominent U waves	Take protective measures when there is a possibility of seizures. • Assess the client's ability to swallow water prior to initiating oral feeding. • Initiate safety measures to prevent injury during seizure activity. • Carefully administer magnesium salts as ordered. Encourage clients to eat magnesium-rich foods if permitted (e.g., whole grains, meat, seafood, and green leafy vegetables). Refer clients to alcohol treatment programs as indicated.
Hypermagnesemia		
Abnormal retention of magnesium, as in • Renal failure • Adrenal insufficiency • Treatment with magnesium salts	Peripheral vasodilation, flushing Nausea, vomiting Muscle weakness, paralysis Hypotension, bradycardia Depressed deep-tendon reflexes Lethargy, drowsiness Respiratory depression, coma Respiratory and cardiac arrest if hypermagnesemia is severe *Laboratory findings:* Serum magnesium above 2.5 mEq/L Electrocardiogram showing prolonged QT interval, prolonged PR interval, widened QRS complexes, tall T waves	Monitor vital signs and level of consciousness when clients are at risk. If patellar reflexes are absent, notify the primary care provider. Advise clients who have renal disease to contact their primary care provider before taking over-the-counter drugs.

Hypocalcemia is a calcium deficit, or a total serum calcium level of less than 8.5 mg/dL or an ionized calcium level of less than 4.0 mg/dL. Severe depletion of calcium can cause tetany with muscle spasms and paresthesias (numbness and tingling around the mouth and hands and feet) and can lead to convulsions. Two signs indicate hypocalcemia: The Chvostek's sign is contraction of the facial muscles that is produced by tapping the facial nerve in front of the ear (Figure 36–7, *A*). Trousseau's sign is a carpal spasm that occurs by inflating a blood pressure cuff on the upper arm to 20 mm Hg greater than the systolic pressure for 2 to 5 minutes (Figure 36–7, *B*). Clients at greatest risk for hypocalcemia are those whose parathyroid glands have been removed. This is frequently associated with total thy-roidectomy or bilateral neck surgery for cancer. Low serum magnesium levels (hypomagnesemia) and chronic alcoholism also increase the risk of hypocalcemia.

Hypercalcemia, or total serum calcium levels greater than 10.5 mg/dL or an ionized calcium level of greater than 5.0 mg/dL, most often occurs when calcium is mobilized from the bony skeleton. This may be due to malignancy or prolonged immobilization.

The risk factors and clinical manifestations related to calcium imbalances are found in Table 36–5.

MAGNESIUM Magnesium (Mg^{2+}) imbalances are relatively common in hospitalized clients, although they may be unrecognized. **Hypomagnesemia** is a magnesium deficiency, or a

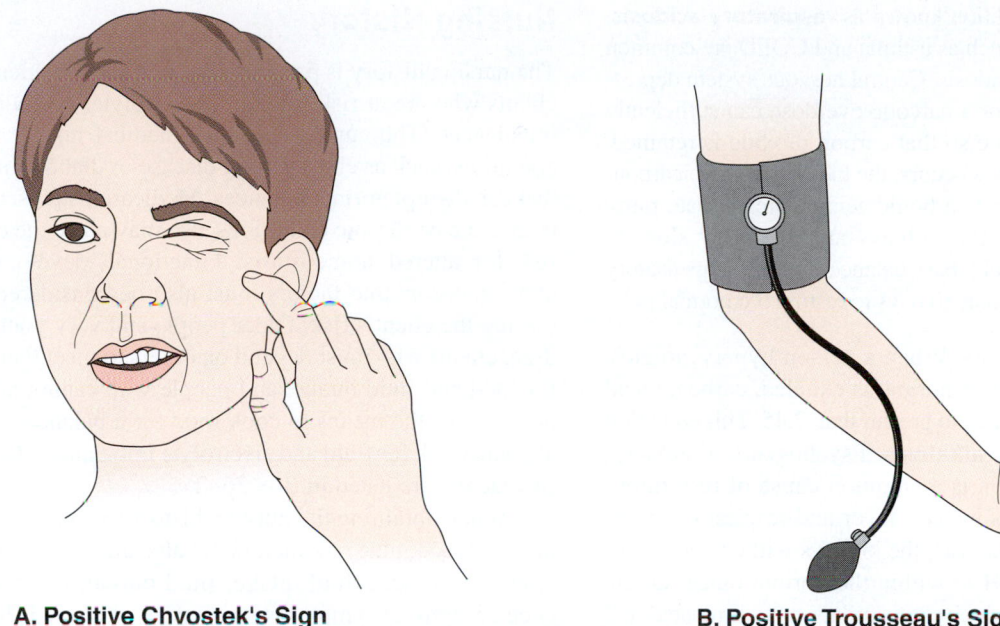

A. Positive Chvostek's Sign

B. Positive Trousseau's Sign

Figure 36–7 ● *A,* Positive Chvostek's sign. *B,* Positive Trousseau's sign.

From Lemone, Priscilla, & Burke, Karen M., *Medical Surgical Nursing: Critical Thinking in Client Care,* 4th ed © 2008. Reproduced with permission of Pearson Education, Inc., Upper Saddle River, New Jersey.

total serum magnesium level of less than 1.5 mEq/L. It occurs more frequently than hypermagnesemia. Chronic alcoholism is the most common cause of hypomagnesemia. Magnesium deficiency also may aggravate the manifestations of alcohol withdrawal, such as delirium tremens (DTs). **Hypermagnesemia** is present when the serum magnesium level rises above 2.5 mEq/L. It is due to increased intake or decreased excretion. It is often iatrogenic, that is, a result of overzealous magnesium therapy. Table 36–5 lists risk factors and manifestations for clients with altered magnesium balance.

CHLORIDE Because of the relationship between sodium ions and chloride ions (Cl^-), imbalances of chloride commonly occur in conjunction with sodium imbalances. **Hypochloremia** is a decreased serum chloride level, in adults a level below 95 mEq/L, and is usually related to excess losses of chloride ion through the GI tract, kidneys, or sweating. Hypochloremic clients are at risk for alkalosis and may experience muscle twitching, tremors, or tetany.

Conditions that cause sodium retention also can lead to a high serum chloride level or **hyperchloremia**, in adults a level above 108 mEq/L. Excess replacement of sodium chloride or potassium chloride are additional risk factors for high serum chloride levels. The manifestations of hyperchloremia include acidosis, weakness, and lethargy, with a risk of dysrhythmias and coma.

PHOSPHATE The phosphate anion PO_4^- is found in both intracellular and extracellular fluid. Most of the phosphorus (P^+) in the body exists as PO_4^-. Phosphate is critical for cellular metabolism because it is a major component of adenosine triphosphate (ATP).

Phosphate imbalances are frequently related to therapeutic interventions for other disorders. Glucose and insulin administration and total parenteral nutrition can cause phosphate to shift into the cells from extracellular fluid compartments, leading to **hypophosphatemia**, defined in adults as a total serum phosphate level less than 2.5 mg/dL. Alcohol withdrawal, acid–base imbalances, and the use of antacids that bind with phosphate in the GI tract are other possible causes of low serum phosphate levels. Manifestations of hypophosphatemia include paresthesias, muscle weakness and pain, mental changes, and possible seizures.

Hyperphosphatemia, defined in adults as a total serum phosphate level greater than 4.5 mg/dL, occurs when phosphate shifts out of the cells into extracellular fluids (e.g., due to tissue trauma or chemotherapy for malignant tumors), in renal failure, or when excess phosphate is administered or ingested. Infants who are fed cow's milk are at risk for hyperphosphatemia, as are people using phosphate-containing enemas or laxatives. Clients who have high serum phosphate levels may experience numbness and tingling around the mouth and in the fingertips, muscle spasms, and tetany.

Acid–Base Imbalances

Acid–base imbalances generally are classified as *respiratory* or *metabolic* by the general or underlying cause of the disorder. Carbonic acid levels are normally regulated by the lungs through the retention or excretion of carbon dioxide, and problems of regulation lead to respiratory acidosis or alkalosis. Bicarbonate and hydrogen ion levels are regulated by the kidneys, and problems of regulation lead to metabolic acidosis or alkalosis. Healthy regulatory systems will attempt to correct acid–base imbalances, a process called **compensation**.

RESPIRATORY ACIDOSIS Hypoventilation and carbon dioxide retention cause carbonic acid levels to increase and the pH to fall below 7.35, a condition known as **respiratory acidosis**. Serious lung diseases such as asthma and COPD are common causes of respiratory acidosis. Central nervous system depression due to anesthesia or a narcotic overdose can sufficiently slow the respiratory rate so that carbon dioxide is retained. When respiratory acidosis occurs, the kidneys retain bicarbonate to restore the normal carbonic acid to bicarbonate ratio. Recall, however, that the kidneys are relatively slow to respond to changes in acid–base balance, so this compensatory response may require hours to days to restore the normal pH.

RESPIRATORY ALKALOSIS When a person hyperventilates, more carbon dioxide than normal is exhaled, carbonic acid levels fall, and the pH rises to greater than 7.45. This condition is termed **respiratory alkalosis**. Psychogenic or anxiety-related hyperventilation is a common cause of respiratory alkalosis. Other causes include fever and respiratory infections. In respiratory alkalosis, the kidneys will excrete bicarbonate to return the pH to within the normal range. Often, however, the cause of the hyperventilation is eliminated and the pH returns to normal before renal compensation occurs.

METABOLIC ACIDOSIS When bicarbonate levels are low in relation to the amount of carbonic acid in the body, the pH falls and **metabolic acidosis** develops. This may develop because of renal failure and the inability of the kidneys to excrete hydrogen ion and produce bicarbonate. It also may occur when too much acid is produced in the body, for example, in diabetic ketoacidosis or starvation when fat tissue is broken down for energy. Metabolic acidosis stimulates the respiratory center, and the rate and depth of respirations increase. Carbon dioxide is eliminated and carbonic acid levels fall, minimizing the change in pH. This respiratory compensation occurs within minutes of the pH imbalance.

METABOLIC ALKALOSIS In **metabolic alkalosis**, the amount of bicarbonate in the body exceeds the normal 20-to-1 ratio. Ingestion of bicarbonate of soda as an antacid is one cause of metabolic alkalosis. Another cause is prolonged vomiting with loss of hydrochloric acid from the stomach. The respiratory center is depressed in metabolic alkalosis, and respirations slow and become more shallow. Carbon dioxide is retained and carbonic acid levels increase, helping balance the excess bicarbonate.

The risk factors and manifestations for acid–base imbalances are listed in Table 36–6.

NURSING MANAGEMENT

ASSESSING

Assessing clients for fluid, electrolyte, and acid–base balance and imbalances is an important nursing care function. Components of the assessment include (a) the nursing history, (b) physical assessment of the client, (c) clinical measurements, and (d) review of laboratory test results.

Nursing History

The nursing history is particularly important for identifying clients who are at risk for fluid, electrolyte, and acid–base imbalances. The current and past medical history reveals conditions such as chronic lung disease or diabetes mellitus that can disrupt normal balances. Medications prescribed to treat acute or chronic conditions also may place the client at risk for altered homeostasis. Functional, developmental, and socioeconomic factors must also be considered in assessing the client's risk. Older people and very young children, clients who must depend on others to meet their needs for food and fluid intake, and people who cannot afford or do not have the means to cook food for a balanced diet are at greater risk for fluid and electrolyte imbalances. Common risk factors are listed in Box 36–2.

When obtaining the nursing history, the nurse needs to not only recognize risk factors but also elicit data about the client's food and fluid intake, fluid output, and the presence of signs or symptoms suggestive of altered fluid and

---

BOX 36–2 Common Risk Factors for Fluid, Electrolyte, and Acid–Base Imbalances

Chronic Diseases and Conditions
- Chronic lung disease (COPD, asthma, cystic fibrosis)
- Heart failure
- Kidney disease
- Diabetes mellitus
- Cushing's syndrome or Addison's disease
- Cancer
- Malnutrition, anorexia nervosa, bulimia
- Ileostomy

Acute Conditions
- Acute gastroenteritis
- Bowel obstruction
- Head injury or decreased level of consciousness
- Trauma such as burns or crushing injuries
- Surgery
- Fever, draining wounds, fistulas

Medications
- Diuretics
- Corticosteroids
- Nonsteroidal anti-inflammatory drugs

Treatments
- Chemotherapy
- IV therapy and total parenteral nutrition
- Nasogastric suction
- Enteral feedings
- Mechanical ventilation

Other Factors
- Age: Very old or very young
- Inability to access food and fluids independently

TABLE 36–6 Acid–Base Imbalances

RISK FACTORS	CLINICAL MANIFESTATIONS	NURSING INTERVENTIONS
Respiratory Acidosis		
Acute lung conditions that impair alveolar gas exchange (e.g., pneumonia, acute pulmonary edema, aspiration of foreign body, near-drowning)	Increased pulse and respiratory rates	Frequently assess respiratory status and lung sounds.
	Headache, dizziness	Monitor airway and ventilation; insert artificial airway and prepare for mechanical ventilation as necessary.
	Confusion, decreased level of consciousness (LOC)	
Chronic lung disease (e.g., asthma, cystic fibrosis, or emphysema)	Convulsions	Administer pulmonary therapy measures such as inhalation therapy, percussion and postural drainage, bronchodilators, and antibiotics as ordered.
Overdose of narcotics or sedatives that depress respiratory rate and depth	Warm, flushed skin	
	Chronic:	
Brain injury that affects the respiratory center	Weakness	
	Headache	Monitor fluid intake and output, vital signs, and arterial blood gases.
Airway obstruction	*Laboratory findings:*	Administer narcotic antagonists as indicated.
Mechanical chest injury	Arterial blood pH less than 7.35	Maintain adequate hydration (2–3 L of fluid per day).
	$PaCO_2$ above 45 mm Hg	
	HCO_3^- normal or slightly elevated in acute; above 26 mEq/L in chronic	
Respiratory Alkalosis		
Hyperventilation due to	Complaints of shortness of breath, chest tightness	Monitor vital signs and ABGs.
• Extreme anxiety		Assist client to breathe more slowly.
• Elevated body temperature	Light-headedness with circumoral paresthesias and numbness and tingling of the extremities	Help client breathe in a paper bag or apply a rebreather mask (to inhale CO_2).
• Overventilation with a mechanical ventilator		
• Hypoxia	Difficulty concentrating	
• Salicylate overdose	Tremulousness, blurred vision	
Brain stem injury	*Laboratory findings (in uncompensated respiratory alkalosis):*	
Fever	Arterial blood pH above 7.45	
Increased basal metabolic rate	$PaCO_2$ less than 35 mm Hg	
Metabolic Acidosis		
Conditions that increase nonvolatile acids in the blood (e.g., renal impairment, diabetes mellitus, starvation)	Kussmaul's respirations (deep, rapid respirations)	Monitor ABG values, intake and output, and LOC.
	Lethargy, confusion	Administer IV sodium bicarbonate carefully if ordered.
Conditions that decrease bicarbonate (e.g., prolonged diarrhea)	Headache	Treat underlying problem as ordered.
	Weakness	
Excessive infusion of chloride-containing IV fluids (e.g., NaCl)	Nausea and vomiting	
	Laboratory findings:	
Excessive ingestion of acids such as salicylates	Arterial blood pH below 7.35	
	Serum bicarbonate less than 22 mEq/L	
Cardiac arrest	$PaCO_2$ less than 38 mm Hg with respiratory compensation	
Metabolic Alkalosis		
Excessive acid losses due to	Decreased respiratory rate and depth	Monitor intake and output closely.
• Vomiting	Dizziness	Monitor vital signs, especially respirations, and LOC.
• Gastric suction	Circumoral paresthesias, numbness and tingling of the extremities	
Excessive use of potassium-losing diuretics		Administer ordered IV fluids carefully.
	Hypertonic muscles, tetany	Treat underlying problem.
Excessive adrenal corticoid hormones due to	*Laboratory findings:*	
• Cushing's syndrome	Arterial blood pH above 7.45	
• Hyperaldosteronism	Serum bicarbonate greater than 26 mEq/L	
Excessive bicarbonate intake from	$PaCO_2$ higher than 45 mm Hg with respiratory compensation	
• Antacids		
• Parenteral $NaHCO_3$		

Current and Past Medical History

- Are you currently seeing a health care provider for treatment of any chronic diseases such as kidney disease, heart disease, high blood pressure, diabetes insipidus, or thyroid or parathyroid disorders?
- Have you recently experienced any acute conditions such as gastroenteritis, severe trauma, head injury, or surgery? If so, describe them.

Medications and Treatments

- Are you currently taking any medications on a regular basis such as diuretics, steroids, potassium supplements, calcium supplements, hormones, salt substitutes, or antacids?
- Have you recently undergone any treatments such as dialysis, parenteral nutrition, or tube feedings or been on a ventilator? If so, when and why?

Food and Fluid Intake

- How much and what type of fluids do you drink each day?
- Describe your diet for a typical day. (Pay particular attention to the client's intake of foods high in sodium content, of protein, and of whole grains, fruits, and vegetables.)
- Have there been any recent changes in your food or fluid intake, for example, as a result of following a weight-loss program?
- Are you on any type of restricted diet?

- Has your food or fluid intake recently been affected by changes in appetite, nausea, or other factors such as pain or difficulty breathing?

Fluid Output

- Have you noticed any recent changes in the frequency or amount of urine output?
- Have you recently experienced any problems with vomiting, diarrhea, or constipation? If so, when and for how long?
- Have you noticed any other unusual fluid losses such as excessive sweating?

Fluid, Electrolyte, and Acid–Base Imbalances

- Have you gained or lost weight in recent weeks?
- Have you recently experienced any symptoms such as excessive thirst, dry skin or mucous membranes, dark or concentrated urine, or low urine output?
- Do you have problems with swelling of your hands, feet, or ankles? Do you ever have difficulty breathing, especially when lying down or at night? How many pillows do you use to sleep?
- Have you recently experienced any of the following symptoms: difficulty concentrating or confusion; dizziness or feeling faint; muscle weakness, twitching, cramping, or spasm; excessive fatigue; abnormal sensations such as numbness, tingling, burning, or prickling; abdominal cramping or distention; heart palpitations?

electrolyte balance. The Assessment Interview provides examples of questions to elicit information regarding fluid, electrolyte, and acid–base balance.

Physical Assessment

Physical assessment to evaluate a client's fluid, electrolyte, and acid–base status focuses on the skin, the oral cavity and mucous membranes, the eyes, the cardiovascular and respiratory systems, and neurologic and muscular status. Data from this physical assessment are used to expand and verify information obtained in the nursing history. Refer to Tables 36–4 through 36–6 for possible abnormal findings related to specific imbalances.

Clinical Measurements

Three simple clinical measurements that the nurse can initiate without a primary care provider's order are daily weights, vital signs, and fluid intake and output.

DAILY WEIGHTS   Daily weight measurements provide a relatively accurate assessment of a client's fluid status. Significant changes in weight over a short time are indicative of acute fluid changes. Each kilogram of weight gained or lost is equivalent to 1 L of fluid gained or lost. Such fluid

gains or losses indicate changes in total body fluid volume rather than in any specific compartment, such as the intravascular compartment. Rapid losses or gains of 5% to 8% of total body weight indicate moderate to severe fluid volume deficits or excesses.

To obtain accurate weight measurements, the nurse should balance the scale before each use and weigh the client (a) at the same time each day, (b) wearing the same or similar clothing, and (c) on the same scale. The type of scale should be documented.

VITAL SIGNS   Changes in vital signs may indicate, or in some cases precede, fluid, electrolyte, and acid–base imbal-

LONG-TERM CARE CONSIDERATIONS
Fluid Imbalance

Regular assessment of weight is particularly important for clients who are at risk for fluid imbalance in long-term care facilities. For these clients, measuring intake and output may be impractical because of lifestyle or problems with incontinence. Regular weight measurement, either daily, every other day, or weekly, provides valuable information about the client's fluid volume status.

ances. Tachycardia is an early sign of hypovolemia. Pulse volume will decrease in FVD and increase in FVE. Irregular pulse rates may occur with electrolyte imbalances. Changes in respiratory rate and depth may cause respiratory acid–base imbalances or act as a compensatory mechanism in metabolic acidosis or alkalosis. Blood pressure may fall significantly with FVD and hypovolemia or increase with FVE. Postural, or orthostatic, hypotension may also occur with FVD and hypovolemia.

FLUID INTAKE AND OUTPUT The measurement and recording of all fluid intake and output (I & O) during a 24-hour period provides important data about the client's fluid and electrolyte balance. Generally, intake and output are measured for hospitalized at-risk clients. To measure fluid intake, nurses convert household measures such as a glass, cup, or soup bowl to metric units. Most agencies provide conversion tables, since the sizes of dishes vary from agency to agency. Such a table is often provided on or with the bedside I & O record. Most agencies have a form for recording I & O, usually a bedside record on which the nurse lists all items measured and the quantities per shift. Some agencies have another form for recording the specifics of intravenous fluids, such as the type of solution, additives, time started, amounts absorbed, and amounts remaining per shift. Fluids to record include oral fluids, ice chips, foods that tend to become liquid at room temperature, tube feedings, parenteral fluids, intravenous medications, catheter or tube irrigants, urinary output, vomitus, liquid feces, tube drainage, and wound drainage. Amount, type, and time of fluid is recorded on the I & O record and totaled at the end of every shift. These totals are recorded on the client's permanent record. I & O may be recorded hourly in intensive care areas. 24 hour totals are usually calculated on night shift.

It is important to inform clients, family members, and all caregivers that accurate measurements of the client's fluid intake and output are required, explaining why and emphasizing the need to use a bedpan, urinal, commode, or in-toilet collection device. Instruct the client not to put toilet tissue into the container with urine. Clients who wish to be involved in recording fluid intake measurements need to be taught how to compute the values and what foods are considered fluids.

To determine whether the fluid output is proportional to fluid intake or whether there are any changes in the client's fluid status, the nurse (a) compares the total 24-hour fluid output measurement with the total fluid intake measurement and (b) compares both to previous measurements. Urinary output is normally equivalent to the amount of fluids ingested; the usual range is 1,500 to 2,000 mL in 24 hours, or 40 to 80 mL per hour (0.5 mL/kg/hour). Clients whose output substantially exceeds intake are at risk for fluid volume deficit. By contrast, clients whose intake substantially exceeds output are at risk for fluid volume excess. In assessing the client's fluid balance, it is important to consider additional factors that may affect intake and output. The client who is extremely diaphoretic or who has rapid, deep respirations has fluid losses that cannot be measured but must be considered in

BOX 36–3	Normal Electrolyte Values for Adults*
Venous Blood	
Sodium	135–145 mEq/L
Potassium	3.5–5.0 mEq/L
Chloride	95–108 mEq/L
Calcium (total)	4.5–5.5 mEq/L or 8.5–10.5 mg/dL
(ionized)	56% of total calcium (2.5 mEq/L or 4.0–5.0 mg/dL)
Magnesium	1.5–2.5 mEq/L or 1.6–2.5 mg/dL
Phosphate (phosphorus)	1.8–2.6 mEq/L or 2.5–4.5 mg/dL
Serum osmolality	280–300 mOsm/kg water

*Normal laboratory values vary from agency to agency.

evaluating fluid status. When there is a significant discrepancy between intake and output or when fluid intake or output is inadequate, this information should be reported to the charge nurse or primary care provider.

Laboratory Tests

Many laboratory studies are conducted to determine the client's fluid, electrolyte, and acid–base status. Some of the more common tests are discussed here.

SERUM ELECTROLYTES Serum electrolyte levels are often routinely ordered for any client admitted to the hospital as a screening test for electrolyte and acid–base imbalances. Serum electrolytes also are routinely assessed for clients at risk in the community, for example, clients who are being treated with a diuretic for hypertension or heart failure. The most commonly ordered serum tests are for sodium, potassium, chloride, magnesium, and bicarbonate ions. Normal values of commonly measured electrolytes are shown in Box 36–3. Some primary care providers use a diagram format for keeping track of the client's electrolytes when documenting in their progress notes. See Figure 36–8.

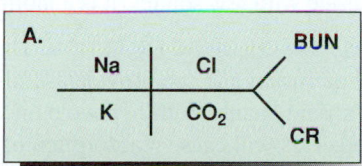

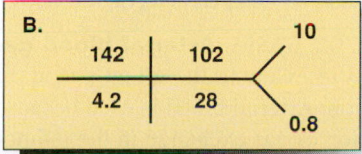

Figure 36–8 ○ **A**, Format for a diagram of serum electrolyte results. **B**, Example that may be seen in a primary care provider's documentation notes.

COMPLETE BLOOD COUNT (CBC) The complete blood count, another basic screening test, includes information about the hematocrit (Hct). The **hematocrit** measures the volume (percentage) of whole blood that is composed of RBCs. Because the hematocrit is a measure of the volume of cells in relation to plasma, it is affected by changes in plasma volume. Thus the hematocrit increases with severe dehydration and decreases with severe overhydration. Normal hematocrit values are 40% to 54% (men) and 37% to 47% (women).

OSMOLALITY *Serum osmolality* is a measure of the solute concentration of the blood. The particles included are sodium ions, glucose, and urea (blood urea nitrogen, or BUN). Serum osmolality can be estimated by doubling the serum sodium, because sodium and its associated chloride ions are the major determinants of serum osmolality. Serum osmolality values are used primarily to evaluate fluid balance. Normal values are 280 to 300 mOsm/kg. An increase in serum osmolality indicates a fluid volume deficit; a decrease reflects a fluid volume excess.

Urine osmolality is a measure of the solute concentration of urine. The particles included are nitrogenous wastes, such as creatinine, urea, and uric acid. Normal values are 500 to 800 mOsm/kg. An increased urine osmolality indicates a fluid volume deficit; a decreased urine osmolality reflects a fluid volume excess.

URINE PH Measurement of urine pH may be obtained by laboratory analysis or by using a dipstick on a freshly voided specimen. Because the kidneys play a critical role in regulating acid–base balance, assessment of urine pH can be useful in determining whether the kidneys are responding appropriately to acid–base imbalances. Normally the pH of the urine is relatively acidic, averaging about 6.0, but a range of 4.6 to 8.0 is considered normal. In metabolic acidosis, urine pH should decrease as the kidneys excrete hydrogen ions; in metabolic alkalosis, the pH should increase.

URINE SPECIFIC GRAVITY **Specific gravity** is an indicator of urine concentration that can be performed quickly and easily by nursing personnel. Normal specific gravity ranges from 1.005 to 1.030 (usually 1.010 to 1.025). When the concentration of solutes in the urine is high, the specific gravity rises; in very dilute urine with few solutes, it is abnormally low.

URINE SODIUM AND CHLORIDE EXCRETION These are indicators of renal perfusion and can provide useful information about a client's fluid status. With hypovolemia, aldosterone will be secreted. This will cause reabsorption of sodium and chloride which will result in decreased levels of sodium and chloride, less than 20 mEq/L each (Elgart, 2004).

ARTERIAL BLOOD GASES **Arterial blood gases (ABGs)** are performed to evaluate the client's acid–base balance and oxygenation. Arterial blood is used because it provides a truer reflection of gas exchange in the pulmonary system than venous blood. Blood gases may be drawn by laboratory technicians, respiratory therapy personnel, or nurses with specialized skills. Because a high-pressure artery is used to obtain blood, it is important to apply pressure to the puncture site for 5 minutes after the procedure to reduce the risk of bleeding or bruising.

Six measurements are commonly used to interpret arterial blood gas tests (Simpson, 2004):

- *pH:* a measure of the relative acidity or alkalinity of the blood. The greater the number of hydrogen ions, the more acidic the solution is. The normal range for pH is narrow, and death may ensue with pH values below 6.8 or above 7.8.
- *PaO_2:* the pressure exerted by oxygen dissolved in the plasma of arterial blood; an indirect measure of blood oxygen content. This measure, representing one of the two forms in which oxygen is transported in the blood, accounts for only about 3% of oxygen content in the blood.
- *$PaCO_2$:* the partial pressure of carbon dioxide in arterial plasma; the respiratory component of acid–base determination. Carbon dioxide is regulated by the lungs, and the $PaCO_2$ is used to determine if an acid–base imbalance is respiratory in origin.
- *Bicarbonate HCO_3^-:* a measure of the metabolic component of acid–base balance.
- *Base excess (BE):* a calculated value of bicarbonate levels, also reflective of the metabolic component of acid–base balance. If the number is preceded by a plus sign, it is a base excess and indicates alkalosis; if preceded by a minus sign, it is a base deficit and indicates acidosis.
- *Oxygen saturation (S_aO_2):* the percentage of hemoglobin saturated (combined) with oxygen. This represents the other form in which oxygen is transported in the blood and accounts for about 97% of the oxygen in the blood.

Normal ABG values are listed in Box 36–4. Changes seen in common acid–base imbalances are summarized in Table 36–7. Note that although the PaO_2 and S_aO_2 are important for assessing respiratory status, they generally do not provide useful information for assessing acid–base balance and so are not included in this table.

When evaluating ABG results to determine acid–base balance, it is important to use a systematic approach such as the one outlined in Box 36–5. Nurses need to assess each

BOX 36–4	**Normal Values of Arterial Blood Gases***
pH	7.35–7.45
PaO_2	80–100 mm Hg
$PaCO_2$	35–45 mm Hg
HCO_3^-	22–26 mEq/L
Base excess	–2 to +2 mEq/L
O_2 saturation	95–98%

*Some normal values will vary according to the kind of test carried out in the laboratory. Nurses are advised to use the normal values issued by the agency when interpreting laboratory results.

TABLE 36–7 **Arterial Blood Gas Values in Common Acid–Base Disorders**

DISORDER		ABG VALUES
Respiratory acidosis	pH	< 7.35
	$PaCO_2$	> 45 mm Hg (excess CO_2 and carbonic acid)
	HCO_3^-	Normal; or > 26 mEq/L with renal compensation
Respiratory alkalosis	pH	> 7.45
	$PaCO_2$	< 35 mm Hg (inadequate CO_2 and carbonic acid)
	HCO_3^-	Normal; or < 22 mEq/L with renal compensation
Metabolic acidosis	pH	< 7.35
	$PaCO_2$	Normal; or < 35 mm Hg with respiratory compensation
Metabolic alkalosis	HCO_3^-	< 22 mEq/L (inadequate bicarbonate)
	pH	> 7.45
	$PaCO_2$	Normal; or > 45 mm Hg with respiratory compensation
	HCO_3^-	> 26 mEq/L (excess bicarbonate)

BOX 36–5 **Interpreting ABGs—Do You Have a Match?**

1. Look at each number separately.
   - Label the pH:
     - If the pH is less than 7.35, the problem is acidosis.
     - If the pH is greater than 7.45, the problem is alkalosis.
   - Label the $PaCO_2$:
     - If the $PaCO_2$ is less than 35 mm Hg, more carbon dioxide is being exhaled than normal and indicates alkalosis.
     - If the $PaCO_2$ is greater than 45 mm Hg, less carbon dioxide is being exhaled than normal and indicates acidosis.
   - Label the bicarbonate:
     - If the HCO_3^- is less than 22 mEq/L, bicarbonate levels are lower than normal, indicating acidosis.
     - If the HCO_3^- is greater than 26 mEq/L, bicarbonate levels are higher than normal, indicating alkalosis.
2. Determine the cause of the acid–base imbalance.
   - Look at the pH—is it acidosis or alkalosis?
3. Determine if the origin of the imbalance is respiratory or metabolic.
   - Check the $PaCO_2$ and HCO_3^-. Which one MATCHES the same acid–base status as the pH?

Example
pH = 7.33 (acidosis)
$PaCO_2$ = 55 (acidosis)
HCO_3 = 29 (alkalosis)
Cause of imbalance (hint: look at pH) = acidosis.
$PaCO_2$ (acidosis) MATCHES the pH (acidosis) = respiratory problem
Client has respiratory acidosis.

4. Look for evidence of compensation.
   - Look at the value that does NOT match the pH:
     - If it (e.g., $PaCO_2$ or HCO_3) is within normal range, there is no compensation.
     - If it (e.g., $PaCO_2$ or HCO_3) is above or below normal range, the body is compensating.

Examples
a. In respiratory acidosis (pH < 7.35, $PaCO_2$ > 45 mm Hg), if the HCO_3^- is greater than 26 mEq/L, the kidneys are retaining bicarbonate to minimize the acidosis: renal compensation.
b. In respiratory alkalosis (pH > 7.45, $PaCO_2$ < 35 mm Hg), if the HCO_3^- is less than 22 mEq/L, the kidneys are excreting bicarbonate to minimize the alkalosis: again, renal compensation.
c. In metabolic acidosis (pH < 7.35, HCO_3^- < 22 mEq/L), if the $PaCO_2$ is less than 35 mm Hg, carbon dioxide is being "blown off" to minimize the acidosis: respiratory compensation.
d. In metabolic alkalosis (pH > 7.45, HCO_3^- > 26 mEq/L), if the $PaCO_2$ is greater than 45 mm Hg, carbon dioxide is being retained to compensate for excess base: again, respiratory compensation.

Note: If the value that doesn't match (e.g., $PaCO_2$ or HCO_3) is above or below normal and the pH is within normal range, the body has completely compensated. Complete compensation takes time to develop and is the result of a chronic condition (e.g., chronic respiratory acidosis with COPD).

measurement individually, then look at the interrelationships to determine what type of acid–base imbalance may be present.

DIAGNOSING

NANDA includes the following diagnostic labels that relate to fluid and acid–base imbalances:

- *Deficient Fluid Volume:* Decreased intravascular, interstitial, and/or intracellular fluid. This refers to dehydration, water loss alone without change in sodium.
- *Excess Fluid Volume:* Increased isotonic fluid retention.
- *Risk for Imbalanced Fluid Volume:* At risk for a decrease, increase, or rapid shift from one to the other of intravascular, interstitial, and/or intracellular fluid. This refers to body fluid loss, gain, or both.
- *Risk for Deficient Fluid Volume:* At risk for experiencing vascular, cellular, or intracellular dehydration.
- *Impaired Gas Exchange:* Excess or deficit in oxygenation and/or carbon dioxide elimination at the alveolar-capillary membrane.

Clinical applications of selected diagnoses are shown in Identifying Nursing Diagnoses, Outcomes, and Interventions and in the Nursing Care Plan and the Concept Map at the end of this chapter.

Fluid, electrolyte, and acid–base imbalances affect many other body areas and as a consequence may be the etiology of other nursing diagnoses, such as

- *Impaired Oral Mucous Membrane* related to fluid volume deficit.
- *Impaired Skin Integrity* related to dehydration and/or edema.
- *Decreased Cardiac Output* related to hypovolemia and/or cardiac dysrhythmias secondary to electrolyte imbalance (K^+ or Mg^{2+}).
- *Ineffective Tissue Perfusion* related to decreased cardiac output secondary to fluid volume deficit or edema.
- *Activity Intolerance* related to hypervolemia.
- *Risk for Injury* related to calcium shift out of bones into extracellular fluids.
- *Acute Confusion* related to electrolyte imbalance.

IDENTIFYING NURSING DIAGNOSES, OUTCOMES, AND INTERVENTIONS   **Clients with Fluid Volume Excess**

Data Cluster Tom Bricker, a 67-year-old pensioner who has a history of heart disease, has experienced a weight gain of 4 to 5 kg (9 to 11 lb) during the past month. He states his rings are too tight to remove, his ankles are swollen, his heart pounds at times, he gets breathless with exertion, and he feels bloated. Physical findings reveal jugular vein distention above 3 cm; delayed emptying of hand veins; bounding pulse (86); pitting edema in feet, ankles, and lower legs; and moist lung sounds (rales/crackles).

NURSING DIAGNOSIS/DEFINITION	SAMPLE DESIRED OUTCOMES*/*DEFINITION*	INDICATORS	SELECTED INTERVENTIONS*/ *DEFINITION*	SAMPLE NIC ACTIVITIES
Excess Fluid Volume/Increased isotonic fluid retention	Fluid Balance [0601]/*Water balance in the intracellular and extracellular compartments of the body*	Not compromised: • 24-hour intake and output • Stable body weight No: • Adventitious breath sounds • Neck vein distention	Fluid Management [4120]/*Promotion of fluid balance and prevention of complications resulting from abnormal or undesired fluid levels*	• Assess location and extent of edema on scale from 1+ to 4+ • Monitor for indications of fluid overload/retention (e.g., crackles, elevated BP, edema, neck vein distention) as appropriate • Maintain accurate intake and output record • Weigh daily and monitor trends • Consult primary care provider if signs and symptoms of fluid volume excess persist or worsen

*The NOC # for desired outcomes and the NIC # for nursing interventions are listed in brackets following the appropriate outcome or intervention. Outcomes, indicators, interventions, and activities selected are only a sample of those suggested by NOC and NIC and should be further individualized for each client.

PLANNING

When planning care the nurse identifies nursing interventions that will assist the client to achieve these broad goals:

- Maintain or restore normal fluid balance.
- Maintain or restore normal balance of electrolytes in the intracellular and extracellular compartments.
- Maintain or restore pulmonary ventilation and oxygenation.
- Prevent associated risks (tissue breakdown, decreased cardiac output, confusion, other neurologic signs).

Goals will vary according to the diagnosis and defining characteristics for each individual. Appropriate preventive and corrective nursing interventions that relate to these must be identified. Specific nursing activities can be selected to meet the client's individual needs. Examples of application of these using NANDA, NIC, and NOC designations are shown in Identifying Nursing Diagnoses, Outcomes, and Interventions and in the Nursing Care Plan and the Concept Map at the end of this chapter. Examples of NIC interventions related to fluid, electrolyte, and acid–base balance include the following:

- Acid–base management
- Electrolyte management
- Fluid monitoring
- Hypovolemia management
- Intravenous (IV) therapy

Specific nursing activities associated with each of these interventions can be selected to meet the individual needs of the client.

Nursing activities to meet goals and outcomes related to fluid, electrolyte, and acid–base imbalances are discussed in the next section. These include (a) monitoring fluid intake and output, cardiovascular and respiratory status, and results of laboratory tests; (b) assessing the client's weight; location and extent of edema, if present; skin turgor and skin status; specific gravity of urine; and level of consciousness and mental status; (c) fluid intake modifications; (d) dietary changes; (e) parenteral fluid, electrolyte, and blood replacement; and (f) other appropriate measures such as administering prescribed medications and oxygen, providing skin care and oral hygiene, positioning the client appropriately, and scheduling rest periods.

IMPLEMENTING

Promoting Wellness

Most people rarely think about their fluid, electrolyte, or acid–base balance. They know it is important to drink adequate fluids and consume a balanced diet, but they may not understand the potential effects when this is not done. Nurses

---

IDENTIFYING NURSING DIAGNOSES, OUTCOMES, AND INTERVENTIONS
Clients with Impaired Gas Exchange

Data Cluster Fred Boysniak was admitted to emergency after being found with an empty bottle of morphine tablets by his bed. He appears very lethargic and stuporous; pulse is 120, respiration 12 and very shallow. Blood gases reveal pH of 7.28, $PaCO_2$ 49 mm Hg, and HCO_3^- 25 mEq/L.

NURSING DIAGNOSIS/DEFINITION	SAMPLE DESIRED OUTCOMES*/*DEFINITION*	INDICATORS	SELECTED INTERVENTIONS*/*DEFINITION*	SAMPLE NIC ACTIVITIES
Impaired Gas Exchange/Excess or deficit in oxygenation and/or carbon dioxide elimination at the alveolar-capillary membrane	Respiratory Status: Ventilation [0403]/*Movement of air in and out of the lungs*	Not compromised • Depth of inspiration • Auscultated breath sounds	Acid–Base Management: Respiratory Acidosis [1913]/*Promotion of acid–base balance and prevention of complications resulting from serum PCO_2 levels higher than desired*	• Monitor respiratory pattern • Monitor ABG levels for decreasing pH level, as appropriate • Monitor neurological status (e.g., level of consciousness and confusion) • Monitor determinants of tissue oxygen delivery (e.g., PaO_2, SaO_2, hemoglobin levels) • Provide mechanical ventilatory support if necessary

*The NOC # for desired outcomes and the NIC # for nursing interventions are listed in brackets following the appropriate outcome or intervention. Outcomes, indicators, interventions, and activities selected are only a sample of those suggested by NOC and NIC and should be further individualized for each client.

can promote clients' health by providing wellness teaching that will help them maintain fluid and electrolyte balance.

Enteral Fluid and Electrolyte Replacement

Fluids and electrolytes can be provided orally in the home and hospital if the client's health permits, that is, if the client is not vomiting, has not experienced an excessive fluid loss, and has an intact gastrointestinal tract and gag and swallow reflexes. Clients who are unable to ingest solid foods may be able to ingest fluids.

FLUID INTAKE MODIFICATIONS Increased fluids (ordered as "push fluids") are often prescribed for clients with actual or potential fluid volume deficits arising, for example, from mild diarrhea or mild to moderate fevers. Guidelines for helping clients increase fluid intake are shown in the Practice Guidelines.

Restricted fluids may be necessary for clients who have fluid retention (fluid volume excess) as a result of renal fail-ure, congestive heart failure, SIADH, or other disease processes. Fluid restrictions vary from "nothing by mouth" to a precise amount ordered by a primary care provider. The restriction of fluids can be difficult for some clients, particularly if they are experiencing thirst. Guidelines for helping clients restrict fluid intake are shown in Practice Guidelines.

DIETARY CHANGES Specific fluid and electrolyte imbalances may require simple dietary changes. For example, clients receiving potassium-depleting diuretics need to be informed about foods with a high potassium content (e.g., bananas, oranges, and leafy greens). Some clients with fluid retention need to avoid foods high in sodium. Most healthy clients can benefit from foods rich in calcium.

ORAL ELECTROLYTE SUPPLEMENTS Some clients can benefit from oral supplements of electrolytes, particularly when a medication is prescribed that affects electrolyte balance, when dietary intake is inadequate for a specific electrolyte, or when fluid and electrolyte losses are excessive as a result of, for example, excessive perspiration.

Helping Clients Restrict Fluid Intake

- Explain the reason for the restricted intake and how much and what types of fluids are permitted orally. Many clients need to be informed that ice chips, gelatin, and ice cream, for example, are considered fluid.
- Help the client decide the amount of fluid to be taken with each meal, between meals, before bedtime, and with medications. For the hospitalized or long-term care client, half the total volume is scheduled during the day shift, when the client is most active, receives two meals, and most oral medications. A large part of the remainder is scheduled for the evening shift to permit fluids with meals and evening visitors.
- Identify fluids or fluid-like substances the client likes and make sure that these are provided, unless contraindicated. A client who is allowed only 200 mL of fluid for breakfast, for example, should receive the type of fluid the client favors.
- Set short-term goals that make the fluid restriction more tolerable. For example, schedule a specified amount of fluid at one or two hourly intervals between meals. Some clients may prefer fluids only between meals if the food provided at mealtime helps relieve thirst.
- Place allowed fluids in small containers such as a 4-ounce juice glass to allow the perception of a full container.
- Periodically offer the client ice chips as an alternative to water, because ice chips when melted are approximately half of the frozen volume.
- Provide frequent mouth care and rinses to reduce the thirst sensation.
- Instruct the client to avoid ingesting or chewing salty or sweet foods (hard candy or gum), because these foods tend to produce thirst. Sugarless gum may be an alternative for some clients.
- Encourage the client when possible to participate in maintaining the fluid intake record.

Corticosteroids and many diuretics can cause too much potassium to be eliminated through the kidneys. For clients taking these medications, potassium supplements may be prescribed. Instruct clients taking oral potassium supplements to take the medication with juice to mask the unpleasant taste and reduce the possibility of gastric distress. Emphasize the importance of taking the medication as prescribed and seeing their primary care provider on a regular basis. Because hyperkalemia can have serious cardiac effects, clients should never increase the amount of potassium being taken without an order to do so. In addition, inform clients that most salt substitutes contain potassium, so it is important to consult with the primary care provider before using salt substitutes.

People who ingest insufficient milk and milk products benefit from calcium supplements. The recommended daily allowance for calcium is 1,000 to 1,500 mg. It is generally recommended that postmenopausal women take 1,500 mg of calcium per day to reduce the risk of osteoporosis. Long-term use of corticosteroid drugs can also cause calcium loss from the bone, and calcium supplements may help reduce this loss. Clients who take supplemental calcium need to maintain a fluid intake of at least 2,500 mL per day (unless contraindicated) to reduce the risk of kidney stones, which are commonly composed of calcium salts.

Although routine supplements for other electrolytes generally are not recommended, clients who have poor dietary habits, who are malnourished, or who have difficulty accessing or eating fresh fruits and vegetables may benefit from electrolyte supplements. A daily multiple vitamin with minerals may achieve the desired goal. People who engage in strenuous activity in a warm environment need to be encouraged to replace water and electrolytes lost through excessive perspiration by consuming a sports drink such as Gatorade or another commercial fluid and electrolyte solution.

Liquid nutritional supplements are often given to clients who are malnourished or have poor eating habits. They are used with frequency in older adults to bolster nutritional status and caloric intake. It is very important to be a "label reader" of the product and to be aware of the contents of the supplement. Some of them are very high in protein and high in potassium, which may be contraindicated in an individual with impaired renal function.

Parenteral Fluid and Electrolyte Replacement

Intravenous (IV) fluid therapy is essential when clients are unable to take food and fluids orally. It is an efficient and effective method of supplying fluids directly into the intravascular fluid compartment and replacing electrolyte losses. Intravenous fluid therapy is usually ordered by the primary care provider. The nurse is responsible for administering and maintaining the therapy and for teaching the client and significant others how to continue the therapy at home if necessary.

INTRAVENOUS SOLUTIONS Intravenous solutions can be classified as isotonic, hypotonic, or hypertonic. Most IV solutions are *isotonic,* having the same concentration of solutes as blood plasma. Isotonic solutions are often used to restore vascular volume. *Hypertonic* solutions have a greater concentration of solutes than plasma; *hypotonic* solutions have a lesser concentration of solutes. Box 36–6 provides examples of IV solutions.

IV solutions can also be categorized according to their purpose. Nutrient solutions contain some form of carbohydrate and water. Water is supplied for fluid requirements and carbohydrate for calories and energy. For example, 1 L of 5% dextrose provides 170 calories. *Nutrient solutions* are useful in preventing dehydration and ketosis but do not provide

BOX 36–6   Selected Intravenous Solutions

Type/Examples

Isotonic Solutions

   0.9% NaCl (normal saline)

   Lactated Ringer's (a balanced electrolyte solution)

   5% dextrose in water (D5W)

Hypotonic Solutions

   0.45% NaCl (half normal saline)

   0.33% NaCl (one-third normal saline)

Hypertonic Solutions

   5% dextrose in normal saline (D5NS)

   5% dextrose in 0.45% NaCl (D5 1/2NS)

   5% dextrose in lactated Ringer's (D5LR)

PRACTICE GUIDELINES   Vein Selection

- Use distal veins of the arm first.
- Use the client's nondominant arm whenever possible.
- Select a vein that is
  a. Easily palpated and feels soft and full.
  b. Naturally splinted by bone.
  c. Large enough to allow adequate circulation around the catheter.
- Avoid using veins that are
  a. In areas of flexion (e.g., the antecubital fossa).
  b. Highly visible, because they tend to roll away from the needle.
  c. Damaged by previous use, phlebitis, infiltration, or sclerosis.
  d. Continually distended with blood, or knotted or tortuous.
  e. In a surgically compromised or injured extremity (e.g., following a mastectomy), because of possible impaired circulation and discomfort for the client.

---

sufficient calories to promote wound healing, weight gain, or normal growth in children. Common nutrient solutions are 5% dextrose in water (D5W) and 5% dextrose in 0.45% sodium chloride (dextrose in half-strength saline).

Electrolyte solutions contain varying amounts of cations and anions. Commonly used solutions are normal saline (0.9% sodium chloride solution), Ringer's solution (which contains sodium, chloride, potassium, and calcium), and lactated Ringer's solution (which contains sodium, chloride, potassium, calcium, and lactate). Lactate is metabolized in the liver to form bicarbonate HCO_3^-. Saline and balanced electrolyte solutions commonly are used to restore vascular volume, particularly after trauma or surgery. They also may be used to replace fluid and electrolytes for clients with continuing losses, for example, because of gastric suction or wound drainage.

Lactated Ringer's solution is an *alkalinizing solution* that may be given to treat metabolic acidosis. *Acidifying solutions,* in contrast, are administered to counteract metabolic alkalosis. Examples of acidifying solutions are 5% dextrose in 0.45% sodium chloride and 0.9% sodium chloride solution.

Volume expanders are used to increase the blood volume following severe loss of blood (e.g., from hemorrhage) or loss of plasma (e.g., from severe burns, which draw large amounts of plasma from the bloodstream to the burn site). Examples of expanders are dextran, plasma, and albumin.

VENIPUNCTURE SITES The site chosen for venipuncture varies with the client's age, the length of time the infusion is to run, the type of solution used, and the condition of veins. For adults, veins in the hand and arm are commonly used; for infants, veins in the scalp and dorsal foot veins are often used. Larger veins are preferred for infusions that need to be given rapidly and for solutions that could be irritating.

The metacarpal, basilic, and cephalic veins are commonly used for intermittent or continuous infusions (Figure 36–9 *B*). The ulna and radius act as natural splints at these sites, and the client has greater freedom of arm movements for activities such as eating. Although the basilic and median cubital veins in the antecubital space are convenient sites for venipuncture, they

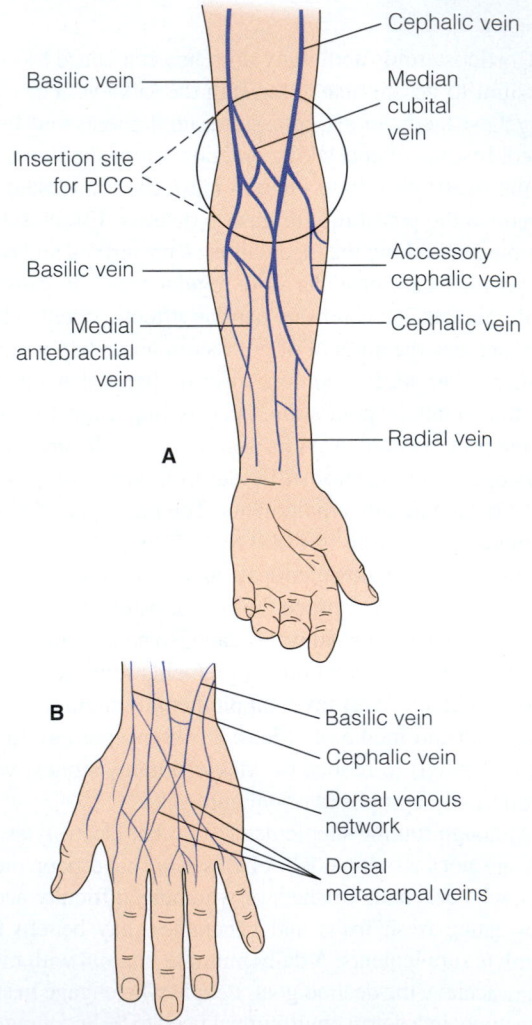

Figure 36–9 ⬤ Commonly used venipuncture sites of the *A,* arm; *B,* hand. *A* also shows the site used for a peripherally inserted central catheter (PICC).

are usually used for blood draws, bolus injections of medication, and insertion sites for a peripherally inserted central catheter line (see Figure 36–9, *A*). See Practice Guidelines for vein selection and general tips for easier IV starts.

When long-term IV therapy or parenteral nutrition is anticipated or the client is receiving IV medications that are damaging to vessels (e.g., chemotherapy), a central venous catheter may be inserted. Central venous catheters usually are inserted into the subclavian or jugular vein, with the distal tip of the catheter resting in the superior vena cava just above the right atrium (Figure 36–10). They may be inserted at the client's bedside or, for longer term access, surgically inserted. Subclavian central venous catheters permit freedom of movement for ambulation; however, there is greater risk of complications, including hemothorax or pneumothorax, cardiac perforation, thrombosis, and infection. Assess the client closely for manifestations such as shortness of breath, chest pain, cough, hypotension, tachycardia, and anxiety after the insertion procedure.

With a peripherally inserted central venous catheter (PICC), the catheter is inserted in the basilic or cephalic vein just above or below the antecubital space of the right arm. The tip of the catheter rests in the superior vena cava. The risk of pneumothorax is eliminated with PICC. These catheters frequently are used for long-term intravenous access when the client will be managing IV therapy at home.

Implantable venous access devices or ports (Figure 36–11) are used for clients with chronic illness who require long-term IV therapy. The device is designed to provide repeated access to the central venous system, avoiding the trauma and complications of multiple venipunctures. Using local anesthesia, implantable ports are surgically placed into a small subcutaneous pocket under the skin, usually on the an-

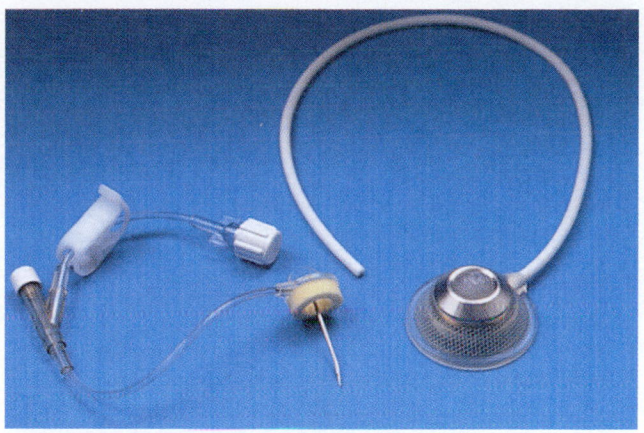

Figure 36–11 ◉ An implantable venous access device (right) and a Huber needle with extension tubing.

terior chest near the clavicle, and no part of the port is exposed. The distal end of the catheter is placed in the subclavian or jugular vein. There are different kinds of implantable venous access devices and they may be tunneled or nontunneled (Rosenthal, 2005b).

Special precautions need to be taken with all central lines and venous access ports to ensure asepsis and catheter patency. Nursing care of clients with these devices is outlined in the Practice Guidelines.

INTRAVENOUS EQUIPMENT Because equipment varies according to the manufacturer, the nurse must become familiar with the equipment used in each particular agency.

Solution containers are available in various sizes (50, 100, 250, 500, or 1,000 mL); the smaller containers are often used to administer medications. Most solutions are currently dispensed in plastic bags. However, glass bottles may need to be used if the administered medications are incompatible with plastic. Glass bottles require an air vent so that air can enter the bottle and replace the fluid that enters the client's vein. Some have a tube inside the bottle that serves as a vent; other containers without air vents require a vent on the administration set. Air vents usually have filters to prevent contamination from the air that enters the container. Air vents are not required for plastic solution bags, because the bags collapse under atmospheric pressure when the solution enters the vein.

It is essential that the solution be sterile and in good condition, that is, clear. Cloudiness, evidence that the container has been opened previously, or leaks indicate possible contamination. Always check the expiration date on the label. Return any questionable or contaminated solutions to the pharmacy or IV therapy department.

Infusion sets usually include an insertion spike, a drip chamber, a roller valve or screw clamp, tubing with secondary ports, and a protective cap over the needle adapter. The insertion spike is kept sterile and inserted into the solution container when the equipment is set up and ready to start. The drip chamber permits a predictable amount of fluid to be delivered. A commonly used drip chamber is the 10 to 20 drops, which delivers macrodrip per milliliter of solution. This information

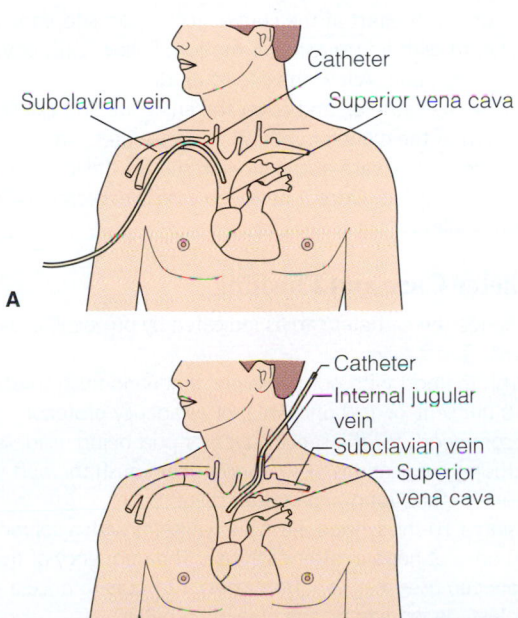

Figure 36–10 ◉ Central venous lines with *A,* subclavian vein insertion, and *B,* left jugular insertion.

General Tips for Easier IV Starts

- Review the client's medical history. In general, you'll want to avoid using an arm affected by hemiplegia or with a dialysis access. Also avoid an arm on the same side as a mastectomy, sites near infections or below previous infiltrations of extravasations, and veins affected by phlebitis.
- Put gravity to work. Dangle the client's arm over the side of the bed to encourage dependent vein filling.
- Make sure the client is comfortable. Pain and anxiety stimulate the sympathetic nervous system and trigger vasoconstriction and vasovagal reactions. Have the client void before you start the IV line, make sure he or she is warm enough, and administer pain medication as ordered before the procedure. Help the patient into a comfortable prone or semi-Fowler position for the IV insertion.
- Warmth encourages vasodilation. Apply warm compresses to the site for 10 to 15 minutes before you attempt venipuncture. Unless contraindicated, the client could take a hot shower or drink warm fluids before IV insertion.
- Avoid hand veins. Because of the risk of nerve injuries, hand veins should be a last choice, especially in older clients whose skin is very thin.
- Choose the right device for the ordered therapy. If the ordered IV medication is irritating to veins and therapy is expected to last more than a few days, consult with the IV nurse or medical team to determine whether the client is a candidate for a midline catheter, a peripherally inserted central catheter, or another type of central venous access device.
- Use the smallest gauge cannula that will accommodate the therapy and allow good venous flow around the catheter tip. For example, for routine hydration or intermittent therapies, use 22- to 27-gauge catheters; for transfusion therapies, 20- to 24-gauge; and for therapy for neonates or clients with very small, fragile veins, 24- to 27-gauge.
- Use good body mechanics. Raise the bed or stretcher to a comfortable working height. Sit, when possible, and keep all equipment within reach. Stabilize the client's hand or arm with your nondominant arm, tucking it under your forearm if necessary to prevent a moving target.
- Display confidence in your own abilities. When you approach the client, don't say, "I'm here to try to start your IV line." Instead, confidently state, "I'm here to insert your IV line."
- If you miss, offer an honest explanation in a matter-of-fact and friendly manner. Think about what you can do to improve your next attempt, and explain what you'll do differently (if anything). Most important, limit your attempts to two. If you're not successful after two tries, ask another nurse or an anesthesia provider to try again a little later.

Note: From "Tailor Your I.V. Insertion Techniques for Special Populations," by K. Rosenthal, 2005a, *Nursing, 35*(5), 39. Copyright © 2005 Lippincott Williams & Wilkins. Reprinted with permission.

Caring for Clients with a Venous Access Device

- On insertion, document the date; the site; the brand, gauge, and catheter length; the location of the catheter tip (verified by x-ray); the length of the external segment; and client teaching. Do not use the access device until correct placement has been verified by x-ray.

Site Care

- Use strict aseptic technique when caring for central lines and long-term venous access devices.
- The frequency of dressing changes may vary from every 3 to 7 days, depending on the site. Dressings also should be changed when loose or soiled.
- Assess the site for any redness, swelling, tenderness, or drainage. Compare the length of the external portion of the catheter with its documented length to assess for possible displacement. Obtain a chest x-ray to determine the catheter tip's position if in doubt. Report and document any position changes or signs of infection.
- Follow agency protocol for cleaning solutions and types of dressings. Isopropyl alcohol or a combination of alcohol and acetone followed by povidone-iodine are commonly used to clean the port site.
- Before accessing the port, clean an area 2 inches in diameter around the site with an alcohol-acetone solution on a sterile cotton swab. Start at the center of the port site, moving outward with a firm, circular motion. Follow with povidone-iodine solution. Allow the site to air dry.
- Secure the catheter, and cover the entry site and external portion of the catheter with an occlusive dressing.
- Provide routine care of the incision site for the implant device until it is healed. Once it heals, no care is necessary when the port is idle.

Catheter Care and Flushing

- Change the catheter cap as indicated by protocol, usually every 3 to 7 days.
- Flush the port with normal saline, a heparin flush solution (10 units/mL or 100 units/mL), or as agency protocol recommends for the specific type of port being used. After infusing medications or solutions, again flush the port with saline before using heparinized saline.
- Using a 10-mL syringe, flush the catheter with a solution of 10 units of heparin after each use. The frequency of flushes between uses may vary from every 12 hours to once a week or less, depending on the type of catheter.
- Remember to flush all lumens for multiple-lumen catheters.
- Use a specially designed needle to access an implanted port. A needle with a 90-degree angle is generally used for

infusions because it is easier to stabilize and more comfortable for the client. Stabilizing the port between the thumb and index finger of the nondominant hand, insert the needle through the center of the port until the resistance of the platform is felt.

- To remove the needle after a treatment, again stabilize the port and use even pressure to withdraw the needle. Maintain positive pressure by withdrawing the needle as the last milliliter of flush solution is being instilled.
- Flush idle implanted ports with heparinized saline in accordance with agency protocol or at least every 8 weeks.

Teaching

Provide clients with the following instructions:

- Do not allow anyone to take a blood pressure on the arm in which a PICC line is inserted.

- Wear a medic-alert tag or bracelet if the device is to be in place for a long period.
- For a PICC, you do not need to restrict activities, except do not immerse the arm in water. Showering is allowed if the site and catheter are covered by an occlusive dressing.
- For an implanted venous port there are no activity restrictions, but remember that the port or catheter tip can become dislodged. Signs of a dislodged catheter tip include pain in the neck or ear on the affected side, swishing or gurgling sounds, or palpitations. Free movement of the port, swelling, or difficulty accessing the port may indicate port dislodgment. Notify the primary care provider should any of these occur or if symptoms of infection develop.

Note: From "Getting a Line on Central Vascular Access Devices," by S. Masoorli & T. Angeles, 2002, *Nursing, 32*(4), pp. 36–43. Copyright © 2005 Lippincott Williams & Wilkins. Reprinted with permission.

---

is found on the package. There are also 60 drops sets, which deliver microdrip per milliliter of solution. The roller valve or screw clamp, which compresses the lumen of the tubing, controls the rate of the flow. The protective cap over the needle adapter maintains the sterility of the end of the tubing so that it can be attached to a sterile needle inserted in the client's vein.

Most infusion sets include one or more injection ports for administering IV medications or secondary infusions. Needleless systems are increasingly used because they reduce the risk of needlestick injury and contamination of the intravenous line. There are various types of needleless systems available, including two-piece prepierced septum and blunt cannula devices, Luer-activated devices, and three-way pressure-activated safety valves (Rosenthal, 2004). With each of these needleless systems, a blunt cannula is inserted into a special injection port or adapter on the IV tubing to administer medications or secondary infusions. Many infusion sets include an in-line filter to trap air, particulate matter, and microbes. A special infusion set may be required if the IV flow rate will be regulated by an infusion pump.

Catheters and needles are commonly used for intravenous infusions. Over-the-needle catheters, also known as angiocaths, are commonly used for adult clients. The plastic catheter fits over a needle used to pierce the skin and vein wall. Once inserted into the vein, the needle is withdrawn and discarded, leaving the catheter in place. IV catheters allow the client more mobility and rarely infiltrate, that is, become dislodged from the vein and allow fluid to flow into interstitial spaces.

Safety devices on IV catheters are now common. With the original over-the-needle catheters, the sharp stylet remained exposed until placed in a sharps container. This resulted in needlestick injuries to nurses. The 2000 Needlestick Safety and Prevention Act requires the use of needle safety devices to prevent exposure to bloodborne pathogens (Wilburn, 2004). The safety devices for IV catheters vary. They can be either an active safety device which requires activation by the nurse or a passive safety device where the safety feature is automatically activated after the stylet is removed from the catheter.

Butterfly, or wing-tipped, needles with plastic flaps attached to the shaft are sometimes used. The flaps are held tightly together to hold the needle securely during insertion; after insertion, they are flattened against the skin and secured with tape.

IV poles are used to hang the solution container. Some poles are attached to hospital beds; others stand on the floor or hang from the ceiling. In the home, plant hangers or robe hooks (even kitchen cabinet knobs or an S-hook over the top of a door) may be used to hang solution containers. The height of most poles is adjustable. The higher the solution container, the greater the force of the solution as it enters the client and the faster the rate of flow.

STARTING AN INTRAVENOUS INFUSION Although the primary care provider is responsible for ordering IV therapy for clients, nurses initiate, monitor, and maintain the prescribed IV infusion. This is true not only in hospitals and long-term care facilities but increasingly in community-based settings such as clinics and clients' homes.

Before starting an infusion, the nurse determines the following:

- The type and amount of solution to be infused
- The exact amount (dose) of any medications to be added to a compatible solution
- The rate of flow or the time over which the infusion is to be completed

If solutions are prepared by the pharmacy or another department, the nurse must verify that the solution supplied exactly matches that which the primary care provider ordered.

Understanding the purpose for the infusion is as important as assessing the client. For example, the nurse may question an order for 5% dextrose in water at 150 mL/h if the client has peripheral edema and other signs of fluid overload.

To perform venipuncture and start an intravenous infusion, see Skill 36–1.

STARTING AN INTRAVENOUS INFUSION

Before preparing the infusion, the nurse first verifies the primary care provider's order indicating the type of solution, the amount to be administered, the rate of flow of the infusion, and any client allergies (e.g., to tape or povidone-iodine).

PURPOSES

- To supply fluid when clients are unable to take in an adequate volume of fluids by mouth
- To provide salts and other electrolytes needed to maintain electrolyte balance

- To provide glucose (dextrose), the main fuel for metabolism
- To provide water-soluble vitamins and medications
- To establish a lifeline for rapidly needed medications

ASSESSMENT

Assess the following:
- Vital signs (pulse, respiratory rate, and blood pressure) for baseline data
- Skin turgor

- Allergy to latex (e.g., tourniquet), tape, or iodine
- Bleeding tendencies
- Disease or injury to extremities
- Status of veins to determine appropriate venipuncture site

PLANNING

Prior to initiating the IV infusion, consider how long the client is likely to have the IV, what kinds of fluids will be infused, and what medications the client will be receiving or is likely to receive. These factors may affect the choice of vein and catheter size.

Delegation

This procedure is done by a registered nurse and, in many states, by a licensed practical nurse or licensed vocational nurse. Check the state's nurse practice act. Due to the use of sterile technique, intravenous infusion therapy is not delegated to unlicensed assistive personnel (UAP). UAP may care for clients receiving IV therapy, and the nurse must ensure that the UAP knows how to perform routine tasks such as bathing and positioning without disturbing the IV. The UAP should also know what complications or adverse signs, such as leakage, should be reported to the nurse. In some states a licensed vocational nurse with special IV therapy training may start intravenous infusions.

EQUIPMENT

- Infusion set
- Sterile parenteral solution
- IV pole
- Adhesive or nonallergenic tape
- Clean gloves
- Tourniquet
- Antiseptic swabs
- Antiseptic ointment (check agency policy)
- Intravenous catheter; see Variation at the end of this procedure for a butterfly (winged-tip) needle
- Sterile gauze dressing or transparent occlusive dressing
- Arm splint, if required
- Towel or pad
- Electronic infusion device or pump (The nurse decides what device is needed as appropriate to the client's condition.)
- IV catheter stabilization device

IMPLEMENTATION

Preparation

1. Prepare the client.
   - Prior to performing the procedure, introduce self and verify the client's identity using agency protocol. Explain the procedure to the client. A venipuncture can cause discomfort for a few seconds, but there should be no discomfort while the solution is flowing. Use a doll to demonstrate for children, and explain the procedure to the parents. Clients often want to know how long the process will last. The primary care provider's order may specify the length of time of the infusion, for example, 3,000 mL over 24 hours.
   - Unless initiating IV therapy is urgent, provide any scheduled care before establishing the infusion to minimize movement of the affected limb during the procedure. Moving the limb after the infusion has been established could dislodge the catheter.
   - Make sure that the client's clothing or gown can be removed over the IV apparatus if necessary. Some agencies provide special gowns that open over the shoulder and down the sleeve for easy removal.

Performance

Perform hand hygiene.
1. Open and prepare the infusion set.
   - Remove tubing from the container and straighten it out.
   - Slide the tubing clamp along the tubing until it is just below the drip chamber to facilitate its access.
   - Close the clamp.
   - Leave the ends of the tubing covered with the plastic caps until the infusion is started. **Rationale:** *This will maintain the sterility of the ends of the tubing.*
2. Spike the solution container.
   - Remove the protective cover from the entry site of the bag.
   - Remove the cap from the spike and insert the spike into the insertion site of the bag or bottle. Follow the manufacturer's instructions.
3. Apply a medication label to the solution container if a medication is added.
   - In many agencies, medications and labels are applied in the pharmacy; if they are not, apply the label upside down on the container.

4. Apply a timing label on the solution container.
   • The timing label may be applied at the time the infusion is started. Follow agency practice. See later discussion of regulating infusion flow rates and Figure 36–12.
5. Hang the solution container on the pole.
   • Adjust the pole so that the container is suspended about 1 m (3 ft) above the client's head. **Rationale:** *This height is needed to enable gravity to overcome venous pressure and facilitate flow of the solution into the vein.*
6. Partially fill the drip chamber with solution.
   • Squeeze the chamber gently until it is half full of solution.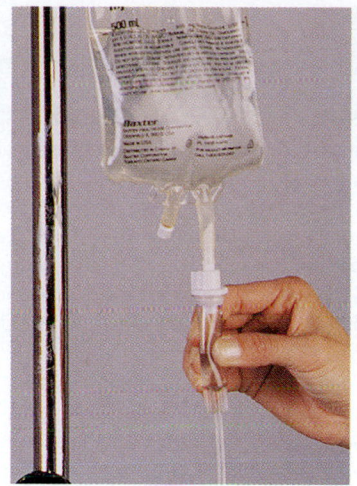
7. Prime the tubing.
   • Remove the protective cap and hold the tubing over a container. Maintain the sterility of the end of the tubing and the cap.
   • Release the clamp and let the fluid run through the tubing until all bubbles are removed. Tap the tubing if necessary with your fingers to help the bubbles move. **Rationale:** *The tubing is primed to prevent the introduction of air into the client. Air bubbles smaller than 0.5 mL usually do not cause problems in peripheral lines.*
   • Reclamp the tubing and replace the tubing cap, maintaining sterile technique.
   • For caps with air vents, do not remove the cap when priming this tubing. **Rationale:** *The flow of solution through the tubing will cease when the cap is moist with one drop of solution.*
   • If an infusion control pump, electronic device, or controller is being used, follow the manufacturer's directions for inserting the tubing and setting the infusion rate.
8. Perform hand hygiene again just prior to client contact.
9. Select the venipuncture site.
   • Use the client's nondominant arm, unless contraindicated (e.g., mastectomy, fistula for dialysis). Identify possible venipuncture sites by looking for veins that are relatively straight, not sclerotic or tortuous, and avoid venous valves. The vein should be palpable, but may not be visible, especially in clients with dark skin. Consider the catheter length; look for a site sufficiently distal to the wrist or elbow that the tip of the catheter will not be at a point of flexion. **Rationale:** *Sclerotic veins may make initiating and maintaining the IV difficult. Joint flexion increases the risk of irritation of vein walls by the catheter.*
   • Check agency protocol about shaving if the site is very hairy. Shaving is not usually recommended *because of the potential for microabrasions, which can increase the risk of infection.*
   • Place a towel or bed protector under the extremity *to protect linens (or furniture if in the home).*
10. Dilate the vein.
   • Place the extremity in a dependent position (lower than the client's heart). **Rationale:** *Gravity slows venous return and distends the veins. Distending the veins makes it easier to insert the needle properly.*
   • Apply a tourniquet firmly 15 to 20 cm (6 to 8 in.) above the venipuncture site. 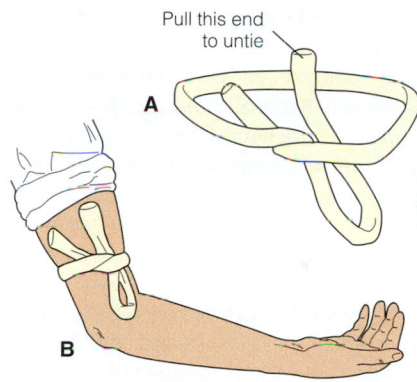 Explain that the tourniquet will feel tight. **Rationale:** *The tourniquet must be tight enough to obstruct venous flow but not so tight that it occludes arterial flow. Obstructing arterial flow inhibits*

① Squeezing the drip chamber.

② Applying a tourniquet.

venous filling. If a radial pulse can be palpated, the arterial flow is not obstructed.
   Use the tourniquet on only one client. This avoids cross-contamination to other clients.
   • If the vein is not sufficiently dilated:
   a. Massage or stroke the vein distal to the site and in the direction of venous flow toward the heart. **Rationale:** *This action helps fill the vein.*
   b. Encourage the client to clench and unclench the fist. **Rationale:** *Contracting the muscles compresses the distal veins, forcing blood along the veins and distending them.*
   c. Lightly tap the vein with your fingertips. **Rationale:** *Tapping may distend the vein.*
   • If the preceding steps fail to distend the vein so that it is palpable, remove the tourniquet and wrap the extremity in a warm, moist towel for 10 to 15 minutes. **Rationale:** *Heat dilates superficial blood vessels, causing them to fill.* Then repeat step 10.
11. Put on clean gloves and clean the venipuncture site. **Rationale:** *Gloves protect the nurse from contamination by the client's blood.*
   • Clean the skin at the site of entry with a topical antiseptic swab (e.g., 2% chlorhexidine, or alcohol). Some institutions may use an anti-infective solution such as povidone-iodine (check agency protocol). Check for

(continued)

STARTING AN INTRAVENOUS INFUSION *(continued)*

allergies to iodine or shellfish before cleansing skin with Betadine or iodine products.

- Use a circular motion, moving from the center outward for several inches. **Rationale:** *This motion carries microorganisms away from the site of entry.*
- Permit the solution to dry on the skin. Povidone-iodine should be in contact with the skin for 1 minute to be effective.

12. Insert the catheter and initiate the infusion.

- If desired and permitted by policy, inject 0.05 mL of 1% lidocaine intradermally over the site where you plan to insert the IV needle. Allow 5 to 10 seconds for the anesthetic to take effect. Transdermal analgesic creams (e.g., ELA-Max, EMLA) may also be used, depending on policy. Allow 30 minutes for the transdermal analgesic to take effect.
- Use the nondominant hand to pull the skin taut below the entry site. **Rationale:** *This stabilizes the vein and makes the skin taut for needle entry. It can also make initial tissue penetration less painful.*
- Holding the over-the-needle catheter at a 15- to 30-degree angle with bevel up, insert the catheter through the skin and into the vein. Sudden lack of resistance is felt as the needle enters the vein. Jabbing, stabbing, or quick thrusting should be avoided because it may cause rupture of delicate veins (Phillips, 2005).
- Once blood appears in the lumen of the needle or you feel the lack of resistance, lower the angle of the catheter until it is almost parallel with the skin, and advance the needle and catheter approximately 0.5 to 1 cm (about 1/4 in.) farther. Holding the needle portion steady, advance the catheter until the hub is at the venipuncture site. The exact technique depends on the type of device used. **Rationale:** *The catheter is advanced to ensure that it, and not just the metal needle, is in the vein.* The exact technique depends on the type of catheter used.
- Release the tourniquet.
- Put pressure on the vein proximal to the catheter to eliminate or reduce blood oozing out of the catheter. Stabilize the hub with thumb and index finger of the nondominant hand.
- Remove the protective cap from the distal end of the tubing and hold it ready to attach to the catheter, maintaining the sterility of the end.
- Carefully remove the needle, engage the needle safety device, and attach the end of the infusion tubing to the catheter hub.
- Initiate the infusion.

13. Tape the catheter.

- Tape the catheter by the "U" method or according to the manufacturer's instructions. Use of a catheter stabilization device is recommended in addition to the use of tape by the Infusion Nurses Society Using three strips of adhesive tape, each about 7.5 cm (3 in.) long:
  a. Place the catheter stabilization device according to the manufacturer's instructions.
  b. Place one strip, sticky side up, under the catheter's hub.

c. Fold each end over so that the sticky sides are against the skin. ❸
d. Place the second strip, sticky side down, over the catheter hub.
e. Place the third strip, sticky side down, over the tubing hub.

14. Dress and label the venipuncture site and tubing according to agency policy.

- Unless there is an allergy, a sterile transparent occlusive dressing is applied. ❹ This permits assessment of the site without disturbing the dressing. This type of dressing can be left on for 72 hours, then changed.
- Discard the tourniquet. Remove soiled gloves and discard appropriately.
- Loop the tubing and secure it with tape. **Rationale:** *Looping and securing the tubing prevent the weight of the tubing or any movement from pulling on the needle or catheter.*
- Label the dressing with the date and time of insertion, type, gauge of catheter used, and your initials.

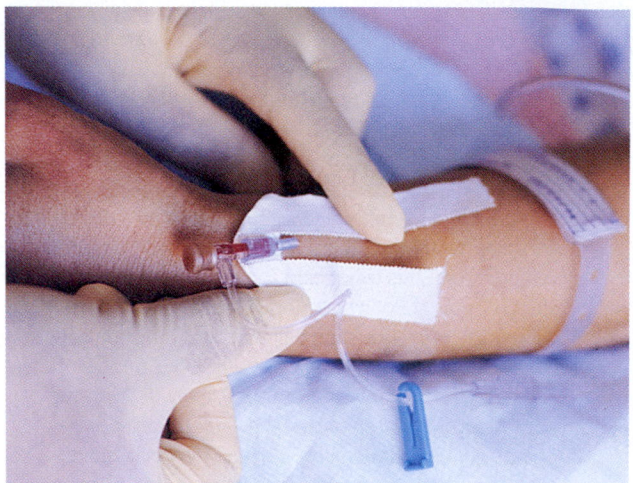

❸ Taping an intravenous catheter by the "U" method.

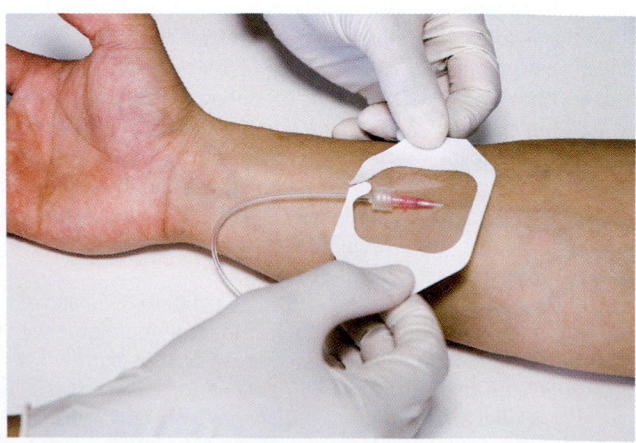

❹ Cover insertion site with transparent dressing.

15. Ensure appropriate infusion flow.
- Apply a padded arm board to splint the joint, as needed.
- Adjust the infusion rate of flow according to the order.

16. Label the IV tubing.
- Label the tubing with the date and time of attachment and your initials. This labeling may also be done when the infusion is started. **Rationale:** *This tubing is labeled to ensure that it is changed at regular intervals (i.e., every 24 to 96 hours according to agency policy).*

17. Document relevant data, including assessments.
- Record the start of the infusion on the client's chart. Some agencies provide a special form for this purpose. Include the date and time of the venipuncture; amount and type of solution used, including any additives (e.g., kind and amount of medications); container number; flow rate; type, length, and gauge of the needle or catheter; venipuncture site, how many attempts were made, and location of each attempt; the type of dressing applied; and the client's general response.

SAMPLE DOCUMENTATION

1/15/2010 0600 Inserted 20 gauge angiocath in (L) forearm on first attempt. IV infusing at 125 mL/hour. Explained reason for IV. Stated understanding. _____ A. Luis, RN

VARIATION: INSERTING A BUTTERFLY (WINGED-TIP) NEEDLE
- Hold the needle, pointed in the direction of the blood flow, at a 30-degree angle, with the bevel up, and pierce the skin beside the vein about 1 cm (1/2 in.) below the site planned for piercing the vein.

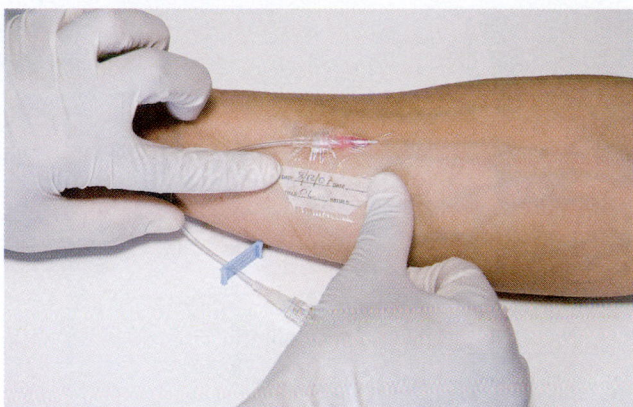

⑤ Taping the butterfly needle by the chevron method.

- Once the needle is through the skin, lower the needle so that it is almost parallel with the skin. **Rationale:** *Lowering the needle reduces the chances of puncturing both sides of the vein.*

Follow the course of the vein, and pierce one side of the vein. Sudden lack of resistance can be felt as blood enters the needle.

- When blood flows back into the needle tubing, insert the needle to its hub.
- Release the tourniquet, attach the infusion, and initiate flow as quickly as possible. **Rationale:** *Attaching the tubing quickly prevents blood from clotting and obstructing the needle.*
- Secure the butterfly needle by taping it securely by the crisscross (chevron) method. **⑤** Place a small gauze square under the needle, if required. **Rationale:** *The gauze keeps the needle in position in the vein.*

EVALUATION

Evaluate the following:
- Skin status at IV site (warm temperature and absence of pain, redness, and swelling)
- Status of dressing

- IV flow rate consistent with that ordered
- Ability to perform self-care activities; understanding of any mobility limitations
- Vital signs compared to baseline level

REGULATING AND MONITORING INTRAVENOUS INFUSIONS

Orders for IV infusions may take several forms: "3,000 mL over 24 hours"; "1,000 mL every 8 hours X 3 bags"; "125 mL/h until oral intake is adequate." The nurse initiating the IV calculates the correct flow rate, regulates the infusion, and monitors the client's responses. Unless an infusion control device is used, the nurse manually regulates the drops per minute of flow using the roller clamp to ensure that the prescribed amount of solution will be infused in the correct time span. If the flow is incorrect, problems such as hypervolemia, hypovolemia, or inadequate medication administration can result.

The number of drops delivered per milliliter of solution varies with different brands and types of infusion sets. This rate, called the drip factor (sometimes called the *drop factor*), generally is printed on the package of the infusion set. Macrodrops commonly have drop factors of 10, 12, 15, or 20 drops/mL; the drop factor for microdrip is always 60 drops/mL.

To calculate flow rates, the nurse must know the volume of fluid to be infused and the specific time for the infusion. Two commonly used methods of indicating flow rates are des-

ignating the number of milliliters to be administered in 1 hour (mL/h) and the number of drops to be given in 1 minute (drops/min). Because l milliliter of fluid displaces 1 cubic centimeter of space, the volume to be infused in the first method may also be designated as cubic centimeters per hour (cc/h).

Milliliters per Hour Hourly rates of infusion can be calculated by dividing the total infusion volume by the total infusion time in hours. For example, if 3,000 mL is infused in 24 hours, the number of milliliters per hour is:

$$\frac{3{,}000 \text{ mL (total infusion volume)}}{24 \text{ h (total infusion time)}} = 125 \text{ mL/h}$$

Nurses need to check infusions at least every hour to ensure that the indicated milliliters per hour have infused and that IV patency is maintained. A strip of adhesive marking the exact time and/or amount to be infused may be taped to the solution container. Some agencies make premarked labels available (Figure 36–12).

Drops per Minute The nurse initiating and monitoring an infusion must regulate the drops per minute to ensure that

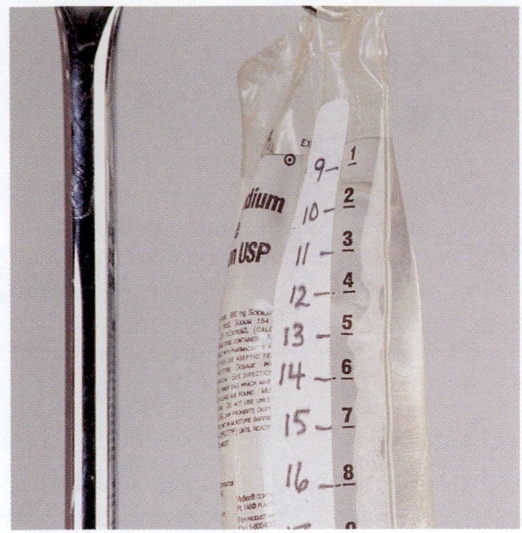

Figure 36–12 ○ Timing label on an intravenous container. The first time marked (0900 hours) would be correct for a bag hung at 0800 hours with a rate of 100 mL per hour.

the prescribed amount of solution will infuse. Drops per minute are calculated by the following formula:

$$\text{Drops per minute} = \frac{\text{Total infusion volume} \times \text{drop factor}}{\text{Total time of infusion in } \textit{minutes}}$$

If the requirements are 1,000 mL in 8 hours and the drip factor is 20 drops/mL, the drops per minute should be:

$$\frac{1,000 \text{ mL} \times 20}{8 \times 60 \text{ min } (480 \text{ min})} = 41 \text{ drops/min}$$

Approximating this rate as 40 drops/min, the nurse regulates the drops per minute by tightening or releasing the IV tubing clamp and counting the drops for 15 seconds, then multiplying that number by 4 (e.g., 10 drops/15 sec).

A number of factors influence flow rate (see Box 36–7).

BOX 36–7 — Factors Influencing Flow Rates

- The position of the forearm. Sometimes a change in the position of the client's arm decreases flow. Slight pronation, supination, extension, or elevation of the forearm on a pillow can increase flow.
- The position and patency of the tubing. Tubing can be obstructed by the client's weight, a kink, or a clamp closed too tightly. The flow rate also diminishes when part of the tubing dangles below the puncture site.
- The height of the infusion bottle. Elevating the height of the infusion bottle a few inches can speed the flow by creating more pressure.
- Possible infiltration or fluid leakage. Swelling, a feeling of coldness, and tenderness at the venipuncture site may indicate infiltration.
- Relationship of the size of the angiocath to the vein. A catheter that is too large may impede the infusion flow.

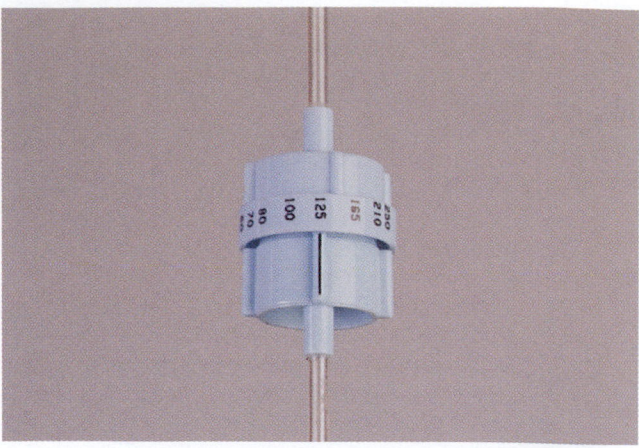

Figure 36–13 ○ The Dial-A-Flo in-line device.

DEVICES TO CONTROL INFUSIONS A number of devices are used to control the rate of an infusion. *Electronic infusion devices* (EIDs) regulate the infusion rate at preset limits. They also have an alarm that is triggered when the solution in the IV bag is low, when there is air in the tubing, or when the tubing is not high enough. The *Dial-A-Flo* in-line device (Figure 36–13) is a regulator that controls the amount of fluid to be administered. Hospitals may stock the Dial-A-Flo for use in situations where a pump is not required, but prevention of fluid overload is important. It is preset at the volume to be infused and can be attached at the time the infusion is set up or when the tubing is changed. Another variation is a *volume-control set*, or *Volutrol*, which is used if the volume of fluid administered is to be carefully controlled. The set, which holds a maximum of 100 mL of solution, is attached below the solution container, and the drip chamber is placed below the set. Volume-control sets are frequently used in pediatric settings, where the volume administered is critical.

CLINICAL ALERT

A flow rate control device should be used when administering IV fluid to older adults or pediatric clients. Both of these age groups are especially at risk for complications of fluid overload, which can occur with rapid infusion of IV fluids.

An infusion pump delivers fluids intravenously by exerting positive pressure on the tubing or on the fluid. In situations where the fluid flow is unrestricted, the pump pressure is comparable to that of gravity flow. However, if restrictions develop (increased venous resistance), the pump can maintain the fluid flow by increasing the pressure applied to the fluid.

A controller, by contrast, operates solely by gravitational force. The delivery pressure depends on the height of the container in relation to the venipuncture site. The container must be at least 76 cm (30 in.) above the venipuncture site for a controller to work. A controller does not have the ability to add pressure to the line and to overcome resistances to fluid flow.

Skill 36–2 outlines the steps involved in monitoring an intravenous infusion.

MONITORING AN INTRAVENOUS INFUSION

PURPOSES
- To maintain the prescribed flow rate
- To prevent complications associated with IV therapy

ASSESSMENT
Assess the following:

- Appearance of infusion site; patency of system
- Type of fluid being infused and rate of flow
- Response of the client

PLANNING
Review the type of equipment used outside the client's room. Read all appropriate materials and confirm the type of tubing, controller, or pump being used.

Delegation
This procedure should be done by the nurse because it is an important part of assessment and complications may occur.

IMPLEMENTATION

Preparation

1. Gather the pertinent data.
   - From the primary care provider's order, determine the type and sequence of solutions to be infused.
   - Determine the rate of flow and infusion schedule.

Performance

1. Ensure that the correct solution is being infused.
   - If the solution in incorrect, slow the rate of flow to a minimum to maintain the patency of the catheter. **Rationale:** *Stopping the infusion may allow a thrombus to form in the IV catheter. If this occurs, the catheter must be removed and another venipuncture performed before the infusion can be resumed.*
   - Change the solution to the correct one. Document and report the error according to agency protocol.
2. Observe the rate of flow every hour.
   - Compare the rate of flow regularly, for example, every hour, against the infusion schedule. **Rationale:** *Infusions that are off schedule can be harmful to a client.*
   - If the rate is too fast, slow it so that the infusion will be completed at the planned time. **Rationale:** *Solution administered too quickly may cause a significant increase in circulating blood volume (which is about 6 L in an adult). Hypervolemia may result in pulmonary edema and cardiac failure. Assess the client for manifestations of hypervolemia and its complications, including dyspnea; rapid, labored breathing; cough; crackles (rales) in the lung bases; tachycardia; and bounding pulses.*
   - If the rate is too slow, check agency practice. Some agencies permit nursing personnel to adjust a rate of flow by a specified amount. Adjustments above this rate require a primary care provider's order. **Rationale:** *Solution that is administered too slowly can supply insufficient fluid, electrolytes, or medication for a client's needs.*
   - If the rate of flow is 150 mL/h or more, check the rate of flow more frequently, for example, every 15 to 30 minutes.
3. Inspect the patency of the IV tubing and catheter.
   - Observe the position of the IV solution. If it is less than 1 m (3 ft) above the IV site, readjust it to the correct height of the pole. **Rationale:** *If the IV bag/bottle is too low, the solution may not flow into the vein because there is insufficient gravitational pressure to overcome the pressure of the blood within the vein.*
   - Observe the drip chamber. If it is less than half full, squeeze the chamber to allow the correct amount of fluid to flow in.
   - Open the drip regulator and observe for a rapid flow of fluid from the solution container into the drip chamber. Then partially close the drip regulator to reestablish the prescribed rate of flow. **Rationale:** *Rapid flow of fluid into the drip chamber indicates patency of the IV line. Closing the drip regulator to the prescribed rate of flow prevents fluid overload.*
   - Inspect the tubing for pinches or kinks or obstructions to flow. Arrange the tubing so that it is lightly coiled and under no pressure. Sometimes the tubing becomes caught under the client's body and the weight blocks the flow.
   - Observe the position of the tubing. If it is dangling below the venipuncture, coil it carefully on the surface of the bed. **Rationale:** *The solution may not flow upward into the vein against the force of gravity.*
   - Lower the solution container below the level of the infusion site and observe for a return flow of blood from the vein. **Rationale:** *A return flow of blood indicates that the needle is patent and in the vein. Blood returns in this instance because venous pressure is greater than the fluid pressure in the IV tubing. Absence of blood return may indicate that the needle is no longer in the vein or that the tip of the catheter is partially obstructed by a thrombus, the vein wall, or a valve in the vein.*
   - Determine whether the bevel of the catheter is blocked against the wall of the vein. If it is blocked, pull back gently, turn it slightly, or carefully raise or lower the angle of insertion slightly, using a sterile gauze pad underneath to protect the skin and change the position of the catheter bevel.
   - If there is leakage, locate the source. If the leak is at the catheter connection, tighten the tubing into the catheter. If the leak cannot be stopped, slow the infusion as much as possible without stopping it, and replace the tubing with a new sterile set. Estimate the amount of solution lost, if it was substantial.

(continued)

SKILL 36–2

MONITORING AN INTRAVENOUS INFUSION *(continued)*

4. Inspect the insertion site for fluid infiltration.
   - When an IV needle becomes dislodged from the vein, fluid flows into interstitial tissues, causing swelling. This is known as *infiltration* and is manifested by localized swelling, coolness, pallor, and discomfort at the IV site.
   - If an infiltration is present, stop the infusion and remove the catheter. Restart the infusion at another site.
   - Apply a warm compress to the site of the infiltration. **Rationale:** *Warmth promotes comfort and vasodilation, facilitating absorption of the fluid from interstitial tissues.*

5. If the infiltration involves a vesicant drug, it is called extravasation and other measures may be indicated. Extravasated vesicant drugs can cause severe tissue injury or destruction. The extravasation of a vesicant drug should be considered an emergency (Hadaway, 2004).
   - Stop the infusion immediately. Disconnect the tubing as close to the catheter hub as possible and attempt to aspirate any drug remaining in the hub. If an injectable antidote is available, the catheter should remain in place.
   - The primary care provider should be notified and if ordered, the antidote administered.
   - The affected arm should be elevated and depending on the drug, heat or cold therapy should be implemented.

6. If infiltration is not evident but the infusion is not flowing, determine whether the needle is dislodged from the vein.
   - Gently pinch the IV tubing adjacent to the needle site. This will cause blood to flow (flash back) into the tubing if the needle is in the vein.
   - Use a sterile syringe of saline to withdraw fluid from the port near the venipuncture site. If blood does not return, discontinue the intravenous solution.

7. Inspect the insertion site for phlebitis (inflammation of a vein).
   - Inspect and palpate the site at least every 8 hours. Phlebitis can occur as a result of injury to a vein, for

example, because of mechanical trauma or chemical irritation. Chemical injury to a vein can occur from intravenous electrolytes (especially potassium and magnesium) and medications. The clinical signs are redness, warmth, and swelling at the intravenous site and burning pain along the course of a vein.
   - If phlebitis is detected, discontinue the infusion, and apply warm compresses to the venipuncture site. Do not use this injured vein for further infusions.

8. Inspect the intravenous site for bleeding.
   - Oozing or bleeding into the surrounding tissues can occur while the infusion is freely flowing but is more likely to occur after the needle has been removed from the vein.
   - Observation of the venipuncture site is extremely important for clients who bleed readily, such as those receiving anticoagulants.

9. Teach the client ways to maintain the infusion system, for example:
   - Avoid sudden twisting or turning movements of the arm with the needle or catheter.
   - Avoid stretching or placing tension on the tubing.
   - Try to keep the tubing from dangling below the level of the needle.
   - Notify a nurse if
     a. The flow rate suddenly changes or the solution stops dripping.
     b. The solution container is nearly empty.
     c. There is blood in the IV tubing.
     d. Discomfort or swelling is experienced at the IV site.

10. Document all relevant information.

EVALUATION
Evaluate the following:
- Amount of fluid infused according to the schedule
- Intactness of IV system
- Appearance of IV site (e.g., dry, tissue infiltration, discomfort)
- Urinary output compared to urinary intake
- Tissue turgor; specific gravity of urine
- Vital signs and lung sounds compared to baseline data

CHANGING INTRAVENOUS CONTAINERS, TUBING, AND DRESSINGS Intravenous solution containers are changed when only a small amount of fluid remains in the neck of the container and fluid still remains in the drip chamber. However, all IV bags should be changed every 24 hours, regardless of how much solution remains, to minimize the risk of contamination. IV tubing is changed every 48 to 96 hours, depending on agency protocol, as is the site dressing. Skill 36–3 provides guidelines for changing an IV solution container, tubing, and the IV site dressing.

SKILL 36–3

CHANGING AN INTRAVENOUS CONTAINER, TUBING, AND DRESSING

PURPOSES
- To maintain the flow of required fluids
- To maintain sterility of the IV system and decrease the incidence of phlebitis and infection
- To maintain patency of the IV tubing
- To prevent infection at the IV site and the introduction of microorganisms into the bloodstream

ASSESSMENT
Assess the following:
- Presence of fluid infiltration, bleeding, or phlebitis at IV site
- Allergy to tape or iodine
- Infusion rate and amount absorbed
- Blockages in IV system
- Appearance of the dressing for integrity, moisture, and need for change
- The date and the time of the previous dressing change

PLANNING
Review primary care provider's orders for changes in fluid administration.

> **Delegation**
> This procedure includes assessment of the IV site and should be completed by a registered nurse. In many states, licensed vocational nurses with IV certification may complete the procedure.

EQUIPMENT
- Container with the correct kind and amount of sterile solution
- Administration set, including sterile tubing and drip chamber
- Timing label
- Sterile gauze square for positioning the needle

For the Dressing
- Clean gloves
- Sterile 2-in. × 2-in. or 4-in. × 4-in. gauze or transparent dressing
- Adhesive remover
- Chlorhexidine swabs
- Alcohol swabs
- Tape
- Towel

IMPLEMENTATION

Preparation
1. Obtain the correct solution container.
   - Read the label of the new container.
   - Verify that you have the correct solution, correct client, correct additives (if any), and correct dose (number of bags or total volume ordered).

Performance
1. Perform hand hygiene.
2. Set up the intravenous equipment with the new container and label all. See Skill 36–1, steps 1 to 8.
   - Apply a timing label to the container.
   - Prime the tubing.
   - Label the tubing.
3. Prepare the IV needle or catheter, tape, and the dressing equipment near the client.
   - Prepare strips of tape as needed for the type of needle or catheter. For the butterfly needle, two or three strips of 1.25-cm (1/2-in.) tape are needed. For a catheter, three strips of 1.25-cm (1/2-in.) tape are needed. These will be used later to secure the needle or catheter without covering the insertion site.
   - Hang the pieces of tape from the edge of a table. **Rationale:** *This places the tape in readiness for use without disrupting the adhesive.* Ensure that the table is clean *to avoid contaminating the tape.*
   - Open all equipment: swabs, dressing and adhesive bandage, and ointment. **Rationale:** *This facilitates access to supplies after gloves are donned.*
   - Place a towel under the extremity. **Rationale:** *This prevents soiling of bed linens.*
   - Apply clean gloves.

4. Remove the soiled dressing and all tape, except the tape holding the catheter or IV needle in place.
   - Remove tape and gauze from the old dressing one layer at a time. **Rationale:** *This prevents dislodgment of the catheter or needle in case tubing becomes entangled between layers of dressing.*
   - Remove adhesive dressings in the direction of the client's hair growth when possible. **Rationale:** *This minimizes discomfort when adhesive is removed from the skin.*
   - Discard the used dressing materials in the appropriate container.
5. Assess the IV site.
   - Inspect the IV site for the presence of infiltration or inflammation. **Rationale:** *Inflammation or infiltration necessitates removal of the IV needle or catheter to avoid further trauma to the tissues.*
   - Go to step 6, or discontinue and relocate the IV site if indicated. See Skill 36–1.
6. Disconnect the used tubing.
   - Place a sterile swab under the hub of the catheter. **Rationale:** *This absorbs any leakage that might occur when the tubing is disconnected.*
   - Clamp the tubing. With the fourth or fifth finger of the nondominant hand, apply pressure to the vein above the end of the catheter. **Rationale:** *This helps prevent blood from coming out of the needle during the change of tubing.*
   - Holding the hub of the catheter with the thumb and index finger of the nondominant hand, loosen the tubing with the dominant hand, using a twisting, pulling motion. **Rationale:** *Holding the catheter firmly but gently maintains its position in the vein.*
   - Remove the used IV tubing.

(continued)

CHANGING AN INTRAVENOUS CONTAINER, TUBING, AND DRESSING *(continued)*

- Place the end of the tubing in the basin or other receptacle.

7. Connect the new tubing, and reestablish the infusion.
   - Continue to hold the catheter and grasp the new tubing with the dominant hand.
   - Remove the protective tubing cap and, maintaining sterility, insert the tubing end securely into the needle hub. Twist it to secure it.
   - Open the clamp to start the solution flowing.

8. Remove the tape securing the needle or catheter.
   - When removing this tape and while cleaning the site, stabilize the needle or catheter hub with one hand. **Rationale:** *This prevents inadvertent dislodgement of the needle or catheter.*

9. Clean the IV site.
   - Start with adhesive remover to remove adhesive residue. **Rationale:** *Removal of adhesive residue facilitates adherence of the new dressing.*
   - Then, using chlorhexidine swabs or alcohol swabs, clean the site, beginning at the catheter or needle and cleaning outward in a 2-in. diameter. **Rationale:** *Cleaning in this manner prevents contamination of the IV site from bacteria on the peripheral skin areas. Antiseptics*

reduce the number of microorganisms present at the site, thus reducing the risk of infection.
   - Follow agency protocol about cleaning procedures.

10. Retape the needle or catheter.
   - For a butterfly needle, apply strips of tape to the wings of the butterfly using the crisscross (chevron) method (Figure 5 in Skill 36–1).
   - For a catheter; apply the tape using the U method (Figure 3 in Skill 36–1).
   - Apply a sterile transparent dressing over the site.
   - Remove gloves.

11. Label the dressing and secure IV tubing.
   - Place the date and time of the dressing change and your initials either on the label provided or directly over the top of the dressing.
   - Secure IV tubing with additional tape as required.

12. Regulate the rate of flow of the solution according to the order on the chart.

13. Document all relevant information.
   - Record the change of the solution container, tubing, and/or dressing in the appropriate place on the client's chart. Also record the fluid intake according to agency practice. Record the number of the container if the containers are numbered at the agency. Also record your assessments.

EVALUATION

Evaluate the following:

- Status of IV site
- Patency of IV system
- Accuracy of flow

When an IV infusion is no longer necessary to maintain the client's fluid intake or to provide a route for medication administration, the infusion is either discontinued and the catheter removed or the catheter is left in place and converted to a saline or heparin lock. If the catheter is removed it should be examined to assure that it is intact and the site should be cleaned and dressed. Converting the IV to a saline or heparin lock maintains IV access for intermittent or PRN medication and fluid administration, while allowing the client the freedom to move about. The patency of the catheter and insertion site must be periodically assessed and flushed to prevent clogging. A specific order must be written to convert the intravenous catheter to a lock.

Blood Transfusions

Intravenous fluids can be effective in restoring intravascular volume; however, they do not affect the oxygen carrying capacity of the blood. When red and white blood cells, platelets, or blood proteins are lost because of hemorrhage or disease, it may be necessary to replace these components to restore the blood's ability to transport oxygen and carbon dioxide, to clot, to fight infection, and to keep extracellular fluid within the intravascular compartment. A blood transfusion is the introduction of whole blood or blood components into the venous circulation.

BLOOD GROUPS   Human blood is commonly classified into four main groups (A, B, AB, and O). The surface of an individual's red blood cells contains a number of proteins known as antigens that are unique for each person. Many blood antigens have been identified, but the antigens A, B,

CULTURALLY COMPETENT CARE   **Blood and Blood Products**

- Jehovah's Witnesses do not receive blood or blood products. Blood volume expanders are acceptable if they are not derivatives of blood.
- Christian Scientists do not ordinarily use blood or blood products.

Note: From Transcultural Concepts in Nursing Care (4th ed.) (pp. 470, 481), by M. M. Andrews and J. S. Boyle, 2003, Philadelphia: Lippincott Williams & Wilkins. Reprinted with permission.

TABLE 36–8	The Blood Groups with Their Constituent Agglutinogens and Agglutinins	
BLOOD TYPES	RBC ANTIGENS (AGGLUTINOGENS)	PLASMA ANTIBODIES (AGGLUTININS)
A	A	B
B	B	A
AB	A and B	—
O	—	A and B

and Rh are the most important in determining blood group or type. Because antigens promote *agglutination* or clumping of blood cells, they are also known as agglutinogens. The A antigen or agglutinogen is present on the RBCs of people with blood group A, the B antigen is present in people with blood group B, and both A and B antigens are found on the RBC surface in people with group AB blood. Neither antigen is present in people with group O blood.

Preformed antibodies to RBC antigens are present in the plasma; these antibodies are often called agglutinins. People with blood group A have B antibodies (agglutinins); A antibodies are present in people with blood group B; and people with blood group O have antibodies to both A and B antigens. People with group AB blood do not have antibodies to either A or B antigens (Table 36–8). When blood is transfused, the blood group of the donor and recipient must match to avoid an antigen-antibody reaction and destruction (hemolysis) of RBCs.

RHESUS (RH) FACTOR The Rh factor antigen is present on the RBCs of approximately 85% of the people in the United States. Blood that contains the Rh factor is known as

Rh-positive (Rh$^+$); when it is not present the blood is said to be Rh-negative (Rh$^-$). In contrast to the ABO blood groups, Rh$^-$ blood does not naturally contain Rh antibodies. However, on exposure to blood containing Rh factor (e.g., an Rh$^-$ mother carrying a fetus with Rh$^+$ blood, or transfusion of Rh$^+$ blood into a client who is Rh$^-$), Rh antibodies develop. Subsequent exposures to Rh$^+$ blood place the client at risk for an antigen-antibody reaction and hemolysis of RBCs.

BLOOD TYPING AND CROSSMATCHING To avoid transfusing incompatible red blood cells, both blood donor and recipient are typed and their blood crossmatched. Blood typing is done to determine the ABO blood group and Rh factor status. This test is also performed on pregnant women and neonates to assess for possible intrauterine exposure of either to an incompatible blood type (particularly Rh factor incompatibilities).

Because blood typing determines only the presence of the major ABO and Rh antigens, crossmatching also is necessary prior to transfusion to identify possible interactions of minor antigens with their corresponding antibodies. RBCs from the donor blood are mixed with serum from the recipient; a reagent (Coombs' serum) is added, and the mixture is examined for visible agglutination. If no antibodies to the donated RBCs are present in the recipient's serum, agglutination does not occur and the risk of transfusion reaction is small.

SELECTION OF BLOOD DONORS Screening of blood donors is rigorous, and requirements change frequently to maintain the safety of blood supplies. Criteria have been established to protect the donor from possible ill effects of donation and to protect the recipient from exposure to diseases transmitted through the blood (Table 36–9). The American Red

TABLE 36–9	Blood Donor Screening
BLOOD DONATION ACCEPTED	BLOOD DONATION DECLINED
• Be in general good health • Be 17–60 years of age • Weigh at least 110 pounds • Pulse 80–100 beats/minute and regular • Temperature should not exceed 99.5 F • Blood pressure 160/90 – 110/60 • Venipuncture site free of lesions, scars, or needle pricks inidicative of addiction to narcotics or frequent blood donation Reasons to Temporarily Refuse Blood Donation • Hypertension • Hypotension • Severe asthma • Anemia • Blood disorders • Brain or spinal surgery • Infectious disease within 4 weeks • Uncontrolled diabetes • Taking Accutane, antibiotics, antiinflammatory drugs (within past 24 hours), or birth control pills	• Ever tested positive for HIV • Have ever injected self with drugs or other substances not prescribed by physician • Any man who has ever had sex with another man – even once • Has hemophilia or other blood clotting disorder and received clotting factor concentrate • Engaged in sex for drugs or money • Lived in Western Europe since 1980 • Held in correctional facility for more than 72 hours in last 12 months • Born in, lived in, or had sex with anyone who lived in or received blood products in Cameroon, Central African Republic, Chad, Congo, Equatorial Guinea, Gabon, Niger, or Nigeria since 1977 • Spent a cumulative 3 months in Great Britain or spent cumulative six months in any part of Europe since 1980 • Are or have ever been in sexual contact with someone in the above list.

This list is not complete and is subject to frequent changes. Reprinted with permission from the American Red Cross. American Red Cross. (2009). *Blood donor requirements*. Retrieved from http://www.bloodbook.com/donr-requir.html

Cross refuses blood donations from people who ever tested positive for HIV, those who use self-injected drugs, men who have had sex with another man, clients with hemophilia or other blood clotting disorders, those who have engaged in sex for money, those held in a correctional facility for more than 72 hours in the last 12 months, people who lived in Western Europe since 1980, and people who have spent a cumulative three months in Great Britain or six months in any part of Europe since 1980. High or low blood pressure may exclude a donor. Low hemoglobin is also cause for temporary deferral of donors. Blood donors are unpaid volunteers. Potential donors are eliminated by a history of hepatitis, HIV infection (or risk factors for HIV infection), heart disease, most cancers, severe asthma, bleeding disorders, or convulsions. Donation may be deferred for people with malaria or who have been exposed to malaria or hepatitis or in situations of pregnancy, surgery, anemia, high or low blood pressure, and certain drugs.

BLOOD AND BLOOD PRODUCTS FOR TRANSFUSION Most clients do not require transfusion of whole blood. It is more common for clients to receive a transfusion of a particular blood component specific to their individual needs. Table 36–10 lists some of the common blood products that may be transfused.

TRANSFUSION REACTIONS Transfusion of ABO- or Rh-incompatible blood can result in a hemolytic transfusion reaction with destruction of the transfused RBCs and subsequent risk of kidney damage or failure. Other forms of transfusion reaction also may occur, including febrile, allergic, circulatory overload, and sepsis. Because the risk of an adverse reaction is high when blood is transfused, clients must be frequently and carefully assessed before and during transfusion. Many reactions become evident within 5 to 15 minutes of initiating the transfusion but they can develop any time during a transfusion; clients are closely monitored during the initial period of the transfusion. Stop the transfusion immediately if signs of a reaction develop. Possible transfusion reactions, their clinical signs, and nursing implications are listed in Table 36–11.

CLINICAL ALERT

Normal saline should always be used when giving a blood transfusion. If the client has an infusion of dextrose, stop that infusion and flush the line with saline prior to initiating the transfusion. Solutions other than saline can cause damage to the blood components.

ADMINISTERING BLOOD Special precautions are necessary when administering blood. When a transfusion is ordered, obtain the blood from the blood bank just before starting the transfusion. Do not store the blood in the refrigerator on the nursing unit; lack of temperature control may damage the blood. Once blood or a blood product is removed from the refrigerator, there is a limited amount of time to administer it (e.g., packed RBCs should not hang for more than 4 hours after being removed from the refrigerator). Follow agency policies for verifying that the unit is correct for the client. The U.S. Food and Drug Administration (FDA) requires blood products to have bar codes to allow for scanning and machine-readable information on blood and blood component container labels to help reduce medication errors (FDA, 2004). Blood is usually administered through a #18- to #20-gauge intravenous needle or catheter; using a smaller needle may slow the infusion and damage blood cells (although a smaller gauge needle may be necessary for small children or clients with small, fragile veins). A Y-type blood

TABLE 36–10   Blood Products for Transfusion

PRODUCT	USE
Whole blood	Not commonly used except for extreme cases of acute hemorrhage. Replaces blood volume and all blood products: RBCs, plasma, plasma proteins, fresh platelets, and other clotting factors.
Packed red blood cells (PRBCs)	Used to increase the oxygen-carrying capacity of blood in anemias, surgery, and disorders with slow bleeding. One unit of PRBCs has the same amount of oxygen-carrying RBCs as a unit of whole blood (Rosenthal, 2004, p. 23). One unit raises hematocrit by approximately 2% to 3%.
Autologous red blood cells	Used for blood replacement following planned elective surgery. Client donates blood for autologous transfusion 4–5 weeks prior to surgery.
Platelets	Replaces platelets in clients with bleeding disorders or platelet deficiency. Fresh platelets most effective. Each unit should increase the average adult client's platelet count by about 5,000 platelets/microliter (Rosenthal, 2004, p. 24).
Fresh frozen plasma	Expands blood volume and provides clotting factors. Does not need to be typed and crossmatched (contains no RBCs). Each unit will increase the level of any clotting factor by 2% to 3% in the average adult (Rosenthal, 2004, p. 26).
Albumin and plasma protein fraction	Blood volume expander; provides plasma proteins.
Clotting factors and cryoprecipitate	Used for clients with clotting factor deficiencies. Each provides different factors involved in the clotting pathway; cryoprecipitate also contains fibrinogen.

TABLE 36–11 **Transfusion Reactions**

REACTION: CAUSE	CLINICAL SIGNS	NURSING INTERVENTION*
Hemolytic reaction: incompatibility between client's blood and donor's blood	Chills, fever, headache, backache, dyspnea, cyanosis, chest pain, tachycardia, hypotension	1. Discontinue the transfusion immediately. **NOTE**: When the transfusion is discontinued, the blood tubing must be removed as well. Use *new* tubing for the normal saline infusion. 2. Maintain vascular access with normal saline, or according to agency protocol. 3. Notify the primary care provider immediately. 4. Monitor vital signs. 5. Monitor fluid intake and output. 6. Send the remaining blood, bag, filter, tubing, a sample of the client's blood, and a urine sample to the laboratory.
Febrile reaction: sensitivity of the client's blood to white blood cells, platelets, or plasma proteins	Fever; chills; warm, flushed skin; headache; anxiety; muscle pain	1. Discontinue the transfusion immediately. 2. Give antipyretics as ordered. 3. Notify the primary care provider. 4. Keep the vein open with a normal saline infusion.
Allergic reaction (mild): sensitivity to infused plasma proteins	Flushing, itching, urticaria, bronchial wheezing	1. Stop or slow the transfusion, depending on agency protocol. 2. Notify the primary care provider. 3. Administer medication (antihistamines) as ordered.
Allergic reaction (severe): antibody–antigen reaction	Dyspnea, chest pain, circulatory collapse, cardiac arrest	1. Stop the transfusion. 2. Keep the vein open with normal saline. 3. Notify the primary care provider immediately. 4. Monitor vital signs. Administer cardiopulmonary resuscitation if needed. 5. Administer medications and/or oxygen as ordered.
Circulatory overload: blood administered faster than the circulation can accommodate	Cough, dyspnea, crackles (rales), distended neck veins, tachycardia, hypertension	1. Place the client upright, with feet dependent. 2. Stop or slow the transfusion. 3. Notify the primary care provider. 4. Administer diuretics and oxygen as ordered.
Sepsis: contaminated blood administered	High fever, chills, vomiting, diarrhea, hypotension	1. Stop the transfusion. 2. Keep the vein open with a normal saline infusion. 3. Notify the primary care provider. 4. Administer IV fluids, antibiotics. 5. Obtain a blood specimen from the client for culture. 6. Send the remaining blood and tubing to the laboratory.

Nurses should follow the agency's protocol regarding interventions. These may vary among agencies.

transfusion set with an in-line or add-on filter is used when administering blood (Figure 36–14). One arm of the administration set connects to the blood; normal saline (0.9% NaCl) is attached to the other arm of the Y-type set. Saline is used to prime the set and flush the needle before administering blood. It also provides a means to keep the vein open should a transfusion reaction occur. No other IV solutions should be administered with blood; they may cause the blood cells to clump or cause clotting. A transfusion should be completed within 4 hours of initiation.

The risk of sepsis increases if blood hangs for a longer period. Blood tubing is changed after every 4 to 6 units per agency policy; new intravenous tubing is used following a transfusion.

Client consent for blood transfusion must be signed before infusion begins. Assess vital signs prior to beginning the infusion and then according to agency policy. Question the client about any previous adverse reactions to blood. Blood administration is never delegated to a UAP due to the complexity of the task. Consult the nurse practice act in your

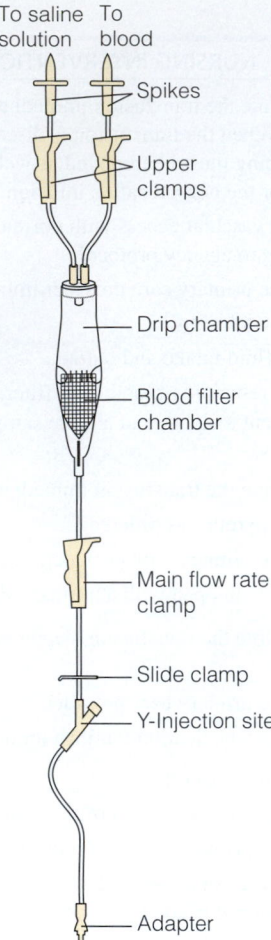

To saline   To
solution   blood

— Spikes

— Upper
  clamps

— Drip chamber

— Blood filter
  chamber

— Main flow rate
  clamp

— Slide clamp

— Y-Injection site

— Adapter

Figure 36–14 ⦿ Schematic of a Y-set for blood administration.

state to determine practical/vocational nurse's scope of practice related to blood transfusions.

Two nurses must check the blood using the blood bag label, the client's identification bracelet, and blood requisition forms. Assure that the blood has not expired. Specifically, check the client's name, identification number, blood type (A, B, AB, or O) and Rh group, the blood donor number, and the expiration date of the blood. Observe the blood for abnormal color, RBC clumping, gas bubbles, and extraneous material. Return outdated or abnormal blood to the blood bank. Use blood administration tubing appropriate for the component to be administered. Gloves should always be worn by the nurse when preparing blood for administration.

When beginning the transfusion adjust the flow rate with the main clamp. Run the blood slowly for the first 5–10 minutes while observing the client closely for clinical signs of reactions. Fifteen minutes after initiating the transfusion, check

the vital signs of the client. If there are no signs of a reaction, establish the required flow rate and assess the client, including vital signs every 30 minutes or more often, depending on the health status, until 1 hour post-transfusion. Most adults can tolerate receiving one unit of blood in 1½ to 2 hours. Do not transfuse a unit of blood for longer than 4 hours. Remind the client to call a nurse immediately if any unusual symptoms are felt during the transfusion. Throughout the transfusion the client should be assessed for manifestations of hypervolemia, status of the infusion site, and any unusual symptoms. If any abnormal symptoms are noted, the blood transfusion should be stopped immediately and new IV fluid and tubing hung to prevent any further blood from infusing. The blood bag and tubing should be sent to the laboratory for investigation of the blood.

When the transfusion is completed, discard the administration set according to agency practice. On the requisition attached to the blood unit, fill in the time the transfusion was completed and the amount transfused. Attach one copy of the requisition to the client's record and another to the empty blood bag. Return the blood bag and requisition to the blood bank.

EVALUATING

Using the overall goals identified in the planning stage of maintaining or restoring fluid balance, maintaining or restoring pulmonary ventilation and oxygenation, maintaining or restoring normal balance of electrolytes, and preventing associated risks of fluid, electrolyte, and acid–base imbalances, the nurse collects data to evaluate the effectiveness of interventions. Examples of desired outcomes for the identified goals are found in Identifying Nursing Diagnoses, Outcomes, and Interventions on pages 1124 and 1125.

If desired outcomes are not achieved, the nurse, client, and support person if appropriate need to explore the reasons before modifying the care plan. For example, if the outcome "Urine output is greater than 1,300 mL per day and within 500 mL of intake" is not achieved, questions to be considered might include:

- Have other outcome measures for the goal of achieving fluid balance been met?
- Does the client understand and comply with planned fluid intake?
- Is all urinary output being measured?
- Are unusual or excessive amounts of fluid being lost by another route (e.g., gastric suction, excessive perspiration, fever, rapid respiratory rate, wound drainage)?
- Are prescribed medications being taken or administered as ordered?

Nursing Care Plan   Deficient Fluid Volume

ASSESSMENT DATA	NURSING DIAGNOSIS	DESIRED OUTCOMES*
Nursing Assessment Merlyn Chapman, a 27-year-old sales clerk, reports weakness, malaise, and flu-like symptoms for 3–4 days. Although thirsty, she is unable to tolerate fluids because of nausea and vomiting, and she has liquid stools 2–4 times per day.	*Deficient Fluid Volume* related to nausea, vomiting, and diarrhea as evidenced by decreased urine output, increased urine concentration, weakness, fever, decreased skin/tongue turgor, dry mucous membranes, increased pulse rate, and decreased blood pressure	Electrolyte & Acid/Base Balance [0600] as evidenced by not compromised: • Serum electrolytes • Muscle strength Fluid Balance [0601] as evidenced by not compromised: • 24-hour intake and output balance • Urine specific gravity • Blood pressure, pulse, and body temperature • Skin turgor • Moist mucous membranes

Physical Examination

Height: 160 cm (5′ 3″)
Weight: 66.2 kg (146 lb)
Mild fever: 38.6°C (101.5°F)
Pulse: 86 BPM
Respirations: 24/minute
Scant urine output
BP: 102/84 mm Hg
Dry oral mucosa, furrowed tongue, cracked lips

Diagnostic Data

Urine specific gravity: 1.035
Serum sodium 155 mEq/L
Serum potassium 3.2 mEq/L
Chest x-ray negative

NURSING INTERVENTIONS*/SELECTED ACTIVITIES	RATIONALE
Electrolyte Management: Hypokalemia [2007]	
Obtain specimens for analysis of altered potassium levels (e.g., serum and urine potassium) as indicated.	*Urine and serum analysis provides information about extracellular levels of potassium. There is no practical way to measure intracellular K[1].*
Administer prescribed supplemental potassium (PO, NG, or IV) per policy.	*Low potassium levels are dangerous and Mrs. Chapman may require supplements.*
Monitor for neurologic and neuromuscular manifestations of hypokalemia (e.g., muscle weakness, lethargy, altered level of consciousness).	*Potassium is a vital electrolyte for skeletal and smooth muscle activity.*
Monitor for cardiac manifestations of hypokalemia (e.g., hypotension, tachycardia, weak pulse, rhythm irregularities).	*Many cardiac rhythm disorders can result from hypokalemia. It is critical to monitor cardiac function with hypokalemia.*
Electrolyte Management: Hypernatremia [2004]	
Obtain specimens for analysis of altered sodium levels (e.g., serum and urine sodium, urine osmolality, and urine specific gravity) as indicated.	*Urine analysis provides information about retention or loss of sodium and the ability of the kidneys to concentrate or dilute urine in response to fluid changes.*
Provide frequent oral hygiene.	*Oral mucous membranes become dry and sticky due to loss of fluid in the interstitial spaces.*
Monitor for neurologic and neuromuscular manifestations of hypernatremia (e.g., lethargy, irritability, seizures, and hyperreflexia).	*Hypernatremia, as a result of low fluid volume, creates a hypertonic vascular space, which causes water to move out of the cells, including brain cells. This accounts for neurologic symptoms.*
Monitor for cardiac manifestations of hypernatremia (e.g., tachycardia, orthostatic hypotension).	*The heart responds to a loss of fluid by increasing the heart rate to compensate with an increase in cardiac output. Low fluid volume leads to a fall in blood pressure.*
Fluid Management [4120]	
Weigh daily and monitor trends.	*Weight helps to assess fluid balance.*
Maintain accurate I & O record.	*Accurate records are critical in assessing the patient's fluid balance.*
Monitor vital signs as appropriate.	*Vital sign changes such as increased heart rate, decreased blood pressure, and increased temperature indicate hypovolemia.*
Give fluids as appropriate.	*As her nausea decreases encourage her oral intake of fluids as tolerated, again to replace lost volume.*
Administer IV therapy as prescribed.	*Mrs. Chapman has signs of severe fluid volume deficit. She will probably require intravenous replacement of fluid. This is especially true because her oral intake is limited because of nausea and vomiting.*

(continued)

Nursing Care Plan Deficient Fluid Volume *(continued)*

EVALUATION

Outcomes met. Mrs. Chapman remained hospitalized for 48 hours. She required fluid replacement of a total of 5 liters. Her blood pressure increased to 122/74, pulse rate decreased to a resting level of 74, and respirations decreased to 12/minute. Her urine output increased as the fluid was replaced and was adequate at > 0.5 mL/kg/hour by the time of discharge. The urine specific gravity was 1.015. Lab work on the day of discharge was: $K+$: 3.8 and $Na+$: 140. She had elastic skin turgor and moist mucous membranes. She was taking oral fluids and was able to discuss symptoms of deficient fluid volume that would necessitate her calling her health care provider.

The NOC # for desired outcomes and the NIC # for nursing interventions and selected activities are listed in brackets following the appropriate outcome or intervention. Outcomes, interventions, and activities selected are only a sample of those suggested by NOC and NIC and should be further individualized for each client.

CRITICAL THINKING QUESTIONS

1. What action would you take if Mrs. Chapman's heart became irregular?

2. Mrs. Chapman is responding inappropriately to your questions; she seems to be confused. What do you think is happening?

3. Offer suggestions for ways to help Mrs. Chapman increase her oral intake.

4. Mrs. Chapman asks why you weigh her every morning. How do you respond?

∞ *See Answers in MyNursingKit.*

CONCEPT MAP   Deficient Fluid Volume

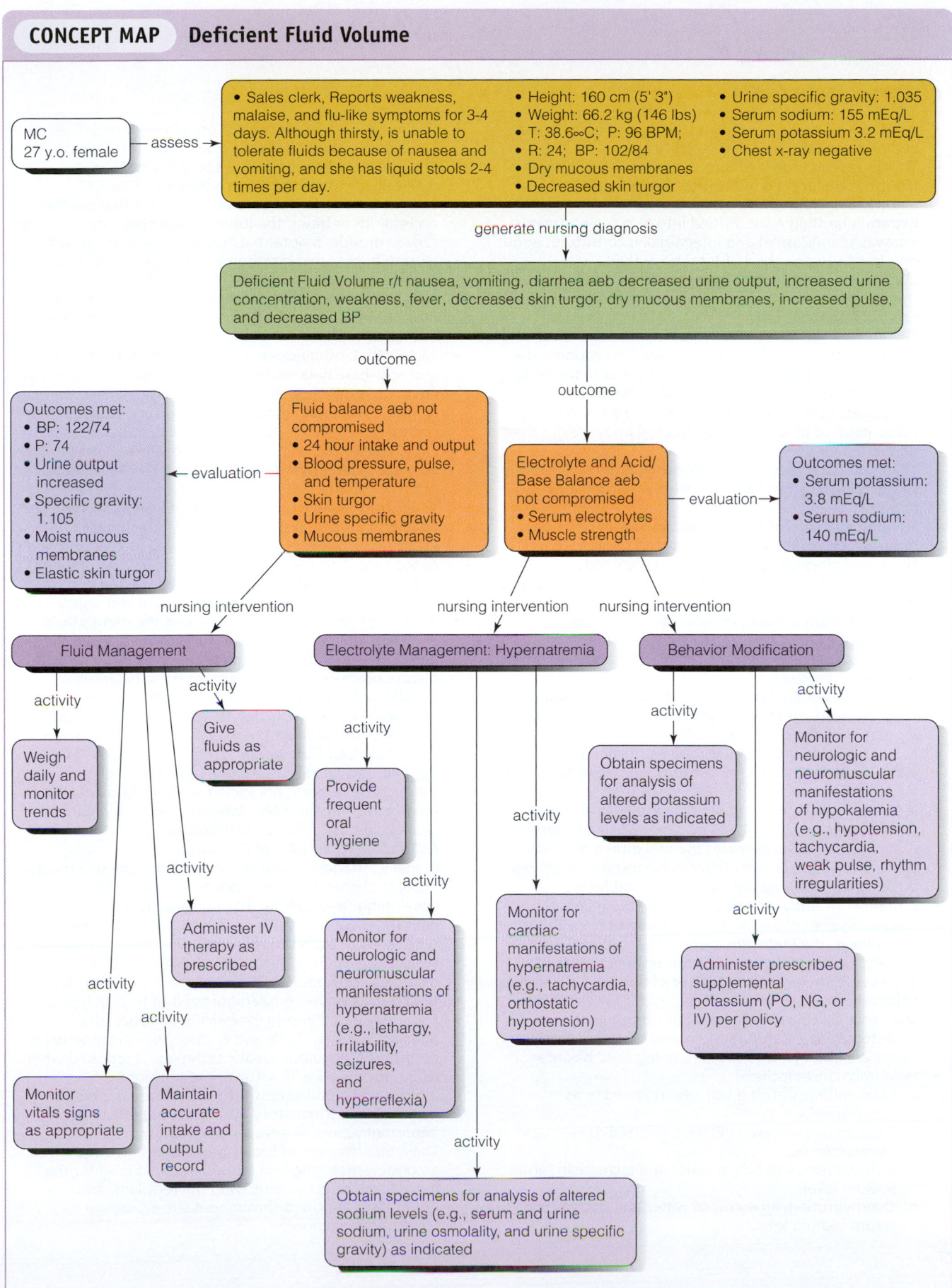

CHAPTER HIGHLIGHTS

- A balance of fluids, electrolytes, acids, and bases in the body is necessary for health and life.
- The body fluid is divided into two major compartments: the intracellular fluid (ICF) inside the cells and extracellular fluid (ECF) outside the cells.
- Extracellular fluid is subdivided into two compartments: intravascular (plasma) and interstitial. It constitutes about one-fourth to one-third of total body fluid.
- ECF is in constant motion throughout the body. It is the transport system that carries nutrients to and waste products from the cells.
- The percentage of total body fluids varies according to the individual's age, body fat, and sex. The younger the person, the higher the proportion of water in the body. The less body fat present, the greater the proportion of body fluid. Postadolescent females have a smaller percentage of fluid in relation to total body weight than do men.
- There are two types of body electrolytes (ions): positively charged ions (cations) and negatively charged ions (anions).
- The principal ions of ECF are sodium and chloride; the principal ions of ICF are potassium and phosphate.
- Fluids and electrolytes move among the body compartments by osmosis, diffusion, filtration, and active transport.
- The major fluid pressures exerted as part of the movement of fluid and electrolytes from one compartment to another are osmotic pressure and hydrostatic pressure.
- The three sources of body fluid are fluids taken orally, food ingested, and the oxidation of food. Fluid intake is regulated by the thirst mechanism.
- Fluid output occurs chiefly through excretion of urine, although body fluid is also lost through sweat, feces, and insensible vapor loss.
- In healthy adults, measurable fluid intake and output should balance (about 1,500 mL per day). The output of urine normally approximates the oral intake of fluids. Water from food and oxidation is balanced by fluid loss through the skin, respiratory process, and feces.
- A number of body systems and organs are involved in regulating the volume and composition of body fluids: the kidneys, the endocrine system, the cardiovascular system, the lungs, and the gastrointestinal system. The kidneys are the primary regulator of fluid and electrolyte balance.
- Substances such as the antidiuretic hormone, the renin-angiotensin-aldosterone system, and the atrial natriuretic factor are also involved in maintaining fluid balance.
- Fluid imbalances include:
  a. Fluid volume deficit (FVD), also referred to as hypovolemia.
  b. Fluid volume excess (FVE), also referred to as hypervolemia.
  c. Dehydration, a deficit in water and increase in serum sodium level.
  d. Overhydration, an excess of water and decrease in serum sodium level.

- The most common electrolyte imbalances are deficits or excesses in sodium, potassium, and calcium.
- The acid–base balance (pH range) of body fluids is maintained within a precise range of 7.35 to 7.45.
- Acid–base balance is regulated by buffers that neutralize excess acids or bases; the lungs, which eliminate or retain carbon dioxide, a potential acid; and the kidneys, which excrete or conserve bicarbonate and hydrogen ions.
- Acid–base imbalance occurs when the normal 20-to-1 ratio of bicarbonate to carbonic acid is upset. Imbalances may be either respiratory or metabolic in origin; either can result in acidosis or alkalosis.
- Factors that influence an individual's fluid, electrolyte, and acid–base balance include age, gender and body size, environmental temperature, and lifestyle. Illness, trauma, surgery, and certain medications can place individuals at risk for fluid, electrolyte, and acid–base imbalances.
- Fluid, electrolyte, and acid–base imbalance is most accurately determined through laboratory examination of blood plasma.
- Assessment relative to fluid, electrolyte, and acid–base balances includes (a) a nursing history; (b) physical examination of the skin, oral cavity, eyes, jugular vein, veins of the hand, and the neurologic system; (c) measurement of body weight, vital signs, and fluid intake and output; and (d) various diagnostic studies of blood and urine.
- A nursing history includes data about the client's fluid and food intake; fluid output; signs of fluid, electrolyte, and acid–base imbalances; and medications, therapies, or disease processes that may disrupt these balances.
- NANDA-approved nursing diagnoses that relate specifically to fluid, electrolyte, and acid–base imbalances include *Deficient Fluid Volume, Excess Fluid Volume, Risk for Imbalanced Fluid Volume, Risk for Deficient Fluid Volume,* and *Impaired Gas Exchange.* Other diagnoses that may be relevant are *Impaired Oral Mucous Membrane, Impaired Skin Integrity, Decreased Cardiac Output, Impaired Tissue Perfusion, Activity Intolerance, Risk for Injury,* and *Acute Confusion.*
- In many instances, fluids and electrolytes can be provided orally to clients who are experiencing or at risk of developing fluid deficits. The nurse needs to establish with the client a 24-hour plan for ingesting the necessary fluids and to respect the client's fluid preferences.
- For clients with fluid retention, fluids may need to be restricted; a schedule and short-term goals that make the fluid restriction more tolerable need to be developed.
- For clients experiencing excessive fluid losses, the administration of fluids and electrolytes intravenously is necessary. Meticulous aseptic technique is required when caring for clients with intravenous infusions.
- Preventing complications such as infiltration, phlebitis, hypervolemia (circulatory overload), and infection is an important aspect of intravenous therapy.
- The administration of blood transfusions involves accurately matching and identifying the blood for the individual, correctly identifying the recipient, and monitoring the client throughout the procedure for transfusion reactions.

THINK ABOUT IT

Refer to the chapter-opening scenario and answer these questions.

1. As the nurse who admits this client to the emergency department, what alterations will you anticipate in this client's vital signs and serum electrolytes?

2. What type of IV fluid would you anticipate will be ordered for this client? Explain your answer.

3. When initiating an IV on this client, what factors will you consider to help you choose the best IV site?

∞ *See suggested responses to Think About It on MyNursingKit.*

TEST YOUR KNOWLEDGE

1. When caring for a client with protein malnutrition, the nurse assesses for which of the following because of the role of protein in normal fluid homeostasis?
1. Increased blood pressure
2. Weak, rapid pulse
3. Edema
4. Jugular vein distention

2. The nurse observes a client hyperventilating and recognizes that this will have what effect on normal acid–base balance?
1. Increase the pH
2. Decrease the pH
3. Increase bicarbonate elimination by the kidney
4. Decrease bicarbonate elimination by the kidney

3. The nurse is volunteering in the first aid tent at a local marathon. Which of the following clients would be at greatest risk for alterations in normal fluid and electrolyte balance?
1. The 21-year-old woman running her first marathon
2. The 25-year-old man running his third marathon on a warm day
3. The 67-year-old experienced male runner who has run in numerous races
4. The 16-year-old male running in his fourth marathon

4. An older client comes to the emergency department experiencing chest pain and shortness of breath. An arterial blood gas is ordered. Which of the following ABG results indicates respiratory acidosis?
1. pH 7.54; $PaCO_2$ 28 mm Hg; HCO_3 22 mEq/L
2. pH 7.32; $PaCO_2$ 46 mm Hg; HCO_3 24 mEq/L
3. pH 7.31; $PaCO_2$ 35 mm Hg; HCO_3 20 mEq/L
4. pH 7.50; $PaCO_2$ 37 mm Hg; HCO_3 28 mEq/L

5. The intake and output (I&O) record of a client with a nasogastric tube that has been attached to suction for 2 days shows greater output than input. Which nursing diagnoses are most applicable? Select all that apply.
1. *Deficient Fluid Volume*
2. *Risk for Deficient Fluid Volume*
3. *Impaired Oral Mucous Membranes*
4. *Impaired Gas Exchange*
5. *Decreased Cardiac Output*

6. Which of the following client statements indicates a need for further teaching regarding treatment for hyperkalemia?
1. "I will eat avocado in my salads."
2. "I will be sure to check my heart rate before I take my digoxin."
3. "I will take my potassium in the morning after eating breakfast."
4. "I will stop using my salt substitute."

7. An older adult man is admitted to the medical unit with a diagnosis of dehydration. Which of the following signs or symptoms are most representative of a sodium imbalance?
1. Hyperreflexia
2. Mental confusion
3. Irregular pulse
4. Muscle weakness

8. The client's arterial blood gas results are: pH 7.32; $PaCO_2$ 58; HCO_3 32. The nurse knows that the client is experiencing which acid–base imbalance?
1. Metabolic acidosis
2. Respiratory acidosis
3. Metabolic alkalosis
4. Respiratory alkalosis

9. A client is admitted to the hospital for hypocalcemia. Nursing interventions relating to which system would have the highest priority?
1. Renal
2. Cardiac
3. Gastrointestinal
4. Neuromuscular

10. The nurse is evaluating the effectiveness of treatment aimed at correcting fluid volume excess. Which of the following would provide the best indication treatment was effective?
1. The client is no longer dyspneic.
2. The client has lost 12 pounds in the past 24 hours.
3. The client no longer displays pitting edema in the ankles.
4. The client's output is greater than intake.

∞ *See answers to Test Your Knowledge in Appendix A.*

REFERENCES AND SELECTED BIBLIOGRAPHY

Allen, K. (2005). Four-step method of interpreting arterial blood gas analysis. *Nursing Times, 101*(1), 42–45.

American Medical Association, American Nurses Association–American Nurses Foundations, Centers for Disease Control and Prevention, Center for Food Safety and Applied Nutrition, Food and Drug Administration, Food Safety and Inspection Service, U.S. Department of Agriculture. (2004). Diagnosis and management of foodborne illnesses: A primer for physicians and other health care professionals. *Morbidity and Mortality Weekly Report, 53* (RR-4), 1–33.

American Red Cross. (2009). *Blood donor requirements.* Retrieved June 17, 2009, from http://www.bloodbook.com/donr-requir.html

Anderson, N. R. (2005). When to use a midline catheter. *Nursing, 35*(4), 28.

Andrews, M. M., & Boyle, J. S. (2003). *Transcultural concepts in nursing care* (4th ed.). Philadelphia: Lippincott Williams & Wilkins.

Astle, S. M. (2005). Restoring electrolyte balance. *RN, 68*(5), 34–39.

Bennett, J. A., Thomas, V., & Riegel, B. (2004). Unrecognized chronic dehydration in older adults. Examining prevalence rate and risk factors. *Journal of Gerontological Nursing, 30*(1), 22–28.

Bulechek, G. M., Butcher, H. K., & Dochterman, J. M. (Eds.). (2008). *Nursing interventions: classification (NIC)* (5th ed.). St. Louis, MO: Mosby.

Bunce, M. (2003). Troubleshooting central lines. *RN, 66*(12), 28–33.

Burger, C. M. (2004). Hyperkalemia: When serum K+ is not okay. *American Journal of Nursing, 104*(10), 66–70.

Burger, C. M. (2004). Hypokalemia: Averting crisis with early recognition and intervention. *American Journal of Nursing, 104*(11), 61–65.

Centers for Disease Control and Prevention. (2002). Guidelines for the prevention of intravascular catheter-related infections. *Morbidity and Mortality Weekly Report, 51*(10), 1–29.

Corbett, J. V. (2008). *Laboratory tests and diagnostic procedures with nursing diagnoses* (7th ed.). Upper Saddle River, NJ: Pearson Prentice Hall.

Deglin, J. H., & Vallerand, A. H. (2008). *Davis's drug guide for nurses* (11th ed.). Philadelphia: Davis.

Dulak, S. B. (2005). Technology today: Smart IV pumps. *RN, 68*(12), 38–43.

Elgart, H. N. (2004). Assessment of fluids and electrolytes. *AACN Clinical Issues, 15*(4), 607–621.

Food and Drug Administration (FDA). (2004). Bar code label requirements for human drug products and biological products. *Federal Register, 69*(38), 9119–9171.

Hadaway, L. C. (2003). Infusing without infecting. *Nursing, 33*(10), 58–64.

Hadaway, L. C. (2004). Preventing and managing peripheral extravasation. *Nursing, 34*(5), 66–67.

Hadaway, L. C. (2005). Reopen the pipeline for I.V. therapy. *Nursing, 35*(8), 54–61.

Hadaway, L. C. (2006). Keeping central line infection at bay. *Nursing, 36*(4), 58–63.

Hayes, D. D. (2004). Balancing act: What happens when sodium and water are off-kilter? *Nursing Made Incredibly Easy, 2*(1), 52–57.

Hayes, D. D. (2004). Magnesium's balancing act. *Nursing Made Incredibly Easy, 2*(4), 44–50.

Hayes, D. D. (2004). Phosphorus: Here, there, everywhere. *Nursing Made Incredibly Easy, 2*(6), 36–41.

Hayes, D. D. (2004). Calcium in the balance. *Nursing Made Incredibly Easy, 2*(2), 46–53.

Hogan, M. A., & Wane, D. (2003). *Fluids, electrolytes, & acid-base balance: Reviews & rationales.* Upper Saddle River, NJ: Prentice Hall.

Just the facts: Fluids & electrolytes. (2005). Philadelphia: Lippincott Williams & Wilkins.

Lynes, D. (2003). Respiratory care skills: An introduction to blood gas analysis. *Nursing Times, 99*(11), 54–55.

Marders, J. (2005). Sounding the alarm for I.V. infiltration. *Nursing, 35*(4), 19–20.

Masoorli, S., & Angeles, T. (2002). Getting a line on central vascular access devices. *Nursing, 32*(4), 36–43.

Moorhead, S., Johnson, M., & Maas, M. L., & Swanson, E. (Eds.). (2008). *Nursing outcomes classification (NOC)* (4th ed.). St. Louis: Mosby.

Moureau, N. L. (2003). Is your skin-prep technique up-to-date? *Nursing, 33*(11), 17.

Moureau, N. L. (2004). Tips for inserting an I.V. in an older patient. *Nursing, 34*(7), 18.

NANDA International. (2009). *NANDA nursing diagnoses: Definitions and classification 2009–2011.* West Sussex, U.K.: Wiley-Blackwell.

Newberry, N. (Ed.). (2009). *Sheehy's emergency nursing* (6th ed.). St. Louis: Mosby.

Phillips, L. D. (2005). *Manual of I.V. therapeutics* (4th ed.). Philadelphia: Davis.

Pruitt, W. C., & Jacobs, M. (2004). Interpreting arterial blood gases: Easy as ABC. *Nursing, 34*(8), 50–53.

Quillen, T. F. (2005). Myths & facts: About hypercalcemia. *Nursing, 35*(7), 74.

Rosenthal, K. (2004). It's not magic! The tricks to cannulating difficult veins. *Nursing Made Incredibly Easy, 2*(2), 4–7.

Rosenthal, K. (2004). The line—for central venous access—forms here. *Nursing Made Incredibly Easy, 2*(5), 4–7.

Rosenthal, K. (2004). What you should know about needleless I.V. systems. *Nursing, 34*(9), 76.

Rosenthal, K. (2004). Avoiding bad blood: Key steps to safe transfusions. *Nursing Made Incredibly Easy, 2*(5), 20–29.

Rosenthal, K. (2005). Documenting peripheral I.V. therapy. *Nursing, 35*(7), 28.

Rosenthal, K. (2005a). Tailor your I.V. insertion techniques for special populations. *Nursing, 35*(5), 37–41.

Rosenthal, K. (2005b). Ports: The gateway to central lines. *Nursing Made Incredibly Easy, 3*(1), 53–56.

Simpson, H. (2004). Interpretation of arterial blood gases: A clinical guide for nurses. *British Journal of Nursing, 13*(9), 522–528.

Spandorfer, P. R., Alessandrini, E. A., Joffe, M. D., Localio, R., & Shaw, K. N. (2005). Oral versus intravenous rehydration of moderately dehydrated children: A randomized, controlled trial. *Pediatrics, 115*(2), 295–301.

Sweeney, J. (2005). What causes sudden hypokalemia? *Nursing, 35*(4), 12.

Sweeney, J. (2005). What causes hyponatremia? *Nursing, 35*(6), 18.

Trimble, T. (2003). Peripheral I.V. starts: Securing and removing the catheter. *Nursing, 33*(9), 26.

Wilburn, S. Q. (2004). Needlestick and sharps injury prevention. *Online Journal of Issues in Nursing, 9*(3), manuscript 4. Retrieved December 11, 2009, from http://www.nursingworld.org/MainMenuCategories/ANAMarketplace/ANAPeriodicals/OJIN/TableofContents/Volume92004/No3Sept04/InjuryPrevention.aspx

Yucha, C. (2004). Renal regulation of acid–base balance. *Nephrology Nursing Journal, 31*(2), 201–208.

CHAPTER 1

1. *Answer: 2 Rationale:* Florence Nightingale contributed to the nursing care of soldiers in the Crimean War. Dorothea Orem developed the theory of self-care needs. Linda Richards was the first American trained nurse, while Mary Mahoney was the first African American professional nurse. *Cognitive Level:* Knowledge *Client Need:* Not Applicable *Nursing Process:* Not Applicable

2. *Answer: 3 Rationale:* Health promotion focuses on maintaining normal status without consideration of diseases. Option 1 is an example of illness prevention. Option 2 is aesthetic (i.e., not needed for health promotion or disease prevention). Option 4 focuses on disease detection. *Cognitive Level:* Application *Client Need:* Health promotion and maintenance *Nursing Process:* Implementation

3. *Answer: 2 Rationale:* The competent nurse has some experience, which allows coordination of multiple complex nursing care demands that can be managed independently. Option 1, the advanced beginner, demonstrates marginally acceptable performance. Option 3, the proficient practitioner, has 3 to 5 years of experience and has developed a holistic understanding of the client. Option 4, the expert practitioner, demonstrates highly skilled intuitive and analytic ability in new situations. *Cognitive Level:* Knowledge *Client Need:* Safe, Effective Care Environment *Nursing Process:* Implementation

4. *Answer: 1 Rationale:* While all of these factors will impact nursing, only aging will impact the supply and demand for nurses. The aging population increases demand while retiring nurses and nurse faculty will impact supply. *Cognitive Level:* Analysis *Client Need:* Safe, Effective Care Environment *Nursing Process:* Planning

5. *Answer: 3 Rationale:* Continuing education refers to formalized experiences designed to enlarge the knowledge or skills of practitioners. The other answers are examples of in-service education, which is designed to upgrade the knowledge or skills of current employees with regard to the specific setting and is usually less formal in presentation. *Cognitive Level:* Analysis *Client Need:* Safe, Effective Care Environment *Nursing Process:* Implementation

6. *Answer: 2 Rationale:* Since the primary purpose of research is to improve the quality of client care, the nurse should determine if published research results are applicable to the nurse's specific client population. Published studies may have flawed designs, data collection, or analysis. Although more than one well-conducted study with similar findings supports usefulness of the results, applicability must still be determined for the specific client population. It is not realistic for the nurse to rerun the data to check the results of the study. *Cognitive Level:* Application *Client Need:* Safe, Effective Care Environment *Nursing Process:* Planning

7. *Answer: 4 Rationale:* The right of self-determination means that subjects feel free of constraints, coercion, or any undue influence to participate in a study. There is no information given to indicate other rights have been violated. *Cognitive Level:* Analysis *Client Need:* Safe, Effective Care Environment *Nursing Process:* Diagnosis

8. *Answer: 1 Rationale:* Practice disciplines are fields of study in which the central focus is performance of a professional role. Time and experience are necessary for developing proficiency in any profession or career. Research and theory development do not have performance as their primary focus. The primary focus of nursing is providing quality service to humans. Team or group practice can be a part of a career in humanities, computer science, or rocket science and is not specific to nursing. *Cognitive Level:* Application *Client Need:* Safe, Effective Care Environment *Nursing Process:* Planning

9. *Answer: 2 Rationale:* A group of related ideas or statements is a conceptual framework. A philosophy is a belief system; a supposition or system of ideas proposed to explain a given phenomenon is a theory; and a paradigm is a pattern of shared understandings and assumptions about reality and the world. *Cognitive Level:* Knowledge *Client Need:* Not Applicable *Nursing Process:* Not Applicable

10. *Answer: 2 Rationale:* Person/client, environment, health, and nursing are relevant when providing care for any client in any setting whether in the hospital, at home, in the community, or in elementary school systems. These elements can be used to understand diseases, conduct and apply research, develop nursing theories, as well as implement the nursing process which is one part of the metaparadigm but does not adequately explain everything encompassed. *Cognitive Level:* Application *Client Need:* Safe, Effective Care Environment *Nursing Process:* Implementation

CHAPTER 2

1. *Answer: 3 Rationale:* This is the best answer because the nurse is assessing the client's level of knowledge following the discussion with the primary care provider. Based on this assessment, the nurse may initiate other actions (e.g., call the primary care provider if the client has many questions). In option 1, the nurse is not assessing

the client to determine if they received enough information to give consent. Option 2 is one way to assess the client's level of knowledge regarding the procedure. However, it is not the best approach because it is a closed-ended question, asking for only a "yes" or "no" response. Option 3 provides more information from the client in his or her own words. The statement in option 4 is true; however, the nurse should first verify if the client received enough information to give consent. After the assessment, this statement may be appropriate but the assessment needs to be done first. *Cognitive Level:* Application *Client Need:* Safe, Effective Care Environment *Nursing Process:* Implementation

2. *Answer: 4 Rationale:* Battery is the willful touching of a person without permission. Another name for an unintentional tort is malpractice. This situation is intentional because the nurse executed the act willfully against the client's wishes and could be pursued as a crime. Assault is the attempt or threat to touch another person unjustifiably or without permission. Invasion of privacy injures the feelings of the person and does not take into consideration how revealing information or exposing the client will affect the client's feelings. *Cognitive Level:* Application *Client Need:* Safe, Effective Care Environment *Nursing Process:* Implementation

3. *Answer: 1 Rationale:* All elements such as duty, foreseeability, causation, harm/injury, and damages must be present for malpractice to be proven. The nurse is a licensed professional responsible for individual actions. Notifying the primary care provider does not exempt the nurse from liability. Since it is apparent the standard of practice was not performed, a breach of duty does exist. Violation/omission of the standard of practice resulted in an excessive dosage. Therefore foreseeability is present; however, no harm occurred to the client. *Cognitive Level:* Analysis *Client Need:* Safe, Effective Care Environment *Nursing Process:* Evaluation

4. *Answer: 4 Rationale:* The UAP must tactfully decline to perform the procedure because a sterile, invasive procedure that places the client at significant risk for infection is generally outside the scope of practice of a UAP, even if supervised by the nurse or permission is given by the client. Even though the UAP is a nursing student, the agency job description should be followed because those are the duties the student was hired to perform. The job description is the standard of care in this situation. *Cognitive Level:* Application *Client Need:* Safe, Effective Care Environment *Nursing Process:* Implementation

5. *Answer: 3 Rationale:* The only person entitled to information without written consent is the client and those providing direct care. The nurse has open access to information regarding assigned clients only. Therefore, the partner/spouse must sign a release form before accessing the medical record and the fact that she is a nurse employee has no legal bearing in this case. *Cognitive Level:* Analysis *Client Need:* Safe, Effective Care Environment *Nursing Process:* Implementation

6. *Answer: 1 Rationale:* A nurse's actions in an ethical dilemma must be defensible according to moral and ethical standards. The nurse may have strong personal beliefs but distancing oneself from the situation does not serve the client. A team is not always required to reach decisions and the nurse is not obligated to follow the client's wishes automatically in every situation, especially when they may have negative consequences for self or others. *Cognitive Level:* Analysis *Client Need:* Safe, Effective Care Environment *Nursing Process:* Planning

7. *Answer: 2 Rationale:* The nurse has an ethical responsibility to act only when actions are safe or risks minimized. This nurse is putting the client at unnecessary risk for a medication error. Many medical practices are controversial but not necessarily unethical (option 1). The nurse should follow the agency policy. Although some may view nurses' strikes as unethical, supporting others who are striking is a personal decision (option 3). Although a client statement in confidence to a nurse may have ethical overtones, it does not automatically constitute an ethical dilemma. Since the assigned health care provider is a member of the team, principles of confidentiality do not include him or her (option 4). *Cognitive Level:* Analysis *Client Need:* Safe, Effective Care Environment *Nursing Process:* Evaluation

8. *Answer: 1 Rationale:* Autonomy is the client's (or surrogate's) right to make his or her own decision. The nurse is obliged to respect a client's or significant others' informed decision. These parents may modify their decision as time goes on and the child's condition, or their feelings, change. This situation is not clearly one of nonmaleficence (do no harm) or beneficence (do good) since there are many aspects of both. If the child appeared to be suffering or an effective treatment was being denied, these principles might apply. Justice (fairness) generally applies when the rights of one client are being balanced against those of another client. *Cognitive Level:* Application *Client Need:* Safe, Effective Care Environment *Nursing Process:* Assessment

9. *Answer: 3 Rationale:* In values clarification, clients are assisted to think about the factors that influence their beliefs and decisions. Any judgmental statement that reflects the rightness or wrongness of the client's thoughts or actions will impede this process. *Cognitive Level:* Analysis *Client Need:* Safe, Effective Care Environment *Nursing Process:* Implementation

10. *Answer: 4 Rationale:* A major role of the client advocate is to mediate between conflicting parties. The nurse needs to assess the situation before offering an intervention. Informing the family is an intervention without assessment. If the primary care provider sends the client home, the nurse has not acted to assist in resolving or reducing the conflict. If the nurse assists in resolving or reducing the conflict, the added expense of an attorney may not be needed. However, legal action should be a last resort. *Cognitive Level:* Analysis *Client Need:* Safe, Effective Care Environment *Nursing Process:* Implementation

CHAPTER 3

1. *Answer: 3 Rationale:* Actions such as diet modification that help to prevent an illness or detect it in its early stages are primary prevention. Treatment of a disease such as antibiotic therapy or surgery is secondary prevention, while rehabilitation efforts following an illness are considered tertiary prevention. *Cognitive Level:* Application *Client Need:* Health Promotion and Maintenance *Nursing Process:* Assessment

2. *Answer: 2 Rationale:* City, county, state, or federal government funds pay for health department and agency activities aimed at the global health of the community. Hospitals may provide a variety of wellness and clinic programs in addition to inpatient services. Surgery may be performed in outpatient surgery centers and physicians' offices in addition to within hospitals. Skilled nursing, extended care, and long-term care facilities provide care to persons of all ages who require rehabilitation or subacute care. This is not necessarily related to insurance coverage for hospital stays. *Cognitive Level:* Analysis *Client Need:* Health Promotion and Maintenance *Nursing Process:* Not Applicable

3. *Answer: 3 Rationale: Nursing's Agenda for Healthcare Reform* (ANA, 1991) called for case management of those with ongoing health care needs. It also proposed that primary care be community based but that essential services be paid for by a combination of public and private funding sources (not just public funds) and be phased in gradually. *Cognitive Level:* Application *Client Need:* Health Promotion and Maintenance *Nursing Process:* Planning

4. *Answer: 2 Rationale:* In community-based health care, clients are cared for according to their geographical locations such as where they live or work, rather than at a major medical center or similar provider setting, which facilitates access. Emphasis is more on client wellness and prevention than on illness and may be paid for through any of the usual forms of insurance or payment (including managed care, private pay, or welfare). *Cognitive Level:* Analysis *Client Need:* Safe, Effective Care Environment *Nursing Process:* Implementation

5. *Answer: 2 Rationale:* In collaboration, each member of the team, including the client, participates in sharing ideas and reaching consensus on the best plan of care. The team is generally led by the health care professional most skilled in the client's specific areas of need. Once the plan is established, it may be implemented by any member of the team or a designate at an appropriate time and place. It not necessarily delegated by the nurse. *Cognitive Level:* Analysis *Client Need:* Safe, Effective Care Environment *Nursing Process:* Implementation.

6. *Answer: 4 Rationale:* Effective discharge planning would have included an assessment of home care needs prior to the client leaving the hospital. The kind of care is determined before the client leaves the current setting. That is why it is called discharge "planning." Following a thorough assessment, the client would be taught self-care strategies and a basic plan of care for the coming days. Obtaining medications and a ride home does not indicate the client possesses the knowledge and skills needed to manage care after discharge. If the client will need care at home, those referrals would be made by the discharge planner and communicated to the client. Option 4 indicates the client knows and accepts these referrals. *Cognitive Level:* Analysis *Client Need:* Safe, Effective Care Environment *Nursing Process:* Evaluation

7. *Answer: 4 Rationale:* The home health nurse more commonly works with single persons or families at one time—addressing their particular needs that may be similar to or different from those of others. The community health nurse will focus on activities that influence the larger group of individuals affected. These include prevention and monitoring of infectious disease plus actions that will promote health for multiple affected persons (e.g., food, water, and shelter). *Cognitive Level:* Comprehension *Client Need:* Safe, Effective Care Environment *Nursing Process:* Implementation

8. *Answer: 1 Rationale:* Assuming the client is medically stable, feeding and bathing are tasks within the aide's abilities. Teaching the client about or adjusting medications (and oxygen is considered a medication) and performing assessments are duties restricted to the registered nurse. *Cognitive Level:* Application *Client Need:* Safe, Effective Care Environment *Nursing Process:* Planning

9. *Answer: 2 Rationale:* The nurse needs to encourage the client to express feelings or thoughts that led to the refusal so that misunderstandings can be clarified and other possible solutions explored. The nurse should apply the principle that all behavior has meaning. Otherwise, the nurse is intervening before assessing the situation. In option 3, that approach did not work the first time. A reason for the refusal needs to be explored. Option 4 is almost a threat and has a paternalistic implication. Clients are entitled to make informed decisions to perform or not perform recommended activities. Notifying the primary care provider is implementing an intervention before the nurse has done an assessment. *Cognitive Level:* Application *Client Need:* Health Promotion and Maintenance *Nursing Process:* Implementation

10. *Answer: 1 Rationale:* If the caregiver's own health is becoming threatened, it may be a sign of overload. It would be appropriate for the caregiver to ask for assistance from others or to ask for clarification of ways he or she can assist the client. Sadness related to a poor prognosis would be a normal and expected response as long as it does not evolve into depression. *Cognitive Level:* Application *Client Need:* Psychosocial Integrity *Nursing Process:* Evaluation

CHAPTER 4

1. *Answer: 3 Rationale:* There is an ongoing shift in the North American population that includes a decreasing

number of Caucasian Americans (formerly the majority population) and increasing numbers of other cultural groups. The birth rate is actually decreasing, immigration has increased, and limited access to health care is a complex issue that is not the major factor here. *Cognitive Level:* Comprehension *Client Need:* Psychosocial Integrity *Nursing Process:* Planning

2. *Answer: 2 Rationale:* Cultural differences may result in various interpretations of a medical regime. Cultural sensitivity results in recognition of the right "not to fit." This is a standard of practice and should be initiated with all clients. Teaching or explaining the effects of lack of adherence would be more appropriate than warning. Asking a person of the same culture to assist may be helpful after the nurse discusses the matter with the client. *Cognitive Level:* Application *Client Need:* Psychosocial Integrity *Nursing Process:* Implementation

3. *Answer: 3 Rationale:* The nurse should indicate that he or she is open to diverse views and practices. Option 1 assumes the client follows this particular cultural practice, which may not be the case. The nurse should assess before intervening. It may be good to learn more about the culture (option 2), but that is not the best starting place to care for the client. Subcultures exist among all cultures. Reading books is helpful, but assessment of individual situations is the best approach. Option 4 reflects an incorrect approach to culturally appropriate care. The nurse needs to assess which customs and practices the individual client performs before drawing conclusions. *Cognitive Level:* Application *Client Need:* Psychosocial Integrity *Nursing Process:* Implementation

4. *Answer: 3 Rationale:* Culturally competent nursing care implies that, within the delivered care, the nurse understands and attends to the total context of the client's situation, including awareness of immigration, stress factors, and cultural differences. Options 1 and 2 do not show that the nurse needs to respect the choices made by the clients. Option 4 shows bias or stereotyping. *Cognitive Level:* Application *Client Need:* Psychosocial Integrity *Nursing Process:* Implementation

5. *Answer: 3 Rationale:* Culture involves socially inherited characteristics of a group. Race usually addresses shared physical characteristics among a group of individuals. *Cognitive Level:* Comprehension *Client Need:* Psychosocial Integrity *Nursing Process:* Implementation

6. *Answer: 4 Rationale:* The nurse should not create stereotypes about the client or make assumptions about what the client's beliefs might be. Instead, the nurse should assess the client to determine the client's cultural beliefs. *Cognitive Level:* Application *Client Need:* Psychosocial Integrity *Nursing Process:* Implementation

7. *Answer: 3 Rationale:* Accepting and accommodating the client's request is the best response. The nurse should understand that many women from the Middle East or Muslim religion may be uncomfortable with a male nurse. Choice 1 might solve the client's situation in the future but would do nothing for the client today.

Choice 2 demonstrates the nurse's defensive response to the client and does not place the client's needs first. Choice 4 requires the client to defend her preferences. *Cognitive Level:* Analysis *Client Need:* Psychosocial Integrity *Nursing Process:* Implementation

8. *Answer: 3 Rationale:* The Jewish religion prohibits the ingestion of meat and dairy products during the same meal. The nurse should ask that the entire meal tray be replaced by the dietary department. The other answers would not resolve the issue properly. *Cognitive Level:* Application *Client Need:* Psychosocial Integrity *Nursing Process:* Implementation

9. *Answer: 1 Rationale:* The nurse should notify the physician of the client's choices and continue to monitor for any problems that may arise to promote safe management of the client's condition. A nurse from the same culture is unnecessary, and discharging the client would be punitive. The nurse does not advocate by insisting the client go against cultural beliefs. *Cognitive Level:* Application *Client Need:* Psychosocial Integrity *Nursing Process:* Implementation

10. *Answer: 1, 4, and 5 Rationale:* Clients from the Hispanic culture may value herbal medicine, use of hot and cold foods, and a caregiver of the same gender. Staring would be seen as causing the evil eye and mourners would not be a common behavior for this culture *Cognitive Level:* Application *Client Need:* Psychosocial Integrity *Nursing Process:* Implementation

CHAPTER 5

1. *Answer: 2 Rationale:* Choices are often related to learned experiences, lifestyle, and values. The client obviously values the business more than physical health. When a person feels strongly enough, a lower level need (rest) can be postponed until a higher level need (success) is met. It is very likely that no one else can meet that need for him and the lower level need must still be met eventually. *Cognitive Level:* Application *Client Need:* Health Promotion and Maintenance *Nursing Process:* Assessment

2. *Answer: 2 Rationale:* Perceived self-efficacy is the confidence the person has for achieving the desired outcome. Option 1 is a person's perceptions about available time, inconvenience, expense, and difficulty performing the activity. Option 3 is the person's perceptions concerning the behaviors, beliefs, or attitudes of others. Option 4 refers to the person's perception of the environment and how it assists or detracts from the healthy behavior. *Cognitive Level:* Application *Client Need:* Health Promotion and Maintenance *Nursing Process:* Planning

3. *Answer: 4 Rationale:* The event causing the highest stress is losing a spouse according to statistics, but it is important to always assess each client's coping strategies in the face of any stressor because differences exist in how people respond to stressors. While the other events may produce stress, none produces as much stress as the

death of a loved one, especially when the death is unexpected or unpredictable. Acute stress increases catecholamine release and can result in illness. *Cognitive Level:* Analysis *Client Need:* Health Promotion and Maintenance *Nursing Process:* Assessment

4. *Answer: 1 Rationale:* Only option 1 provides a strategy for the action stage of change. Option 2 is a strategy for the contemplation stage, option 3 is a strategy for the preparation stage, and option 4 is a strategy for the maintenance stage. *Cognitive Level:* Application *Client Need:* Health Promotion and Maintenance *Nursing Process:* Implementation

5. *Answer: 4 Rationale:* Change is a complex process and a nurse should not give up or assume that the client doesn't want to change. People often resist a tough approach because it can make them feel cornered. This approach may work for some people but not for everyone. The goal of teaching is to try to help the client become the expert as well. *Cognitive Level:* Application *Client Need:* Health Promotion and Maintenance *Nursing Process:* Implementation

6. *Answer: 3 Rationale:* Frustration is an example of an emotion. The client who chooses healthy foods (option 1) represents the physical component, taking parenting classes enhances the intellectual component (option 2), and the bowling league (option 4) enhances both the physical and social components. *Cognitive Level:* Comprehension *Client Need:* Health Promotion and Maintenance *Nursing Process:* Assessment

7. *Answer: 2 Rationale:* The mother has taken on the sick role by expecting to be excused from her usual role responsibilities. The sick role states that persons are not answerable for their illness, contrary to the obese client's perspective. In the sick role, the client tries to get better as opposed to the man who misses his physical therapy appointments. The older adult is not following the sick role expectation to rely on competent help. *Cognitive Level:* Application *Client Need:* Health Promotion and Maintenance, and Physiological Adaptation *Nursing Process:* Assessment

8. *Answer: 3 Rationale:* Although the effectiveness of alternative therapies is sometimes not scientifically established, many people report significant benefit from them for a wide variety of conditions. Alternative therapies often cost less, but this is not always the case. Clients often seek alternative therapies because traditional therapies are ineffective, but some seek them as primary therapies before trying traditional therapy. Both forms of therapy may utilize products from nature. *Cognitive Level:* Application *Client Need:* Physiological Integrity *Nursing Process:* Implementation

9. *Answer: 1 Rationale:* Spirituality gives us purpose and meaning in life; involves a relationship with oneself, others, and a higher power; and involves finding significant meaning in the entirety of life. Spirituality is a much broader concept than religion and religious services. Responsibility to life patterns is a concept of hu-

manism. *Cognitive Level:* Application *Client Need:* Psychological Integrity *Nursing Process:* Planning

10. *Answer: 2 Rationale:* Healing environments help empower clients to make healthy decisions. They are not dependent on technology or physicians' orders. Aquariums are environmental interventions, not a general approach to clients. *Cognitive Level:* Application *Client Need:* Health Promotion

CHAPTER 6

1. *Answer: 2 Rationale:* The nurse has inferred and concluded something that is beyond the available information (and in this case is not accurate). The prescription and the diarrhea are facts. It would be judgment and opinion if the nurse stated that the laxative would make the diarrhea worse and should not be given. (Note: Critical thinking will cause this nurse to examine the assumptions made and gather more data before acting.) *Cognitive Level:* Analysis *Client Need:* Safe, Effective Care Environment *Nursing Process:* Evaluation

2. *Answer: 1 Rationale:* The nurse recognizes that many factors could interfere with the client eating—such as that the food presented is not culturally appropriate. These assumptions must be clarified. Options 2 and 3 reach conclusions not supported by the facts. In option 4, the nurse has made a judgment or has an opinion that may not be accurate. Also, the nurse is acting without assessment. Implementation should be preceded by assessment. *Cognitive Level:* Application *Client Need:* Physiological Integrity *Nursing Process:* Planning

3. *Answer: 4 Rationale:* The critical-thinking approach should include perseverance until a reasonable solution or answer is determined. Giving in (option 1), overquestioning self or poor trust in one's own beliefs (option 2), or bypassing normal hierarchies of authority (option 3) violate the desirable attitudes of integrity, intellectual courage, and confidence in reason. *Cognitive Level:* Application *Client Need:* Safe, Effective Care Environment *Nursing Process:* Implementation

4. *Answer: 1 Rationale:* The scientific method uses a research study-based approach to problem solving. Trial and error and intuition would involve unstructured approaches resulting in less predictable results. The nursing process generally uses application of known interventions, previously determined by the scientific (research) process. *Cognitive Level:* Application *Client Need:* Safe, Effective Care Environment *Nursing Process:* Planning

5. *Answer: 4 Rationale:* It is important to project what problems might interfere with the plan and have appropriate responses prepared to prevent the interferences. The purpose for the decision should have been clear enough at the outset as to not require reexamination at this point (option 1). Clients and families should be consulted early—in the purpose-setting and criteria-setting steps (option 2). Criteria should not be set until all

significant participants have an opportunity to present their point of view. Considering various means for reaching the outcomes is the same as examining alternatives (option 3). *Cognitive Level:* Application *Client Need:* Safe, Effective Care Environment *Nursing Process:* Planning

6. *Answer: 3 Rationale:* Critical thinkers first gather data for analysis before acting, so the first step would be to assess the client further in order to determine where the client's anxiety is originating from. Calling the physician before assessing the client would limit the amount of data and information the nurse could provide and may not be necessary depending on the cause of the anxiety (option 1). Assuming that the client's anxiety is related to insufficient knowledge would not demonstrate critical thinking because the nurse has formed an opinion with inadequate information (option 2). Creating a nursing diagnosis also must be preceded by an assessment for the cause of the anxiety. If the anxiety is easily removed once the cause is determined, there may be no need for adding the nursing diagnosis (option 4). *Cognitive Level:* Analysis *Client Need:* Psychosocial Integrity *Nursing Process:* Assessment

7. *Answer: 4 Rationale:* Critical thinking requires the gathering of information that can be analyzed to come to the correct conclusion. In this situation the student should find out what behavior is causing the instructor to make the suggestion because the student cannot change what he or she does not understand. Capitulating and agreeing with the instructor without fully understanding the advice, arguing, or becoming defensive does not involve critical thinking and will be less productive than exploring the rationale behind the instructor's comment. *Cognitive Level:* Analysis *Client Need:* Safe, Effective Care Environment *Nursing Process:* Implementation

8. *Answer: 2, 3 Rationale:* When the client complains of shortness of breath the nurse recognizes this as an indication of inadequate oxygen intake but is unable to accurately determine the cause until further data are gathered including respiratory rate, breath sounds, oxygen saturation, and gathering information from the client regarding when this started, any other symptoms, and a more complete explanation of what the client means by the term "short of breath." Only by gathering all important information can the nurse determine if the cause is lack of deep breathing, excessive narcotic administration, or some other cause. To treat the problem and notify the physician before gathering all the necessary data would be ineffective. *Cognitive Level:* Analysis *Client Need:* Physiological Integrity *Nursing Process:* Assessment

9. *Answer: 2 Rationale:* The student would demonstrate responsibility by arriving in clinical well rested and alert to improve their performance. Responsibility does not require the purchase of the most expensive stethoscope because less expensive stethoscopes can function adequately. Reviewing all of their notes would be productive if studying for a test, but it is ineffective when preparing for clinical, although reading the client's medical record

and researching information regarding the client's condition would be helpful. Waiting until the morning of clinical to determine where and when they are to report would be inappropriate because this information should be known ahead of time. *Cognitive Level:* Application *Client Need:* Safe, Effective Care Environment *Nursing Process:* Planning

10. *Answer: 2 Rationale:* Critical thinking will lead the nurse to realize the situation cannot be adequately managed alone and the priority is to call for help. Only after other help has been summoned can CPR be started, while someone else gets the crash cart. The nurse has already assessed the client if it is known there is no pulse and the client is not breathing. *Cognitive Level:* Application *Client Need:* Physiological Integrity *Nursing Process:* Planning

CHAPTER 7

1. *Answer: 2 Rationale:* Primary data come from the client (option 4), whereas secondary data come from any other source (chart, family). Subjective data are covert (reported or an opinion), whereas objective data can be measured or validated (weight—option 1, edema—option 3). If the spouse had stated that the client had eaten only toast and tea, this would be secondary objective (measured) data. *Cognitive Level:* Application *Client Need:* Safe, Effective Care Environment *Nursing Process:* Assessment

2. *Answer: 3 Rationale:* Eliciting feelings requires an open-ended question that does more than seek factual information (option 1) and cannot be answered with a single word (option 2). The family can provide indirect information about the client but is not most likely to provide the most accurate information (option 4). *Cognitive Level:* Analysis *Client Need:* Psychosocial Integrity *Nursing Process:* Assessment

3. *Answer: 2 Rationale:* Because the venous return is impaired, fluid is static, resulting in swelling. Therefore, decreased venous return is the cause (etiology) of the problem. The etiology usually follows the term "related to." *Excess Fluid Volume* is the nursing diagnosis, and edema of the lower extremity is the sign/symptom or critical attribute. The cause is known. *Cognitive Level:* Application *Client Need:* Safe, Effective Care Environment *Nursing Process:* Diagnosis

4. *Answer: 1 Rationale:* A collaborative, or multidisciplinary, problem is indicated when both nursing interventions and those interventions requiring another member of the health care team are needed to prevent or treat the problem. If nursing care alone (whether that care involves independent or dependent nursing actions) can treat the problem, a nursing diagnosis is indicated. If medical care alone can treat the problem, a medical diagnosis is indicated. *Cognitive Level:* Application *Client Need:* Safe, Effective Care Environment *Nursing Process:* Diagnosis

5. *Answer: 2 Rationale:* The client's nausea, especially when reported lack of bowel sounds is considered, may

indicate a paralytic ileus. Further assessment and consultation with the client is needed to determine cause and severity but this would be the nurse's highest priority. Postoperative nausea to the level of inhibiting oral intake has the greatest likelihood of leading to complications and requires nursing intervention now. The client's pain level is within acceptable limits and pain management interventions are effective. The client's activity level is not addressed in enough detail to know if it is a concern. Wound infection can occur but there are no data to indicate the presence of this risk at this time. *Cognitive Level:* Analysis *Client Need:* Physiological Integrity *Nursing Process:* Planning

6. *Answer: 3 Rationale:* The goal or outcome should state the opposite of the nursing diagnosis stem, and thus healthy, intact skin is the reverse condition of impaired skin integrity. Turning in bed, applying lotion, and using a special mattress are all interventions that may result in achieving the goal, but they are not the end result the nurse is working toward. *Cognitive Level:* Application *Client Need:* Physiological Integrity *Nursing Process:* Planning

7. *Answer: 3 Rationale:* Although there may be standard policies or routines for measuring intake and output, the nursing intervention should specify if this is to be done "routinely" or at specific intervals (e.g., q4h). Critical thinking indicates when intake and output should be monitored more frequently than ordered. *Cognitive Level:* Application *Client Need:* Physiological Integrity *Nursing Process:* Planning

8. *Answer: 3 Rationale:* The first step of implementing is reassessing the client to determine that the activity is still indicated and safe. The next action would be to determine if assistance is required, and then implement the intervention (delegating if appropriate), and last document the intervention. *Cognitive Level:* Application *Client Need:* Safe, Effective Care Environment *Nursing Process:* Implementation

9. *Answer: 2 Rationale:* There is no reason to delete or modify the nursing diagnosis or demote its priority since the risk factors that prompted it are still present. *Cognitive Level:* Analysis *Client Need:* Safe, Effective Care Environment *Nursing Process:* Evaluation

10. *Answer: 2 Rationale:* Because this assessment focuses on how care is provided, it is a process evaluation. A structure evaluation would focus on the setting (e.g., how well equipment functions), and outcome evaluations focus on changes in client status (e.g., whether reported satisfaction levels vary with type of person who answers the call light). An audit would be a chart or document review. *Cognitive Level:* Analysis *Client Need:* Safe, Effective Care Environment *Nursing Process:* Evaluation

CHAPTER 8

1. *Answer: 3 Rationale:* Control over who has access to confidential computerized data is the greatest concern.

Computer hackers can bypass codes and gain access to personal information, which could result in identity theft. The benefits often outweigh cost. Computerized data can be much more accurate than paper and pencil. Due to ease of making copies and backups, electronic data can last forever. *Cognitive Level:* Analysis *Client Need:* Safe, Effective Care Environment *Nursing Process:* Implementation

2. *Answer: 1 Rationale:* Each website is different and the nurse is compelled to evaluate the site and the treatment to determine if it is safe and appropriate for the client. Some websites are used for advertising but many are sponsored by legitimate organizations such as the National Cancer Institute (option 4). They often report results of extensive research that may be valid upon careful examination (option 2). One of the most important purposes of posting treatment information and results on the Internet is so that many different people can determine if the treatment is useful for other clients (option 3). *Cognitive Level:* Application *Client Need:* Health Promotion and Maintenance *Nursing Process:* Implementation

3. *Answer: 3 Rationale:* The nurse should always log off of the computer when not directly in front of the screen to prevent unauthorized access to not only that client's information but also other information to which the nurse has access when logged in. All of the other answers endanger the client's confidentiality. *Cognitive Level:* Application *Client Need:* Safe, Effective Care Environment *Nursing Process:* Implementation

4. *Answer: 4 Rationale:* It is the most complete answer. The client's record is a legal record and should not be altered with correcting liquid. You may see "error" written above a mistake even though many authors suggest not writing it. It is important to also put your name or initials next to the words of the mistaken entry. *Cognitive Level:* Application *Client Need:* Safe, Effective Care Environment *Nursing Process:* Implementation

5. *Answer: 4 Rationale:* Option 4 is the "best" answer although it could be more complete by adding the response of the primary care provider and the client's response to this blood pressure. Option 1 is too vague because it is not clear if the nurse found the client or was present when the client fell. Also, there is no need to write the word *client* because it is the client's chart. Option 2 is judgmental, revealing a negative attitude toward the person. It would be better to describe specific signs and symptoms such as staggering, slurred speech, and smell of alcohol on breath. Option 3 is too general and can be more specific by charting "2 cm × 3 cm purplish bruise on mid-inner thigh along with color." *Cognitive Level:* Analysis *Client Need:* Safe, Effective Care Environment *Nursing Process:* Evaluation

6. *Answer: 2 Rationale:* The graphic record provides the trend of the vital signs. Option 1, verbal information, is not appropriate for validating assessment data that is objective. This is more appropriate for subjective data. The medication record would not include documentation

of blood pressure ranges but may be consulted if the client is found to have a history of hypertension to determine existing treatment plan (option 3). The progress notes (option 4) provide information about how the client is progressing. It may or may not have information about the client's BP. *Cognitive Level:* Application *Client Need:* Safe, Effective Care Environment *Nursing Process:* Assessment

7. *Answer: 1, 2, and 4 Rationale:* When reporting on the client it is appropriate to report the reason for admission, when the client was last medicated for pain (although the student should always check the MAR to determine if the client was medicated since receiving report), and provide priorities of care due soon after report is received. Option 3 is incorrect as it could be a HIPAA violation if others hear health protected information. Option 5 is not needed unless it is a concern and it would not be done for every client. *Cognitive Level:* Analysis *Client Need:* Safe, Effective Care Environment *Nursing Process:* Implementation

8. *Answer: 2, 3 and 5 Rationale:* Options 2, 3, and 5 are all appropriate, listing the required information and avoiding use of inappropriate abbreviations. Option 1: MS is on the "Do Not Use" list of abbreviations—the nurse needs to write out morphine sulfate. Option 4 has three errors— should not have a trailing zero after the decimal point; u and SQ are both on the "Do Not Use" abbreviation list. *Cognitive Level:* Analysis *Client Need:* Safe, Effective Care Environment *Nursing Process:* Implementation

9. *Answer: 1 Rationale:* Option 1 is the most specific, nonassuming, and nonjudgmental charting. Option 2 draws conclusions by saying they are cigarette burns and could be more specific by describing the lesions in more detail. Option 3 is jumping to a conclusion of elder abuse, and option 4 is also making an assumption that the lesions are from cigarette burns. *Cognitive Level:* Analysis *Client Need:* Safe, Effective Care Environment *Nursing Process:* Evaluation

10. *Answer: 1 Rationale:* Option 1 describes the rationale for the most important reason nurses document in the client's record: because it is client focused and places the client at the center of nursing behavior, as it should in all situations. Option 2 implies that lawsuit avoidance is a primary purpose of documentation and, while good documentation contributes to lawsuit claims, it is not a driving purpose of documentation. Options 3 and 4 place responsibility for documentation on the facility when it is actually dictated by professional expectations. *Cognitive Level:* Analysis *Client Need:* Safe, Effective Care Environment *Nursing Process:* Implementation.

CHAPTER 9

1. *Answer: 4 Rationale:* Growth reflects physical changes, while development is increasing levels of function and skills. While growth generally occurs only in childhood, development occurs throughout the lifespan. Options 1, 2, and 3, cover only one aspect of the definition of growth and development, while option 4 addresses all components. *Cognitive Level:* Knowledge *Client Need:* Safe, Effective Care Environment *Nursing Process:* Assessment

2. *Answer: 1 Rationale:* This child is in Piaget's intuitive thought phase with egocentric thinking. Erickson identifies the stage of psychosocial development as industry versus inferiority. As a result, this child's anxiety and learning needs will best be met by allowing him to explore the equipment while the nurse explains its function in terms the child can comprehend. His imagination is not out of control (option 2) but is reasonable for this stage of development. While an age-appropriate approach is needed to help him understand, he is not too young to understand. He is past the need for fantasy, and threatening him (option 4) is not appropriate. *Cognitive Level:* Analysis *Client Need:* Psychosocial Integrity *Nursing Process:* Implementation

3. *Answer: 4 Rationale:* The child's health, nutrition, and genetics are all unknown factors that may or may not be playing a role in his development. However, the frequent movement from home to home often seen with foster children does not provide the best environment for development and is most likely the cause of the child's developmental delays. *Cognitive Level:* Analysis *Client Need:* Psychosocial Integrity *Nursing Process:* Assessment

4. *Answer: 1 Rationale:* During the phase of concrete operations, children change from egocentric interactions (option 2) to cooperative interactions, increasing their concepts associated with specific objects (option 1). They begin to understand cause-and-effect relationships but are not yet able to operate using abstract principles (option 3). Riding a bike is more dependent on physical growth, including balance, than cognitive changes. *Cognitive Level:* Analysis *Client Need:* Psychosocial Integrity *Nursing Process:* Assessment

5. *Answer: 2, 3 Rationale:* Moral development is highly individualized and continues throughout adulthood. Some people advance through the stages of moral development to the last stage, while others become stuck in lower phases and never develop further. Because of its highly individualized development, morality is not related to spirituality or age, nor does it remain stagnant but has the possibility of moving backwards or forward through the stages. *Cognitive Level:* Comprehension *Client Need:* Psychosocial Integrity *Nursing Process:* Assessment

6. *Answer: 1 Rationale:* Because the most important group to adolescents is their peers, encouraging peer interaction will be most helpful. It may be necessary for the nurse to explain to visting peers any alteration in the client's appearance in order to reduce anxiety over body image during their visit. Need or desire for parenteral rooming in varies by child, and the client should make the choice. She most likely will be unable to go to the recreation room during most of her hospital stay, so

finding appropriate diversional activities will be an important activity for the nurse. Pain management will likely include narcotics, so she may not be able to keep up with her homework at this time, but this may be an important factor to consider when she is at home recovering on less mind-altering medications. *Cognitive Level:* Application *Client Need:* Psychosocial Integrity *Nursing Process:* Implementation

7. *Answer: 2 Rationale:* Children begin shedding teeth at about age 6–7 and continue through the school-age years. Birth weight triples by about 12 months, and children enter school weighing about 45 pounds, gaining 5–7 pounds per year. There are significant physical changes during the school age years, and fat deposits do not normally appear until puberty. *Cognitive Level:* Comprehension *Client Need:* Physiological Integrity *Nursing Process:* Assessment

8. *Answer: 3 Rationale:* The child is demonstrating regression, when behavior reverts back to previous developmental levels, as a result of the emotional distress related to hospitalization. It is important for the mother to understand this behavior is temporary and will fade once the child is home and feels safe. It is neither a result of bladder injury nor attention seeking. A psychiatric consult is not needed, and the issue will resolve after discharge when the child feels safe again. *Cognitive Level:* Application *Client Need:* Psychosocial Integrity *Nursing Process:* Implementation

9. *Answer: 1. Rationale.* During puberty it is normal for weight to increase and fatty deposits to be noted. Because teens often become self-conscious of these changes, the best course of action for the nurse would be to provide reassurance that this is normal and that there is no need for weight control measures. *Cognitive Level:* Analysis *Client Need:* Physiological Integrity *Nursing Process:* Implementation

10. *Answer: 1 Rationale:* The priority teaching for the parents of this child is the importance of observing the child closely at all times when near or in the swimming pool. Even children who know how to swim can drown if they are in a crowded pool or get involved in horseplay. Introducing fear of swimming would be counterproductive. It takes only a few inches of water for a child to drown, so a kiddy pool would not prevent potential injury. *Cognitive Level:* Application *Client Need:* Health Promotion and Maintenance *Nursing Process:* Implementation

CHAPTER 10

1. *Answer: 2 Rationale:* Grieving is a normal behavior after the death of a loved one, and the behaviors listed in the other answers would indicate signs of normal grieving such as sharing photographs (option 1), visiting the cemetery (option 3), or attending mass daily (option 4). When the behavior becomes extreme, and signs of self-neglect

are obvious, ineffective coping may be a problem. Then it would be the responsibility of the nurse to be attentive to the problem and engage appropriate resources for her, if needed. *Cognitive Level:* Application *Client Need:* Psychosocial Integrity *Nursing Process:* Assessment

2. *Answer: 3 Rationale:* Since the hearing loss occurs in the ability to distinguish high-pitched tones, speaking in a low and distinctive voice tone is the most appropriate method of communicating with the clients. Hearing loss in the older adult includes a loss of the ability to discern higher frequencies, and speaking slowly at a particular volume is not the best way to communicate with the clients (option 1). The stem indicates the clients have noticeable hearing loss, but does not indicate the clients are deaf; large lettering is appropriate if the client has a visual problem (option 2); hearing aids are not usually effective when the problem is related to neural damage (option 4). *Cognitive Level:* Analysis *Client Need:* Health Promotion and Maintenance *Nursing Process:* Assessment

3. *Answer: 2 Rationale:* Reminiscence about past life events, doing a "life review" of past experiences, especially if they were positive, is considered to be a normal psychosocial activity of older adults. It helps them focus on past accomplishments and contributions to society, thus increasing their self-concept. If behavioral or significant memory problems had been noted, then a geriatric psychiatric consult would be appropriate (option 1), but not in this situation. Other activities and conversations should certainly be encouraged, but not to the point of demeaning the importance of his life stories options 3 and 4). *Cognitive Level:* Application *Client Need:* Health Promotion and Maintenance *Nursing Process:* Assessment

4. *Answer: 3 and 4 Rationale:* When clients with dementia become agitated, the main interventions are to decrease stimuli. Distracting them, staying with them, and the use of a calm, gentle manner will usually decrease the agitation. Touching must be done in a gentle way, not to surprise or alarm them. Allowing her to continue pacing or leaving her alone places the client in danger (options 1 and 2). Lying about her location is both dishonest and damaging to the nurse/client relationship (option 2). Providing complex explanations will not be effective for this client (option 5). *Cognitive Level:* Application *Client Need:* Psychosocial Integrity *Nursing Process:* Implementation

5. *Answer: 3 Rationale:* This option will provide the nurse with the most information for potential intervention. Urinary incontinence is not normal and it is something the nurse should investigate and not just accept at face value (option 1). Elimination of the catheter will reduce the risk for infection and should not be placed to avoid incontinence (option 2). More information is needed before the promise of getting the client to the bathroom in time can be made (Option 4). *Cognitive Level:* Analysis *Client Need:* Physiological Integrity *Nursing Process:* Assessment

6. *Answer: 1 Rationale:* The client has loss of muscle strength. Strengthening exercises will improve his mobility and lessen the possibility of a fall. Option 2: There is no indication the client is to be limited in his mobility, just assisted to be safer when standing. Option 3: Praise should come after the proper intervention is implemented and a plan is in place so that the praise is focused toward a goal to resolve the problem. Option 4 resolves the problem immediately but does nothing to resolve the underlying problem and uses a dangerous method of helping the client that can result in injury to both the client and the nurse. *Cognitive Level:* Application *Client Need:* Safe, Effective Care Environment *Nursing Process:* Implementation

7. *Answer: 4 Rationale:* Sexual activity is possible for older adults although the responses are slower. Option 1: The clients would need a health history and physical assessment of the cardiovascular system before drawing this conclusion. Option 2: With the introduction of Viagra, and similar medications, older men are more able to perform than in the past. Option 3: Older men's interest tends to decline, but it is not known whether it is related to impotence; apparently this older adult is interested in sexual activity. *Cognitive Level:* Analysis *Client Need:* Health Promotion and Maintenance *Nursing Process:* Implementation

8. *Answer: 3 Rationale:* Presbyopia is loss of near vision related to aging. Option 1 is loss of hearing ability related to aging. Option 2 is dry mouth related to a decrease in saliva, and option 4 is a decrease in the motility of the esophagus related to aging. *Cognitive Level:* Application *Client Need:* Health Promotion and Maintenance *Nursing Process:* Assessment

9. *Answer: 2 Rationale:* Genetics, interests, careers, marital status, and economic status vary as much among older adults as among other age groups so they are as individual as those in any other stage of development. There is no reason to expect all older adults to experience physical changes at the same rate because so many factors are contributory (option 1). Independence is to be encouraged for as long as possible, and not all older adults require long-term care (option 3). Older adults are often vital contributing members of society with a great deal to share with those from other generations (option 4). *Cognitive Level:* Application *Client Need:* Health Promotion and Maintenance *Nursing Process:* Assessment

10. *Answer: 4 Rationale:* Older adult clients often want to maintain their autonomy even if they have to struggle somewhat so the nurse should encourage the client's need to perform self-care as much as possible and avoid trying to do everything for the client (option 1). There is no reason to believe incontinence pads will be needed based on the scenario provided (option 2) as this is not a normal part of the aging process. The client's need for spiritual support would need to be assessed before making the assumption that a spiritual leader should be called. *Cognitive Level:* Application *Client Need:* Psychosocial Integrity *Nursing Process:* Planning

CHAPTER 11

1. *Answer: 1 Rationale:* Grandparents, aunts, and uncles are considered extended family members. Parents and spouse are considered immediate family members (option 2). Children who no longer live at home are considered immediate family members (option 3). Roommates and close family friends may be considered extended family members if there are not grandparents, aunts, and uncles (option 4). *Cognitive Level:* Analysis *Client Need:* Psychosocial Integrity *Nursing Process:* Assessment

2. *Answer: 4 Rationale:* The father picks up the child and provides feedback that the child's behavior was effective in keeping him home longer. Input is the child's crying, which serves as throughput for the father to think about his behavior, and output is the child stopping crying. *Cognitive Level:* Application *Client Need:* Psychosocial Integrity *Nursing Process:* Assessment

3. *Answer: 1 Rationale:* The health history of the client's current living partners is critical information since many illnesses are communicable or environmental so knowledge about blood relatives is critical. The nurse also validates that family is whoever the client says they are and obtains information on these family members. Limiting only the information pertaining to blood relatives eliminates vital information about the client's current living history and their definition of family (option 2). Leaving the section blank eliminates all important information from the family history (option 3). Neither the history nor the physical exam is more important than the other—both are necessary for a complete plan of care. *Cognitive Level:* Application *Client Need:* Psychosocial Integrity *Nursing Process:* Assessment

4. *Answer:* A visual representation of family members by gender, age, health status, and lines of relationships through the generations is referred to as a genogram. *Cognitive Level:* Knowledge *Client Need:* Psychosocial Integrity *Nursing Process:* Assessment

5. *Answer: 1, 2, and 4 Rationale:* It is essential that the nurse determine the duration of the illness (option 1), the meaning of the illness to the family and its significance to family systems (option 2), and the financial impact of the illness in order to completely assess the impact of the illness on the family as a whole (option 4). Duration of the illness will determine the degree of disruption and adaptation required. These factors affect the members of the family in addition to the ill client. Option 3: Coping mechanisms used by other families with similar illnesses may not be relevant since families vary greatly in their makeup and function patterns. Option 5: Knowing the incidence of the illness in the community at large is an important factor for the community health nurse in exploring epidemiological issues such as prevention strategies and public health policies but is not as relevant for assisting the particular family. *Cognitive Level:* Comprehension *Client Need:* Psychosocial Integrity *Nursing Process:* Assessment

6. *Answer: 1 Rationale:* Presenting to the clinic indicates the family is ready to face the health challenges caused by the previous activities and is seeking information to help them do so. There is no evidence that the adult child or parent is experiencing disabling coping (option 2). Impaired Parenting applies when the parent is unable to care for a child rather than the reverse (option 3). Although some strain may be experienced by the child, evidence does not indicate this problem, so Caregiver Role Strain is not indicated (option 4). *Cognitive Level:* Analysis *Client Need:* Psychosocial Integrity *Nursing Process:* Diagnosis

7. *Answer: 3 Rationale:* Establishing trust allows for effective communication and confirms that there is mutual commitment to the goals. A trusting relationship is important for communication as well as accepting and implementing a plan. Meetings with the family as a group may or may not be indicated depending on the situation and is not a given fact (option 1). While considering the cost of health care may be important it is not a factor at the stage of finalizing a care plan (option 3). A detailed history and examination of each family member should have been performed before finalizing a plan of care or beginning implementation (option 4). *Cognitive Level:* Application *Client Need:* Psychosocial Integrity *Nursing Process:* Planning

8. *Answer: 4 Rationale:* The focus of activity on personal purposes does not promote effective family functioning. A family system that functions efficiently focuses primarily on purposes involving the total system and allows input from the outside, personal boundaries are well-defined, and family members are interdependent. *Cognitive Level:* Analysis *Client Need:* Psychosocial Integrity *Nursing Process:* Evaluation

9. *Answer: 3 Rationale:* Research indicates that children from adolescent families are at increased risk of teen pregnancy as well as social and health problems as a result of the immaturity of the parent or parents. There would be no reason to anticipate increased incidence of teen pregnancy from a gay or lesbian, blended, or intragenerational family compared to the general population. *Cognitive Level:* Analysis *Client Need:* Psychosocial Integrity *Nursing Process:* Assessment

10. *Answer: 1 Rationale:* The structural–functional theory focuses on family structure and function including membership of the family and the relationship among members. Roles of family members are included in learning family membership (option 2). Family goals and harmony within the family cannot be addressed until an understanding of members and functions is gained. *Cognitive Level:* Application *Client Need:* Psychosocial Integrity *Nursing Process:* Assessment

CHAPTER 12

1. *Answer: 2 Rationale:* This assessment activity gathers more information to help the nurse know the client's usual self-care practices. Option 1 aims to provide comfort. Option 3 is a therapeutic, not an assessment, activity. Option 4 does not meet the aim of knowing the client. *Cognitive Level:* Application *Client Need:* Psychosocial Integrity *Nursing Process:* Implementation

2. *Answer: 1 Rationale:* Teaching the client to make self-care decisions at home empowers him to care for his illness. Teaching almost always fits into the category of empowerment, while compassion (option 2) is shown by listening to a client's feelings or consoling the client who is upset, for example. Knowing the client involves assessment and learning more about the client's health care activities, among other things. Nursing presence is demonstrated by the nurse being with the client whether giving moral support or delivering care. *Cognitive Level:* Application *Client Need:* Health Promotion and Maintenance *Nursing Process:* Implementation

3. *Answer: 3 Rationale:* Mayeroff defines patience as "allowing the other to grow in his own way and time." Knowing means understanding the client's needs and how to respond; humility is acknowledging that there is always more to learn and learning may come from any source. Courage is the sense of going into the unknown, informed by insight from past experiences. *Cognitive Level:* Knowledge *Client Need:* Psychosocial Integrity *Nursing Process:* Planning

4. *Answer: 1 Rationale:* Since Leininger's theory addresses cultural elements relevant to nursing, only the option impacting culture is correct. The other options have nothing to do with cultural diversity and universality. *Cognitive Level:* Analysis *Client Need:* Psychosocial Integrity *Nursing Process:* Evaluation

5. *Answer: 3 Rationale:* This represents an ethical dilemma. The other options are ways of knowing less clearly related to the situation. *Cognitive Level:* Application *Client Need:* Psychosocial Integrity *Nursing Process:* Assessment

6. *Answer: 1 Rationale:* The nurse's presence is most significant in this situation. Assessment (option 2), knowing the client (option 3), and empowering the client (option 4) are not the focus of the nurse's action. *Cognitive Level:* Application *Client Need:* Psychosocial Integrity *Nursing Process:* Implementation

7. *Answer: 2 Rationale:* This describes the model for the theory of bureaucratic caring. Nursing as caring (option 1) is Boykin and Schoenhofer's theory suggesting that the purpose of the discipline and profession of nursing is to know persons and nurture them as persons living in caring and growing in caring. Option 3 describes M. Simone Roach's theory that caring is a philosophical concept and the human mode of being, or the "most common, authentic criterion of humanness." Option 4 describes Watson's theory that views caring as the essence and the moral ideal of nursing. *Cognitive Level:* Knowledge *Client Need:* Psychosocial Integrity *Nursing Process:* Assessment

8. *Answer: 1 Rationale:* Empirical knowing is gained from studying scientific models and theories. Aesthetic knowing

arises from application in practice (option 2). Personal knowing arises from self-examination (option 3). Ethical knowing arises from confronting conflicting values (option 4). *Cognitive Level:* Application *Client Need:* Safe, Effective Care Environment *Nursing Process:* Planning

9. *Answer: 4 Rationale:* Meditation involves the described behaviors. Storytelling involves communication with others (option 1). Yoga combines various postures with breathing practices (option 2). Music therapy involves listening to music (option 3). *Cognitive Level:* Analysis *Client Need:* Health promotion and maintenance *Nursing Process:* Implementation

10. *Answer: 3 Rationale:* This is the recommendation for a healthy lifestyle. Option 1: More sustained activity has more positive physiological benefits. Options 2 and 4: This amount of activity exceeds baseline requirements and may be more difficult to maintain. *Cognitive Level:* Application *Client Need:* Health Promotion and Maintenance *Nursing Process:* Implementation

CHAPTER 13

1. *Answer: 3 Rationale:* Nonverbal, gentle touch is an important tool; overstimulation may affect the client in a negative way. Option 1: Written communication requires a higher level of consciousness than verbal. Option 2: The client does not have a hearing problem but the ability to interpret and understand communication. Option 4: Lack of facial expression may increase fear. *Cognitive Level:* Application *Client Need:* Psychosocial Integrity *Nursing Process:* Implementation

2. *Answer: 2, 3, and 4 Rationale:* The purpose of the helping relationship is to help clients manage their problems in living more effectively, develop unused or underused opportunities more fully, and help clients become better at helping themselves in their everyday lives. The nurse cannot solve all of the client's problems nor does the nurse want to be a friend to the client. *Cognitive Level:* Application *Client Need:* Health Promotion and Maintenance *Nursing Process:* Planning

3. *Answer:* Options 1 and 3 are listening behaviors; the others are barriers to listening. The nurse does not encourage compliance but rather explores the client's needs in order to create a plan of care that is in keeping with the client's needs and lifestyle. *Cognitive Level:* Application *Client Need:* Psychosocial Integrity *Nursing Process:* Implementation

4. *Answer: 1 Rationale:* Respect is correct because the nurse is validating the client's feeling. It is not genuineness (option 2) because the nurse is giving information versus being genuine. Concreteness (option 3) is giving a specific example. The nurse is not confronting (option 4) but supporting through respect for the client's feelings. *Cognitive Level:* Application *Client Need:* Psychosocial Integrity *Nursing Process:* Implementation

5. *Answer: 2 Rationale:* Because anxiety and low self-esteem precede powerlessness, which results in indecisiveness, it is the most correct answer; nursing management always deals with the client's current display of needs. Options 1 and 3: Anxiety and low self-esteem may cause a sense of powerlessness that results in indecisiveness. Option 4: There is no evidence that the client's social interactions are less than adequate. *Cognitive Level:* Application *Client Need:* Psychosocial Integrity *Nursing Process:* Diagnosis

6. *Answer: 2 and 3 Rationale:* Assessing possible visual or hearing problems allows the nurse to provide appropriate interventions (e.g., inserting hearing aid). Communicating what will be occurring at a stressful time helps the client feel more secure and can reduce anxiety. Option 1 is not the best answer as the client could say yes/no or nod the head and the nurse will not know if the client fully understands. It would be better to ask the client to tell you where he or she is. Option 4 is important to do; however, immediately after surgery is not the best time as the client may be in pain and/or groggy from the anesthesia. Speaking loudly can be very irritating to the client, whether or not the client has a hearing deficit. Speak clearly in a normal tone of voice. *Cognitive Level:* Application *Client Need:* Psychosocial Integrity *Nursing Process:* Implementation

7. *Answer: 3 Rationale:* Option 3 does not introduce the nurse's bias but allows the client to speak for herself. All of the other options are forms of elderspeak and are not only incorrect but also disrespectful. *Cognitive Level:* Analysis *Client Need:* Psychosocial Integrity *Nursing Process:* Implementation

8. *Answer: 4 Rationale:* Option 4 is a therapeutic technique using an open-ended question that allows the client to elaborate. The other options are barriers to communication. In option 1 the client did not ask about the abilities of the surgeon and the response is not focused on the client. Option 2 is changing the subject, and option 3 is giving advice, both of which are not therapeutic and are incorrect. *Cognitive Level:* Analysis *Client Need:* Psychosocial Integrity *Nursing Process:* Implementation

9. *Answer: 2 Rationale:* Option 2 uses an "I" statement which is assertive communication and is clear and direct. The message includes only the necessary information. Option 1 contains inflammatory language ("ineffective" and "you prescribed"). Options 3 and 4 do not provide the health care provider with specific information and could stimulate defensive behaviors. *Cognitive Level:* Analysis *Client Need:* Safe, Effective Care Environment *Nursing Process:* Assessment.

10. *Answer: 1 Rationale:* It encourages the client to verbalize and choose the topic of the conversation. Option 2 is used when the nurse is unsure of the message and asks the client to repeat or restate the message. Option 3 is used to help a client differentiate the real from the unreal, and there is no information available to indicate this is a concern in this situation. Option 4 is used at the end of an

interview or teaching session. *Cognitive Level:* Application *Client Need:* Psychosocial Integrity *Nursing Process:* Assessment

CHAPTER 14

1. *Answer: 2 Rationale:* Only option one deals with the affective, or feeling, domain of Bloom's taxonomy. Options 1 and 3 are psychomotor, and 4 is under the cognitive domain. *Cognitive Level:* Comprehension *Client Need:* Health Promotion and Maintenance *Nursing Process:* Implementation

2. *Answer: 3 Rationale:* Learning is faster and retention better when the learner is actively involved. Options 1 and 2 are passive learning strategies. Option 4 promotes affective learning about adapting to a chronic health condition and is important. However, the question asks about learning diet information. *Cognitive Level:* Application *Client Need:* Physiological Integrity *Nursing Process:* Implementation

3. *Answer: 2 Rationale:* The client most ready to learn is experiencing or has recently experienced the least amount of stress or is the least preoccupied with other concerns. There will be no separation anxiety because the parents are present. The story book may allow the child to learn information about the hospital and ask questions. The client in option 1 will be preoccupied by his diagnosis. The client in option 3 is most likely still in pain and cognition is likely impaired by the medication administered. The client in option 4 may be too tired after his physical therapy treatment. *Cognitive Level:* Application *Client Need:* Psychosocial Integrity *Nursing Process:* Assessment

4. *Answer: 1 Rationale:* Individuals learn in various ways, such as visually, group learning, auditory, participatory, etc. The individual knows how learning has occurred in the past. Option 2 is a component of the implementation phase of teaching, and the question is asking how to assess a client's style of learning. Options 3 and 4 involve others and it is best to ask the client. *Cognitive Level:* Knowledge *Client Need:* Health Promotion and Maintenance *Nursing Process:* Assessment

5. *Answer: 3 Rationale:* Option 1 is an old diagnosis, which has been changed. Option 2 is a wellness nursing diagnosis; the data would need to address that the client is seeking health information and why, in order to be the correct answer. The diagnosis of *Noncompliance* is associated with the intent to comply, but situational factors make it difficult. The data in the question do not support option 4. *Cognitive Level:* Knowledge *Client Need:* Physiological Integrity *Nursing Process:* Diagnosis

6. *Answer: 2 and 3 Rationale:* Both options 2 and 3 are open-ended questions that will give the client the opportunity to ask questions. Options 1 and 4 are closed-ended (yes/no) questions. A "no" answer may cause a discussion but it will be difficult for the nurse to assess

if it is the information the client really wants to know. Option 5 is falsely reassuring and doesn't seek the client's input at all, thereby closing the line of communication. *Cognitive Level:* Application *Client Need:* Psychosocial Integrity *Nursing Process:* Assessment

7. *Answer: 1, 2, 3, and 4 Rationale:* Option 5 includes a request to be allowed to read the brochure so it is unlikely, but not impossible, this client has an illiteracy problem, although the nurse can assess literacy further when determining how much of the pamphlet the client read and understood. All of the other statements could indicate a low literacy skill. The nurse will need to assess which teaching strategies will be most appropriate and will also need to carefully evaluate if the client has learned the skill and necessary information. *Cognitive Level:* Analysis *Client Need:* Physiological Integrity *Nursing Process:* Assessment

8. *Answer: 3 Rationale:* All are important factors to assess. The priority, however, would be the potential economic factor as the medications can be very expensive and the client may not take them if he or she cannot afford them. *Cognitive Level:* Application *Client Need:* Physiological Integrity *Nursing Process:* Assessment

9. *Answer: 3 Rationale:* This option is the easiest for the nurse to evaluate. Option 1 is difficult to evaluate because "understand" is too vague. Option 2 refers more to an affective outcome and the question is asking about a cognitive outcome. Option 4 is telling more about the husband than the client. *Cognitive Level:* Analysis *Client Need:* Health Promotion and Maintenance *Nursing Process:* Evaluation

10. *Answer: 2 Rationale:* This is the only option that clearly reflects the teaching process, evaluation method, and the response of the client indicating evidence of learning. "Seemed to understand" (option 1) is meaningless—either she did or did not understand; if the nurse is uncertain of understanding, further evaluation is needed. Option 3 does not evaluate learning and is inadequate teaching. Option 4 indicates the nurse provided answers only to questions asked, which is often far less than what the client needs to know. *Cognitive Level:* Analysis *Client Need:* Physiological Integrity *Nursing Process:* Evaluation

CHAPTER 15

1. *Answer: 1 Rationale:* This is a situation in which urgent decisions are needed, and one person provides instructions without input from others (authoritarian). This is especially appropriate if the rest of the group is not functioning at an appropriate level. Option 2 would be found in shared governance structures when the risks are low and there is time for collaboration. Option 3 is most effective in groups with high levels of professional and personal maturity and where cooperation and coordination are not significant. Option 4 involves the rigid use of rules; since managing casualties is a highly unpredictable

activity, enforcement of rules is not appropriate. *Cognitive Level:* Analysis *Client Need:* Safe, Effective Care Environment *Nursing Process:* Planning

2. **Answer: 1 Rationale:** Transformational leaders are creative and use collaboration and group empowerment. Subgroups or task forces (option 2) would be found in shared governance structures (democratic leadership). Transactional leaders use rewards such as paying the cost of continuing education as incentives. Situational leaders vary their approach depending on the context. *Cognitive Level:* Comprehension *Client Need:* Safe, Effective Care Environment *Nursing Process:* Implementation

3. **Answer: 2 Rationale:** The manager is responsible for evaluating the staff (accountable) but has no authority to terminate staff who do not meet the standards or to promote staff with outstanding performance. In option 1, the manager has authority to carry out the reduction but is not accountable because the actions were delegated and not initiated independently. In option 3, the manager has only responsibility; in option 4, both authority and accountability. *Cognitive Level:* Analysis *Client Need:* Safe, Effective Care Environment *Nursing Process:* Planning

4. **Answer: 3 Rationale:** A fresh postoperative client is, by definition, in a somewhat unstable condition, and the nurse must assess and supervise this initial transfer. A UAP should be able to perform the transfer safely with a new wheelchair or older adult client; the scenario does not indicate that the wheelchair had special features. Age does not determine the need for assistance. The task is simple and can be easily recalled safely after an absence. *Cognitive Level:* Analysis *Client Need:* Safe, Effective Care Environment *Nursing Process:* Planning

5. **Answer: 4 Rationale:** Interaction between the two groups may lead to a compromise. Option 1: Although explaining the reasons for the desired change is useful, overemphasis on the rationale may not be useful since resistance is often more emotional than rational. Option 2: This situation does not meet the criteria for an autocratic leadership style. There is no urgency and the task primarily involves the staff. Option 3: If the manager were not solidly committed to the proposal, it should not have been introduced, resulting in unnecessary disturbance; the manager should be open to modification of the proposal if justified. *Cognitive Level:* Application *Client Need:* Safe, Effective Care Environment *Nursing Process:* Implementing

6. **Answer: 1 Rationale:** Leadership includes influencing others to work together to accomplish a common goal, and the goal can be positive or negative. In this instance the nurse is leading the staff toward dissatisfaction and resentment, but the nurse is still is leading. Option 2 indicates a nurse with a good work ethic but no indication of influencing others other than by providing a good role model. Option 3 demonstrates a nurse who attempts to take a leadership position but is not influencing others because of poor planning. Option 4 is a nurse in a leadership role who is not displaying leadership

skills as indicated by the staff's poor perception of the manager as a member of the team. *Cognitive Level:* Analysis *Client Need:* Safe, Effective Care Environment *Nursing Process:* Assessment

7. **Answer: 4 Rationale:** The nurse the staff identify as a good resource is acting as an informal leader, helping nurses to problem solve issues that arise on the shift. The other nurses are in formal positions of authority. *Cognitive Level:* Application *Client Need:* Safe, Effective Care Environment *Nursing Process:* Assessment

8. **Answer: 2 Rationale:** When numerous committees are created to contribute to the management of a nursing unit or facility, the leadership style anticipated is democratic, which encourages group discussion and decision making. Autocratic leadership makes decisions for the group without the use of the group's creativity or self-motivation. Laissez-faire leadership encourages a hands-off approach from the leader. In this example, the nurse manager will oversee committee decision making to assure that client care is optimized. Bureaucratic leaders do not trust themselves or others to make decisions and rely on the organization's rules. *Cognitive Level:* Analysis *Client Need:* Safe, Effective Care Environment *Nursing Process:* Planning

9. **Answer: 2 Rationale:** This is a middle management position because the nurse will supervise first-level managers such as charge nurses or assistant unit managers. Upper-level managers are executives, such as the director of nursing or chief nurse manager. *Cognitive Level:* Application *Client Need:* Safe, Effective Care Environment *Nursing Process:* Assessment

10. **Answer: 1, 2, 3, 5 Rationale:** The nurse functioning as a staff nurse has the authority to provide client care, is accountable for the performance of that care, is responsible for providing high-quality care, and has an obligation to the client to provide the best care possible to the client. The nurse is not entitled, which implies a right accorded by law. While the law requires every nurse to maintain licensure to demonstrate competence, the license can be removed if care is not safely provided. *Cognitive Level:* Application *Client Need:* Safe, Effective Care Environment *Nursing Process:* Planning

CHAPTER 16

1. **Answer: 2 Rationale:** Although the temperature is lower than expected for a morning temperature, it would be best to determine the client's previous temperature range because this may be normal for this client. Only if the temperature is out of range is it necessary to retake the reading using a different thermometer (option 3) and there would be no need to wait 15 minutes (option 1). The temperature would be documented after determining accuracy of the reading (option 4). *Cognitive Level:* Application *Client Need:* Health Maintenance and Promotion *Nursing Process:* Assessment

2. *Answer: 3 Rationale:* The apical rate would confirm the rate and determine the actual cardiac rhythm for a client with an abnormal rhythm; a radial pulse would reveal only the heart rate and suggest an arrhythmia. For clients in shock, use the carotid or femoral pulse (option 1). The radial pulse is adequate for determining change in orthostatic heart rate (option 2). The radial pulse is appropriate for routine postoperative vital sign checks for clients with regular pulses (option 4). *Cognitive Level:* Comprehension *Client Need:* Health Maintenance and Promotion *Nursing Process:* Planning

3. *Answer: 4 Rationale:* Since the client's needs are always considered first, the measurement should be delayed until the phone call is completed. Option 1: Respirations should be measured for 30 seconds to 1 minute and are affected by talking, so measurement while on the phone would be inaccurate. Option 2: There needs to be an important reason for interrupting the client and since this client is not in distress no truly important reason exists. Option 3: It is inappropriate to wait and listen to the client's conversation. *Cognitive Level:* Comprehension *Client Need:* Health Maintenance and Promotion *Nursing Process:* Planning

4. *Answer: 2 Rationale:* If the cuff is inflated to about 30 mm Hg over previous systolic pressure, that would be 168. To ensure that the diastolic has been determined, the cuff should be released slowly until the mid-60s mm Hg (and then completely) for someone with a previous reading of 74. The cuff should be deflated at a rate of 2 to 3 mm per second. Thus, a range of 90 mm Hg will require 30 to 45 seconds. *Cognitive Level:* Analysis *Client Need:* Health Maintenance and Promotion *Nursing Process:* Implementation

5. *Answer: 1 Rationale:* Vital signs measurement may be delegated to UAP if the client is in stable condition, the findings are expected to be predictable, and the technique requires no modification. Only the preoperative client meets these requirements. The client receiving blood (option 2) and the client with asthma (option 3) are not considered stable. In addition, UAP are not delegated to take apical pulse measurements for the client with an irregular pulse as would be the case with the client newly started on antiarrhythmic medication (option 3). *Cognitive Level:* Application *Client Need:* Health Maintenance and Promotion *Nursing Process:* Planning

6. *Answer: 3, 4, and 5 Rationale:* For this client, the nurse could take an axillary, tympanic, or temporal artery temperature. Due to the facial drooping and difficulty swallowing, the oral route is not recommended. Although the rectal route could be used, it would require unnecessary moving and positioning of a client who cannot assist, would expose the client to potential embarrassment, and would not provide a significant advantage over the other routes. *Cognitive Level:* Application *Client Need:* Health Maintenance and Promotion *Nursing Process:* Assessment

7. *Answer: 4 Rationale:* The posterior tibial and pedal pulses in the foot are considered peripheral and at least one of them should be palpable in normal individuals. Option 1: A bounding radial pulse is more indicative that perfusion exists. Options 2 and 3: Apical and carotid pulses are central and not peripheral. *Cognitive Level:* Analysis *Client Need:* Health Promotion and Maintenance *Nursing Process:* Diagnosing

8. *Answer: 3 Rationale:* Dyspnea, difficult or labored breathing, is commonly related to inadequate oxygenation. Therefore, the client is likely to experience shortness of breath, that is, a sense that none of the breaths provide enough oxygen and an immediate second breath is needed. Shallow respirations (option 1) are seen in tachypnea (rapid breathing). Wheezing (option 2) is a high-pitched breathing sound that may or may not occur with dyspnea. The medical term for coughing up blood is hemoptysis (option 4) and is unrelated to dyspnea. *Cognitive Level:* Application *Client Need:* Health Promotion and Maintenance *Nursing Process:* Evaluating

9. *Answer:* This blood pressure should be recorded as 180/105/95 using the systolic/1st diastolic/2nd diastolic convention. *Rationale:* Phase 1 first sound is a clear tapping when deflation of the cuff begins. Phase 2 has a muffled, swishing sound. In phase 3, blood is flowing freely via an increasingly open artery; sounds are more crisp and more intense but softer than phase 1. Phase 4 sounds become muffled and have a soft blowing quality. In phase 5 the last sound is heard followed by silence. *Cognitive Level:* Analysis *Client Need:* Health Promotion and Maintenance *Nursing Process:* Assessment

10. *Answer: 4 Rationale:* The SpO_2 in this case is 97%. Option 1 indicates the systolic blood pressure of 121 mm Hg, option 2 the mean arterial pressure of 95 mm Hg, option 3 the pulse of 87, and option 5 the diastolic blood pressure of 84 mm Hg. In addition, the client's temperature is shown. *Cognitive Level:* Comprehension *Client Need:* Health Maintenance and Promotion *Nursing Process:* Assessment

CHAPTER 17

1. *Answer: 2 Rationale:* Resonance is a normal sound over the lung. Tympany (option 1) would be heard over the stomach (air filled), hyperresonance (option 3) is never a normal finding, and dullness (option 4) would be heard below (not above) the 10th intercostal space. *Cognitive Level:* Knowledge *Client Need:* Health Promotion and Maintenance *Nursing Process:* Evaluating

2. *Answer: 4 Rationale:* The client should sit for examination of the head and neck. For palpation of the abdomen, genitals, and breast, the client should be supine (options 1, 2, and 3). *Cognitive Level:* Application *Client Need:* Health Promotion and Maintenance *Nursing Process:* Planning

3. *Answer: 1 Rationale:* A bruit suggests abnormal turbulence in the aorta, and the primary care provider must be notified. In order for absence of bowel sounds to be

considered abnormal, they must be silent for 3 to 5 minutes (option 2). Continuous bowel sounds are normally heard over the ileocecal valve following meals (option 3). Bowel sounds are more commonly irregular than they are regular (option 4). *Cognitive Level:* Comprehension *Client Need:* Health Promotion and Maintenance *Nursing Process:* Evaluating

4. *Answer: 1 Rationale:* If a pedal pulse, which is more distal than the popliteal, is present, then adequate arterial circulation to the leg is present even though the popliteal artery has not been located. Another option, not provided in the question, would be to perform Doppler ultrasound to see if popliteal pulses could be heard. Presence of a femoral pulse would not provide confirmation that arterial flow exists below that point (option 2). Taking a thigh BP requires locating the popliteal pulse (option 3). Since the purpose of finding the popliteal pulse is to provide information about arterial circulation to the leg, checking the distal pulse before requesting assistance from another nurse is appropriate (option 4). *Cognitive Level:* Analysis *Client Need:* Health Promotion and Maintenance *Nursing Process:* Planning

5. *Answer: 2 Rationale:* Visual acuity often lessens with age. Facial hair is likely to become coarser, not finer (option 1). The sense of smell becomes less, rather than more acute (option 3). The respiratory rate and rhythm should be regular at rest (option 4). However, both may change quickly with activity and be slow to return to the resting level. *Cognitive Level:* Analysis *Client Need:* Health Promotion and Maintenance *Nursing Process:* Evaluating

6. Answers include any 5 of the following: color, turgor, temperature, moisture, lesions, odor, and edema. *Cognitive Level:* Knowledge *Client Need:* Health Promotion and Maintenance *Nursing Process:* Assessing

7. *Answer: 3 Rationale:* Recent memory includes events of the current day. Recalling a series of numbers tests immediate recall (option 1). Recalling childhood events tests remote (long-term) memory (option 2) and subtracting backwards from 100 tests attention span and calculation skills (option 4). *Cognitive Level:* Application *Client Need:* Health Promotion and Maintenance *Nursing Process:* Planning

8. *Answer: 4 Rationale:* Row 6 indicates normal vision of 20/20. If the client can only read to line 4, vision is impaired and could lead to falls or other injuries. This impaired vision is not related to deficient knowledge (option 1) or memory (option 2) and may or may not be related to circulation as there are many causes of alterations in vision (option 3). *Cognitive Level:* Analysis *Client Need:* Health Promotion and Maintenance *Nursing Process:* Diagnosing

9. *Answer: 3 Rationale:* Use the pads of two fingers and a gentle rotating motion over the nodes. None of the other options is proper palpation of lymph nodes and would yield unreliable results (options 1, 2, and 4). *Cognitive Level:* Application *Client Need:* Health Promotion and Maintenance *Nursing Process:* Implementing

10. *Answer: 4 and 5 Rationale:* Of the terms listed, only equal and firm are normal findings. Atrophied, contractured, and crepitation are abnormal findings (options 1, 2, and 3). Review the terms in the glossary to go over their meanings. *Cognitive Level:* Comprehension *Client Need:* Health Promotion and Maintenance *Nursing Process:* Evaluating

CHAPTER 18

1. *Answer: 3 Rationale:* During the transduction phase, tissue injury triggers the release of biochemical mediators such as prostaglandin. Ibuprofen works by blocking the production of prostaglandin. The coanalgesic medication in option 1 would affect the modulation phase because coanalgesics inhibit the reuptake of norepinephrine and serotonin, which increases the modulation phase that helps inhibit painful ascending stimuli. In option 2, opioids block the release of neurotransmitters, particularly substance P, which stops the pain at the spinal level that occurs during the transmission phase. In option 4, distraction is best used during the perception phase when the client becomes conscious of the pain. Distraction (e.g., music, guided imagery, TV) can help direct the client's attention away from the pain. *Cognitive Level:* Application *Client Need:* Physiological Integrity *Nursing Process:* Implementation

2. *Answer: 3 Rationale:* Pain threshold is the least amount of stimuli that is needed for a person to label a sensation as pain. The client first notices the pain at a 3 so this would be the client's pain threshold. Pain tolerance level is exceeded when the client is no longer able to tolerate the pain and it interferes with normal functioning, which would be at the level of 5. *Cognitive Level:* Analysis *Client Need:* Physiological Integrity: basic care and comfort *Nursing Process:* Assessment

3. *Answer: 3 Rationale:* A rating of 6 is considered moderate–severe and demands immediate attention. Mild pain is rated 1–3, moderate pain is 4–6, and severe pain is 7–10. *Cognitive Level:* Application *Client Need:* Physiological Integrity *Nursing Process:* Assessment

4. *Answer: 1 Rationale:* This indicates an increasing level of sedation, which can be an early sign of impending respiratory depression. Option 2 is slightly elevated but not as significant as option 1. Option 3 can indicate increasing sedation; however, option 1 describes a higher level of sedation and the need to monitor the client closely for potential complications. Option 4 indicates pain management that may be tolerable for the client. *Cognitive Level:* Application *Client Need:* Physiological Integrity: Basic Care and Comfort *Nursing Process:* Planning

5. *Answer: 4 Rationale:* The client's perception/intensity rating of his pain is the most important even though other signs may suggest he is not having pain. His pain rating warrants a higher dose of the as-needed (prn) morphine. With option 1, you would be undermedicating the client

based on the most important data when assessing a client's pain, his perception or rating of the pain. Option 2: Research shows that few clients become addicted, plus there is no information to indicate signs of addiction. This answer, based on the data, would be undermedicating the client. Option 3 does not address the intensity as well as 4. *Cognitive Level:* Analysis *Client Need:* Physiological Integrity *Nursing Process:* Evaluation

6. *Answer: 4 Rationale:* Options 2 and 3 are subcategories of physiological pain. A clue to the answer is that the client has diabetes, which often leads to diabetic peripheral neuropathy. *Cognitive Level:* Analysis *Client Need:* Physiological Integrity *Nursing Process:* Assessment

7. *Answer: 2, 4, and 5 Rationale:* Massage, heat, and cold are topical therapies that can "close" the gates and inhibit the transmission of further pain. Client education and anticipatory guidance address the client's mood and goals which can also inhibit further pain by reducing fear and anxiety. Options 1 and 3 are pharmacological interventions which are important; however, they inhibit the pain during the transmission phase of nociception. *Cognitive Level:* Application *Client Need:* Physiological Integrity *Nursing Process:* Implementation

8. *Answer: 2 Rationale:* The words "pain" or "complain" may have emotional or sociocultural meanings. It is better to ask clients if they are having any discomfort—they can then elaborate in their own words. Option 3 is too general and expects clients to report their pain without being asked. *Cognitive Level:* Application *Client Need:* Safe, Effective Care Environment *Nursing Process:* Assessment

9. *Answer: 3 and 5 Rationale:* Older clients may withhold complaints of pain because it may indicate a worsening of their condition that may threaten their independence. Older adults may describe pain differently—using words other than "pain." Although many perceive pain as a natural outcome of aging, pain is not a natural part of aging. Pain perception may decrease and narcotics can be used with careful monitoring by the nurse. *Cognitive Level:* Comprehension *Client Need:* Physiological Integrity *Nursing Process:* Planning

10. *Answer: 1 Rationale:* Based on the information provided, the nurse needs to gather more information about the client's understanding about the effects of pain on recovery and if the client has misconceptions about pain. Option 2 usually pertains more to chronic pain and fatigue. Options 3 and 4 could be true but the priority is option 1. Movement enhances respiratory, cardiovascular, and gastrointestinal recovery from general anesthesia and the outcomes associated with a surgical procedure. *Cognitive Level:* Analysis *Client Need:* Physiological Integrity *Nursing Process:* Diagnosis

CHAPTER 19

1. *Answer: 2 Rationale:* Blocking the movement of the organism from the reservoir will succeed in preventing the

infection of any other persons. Since the carrier person is the reservoir and the condition is chronic, it is not possible to eliminate the reservoir. Blocking the entry into a host or decreasing the susceptibility of the host will be effective for only that one single individual and, thus, is not as effective as blocking exit from the reservoir. *Cognitive Level:* Comprehension *Client Need:* Safe, Effective Care Environment *Nursing Process:* Planning

2. *Answer: 1 Rationale:* Since the hands are frequently in contact with clients and equipment, they are the most obvious source of transmission. Regular and routine hand cleansing is the most effective way to prevent movement of potentially infective materials. PPE (gloves and masks) is indicated for situations requiring standard precautions. Isolation precautions are used for clients with known communicable diseases. Routine use of antibiotics is not effective and can be harmful due to the incidence of superinfection and development of resistant organisms. *Cognitive Level:* Application *Client Need:* Safe, Effective Care Environment *Nursing Process:* Implementing

3. *Answer: 3 Rationale:* Standard precautions include all aspects of contact precautions with the exception of placing the client in a private room. A mask is indicated when working over a sterile wound rather than an infected one. Disposable food trays are not necessary for clients with infected wounds unlikely to contaminate the client's hands. Sterile technique (surgical asepsis) is not indicated for all contact with the client. The nurse would utilize clean technique when dressing the wound to prevent introduction of additional microbes. *Cognitive Level:* Application *Client Need:* Safe, Effective Care Environment *Nursing Process:* Implementing

4. *Answer: 1 Rationale:* Unless overly contaminated by material that has splashed in the nurse's face and cannot be effectively rinsed off, goggles may be worn repeatedly. Since gowns are at high risk for contamination, they should be used only once and then discarded or washed. Surgical masks and gloves are never washed or reused. *Cognitive Level:* Comprehension *Client Need:* Safe, Effective Care Environment *Nursing Process:* Implementing

5. *Answer: 4 Rationale:* It should not be necessary to unroll this small edge of the cuff. The most important consideration is the sterility of the fingers and hand that will be used to perform the sterile procedure. The rolled-under portion is now contaminated and should not be unrolled by the nurse or colleague since it would then touch the remaining sterile portion of the glove. *Cognitive Level:* Application *Client Need:* Safe, Effective Care Environment *Nursing Process:* Implementing

6. *Answer: 2, 3, and 4 Rationale:* All adults should receive a tetanus booster every 10 years (or sooner if injured). Flu shots are recommended for all adults over age 50. Only persons at risk need to receive hepatitis B and A vaccine. The client's report of infection with rubella does not guarantee immunity, which can be

confirmed only through a blood test for antibody titer. *Cognitive Level:* Knowledge *Client Need:* Safe, Effective Care Environment *Nursing Process:* Assessing

7. *Answer:* Because a malnourished client with a wound is less able to resist an infection, Risk for Infection is the most likely nursing diagnosis. Others may include Pain or Imbalanced Nutrition but they are less focused on the immediate health risk. *Cognitive Level:* Application *Client Need:* Safe, Effective Care Environment *Nursing Process:* Diagnosing

8. *Answer: 2 Rationale:* Raw foods touched by human hands can carry significant infectious organisms and must be washed or peeled. Antimicrobial soap is not indicated for regular use and may lead to resistant organisms. Hand cleansing should occur as needed, not on a timed schedule. Hot water can dry and harm skin, increasing the risk of infection. Clients should learn all the signs of inflammation and infection (e.g., redness, swelling, pain, heat) and not rely on the presence of pus to indicate this. Persons should not share washcloths or towels. *Cognitive Level:* Analysis *Client Need:* Safe, Effective Care Environment *Nursing Process:* Evaluating

9. *Answer: 1 Rationale:* Sterile objects are considered unsterile if placed lower than the waist. Only area 1 in this situation would be considered sterile. Above the neck, higher than 2 inches above the elbow, below the waist/table, and the back are all considered unsterile. *Cognitive Level:* Application *Client Need:* Physiologic Integrity *Nursing Process:* Planning

10. *Answer: 3 Rationale:* All items within 1 inch of the edge of the sterile field are considered contaminated because the edge of the field is in contact with unsterile areas. When hands are ungloved, forceps tips are to be held downward to prevent fluid from becoming contaminated by the hands and then returned to the sterile field. Fields should be established immediately before use to prevent accidental contamination when not observed closely. Reaching over a sterile field increases the chances of dropping an unsterile item onto or touching the sterile field. *Cognitive Level:* Application *Client Need:* Safe, Effective Care Environment *Nursing Process:* Evaluating

CHAPTER 20

1. *Answer: 2 Rationale:* The client's hematocrit is significantly low and can result in hypoxia or even death because it reflects number of red cells to serum. Red blood cells participate in oxygenation. All of the other options are within normal range. *Cognitive Level:* Application *Client Need:* Physiological Integrity *Nursing Process:* Implementation

2. *Answer: 3 Rationale:* Communication of the test to all staff is likely to result in completing the collection. Option 1 is incorrect because you want to discard the first voiding. A clean receptacle, not a sterile one, is used to collect the urine; the purpose of the test will determine

if refrigeration is needed because not all 24-hour urine specimens require refrigeration. *Cognitive Level:* Application *Client Need:* Physiological Integrity *Nursing Process:* Implementation

3. *Answer: 2 Rationale:* Only the KUB looks at the entire urinary system; it is an x-ray of the kidneys, ureters, and bladder. An IVP and retrograde pyelography use injections of contrast media; they look at kidney function. A cystoscopy uses a lighted instrument (cystoscope) inserted through the urethra resulting in direct visualization of the urethra and bladder. *Cognitive Level:* Application *Client Need:* Physiological Integrity *Nursing Process:* Assessment

4. *Answer: 4 Rationale:* A nuclear scan demonstrates ability of tissue to absorb the chemical injected into the bloodstream. All of the other answers provide anatomical information. *Cognitive Level:* Comprehension *Client Need:* Physiological Integrity *Nursing Process:* Assessment

5. *Answer: 3 Rationale:* Bone marrow aspiration includes deep penetration into soft tissue and large bones such as the sternum and iliac crest, resulting in an increased risk for bleeding. Option 1 pertains to a liver biopsy, 2 to a thoracentesis, and 4 a lumbar puncture. *Cognitive Level:* Application *Client Need:* Physiological Integrity *Nursing Process:* Implementation

6. *Answer: 1 and 4 Rationale:* ALT is an enzyme that contributes to protein and carbohydrate metabolism. An increase in the enzyme indicates damage to liver. The liver contributes to the metabolism of protein, which results in the production of ammonia. If the liver is damaged, the ammonia level will increase. Myoglobin, cholesterol, and BNP are relevant for heart disease but irrelevant to the liver. *Cognitive Level:* Application *Client Need:* Physiological Integrity *Nursing Process:* Assessment

7. *Answer: 3 Rationale:* Only the glycosylated hemoglobin (option 3) gives information related to blood glucose levels over the past 3 months. Options 1 and 2 will provide information about the current blood glucose level but will contribute no data related to glucose levels over the last 3 months. Option 4 is used to make a determination of the diagnosis diabetes. *Cognitive Level:* Knowledge *Client Need:* Physiological Integrity *Nursing Process:* Planning

8. *Answer: 2, 3, and 5 Rationale:* The reagent is placed on the back of the card holding the stool smear. The specimen should be collected from two different sites so as not to test only one area of the stool. If positive, the test will turn blue. Vitamin C intake can produce a false positive. A pink color would be considered negative and does not require verification. *Cognitive Level:* Application *Client Need:* Physiological Integrity *Nursing Process:* Planning

9. *Answer: 2 Rationale:* A thoracentesis puncture site is usually on the posterior chest, so the client is positioned leaning forward in order to separate the ribs, allowing for exposure of the site. The site would not be exposed when supine in the Trendelenburg position. Vital sign changes

and pain are not commonly associated with this procedure; monitoring the client is the nurse's responsibility because it requires assessments beyond the capability of the UAP. *Cognitive Level:* Analysis *Client Need:* Physiological Integrity *Nursing Process:* Planning

10. *Answer: 2, 4, and 5 Rationale:* A sputum specimen is often collected in the morning. "Spit" is usually saliva—the client needs to cough up or expectorate mucus or sputum. Once collected the specimen should be taken to the lab immediately to maintain the integrity of the pathogens in the specimen if present. Because a false negative is possible, the specimen is collected on 3 consecutive days. *Cognitive Level:* Application *Client Need:* Physiological Integrity *Nursing Process:* Planning

CHAPTER 21

1. *Answer: 3, 1, 4, 2 Rationale:* The first and most important step to take is to protect the clients from the fire. Only after clients in immediate danger are protected should the fire be reported. While help is on the way, the fire can be contained by closing doors. This step can be performed by some staff members while another is assigned to report the fire. The fire may be extinguished by the staff if it is small and easily extinguished. Larger fires will be extinguished by the fire department. *Cognitive Level:* Comprehension *Client Need:* Safe, Effective Care Environment *Nursing Process:* Implementation

2. *Answer: 1 Rationale:* Young and middle-aged adults are most likely to be injured by motor vehicle accidents. Option 2 is the leading cause for school-age children, option 3 is the leading cause for older adults, and option 4 relates to adolescents. *Cognitive Level:* Analysis *Client Need:* Safe, Effective Care Environment *Nursing Process:* Assessment

3. *Answer: 3 Rationale:* A bedside commode decreases the number of steps required to reach the toilet. Leaving the light on would assist the client in locating the bathroom, but would not reduce the risk of falling when rushing to the bathroom. The nurse cannot withhold a client's medication without consultation with the physician. Rails up would increase the risk of falls as well as falling from a greater distance. *Cognitive Level:* Application *Client Need:* Safe, Effective Care Environment *Nursing Process:* Implementation

4. *Answer: 3 Rationale:* Remember that toddlers are active, like to explore, and are unable to use discretion about what they place in their mouths, placing them at risk for poisoning (e.g., lead poisoning, toxic substances under the sink or in a drawer). The risk for suffocation (option 1) could happen but is more likely with a newborn or infant, which is the reason parents are taught not to prop the bottle, to cut food in small pieces, and to use toys with no small detachable pieces. Option 2 is too vague to address risks associated with a specific group of clients. Option 4 is more applicable to the older adult who is on total bed rest. *Cognitive Level:* Analysis *Client Need:* Safe, Effective Care Environment *Nursing Process:* Diagnosis

5. *Answer: 4 Rationale:* A bed exit safety monitoring device is an intervention that can allow the client to feel independent and also alert the nurse and nursing staff when the client needs assistance. It is the most realistic answer that promotes client safety. Option 1 can increase agitation and confusion and removes the client's independence. Option 2 would help but transfers the responsibility to the family member. Option 3: The client could fall during the unobserved intervals and is also not a realistic time management strategy for the nurse. *Cognitive Level:* Analysis *Client Need:* Safe, Effective Care Environment *Nursing Process:* Implementation

6. *Answer: 2 and 5 Rationale:* Padding the side rails and maintaining oral suction equipment will keep the client safe in the event of another seizure. Option 1 is incorrect because attempting to insert something into the client's mouth during a seizure is likely to cause more injury. Options 3 and 4 are more relevant after the cause of the seizure is known and a determination is made as to the ability to resolve the issue. These steps are taken if recurrent seizures are anticipated. *Cognitive Level:* Application *Client Need:* Safe, Effective Care Environment *Nursing Process:* Planning

7. *Answer: 4 Rationale:* Placing the bed in the lowest position helps to prevent injury by making it easier for the client to get out of bed, as well as reducing the distance he or she will fall in the event of an accident. Option 1 can cause a fall with injury because the client may fall from a higher distance when trying to get over the rail. Review of medications is a valid step to reduce risks of falls but is a lower priority than lowering the height of the bed. Certain medications can increase a risk of a fall (e.g., tranquilizers, analgesics). The nurse would discuss this with the primary care provider. Option 3 would help the nurse assess if a client is at risk for a fall, but once the risk for falls is identified it would not be useful in reducing risk. *Cognitive Level:* Analysis *Client Need:* Safe, Effective Care Environment *Nursing Process:* Implementation

8. *Answer: 3, 4, and 5 Rationale:* Reviewing near misses could identify flaws in the system or practices that placed the client at risk. Communication among staff and with clients will increase efficiency and help to prevent errors. Documenting medication administration immediately prevents accidental overdosage. Options 1 and 2: No facility would hire anyone but competent nurses, and even they can make a medication error if safety is not given a high priority. Multitasking increases the risk of errors, so regardless of the nurse's abilities it is important to give every task the nurse's full attention. *Cognitive Level:* Comprehension *Client Need:* Safe, Effective Care Environment *Nursing Process:* Planning

9. *Answer: 3 Rationale:* Suicide and homicide are two leading causes of death among teenagers, and adolescent

males commit suicide at a higher rate than adolescent females. Options 1, while true, does not address safety concerns. Option 2 is less likely to be a concern with male adolescents than female adolescents and is not the highest priority. Option 4 is not true because while driver's education is helpful, it does not ensure safe practices. *Cognitive Level:* Analysis *Client Need:* Health Promotion and Maintenance *Nursing Process:* Planning

10. *Answer: 1, 3, 4, and 5 Rationale:* Standards require documentation of the necessity of the restraints. Range of motion prevents joint stiffness and pain from disuse. Orienting the client helps the nurse determine the necessity of the restraint. The restraints must be assessed to assure circulation is not compromised if they are tied too tightly. Option 2 is inappropriate because it can cause injury if the side rail is lowered without untying the restraint. *Cognitive Level:* Analysis *Client Need:* Safe, Effective Care Environment *Nursing Process:* Implementation

CHAPTER 22

1. *Answer: 3 Rationale:* The client fits the descriptors for semi-dependent functional level because, while not totally independent, the client is able to perform most self-care with some assistance. *Cognitive Level:* Application *Client Need:* Physiological Integrity *Nursing Process:* Assessment

2. *Answer: 3 Rationale:* The client will be positioned in a side-lying position with the head of the bed lowered because the client is at risk for aspiration. The absence of gag reflex lets the nurse know that the client has no natural defense (cough) and is at a higher risk for aspiration. All other answers are assessments more appropriate prior to bathing the client. *Cognitive Level:* Application *Client Need:* Physiological Integrity *Nursing Process:* Assessment

3. *Answer: 2 Rationale:* A lotion will help moisten the skin. Perfumed lotions contain alcohol, which is drying to the skin. Soaking the feet for a long time or frequently also causes dry skin. Applying foot powder is appropriate to prevent or control unpleasant foot odor. Elastic stockings may decrease circulation. *Cognitive Level:* Application *Client Need:* Physiological Integrity *Nursing Process:* Implementation

4. *Answer: 1 Rationale:* Check that the battery is in the hearing aid. Turn off the hearing aid and make sure the volume is turned all the way down because a too loud volume is distressing. An in-the-ear hearing aid is cleaned with a damp cloth. Make sure the device is functioning. Removing cerumen without a prescription is beyond the UAP scope of practice as well as the nurse. Hearing aids are cleansed with a moist cloth. *Cognitive Level:* Application *Client Need:* Physiological Integrity *Nursing Process:* Implementation

5. *Answer: 4 Rationale:* Both the placement of the linens for a surgical bed and placing the bed in a high position facilitate the client's transfer from a stretcher into the bed. The linens for a closed bed are drawn up to the top of the bed and under the pillows. *Cognitive Level:* Knowledge *Client Need:* Physiological Integrity *Nursing Process:* Implementation

6. *Answer: 1, 2, and 4 Rationale:* Keeping the client covered avoids cooling of the skin, maintains privacy, and will help to reduce distress during the bath. Singing or talking to the client reduces the client's anxiety related to the bath. Be organized to allow movement from one part of the bath to the next without interruption, which could lengthen the time required for bathing the client and increase client anxiety. Moving quickly may agitate the client. Protesting, screaming, and crying are not normal and are reasons to stop the bath and approach again later. *Cognitive Level:* Application *Client Need:* Physiological Integrity *Nursing Process:* Implementation

7. *Answer: 4 Rationale:* It is important to retract the foreskin to remove the smegma that collects under the foreskin and can cause bacterial growth. The other steps are appropriate and correct. *Cognitive Level:* Analysis *Client Need:* Physiological Integrity *Nursing Process:* Evaluation

8. *Answer: 1, 3, and 5 Rationale:* If the bottle is given during naps or bed time, the solution has continuous contact with the toddler's teeth, which increases risk of dental carries. The first visit to the dentist should be long before starting school and is frequently recommended by age 2. The developmental level warrants supervision. Over 50% of older adults have their own teeth and are at risk for periodontal disease. *Cognitive Level:* Application *Client Need:* Health Promotion and Maintenance *Nursing Process:* Planning

9. *Answer: 2 Rationale:* The client needs to avoid walking barefoot as that could cause injury, which may result in an infection. Also, neurological impairment is likely, which may result in decreased sensation and an inability to feel an injury. The other statements indicate understanding of correct foot care. *Cognitive Level:* Analysis *Client Need:* Health Promotion and Maintenance *Nursing Process:* Evaluation

10. *Answer: 1 Rationale:* Fowler's is a sitting position, which should ease the client's breathing. The head of the bed (HOB) in semi-Fowler's is only semi-elevated. The HOB is lowered in the Trendelenburg position increasing blood flow to the brain but putting increased pressure on the diaphragm. While the HOB is raised in the reverse Trendelenburg position, it is a straight tilt and may not be as comfortable as Fowler's. *Cognitive Level:* Application *Client Need:* Safe, Effective Care Environment *Nursing Process:* Implementation

CHAPTER 23

1. *Answer: 2 Rationale:* The medication should be held until it can be clarified that the drug is the correct medication

in the correct dosage and that the client is ordered this particular medication. Whenever there is any doubt, the medication administration process should be interrupted until the question is clarified. While some generic medications come in different colors, until the nurse can determine this is the case, the medication should not be administered. "Maybe" is not acceptable—the doctor may have ordered a new medication, but the nurse must check to make sure that is the case before administration. Medications should never be left unattended. Do not leave medications at the bedside. *Cognitive Level:* Application *Client Need:* Physiological Integrity *Nursing Process:* Implementation

2. *Answer: 4 Rationale:* The dosage is missing from this order. All of the other orders are acceptable with all information provided. *Cognitive Level:* Application *Client Need:* Physiological Integrity *Nursing Process:* Evaluation

3. *Answer: 2 Rationale:* Five milliliters is too great an amount to inject into one site. The nurse needs to divide the amount into two 2.5-mL injections. A 3-mL syringe could be used. The length of the needle will depend on the muscle development of the client. The nurse needs to assess the client. The presumption, based on the information provided, is that this client's muscle mass is within normal limits. The needle length would need to be 1 1/2 inches because the medication is ordered to be given "deep IM." This also suggests that the medication should be given in the preferred site for IM injections—the ventrogluteal site—because it provides the greatest thickness of gluteal muscle. The gauge of the needle for an IM injection into the ventrogluteal muscle can range between #20 and #23. The nurse needs to assess the viscosity of the medication. Smaller gauges (e.g., #23) produce less tissue trauma; however, viscous solutions may require a larger gauge (e.g., #20–#21). *Cognitive Level:* Analysis *Client Need:* Physiological Integrity *Nursing Process:* Implementation

4. *Answer: 3 Rationale:* The type of syringe for subcutaneous injections depends on the medication to be given. This situation does not indicate that the medication is insulin and, thus, another syringe is needed. Generally a 1-mL syringe is used for most subcutaneous injections. Generally, a #20 to #23 gauge needle is used for IM injections. Needle size and length are based on the client's body mass, the intended angle of insertion, and the site of the injection. Generally, a #25-gauge, 5/8-inch needle is used for adults of normal weight and the needle is inserted at a 45-degree angle. Because 2 inches of tissue can be grasped or pinched at the site of the injection, the nurse should administer the medication at a 90-degree angle to ensure the medication reaches subcutaneous tissue. *Cognitive Level:* Analysis *Client Need:* Physiological Integrity *Nursing Process:* Implementation

5. *Answer: 1 Rationale:* A tuberculin test is given by intradermal injection. A tuberculin syringe is used because the dosage will most likely be 0.1 mL. A short, fine needle is needed to avoid entering the subcuta-

neous tissue. The needle should have a short bevel and usually be between #25 and #27 gauge. The needle should be between 1/4- to 5/8-inch long. *Cognitive Level:* Analysis *Client Need:* Physiological Integrity *Nursing Process:* Implementation

6. *Answer: 1 Rationale:* If the nurse goes by the amount of the medication (0.5 mL) only, the deltoid muscle would be considered the best site. However, the question indicates the client is elderly and emaciated, which often results in diminished or atrophied muscles. The nurse should consider the ventrogluteal site because that site will have the most muscle mass. The abdomen and outer aspect of the upper arm are subcutaneous, not IM, sites. *Cognitive Level:* Analysis *Client Need:* Physiological Integrity *Nursing Process:* Implementation

7. *Answer: 1 Rationale:* Due to renal insufficiency, the dose of the medication would need to be decreased in order to avoid accumulation of the medication and the risk of toxicity. *Cognitive Level:* Application *Client Need:* Physiological Integrity *Nursing Process:* Assessment

8. *Answer: 2 Rationale:* In order to straighten the ear canal in children less than 3 years of age, the ear must be pulled down and back. In individuals over 3 years of age, the ear is pulled up and back. *Cognitive Level:* Application *Client Need:* Physiological Integrity *Nursing Process:* Implementation

9. *Answer:* 0.375 or rounded to 0.38 mL *Rationale:* After converting to like numbers, the formula would be set up as follows:

400 micrograms = 1 mL
150 micrograms = X mL
Cross multiply (400 X = 150)
Divide by 400
X = 0.375

Cognitive Level: Application *Client Need:* Physiological Integrity *Nursing Process:* Implementation

10. *Answer: 3, 4, 1, 5, 2, 6, 7, 8 Rationale:* This is the correct order for this skill—first the nurse prepares the insulin, assesses the skin, and cleanses the skin. The nurse would then pinch the skin, insert the needle, inject the medication, count to 5, and remove the syringe. *Cognitive Level:* Application *Client Need:* Physiological Integrity *Nursing Process:* Implementation

CHAPTER 24

1. *Answer: 2 Rationale:* A score ranging from 15 to 18 is considered at risk and a turning schedule is appropriate. Option 1 requires a score above 18 (normal and ongoing assessment is indicated). Option 3, moderate risk, for which a transparent barrier would be appropriate, is applied to persons with scores of 13 to 14. Option 4, very high risk, is assigned for those with a score of 9 or less. *Cognitive Level:* Application *Client Need:* Safe, Effective Care Management *Nursing Process:* Implementing

2. *Answer: 3 Rationale:* The 59-year-old client diagnosed with terminal bowel cancer is at greatest risk because he has poor circulation, impaired nutrition, a draining wound that would keep the skin moist, increasing concerns about skin breakdown, and most likely has reduced perfusion. While the other clients have risk factors, this client has the greatest number of risk factors putting him at greatest risk for skin breakdown. *Cognitive Level:* Analysis *Client Need:* Physiological Integrity *Nursing Process:* Assessment

3. *Answer: 3 Rationale:* Hydrocolloid dressings protect shallow ulcers and maintain an appropriate healing environment. Alginates (option 1) are used for wounds with significant drainage; dry gauze (option 2) will stick to new granulation tissue, causing more damage. A dressing is needed to protect the wound and enhance healing. *Cognitive Level:* Application *Client Need:* Physiological Integrity *Nursing Process:* Implementing

4. *Answer: 1 Rationale:* The heating pad needs to be removed. After 30 minutes of heat application, the blood vessels in the area will begin to exhibit the rebound effect resulting in vasoconstriction. Lowering the temperature, but still delivering heat—dry or moist—will not prevent the rebound effect. The visual appearance of the site on inspection (option 3) does not indicate if rebound is occurring. *Cognitive Level:* Analysis *Client Need:* Physiological Integrity *Nursing Process:* Planning

5. *Answer: 3 Rationale:* Immobile and dependent persons should be repositioned at least every 2 hours, not every 4, so this client or family member requires further teaching. Warm water and moisturizing damp skin are correct techniques for skin care. Red areas that do not return to normal skin color should be reported. It would also be correct to use a foam pad to help relieve pressure. *Cognitive Level:* Analysis *Client Need:* Physiological Integrity *Nursing Process:* Evaluating

6. *Answer:* Potential pressure ulcer sites for side-lying clients include ankles, knees, trochanters, ilia, shoulders, and ears. *Rationale:* These are the primary pressure points that come in contact with the mattress. *Cognitive Level:* Knowledge *Client Need:* Health Promotion and Maintenance *Nursing Process:* Assessing

7. *Answer: 2 Rationale:* This client has an actual impairment of the integrity of the skin due to the rash and the scratching so is no longer "at risk." Because the damage is at the skin level, it is not impaired tissue integrity (option 3) since that would involve deeper tissues. Surface excoriation is also not prone to becoming infected. *Cognitive Level:* Analysis *Client Need:* Physiological Integrity *Nursing Process:* Diagnosing

8. *Answer: 1, 3, and 4 Rationale:* Risk factors for pressure ulcers include low-protein diet, lengthy surgical procedures, and fever. Protein is needed for adequate skin health and healing. During surgery, the client is on a hard surface and may not be well protected from pressure on bony prominences. Fever increases skin moisture, which can lead to skin breakdown, plus the stress

on the body from the cause of the fever could impair circulation and skin integrity. Insomnia (option 2) would generally involve restless sleeping which transfers pressure to different parts of the body and would reduce the chances of skin breakdown. A waterbed (option 5) distributes pressure more evenly than a regular mattress and, thus, actually reduces the chances of skin breakdown. *Cognitive Level:* Application *Client Need:* Physiological Integrity *Nursing Process:* Planning

9. *Answer: 1, 2, and 4 Rationale:* To irrigate a wound, the nurse uses clean gloves to remove the old dressing and to hold the basin collecting the irrigating fluid plus sterile gloves to apply the new dressing. A 60-mL syringe is the correct size to hold the volume of irrigating solution plus deliver safe irrigating pressure. The irrigation fluid should be room or body temperature—certainly not refrigerated—but it should never be microwaved because of the increased risk of burning the client. *Cognitive Level:* Comprehension *Client Need:* Physiological *Nursing Process:* Planning

10. *Answer: 2 Rationale:* The knot of the triangle sling must be kept off the spinal processes as this would be uncomfortable and put unnecessary pressure on the vertebrae. The elbow should be flexed slightly less than 80 degrees (not > 90 as in option 1) so the hand is above the elbow to prevent dependent swelling. The sling must extend past the wrist in order to support the hand. Although the sling must be removed to check for circulation and skin integrity, every 2 hours (option 4) is unnecessarily frequent and impractical. *Cognitive Level:* Comprehension *Client Need:* Physiological Integrity *Nursing Process:* Implementation

CHAPTER 25

1. *Answer: 3 Rationale:* These tests are specific to liver function. Option 1 evaluates fluid and electrolyte status. Option 2 evaluates renal status; option 4 evaluates nutritional status. *Cognitive Level:* Analysis *Client Need:* Physiological Integrity *Nursing Process:* Assessment

2. *Answer: 2 Rationale:* Anticipatory grieving is the state in which an individual experiences reactions in response to an expected significant loss. The definition for option 1 is "confusion in mental picture of one's self" and is often characterized by negative responses such as shame, embarrassment, guilt, or revulsion. Option 3, fear, is usually characterized by feelings of dread, fright, apprehension, or alarm. Ineffective coping, option 4, is usually characterized by verbalization of inability to cope or ask for help, inappropriate use of defense mechanisms, or inability to meet role expectations. *Cognitive Level:* Application *Client Need:* Psychological Integrity *Nursing Process:* Diagnosis

3. *Answer: 4 Rationale:* Option 1 is incorrect because of the ASA guidelines for preoperative fasting. Option 2 is

incorrect because clients are taught how to cough and also how to splint their incision to prevent complications. Option 3 is incorrect because anticoagulants are discontinued a few days before surgery to avoid excessive bleeding postoperatively. *Cognitive Level:* Application *Client Need:* Physiological Integrity *Nursing Process:* Evaluation

4. *Answer: 2 Rationale:* The symptoms describe decreased cardiac output and not any of the other listed complications. *Cognitive Level:* Application *Client Need:* Physiological Integrity *Nursing Process:* Assessment

5. *Answer: 3 Rationale:* Options 1 and 2 are incorrect because the client is still recovering from the anesthesia used during surgery. Option 4 is incorrect because pain usually decreases after the second or third postoperative day. *Cognitive Level:* Application *Client Need:* Physiological Integrity *Nursing Process:* Implementation

6. *Answer:* Splinting *Rationale:* If the incision is painful when the client coughs, splinting the abdomen may reduce the pain while coughing. *Cognitive Level:* Knowledge *Client Need:* Physiological Integrity *Nursing Process:* Implementation

7. *Answer: 4 Rationale:* The tongue can obstruct the airway in a semi-conscious client. Repositioning in the side-lying position with the face slightly down will help prevent occlusion of the pharynx and also allow drainage of mucus out of the mouth. A pillow under the head increases the risk of aspiration or airway obstruction. Since the problem is airway obstruction, actions to promote an open airway are most appropriate. The nurse would want to keep the airway in place. The problem is obstruction, not percentage of available oxygen. *Cognitive Level:* Application *Client Need:* Physiological Integrity *Nursing Process:* Implementation

8. *Answer: 1 and 3 Rationale:* The nurse would also assess bowel sounds—for presence and degree of activity. Anesthetics, narcotics, fasting, and inactivity all inhibit peristalsis. Oral fluids and food are started after the return of peristalsis. The client may feel hungry but peristalsis may not be present. The other options are important but not related specifically to advancing the client's diet. *Cognitive Level:* Application *Client Need:* Physiological Integrity *Nursing Process:* Assessment

9. *Answer:* Safety *Rationale:* The client's protective reflexes are compromised, especially with general anesthesia. Thus the perioperative nurse needs to maintain the client's safety during surgery. *Cognitive Level:* Analysis *Client Need:* Safe, Effective Care Environment *Nursing Process:* Planning

10. *Answer: 2, 3, and 5 Rationale:* Sterile technique is used. The suture material that is visible is in contact with bacteria and must not be pulled beneath the skin during removal. Removal of alternate sutures prevents dehiscence. *Cognitive Level:* Application *Client Need:* Physiological Integrity *Nursing Process:* Implementation

CHAPTER 26

1. *Answer: 4 Rationale:* A sudden, unexpected admission for surgery may involve many experiences (e.g., lab work, x-rays, signing of forms) while the client is in pain or some form of discomfort. The time for orientation will thus be lessened. After surgery, the client may be in pain and possibly in a critical care setting. Options 1 and 2 reflect a greater risk for sensory deprivation, and 3 is a normal activity for a teenager. *Cognitive Level:* Application *Client Need:* Psychosocial Integrity *Nursing Process:* Evaluation

2. *Answer: 3 Rationale:* The transfer to a different setting can change the amount or patterning of incoming stimuli accompanied by a diminished, exaggerated, distorted, or impaired response to such stimuli. Options 1 and 2: There is no evidence of long-standing or progressive deterioration of intellect and personality. Option 4: Disturbed Thought Processes is applied when cognitive abilities (e.g., dementia) interfere with the ability to accurately interpret stimuli. *Cognitive Level:* Application *Client Need:* Psychosocial Integrity *Nursing Process:* Diagnosis

3. *Answer: 2 Rationale:* Because of the paraplegia (paralysis of lower body), the client is unable to feel discomfort. The client will be taught to lift self using chair arms every 10 minutes if possible. Option 1 is an actual problem versus a potential problem. In option 3, the client wears glasses that help correct the poor vision. Option 4 is more of a Risk for Injury diagnosis. *Cognitive Level:* Application *Client Need:* Psychosocial Integrity *Nursing Process:* Diagnosis

4. *Answer: 2 Rationale:* This client could use an assistive device that flashes a light when the doorbell rings. Option 1 relates to safety of the environment rather than sensory alteration. Options 3 and 4 reflect how the client adapts to the sensory alteration. *Cognitive Level:* Analysis *Client Need:* Safe, Effective Care Environment *Nursing Process:* Evaluation

5. *Answer: 4 Rationale:* Option 4 is the only response that helps orient the client and treats the client with respect. *Cognitive Level:* Application *Client Need:* Psychosocial Integrity *Nursing Process:* Implementation

6. *Answer: 1, 3, and 4 Rationale:* Options 2 and 5 relate to interventions for a client with a hearing impairment. *Cognitive Level:* Application *Client Need:* Psychosocial Integrity *Nursing Process:* Implementation

7. *Answer: 3 Rationale:* A disorganized, cluttered environment increases confusion. Option 1: Keeping the room well lit during waking hours promotes adequate sleep at night. It is important to eliminate unnecessary noise (option 2). Client does not meet the standard criteria for restraint application (option 4). *Cognitive Level:* Application *Client Need:* Safe, Effective Care Environment *Nursing Process:* Implementation

8. *Answer: 2, 4, and 5 Rationale:* Options 1 and 3 are clinical signs of sensory overload. *Cognitive Level:*

Knowledge *Client Need:* Psychosocial Integrity *Nursing Process:* Assessment

9. *Answer: 1, 3, 4, and 5 Rationale:* While discharge planning is essential to all clients, it is not part of assessing for sensory-perceptual functioning and is an intervention, not an assessment. Knowing the client's history, performing a thorough physical to test for sensory deficits, and learning more about the client's environment and social network will assist the nurse in making a risk assessment. *Cognitive Level:* Application *Client Need:* Physiological Integrity *Nursing Process:* Assessment

10. *Answer: 1 Rationale:* The amplified telephone helps with hearing and provides a means for communicating with others. Option 2 refers to a tactile impairment. Option 3 relates to a visual impairment, and option 4 an olfactory impairment. *Cognitive Level:* Application *Client Need:* Psychosocial Integrity *Nursing Process:* Planning

CHAPTER 27

1. *Answer: 1 Rationale:* Sally has an inappropriate view of her physical self, which is body image. Personal identity is a sense of uniqueness; self-expectation consists of those things one believes the self should be able to do; and core self-concept includes the most vital central beliefs about one's identity. *Cognitive Level:* Application *Client Need:* Psychosocial Integrity *Nursing Process:* Diagnosing

2. *Answer: 3 Rationale:* This is role conflict—several different roles are competing for the person's time, energy, and abilities. Role ambiguity results when there are unclear expectations of the role. Role strain exists when there are feelings of inadequacy in performing a role. Role enhancement is a nursing intervention. *Cognitive Level:* Comprehension *Client Need:* Psychosocial Integrity *Nursing Process:* Diagnosing

3. *Answer: 2 Rationale:* This is a realistic and measurable outcome. Restored self-esteem is vague and not measurable. Teaching is an intervention, not an outcome. Describes preoccupation with altered self, relates to body image rather than self-esteem. *Cognitive Level:* Application *Client Need:* Psychosocial Integrity *Nursing Process:* Planning

4. *Answer: 1 Rationale:* This response encourages the client to say more and focuses on the positive. Option 2 is condescending and closes the discussion. Both options 3 and 4 ignore the emotional component of the client's statement and do not address the person's feelings of worthlessness. *Cognitive Level:* Application *Client Need:* Psychosocial Integrity *Nursing Process:* Implementing

5. *Answer: 4 Rationale:* A person who follows the crowd is demonstrating unsuccessful resolution of the task of identity versus role confusion. Successful resolution would result in assertion of independence. Inability to express desires is symptomatic of unresolved autonomy versus shame and doubt in toddlerhood, while difficulty being a team player suggests unresolved early school-age industry versus inferiority. *Cognitive Level:* Comprehension *Client Need:* Psychosocial Integrity *Nursing Process:* Assessing

6. *Answer: 3 Rationale:* Self-awareness consists of the relation between own and others' perceptions of the person. The other options reflect only how the nurse sees him/herself. *Cognitive Level:* Analysis *Client Need:* Psychosocial Integrity *Nursing Process:* Evaluating

7. *Answer: 1 Rationale:* A person who perceives herself primarily in terms of relationships with others must have this considered in planning care. Although it may seem important for her to develop outside interests, she may not be able to do this, especially with a new diagnosis of a chronic condition. It is not mandatory for the family to be present during care planning, although items impacting their lives should be validated with them before the plan is finalized. Psychological counseling is not automatically indicated unless her role performance is unhealthy. *Cognitive Level:* Analysis *Client Need:* Psychosocial Integrity *Nursing Process:* Planning

8. *Answer: 2 and 5 Rationale:* A person with chronic low self-esteem often is able to only make negative statements about self and tends to exaggerate his or her own weaknesses without seeing the positive attributes. The client would have difficulty confronting authority (option 1). Option 3 relates to role performance, not self-esteem issues. The client could have difficulty achieving even common/realistic goals and is unlikely to evaluate him- or herself highly enough to set unrealistic goals. *Cognitive Level:* Application *Client Need:* Psychosocial Integrity *Nursing Process:* Diagnosing

9. *Answer: 2 and 3 Rationale:* Clients with poor self-concept should be encouraged to recognize their strengths by learning how to talk positively about self while minimizing negative self-talk. They should not be encouraged to compare themselves with others because they will be unable to assess themselves accurately and comparisons will invariably result in feeling they are less than competent. Having them care for others can be a very therapeutic intervention and they should be given realistic and normal levels of expectations for their behavior. *Cognitive Level:* Application *Client Need:* Psychosocial Integrity *Nursing Process:* Implementing

10. *Answer: 4 Rationale:* The social self is how one is perceived by others and is difficult, if not impossible, to influence since the client does not control the viewpoints of other persons. With planning, the number of the client's resources can be increased, self-knowledge improved, and core self-concept broadened since these are within the client's control. *Cognitive Level:* Analysis *Client Need:* Psychosocial Integrity *Nursing Process:* Planning

CHAPTER 28

1. *Answer: 4 Rationale:* Clients may feel a great deal of shame and discomfort regarding sexuality, particularly if the nurse is younger than they are. Most people assume that providers have a great deal of information (option 1). Many clients have questions and concerns but may not know how to discuss the topic (option 2). While talking with someone of the same gender may make it easier for some women, it is not a requirement for assessment and intervention (option 3). *Cognitive Level:* Analysis *Client Need:* Health Promotion and Maintenance *Nursing Process:* Planning

2. *Answer: 2 Rationale:* Transsexuals' anatomical gender is not the same gender as they feel themselves to be. Option 1 is the definition of intersex. Option 3 is the definition of bisexuality. Transsexuality is a lifelong belief and not altered by an acute condition (option 4). *Cognitive Level:* Comprehension *Client Need:* Health Promotion and Maintenance *Nursing Process:* Implementing

3. *Answer: 4 Rationale:* Masturbation is a normal activity for most people and assists with self-exploration of sexuality and has no relationship to mental health (option 1). There is no evidence that masturbation interferes with academics (option 2). Individuals masturbate at all ages of life (option 3). *Cognitive Level:* Comprehension *Client Need:* Health Promotion and Maintenance *Nursing Process:* Implementing

4. *Answer: 2 Rationale:* Orgasmic response and sex drive are often inhibited by antidepressants. If the depression lifts, there may be an improvement but the focus in option 1 is on the partner rather than where it should be—on the client. Retrograde ejaculation is associated with removal of the prostate (option 2). Skin hypersensitivity is not a side effect of antidepressant medications (option 4). *Cognitive Level:* Application *Client Need:* Health Promotion and Maintenance *Nursing Process:* Planning

5. *Answer: 4 Rationale:* More information is needed before intervening. Also, the client needs the opportunity to express her feelings. Option 1 is an unprofessional response and false reassurance. The ANA Code of Ethics indicates that clients are entitled to a timely and appropriate response to their needs. Option 2 suggests postponing the discussion and that the physician is the better person to deal with her concerns, which is untrue. Option 3 represents feeding into her negative self-concept and inappropriate self-disclosure. *Cognitive Level:* Application *Client Need:* Health Promotion and Maintenance *Nursing Process:* Implementing

6. *Answer: 1 Rationale:* Dyspareunia is painful intercourse. Knowledge of the partner's awareness will contribute to resolution. Involuntary vaginal spasms are called vaginismus (option 2). Painful menstruation is called dysmenorrhea (option 3). Breast swelling can occur during portions of the menstrual cycle but is unrelated to painful intercourse (option 4). *Cognitive Level:* Analysis *Client Need:* Health Promotion and Maintenance *Nursing Process:* Assessing

7. *Answer: 3 Rationale:* Antihypertensive medications are known to affect sexual functioning in several different ways, so some focused history questions would be indicated. There is no evidence of a relationship between sexual functioning and anti-inflammatories, hypnotics, or antihistamines (options 2, 3, and 4). However, the underlying condition that leads the client to take other medications could be important. Side effects of any medication could impact sexual interest or energy level, which reinforces the importance of including sexual health history with all clients. *Cognitive Level:* Application *Client Need:* Health Promotion and Maintenance *Nursing Process:* Assessing

8. *Answer: 2 Rationale:* LI includes instructing clients regarding when sexual activity is safe or unsafe. P involves giving permission to be sexual beings and to discuss issues (option 1). SS includes specific suggestions that help clients promote optimal functioning (option 3). Intensive therapy (IT) requires special skills offered by a nurse specialist or sex therapist (option 4). *Cognitive Level:* Analysis *Client Need:* Health Promotion and Maintenance *Nursing Process:* Implementing

9. *Answer: 4 Rationale:* A change in sexual frequency is not abnormal but may suggest an opportunity for enhanced knowledge if he desires. It does not suggest pathology or disturbed body image (option 1 and 2). It would be incorrect to assume his lifestyle is sedentary merely because the frequency of his sexual activity has decreased. Further assessment of the reason for the decrease in sexual activity is indicated (option 3). *Cognitive Level:* Application *Client Need:* Health Promotion and Maintenance *Nursing Process:* Diagnosing

10. *Answer: 3 Rationale:* The key term is ineffective. If the suggestions given by the nurse are ineffective in reaching the desired goals, the client may require intervention from someone with more specialized skills. Verbalizing constructive methods of exploring and modifying sexual activity are healthy responses and do not require a more skilled therapist (option 1 and 4). Sex support groups can be an effective means of coping with dysfunction (option 2). *Cognitive Level:* Comprehension *Client Need:* Health Promotion and Maintenance *Nursing Process:* Evaluating

CHAPTER 29

1. *Answer: 4 Rationale:* Options 1 and 2 involve assessment and diagnosis, not planning. Option 3, simply keeping the client busy, does not necessarily contribute to feeling fulfilled or purposeful. *Cognitive Level:* Application *Client Need:* Psychosocial Integrity *Nursing Process:* Planning

2. *Answer: 3 Rationale:* The best initial response is to assess. Option 1 may be interpreted as distancing by the client. Option 2 inserts the nurse's experience, which is generally inappropriate. Option 4 is not appropriate for someone in

spiritual distress. *Cognitive Level:* Analysis *Client Need:* Psychosocial Integrity *Nursing Process:* Evaluation

3. *Answer: 3 Rationale:* The key term is full. Option 1 would be inadequate; option 2 is only partial presencing; and option 4 is transcendent presencing. *Cognitive Level:* Knowledge *Client Need:* Psychosocial Integrity *Nursing Process:* Implementation

4. *Answer: 3 Rationale:* This client portrays no distress or risk for distress (option 1 and 2), but rather the potential for enhanced spiritual health as a result of the transformative illness experience. Option 4 is not a valid diagnosis. *Cognitive Level:* Application *Client Need:* Psychosocial Integrity *Nursing Process:* Diagnosis

5. *Answer: 4 Rationale:* Assessment is always the first step of the process of spiritual caregiving or any nursing activity. The other options may not respect the spiritual beliefs of either the nurse or the client. While an assessment may lead the nurse to share personal beliefs, these are never urged on the client. *Cognitive Level:* Application *Client Need:* Psychosocial Integrity *Nursing Process:* Implementation

6. *Answer: 3 Rationale:* Many older adults are religious and spiritually aware. The other answers are disputed by recent research evidence. *Cognitive Level:* Knowledge *Client Need:* Psychosocial Integrity *Nursing Process:* Implementation

7. *Answer: 3 Rationale:* The other options are potentially uncaring or unethical. Jehovah's Witnesses have a well-developed network of representatives who can be called to explain and explore medical options with their fellow believers and medical staff. *Cognitive Level:* Analysis *Client Need:* Psychosocial Integrity *Nursing Process:* Evaluation

8. *Answer: 2 Rationale:* Residing in the SNF likely will curb the client's participation in her church. It is not known if the relocation or an alteration in religious practice will affect her spiritual well-being in either a negative or positive way. *Cognitive Level:* Application *Client Need:* Psychosocial Integrity *Nursing Process:* Diagnosis

9. *Answer: 2 Rationale:* The other options are appropriate for a more specific assessment, if the screening suggests it is necessary. A nurse does not have time or authority to conduct a complete spiritual assessment for every client. What is important for the nurse to assess, however, is how the client's spiritual beliefs and practices may affect the response to illness and how the health care team can support spiritual health. *Cognitive Level:* Application *Client Need:* Psychosocial Integrity *Nursing Process:* Assessment

10. *Answer: 1 Rationale:* Although the mother is arguably angry (options 2 and 3), it is unknown whether this anger is impairing her religiosity or her coping. More data are needed before determining that either option 2 or 3 is the best diagnosis. The mother is experiencing distress versus being at risk for it (option 4). *Cognitive Level:* Application *Client Need:* Psychosocial Integrity *Nursing Process:* Diagnosis

CHAPTER 30

1. *Answer: 4 Rationale:* Wearing glasses is another example of beginning a new strategy to assist with what will be a lifelong health need even though it is not necessarily a desired change. Interviewing for a job (option 1) is a very short-lived situational stressor. Coping strategies effective while a teenager may not be relevant at age 50 (option 2). Experiencing the stress of a divorce is a social/role stressor quite different from that of a health problem and would not be as predictive of the client's coping strategies related to health (option 3). *Cognitive Level:* Analysis *Client Need:* Psychosocial Integrity *Nursing Process:* Assessing

2. *Answer: 3 Rationale:* With stress, respirations increase, pupils dilate, peripheral blood vessels constrict, and the heart rate increases. *Cognitive Level:* Application *Client Need:* Psychosocial Integrity Integrative Process *Nursing Process:* Assessing

3. *Answer: 2 Rationale:* It is too soon for Caregiver Role Strain to be an appropriate nursing diagnosis—especially since the child is not at home. Ineffective Denial and Fear are common reactions to this type of threat. The father demonstrates Compromised Family Coping by his difficulty in being supportive. *Cognitive Level:* Application *Client Need:* Psychosocial Integrity *Nursing Process:* Diagnosing

4. *Answer: 1, 2, and 3 Rationale:* Correct answers include abbreviated (normal grief that is briefly experienced), anticipatory grief (experienced before the loss/death but appropriate), and disenfranchised grief (the emotions are felt privately, just not expressed in public). Unhealthy/abnormal types of grief include complicated grief in several different forms: Unresolved grief is extended in length and severity. With inhibited grief, symptoms are suppressed, and other effects, including somatic, are experienced instead. *Cognitive Level:* Knowledge *Client Need:* Psychosocial Integrity *Nursing Process:* Diagnosing

5. *Answer: 2 Rationale:* When possible, modifications of policy that demonstrate respect for individual differences should be explored. The primary care provider is in no position to modify the implementation of hospital policy. Utilizing an empty room and a staff member for a deceased client is an inappropriate use of resources. *Cognitive Level:* Analysis *Client Need:* Psychosocial Integrity *Nursing Process:* Planning

6. *Answer: 1 Rationale:* This statement acknowledges the family's grief simply. Avoid statements that may be interpreted as overly impersonal (option 2), false support (option 3), or harsh (option 4). *Cognitive Level:* Application *Client Need:* Psychosocial Integrity *Nursing Process:* Implementing

7. *Answer: 4 Rationale:* Adaptive responses indicate the client can put the loss into perspective and begin to develop strategies for coping with the loss. Although the other options are responses the client might likely give and feel, and are not pathologic, they do not demonstrate

movement toward a goal of adaptation nor problem solving. *Cognitive Level:* Application *Client Need:* Psychosocial Integrity *Nursing Process:* Evaluating

8. *Answer: 1 Rationale:* Mild anxiety enhances perception, learning, and productive abilities. Moderate anxiety narrows perception while severe anxiety consumes most of the person's energy and decreases perception still further making it difficult to focus. Panic is overpowering and causes the person to lose control. *Cognitive Level:* Application. *Client Need:* Psychosocial Integrity *Nursing Process:* Assessment

9. *Answer: 3 Rationale:* Incontinence of urine, diminished sensation, and absent gag reflex can occur secondary to a number of issues and do not indicate death by themselves. However, the client with numerous symptoms added together increase the likelihood of impending death. *Cognitive Level:* Application. *Client Need:* Physiological Adaptation: Physiological integrity. *Nursing Process:* Assessment

10. *Answer: 3 Rationale:* Looking for alternate means to allow this client to see his dog without breaking hospital rules and placing other clients in potential danger would be best. It is unlikely that pictures or talking to the dog on the phone will satisfy this client's need to say good-bye. *Cognitive Level:* Analysis *Client Need:* Psychosocial Integrity *Nursing Process:* Planning

CHAPTER 31

1. *Answer: 2 Rationale:* A key word in the question is "base," and the feet provide this foundation. Leaning backward actually decreases balance, and tensing abdominal muscles alone or bending the knees does not affect the base of support. *Cognitive Level:* Application *Client Need:* Health Promotion and Maintenance *Nursing Process:* Implementation

2. *Answer: 1, 3, and, 5 Rationale:* Isotonic exercise increases muscle tone, mass, and strength and maintains joint flexibility and circulation. During isotonic exercise, both heart rate and cardiac output quicken to increase blood flow to all parts of the body. Little or no change in blood pressure occurs. *Cognitive Level:* Knowledge *Client Need:* Physiological Integrity *Nursing Process:* Planning

3. *Answer: 1 Rationale:* Vital signs that do not return to baseline 5 minutes after exercising indicate intolerance of exercise at that time. This is a real problem, not "at risk for." There is no evidence that the client requires assistance (impaired mobility) or is immobile (disuse syndrome). *Cognitive Level:* Analysis *Client Need:* Physiological Integrity *Nursing Process:* Diagnosis

4. *Answer: 2 Rationale:* The benzodiazepines (e.g., Valium) impair the function of the central nervous system, resulting in unstable ambulation or movement and should be questioned, particularly if the client has pre-existing risks for falls. Sinemet is often prescribed to clients with Parkinson's disease and would improve muscle activity and reduces their risk of falling. Elavil is an antidepressant and does not usually affect coordination or increase the risk of falling. Lasix is a diuretic that would increase the risk of falling only if electrolytes were not adequately monitored and balanced. *Cognitive Level:* Analysis *Client Need:* Safe, Effective Care Environment *Nursing Process:* Planning

5. *Answer: 4 Rationale:* Placing the client in a safe position is the best strategy. Leaving the client to find help or having the client continue to ambulate back to the room creates unsafe conditions as the client may faint before help is found or the client is able to return to her room. Rapid, shallow breathing (hyperventilation) may increase dizziness. *Cognitive Level:* Application *Client Need:* Safe, Effective Care Environment *Nursing Process:* Implementation

6. *Answer: 2 Rationale:* The reddened area of the skin is an indication of early skin damage and will advance to skin breakdown if not corrected. The other options are within normal limits. *Cognitive Level:* Application *Client Need:* Physiological Integrity *Nursing Process:* Planning

7. *Answer: 2 Rationale:* This is the brainstem, where the reticular formation (and RAS) is located and which integrates sensory information from the peripheral nervous system and relays the information to the cerebral cortex. An intact cerebral cortex and reticular formation are necessary for the regulation of sleep and waking states. *Cognitive Level:* Application *Client Need:* Physiological Integrity *Nursing Process:* Implementation

8. *Answer: 4 Rationale:* Most clients with sleep apnea report excessive daytime sleepiness. If they don't volunteer this, clients should be asked if they fall asleep or struggle to stay awake at work. Although cardiac arrhythmias may occur, they are usually detectable only during a sleep study, and thus the client would not be aware of them. Nasal obstruction is rarely the cause of sleep apnea or a complaint of clients with sleep apnea. There are many causes of chest pain, and this is unlikely to be something reported by clients with sleep apnea unless they have underlying cardiac disease. *Cognitive Level:* Analysis *Client Need:* Physiological Integrity *Nursing Process:* Assessment

9. *Answer: 4 Rationale:* Suddenly stopping barbiturate sleeping pills can precipitate a dangerous withdrawal. Doses should be tapered gradually and the tapering process supervised by the client's primary care provider. *Cognitive Level:* Analysis *Client Need:* Physiological Integrity *Nursing Process:* Implementation

10. *Answer: 1 Rationale:* Preschool children require 10 to 12 hours of sleep/night. Young children often rise early, so it is more appropriate to put the child to bed earlier in the evening. If adequate nighttime sleep is obtained, naps are not required. *Cognitive Level:* Analysis *Client Need:* Health Promotion and Maintenance *Nursing Process:* Implementation

CHAPTER 32

1. *Answer: 2 Rationale:* A BMI of 31 to 40 indicates moderate to severe obesity. A BMI of less than 20 indicates underweight. BMI is calculated using the client's weight in kilograms/(height meters). The client is not at risk for imbalance since it already exists. There is no evidence to support a diagnosis of Deficient Knowledge. *Cognitive Level:* Application *Client Need:* Health Promotion and Maintenance *Nursing Process:* Diagnosing

2. *Answer: 4 Rationale:* This client needs more grains in the diet. The food pyramid indicates that the client should have 6 to 7 oz grains per day, 3 cups/week dark green vegetables, 2 cups/week orange vegetables, 3 cups/week legumes, 3 cups/week starchy vegetables, 1.5 to 2 cups fruit per day, 5 to 6 oz meat and beans per day, and 3 cups milk, yogurt, and cheese per day. *Cognitive Level:* Application *Client Need:* Health Promotion and Maintenance *Nursing Process:* Planning

3. *Answer: 2, 3, 4, 6, and 8 Rationale:* A full liquid diet contains only liquids or foods that turn to liquid at body temperature. Pudding, juices, hard candy, Cream of Wheat cereal, and fruit smoothies are permitted on a full liquid diet. Scrambled eggs, mashed potatoes, and oatmeal cereal are not permitted until the client advances to a soft diet. *Cognitive Level:* Application *Client Need:* Physiological Integrity *Nursing Process:* Implementing

4. *Answer: 3 Rationale:* Gastric secretions are acidic as evidenced by a pH of less than 6. Improper tube placement would not necessarily impact the client's ability to speak. Gagging during insertion is common and does not indicate that the tube is or is not in the stomach. Ability to easily instill fluid into the tube does not relate to its placement. The lungs would offer no resistance to the flow of liquid. *Cognitive Level:* Application *Client Need:* Physiological Integrity *Nursing Process:* Evaluating

5. *Answer: 1 Rationale:* For proper flow, the feeding container hangs 1 foot above the tube insertion. Feedings may be administered if there is less than 90 to 100 mL of residual volume (unless agency policy specifies otherwise). To prevent or reduce the risk of aspiration, the client should be placed in Fowler's position during feeding. The feeding should be warmed to room temperature before administration to decrease cramping and diarrhea. *Cognitive Level:* Application *Client Need:* Physiological Integrity *Nursing Process:* Implementing

6. *Answer: 1 Rationale:* The Dietary Guidelines recommend 30 minutes of physical activity on most days of the week to achieve optimal weight. Some persons benefit from a low-carbohydrate diet, but no particular diet is the solution for all persons. A reasonable diet emphasizes balance and portion control rather than forbidding or requiring any specific foods. Fresh and chemical-free foods may be healthier than preserved foods but do not automatically assist with weight loss. *Cognitive Level:* Analysis *Client Need:* Health Promotion and Maintenance *Nursing Process:* Evaluating

7. *Answer: 3 Rationale:* Always inquire into the client's favorite foods when planning a diet. Dairy may not be indicated for this client due to the high incidence of lactose intolerance in individuals of Asian heritage. Beer can be a source of calories and, in moderation, is not harmful and may maintain the client's satisfaction with the dietary changes. The nurse will need to assess the ability to swallow beer safely, however. Calories from lipid sources should be kept below 35% and, when enhanced wound healing is indicated (not so with a stroke), increased protein and carbohydrates are needed rather than fats. *Cognitive Level:* Application *Client Need:* Health Promotion and Maintenance *Nursing Process:* Planning

8. *Answer:* This client has lost 13 pounds, which is 6.7%: (195–182)/195. If the weight loss has been steady over the past 2 months, that would indicate a 3.3% loss per month. Less than 5% loss in 1 month is not significant but if this loss continues, the client will reach a 10% loss in 3 months, which is a severe loss. A more detailed assessment is indicated to determine the client's nutritional status. *Cognitive Level:* Application *Client Need:* Health Promotion and Maintenance *Nursing Process:* Assessing

9. *Answer: 2 Rationale:* A small-bore nasal feeding tube tip is most commonly placed in the stomach. Option 1 indicates the esophagus. A tube tip placed there can lead to aspiration. Option 3 indicates the post-pyloric duodenum. Small-bore nasal tubes can be advanced to this location if desired but is less common than gastric placement. Option 4 indicates the jejunum where feeding tubes can be placed but usually not from a nasally placed tube. *Cognitive Level:* Comprehension *Client Need:* Physiological Integrity *Nursing Process:* Evaluating

10. *Answer: 4 Rationale:* 3 ounces tuna + 2 slices whole wheat bread = 3.1 mg Fe; 1 ounce cheese = ~200 mg Ca++; pear = 4.2 gm fiber. Option 1: 1/3 cup raisins = 1.75 mg Fe; 3 ounces cottage cheese = 90 mg Ca++; 1 banana = 2.1 gm fiber. Option 3: 1/2 cup spaghetti + 2 ounces ground beef = 2.3 mg Fe; 1/2 cup ice cream = 97 mg Ca++; 1/2 cup lima beans = 3.2 gm fiber. Option 2: 3 ounces chicken + 1/2 cup peanuts = 2.9 mg Fe; 1/2 cup broccoli = ~158 mg Ca++; 1/2 cup broccoli = 2.4 gm fiber. *Cognitive Level:* Application *Client Need:* Health Promotion and Maintenance *Nursing Process:* Implementing

CHAPTER 33

1. *Answer: 4. Rationale:* The capacity of the bladder may decrease with age but the muscle is weaker and can cause urine to be retained. Older adults do not ignore the urge to void and may have difficulty in getting to the toilet in time. The kidney becomes less able to concentrate urine with age. *Cognitive Level:* Knowledge *Client Need:* Physiological Integrity *Nursing Process:* Assessment

2. *Answer: 1, 2, and 4 Rationale:* The perineum may become irritated by the frequent contact with urine. Normal fluid intake is at least 1,500 mL/day and clients often decrease their intake to try to minimize urine leakage. Urinary tract infections can contribute to incontinence. Antihistamines can cause urinary retention rather than incontinence (option 3) and childhood traumas are unlikely to be the cause of incontinence (option 5). *Cognitive Level:* Analysis *Client Need:* Physiological Integrity *Nursing Process:* Assessment

3. *Answer: 2 Rationale:* The penis and condom should be checked one-half hour after application to ensure that it is not too tight. A 1-inch space should be left between the penis and the end of the condom. The condom is changed every 24 hours, and the tubing is taped to the leg or attached to a leg bag. An indwelling catheter is taped to the lower abdomen or upper thigh. *Cognitive Level:* Application *Client Need:* Safe, Effective Care Environment *Nursing Process:* Implementation

4. *Answer: 1 Rationale:* The catheter in the vagina is contaminated and cannot be reused. If left in place, it may help avoid mistaking the vaginal opening for the urinary meatus when the nurse obtains a new sterile catheter and prepares to insert it into the urinary meatus. A single failure to catheterize the meatus does not indicate that another nurse is needed although sometimes a second nurse can be helpful with visualizing the meatus. *Cognitive Level:* Application *Client Need:* Safe, Effective Care Environment *Nursing Process:* Implementation

5. *Answer: 3 Rationale:* Soaking in a bathtub can increase the risk of exposure to bacteria. The bag should be below the level of the bladder to promote proper drainage. Intake of cranberry juice creates an environment nonconducive to infection. Clean technique is appropriate for touching the exterior portions of the system. *Cognitive Level:* Analysis *Client Need:* Health Promotion and Maintenance *Nursing Process:* Evaluation

6. *Answer: 4 Rationale:* The key phrase is the urge to void. Option 1: occurs when the client coughs, sneezes, or jars the body resulting in accidental loss of urine. Option 2: absence of control. Option 3: involuntary loss of urine related to impaired function. *Cognitive Level:* Application *Client Need:* Physiological Integrity *Nursing Process:* Diagnosis

7. *Answer: 2 and 4 Rationale:* Symptoms of UTI should be reviewed with the client to promote prompt reporting if symptoms return and validates the diagnosis. Cotton underwear promotes appropriate exposure to air, resulting in decreased bacterial growth. In option 1, increased fluids decrease concentration and irritation. In option 3, the client should wipe the perineal area from front to back to prevent spread of bacteria from rectal area to urethra. In option 5, showers reduce exposure of area to bacteria. *Cognitive Level:* Application *Client Need:* Health Promotion and Maintenance *Nursing Process:* Implementation

8. *Answer: 2 Rationale:* The Kock pouch uses a portion of the ileum to form a reservoir for urine, and nipple valves are formed to close as the pouch fills with urine, preventing leakage and reflux of urine back toward the kidneys. The client empties the pouch by inserting a clean catheter approximately every 4 hours. The ileal conduit and vesicostomy (options 1 and 4) are incontinent urinary diversions, and clients are required to use an external ostomy appliance to contain the urine. Clients with a neobladder can control their voiding (option 3). *Cognitive Level:* Analysis *Client Need:* Health Promotion and Maintenance *Nursing Process:* Assessment

9. *Answer: 3 Rationale:* Since the bladder muscles will not contract to increase the intra-bladder pressure to promote urination, the process is initiated manually. To promote continence, bladder contractions are required for habit training, bladder training, and increasing the tone of the pelvic muscles. *Cognitive Level:* Application *Client Need:* Physiological Integrity *Nursing Process:* Implementation

10. *Answer: 2 and 5 Rationale:* It is important for the client to inhibit the urge-to-void sensation when a premature urge is experienced. Pelvic muscle exercises help to control the urge to void. Some clients may need diapers but this is not the BEST indicator of a successful program. Citrus juices may irritate the bladder. Carbonated beverages increase diuresis, increasing the risk of incontinence. *Cognitive Level:* Application *Client Need:* Health Promotion and Maintenance *Nursing Process:* Evaluation

CHAPTER 34

1. *Answer: 1 Rationale:* Habitually ignoring the urge to defecate can lead to constipation through loss of the natural urge and the accumulation of feces. Diarrhea will not result—if anything, there is increased opportunity for water reabsorption because the stool remains in the colon, leading to firmer stool (option 2). Ignoring the urge shows a strong voluntary sphincter, not a weak one that could result in incontinence (option 3). Hemorrhoids would occur only if severe drying out of the stool occurs and, thus, repeated need to strain to pass stool (option 4). *Cognitive Level:* Comprehension *Client Need:* Physiological Integrity *Nursing Process:* Implementation

2. *Answer: 2 Rationale:* The standard of practice in assisting older adults to maintain normal function of the gastrointestinal tract is regular ingestion of a well-balanced diet, adequate fluid intake, and regular exercise. If the bowel pattern is not regular with these activities, this abnormality should be reported. Stimulant laxatives can be very irritating and are not the preferred treatment for occasional constipation in older adults. In addition, a normal stool pattern for an older adult may not be daily elimination. *Cognitive Level:* Analysis *Client Need:* Physiological Integrity *Nursing Process:* Evaluation

3. *Answer: 4 Rationale:* Small-volume enemas along with other preparations are used to prepare the client for this

procedure. An oil retention enema is used to soften hard stool (option 1). Return flow enemas help expel flatus (option 2). Because of the risk of loss of fluid and electrolytes, high, large-volume enemas are seldom used (option 3). *Cognitive Level:* Analysis *Client Need:* Health Promotion and Maintenance *Nursing Process:* Planning

4. *Answer: 3 Rationale:* An established stoma should be dark pink like the color of the buccal mucosa and is slightly raised above the abdomen. The skin under the appliance may remain pink/red for a while after the adhesive is pulled off. Feces from an ascending ostomy are very liquid, less so from a transverse ostomy, and more solid from a descending or sigmoid stoma. *Cognitive Level:* Application *Client Need:* Physiological Integrity *Nursing Process:* Assessment

5. *Answer: 2 Rationale:* Once the cause of diarrhea has been identified and corrected, the client should return to his or her previous elimination pattern. This is not an example of an allergy to the antibiotic but a common consequence of overgrowth of bowel organisms not killed by the drug. Antidiarrheal medications are usually prescribed according to the number of stools, not routinely around the clock. Increasing intake of soluble fiber such as oatmeal or potatoes may help absorb excess liquid and decrease the diarrhea, but insoluble fiber will not. *Cognitive Level:* Analysis *Client Need:* Physiological Integrity *Nursing Process:* Planning

6. *Answer: 2 Rationale:* The client has assessment findings consistent with complications of surgery. Option 1: Irrigating the stoma is a dependent nursing action, and is also intervention without appropriate assessment. Option 3: Assessing the peristomal skin area is an independent action, but administering an antiemetic is an intervention without appropriate assessment. Antiemetics are generally ordered to treat immediate postop nausea, not several days postop. Option 4: Administering a bulk-forming laxative to a nauseated postoperative client is contraindicated. *Cognitive Level:* Analysis *Client Need:* Physiological Integrity *Nursing Process:* Implementation

7. *Answer: 3 Rationale:* This provides relief of postoperative flatus, stimulating bowel motility. Options 1, 2, and 4 manage constipation and do not provide flatus relief. *Cognitive Level:* Application *Client Need:* Physiological Integrity *Nursing Process:* Implementation

8. *Answer: 3 Rationale:* Bleeding into the upper GI tract is black and tarry. Option 1 can be a sign of malabsorption in an infant, option 2 is normal stool, and option 4 is characteristic of an obstructive condition of the rectum. *Cognitive Level:* Analysis *Client Need:* Health Promotion and Maintenance *Nursing Process:* Assessment

9. *Answer: 1, 3, 4, and 5 Rationale:* Option 1 is the most appropriate because the client is unable to control when stool evacuation will occur. In option 3, client thoughts about self may be altered if unable to control stool evacuation. In option 4, client may not feel as comfortable around others due to anxiety of an embarrassing incontinence episode. In option 5, increased tissue contact

with fecal material may result in impairment. Option 2 is more appropriate for a client with diarrhea. Incontinence is the inability to control feces of normal consistency. *Cognitive Level:* Analysis *Client Need:* Physiological Integrity *Nursing Process:* Diagnosis

10. *Answer: 5 Rationale:* Option 5 is a sigmoidostomy site. Option 1 is an ileostomy site, option 2 is ascending colostomy, option 3 is transverse colostomy, and option 4 is descending colostomy. *Cognitive Level:* Application *Client Need:* Physiological Integrity *Nursing Process:* Assessment

CHAPTER 35

1. *Answer: 1 Rationale:* Clients with chronic obstructive pulmonary disease may have only low levels of supplemental oxygen, generally not over 2 liters per minute, because their motivation to breathe comes from mild hypoxemia. Elimination of this hypoxemia will eliminate their drive to breathe and could result in apnea. *Cognitive Level:* Application *Client Need:* Safe, Effective Care Environment *Nursing Process:* Implementation

2. *Answer: 2 Rationale:* Proper use of an SMI requires the client to take slow, steady inhalations, every hour or two, 5 to 10 breaths each time. The device measures inspiration, not expiration. Only the mouthpiece can be successfully rinsed or wiped. The device should not be submerged in water. *Cognitive Level:* Analysis *Client Need:* Health Promotion and Maintenance *Nursing Process:* Evaluation

3. *Answer: 2 Rationale:* The tube should be reconnected to the water seal as quickly as possible. Assisting the client back to bed and assessing the client's lungs are possible actions after the system is reconnected, but these should not be performed until the tube is reconnected to the water seal. Coughing forcibly is not appropriate. *Cognitive Level:* Application *Client Need:* Safe, Effective Care Environment *Nursing Process:* Implementation

4. *Answer: 1 Rationale:* Anemia is a condition of decreased red blood cells and decreased hemoglobin. Hemoglobin is how the oxygen molecules are transported to the tissues. A client with anemia does not have adequate oxygen-carrying capacity to oxygenate the tissues. Option 2 would depend on where the infection is located. Option 3: A fractured rib would interrupt transport of oxygen from the atmosphere to the airways. Option 4: Damage to the medulla would interfere with neural stimulation of the respiratory system and could impact passage of air from the atmosphere to the airways. *Cognitive Level:* Application *Client Need:* Physiological integrity *Nursing Process:* Planning

5. *Answer: 1 Rationale:* Postural drainage results in expectoration of large amounts of mucus. Clients sometimes ingest part of the secretions. The secretions may also produce an unpleasant taste in the oral cavity,

which could result in nausea/vomiting. This procedure should be done on an empty stomach to reduce risks of nausea and vomiting as well as client discomfort. *Cognitive Level:* Application *Client Need:* Physiological Integrity *Nursing Process:* Planning

6. *Answer: 3 Rationale:* Capillary refill is an assessment of capillary blood flow and thus tissue perfusion. Symmetrical chest expansion (option 1) is an assessment of respiratory function, and pursed-lip breathing (option 2) is a technique used to assist clients with obstructive lung diseases to keep alveoli open during respirations. Activity intolerance (option 4) can occur because of low cardiac output (e.g., heart failure). Activity tolerance would indicate adequate tissue perfusion but activity intolerance could be secondary to factors other than tissue perfusion so is not a primary measure of perfusion. *Cognitive Level:* Application *Client Need:* Physiological Integrity *Nursing Process:* Evaluation

7. *Answer: 3 and 5 Rationale:* These are enzymes that are released into the blood from the damaged cardiac tissues when there is hypoxia and myocardial damage. Option 1 reflects renal function. Option 2 reflects number of red blood cells. Option 4 reflects glucose levels. *Cognitive Level:* Application *Client Need:* Physiological Integrity *Nursing Process:* Planning

8. *Answer: 3 Rationale:* Very rapid heart rates do not allow adequate time for the ventricles to fill, causing cardiac output to fall. Option 1 is normal. Option 2 is a normal cardiac output of 4900 mL/min. The formula is SV × HR = CO is about 5 L/min. Option 4: Positive inotropic drugs (e.g., digoxin) increase contractility of the cardiac muscle and thus increase stroke volume, which increases cardiac output. *Cognitive Level:* Analysis *Client Need:* Physiological Integrity *Nursing Process:* Assessment

9. *Answer: 4 Rationale:* The three cardinal signs of cardiac arrest are absence of heart beat, cessation of breathing (apnea), and the absence of cerebral circulation reflected in dilated pupils. *Cognitive Level:* Application *Client Need:* Physiological Integrity *Nursing Process:* Implementation

10. *Answer: 1, 3, and 5 Rationale:* Option 1: An example of ineffective tissue perfusion is a decrease in arterial circulation in the legs related to atherosclerosis. Option 3: Examples of decreased cardiac output are clients with MI, heart failure, or tachycardia. Option 5: Not enough blood is being pumped by the heart to meet the demands of the body. Activity intolerance is when the client doesn't have physiological energy for ADLs. Common reasons can be anemias and heart failure. Options 2 and 4: Acute confusion and sleep pattern disturbance are not directly related to cardiovascular disease, although some clients may display these symptoms if perfusion is acutely compromised. *Cognitive Level:* Application *Client Need:* Physiological Integrity *Nursing Process:* Diagnosing

CHAPTER 36

1. *Answer: 3 Rationale:* Protein molecules help to maintain fluid within the intravascular space. Clients who are protein malnourished are at greater risk for edema because fluid is drawn out of the intravascular space. The other options are related to fluid imbalances. *Cognitive Level:* Analysis *Client Need:* Physiological Integrity *Nursing Process:* Assessment

2. *Answer: 1 Rationale:* Hyperventilation causes excessive carbon dioxide loss, resulting in respiratory alkalosis, or an increase in pH. Because the kidneys are slower to respond to pH changes, and hyperventilation is a short-term problem, kidney response is usually not impacted. *Cognitive Level:* Analysis *Client Need:* Physiological Integrity *Nursing Process:* Planning

3. *Answer: 3 Rationale:* Older adults have less body fluids and diminished thirst responses, which put this client at greatest risk. Other options are clients with only one risk factor and reduced risk. *Cognitive Level:* Analysis *Client Need:* Physiological Integrity *Nursing Process:* Planning

4. *Answer: 2 Rationale:* Because of the retention of CO_2, the clinical profile of respiratory acidosis includes decreased pH < 7.35, $PaCO_2$ > 42 mm Hg with varying levels of HCO_3 related to hypoventilation. Option 1 is respiratory alkalosis which occurs because of blowing off of CO_2 resulting in a decreased level of acid and retention or production of bicarbonate resulting in pH > 7.45, $PaCO_2$ < 38 mm Hg, HCO_3 > 26 mEq/mL related to hyperventilation. Option 3: Metabolic acidosis occurs because of a gain of hydrogen ions or a loss of HCO_3 with a pH < 7.35, normal $PaCO_2$ 35–45 mm Hg, and HCO_3 < 22 mEq/mL, often caused by diarrhea, bicarbonate infusion, or retention related to kidney failure. Option 4: Metabolic alkalosis caused by gain of bicarbonate or loss of hydrogen ions related to vomiting, gastric suction, or loss of upper gastrointestinal secretions by various other methods. *Cognitive Level:* Application *Client Need:* Physiological Integrity *Nursing Process:* Assessment

5. *Answer: 1, 3, and 5 Rationale:* Options 1, 3, and 5 relate to fluid volume deficit. The data indicate an actual problem, which excludes option 2. Option 4 relates more to fluid volume excess. *Cognitive Level:* Analysis *Client Need:* Physiological Integrity *Nursing Process:* Nursing Diagnosis

6. *Answer: 4 Rationale:* Salt substitutes contain potassium. The client can still use it within reason. Avocado is higher in potassium than most foods. Hypokalemia can potentiate digoxin toxicity and checking the pulse will help the client to avoid this; it is important to take potassium with food to avoid gastric upset. *Cognitive Level:* Application *Client Need:* Physiological Integrity *Nursing Process:* Evaluation

7. *Answer: 2 Rationale:* Sodium contributes to the function of neural tissue. Because calcium contributes the function of voluntary muscle contraction, options 1 and 4 are more appropriate for calcium imbalances. Because

potassium and calcium contribute to cardiac function, irregular pulse is more likely to be associated with those alterations. ***Cognitive Level:*** Application ***Client Need:*** Physiological Integrity ***Nursing Process:*** Assessment

8. ***Answer: 2 Rationale:*** Because of CO_2 retention the $PaCO_2$ is elevated. CO_2 is involved in production of acid which will result in a decreased pH. HCO_3 will vary. Option 1: Metabolic acidosis involves a loss of bicarbonate but no retention of CO_2. Option 3: Metabolic alkalosis involves a loss of acid or retention of HCO_3, but no retention of CO_2. Option 4: Respiratory alkalosis involves a loss of CO_2 resulting in an increased pH. ***Cognitive Level:*** Application ***Client Need:*** Physiological Integrity ***Nursing Process:*** Assessment

9. ***Answer: 4 Rationale:*** The major clinical signs and symptoms of hypocalcemia are due to increased neuromuscular activity. ***Cognitive Level:*** Analysis ***Client Need:*** Physiological Integrity ***Nursing Process:*** Implementation

10. ***Answer: 2 Rationale:*** The best indicator of the effectiveness of treatment for fluid volume alterations is changes in weight. Dyspnea will generally subside as soon as fluid volumes begin to decline, while absence of pitting edema will be a later change. Output can be greater than intake but may not be high enough to make a significant improvement in the client's overall fluid status. ***Cognitive Level:*** Analysis ***Client Need:*** Physiological Integrity ***Nursing Process:*** Evaluation

GLOSSARY

A

24-hour food recall   client recall of all the food and beverages consumed during a typical 24-hour period

Abdominal paracentesis   removal of fluids from the peritoneal cavity

Absorption   the process by which a drug passes into the bloodstream

Accommodation   a process of change whereby cognitive processes mature sufficiently to allow a person to solve problems that were previously unsolvable

Accountability   the ability and willingness to assume responsibility for one's actions and to accept the consequences of one's behavior

Acculturation   the involuntary process that occurs when people adapt to or borrow traits from another culture

Accuracy   how close data measurements are to their true value

Acid   a substance that releases hydrogen ions (H+) in solution

Acidosis   a condition that occurs with increases in blood carbonic acid or with decreases in blood bicarbonate; blood pH below 7.35

Acquired immunity   *see* Passive immunity

Action stage   occurs when a person actively implements behavioral and cognitive strategies to interrupt previous behavior patterns and adopt new ones; this stage requires a great commitment of time and energy

Active euthanasia   actions that directly bring about the client's death with or without consent

Active immunity   a resistance of the body to infection in which the host produces its own antibodies in response to natural or artificial antigens

Active ROM exercises   isotonic exercises in which the client moves each joint in the body through its complete range, maximally stretching all muscle groups within each plane over the joint

Active transport   movement of substances across cell membranes against the concentration gradient

Activity theory   the best way to age is to stay active physically and mentally

Activity tolerance   the type and amount of exercise or daily activities an individual is able to perform

Activity-exercise pattern   refers to a person's pattern of exercise, activity, leisure, and recreation

Actual loss   can be identified by others and can arise either in response to or in anticipation of a situation

Acupressure   a form of healing in which the therapist exerts finger pressure on specific sites

Acupuncture   a form of healing in which the therapist applies needles to stimulate specific sites of the body

Acute confusion   also called *delirium;* abrupt onset of confusion and a reversible cause

Acute illness   typically characterized by severe symptoms of relatively short duration

Acute infection   those that generally appear suddenly or last a short time

Acute pain   pain that lasts only through the expected recovery period (less than 6 months), whether it has a sudden or slow onset and regardless of the intensity

Adaptation   the process of modifying to meet new, changing, or different conditions

Adaptive mechanism   learned behaviors that assist an individual to adjust to the environment

Adherence   the extent to which an individual's behavior (for example, taking medications, following diets, or making lifestyle changes) coincides with medical or health advice; commitment or attachment to a regimen

Adolescence   the period during which a person becomes physically and psychologically mature and acquires a personal identity

Adolescent growth spurt   the period during puberty when sudden and dramatic physical changes occur

Adult day care   a day care center that provides health and social services to the older person

Advance health care directive   a variety of legal and lay documents that allow persons to specify aspects of care they wish to receive should they become unable to make or communicate their preferences

Adventitious breath sounds   abnormal or acquired breath sounds

Adverse effects   more severe side effects that may justify the discontinuation of a drug

Advocate   individual who pleads the cause of another or argues or pleads for a cause or proposal

Aerobic   living only in the presence of oxygen

Aerobic exercise   any activity during which the body takes in more or an equal amount of oxygen than it expends

Aesthetic knowing   providing care and meeting the needs of clients through creativity and style

Afebrile   absence of a fever

Affective domain   known as the "feeling" domain and is divided into categories that specify the degree of a person's depth of emotional response to tasks; includes feelings, emotions, interests, attitudes, and appreciations

Afterload   the resistance against which the heart must pump to eject blood into the circulation

Ageism   deep and profound prejudice in American society against older adults

Agglutinins   specific antibodies formed in the blood

Agglutinogens   a substance that acts as an antigen and stimulates the production of agglutinins

Agnostic a person who doubts the existence of God or a supreme being or believes the existence of God has not been proved

Agonist a drug that interacts with a receptor to produce a response

Agonist analgesic full agonists which are pure opioid drugs that bind tightly to mu receptor sites, producing maximum pain inhibition, an agonist effect

Agonist-antagonist analgesic mixed agonist-antagonist drugs that can act like opioids and relieve pain (agonist effect) when given to a client who has not taken any pure opioids

Airborne precautions methods used to reduce exposure to infectious agents transmitted by airborne droplet nuclei smaller than 5 microns

Alarm reaction the initial reaction of the body to stress, which alerts the body's defenses

Algor mortis the gradual decrease of the body's temperature after death

Alkalosis a condition that occurs with increases in blood bicarbonate or decreases in blood carbonic acid; blood pH above 7.45

Allodynia where nonpainful stimuli (e.g., contact with linen, water, or wind) produces pain or dysthesia, which is an unpleasant abnormal sensation

Allopathic medicine term used to describe Western medical practice

Alopecia the loss of scalp hair (baldness) or body hair

Alternative medicine an unrelated group of nonorthodox practices, often with explanatory systems that do not follow conventional biomedical explanations

Alzheimer's disease disease that involves progressive dementia, memory loss, and inability to care for self

Amblyopia reduced visual acuity in one eye

Ambulation the act of walking

Ampule a small glass container for individual doses of liquid medications

Anabolism a process in which simple substances are converted by the body's cells into more complex substances (e.g., building tissue, positive nitrogen balance)

Anaerobic living only in the absence of oxygen

Anaerobic exercise involves activity in which the muscles cannot draw out enough oxygen from the bloodstream; used in endurance training

Anal stimulation stimulation applied to anus for sexual pleasure

Anaphylactic reaction a severe allergic reaction that usually occurs immediately after the administration of a drug

Andragogy the art and science of helping adults learn

Androgyny belief that most characteristics and behaviors are human qualities and not limited to a gender

Anemia a condition in which the blood is deficient in red blood cells or hemoglobin

Anger an emotional state consisting of a subjective feeling of animosity or strong displeasure

Angiography a diagnostic procedure enabling x-ray visual examination of the vascular system after injection of a radiopaque dye

Angle of Louis the junction between the body of the sternum and the manubrium; the starting point for locating the ribs anteriorly

Animal-assisted therapy the use of specifically selected animals as a treatment modality in health and human service settings

Anions ions that carry a negative charge; includes chlorine (Cl^-), bicarbonate (HCO_3^-), phosphate (HPO_4^{2-}), and sulfate (SO_4^-)

Ankylosed permanently immobile joints

Anorexia lack of appetite

Anorexia nervosa a disease characterized by a prolonged inability or refusal to eat, rapid weight loss, and emaciation in persons who continue to believe they are fat

Anoscopy visual examination of the anal canal using an anoscope (a lighted instrument)

Answer (legal) a written response made by the defendant

Antagonist drug that inhibits cell function by occupying the drug's receptor sites

Antibodies immunoglobulins, part of the body's plasma proteins, defend primarily against the extracellular phases of bacterial and viral infections

Anticipatory grief grief experienced in advance of the event

Anticipatory loss the experience of loss before the loss actually occurs

Antigen a substance capable of inducing the formation of antibodies

Antihelix the anterior curve of the auricle's upper aspect

Antiseptics agents that inhibit the growth of some microorganisms

Anuria the failure of the kidneys to produce urine, resulting in a total lack of urination or output of less than 100 mL per day in an adult

Anxiety a state of mental uneasiness, apprehension, or dread producing an increased level of arousal caused by an impending or anticipated threat to self or significant relationships

Apgar scoring system a scoring system to assess newborn babies

Aphasia any defects in or loss of the power to express oneself by speech, writing, or signs, or to comprehend spoken or written language due to disease or injury of the cerebral cortex

Apical pulse a central pulse located at the apex of the heart

Apical-radial pulse measurement of the apical beat and the radial pulse at the same time

Apnea a complete absence of respirations

Apocrine glands sweat glands located largely in the axillae and anogenital areas; they begin to function at puberty under the influence of androgens

Approximated   closed tissue surfaces

Aromatherapy   therapeutic use of essential oils of plants in which odor or fragrance plays an important part

Arrhythmia   a pulse with an abnormal rhythm

Arterial blood gases   specimen of arterial blood that assesses oxygenation, ventilation, and acid–base status

Arterial blood pressure   the measure of the pressure exerted by the blood as it pulsates through the arteries

Arteriosclerosis   a condition in which the elastic and muscular tissues of the arteries are replaced with fibrous tissue

Ascites   the accumulation of fluid in the abdominal cavity

Asepsis   freedom from infection or infectious material

Asphyxiation   lack of oxygen due to interrupted breathing

Aspiration   the withdrawal of fluid that has abnormally collected (e.g., pleural cavity, abdominal cavity) or to obtain a specimen (e.g., cerebral spinal fluid)

Assault   an attempt or threat to touch another person unjustifiably

Assessing   the process of collecting, organizing, validating, and recording data (information) about a client's health status

Assignment   a downward or lateral transfer of both the responsibility and accountability of an activity from one individual to another

Assimilation   the process by which an individual develops a new cultural identity and becomes like the members of the dominant culture

Assisted living   facility with various degrees of personal care assistance designed to meet the needs of an older person

Assisted suicide   a form of active euthanasia in which clients are given the means to kill themselves

Assumption   taking something for granted or making a logical leap to reach a conclusion without proof, resulting in a conclusion that may be true or false

Astigmatism   an uneven curvature of the cornea that prevents horizontal and vertical rays from focusing on the retina

Atelectasis   a condition that occurs when ventilation is decreased and pooled secretions accumulate in a dependent area of a bronchiole and block it

Atheist   one who denies the existence of God

Atherosclerosis   buildup of fatty plaque within the arteries

Atria   two upper hollow chambers of the heart

Atrioventricular (AV) node   conduction pathways that slightly delay transmission of the impulse from the atria to the ventricles of the heart

Atrioventricular (AV) valves   between the atria and ventricles of the heart, the tricuspid valve on the right and the bicuspid or mitral valve on the left

Atrophy   wasting away; decrease in size of organ or tissue (e.g., muscle)

Attentive listening   listening actively, using all senses, as opposed to listening passively with just the ear

Attitudes   mental stance that is composed of many different beliefs; usually involving a positive or negative judgment toward a person, object, or idea

Audit   examination or review of records

Auditory   related to or experienced through hearing

Auricle   flap of the ear

Auscultation   the process of listening to sounds produced within the body

Auscultatory gap   the temporary disappearance of sounds normally heard over the brachial artery when the sphygmomanometer cuff pressure is high and the sounds reappear at a lower level

Authoritarian leader   the individual who makes decisions for the group

Authority   the power given by an organization to direct the work of others; the right to act

Autoantigen   an antigen that originates in a person's own body

Autocratic leader   *see* Authoritarian leader

Automaticity   an electrical impulse and contraction independent of the nervous system and generated by the cardiac muscle

Autonomy   the state of being independent and self-directed, without outside control, to make one's own decisions

Autopsy   an examination of the body after death to determine the cause of death and to learn more about a disease process

Awareness   the ability to perceive environmental stimuli and body reactions and to respond appropriately through thought and action

Ayurveda   Indian system of medicine where illness is viewed as a state of imbalance among the body's systems

B

Baby Boomers   generation that includes those born in years 1945–1964

Bacteremia   bacteria in the blood

Bacteria   the most common infection-causing microorganisms

Bactericidal   bacteria-killing action

Balance   concept of equilibrium between mental, physical, emotional, spiritual, and environmental components to achieve optimum wellness

Bandage   a strip of cloth used to wrap some part of the body

Basal metabolic rate (BMR)   the rate of energy utilization in the body required to maintain essential activities such as breathing

Base of support   the area on which an object rests

Bases   (alkalis) have low hydrogen ion concentration and can accept hydrogen ions in solution

Battery   (legal) the willful or negligent touching of a person (or the person's clothes or even something the person is carrying), which may or may not cause harm

Bed rest strict confinement to bed (complete bed rest), or the client may be allowed to use a bedside commode or have bathroom privileges

Bedpan a receptacle for urine and feces for clients who are restricted to bed

Behaviorist theory includes the careful identification of what is to be taught and the immediate identification of and reward for correct responses

Beliefs interpretations or conclusions that one accepts as true

Beneficence the moral obligation to do good or to implement actions that benefit clients and their support persons

Bereavement a subjective response of a person who has experienced the loss of a significant other through death

Bevel the slanted part at the tip of a needle

Bicultural used to describe a person who crosses two cultures, lifestyles, and sets of values

Bier block *see* Intravenous block

Binder a type of bandage applied to large body areas (abdomen or chest) or for a specific body part (arm sling); used to provide support

Bioelectromagnetics science that studies how living organisms interact with electromagnetic fields

Bioethics ethical rules or principles that govern right conduct concerning life

Biofeedback a stress management technique that brings under conscious control bodily processes normally thought to be beyond voluntary command

Biological rhythms *see* Biorhythms

Biomedical health belief *see* Scientific health belief

Biomedicine term used to describe Western medical practice

Biopsy the removal and examination of tissue from the living body

Biorhythms inner rhythms that appear to control a variety of biologic processes

Bioterrorism intentional attack using biological weapons such as viruses, bacteria, or other germs

Biotransformation process by which a drug is converted to a less active form; also called *detoxification*

Biot's respirations shallow breaths interrupted by apnea

Bladder training client postpones voiding, resists or inhibits the sensation of urgency, and voids according to a timetable rather than according to the urge to void

Blanch test a test during which the client's fingertip is temporarily pinched to assess capillary refill and peripheral circulation

Blood chemistry a number of tests performed on blood serum (the liquid portion of the blood)

Blood pressure (BP) the force exerted on arterial walls by blood flowing within the vessel

Blood urea nitrogen (BUN) a measure of blood level of urea, the end product of protein metabolism

Bloodborne pathogens those microorganisms carried in blood and body fluids that are capable of infecting other

persons with serious and difficult-to-treat viral infections, namely, hepatitis B virus, hepatitis C virus, and HIV

Body image how a person perceives the size, appearance, and functioning of his or her body and its parts

Body mass index (BMI) indicates whether weight is appropriate for height

Body substance isolation (BSI) generic infection control precautions for all clients except those with diseases transmitted through the air

Body temperature the balance between the heat produced by the body and the heat lost from the body

Bodymind a state of integration that includes body, mind, and spirit

Boomerang kids slang term used for young adults who move back into their parents' homes after an initial period of independent living

Bottle mouth syndrome describes the decay of an infant's teeth caused by constant contact with sweet liquid from a bottle

Boundary the real or imaginary lines that differentiate one system from another system or a system from its environment

Bowel (fecal) incontinence loss of voluntary ability to control fecal and gaseous discharges through the anal sphincter

Bradycardia abnormally slow pulse rate, less than 60 beats per minute

Bradypnea abnormally slow respiratory rate, usually less than 10 respirations per minute

Brand name the name given to a drug by the drug's manufacturer

Breach of duty a standard of care that is expected in the specific situation but that the nurse did not observe; this is the failure to act as a reasonable, prudent nurse under the circumstances

Bronchoscopy visual examination of the bronchi using a bronchoscope

Bruit a blowing or swishing sound created by turbulence of blood flow

Buccal pertaining to the cheek

Buffers prevent excessive changes in pH by removing or releasing hydrogen ions

Bulimia an uncontrollable compulsion to eat large amounts of food and then expel it by self-induced vomiting or by taking laxatives

Bundle of His the right and left bundle branches of the ventricular conduction pathways

Burden of proof the duty of proving an assertion

Bureaucratic leader does not trust self or others to make decisions and instead relies on the organization's rules, policies, and procedures to direct the group's work efforts

Burn results from excessive exposure to thermal, chemical, electric, or radioactive agents

Burnout a complex syndrome of behaviors that can be likened to the exhaustion stage of the general adaptation syndrome; an overwhelming feeling that can lead to physical and emotional depletion, a negative attitude and self-concept, and feelings of helplessness and hopelessness

C

Calculi   renal stones

Callus   a thickened portion of the skin

Caloric value   the amount of energy that nutrients or foods supply to the body

Calorie (c, cal, kcal)   a unit of heat energy equivalent to the amount of heat required to raise the temperature of 1 kg of water 1°C

Cancer pain   pain associated with cancers; can be related or unrelated to the disease or its treatment

Cannula   a tube with a lumen (channel) that is inserted into a cavity or duct and is often fitted with a trocar during insertion

Carbon monoxide   an odorless, colorless, tasteless gas that is very toxic

Cardiac arrest   the cessation of heart function

Cardiac output (CO)   the amount of blood ejected by the heart with each ventricular contraction

Cardinal signs   *see* Vital signs

Caregiver   a role that has traditionally included those activities that assist the client physically and psychologically

Caregiver burden   responses to long-term stress, such as chronic fatigue, sleeping difficulties, and high blood pressure, in family members who undertake the care of a person in the home for a long period

Caregiver role strain   physical, emotional, social, and financial burdens that can seriously jeopardize the caregiver's own health and well-being

Caries   tooth cavities

Caring   intentional action that conveys physical and emotional security and genuine connectedness with another person or group of people

Caring practice   nursing care that includes connection, mutual recognition, and involvement

Carminative   an agent that promotes the passage of flatus from the colon

Carrier   a person or animal that harbors a specific infectious agent and serves as a potential source of infection, yet does not manifest any clinical signs of disease

Case management   a method for delivering nursing care in which the nurse is responsible for a caseload of clients across the health care continuum

Case manager   a nurse who works with the multidisciplinary health care team to measure the effectiveness of the case management plan and monitor outcomes

Catabolism   a process in which complex substances are broken down into simpler substances (e.g., breakdown of tissue)

Cataracts   opacity of the lens or capsule of the eye

Cathartics   drugs that induce defecation

Cations   ions that carry a positive charge; includes sodium (Na^+), potassium (K^+), calcium (Ca^{2+}), and magnesium (Mg^{2+})

Causation   a fact that must be proven that the harm occurred as a direct result of the nurse's failure to follow the standard of care and the nurse could have (or should have) known that failure to follow the standard of care could result in such harm

Cell-mediated defenses   *see* Cellular immunity

Cellular immunity   also known as cell-mediated defenses, occur through the T-cell system

Center of gravity   the point at which the mass (weight) of the body is centered

Central neuropathic pain   pain resulting from malfunctioning nerves in the central nervous system

Central processing unit (CPU)   the processor/microprocessor that performs the computer program instructions, located in the box that contains the computer hardware

Central venous catheter   catheter that is usually inserted into the subclavian or jugular vein, with the distal tip of the catheter resting in the superior vena cava just above the right atrium

Cephalocaudal   proceeding in the direction from head to toe

Cerebral death   the higher brain center or cerebral cortex is irreversibly destroyed

Cerumen   the wax-like substance secreted by glands in the external ear canal

Change   process of making something different from what it was

Change agents   persons (or groups) who initiate change or who assist others in making modifications in themselves or in the system

Change-of-shift report   a report given to nurses on the next shift

Charismatic leader   characterized by an emotional relationship between the leader and the group members; personality of the leader evokes strong feelings of commitment to both the leader and the leader's cause and beliefs

Chart   a formal, legal document that provides evidence of a client's care

Charting   the process of making an entry on a client record

Charting by exception (CBE)   a documentation system in which only significant findings or exceptions to norms are recorded

Chemical name   the name by which a chemist knows a drug; describes the constituents of the drug precisely

Chemical restraints   medications used to control socially disruptive behavior

Chemical thermogenesis   the stimulation of heat production in the body through increased cellular metabolism caused by increases in thyroxine output

Cheyne-Stokes respirations   rhythmic waxing and waning of respirations from very deep breathing to very shallow breathing with periods of temporary apnea, often associated with cardiac failure, increased intracranial pressure, or brain damage

Chiropractic from the Greek meaning "done by hand"; involves adjustments of the spine and joints and is grounded in the assumption that maintaining the alignment of the spine and joints facilitates the flow of energy throughout the body, including the nervous, circulatory, respiratory, gastrointestinal, and limbic systems

Cholesterol a lipid that does not contain fatty acid but possesses many of the chemical and physical properties of other lipids

Chronic illness illness that lasts for an extended period of time, usually greater than 6 months

Chronic infection infection that occurs slowly, over a very long period, and may last months or years

Chronic pain prolonged pain, usually recurring or persisting over 6 months or longer, and interferes with functioning

Chyme digested products that leave the stomach through the small intestine and then pass through the ileocecal valve

Circulating immunity *see* Humoral immunity

Circulating nurse assists scrub nurses and surgeons during surgery

Civil action deals with the relationship between individuals in society

Civil law the body of law that deals with relationships among private individuals; also known as *private law*

Clara Barton a schoolteacher who volunteered as a nurse during the Civil War. Most notably, she organized the American Red Cross, which linked with the International Red Cross when the U.S. Congress ratified the Geneva Convention in 1882

Clarity seeing something clearly without bias or judgment

Clean free of potentially infectious agents

Clean voided specimen urine specimens for routine urinalysis

Clean-catch specimen urine specimens for urine culture

Cleaning bath a type of bath given chiefly for hygiene purposes

Client a person who engages the advice or services of another person who is qualified to provide this service

Client advocate nursing role of pleading the cause of a client

Client record *see* Chart

Climacteric the point in development when reproduction capacity in the female terminates (menopause) and the sexual activity of the male decreases (andropause)

Clinical aromatherapy the controlled use of essential oils for specific measurable outcomes

Clinical judgment considering all relevant aspects of collected data about a client to reach a decision about the meaning of the data and the proper response

Clinical reasoning the thinking process that allows nurses to logically draw conclusions and make a clinical judgment

Closed awareness a type of awareness in which the client is unaware of impending death

Closed questions restrictive question requiring only a short answer

Closed system system that does not exchange energy, matter, or information with its environment

Closed wound drainage system consists of a drain connected to either an electric suction or a portable drainage suction, such as a Hemovac or Jackson-Pratt

Clubbing elevation of the proximal aspect of the nail and softening of the nail bed

Co-analgesic medication that is not classified as a pain medication; however, it has properties that may reduce pain alone, or in combination with other analgesics; relieve other discomforts; potentiate the effect of pain medication; or reduce the pain medication's side effects

Cochlea a seashell-shaped structure found in the inner ear; essential for sound transmission and hearing

Code blue emergency announcing cardiac/respiratory arrest and initiating interventions

Code of ethics a formal statement of a group's ideals and values; a set of ethical principles shared by members of a group, reflecting their moral judgments and serving as a standard for professional actions

Cognitive development refers to the manner in which people learn to think, reason, and use language

Cognitive domain the "thinking" domain, includes six intellectual abilities and thinking processes beginning with knowing, comprehending, and applying to analysis, synthesis, and evaluation

Cognitive skills intellectual skills that include problem solving, decision making, critical thinking, and creativity

Cognitive theory recognition of developmental levels of learners, and acknowledgments of the learner's motivation and environment

Coinsurance an insurance plan in which the client pays a percentage of the payment and some other group (e.g., employer, government) pays the remaining percentage

Collaboration a collegial working relationship with another health care provider in the provision of client care

Collaborative care plans *see* Critical pathways

Collaborative interventions actions the nurse carries out in collaboration with other health team members, such as physical therapists, social workers, dietitians, and physicians

Collagen a protein found in connective tissue; a whitish protein substance that adds tensile strength to a wound

Colloid osmotic pressure a pulling force exerted by colloids that help maintain the water content of blood

Colloids substances such as large protein molecules that do not readily dissolve into true solutions

Colonization the presence of organisms in body secretions or excretions in which strains of bacteria become resident flora but do not cause illness

Colonoscopy visual examination of the interior of the colon with a colonoscope

Colostomy an opening into the colon (large bowel)

Commode a portable, chairlike structure used as a toilet

Common law the body of principles that evolves from court decisions

Communicable disease a disease that can spread from one person to another

Communication a two-way process involving the sending and receiving of messages

Communicator nurses identify client problems and then communicate these verbally or in writing to other members of the health team

Community a collection of people who share some attribute of their lives

Community health nursing the synthesis of nursing and public health practice as applied to promoting and preserving the health of populations

Community nursing centers (CNCs) provide primary care to specific populations and are staffed by nurse practitioners and community health nurses

Community-based health care (CBHC) a system that provides health-related services within the context of people's daily lives; that is, in places where people spend their time in the community

Community-based nursing (CBN) nursing care directed toward a specific population or group within the community; primary, secondary, or tertiary care may be provided to individuals or groups

Compensation defense mechanism in which a person substitutes an activity for one that he or she would prefer doing or cannot do

Compensatory counterbalancing

Complaint (legal) a document filed by a plaintiff

Complementary and alternative medicine (CAM) those practices that do not form part of the dominant system for managing health and disease

Complementary medicine *see* Alternative medicine

Complementary therapies therapeutic practices that are not currently considered an integral part of conventional allopathic medical practice

Complete blood count (CBC) specimens of venous blood; includes hemoglobin and hematocrit measurements, erythrocyte (RBC) count, leukocyte (WBC) count, red blood cell indices, and a differential white cell count

Complete proteins a protein that contains all of the essential amino acids as well as many nonessential ones

Compliance the extent to which an individual's behavior coincides with medical or health advice

Complicated grief pathologic grief; exists when coping strategies are maladaptive

Compress a moist gauze dressing applied frequently to an open wound, sometimes medicated

Compromised host any person at increased risk for an infection

Computed tomography (CT) a painless, noninvasive x-ray procedure that has the unique capability of distinguishing minor differences in the density of tissues

Computer-based patient records (CPRs) electronic client data retrievable by caregivers, administrators, accreditors, and other persons who require the data

Concept map a visual tool in which ideas or data are enclosed in circles or boxes of some shape and relationships between these are indicated by connecting lines or arrows

Concepts abstract ideas or mental images of phenomena or reality

Conceptual framework a group of related concepts

Conceptual model a graphic illustration of the relationships among concepts

Conclusion ending or end point; the final decision, determination, or result

Concurrent audit evaluation of a client's health care while the client is still receiving care from the agency

Conduction the transfer of heat from one molecule to another in direct contact

Conduction hearing loss the result of interrupted transmission of sound waves through the outer and middle ear structures

Confidentiality any information a subject relates will not be made public or available to others without the subject's consent

Congruent communication the verbal and nonverbal aspects of the message match

Conjunctivitis inflammation of the bulbar and palpebral conjunctiva

Conscious sedation a minimal depression of level of consciousness during which the client retains the ability to consciously maintain a patent airway and respond appropriately to verbal and physical stimuli

Consequence-based (teleological) theories the ethics of judging whether an action is moral

Constant fever a state in which the body temperature fluctuates minimally but always remains above normal

Constipation passage of small, dry, hard stool or passage of no stool for an abnormally long time

Consultative leader *see* Democratic leader

Consumer an individual, a group of people, or a community that uses a service or commodity

Contact precautions methods used to reduce exposure to infectious agents easily transmitted by direct client contact or by contact with items in the client's environment

Contemplation stage stage in which a person acknowledges having a problem, seriously considers changing a specific behavior, actively gathers information, and verbalizes plans to change the behavior in the near future

Continuing education (CE) formalized experiences designed to enlarge the knowledge or skills of practitioners

Continuity of care the coordination of health care services by health care providers for clients moving from one health care setting to another and between and among health care professionals

Continuity theory   people maintain their values, habits, and behavior in old age

Contract   a written or verbal agreement between two or more people to do or not do some lawful act

Contract law   the enforcement of agreements among private individuals or the payment of compensation for failure to fulfill the agreement

Contractility   the inherent ability of cardiac muscle fibers to shorten or contract

Contractual obligations   duty of care established by the presence of an expressed or implied contract

Contractual relationships   vary among practice settings; may be as an independent or employer-employee relationship

Contracture   permanent shortening of a muscle and subsequent shortening of tendons and ligaments

Convection   the dispersion of heat by air currents

Conventional medicine   term used to describe Western medical practice

Coordinating   the process of ensuring that plans are carried out and evaluating outcomes

Coping   dealing with change

Coping mechanism   an innate or acquired way of responding to a changing environment or specific problem or situation

Coping strategy   *see* Coping mechanism

Core self-concept   the beliefs and images that are most vital to the person's identity

Core temperature   the temperature of the deep tissues of the body (e.g., thorax, abdominal cavity); relatively constant at 37°C (98.6°F)

Corn   a conical, circular, painful, raised area on the toe or foot

Coronary arteries   a network of vessels known as the coronary circulation

Coroner   a public official, not necessarily a physician, appointed or elected to inquire into the causes of death

Costal (thoracic) breathing   use of the external intercostal muscles and other accessory muscles, such as the sternocleidomastoid muscles

Counseling   the process of helping a client to recognize and cope with stressful psychologic or social problems, to develop improved interpersonal relationships, and to promote personal growth

Countershock phase   second part of the alarm reaction in which the changes the body experienced during the shock phase are reversed

Covert data (systems, subjective data)   information (data) apparent only to the person affected that can be described or verified only by that person

Creatine kinase (CK)   enzyme that is released into the blood during a myocardial infarction (MI)

Creatinine   a nitrogenous waste that is excreted in the urine

Creatinine clearance   a test uses 24-hour urine and serum creatinine levels to determine the glomerular filtration rate, a sensitive indicator of renal function

Creativity   thinking that results in the development of new ideas and products

Credentialing   the process of determining and maintaining competence in practice; includes licensure, registration, certification, and accreditation

Credé's maneuver   manual exertion of pressure on the bladder to force urine out

Crepitation   (1) a dry, crackling sound like that of crumpled cellophane, produced by air in the subcutaneous tissue or by air moving through fluid in the alveoli of the lungs; (2) a crackling, grating sound produced by bone rubbing against bone

Crime   an act committed in violation of public (criminal) law and punishable by a fine and/or imprisonment

Criminal actions   deal with disputes between an individual and the society as a whole

Criminal law   deals with actions against the safety and welfare of the public

Crisis counseling   therapy focused on solving immediate problems involving individuals, groups, or families in crisis

Crisis intervention   a short-term helping process of assisting clients to work through a crisis to its resolution and restore their precrisis level of functioning

Critical analysis   a set of questions one can apply to a particular situation or idea to determine essential information and ideas and discard superfluous information and ideas

Critical pathways   multidisciplinary guidelines for client care based on specific medical diagnoses designed to achieve predetermined outcomes

Critical theory   describes theories that help elucidate how social structures affect a wide variety of human experiences from art to social practices

Critical thinking   a cognitive process that includes creativity, problem solving, and decision making

Cross-dresser   Individual of one gender (typically male) who dresses in clothing specific to the opposite gender

Crystalloids   salts that dissolve readily into true solutions

Cues   any piece of information or data that influences decisions

Cultural care deprivation   lack of culturally assistive, supportive, or facilitative acts

Cultural deprivation   *see* Cultural care deprivation

Culturally appropriate   application of underlying background knowledge that must be possessed to provide a given client with the best possible health care

Culturally competent   within the delivered care the nurse understands and attends to the total context of the client's situation and uses a complex combination of knowledge, attitudes, and skills

Culturally sensitive   care that demonstrates basic knowledge of and constructive attitudes toward the health traditions observed among the diverse cultural groups found in the setting

Culture   a world view and set of traditions used and transmitted from generation to generation by a particular group, includes related attitudes and institutions

Culture shock a disorder that occurs in response to transition from one cultural setting to another

Cultures laboratory cultivations of microorganisms in a special growth medium

Cumulative effect the increasing response to repeated doses of a drug that occurs when the rate of administration exceeds the rate of metabolism or excretion

Curanderismo cultural healing tradition found in Latin America that uses Western medicine beliefs, treatments, and practices at three levels of care: material level, spiritual level, and mental level

Cyanosis bluish discoloration of the skin and mucous membranes caused by reduced oxygen in the blood

Cystoscope a lighted instrument used to visualize the interior of the urinary bladder

Cystoscopy visual examination of the urinary bladder with a cystoscope

D

Dacryocystitis inflammation of the lacrimal sac

Damages if malpractice caused the injury, the nurse is held liable for damages that may be compensated

Dandruff a dry or greasy, scaly material shed from the scalp

Data information

Data warehousing the accumulation of large amounts of data that are stored over time

Database all information about a client, includes nursing health history and physical assessment, physician's history, physical examination, and laboratory and diagnostic test results

Debridement removal of infected and necrotic tissue

Decision (legal) outcome made by a judge

Decision making the process of establishing criteria by which alternative courses of action are developed and selected

Decode to relate the message perceived to the receiver's storehouse of knowledge and experience and to sort out the meaning of the message

Decubitus ulcers *see* Pressure ulcers

Deductive reasoning making specific observations from a generalization

Defamation (legal) a communication that is false, or made with careless disregard for the truth, and results in injury to the reputation of another

Defecation expulsion of feces from the rectum and anus

Defendant (legal) person against whom a plaintiff files a complaint

Defense mechanism any reaction that serves to protect against something physically or psychologically harmful

Defining characteristics client signs and symptoms that must be present to validate a nursing diagnosis

Dehiscence the partial or total rupturing of a sutured wound; usually involves an abdominal wound in which the layers below the skin also separate

Dehydration insufficient fluid in the body

Delegation the transfer of responsibility for the performance of an activity from one person to another while retaining accountability for the outcome

Delirium also called *acute confusion;* abrupt onset of confusion and a reversible cause

Demand feeding child is fed when hungry

Dementia a global impairment of cognitive function that usually is progressive and may be permanent; interferes with normal social and occupational activities

Democratic leader encourages group discussion and decision making

Demography the study of population, including statistics about distribution by age and place of residence, mortality, and morbidity

Dental caries tooth decay

Denver Developmental Screening Test (DDST) a screening test used to assess children from birth to 6 years of age

Dependence the need for a substance, person, or act in order to prevent a psychophysiological response; *also see* drug dependence

Dependent functions with regard to medical diagnoses, physician-prescribed therapies and treatments nurses are obligated to carry out

Dependent interventions those activities carried out on the order of a physician, under a physician's supervision, or according to specified routines

Dependent variable the behavior, characteristic, or outcome that the researcher wishes to explain or predict

Depression feelings of sadness and dejection, often accompanied by physiologic change such as decreased functional activity

Descriptive statistics procedures that summarize large volumes of data; used to describe and synthesize data, showing patterns and trends

Desire phase part of the response cycle, which starts in the brain, with conscious sexual desires

Desired effect *see* Therapeutic effect

Desired outcomes the client's positive response to treatment, the response that care is aimed at obtaining

Detoxification *see* Biotransformation

Detrusor muscle the smooth muscle layers of the bladder

Development an individual's increasing capacity and skill in functioning, related to growth

Developmental stage level of achievement for a particular segment of a person's life

Developmental task skill or behavior pattern learned during stages of development

Diagnosis a statement or conclusion concerning the nature of some phenomenon

Diagnosis-related groups (DRGs) a Medicare payments system to hospitals and physicians that establishes fees according to diagnosis

Diagnostic labels title used in writing a nursing diagnosis; taken from the North American Nursing

Diagnosis Association (NANDA) standardized taxonomy of terms

Dialysis   a technique by which fluids and molecules pass through a semipermeable membrane according to the rules of osmosis

Diaphragmatic (abdominal) breathing   contraction and relaxation of the diaphragm, observed by the movement of the abdomen, which occurs as a result of the diaphragm's contraction and downward movement

Diarrhea   defecation of liquid feces and increased frequency of defecation

Diastole   the period during which the ventricles relax

Diastolic pressure   the pressure of the blood against the arterial walls when the ventricles of the heart are at rest

Diet history   a comprehensive assessment of a client's food intake that involves an extensive interview by a nutritionist or dietitian

Differentiated practice   a system in which the best possible use of nursing personnel is based on their educational preparation and resultant skill sets

Diffusion   the mixing of molecules or ions of two or more substances as a result of random motion

Directing   a management function that involves communicating the task to be completed and providing guidance and supervision

Directive interview   a highly structured interview that uses closed questions to elicit specific information

Dirty   denotes the likely presence of microorganisms, some of which may be capable of causing infection

Disaccharides   sugars that are composed of double molecules

Discharge planning   the process of anticipating and planning for client needs after discharge

Discovery   (legal) pretrial activities to gain all of the facts of a situation

Discrimination   the differential treatment of individuals or groups

Discussion   an informal oral consideration of a subject by two or more health care personnel to identify a problem or establish strategies to resolve a problem

Disease   an alteration in body function resulting in a reduction of capacities or shortening of the normal life span

Disease prevention   behavior motivated by a desire to actively avoid illness, detect it early, or maintain functioning within the constraints of illness (also called *health protection*)

Disengagement theory   aging involves mutual withdrawal (disengagement) between the older person and others in the elderly person's environment

Disinfectants   agents that destroy pathogens other than spores

Dissatisfaction problems   dissatisfaction with sexual encounters despite desire, arousal, and orgasm

Distance learning   learning in which people communicate effectively across long distances

Distribution   the transportation of a drug from its site of absorption to its site of action

Diuresis   the production of large amounts of urine by the kidneys without an increased fluid intake

Diuretics   agents that increase urine secretion

Diversity   the fact or state of being different

Documenting   *see* Charting or Recording

Do-not-resuscitate (DNR) order   a physician's order that specifies no effort be made to resuscitate the client with terminal or irreversible illness in the event of a respiratory or cardiac arrest

Dorothea Dix   woman leader who provided nursing care during the Civil War

Dorsal (supine) position   a back-lying position without a pillow

Dorsal recumbent position   a back-lying position with the head and shoulders slightly elevated

Drip factor (drop factor)   the number of drops per milliliter of solution delivered for a particular drip chamber

Droplet nuclei   residue of evaporated droplets that remains in the air for long periods of time

Droplet precautions   methods used to reduce exposure to infectious agents transmitted by particle droplets larger than 5 microns

Drug   a chemical compound taken for disease prevention, diagnosis, cure, or relief or to affect the structure or function of the body

Drug abuse   excessive intake of a substance either continually or periodically

Drug allergy   an immunologic reaction to a drug

Drug dependence   inability to keep the intake of a drug or substance under control

Drug habituation   a mild form of psychologic dependence on a drug

Drug half-life (Elimination half-life)   the time required for the elimination process to reduce the concentration of a drug to one-half what it was at initial administration

Drug interaction   the beneficial or harmful interaction of one drug with another drug

Drug tolerance   a condition in which successive increases in the dosage of a drug are required to maintain a given therapeutic effect

Drug toxicity   the quality of a drug that exerts a deleterious effect on an organism or tissue

Dullness   a thudlike sound produced during percussion by dense tissue of body organs such as the liver, spleen, or heart

Durable medical equipment (DME) Equipment   used for health care by the client at home that is multi-use and not disposable after one use

Duration   the length of time that a sound is heard

Duty   the nurse must have (or should have had) a relationship with the client that involves providing care and following an acceptable standard of care

Dysesthesia   unpleasant abnormal sensation

Dysmenorrhea   painful menstruation

Dyspareunia   difficult or painful intercourse

Dysphagia   difficulty or inability to swallow

Dyspnea   difficult or labored breathing

Dysrhythmia   a pulse with an irregular rhythm

Dysuria   painful or difficult voiding

E

Eccrine glands   glands that produce sweat; found over most of the body

Echocardiogram   a noninvasive test that uses ultrasound to visualize structures of the heart and evaluate left ventricular function

Ectoderm   the outer layer of tissue formed in the second week of life

Edema   the presence of excess interstitial fluid in the body

Effectiveness   a measure of the quality or quantity of services provided

Efficiency   a measure of the resources used in the provision of nursing services

Effleurage   a stroking massage technique

Ego   includes consciousness and memory, which serve to mediate between primitive instinctual drives (id), internal social prohibitions (superego), and reality

Ego defense mechanisms   (Freud) mental mechanisms that develop as the personality attempts to defend itself, establish compromises among conflicting impulses, and allay inner tensions

Ejaculation   expulsion of seminal fluid and sperm

Elasticity of the arterial wall   expansibility or stretching of the vessels

Elderspeak   speech style similar to babytalk; gives the message of dependence and incompetence to older adults

Elective surgery   performed when surgical intervention is the preferred treatment for a condition that is not imminently life threatening or to improve the client's life

Electric shock   occurs when a current travels through the body to the ground rather than through electric wiring, or from static electricity that builds up on the body

Electrocardiogram (ECG, EKG)   a graph of the electric activity of the heart

Electrocardiography   provides a graphic recording of the heart's electrical activity

Electroencephalogram (EEG)   a graph of the electrical activity of the brain

Electromyogram (EMG)   a graph of the electrical activity of muscles

Electro-oculogram (EOG)   a graph of the electrical activity of eye to eye movement

Electrolytes   chemical substances that develop an electric charge and are able to conduct an electric current when placed in water; ions

Electronic communication   communication involving computers and technology (i.e., e-mail)

Electronic medical records (EMRs)   *see* Computer-based patient records (CPRs)

Elimination half-life   *see* Drug half-life

Embolus   a blood clot (or a substance such as air) that has moved from its place of origin and is causing obstruction to circulation elsewhere (plural: *emboli*)

Embryonic phase   the phase during which the fertilized ovum develops into an organism with most of the features of a human

Emergency surgery   surgery that is performed immediately to preserve function or the life of the client

Emmetropic   normal refraction so that the eyes focus images on the retina

Empathy   the ability to discriminate what the other person's world is like and to communicate to the other this understanding in a way that shows that the helper understands the client's feelings and the behavior and experience underlying these feelings

Emphysema   a chronic pulmonary condition in which the alveoli are dilated and distended

Empirical data   information collected from the observable world

Empirical knowing   knowledge that comes from science; ranges from factual, observable phenomena to theoretical analysis

Encoding   involves the selection of specific signs or symbols (codes) to transmit the message, such as which language and words to use, how to arrange the words, and what tone of voice and gestures to use

Endocardium   a layer of the heart wall lining the inside of the heart's chambers and great vessels

Endoderm   the inner layer of tissue formed in the second week of life

End-of-life care   care provided in the final weeks before death

Endogenous   developing from within

Enema   a solution introduced into the rectum and sigmoid colon to remove feces and/or flatus

Energy   the force that integrates the body, mind, and spirit

Enteral   through the gastrointestinal system

Entoderm   *see* Endoderm

Enuresis   bed-wetting; involuntary passing of urine in children after bladder control is achieved

Environment   all of the conditions, circumstances, and influences surrounding and affecting the development of an organism or person

Enzymes   biologic catalysts that speed up chemical reactions

Epicardium   the visceral pericardium adhering to the surface of the heart, forming the heart's outermost layer

Epidural   commonly used route for parenteral administration into the epidural space (the area inside the spinal column but outside the dura mater)

Epidural anesthesia   the injection of an anesthetic agent into the epidural space

Equianalgesia   equal analgesia; used when referring to the doses of various opioid analgesics that provide approximately the same pain relief

Equilibrium   a state of balance

Erectile dysfunction   the inability to achieve or maintain an erection sufficient for sexual satisfaction for oneself or one's partner

Erythema a redness associated with a variety of skin rashes

Erythrocytes red blood cells, or RBCs

Eschar thick necrotic tissue produced by burning, by a corrosive application, or by death of tissue associated with loss of vascular supply, bacterial invasion, and putrefaction

Essential amino acids amino acids that cannot be manufactured in the body and must be supplied as part of the protein ingested in the diet

Ethical knowing knowledge that focuses on matters of obligation or what ought to be done

Ethics the rules or principles that govern right conduct

Ethnic belonging to a specific group of individuals who share a common social and cultural heritage

Ethnocentrism the belief that one's own culture or way of life is better than that of others

Ethnography research that provides a framework to focus on the culture of a group of people

Ethnopharmacology study of the effect of ethnicity on responses to prescribed medicines

Etiology the causal relationship between a problem and its related or risk factors

Eupnea normal, quiet breathing

Eustachian tube the part of the middle ear that connects the middle ear to the nasopharynx; stabilizes air pressure between the external atmosphere and the middle ear

Euthanasia the act of painlessly putting to death persons suffering from incurable or distressing disease

Evaluating a planned ongoing, purposeful activity in which clients and health care professionals compare expected outcomes to actual outcomes

Evaluation statement a statement that consists of two parts: a conclusion and supporting data

Evidence-based practice (EBP) the use of some form of substantiation in making clinical decisions

Evisceration extrusion of the internal organs

Exacerbation the period during a chronic illness when symptoms reappear after remission

Excitement/plateau phase part of the response cycle, involves vasocongestion and myotonia

Excoriation loss of the superficial layers of the skin

Excretion elimination of a waste product produced by the body cells from the body

Exercise a type of physical activity; a planned, structured, and repetitive bodily movement done to improve or maintain one or more components of physical fitness

Exhalation (expiration) the movement of gases from the lungs to the atmosphere

Exogenous developing from outside sources

Exophthalmus a protrusion of the eyeballs with elevation of the upper eyelids, resulting in a startled or staring expression

Expectorate to cough and spit up mucus or other materials

Expert witness one who has special training, experience, or skill in a relevant area and is allowed by the court to offer an opinion on some issue within that area of expertise

Expiration *see* Exhalation

Express consent an oral or written agreement

Extended family family that includes the relatives of the nuclear family (e.g., grandparents, aunts, uncles)

External auditory meatus the entrance to the ear canal

Extinction the failure to perceive touch on one side of the body when two symmetric areas of the body are touched simultaneously

Extracellular fluid (ECF) fluid found outside the body cells

Exudate material, such as fluid and cells, that has escaped from blood vessels during the inflammatory process and is deposited in tissue or on tissue surfaces

F

Fabiola a wealthy Roman matron; viewed by some as the patron saint of early nursing who used her position and wealth to establish hospitals for the sick

Fad a widespread but short-lived interest, or a practice followed with considerable zeal

Failure to thrive a unique syndrome in which an infant falls below the fifth percentile for weight and height on a standard growth chart or is falling in percentiles on a growth chart

Faith an active "mode of being-in-relation" to another or others in which we invest commitment, belief, love, and hope

False imprisonment the unlawful restraint or detention of another person against his or her wishes

Family the basic unit of society that consists of those individuals, male or female, youth or adult, legally or not legally related, genetically or not genetically related, who are considered by others to represent their significant persons

Family-centered nursing nursing that considers the health of the family as a unit in addition to the health of individual family members

Fats lipids that are solid at room temperature

Fat-soluble vitamins A, D, E, and K vitamins that the body can store

Fatty acids the basic structural units of most lipids made up of carbon chains and hydrogen

Fear an emotional response to an actual, present danger

Feasibility the availability of time as well as the material and human resources needed to investigate a research problem or question

Febrile pertaining to a fever; feverish

Fecal impaction a mass or collection of hardened, putty-like feces in the folds of the rectum

Fecal incontinence *see* Bowel incontinence

Feces (stool) body wastes and undigested food eliminated from the bowel

Feedback the response or message that the receiver returns to the sender during communication

Felony   a crime of a serious nature, such as murder, punishable by a term in prison

Female orgasmic disorder   when the female sexual response stops before orgasm occurs

Female sexual arousal disorder   when lack of vaginal lubrication causes discomfort or pain during intercourse

Fetal phase   characterized by a period of rapid growth in the size of the fetus; both genetic and environmental factors affect its growth

Fever   elevated body temperature

Fever spike   a temperature that rises to fever level rapidly following a normal temperature and then returns to normal within a few hours

Fibrin   an insoluble protein formed from fibrinogen during the clotting of blood

Fidelity   a moral principle that obligates the individual to be faithful to agreements and responsibilities one has undertaken

Fifth vital sign   pain assessment

Filtration   process whereby fluid and solutes move together across a membrane from one compartment to another

Filtration pressure   the pressure in a compartment that results in the movement of fluid and substances dissolved in fluid out of the compartment

First-level manager   a manager responsible for managing the work of nonmanagerial personnel and the day-to-day activities of a specific work group or groups

Fissures   deep grooves that occur as a result of dryness and cracking of the skin

Fixation   immobilization or the inability of the personality to proceed to the next developmental stage because of anxiety

Flaccid   weak or lax

Flatness   an extremely dull sound produced, during percussion, by very dense tissue, such as muscle or bone

Flatulence   the presence of excessive amounts of gas in the stomach or intestines

Flatus   gas or air normally present in the stomach or intestines

Florence Nightingale   considered the founder of modern nursing, she was influential in developing nursing education, practice, and administration

Flow sheet   a record of the progress of specific or specialized data such as vital signs, fluid balance, or routine medications; often charted in graph form

Fluid volume deficit   (hypovolemia) loss of both water and electrolytes in similar proportions from the extracellular fluid

Fluid volume excess (FVE)   (hypervolemia) retention of both water and sodium in similar proportions to normal extracellular fluid (ECF)

Focus charting   a method of charting that uses key words or foci to describe what is happening to the client

Folk medicine   beliefs and practices relating to illness prevention and healing that derive from cultural traditions rather than from modern medicine's scientific base

Fontanels   unossified membranous gaps in the bone structure of the skull of a newborn that make molding of the head possible

Food diary   a detailed record of measured amounts (portion sizes) of all food and fluids a client consumes during a specified period, usually 3 to 7 days

Food frequency record   a checklist that indicates how often general food groups or specific foods are eaten

Foot drop   plantar flexion contracture

Foreseeability   a link that must exist between the nurse's act and the injury suffered

Formal leader   an appointed leader selected by an organization and given official authority to make decisions and act

Formal nursing care plan   a written or computerized guide that organizes information about the client's care

Fowler's position   a bed-sitting position with the head of the bed raised to 45 degrees

Friction   rubbing; the force that opposes motion

Full disclosure   a basic right, which means that deception, either by withholding information about a client's participation in a study or by giving the client false or misleading information about what participating in the study will involve, must not occur

Functional strength   ability of the body to perform work

Fungi   infection-causing microorganisms that include yeasts and molds

G

Gait   the way a person walks

Gastrocolic reflex   increased peristalsis of the colon after food has entered the stomach

Gastrostomy   an opening through the abdominal wall into the stomach

Gastrostomy tube   a tube that is surgically placed directly into the client's stomach and provides a route for administering nutrition and medications

Gauge   diameter of a shaft

Gender   indicates biologic male or female status

Gender identity   a person's sense of being masculine or feminine, as distinct from being male or female

Gender-role behavior   outward expression of a person's sense of maleness or femaleness

General adaptation syndrome (GAS)   (Selye) a general arousal response of the body to a stressor characterized by certain physiologic events and dominated by the sympathetic nervous system

General anesthesia   the induced loss of all sensation and consciousness

Generation X   generation that includes those born in years 1965–1978

Generation Y   generation that includes those born in years 1979–2000

Generativity   concern for establishing and guiding the next generation

Generic name   a drug name not protected by trademark and usually describing the chemical structure of the drug

Genital intercourse   penile/vaginal intercourse (coitus)

Geragogy   the term used to describe the process involved in stimulating and helping elderly persons to learn

Geriatrics   medical care of the elderly

Gerontology   the study of aging and older adults

Gingival   of or relating to the gums

Gingivitis   red, swollen gingiva (gums)

Glaucoma   a disturbance in the circulation of aqueous fluid; causes an increase in intraocular pressure

Global self   refers to the collective beliefs and images one holds about oneself; the most complete description that individuals can give of themselves at any one time

Global self-esteem   how much one likes one's perceived self as a whole

Glomerulus   a tuft of capillaries in the kidney surrounded by Bowman's capsule

Glossitis   inflammation of the tongue

Glycerides   the most common form of lipids consisting of a glycerol molecule with up to three fatty acids

Glycogen   the chief carbohydrate stored in the body, particularly in the liver and muscles

Glycogenesis   the process of glycogen formation

Goals/desired outcomes   a part of a care plan that describes, in terms of observable client responses, what the nurse hopes to achieve by implementing the nursing interventions

Goniometer   a device used to measure the angle of a joint in degrees

Governance   the establishment and maintenance of social, political, and economic arrangements by which practitioners control their practice, self-discipline, working conditions, and professional affairs

Grand theories   articulate a broad range of the significant relationships among the concepts of a discipline

Granulation tissue   young connective tissue with new capillaries formed in the wound healing process

Grief   emotional suffering often caused by bereavement

Gross negligence   involves extreme lack of knowledge, skill, or decision making that the person clearly should have known would put others at risk for harm

Grounded theory   research to understand social structures and social processes; this method focuses on the generation of categories or hypotheses that explain patterns of behavior of people in the study

Group   two or more people with shared purposes and goals

Group dynamics   forces that determine the behavior of the group and the relationships among the group members

Growth   physical change and increase in size

Guaiac test   a test performed for occult (hidden) blood to detect gastrointestinal bleeding not visible to the eye

Guided imagery   state of focused attention that encourages changes in attitudes, behavior, and physiologic reactions

Gustatory   referring to the sense of taste

H

Habit training   attempts to keep clients dry by having them void at regular intervals; also referred to as *timed voiding* or *scheduled toileting*

Habituation   a tolerance built to a substance from recurrent use (e.g., drug tolerance); a decline and eventual elimination of a conditioned response by repeating the stimulus (negative or positive) whenever the response occurs

Half-life   *see* Drug half-life

Hardware   the physical parts of a computer

Harm   (Injury) the client or plaintiff must demonstrate some type of harm or injury (physical, financial, or emotional) as a result of the breach of duty owed the client; the plaintiff will be asked to document physical injury, medical costs, loss of wages, "pain and suffering," and any other damages

Harriet Tubman   known as "the Moses of Her People" for her work with the Underground Railroad; during the Civil War she nursed the sick and suffering of her own race

Haustra   pouches that form in the large intestine when the longitudinal muscles are shorter than the colon

Haustral churning   (shuffling) movement of the chyme back and forth within the haustra in the large intestine

Health   well-being involving the physical, psychological, social, and spiritual aspects of a person allowing them to compensate for environmental changes, the absence of disease, or other abnormality

Health behaviors   the actions a person takes to understand his or her health state, maintain an optimal state of health, prevent illness and injury, and reach his or her maximum physical and mental potential

Health beliefs   concepts about health that an individual believes are true

Health care proxy   a legal statement that appoints a proxy to make medical decisions for the client in the event the client is unable to do so

Health care system   the totality of services offered by all health disciplines

Health literacy   ability to read, understand, and act on provided health information

Health maintenance organization (HMO)   a group health care agency that provides basic and supplemental health maintenance and treatment services to voluntary enrollees

Health promotion   any activity undertaken for the purpose of achieving a higher level of health and well-being

Health protection   behavior motivated by a desire to actively avoid illness, detect it early, or maintain functioning within the constraints of illness

Health risk assessment (HRA)   an assessment and educational tool that indicates a client's risk for disease or injury during the next 10 years by comparing the client's risk with the mortality risk of the corresponding age, sex, and racial group

Health status   the health of a person at a given time

Heart failure   a condition that develops if the heart cannot keep up with the body's need for oxygen and nutrients to the tissues; usually occurs because of myocardial infarction, but it may also result from chronic overwork of the heart

Heart-lung death   the traditional clinical signs of death: cessation of the apical pulse, respirations, and blood pressure

Heat balance   the state a person is in when the amount of heat produced by the body exactly equals the amount of heat lost

Heat exhaustion   condition that is the result of excessive heat and dehydration

Heat stroke   life-threatening condition with body temperature greater than 106°F

Heimlich maneuver   subdiaphragmatic abdominal thrusts used to clear an obstructed airway

Helix   the posterior curve of the auricle's upper aspect

Helping relationships   the nurse–client relationship

Hematocrit   the proportion of red blood cells (erythrocytes) to the total blood volume

Hematoma   a collection of blood in a tissue, organ, or space due to a break in the wall of a blood vessel

Hemoglobin (Hg)   the red pigment in red blood cells that carries oxygen

Hemoglobin A_{1C}   measurement of blood glucose that is bound to hemoglobin

Hemolytic transfusion reaction   destruction of red blood cells as a result of transfusion of incompatible blood

Hemoptysis   the presence of blood in the sputum

Hemorrhage   excessive loss of blood from the vascular system

Hemorrhagic exudate   *see* Sanguineous exudate

Hemorrhoids   distended veins in the rectum

Hemostasis   cessation of bleeding

Hemothorax   a collection of blood in the pleural cavity

Herbal medicine   treating illness with herbs

Heritage   something that is handed down from generation to generation; it includes far more than material possessions, also including traditions and customs

Heritage consistency   the degree to which one's lifestyle reflects his or her respective tribal culture

Heritage inconsistency   the observance of the beliefs and practices of one's acculturated belief system

Hernia   a protrusion (such as of the intestine through the inguinal wall or canal)

High Fowler's position   a bed-sitting position in which the head of the bed is elevated 90 degrees

Higher brain death   *see* Cerebral death

Hirsutism   abnormal hairiness, particularly in women

Holism   all living organisms are seen as interacting, unified wholes that are more than the sums of their parts

Holistic health   a model of health based on the belief that the whole is more than the sum of its parts

Holistic health belief   holds that the forces of nature must be maintained in balance or harmony

Holistic health care   a system that considers all components of health: health promotion, health maintenance, health education and illness prevention, and restorative–rehabilitative care

Holistic nursing   nursing practice that has as its goal the healing of the whole person

Holy day   a day set aside for special religious observance

Homans' sign   calf pain produced by dorsiflexion of the foot

Home care   providing care in the client's home

Home health nursing   services and products provided to clients in their homes that are needed to maintain, restore, or promote their physical, psychologic, and social well-being

Homeopathy   an alternative therapy based on the theory that the cure for the disease lies in the disease itself; thus, treatment is with highly diluted amounts of substances that at a higher concentration would produce the same symptoms as the disease

Homeostasis   the tendency of the body to maintain a state of balance or equilibrium while continually changing; a mechanism in which deviations from normal are sensed and counteracted

Hope   a multidimensional concept that includes perceiving realistic expectations and goals, having motivation to achieve goals, anticipating outcomes, establishing trust and interpersonal relationships, relying on internal and external resources, having determination to endure, and being oriented to the future

Hordeolum (sty)   a redness, swelling, and tenderness of the hair follicle and glands that empty at the edge of the eyelids

Horticultural therapy   also called *gardening* or *healing garden;* adjunct therapy to occupational and physical therapy that may involve viewing nature, visiting a healing garden or wander garden, or actively gardening

Hospice   the delivery of care for terminally ill clients either in health care facilities or in the client's home

Hospice nursing   care frequently given to terminally ill clients in their home; often considered a subspecialty of public health nursing

Hospital information system (HIS)   computer software program suite used to manage client, financial, and administrative data

Hub   the part of a needle that fits onto a syringe

Humanism   learning that focuses on the feelings and attitudes of learners, the importance of the individual in identifying learning needs and taking responsibility for them, and the self-motivation of the learners to work toward self-reliance and independence

Humanist   a perspective that includes propositions such as the mind and body are indivisible, people have the power to solve their own problems, and people are responsible for their lives and well-being

Humidifiers   devices that add water vapor to inspired air

Humoral immunity   antibody-mediated defense; resides ultimately in the B lymphocytes and is mediated by the antibodies produced by B cells

Hydrostatic pressure   the pressure a liquid exerts on the sides of the container that holds it; also called *filtration force*

Hygiene   the science of health and its maintenance

Hyperalgesia   extreme sensitivity to pain

Hypercalcemia   an excess of calcium in the blood plasma

Hypercapnia   a condition in which carbon dioxide accumulates in the blood

Hypercarbia   *see* Hypercapnia

Hyperchloremia   an excess of chloride in the blood plasma

Hyperemia   increased blood flow to an area

Hyperinflation   giving the client breaths that are 1 to 1.5 times the tidal volume through the ventilator circuit or via a manual resuscitation bag

Hyperkalemia   an excess of potassium in the blood plasma

Hypermagnesemia   an excess of magnesium in the blood plasma

Hypernatremia   an excess of sodium in the blood plasma

Hyperopia   abnormal refraction in which light rays focus behind the retina, farsightedness

Hyperoxygenation   done with a manual resuscitation bag or through a ventilator; increases oxygen flow (usually to 100%) before suctioning and between suction attempts

Hyperpathia   heightened response to a painful stimulus; hyperalgesia

Hyperphosphatemia   an excess of phosphate in the blood plasma

Hyperpyrexia   *see* Hyperthermia

Hyperresonance   an abnormal booming sound produced during percussion of the lungs

Hypersomnia   excessive sleep

Hypertension   an abnormally high blood pressure; over 140 mm Hg systolic and/or 90 mm Hg diastolic

Hyperthermia   an extremely high body temperature (e.g., 41°C [105.8°F])

Hypertonic   solutions that have a higher osmolality than body fluids

Hypertrophy   enlargement of a muscle or organ

Hyperventilation   very deep, rapid respirations

Hypervolemia   increased blood volume

Hypnotherapy   application of hypnosis (trance state or altered state of consciousness) to a medical or psychologic disorder

Hypoactive sexual desire disorder   involves a persistent or recurring absence of sexual thoughts or disinterest in sexual activity

Hypocalcemia   deficiency of calcium in the blood plasma

Hypochloremia   deficiency of chloride in the blood plasma

Hypodermic   under the skin

Hypodermic syringe   a type of syringe that comes in 2-, 2.5-, and 3-mL sizes; the syringe usually has two scales marked on it: the minim and the milliliter

Hypokalemia   deficiency of potassium in the blood plasma

Hypomagnesemia   deficiency of magnesium in the blood plasma

Hyponatremia   deficiency of sodium in the blood plasma

Hypophosphatemia   deficiency of phosphate in the blood plasma

Hypotension   an abnormally low blood pressure; less than 100 mm Hg systolic in an adult

Hypothalamic integrator   the center in the brain that controls the core temperature; located in the preoptic area of the hypothalamus

Hypothermia   a core body temperature below the lower limit of normal

Hypothesis   a prediction of the relationship among two or more variables

Hypotonic   solutions that have a lower osmolality than body fluids

Hypoventilation   very shallow respirations

Hypovolemia   an abnormal reduction in blood volume

Hypoxemia   reduced oxygen in the blood

Hypoxia   insufficient oxygen anywhere in the body

I

Iatrogenic disease   disease caused unintentionally by medical therapy

Iatrogenic infections   infections that are the direct result of diagnostic or therapeutic procedures

Id   the source of instinctive and unconscious psychologic urges

Ideal body weight (IBW)   the optimal weight recommended for optimal health

Ideal self   how we would prefer to be; the individual's perception of how one should behave based on certain personal standards, aspirations, goals, or values

Identification   perceiving one's self as similar to and behaving like another person

Idiosyncratic effect   a different, unexpected, or individual effect from the normal one usually expected from a medication; the occurrence of unpredictable and unexplainable symptoms

Ileal conduit   channel created when a segment of the ileum is removed and the intestinal ends reattached

Ileostomy   an opening into the ileum (small bowel)

Illicit drugs   drugs that are sold illegally; street drugs

Illness   a highly personal state in which the person feels unhealthy or ill, may or may not be related to disease

Illness behavior   the course of action a person takes to define the state of his or her health and pursue a remedy

Imagery   the internal experience of memories, dreams, fantasies, and visions that serve as a bridge connecting body, mind, and spirit

Imagination   an important part of preschoolers' life (the preschooler has an active imagination and fantasizes in play)

Imitation   copying the behaviors and attitudes of another person

Immobility   prescribed or unavoidable restriction of movement in any area of a person's life

Immune defenses   *see* Specific (immune) defenses

Immunity   a specific resistance of the body to infection; it may be natural, or resistance may develop after exposure to a disease agent

Immunoglobulins   *see* Antibodies

Impaired nurse   a nurse whose practice has deteriorated because of chemical abuse

Implementing   the phase of the nursing process in which the nursing care plan is put into action

Implication   something that is not stated but is referred, ascribed, or attributed to that can result in either true or false clinical judgment; for example, the client's not wearing a wedding ring implies he or she is not married

Implied consent   consent that is assumed in an emergency when consent cannot be obtained from the client or a relative

Implied contract   a contract that has not been explicitly agreed to by the parties but that the law nevertheless considers to exist

Incentive spirometers   devices that measure the flow of air inhaled through the mouthpiece

Incomplete proteins   protein that lacks one or more essential amino acids; usually derived from vegetables

Incus   the anvil bone of the middle ear

Independent variable   the presumed cause or influence on the dependent variable

Independent functions   areas of health care unique to nursing, separate and distinct from medical management

Independent interventions   activities that the nurse is licensed to initiate as a result of the nurse's own knowledge and skills

Independent practice associations (IPAs)   provide care in offices; clients pay a fixed prospective payment and IPA pays the provider; earnings or losses are assumed by the IPA

Indicator   an observable patient state, behavior, or self-reported perception or evaluation; similar to desired outcomes in traditional language

Individualized care plan   a plan tailored to meet the unique needs of a specific client—needs that are not addressed by the standardized plan

Individualized exercise prescription   exercise mode and dose tailored to a specific individual to ensure greater adherence to the exercise program

Inductive reasoning   making generalizations from specific data

Infection   the disease process produced by microorganisms

Inferences   interpretations or conclusions made based on cues or observed data

Inflammation   local and nonspecific defensive tissue response to injury or destruction of cells

Influence   an informal strategy used to gain the cooperation of others without exercising formal authority

Informal nursing care plan   a strategy for action that exists in the nurse's mind

Informal leader   an individual selected by the group as its leader because of seniority, age, special abilities, or charisma

Informed consent   a client's agreement to accept a course of treatment or a procedure after receiving complete information, including the risks of treatment and facts relating to it, from the physician

Infrared photoenergy therapy   treatment to improve sensory impairment associated with peripheral neuropathy

Ingestion   the act of taking in food or medication

Ingrown toenail   the growing inward of the nail into the soft tissues around it, most often results from improper nail trimming

Inhalation   (inspiration) the act of breathing in; the intake of air or other substances into the lungs

Inhibiting effect   the decreased effect of one or both drugs

Injury   *see* Harm

Input   consists of information, material, or energy that enters a system

Inquest   a legal inquiry into the cause or manner of a death

Insensible fluid loss   fluid loss that is not perceptible to the individual

Insensible heat loss   heat loss that occurs from evaporation (vaporization) of moisture from the respiratory tract, mucosa of the mouth, and the skin

Insensible water loss   continuous and unnoticed water loss

In-service education   education that is designed to upgrade the knowledge or skills of employees

Insomnia   inability to obtain a sufficient quality or quantity of sleep

Inspection   the visual examination, that is, assessment by using the sense of sight

Inspiration   *see* Inhalation

Insulin syringe   similar to a hypodermic syringe, but the scale is specially designed for insulin: a 100-unit calibrated scale intended for use with U-100 insulin

Integrated delivery system (IDS)   a system that incorporates acute care services, home health care, extended and skilled care facilities, and outpatient services

Integrated health care system   one that makes all levels of care available in an integrated form—primary care, secondary care, and tertiary care

Intellectual standard   process of thinking that results in reasonable, rational thoughts, involving clarity, accuracy, relevance, logicalness, breadth, precision, significance, completeness, fairness, and depth

Intensity   the loudness or softness of a sound, amplitude

Intention tremor   involuntary trembling when an individual attempts a voluntary movement

Intermittent fever   a body temperature that alternates at regular intervals between periods of fever and periods of normal or subnormal temperatures

Internet   a worldwide computer network

Interpersonal skills   all verbal and nonverbal activities people use when communicating directly with one another

Interpretation   analysis of data to reach a specific conclusion; a mental representation of the meaning or significance of something

Interpreter   an individual who mediates spoken communication between people speaking different languages without adding, omitting, or distorting meaning or editorializing

Intersex   ambiguous gender

Interstate compact   an agreement between two or more states

Interstitial fluid   fluid that surrounds the cells, includes lymph

Interview   a planned communication; a conversation with a purpose

Intimacy   a close friendship

Intracellular fluid (ICF)   fluid found within the body cells, also called *cellular fluid*

Intractable pain   pain that is resistant to cure or relief

Intradermal   under the epidermis (into the dermis)

Intradermal (ID) injection   the administration of a drug into the dermal layer of the skin just beneath the epidermis

Intramuscular   into the muscle

Intramuscular (IM) injections   injections into muscle tissue that are absorbed more quickly than subcutaneous injections because of the greater blood supply to the body muscles

Intraoperative phase   begins when the client is transferred to the operating table and ends when the client is admitted to the postanesthesia care unit

Intrapleural pressure   pressure in the pleural cavity surrounding the lungs

Intrapulmonary pressure   pressure within the lungs

Intraspinal   into the spinal cord

Intrathecal   *see* Intraspinal

Intravascular fluid   plasma

Intravenous   within a vein

Intravenous block   anesthesia used most often for procedures involving the arm, wrist, and hand

Intravenous pyelography (IVP)   x-ray filming of the kidney and ureters after injection of a radiopaque material into the vein

Introjection   the assimilation of the attributes of others

Intuition   the understanding or learning of things without the conscious use of reasoning

Invasion of privacy   a direct wrong of a personal nature, it injures the feelings of the person and does not take into account the effect of revealed information on the standing of the person in the community

Ions   atoms or group of atoms that carry a positive or negative electric charge; electrolytes

Iron deficiency anemia   a form of anemia caused by inadequate supply of iron for synthesis of hemoglobin

Irrigation (lavage)   a flushing or washing-out of a body cavity, organ, or wound with a specified solution that may or may not be medicated

Ischemia   deficiency of blood supply caused by obstruction of circulation to the body part

Isokinetic (resistive) exercises   muscle contraction or tension against resistance

Isolation   practices that prevent the spread of infection and communicable disease

Isometric (static or setting) exercise   tensing of a muscle against an immovable outer resistance that does not change muscle length or produce joint motion

Isotonic   solutions that have the same osmolality as body fluids

Isotonic (dynamic) exercise   exercise in which muscle tension is constant and the muscle shortens to produce muscle contraction and active movement

J

Jaundice   a yellowish color of the sclera, mucous membranes, and/or skin

Jejunostomy   an opening through the abdominal wall into the jejunum

Justice   fairness

K

Kardex   the trade name for a method that makes use of a series of cards to concisely organize and record client data and instructions for daily nursing care—especially care that changes frequently and must be kept up to date

Keloid   a hypertrophic scar containing an abnormal amount of collagen

Kidneys/ureters/bladder (KUB)   x-ray of the kidneys, ureters, and bladder

Kilocalorie (kcal)   *see* Calorie

Kilojoule (kJ)   a metric measurement referring to the amount of energy required when a force of 1 newton (N) moves 1 kg of weight 1 m of distance

Kinesthetic   refers to awareness of the position and movement of body parts

Knights of Saint Lazarus   an order of knights that dedicated themselves to the care of people with leprosy, syphilis, and chronic skin conditions

Korotkoff's sounds   a series of five sounds produced by blood within the artery with each ventricular contraction

Kosher   acceptable or prepared according to Jewish law

Kussmaul's breathing   hyperventilation that accompanies metabolic acidosis in which the body attempts to compensate (give off excess body acids) by blowing off carbon dioxide through deep and rapid breathing

Kyphosis   excessive convex curvature of the thoracic spine

L

Laissez-faire (nondirective, permissive) leader   recognizes the group's need for autonomy and self-regulation

Lanugo   the fine, woolly hair or down on the shoulders, back, sacrum, and earlobes of the unborn child that may remain for a few weeks after birth

Large calorie (Calorie, kilocalorie [kcal])   *see* Calorie

Laryngoscopy   visual examination of the larynx with a laryngoscope

Lateral position   a side-lying position

Lavage   an irrigation or washing of a body organ, such as the stomach

Lavinia L. Dock   a nursing leader and suffragist who was active in the protest movement for women's rights that resulted in the U.S. Constitution amendment allowing women to vote in 1920

Law   a rule made by humans that regulates social conduct in a formally prescribed and binding manner

Laxatives   medications that stimulate bowel activity and assist fecal elimination

Leader   a person who influences others to work together to accomplish a specific goal

Leadership style   describes traits, behaviors, motivations, and choices used by individuals to effectively influence others

Leading question   a question that influences the client to give a particular answer

Learning   a change in human disposition or capability that persists over a period of time and cannot be solely accounted for by growth

Learning need   a desire or a requirement to know something that is currently unknown to the learner

Leukocytes   white blood cells

Leukocytosis   an increase in the number of white blood cells

Liability   the quality or state of being legally responsible for one's obligations and action and to make financial restitution for wrongful acts

Libel   defamation by means of print, writing, or pictures

Libido   urge or desire for sexual activity

License   a legal permit granted to individuals to engage in the practice of a profession and to use a particular title

Licensed vocational (practical) nurse (LVN/LPN)   a nurse who practices under the supervision of a registered nurse, providing basic direct technical care to clients

Lifestyle   the values and behaviors adopted by a person in daily life

Lift   an abnormal anterior movement of the chest related to enlargement of the right ventricle

Lillian Wald   founder of the Henry Street Settlement and Visiting Nurse Service, which provided nursing and social services and organized educational and cultural activities; considered the founder of public health nursing

Linda Richards   America's first trained nurse

Line of gravity   an imaginary vertical line running through the center of gravity

Lipids   organic substances that are greasy and insoluble in water but soluble in alcohol or ether

Lipoproteins   soluble compounds made up of various lipids

Litigation   the action of a lawsuit

Living will   a document that states medical treatments(s) the client chooses to omit or refuse in the event that the client is unable to make these decisions

Livor mortis   discoloration of the skin caused by breakdown of the red blood cells; occurs after blood circulation has ceased; appears in the dependent areas of the body

Lobule   earlobe

Local adaptation syndrome (LAS)   the reaction of one organ or body part to stress

Local anesthesia   an anesthetic agent used for minor surgical procedures that is injected into a specific area

Local area network (LAN)   personal computers (PCs) linked directly to nearby PCs and servers by wires or wireless communication devices

Local infection   an infection that is limited to the specific part of the body where the microorganisms remain

Locus of control (LOC)   a concept about whether clients believe their health status is under their own or others' control

Logic, logical   correct reasoning using inductive or deductive thinking in order to reach a conclusion or judgment

Logrolling   a technique used to turn a client whose body must at all times be kept in straight alignment (like a log)

Long-term memory   the repository for information stored for periods longer than 72 hours and usually weeks and years

Lordosis   an exaggerated concavity in the lumbar region of the vertebral column

Loss   an actual or potential situation in which a valued ability, object, or person is inaccessible or changed so that it is perceived as no longer valuable

Low Fowler's position   a bed-sitting position in which the head of the bed is elevated between 15 and 45 degrees, with or without knee flexion

Lumbar puncture   a procedure where cerebrospinal fluid (CSF) is withdrawn through a needle that is inserted into the subarachnoid space of the spinal canal between the third and fourth lumbar vertebrae or between the fourth and fifth lumbar vertebrae

Lung compliance   expansibility of the lung

Lung recoil   the tendency of lungs to collapse away from the chest wall

Lung scan   records the emissions from radioisotopes that indicate how well gas and blood are traveling through the lungs; also known as a *V/Q* (ventilation/perfusion) *scan*

M

Maceration   the wasting away or softening of a solid as if by the action of soaking; often used to describe degenerative changes and eventual disintegration

Macrominerals   any of the minerals that people require daily in amounts over 100 mg

Macronutrients   refers to carbohydrates, fats, and protein because they are needed in large amounts (e.g., hundreds of grams) to provide energy

Magico-religious health belief   a belief system in which people attribute the fate of the world and those in it to the actions of God, the gods, or other supernatural forces for good or evil

Magnetic resonance imaging (MRI)   a noninvasive diagnostic scanning technique in which the client is placed in a magnetic field

Maintenance stage   stage at which a person integrates newly adopted behavior patterns into his or her lifestyle

Major surgery   surgery that involves a high degree of risk for a variety of reasons; it may be complicated or prolonged; large losses of blood may occur; vital organs may be involved; postoperative complications may occur

Male erectile disorder   when a man has erection problems during 25% or more of his sexual interactions

Male orgasmic disorder   disorder where a man can maintain an erection but has difficulty ejaculating

Malleus   hammer bone of the middle ear

Malnutrition   a disorder of nutrition; insufficient nourishment of the body cells

Malpractice   the negligent acts of persons engaged in professions or occupations in which highly technical or professional skills are employed

Managed care   a method of organizing care delivery that emphasizes communication and coordination of care among all health care team members

Management information system (MIS)   software designed to facilitate the organization and application of data used to manage an organization or department

Manager   one who is appointed to a position in an organization that gives the power to guide and direct the work of others

Mandated reporters   a role of the nurse in which he or she identifies and assesses cases of violence against others, and in every case the situation must be reported to the proper authorities

Manometer   an instrument used to measure the pressure of fluids or gases

Manslaughter   second-degree murder

Manubrium   the handle-like superior part of the sternum that joins with the clavicles

Margaret Higgins Sanger   considered the founder of Planned Parenthood, was imprisoned for opening the first birth control information clinic in Baltimore in 1916

Mary Breckinridge   a nurse who practiced midwifery in England, Australia, and New Zealand; founded the Frontier Nursing Service in Kentucky in 1925 to provide family-centered primary health care to rural populations

Mary Mahoney   first African American professional nurse

Mass peristalsis   involves a wave of powerful muscular contraction that moves over large areas of the colon; usually occurs after eating

Mastoid   a bony prominence behind the ear

Masturbation   sexual self-stimulation

Maturity   the state of maximal function and integration; the state of being fully developed

Mean   a measure of central tendency, computed by summing all scores and dividing by the number of subjects; commonly symbolized as X or M

Measures of central tendency   measures that describe the center of a distribution of data, denoting where most of the subjects lie; include the mean, median, and mode

Measures of variability   measures that indicate the degree of dispersion or spread of the data; include range, variance, and standard deviation

Meatus   an opening, passage, or channel

Meconium   the first fecal material passed by the newborn, normally up to 24 hours after birth

Median   a measure of central tendency, representing the exact middle score or value in a distribution of scores; the median is the value above and below which 50% of the scores lie

Medicaid   a U.S. federal public assistance program paid out of general taxes and administered through the individual states to provide health care for those who require financial assistance

Medical asepsis   all practices intended to confine a specific microorganism to a specific area, limiting the number, growth, and spread of microorganisms

Medical examiner   a physician who usually has advanced education in pathology or forensic medicine who determines causes of death

Medicare   a national and state health insurance program for U.S. residents older than 65 years of age

Medication   a substance administered for the diagnosis, cure, treatment, or relief of a symptom or for prevention of disease

Medication reconciliation   comparison of medications client is taking to physician's admission, transfer, and/or discharge orders

Meditation   mental exercise that directs the mind to think inwardly by closing the sense organs to external stimulation

Menarche   onset of menstruation

Meniscus   the crescent-shaped upper surface of a column of fluid

Menopause   cessation of menstruation

Menstruation   the monthly discharge of blood through the vagina occurring in nonpregnant women from puberty to menopause

Mentor   a person who serves as an experienced guide, adviser, or advocate and assumes responsibility for promoting the growth and professional advancement of a less experienced individual

Mesoderm   middle layer of the embryonic tissue that forms during the first 3 weeks of life

Metabolic acidosis   a condition characterized by a deficiency of bicarbonate ions in the body in relation to the amount of carbonic acid in the body; the pH falls to less than 7.35

Metabolic alkalosis   a condition characterized by an excess of bicarbonate ions in the body in relation to the amount of carbonic acid in the body; the pH rises to greater than 7.45

Metabolism   the sum of all physical and chemical processes by which a living substance is formed and maintained and by which energy is made available for use by the organism

Metabolites   end products or enzymes

Metaparadigm   originates from the Greek *meta*, meaning "with," and *paradigm*, meaning "pattern"; based on four theoretical concepts of nursing: person, environment, health, and nursing

Metered-dose inhaler (MDI)   a handheld nebulizer, which is a pressurized container of medication that can be used by the client to release the medication through a mouthpiece

Microminerals   a vitamin or mineral

Micronutrients   vitamins and minerals that are needed in small amounts (e.g., milligrams or micrograms) to metabolize energy-providing nutrients

Micturition   *see* Urination

Mid-arm circumference (MAC)   a measure of fat, muscle, and skeleton

Mid-arm muscle circumference (MAMC)   calculated by using reference tables or by using a formula that incorporates the triceps skinfold and the MAC

Middle-level manager   a manager who supervises a number of first-level managers and is responsible for the activities in the departments supervised

Midlevel theories   focus on exploration of concepts such as pain, self-esteem, learning, and hardiness

Midstream urine specimen   *see* Clean-catch specimen

Milliequivalent   one-thousandth of an equivalent, which is the chemical combining power of a substance

Minerals   a substance found in organic compounds, as inorganic compounds and as free ions

Minor surgery   surgery that involves little risk, produces few complications, and is often performed in a "day surgery" facility

Miosis   constricted pupils

Misdemeanor   a legal offense usually punishable by a fine or a short-term jail sentence, or both

Mixed hearing loss   a combination of conduction and sensorineural loss

Mobility   ability to move about freely, easily, and purposefully in the environment

Mode   the score or value that occurs most frequently in a distribution of scores

Modeling   observing the behavior of people who have successfully achieved a goal that one has set for oneself and, through observing, acquiring ideas for behavior and coping strategies

Monosaccharides   sugars that are composed of single molecules

Monotheism   belief in the existence of one God

Monounsaturated fatty acids   a fatty acid with one double bond

Moral   relating to right and wrong

Moral behavior   the way a person perceives the requirements necessary for people to live together and how he or she responds to them

Moral development   process of learning to tell the difference between right and wrong and of learning what ought and ought not to be done

Moral rules   specific prescriptions for actions

Morality   a doctrine or system denoting what is right and wrong in conduct, character, or attitude

Mortician   a person trained in the care of the dead; also called an *undertaker*

Motivation   the desire to learn

Mourning   the process through which grief is eventually resolved or altered

Multidisciplinary care plan   a standardized plan that outlines the care required for clients with common, predictable—usually medical—conditions

Music therapy   the behavioral science concerned with the systematic application of music to produce relaxation and desired changes in emotions, behavior, and physiology

Mutual pretense   a type of awareness in which the client, family, and health personnel know that the prognosis is terminal but do not talk about it and make an effort not to raise the subject

Mutual recognition model   a regulatory model developed by the National Council of State Boards of Nursing (NCSBN), which allows for multistate licensure

Mydriasis   enlarged pupils

Myocardial infarction (MI)   heart attack; cardiac tissue necrosis owing to obstruction of blood flow to the heart

Myocardium   a layer of the heart wall; cardiac muscle cells that form the bulk of the heart and contract with each beat

Myopia   abnormal refraction in which light rays focus in front of the retina (nearsightedness)

N

Narcolepsy   an uncontrollable desire for sleep or attacks of sleep during the day

Narrative charting   a descriptive record of client data and nursing interventions, written in sentences and paragraphs

Nasoenteric tube   a tube inserted through one of the nostrils, down the nasopharynx, and into the alimentary tract

Nasogastric tube   a tube inserted by way of the nasopharynx and placed into the client's stomach for the purpose of feeding the client or to remove gastric secretions

Naturopathic medicine   practice that focuses on nutrition, herbs, homeopathy, acupuncture, hydrotherapy, physical medicine, counseling, and minor surgical interventions

Naturopathy   study of nutrition, herbs, homeopathy, acupuncture, hydrotherapy, physical medicine, counseling, and minor surgical interventions

Negative feedback   feedback that inhibits change

Negligence   failure to behave in a reasonable and prudent manner; an unintentional tort

Nephrostomy   diversion of urine from a kidney to a stoma

Nerve block   chemical interruption of a nerve pathway effected by injecting a local anesthetic

Network   linkages

Networking   a process by which people develop linkages throughout the profession to communicate, share ideas and information, and offer support and direction to each other

Neurectomy   surgery in which peripheral or cranial nerves are interrupted to alleviate localized pain

Neurogenic bladder   interference with the normal mechanisms of urine elimination in which the client does not perceive bladder fullness and is unable to control the urinary sphincters; the result of impaired neurologic function

Neuropathic pain   the result of a disturbance of the peripheral or central nervous system that results in pain that may or may not be associated with an ongoing tissue-damaging process

Neutral question   a question that does not direct or pressure a client to answer in a certain way

Nitrogen balance   a measure of the degree of protein anabolism and catabolism; net result of intake and loss of nitrogen

Nociception   the physiologic processes related to pain perception

Nociceptor   a pain receptor

Nocturia   voiding two or more times at night

Nocturnal emissions   orgasm and emission of semen during sleep

Nocturnal enuresis   involuntary urination at night

Nocturnal frequency   the need for older adults to arise during the night to urinate

Nondirective interview   an interview using open-ended questions and empathetic responses to build rapport and learn client concerns

Nondirective leader   see Laissez-faire (nondirective, permissive) leader

Nonessential amino acids   an amino acid that the body can manufacture

Nonmaleficence   the duty to do no harm

Nonspecific defenses   bodily defenses that protect a person against all microorganisms, regardless of prior exposure

Nonsteroidal anti-inflammatory drugs (NSAIDs)   drugs that relieve pain by acting on the peripheral nerve endings to inhibit the formation of the prostaglandins that tend to sensitize nerves to painful stimuli; have analgesic, antipyretic, and anti-inflammatory effects; include aspirin and ibuprofen

Nonverbal communication   communication other than words, including gestures, posture, and facial expressions

Norm   an ideal or fixed standard; an expected standard of behavior of group members

Normocephalic   normal head size

Normocephaly   normal head circumference at birth; usually 35 cm (14 in.)

Nosocomial infections   infections associated with the delivery of health care services in a health care facility

NPO   from the Latin *nil per os* meaning "nothing by mouth"

NREM (non-REM) sleep   a deep restful sleep rate; also called *slow wave sleep*

Nuclear family   a family of parents and their offspring

Nurse informaticist   an expert who combines computer, information, and nursing science to develop policies and procedures that promote effective use of computerized records by nurses and other health care professionals

Nursing   the attributes, characteristics, and actions of the nurse providing care on behalf of, or in conjunction with, the client

Nursing diagnosis   the nurse's clinical judgment about individual, family, or community responses to actual and potential health problems/life processes to provide the basis for selecting nursing interventions to achieve outcomes for which the nurse is accountable

Nursing ethics   ethical issues that occur in nursing practice

Nursing informatics   the science of using computer information systems in the practice of nursing

Nurse informaticist   expert who combines computer, information, and nursing science

Nursing intervention   any treatment, based on clinical judgment and knowledge, that a nurse performs to enhance patient/client outcomes

Nursing Interventions Classification (NIC)   a taxonomy of nursing actions each of which includes a label, a definition, and a list of activities

Nursing Outcomes Classification (NOC)   a taxonomy for describing client outcomes that respond to nursing interventions

Nursing process   a systematic rational method of planning and providing nursing care

Nutrients   organic or inorganic substances found in food

Nutrition   the sum of all interactions between an organism and the food it consumes

Nutritive value   the nutrient content of a specified amount of food

Nystagmus   rapid involuntary rhythmic eye movement

O

Obese (obesity)   when body mass index (BMI) is greater than 30 kg/m²

Objective data   information (data) that is detectable by an observer or can be tested against an accepted standard; can be seen, heard, felt, or smelled

Obligatory losses   essential fluid losses required to maintain body functioning

Occult blood   hidden blood

Occupational exposure   skin, eye, mucous membrane, or parenteral contact with blood or other potentially infectious materials that may result from the performance of an employee's duties

Official name   the name under which a drug is listed in one of the official publications (e.g., the *United States Pharmacopeia*)

Oils   lipids that are liquid at room temperature

Olfactory   related to smell

Oliguria   production of abnormally small amounts of urine by the kidney

Oncotic pressure   *see* Colloid osmotic pressure

One-point discrimination   the ability to sense whether one or two areas of the skin are being stimulated by pressure

Online   connected to a computer network

Onset of action   the time after drug administration when the body initially responds to the drug

Open awareness   a type of awareness in which a client and people around know about the impending death

Open system   system in which energy, matter, and information move into and out of the system through the system boundary

Open-ended questions   questions that specify only the broad topic to be discussed and invite clients to discover and explore their thoughts and feelings about the topic

Operational definitions   definitions that specify the instruments or procedures by which concepts will be measured

Ophthalmic   referring to the eye

Opportunistic pathogen   a microorganism causing disease only in a susceptible individual

Oral   referring to the mouth

Oral-genital sex   oral stimulation of either female or male genitals

Organizing   determining responsibilities, communicating expectations, and establishing the chain of command for authority and communication

Orgasmic phase   part of the response cycle, the involuntary climax of sexual tension, accompanied by physiologic and psychologic release

Orthopnea   ability to breathe only when in an upright position (sitting or standing)

Orthopneic position   a sitting position that relieves respiratory difficulty; the client leans over and is supported by an overbed table across the lap

Orthostatic hypotension   decrease in blood pressure related to positional or postural changes from lying to sitting or standing positions

Osmolality   the concentration of solutes in body fluids

Osmosis   passage of a solvent through a semipermeable membrane from an area of lesser solute concentration to one of greater solute concentration

Osmotic pressure   pressure exerted by the number of nondiffusible particles in a solution; the amount of pressure needed to stop the flow of water across a membrane

Ossicles   the three middle ear bones of sound transmission

Osteoporosis   demineralization of the bone

Ostomy   a suffix denoting the formation of an opening or outlet such as an opening on the abdominal wall for the elimination of feces or urine

Otic   referring to the ear

Otoscope   an instrument used to examine the ears

Outcome evaluation   focuses on demonstrable changes in the client's health status as result of nursing care

Output   energy, matter, or information from a system given out by the system as a result of its processes

Overhydration   occurs when water is gained in excess of electrolytes, resulting in low serum osmolality and low serum sodium levels, also known as *hypo-osmolar imbalance* or *water intoxication*

Overnutrition   a caloric intake in excess of daily energy requirements, resulting in storage of energy in the form of adipose tissue

Overweight   a BMI of 26–30 kg/m²

Oxyhemoglobin   the compound of oxygen and hemoglobin

P

Pace   number of steps taken per minute or the distance taken in one step when walking

Packing   filling an open wound or cavity with a material such as gauze

Pain   whatever the experiencing person says it is, existing whenever he or she says it does

Pain management   assisting the client to reduce the level of discomfort experienced to an acceptable level as reported by the client, using both pharmacological and nonpharmacological measures

Pain threshold   the amount of pain stimulation a person requires before feeling pain

Pain tolerance   the maximum amount and duration of pain that an individual is willing to endure

Palliative care   symptom care of clients for whom disease no longer responds to cure-focused treatment

Pallor   the absence of underlying red tones in the skin; may be most readily seen in the buccal mucosa

Palpation   the examination of the body using the sense of touch

Papanicolaou (Pap) test   a method of taking a sample of cervical cells for microscopic examination to detect malignancy

Paradigm   a pattern of shared understandings and assumptions about reality and the world

Parasites   microorganisms that live in or on another from which it obtains nourishment

Parasomnia   a cluster or pattern of waking behavior that appears during sleep, such as somnambulism (sleepwalking), sleeptalking, and enuresis (bed-wetting)

Parenteral   drug administration occurring outside the alimentary tract; injected into the body through some route other than the alimentary canal (e.g., intramuscularly)

Paresis   slight or incomplete paralysis

Parotitis   inflammation of the parotid salivary gland

Partial pressure   the pressure exerted by each individual gas in a mixture according to its percentage concentration in the mixture

Partially complete proteins   proteins that contain less than the required amount of one or more essential amino acids; cannot alone support continued growth

Participative leader   *see* Democratic leader

Passive euthanasia   allowing a person to die by withholding or withdrawing measures to maintain life

Passive (Acquired) immunity   a resistance of the body to infection in which the host receives natural or artificial antibodies produced by another source

Passive ROM exercises   another person moves each of a client's joints through its complete range of movement, maximally stretching all muscle groups within each plane over each joint

Pathogenicity   the ability to produce disease; a pathogen is a microorganism that causes disease

Pathologic fractures   spontaneous fractures to which elderly persons are prone

Patient   a person who is waiting for or undergoing medical treatment and care

Patient-controlled analgesia (PCA)   a pain management technique that allows the client to take an active role in managing pain

Patient-focused care   delivery model that brings all services and care providers to the client

Patient Self-Determination Act (PSDA)   legislation requiring that every competent adult be informed in writing on admission to a health care institution about his or her rights to accept or refuse medical care and to use advance directives

Peak level   indicates the highest concentration of the drug in the blood serum

Peak plasma level   the concentration of a drug in the blood plasma that occurs when the elimination rate equals the rate of absorption

Pedagogy   the discipline concerned with helping children learn

Pediculosis   infestation with head lice

Peer groups   assume great importance and have a number of functions: provide a sense of belonging, pride, social learning, and sexual roles; most peer groups have well-defined, sex-specific modes of acceptable behavior and in adolescence, the peer groups change with age

Penrose drain   a flexible rubber drain

Perceived loss   the loss experienced by a person that cannot be verified by others

Perception   the ability to interpret the environment through the senses

Percutaneous   through the skin

Percussion   a method in which the body surface is struck to elicit sounds that can be heard or vibrations that can be felt

Percutaneous endoscopic gastrostomy (PEG)   feeding catheter inserted into the stomach through the skin and subcutaneous tissues of the abdomen

Percutaneous endoscopic jejunostomy (PEJ)   feeding catheter inserted into the jejunum through the skin and subcutaneous tissues of the abdomen

Perfusion   passage of blood constituents through the vessels of the circulatory system

Pericardium   double layer of fibroserous membrane of the heart; the parietal, or outermost, pericardium serves to protect the heart and anchor it to surrounding structures

Peridural anesthesia   *see* Epidural anesthesia

Periodontal disease   disorder of the supporting structures of the teeth

Perioperative period   refers to the three phases of surgery: preoperative, intraoperative, and postoperative

Peripheral pulse   a pulse located in the periphery of the body (e.g., foot, wrist)

Peripheral vascular resistance (PVR)   impedance or opposition to blood flow to the tissues; determined by viscosity, or thickness, of the blood; blood vessel length; blood vessel diameter

Peripherally inserted central venous catheter (PICC)   catheter inserted in the basilic or cephalic vein just above or below the antecubital space

Peripheral neuropathic pain   pain (e.g., phantom limb pain, postherpetic neuralgia, carpal tunnel syndrome) that follows damage and/or sensitization of peripheral nerves

Peripherals   at the edge or outward boundary

Peristalsis   wavelike movements produced by circular and longitudinal muscle fibers of the intestinal walls; the movement propels the intestinal contents onward

Permissive leader   *see* Laissez-faire leader

Personal computers (PCs)   individual microcomputer systems referred to as a desktop, portable, laptop, notebook, or handheld computer

Personal knowing   promotes wholeness and integrity in the personal encounter to achieve engagement

Personal space   the distance people prefer in interactions with others

Personal values   values internalized from the society or culture in which one lives

Personality   the outward expression of the inner self

PES format   the three essential components of nursing diagnostic statements including the terms describing the *problem*, the *etiology* of the problem, and the defining characteristics or cluster of *signs* and *symptoms*

pH   a measure of the relative alkalinity or acidity of a solution; a measure of the concentration of hydrogen ions

Phagocytes   cells that ingest microorganisms, other cells, and foreign particles

Pharmacist   a person licensed to prepare and dispense drugs and prescriptions

Pharmacodynamics   the process by which a drug alters cell physiology

Pharmacogenetics   process by which the effect of a drug is influenced by genetic variations such as gender, size, and body composition

Pharmacokinetics   the study of the absorption, distribution, biotransformation, and excretion of drugs

Pharmacology   the scientific study of the actions of drugs on living animals and humans

Pharmacopoeia   a book containing a list of drug products used in medicine, including their descriptions and formulas

Pharmacy   the art of preparing, compounding, and dispensing drugs; also refers to the place where drugs are prepared and dispensed

Phenomenology   research that investigates people's life experiences and how they interpret those experiences

Philosophy   an early effort to define phenomena that serves as the basis for later theoretical formulations

Phlebotomist   a person from a laboratory who performs venipuncture, collecting the blood specimen for the tests ordered by the physician

Physical activity   bodily movement produced by skeletal muscles that requires energy expenditure and produces progressive health benefits

Physical restraints   any manual method or physical or mechanical device, material, or equipment attached to the client's body that restrict the client's movement

Physiologic dependence   biochemical changes occurring in the body as a result of excessive use of a drug

Physiologic pain   pain experienced when an intact properly functioning nervous system sends signals that tissues are damaged

PIE   an acronym for a charting model that follows a recording sequence of *problems*, *interventions*, and *evaluation* of the effectiveness of the interventions

Piggyback   secondary IV setup where the second IV set connects the second container to the tubing of the primary container at the upper port

Pilates   method of physical movement and exercise designed to stretch, strengthen, and balance the body, in particular the core of the body

Pinna   *see* Auricle

Pitch   the frequency or number of vibrations heard during auscultation

Pitting edema   edema in which firm finger pressure on the skin produces an indentation (pit) that remains for several seconds

Placebo   any form of treatment (e.g., medication) that produces an effect in the client because of its intent rather than its chemical or physical properties

Placenta   a flat, disc-shaped organ that is highly vascular and normally forms in the upper segment of the endometrium of the uterus; exchanges nutrients and gases between the fetus and the mother

Plaintiff   a person claiming infringement of legal rights by one or more persons

Planned change   an intended, purposive attempt by an individual, group, organization, or larger social system to influence its own status quo or that of another organism or situation

Planning   an ongoing process that involves (a) assessing a situation, (b) establishing goals and objectives based on assessment of a situation or future trends, and (c) developing a plan of action that identifies priorities, delineates who is responsible, determines deadlines, and describes how the intended outcome is to be achieved and evaluated

Plantar wart   a wart on the sole of the foot

Plaque   an invisible soft film consisting of bacteria, molecules of saliva, and remnants of epithelial cells and leukocytes that adhere to the enamel surface of teeth

Plasma   the fluid portion of the blood in which the blood cells are suspended

Plateau   a maintained concentration of a drug in the plasma during a series of scheduled doses

Pleximeter   in percussion, the middle finger of the nondominant hand placed firmly on the client's skin

Plexor   in percussion, the middle finger of the dominant hand or a percussion hammer used to strike the pleximeter

Pneumothorax   collection of air in the pleural space

Point of maximal impulse (PMI)   the point where the apex of the heart touches the anterior chest wall

Policies   rules developed to govern the handling of frequently occurring situations

Polycythemia   a condition in which clients with chronic hypoxia may develop higher than normal counts of red blood cells

Polydipsia   excessive thirst

Polypnea   abnormally fast respirations

Polysaccharides   a branched chain of dozens, sometimes hundreds, of glucose molecules; starches

Polysomnography   a cluster or pattern of waking behavior that appears during sleep, such as somnambulism (sleepwalking), sleeptalking, and enuresis (bed-wetting)

Polytheism   the belief in more than one God

Polyunsaturated fatty acids   fatty acid with more than one double bond (or many carbons not bonded to a hydrogen atom)

Polyuria   *see* Diuresis

Population includes all possible members of a group who meet the criteria for a study

Positive feedback feedback that stimulates change

Positive reinforcement giving rewards such as praise for a learner's achievements

Positron emission tomography (PET) a noninvasive radiologic study that involves the injection or inhalation of a radioisotope

Possible nursing diagnosis one in which evidence about a health problem is incomplete or unclear

Postmortem examination *see* Autopsy

Postoperative phase begins with the admission of the client to the postanesthesia area and ends when healing is complete

Postural drainage the drainage, by gravity, of secretions from various lung segments

Potency the strength or power of something; when used in reference to medications, potency is a comparison rather than an absolute expression of drug activity because it depends on both affinity and efficacy

Potentiating effect the increased effect of one or both drugs

Power the amount of controlling influence something or someone has to control or override something else

Practice discipline field of study in which the central focus is performance of professional role (nursing, teaching, management, making music)

Prayer human communication with divine and spiritual entities

Preceptor an experienced nurse who assists the novice nurse in improving nursing skill and judgment

Precision accuracy as reflected by the ability to reproduce the same outcome

Precontemplation stage a person typically denies having a problem and instead views others as having a problem and therefore wants to change the other person's behavior

Precordium an area of the chest overlying the heart

Preemptive analgesia the administration of analgesics prior to an invasive or operative procedure in order to treat pain before it occurs

Preferred provider arrangements (PPAs) similar to PPOs, but PPAs can contract with individual health care providers; the plan can be limited or unlimited

Preferred provider organization (PPO) a group of physicians or a hospital that provides companies with health services at a discounted rate

Prefilled unit-dose system injectable medications that are disposable and are available as (a) prefilled syringes ready for use or (b) prefilled sterile cartridges and needles that require the attachment of a reusable holder (injection system) before use

Prejudice a negative belief or preference that is generalized about a group and that leads to "prejudgment"

Preload the degree to which muscle fibers in the ventricle are stretched at the end of diastole

Preoperative phase begins when the decision to have surgery is made and ends when the client is transferred to the operating table

Preparation stage occurs when the person undertakes cognitive and behavioral activities that prepare the person for change

Presbycusis loss of hearing related to aging

Presbyopia loss of elasticity of the lens and thus loss of ability to see close objects as a result of the aging process

Prescription the written direction for the preparation and administration of a drug

Presencing being present, being there, or just being with a client

Pressure a compressing downward force on a body area

Pressure ulcers any lesion caused by unrelieved pressure that results in damage to underlying tissue; formerly called decubitus ulcers, bed sores, pressure sores

Primary care (PC) the point of entry into the health care system at which initial health care is given

Primary health care (PHC) essential health care based on practical, scientifically sound and socially acceptable methods and technology made universally accessible to individuals and families in the community through their full participation and at a cost that the community and country can afford to maintain at every stage of their development in the spirit of self-reliance and self-determination

Primary intention healing tissue surfaces are approximated (closed) and there is minimal or no tissue loss, formation of minimal granulation tissue and scarring

Primary nursing a method of delivering client care that emphasizes continuity of care by assigning one nurse to be responsible for a client's care 24 hours a day 7 days a week

Primary prevention activities directed toward the protection from or avoidance of potential health risks

Primary sexual characteristics relate to the organs necessary for reproduction, such as the testes, penis, vagina, and uterus

Principles-based (deontological) theories emphasize individual rights, duties, and obligations

Priority setting the process of establishing a preferential order for nursing strategies

Private (civil) law the body of law that deals with relationships between private individuals

Prn order "as needed order"; permits the nurse to give a medication when, in the nurse's judgment, the client requires it

Problem solving obtaining information that clarifies the nature of the problem and suggests possible solutions

Problem-oriented medical record (POMR) data about the client are recorded and arranged according to the client's problems, rather than according to the source of the information

Problem-oriented record (POR) *see* Problem-oriented medical record (POMR)

Procedures   steps used in carrying out policies or activities

Process evaluation   a component of quality assurance that focuses on how care was given

Process recording   the verbatim (word-for-word) account of a conversation

Proctoscopy   the viewing of the rectum

Proctosigmoidoscopy   the viewing of the rectum and sigmoid colon

Productivity   in health care, frequently measured by the amount of nursing resources used per client or in terms of required versus actual hours of care provided

Profession   an occupation that requires extensive education or a calling that requires special knowledge, skill, and preparation

Professional values   values acquired during socialization into nursing from codes of ethics, nursing experiences, teachers, and peers

Professionalism   a set of attributes, a way of life that implies responsibility and commitment

Professionalization   the process of becoming professional; acquiring characteristics considered to be professional

Progress notes   chart entries made by a variety of methods and by all health professionals involved in a client's care for the purpose of describing a client's problems, treatments, and progress toward desired outcomes

Prompted voiding   supplements habit training by encouraging the client to try to use the toilet (prompting) and reminding the client when to void

Prone position   face-lying position, with or without a small pillow

Proprioception   awareness of posture, movement, and changes in equilibrium; knowledge of position, weight, and resistance of objects in relation to body

Proprioceptors   sensory receptors that are sensitive to movement and the position of the body

Protein-calorie malnutrition   problem of clients with long-term deficiencies in caloric intake; characteristics include depressed visceral proteins (e.g., albumin), weight loss, and visible muscle and fat wasting

Protocols   a predetermined and preprinted plan specifying the procedure to be followed in a particular situation

Proxemics   the study of distance between people in their interactions

Psychologic dependence   a state of emotional reliance on a drug to maintain one's well-being; a feeling of need or craving for a drug

Psychologic homeostasis   emotional or psychologic balance or state of mental well-being

Psychomotor domain   the "skill" domain; includes motor skills such as giving an injection

Puberty   the first stage of adolescence in which sexual organs begin to grow and mature

Public law   refers to the body of law that deals with relationships between individuals and the government and governmental agencies

Pulse   the wave of blood within an artery that is created by contraction of the left ventricle of the heart

Pulse deficit   the difference between the apical pulse and the radial pulse

Pulse oximeter   a noninvasive device that measures the arterial blood oxygen saturation by means of a sensor attached to the finger

Pulse pressure   the difference between the systolic and the diastolic blood pressure

Pulse rhythm   the pattern of the beats and intervals between the beats

Pulse volume   the strength or amplitude of the pulse, the force of blood exerted with each heart beat

Pureed diet   a modification of the soft diet; liquid may be added to the food, which is then blended to a semisolid consistency

Purkinje fibers   fibers of the ventricular conduction pathways that terminate in ventricular muscle, stimulating contraction

Purulent exudates   an exudate consisting of leukocytes, liquefied dead tissue debris, and dead and living bacteria

Pus   a thick liquid associated with inflammation and composed of cells, liquid, microorganisms, and tissue debris

Pyogenic bacteria   bacteria that produce pus

Pyorrhea   purulent periodontal disease

Pyrexia   a body temperature above the normal range, fever

Q

Qi   body's vital energy reflexology

Qi gong   breathing and mental exercises combined with body movements

Qualifiers   words that have been added to some NANDA labels to give additional meaning to the diagnostic statement

Quality improvement   an organizational commitment and approach used to continuously improve all processes in the organization with the goal of meeting and exceeding customer expectations and outcomes; also known as *total quality management* (TQM) and *continuous quality improvement* (CQI)

Quality-assurance (QA) program   an ongoing systematic process designed to evaluate and promote excellence in the health care provided to clients

R

Race   classification of people according to shared biologic characteristics and physical features

Radiation   the transfer of heat from the surface of one object to the surface of another without contact between the two objects

Radiopharmaceutical   a pharmaceutical (targeted to a specific organ) labeled with a radioisotope, administered through various routes, to determine hyperfunction or hypofunction of the organ

Random access memory (RAM)   data and instructions stored on chips; RAM storage is temporary and cleared when the computer is turned off

Range   a measure of variability, consisting of the difference between the highest and lowest values in a distribution of scores

Range of motion (ROM)   the degree of movement possible for each joint

Rapport   a relationship between two or more people of mutual trust and understanding

Rationale   the scientific reason for selecting a specific action

RBC indices   may be performed as part of the CBC to evaluate the size, weight, and hemoglobin concentration of red blood cells

Reactive hyperemia   a bright red flush on the skin occurring after pressure is relieved

Readiness   behaviors or cues that reflect a learner's motivation to learn at a specific time

Reagent   substance used in a chemical reaction to detect a specific substance

Reasoning   thinking that is both coherent and logical and can be inductive or deductive

Recent memory   deals with activities of the recent past of minutes to a few hours

Receptor   a location on the surface of a cell membrane or within a cell (usually a protein) to which a drug chemically binds

Reconstitution   the technique of adding a solvent to a powdered drug to prepare it for injection

Record   a written communication providing formal, legal documentation of a client's progress

Recording   the process of making written entries about a client on the medical record

Red blood cell (RBC) count   number of red blood cells per cubic millimeter of whole blood

Red blood cell (RBC) indices   evaluate size, weight, and hemoglobin concentrations of RBCs

Referred pain   pain perceived to be in one area but whose source is another area

Reflection   thinking from a critical point of view, analyzing why one acted in a certain way, and assessing the results of one's actions

Reflex   an automatic response of the body to a stimulus

Reflexology   a treatment based on massage of the feet to relieve symptoms in other parts of the body

Reflux   backward flow

Regeneration   renewal, regrowth, the replacement of destroyed tissue cells by cells that are identical or similar in structure and function

Regional anesthesia   the temporary interruption of the transmission of nerve impulses to and from a specific area or region of the body; the client loses sensation in an area of the body but remains conscious

Registry   private duty agency which contracts with individual practioners

Regression   a defense mechanism in which one adapts behavior that was comforting earlier in life to overcome the discomfort and insecurity of the present situation

Regurgitation   the spitting up or backward flow of undigested food

Relapsing fever   the occurrence of short febrile periods of a few days interspersed with periods of 1 or 2 days of normal temperature

Relationship-based (caring) theories   stress courage, generosity, commitment, and the need to nurture and maintain relationships

Relaxation response   physiologic state achieved through deep relaxation breathing

Relevance   how strongly something relates to the matter at hand

Reliability   the degree to which an instrument produces consistent results on repeated use

Religion   an organized system of worship

REM sleep   sleep during which the person experiences *rapid eye movements*

Remission   a period during a chronic illness when there is a lessening of severity or cessation of symptoms

Remittent fever   the occurrence of a wide range of temperature fluctuations, more than 2°C (3.6°F) over the 24-hour period, all of which are above normal

Renin-angiotensin-aldosterone system   system initiated by specialized receptors in the juxtaglomerular cells of the kidney nephrons that respond to changes in renal perfusion

Report   whether oral or written, it should be concise, including pertinent information but no extraneous detail

Repression   a defense mechanism in which painful thoughts, experiences, and impulses are removed from awareness

Res ipsa loquitur   "the thing that speaks for itself"; a legal doctrine that relates to negligence in which the harm cannot be traced to a specific health care provider or standard but does not normally occur unless there has been a negligent act

Researchability   the problem can be subjected to scientific investigation

Reservoir   a source of microorganisms

Resident flora   microorganisms that normally reside on the skin and mucous membranes, and inside the respiratory and gastrointestinal tracts

Residual urine   the amount of urine remaining in the bladder after a person voids

Resolution phase   the part of the response cycle period of return to the unaroused state, which may last 10 to 15 minutes after orgasm, or longer if there is no orgasm

Resonance   a low-pitched, hollow sound produced over normal lung tissue when the chest is percussed

Respiration   the act of breathing; transport of oxygen from the atmosphere to the body cells and transport of carbon dioxide from the cells to the atmosphere

Respiratory acidosis   (hypercapnia) a state of excess carbon dioxide in the body

Respiratory alkalosis   a state of excessive loss of carbon dioxide from the body

Respiratory character   *see* Respiratory quality

Respiratory membrane   where gas exchange occurs between the air on the alveolar side and the blood on the capillary side; the alveolar and capillary walls form the respiratory membrane

Respiratory quality   refers to those aspects of breathing that are different from normal, effortless breathing, includes the amount of effort exerted to breathe and the sounds produced by breathing

Respiratory rhythm   refers to the regularity of the expirations and the inspirations

Respondeat superior   a legal term meaning "let the master answer"; the employer assumes responsibility for the conduct of the employee and can also be held responsible for malpractice by the employee

Responsibility   the specific accountability or liability associated with the performance of duties of a particular role

Resting energy expenditure (REE)   the amount of energy required to maintain basic body functions

Resting tremor   a tremor that is apparent when the client is at rest and diminishes with activity

Restraints   protective devices used to limit physical activity of the client or a part of the client's body

Retrograde pyelography   radiographic study of the urinary tract where contrast medium is instilled directly into the kidney pelvis via the urethra, bladder, and ureters

Retrospective audit   evaluation of a client's record after discharge from an agency

Review of systems   *see* Screening examination

Rhizotomy   interruption of the anterior or posterior nerve root between the ganglion and the cord; generally performed on cervical nerve roots to alleviate pain of the head and neck

Right   (legal) a privilege or fundamental power to which an individual is entitled unless it is revoked by law or given up voluntarily

Right of self-determination   subjects feel free from constraints, coercion, or any undue influence to participate in a study

Rigor mortis   the stiffening of the body that occurs after death

Risk factors   factors that cause a client to be vulnerable to developing a health problem

Risk management   having in place a system to reduce danger to clients and staff

Risk nursing diagnosis   clinical judgment that a problem does not exist, but the presence of risk factors indicates that a problem is likely to develop unless nurses intervene

Risk of harm   exposure to the possibility of injury going beyond everyday situations

Role   the set of expectations about how a person occupying a specific position behaves

Role ambiguity   unclear role expectations; people do not know what to do or how to do it and are unable to predict the reactions of others to their behavior

Role conflict   a clash between the beliefs or behaviors imposed by two or more roles fulfilled by one person

Role development   involves socialization into a particular role

Role mastery   performance of role behaviors that meet social expectations

Role model   providing an example of acceptable behavior(s) through demonstration

Role performance   what a person does in a particular role in relation to the behaviors expected of that role

Role strain   a generalized state of frustration or anxiety experienced with the stress of role conflict and ambiguity

Root cause analysis   process for identifying factors that bring about deviations in practices that lead to an event

S

S_1 the first heart sound; occurs when the atrioventricular valves (mitral and tricuspid) close

S_2 the second heart sound; occurs when the semilunar valves (aortic and pulmonic) close

Safety monitoring device   a position-sensitive switch that triggers an audio alarm when a client attempts to get out of the bed or chair

Sairy Gamp   a character in the Charles Dickens book *Martin Chizzlewit* who represented the negative image of nurses in the early 1800s

Saliva   the clear liquid secreted by the salivary glands in the mouth, sometimes referred to as *spit*

Sample   segment of the population from whom data will actually be collected

Sanguineous exudate   an exudate containing large amounts of red blood cells

Sarcopenia   steady decrease in muscle fibers

Saturated fatty acids   those in which all carbon atoms are filled to capacity (i.e., saturated) with hydrogen

Scabies   a contagious skin infestation caused by an arachnid, the itch mite

Scald   a burn from a hot liquid or vapor, such as steam

Scientific health belief   based on the belief that life and life processes are controlled by physical and biochemical processes that can be manipulated by humans

Screening examination   (review of systems) a brief review of essential functioning of various body parts or systems

Scrub person   person who assists the surgeon

Sebaceous glands   active under the influence of androgens in both males and females, which secrete sebum and become most active on the face, neck, shoulder, upper back, and chest; are often the cause of an increased incidence of acne

Sebum the oily, lubricating secretion of sebaceous glands in the skin

Secondary intention healing wound in which the tissue surfaces are not approximated and there is extensive tissue loss; formation of excessive granulation tissue and scarring

Secondary prevention activities designed for early diagnosis and treatment of disease or illness

Secondary sexual characteristics physical characteristics that differentiate the male from the female but do not relate directly to reproduction

Seizure a sudden onset of a convulsion or other paroxysmal motor or sensory activity

Seizure precautions safety measures taken by the nurse to protect clients from injury should they have a seizure

Selectively permeable cell membranes that allow substances to move across them with varying degrees of ease

Self-awareness the relationship between one's perception of oneself and others' perceptions of oneself

Self-concept the collection of ideas, feelings, and beliefs one has about oneself

Self-esteem the value one has for oneself; self-confidence

Self-regulation homeostatic mechanisms that come into play automatically in the healthy person

Semicircular canals in the inner ear; contain the organs of equilibrium

Semi-Fowler's position *see* Low Fowler's position

Semilunar valves crescent moon-shaped valves between the cardiac ventricles and the pulmonary artery (pulmonic valve) and the aorta (aortic valve)

Sensorineural hearing loss the result of damage to the inner ear, the auditory nerve, or the hearing center in the brain

Sensoristasis the need for sensory stimulation

Sensory deficit partial or complete impairment of any sensory organ

Sensory deprivation insufficient sensory stimulation for a person to function

Sensory memory momentary perception of stimuli by the senses

Sensory overload an overabundance of sensory stimulation

Sensory perception the organization and translation of stimuli into meaningful information

Sensory reception process of receiving environmental stimuli

Sentinel event an unexpected occurrence involving death or serious physical or psychological injury, or the risk thereof

Separation anxiety the fear and frustration experienced by young children that comes with parental absences

Sepsis the presence of pathogenic organisms or their toxins in the blood or body tissues

Septicemia occurs when bacteremia results in systemic infection

Septum a dividing structure such as that between the cardiac chambers or between the two sides of the nose

Serosanguineous exudate inflammatory material consisting of a combination of clear and blood-tinged drainage

Serous exudates inflammatory material composed of serum (clear portion of blood) derived from the blood and serous membranes of the body such as the peritoneum, pleura, pericardium, and meninges; watery in appearance and has few cells

Serum osmolality a measure of the solute concentration of the blood

Sexual aversion disorder severe distaste for sexual activity or thought of sexual activity

Sexual health the integration of the somatic, emotional, intellectual, and social aspects of sexuality, in ways that are positively enriching and that enhance personality, communication, and love

Sexual orientation the preference of a person for one sex or the other

Sexual pain disorders include dyspareunia, vaginismus, and genital pain

Sexual self-concept how one values oneself as a sexual being

Shaft the part of a needle that is attached to the hub

Shaken baby syndrome (SBS) violent shaking of the infant by the arms or shoulders causing a whiplash, which can lead to severe injury in infants

Shared governance a method that aims to distribute decision making among a group of people

Shared leadership a contemporary theory of leadership that recognizes the leadership capabilities of each member in a professional group and assumes that appropriate leadership will emerge in relation to the challenges that confront the group

Shearing force a combination of friction and pressure that, when applied to the skin, results in damage to the blood vessels and tissues

Shock phase first part of the alarm reaction in which the stressor may be perceived consciously or unconsciously by the person

Short-term memory information held in the brain for immediate use or what one has in mind at a given moment

Shroud a large piece of plastic or cotton material used to enclose a body after death

Side effect the secondary effect of a drug that is unintended; usually predictable and may be either harmless or potentially harmful

Significance the potential to contribute to nursing science by enhancing client care, testing or generating a theory, or resolving a day-to-day clinical problem

Sims' position side-lying position with lowermost arm behind the body and uppermost leg flexed

Single order   common medication order that is a "one-time order"; medication is to be given once at a specified time

Sinoatrial (SA or sinus) node   the primary pacemaker of the heart located where the superior vena cava enters the right atrium

Situational leader   adapts style according to consideration of the staff members' abilities, knowledge of the nature of the task to be done, and sensitivity to the context or environment in which the task takes place

Sitz bath   used to soak a client's pelvic area; also referred to as a *hip bath*

Skinfold measurement   an indicator of the amount of body fat, the main form of stored energy

Slander   defamation by the spoken word, stating unprivileged (not legally protected) or false words by which a reputation is damaged

Sleep   an altered state of consciousness in which the individual's perception of and reaction to the environment are decreased

Sleep apnea   periodic cessation of breathing during sleep

Sleep architecture   basic organization of normal sleep

Sleep hygiene   refers to interventions used to promote sleep

Small calorie (c, cal)   the amount of heat required to raise the temperature of 1 g of water 1°C

SOAP   an acronym for a charting method that follows a recording sequence of *subjective* data, *objective* data, *assessment*, and *planning*

Socialization   a process by which a person learns the ways of a group or society in order to become a functioning participant

Socratic questioning   a technique one can use to look beneath the surface, recognize and examine assumptions, search for inconsistencies, examine multiple points of view, and differentiate what one knows from what one merely believes

Sojourner Truth   an abolitionist, Underground Railroad agent, preacher, and women's rights advocate, she was a nurse for more than 4 years during the Civil War and worked as a nurse and counselor for the Freedman's Relief Association after the war

Solutes   substances dissolved in a liquid

Solvent   the liquid in which a solute is dissolved

Somatic pain   pain that originates in the skin, muscles, bone, or connective tissue

Somnology   the study of sleep

Sordes   accumulation of foul matter (food, microorganisms, and epithelial elements) on the teeth and gums

Source-oriented clinical record   a record in which each person or department makes notations in a separate section or sections of the client's chart

Spastic   describing the sudden, prolonged involuntary muscle contractions of clients with damage to the central nervous system

Specific defenses   immune functions directed against identifiable bacteria, viruses, fungi, or other infectious agents

Specific gravity   the weight or degree of concentration of a substance compared with that of an equal volume of another, such as distilled water, taken as a standard

Specific self-esteem   how much one approves of a certain part of oneself

Spinal anesthesia   anesthesia produced by injecting an anesthetic agent into the subarachnoid space surrounding the spinal cord; also referred to as a *subarachnoid block (SAB)*

Spinal cord stimulation (SCS)   involves the insertion of a cable that allows the placement of an electrode directly on the spinal cord and is used with nonmalignant pain that has not been controlled with less invasive therapies

Spiritual distress   a disturbance in or a challenge to a person's belief or value system that provides strength, hope, and meaning to life

Spiritual health   *see* Spiritual well-being

Spiritual well-being   a feeling of inner peace and of being generally alive, purposeful, and fulfilled; the feeling is rooted in spiritual values and/or specific religious beliefs

Spirituality   belief in or relationship with some higher power, creative force, driving being, or infinite source of energy

Spreadsheet   programs that manipulate primarily numbers

Sputum   the mucous secretion from the lungs, bronchi, and trachea

Stage of exhaustion   the third stage in the adaptation syndromes that occurs when the adaptation that the body made during the second stage cannot be maintained

Stage of resistance   the second stage in the adaptation syndromes when the body's adaptation takes place

Standard   a generally accepted rule, model, pattern, or measure

Standard deviation   the most frequently used measure of variability, indicating the average to which scores deviate from the mean; commonly symbolized as SD or S

Standardized care plan   formal plan that specifies the nursing care for groups of clients with common needs (e.g., all clients with myocardial infarction)

Standards of care   the skills and learning commonly possessed by members of a profession

Standards of practice   descriptions of the responsibilities for which nurses are accountable

Standards of professional performance   as set by the American Nurses Association (ANA), describe behaviors expected in the professional nursing role

Standing order   a written document about policies, rules, regulations, or orders regarding client care; gives nurses the authority to carry out specific actions under certain circumstances

Stapes   stirrups bone of the middle ear

Stat order   common medication order which indicates that the medication is to be given immediately and only once

Statistically significant   term applied after data have been analyzed to determine whether the results had a probability less than 0.05, which is considered the acceptable level of significance

Statutory law   a law enacted by any legislative body

Steatorrhea   an excessive amount of fat in the stool, which can indicate faulty absorption of fat from the small intestine

Stereognosis   the ability to recognize objects by touching and manipulating them

Stereotyping   assuming that all members of a culture or ethnic group are alike

Sterile field   a specified area that is considered free from microorganisms

Sterile technique   practices that keep an area or object free of all microorganisms

Sterilization   a process that destroys all microorganisms, including spores and viruses

Sternum   the breastbone

Stimulus-based stress model   stress is defined as a stimulus, life event, or set of circumstances that arouses physiologic and/or psychologic reactions that may increase the individual's vulnerability to illness

Stoma   an artificial opening in the abdominal wall; it may be permanent or temporary

Stool   *see* Feces

Strabismus   squinting or crossing of the eyes; uncoordinated eye movements

Stress   an event or set of circumstances causing a disrupted response; the disruption caused by a noxious stimulus or stressor

Stress electrocardiography   uses ECGs to assess a client's response to an increased cardiac workload during exercise

Stressor   any factor that produces stress or alters the body's equilibrium

Stridor   a harsh, crowing sound made on inhalation caused by constriction of the upper airway

Strike   an organized work stoppage by a group of employees to express a grievance, enforce a demand for changes in condition of employment, or solve a dispute with management

Stroke volume (SV)   the amount of blood ejected with each cardiac contraction

Structure evaluation   focuses on the setting in which care is given

Subarachnoid block (SAB)   *see* Spinal anesthesia

Subculture   usually composed of people who have a distinct identity and yet are related to a larger cultural group

Subcutaneous   beneath the layers of the skin; hypodermic

Subjective data   data that are apparent only to the person affected; can be described or verified only by that person

Sublingual   under the tongue

Subsystems   system components

Suctioning   the aspiration of secretions by a catheter connected to a suction machine or wall outlet

Sudden infant death syndrome (SIDS)   the sudden and unexpected death of an infant

Sudoriferous sweat glands   glands of the dermis that secrete sweat

Superego   the conscience of personality; the source of feelings of guilt, shame, and inhibition

Supine position   *see* Dorsal position

Supplemental Security Income (SSI)   special payments for people with disabilities, those who are blind, and people who are not eligible for Social Security; these payments are not restricted to health care costs

Suppositories   solid, cone-shaped, medicated substances inserted into the rectum, vagina, or urethra

Suppuration   the formation of pus

Suprapubic catheter   catheter inserted through the abdominal wall above the symphysis pubis into the urinary bladder

Suprasystem   the system above another system

Surface anesthesia   *see* Topical anesthesia

Surface temperature   the temperature of tissue, the subcutaneous tissue, and fat

Surfactant   a surface-active agent (e.g., soap or a synthetic detergent); in pulmonary physiology, a mixture of phospholipids secreted by alveolar cells into the alveoli and respiratory air passages that reduces the surface tension of pulmonary fluids and thus contributes to the elastic properties of pulmonary tissue

Surgical asepsis   *see* Sterile technique

Suture   a thread used to sew body tissues together

Sutures   junction lines of the skull bones

Sweat glands   *see* Sudoriferous glands

Sympathectomy   severance of the pathways of the sympathetic division of the autonomic nervous system; eliminates vasospasm, improves peripheral blood supply, and is effective in treating painful vascular disorders

Sympathetically maintained pain   pain that occurs with abnormal connections between pain fibers and the sympathetic nervous system

Symptoms   *see* Covert data

Syndrome diagnosis   a diagnosis that is associated with a cluster of other diagnoses

Synergistic   when two different drugs increase the action of one or another drug

System   a set of interacting identifiable parts or components

Systemic infection   occurs when pathogens spread and damage different parts of the body

Systole   the period during which the ventricles contract

Systolic pressure   the pressure of the blood against the arterial walls when the ventricles of the heart contract

T

T'ai chi   discipline that combines physical fitness, meditation, and self-defense

Tachycardia   an abnormally rapid pulse rate; greater than 100 beats per minute

Tachypnea   abnormally fast respirations; usually more than 24 respirations per minute

Tactile   related to touch

Tandem   secondary IV setup in which the second container is attached to the line of the first container at the lower, secondary port

Tartar   a visible, hard deposit of plaque and dead bacteria that forms at the gum lines

Taxonomy   a classification system or set of categories, such as nursing diagnoses, arranged on the basis of a single principle or consistent set of principles

Teacher   a nurse who helps clients learn about their health and the health care procedures they need to perform to restore or maintain their health

Teaching   system of activities intended to produce learning

Team nursing   the delivery of individualized nursing care to clients by a team led by a professional nurse

Technical skills   "hands-on" skills such as those required to manipulate equipment, administer injections, and move or reposition patients

Telecommunications   the transmission of information from one site to another, using equipment to transmit information in the forms of signs, signals, words, or pictures by cable, radio, or other systems

Telemedicine   technology used to transmit electronic medical data about clients to persons at distant locations

Temperament   the way individuals respond to their external and internal environment

Teratogen   anything that adversely affects normal cellular development in the embryo or fetus

Termination stage   the ultimate goal where the individual has complete confidence that the problem is no longer a temptation or threat

Territoriality   a concept of the space and things that individuals consider their own

Tertiary intention   healing that occurs in wounds left open for 3 to 5 days and then closed with sutures, staples, or adhesive skin closures

Tertiary prevention   activities designed to restore individuals with disabilities to their optimal level of functioning

Theory   a system of ideas that is proposed to explain a given phenomenon (e.g., theory of gravity)

Therapeutic baths   given for physical effects, such as to soothe irritated skin or to treat an area (e.g., the perineum)

Therapeutic communication   an interactive process between nurse and client that helps the client overcome temporary stress, to get along with other people, to adjust to the unalterable, and to overcome psychologic blocks that stand in the way of self-realization

Therapeutic effect   the primary effect intended of a drug; reason the drug is prescribed

Third space syndrome   fluid shifts from the vascular space into an area where it is not readily accessible as extracellular fluid

Thoracentesis   insertion of a needle into the pleural cavity for diagnostic or therapeutic purposes

Thrill   a vibrating sensation over a blood vessel that indicates turbulent blood flow

Thrombophlebitis   inflammation of a vein followed by formation of a blood clot

Thrombus   a solid mass of blood constituents in the circulatory system; a clot (plural: *thrombi*)

Throughput   a transformation that occurs after input is absorbed by the system and is then processed in a way that is useful to the system

Ticks   small gray-brown parasites that bite into tissue and suck blood and transmit several diseases to people, in particular Rocky Mountain spotted fever, Lyme disease, and tularemia.

Tidal volume   the volume of air that is normally inhaled and exhaled

Tinea pedis   athlete's foot (ringworm of the foot), which is caused by a fungus

Tissue perfusion   passage of fluid (e.g., blood) through a specific organ or body part

Tolerance   the respect, appreciation, and acceptance of diversity in others without bias or judgment

Top-level manager   organizational executive primarily responsible for establishing goals and developing strategic plans

Topical   applied externally (e.g., to the skin or mucous membranes)

Topical anesthesia   (surface anesthesia) applied directly to the skin and mucous membranes, open skin surfaces, wounds, and burns

Torr   millimeters of mercury

Tort   a civil wrong committed against a person or a person's property

Tort law   law that defines and enforces duties and rights among private individuals that are not based on contractual agreements

Trade name   name given a drug by the manufacturer

Traditional   observance of the beliefs and practices of one's heritage or cultural belief system

Traditional Chinese medicine (TCM)   based on the premise that the body's vital energy circulates through pathways or meridians and can be accessed and manipulated through specific anatomical points along the surface of the body

Tragus   the cartilaginous protrusion at the entrance to the ear canal

Transactional leader   a contemporary theory of leadership in which resources are exchanged as an incentive for loyalty and performance

Transactional stress theory   a theory that encompasses a set of cognitive, affective, and adaptive (coping) responses that arise out of person–environment transactions; the person and the environment are inseparable and affect each other

Transcellular fluid   compartment of extracellular fluids; includes cerebrospinal, pericardial, pancreatic, pleural, intraocular, biliary, peritoneal, and synovial fluids

Transcendence a person's recognition that there is something other or greater than the self and a seeking and valuing of that greater other, whether it is an ultimate being, force, or value

Transcultural nursing providing care within the differences and similarities of the beliefs, values, and patterns of cultures

Transcutaneous electrical nerve stimulation (TENS) a noninvasive, nonanalgesic pain control technique that allows the client to assist in the management of acute and chronic pain

Transdermal patch a particular type of topical or dermatologic medication delivery system

Transformational leader leader who fosters creativity, risk taking, commitment, and collaboration by empowering the group to share in the organization's vision

Transgenderism gradation of human characteristics that run from female to male

Translator a person who converts written material (such as patient education pamphlets) from one language into another

Transsexual individual who feels his or her sexual anatomy is not consistent with his or her gender identity

Tremor an involuntary trembling of a limb or body part

Trial the period during which all relevant facts are presented to a jury or judge

Triangular fossa a depression of the antihelix

Triglycerides substances that have three fatty acids; they account for more than 90% of the lipids in food and in the body

Trigone a triangular area at the base of the bladder marked by the ureter openings at the posterior corners and the opening of the urethra at the anterior corner

Trimesters the 3-month periods during pregnancy marking certain landmarks for developmental changes in mother and the fetus; three trimesters occur during a pregnancy

Tripod (triangle) position the proper standing position with crutches; crutches are placed about 15 cm (6 in.) in front of the feet and out laterally about 15 cm (6 in.), creating a wide base of support

Trocar a sharp pointed instrument that fits inside a cannula and is used to pierce body tissues

Troponin enzyme that is released into the blood during a myocardial infarction (MI)

Trough level represents the lowest concentration of a drug in the blood serum

Tuberculin syringe originally designed to administer tuberculin; a narrow syringe, calibrated in tenths and hundredths of a milliliter (up to 1 mL) on one scale and in sixteenths of a minim (up to 1 minim) on the other scale

Two-point discrimination *see* One-point discrimination

Tympanic membrane the eardrum

Tympany a musical or drumlike sound produced during percussion over an air-filled stomach and abdomen

U

Ultrasonography the use of ultrasound to produce an image of an organ or tissue

Unconscious mind the mental life of a person of which the person is unaware

Undernutrition an intake of nutrients insufficient to meet daily energy requirements because of inadequate food intake or improper digestion and absorption of food

Undertaker *see* Mortician

Universal precautions (UP) techniques to be used with all clients to decrease the risk of transmitting unidentified pathogens; currently, Standard Precautions incorporate UP and BSI

Unplanned change haphazard change that occurs without control by any person or group

Unprofessional conduct one of the grounds for action against the nurse's license; includes incompetence or gross negligence, conviction of practicing without a license, falsification of client records, and illegally obtaining, using, or possessing controlled substances

Unsaturated fatty acid a fatty acid that could accommodate more hydrogen atoms than it currently does

Upper-level managers organizational executives who are primarily responsible for establishing goals and developing strategic plans

Urea a substance found in urine, blood, and lymph; the main nitrogenous substance in blood

Ureterostomy type of urinary diversion that involves surgery of the ureters

Urgency the feeling that one must urinate

Urinary frequency the need to urinate often

Urinary hesitancy a delay and difficulty in initiating voiding; often associated with dysuria

Urinary incontinence a temporary or permanent inability of the external sphincter muscles to control the flow of urine from the bladder

Urinary reflux backward flow of urine

Urinary retention the accumulation of urine in the bladder and inability of the bladder to empty itself

Urinary stasis stagnation of urinary flow

Urination (micturition, voiding) the process of emptying the bladder

Urine osmolality a measure of the solute concentration of urine, a more exact measurement of urine concentration than specific gravity

Utilitarianism a specific, consequence-based, ethical theory that judges as right the action that does the most good and least amount of harm for the greatest number of persons; often used in making decisions about the funding and delivery of health care

Utility   *see* Utilitarianism

V

Vaginismus   involuntary spasm of outer one-third of vaginal muscles; makes penetration of vagina painful

Validation   the determination that the diagnosis accurately reflects the problem of the client, that the methods used for data gathering were appropriate, and that the conclusion or diagnosis is justified by the data

Validity   the degree to which an instrument measures what it is intended to measure

Valsalva maneuver   forceful exhalation against a closed glottis, which increases intrathoracic pressure and thus interferes with venous blood return to the heart

Value set   all of the values (e.g., personal, professional, religious) that a person holds

Value system   the organization of a person's values along a continuum of relative importance

Values   something of worth; a belief held dearly by a person

Values clarification   a process by which individuals define their own value

Vaporization   continuous evaporation of moisture from the respiratory tract and from the mucosa of the mouth and from the skin

Variance   a variation or deviation from a critical pathway; goals not met or interventions not performed according to the time frame

Vasoconstriction   a decrease in the caliber (lumen) of blood vessels

Vasodilation   an increase in the caliber (lumen) of blood vessels

Vector-borne transmission   a vector is an animal or flying or crawling insect that serves as an intermediate means of transporting the infectious agent

Vehicle-borne transmission   a vehicle is any substance that serves as an intermediate means to transport and introduce an infectious agent into a susceptible host through a suitable portal of entry

Venipuncture   puncture of a vein for collection of a blood specimen or for infusion of therapeutic solutions

Ventilation   the movement of air in and out of the lungs; the process of inhalation and exhalation

Ventricles   two lower chambers of the heart

Veracity   a moral principle that holds that one should tell the truth and not lie

Verbal communication   use of verbal language to send and receive messages

Verdict   the outcome made by a jury

Vernix caseosa   a protective covering that develops over the unborn fetus's skin; a white, cheese-like substance that adheres to the skin and can become 1/8-inch thick by birth

Vesicostomy   surgical production of an opening into the bladder

Vestibule   contains the organs of equilibrium; found in the inner ear

Vestibulitis   severe pain on touch or attempted vaginal entry

Vial   a medication container with a sealed rubber cap, for single or multiple doses

Vibration   a series of vigorous quiverings produced by hands that are placed flat against the chest wall to loosen thick secretions

Virulence   ability to produce disease

Viruses   nucleic acid-based infectious agents

Visceral   internal organs

Visceral pain   results from stimulation of pain receptors in the abdominal cavity, cranium, and thorax

Viscous   thick, sticky

Vision   the mental image of a possible and desirable future state

Visiting nursing   delivery of services in the client's home

Visual   related to sight

Visual acuity   the degree of detail the eye can discern in an image

Visual fields   the area an individual can see when looking straight ahead

Vital capacity   the maximum amount of air that can be exhaled after a maximum inhalation

Vital signs   measurements of physiologic functioning, specifically body temperature, pulse, respirations, and blood pressure; may include pain and pulse oximetry

Vitamin   an organic compound that cannot be manufactured by the body and is needed in small quantities to catalyze metabolic processes

Vitiligo   patches of hypopigmented skin, caused by the destruction of melanocytes in the area

Voiding   *see* Urination

Volume control infusion set   small fluid containers (100 to 150 mL in size) attached below the primary infusion container so that the medication is administered through the client's IV line

Volume expanders   used to increase the blood volume following severe loss of blood (e.g., from hemorrhage) or loss of plasma (e.g., from severe burns, which draw large amounts of plasma from the bloodstream to the burn site)

Vulvodynia   constant and unremitting burning of vulva

W

Water-soluble vitamins   vitamins that the body cannot store, so people must get a daily supply in the diet; include C and B-complex vitamins

Well-being   a subjective perception of balance, harmony, and vitality

Wellness a state of well-being; engaging in attitudes and behaviors that enhance quality of life and maximize personal potential

Wellness diagnosis (NANDA) describes human responses to levels of wellness in an individual, family, or community that have a readiness for enhancement

White blood cells (WBCs) body cells that are part of the body's defense against infection and disease

Wide area network (WAN) computers linked across large distances

World Wide Web (WWW) refers to the complex links among webpages or websites, accessed through "addresses" called *universal resource locators* (URLs)

X

Xenophobia the fear or dislike of people different from one's self

Xerostomia dry mouth

Y

Yoga a type of meditation that is a system of exercises for attaining bodily or mental control and well-being

INDEX

Page numbers followed by *f* indicate figures and those followed by *t* indicate tables, boxes, or special features. The titles of special features (e.g., Lifespan Considerations; Nursing Care Plans; Skills) are also capitalized.

Special Features